Merriam-Webster's Medical Dictionary

Merriam-Webster's Medical Dictionary

Merriam-Webster, Incorporated
Springfield, Massachusetts, U.S.A.

A GENUINE MERRIAM-WEBSTER

The name *Webster* alone is no guarantee of excellence. It is used by a number of publishers and may serve mainly to mislead an unwary buyer.

Merriam-Webster™ is the name you should look for when you consider the purchase of dictionaries or other fine reference books. It carries the reputation of a company that has been publishing since 1831 and is your assurance of quality and authority.

ISBN 978-0-87779-294-9

MADE IN THE UNITED STATES OF AMERICA

6th Printing Quad Graphics Martinsburg, WV January 2020

CONTENTS

PREFACE

This new edition of MERRIAM-WEBSTER'S MEDICAL DICTIONARY follows the tradition established in earlier editions in providing a concise guide to the essential language of medicine. This dictionary contains features that are standard for most desk dictionaries of the English language but are often missing from medical dictionaries. For example, users of this book will find how to pronounce *CABG, 5-HT,* and *NSAID;* how to spell and pronounce the plurals of *dermatitis, larynx,* and *papilloma;* where to divide *colonoscopy* and *staphylococcal* at the end of a line; and whether a word such as *fungicide, fungicidal,* or *fungicidally* functions as a noun, adjective, or adverb.

The 39,000 vocabulary entries include the most commonly used words of human and veterinary medicine. The reader will find entries for human diseases such as *cystic fibrosis, Lyme disease,* and *type 1 diabetes* and also for those of domestic animals, such as *heartworm* of dogs, *panleukopenia* of cats, and *azoturia* of horses. Over 1,000 new terms that a patient or health-care consumer is likely to encounter have been added for this edition and include *autism spectrum disorder, channelopathy, chemo brain, deep brain stimulation, gateway drug, hyperbaric oxygen therapy, obesogenic, prebiotic, thoracic outlet syndrome,* and *traumatic brain injury.* New entries relating to the fields of psychology and psychiatry include *factitious disorder, gender dysphoria, hypoactive sexual desire disorder,* and *pareidolia.* Newly entered terms of public-health concern include *C. diff, MERS, superbug,* and *vancomycin-resistant enterococcus.* Every word used in a definition in this book appears as a boldface vocabulary entry either in this dictionary or in its companion general paperback, *The Merriam-Webster Dictionary.*

This dictionary is designed to serve as an interface between the language of doctor and the language of patient, between sports medicine and the sports page, between the technical New Latin names of plants and animals and their common names, and between the old and the new in medical terminology. The user of this dictionary will find, for example, that the *abs, glutes, lats,* and *pecs* of the physical fitness enthusiast are the *abdominals, glutei, latissimi dorsi,* and *pectorales* of the anatomist. In medical literature or the medical records of a patient, a more technical term may often be used in place of a familiar one. *Heart attack* may be called *myocardial infarction, hives* may be called *urticaria,* and *ministroke* may be called *transient ischemic attack.* Both the technical and familiar terms are entered in this dictionary with mention of synonymous terminology. Because a disease or medical condition may acquire multiple names over time, this dictionary enters all generally recognized names with mention of synonymy. At the entry *stroke,* for example, the dictionary user will find *apoplexy, brain attack, cerebral accident,* and *cerebrovascular accident* all listed at the end of the definition as other names for *stroke.* Additionally, each of these terms is entered with indication of synonymy.

This 2016 edition includes many new additions to the dictionary's coverage of the most commonly used and recognized drugs. Entry of a generic drug name is often accompanied by entry of the related trademark. When a trademark for a drug is entered in this dictionary, it is also mentioned in a cross-reference following the definition of its generic equivalent, so that, for example, from either of the entries for *atorvastatin* and *Lipitor, fluoxetine* and *Prozac,* or *sildenafil* and *Viagra,* the reader can determine which is a generic name and which is a proprietary name for the same drug. Over 600 active trademarks are currently entered along with numerous trademarks whose registration has expired. In cases where the name of an expired trademark still has frequent mention in current sources, dictionary entry has been retained but the functional label has been changed from *trademark* to *noun* and a usage note indicating former trademark status has been appended to the entry. No entry in this dictionary, however, should be regarded as affecting the validity of any trademark or service mark.

A useful feature of this book is that words occurring only as part of compound terms are entered at their own place in alphabetical sequence with a cross-reference to the compound terms themselves. Thus, *herpetiformis* has a cross-reference to *dermatitis herpetiformis, basale* has a cross-reference to *stratum basale,* and *longus* is followed by a list of 11 compound terms of which it is part. This cross-reference feature may help the reader unfamiliar with medical terminology to find the place of definition of compound terms.

The biographical information following words derived from the names of persons includes the person's name, birth and death dates, nationality, and occupation or status. The reader can learn that *Asperger's syndrome* was named after the Austrian psychiatrist *Hans Asperger,* that *Hodgkin's lymphoma* was named after the British physician *Thomas Hodgkin,* and that *Tommy John surgery* (more technically known as *ulnar collateral ligament reconstruction*) was named after the American baseball player *Thomas Edward John.* Such information is entered only for historical figures, not for fictional or mythical characters.

It is the intent of the editors that this dictionary serve the purposes of all those who seek information about medical English especially as it is currently spoken and written, whether in the context of a clinical setting, in a magazine or newspaper article, in a television commercial or medical drama, or from the perspective of medical lexicography as an art and science.

Merriam-Webster's Medical Dictionary is the result of the collective effort by the staff of Merriam-Webster, Incorporated. This new edition builds on previous editions prepared by Roger W. Pease, Jr., Ph.D., Christopher C. Connor, and myself. For the 2016 and 2006 editions, Joshua S. Guenter, Ph.D., was responsible for pronunciations, building on the previous work of Brian M. Sietsema, Ph.D. Biographical information was researched for this and previous editions by Michael G. Belanger. Cross-reference work for the 2016 edition was performed by Emily A. Vezina, building on the previous work of Adrienne M. Scholz, Maria A. Sansalone, and Donna L. Rickerby. For this edition, Daniel B. Brandon was responsible for the handling of the electronic data files, and the task of proofreading was done by editors Brandon, Connor, and Scholz and by Serenity H. Carr, Allison M. DeJordy, Benjamin T. Korzec, Neil S. Serven, and Paul S. Wood. Emily A. Vezina managed production, and Madeline L. Novak coordinated all editorial operations.

Joan I. Narmontas
Editor

EXPLANATORY NOTES

This section provides information on the conventions used throughout the dictionary, from the styling of entries and pronunciation to how we present information on usage and meaning. An understanding of the information contained in these notes will make the dictionary both easier and more rewarding to use.

ENTRIES

MAIN ENTRIES

A boldface letter or a combination of such letters, including punctuation marks and diacritics where needed, that is set flush with the left-hand margin of each column of type is a main entry or entry word. The main entry may consist of letters set solid, of letters joined by a hyphen, or of letters separated by one or more spaces:

al•ler•gy . . . *n*
[1]**an•ti–in•flam•ma•to•ry** . . . *adj*
blood vessel *n*
non–A, non–B hepatitis . . . *n*

The material in lightface type that follows each main entry explains its inclusion in the dictionary.

Variation in the styling of compound words in English is frequent and widespread. It is often completely acceptable to choose freely among open, hyphenated, and closed alternatives. To save space for other information, this dictionary usually limits itself to a single styling for a compound. When a compound is widely used and one styling predominates, that styling is shown. When a compound is uncommon or when the evidence indicates that two or three stylings are approximately equal in frequency, the styling shown is based on the treatment of parallel compounds.

ORDER OF MAIN ENTRIES

The main entries follow one another in alphabetical order letter by letter without regard to intervening spaces or hyphens: *luteinizing hormone* follows *luteinization* and *heart-healthy* follows *heart failure*. Words that often begin with the abbreviation *St.* in common usage have the abbreviation spelled out: *Saint Anthony's fire, Saint Vitus' dance.*

Full words come before parts of words made up of the same letters. Parts of words with no hyphen in front but followed by a hyphen come before parts of words preceded by a hyphen. Solid words come first and are followed by hyphenated compounds and then by open compounds. Lowercase entries come before entries that begin with a capital letter:

path *abbr*
path- . . . *comb form*

-path . . . *n comb form*
work·up . . . *n*
work up . . . *vb*
tri·chi·na . . . *n*
Trichina *n*

Entries containing an Arabic numeral within or at the end of the word are alphabetized as if the number were spelled out: *glucose phosphate* comes after *glucose-1-phosphate* and before *glucose-6-phosphate*, while *LD50* is between *LD* and *LDH*. Some chemical terms are preceded by one or more Arabic numerals or by a chemical prefix abbreviated to a Roman or Greek letter or by a combination of the two usually set off by a hyphen. In general, the numerical or abbreviated prefix is ignored in determining the word's alphabetical place: *N-allylnormorphine* is entered in the letter *a*, *5-hydroxytryptamine* in the letter *h*, and *β2-microglobulin* in the letter *m*. However, if the prefix is spelled out, it is used in alphabetizing the word: *beta globulin* is entered in the letter *b*, and *levo-dihydroxyphenylalanine* in the letter *l*. In a few cases, entries have been made at more than one place to assist the reader in finding the place of definition, especially when the prefix has variants: *gamma-aminobutyric acid*, defined in the letter *g*, is often written with a Greek letter as *γ-aminobutyric acid*, and an entry has been made in the letter *a* to direct the reader to the place of definition.

If the names of two chemical substances differ only in their prefixes, the terms are alphabetized first by the main part of the word and then in relation to each other according to the prefix: *L-PAM* immediately precedes *2-PAM* in the letter *p*.

HOMOGRAPHS

When main entries are spelled alike, they are distinguished by superscript numerals preceding each word:

[1]**ano·rex·ic** . . . *adj*
[2]**anorexic** *n*
[1]**di·et** . . . *n*
[2]**diet** *vb*
[3]**diet** *adj*

Although homographs are spelled alike, they may differ in pronunciation, derivation, or functional classification (as part of speech). The order of homographs is historical: the one first used in English is entered first. In this dictionary abbreviations and symbols are listed last in a series of homographs and are not given superscripts. Abbreviations appear before symbols when both are present.

END-OF-LINE DIVISION

The centered dots within entry words indicate division points at which a hyphen may be put at the end of a line of print or writing. Centered dots are not shown after a single initial letter or before a single terminal letter because printers seldom cut off a single letter:

abort . . . *vb*
body . . . *n*

Nor are they shown at second and succeeding homographs unless these differ among themselves in division or pronunciation:

[1]**mu·tant** . . . *adj*
[2]**mutant** *n*
[1]**pre·cip·i·tate** \pri-ˈsi-pə-ˌtāt\ *vb*
[2]**pre·cip·i·tate** \pri-ˈsi-pə-tət, -ˌtāt\ *n*

There are acceptable alternative end-of-line divisions just as there are acceptable variant spellings and pronunciations. No more than one division is, however, shown for an entry in this dictionary.

Many words have two or more common pronunciation variants, and the same end-of-line division is not always appropriate for each of them. The division *ho·me·op·a·thy,* for example, best fits the variant \ˌhō-mē-ˈä-pə-thē\ whereas the division *hom·e·op·a·thy* best fits the variant \ˌhä-mē-ˈä-pə-thē\. In instances like this, the division falling farther to the left is used, regardless of the order of the pronunciations:

ho·me·op·a·thy \ˌhō-mē-ˈä-pə-thē, ˌhä-\

A double hyphen at the end of a line in this dictionary stands for a hyphen that belongs at that point in a hyphenated word and that is retained when the word is written as a unit on one line:

DNA polymerase *n* : any of several polymerases that promote replication . . . of DNA usu. using single= stranded DNA as a template

VARIANTS

When a main entry is followed by the word *or* and another spelling, the two spellings are equal variants:

[1]**neu·tro·phil** . . . *or* **neu·tro·phil·ic**

If two variants joined by *or* are out of alphabetical order, they remain equal variants. The one printed first is, however, slightly more common than the second:

phys·i·o·log·i·cal . . . *or* **phys·i·o·log·ic**

When another spelling is joined to the main entry by the word *also*, the spelling after *also* is a secondary variant and occurs less frequently than the first:

lip·id . . . *also* **lip·ide**

If there are two secondary variants, the second is joined to the first by *or*. Once the word *also* is used to signal a secondary variant, all following variants are joined by *or:*

taen- *or* **taeni-** *also* **ten-** *or* **teni-**

A variant whose own alphabetical place is at some distance from the main entry is also entered at its own place with a cross-reference to the main entry. Such variants at consecutive or nearly consecutive entries are listed together:

tendonitis *var of* TENDINITIS

anchylose, anchylosis *var of* ANKYLOSE, ANKYLOSIS

Variants having a usage label (as *Brit* or *chiefly Brit*) appear only at their own alphabetical places:

-aemia *also* **-haemia** *chiefly Brit var of* -EMIA

anae·mia *chiefly Brit var of* ANEMIA

haem- *or* **haemo-** *chiefly Brit var of* HEM-

hae·mo·glo·bin *chiefly Brit var of* HEMOGLOBIN

When long lists of such variants would be generated by entering all those at consecutive entries, only one or a few are given. The rest can be deduced by analogy with those which are entered. For example, the chiefly British variant *haemoglobinaemia* is formed analogously with *haemoglobin* and *anaemia* (it might also be recognized from the combining forms *-aemia* and *haem-* or *haemo-*).

RUN-ON ENTRIES

A main entry may be followed by one or more derivatives or by a homograph with a different functional label. These are run-on entries. Each is introduced by a boldface dash and each has a functional label. They are not defined, however, since their meanings can readily be derived from the meaning of the root word:

healthy . . . *adj* . . . — **health•i•ly** . . . *adv* — **health•i•ness** . . . *n*
drift . . . *n* . . . — **drift** *vb*

A main entry may be followed by one or more phrases containing the entry word. These are also run-on entries. Each is introduced by a boldface dash but there is no functional label. They are, however, defined since their meanings are more than the sum of the meanings of their elements:

²couch *n* . . . — **on the couch** : . . .
risk . . . *n* . . . — **at risk** : . . .

A run-on entry is an independent entry with respect to function and status. Labels at the main entry do not apply unless they are repeated.

PRONUNCIATION

The matter between a pair of reversed virgules \ \ following the entry word indicates the pronunciation. The symbols used are listed in the chart printed on the page facing the first page of the dictionary proper and on the inside of the back cover.

SYLLABLES

A hyphen is used in the pronunciation to show syllabic division. These hyphens sometimes coincide with the centered dots in the entry word that indicate end-of-line division; sometimes they do not:

ab•scess \ˈab-ˌses\
met•ric \ˈme-trik\

STRESS

A high-set mark \ˈ\ indicates primary (strongest) stress or accent; a low-set mark \ˌ\ indicates secondary (medium) stress or accent:

ear•ache \ˈir-ˌāk\

The stress mark stands at the beginning of the syllable that receives the stress.

VARIANT PRONUNCIATIONS

The presence of variant pronunciations indicates that not all educated speakers pronounce words the same way. A second-place variant is not to be regarded as less acceptable than the pronunciation that is given first. It may, in fact, be used by as many educated speakers as the first variant, but the requirements of the printed page are such that one must precede the other:

oral \ˈōr-əl, ˈär-\
um•bi•li•cus \ˌəm-bə-ˈlī-kəs, ˌəm-ˈbi-li-\

PARENTHESES IN PRONUNCIATIONS

Symbols enclosed by parentheses represent elements that are present in the pronunciation of some speakers but are absent from the pronunciation of other speakers:

de•sen•si•tize \(ˌ)dē-ˈsen-sə-tīz\
RNA \ˌär-(ˌ)en-ˈā\

PARTIAL AND ABSENT PRONUNCIATIONS

When a main entry has less than a full pronunciation, the missing part is to be supplied from a pronunciation in a preceding entry or within the same pair of reversed virgules:

psy•chol•o•gy \-jē\
vit•i•li•go \ˌvi-tə-ˈlī-ˌgō, -ˈlē-\

The pronunciation of the first two syllables of *psychology* is found at the main entry *psychologist:*

psy•chol•o•gist \sī-ˈkä-lə-jist\

The hyphens before and after \-ˈlē-\ in the pronunciation of *vitiligo* indicate that both the first and the last parts of the pronunciation are to be taken from the immediately preceding pronunciation.

When a variation of stress is involved, a partial pronunciation may be terminated at the stress mark which stands at the beginning of a syllable not shown:

li•gate \ˈlī-ˌgāt, lī-ˈ\

In general, no pronunciation is indicated for open compounds consisting of two or more English words that have own-place entry:

lateral collateral ligament *n*

A pronunciation is shown, however, for any unentered element of an open compound:

Meiss•ner's corpuscle \ˈmīs-nərz-\
hyperemesis grav•i•dar•um \-ˌgra-və-ˈdar-əm\

Only the first entry in a sequence of numbered homographs is given a pronunciation if their pronunciations are the same:

[1]sig•moid \ˈsig-ˌmȯid\ *adj*
[2]sigmoid *n*

The pronunciation of unpronounced derivatives run on at a main entry is a combination of the pronunciation at the main entry and the pronunciation of the suffix or final element.

ABBREVIATIONS, ACRONYMS, & SYMBOLS

Pronunciations are not usually shown for entries with the functional labels *abbr* or *symbol* since they are usually spoken by saying the individual letters in sequence or by giving the expansion. The pronunciation is given only if there is an unusual and unexpected way of saying the abbreviation or symbol:

ICU *abbr* intensive care unit
Al *symbol* aluminum
CABG \'ka-bij\ *abbr* coronary artery bypass graft

Acronyms (as *DNA* and *HEPA*) and compounds (as *ACE inhibitor*) consisting of an acronym and a word element which have one of the traditional parts of speech labels (usually *n, adj, adv,* or *vb* in this book) are given a pronunciation even when the word is spoken by pronouncing the letters in sequence:

DNA \ˌdē-(ˌ)en-'ā\ *n*
ACE inhibitor \'ās-, ˌā-(ˌ)sē-'ē-\ *n*
HEPA \'he-pə\ *adj*

FUNCTIONAL LABELS

An italic label indicating a part of speech or some other functional classification follows the pronunciation or, if no pronunciation is given, the main entry. Of the eight traditional parts of speech, five appear in this dictionary as follows:

healthy . . . *adj*
psy•cho•log•i•cal•ly . . . *adv*
hos•pi•tal . . . *n*
per . . . *prep*
pre•scribe . . . *vb*

Other italic labels used to indicate functional classifications that are not traditional parts of speech include:

tid *abbr*
pleur- *or* **pleuro-** *comb form*
-poi•e•sis . . . *n comb form*
-poi•et•ic . . . *adj comb form*
dys- *prefix*
-lyt•ic . . . *adj suffix*
-i•a•sis . . . *n suffix*
Rolf•ing . . . *service mark*
Ca *symbol*
Val•ium . . . *trademark*

Two functional labels are sometimes combined:

calm•ative . . . *n or adj*
cold turkey *n* . . . — **cold–turkey** *adv or vb*

INFLECTED FORMS

The inflected forms recorded in this dictionary include the plurals of nouns; the past tense, the past participle when it differs from the past tense, and the present participle of verbs; and the comparative and superlative forms of adjectives and adverbs. When these inflected forms are created in a manner considered regular in English (as by adding *-s* or *-es* to nouns, *-ed* and *-ing* to verbs, and *-er* and *-est* to adjectives and adverbs) and when it seems that there is nothing about the formation to give the dictionary user doubts, the inflected form is not shown in order to save space for information more likely to be sought.

If the inflected form is created in an irregular way or if the dictionary user is likely to have doubts about it (even if it is formed regularly), the inflected form is shown in boldface either in full or, especially when the word has three or more syllables, cut back to a convenient and easily recognizable point.

The inflected forms of nouns, verbs, adjectives, and adverbs are shown in this dictionary when suffixation brings about a change in final *y* to *i*, when the word ends in *-ey*, when there are variant inflected forms, and when the dictionary user might have doubts about the spelling of the inflected form:

scaly . . . *adj* **scal•i•er; -est**
[2]**atrophy** . . . *vb* **-phied; -phy•ing**
kid•ney . . . *n, pl* **kidneys**
sar•co•ma . . . *n, pl* **-mas** *also* **-ma•ta**
[1]**burn** . . . *vb* **burned** . . . *or* **burnt** . . . ; **burn•ing**
sta•tus . . . *n, pl* **sta•tus•es**

A plural is also shown for a noun when it ends in a consonant plus *o* or in a double *oo,* and when its plural is identical with the singular. Many nouns in medical English have highly irregular plurals modeled after their language of origin. Sometimes more than one element of a compound term is pluralized:

ego . . . *n, pl* **egos**
HMO . . . *n, pl* **HMOs**
tat•too . . . *n, pl* **tattoos**
[1]**pu•bes** . . . *n, pl* **pubes**
en•ceph•a•li•tis . . . *n, pl* **-lit•i•des**
cor pul•mo•na•le . . . *n, pl* **cor•dia pul•mo•na•lia**

Nouns that are plural in form and that are regularly used with a plural verb are labeled *n pl:*

in•nards . . . *n pl*

If nouns that are plural in form are regularly used with a singular verb, they are labeled *n* or if they are used with either a singular or plural verb, they are labeled *n sing or pl:*

rick•ets . . . *n*
blind stag•gers . . . *n sing or pl*

The inflected forms of verbs, adjectives, and adverbs are also shown whenever suffixation brings about a doubling of a final consonant, elision of a final *e,* or a radical change in the base word itself. The principal parts of a verb are shown when a final *-c* changes to *-ck* in suffixation:

re•fer . . . *vb* **re•ferred; re•fer•ring**
hot . . . *adj* **hot•ter; hot•test**
op•er•ate . . . *vb* **-at•ed; -at•ing**
sane . . . *adj* **san•er; san•est**
[1]**break** . . . *vb* **broke** . . . ; **bro•ken** . . . ; **break•ing**
[1]**ill** . . . *adj* **worse** . . . ; **worst**
mim•ic . . . *vb* **mim•icked** . . . ; **mim•ick•ing**

Inflected forms are not shown at undefined run-ons.

CAPITALIZATION

Most entries in this dictionary begin with a lowercase letter, indicating that the word is not ordinarily capitalized. A few entries have an italic label *often cap,* indicating that the word is as likely to begin with a capital letter as not and is equally acceptable either way. Some entries begin with an uppercase letter, which indicates that the word is usually capitalized:

pan•cre•as . . . *n*
braille . . . *n, often cap*
Gol•gi apparatus . . . *n*

The capitalization of entries that are open or hyphenated compounds is similarly indicated by the form of the entry or by an italic label:

heart attack *n*
[1]**neo–Freud•ian** . . . *adj, often cap N*
Agent Orange . . . *n*

Many acronyms are written entirely or partly in capitals, and this fact is shown by the form of the entry or by an italic label:

DNA . . . *n*
mRNA . . . *n*
cgs *adj, often cap C&G&S*

A word that is capitalized in some senses and lowercase in others shows variations from the form of the main entry by the use of italic labels at the appropriate senses:

strep•to•coc•cus . . . *n* **1** *cap*
pill . . . *n* . . . **2** *often cap*

ATTRIBUTIVE NOUNS

The italicized label *often attrib* placed after the functional label *n* indicates that the noun is often used as an adjective equivalent in attributive position before another noun:

> **blood** . . . *n, often attrib*
> **hos•pi•tal** . . . *n, often attrib*

Examples of the attributive use of these nouns are *blood clot, blood disorder, hospital patient,* and *hospital ward.*

While any noun may occasionally be used attributively before another noun, the label *often attrib* is limited to those having broad attributive use. This label is not used when an adjective homograph (as *serum*) is entered. And it is not used at open compounds that are used attributively with an inserted hyphen.

ETYMOLOGY

Etymologies showing the origin of particular words are given in this dictionary only for some abbreviations and acronyms and for all eponyms.

If an entry for an abbreviation is followed by the expansion from which it is derived, no etymology is given. However, if the abbreviation is derived from a phrase in a foreign language or in English that is not mentioned elsewhere in the entry, that phrase and its language of origin (if other than English) are given in square brackets following the functional label:

> **IFN** *abbr* interferon
> **bid** *abbr* [Latin *bis in die*] twice a day

Words derived from the names of persons are called eponyms. Eponymous entries in this dictionary that are derived from the names of one or more real persons are followed by the last name, personal name, birth and death dates where known, nationality, and occupation or status of the person (or persons) from whose name the term is derived:

> **pas•teu•rel•la** . . . *n* . . .
> **Pas•teur** . . . , **Louis (1822–1895),** French chemist and bacteriologist.

Doubtful dates are followed by a question mark, and approximate dates are preceded by *ca* (circa). In some instances only the years of principal activity are given, preceded by the abbreviation *fl* (flourished):

> **Ka•wa•sa•ki disease** . . . *n* . . .
> **Kawasaki, Tomisaku (*fl* 1961),** Japanese pediatrician.

If a series of main entries is derived from the name of one person, the data usually follow the first entry. The dictionary user who turns, for example, to *pasteurellosis, pasteurization,* or *Pasteur treatment* and seeks biographical information is expected to glance back to the first entry in the sequence, *pasteurella.*

If an eponymous entry is defined by a synonymous cross-reference to the entry where the biographical data appear, no other cross-reference is made. However, if the definition of an eponymous entry contains no clue as to the location of the data, the name of the individual is given following the entry and a directional cross-reference is made to the appropriate entry:

> **gland of Bartholin** *n* : BARTHOLIN'S GLAND
> **Ro•lan•dic area** . . . *n* : the motor area of the cerebral cortex lying just anterior to the central sulcus . . .
> **L. Rolando** — see FISSURE OF ROLANDO

The data for C. T. Bartholin can be found at *Bartholin's gland* and that for Luigi Rolando at *fissure of Rolando.*

USAGE

USAGE LABELS

Status labels are used in this dictionary to signal that a word or a sense of a word is restricted in usage.

A word or sense limited in use to a specific region of the English-speaking world has an appropriate label. The adverb *chiefly* precedes a label when the word has some currency outside the specified region, and a double label is used to indicate currency in each of two specific regions:

red bug . . . *n, Southern & Midland*
ap•pen•di•cec•to•my . . . *n* . . . *Brit*
fru•se•mide . . . *n, chiefly Brit*

The stylistic label *slang* is used with words or senses that are especially appropriate in contexts of extreme informality, that usually have a currency not limited to a particular region or area of interest, and that are composed typically of shortened forms or extravagant or facetious figures of speech. Words with the label *slang* are entered if they have been or in the opinion of the editors are likely to be encountered in communicating with patients especially in emergencies. A few words from the huge informal argot of medicine are entered with the label *med slang* because they have appeared in general context or have been the subject of discussion in medical journals:

ben•ny . . . *n* . . . *slang*
go•mer . . . *n, med slang*

Subject orientation is generally given in the definition; however, a guide phrase is sometimes used to indicate a specific application of a word or sense:

[1]drug . . . *n* **1** . . . **b** *according to the Food, Drug, and Cosmetic Act*
erupt . . . *vb* **1** *of a tooth*

ILLUSTRATIONS OF USAGE

Definitions are sometimes followed by verbal illustrations that show a typical use of the word in context. These illustrations are enclosed in angle brackets, and the word being illustrated is usually replaced by a lightface swung dash. The swung dash stands for the boldface entry word, and it may be followed by an italicized suffix:

ab•er•rant . . . *adj* . . . **2** . . . ⟨~ salivary tissue⟩
pinch . . . *vb* . . . ⟨a ~*ed* nerve caused by entrapment⟩

The swung dash is not used when the form of the boldface entry word is changed in suffixation, and it is not used for open compounds:

tu•ber•os•i•ty . . . *n* . . . ⟨ischial *tuberosities*⟩
tie off *vb* . . . ⟨*tie off* a bleeding vessel⟩

USAGE NOTES

Definitions are sometimes followed by usage notes that give supplementary information about such matters as idiom, syntax, semantic relationship, and status. For trademarks and service marks, a usage note is used in place of a definition. A usage note is introduced by a lightface dash:

pill . . . *n* . . . **2** . . . : . . . — usu. used with *the*
bug . . . *n* **1 a** : . . . — not used technically

> **hs** *abbr* . . . — used esp. in writing prescriptions
>
> **pec** . . . *n* . . . — usu. used in pl.
>
> **Val·ium** . . . *trademark* — used for a preparation of diazepam

Sometimes a usage note calls attention to one or more terms that mean the same thing as the main entry:

> **HIV** . . . *n* : either of two retroviruses that infect and destroy helper T cells of the immune system causing the marked reduction in their numbers that is diagnostic of AIDS — called also *AIDS virus, human immunodeficiency virus*

The called-also terms are shown in italic type. If the called-also term falls alphabetically at some distance from the principal entry, the called-also term is entered in alphabetical sequence with the sole definition being a synonymous cross-reference to the entry where it appears in the usage note:

> **AIDS virus** *n* : HIV
>
> **human immunodeficiency virus** *n* : HIV

Two or more usage notes are separated by a semicolon:

> **parathyroid hormone** *n* : a hormone of the parathyroid gland . . . — abbr. *PTH;* called also *parathormone*

SENSE DIVISION

A boldface colon is used in this dictionary to introduce a definition:

> **pul·mo·nary** . . . *adj* : relating to, functioning like, associated with, or carried on by the lungs

It is also used to separate two or more definitions of a single sense:

> **mal·func·tion** . . . *vb* : to function imperfectly or badly : fail to operate in the normal or usual manner

Boldface Arabic numerals separate the senses of a word that has more than one sense:

> **nerve** . . . *n* **1** : any of the filamentous bands of nervous tissue that connect parts of the nervous system with other organs . . . **2 nerves** *pl* : a state or condition of nervous agitation or irritability **3** : the sensitive pulp of a tooth

Boldface lowercase letters separate the subsenses of a word:

> [1]**dose** . . . *n* **1 a** : the measured quantity of a therapeutic agent to be taken at one time **b** : the quantity of radiation administered or absorbed **2** : a gonorrheal infection

Lightface numerals in parentheses indicate a further division of subsenses:

> **ra·di·a·tion** . . . *n* . . . **2 a** : . . . **b** (1) : the process of emitting radiant energy . . . (2) : the combined processes of emission, transmission, and absorption of radiant energy

A lightface colon following a definition and immediately preceding two or more subsenses indicates that the subsenses are subsumed by the preceding definition:

> **nasal spine** *n* : any of several median bony processes adjacent to the nasal passages: as **a** : ANTERIOR NASAL SPINE **b** : POSTERIOR NASAL SPINE
>
> **extensor ret·i·nac·u·lum** . . . *n* **1** : either of two fibrous bands of fascia crossing the front of the ankle: **a** : a lower band . . . **b** : an upper band . . .

The word *as* may or may not follow the lightface colon. Its presence (as at *nasal spine*) indicates that the following subsenses are typical or significant examples. Its absence (as at *extensor retinaculum*) indicates that the subsenses which follow are exhaustive.

Sometimes a particular semantic relationship between senses is suggested by the use of one of four italic sense dividers: *esp, specif, also,* or *broadly*. The sense divider *esp* (for *especially*) is used to introduce the most common meaning subsumed in the more general preceding definition. The sense divider *specif* (for *specifically*) is used to introduce a common but highly restricted meaning subsumed in the more general preceding definition. The sense divider *also* is used to introduce a meaning that is closely related to but may be considered less important than the preceding sense. The sense divider *broadly* is used to introduce an extended or wider meaning of the preceding definition.

The order of senses within an entry is historical: the sense known to have been first used in English is entered first. This is not to be taken to mean, however, that each sense of a multisense word developed from the immediately preceding sense. It is altogether possible that sense 1 of a word has given rise to sense 2 and sense 2 to sense 3, but frequently sense 2 and sense 3 may have arisen independently of one another from sense 1.

Information coming between the entry word and the first definition of a multisense word applies to all senses and subsenses. Information applicable only to some senses or subsenses is given between the appropriate boldface numeral or letter and the symbolic colon.

> **bur** . . . *n* **1** *usu* **burr**
>
> **chla•myd•ia** . . . *n* **1** *cap* . . . **2** *pl* **-iae** *also* **-ias**

NAMES OF PLANTS, ANIMALS, & MICROORGANISMS

The most familiar names of living and formerly living things are the common or vernacular names (as *mosquito, poison ivy,* and *AIDS virus*) that are determined by popular usage.

In contrast, the scientific names of biological classification are governed by four highly prescriptive, internationally recognized codes of nomenclature for zoology, botany, bacteriology, and virology. These systems of names classify each kind of organism into a hierarchy of groups—taxa—with each kind of organism having one—and only one—correct name and belonging to one—and only one—taxon at each level of classification in the hierarchy.

The taxonomic names of biological nomenclature are used in this dictionary in the definitions of the common names of plants, animals, and microorganisms and in the definitions of diseases and products relating to specific plants, animals, and microorganisms when those organisms do not have entries of their own. Some genus names appear as dictionary entries in the book but they are the only taxonomic names that have their own entries. Taxonomic names that are not given own-place entry will appear only within parentheses when used in a definition:

> **dust mite** *n* : any of various mites (esp. family Pyroglyphidae) commonly found in dust . . .

If a genus name is used in a definition and is not inside parentheses, there is an entry for it at its own alphabetical place:

> **Rocky Mountain spotted fever** *n* : an acute bacterial disease . . . that is caused by a bacterium of the genus *Rickettsia* (*R. rickettsii*) usu. transmitted by ixodid ticks and esp. by the American dog tick and Rocky Mountain wood tick

The use of the genus name *Rickettsia* outside of parentheses indicates that a definition of this genus is entered at its own place. The scientific names of the *American dog tick* and *Rocky Mountain wood tick* will be found at the entries for these organisms. The name of the family (Ixodidae) to which the two ticks belong will be found in parentheses at the entry for *ixodid.*

Many common names are derived directly from the names of taxa, and especially genera, with little or no modification. The genus name (as *Acarus* or *Chlamydia* or *Lentivirus*) is capitalized and italicized but is never pluralized. In contrast, the common or vernacular name (as acarus or chlamydia or lentivirus) is not usually capitalized or italicized but does take a plural (as acari or chlamydiae or lentiviruses). In many cases both the systematic taxonomic name and the common name derived from it are entered in this dictionary:

> **giar•dia** . . . *n* **1** *cap* : a genus of flagellate protozoans inhabiting the intestines of various mammals and including one (*G. lamblia*) that is associated with diarrhea in humans **2** : any flagellate of the genus *Giardia*
>
> **strep•to•coc•cus** . . . *n* **1** *cap* : a genus of . . . gram-positive bacteria (family Streptococcaceae) that . . . include important pathogens of humans and domestic animals **2** *pl* **-coc•ci** . . . : any bacterium of the genus *Streptococcus*; *broadly* : a coccus occurring in chains
>
> **han•ta•vi•rus** . . . *n* **1** *cap* : a genus of bunyaviruses that . . . include viruses causing hantavirus pulmonary syndrome and hemorrhagic fever with renal syndrome **2** : any virus of the genus *Hantavirus*

LINNAEAN NOMENCLATURE OF PLANTS, ANIMALS, & BACTERIA

The nomenclatural codes for botany, zoology, and bacteriology follow the binomial nomenclature of Swedish botanist Carolus Linnaeus (1707–1778), who employed a New Latin vocabulary for the names of organisms and the ranks in the hierarchy of classification.

The fundamental taxon is the genus. It includes a group of closely related kinds of plants (as the genus *Digitalis,* which contains the foxgloves), a group of closely related kinds of animals (as the genus *Micrurus,* which includes the venomous coral snakes of the southern U.S.), or a group of closely related kinds of bacteria (as the genus *Borrelia,* which includes the causative agents of relapsing fever and Lyme disease). The genus name is an italicized and capitalized singular noun.

The unique name of each kind of organism or species in the Linnaean system of classification is the binomial or species name which consists of two parts: a genus name and an italicized lowercase word—the specific epithet—denoting the species. The name for a variety or subspecies—the trinomial, variety name, or subspecies name—adds a similar varietal or subspecific epithet. For example, the head louse (*Pediculus humanus capitis*) and the body louse (*Pediculus humanus humanus*) are subspecies of a species (*Pediculus humanus*) infesting humans.

The genus name in a binomial may be abbreviated to its initial letter if it has been previously spelled out in full within the same text. In this dictionary, a genus name will be found abbreviated before a specific epithet when the genus is spelled out in full earlier within the same sense or within a group of senses that fall under a single boldface sense number:

> **scar•let fever** . . . *n* : an acute contagious febrile disease caused by Group A bacteria of the genus *Streptococcus* (esp. various strains of *S. pyogenes*) . . .

In Linnaean nomenclature, the names of taxa higher than the genus (as family, order, and class) are capitalized plural nouns that are often used with singular verbs and are not abbreviated in normal use. They are not italicized.

Sometimes two or more different New Latin names can be found used in current literature for the same organism or group. This may happen, for example, when old monographs and field guides are kept in print after name changes occur or when there are legitimate differences of opinion about the validity of the names. To help the reader in recognizing an organism or group in such cases, some alternate names are shown as synonyms in this dictionary:

> **Ro•cha•li•maea** . . . *n, syn of* BARTONELLA
>
> **plague** . . . *n* . . . **2** : a virulent contagious febrile disease that is caused by a bacterium of the genus *Yersinia* (*Y. pestis* syn. *Pasteurella pestis*) . . .

VIRUS NOMENCLATURE

The system of virus classification and nomenclature in this dictionary follows the system set forth by the International Committee on Taxonomy of Viruses (ICTV), a committee of the Virology Division of the International Union of Microbiological Societies. The ICTV rules governing virus taxonomy were first formalized in 2000 in the *7th Report of the ICTV* and have continued to be updated in subsequent reports.

The code of virus nomenclature is independent of the Linnaean systems governing the taxonomy of plants, animals, and bacteria and differs in the way names are constructed and written. The names for species, genera, and families of viruses appear in italics and are preceded by the name of the taxon ("species," "genus," or "family") in roman before the italicized name. No two valid taxa in virus classification are permitted to have the same name even if they are assigned to different higher taxa. Thus, each valid taxonomic name is unique no matter where it occurs in the taxonomic hierarchy.

In the nomenclature of viruses, the names of all valid taxa at the species or higher level are written in italics. The name of a species consists of an italicized phrase in which the first word is capitalized, other words are lowercase unless derived from a proper name, and the last word is *virus* or ends in *-virus,* sometimes followed by a number or letter or combination of both (as in species *Human herpesvirus 3,* the causative agent of chicken pox). The name of a genus is a single capitalized word ending in *-virus* sometimes followed by a capital letter (as in genus *Influenzavirus A* which contains species *Influenza A virus*). The name of a family is a single capitalized word ending in *-viridae* (as in family *Herpesviridae* or family *Poxviridae*):

> **small•pox** . . . *n* : an acute contagious febrile disease of humans that is caused by a poxvirus of the genus *Orthopoxvirus* (species *Variola virus*) . . .
>
> **pox•vi•rus** . . . *n* : any of a family (*Poxviridae*) of large brick-shaped or ovoid double-stranded DNA viruses . . .

Italics are not used for the names of strains or subtypes or for synonyms or former names that are no longer valid:

> **pa•po•va•vi•rus** . . . *n* : any of a former family (Papovaviridae) that included the papillomaviruses and polyomaviruses

The rejected family name Papovaviridae is written in roman. The names of the two valid families (*Papillomaviridae* and *Polyomaviridae*) into which the family Papovaviridae has been split are mentioned in parentheses at the entries for *papillomavirus* and *polyomavirus.*

CROSS-REFERENCE

Four different kinds of cross-references are used in this dictionary: directional, synonymous, cognate, and inflectional. In each instance the cross-reference is readily recognized by the lightface small capitals in which it is printed.

A cross-reference usually following a lightface dash and beginning with *see* or *compare* is a directional cross-reference. It directs the dictionary user to look elsewhere for further information. A *compare* cross-reference is regularly appended to a definition; a *see* cross-reference may stand alone:

heart attack *n* . . . — compare ANGINA PECTORIS, CORONARY INSUFFICIENCY, HEART FAILURE 1

iron . . . *n* **1** . . . — symbol *Fe;* see ELEMENT table

mammary artery — see INTERNAL MAMMARY ARTERY

A *see* cross-reference may be used to indicate the place of definition of an entry containing one or more Arabic numerals or abbreviated chemical prefixes that might cause doubt. Examples of chemical names are given above at "Order of Main Entries." The entry below follows the entry for the abbreviation *GP:*

G_1 phase, G_2 phase — see entries alphabetized as G ONE PHASE, G TWO PHASE

A *see* cross-reference may follow a main entry that consists of a single word which does not stand alone but appears only in a compound term or terms; the *see* cross-reference at such entries indicates the compound term or terms in which the single word appears:

herpetiformis — see DERMATITIS HERPETIFORMIS

dorsi — see ILIOCOSTALIS DORSI, LATISSIMUS DORSI, LONGISSIMUS DORSI

A *see* cross-reference may appear after the definition of the name of a generic drug to refer the reader to a trademark used for a preparation of the drug:

di•az•e•pam . . . *n* . . . — see VALIUM

A cross-reference following a boldface colon is a synonymous cross-reference. It may stand alone as the only definition for an entry or for a sense of an entry; it may follow an analytical definition; or it may be one of two synonymous cross-references separated by a comma:

serum hepatitis *n* **:** HEPATITIS B

liv•id . . . *adj* **:** discolored by bruising **:** BLACK-AND-BLUE

af•fec•tion . . . *n* . . . **2** . . . **b :** DISEASE, MALADY

A synonymous cross-reference indicates that a definition at the entry cross-referred to can be substituted as a definition for the entry or the sense or subsense in which the cross-reference appears.

A cross-reference following an italic *var of* is a cognate cross-reference:

procaryote *var of* PROKARYOTE

ma•noeu•vre *chiefly Brit var of* MANEUVER

A cross-reference following an italic label that identifies an entry as an inflected form is an inflectional cross-reference. Inflectional cross-references appear only when the inflected form falls alphabetically at some distance from the main entry:

corpora *pl of* CORPUS

broke *past of* BREAK

When guidance seems needed as to which one of several homographs or which sense of a multisense word is being referred to, a superscript numeral may precede the cross-reference or a sense number may follow it or both:

ossa *pl of* [1]OS
lateral cuneiform bone *n* : CUNEIFORM BONE 1c

COMBINING FORMS, PREFIXES, & SUFFIXES

An entry that begins or ends with a hyphen is a word element that forms part of an English compound:

pharmaco- *comb form* . . . ⟨*pharmaco*logy⟩
dys- *prefix* **1** : . . . ⟨*dys*plasia⟩
-i·a·sis . . . *n suffix, pl* **-i·a·ses** . . . ⟨ameb*iasis*⟩

Combining forms, prefixes, and suffixes are entered in this dictionary for two reasons: to make understandable the meaning of many undefined run-ons and to make recognizable the meaningful elements of words that are not entered in the dictionary.

ABBREVIATIONS & SYMBOLS

Abbreviations and symbols for chemical elements are included as main entries in the vocabulary:

RQ *abbr* respiratory quotient
Al *symbol* aluminum

Abbreviations are entered without periods and have been normalized to one form of capitalization. In practice, however, there is considerable variation, and stylings other than those given in this dictionary are often acceptable.

The more common abbreviations and the symbols of chemical elements also appear after the definition at the entries for the terms they represent:

respiratory quotient *n* : . . . — abbr. *RQ*

Symbols that are not capable of being alphabetized are included in a separate section in the back of this book headed "Signs and Symbols."

ABBREVIATIONS USED IN THIS WORK

abbr	abbreviation
AD	anno Domini
adj	adjective
adv	adverb
attrib	attributive
b	born
BC	before Christ
Brit	British
C	Celsius
ca	circa
cap	capitalized
comb	combining
d	died
esp	especially
F	Fahrenheit
fl	flourished
n	noun
No	North
n pl	noun plural
occas	occasionally
orig	originally
part	participle
pl	plural
pres	present
prob	probably
sing	singular
So	South
SoAfr	South African
specif	specifically
spp	species (*pl*)
syn	synonym
U.S.	United States
usu	usually
var	variant
vb	verb

PRONUNCIATION SYMBOLS

ə	abut, collect, suppose
ˈə, ˌə	humdrum
^{ə}	(in ^{ə}l, ^{ə}n) battle, cotton; (in l^{ə}, m^{ə}, r^{ə}) French table, prisme, titre
ər	further
a	map, patch
ā	day, fate
ä	bother, cot, father
ȧ	a sound between \a\ and \ä\, as in an Eastern New England pronunciation of aunt, ask
au̇	now, out
b	baby, rib
ch	chin, catch
d	did, adder
e	set, red
ē	beat, easy
f	fifty, cuff
g	go, big
h	hat, ahead
hw	whale
i	tip, banish
ī	site, buy
j	job, edge
k	kin, cook
k̲	German Bach, Scots loch
l	lily, cool
m	murmur, dim
n	nine, own
^{n}	indicates that a preceding vowel is pronounced through both nose and mouth, as in French bon \bō^{n}\
ŋ	sing, singer, finger, ink
ō	bone, hollow
ȯ	saw
œ	French bœuf, German Hölle
œ̄	French feu, German Höhle
ȯi	toy
p	pepper, lip
r	rarity
s	source, less
sh	shy, mission
t	tie, attack
th	thin, ether
t̲h̲	then, either
ü	boot, few \ˈfyü\
u̇	put, pure \ˈpyu̇r\
ue	German füllen
ue̅	French rue, German fühlen
v	vivid, give
w	we, away
y	yard, cue \ˈkyü\
^{y}	indicates that a preceding \l\, \n\, or \w\ is modified by having the tongue approximate the position for \y\, as in French digne \dēn^{y}\
z	zone, raise
zh	vision, pleasure
\	slant line used in pairs to mark the beginning and end of a transcription: \ˈpen\
ˈ	mark at the beginning of a syllable that has primary (strongest) stress: \ˈshə-fəl-ˌbōrd\
ˌ	mark at the beginning of a syllable that has secondary (next-strongest) stress: \ˈshə-fəl-ˌbōrd\
-	mark of syllable division in pronunciations (the mark of end-of-line division in boldface entries is a centered dot ·)
( )	indicate that what is symbolized between sometimes occurs and sometimes does not occur in the pronunciation of the word: **bak·ery** \ˈbā-k(ə-)rē\ = \ˈbā-kə-rē, ˈbā-krē\

A \ˈā\ *n* : one of the four ABO blood groups characterized by the presence of antigens designated by the letter A and by the presence of antibodies against the antigens present in the B blood group

A *abbr* **1** adenine **2** ampere

Å *symbol* angstrom

a- *or* **an-** *prefix* : not : without ⟨*a*sexual⟩ — *a-* before consonants other than *h* and sometimes even before *h*, *an-* before vowels and usu. before *h* ⟨*a*chromatic⟩ ⟨*an*hydrous⟩

aa *or* **āā** *abbr* [Latin *ana*] of each — used at the end of a list of two or more substances in a prescription to indicate that equal quantities of each are to be taken

AA *abbr* Alcoholics Anonymous

AAFP *abbr* American Academy of Family Physicians

AAMC *abbr* Association of American Medical Colleges

AAT *abbr* alpha-1-antitrypsin

ab \ˈab\ *n* : ABDOMINAL — usu. used in pl. ⟨highly developed ∼*s*⟩

AB \ˈā-ˈbē\ *n* : the one of the four ABO blood groups characterized by the presence of antigens designated by the letters A and B and by the absence of antibodies against these antigens

ab- *prefix* : from : away : off ⟨*ab*oral⟩

ABA *abbr* applied behavior analysis

abac•a•vir \ə-ˈba-kə-ˌvir\ *n* : an antiviral drug taken orally in the form of its sulfate $(C_{14}H_{18}N_6O)_2{\cdot}H_2SO_4$ in combination with other antiretroviral drugs to treat HIV infection

abac•te•ri•al \ˌā-(ˌ)bak-ˈtir-ē-əl\ *adj* : not caused by or characterized by the presence of bacteria ⟨∼ prostatitis⟩

A band *n* : one of the cross striations in striated muscle that contain myosin filaments and appear dark under the light microscope and light in polarized light

aba•sia \ə-ˈbā-zhə, -zhē-ə\ *n* : inability to walk caused by a defect in muscular coordination — compare ASTASIA

aba•tac•ept \ˌab-ə-ˈta-ˌsept\ *n* : a protein drug that inhibits the activation of T cells and is administered by injection to treat rheumatoid arthritis — see ORENCIA

Ab•be flap \ˈa-bē-\ *n* : lip reconstruction that involves surgically grafting a flap of tissue that is one-half the width of the defect from one lip to the other using a pedicle with an arterial supply

Abbe, Robert (1851–1928), American surgeon.

ab•cix•i•mab \ˌab-ˈsik-si-mab\ *n* : an anticlotting drug that inhibits platelet aggregation — see REOPRO

abdom *abbr* abdomen; abdominal

ab•do•men \ˈab-də-mən, (ˌ)ab-ˈdō-\ *n* **1 a** : the part of the body between the thorax and the pelvis with the exception of the back — called also *belly* **b** : the cavity of this part of the trunk lined by the peritoneum, enclosed by the body walls, the diaphragm, and the pelvic floor, and containing the visceral organs (as the stomach, intestines, and liver) **c** : the portion of this cavity between the diaphragm and the brim of the pelvis **2** : the posterior often elongated region of the body behind the thorax in arthropods

abdomin- *or* **abdomino-** *comb form* **1** : abdomen ⟨*abdomino*plasty⟩ **2** : abdominal and ⟨*abdomino*perineal⟩

[1]**ab•dom•i•nal** \ab-ˈdä-mən-ᵊl\ *adj* **1** : of, belonging to, or affecting the abdomen **2** : performed by entry through the abdominal wall — **ab•dom•i•nal•ly** *adv*

[2]**abdominal** *n* : an abdominal muscle — usu. used in pl.

abdominal aorta *n* : the portion of the aorta between the diaphragm and the bifurcation into the right and left common iliac arteries

abdominal cavity *n* : ABDOMEN 1b

abdominal hernia *n* : any of various hernias (as an inguinal hernia or umbilical hernia) in which an anatomical part (as a section of the intestine) protrudes through an opening, tear, or weakness in the abdominal wall musculature

abdominal reflex *n* : contraction of the muscles of the abdominal wall in response to stimulation of the overlying skin

abdominal region *n* : any of the nine areas into which the abdomen is divided by four imaginary planes of which two are vertical passing through the middle of the inguinal ligament on each side and two are horizontal passing respectively through the junction of the ninth rib and costal cartilage and through the top of the iliac crest — see EPIGASTRIC 2b, HYPOCHONDRIAC 2b, HYPOGASTRIC 1, ILIAC 2, LUMBAR 2, UMBILICAL 2

abdominis — see OBLIQUUS EXTERNUS ABDOMINIS, OBLIQUUS INTERNUS ABDOMINIS, RECTUS ABDOMINIS, TRANSVERSUS ABDOMINIS

ab•dom•i•no•pel•vic \(ˌ)ab-ˌdä-mə-nō-ˈpel-vik\ *adj* : relating to or being the abdominal and pelvic cavities

ab•dom•i•no•per•i•ne•al \-ˌper-ə-ˈnē-əl\ *adj* : relating to the abdominal and perineal regions

abdominoperineal resection *n* : resection of a part of the lower bowel together with adjacent lymph nodes through abdominal and perineal incisions

ab·dom·i·no·plas·ty \ab-ˈdä-mə-nō-ˌplas-tē\ *n, pl* **-ties** : cosmetic surgery of the abdomen that typically involves the removal of excess skin and fat and tightening of the abdominal muscles — called also *tummy tuck*

ab·du·cens nerve \ab-ˈdü-ˌsenz-, -ˈdyü-\ *n* : either of the sixth pair of cranial nerves that are motor nerves, arise beneath the floor of the fourth ventricle, and supply the lateral rectus muscle of each eye — called also *abducens, sixth cranial nerve*

ab·du·cent nerve \-sənt-\ *n* : ABDUCENS NERVE

ab·duct \ab-ˈdəkt *also* ˈab-ˌ\ *vb* : to draw or spread away (as a limb or the fingers) from a position near or parallel to the median axis of the body or from the axis of a limb — **ab·duc·tion** \ab-ˈdək-shən\ *n*

ab·duc·tor \ab-ˈdək-tər\ *n, pl* **ab·duc·to·res** \ˌab-ˌdək-ˈtōr-(ˌ)ēz\ *or* **abductors** : a muscle that draws a part away from the median line of the body or from the axis of an extremity

abductor dig·i·ti min·i·mi \-ˈdi-jə-(ˌ)tē-ˈmi-nə-(ˌ)mē\ *n* **1** : a muscle of the hand that abducts the little finger and flexes the phalanx nearest the hand **2** : a muscle of the foot that abducts the little toe

abductor hal·lu·cis \-ˈhal-yə-səs; -ˈha-lə-səs, -kəs\ *n* : a muscle of the foot that abducts the big toe

abductor pol·li·cis brev·is \-ˈpä-lə-səs-ˈbre-vəs, -lə-kəs-\ *n* : a thin flat muscle of the hand that abducts the thumb at right angles to the plane of the palm

abductor pollicis lon·gus \-ˈlȯŋ-gəs\ *n* : a muscle of the forearm that abducts the thumb and wrist

aberrans — see VAS ABERRANS OF HALLER

ab·er·rant \a-ˈber-ənt; ˈa-bə-rənt, -ˌber-ənt\ *adj* **1** : straying from the right or normal way ⟨~ behavior⟩ **2** : deviating from the usual or natural type : ATYPICAL 1 ⟨~ salivary tissue⟩

ab·er·ra·tion \ˌa-bə-ˈrā-shən\ *n* **1** : failure of a mirror, refracting surface, or lens to produce exact point-to-point correspondence between an object and its image **2** : unsoundness or disorder of the mind **3** : an aberrant organ or individual — **ab·er·ra·tion·al** \-sh(ə-)nəl\ *adj*

ab·er·rom·e·ter \ˌa-bə-ˈrä-mə-tər\ *n* : a machine that detects and measures structural imperfections in the eyeball — **ab·er·rom·e·try** \ˌa-bə-ˈrä-mə-trē\ *n*

A–be·ta \ˈā-ˈbā-tə\ *n* : BETA-AMYLOID

abe·ta·li·po·pro·tein·emia \ˌā-ˌbā-tə-ˌlī-pə-ˌprō-tē-ˈnē-mē-ə, -ˌli-pə-, -ˌprō-tē-ə-ˈnē-\ *n* : a rare genetic disorder in which the body is unable to absorb dietary fats and fat-soluble vitamins (as vitamin A and E) because of an absence of apolipoprotein B-containing lipoproteins (as chylomicrons) in the blood and that is inherited as an autosomal recessive trait — called also *Bassen-Kornzweig syndrome*

abey·ance \ə-ˈbā-əns\ *n* : temporary inactivity or suspension

ABFP *abbr* American Board of Family Practice

ABG *abbr* arterial blood gas

ABI *abbr* **1** acquired brain injury **2** ankle-brachial index

Abil·i·fy \ə-ˈbi-lə-ˌfī\ *trademark* — used for a preparation of aripiprazole

abi·ot·ro·phy \ˌā-(ˌ)bī-ˈä-trə-fē\ *n, pl* **-phies** : degeneration or loss of function or vitality in an organism or in cells or tissues not due to any apparent injury

ab·late \a-ˈblāt\ *vb* **ab·lat·ed; ab·lat·ing** : to remove or destroy esp. by cutting — **ablative** *adj*

ab·la·tion \a-ˈblā-shən\ *n* : the process of ablating; *esp* : surgical removal

ab·la·tio pla·cen·tae \a-ˈblā-shē-ō-plə-ˈsen-(ˌ)tē\ *n* : ABRUPTIO PLACENTAE

abled \ˈā-bəld\ *adj* : capable of unimpaired function — compare DIFFERENTLY ABLED

¹ab·nor·mal \(ˌ)ab-ˈnȯr-məl\ *adj* : deviating from the normal or average ⟨~ behavior⟩ ⟨~ development⟩ — **ab·nor·mal·ly** *adv*

²abnormal *n* : an abnormal person

ab·nor·mal·i·ty \ˌab-nȯr-ˈma-lə-tē\ *n, pl* **-ties** **1** : the quality or state of being abnormal **2** : something abnormal

abnormal psychology *n* : a branch of psychology concerned with mental and emotional disorders (as neuroses and psychoses) and with certain incompletely understood normal phenomena (as dreams)

ABO blood group \ˌā-(ˌ)bē-ˈō-\ *n* : one of the four blood groups A, B, AB, or O comprising the ABO system

ABO group *n* **1** : ABO SYSTEM **2** : ABO BLOOD GROUP

ab·oral \(ˌ)a-ˈbōr-əl, -ˈbȯr-\ *adj* : situated opposite to or away from the mouth — **aborally** *adv*

abort \ə-ˈbȯrt\ *vb* **1** : to cause or undergo abortion **2** : to stop in the early stages ⟨~ a disease⟩ — **abort·er** *n*

¹abor·ti·fa·cient \ə-ˌbȯr-tə-ˈfā-shənt\ *adj* : inducing abortion

²abortifacient *n* : an agent (as a drug) that induces abortion

abor·tion \ə-ˈbȯr-shən\ *n* **1** : the termination of a pregnancy after, accompanied by, resulting in, or closely followed by the death of the embryo or fetus: **a** : spontaneous expulsion of a human fetus during the first 12 weeks of gestation — compare MISCARRIAGE **b** : induced expulsion of a human fetus **c** : expulsion of a fetus of a domestic animal often due to infection at any time before completion of pregnancy **2** : arrest of development of an organ so that it remains imperfect or is absorbed **3** : the arrest of a disease in its earliest stage

abor·tion·ist \-sh(ə-)nist\ *n* : one who induces abortion

abortion pill *n* **:** a drug taken orally to induce abortion esp. early in pregnancy; *esp* **:** MIFEPRISTONE

abor·tive \ə-ˈbȯr-tiv\ *adj* **1 :** imperfectly formed or developed **:** RUDIMENTARY **2 a :** ABORTIFACIENT **b :** cutting short ⟨~ treatment of pneumonia⟩ **c :** failing to develop completely or typically

abor·tus \ə-ˈbȯr-təs\ *n* **:** an aborted fetus; *specif* **:** a human fetus less than 12 weeks old or weighing at birth less than 17 ounces

ABO system \ˌā-(ˌ)bē-ˈō-\ *n* **:** the basic system of antigens of human blood behaving in heredity as an allelic unit to produce any of the ABO blood groups

aboulia *var of* ABULIA

ABP *abbr* **1** ambulatory blood pressure **2** arterial blood pressure

ABPP *abbr* American Board of Professional Psychology

abrade \ə-ˈbrād\ *vb* **abrad·ed; abrad·ing :** to irritate or roughen by rubbing **:** CHAFE

abra·sion \ə-ˈbrā-zhən\ *n* **1 :** wearing, grinding, or rubbing away by friction **2 a :** the rubbing or scraping of the surface layer of cells or tissue from an area of the skin or mucous membrane; *also* **:** a place so abraded **b :** the mechanical wearing away of the tooth surfaces by chewing

[1]**abra·sive** \ə-ˈbrā-siv, -ziv\ *adj* **:** tending to abrade ⟨an ~ substance⟩ — **abra·sive·ness** *n*

[2]**abrasive** *n* **:** a substance used for abrading, smoothing, or polishing

ab·re·ac·tion \ˌa-brē-ˈak-shən\ *n* **:** the expression and emotional discharge of unconscious material (as a repressed idea or emotion) by verbalization esp. in the presence of a therapist — **ab·re·act** \-ˈakt\ *vb* — **ab·re·ac·tive** \-ˈak-tiv\ *adj*

ab·rup·tion \a-ˈbrəp-shən\ *n* **:** a sudden breaking off **:** detachment of portions from a mass ⟨placental ~⟩

ab·rup·tio pla·cen·tae \ə-ˈbrəp-shē-ˌō-plə-ˈsen-(ˌ)tē, -tē-ˌō-\ *n* **:** premature detachment of the placenta from the wall of the uterus — called also *ablatio placentae*

abs \ˈabz\ *pl of* AB

ab·scess \ˈab-ˌses\ *n, pl* **ab·scess·es** \ˈab-sə-ˌsēz, -(ˌ)se-səz\ **:** a localized collection of pus surrounded by inflamed tissue — **ab·scessed** \-ˌsest\ *adj*

ab·scis·sion \ab-ˈsi-zhən\ *n* **:** the act or process of cutting off **:** ABLATION

ab·sco·pal \ab-ˈskō-pəl\ *adj* **:** relating to or being an effect on a nonirradiated part of the body that results from irradiation of another part

ab·sence epilepsy \ˈab-səns-\ *n* **:** epilepsy characterized by the presence of absence seizures: as **a :** CHILDHOOD ABSENCE EPILEPSY **b :** JUVENILE ABSENCE EPILEPSY

absence seizure *n* **:** a nonconvulsive generalized seizure that is marked by the temporary impairment of consciousness usu. manifested as a blank facial expression often accompanied by repetitive movements (as smacking of the lips or blinking of the eyelids), that begins and ends abruptly, and is usu. unremembered afterward, and that is characteristic of childhood and juvenile absence epilepsies — called also *petit mal, petit mal seizure*

ab·so·lute \ˌab-sə-ˈlüt\ *adj* **1 :** pure or relatively free from mixture ⟨~ alcohol⟩ **2 :** relating to, measured on, or being a temperature scale based on absolute zero ⟨~ temperature⟩

absolute humidity *n* **:** the amount of water vapor present in a unit volume of air — compare RELATIVE HUMIDITY

absolute refractory period *n* **:** the period immediately following the firing of a nerve fiber when it cannot be stimulated no matter how great a stimulus is applied — called also *absolute refractory phase;* compare RELATIVE REFRACTORY PERIOD

absolute zero *n* **:** a theoretical temperature characterized by complete absence of heat and equivalent to exactly −273.15°C or −459.67°F

ab·sorb \əb-ˈsȯrb, -ˈzȯrb\ *vb* **1 :** to take up esp. by capillary, osmotic, solvent, or chemical action **2 :** to transform (radiant energy) into a different form usu. with a resulting rise in temperature — **ab·sorb·able** \əb-ˈsȯr-bə-bəl, -ˈzȯr-\ *adj* — **ab·sorb·er** *n*

ab·sor·bent *also* **ab·sor·bant** \-bənt\ *adj* **:** able to absorb — **ab·sor·ben·cy** \-bən-sē\ *n* — **absorbent** *also* **absorbant** *n*

ab·sorp·ti·om·e·try \əb-ˌsȯrp-shē-ˈäm-ə-trē\ *n, pl* **-tries :** measurement of the amount of radiation absorbed (as by living tissue) esp. to determine density — see DUAL-ENERGY X-RAY ABSORPTIOMETRY

ab·sorp·tion \əb-ˈsȯrp-shən, -ˈzȯrp-\ *n* **:** the process of absorbing or of being absorbed — compare ADSORPTION — **ab·sorp·tive** \-tiv\ *adj*

ab·stain \ab-ˈstān\ *vb* **:** to refrain deliberately and often with an effort of self-denial from an action or practice — **ab·stain·er** *n*

ab·sti·nence \ˈab-stə-nəns\ *n* **:** the act or practice of abstaining esp. from engagement in sexual intercourse or consumption of intoxicating beverages — **ab·sti·nent** \-nənt\ *adj*

ab·stract \ˈab-ˌstrakt\ *n* **1 :** a written summary of the key points esp. of a scientific paper **2 :** a pharmaceutical preparation made by mixing a powdered solid extract of a vegetable substance with lactose in such proportions that one part of the final product represents two parts of the original drug from which the extract was made — **ab·stract** \ˈab-ˌstrakt, ab-ˈ\ *vb*

abu·lia *or* **abou·lia** \ā-ˈbü-lē-ə, ə-, -ˈbyü-\ *n* : abnormal lack of ability to act or to make decisions that is characteristic of certain psychotic and neurotic conditions — **abu·lic** *also* **abou·lic** \-lik\ *adj*

[1]**abuse** \ə-ˈbyüs\ *n* **1** : improper or excessive use or treatment ⟨drug ~⟩ **2** : physical maltreatment: as **a** : the act of violating sexually : RAPE **b** *under some statutes* : rape or indecent assault not amounting to rape

[2]**abuse** \ə-ˈbyüz\ *vb* **abused; abus·ing 1** : to put to a wrong or improper use ⟨~ drugs⟩ **2** : to treat so as to injure or damage ⟨~ a child⟩ **3 a** : MASTURBATE **b** : to subject to abuse and esp. to rape or indecent assault — **abus·able** \-ˈbyü-zə-bəl\ *adj* — **abus·er** *n*

abut·ment \ə-ˈbət-mənt\ *n* : a tooth or part of a dental implant to which a prosthetic appliance (as a bridge) is attached for support

ABVD \ˌā-ˌbē-ˌvē-ˈdē\ *n* : a chemotherapy drug regimen of doxorubicin, bleomycin, vinblastine, and dacarbazine that is used to treat Hodgkin's lymphoma

ac *abbr* **1** acute **2** [Latin *ante cibum*] before meals — used in writing prescriptions

Ac *symbol* actinium

aca·cia \ə-ˈkā-shə\ *n* : GUM ARABIC

acal·cu·lia \ˌā-ˌkal-ˈkyü-lē-ə\ *n* : lack or loss of the ability to perform simple arithmetic tasks

acal·cu·lous \ā-ˈkal-kyə-ləs\ *adj* : not affected with, caused by, or associated with gallstones ⟨an ~ gallbladder⟩

acam·pro·sate \ə-ˈkam-prə-ˌsāt\ *n* : a drug $C_{10}H_{20}N_2O_8S_2Ca$ taken orally to maintain abstinence from alcohol during treatment of alcohol dependence — called also *acamprosate calcium*

acanth- *or* **acantho-** *comb form* **1** : spine : prickle : projection ⟨*acantho*cyte⟩ **2** : prickle cell layer ⟨*acantho*ma⟩

acanth·amoe·ba \ə-ˌkanth-ə-ˈmē-bə\ *n* **1** *cap* : a genus of amoebas (family Acanthamoebidae) found esp. in soil and freshwater and including several which cause infections of the skin, respiratory tract, eyes, and brain **2** : any amoeba of the genus *Acanthamoeba*

acan·tho·ceph·a·lan \ə-ˌkan-thə-ˈse-fə-lən\ *n* : any of a small phylum (Acanthocephala) of unsegmented parasitic worms that have a proboscis bearing hooks by which attachment is made to the intestinal wall of the host — **acanthocephalan** *adj*

acan·tho·cyte \ə-ˈkan-thə-ˌsīt\ *n* : an abnormal red blood cell having unevenly spaced and variously shaped cytoplasmic projections — called also *spur cell*

acan·tho·cy·to·sis \ə-ˌkan(t)-thə-ˌsī-ˈtō-səs\ *n, pl* **-to·ses** \-ˈtō-ˌsēz\ **1** : the presence of acanthocytes in the blood **2** : the abnormal state marked by the presence of acanthocytes in the blood; *esp* : ABETALIPOPROTEINEMIA

ac·an·thol·y·sis \ˌak-ˌan-ˈthäl-ə-səs, ˌā-ˌkan-, ˌak-ən-\ *n, pl* **-y·ses** \-ə-ˌsēz\ : loss of coherence between keratinocytes of the epidermis characteristic of various conditions (as pemphigus) marked by vesicular eruption — **acan·tho·lyt·ic** \ə-ˌkan-thə-ˈlit-ik\ *adj*

ac·an·tho·ma \ˌa-(ˌ)kan-ˈthō-mə, ˌā-\ *n, pl* **-mas** \-məz\ *also* **-ma·ta** \-mə-tə\ : a tumor originating in the skin through excessive growth of skin cells esp. of the stratum spinosum

ac·an·tho·sis \-ˈthō-səs\ *n, pl* **-tho·ses** \-ˌsēz\ : a benign overgrowth of the stratum spinosum of the skin — **ac·an·thot·ic** \-ˈthä-tik\ *adj*

acanthosis ni·gri·cans \-ˈni-grə-ˌkanz, -ˈnī-\ *n* : a skin condition that is marked by dark discoloration and velvety thickening of the skin esp. of body folds and creases and is often associated with obesity, insulin resistance, hormonal irregularity, or medication use but may rarely occur as a sign of cancer

acap·nia \ə-ˈkap-nē-ə, (ˌ)ā-\ *n* : a condition of carbon dioxide deficiency in blood and tissues

acar- *or* **acari-** *or* **acaro-** *comb form* : mite ⟨*acar*iasis⟩ ⟨*acari*cide⟩

acar·bose \ā-ˈkär-ˌbōs\ *n* : an antidiabetic drug $C_{25}H_{43}NO_{18}$ taken orally in the treatment of type 2 diabetes

acar·di·ac \(ˈ)ā-ˈkär-dē-ˌak\ *adj* : lacking a heart; *also* : marked by the presence of an acardiac fetus ⟨~ pregnancies⟩

ac·a·ri·a·sis \ˌa-kə-ˈrī-ə-səs\ *n, pl* **-a·ses** \-ˌsēz\ : infestation with or disease caused by mites

acar·i·cide \ə-ˈkar-ə-ˌsīd\ *n* : a pesticide that kills mites and ticks — **acar·i·cid·al** \ə-ˌkar-ə-ˈsīd-ᵊl\ *adj*

ac·a·rid \ˈa-kə-rəd\ *n* : any of an order (Acari syn. Acarina) of arachnids comprising the mites and ticks; *esp* : any of a family (Acaridae) of mites that feed on organic substances and sometimes cause dermatitis in persons repeatedly exposed to infested products — compare GROCER'S ITCH — **acarid** *adj*

ac·a·rine \ˈa-kə-ˌrīn, -ˌrēn, -rən\ *adj* : of, relating to, or caused by mites or ticks ⟨~ dermatitis⟩ — **acarine** *n*

ac·a·rus \ˈa-kə-rəs\ *n, pl* **-ri** \-ˌrī, -ˌrē\ : MITE; *esp* : one of a formerly extensive genus (*Acarus*)

ac·cel·er·ate \ik-ˈse-lə-ˌrāt, ak-\ *vb* **-at·ed; -at·ing** : to speed up; *also* : to undergo or cause to undergo acceleration

ac·cel·er·a·tion \ik-ˌse-lə-ˈrā-shən, ak-\ *n* **1** : the act or process of accelerating : the state of being accelerated **2** : change of velocity; *also* : the rate of this change **3** : advancement in mental growth or achievement beyond the average for one's age

ac·cel·er·a·tor \ik-ˈse-lə-ˌrā-tər, ak-\ *n* : a muscle or nerve that speeds the performance of an action

accelerator globulin *n* : FACTOR V

accelerator nerve *n* : a nerve whose impulses increase the rate of the heart

ac·cep·tor \ik-ˈsep-tər, ak-\ *n* : an atom, molecule, or subatomic particle capable of receiving another entity (as an electron) esp. to form a compound — compare DONOR 2

[1]**ac·ces·so·ry** \ik-ˈse-sə-rē, ak-, -ˈses-rē\ *adj* **1** : aiding, contributing, or associated in a secondary way: as **a** : being or functioning as a vitamin **b** : associated in position or function with something (as an organ or lesion) usu. of more importance **2** : SUPERNUMERARY ⟨~ spleens⟩

[2]**accessory** *n, pl* **-ries** : ACCESSORY NERVE

accessory hemiazygos vein *n* : a vein that drains the upper left side of the thoracic wall, descends along the left side of the spinal column, and empties into the azygos or hemiazygos veins near the middle of the thorax

accessory nerve *n* : either of a pair of motor nerves that are the 11th cranial nerves, arise from the medulla and the upper part of the spinal cord, and supply chiefly the pharynx and muscles of the upper chest, back, and shoulders — called also *accessory, spinal accessory nerve*

accessory olivary nucleus *n* : any of several small masses or layers of gray matter that are situated adjacent to the inferior olive and of which there are typically two on each side

accessory pancreatic duct *n* : a duct of the pancreas that branches from the chief pancreatic duct and opens into the duodenum above it — called also *duct of Santorini*

ac·ci·dent \ˈak-sə-dənt, -ˌdent\ *n* **1** : an unfortunate event resulting from carelessness, unawareness, ignorance, or a combination of causes **2** : an unexpected bodily event of medical importance esp. when injurious ⟨a cerebrovascular ~⟩ **3** : an unexpected happening causing loss or injury which is not due to any fault or misconduct on the part of the person injured but for which legal relief may be sought — **ac·ci·den·tal** \ˌak-sə-ˈdent-^{ə}l\ *adj* — **ac·ci·den·tal·ly** \-ˈdent-lē, -^{ə}l-ē\ *also* **ac·ci·dent·ly** \-ˈdent-lē\ *adv*

accident–prone *adj* **1** : having a greater than average number of accidents **2** : having personality traits that predispose to accidents

ac·cli·mate \ˈa-klə-ˌmāt; ə-ˈklī-mət, -ˌmāt\ *vb* **-mat·ed; -mat·ing** : ACCLIMATIZE

ac·cli·ma·tion \ˌa-klə-ˈmā-shən, -ˌklī-\ *n* : acclimatization esp. by physiological adjustment of an organism to environmental change

ac·cli·ma·tize \ə-ˈklī-mə-ˌtīz\ *vb* **-tized; -tiz·ing** : to adapt to a new temperature, altitude, climate, environment, or situation — **ac·cli·ma·ti·za·tion** \ə-ˌklī-mə-tə-ˈzā-shən\ *n*

ac·com·mo·date \ə-ˈkä-mə-ˌdāt\ *vb* **-dat·ed; -dat·ing** : to adapt oneself; *also* : to undergo visual accommodation — **ac·com·mo·da·tive** \-ˌdā-tiv\ *adj*

ac·com·mo·da·tion \ə-ˌkä-mə-ˈdā-shən\ *n* : an adaptation or adjustment esp. of a bodily part (as an organ): as **a** : the automatic adjustment of the eye for seeing at different distances effected chiefly by changes in the convexity of the crystalline lens **b** : the range over which such adjustment is possible

ac·couche·ment \ˌa-ˌküsh-ˈmä^n, ə-ˈküsh-ˌ\ *n* : the time or act of giving birth

ac·cre·tio cor·dis \ə-ˈkrē-shē-ō-ˈkȯr-dəs\ *n* : adhesive pericarditis in which there are adhesions extending from the pericardium to the mediastinum, pleurae, diaphragm, and chest wall

ac·cre·tion \ə-ˈkrē-shən\ *n* : the process of growth or enlargement; *esp* : increase by external addition or accumulation — compare APPOSITION 1 — **ac·cre·tion·ary** \-shə-ˌner-ē\ *adj*

accumbens — see NUCLEUS ACCUMBENS

Ac·cu·pril \ˈa-kyü-ˌpril\ *trademark* — used for a preparation of the hydrochloride of quinapril

Ac·cu·tane \ˈa-kyü-ˌtān\ *trademark* — used for a preparation of isotretinoin

Ace \ˈās\ *trademark* — used for a bandage with elastic properties

ac·e·bu·to·lol \ˌa-sə-ˈbyü-tə-ˌlȯl\ *n* : a beta-blocker taken orally in the form of its hydrochloride $C_{18}H_{28}N_2O_4 \cdot HCl$ to treat hypertension and ventricular arrhythmia — see SECTRAL

ACE inhibitor \ˈās-, ˌā-(ˌ)sē-ˈē-\ *n* : any of a group of antihypertensive drugs (as captopril) that relax arteries and promote renal excretion of salt and water by inhibiting the activity of angiotensin converting enzyme

acel·lu·lar \(ˌ)ā-ˈsel-yə-lər\ *adj* **1** : containing no cells ⟨~ vaccines⟩ **2** : not divided into cells : consisting of a single complex cell ⟨~ protozoans⟩

acen·tric \(ˌ)ā-ˈsen-trik\ *adj* : lacking a centromere ⟨~ chromosomes⟩

ace·phal·gic \ˌā-sə-ˈfal-jik\ *adj, of a migraine* : characterized by visual sensations (as flashing or flickering lights) without an accompanying headache

ace·sul·fame–K \ˈā-sē-ˌsəl-ˌfām-ˈkā\ *n* : a white crystalline powder $C_4H_4KNO_4S$ that is much sweeter than sucrose and is used as a noncaloric sweetener — called also *acesulfame potassium*

acetabular notch \-ˈnäch\ *n* : a notch in the rim of the acetabulum through which blood vessels and nerves pass

ac•e•tab•u•lo•plas•ty \ˌa-sə-ˈta-byə-(ˌ)lō-ˌplas-tē\ *n, pl* **-ties** : plastic surgery on the acetabulum intended to restore its normal state

ac•e•tab•u•lum \-ˈta-byə-ləm\ *n, pl* **-lums** *or* **-la** \-lə\ : the cup-shaped socket in the hip bone — **ac•e•tab•u•lar** \-lər\ *adj*

ac•et•al•de•hyde \ˌa-sə-ˈtal-də-ˌhīd\ *n* : a volatile water-soluble irritating liquid aldehyde C_2H_4O used chiefly in organic synthesis

acet•amin•o•phen \ə-ˌsē-tə-ˈmi-nə-fən, -ˌset-, -ˈmē-, ˌa-sə-tə-\ *n* : a crystalline compound $C_8H_9NO_2$ used in medicine instead of aspirin to relieve pain and fever — called also *paracetamol;* see LIQUIPRIN, TYLENOL

ac•et•an•i•lide *or* **ac•et•an•i•lid** \ˌa-sə-ˈtan-ᵊl-ˌīd, -əd\ *n* : a white crystalline compound C_8H_9NO used esp. to relieve pain or fever

ac•e•tate \ˈa-sə-ˌtāt\ *n* : a salt or ester of acetic acid

ac•et•azol•amide \ˌa-sə-tə-ˈzō-lə-ˌmīd, -ˈzä-, -məd\ *n* : a diuretic drug $C_4H_6N_4O_3S_2$ used esp. to treat edema associated with congestive heart failure, control epileptic seizures, prevent and treat altitude sickness, and treat glaucoma

ace•tic acid \ə-ˈsē-tik-\ *n* : a colorless pungent acid $C_2H_4O_2$ that is the chief acid of vinegar and is used occas. in medicine as an astringent and styptic

ace•to•ace•tic acid \ˌa-sə-(ˌ)tō-ə-ˌsē-tik-, ə-ˌsē-tō-\ *n* : an unstable acid $C_4H_6O_3$ that is one of the ketone bodies found in abnormal amounts in the blood and urine in certain conditions of impaired metabolism (as in starvation and diabetes mellitus) — called also *diacetic acid*

ace•to•hex•amide \ˌa-sə-tō-ˈhek-sə-məd, ə-ˌsē-tō-, -ˌmīd\ *n* : a sulfonylurea drug $C_{15}H_{20}N_2O_4S$ used in the oral treatment of some of the milder forms of type 2 diabetes in adults to lower the level of glucose in the blood

ace•to•hy•drox•am•ic acid \ˌa-sə-tō-ˌhī-ˌdräk-ˌsa-mik-, ə-ˌsē-tō-\ *n* : a synthetic compound $C_2H_5NO_2$ taken orally to reduce ammonia levels in the urine in the treatment of urinary tract infections and associated kidney stones

ace•to•me•roc•tol \ˌa-sə-(ˌ)tō-mə-ˈräk-ˌtól, ə-ˌsē-tō-, -ˌtōl\ *n* : a white crystalline mercury derivative $C_{16}H_{24}HgO_3$ of phenol used in solution as a topical antiseptic

ac•e•ton•ae•mia *chiefly Brit var of* ACETONEMIA

ac•e•tone \ˈa-sə-ˌtōn\ *n* : a volatile fragrant flammable liquid ketone C_3H_6O found in abnormal quantities in diabetic urine

acetone body *n* : KETONE BODY

ac•e•ton•emia \ˌa-sə-tō-ˈnē-mē-ə\ *n* : KETOSIS 2; *also* : KETONEMIA 1

acetonide — see FLUOCINOLONE ACETONIDE

ac•e•ton•uria \ˌa-sə-tō-ˈnúr-ē-ə, -ˈnyúr-\ *n* : KETONURIA

ace•to•phe•net•i•din \ˌa-sə-(ˌ)tō-fə-ˈne-tə-dən, ə-ˌsē-tō-\ *n* : PHENACETIN

ace•tyl \ə-ˈsēt-ᵊl, ˈa-sət-; ˈa-sə-ˌtēl\ *n* : the radical CH_3CO of acetic acid

acet•y•lase \ə-ˈset-ᵊl-ˌās\ *n* : any of a class of enzymes that accelerate the synthesis of esters of acetic acid

acet•y•late \ə-ˈset-ᵊl-ˌāt\ *vb* **-lat•ed; -lat•ing** : to introduce the acetyl radical into (a compound) — **acet•y•la•tion** \-ˌset-ᵊl-ˈā-shən\ *n*

ace•tyl•cho•line \ə-ˌset-ᵊl-ˈkō-ˌlēn, -ˌsēt-; ˌa-sə-ˌtēl-\ *n* : a neurotransmitter $[C_7H_{16}NO_2]^+$ released at autonomic synapses and neuromuscular junctions, active in the transmission of nerve impulses, and formed enzymatically in the tissues from choline

ace•tyl•cho•lin•es•ter•ase \-ˌkō-lə-ˈnes-tə-ˌrās, -ˌrāz\ *n* : an enzyme that occurs chiefly in cholinergic nerve endings and promotes the hydrolysis of acetylcholine : CHOLINESTERASE 1

acetyl CoA \-ˌkō-ˈā\ *n* : ACETYL COENZYME A

acetyl coenzyme A *n* : a compound $C_{25}H_{38}N_7O_{17}P_3S$ formed as an intermediate in metabolism and active as a coenzyme in biological acetylations

ace•tyl•cys•te•ine \ə-ˌsēt-ᵊl-ˈsis-tə-ˌēn, -ˌset-; ˌa-sə-ˌtēl-, ˌa-sət-ᵊl-\ *n* : a mucolytic agent $C_5H_9NO_3S$ used esp. to reduce the viscosity of abnormally viscid respiratory tract secretions — see MUCOMYST

ace•tyl•phenyl•hy•dra•zine \-ˌfen-ᵊl-ˈhī-drə-ˌzēn, -ˌfēn-\ *n* : a compound $C_8H_{10}ON_2$ used in the symptomatic treatment of polycythemia

ace•tyl•sa•lic•y•late \ə-ˌsēt-ᵊl-sə-ˈli-sə-ˌlāt\ *n* : a salt or ester of acetylsalicylic acid

ace•tyl•sal•i•cyl•ic acid \ə-ˈsēt-ᵊl-ˌsa-lə-ˌsi-lik-\ *n* : ASPIRIN 1

AcG *abbr* [*ac*celerator *g*lobulin] factor V

ACh *abbr* acetylcholine

acha•la•sia \ˌā-kə-ˈlā-zhē-ə, -zhə\ *n* : failure of a ring of muscle (as a sphincter) to relax

¹**ache** \ˈāk\ *vb* **ached; ach•ing** : to suffer a usu. dull persistent pain

²**ache** *n* **1** : a usu. dull persistent pain **2** : a condition marked by aching

achieve•ment age \ə-ˈchēv-mənt-\ *n* : the level of an individual's educational achievement as measured by a standardized test and expressed as the age for which the test score would be the average score

achievement test *n* : a standardized test for measuring the skill or knowledge attained by an individual in one or more fields of work or study

Achil•les reflex \ə-ˈki-lēz-\ *n* : ANKLE JERK

Achilles tendon *n* : the strong tendon joining the muscles in the calf of the leg to the bone of the heel — called also *tendon of Achilles*

achlor•hy•dria \ˌā-ˌklōr-ˈhī-drē-ə\ *n* : absence of hydrochloric acid from the gastric juice — compare HYPERCHLORHYDRIA, HYPOCHLORHYDRIA — **achlor•hy•dric** \-ˈhī-drik\ *adj*

acho•lia \(ˌ)ā-ˈkō-lē-ə, -ˈkä-\ *n* : deficiency or absence of bile

achol•ic \(ˌ)ā-ˈkä-lik\ *or* **acho•lous** \-ˈkō-ləs\ *adj* : exhibiting deficiency of bile ‹~ stools›

achol•uria \ˌā-kō-ˈlu̇r-ē-ə, -kä-, -lyu̇r-\ *n* : absence of bile pigment from the urine — **achol•uric** \-ˈlu̇r-ik, -ˈlyu̇r-\ *adj*

achon•dro•gen•e•sis \ˌā-ˌkän-drə-ˈje-nə-səs\ *n* : a rare disorder of fetal bone and cartilage in which infants are typically stillborn or die shortly after birth

achon•dro•pla•sia \ˌā-ˌkän-drə-ˈplā-zhē-ə, -zhə\ *n* : a genetic disorder that is marked by abnormally slow conversion of cartilage to bone during development, results in a form of dwarfism characterized by a usu. normal torso and shortened limbs, and is usu. inherited as an autosomal dominant — **achon•dro•plas•tic** \-ˈplas-tik\ *adj or n*

achromat- *or* **achromato-** *comb form* : uncolored except for shades of black, gray, and white ‹*achromatopsia*›

ach•ro•mat•ic \ˌa-krə-ˈma-tik\ *adj* **1** : not readily colored by the usual staining agents **2** : possessing or involving no hue : being or involving only black, gray, or white ‹~ visual sensations› — **ach•ro•mat•i•cal•ly** \-ti-k(ə-)lē\ *adv* — **ach•ro•mat•ism** \(ˌ)ā-ˈkrō-mə-ˌti-zəm, a-\ *n*

achro•ma•top•sia \ˌā-ˌkrō-mə-ˈtäp-sē-ə\ *n* : a visual defect that is marked by total color blindness in which the colors of the spectrum are seen as tones of white, gray, and black, by poor visual acuity, and by extreme sensitivity to bright light

achro•mia \(ˌ)ā-ˈkrō-mē-ə\ *n* : absence of normal pigmentation esp. in red blood cells and skin

achy \ˈā-kē\ *adj* **ach•i•er; ach•i•est** : affected with aches — **ach•i•ness** *n*

achy•lia \(ˌ)ā-ˈkī-lē-ə\ *n* : ACHYLIA GASTRICA — **achy•lous** \(ˌ)ā-ˈkī-ləs\ *adj*

achylia gas•tri•ca \-ˈgas-tri-kə\ *n* **1** : partial or complete absence of gastric juice **2** : ACHLORHYDRIA

[1]**ac•id** \ˈa-səd\ *adj* **1** : sour, sharp, or biting to the taste **2 a** : of, relating to, or being an acid; *also* : having the reactions or characteristics of an acid ‹an ~ solution› **b** *of salts and esters* : derived by partial exchange of replaceable hydrogen ‹~ sodium carbonate $NaHCO_3$› **c** : marked by or resulting from an abnormally high concentration of acid ‹~ indigestion› — not used technically

[2]**acid** *n* **1** : a sour substance; *specif* : any of various typically water-soluble and sour compounds that in solution are capable of reacting with a base to form a salt, redden litmus, and have a pH less than 7, and that are hydrogen-containing molecules or ions able to give up a proton to a base or are substances able to accept a pair of electrons from a base **2** : LSD

ac•i•dae•mia *chiefly Brit var of* ACIDEMIA

acid–base balance \ˈa-səd-ˈbās-\ *n* : the state of equilibrium between proton donors and proton acceptors in the buffering system of the blood that is maintained at approximately pH 7.35 to 7.45 under normal conditions in arterial blood

ac•i•de•mia \ˌa-sə-ˈdē-mē-ə\ *n* : a condition in which the hydrogen-ion concentration in the blood is increased

acid–fast \ˈa-səd-ˌfast\ *adj* : not easily decolorized by acids (as when stained) — used esp. of bacteria

acid•ic \ə-ˈsi-dik, a-\ *adj* **1** : acid-forming **2** : ACID

acid•i•fy \-də-ˌfī\ *vb* **-fied; -fy•ing** **1** : to make acid **2** : to convert into an acid — **acid•i•fi•ca•tion** \ə-ˌsi-də-fə-ˈkā-shən, a-\ *n* — **acid•i•fi•er** \ə-ˈsi-də-ˌfī-ər, a-\ *n*

acid•i•ty \ə-ˈsi-də-tē, a-\ *n, pl* **-ties** **1** : the quality, state, or degree of being sour or chemically acid **2** : the quality or state of being excessively or abnormally acid : HYPERACIDITY

acid maltase deficiency *n* : POMPE DISEASE

acid•o•gen•ic \ə-ˌsi-də-ˈje-nik, ˌa-sə-dō-\ *adj* : acid-forming

[1]**acid•o•phil** \ə-ˈsi-də-ˌfil, a-\ *also* **acid•o•phile** \-ˌfīl\ *adj* : ACIDOPHILIC 1

[2]**acidophil** *also* **acidophile** *n* : a substance, tissue, or organism that stains readily with acid stains

acid•o•phil•ic \-ˈfi-lik\ *adj* **1** : staining readily with acid stains **2** : preferring or thriving in a relatively acid environment ‹~ bacteria›

ac•i•doph•i•lus \ˌa-sə-ˈdä-fə-ləs\ *n* : a lactobacillus (*Lactobacillus acidophilus*) that is added esp. to dairy products (as yogurt and milk) or prepared as a dietary supplement, is part of the normal intestinal and vaginal flora, and is used therapeutically esp. to promote intestinal health; *also* : a preparation containing such bacteria

ac•i•do•sis \ˌa-sə-ˈdō-səs\ *n, pl* **-do•ses** \-ˌsēz\ : an abnormal condition of reduced alkalinity of the blood and tissues marked by sickly sweet breath, headache, nausea and vomiting, and visual disturbances and usu. a result of excessive acid production — compare ALKALOSIS, KETOSIS 1 — **ac•i•dot•ic** \-ˈdä-tik\ *adj*

acid phosphatase *n* : a phosphatase (as the phosphomonoesterase from the prostate gland) active in acid medium

acid pump *n* : PROTON PUMP
acid reflux *n* : GASTROESOPHAGEAL REFLUX
acid•u•late \ə-ˈsi-jə-ˌlāt\ *vb* **-lat•ed; -lat•ing** : to make acid or slightly acid — **acid•u•la•tion** \-ˌsi-jə-ˈlā-shən\ *n*
ac•id•uria \ˌa-sə-ˈdu̇r-ē-ə, -ˈdyu̇r-\ *n* : the condition of having acid in the urine esp. in abnormal amounts — see AMINOACIDURIA
ac•id•uric \ˌa-sə-ˈdu̇r-ik, -ˈdyu̇r-\ *adj* : tolerating a highly acid environment; *also* : ACIDOPHILIC 2
ac•i•nar \ˈa-sə-nər, -ˌnär\ *adj* : of, relating to, or comprising an acinus ⟨pancreatic ~ cells⟩
ac•i•ne•to•bac•ter \ˌa-sə-ˈnē-tō-ˌbak-tər\ *n* **1** *cap* : a genus of nonmotile gram-negative rod-shaped bacteria (family Moraxellaceae) that occur in soil and water and are associated with opportunistic infections esp. of the skin, lungs, and urinary tract **2** : a bacterium of the genus *Acinetobacter*
acin•ic \ə-ˈsi-nik\ *adj* : ACINAR
ac•i•nous \ˈa-sə-nəs, ə-ˈsī-nəs\ *adj* : consisting of or containing acini
aci•nus \ˈa-sə-nəs, ə-ˈsī-\ *n, pl* **aci•ni** \-ˌnī\ : any of the small sacs that terminate the ducts of some exocrine glands and are lined with secretory cells
Acip•Hex \ˈas-ə-ˌfeks\ *trademark* — used for a preparation of the sodium salt of rabeprazole
ac•i•tret•in \ˌa-sə-ˈtre-tᵊn\ *n* : a retinoid drug $C_{21}H_{26}O_3$ taken orally to treat severe psoriasis — see SORIATANE
ackee *var of* AKEE
ACL \ˌā-(ˌ)sē-ˈel\ *n* : ANTERIOR CRUCIATE LIGAMENT
ACLS *abbr* advanced cardiac life support
ac•ne \ˈak-nē\ *n* : a disorder of the skin caused by inflammation of the skin glands and hair follicles; *specif* : a form found chiefly in adolescents and marked by pimples esp. on the face — **ac•ned** \-nēd\ *adj*
ac•ne•gen•ic \ˌak-ni-ˈje-nik\ *adj* : producing or increasing the severity of acne ⟨the ~ effect of some hormones⟩
ac•ne•i•form \ˈak-nē-ə-ˌfȯrm, ak-ˈnē-\ *or* **ac•ne•form** \ˈak-nē-ˌfȯrm\ *adj* : resembling acne ⟨an ~ eruption⟩
ac•ne ro•sa•cea \ˌak-nē-rō-ˈzā-shē-ə, -shə\ *n, pl* **ac•nae ro•sa•ce•ae** \ˌak-nē-rō-ˈzā-shē-ˌē\ : ROSACEA
acne ur•ti•ca•ta \-ˌər-tə-ˈkā-tə\ *n* : a chronic inflammatory condition of the skin that resembles acne and typically affects middle-aged women
acne vul•gar•is \-ˌvəl-ˈgar-əs\ *n, pl* **acnae vul•gar•es** \-ˈgar-ˌēz\ : a chronic acne involving mainly the face, chest, and shoulders that is common in adolescents and is marked by the intermittent formation of papular or pustular lesions often resulting in scarring
ACNM *abbr* American College of Nurse-Midwives
ACOG *abbr* American College of Obstetricians and Gynecologists
acous•tic \ə-ˈkü-stik\ *or* **acous•ti•cal** \-sti-kəl\ *adj* : of or relating to the sense or organs of hearing, to sound, or to the science of sounds — **acous•ti•cal•ly** \-k(ə-)lē\ *adv*
acoustic meatus *n* : AUDITORY CANAL
acoustic nerve *n* : AUDITORY NERVE
acoustic neuroma *n* : a nonmalignant usu. slow-growing tumor involving the Schwann cells of the vestibular nerve that may be life-threatening if not treated
acoustic tubercle *n* : a pear-shaped prominence on the inferior cerebellar peduncle including the dorsal nucleus of the cochlear nerve
ACP *abbr* American College of Physicians
ac•quain•tance rape \ə-ˈkwānt-ᵊn(t)s-\ *n* : rape committed by someone known to the victim
ac•quired \ə-ˈkwīrd\ *adj* **1** *of a disease or medical condition* : developed or originating after birth : not congenital or hereditary — compare CONGENITAL 2, FAMILIAL, GENETIC 2, HEREDITARY **2** : being or relating to a physical or behavioral trait arising in response to the action of the environment on the organism
acquired brain injury *n* : injury to the brain (as from stroke or a blow to the head) that is not congenital, hereditary, or degenerative and that causes temporary or permanent symptoms (as memory loss, poor concentration, irritability, depression, headaches, fatigue, or impaired coordination) — abbr. *ABI;* see TRAUMATIC BRAIN INJURY
acquired immune deficiency syndrome *n* : AIDS
acquired immunity *n* : immunity that develops after exposure to a suitable agent (as by an attack of a disease or by injection of antigens) — compare ACTIVE IMMUNITY, INNATE IMMUNITY, PASSIVE IMMUNITY
acquired immunodeficiency syndrome *n* : AIDS
acr- *or* **acro-** *comb form* **1** : top : peak : summit ⟨*acro*cephaly⟩ **2** : height ⟨*acro*phobia⟩ **3** : extremity of the body ⟨*acro*cyanosis⟩
Ac•re•mo•ni•um \ˌak-ri-ˈmō-nē-əm\ *n* : a genus of chiefly saprophytic filamentous fungi that includes several forms (as *A. killense* and *A. falciforme*) causing infections (as pneumonia) esp. in immunocompromised individuals
ac•rid \ˈa-krəd\ *adj* : irritatingly sharp and harsh or unpleasantly pungent in taste or odor — **ac•rid•ly** *adv*
ac•ri•dine \ˈa-krə-ˌdēn\ *n* : a colorless crystalline compound $C_{13}H_9N$ occurring in coal tar and used in dye and pharmaceutical manufacturing
ac•ri•fla•vine \ˌa-krə-ˈflā-ˌvēn, -vən\ *n* : a yellow acridine dye $C_{14}H_{14}N_3Cl$

used often in the form of its reddish-brown hydrochloride as an antiseptic esp. for wounds

ac•ro•cen•tric \ˌa-krō-ˈsen-trik\ *adj* : having the centromere situated so that one chromosomal arm is much shorter than the other — compare METACENTRIC, TELOCENTRIC — **acrocentric** *n*

ac•ro•ceph•a•lo•syn•dac•ty•ly \-ˌse-fə-(ˌ)lō-sin-ˈdak-tə-lē\ *n, pl* **-lies** : any of several congenital genetic syndromes (as Apert syndrome) marked by premature closure of the cranial sutures, malformation of the skull with facial anomalies and often webbed or fused fingers and toes

ac•ro•ceph•a•ly \ˌa-krə-ˈse-fə-lē\ *n, pl* **-lies** *also* **-lias** : OXYCEPHALY

ac•ro•chor•don \ˌa-krə-ˈkȯr-ˌdän\ *n* : SKIN TAG

ac•ro•cy•a•no•sis \ˌa-krō-ˌsī-ə-ˈnō-səs\ *n, pl* **-no•ses** \-ˌsēz\ : a vascular disorder of the hands and feet involving abnormal contraction of the arteriolar walls intensified by exposure to cold and resulting in bluish mottled skin, chilling, and sweating of the affected parts — **ac•ro•cy•a•not•ic** \-ˈnä-tik\ *adj*

ac•ro•der•ma•ti•tis \ˌa-krō-ˌdər-mə-ˈtī-təs\ *n* : inflammation of the skin of the extremities

acrodermatitis chron•i•ca atroph•i•cans \-ˌkrä-ni-kə-a-ˈträ-fi-ˌkanz\ *n* : a chronic skin condition of the extremities that is a late manifestation of Lyme disease and is marked by bluish-red lesions and localized swelling followed months or years later by thin wrinkled atrophied skin usu. with ulcerations

acrodermatitis en•tero•path•i•ca \-ˌen-tə-rō-ˈpa-thi-kə\ *n* : a disorder of zinc absorption inherited as a recessive autosomal trait that is marked by symptoms of zinc deficiency (as diarrhea, hair loss, and skin lesions) and can be controlled with lifelong oral zinc supplementation

ac•ro•dyn•ia \ˌa-krō-ˈdi-nē-ə\ *n* : a disease of infants and young children that is an allergic reaction to mercury, is characterized by dusky pink discoloration of hands and feet with local swelling and intense itching, and is accompanied by insomnia, irritability, and sensitivity to light — called also *erythredema, pink disease, Swift's disease* — **ac•ro•dyn•ic** \-ˈdi-nik\ *adj*

[1]**ac•ro•me•gal•ic** \ˌa-krō-mə-ˈga-lik\ *adj* : exhibiting acromegaly

[2]**acromegalic** *n* : one affected with acromegaly

ac•ro•meg•a•ly \ˌa-krō-ˈme-gə-lē\ *n, pl* **-lies** : chronic hyperpituitarism that is characterized by a gradual and permanent enlargement of the flat bones (as the lower jaw) and of the hands and feet, abdominal organs, nose, lips, and tongue and that develops after ossification is complete — compare GIGANTISM

ac•ro•me•so•me•lic dysplasia \ˌa-krō-ˌme-zə-ˌmē-lik-, -ˌmē-zə-\ *n* : a rare disorder of bone and cartilage development that is a form of dwarfism inherited as an autosomal recessive trait in which the trunk is of normal proportion but the forearms and lower legs are extremely short — called also *acromesomelic dwarfism*

acro•mi•al \ə-ˈkrō-mē-əl\ *adj* : of, relating to, or situated near the acromion

acromial process *n* : ACROMION

ac•ro•mi•cria \ˌa-krō-ˈmi-krē-ə, -ˈmī-\ *n* : abnormal smallness of the extremities

acromio- *comb form* : acromial and <*acromio*clavicular>

acro•mio•cla•vic•u•lar \ə-ˌkrō-mē-(ˌ)ō-klə-ˈvi-kyə-lər\ *adj* : relating to, being, or affecting the joint connecting the acromion and the clavicle

acro•mi•on \ə-ˈkrō-mē-ˌän, -ən\ *n* : the outer end of the spine of the scapula that protects the glenoid cavity, forms the outer angle of the shoulder, and articulates with the clavicle — called also *acromial process, acromion process*

acro•mi•on•ec•to•my \ə-ˌkrō-mē-ˌän-ˈek-tə-mē, -mē-ə-ˈnek-\ *n, pl* **-mies** : partial or total surgical excision of the acromion

ac•ro•mio•plas•ty \ə-ˌkrō-mē-ō-ˈplas-tē\ *n, pl* **-ties** : surgical cutting, shaping, and smoothing of the front or lower surface of the acromion to relieve compression of the rotator cuff

acro•pa•chy \ˈa-krō-ˌpa-kē, ə-ˈkrä-pə-kē\ *n, pl* **-pa•chies** : an uncommon condition associated with autoimmune dysfunction of the thyroid gland (as in Graves' disease) that is marked esp. by swelling and clubbing of fingers and toes and periostitis of the hands and feet

ac•ro•par•es•the•sia \ˌa-krō-ˌpar-əs-ˈthē-zhē-ə, -zhə\ *n* : a condition of burning, tingling, or pricking sensations or numbness in the extremities present on awaking and of unknown cause or produced by compression of nerves during sleep

acrop•a•thy \ə-ˈkrä-pə-thē\ *n, pl* **-thies** : a disease affecting the extremities

ac•ro•phobe \ˈa-krə-ˌfōb\ *n* : a person affected with acrophobia

ac•ro•pho•bia \ˌa-krə-ˈfō-bē-ə\ *n* : abnormal or pathological fear of heights — **ac•ro•pho•bic** \-bik\ *adj*

ac•ro•sclero•der•ma \ˌa-krō-ˌskler-ə-ˈdər-mə\ *n* : scleroderma affecting the extremities, face, and chest

ac•ro•scle•ro•sis \ˌa-krō-sklə-ˈrō-səs\ *n, pl* **-ro•ses** \-ˌsēz\ : ACROSCLERODERMA

ac•ro•some \ˈa-krə-ˌsōm\ *n* : an anterior prolongation of a spermatozoon that releases egg-penetrating enzymes — **ac•ro•so•mal** \ˌa-krə-ˈsō-məl\ *adj*

ac•ry•late \ˈak-rə-ˌlāt\ *n* : a salt or ester of acrylic acid

acryl•ic \ə-ˈkri-lik\ *adj* : of or relating to acrylic acid or its derivatives

acrylic acid *n* : a synthetic unsaturated liquid acid $C_3H_4O_2$ that polymerizes readily

ACSW *abbr* Academy of Certified Social Workers

ACTH \ˌā-ˌsē-(ˌ)tē-ˈāch\ *n* : a protein hormone of the anterior lobe of the pituitary gland that stimulates the adrenal cortex — called also *adrenocorticotropic hormone*

Ac•ti•fed \ˈak-tə-ˌfed\ *trademark* — used for a preparation of the maleate of chlorpheniramine and the hydrochloride of phenylephrine

ac•ti•graph \ˈak-tə-ˌgraf\ *n* : a small device usu. worn on the wrist that records the activity level of the body by sensing physical movement and is used esp. to measure the amount and quality of sleep — **ac•tig•ra•phy** \ak-ˈti-grə-fē\ *n*

ac•tin \ˈak-tən\ *n* : a cellular protein found esp. in microfilaments (as those comprising myofibrils) and active in muscular contraction, cellular movement, and maintenance of cell shape — see F-ACTIN, G-ACTIN

actin- *or* **actini-** *or* **actino-** *comb form* **1** : of, utilizing, or caused by actinic radiation (as X-rays) ⟨*actino*therapy⟩ **2** : actinomycete ⟨*actino*mycosis⟩

ac•tin•ic \ak-ˈti-nik\ *adj* : of, relating to, resulting from, or exhibiting chemical changes produced by radiant energy esp. in the visible and ultraviolet parts of the spectrum

actinic keratosis *n* : a rough scaly pink or white growth that occurs on the surface of the skin in areas frequently exposed to sunlight and that may develop into squamous cell carcinoma

ac•tin•i•um \ak-ˈti-nē-əm\ *n* : a radioactive trivalent metallic element — symbol *Ac;* see ELEMENT table

ac•ti•no•bac•il•lo•sis \ˌak-tə-(ˌ)nō-ˌba-sə-ˈlō-səs, ak-ˌti-nō-\ *n, pl* **-lo•ses** \-ˌsēz\ : a disease that affects domestic animals and sometimes humans, resembles actinomycosis, and is caused by a bacterium of the genus *Actinobacillus* (*A. lignieresi*)

ac•ti•no•ba•cil•lus \-bə-ˈsi-ləs\ *n* **1** *cap* : a genus of aerobic gram-negative parasitic bacteria (family Pasteurellaceae) — see ACTINOBACILLOSIS **2** *pl* **-li** \-ˌlī\ : a bacterium of the genus *Actinobacillus*

ac•ti•no•my•ces \ˌak-tə-(ˌ)nō-ˈmī-ˌsēz, ak-ˌti-nō-\ *n* **1** *cap* : a genus of filamentous or rod-shaped gram-positive bacteria (family Actinomycetaceae) that includes usu. commensal and sometimes pathogenic forms inhabiting mucosal surfaces esp. of the oral cavity — compare ACTINOMYCOSIS **2** *pl* **actinomyces** : a bacterium of the genus *Actinomyces*

ac•ti•no•my•cete \-ˈmī-ˌsēt, -mī-ˈsēt\ *n* : any of an order (Actinomycetales) of filamentous or rod-shaped bacteria (as the actinomyces or streptomyces)

ac•ti•no•my•cin \-ˈmīs-ᵊn\ *n* : any of various mostly toxic polypeptide antibiotics isolated from soil bacteria (esp. *Streptomyces antibioticus*)

actinomycin D *n* : DACTINOMYCIN

ac•ti•no•my•co•sis \ˌak-tə-nō-ˌmī-ˈkō-səs\ *n, pl* **-co•ses** \-ˌsēz\ : infection with or disease caused by actinomycetes

ac•ti•no•spec•ta•cin \ˌak-tə-(ˌ)nō-ˈspek-tə-sən, ak-ˌti-nō-\ *n* : SPECTINOMYCIN

ac•ti•no•ther•a•py \-ˈther-ə-pē\ *n, pl* **-pies** : application for therapeutic purposes of the chemically active rays of the electromagnetic spectrum (as ultraviolet light or X-rays)

ac•tion \ˈak-shən\ *n* **1** : the process of exerting a force or bringing about an effect that results from the inherent capacity of an agent **2** : a function or the performance of a function of the body (as defecation) or of one of its parts ⟨heart ~⟩ **3** : an act of will **4** *pl* : BEHAVIOR ⟨aggressive ~*s*⟩

action potential *n* : a momentary reversal in the potential difference across a plasma membrane (as of a nerve cell or muscle fiber) that occurs when a cell has been activated by a stimulus — compare RESTING POTENTIAL

Ac•tiq \ˌak-ˈtēk\ *trademark* — used for a preparation of the citrate of fentanyl

Ac•ti•vase \ˈak-tə-ˌvās\ *trademark* — used for a preparation of alteplase

ac•ti•vate \ˈak-tə-ˌvāt\ *vb* **-vat•ed; -vat•ing** : to make active or more active: as **a** : to convert into a biologically active derivative or form ⟨*activated* plasminogen⟩ **b** : to make or become biologically or molecularly active ⟨neurons *activated* by dopamine⟩ ⟨~ protein synthesis⟩ — **ac•ti•va•tion** \ˌak-tə-ˈvā-shən\ *n*

ac•ti•vat•ed charcoal *n* : a highly adsorbent fine black odorless tasteless powdered charcoal used in medicine esp. as an antidote in many forms of poisoning and as an antiflatulent

ac•ti•va•tor \ˈak-tə-ˌvā-tər\ *n* **1** : a substance that increases the activity of an enzyme **2** : a substance given off by developing tissue that stimulates differentiation of adjacent tissue; *also* : a structure giving off such a stimulant

ac•tive \ˈak-tiv\ *adj* **1** : capable of acting or reacting esp. in some specific way ⟨an ~ enzyme⟩ **2** : tending to progress or to cause degeneration ⟨~ tuberculosis⟩ **3** : exhibiting optical activity **4** : requiring the expenditure of energy **5** : producing active immunity — **ac•tive•ly** *adv*

active immunity *n* : usu. long-lasting immunity that is acquired through production of antibodies and memory cells within the organism in response to the presence of antigens — compare ACQUIRED IMMUNITY, INNATE IMMUNITY, PASSIVE IMMUNITY

active placebo *n* : a substance used esp. in clinical drug trials that has no therapeutic effect on the condition being treated but may produce side effects (as drowsiness or nausea) similar to those of the drug whose effectiveness is being tested

active site *n* : a region esp. of a protein (as an enzyme) where catalytic activity takes place and whose shape permits the binding only of a specific reactant molecule

active transport *n* : movement of a chemical substance by the expenditure of energy against a gradient in concentration or electrical potential across a plasma membrane

ac•tiv•i•ty \ak-ˈti-və-tē\ *n, pl* **-ties** **1** : natural or normal function ⟨digestive ~⟩ **2** : the characteristic of acting chemically or of promoting a chemical reaction ⟨the ~ of a catalyst⟩

ac•to•my•o•sin \ˌak-tə-ˈmī-ə-sən\ *n* : a viscous contractile complex of actin and myosin concerned together with ATP in muscular contraction

Ac•to•nel \ˈak-tə-ˌnel\ *trademark* — used for a preparation of the sodium salt of risedronate

Ac•tos \ˈak-ˌtōz\ *trademark* — used for a preparation of the hydrochloride of pioglitazone

act out *vb* **1** : to express (as an impulse or a fantasy) directly in overt behavior without modification to comply with social norms **2** : to behave badly or in a socially unacceptable often self-defeating manner esp. as a means of venting painful emotions (as fear or frustration)

acu- *comb form* **1** : performed with a needle ⟨*acu*puncture⟩ **2** : applied to selected areas of the body (as in acupuncture) ⟨*acu*pressure⟩

acu•ity \ə-ˈkyü-ə-tē\ *n, pl* **-ities** : keenness of sense perception ⟨~ of hearing⟩ — see VISUAL ACUITY

acuminata — see CONDYLOMA ACUMINATUM, VERRUCA ACUMINATA

acuminatum — see CONDYLOMA ACUMINATUM

acu•pres•sure \ˈa-kyů-ˌpre-shər\ *n* : the application of pressure (as with the fingertips) to the same points on the body stimulated in acupuncture that is used for its therapeutic effects — see SHIATSU — **acu•pres•sur•ist** \-ˌpre-shə-rist\ *n*

acu•punc•ture \-ˌpəŋk-chər\ *n* : an orig. Chinese practice of inserting fine needles through the skin at specific points esp. to cure disease, relieve pain, or promote healing — **acu•punc•tur•ist** \-chə-rist\ *n*

-acusis *n comb form* : hearing ⟨dipl*acusis*⟩ ⟨hyper*acusis*⟩

acustica — see MACULA ACUSTICA

acuta — see PITYRIASIS LICHENOIDES ET VARIOLIFORMIS ACUTA

acute \ə-ˈkyüt\ *adj* **1** : sensing or perceiving accurately, clearly, effectively, or sensitively ⟨~ vision⟩ **2 a** : characterized by sharpness or severity of sudden onset ⟨~ pain⟩ ⟨an ~ infection⟩ **b** : having a sudden onset, sharp rise, and short course ⟨~ illness⟩ — compare CHRONIC 2 **c** : ACUTE CARE ⟨an ~ hospital⟩ — **acute•ly** *adv* — **acute•ness** *n*

acute abdomen *n* : an acute internal abdominal condition requiring immediate operation

acute alcoholism *n* : alcohol poisoning resulting from the usu. rapid excessive consumption of alcoholic beverages that is characterized by depression of central nervous system functioning leading to slurred speech, muscle incoordination, and drowsiness or loss of consciousness

acute care *adj* : providing or concerned with short-term usu. immediate medical care (as for serious illness or traumatic injury) — **acute care** *n*

acute disseminated encephalomyelitis *n* : an acute inflammation of the brain and spinal cord that is thought to be the result of an immune response following infectious illness or vaccination — abbr. *ADEM*

acute febrile neutrophilic dermatosis *n* : SWEET'S SYNDROME

acute lymphoblastic leukemia *n* : lymphocytic leukemia that is marked by an abnormal increase in the number of lymphoblasts, that is characterized by rapid onset and progression, and that occurs chiefly during childhood — abbr. *ALL;* compare CHRONIC LYMPHOCYTIC LEUKEMIA

acute lymphocytic leukemia *n* : ACUTE LYMPHOBLASTIC LEUKEMIA

acute mountain sickness *n* : altitude sickness that is experienced usu. within several hours to one day of ascending above 8000 to 10,000 feet (about 2500 to 3000 meters) and that is marked by headache, nausea, loss of appetite, vomiting, insomnia, dizziness, and fatigue — abbr. *AMS*

acute myelogenous leukemia *n* : myelogenous leukemia of rapid onset and progression that is marked by an abnormal increase in the number of myeloblasts esp. in bone marrow and blood and that occurs chiefly in adulthood — abbr. *AML;* called also *acute myeloid leukemia;* compare CHRONIC MYELOGENOUS LEUKEMIA

acute myocardial infarction *n* : HEART ATTACK — abbr. *AMI*

acute necrotizing ulcerative gingivitis *n* : a severe form of gingivitis that is marked esp. by painful bleeding gums with gray ulceration and necrosis accompanied by bad breath and fever and is associated with the proliferation of microorganisms (as *Fusobacterium nucleatum* and *Treponema vincentii*) which are normally part of the oral flora — called also *necrotizing ulcerative gingivitis, trench mouth, Vincent's infection*

acute nonlymphocytic leukemia *n* : any of several forms of mylogenous leukemia marked by an abnormal increase in the number of immature white blood cells that are not of the same lineage as B cells and T cells; *esp* : ACUTE MYELOGENOUS LEUKEMIA

acute otitis media *n* : bacterial or viral infection of the middle ear that is of rapid onset and is marked esp. by inflammation, earache, fever, fluid in the middle ear, and sometimes rupture of the tympanic membrane — abbr. *AOM*

acute respiratory distress syndrome *n* : respiratory failure of sudden onset in adults or children that follows injury to the endothelium of the lung (as in sepsis, chest trauma, or pneumonia) resulting in accumulation of protein-rich fluid and alveoli collapse — abbr. *ARDS;* called also *adult respiratory distress syndrome*

acy•a•not•ic \ˌā-ˌsī-ə-ˈnä-tik\ *adj* : characterized by the absence of cyanosis ⟨~ patients⟩ ⟨~ heart disease⟩

acy•clo•vir \ˌā-ˈsī-klō-ˌvir\ *n* : a cyclic nucleoside $C_8H_{11}N_5O_3$ used esp. to treat shingles, genital herpes, and chicken pox — see ZOVIRAX

ac•yl \ˈa-səl, -ˌsēl; ˈā-səl\ *n* : a radical derived usu. from an organic acid by removal of the hydroxyl from all acid groups

Ac•zone \ˈak-ˌzōn\ *trademark* — used for a topical preparation of dapsone

AD *abbr* **1** Alzheimer disease; Alzheimer's disease **2** atopic dermatitis **3** [Latin *auris dextra*] right ear — used esp. in audiology and in writing medical prescriptions

ADA *abbr* **1** adenosine deaminase **2** American Dental Association **3** American Diabetes Association **4** American Dietetic Association **5** Americans with Disabilities Act

adac•tyl•ia \ˌā-ˌdak-ˈti-lē-ə\ *n* : congenital lack of fingers or toes

Ad•a•lat \ˈad-ə-ˌlat\ *trademark* — used for a preparation of nifedipine

ada•lim•u•mab \ˌād-ə-ˈlim-yu̇-ˌmab\ *n* : an immunosuppressive drug that is a monoclonal antibody administered by subcutaneous injection to treat the symptoms of various autoimmune diseases (as rheumatoid arthritis and Crohn's disease) — see HUMIRA

ad•a•man•ti•no•ma \ˌa-də-ˌmant-ᵊn-ˈō-mə\ *n, pl* **-mas** *also* **-ma•ta** \-mə-tə\ : AMELOBLASTOMA

Ad•am's ap•ple \ˈa-dəmz-ˈa-pəl\ *n* : the projection in the front of the neck that is formed by the thyroid cartilage

ad•ams•ite \ˈa-dəm-ˌzīt\ *n* : a yellow crystalline arsenical $C_{12}H_9AsClN$ used as a respiratory irritant in tear gas

Adams, Roger (1889–1971), American chemist.

Adams–Stokes syndrome *n* : STOKES-ADAMS SYNDROME

R. Adams — see STOKES-ADAMS SYNDROME

J. Stokes — see CHEYNE-STOKES RESPIRATION

adap•a•lene \ə-ˈdap-ə-ˌlēn\ *n* : a retinoid $C_{28}H_{28}O_3$ applied topically to the skin in the treatment of acne vulgaris — see DIFFERIN, EPIDUO

adapt \ə-ˈdapt\ *vb* : to make or become fit often by modification — **ad•ap•ta•tion** \ˌa-ˌdap-ˈtā-shən\ *n*

adap•tive \ə-ˈdap-tiv\ *adj* **1** : capable of adapting **2 a** : used to assist a person with a disability in performing a task or activity : ASSISTIVE ⟨~ devices⟩ **b** : engaged in by disabled persons with the aid of specialized equipment or techniques ⟨~ sports⟩

adap•to•gen \ə-ˈdap-tə-jən\ *n* : a nontoxic substance and esp. a plant extract held to increase the body's ability to resist the damaging effects of stress and promote or restore normal physiological functioning — **adap•to•gen•ic** \ə-ˌdap-tə-ˈje-nik\ *adj*

Ad•cir•ca \ad-ˈsər-kə\ *trademark* — used for a preparation of tadalafil

ADD *abbr* attention deficit disorder

ad•der \ˈa-dər\ *n* **1** : the common venomous European viper of the genus *Vipera* (*V. berus*); *broadly* : a terrestrial viper (family Viperidae) **2** : any of several No. American snakes that are harmless but are popularly believed to be venomous

Ad•der•all \ˈa-də-ˌrȯl\ *trademark* — used for a preparation of amphetamine and dextroamphetamine salts

[1]ad•dict \ə-ˈdikt\ *vb* : to cause (a person) to become physiologically dependent upon a substance

[2]ad•dict \ˈa-(ˌ)dikt\ *n* : one who is addicted to a substance

ad•dic•tion \ə-ˈdik-shən\ *n* : compulsive physiological need for and use of a habit-forming substance (as heroin, nicotine, or alcohol) characterized by tolerance and by well-defined physiological symptoms upon withdrawal; *broadly* : persistent compulsive use of a substance known by the user to be physically, psychologically, or socially harmful — compare HABITUATION — **ad•dic•tive** \-ˈdik-tiv\ *adj*

Ad•dis count \ˈa-dis-ˌkau̇nt\ *n* : a technique for the quantitative determination of cells, casts, and protein in a 12-hour urine sample used in the diagnosis and treatment of kidney disease

Addis, Thomas (1881–1949), American physician.

Ad•di•so•ni•an \ˌa-də-ˈsō-nē-ən, -nyən\ *adj* : of, relating to, or affected with Addison's disease ⟨~ crisis⟩

Addison, Thomas (1793–1860), English physician.

addisonian anemia *n, often cap 1st A* : PERNICIOUS ANEMIA

Addison's disease *n* : a rare disease marked by deficient secretion of adrenocortical hormones (as cortisol) that is characterized by fatigue, muscle weakness, weight loss, nausea, diarrhea, low blood pressure, irritability or depression, and brownish pigmentation of the skin and is caused by progressive destruction of the adrenal glands (as by an autoimmune response or infection)

[1]**ad•di•tive** \ˈa-də-tiv\ *adj* : characterized by, being, or producing effects (as drug responses or gene products) that when the causative factors act together are the sum of their individual effects — **ad•di•tive•ly** *adv* — **ad•di•tiv•i•ty** \ˌa-də-ˈti-və-tē\ *n*

[2]**additive** *n* : a substance added to another in relatively small amounts to effect a desired change in properties ⟨food ~*s* that improve flavor⟩

ad•duct \ə-ˈdəkt, a-\ *vb* : to draw (as a limb) toward or past the median axis of the body; *also* : to bring together (similar parts) ⟨~ the fingers⟩ — **ad•duc•tion** \ə-ˈdək-shən, a-\ *n*

ad•duc•tor \-ˈdək-tər\ *n* **1** : any of three powerful triangular muscles that contribute to the adduction of the human thigh: **a** : one arising from the superior ramus of the pubis and inserted into the middle third of the linea aspera — called also *adductor longus* **b** : one arising from the inferior ramus of the pubis and inserted into the iliopectineal line and the upper part of the linea aspera — called also *adductor brevis* **c** : one arising from the inferior ramus of the pubis and the ischium and inserted behind the first two into the linea aspera — called also *adductor magnus* **2** : any of several muscles other than the adductors of the thigh that draw a part toward the median line of the body or toward the axis of an extremity

adductor brev•is \-ˈbre-vəs\ *n* : ADDUCTOR 1b

adductor hal•lu•cis \-ˈhal-yə-sis; -ˈha-lə-səs, -kəs\ *n* : a muscle of the foot that adducts and flexes the big toe and helps to support the arch of the foot — called also *adductor hallucis muscle*

adductor lon•gus \-ˈlȯŋ-gəs\ *n* : ADDUCTOR 1a

adductor mag•nus \-ˈmag-nəs\ *n* : ADDUCTOR 1c

adductor pol•li•cis \-ˈpä-lə-səs, -kəs\ *n* : a muscle of the hand with two heads that adducts the thumb by bringing it toward the palm — called also *adductor pollicis muscle*

adductor tubercle *n* : a tubercle on the proximal part of the medial epicondyle of the femur that is the site of insertion of the adductor magnus

Add•yi \ˈad-ē\ *trademark* — used for a preparation of flibanserin

adef•o•vir \ə-ˈde-fə-ˌvir\ *n* : an antiviral drug $C_{20}H_{32}N_5O_8P$ taken orally in the treatment of hepatitis B — called also *adefovir di•pi•vox•il* \-ˌdī-pə-ˈväk-səl\; see HESPERA

ADEM *abbr* acute disseminated encephalomyelitis

aden- *or* **adeno-** *comb form* : gland : glandular ⟨*aden*itis⟩ ⟨*adeno*myoma⟩

ad•e•nine \ˈad-ᵊn-ˌēn\ *n* : a purine base $C_5H_5N_5$ that codes hereditary information in the genetic code in DNA and RNA — compare CYTOSINE, GUANINE, THYMINE, URACIL

adenine arabinoside *n* : VIDARABINE

ad•e•ni•tis \ˌad-ᵊn-ˈī-təs\ *n* : inflammation of a gland; *esp* : LYMPHADENITIS

ad•e•no•ac•an•tho•ma \ˌad-ᵊn-(ˌ)ō-ˌa-ˌkan-ˈthō-mə\ *n, pl* **-mas** *also* **-ma•ta** \-mə-tə\ : an adenocarcinoma with epithelial cells differentiated and proliferated into squamous cells

ad•e•no•car•ci•no•ma \-ˌkärs-ᵊn-ˈō-mə\ *n, pl* **-mas** *also* **-ma•ta** \-mə-tə\ : a malignant tumor originating in glandular epithelium — **ad•e•no•car•ci•no•ma•tous** \-mə-təs\ *adj*

ad•e•no•fi•bro•ma \-ˌfī-ˈbrō-mə\ *n, pl* **-mas** *also* **-ma•ta** \-mə-tə\ : a benign tumor of glandular and fibrous tissue

ad•e•no•hy•poph•y•sis \-hī-ˈpä-fə-səs\ *n, pl* **-y•ses** \-ˌsēz\ : the anterior part of the pituitary gland that is derived from the embryonic pharynx and is primarily glandular in nature — called also *anterior lobe, anterior pituitary;* compare NEUROHYPOPHYSIS — **ad•e•no•hy•poph•y•se•al** \-(ˌ)hī-ˌpä-fə-ˈsē-əl\ *or* **ad•e•no•hy•po•phys•i•al** \-ˌhī-pə-ˈfi-zē-əl\ *adj*

[1]**ad•e•noid** \ˈad-ᵊn-ˌȯid, ˈad-ˌnȯid\ *adj* **1** : of, like, or relating to glands or glandular tissue; *esp* : like or belonging to lymphoid tissue **2** : of or relating to the adenoids **3 a** : of, relating to, or affected with abnormally enlarged adenoids **b** : characteristic of one affected with abnormally enlarged adenoids ⟨~ facies⟩

[2]**adenoid** *n* **1** : an abnormally enlarged mass of lymphoid tissue at the back of the pharynx characteristically obstructing the nasal and ear passages and inducing mouth breathing, a nasal voice, postnasal discharge, and dullness of facial expression — usu. used in pl. **2** : PHARYNGEAL TONSIL

ad•e•noi•dal \ˌad-ᵊn-ˈȯid-ᵊl\ *adj* : exhibiting the characteristics (as snoring, mouth breathing, and a nasal voice) of one affected with abnormally enlarged adenoids : ADENOID — not usu. used technically

ad•e•noid•ec•to•my \ˌad-ᵊn-ˌȯi-ˈdek-tə-mē\ *n, pl* **-mies** : surgical removal of the adenoids

ad•e•noid•itis \ˌad-ᵊn-ˌȯi-ˈdī-təs\ *n* : inflammation of the adenoids

ad•e•no•lym•pho•ma \ˌad-ᵊn-(ˌ)ō-lim-ˈfō-mə\ *n, pl* **-mas** *also* **-ma•ta** \-mət-ə\ : a benign tumor of the salivary glands and usu. of the parotid gland — called also *Warthin's tumor*

ad•e•no•ma \ˌad-ᵊn-ˈō-mə\ *n, pl* **-mas** *also* **-ma•ta** \-mə-tə\ : a benign tumor

of a glandular structure or of glandular origin — **ad·e·no·ma·tous** \-mə-təs\ *adj*
ad·e·no·ma·toid \ˌad-ᵊn-ˈō-mə-ˌtȯid\ *adj* : relating to or resembling an adenoma ⟨an ∼ tumor⟩
ad·e·no·ma·to·sis \ˌad-ᵊn-ˌō-mə-ˈtō-səs\ *n, pl* **-to·ses** \-ˌsēz\ : a condition marked by multiple growths consisting of glandular tissue
adenomatous polyposis coli *n* : FAMILIAL ADENOMATOUS POLYPOSIS
ad·e·no·my·o·ma \ˌad-ᵊn-(ˌ)ō-ˌmī-ˈō-mə\ *n, pl* **-mas** *also* **-ma·ta** \-mə-tə\ : a benign tumor composed of muscular and glandular elements
ad·e·no·my·o·sis \-ˌmī-ˈō-səs\ *n, pl* **-o·ses** \-ˌsēz\ : endometriosis esp. when the endometrial tissue invades the myometrium
ad·e·nop·a·thy \ˌad-ᵊn-ˈä-pə-thē\ *n, pl* **-thies** : any disease or enlargement involving glandular tissue; *esp* : one involving lymph nodes
aden·o·sine \ə-ˈde-nə-ˌsēn, -sən\ *n* : a nucleoside $C_{10}H_{13}N_5O_4$ that is a constituent of RNA yielding adenine and ribose on hydrolysis
adenosine deaminase *n* : an enzyme which catalyzes the conversion of adenosine to inosine and whose deficiency causes a form of severe combined immunodeficiency disease as a result of the accumulation of toxic metabolites which inhibit DNA synthesis — abbr. *ADA*
adenosine diphosphate *n* : ADP
adenosine mo·no·phos·phate \-ˌmä-nə-ˈfäs-ˌfāt, -ˌmō-\ *n* : AMP
adenosine phosphate *n* : any of three phosphates of adenosine: **a** : AMP **b** : ADP **c** : ATP
adenosine 3',5'–monophosphate \-ˈthrē-ˈfīv-\ *n* : CYCLIC AMP
adenosine tri·phos·pha·tase \-trī-ˈfäs-fə-ˌtās, -ˌtāz\ *n* : ATPASE
adenosine tri·phos·phate \-trī-ˈfäs-ˌfāt\ *n* : ATP
ad·e·no·sis \ˌad-ᵊn-ˈō-səs\ *n, pl* **-no·ses** \-ˌsēz\ : a disease of glandular tissue; *esp* : one involving abnormal proliferation or occurrence of glandular tissue ⟨vaginal ∼⟩
S–aden·o·syl·me·thi·o·nine *also* **aden·o·syl·me·thi·o·nine** \(ˌes)-ə-ˌde-nə-ˌsil-mə-ˈthī-ə-ˌnēn\ *n* : the active form of methionine $C_{15}H_{22}N_6O_5S$ that acts as a methyl group donor (as in the formation of creatine) and is an intermediate in the formation of homocysteine — see SAME
ad·e·not·o·my \ˌad-ᵊn-ˈä-tə-mē\ *n, pl* **-mies** : the operation of dissecting, incising, or removing a gland and esp. the adenoids
ad·e·no·vi·rus \ˌad-ᵊn-ō-ˈvī-rəs\ *n* : any of a family (*Adenoviridae*) of double-stranded DNA viruses that cause infections of the respiratory system, conjunctiva, and gastrointestinal tract and include some capable of inducing malignant tumors in experimental animals — **ad·e·no·vi·ral** \-rəl\ *adj*
ad·e·nyl·ic acid \ˌad-ᵊn-ˈi-lik-\ *n* : AMP
ADH *abbr* **1** alcohol dehydrogenase **2** antidiuretic hormone
ADHD *abbr* attention deficit hyperactivity disorder
ad·here \ad-ˈhir\ *vb* **ad·hered; ad·her·ing 1** : to hold fast or stick by or as if by gluing, suction, grasping, or fusing **2** : to become joined (as in pathological adhesion) — **ad·her·ence** \-ˈhir-ᵊns\ *n*
ad·he·sion \ad-ˈhē-zhən\ *n* **1** : the action or state of adhering; *specif* : a sticking together of substances **2 a** : the abnormal union of surfaces normally separate by the formation of new fibrous tissue resulting from an inflammatory process; *also* : the newly formed uniting tissue ⟨pleural ∼*s*⟩ **b** : the union of wound edges esp. by first intention
[1]**ad·he·sive** \-ˈhē-siv, -ziv\ *adj* **1 a** : tending to adhere or cause adherence **b** : prepared for adhering **2** : characterized by adhesions — **ad·he·sive·ly** *adv*
[2]**adhesive** *n* **1** : a substance that bonds two materials together by adhering to the surface of each **2** : ADHESIVE TAPE
adhesive capsulitis *n* : FROZEN SHOULDER
adhesive pericarditis *n* : pericarditis in which adhesions form between the two layers of pericardium
adhesive tape *n* : tape coated on one side with an adhesive mixture; *esp* : one used for covering wounds
Ad·ie's syndrome \ˈa-dēz-\ *or* **Ad·ie syndrome** \-dē-\ *n* : a neurological disorder that is characterized esp. by an abnormally dilated pupil, absent or diminished light reflexes of the eye, abnormal visual accommodation, and usu. impaired reflex activity of the arms or legs, most commonly affects women between the ages of 20 to 50, and is caused by damage to the ciliary ganglion — called also *Holmes-Adie syndrome*
Adie \ˈā-dē\, **William John (1886–1935)**, British neurologist.
adip- *or* **adipo-** *comb form* : fat : fatty tissue ⟨*adipo*cyte⟩
ad·i·po·cere \ˈa-də-pə-ˌsir\ *n* : a waxy or fatty brownish substance produced by chemical changes affecting dead body fat and muscle long buried or immersed in moisture
ad·i·po·cyte \ˈa-də-pə-ˌsīt\ *n* : FAT CELL
ad·i·pose \ˈa-də-ˌpōs\ *adj* : of or relating to fat; *broadly* : FAT
adipose tissue *n* : connective tissue in which fat is stored and which has the cells distended by droplets of fat
ad·i·pos·i·ty \ˌa-də-ˈpä-sə-tē\ *n, pl* **-ties** : the quality or state of being fat : OBESITY
ad·i·po·so·gen·i·tal dystrophy \ˌa-də-ˌpō-sō-ˈje-nət-ᵊl-\ *n* : a combination of obesity, retarded development of the

sex glands, and changes in secondary sex characteristics that results from impaired function or disease of the pituitary gland and hypothalamus — called also *Fröhlich's syndrome*

adiposus — see PANNICULUS ADIPOSUS

adip•sia \ā-ˈdip-sē-ə, ə-\ *n* : absence of thirst; *also* : abnormal abstinence from the intake of fluids

ad•i•tus \ˈa-də-təs\ *n, pl* **aditus** *or* **ad•i•tus•es** : a passage or opening for entrance

ad•junct \ˈa-ˌjəŋkt\ *n* : ADJUVANT b

ad•junc•tive \ə-ˈjəŋk-tiv, a-\ *adj* : involving the medical use of an adjunct ⟨~ therapy⟩ — **ad•junc•tive•ly** *adv*

ad•just \ə-ˈjəst\ *vb* **1** : to bring about orientation or adaptation of (oneself) **2** : to achieve mental and behavioral balance between one's own needs and the demands of others — **ad•just•ment** \-mənt\ *n*

ad•just•ed *adj* : having achieved an often specified and usu. harmonious relationship with the environment or with other individuals

adjustment disorder *n* : any of a group of psychological disorders characterized by emotional or behavioral symptoms that occur in response to a specific stressor (as divorce or unemployment)

[1]**ad•ju•vant** \ˈa-jə-vənt\ *adj* **1** : serving to aid or contribute **2** : assisting in the prevention, amelioration, or cure of disease ⟨~ chemotherapy following surgery⟩

[2]**adjuvant** *n* : one that helps or facilitates: as **a** : an ingredient (as in a prescription) that facilitates or modifies the action of the principal ingredient **b** : something (as a drug or method) that enhances the effectiveness of a medical treatment **c** : a substance enhancing the immune response

ADL *abbr* activities of daily living

Ad•le•ri•an \ad-ˈlir-ē-ən, äd-\ *adj* : of, relating to, or being a theory and technique of psychotherapy emphasizing the importance of feelings of inferiority, a will to power, and overcompensation in neurotic processes

Ad•ler \ˈäd-lər\, **Alfred (1870–1937),** Austrian psychiatrist.

ad lib \(ˌ)ad-ˈlib\ *adv* : without restraint or imposed limit : as much or as often as is wanted — often used in writing prescriptions

ad li•bi•tum \(ˌ)ad-ˈli-bə-təm\ *adv* : AD LIB ⟨rats fed *ad libitum*⟩

ad•min•is•ter \əd-ˈmi-nə-stər\ *vb* **ad•min•is•tered; ad•min•is•ter•ing** : to give (as medicine) remedially — **ad•min•is•tra•tion** \ad-ˌmi-nə-ˈstrā-shən\ *n*

ad•mit \əd-ˈmit\ *vb* **ad•mit•ted; ad•mit•ting** : to accept into a medical facility (as a hospital) as an inpatient

ad•nexa \ad-ˈnek-sə\ *n pl* : conjoined, subordinate, or associated anatomic parts ⟨the uterine ~ include the ovaries and fallopian tubes⟩ — **ad•nex•al** \-səl\ *adj*

ad•nex•i•tis \ˌad-ˌnek-ˈsī-təs\ *n* : inflammation of adnexa

ad•o•les•cence \ˌad-ᵊl-ˈes-ᵊns\ *n* **1** : the state or process of growing up **2** : the period of life from puberty to maturity

ad•o•les•cent \-ᵊnt\ *n* : one in the state of adolescence — **adolescent** *adj* — **ad•o•les•cent•ly** *adv*

adop•tive immunotherapy \ə-ˈdäp-tiv-\ *n* : treatment esp. for cancer in which lymphocytes removed from a patient are cultured with interleukin-2 (as to generate lymphokine-activated killer cells or induce proliferation of tumor-infiltrating lymphocytes) and are returned to the patient's body to mediate tumor regression

ADP \ˌā-(ˌ)dē-ˈpē\ *n* : a nucleotide $C_{10}H_{15}N_5O_{10}P_2$ composed of adenosine and two phosphate groups that is formed in living cells as an intermediate between ATP and AMP and that is reversibly converted to ATP for the storing of energy by the addition of a high-energy phosphate group — called also *adenosine diphosphate*

adren- *or* **adreno-** *comb form* **1 a** : adrenal glands ⟨*adreno*cortical⟩ **b** : adrenal and ⟨*adreno*genital⟩ **2** : adrenaline ⟨*adren*ergic⟩

[1]**ad•re•nal** \ə-ˈdrēn-ᵊl\ *adj* : of, relating to, or derived from the adrenal glands or their secretion — **ad•re•nal•ly** *adv*

[2]**adrenal** *n* : ADRENAL GLAND

ad•re•nal•ec•to•my \ə-ˌdrēn-ᵊl-ˈek-tə-mē\ *n, pl* **-mies** : surgical removal of one or both adrenal glands

adrenal gland *n* : either of a pair of complex endocrine organs near the anterior medial border of the kidney consisting of a mesodermal cortex that produces glucocorticoid, mineralocorticoid, and androgenic hormones and an ectodermal medulla that produces epinephrine and norepinephrine — called also *adrenal, suprarenal gland*

Adren•a•lin \ə-ˈdren-ᵊl-ən\ *trademark* — used for a preparation of levorotatory epinephrine

adren•a•line \ə-ˈdren-ᵊl-ən\ *n* : EPINEPHRINE

ad•ren•er•gic \ˌa-drə-ˈnər-jik\ *adj* **1** : liberating or activated by adrenaline or a substance like adrenaline — compare CHOLINERGIC 1, NORADRENERGIC **2** : resembling adrenaline esp. in physiological action — **ad•ren•er•gi•cal•ly** \-ji-k(ə-)lē\ *adv*

ad•re•no•cep•tor \ə-ˈdrē-nə-ˌsep-tər\ *n* : any of a group of cell receptors that are activated by epinephrine or norepineprhine : an adrenergic receptor — called also *adrenoreceptor*

ad•re•no•cor•ti•cal \ə-ˌdrē-nō-ˈkȯr-ti-kəl\ *adj* : of, relating to, or derived from the cortex of the adrenal glands

ad•re•no•cor•ti•coid \-ˌkȯid\ *n* : ADRENOCORTICOSTEROID — **adrenocorticoid** *adj*

ad•re•no•cor•ti•co•ste•roid \-ˈstir-ˌȯid, -ˈster-\ *n* : a steroid hormone (as cortisone or aldosterone) obtained from, resembling, or having physiological effects like those of the adrenal cortex : CORTICOSTEROID

ad•re•no•cor•ti•co•tro•pic \-ˈtrō-pik, -ˈträ-\ *also* **ad•re•no•cor•ti•co•tro•phic** \-ˈtrō-fik, -ˈträ-\ *adj* : acting on or stimulating the adrenal cortex

adrenocorticotropic hormone *n* : ACTH

ad•re•no•cor•ti•co•tro•pin \-ˈtrō-pən\ *also* **ad•re•no•cor•ti•co•tro•phin** \-fən\ *n* : ACTH

adre•no•gen•i•tal syndrome \ə-ˌdrē-nō-ˈje-nət-ᵊl-, -ˌdre-\ *n* : CUSHING'S SYNDROME

adre•no•leu•ko•dys•tro•phy \-ˌlü-kō-ˈdis-trə-fē\ *n, pl* **-phies** : a rare demyelinating disease of the central nervous system that is inherited as an X-linked recessive trait chiefly affecting males in childhood and that is characterized by progressive blindness, deafness, tonic spasms, and mental deterioration — abbr. *ALD;* called also *Schilder's disease*

adre•no•lyt•ic \ə-ˌdrēn-ᵊl-ˈi-tik, -ˌdren-\ *adj* : blocking the release or action of adrenaline at nerve endings

adre•no•med•ul•lary \ə-ˌdrē-nō-ˈmed-ᵊl-ˌer-ē, -ˌdre-, -ˈme-jə-ˌler-; -mə-ˈdə-lə-rē\ *adj* : relating to or derived from the medulla of the adrenal glands

adre•no•re•cep•tor \ə-ˌdrē-nō-ri-ˈsep-tər, -ˌdre-\ *n* : ADRENOCEPTOR

adre•no•ste•rone \ə-ˌdrē-nō-stə-ˈrōn, -ˌdre-; ˌa-drə-ˈnäs-tə-ˌ\ *n* : a crystalline steroid $C_{19}N_{24}O_3$ obtained from the adrenal cortex and having androgenic activity

Adria•my•cin \ˌā-drē-ə-ˈmīs-ᵊn, ˌa-\ *trademark* — used for a preparation of the hydrochloride of doxorubicin

ad•sorb \ad-ˈsȯrb, -ˈzȯrb\ *vb* : to take up and hold by adsorption — **ad•sorb•able** \-ˈsȯr-bə-bəl, -ˈzȯr-\ *adj*

ad•sor•bent \-bənt\ *adj* : having the capacity or tendency to adsorb — **adsorbent** *n*

ad•sorp•tion \ad-ˈsȯrp-shən, -ˈzȯrp-\ *n* : the adhesion in an extremely thin layer of molecules (as of gases) to the surfaces of solid bodies or liquids with which they are in contact — compare ABSORPTION — **ad•sorp•tive** \-ˈsȯrp-tiv, -ˈzȯrp-\ *adj*

adult \ə-ˈdəlt, ˈa-ˌdəlt\ *n* **1** : one that has arrived at full development or maturity esp. in size, strength, or intellectual capacity **2** : a human male or female after a specific age (as 21) — **adult** *adj* — **adult•hood** \ə-ˈdəlt-ˌhu̇d\ *n*

adul•ter•ate \ə-ˈdəl-tə-ˌrāt\ *vb* **-at•ed; -at•ing** : to make impure by the addition of a foreign or inferior substance — **adul•ter•ant** \-rənt\ *n or adj* — **adul•ter•a•tion** \-ˈrā-shən\ *n*

adult–on•set diabetes *n* : TYPE 2 DIABETES

adult respiratory distress syndrome *n* : ACUTE RESPIRATORY DISTRESS SYNDROME

adult T-cell leukemia *n* : a lymphoproliferative disease that is marked by high counts of malignant T cells, skin lesions, hypercalcemia, and enlargement of the liver, spleen, and lymph nodes and is associated with the retrovirus HTLV-I — abbr. *ATL;* called also *adult T-cell leukemia/lymphoma*

Ad•vair \ˈad-ˌver\ *trademark* — used for a preparation of fluticasone propionate and a salt of salmeterol

ad•vance di•rec•tive \əd-ˈvan(t)s-də-ˈrek-tiv\ *n* : a legal document (as a living will) signed by a competent person to provide guidance for health-care decisions in the event that the person becomes incompetent to make such decisions

ad•vance•ment \əd-ˈvans-mənt\ *n* : detachment of a muscle or tendon from its insertion and reattachment (as in the surgical correction of strabismus) at a more advanced point from its insertion ⟨flexor tendon ~⟩

advancement flap *n* : a flap of tissue stretched and sutured in place to cover a defect at a nearby position

ad•ven•ti•tia \ˌad-vən-ˈti-shə, -ven-\ *n* : the outer layer that makes up a tubular organ or structure and esp. a blood vessel, is composed of collagenous and elastic fibers, and is not covered with peritoneum — called also *tunica adventitia* — **ad•ven•ti•tial** \-shəl\ *adj*

ad•ven•ti•tious \-shəs\ *adj* : arising sporadically or in other than the usual location

Ad•vil \ˈad-(ˌ)vil\ *trademark* — used for a preparation of ibuprofen

ady•na•mia \ˌā-dī-ˈna-mē-ə, ˌa-də-, -ˈnā-\ *n* : asthenia caused by disease

ady•nam•ic \ˌā-(ˌ)dī-ˈna-mik, ˌa-də-\ *adj* : characterized by or causing a loss of strength or function ⟨~ ileus⟩

AED *abbr* automated external defibrillator; automatic external defibrillator

ae•des \ā-ˈē-(ˌ)dēz\ *n* **1** *cap* : a large cosmopolitan genus of mosquitoes that includes vectors of some diseases (as yellow fever and dengue) **2** *pl* **aedes** : any mosquito of the genus *Aedes* — **ae•dine** \-ˌdīn, -ˌdēn\ *adj*

ae•goph•o•ny *chiefly Brit var of* EGOPHONY

aelurophobe, aelurophobia *var of* AILUROPHOBE, AILUROPHOBIA

-aemia *also* **-haemia** *chiefly Brit var of* -EMIA

aer- *or* **aero-** *comb form* **1** : air : atmosphere ⟨*aer*ate⟩ ⟨*aero*bic⟩ **2** : gas ⟨*aero*sol⟩ **3** : aviation ⟨*aero*medicine⟩

aer•ate \ˈar-ˌāt, ˈa-ər-\ *vb* **aer•at•ed; aer•at•ing** **1** : to supply (the blood) with oxygen by respiration **2** : to supply or impregnate (as a liquid) with air — **aer•a•tion** \ˌar-ˈā-shən, ˌa-ər-\ *n*

aero•al•ler•gen \ar-ō-ˈal-ər-jən\ *n* : an allergen carried in the air

aer•obe \ˈar-ˌōb, ˈa-ər-\ *n* : an organism (as a bacterium) that lives only in the presence of oxygen

aer•o•bic \ˌar-ˈō-bik, ˌa-ər-\ *adj* **1** : living, active, or occurring only in the presence of oxygen ⟨~ respiration⟩ **2** : of, relating to, or induced by aerobes **3 a** : of, relating to, or being activity which increases the body's demand for oxygen thereby resulting in a marked temporary increase in respiration and heart rate ⟨~ exercise⟩ **b** : of or relating to the body's ability to consume oxygen during exercise ⟨~ capacity⟩ **c** : relating to, resulting from, or used in aerobics or aerobic activity — **aer•o•bi•cal•ly** \-bi-k(ə-)lē\ *adv*

aer•o•bics \-biks\ *n pl* **1** : a system of physical conditioning involving exercises (as running, walking, swimming, or calisthenics) strenuously performed so as to cause marked temporary increase in respiration and heart rate — used with a sing. or pl. verb **2** : aerobic exercises

aero•bi•ol•o•gy \ˌar-ō-bī-ˈä-lə-jē\ *n, pl* **-gies** : the science dealing with the occurrence, transportation, and effects of airborne materials or microorganisms (as viruses or pollen)

aero•di•ges•tive \ˌer-ō-dī-ˈje-stiv, -də-\ *adj* : of, relating to, including, or affecting both the respiratory and digestive tracts

aer•odon•tal•gia \ˌar-ō-dän-ˈtal-jē-ə, -jə\ *n* : toothache resulting from atmospheric decompression

aero•em•bo•lism \-ˈem-bə-ˌli-zəm\ *n* : decompression sickness esp. when caused by rapid ascent to high altitudes and resulting exposure to rapidly lowered air pressure — called also *air bends*

aero•med•i•cine \ˌar-ō-ˈme-də-sən\ *n* : a branch of medicine that deals with the diseases and disturbances arising from flying and the associated physiological and psychological problems — **aero•med•i•cal** \-ˈme-di-kəl\ *adj*

aero–oti•tis \ˌar-ə-wō-ˈtī-təs\ *n* : AERO-OTITIS MEDIA

aero–otitis me•dia \-ˈmē-dē-ə\ *n* : the traumatic inflammation of the middle ear resulting from differences between atmospheric pressure and pressure in the middle ear

aero•pha•gia \ˌar-ō-ˈfā-jē-ə, -jə\ *also* **aer•oph•a•gy** \ˌar-ˈä-fə-jē, ˌa-ər-\ *n, pl* **-gias** *also* **-gies** : the swallowing of air esp. in hysteria

aero•pho•bia \ˌar-ō-ˈfō-bē-ə\ *n* **1** : abnormal or excessive fear of drafts or of fresh air **2** : fear or strong dislike of flying — **aero•pho•bic** \-bik\ *adj*

aero•sol \ˈar-ə-ˌsäl, -ˌsȯl\ *n* **1** : a suspension of fine solid or liquid particles in gas ⟨smoke is an ~⟩ **2** : a substance (as a medicine) dispensed from a pressurized container as an aerosol; *also* : the container for this

aero•sol•i•za•tion \ˌar-ə-ˌsä-lə-ˈzā-shən, -ˌsȯ-\ *n* : dispersal (as of a medicine) in the form of an aerosol — **aero•sol•ize** \ˈar-ə-ˌsä-ˌlīz, -ˌsȯ-\ *vb* — **aero•sol•iz•er** *n*

aero•space medicine \ˈar-ō-ˌspās-\ *n* : a medical specialty concerned with the health and medical problems of flight personnel both in the earth's atmosphere and in space

aer•oti•tis \ˌar-ō-ˈtī-təs\ *n* : AERO-OTITIS MEDIA

Aes•cu•la•pi•an staff \ˌes-kyə-ˈlā-pē-ən-\ *n* : STAFF OF AESCULAPIUS

aetio- *chiefly Brit var of* ETIO-

ae•ti•o•log•ic, ae•ti•ol•o•gy, ae•ti•o•patho•gen•e•sis *chiefly Brit var of* ETIOLOGIC, ETIOLOGY, ETIOPATHOGENESIS

AF *abbr* atrial fibrillation

afe•brile \(ˌ)ā-ˈfe-ˌbrīl *also* -ˈfē-\ *adj* : free from fever : not marked by fever

[1]**af•fect** \ˈa-ˌfekt\ *n* : the conscious subjective aspect of an emotion considered apart from bodily changes

[2]**af•fect** \ə-ˈfekt, a-\ *vb* : to produce an effect upon; *esp* : to produce a material influence upon or alteration in

af•fec•tion \ə-ˈfek-shən\ *n* **1** : the action of affecting : the state of being affected **2 a** : a bodily condition **b** : DISEASE, MALADY ⟨a pulmonary ~⟩

af•fec•tive \a-ˈfek-tiv\ *adj* : relating to, arising from, or influencing feelings or emotions : EMOTIONAL ⟨~ symptoms⟩ — **af•fec•tive•ly** *adv* — **af•fec•tiv•i•ty** \ˌa-ˌfek-ˈti-və-tē\ *n*

affective disorder *n* : MOOD DISORDER

[1]**af•fer•ent** \ˈa-fə-rənt, -ˌfer-ənt\ *adj* : bearing or conducting inward; *specif* : conveying impulses toward the central nervous system — compare EFFERENT — **af•fer•ent•ly** *adv*

[2]**afferent** *n* : an afferent anatomical part (as a nerve)

af•fin•i•ty \ə-ˈfin-ət-ē\ *n, pl* **-ties** : an attractive force between substances that causes them to enter into and remain in chemical combination

affinity chromatography *n* : chromatography in which a macromolecule (as a protein) is isolated and purified by passing it in solution through a column treated with a substance having a ligand for which the macromolecule has an affinity

A–fib \ˈā-ˈfib\ *n* : ATRIAL FIBRILLATION

afi•brin•o•gen•emia \ˌā-(ˌ)fī-ˌbri-nə-jə-ˈnē-mē-ə\ *n* : an abnormality of blood clotting caused by usu. congenital absence of fibrinogen in the blood

Afin•i•tor \ə-ˈfin-ə-ˌtȯr\ *trademark* — used for a preparation of everolimus

af•la•tox•in \ˌa-flə-ˈtäk-sən\ *n* : any of several carcinogenic mycotoxins that are produced esp. in stored agricultural crops (as peanuts) by molds (as *Aspergillus flavus*)

Aflur·ia \ə-ˈflu̇r-ē-ə\ *trademark* — used for a vaccine against influenza administered as an intramuscular injection
AFP *abbr* alpha-fetoprotein
African horse sickness *n* : an often fatal disease esp. of horses that is caused by a reovirus of the genus *Orbivirus* (species *African horse sickness virus*), is endemic in sub-Saharan Africa, is marked by fever, edematous swellings, and internal hemorrhage, and is transmitted esp. by biting flies of the genus *Culicoides*
Af·ri·can·ized bee \ˈa-fri-kə-ˌnīzd-\ *n* : a honeybee that originated in Brazil as a hybrid between an aggressive African subspecies (*Apis mellifera scutellata*) and European honeybees and has spread to Mexico and the southernmost U.S. — called also *Africanized honeybee, killer bee*
African sleeping sickness *n* : SLEEPING SICKNESS 1
African swine fever *n* : highly contagious usu. fatal disease that affects only swine, resembles but is more severe than hog cholera, and is caused by a double-stranded DNA virus (species *African swine fever virus* of the genus *Asfivirus,* family *Asfarviridae*) — called also *swine fever*
African trypanosomiasis *n* : any of several trypanosomiases caused by African trypanosomes; *esp* : SLEEPING SICKNESS 1
af·ter·birth \ˈaf-tər-ˌbərth\ *n* : the placenta and fetal membranes that are expelled after delivery
af·ter·care \-ˌkar\ *n* : the care, treatment, help, or supervision given to persons discharged from an institution (as a hospital or prison)
af·ter·ef·fect \ˈaf-tər-i-ˌfekt\ *n* **1** : an effect that follows its cause after an interval **2** : a secondary result esp. in the action of a drug coming on after the subsidence of the first effect
af·ter·im·age \-ˌi-mij\ *n* : a usu. visual sensation occurring after stimulation by its external cause has ceased — called also *aftersensation, aftervision*
af·ter·load \ˈaf-tər-ˌlōd\ *n* : the force against which a ventricle contracts that is contributed to by the vascular resistance esp. of the arteries and by the physical characteristics (as mass and viscosity) of the blood
af·ter·pain \-ˌpān\ *n* : pain that follows its cause only after a distinct interval
af·ter·taste \-ˌtāst\ *n* : persistence of a sensation (as of flavor or an emotion) after the stimulating agent or experience has gone
af·to·sa \af-ˈtō-sə, -zə\ *n* : FOOT-AND-MOUTH DISEASE
Ag *symbol* [Latin *argentum*] silver
aga·lac·tia \ˌā-gə-ˈlak-shē-ə, -shə, -tē-ə\ *n* : the failure of the secretion of milk from any cause other than the normal ending of the lactation period — **aga·lac·tic** \-ˈlak-tik\ *adj*
agam·ma·glob·u·lin·emia \(ˌ)ā-ˌga-mə-ˌglä-byə-lə-ˈnē-mē-ə\ *n* : a pathological condition in which the body forms few or no gamma globulins or antibodies — compare DYSGAMMAGLOBULINEMIA
agan·gli·on·ic \(ˌ)ā-ˌgaŋ-glē-ˈä-nik\ *adj* : lacking ganglia
agar \ˈä-gər\ *n* **1** : a gelatinous extract of a red alga (as of the genera *Gelidium, Gracilaria,* and *Eucheuma*) used esp. in culture media or as a gelling and stabilizing agent in foods **2** : a culture medium containing agar
agar–agar \ˌä-gər-ˈä-gər\ *n* : AGAR
aga·rose \ˈa-gə-ˌrōs, ˈä-, -ˌrōz\ *n* : a polysaccharide obtained from agar that is used esp. as a supporting medium in gel electrophoresis
¹age \ˈāj\ *n* **1 a** : the part of life from birth to a given time ⟨a child 10 years of ~⟩ **b** : the time or part of life at which some particular event, qualification, or capacity arises, occurs, or is lost ⟨of reproductive ~⟩ **c** : an advanced stage of life **2** : an individual's development measured in terms of the years requisite for like development of an average individual — see BINET AGE, MENTAL AGE
²age *vb* **aged; ag·ing** *or* **age·ing** : to grow old or cause to grow old
agen·e·sis \(ˌ)ā-ˈje-nə-səs\ *n, pl* **-e·ses** \-ˌsēz\ : lack or failure of development (as of a body part)
agent \ˈā-jənt\ *n* **1** : something that produces or is capable of producing an effect **2** : a chemically, physically, or biologically active principle — see OXIDIZING AGENT, REDUCING AGENT
Agent Orange \-ˈȯr-inj\ *n* : an herbicide widely used as a defoliant in the Vietnam War that is composed of 2,4-D and 2,4,5-T and contains dioxin as a contaminant
age–related macular degeneration *n* : macular degeneration that affects the elderly in either a slowly progressing form marked esp. by the accumulation of yellow deposits in and thinning of the macula or in a rapidly progressing form marked by scarring produced by bleeding and fluid leakage below the macula — abbr. *AMD*
age spots *n pl* : benign flat spots evenly covered with darker pigment that occur on sun-exposed skin esp. of persons aged 50 and over — called also *lentigo senilis, liver spots*
ageu·sia \ə-ˈgyü-zē-ə, (ˌ)ā-, -ˈjü-, -sē-\ *n* : absent or impaired sense of taste — **ageu·sic** \-zik, -sik\ *adj*
ag·glu·ti·na·bil·i·ty \ə-ˌglüt-ᵊn-ə-ˈbi-lə-tē\ *n, pl* **-ties** : capacity to be agglutinated — **ag·glu·ti·na·ble** \-ˈglüt-ᵊn-ə-bəl\ *adj*
¹ag·glu·ti·nate \ə-ˈglüt-ᵊn-ˌāt\ *vb* **-nat·ed; -nat·ing** : to undergo or cause to undergo agglutination
²ag·glu·ti·nate \-ᵊn-ət, -ᵊn-ˌāt\ *n* : a clump of agglutinated material

ag·glu·ti·na·tion \ə-ˌglüt-ᵊn-ˈā-shən\ *n* : a reaction in which particles (as red blood cells or bacteria) suspended in a liquid collect into clumps and which occurs esp. as a serological response to a specific antibody — **ag·glu·ti·na·tive** \ə-ˈglüt-ᵊn-ˌā-tiv, -ə-tiv\ *adj*

agglutination test *n* : any of several tests based on the ability of a specific serum to cause agglutination of a suitable system and used in the diagnosis of infections, the identification of microorganisms, and in blood typing — compare WIDAL TEST

ag·glu·ti·nin \ə-ˈglüt-ᵊn-ən\ *n* : a substance (as an antibody) producing agglutination

ag·glu·ti·no·gen \ə-ˈglüt-ᵊn-ə-jən\ *n* : an antigen that stimulates production of an agglutinin — **ag·glu·ti·no·gen·ic** \-ˌglüt-ᵊn-ə-ˈje-nik\ *adj*

ag·gra·vate \ˈag-rə-ˌvāt\ *vb* **-vat·ed; -vat·ing** **1** : to make worse, more serious, or more severe **2** : to produce inflammation in : IRRITATE

ag·gre·gate \ˈa-gri-ˌgāt\ *vb* **-gat·ed; -gat·ing** : to collect or gather into a mass or whole — **ag·gre·gate** \-gət\ *adj or n* — **ag·gre·ga·tion** \a-gri-ˈgā-shən\ *n*

Ag·gre·nox \ˈag-ri-ˌnäks\ *trademark* — used for a preparation of aspirin and dipyridamole

ag·gres·sion \ə-ˈgre-shən\ *n* : hostile, injurious, or destructive behavior or outlook

ag·gres·sive \ə-ˈgre-siv\ *adj* **1** : tending toward or exhibiting aggression ⟨~ behavior⟩ **2** : growing, developing, or spreading rapidly ⟨~ bone tumors⟩ **3** : more severe, intensive, or comprehensive than usual esp. in dosage or extent ⟨~ chemotherapy⟩ — **ag·gres·sive·ly** *adv* — **ag·gres·sive·ness** *n* — **ag·gres·siv·i·ty** \ˌa-ˌgre-ˈsi-və-tē\ *n*

agitans — see PARALYSIS AGITANS

agitated depression *n* : a depressive disorder characterized esp. by restlessness, overactivity, and anxiety

ag·i·ta·tion \ˌaj-ə-ˈtā-shən\ *n* : a state of excessive psychomotor activity accompanied by increased tension and irritability — **ag·i·tat·ed** \ˈaj-ə-ˌtāt əd\ *adj*

agly·cone \ˌa-ˈglī-ˌkōn\ *also* **agly·con** \-ˌkän\ *n* : an organic compound (as a phenol or alcohol) combined with the sugar portion of a glycoside

ag·na·thia \ag-ˈnā-thē-ə, (ˌ)āg-, -ˈna-thē-\ *n* : the congenital complete or partial absence of one or both jaws

ag·no·gen·ic \ˌag-nō-ˈje-nik\ *adj* : of unknown cause ⟨~ metaplasia⟩

ag·no·sia \ag-ˈnō-zhə, -shə\ *n* : loss or diminution of the ability to recognize familiar objects or stimuli usu. as a result of brain damage — see VISUAL AGNOSIA

-agogue *n comb form* : substance that promotes the secretion or expulsion of ⟨chol*agogue*⟩ ⟨emmen*agogue*⟩

ag·o·nal \ˈa-gən-ᵊl\ *adj* : of, relating to, or associated with agony and esp. the death agony — **ag·o·nal·ly** *adv*

ag·o·nist \ˈa-gə-nist\ *n* **1** : a muscle that on contracting is automatically checked and controlled by the opposing simultaneous contraction of another muscle — called also *agonist muscle, prime mover;* compare ANTAGONIST a, SYNERGIST **2** : a chemical substance (as a drug) capable of combining with a receptor on a cell and initiating the same reaction or activity typically produced by the binding of an endogenous substance ⟨binding of adrenergic ~*s*⟩ — compare ANTAGONIST b

ag·o·ny \ˈa-gə-nē\ *n, pl* **-nies** **1** : intense pain of mind or body **2** : the struggle that precedes death

ag·o·ra·pho·bia \ˌa-gə-rə-ˈfō-bē-ə\ *n* : abnormal fear of being helpless in a situation from which escape may be difficult or embarrassing that is characterized initially often by panic or anticipatory anxiety and finally by avoidance of open or public places

[1]**ag·o·ra·pho·bic** \-ˈfō-bik\ *adj* : of, relating to, or affected with agoraphobia

[2]**agoraphobic** *or* **ag·o·ra·phobe** \ˈa-gə-rə-ˌfōb\ *also* **ag·o·ra·pho·bi·ac** \ˌa-gə-rə-ˈfō-bē-ˌak\ *n* : a person affected with agoraphobia

-agra *n comb form* : seizure of pain ⟨pell*agra*⟩ ⟨pod*agra*⟩

agram·ma·tism \(ˌ)ā-ˈgra-mə-ˌti-zəm\ *n* : the pathological inability to use words in grammatical sequence

agran·u·lo·cyte \(ˌ)ā-ˈgran-yə-lō-ˌsīt\ *n* : a leukocyte without cytoplasmic granules — compare GRANULOCYTE

agran·u·lo·cyt·ic angina \ˌā-ˌgran-yə-lō-ˈsi-tik-\ *n* : AGRANULOCYTOSIS

agran·u·lo·cy·to·sis \ˌā-ˌgran-yə-lō-ˌsī-ˈtō-səs\ *n, pl* **-to·ses** \-ˌsēz\ : an acute blood disorder that is marked by a decrease of circulating granulocytes (as neutrophils) and is characterized esp. by weakness, chills, swollen neck, sore throat, mouth ulcers, and jaundice and is usu. an acquired condition occurring as a side effect of certain drugs or chemotherapy or sometimes as a complication of a medical condition (as aplastic anemia) — called also *agranulocytic angina, granulocytopenia*

agraph·ia \(ˌ)ā-ˈgra-fē-ə\ *n* : the pathological loss of the ability to write — **agraph·ic** \-fik\ *adj*

Ag·ry·lin \ˈag-rə-lin\ *trademark* — used for a preparation of the hydrochloride of anagrelide

ague \ˈā-(ˌ)gyü\ *n* **1** : a fever (as malaria) marked by paroxysms of chills, fever, and sweating that recur at regular intervals **2** : a fit of shivering : CHILL

agy·ria \ˌā-ˈjī-rē-ə\ *n* : severe lissencephaly marked by the absence of cerebral convolutions; *broadly*

: LISSENCEPHALY — compare PACHYGYRIA

AHA \ā-(ˌ)āch-ˈā\ *n* : ALPHA HYDROXY ACID

AHA *abbr* **1** American Heart Association **2** American Hospital Association

AHF *abbr* **1** antihemophilic factor **2** [*anti*hemophilic *f*actor] factor VIII

AHG *abbr* antihemophilic globulin

AI *abbr* artificial insemination

aich•mo•pho•bia \ˌāk-mə-ˈfō-bē-ə, -mō-\ *n* : a morbid fear of sharp or pointed objects (such as scissors or a needle) — called also *belonephobia*

aid \ˈād\ *n* **1** : the act of helping or treating; *also* : the help or treatment given **2** : an assisting person or group ⟨a laboratory ~⟩ **3** : something by which assistance is given : an assisting device; *esp* : HEARING AID

AID *abbr* artificial insemination by donor

aide \ˈād\ *n* : a person who acts as an assistant — see NURSE'S AIDE

AIDS \ˈādz\ *n* : a disease of the immune system that is characterized cytologically esp. by a reduction of CD4-bearing helper T cells to 20 percent or less of normal resulting in susceptibility to life-threatening conditions (as Pneumocystis carinii pneumonia) and to some (as Kaposi's sarcoma) that become life-threatening and that is caused by infection with HIV commonly transmitted in infected blood esp. during illicit intravenous drug use and in bodily secretions (as semen) during sexual intercourse — called also *acquired immune deficiency syndrome, acquired immunodeficiency syndrome*

AIDS–related complex *n* : a group of symptoms (as fever, weight loss, and lymphadenopathy) that is associated with the presence of antibodies to HIV and is followed by the development of AIDS in a certain proportion of cases — abbr. *ARC*

AIDS virus *n* : HIV

AIH *abbr* artificial insemination by husband

ail \ˈāl\ *vb* **1** : to affect with a disease or physical or emotional pain or discomfort **2** : to become affected with pain or discomfort : to suffer ill health

ail•ment \ˈāl-mənt\ *n* : a bodily disorder or chronic disease

ai•lu•ro•phobe \ī-ˈlu̇r-ə-ˌfōb, ā-\ *or* **ae•lu•ro•phobe** \ē-\ *n* : a person who hates or fears cats

ai•lu•ro•pho•bia *or* **ae•lu•ro•pho•bia** \-ˌlu̇r-ə-ˈfō-bē-ə\ *n* : abnormal fear of cats

air \ˈar\ *n* : a mixture of invisible odorless tasteless gases that surrounds the earth, that is composed by volume chiefly of 78 percent nitrogen, 21 percent oxygen, 0.9 percent argon, 0.03 percent carbon dioxide, varying amounts of water vapor, and minute amounts of rare gases (as helium), and that has a pressure at sea level of about 14.7 pounds per square inch

air ambulance *n* : an aircraft and esp. a helicopter equipped for transporting the injured or sick

air bends *n pl* : AEROEMBOLISM

air•borne \ˈar-ˌbōrn\ *adj* : carried or transported by the air ⟨~ allergens⟩

Air•cast \ˈar-ˌkast\ *trademark* — used for a pneumatic brace

air embolism *n* : obstruction of the circulation by air that has gained entrance to veins usu. through wounds — compare AEROEMBOLISM

air hunger *n* : deep labored breathing at a rapid rate (as in acidosis); *also* : KUSSMAUL BREATHING

air passage *n* : an anatomical part (as the pharynx and bronchial tubes) involved in respiration

air sac *n* : ALVEOLUS b

air•sick \ˈar-ˌsik\ *adj* : affected with motion sickness associated with flying — **air•sick•ness** *n*

air•way \-ˌwā\ *n* : a passageway for air into or out of the lungs; *specif* : a device passed into the trachea by way of the mouth or nose or through an incision to maintain a clear respiratory passageway (as during anesthesia)

aka•thi•sia \ˌā-ka-ˈthi-zhē-ə, -zhə, ˌa-, -ˈthē-\ *n* : a condition characterized by uncontrollable motor restlessness

ak•ee *or* **ack•ee** \ˈa-kē, a-ˈkē\ *n* : the fruit of an African tree (*Blighia sapida* of the family Sapindaceae) that has edible flesh when ripe but is poisonous when immature or overripe

aki•ne•sia \ˌā-kī-ˈnē-zhē-ə, -zhə\ *n* : loss or impairment of voluntary activity (as of a muscle) — **aki•net•ic** \ˌā-kə-ˈne-tik, -kī-\ *adj*

Al *symbol* aluminum

ala \ˈā-lə\ *n, pl* **alae** \-ˌlē\ : a wing or a winglike anatomic process or part; *esp* : ALA NASI

ALA *abbr* aminolevulinic acid

alaeque — see LEVATOR LABII SUPERIORIS ALAEQUE NASI

ala na•si \-ˈnā-ˌsī, -ˌzī\ *n, pl* **alae na•si** \-ˌsī, -ˌzī\ : the expanded outer wall of cartilage on each side of the nose

al•a•nine \ˈa-lə-ˌnēn\ *n* : a simple nonessential crystalline amino acid $C_3H_7NO_2$ formed esp. by the hydrolysis of proteins

alanine aminotransferase *n* : an enzyme which promotes transfer of an amino group from glutamic acid to pyruvic acid and which when present in abnormally high levels in the blood is a diagnostic indication of liver disease or damage — abbr. *ALT;* called also *alanine transaminase, glutamic-pyruvic transaminase*

alar cartilage \ˈā-lər-\ *n* : one of the pair of lower lateral cartilages of the nose

alar ligament *n* : either of a pair of strong rounded fibrous cords of which one arises on each side of the cranial part of the dens, passes obliquely and laterally upward, and inserts on the medial side of a condyle of the occipital bone — called also *check ligament*

alarm reaction *n* : the initial reaction of an organism (as increased hormonal activity) to stress

alas•trim \ˈa-lə-ˌstrim, ˌa-lə-ˈ; ə-ˈlas-trəm\ *n* : VARIOLA MINOR

alba — see LINEA ALBA, MATERIA ALBA, PHLEGMASIA ALBA DOLENS

al•ben•da•zole \ˌal-ˈben-də-ˌzōl\ *n* : an anthelmintic drug $C_{12}H_{15}N_3O_2S$ used esp. to treat infections of humans and domestic animals caused by larvae of various tapeworms and nematodes

Al•bers–Schön•berg disease \ˈal-bərz-ˈshərn-ˌbərg-, -ˈshōn-\ *n* : OSTEOPETROSIS

Albers–Schönberg, Heinrich Ernst (1865–1921), German radiologist.

albicans, albicantia — see CORPUS ALBICANS

albicantes — see LINEAE ALBICANTES

al•bi•nism \ˈal-bə-ˌni-zəm, al-ˈbī-\ *n* : the condition of an albino — **al•bi•nis•tic** \ˌal-bə-ˈnis-tik\ *adj*

al•bi•no \al-ˈbī-(ˌ)nō\ *n, pl* **-nos** : an organism exhibiting deficient pigmentation; *esp* : a human being who is congenitally deficient in pigment and usu. has a milky or translucent skin, white or colorless hair, and eyes with pink or blue iris and deep-red pupil — **al•bin•ic** \-ˈbi-nik\ *adj*

al•bi•not•ic \ˌal-bə-ˈnä-tik\ *adj* **1** : of, relating to, or affected with albinism **2** : tending toward albinism

albuginea — see TUNICA ALBUGINEA

al•bu•men \al-ˈbyü-mən; ˈal-ˌbyü-, -byə-\ *n* **1** : the white of an egg **2** : ALBUMIN

al•bu•min \al-ˈbyü-mən; ˈal-ˌbyü-, -byə-\ *n* : any of various heat-coagulable water-soluble proteins found esp. in blood, muscle, the whites of eggs, milk, and some plant seeds

¹al•bu•min•oid \-mə-ˌnȯid\ *adj* : resembling albumin

²albuminoid *n* **1** : PROTEIN 1 **2** : SCLEROPROTEIN

al•bu•min•uria \al-ˌbyü-mə-ˈnu̇r-ē-ə, -ˈnyu̇r-\ *n* : the presence of albumin in the urine that is usu. a symptom of disease of the kidneys but sometimes a response to other diseases or physiological disturbances of benign nature — **al•bu•min•uric** \-ˈnu̇r-ik, -ˈnyu̇r-\ *adj*

al•bu•te•rol \al-ˈbyü-tə-ˌrȯl\ *n* : a beta-agonist bronchodilator used in the form of its sulfate $(C_{13}H_{21}NO_3)_2 \cdot H_2SO_4$ to treat bronchospasm associated esp. with asthma and chronic obstructive pulmonary disease — called also *salbutamol;* see COMBIVENT, PROVENTIL, VENTOLIN

alcaptonuria *var of* ALKAPTONURIA

al•co•hol \ˈal-kə-ˌhȯl\ *n* **1 a** : ethanol esp. when considered as the intoxicating agent in fermented and distilled liquors **b** : drink (as whiskey or beer) containing ethanol **c** : a mixture of ethanol and water that is usu. 95 percent ethanol **2** : any of various compounds that are analogous to ethanol in constitution and that are hydroxyl derivatives of hydrocarbons

alcohol dehydrogenase *n* : any of various dehydrogenases that catalyze reversibly the conversion between an alcohol and an aldehyde or ketone that in humans are zinc-containing enzymes found esp. in the liver and gastric mucosa which catalyze the oxidation of an alcohol (as ethanol) to an aldehyde (as acetaldehyde) in the presence of NAD — abbr. *ADH*

¹al•co•hol•ic \ˌal-kə-ˈhȯ-lik, -ˈhä-\ *adj* **1 a** : of, relating to, or caused by alcohol ⟨~ hepatitis⟩ **b** : containing alcohol **2** : affected with alcoholism — **al•co•hol•i•cal•ly** \-li-k(ə-)lē\ *adv*

²alcoholic *n* : one affected with alcoholism

al•co•hol•ism \ˈal-kə-ˌhȯ-ˌli-zəm, -kə-hə-\ *n* **1** : continued excessive or compulsive use of alcoholic drinks **2 a** : poisoning by alcohol **b** : a chronic, progressive, potentially fatal disorder marked by excessive and usu. compulsive drinking of alcohol that leads to psychological and physical dependence or addiction and is typically characterized by impaired ability to work and socialize, tendency to drink alone and engage in violent behavior, alcohol-related illness (as hepatitis or cirrhosis of the liver), and moderate to severe withdrawal symptoms upon detoxification

ALD *abbr* adrenoleukodystrophy

al•de•hyde \ˈal-də-ˌhīd\ *n* : ACETALDEHYDE; *broadly* : any of various reactive compounds (as acetaldehyde) containing the group CHO — **al•de•hy•dic** \ˌal-də-ˈhī-dik\ *adj*

al•dose \ˈal-ˌdōs, -ˌdōz\ *n* : a sugar containing one aldehyde group per molecule

al•do•ste•rone \al-ˈdäs-tə-ˌrōn; ˌal-dō-ˈstir-ˌōn, -stə-ˈrōn\ *n* : a steroid hormone $C_{21}H_{28}O_5$ of the adrenal cortex that functions in the regulation of the salt and water balance of the body

al•do•ste•ron•ism \al-ˈdäs-tə-ˌrō-ˌni-zəm, ˌal-dō-stə-ˈrō-\ *n* : a condition that is characterized by excessive secretion of aldosterone and typically by loss of body potassium, muscular weakness, and elevated blood pressure — called also *hyperaldosteronism*

al•drin \ˈȯl-drən, ˈal-\ *n* : an exceedingly poisonous insecticide $C_{12}H_6Cl_6$

K. Alder — see DIELDRIN

alen•dro•nate \ə-ˈlen-drə-ˌnāt\ *n* : a hydrated bisphosphonate sodium salt $C_4H_{12}NNaO_7P_2 \cdot 3H_2O$ used to inhibit bone resorption esp. in the treatment of osteoporosis and Paget's disease of bone — called also *alendronate sodium;* see FOSAMAX

aleu•ke•mia \ˌā-lü-ˈkē-mē-ə\ *n* : leukemia in which the circulating leukocytes are normal or decreased in number; *esp* : ALEUKEMIC LEUKEMIA

aleu•ke•mic \-ˈkē-mik\ *adj* : not marked by increase in circulating white blood cells

aleukemic leukemia *n* : leukemia resulting from changes in the tissues forming white blood cells and characterized by a normal or decreased number of white blood cells in the circulating blood — called also *aleukemic myelosis*

Aleve \ə-ˈlēv\ *trademark* — used for a preparation of the sodium salt of naproxen

Al•ex•an•der technique \ˌal-ig-ˈzan-dər-\ *n, often cap T* : a technique for positioning and moving the body that is believed to reduce tension

Alexander, Frederick Matthias (1869–1955), Australian elocutionist.

alex•ia \ə-ˈlek-sē-ə\ *n* : aphasia characterized by loss of ability to read — **alex•ic** \-ˈlek-sik\ *adj*

alex•in \ə-ˈlek-sən\ *n* : COMPLEMENT 2 — **al•ex•in•ic** \ˌa-ˌlek-ˈsi-nik\ *adj*

alex•i•thy•mia \ə-ˌleks-i-ˈthī-mē-ə\ *n* : inability to express or describe one's feelings — **alex•i•thy•mic** \-ˈthī-mik\ *adj*

ALG *abbr* antilymphocyte globulin; antilymphocytic globulin

alg- *or* **algo-** *comb form* : pain ⟨*algo*lagnia⟩

al•ga \ˈal-gə\ *n, pl* **al•gae** \ˈal-(ˌ)jē\ *also* **algas** : a plant or plantlike chiefly aquatic usu. chlorophyll-containing nonvascular organism (as a seaweed) — see BROWN ALGA, RED ALGA — **al•gal** \-gəl\ *adj*

al•ge•sia \al-ˈjē-zē-ə, -ˈjē-zhə\ *n* : sensitivity to pain — **al•ge•sic** \-ˈjē-zik, -sik\ *adj*

-al•gia \ˈal-jə, -jē-ə\ *n comb form* : pain ⟨neur*algia*⟩

al•gi•cide *or* **al•gae•cide** \ˈal-jə-ˌsīd\ *n* : an agent used to kill algae — **al•gi•cid•al** \ˌal-jə-ˈsīd-ᵊl\ *adj*

al•gin•ic acid \(ˌ)al-ˈji-nik-\ *n* : an insoluble colloidal polysaccharide $(C_6H_8O_6)_n$ that is obtained from brown seaweeds and is used medically esp. to relieve the symptoms (as burning) of excess stomach acid

al•go•gen•ic \ˌal-gō-ˈje-nik\ *adj* : producing pain

al•go•lag•nia \ˌal-gō-ˈlag-nē-ə\ *n* : a perversion (as masochism or sadism) in which pleasure and esp. sexual gratification is obtained by inflicting or suffering pain — **al•go•lag•nic** \-nik\ *adj*

al•gol•o•gy \al-ˈgäl-ə-jē\ *n* : a medical specialty concerned with the study and treatment of pain

al•gor mor•tis \ˈal-ˌgȯr-ˈmȯr-təs\ *n* : the gradual cooling of the body following death

ali- *comb form* : wing or winglike part ⟨*ali*sphenoid⟩

alien•ate \ˈā-lē-ə-ˌnāt, ˈāl-yə-\ *vb* **-at•ed; -at•ing** : to make unfriendly, hostile, or indifferent where attachment formerly existed

alien•a•tion \ˌā-lē-ə-ˈnā-shən, ˌāl-yə-\ *n* : a withdrawing or separation of a person or a person's affections from an object or position of former attachment

al•i•men•ta•ry \ˌa-lə-ˈmen-tə-rē, -ˈmen-trē\ *adj* : of, concerned with, or relating to nourishment or to the function of nutrition : NUTRITIVE

alimentary canal *n* : DIGESTIVE TRACT

alimentary system *n* : DIGESTIVE SYSTEM

alimentary tract *n* : DIGESTIVE TRACT

al•i•men•ta•tion \ˌa-lə-mən-ˈtā-shən, -ˌmen-\ *n* : the act or process of affording nutriment or nourishment

Alim•ta \ə-ˈlim-tə\ *trademark* — used for a preparation of pemetrexed

al•i•phat•ic \ˌa-lə-ˈfa-tik\ *adj* : of, relating to, or being an organic compound (as an alkane or alkene) having an open-chain structure

[1]**al•i•quot** \ˈa-lə-ˌkwät\ *adj* : being an equal fractional part (as of a solution) — **aliquot** *n*

[2]**aliquot** *vb* : to divide (as a solution) into equal parts

[1]**ali•sphe•noid** \ˌā-ləs-ˈfē-ˌnȯid, ˌa-\ *adj* : belonging or relating to or forming the wings of the sphenoid or the pair of bones that fuse with other sphenoidal elements to form the greater wings of the sphenoid in the adult

[2]**alisphenoid** *n* : an alisphenoid bone; *esp* : GREATER WING

alive \ə-ˈlīv\ *adj* : having life : not dead or inanimate

al•ka•lae•mia *chiefly Brit var of* ALKALEMIA

al•ka•le•mia \ˌal-kə-ˈlē-mē-ə\ *n* : a condition in which the hydrogen ion concentration in the blood is decreased

al•ka•li \ˈal-kə-ˌlī\ *n, pl* **-lies** *or* **-lis** : a substance having marked basic properties — compare BASE

alkali disease *n* : selenosis of livestock

al•ka•line \ˈal-kə-lən, -ˌlīn\ *adj* : of, relating to, containing, or having the properties of an alkali or alkali metal : BASIC; *esp, of a solution* : having a pH of more than 7 — **al•ka•lin•i•ty** \ˌal-kə-ˈli-nə-tē\ *n*

alkaline phosphatase *n* : any of the phosphatases active chiefly in alkaline medium and occurring in esp. high concentrations in bone, the liver, the kidneys, and the placenta

al•ka•lin•ize \ˈal-kə-lə-ˌnīz\ *vb* **-ized; -iz•ing** : to make alkaline — **al•ka•lin•i•za•tion** \ˌal-kə-ˌli-nə-ˈzā-shən, -lə-\ *n*

alkali reserve *n* : the concentration of one or more basic ions or substances in a fluid medium that buffer its pH by neutralizing acid; *esp* : the concentration of bicarbonate in the blood

al•ka•lize \ˈal-kə-ˌlīz\ *vb* **-lized; -liz•ing** : ALKALINIZE — **al•ka•li•za•tion** \ˌal-kə-lə-ˈzā-shən\ *n*

al•ka•liz•er \ˈal-kə-ˌlī-zər\ *n* : an alkalinizing agent

al•ka•loid \ˈal-kə-ˌlȯid\ *n* : any of numerous usu. colorless, complex, and bitter organic bases (as morphine or caffeine) containing nitrogen and usu. oxygen that occur esp. in seed plants — **al•ka•loi•dal** \ˌal-kə-ˈlȯid-ᵊl\ *adj*

al•ka•lo•sis \ˌal-kə-ˈlo-səs\ *n, pl* **-lo•ses** \-ˌsēz\ : an abnormal condition of increased alkalinity of the blood and tissues — compare ACIDOSIS, KETOSIS — **al•ka•lot•ic** \ˌal-kə-ˈlä-tik\ *adj*

al•kane \ˈal-ˌkān\ *n* : any of a series of aliphatic hydrocarbons C_nH_{2n+2} (as methane) in which each carbon is bonded to four other atoms

al•kap•ton•uria *or* **al•cap•ton•uria** \(ˌ)al-ˌkap-tə-ˈnu̇r-ē-ə, -ˈnyu̇r-\ *n* : a rare metabolic disease that is marked by the accumulation of homogentisic acid in the tissues and urine due to an enzyme deficiency, is characterized esp. by early-onset osteoarthritis, blackened urine, and dark pigmentation of the skin and cartilage, and is inherited as a recessive trait — **al•kap•ton•uric** *or* **al•cap•ton•uric** \-ˈnu̇r-ik, ˈ-nyu̇r-\ *n or adj*

al•kene \ˈal-ˌkēn\ *n* : any of numerous unsaturated hydrocarbons having one double bond; *specif* : any of a series of open-chain hydrocarbons C_nH_{2n}

[1]**al•kyl** \ˈal-kəl\ *adj* : having a monovalent organic group and esp. one C_nH_{2n+1} (as methyl) derived from an alkane (as methane)

[2]**alkyl** *n* : a compound of one or more alkyl groups with a metal

al•kyl•ate \ˈal-kə-ˌlāt\ *vb* **-at•ed; -at•ing** : to introduce one or more alkyl groups into (a compound) — **al•kyl•a•tion** \ˌal-kə-ˈlā-shən\ *n*

alkylating agent *n* : a substance that causes replacement of hydrogen by an alkyl group; *specif* : one with mutagenic activity that inhibits cell division and growth and is used to treat some cancers

ALL *abbr* acute lymphoblastic leukemia; acute lymphocytic leukemia

all- *or* **allo-** *comb form* **1** : other : different : atypical ⟨*all*ergy⟩ ⟨*allo*pathy⟩ **2** *allo-* : isomeric form or variety of (a specified chemical compound) ⟨*allo*purinol⟩

al•lan•to•ic \ˌa-lən-ˈtō-ik, -ˌlan-\ *adj* : relating to, contained in, or characterized by an allantois

al•lan•to•in \ə-ˈlan-tə-wən\ *n* : a crystalline oxidation product $C_4H_6N_4O_3$ of uric acid used to promote healing of local wounds and infections

al•lan•to•is \ə-ˈlan-tə-wəs\ *n, pl* **al•lan•to•ides** \ˌa-lən-ˈtō-ə-ˌdēz, -ˌlan-\ : a vascular fetal membrane that is formed as a pouch from the hindgut and that in placental mammals is intimately associated with the chorion in formation of the placenta

Al•le•gra \ə-ˈleg-rə, -ˈlā-grə\ *trademark* — used for a preparation of the hydrochloride of fexofenadine

al•lele \ə-ˈlēl\ *n* **1** : any of the alternative forms of a gene that may occur at a given locus **2** : either of a pair of alternative Mendelian characters (as ability versus inability to taste the chemical phenylthiocarbamide) — **al•le•lic** \-ˈlē-lik, -ˈle-\ *adj* — **al•lel•ism** \-ˈlē-ˌli-zəm, -ˈle-\ *n*

allelo- *comb form* : alternative ⟨*allelo*morph⟩

al•le•lo•morph \ə-ˈle-lə-ˌmȯrf, -ˈlē-\ *n* : ALLELE — **al•le•lo•mor•phic** \ə-ˌle-lə-ˈmȯr-fik, -ˌlē-\ *adj* — **al•le•lo•mor•phism** \ə-ˈle-lə-ˌmȯr-ˌfi-zəm, -ˈlē-\ *n*

al•ler•gen \ˈa-lər-jən\ *n* : a substance that induces allergy

al•ler•gen•ic \ˌa-lər-ˈje-nik\ *adj* : having the capacity to induce allergy ⟨~ proteins⟩ ⟨~ foods⟩ — **al•ler•ge•nic•i•ty** \-jə-ˈni-sə-tē\ *n*

al•ler•gic \ə-ˈlər-jik\ *adj* **1** : of, relating to, or characterized by allergy ⟨an ~ reaction⟩ **2** : affected with allergy : subject to an allergic reaction — **al•ler•gic•al•ly** \ə-ˈlər-ji-k(ə-)lē\ *adv*

allergic contact dermatitis *n* : an allergic response following direct contact of an allergen (as latex, nickel, or poison ivy) with the skin that is typically marked by an itchy red rash often accompanied by swelling and watery blisters — compare IRRITANT CONTACT DERMATITIS

allergic encephalomyelitis *n* : encephalomyelitis produced by an allergic response following introduction of an antigen into the body; *specif* : EXPERIMENTAL ALLERGIC ENCEPHALOMYELITIS

allergic granulomatosis *n* : CHURG-STRAUSS SYNDROME

allergic rhinitis *n* : rhinitis caused by exposure to an allergen; *esp* : HAY FEVER

al•ler•gist \-jist\ *n* : a specialist in allergy

al•ler•goid \ˈa-lər-ˌgȯid\ *n* : an allergen (as pollen) that has been chemically modified and is used esp. in immunotherapy to treat allergies by lessening the immune response

al•ler•gol•o•gy \ˌa-lər-ˈgä-lə-jē\ *n, pl* **-gies** : a branch of medicine concerned with allergy — **al•ler•gol•o•gist** \ˌal-ər-ˈgäl-ə-jist\ *n*

al•ler•gy \ˈa-lər-jē\ *n, pl* **-gies** **1** : altered bodily reactivity (as hypersensitivity) to an antigen in response to a first exposure **2** : exaggerated or pathological reaction (as by sneezing, difficult breathing, itching, or skin rashes) to substances, situations, or physical states that are without comparable effect on the average individual **3** : medical practice concerned with allergies

allergy shot *n* : an injection containing very small amounts of allergen (as mold or grass pollen) to which an individual is sensitive that is given at regular intervals usu. over a period of several years to desensitize the immune system and reduce allergic symptoms

al•le•thrin \ˈa-lə-thrən\ *n* : a light yellow oily insecticide $C_{19}H_{26}O_3$

al•le•vi•ate \ə-ˈlē-vē-ˌāt\ *vb* **-at•ed; -at•ing** : to make (as symptoms) less severe or more bearable — **al•le•vi•a•tion** \-ˌlē-vē-ˈā-shən\ *n*

al•le•vi•a•tive \ə-ˈlē-vē-ˌā-tiv\ *adj* : tending to alleviate : PALLIATIVE ⟨a medicine that is ~ but not curative⟩

Al•li \ˈa-ˌlī\ *trademark* — used for a preparation of orlistat

al•li•cin \ˈa-lə-sən\ *n* : a pungent compound $C_6H_{10}OS_2$ imparting the distinctive smell to garlic and possessing antimicrobial properties

al•lied health \ˈa-ˌlīd-\ *n* : a broad field of health-care professions made up of trained individuals (as physical therapists, dental hygienists, and audiologists) who are typically licensed or certified but are not physicians, dentists, or nurses

allo- — see ALL-

al•lo•an•ti•body \ˌa-lō-ˈan-ti-ˌbä-dē\ *n, pl* **-bod•ies** : an antibody produced following introduction of an alloantigen into the system of an individual of a species lacking that particular antigen — called also *isoantibody*

al•lo•an•ti•gen \ˌa-lō-ˈan-tə-jən\ *n* : a genetically determined antigen present in some but not all individuals of a species (as those of a particular blood group) and capable of inducing the production of an alloantibody by individuals which lack it — called also *isoantigen* — **al•lo•an•ti•gen•ic** \-ˌan-tə-ˈje-nik\ *adj*

al•lo•bar•bi•tal \ˌa-lə-ˈbär-bə-ˌtȯl\ *n* : a white crystalline barbiturate $C_{10}H_{12}N_2O_3$ used as a sedative and hypnotic

al•lo•bar•bi•tone \-ˌtōn\ *n, chiefly Brit* : ALLOBARBITAL

al•lo•cor•tex \-ˈkȯr-ˌteks\ *n* : ARCHIPALLIUM

Al•lo•der•ma•nys•sus \-ˌdər-mə-ˈni-səs\ *n* : a genus of bloodsucking mites parasitic on rodents including one (*A. sanguineus*) implicated as a vector of rickettsialpox in humans

al•lo•dyn•ia \ˌal-ə-ˈdin-ē-ə\ *n* : pain resulting from a stimulus (as a light touch of the skin) which would not normally provoke pain; *also* : a condition marked by allodynia

al•lo•ge•ne•ic \ˌa-lō-jə-ˈnē-ik\ *also* **al•lo•gen•ic** \-ˈje-nik\ *adj* : involving, derived from, or being individuals of the same species that are sufficiently unlike genetically to interact antigenically ⟨~ skin grafts⟩ — compare SYNGENEIC, XENOGENEIC

al•lo•graft \ˈa-lə-ˌgraft\ *n* : a homograft between allogeneic individuals — **allograft** *vb*

al•lo•im•mu•ni•za•tion \ˌa-lō-ˌi-myə-nə-ˈzā-shən\ *n* : ISOIMMUNIZATION

al•lo•iso•leu•cine \ˌa-lō-ˌī-sə-ˈlü-ˌsēn\ *n* : either of two stereoisomers of isoleucine of which one is present in bodily fluids of individuals affected with maple syrup urine disease

al•lo•path \ˈa-lə-ˌpath\ *n* : one who practices allopathy

al•lop•a•thy \ə-ˈlä-pə-thē, a-\ *n, pl* **-thies** **1** : a system of medical practice that aims to combat disease by using remedies (as drugs or surgery) which produce effects different from or incompatible with those produced by the disease treated — compare HOMEOPATHY **2** : a system of medical practice making use of all measures that have proved of value in treatment of disease — **al•lo•path•ic** \ˌa-lə-ˈpa-thik\ *adj* — **al•lo•path•i•cal•ly** \-thi-k(ə-)lē\ *adv*

al•lo•pu•ri•nol \ˌa-lō-ˈpyu̇r-ə-ˌnȯl, -ˌnōl\ *n* : a drug $C_3H_4N_4O$ used to promote excretion of uric acid esp. in the treatment of gout

al•lo•re•ac•tive \ˌa-lō-rē-ˈak-tiv\ *adj* : reacting in response to a transplanted allograft ⟨~ T cells⟩ — **al•lo•re•ac•tiv•i•ty** \ˌa-lō-(ˌ)rē-ˌak-ˈti-və-tē\ *n*

all–or–none *adj* : marked either by complete operation or effect or by none at all ⟨~ nerve impulse⟩

all–or–none law *n* : a principle in physiology: in any single nerve or muscle fiber the response to a stimulus above threshold level is maximal and independent of the intensity of the stimulus

all–or–noth•ing *adj* : ALL-OR-NONE

al•lo•ste•ric \ˌa-lō-ˈster-ik, -ˈstir-\ *adj* : of, relating to, or being a change in the shape and activity of a protein that results from combination with another substance at a point other than the chemically active site — **al•lo•ste•ri•cal•ly** \-i-k(ə-)lē\ *adv*

al•lo•trans•plant \ˌa-lō-trans-ˈplant\ *vb* : to transplant between genetically different individuals — **al•lo•trans•plant** \-ˈtrans-ˌ\ *n* — **al•lo•trans•plan•ta•tion** \-ˌtrans-ˌplan-ˈtā-shən\ *n*

al•lo•type \ˈa-lə-ˌtīp\ *n* : an alloantigen that is part of a plasma protein (as an antibody) — compare IDIOTYPE, ISOTYPE — **al•lo•typ•ic** \ˌa-lə-ˈti-pik\ *adj* — **al•lo•typ•i•cal•ly** \-pi-k(ə-)lē\ *adv* — **al•lo•typy** \ˈa-lə-ˌtī-pē\ *n*

al•lox•an \ə-ˈläk-sən\ *n* : a crystalline compound $C_4H_2N_2O_4$ causing diabetes mellitus when injected into experimental animals — called also *mesoxalylurea*

al•loy \ˈa-ˌlȯi, ə-ˈlȯi\ *n* : a metal and a nonmetal united usu. by fusion; *also* : the state of union of the components — **al•loy** \ə-ˈlȯi, ˈa-ˌlȯi\ *vb*

al•lo•zyme \ˈa-lə-ˌzīm\ *n* : any of the variants of an enzyme that are determined by alleles at a single genetic locus — **al•lo•zy•mic** \ˌa-lə-ˈzī-mik\ *adj*

all–trans–retinoic acid *n* : TRETINOIN

allyl iso•thio•cy•a•nate \ˈa-ləl-ˌī-sō-ˌthī-ə-ˈsī-ə-ˌnāt, -nət\ *n* : a pungent irritating liquid C_4H_5NS that is the main component of mustard oil and is used medically as a counterirritant

N–al•lyl•nor•mor•phine \ˌen-ˌal-əl-ˌnȯr-ˈmȯr-ˌfēn\ *n* : NALORPHINE

al•oe \ˈa-(ˌ)lō\ *n* **1** *cap* : a large genus of succulent chiefly southern African plants of the lily family (Liliaceae) **2** : a plant of the genus *Aloe* **3** : the dried juice of the leaves of various aloes used esp. formerly as a purgative and tonic — usu. used in pl. with a sing. verb **4** : ALOE VERA

aloe vera \-ˈver-ə, -ˈvir-\ *n* : an aloe (*Aloe barbadensis* syn. *A. vera*) whose leaves furnish a gelatinous emollient extract used esp. in cosmetics and skin creams; *also* : such an extract or a preparation composed primarily of such an extract

alo•gia \(ˈ)ā-ˈlō-j(ē-)ə\ *n* : inability to speak : difficulty in speaking

al•o•in \ˈa-lə-wən\ *n* : a bitter yellow cathartic obtained from the aloe and containing one or more glycosides

al•o•pe•cia \ˌa-lə-ˈpē-shē-ə, -shə\ *n* : partial or complete loss of hair : BALDNESS — **al•o•pe•cic** \-ˈpē-sik\ *adj*

alopecia ar•e•a•ta \-ˌar-ē-ˈā-tə, -ˈä-\ *n* : sudden loss of hair in circumscribed patches with little or no inflammation

alopecia to•tal•is \-tō-ˈta-ləs\ *n* : the complete and usu. sudden loss of hair from the scalp

alopecia uni•ver•sa•lis \-ˌyü-nə-vər-ˈsa-ləs\ *n* : the complete and usu. sudden loss of hair from the scalp, face, and body

¹al•pha \ˈal-fə\ *n* **1** : the 1st letter of the Greek alphabet — symbol Α or α **2** : ALPHA PARTICLE **3** : ALPHA WAVE

²alpha *or* **α-** *adj* **1** : of or relating to one of two or more closely related chemical substances ⟨the *alpha* chain of hemoglobin⟩ — used somewhat arbitrarily to specify ordinal relationship or a particular physical form **2** : closest in position in the structure of an organic molecule to a particular group or atom; *also* : occurring at or having a structure characterized by such a position ⟨α-substitution⟩

al•pha–ad•ren•er•gic \ˈal-fə-ˌa-drə-ˈnər-jik\ *adj* : of, relating to, or being an alpha receptor ⟨~ agonists⟩

al•pha–ad•re•no•cep•tor \-ə-ˈdrē-nə-ˌsep-tər\ *also* **al•pha–ad•re•no•re•cep•tor** \-ri-ˌsep-tər\ *n* : ALPHA-RECEPTOR

al•pha–ami•no acid *or* **α–ami•no acid** \-ə-ˈmē-nō-\ *n* : any of the more than 20 amino acids that have an amino group in the alpha position with most having the general formula $RCH(NH_2)COOH$, that are synthesized in plant and animal tissues, that are building blocks of proteins from which they can be obtained by hydrolysis, and that play an important role in metabolism, growth, maintenance, and repair of tissue

al•pha–block•er \-ˌbläk-ər\ *n* : any of a group of drugs (as doxazosin and terazosin) that combine with and block the activity of an alpha-receptor to relax smooth muscle and are used esp. to treat hypertension and benign prostatic hyperplasia

alpha cell *n* : an acidophilic glandular cell (as of the pancreas or the adenohypophysis) — compare BETA CELL

alpha chain disease *n* : IMMUNOPROLIFERATIVE SMALL INTESTINAL DISEASE

alpha–fetoprotein *or* **α–fetoprotein** *n* : a fetal blood protein present abnormally in adults with some forms of cancer (as of the liver) and normally in the amniotic fluid of pregnant women with very low levels tending to be associated with Down syndrome in the fetus and very high levels with neural tube defects (as spina bifida) in which the tube remains open

Al•pha•gan \ˈal-fə-ˌgan\ *trademark* — used for an ophthalmic solution containing brimonidine

alpha globin *also* **α–globin** *n* : the chain of hemoglobin that is designated alpha and when deficient or defective causes alpha-thalassemia — compare BETA GLOBIN

alpha globulin *n* : any of several globulins of plasma or serum that have at alkaline pH the greatest electrophoretic mobility next to albumin — compare BETA GLOBULIN, GAMMA GLOBULIN

al•pha–he•lix *or* **α–he•lix** \ˌal-fə-ˈhē-liks\ *n* : the coiled structural arrangement of many proteins consisting of a single chain of amino acids stabilized by hydrogen bonds — compare BETA-SHEET, DOUBLE HELIX — **al•pha–he•li•cal** \-ˈhe-li-kəl, -ˈhē-\ *adj*

alpha hydroxy acid *n* : a carboxylic acid (as glycolic acid or lactic acid) occurring in natural products (as fruit or yogurt) and used in cosmetics for its exfoliating effect on the surface layer of the skin — called also *AHA*, *alpha hydroxy*

alpha interferon *n* : an interferon produced by white blood cells that inhibits viral replication, suppresses cell proliferation, and regulates immune response and is used in a form obtained from recombinant DNA to treat various diseases — called also *interferon alpha*

al•pha–ke•to•glu•tar•ic acid *or* **α–ketoglutaric acid** \-ˌkē-tō-glü-ˈtar-ik-\ *n* : the alpha keto isomer of ketoglutaric acid formed in various metabolic processes (as the Krebs cycle)

alpha–lipoprotein *or* **α–lipoprotein** *n* : HDL

al•pha–1–an•ti•tryp•sin \-ˌwən-ˌan-ti-ˈtrip-sən, -ˌtī-\ *n* : a trypsin-inhibiting serum protein whose deficiency is associated with the development of emphysema — abbr. *AAT*

alpha particle *n* : a positively charged nuclear particle identical with the nucleus of a helium atom that consists of two protons and two neutrons and is ejected at high speed in certain radioactive transformations

al·pha–re·cep·tor \ˈal-fə-ri-ˌsep-tər\ *n* : any of a group of receptors that are present on cell surfaces of some effector organs and tissues innervated by the sympathetic nervous system and that mediate certain physiological responses (as vasoconstriction, relaxation of intestinal muscle, and contraction of most smooth muscle) when bound by specific adrenergic agents — compare BETA-RECEPTOR

5–al·pha–re·duc·tase *also* **5α–re·duc·tase** \ˈfīv-ˈal-fə-ri-ˈdək-ˌtās, -ˌtāz\ *n* : an enzyme that catalyzes the conversion of testosterone to dihydrotestosterone

5–alpha–reductase deficiency *n* : a genetic disorder in which males exhibit external genitalia that typically resembles that of females but in which some secondary sex characteristics (as an increase in muscle mass and descending of the testes) develop during puberty, that is caused by a deficiency of 5-alpha-reductase during embryogenesis, and that is inherited as an autosomal recessive trait

alpha state *n* : a state of wakeful relaxation that is associated with increased alpha wave activity

al·pha–sy·nu·clein *or* **α–synuclein** \ˌal-fə-si-ˈn(y)ü-klē-ən\ *n* : a protein that is found primarily in neurons and accumulates to form Lewy bodies in people affected with Parkinson's disease and some forms of dementia

al·pha–thal·as·se·mia *also* **α–thalassemia** \ˌal-fə-ˌtha-lə-ˈsē-mē-ə\ *n* : thalassemia in which the hemoglobin chains designated alpha are affected causing a condition that is either asymptomatic, is marked by mild anemia or by hemolytic anemia and enlargement of the spleen, or is fatal during fetal development or early infancy — compare BETA-THALASSEMIA

al·pha–to·coph·er·ol \ˌal-fə-tō-ˈkä-fə-ˌrȯl, -ˌrōl\ *n* : a tocopherol $C_{29}H_{50}O_2$ with high vitamin E potency

al·pha·vi·rus \ˈal-fə-ˌvī-rəs\ *n* **1** *cap* : a genus of togaviruses transmitted by arthropods and esp. mosquitoes and including the Mayaro virus, Semliki Forest virus, Sindbis virus, and the causative agents of chikungunya and equine encephalitis **2** : any virus of the genus *Alphavirus*

alpha wave *n* : an electrical rhythm of the brain with a frequency of 8 to 13 cycles per second that is often associated with a state of wakeful relaxation — called also *alpha, alpha rhythm*

Al·port syndrome \ˈal-ˌpȯrt-\ *or* **Alport's syndrome** *n* : a genetic kidney disorder that is characterized esp. by blood in the urine, hearing loss, eye abnormalities, and progressive renal failure, is usu. inherited as an X-linked trait, and is typically more severe in males

Alport, Arthur Cecil (1880–1959), British physician.

al·praz·o·lam \al-ˈpraz-ə-ˌlam\ *n* : a benzodiazepine tranquilizer $C_{17}H_{13}ClN_4$ used esp. in the treatment of mild to moderate anxiety — see XANAX

al·pren·o·lol \al-ˈpre-nə-ˌlȯl, -ˌlōl\ *n* : a beta-blocker that has been used in the form of its hydrochloride $C_{15}H_{23}NO_2 \cdot HCl$ esp. to treat cardiac arrhythmias

al·pros·ta·dil \al-ˈpräs-tə-dil\ *n* : a prostaglandin $C_{20}H_{34}O_5$ that promotes vasodilation and is used esp. to treat erectile dysfunction — called also *prostaglandin* E_1

Al·rex \ˈal-ˌreks\ *trademark* — used for a preparation of loteprednol

ALS *abbr* **1** advanced life support **2** amyotrophic lateral sclerosis **3** antilymphocyte serum; antilymphocytic serum

al·ser·ox·y·lon \ˌal-sə-ˈräk-sə-ˌlän\ *n* : a complex extract from a rauwolfia (*Rauvolfia serpentina*) that has a physiological action resembling but milder than that of reserpine

ALT *abbr* alanine aminotransferase; alanine transaminase

Al·tace \ˈal-ˌtās\ *trademark* — used for a preparation of ramipril

al·te·plase \ˈal-tə-ˌplās\ *n* : a recombinant form of tissue plasminogen activator that is used to prevent damage to heart muscle following a heart attack and to reduce neurological damage following ischemic stroke — see ACTIVASE

al·ter \ˈȯl-tər\ *vb* **al·tered; al·ter·ing** : CASTRATE, SPAY

al·ter·ative \ˈȯl-tə-ˌrā-tiv, -rə-\ *n* : a drug used empirically to alter favorably the course of an ailment

altered state of consciousness *n* : any of various states of awareness that deviate from and are usu. clearly demarcated from ordinary waking consciousness

al·ter·nans \ˈȯl-tər-ˌnanz\ *n* : alternation in the pattern of activity (as that produced by the heartbeat) — see PULSUS ALTERNANS

al·ter·nate host \ˈȯl-tər-nət-\ *n* : INTERMEDIATE HOST 1

alternating personality *n* : MULTIPLE PERSONALITY DISORDER

al·ter·na·tive \ȯl-ˈtər-nət-iv\ *adj* : of, relating to, or based on alternative medicine ⟨~ therapies⟩

alternative insemination *n* : ARTIFICIAL INSEMINATION

alternative medicine *n* : any of various systems of healing or treating disease (as chiropractic, homeopathy, or Ayurveda) not included in the traditional medical school curricula taught in the U.S. and Britain — called also *alternative healing*

altitude sickness *n* : the effects (as nosebleed, nausea, or cerebral edema) of oxygen deficiency developed at high altitudes with reduced atmospheric pressure

al•um \ˈa-ləm\ *n* : a potassium aluminum sulfate $KAl(SO_4)_2 \cdot 12H_2O$ or an ammonium aluminum sulfate $NH_4Al(SO_4)_2\ 12H_2O$ used esp. as an emetic and as an astringent

alu•mi•na \ə-ˈlü-mə-nə\ *n* : an oxide of aluminum Al_2O_3 that in hydrated forms is used in antacids — called also *aluminum oxide*

al•u•min•i•um \ˌal-yu̇-ˈmi-nē-əm\ *n, chiefly Brit* : ALUMINUM

alu•mi•num \ə-ˈlü-mə-nəm\ *n, often attrib* : a bluish silver-white malleable ductile trivalent metallic element — symbol *Al;* see ELEMENT table

aluminum chloride *n* : a deliquescent compound $AlCl_3$ or Al_2Cl_3 that is used as a topical astringent and antiseptic on the skin, and in some deodorants to control sweating

aluminum hydroxide *n* : any of several white gelatinous or crystalline hydrates $Al_2O_3 \cdot nH_2O$ of alumina; *esp* : one $Al_2O_3 \cdot 3H_2O$ or $Al(OH)_3$ used in medicine as an antacid

aluminum oxide *n* : ALUMINA

aluminum sulfate *n* : a colorless salt $Al_2(SO_4)_3$ that is a powerful astringent and is used as a local antiperspirant and in water purification

Al•u•pent \ˈa-lü-ˌpent\ *trademark* — used for a preparation of the sulfate of metaproterenol

alvei *pl of* ALVEUS

alveol- *or* **alveolo-** *comb form* : alveolus ⟨*alveol*ectomy⟩

al•ve•o•lar \al-ˈvē-ə-lər\ *adj* : of, relating to, resembling, or having alveoli; *esp* : of, relating to, or constituting the part of the jaws where the teeth arise, the air-containing cells of the lungs, or glands with secretory cells about a central space

alveolar arch *n* : the arch of the upper or lower jaw formed by the alveolar processes

alveolar artery *n* : any of several arteries supplying the teeth; *esp* : POSTERIOR SUPERIOR ALVEOLAR ARTERY — compare INFERIOR ALVEOLAR ARTERY

alveolar canals *n pl* : the canals in the jawbones for the passage of the dental nerves and associated vessels

alveolar duct *n* : one of the somewhat enlarged terminal sections of the bronchioles that branch into the terminal alveoli

alveolar nerve — see INFERIOR ALVEOLAR NERVE, SUPERIOR ALVEOLAR NERVE

alveolar process *n* : the bony ridge or raised thickened border on each side of the upper or lower jaw that contains the sockets of the teeth — called also *alveolar ridge*

alveolar vein — see INFERIOR ALVEOLAR VEIN; POSTERIOR SUPERIOR ALVEOLAR VEIN

al•ve•o•lec•to•my \al-ˌvē-ə-ˈlek-tə-mē, ˌal-vē-\ *n, pl* **-mies** : surgical excision of a portion of an alveolar process usu. as an aid in fitting dentures

al•ve•o•li•tis \al-ˌvē-ə-ˈlī-təs, ˌal-vē-\ *n* : inflammation of one or more alveoli esp. of the lung

al•ve•o•lo•plas•ty \al-ˈvē-ə-(ˌ)lō-ˌplas-tē\ *or* **al•veo•plas•ty** \ˈal-vē-ō-\ *n, pl* **-ties** : surgical shaping of the dental alveoli and alveolar processes esp. after extraction of several teeth or in preparation for dentures

al•ve•o•lus \al-ˈvē-ə-ləs\ *n, pl* **-li** \-ˌlī, -(ˌ)lē\ : a small cavity or pit: as **a** : a socket for a tooth **b** : any of the small thin-walled air-containing compartments of the lungs that are typically arranged into saclike clusters into which an alveolar duct terminates and from which respiratory gases are exchanged with the pulmonary capillaries **c** : an acinus of a compound gland **d** : any of the pits in the wall of the stomach into which the glands open

Al•ves•co \al-ˈve-skō\ *trademark* — used for a preparation of ciclesonide for oral inhalation

al•ve•us \ˈal-vē-əs\ *n, pl* **al•vei** \-vē-ˌī, -ˌē\ : a thin layer of medullary nerve fibers on the ventricular surface of the hippocampus

Alz•hei•mer's disease \ˈälts-ˌhī-mərz-, ˈalts-\ *also* **Alzheimer disease** *n* : a degenerative brain disease of unknown cause that is the most common form of dementia, that usu. starts in late middle age or in old age, that results in progressive memory loss, impaired thinking, disorientation, and changes in personality and mood, and that is marked histologically by the degeneration of brain neurons esp. in the cerebral cortex and by the presence of neurofibrillary tangles and plaques containing beta-amyloid — abbr. *AD;* called also *Alzheimer's*

Alzheimer, Alois (1864–1915), German neurologist.

Am *symbol* americium

AMA *abbr* **1** against medical advice **2** American Medical Association

am•a•crine cell \ˈa-mə-ˌkrīn-, (ˌ)ā-ˈma-ˌkrīn-\ *n* : a unipolar nerve cell found in the retina, in the olfactory bulb, and in close connection with the Purkinje cells of the cerebellum

amal•gam \ə-ˈmal-gəm\ *n* : an alloy of mercury with another metal that is solid or liquid at room temperature according to the proportion of mercury present and is used esp. in making tooth cements

am•a•ni•ta \ˌa-mə-ˈnī-tə, -ˈnē-\ *n* **1** *cap* : a genus of widely distributed white-spored basidiomycetous fungi (family Amanitaceae) that includes some deadly poisonous forms (as the death cap) **2** : a fungus of the genus *Amanita*

am•a•ni•tin \-ˈnit-ᵊn, -ˈnēt-\ *n* : a highly toxic cyclic peptide produced by the death cap that selectively inhibits mammalian RNA polymerase

aman·ta·dine \ə-ˈman-tə-ˌdēn\ *n* : a drug administered orally esp. in the form of its hydrochloride $C_{10}H_{17}N \cdot HCl$ to prevent viral infection (as by the virus causing influenza A) and in the treatment of Parkinson's disease — see SYMMETREL

Am·a·ran·thus \ˌa-mə-ˈran-thəs\ *n* : a genus of herbs (family Amaranthaceae) including some which produce pollen that is a hay fever allergen

amas·tia \(ˌ)ā-ˈmas-tē-ə\ *n* : the absence or underdevelopment of the mammary glands

am·au·ro·sis \ˌa-mȯ-ˈrō-səs\ *n, pl* **-ro·ses** \-ˌsēz\ : partial or complete loss of sight occurring esp. without an externally perceptible change in the eye — **am·au·rot·ic** \-ˈrä-tik\ *adj*

amaurosis fu·gax \-ˈfü-ˌgaks, -ˈfyü-\ *n* : temporary partial or complete loss of sight in one eye that is typically caused by an abrupt reduction in blood flow to an eye

amaurotic idiocy *n, dated, now usu. offensive* : any of several recessive genetic conditions characterized by the accumulation of lipid-containing cells in the viscera and nervous system, intellectual disability, and impaired vision or blindness; *esp* : TAY-SACHS DISEASE

ambi- *prefix* : both ⟨*ambi*valence⟩ ⟨*ambi*sexuality⟩

am·bi·dex·ter·i·ty \ˌam-bi-(ˌ)dek-ˈster-ə-tē\ *n, pl* **-ties** : the quality or state of being ambidextrous

am·bi·dex·trous \ˌam-bi-ˈdek-strəs\ *adj* : using both hands with equal ease — **am·bi·dex·trous·ly** *adv*

Am·bi·en \ˈam-bē-ˌen\ *trademark* — used for a preparation of the tartrate of zolpidem

am·bi·ent \ˈam-bē-ənt\ *adj* : surrounding on all sides ⟨~ air pollution⟩

ambiguus — see NUCLEUS AMBIGUUS

am·bi·sex·u·al \ˌam-bi-ˈsek-shə-wəl\ *adj* : BISEXUAL — **ambisexual** *n* — **am·bi·sex·u·al·i·ty** \-ˌsek-shə-ˈwa-lə-tē\ *n*

am·biv·a·lence \am-ˈbi-və-ləns\ *n* : simultaneous and contradictory attitudes or feelings (as attraction and repulsion) toward an object, person, or action — **am·biv·a·lent** \-lənt\ *adj* — **am·biv·a·lent·ly** *adv*

am·biv·a·len·cy \-lən-sē\ *n, pl* **-cies** : AMBIVALENCE

am·bi·vert \ˈam-bi-ˌvərt\ *n* : a person having characteristics of both extrovert and introvert

ambly- *or* **amblyo-** *comb form* : connected with amblyopia ⟨*amblyo*scope⟩

Am·bly·om·ma \ˌam-blē-ˈä-mə\ *n* : a genus of ixodid ticks including the lone star tick (*A. americanum*)

am·bly·ope \ˈam-blē-ˌōp\ *n* : an individual affected with amblyopia

am·bly·opia \ˌam-blē-ˈō-pē-ə\ *n* : dimness of sight esp. in one eye without apparent change in the eye structures — called also *lazy eye, lazy-eye blindness* — **am·bly·opic** \-ˈō-pik, -ˈä-\ *adj*

am·bly·o·scope \ˈam-blē-ə-ˌskōp\ *n* : an instrument for training amblyopic eyes to function properly

Am·bro·sia \am-ˈbrō-zhə, -zhē-ə\ *n* : a genus of mostly American composite herbs that includes the ragweeds

Am·bu \ˈam-ˌbü\ *trademark* — used for an artificial-respiration device consisting of a bag that is squeezed by hand

am·bu·lance \ˈam-byə-ləns\ *n* : a vehicle equipped for transporting the injured or sick

am·bu·lant \ˈam-byə-lənt\ *adj* : walking or in a walking position; *specif* : AMBULATORY ⟨an ~ patient⟩

am·bu·late \-ˌlāt\ *vb* **-lat·ed; -lat·ing** : to move from place to place — **am·bu·la·tion** \ˌam-byə-ˈlā-shən\ *n*

am·bu·la·to·ry \ˈam-byə-lə-ˌtōr-ē\ *adj* **1** : of, relating to, or adapted to walking ⟨~ exercise⟩ **2 a** : able to walk about and not bedridden ⟨~ patients⟩ **b** : performed on or involving a patient who is able to walk about ⟨~ therapy⟩ **c** : performed on or provided to an outpatient ⟨~ care⟩; *also* : relating to or intended for outpatient care ⟨~ surgical centers⟩ **d** : performed on or worn by a patient during the course of normal daily activities (as working and sleeping) ⟨~ blood pressure monitors⟩; *also* : obtained by ambulatory monitoring ⟨24-hour ~ blood pressure⟩ — **am·bu·la·to·ri·ly** \ˌam-byə-lə-ˈtōr-ə-lē\ *adv*

AMD *abbr* age-related macular degeneration

ameba, ameboid *var of* AMOEBA, AMOEBOID

am·e·bi·a·sis *or* **am·oe·bi·a·sis** \ˌa-mi-ˈbī-ə-səs\ *n, pl* **-a·ses** \-ˌsēz\ : infection with or disease caused by amoebas (esp. *Entamoeba histolytica*)

ame·bic *or* **amoe·bic** \ə-ˈmē-bik\ *adj* **1** : resembling or relating to an amoeba **2** *usu amebic* : caused by amoebas

amebic abscess *or* **amoebic abscess** *n* : a specific purulent invasive lesion commonly of the liver caused by parasitic amoebas (esp. *Entamoeba histolytica*)

amebic dysentery *or* **amoebic dysentery** *n* : acute human intestinal amebiasis caused by a common amoeba of the genus *Entamoeba* (*E. histolytica*) and marked by dysentery, abdominal pain, and erosion of the intestinal wall

ame·bi·cide *or* **amoe·bi·cide** \ə-ˈmē-bə-ˌsīd\ *n* : a substance used to kill or capable of killing amoebas and esp. parasitic amoebas — **ame·bi·cid·al** *or* **amoe·bi·cid·al** \ə-ˌmē-bə-ˈsīd-ᵊl\ *adj*

ame·bo·cyte *or* **amoe·bo·cyte** \ə-ˈmē-bə-ˌsīt\ *n* : a cell (as a phagocyte) having amoeboid form or movements

amel·a·not·ic \ˌā-ˌmē-lə-ˈnä-tik\ *adj* : containing little or no melanin

: lacking pigmentation ⟨~ melanoma⟩

ame•lia \ə-ˈmē-lē-ə, (ˌ)ā-\ *n* : congenital absence of one or more limbs

am•e•lo•blast \ˈa-mə-lō-ˌblast\ *n* : any of a group of columnar cells that produce and deposit enamel on the surface of a developing tooth — **am•e•lo•blas•tic** \ˌa-mə-lō-ˈblas-tik\ *adj*

am•e•lo•blas•to•ma \ˌa-mə-lō-blas-ˈtō-mə\ *n, pl* **-mas** *also* **-ma•ta** \-mə-tə\ : a tumor of the jaw derived from remnants of the embryonic rudiment of tooth enamel — called also *adamantinoma*

am•e•lo•den•tin•al \-ˈden-ˌtēn-ᵊl, -den-ˈtēn-\ *adj* : of or relating to enamel and dentin

am•e•lo•gen•e•sis \-ˈje-nə-səs\ *n, pl* **-e•ses** \-ˌsēz\ : the process of forming tooth enamel

amelogenesis im•per•fec•ta \-ˌim-(ˌ)pər-ˈfek-tə\ *n* : faulty development of tooth enamel that is genetically determined

amen•or•rhea \ˌā-ˌme-nə-ˈrē-ə, ˌä-\ *n* : abnormal absence or suppression of menstruation — **amen•or•rhe•ic** \-ˈrē-ik\ *adj*

Amerge \ə-ˈmərj\ *trademark* — used for a preparation of naratriptan

American cockroach *n* : a free-flying cockroach (*Periplaneta americana*) that is a common domestic pest

American dog tick *n* : a common No. American ixodid tick of the genus *Dermacentor* (*D. variabilis*) esp. of dogs and humans that is an important vector of Rocky Mountain spotted fever and tularemia — called also *dog tick*

American trypanosomiasis *n* : CHAGAS DISEASE

am•er•i•ci•um \ˌa-mə-ˈri-shē-əm, -sē-\ *n* : a radioactive metallic element produced by bombardment of plutonium with high-energy neutrons — symbol *Am;* see ELEMENT table

Ames test \ˈāmz-\ *n* : a test for identifying potential carcinogens by studying the frequency with which they cause histidine-producing genetic mutants in bacterial colonies of the genus *Salmonella* (*S. typhimurium*) initially lacking the ability to synthesize histidine — called also *Ames assay*

Ames, Bruce Nathan (*b* 1928), American biochemist.

ameth•o•caine \ə-ˈme-thə-ˌkān\ *n* : TETRACAINE

am•e•thop•ter•in \ˌa-mə-ˈthäp-tə-rən\ *n* : METHOTREXATE

am•e•tro•pia \ˌa-mə-ˈtrō-pē-ə\ *n* : an abnormal refractive eye condition (as myopia, hyperopia, or astigmatism) in which images fail to focus upon the retina — **am•e•tro•pic** \-ˈtrō-pik, -ˈträ-\ *adj*

AMH *abbr* anti-Mullerian hormone

AMI *abbr* acute myocardial infarction

Am•i•car \ˈa-mi-ˌkär\ *trademark* — used for a preparation of aminocaproic acid

am•ide \ˈam-ˌīd, -əd\ *n* : an organic compound derived from ammonia or an amine by replacement of an atom of hydrogen with an acyl group

am•i•done \ˈa-mə-ˌdōn\ *n* : METHADONE

am•i•ka•cin \ˌa-mi-ˈkā-sᵊn\ *n* : a semisynthetic aminoglycoside antibiotic that is administered intravenously or intramuscularly in the form of its sulfate $C_{22}H_{43}N_5O_{13}\cdot 2H_2SO_4$ chiefly to treat serious bacterial infections

amil•o•ride \ə-ˈmi-lə-ˌrīd\ *n* : a diuretic $C_6H_8ClN_7O$ that promotes sodium excretion and potassium retention

amine \ə-ˈmēn, ˈa-ˌmēn\ *n* : any of a class of organic compounds derived from ammonia by replacement of hydrogen atoms with alkyl groups

ami•no \ə-ˈmē-(ˌ)nō\ *adj* : relating to, being, or containing an amine group — often used in combination

amino acid *n* : an organic acid containing the amino group NH_2; *esp* : ALPHA-AMINO ACID

ami•no•ac•i•de•mia \ə-ˌmē-nō-ˌa-sə-ˈdē-mē-ə\ *n* : a condition in which the concentration of amino acids in the blood is abnormally increased

ami•no•ac•id•uria \-ˌa-sə-ˈdu̇r-ē-ə, -ˈdyu̇r-\ *n* : a condition in which one or more amino acids are excreted in excessive amounts

ami•no•ben•zo•ic acid \ə-ˌmē-nō-ben-ˈzō-ik-\ *n* : any of three crystalline derivatives $C_7H_7NO_2$ of benzoic acid; *esp* : PARA-AMINOBENZOIC ACID

γ–aminobutyric acid *var of* GAMMA-AMINOBUTYRIC ACID

ami•no•ca•pro•ic acid \ə-ˌmē-nō-kə-ˌprō-ik-\ *n* : a drug $C_6H_{13}NO_2$ that inhibits the breakdown of fibrin and is used to control bleeding (as during surgery) esp. in cases where blood clots are broken down too quickly — see AMICAR

ami•no•glu•teth•i•mide \-glü-ˈte-thə-ˌmīd\ *n* : a drug $C_{13}H_{16}N_2O_2$ that inhibits the production of steroids by the adrenal cortex and is used chiefly in the treatment of Cushing's disease

ami•no•gly•co•side \-ˈglī-kə-ˌsīd\ *n* : any of a group of antibiotics (as streptomycin and neomycin) that inhibit bacterial protein synthesis and are active esp. against gram-negative bacteria

ami•no•lev•u•lin•ic acid \ə-ˌmē-nō-ˌlev-yə-ˌli-nik-\ *also* **5–aminolevulinic acid** : a drug applied to the face and scalp in the form of its hydrochloride $C_5H_9NO_3\cdot HCl$ to make the skin sensitive to light in photodynamic treatment esp. of actinic keratoses — abbr. *ALA;* see LEVULAN

ami•no•pep•ti•dase \ə-ˌmē-nō-ˈpep-tə-ˌdās, -ˌdāz\ *n* : an enzyme that hydrolyzes peptides

am·i·noph·yl·line \ˌa-mə-ˈnä-fə-lən\ *n* : a theophylline derivative $C_{16}H_{24}N_{10}O_4$ used esp. to stimulate the heart in congestive heart failure and to dilate the air passages in respiratory disorders — called also *theophylline ethylenediamine*

β–ami·no·pro·pio·ni·trile \ˌbā-tə-ə-ˌmē-nō-ˌprō-pē-ō-ˈnī-trəl, -ˌtrīl\ *n* : a potent lathyrogen $C_3H_6N_2$

am·i·nop·ter·in \ˌa-mə-ˈnäp-tə-rən\ *n* : a derivative $C_{19}H_{20}N_8O_5$ of glutamic acid that is a folic acid antagonist and has been used as a rodenticide and antileukemic agent

ami·no·py·rine \ə-ˌmē-nō-ˈpīr-ˌēn\ *n* : a compound $C_{13}H_{17}N_3O$ formerly used to relieve pain and fever but now largely abandoned because of the occurrence of fatal agranulocytosis as a side effect in some users

ami·no·sal·i·cyl·ic acid \ə-ˌmē-nō-ˌsa-lə-ˈsi-lik-\ *n* : any of four isomeric derivatives $C_7H_7O_3N$ of salicylic acid that have a single amino group; *esp* : PARA-AMINOSALICYLIC ACID

ami·no·thi·a·zole \ə-ˌmē-nō-ˈthī-ə-ˌzōl\ *n* : a heterocyclic amine $C_3H_4N_2S$ that has been used as a thyroid inhibitor to treat hyperthyroidism

ami·no·trans·fer·ase \-ˈtrans-fə-ˌrās, -ˌrāz\ *n* : TRANSAMINASE

ami·o·da·rone \ə-ˈmē-ō-də-ˌrōn\ *n* : a drug administered in the form of its hydrochloride $C_{25}H_{29}I_2NO_3{\cdot}HCl$ to treat ventricular arrhythmias

Am·i·ti·za \ˌam-ə-ˈtī-zə\ *trademark* — used for a preparation of lubiprostone

am·i·trip·ty·line \ˌa-mə-ˈtrip-tə-ˌlēn\ *n* : a tricyclic antidepressant drug used in the form of its hydrochloride $C_{20}H_{23}N{\cdot}HCl$ to prevent migraines and to treat neuropathic pain, bulimia, and depression

AML *abbr* acute myelogenous leukemia; acute myeloid leukemia

am·lo·di·pine \am-ˈlō-də-ˌpēn\ *n* : a calcium channel blocker administered in the form of its salt $C_{20}H_{25}ClN_2O_5{\cdot}C_6H_5SO_3H$ to treat hypertension and angina pectoris — see AZOR, CADUET, EXFORGE, LOTREL, NORVASC, TRIBENZOR

am·mo·nia \ə-ˈmō-nyə\ *n* **1** : a pungent colorless gaseous alkaline compound NH_3 that is very soluble in water and can easily be condensed to a liquid by cold and pressure **2** : AMMONIA WATER

am·mo·ni·a·cal \ˌa-mə-ˈnī-ə-kəl\ *also* **am·mo·ni·ac** \ə-ˈmō-nē-ˌak\ *adj* : of, relating to, containing, or having the properties of ammonia

ammonia water *n* : a water solution of ammonia — called also *spirit of hartshorn*

am·mo·ni·um \ə-ˈmō-nē-əm\ *n* : an ion $NH_4{}^+$ derived from ammonia by combination with a hydrogen ion

ammonium carbonate *n* : a carbonate of ammonium; *specif* : the commercial mixture of the bicarbonate and carbamate used esp. in smelling salts

ammonium chloride *n* : a white crystalline volatile salt NH_4Cl that is used in dry cells and as an expectorant — called also *sal ammoniac*

ammonium nitrate *n* : a colorless crystalline salt $N_2H_4NO_3$ used in veterinary medicine as an expectorant and urinary acidifier

ammonium sulfate *n* : a colorless crystalline salt $(NH_4)_2SO_4$ used in medicine as a local analgesic

am·ne·sia \am-ˈnē-zhə\ *n* **1** : loss of memory sometimes including the memory of personal identity due to brain injury, shock, fatigue, repression, or illness or sometimes induced by anesthesia **2** : a gap in one's memory

am·ne·si·ac \am-ˈnē-zhē-ˌak, -zē-\ *also* **am·ne·sic** \-zik, -sik\ *n* : a person affected with amnesia

am·ne·sic \am-ˈnē-zik, -sik\ *also* **am·ne·si·ac** \-zhē-ˌak, -zē-\ *adj* : of, relating to, or causing amnesia ⟨an ~ trauma⟩; *also* : affected with or caused by amnesia ⟨an ~ patient⟩

amnesic shellfish poisoning *n* : shellfish poisoning that is characterized by gastrointestinal and neurological symptoms (as vomiting, abdominal cramps, headache, and short-term memory loss) and sometimes death and is caused by domoic acid ingested in contaminated shellfish — called also *amnestic shellfish poisoning*

am·nes·tic \am-ˈnes-tik\ *adj* : AMNESIC; *also* : causing amnesia ⟨~ agents⟩

amnii — see LIQUOR AMNII

am·nio \ˈam-nē-ō\ *n* : AMNIOCENTESIS

amnio- *comb form* : amnion ⟨*amnio*centesis⟩

am·nio·cen·te·sis \ˌam-nē-ō-(ˌ)sen-ˈtē-səs\ *n, pl* **-te·ses** \-ˌsēz\ : the surgical insertion of a hollow needle through the abdominal wall and into the uterus of a pregnant female to obtain amniotic fluid esp. to examine the fetal chromosomes for an abnormality and for the determination of sex

am·ni·og·ra·phy \ˌam-nē-ˈä-grə-fē\ *n, pl* **-phies** : radiographic visualization of the uterine cavity, placenta, and fetus after injection of a radiopaque substance into the amnion

am·nio·in·fu·sion \ˌam-nē-ō-in-ˈfyü-zhən\ *n* : the introduction of sterile saline or lactated Ringer's solution into the amniotic cavity via the uterine cervix esp. to increase the volume of amniotic fluid (as during labor)

am·ni·on \ˈam-nē-ˌän, -ən\ *n, pl* **amnions** *or* **am·nia** \-nē-ə\ : a thin membrane forming a closed sac about the embryos of reptiles, birds, and mammals and containing the amniotic fluid

am·ni·o·nit·is \ˌam-nē-ə-ˈnī-təs\ *n* : inflammation of the amnion typically due to infection; *also* : CHORIOAMNIONITIS

am•nio•scope \ˈam-nē-ə-ˌskōp\ *n* : an endoscope for observation of the amnion and its contents

am•ni•os•co•py \ˌam-nē-ˈäs-kə-pē\ *n, pl* **-pies** : visual observation of the amnion and its contents by means of an endoscope

am•ni•ote \ˈam-nē-ˌōt\ *n* : any of a group (Amniota) of vertebrates that undergo embryonic development within an amnion and include the birds, reptiles, and mammals — **amniote** *adj*

am•ni•ot•ic \ˌam-nē-ˈä-tik\ *adj* **1** : of or relating to the amnion **2** : characterized by the development of an amnion

amniotic band *n* : strands of amniotic tissue that are formed by premature rupture of the amnion and that become entangled esp. in the extremities of the developing fetus

amniotic band syndrome *n* : the highly variable group of physical abnormalities that can result from the formation of amniotic bands

amniotic cavity *n* : the fluid-filled space between the amnion and the fetus

amniotic fluid *n* : the serous fluid in which the embryo is suspended within the amnion

amniotic sac *n* : AMNION

am•ni•ot•o•my \ˌam-nē-ˈä-tə-mē\ *n, pl* **-mies** : intentional rupture of the amnion chiefly to induce or facilitate labor

amo•bar•bi•tal \ˌa-mō-ˈbär-bə-ˌtȯl\ *n* : a barbiturate used esp. in the form of its sodium salt $C_{11}H_{17}N_2NaO_3$ as a hypnotic and sedative — called also *amylobarbitone;* see AMYTAL, TUINAL

amo•di•a•quine \ˌa-mə-ˈdī-ə-ˌkwin, -ˌkwēn\ *also* **amo•di•a•quin** \-ˌkwin\ *n* : a compound derived from quinoline and used in the form of its dihydrochloride $C_{20}H_{22}ClN_3O{\cdot}2HCl{\cdot}2H_2O$ as an antimalarial

amoe•ba \ə-ˈmē-bə\ *n* **1** *cap* : a genus of protozoans with lobed pseudopodia that lack permanent organelles or supporting structures and are found in fresh and salt water and moist terrestrial environments **2** *also* **ameba** *pl* **-bas** *or* **-bae** \-(ˌ)bē\ : a protozoan of the genus *Amoeba; broadly* : an amoeboid protozoan

amoebiasis, amoebic, amoebicide, amoebocyte *var of* AMEBIASIS, AMEBIC, AMEBICIDE, AMEBOCYTE

amoe•boid *or* **ame•boid** \ə-ˈmē-ˌbȯid\ *adj* : resembling an amoeba specif. in moving or changing in shape by means of protoplasmic flow

Amoe•bo•tae•nia \ə-ˌmē-(ˌ)bō-ˈtē-nē-ə\ *n* : a genus of tapeworms (family Dilepididae) parasitic in the intestines of poultry

amor•phous \ə-ˈmȯr-fəs\ *adj* **1** : having no apparent shape or organization **2** : having no real or apparent crystalline form

amox•a•pine \ə-ˈmäk-sə-ˌpēn\ *n* : a tricyclic antidepressant drug $C_{17}H_{16}ClN_3O$

amox•i•cil•lin \ə-ˌmäk-sē-ˈsi-lən\ *n* : a semisynthetic penicillin $C_{16}H_{19}N_3O_5S$ derived from ampicillin — see AMOXIL, AUGMENTIN, TRIMOX

Amox•il \ə-ˈmäk-sil\ *trademark* — used for a preparation of amoxicillin

amox•y•cil•lin \ə-ˌmäk-sē-ˈsi-lən\ *Brit var of* AMOXICILLIN

AMP \ˌā-(ˌ)em-ˈpē\ *n* : a nucleotide $C_{10}H_{12}N_5O_3H_2PO_4$ that is composed of adenosine and one phosphate group and is reversibly convertible to ADP and ATP in metabolic reactions — called also *adenosine monophosphate;* compare CYCLIC AMP

am•pere \ˈam-ˌpir, -ˌper\ *n* : a unit of electric current equivalent to a steady current produced by one volt applied across a resistance of one ohm

Am•père \äⁿ-per\, **André Marie (1775–1836)**, French physicist.

am•phet•amine \am-ˈfe-tə-ˌmēn, -mən\ *n* : a racemic sympathomimetic amine $C_9H_{13}N$ or one of its derivatives (as dextroamphetamine or methamphetamine) that is a stimulant of the central nervous system, is frequently abused illicity often leading to dependence, and is used clinically esp. in the form of its sulfate $C_9H_{13}N{\cdot}H_2SO_4$ to treat attention deficit disorder and narcolepsy and formerly as a short-term appetite suppressant — see ADDERALL

amphi- *or* **amph-** *prefix* : on both sides : of both kinds : both ⟨*amphi*mixis⟩

am•phi•ar•thro•sis \ˌam-fē-(ˌ)är-ˈthrō-səs\ *n, pl* **-thro•ses** \-ˌsēz\ : a slightly movable articulation (as a symphysis or a syndesmosis)

am•phi•bol•ic \ˌam-fə-ˈbä-lik\ *adj* : having an uncertain or irregular outcome — used of stages in fevers or the critical period of disease when prognosis is uncertain

am•phi•mix•is \ˌam-fə-ˈmik-səs\ *n, pl* **-mix•es** \-ˌsēz\ : the union of gametes in sexual reproduction

am•phi•path•ic \ˌam-fə-ˈpa-thik\ *adj* : AMPHIPHILIC — **am•phi•path** \ˈam-fə-ˌpath\ *n*

am•phi•phil•ic \ˌam-fə-ˈfi-lik\ *adj* : of, relating to, consisting of, or being one or more molecules (as of a glycolipid or sphingolipid) in a biological membrane having a polar water-soluble terminal group attached to a water-insoluble hydrocarbon chain — **am•phi•phile** \ˈam-fə-ˌfīl\ *n*

am•phi•stome \ˈam-fi-ˌstōm\ *n* : any of a suborder (Amphistomata) of digenetic trematodes — compare GASTRODISCOIDES — **amphistome** *adj*

am•phor•ic \am-ˈfȯr-ik\ *adj* : resembling the sound made by blowing across the mouth of an empty bottle ⟨~ breathing⟩ ⟨~ sounds⟩

am·pho·ter·i·cin B \ˌam-fə-ˈter-ə-sən-\ *n* : an antifungal antibiotic obtained from a soil actinomycete (*Streptomyces nodosus*) and used esp. to treat systemic fungal infections

am·pi·cil·lin \ˌam-pə-ˈsi-lən\ *n* : a penicillin $C_{16}H_{19}N_3O_4S$ that is effective against gram-negative and gram-positive bacteria and is used to treat infections of the urinary, respiratory, and intestinal tracts — see PENBRITIN

am·pli·fi·ca·tion \ˌam-plə-fə-ˈkā-shən\ *n* **1** : an act, example, or product of amplifying **2** : a usu. massive replication of genetic material and esp. of a gene or DNA sequence (as in a polymerase chain reaction)

am·pli·fy \ˈam-plə-ˌfī\ *vb* **-fied; -fy·ing** **1** : to make larger or greater (as in amount or intensity) **2** : to cause (a gene or DNA sequence) to undergo amplification

am·pule *or* **am·poule** *also* **am·pul** \ˈam-ˌpyül, -pül\ *n* **1** : a hermetically sealed small bulbous glass vessel that is used to hold a solution for esp. hypodermic injection **2** : a vial resembling an ampule

am·pul·la \am-ˈpu̇-lə, ˈam-ˌpyü-lə\ *n, pl* **-lae** \-ˌlē\ : a saccular anatomic swelling or pouch: as **a** : the dilatation containing a patch of sensory epithelium at one end of each semicircular canal of the ear **b** : one of the dilatations of the milk-carrying tubules of the mammary glands that serve as reservoirs for milk **c** (1) : the middle portion of the fallopian tube (2) : the distal dilatation of a vas deferens near the opening of the duct leading from the seminal vesicle **d** : a terminal dilatation of the rectum just before it joins the anal canal

ampulla of Va·ter \-ˈfä-tər\ *n* : a trumpet-mouthed dilatation of the duodenal wall at the opening of the fused pancreatic and common bile ducts — called also *papilla of Vater*

Vater, Abraham (1684–1751), German anatomist.

ampullaris — see CRISTA AMPULLARIS

am·pul·la·ry \am-ˈpu̇-lə-rē\ *also* **am·pul·lar** \-ˈpu̇-lər\ *adj* : resembling or relating to an ampulla

am·pu·tate \ˈam-pyə-ˌtāt\ *vb* **-tat·ed; -tat·ing** : to cut (as a limb) from the body — **am·pu·ta·tion** \ˌam-pyə-ˈtā-shən\ *n*

amputation neuroma *n* : NEUROMA 2

am·pu·tee \ˌam-pyə-ˈtē\ *n* : one that has had a limb amputated

Am·rix \ˈam-ˌriks\ *trademark* — used for a preparation of cyclobenzaprine

AMS *abbr* acute mountain sickness

Am·sler grid \ˈäm-zlər-\ *n* : a pattern of uniformly spaced horizontal and perpendicular lines with a dot at the center that is viewed with one eye covered for the purposes of detecting defects in the central visual field

Amsler, Marc (1891–1968), Swedish ophthalmologist.

amygdal- *or* **amygdalo-** *comb form* **1** : almond ⟨*amygdal*in⟩ **2** : amygdala ⟨*amygdal*ectomy⟩ ⟨*amygdalo*tomy⟩

amyg·da·la \ə-ˈmig-də-lə\ *n, pl* **-lae** \-ˌlē, -ˌlī\ : the one of the four basal ganglia in each cerebral hemisphere that is part of the limbic system and consists of an almond-shaped mass of gray matter in the roof of the lateral ventricle — called also *amygdaloid body, amygdaloid nucleus*

amyg·da·lar \ə-ˈmig-də-lər\ *adj* : of, relating to, or affecting the amygdala : AMYGDALOID

amyg·da·lec·to·my \ə-ˌmig-də-ˈlek-tə-mē\ *n, pl* **-mies** : surgical removal of the amygdala — **amyg·da·lec·to·mized** \-tə-ˌmīzd\ *adj*

amyg·da·lin \ə-ˈmig-də-lən\ *n* : a white crystalline cyanogenic glucoside $C_{20}H_{27}NO_{11}$ found esp. in the seeds of the apricot, peach, and bitter almond

amyg·da·loid \-ˌlȯid\ *adj* **1** : almond-shaped **2** : of, relating to, or affecting the amygdala : AMYGDALAR ⟨~ lesions⟩

amygdaloid body *n* : AMYGDALA

amygdaloid nucleus *n* : AMYGDALA

amyg·da·lot·o·my \ə-ˌmig-də-ˈlä-tə-mē\ *n, pl* **-mies** : destruction of part of the amygdala (as for the control of epilepsy) esp. by surgical incision

amyl- *or* **amylo-** *comb form* : starch ⟨*amyl*ase⟩

am·y·lase \ˈa-mə-ˌlās, -ˌlāz\ *n* : any of a group of enzymes (as amylopsin) that catalyze the hydrolysis of starch and glycogen or their intermediate hydrolysis products

am·y·lin \ˈa-mə-lən\ *n* : a pancreatic hormone secreted with insulin that inhibits glucose synthesis stimulated by insulin in skeletal muscles — called also *islet amyloid polypeptide*

am·yl nitrite \ˈa-məl-\ *n* : a pale yellow pungent flammable liquid ester $C_5H_{11}NO_2$ that is used chiefly in medicine as a vasodilator esp. in treating angina pectoris and illicitly as an aphrodisiac — called also *isoamyl nitrite;* compare POPPER

am·y·lo·bar·bi·tone \ˌa-mə-lō-ˈbär-bə-ˌtōn\ *n, Brit* : AMOBARBITAL

am·y·loid \ˈa-mə-ˌlȯid\ *n* : a waxy translucent substance consisting primarily of protein that is deposited in some animal organs and tissue under abnormal conditions (as in Alzheimer's disease) — see BETA-AMYLOID — **amyloid** *adj*

amyloid beta *n* : BETA-AMYLOID — called also *amyloid beta peptide, amyloid beta protein*

am·y·loid·osis \ˌa-mə-ˌlȯi-ˈdō-səs\ *n, pl* **-o·ses** \-ˌsēz\ : a disorder characterized by the deposition of amyloid in organs or tissues of the animal body — see PARAMYLOIDOSIS

amyloid precursor protein *n* : a transmembrane protein from which beta-amyloid is derived by proteolytic cleavage by secretases

am·y·lop·sin \ˌa-mə-ˈläp-sən\ *n* : the amylase of the pancreatic juice
am·y·lum \ˈa-mə-ləm\ *n* : STARCH
amyo·to·nia \ˌā-ˌmī-ə-ˈtō-nē-ə\ *n* : deficiency of muscle tone
amyotonia con·gen·i·ta \-kən-ˈje-nə-tə\ *n* : a congenital disease of infants characterized by flaccidity of the skeletal muscles
amyo·tro·phia \ˌā-ˌmī-ə-ˈtrō-fē-ə\ *or* **amy·ot·ro·phy** \-ˌmī-ˈä-trə-fē\ *n, pl* **-phi·as** *or* **-phies** : atrophy of a muscle — **amyo·tro·phic** \-ˌmī-ə-ˈträ-fik, -ˈtrō-\ *adj*
amyotrophic lateral sclerosis *n* : a rare fatal progressive degenerative disease that affects pyramidal motor neurons, usu. begins in middle age, and is characterized esp. by increasing and spreading muscular weakness — abbr. *ALS;* called also *Lou Gehrig's disease*
Am·y·tal \ˈa-mə-ˌtȯl\ *trademark* — used for a preparation of amobarbital
an- *var of* A-, ANA-
ana \ˈa-nə\ *adv* : of each an equal quantity — used in prescriptions
ana- *or* **an-** *prefix* : up : upward ⟨*ana*bolism⟩
ANA *abbr* **1** American Nurses Association **2** antinuclear antibodies; antinuclear antibody
anabolic steroid *n* : any of a group of usu. synthetic hormones that are derivatives of testosterone, are used medically esp. to promote tissue growth, and are sometimes abused by athletes to increase the size and strength of their muscles and improve endurance
anab·o·lism \ə-ˈna-bə-ˌli-zəm\ *n* : the constructive part of metabolism concerned esp. with macromolecular synthesis — compare CATABOLISM — **an·a·bol·ic** \ˌa-nə-ˈbä-lik\ *adj*
an·acid·i·ty \ˌa-nə-ˈsi-də-tē\ *n, pl* **-ties** : ACHLORHYDRIA
an·a·clit·ic \a-nə-ˈkli-tik\ *adj* : of, relating to, or characterized by the direction of love toward an object (as the mother) that satisfies nonsexual needs (as hunger)
anac·ro·tism \ə-ˈna-krə-ˌti-zəm\ *n* : an abnormality of the blood circulation characterized by a secondary notch in the ascending part of a sphygmographic tracing of the pulse — **an·a·crot·ic** \ˌa-nə-ˈkrä-tik\ *adj*
anae·mia *chiefly Brit var of* ANEMIA
an·aer·obe \ˈa-nə-ˌrōb, (ˌ)a-ˈnar-ˌōb\ *n* : an anaerobic organism
an·aer·o·bic \ˌa-nə-ˈrō-bik, ˌa-ˌnar-ˈō-\ *adj* **1 a** : living, active, or occurring in the absence of free oxygen ⟨~ respiration⟩ **b** (1) : of, relating to, or being activity in which the body incurs an oxygen debt ⟨an ~ workout⟩ (2) : of or relating to the body's ability to incur an oxygen debt ⟨~ thresholds⟩ **2** : relating to or induced by anaerobes — **an·aer·o·bi·cal·ly** \-bi-k(ə-)lē\ *adv*
an·aes·the·sia, an·aes·the·si·ol·o·gist, an·aes·the·si·ol·o·gy, an·aes·the·tic, an·aes·the·tist, an·aes·the·tize *chiefly Brit var of* ANESTHESIA, ANESTHESIOLOGIST, ANESTHESIOLOGY, ANESTHETIC, ANESTHETIST, ANESTHETIZE
Anaf·ra·nil \ə-ˈna-frə-ˌnil\ *trademark* — used for a preparation of the hydrochloride of clomipramine
an·a·gen \ˈa-nə-ˌjen\ *n* : the active phase of the hair growth cycle preceding catagen and telogen
anag·re·lide \ə-ˈnag-rə-ˌlīd\ *n* : a phosphodiesterase inhibitor administered esp. in the form of its hydrochloride $C_{10}H_7Cl_2N_3O·HCl$ to treat thrombocytosis — see AGRYLIN
an·a·kin·ra \ˌa-nə-ˈkin-rə\ *n* : a drug that blocks the activity of interleukin-1 and is administered by subcutaneous injection in the treatment of rheumatoid arthritis — see KINERET
anal \ˈān-ᵊl\ *adj* **1** : of, relating to, or situated near the anus ⟨the ~ opening⟩ ⟨~ fissures⟩ **2 a** : of, relating to, or characterized by the stage of psychosexual development in psychoanalytic theory during which the child derives libidinal gratification from the expulsion and retention of the feces **b** : of, relating to, or characterized by personality traits (as orderliness and frugality) considered typical of fixation at the anal stage of development : ANAL-RETENTIVE — compare GENITAL 3, ORAL 2, PHALLIC 2 — **anal·ly** *adv*
anal *abbr* **1** analysis **2** analytic **3** analyze
anal canal *n* : the terminal section of the rectum
[1]**an·a·lep·tic** \ˌa-nə-ˈlep-tik\ *adj* : of, relating to, or acting as an analeptic
[2]**analeptic** *n* : a restorative agent; *esp* : a drug that acts as a stimulant on the central nervous system
anal eroticism *n* : the experiencing of pleasurable sensations or sexual excitement associated with or symbolic of stimulation of the anus — called also *anal erotism* — **anal erotic** *adj*
an·al·ge·sia \ˌan-ᵊl-ˈjēzhə, -zhē-ə, -zē-\ *n* : insensibility to pain without loss of consciousness
[1]**an·al·ge·sic** \-ˈjē-zik, -sik\ *adj* : relating to, characterized by, or producing analgesia
[2]**analgesic** *n* : an agent for producing analgesia
an·al·get·ic \-ˈje-tik\ *n or adj* : ANALGESIC
anal·i·ty \ā-ˈna-lə-tē\ *n, pl* **-ties** : an anal psychological state, stage, or quality
anal·o·gous \ə-ˈna-lə-gəs\ *adj* : having similar function but a different structure and origin ⟨~ organs⟩
an·a·logue *or* **an·a·log** \ˈan-ᵊl-ˌȯg, -ˌäg\ *n* **1** : an organ similar in function to an organ of another species but different in structure and origin **2** *usu* *analog* : a chemical compound that is structurally similar to another but

differs slightly in composition (as in the replacement of one atom by an atom of a different element)

anal•o•gy \ə-ˈna-lə-jē\ *n, pl* **-gies** : functional similarity between anatomical parts without similarity of structure and origin — compare HOMOLOGY 1

anal–re•ten•tive \ˈān-ᵊl-ri-ˈten-tiv\ *adj* : exhibiting or typifying personality traits (as frugality and obstinacy) held to be psychological consequences of toilet training : ANAL 2b — **anal retentive** *n* — **anal retentiveness** *n*

anal sadism *n* : the personality traits (as aggressiveness, negativism, and destructiveness) typical of the anal stage of development — **anal–sa•dis•tic** \ˌān-ᵊl-sə-ˈdis-tik\ *adj*

anal sphincter *n* : either of two sphincters controlling the closing of the anus: **a** : an outer sphincter of striated muscle surrounding the anus immediately beneath the skin — called also *external anal sphincter, sphincter ani externus* **b** : an inner sphincter formed by thickening of the circular smooth muscle of the rectum — called also *internal anal sphincter, sphincter ani internus*

anal verge \-ˈvərj\ *n* : the lower edge of the anal canal that marks the junction of the anal canal and the external hair-bearing skin

anal•y•sand \ə-ˈna-lə-ˌsand\ *n* : one who is undergoing psychoanalysis

an•a•lyse *Brit var of* ANALYZE

anal•y•sis \ə-ˈna-lə-səs\ *n, pl* **-y•ses** \-ˌsēz\ **1** : separation of a whole into its component parts **2 a** : the identification or separation of ingredients of a substance **b** : a statement of the constituents of a mixture **3** : PSYCHOANALYSIS

an•a•lyst \ˈan-ᵊl-ist\ *n* : PSYCHOANALYST

an•a•lyt•ic \ˌan-ᵊl-ˈi-tik\ *or* **an•a•lyt•i•cal** \-ti-kəl\ *adj* **1** : of or relating to analysis; *esp* : separating something into component parts or constituent elements **2** : PSYCHOANALYTIC — **an•a•lyt•i•cal•ly** \-ti-k(ə-)lē\ *adv*

analytic psychology *n* : a modification of psychoanalysis due to C. G. Jung that adds to the concept of the personal unconscious a collective unconscious and advocates that psychotherapy be conducted in terms of the patient's present-day conflicts and maladjustments

an•a•lyze \ˈan-ᵊl-ˌīz\ *vb* **-lyzed; -lyz•ing** **1** : to study or determine the nature and relationship of the parts of by analysis; *esp* : to examine by chemical analysis **2** : PSYCHOANALYZE

an•am•ne•sis \ˌa-ˌnam-ˈnē-səs\ *n, pl* **-ne•ses** \-ˌsēz\ **1** : a recalling to mind **2** : a preliminary case history of a medical or psychiatric patient

an•am•nes•tic \-ˈnes-tik\ *adj* **1** : of or relating to anamnesis **2** : of or relating to a secondary response to an immunogenic substance after serum antibodies can no longer be detected in the blood

ana•phase \ˈa-nə-ˌfāz\ *n* : the stage of mitosis and meiosis in which the chromosomes move toward the poles of the spindle — **ana•pha•sic** \ˌa-nə-ˈfā-zik\ *adj*

an•aph•ro•dis•i•ac \-ˈdē-zē-ˌak, -ˈdi-\ *adj* : of, relating to, or causing absence or impairment of sexual desire — **anaphrodisiac** *n*

ana•phy•lac•tic \ˌa-nə-fə-ˈlak-tik\ *adj* : of, relating to, affected by, or causing anaphylaxis or anaphylactic shock — **ana•phy•lac•ti•cal•ly** \-ti-k(ə-)lē\ *adv*

anaphylactic shock *n* : an often severe and sometimes fatal systemic reaction in a susceptible individual upon a second exposure to a specific antigen (as wasp venom or penicillin) after previous sensitization that is characterized esp. by respiratory symptoms, fainting, itching, and hives

ana•phy•lac•toid \ˌa-nə-fə-ˈlak-ˌtȯid\ *adj* : resembling anaphylaxis or anaphylactic shock

ana•phy•lax•is \ˌa-nə-fə-ˈlak-səs\ *n, pl* **-lax•es** \-ˌsēz\ **1** : hypersensitivity (as to foreign proteins or drugs) resulting from sensitization following prior contact with the causative agent **2** : ANAPHYLACTIC SHOCK

an•a•pla•sia \ˌa-nə-ˈplā-zhē-ə, -zē-\ *n* : reversion of cells to a more primitive or undifferentiated form

an•a•plas•ma \ˌa-nə-ˈplaz-mə\ *n* **1** *cap* : a genus of parasitic gram-negative nonmotile bacteria (family Anaplasmataceae) that are transmitted chiefly by ticks and biting flies and infect the red blood cells of humans and animals — see ANAPLASMOSIS **2** *pl* **-mas** *or* **-ma•ta** \-mə-tə\ : any bacterium of the genus *Anaplasma*

an•a•plas•mo•sis \-ˌplaz-ˈmō-səs\ *n, pl* **-mo•ses** \-ˌsēz\ : infection with or a disease caused by tick-borne bacteria of the genus *Anaplasma*: as **a** : a disease of humans that is typically marked by fever, headache, chills, muscle aches, and fatigue and is caused by a bacterium (*A. phagocytophilum* syn. *Ehrlichia phagocytophila*) infecting granulocytes — called also *ehrlichiosis, human granulocytic anaplasmosis, human granulocytic ehrlichiosis* **b** : an often fatal disease of cattle caused by a bacterium (*A. marginale*) which infects and destroys red blood cells — called also *gall sickness*

an•a•plas•tic \ˌa-nə-ˈplas-tik\ *adj* : characterized by, composed of, or being cells which have reverted to a relatively undifferentiated state

an•a•plas•tol•o•gy \-ˌplas-ˈtä-lə-jē\ *n, pl* **-gies** : a branch of medical technology concerned with the design, preparation, and fitting of usu. non-weight-bearing highly realistic prosthetic devices (as an artificial eye or finger) to individual specifications and with the study of the materials from which they are fabricated — **an•a•plas•tol•o•gist** \-jist\ *n*

an•ar•thria \a-ˈnär-thrē-ə\ *n* : inability to articulate remembered words as a result of a brain lesion — compare APHASIA

an•a•sar•ca \ˌa-nə-ˈsär-kə\ *n* : generalized edema with accumulation of serum in the connective tissue

anas•to•mose \ə-ˈnas-tə-ˌmōz, -ˌmōs\ *vb* **-mosed; -mos•ing** : to connect, join, or communicate by anastomosis

anas•to•mo•sis \ə-ˌnas-tə-ˈmō-səs, ˌa-nəs-\ *n, pl* **-mo•ses** \-ˌsēz\ **1 a** : a communication between or coalescence of blood vessels **b** : the surgical union of parts and esp. hollow tubular parts **2** : a product of anastomosis; *esp* : a network (as of channels or branches) produced by anastomosis — **anas•to•mot•ic** \-ˈmä-tik\ *adj*

anas•tro•zole \ə-ˈnas-trə-ˌzōl\ *n* : a nonsteroidal aromatase inhibitor $C_{17}H_{19}N_5$ that is administered orally to treat breast cancer in postmenopausal women — see ARIMIDEX

anat *abbr* anatomic; anatomical; anatomy

an•a•tom•ic \ˌa-nə-ˈtä-mik\ *or* **an•a•tom•i•cal** \-mi-kəl\ *adj* **1** : of or relating to anatomy **2** : STRUCTURAL 1 ⟨an ~ obstruction⟩ — **an•a•tom•i•cal•ly** \-mi-k(ə-)lē\ *adv*

Anatomica — see BASLE NOMINA ANATOMICA, NOMINA ANATOMICA

anatomical dead space *n* : the dead space in that portion of the respiratory system which is external to the alveoli and includes the air-conveying ducts from the nostrils to the terminal bronchioles — compare PHYSIOLOGICAL DEAD SPACE

anatomical position *n* : the normal position of the human body when active

anat•o•mist \ə-ˈna-tə-mist\ *n* : a specialist in anatomy

anat•o•my \ə-ˈna-tə-mē\ *n, pl* **-mies 1** : a branch of morphology that deals with the structure of organisms — compare PHYSIOLOGY 1 **2** : a treatise on anatomic science or art **3** : the art of separating the parts of an organism in order to ascertain their position, relations, structure, and function : DISSECTION **4** : structural makeup esp. of an organism or any of its parts

ana•tox•in \ˌa-nə-ˈtäk-sən\ *n* : TOXOID

ANC *abbr* absolute neutrophil count

ANCA *abbr* antineutrophil cytoplasmic antibody; antineutrophilic cytoplasmic antibody

anchyl- *or* **anchylo-** — see ANKYL-

anchylose, anchylosis *var of* ANKYLOSE, ANKYLOSIS

an•cil•lary \ˈan-sə-ˌler-ē\ *adj* : being auxiliary or supplementary

an•co•ne•us \aŋ-ˈkō-nē-əs\ *n, pl* **-nei** \-nē-ˌī\ : a small triangular extensor muscle that is superficially situated behind and below the elbow joint and that extends the forearm — called also *anconeus muscle*

An•cy•los•to•ma \ˌaŋ-ki-ˈläs-tə-mə, ˌan-sə-\ *n* : a genus of hookworms (family Ancylostomatidae) that are intestinal parasites of mammals

an•cyl•o•stome \aŋ-ˈki-lə-ˌstōm, -ˈsi-\ *or* **an•kyl•o•stome** \-ˈki-\ *n* : any of the genus *Ancylostoma* of hookworms

an•cy•lo•sto•mi•a•sis \ˌaŋ-ki-lō-stə-ˈmī-ə-səs, ˌan-sə-\ *or* **an•ky•lo•sto•mi•as•is** \-ki-lō-\ *n, pl* **-a•ses** \-ˌsēz\ : infestation with or disease caused by hookworms; *esp* : an anemic state due to blood loss from the feeding of hookworms in the small intestine — called also *hookworm disease*

andr- *or* **andro-** *comb form* **1** : male ⟨*andro*gen⟩ **2** : male and ⟨*andro*gynous⟩

an•dro \an-drō\ *n* : ANDROSTENEDIONE

An•dro•derm \ˈan-drō-ˌdərm\ *trademark* — used for a preparation of testosterone administered as a skin patch

An•dro•gel \ˈan-drō-ˌjel\ *trademark* — used for a topical preparation of testosterone

an•dro•gen \ˈan-drə-jən\ *n* : a male sex hormone (as testosterone) — **an•dro•gen•ic** \ˌan-drə-ˈje-nik\ *adj*

androgen deprivation therapy *n* : therapy for prostate cancer that severely reduces the body's production of androgens and esp. testosterone through the administration of drugs (as flutamide and leuprolide) or through surgical removal of the testicles

androgenetic alopecia \ˌan-drə-jə-ˈnet-ik-\ *n* : hereditary androgen-dependent hair loss typically marked by moderate to severe hair loss on the temples and crown in men and diffuse thinning on the crown in women — see MALE-PATTERN BALDNESS

androgen insensitivity syndrome *n* : a genetic disorder inherited as an X-linked recessive trait that causes complete or partial insensitivity to androgens in the body and results in a female physical appearance, the X and Y chromosomes of a male, external genitalia that are female or ambiguous, no uterus, and usu. normal but undescended testes — called also *testicular feminization, testicular feminization syndrome*

an•drog•e•nize \an-ˈdrä-jə-ˌnīz\ *vb* **-nized; -niz•ing** : to treat or influence with male sex hormone esp. in excessive amounts — **an•drog•e•ni•za•tion** \an-ˌdräj-ə-nə-ˈzā-shən\ *n*

an•drog•y•nous \an-ˈdrä-jə-nəs\ *adj* : having the characteristics or nature of both male and female — **an•drog•y•ny** \-nē\ *n*

an•droid \ˈan-ˌdrȯid\ *adj* **1** *of the pelvis* : having the angular form and narrow outlet typical of the human male —

compare ANTHROPOID, GYNECOID, PLATYPELLOID **2** : relating to or characterized by the distribution of body fat chiefly in the abdominal region ⟨~ obesity⟩ — compare GYNECOID

an•drol•o•gist \an-ˈdräl-ə-jəst\ *n* : a specialist in andrology

an•dro•lo•gy \an-ˈdrä-lə-jē\ *n, pl* **-gies** : a branch of medicine concerned with male diseases and esp. with those affecting the reproductive system

an•drom•e•do•tox•in \an-ˌdrä-mə-dō-ˈtäk-sən\ *n* : a toxic compound $C_{31}H_{50}O_{10}$ found in various plants of the heath family (Ericaceae)

an•dro•pause \ˈan-drə-ˌpȯz\ *n* : a gradual and highly variable decline in the production of androgenic hormones and esp. testosterone in the human male together with its associated effects that is held to occur during and after middle age but is often difficult to discriminate from the effects of confounding factors (as chronic illness or stress) that can depress testosterone levels — called also *male climacteric, male menopause, viropause*

an•dro•stene•diol \ˌan-drə-ˌstēn-ˈdī-ˌȯl, -ˈstēn-dē-ˌȯl\ *n* : any of several isomers of androstenedione that are synthesized from dehydroepiandrosterone and are precursors of testosterone

an•dro•stene•di•one \ˌan-drə-ˌstēn-ˈdī-ˌōn, -ˈstēn-dē-ˌōn\ *n* : a steroid sex hormone $C_{19}H_{26}O_2$ that is secreted by the testis, ovary, and adrenal cortex and is a precursor of testosterone and estrogen

an•dros•ter•one \an-ˈdräs-tə-ˌrōn\ *n* : an androgenic hormone that is a hydroxy ketone $C_{19}H_{30}O_2$ found in human urine

Anec•tine \ə-ˈnek-tən\ *trademark* — used for a preparation of succinylcholine

ane•mia \ə-ˈnē-mē-ə\ *n* **1** : a condition in which the blood is deficient in red blood cells, in hemoglobin, or in total volume — see APLASTIC ANEMIA, HYPERCHROMIC ANEMIA, HYPOCHROMIC ANEMIA, MEGALOBLASTIC ANEMIA, MICROCYTIC ANEMIA, PERNICIOUS ANEMIA, SICKLE CELL ANEMIA **2** : ISCHEMIA — **ane•mic** \ə-ˈnē-mik\ *adj* — **ane•mi•cal•ly** \-mi-k(ə-)lē\ *adv*

an•en•ceph•a•lus \ˌan-(ˌ)en-ˈse-fə-ləs\ *n, pl* **-li** \-ˌlī\ : ANENCEPHALY

an•en•ceph•a•ly \ˌan-(ˌ)en-ˈse-fə-lē\ *n, pl* **-lies** : congenital absence of all or a major part of the brain — **an•en•ce•phal•ic** \-ˌen-sə-ˈfa-lik\ *adj or n*

aneph•ric \(ˌ)a-ˈne-frik, (ˌ)ā-\ *adj* : lacking kidneys : without functioning kidneys

aner•gia \(ˈ)a-ˈnər-j(ē-)ə\ *n* : lack of energy

an•er•gy \ˈa-(ˌ)nər-jē\ *n, pl* **-gies** : a condition in which the body's immune system fails to react to an antigen : immunologic hyporesponsiveness — **an•er•gic** \-jik\ *adj*

an•es•the•sia \ˌa-nəs-ˈthē-zhə\ *n* **1** : loss of sensation esp. to touch usu. resulting from a lesion in the nervous system or from some other abnormality **2** : loss of sensation and usu. of consciousness without loss of vital functions artificially produced by the administration of one or more agents that block the passage of pain impulses along nerve pathways to the brain

an•es•the•si•ol•o•gist \ˌa-nəs-ˌthē-zē-ˈä-lə-jist\ *n* : ANESTHETIST; *specif* : a physician specializing in anesthesiology

an•es•the•si•ol•o•gy \-jē\ *n, pl* **-gies** : a branch of medical science dealing with anesthesia and anesthetics

[1]**an•es•thet•ic** \ˌa-nəs-ˈthe-tik\ *adj* **1** : capable of producing anesthesia ⟨~ agents⟩ **2** : of, relating to, or caused by anesthesia ⟨an ~ effect⟩ — **an•es•thet•i•cal•ly** \-ti-k(ə-)lē\ *adv*

[2]**anesthetic** *n* : a substance that produces anesthesia

anes•the•tist \ə-ˈnes-thə-tist\ *n* : one who administers anesthetics — compare ANESTHESIOLOGIST

anes•the•tize \-ˌtīz\ *vb* **-tized; -tiz•ing** : to subject to anesthesia — **anes•the•ti•za•tion** \ə-ˌnes-thə-tə-ˈzā-shən\ *n*

an•es•trous \(ˌ)a-ˈnes-trəs\ *adj* **1** : not exhibiting estrus **2** : of or relating to anestrus

an•es•trus \-trəs\ *n* : the period of sexual quiescence between two periods of sexual activity in cyclically breeding mammals — compare ESTRUS

an•eu•ploid \ˈan-yu̇-ˌploid\ *adj* : having or being a chromosome number that is not an exact multiple of the usu. haploid number — **aneuploid** *n* — **an•eu•ploi•dy** \-ˌplȯi-dē\ *n*

an•eu•rine \ˈan-yə-ˌrēn, (ˌ)ā-ˈnyu̇r-ˌēn\ *n* : THIAMINE

an•eu•rysm *also* **an•eu•rism** \ˈan-yə-ˌri-zəm\ *n* : an abnormal blood-filled dilatation of a blood vessel and esp. an artery resulting from disease of the vessel wall — **an•eu•rys•mal** *also* **an•eu•ris•mal** \ˌan-yə-ˈriz-məl\ *adj* — **an•eu•rys•mal•ly** *adv*

ANF *abbr* atrial naturetic factor

angel dust *n* : PHENCYCLIDINE

An•gel•man syndrome \ˈaŋ-jəl-mən-\ *also* **An•gel•man's syndrome** \-mənz-\ *n* : a genetic disorder characterized by severe intellectual disability, seizures, ataxic gait, jerky movements, lack of speech, microcephaly, and frequent smiling and laughter

Angelman, Harry (1915–1996), British pediatrician.

angi- *or* **angio-** *comb form* **1** : blood or lymph vessel ⟨*angio*ma⟩ ⟨*angio*genesis⟩ **2** : blood vessels and ⟨*angio*cardiography⟩

-angia *pl of* -ANGIUM

an·gi·i·tis \ˌan-jē-ˈī-təs\ *n, pl* **-it·i·des** \-ˈi-tə-ˌdēz\ : VASCULITIS

an·gi·na \an-ˈjī-nə, ˈan-jə-\ *n* : a disease marked by spasmodic attacks of intense suffocative pain: as **a** : a severe inflammatory or ulcerated condition of the mouth or throat ⟨diphtheritic ~⟩ — see LUDWIG'S ANGINA, VINCENT'S ANGINA **b** : ANGINA PECTORIS — **an·gi·nal** \an-ˈjīn-ᵊl, ˈan-jən-\ *adj*

angina pec·to·ris \-ˈpek-tə-rəs\ *n* : a disease that is marked esp. by brief sudden attacks of chest pain or discomfort caused by deficient oxygenation of the heart muscles usu. due to impaired blood flow to the heart and that typically occurs at the same time with coronary heart disease and is often precipitated by physical exertion or emotional stress — see UNSTABLE ANGINA; compare CORONARY INSUFFICIENCY, HEART ATTACK, HEART FAILURE 1

an·gi·nose \ˈan-jə-ˌnōs, an-ˈjī-\ *or* **an·gi·nous** \(ˌ)an-ˈjī-nəs, ˈan-jə-\ *adj* : relating to angina or angina pectoris

an·gio·car·dio·gram \ˌan-jē-ō-ˈkär-dē-ə-ˌgram\ *n* : a radiograph of the heart and its blood vessels prepared by angiocardiography

an·gio·car·di·og·ra·phy \-ˌkär-dē-ˈä-grə-fē\ *n, pl* **-phies** : the radiographic visualization of the heart and its blood vessels after injection of a radiopaque substance — **an·gio·car·dio·graph·ic** \-dē-ə-ˈgra-fik\ *adj*

an·gio·dys·pla·sia \ˌan-jē-ō-dis-ˈplā-zh(ē-)ə\ *n* : an abnormal condition of blood vessels of the gastrointestinal tract and esp. the intestine in which vessels are thin, fragile, and enlarged

an·gio·ede·ma \ˌan-jē-ō-i-ˈdē-mə\ *n, pl* **-mas** *also* **-ma·ta** \-mə-tə\ : an often painful acute or chronic disorder that affects the mucous membranes and deepest layers of the skin along with underlying tissue esp. of the lips, mouth, throat, eyes, hands, and feet, is marked chiefly by rapid swelling from fluid leaking out of blood vessels, and may be caused by an allergic reaction (as to food or drugs), sometimes occurs as a hereditary condition, and is often of unknown cause — called also *angioneurotic edema, giant urticaria, Quincke's disease, Quincke's edema*

an·gio·fi·bro·ma \ˌan-jē-ō-fī-ˈbrō-mə\ *n, pl* **-mas** *also* **-ma·ta** \-mə-tə\ : a noncancerous tumor that is composed of fibrous tissue and blood vessels and occurs chiefly in the nasal cavities and upper pharynx

an·gio·fol·lic·u·lar lymph node hyperplasia \ˌan-jē-ō-fə-ˈlik-yə-lər-, -fä-\ *n* : CASTLEMAN'S DISEASE — called also *angiofollicular hyperplasia*

an·gio·gen·e·sis \-ˈje-nə-səs\ *n, pl* **-e·ses** \-ˌsēz\ : the formation and differentiation of blood vessels

an·gio·gram \ˈan-jē-ə-ˌgram\ *n* **1** : a radiograph made by angiography **2** : ANGIOGRAPHY

an·gi·og·ra·phy \ˌan-jē-ˈä-grə-fē\ *n, pl* **-phies** : the radiographic visualization of the blood vessels after injection of a radiopaque substance — **an·gi·og·ra·pher** \-fər\ *n* — **an·gio·graph·ic** \ˌan-jē-ə-ˈgra-fik\ *adj* — **an·gio·graph·i·cal·ly** \-fi-k(ə-)lē\ *adv*

an·gio·im·mu·no·blas·tic T–cell lymphoma \ˌan-jē-ō-ˌim-yə-nō-ˈblas-tik-, -im-ˌyü-nō-\ *n* : an uncommon and often fatal non-Hodgkin lymphoma that arises from T cells and is characterized esp. by fever, weight loss, enlarged lymph nodes, night sweats, skin rash, and the proliferation of small abnormal blood vessels — called also *angioimmunoblastic lymphadenopathy, angioimmunoblastic lymphadenopathy with dysproteinemia, immunoblastic lymphadenopathy*

an·gio·in·va·sive \ˌan-jē-ō-in-ˈvā-siv, -ziv\ *adj* : marked by or causing infiltration of blood vessels ⟨~ pulmonary aspergillosis⟩

an·gio·ker·a·to·ma \ˌan-jē-ō-ˌker-ə-ˈtō-mə\ *n, pl* **-mas** *also* **-ma·ta** \-mə-tə\ : a small dark red or bluish benign skin lesion that is composed of dilated capillaries in the upper dermis with accompanying overgrowth of the epidermis and that typically appears singly or in clusters as a raised spot with a scaly or wart-like surface; *also* : a condition marked by the presence of angiokeratomas

an·gi·ol·o·gy \ˌan-jē-ˈä-lə-jē\ *n, pl* **-gies** : the study of blood vessels and lymphatics

an·gi·o·ma \ˌan-jē-ˈō-mə\ *n, pl* **-mas** *also* **-ma·ta** \-mə-tə\ : a tumor (as a hemangioma) composed chiefly of blood vessels or lymphatic vessels — **an·gi·o·ma·tous** \-mə-təs\ *adj*

an·gi·o·ma·to·sis \ˌan-jē-(ˌ)ō-mə-ˈtō-səs\ *n, pl* **-to·ses** \-ˌsēz\ : a condition characterized by the formation of multiple angiomas

an·gio·myo·li·po·ma \ˌan-jē-ō-ˌmī-ə-lī-ˈpō-mə, -li-\ *n, pl* **-mas** *also* **-ma·ta** \-mə-tə\ : a benign tumor composed of blood vessels, smooth muscle, and fat that occurs esp. in the kidney and is often asymptomatic but may cause pain or blood in the urine

an·gio·neu·rot·ic edema \-nu̇-ˌrä-tik, -nyu̇-\ *n* : ANGIOEDEMA

an·gi·op·a·thy \ˌan-jē-ˈä-pə-thē\ *n, pl* **-thies** : a disease of the blood or lymph vessels

an·gio·plas·ty \ˈan-jē-ə-ˌplas-tē\ *n, pl* **-ties** : surgical repair or recanalization of a blood vessel; *esp* : BALLOON ANGIOPLASTY

an·gio·poi·e·tin \ˌan-jē-ə-ˈpȯi-ə-tən\ *n* : a protein that binds chiefly to a receptor on endothelial cells and promotes the maturation and stability of blood vessels

an·gio·sar·co·ma \ˌan-jē-ō-sär-ˈkō-mə\ *n, pl* **-mas** *also* **-ma·ta** \-mə-tə\ : a rare malignant vascular tumor (as of the liver or breast)
an·gio·scope \ˈan-jē-ə-ˌskōp\ *n* : a flexible endoscope that is used to visually examine the interior of a blood vessel — **an·gi·os·co·py** \ˌan-jē-ˈä-skə-pē\ *n*
an·gio·spasm \ˈan-jē-ō-ˌspa-zəm\ *n* : spasmodic contraction of the blood vessels with increase in blood pressure — **an·gio·spas·tic** \ˌan-jē-ō-ˈspas-tik\ *adj*
an·gio·ten·sin \ˌan-jē-ō-ˈten-sən\ *n* **1** : either of two forms of a kinin of which one has marked physiological activity and the other is its physiologically inactive precursor; *esp* : ANGIOTENSIN II **2** : a synthetic amide derivative of angiotensin II used to treat some forms of hypotension
an·gio·ten·sin·ase \ˌan-jē-ō-ˈten-sə-ˌnās, -ˌnāz\ *n* : any of several enzymes in the blood that hydrolyze angiotensin — called also *hypertensinase*
angiotensin converting enzyme *n* : a proteolytic enzyme that converts angiotensin I to angiotensin II — see ACE INHIBITOR
angiotensin converting enzyme inhibitor *n* : ACE INHIBITOR
an·gio·ten·sin·o·gen \-ten-ˈsi-nə-jən\ *n* : a glycoprotein formed chiefly in the liver that is cleaved by renin to produce angiotensin I — called also *hypertensinogen*
angiotensin I \-ˈwən\ *n* : the physiologically inactive form of angiotensin that is composed of 10 amino-acid residues, is derived from angiotensinogen, and is converted by angiotensin converting enzyme to angiotensin II
angiotensin–receptor blocker *n* : any of a class of drugs (as losartan and valsartan) that block the effects of angiotensin II and are used esp. to treat hypertension — abbr. *ARB*
angiotensin II \-ˈtü\ *n* : a protein with vasoconstrictive activity that increases blood pressure, stimulates the release of aldosterone, is composed of a chain of eight amino-acid residues, and is the physiologically active form of angiotensin
an·gio·to·nin \-ˈtō-nən\ *n* : ANGIOTENSIN
-angium *n comb form, pl* **-angia** : vessel : receptacle ⟨mes*angium*⟩
an·gle \ˈaŋ-gəl\ *n* **1** : a corner whether constituting a projecting part or a partially enclosed space **2** : the figure formed by two lines extending from the same point
an·gle·ber·ry \ˈaŋ-gəl-ˌber-ē\ *n, pl* **-ries** : a papilloma or warty growth of the skin or mucous membranes of cattle and sometimes horses often occurring in great numbers
angle–closure glaucoma *n* : glaucoma in which the drainage channel for the aqueous humor is blocked by the iris — called also *closed-angle glaucoma, narrow-angle glaucoma;* compare OPEN-ANGLE GLAUCOMA
angle of the jaw *n* : GONIAL ANGLE
angle of the mandible *n* : GONIAL ANGLE
ang·strom \ˈaŋ-strəm\ *n* : a unit of length equal to one ten-billionth of a meter
Ångström, Anders Jonas (1814–1874), Swedish astronomer and physicist.
angstrom unit *n* : ANGSTROM
an·gu·lar \ˈaŋ-gyə-lər\ *adj* **1 a** : having an angle or angles **b** : forming an angle or corner : sharp-cornered **2** : relating to or situated near an anatomical angle; *specif* : relating to or situated near the inner angle of the eye — **an·gu·lar·i·ty** \ˌaŋ-gyü-ˈlar-ə-tē\ *n* — **an·gu·lar·ly** *adv*
angular artery *n* : the terminal part of the facial artery that passes up alongside the nose to the inner angle of the orbit
angular gyrus *n* : the cerebral gyrus of the posterior part of the external surface of the parietal lobe that arches over the posterior end of the sulcus between the superior and middle gyri of the temporal lobe — called also *angular convolution*
angularis — see INCISURA ANGULARIS
angular vein *n* : a vein that comprises the first part of the facial vein and runs obliquely down at the side of the upper part of the nose
an·gu·la·tion \ˌaŋ-gyə-ˈlā-shən\ *n* : an angular position, formation or shape; *esp* : an abnormal bend or curve in an organ — **an·gu·late** \ˈaŋ-gyə-ˌlāt\ *vb*
anguli — see LEVATOR ANGULI ORIS
an·gu·lus \ˈaŋ-gyə-ləs\ *n, pl* **an·gu·li** \-ˌlī, -ˌlē\ : an anatomical angle; *also* : an angular part or relationship
an·he·do·nia \ˌan-hē-ˈdō-nē-ə\ *n* : a psychological condition characterized by inability to experience pleasure in acts which normally produce it — compare ANALGESIA — **an·he·don·ic** \-ˈdä-nik\ *adj*
an·hi·dro·sis *also* **an·hy·dro·sis** \ˌan-hi-ˈdrō-səs, -hī-\ *n, pl* **-dro·ses** \-ˌsēz\ : abnormal deficiency or absence of sweating
[1]**an·hi·drot·ic** *also* **an·hy·drot·ic** \-ˈdrä-tik\ *adj* **1** : tending to check sweating **2** : marked by anhidrosis
[2]**anhidrotic** *also* **anhydrotic** *n* : an anhidrotic agent
anhydr- *or* **anhydro-** *comb form* : lacking water ⟨*anhydr*emia⟩
an·hy·dre·mia \ˌan-(ˌ)hī-ˈdrē-mē-ə\ *n* : an abnormal reduction of water in the blood
an·hy·dro·hy·droxy·pro·ges·ter·one \an-ˌhī-drō-ˌhī-ˌdräk-sē-prō-ˈjes-tə-ˌrōn\ *n* : ETHISTERONE
an·hy·drous \(ˌ)an-ˈhī-drəs\ *adj* : free from water and esp. water that is

chemically combined in a crystalline substance ⟨~ ammonia⟩

ani *pl of* ANUS

ani — see LEVATOR ANI, PRURITUS ANI

an·ic·ter·ic \ˌa-(ˌ)nik-ˈter-ik\ *adj* : not accompanied or characterized by jaundice ⟨~ hepatitis⟩

anid·u·la·fun·gin \ə-ˌnid-yə-lə-ˈfən-jən, -ˌni-jə-\ *n* : a semisynthetic antifungal agent $C_{58}H_{73}N_7O_{17}$ administered intravenously to treat candida infections — see ERAXIS

an·i·line \ˈan-ᵊl-ən\ *n* : an oily liquid poisonous amine $C_6H_5NH_2$ used chiefly in organic synthesis (as of dyes and pharmaceuticals) — **aniline** *adj*

ani·lin·gus \ˌā-ni-ˈliŋ-gəs\ *or* **ani·linc·tus** \-ˈliŋk-təs\ *n* : erotic stimulation achieved by contact between mouth and anus

an·i·ma \ˈa-nə-mə\ *n* : an individual's true inner self that in the analytic psychology of C. G. Jung reflects archetypal ideals of conduct; *also* : an inner feminine part of the male personality — compare ANIMUS, PERSONA

animal heat *n* : BODY HEAT

animal model *n* : an animal similar to humans (as in its physiology) that is used in medical research to obtain results that can be extrapolated to human medicine; *also* : a pathological or physiological condition that occurs in such an animal and is similar to one occurring in humans

animal starch *n* : GLYCOGEN

an·i·mate \ˈa-nə-mət\ *adj* **1** : possessing or characterized by life **2** : of or relating to animal life as opposed to plant life

an·i·mus \ˈa-nə-məs\ *n* : an inner masculine part of the female personality in the analytic psychology of C. G. Jung — compare ANIMA

an·ion \ˈa-ˌnī-ən\ *n* : the ion in an electrolyzed solution that migrates to the anode; *broadly* : a negatively charged ion — **an·ion·ic** \ˌa-(ˌ)nī-ˈä-nik\ *adj* — **an·ion·i·cal·ly** \-ni-k(ə-)lē\ *adv*

an·irid·ia \ˌa-ˌnī-ˈri-dē-ə\ *n* : congenital or traumatically induced absence or defect of the iris

anis- *or* **aniso-** *comb form* : unequal ⟨*anis*eikonia⟩ ⟨*aniso*cytosis⟩

an·i·sa·ki·a·sis \ˌa-nə-sə-ˈkī-ə-sis\ *n* : intestinal infection that is caused by the larvae of a nematode (esp. *Anisakis simplex* and *Pseudoterranova decipiens*), is marked by severe abdominal pain, nausea, and vomiting, and is usu. contracted by eating raw or undercooked fish

an·is·ei·ko·nia \ˌa-ˌnī-ˌsī-ˈkō-nē-ə\ *n* : a defect of binocular vision in which the two retinal images of an object differ in size — **an·is·ei·kon·ic** \-ˈkä-nik\ *adj*

an·iso·co·ria \ˌa-ˌnī-sō-ˈkōr-ē-ə\ *n* : inequality in the size of the pupils of the eyes

an·iso·cy·to·sis \-ˌsī-ˈtō-səs\ *n, pl* **-to·ses** \-ˌsēz\ : variation in size of cells and esp. of the red blood cells (as in pernicious anemia) — **an·iso·cy·tot·ic** \-ˈtä-tik\ *adj*

an·iso·me·tro·pia \ˌa-ˌnī-sə-mə-ˈtrō-pē-ə\ *n* : unequal refractive power in the two eyes — **an·iso·me·tro·pic** \-ˈträ-pik, -ˈtrō-\ *adj*

an·i·strep·lase \ˌa-ni-ˈstrep-lās\ *n* : a thrombolytic complex of plasminogen and streptokinase that has been used esp. to treat heart attack — called also *APSAC*

an·kle \ˈaŋ-kəl\ *n* **1** : the joint between the foot and the leg that constitutes in humans a ginglymus joint between the tibia and fibula above and the talus below — called also *ankle joint* **2** : the region of the ankle joint

an·kle·bone \-ˌbōn\ *n* : TALUS 1

ankle–brachial index *n* : a measure of the difference in the systolic blood pressure of the arm and ankle calculated by dividing the blood pressure of the ankle by that of the arm with a number below .9 indicating narrowing or blockage of leg arteries — abbr. *ABI*

ankle jerk *n* : a reflex downward movement of the foot produced by a spasmodic contraction of the muscles of the calf in response to sudden extension of the leg or the striking of the Achilles tendon above the heel — called also *Achilles reflex*

ankle joint *n* : ANKLE 1

ankyl- *or* **ankylo-** *also* **anchyl-** *or* **anchylo-** *comb form* : stiffness : immobility ⟨*ankyl*osis⟩

an·ky·lo·glos·sia \ˌaŋ-kə-(ˌ)lō-ˈglä-sē-ə, -ˈglo-\ *n* : limited normal movement of the tongue chiefly due to an abnormally shortened frenulum : TONGUE-TIE

an·ky·lose *also* **an·chy·lose** \ˈaŋ-ki-ˌlōs, -ˌlōz\ *vb* **-losed; -los·ing** **1** : to unite or stiffen by ankylosis **2** : to undergo ankylosis

ankylosing spondylitis *n* : a chronic inflammatory disease that affects the spine and sacroiliac joints and often other joints (as of the shoulder) and that is marked esp. by pain and stiffness — abbr. *AS;* called also *Marie-Strümpell disease, rheumatoid spondylitis*

an·ky·lo·sis *also* **an·chy·lo·sis** \ˌaŋ-ki-ˈlō-səs\ *n, pl* **-lo·ses** \-ˌsēz\ : stiffness or fixation of a joint by disease or surgery — **an·ky·lot·ic** *also* **an·chy·lot·ic** \-ˈlä-tik\ *adj*

ankylostome, ankylostomiasis *var of* ANCYLOSTOME, ANCYLOSTOMIASIS

an·la·ge \ˈän-ˌlä-gə\ *n, pl* **-gen** \-gən\ *also* **-ges** \-əz\ : the foundation of a subsequent development; *esp* : PRIMORDIUM

an·neal \ə-ˈnēl\ *vb* **1** : to heat and then cool (double-stranded nucleic acid) in order to separate strands and induce combination at lower temperatures esp. with complementary strands **2** : to be capable of combining with complementary nucleic acid by a process of heating and cooling

an·ne·lid \ˈan-ᵊl-əd\ *n* : any of a phylum (Annelida) of usu. elongated segmented invertebrates (as earthworms and leeches) — **annelid** *adj*

an·nu·lar \ˈan-yə-lər\ *adj* : of, relating to, or forming a ring

annulare — see GRANULOMA ANNULARE

annular ligament *n* : a ringlike ligament or band of fibrous tissue encircling a part: as **a** : a strong band of fibers surrounding the head of the radius and retaining it in the radial notch of the ulna **b** : a ring attaching the base of the stapes to the oval window

an·nu·lo·plas·ty \ˈan-yə-(ˌ)lō-ˌpla-stē\ *n, pl* **-ties** : surgical treatment of a ringlike anatomical part; *specif* : surgical repair of a heart valve that typically involves reducing the diameter of the valve's fibrous ring

an·nu·lus *also* **an·u·lus** \ˈan-yə-ləs\ *n, pl* **-li** \-ˌlī\ *also* **-lus·es** : a ringlike part, structure, or marking; *esp* : any of various ringlike anatomical parts

annulus fi·bro·sus \-fī-ˈbrō-səs, -fi-\ *n* : a ring of fibrous tissue (as that surrounding a heart valve); *esp* : the outer portion of an intervertebral disk that surrounds the nucleus pulposus and is composed chiefly of layers of collagen fibers

[1]**ano-** *prefix* : upward ⟨*ano*opsia⟩

[2]**ano-** *comb form* **1** : anus ⟨*ano*scope⟩ **2** : anus and ⟨*ano*rectal⟩

ano·ci·as·so·ci·a·tion \ə-ˌnō-sē-ə-ˌsō-sē-ˈā-shən, a-, -ˌsō-shē-\ *n* : a method of preventing shock incident to surgery by preventing communication between the area of operation and the nervous system (as by means of a local anesthetic)

ano·derm \ˈā-nō-ˌdərm\ *n* : the epithelium lining the anal canal

an·odon·tia \ˌa-nō-ˈdän-chə, -chē-ə\ *n* : an esp. congenital absence of teeth

[1]**an·o·dyne** \ˈa-nə-ˌdīn\ *adj* : serving to ease pain

[2]**anodyne** *n* : a drug that allays pain

ano·gen·i·tal \ˌā-nō-ˈje-nə-tᵊl\ *adj* : of, relating to, or involving the genital organs and the anus ⟨an ~ infection⟩

anom·a·lo·scope \ə-ˈnä-mə-lə-ˌskōp\ *n* : an optical device designed to test color vision

anom·a·lous \ə-ˈnä-mə-ləs\ *adj* : deviating from normal; *specif* : having abnormal vision with respect to a particular color but not color-blind

anom·a·ly \ə-ˈnä-mə-lē\ *n, pl* **-lies** : a deviation from normal esp. of a bodily part

ano·mia \ə-ˈnä-mē-ə, -ˈnō-\ *n* : ANOMIC APHASIA

ano·mic \ə-ˈnä-mik, ā-, -ˈnō-\ *adj* : relating to or characterized by anomie

anomic aphasia *n* : an impairment of language that is marked by difficulty or inability in finding the proper word and esp. the name of objects and typically results from an injury to the brain (as from a stroke) — called also *nominal aphasia*

an·o·mie *also* **an·o·my** \ˈa-nə-mē\ *n* : personal unrest, alienation, and anxiety that comes from a lack of purpose or ideals

an·onych·ia \ˌa-nə-ˈni-kē-ə\ *n* : congenital absence of the nails

ano·op·sia \ˌa-nō-ˈäp-sē-ə\ *or* **an·op·sia** \ə-ˈnäp-\ *n* : upward strabismus

anoph·e·les \ə-ˈnä-fə-ˌlēz\ *n* **1** *cap* : a genus of mosquitoes that includes all mosquitoes that transmit malaria to humans **2** : any mosquito of the genus *Anopheles* — **anopheles** *adj* — **an·oph·e·line** \-ˌlīn\ *adj or n*

an·oph·thal·mia \ˌa-näf-ˈthal-mē-ə, -äp-\ *n* : congenital absence of the eyes — **an·oph·thal·mic** \-ˈthal-mik\ *adj*

an·oph·thal·mos \-ˈthal-məs\ *n* **1** : ANOPHTHALMIA **2** : an individual born without eyes

an·opia \ə-ˈnō-pē-ə, a-\ *n* : a defect of vision; *esp* : HEMIANOPIA

ano·plas·ty \ˈā-nə-ˌplas-tē, ˈa-\ *n, pl* **-ties** : a plastic surgery on the anus (as for stricture)

An·op·lo·ceph·a·la \ˌa-nə-(ˌ)plō-ˈse-fə-lə\ *n* : a genus of taenioid tapeworms including some parasites of horses

anopsia *var of* ANOOPSIA

an·or·chid·ism \ə-ˈnȯr-ki-ˌdi-zəm, a-\ *n* : congenital absence of one or both testes

ano·rec·tal \ˌā-nō-ˈrekt-ᵊl, ˌa-nə-\ *adj* : of, relating to, or involving both the anus and rectum ⟨~ surgery⟩

[1]**an·o·rec·tic** \ˌa-nə-ˈrek-tik\ *also* **an·o·ret·ic** \-ˈre-tik\ *adj* **1 a** : lacking appetite **b** : ANOREXIC 2 **2** : causing loss of appetite ⟨~ drugs⟩

[2]**anorectic** *also* **anoretic** *n* **1** : an anorectic agent **2** : ANOREXIC

an·orex·ia \ˌa-nə-ˈrek-sē-ə, -ˈrek-shə\ *n* **1** : loss of appetite esp. when prolonged **2** : ANOREXIA NERVOSA

anorexia ner·vo·sa \-(ˌ)nər-ˈvō-sə, -zə\ *n* : a serious eating disorder primarily of young women in their teens and early twenties that is characterized esp. by a pathological fear of weight gain leading to faulty eating patterns, malnutrition, and usu. excessive weight loss

[1]**ano·rex·i·ant** \ˌa-nə-ˈrek-sē-ənt, -ˈrek-shənt\ *n* : a drug that suppresses appetite

[2]**anorexiant** *adj* : ANORECTIC 2

[1]**ano·rex·ic** \-ˈrek-sik\ *adj* **1** : ANORECTIC 1a, 2 **2** : relating to, characteristic of, or affected with anorexia nervosa

[2]**anorexic** *n* : a person affected with anorexia nervosa

an·orex·i·gen \ˌa-nə-ˈrek-sə-jən, -nō-\ *n* : a drug that suppresses the appetite : ANORECTIC

ano·rex·i·gen·ic \-ˌrek-sə-ˈje-nik\ *adj* : ANORECTIC 2

an·or·gas·mia \ˌa-nȯr-ˈgaz-mē-ə\ *n* : sexual dysfunction characterized by failure to achieve orgasm — **an·or·gas·mic** \-mik\ *adj*

ano·scope \ˈā-nə-ˌskōp\ *n* : an instrument for facilitating visual examination of the anal canal

ano·sco·py \ā-ˈnäs-kə-pē, ə-\ *n, pl* **-pies** : visual examination of the anal canal with an anoscope — **ano·scop·ic** \ˌā-nə-ˈskä-pik\ *adj*

an·os·mia \a-ˈnäz-mē-ə\ *n* : loss or impairment of the sense of smell — **an·os·mic** \-mik\ *adj*

ano·sog·no·sia \ˌa-nō-ˌsäg-ˈnō-zh(ē-)ə\ *n* : an inability or refusal to recognize a defect or disorder that is clinically evident — see ANTON'S SYNDROME

ano·vag·i·nal \ˌā-nō-ˈva-jən-ᵊl\ *adj* : connecting the anal canal and the vagina ⟨a congenital ~ fistula⟩

an·ovu·la·tion \ˌa-ˌnä-vyə-ˈlā-shən, -ˌnō-\ *n* : failure or absence of ovulation

an·ovu·la·to·ry \(ˌ)a-ˈnä-vyə-lə-ˌtōr-ē, -ˈnō-\ *adj* **1** : not involving or associated with ovulation ⟨~ bleeding⟩ **2** : suppressing ovulation ⟨~ drugs⟩

an·ox·emia \ˌa-ˌnäk-ˈsē-mē-ə\ *n* : a condition of subnormal oxygenation of the arterial blood — **an·ox·emic** \-mik\ *adj*

an·ox·ia \ə-ˈnäk-sē-ə, a-\ *n* : hypoxia esp. of such severity as to result in permanent damage — **an·ox·ic** \-sik\ *adj*

ANP *abbr* atrial natriuretic peptide

ANS *abbr* autonomic nervous system

an·sa \ˈan-sə\ *n, pl* **an·sae** \-ˌsē\ : a loop-shaped anatomical structure

ansa cer·vi·ca·lis \-ˌsər-və-ˈka-ləs, -ˈkā-\ *n* : a nerve loop from the upper cervical nerves that accompanies the hypoglossal nerve and innervates the infrahyoid muscles

ansa hy·po·glos·si \-ˌhī-pə-ˈglä-ˌsī, -ˈglȯ-, -(ˌ)sē\ *n* : ANSA CERVICALIS

An·said \ˈan-sed\ *trademark* — used for a preparation of flurbiprofen

ansa sub·cla·via \-ˌsəb-ˈklā-vē-ə\ *n* : a nerve loop of sympathetic fibers passing around the subclavian artery

anserinus — see PES ANSERINUS

ant- — see ANTI-

Ant·a·buse \ˈan-tə-ˌbyüs\ *trademark* — used for a preparation of disulfiram

[1]**ant·ac·id** \(ˌ)ant-ˈa-səd\ *also* **an·ti·ac·id** \ˌan-tē-ˈa-səd, -ˌtī-\ *adj* : tending to counteract acidity

[2]**antacid** *also* **antiacid** *n* : an agent (as an alkali or absorbent) that counteracts or neutralizes acidity

an·tag·o·nism \an-ˈta-gə-ˌni-zəm\ *n* : opposition in physiological action: **a** : opposing action in the effect of contraction of muscles **b** : interaction of two or more substances such that the action of any one of them on living cells or tissues is lessened — compare SYNERGISM — **an·tag·o·nize** \an-ˈta-gə-ˌnīz\ *vb*

an·tag·o·nist \-nist\ *n* : an agent that acts in physiological opposition: as **a** : a muscle that contracts with and limits the action of an agonist with which it is paired — called also *antagonistic muscle;* compare AGONIST 1, SYNERGIST 2 **b** : a chemical substance that opposes the action on the nervous system of a drug or a substance occurring naturally in the body by combining with and blocking its nervous receptor — compare AGONIST 2

an·tag·o·nis·tic \(ˌ)an-ˌta-gə-ˈnis-tik\ *adj* **1** : characterized by or resulting from antagonism **2** : relating to or being muscles that are antagonists — **an·tag·o·nis·ti·cal·ly** \-ti-k(ə-)lē\ *adv*

an·tal·gic \an-ˈtal-jik\ *adj* **1** : marked by or being an unnatural position or movement assumed by someone to minimize or alleviate pain or discomfort (as in the leg or back) **2** : relieving pain : ANALGESIC

An·tara \an-ˈter-ə\ *trademark* — used for a preparation of fenofibrate

ante- *prefix* **1** : anterior : forward ⟨*ante*hyophysis⟩ **2 a** : prior to : earlier than ⟨*ante*partum⟩ **b** : in front of ⟨*ante*brachium⟩

an·te·bra·chi·um *or* **an·ti·bra·chi·um** \ˌan-ti-ˈbrā-kē-əm\ *n, pl* **-chia** \-kē-ə\ : the part of the arm or forelimb between the brachium and the carpus : FOREARM

an·te·cu·bi·tal \ˌan-ti-ˈkyü-bət-ᵊl\ *adj* : of or relating to the inner or front surface of the forearm

antecubital fossa *n* : a triangular cavity of the elbow joint that contains a tendon of the biceps, the median nerve, and the brachial artery

an·te·flex·ion \ˌan-ti-ˈflek-shən\ *n* : a displacement forward of an organ (as the uterus) so that its axis is bent upon itself

an·te·grade \ˈan-ti-ˌgrād\ *adj* : ANTEROGRADE 1

an·te·mor·tem \-ˈmȯr-təm\ *adj* : preceding death

an·te·na·tal \-ˈnāt-ᵊl\ *adj, chiefly Brit* : PRENATAL ⟨~ diagnosis of birth defects⟩ — **an·te·na·tal·ly** *adv*

an·te·par·tum \-ˈpär-təm\ *adj* : relating to the period before parturition : before childbirth ⟨~ care⟩

an·te·ri·or \an-ˈtir-ē-ər\ *adj* **1** : relating to or situated near or toward the head or toward the part in headless animals most nearly corresponding to the head **2** : situated toward the front of the body : VENTRAL — used in human anatomy because of the upright posture of humans — **an·te·ri·or·ly** *adv*

anterior cerebral artery *n* : CEREBRAL ARTERY a

anterior chamber *n* : a space in the eye bounded in front by the cornea and in back by the iris and middle part of the lens — compare POSTERIOR CHAMBER

anterior circumflex humeral artery *n* : ANTERIOR HUMERAL CIRCUMFLEX ARTERY

anterior column *n* : VENTRAL HORN
anterior commissure *n* : a band of nerve fibers crossing from one side of the brain to the other just anterior to the third ventricle
anterior communicating artery *n* : COMMUNICATING ARTERY a
anterior corticospinal tract *n* : VENTRAL CORTICOSPINAL TRACT
anterior cruciate ligament *n* : a cruciate ligament of each knee that attaches the front of the tibia with the back of the femur and functions esp. to prevent hyperextension of the knee and is subject to injury esp. by tearing — called also *ACL*
anterior facial vein *n* : FACIAL VEIN
anterior fontanel *n* : the fontanel occurring at the meeting point of the coronal and sagittal sutures
anterior funiculus *n* : VENTRAL FUNICULUS
anterior gray column *n* : VENTRAL HORN
anterior horn *n* **1** : VENTRAL HORN **2** : the cornu of the lateral ventricle of each cerebral hemisphere that curves outward and forward into the frontal lobe — compare INFERIOR HORN, POSTERIOR HORN 2
anterior humeral circumflex artery *n* : an artery that branches from the axillary artery in the shoulder, curves around the front of the humerus, and is distributed esp. to the shoulder joint, head of the humerus, biceps brachii, and deltoid muscle — called also *anterior circumflex humeral artery;* compare POSTERIOR HUMERAL CIRCUMFLEX ARTERY
anterior inferior cerebellar artery *n* : an artery that arises from the basilar artery and divides into branches distributed to the anterior parts of the inferior surface of the cerebellum
anterior inferior iliac spine *n* : a projection on the anterior margin of the ilium that is situated below the anterior superior iliac spine and is separated from it by a notch — called also *anterior inferior spine*
anterior intercostal artery *n* : INTERCOSTAL ARTERY a
anterior jugular vein *n* : JUGULAR VEIN c
anterior lingual gland *n* : either of two mucus-secreting glands of the tip of the tongue
anterior lobe *n* : ADENOHYPOPHYSIS
anterior median fissure *n* : a groove along the anterior midline of the spinal cord that incompletely divides it into symmetrical halves — called also *ventral median fissure*
anterior nasal spine *n* : the nasal spine that is formed by the union of processes of the two premaxillae
anterior pillar of the fauces *n* : PALATOGLOSSAL ARCH
anterior pituitary *n* : ADENOHYPOPHYSIS — called also *anterior pituitary gland*
anterior root *n* : VENTRAL ROOT
anterior sacrococcygeal muscle *n* : SACROCOCCYGEUS VENTRALIS
anterior spinal artery *n* : SPINAL ARTERY a
anterior spinothalamic tract *n* : SPINOTHALAMIC TRACT a
anterior superior iliac spine *n* : a projection at the anterior end of the iliac crest — called also *anterior superior spine*
anterior synechia *n* : SYNECHIA a
anterior temporal artery *n* : TEMPORAL ARTERY 3a
anterior tibial artery *n* : TIBIAL ARTERY b
anterior tibial nerve *n* : DEEP PERONEAL NERVE
anterior tibial vein *n* : TIBIAL VEIN b
anterior triangle *n* : a triangular region that is a landmark in the neck and has its apex at the sternum pointing downward — compare POSTERIOR TRIANGLE
anterior ulnar recurrent artery *n* : ULNAR RECURRENT ARTERY a
antero- *comb form* : anterior and : extending from front to ⟨*antero*lateral⟩ ⟨*antero*posterior⟩
an•tero•grade \ˈan-tə-(ˌ)rō-ˌgrād\ *adj* **1** : occurring or performed in the normal or forward direction of conduction or flow: as **a** : occurring along nerve cell processes away from the cell body ⟨~ axonal transport⟩ **b** : occurring in the normal direction or path of blood circulation ⟨restoration of ~ flow⟩ — compare RETROGRADE 2 **2** : affecting memories for a period of time immediately following a precipitating event (as alcohol intoxication or traumatic brain injury) and esp. from the time of onset to the present — compare RETROGRADE 3 ⟨~ amnesia⟩
an•tero•in•fe•ri•or \ˌan-tə-(ˌ)rō-in-ˈfir-ē-ər\ *adj* : located in front and below ⟨the ~ aspect of the femur⟩ — **an•tero•in•fe•ri•or•ly** *adv*
an•tero•lat•er•al \-ˈla-tə-rəl, -trəl\ *adj* : situated or occurring in front and to the side — **an•tero•lat•er•al•ly** *adv*
anterolateral ligament *n* : a ligament that connects the lateral epicondyle of the femur with the front and outer side of the tibia near the lateral meniscus of the knee and is thought to stabilize the knee by controlling internal rotation of the tibia
an•tero•me•di•al \-ˈmē-dē-əl\ *adj* : located in front and toward the middle
an•tero•pos•te•ri•or \-pō-ˈstir-ē-ər, -pä-\ *adj* : concerned with or extending along a direction or axis from front to back or from anterior to posterior — **an•tero•pos•te•ri•or•ly** *adv*
an•tero•sep•tal \ˌan-tə-(ˌ)rō-ˈsep-tᵊl\ *adj* : located in front of a septum and esp. the interventricular septum ⟨~ infarct⟩
an•tero•su•pe•ri•or \-su̇-ˈpir-ē-ər\ *adj* : located in front and above — **an•tero•su•pe•ri•or•ly** *adv*

an·tero·ven·tral \ˌan-tə-(ˌ)rō-ˈven-trəl\ *adj* : located in front and toward the lower surface — **an·tero·ven·tral·ly** *adv*
an·te·ver·sion \ˌan-ti-ˈvər-zhən, -shən\ *n* : a condition of being anteverted — used esp. of the uterus
an·te·vert \ˈan-ti-ˌvərt, ˌan-ti-ˈ\ *vb* : to displace (a body organ) so that the whole axis is directed farther forward than normal
anth- — see ANTI-
anthelix *var of* ANTIHELIX
[1]**an·thel·min·tic** \ˌant-ˌhel-ˈmin-tik, ˌan-ˌthel-\ *also* **an·thel·min·thic** \-ˈmin-thik\ *adj* : expelling or destroying parasitic worms (as tapeworms) esp. of the intestine
[2]**anthelmintic** *also* **anthelminthic** *n* : an anthelmintic drug
-anthem *or* **-anthema** *n comb form, pl* **-anthems** *or* **-anthemata** : eruption : rash ⟨en*anthem*⟩ ⟨ex*anthema*⟩
anthrac- *or* **anthraco-** *comb form* : carbon : coal ⟨*anthraco*sis⟩
an·thra·co·sil·i·co·sis \ˌan-thrə-(ˌ)kō-ˌsi-lə-ˈkō-səs\ *also* **an·thra·sil·i·co·sis** \ˌan-thrə-ˌsi-\ *n, pl* **-co·ses** \-ˌsēz\ : massive fibrosis of the lungs resulting from inhalation of carbon and quartz dusts
an·thra·co·sis \ˌan-thrə-ˈkō-səs\ *n, pl* **-co·ses** \-ˌsēz\ : black discoloration of bronchi from carbon pigment that typically causes deformation and obstruction, may be asymptomatic or cause respiratory symptoms (as cough and labored breathing), and is often associated with the inhalation of coal dust and wood smoke — **an·thra·cot·ic** \-ˈkä-tik\ *adj*
an·thra·cy·cline \ˌan-thrə-ˈsī-ˌklēn\ *n* : any of a class of antineoplastic drugs (as doxorubicin) derived from an actinomycete of the genus *Streptomyces* (esp. *S. peucetius*)
an·thra·lin \ˈan-thrə-lən\ *n* : a yellowish-brown compound $C_{14}H_{10}O_3$ used to treat skin diseases (as psoriasis) — called also *dithranol*
an·thrax \ˈan-ˌthraks\ *n, pl* **-thra·ces** \-thrə-ˌsēz\ : an infectious disease of warm-blooded animals (as cattle and sheep) caused by a spore-forming bacterium (*Bacillus anthracis*), transmissible to humans esp. by the handling of infected products (as wool), and characterized by cutaneous ulcerating nodules or by often fatal lesions in the lungs; *also* : the bacterium causing anthrax
anthrop- *or* **anthropo-** *comb form* : human being ⟨*anthropo*philic⟩
an·thro·poid \ˈan-thrə-ˌpȯid\ *adj, of the pelvis* : having a relatively great anteroposterior dimension — compare ANDROID, GYNECOID, PLATYPELLOID
an·thro·pom·e·try \ˌan-thrə-ˈpä-mə-trē\ *n, pl* **-tries** : the study of human body measurements esp. on a comparative basis — **an·thro·po·met·ric** \-pə-ˈme-trik\ *adj*
an·thro·po·phil·ic \ˌan-thrə-(ˌ)pō-ˈfi-lik\ *also* **an·thro·poph·i·lous** \-ˈpä-fə-ləs\ *adj* : attracted to humans esp. as a source of food ⟨~ mosquitoes⟩
anti- *or* **ant-** *or* **anth-** *prefix* **1** : opposing in effect or activity ⟨*anti*histamine⟩ **2** : serving to prevent, cure, or alleviate ⟨*anti*anxiety⟩
antiacid *var of* ANTACID
an·ti–ac·ne \ˌan-tē-ˈak-nē, -tī-\ *adj* : alleviating the symptoms of acne ⟨~ creams⟩
an·ti·ag·ing \-ˈāj-iŋ\ *adj* : used or tending to prevent or lessen the effects of aging ⟨~ skin creams⟩
an·ti–AIDS \-ˈādz\ *adj* : used to treat or delay the development of AIDS ⟨the ~ drug AZT⟩
an·ti·al·ler·gic \-ə-ˈlər-jik\ *also* **an·ti·al·ler·gen·ic** \-ˌa-lər-ˈje-nik\ *adj* : ANTI-ALLERGY — **antiallergic** *also* **antiallergenic** *n*
anti–allergy \-ˈa-lər-jē\ *adj* : relieving, controlling, or preventing allergic symptoms ⟨~ medications⟩
an·ti·an·a·phy·lax·is \-ˌa-nə-fə-ˈlak-səs\ *n, pl* **-lax·es** \-ˌsēz\ : the state of desensitization to an antigen
an·ti·an·dro·gen \-ˈan-drə-jən\ *n* : a substance that tends to inhibit the production, activity, or effects of a male sex hormone — **an·ti·an·dro·gen·ic** \-ˌan-drə-ˈje-nik\ *adj*
an·ti–ane·mia \-ə-ˈnē-mē-ə\ *adj* : ANTIANEMIC
an·ti·ane·mic \-ə-ˈnē-mik\ *adj* : effective in or relating to the prevention or correction of anemia
an·ti·an·gi·nal \-an-ˈjīn-ᵊl, -ˈan-jən-ᵊl\ *adj* : used or tending to prevent or relieve angina pectoris ⟨~ drugs⟩
an·ti·an·gio·gen·e·sis \-ˌan-jē-ō-ˈjen-ə-səs\ *n, pl* **-e·ses** \-ˌsēz\ : the prevention or inhibition of angiogenesis — **an·ti·an·gio·gen·ic** \-ˈjen-ik\ *adj*
an·ti·an·ti·body \ˌan-tē-ˈan-ti-ˌbä-dē, ˌan-ˌtī-\ *n, pl* **-bod·ies** : an antibody with specific immunologic activity against another antibody
an·ti·anx·i·ety \-(ˌ)aŋ-ˈzī-ə-tē\ *adj* : tending to prevent or relieve anxiety
[1]**an·ti·ar·rhyth·mic** \-(ˌ)ā-ˈrith-mik\ *adj* : controlling, inhibiting, or preventing cardiac arrhythmia ⟨an ~ agent⟩
[2]**antiarrhythmic** *n* : an antiarrhythmic agent (as a beta-blocker)
[1]**an·ti·ar·thrit·ic** \-är-ˈthri-tik\ *or* **an·ti·ar·thri·tis** \-ˈthrī-təs\ *adj* : tending to relieve or prevent arthritic symptoms
[2]**antiarthritic** *n* : an antiarthritic agent
an·ti–asth·ma \-ˈaz-mə\ *or* **an·ti·asth·ma·tic** \-az-ˈma-tik\ *adj* : used to relieve the symptoms of asthma
antiasthmatic *n* : an anti-asthma drug
[1]**an·ti·bac·te·ri·al** \ˌan-ti-bak-ˈtir-ē-əl, ˌan-ˌtī-\ *adj* : directed or effective against bacteria
[2]**antibacterial** *n* : an antibacterial agent
an·ti·bi·o·sis \ˌan-ti-bī-ˈō-səs, ˌan-ˌtī-; ˌan-ti-bē-\ *n, pl* **-o·ses** \ˌsēz\ : antagonistic association between organisms to the detriment of one of them or

between one organism and a metabolic product of another

[1]**an·ti·bi·ot·ic** \-bī-ˈä-tik, -bē-\ *adj* **1** : tending to prevent, inhibit, or destroy life **2** : of or relating to antibiotics or to antibiosis — **an·ti·bi·ot·i·cal·ly** \-ti-k(ə-)lē\ *adv*

[2]**antibiotic** *n* : a substance produced by or a semisynthetic substance derived from a microorganism and able in dilute solution to inhibit or kill another microorganism

antibiotic lock *n* : a technique in which a concentrated antibiotic solution is instilled and kept within a patient's catheter for a prolonged period (as 10 to 12 hours) to prevent or treat a catheter-related infection

an·ti·bleed·ing \-ˈblēd-iŋ\ *adj* : slowing, stopping, or preventing bleeding or hemorrhage

an·ti·body \ˈan-ti-ˌbä-dē\ *n, pl* **-bod·ies** : any of a large number of proteins of high molecular weight that are produced normally by specialized B cells after stimulation by an antigen and act specif. against the antigen in an immune response, that are produced abnormally by some cancer cells, and that typically consist of four subunits including two heavy chains and two light chains — called also *immunoglobulin*

antibrachium *var of* ANTEBRACHIUM

an·ti·can·cer \ˌan-ti-ˈkan-sər, ˌan-ˌtī-\ *adj* : used against or tending to arrest cancer ⟨~ drugs⟩ ⟨~ activity⟩

an·ti·car·cin·o·gen \-kär-ˈsi-nə-jən, -ˈkärs-ᵊn-ə-ˌjen\ *n* : an anticarcinogenic agent

an·ti·car·ci·no·gen·ic \-ˌkärs-ᵊn-ō-ˈjenik\ *adj* : tending to inhibit or prevent the activity of a carcinogen or the development of carcinoma

an·ti·car·dio·lip·in antibody \-ˌkärd-ē-ō-ˈlip-ən-\ *n* : an antibody that is directed against phospholipids and esp. cardiolipin and that is associated with increased risk for recurring arterial and venous thromboses

an·ti·car·ies \ˌan-ti-ˈkar-ēz, ˌan-ˌtī-\ *adj* : ANTICAVITY

an·ti·car·io·genic \-ˌkar-ē-ō-ˈjen-ik\ *adj* : ANTICAVITY

an·ti·cav·i·ty \-ˈka-vət-ē\ *adj* : tending to prevent tooth decay or the formation of cavities

an·ti·chla·myd·i·al \-klə-ˈmi-dē-əl\ *adj* : destroying or inhibiting the growth of chlamydia

an·ti·cho·les·ter·ol \-kə-ˈles-tə-ˌrōl, -ˌrȯl\ *adj* : tending to reduce the level of cholesterol in the blood ⟨~ drugs⟩

[1]**an·ti·cho·lin·er·gic** \-ˌkō-lə-ˈnər-jik\ *adj* : opposing or blocking the physiological action of acetylcholine

[2]**anticholinergic** *n* : a drug having an anticholinergic action

an·ti·cho·lin·es·ter·ase \-ˈnes-tə-ˌrās, -ˌrāz\ *n* : any substance (as neostigmine) that inhibits a cholinesterase by combination with it

an·tic·i·pa·tion \(ˌ)an-ˌti-sə-ˈpā-shən\ *n* **1** : occurrence (as of a symptom) before the normal or expected time **2** : mental attitude that influences a later response — **an·tic·i·pate** \an-ˈti-sə-ˌpāt\ *vb*

an·ti·clot·ting \ˌan-ti-ˈklä-tiŋ, ˌan-ˌtī-\ *adj* : inhibiting the clotting of blood

[1]**an·ti·co·ag·u·lant** \-kō-ˈa-gyə-lənt\ *adj* : of, relating to, or utilizing anticoagulants ⟨~ therapy⟩

[2]**anticoagulant** *n* : a substance that hinders coagulation and esp. coagulation of the blood : BLOOD THINNER

an·ti·co·ag·u·la·tion \-kō-ˌa-gyə-ˈlā-shən\ *n* : the process of hindering the clotting of blood esp. by treatment with an anticoagulant — **an·ti·co·ag·u·late** \-kō-ˈa-gyə-ˌlāt\ *vb* — **an·ti·co·ag·u·la·to·ry** \-lə-ˌtōr-ē\ *adj*

an·ti·co·ag·u·lat·ive \-ˈa-gyə-ˌlā-tiv\ *adj* : ANTICOAGULANT ⟨~ activity⟩

an·ti·co·ag·u·lin \-gyə-lən\ *n* : a substance (as one in snake venom) that retards clotting of vertebrate blood

an·ti·co·don \ˌan-ti-ˈkō-ˌdän\ *n* : a triplet of nucleotide bases in transfer RNA that identifies the amino acid carried and binds to a complementary codon in messenger RNA during protein synthesis at a ribosome

an·ti·com·ple·ment \-ˈkäm-plə-mənt\ *n* : a substance that interferes with the activity of complement — **an·ti·com·ple·men·ta·ry** \-ˌkäm-plə-ˈmen-tə-rē, -men-trē\ *adj*

[1]**an·ti·con·vul·sant** \-kən-ˈvəl-sənt\ *also* **an·ti·con·vul·sive** \-siv\ *n* : an anticonvulsant drug

[2]**anticonvulsant** *also* **anticonvulsive** *adj* : used or tending to control or prevent convulsions (as in epilepsy)

anticus — see SCALENUS ANTICUS, SCALENUS ANTICUS SYNDROME, TIBIALIS ANTICUS

an·ti–dan·druff \-ˈdan-drəf\ *adj* : tending to treat or prevent dandruff ⟨an ~ shampoo⟩

[1]**an·ti·de·pres·sant** \-di-ˈpres-ᵊnt\ *also* **an·ti·de·pres·sive** \-ˈpre-siv\ *adj* : used or tending to relieve or prevent psychological depression

[2]**antidepressant** *also* **antidepressive** *n* : a drug used to treat psychological depression — called also *energizer, psychic energizer;* see TRICYCLIC ANTIDEPRESSANT

[1]**an·ti·di·a·bet·ic** \-ˌdī-ə-ˈbe-tik\ *n* : an antidiabetic drug

[2]**antidiabetic** *adj* : tending to relieve diabetes ⟨~ drugs⟩

[1]**an·ti·di·ar·rhe·al** \-ˌdī-ə-ˈrē-əl\ *adj* : tending to prevent or relieve diarrhea

[2]**antidiarrheal** *n* : an antidiarrheal agent

an·ti·di·ure·sis \-ˌdī-yu̇-ˈrē-səs\ *n, pl* **-ure·ses** \-ˌsēz\ : reduction in or suppression of the excretion of urine

[1]**an·ti·di·uret·ic** \-ˈre-tik\ *adj* : tending to oppose or check excretion of urine

[2]**antidiuretic** *n* : an antidiuretic substance
antidiuretic hormone *n* : VASOPRESSIN
an•ti•do•pa•mi•ner•gic \-ˌdō-pə-ˌmē-ˈnər-jik\ *adj* : inhibiting or blocking the activity of dopamine or related substances
an•ti•dote \ˈan-ti-ˌdōt\ *n* : a remedy that counteracts the effects of poison — **an•ti•dot•al** \ˌan-ti-ˈdōt-ᵊl\ *adj* — **an•ti•dot•al•ly** *adv*
an•ti•dro•mic \ˌan-ti-ˈdrä-mik, -ˈdrō-\ *adj* **1** : proceeding or conducting in a direction opposite to the usual one — used esp. of a nerve impulse or fiber ⟨~ action potentials⟩ **2** : characterized by antidromic conduction ⟨~ tachycardia⟩ — **an•ti•dro•mi•cal•ly** \-mi-k(ə-)lē\ *adv*
[1]**an•ti•dys•en•ter•ic** \ˌan-ti-ˌdis-ᵊn-ˈter-ik, ˌan-ˌtī-\ *adj* : tending to relieve or prevent dysentery
[2]**antidysenteric** *n* : an antidysenteric agent
[1]**an•ti•emet•ic** \-ə-ˈme-tik\ *adj* : used or tending to prevent or treat nausea and vomiting ⟨~ drugs⟩
[2]**antiemetic** *n* : an antiemetic agent
[1]**an•ti•ep•i•lep•tic** \-ˌe-pə-ˈlep-tik\ *adj* : tending to control or prevent epileptic seizures ⟨~ drugs⟩
[2]**antiepileptic** *n* : an antiepileptic drug
an•ti•es•tro•gen \-ˈes-trə-jən\ *n* : a substance that inhibits the physiological action of an estrogen — **an•ti•es•tro•gen•ic** \-ˌes-trə-ˈje-nik\ *adj*
an•ti•fer•til•i•ty \-(ˌ)fər-ˈti-lə-tē\ *adj* : having the capacity or tending to reduce or destroy fertility : CONTRACEPTIVE ⟨~ agents⟩
an•ti•fi•bril•la•to•ry \-ˈfi-brə-lə-ˌtōr-ē, -ˈfī-\ *adj* : tending to suppress or prevent cardiac fibrillation
an•ti•fi•bri•no•ly•sin \-ˌfī-brən-ᵊl-ˈīs-ᵊn\ *n* : an antibody that acts specif. against fibrinolysins of hemolytic streptococci and that is used chiefly in some diagnostic tests — **an•ti•fi•bri•no•ly•sis** \-ˈī-səs\ *n* — **an•ti•fi•bri•no•lyt•ic** \-ˈi-tik\ *adj*
an•ti•fi•lar•i•al \-fə-ˈlar-ē-əl, -ˈler-\ *adj* : tending to destroy filarial worms or to inhibit their growth; *also* : produced in response to filarial infection ⟨~ antibodies⟩ — **antifilarial** *n*
[1]**an•ti•flat•u•lent** \-ˈfla-chə-lənt\ *adj* : preventing or relieving flatulence
[2]**antiflatulent** *n* : an antiflatulent agent
an•ti•flu \-ˈflü\ *adj* : used to prevent influenza ⟨an ~ drug⟩
an•ti•fo•late \-ˈfō-ˌlāt\ *n* : a drug (as methotrexate or sulfamethoxazole) that interferes with folate activity and is used chiefly as an anticancer, antibacterial, and antimalarial agent
[1]**an•ti•fun•gal** \ˌan-ti-ˈfəŋ-gəl, ˌan-ˌtī-\ *adj* : destroying fungi or inhibiting their growth : FUNGICIDAL, FUNGISTATIC
[2]**antifungal** *n* : an antifungal agent
an•ti•gen \ˈan-ti-jən\ *n* : any substance foreign to the body that evokes an immune response either alone or after forming a complex with a larger molecule (as a protein) and that is capable of binding with a product (as an antibody or T cell) of the immune response — **an•ti•gen•ic** \ˌan-ti-ˈje-nik\ *adj* — **an•ti•gen•i•cal•ly** \-ni-k(ə-)lē\ *adv*
an•ti•gen•emia \ˌan-ti-jə-ˈnē-mē-ə\ *n* : the condition of having an antigen present in the blood
antigenic determinant *n* : EPITOPE
an•ti•gen•ic•i•ty \-ˈni-sə-tē\ *n, pl* **-ties** : the capacity to act as an antigen
antigen–presenting cell *n* : any of various cells (as a macrophage or a B cell) that take up an antigen and process it into a form recognized by and serving to activate a specific helper T cell — abbr. *APC*
an•ti•glau•co•ma \-glau̇-ˈkō-mə, glȯ-\ *adj* : used to prevent or treat glaucoma ⟨~ eye drops⟩
an•ti•glob•u•lin \ˌan-ti-ˈglä-byə-lən, ˌan-ˌtī-\ *n* : an antibody that combines with and precipitates globulin
an•ti•go•nad•o•trop•ic \-gō-ˌna-də-ˈträ-pik\ *adj* : tending to inhibit the physiological activity of gonadotropic hormones
an•ti•go•nad•o•tro•pin \-ˈtrō-pən\ *n* : an antigonadotropic substance
an•ti•he•lix \-ˈhē-liks\ *also* **ant•he•lix** \(ˈ)ant-\ *n, pl* **-li•ces** \-ˈhe-lə-ˌsēz, -ˈhē-\ *or* **-lix•es** \-ˈhē-lik-səz\ : the curved elevation of cartilage within or in front of the helix
an•ti•hel•min•thic \-hel-ˈmin(t)-thik\ *adj* : ANTHELMINTIC
an•ti•he•mo•phil•ic factor \-ˌhē-mə-ˈfi-lik-\ *n* : FACTOR VIII — called also *antihemophilic globulin*
an•ti•hem•or•rhag•ic \-ˌhe-mə-ˈra-jik\ *adj* : tending to prevent or arrest hemorrhage
an•ti–her•pes \-ˈhər-(ˌ)pēz\ *adj* : acting against a herpesvirus or the symptoms caused by infection with it ⟨the ~ drug acyclovir⟩
an•ti•hi•drot•ic \-hi-ˈdrä-tik, -hī-\ *adj* : ANHIDROTIC — **antihidrotic** *n*
[1]**an•ti•his•ta•mine** \-ˈhis-tə-ˌmēn, -mən\ *adj* : tending to block or counteract the physiological action of histamine
[2]**antihistamine** *n* : any of various compounds that oppose the actions of histamine and are used esp. for treating allergic reactions (as hay fever), cold symptoms, and motion sickness
an•ti•his•ta•min•ic \-ˌhis-tə-ˈmi-nik\ *adj or n* : ANTIHISTAMINE
an•ti–HIV \-ˌā-ˌchī-ˈvē\ *adj* : acting, used, or effective against HIV infection
an•ti•hor•mon•al \-hȯr-ˈmōn-ᵊl\ *adj* : blocking or inhibiting the effect or production of a hormone : of, relating to, or utilizing antihormones ⟨~ therapy⟩
[1]**an•ti•hor•mone** \-ˈhȯr-ˌmōn\ *n* : a substance (as tamoxifen) that blocks the action or inhibits the production of a hormone

²**antihormone** *adj* : ANTIHORMONAL

an•ti–HPV \-ˌāch-(ˌ)pē-ˈvē\ *adj* : acting against or preventing infection with human papillomavirus

an•ti•hu•man \-ˈhyü-mən, -ˈyü-\ *adj* : reacting strongly with human antigens ⟨~ antibodies⟩

an•ti•hy•per•gly•ce•mic \-ˌhī-pər-glī-ˈsē-mik\ *adj* : counteracting the accumulation of excess sugar in the blood : HYPOGLYCEMIC 2

an•ti•hy•per•lip•id•emic \-ˌhī-pər-ˌli-pə-ˈdē-mik\ *adj* : acting to prevent or counteract the accumulation of lipids in the blood ⟨an ~ drug⟩

¹**an•ti•hy•per•ten•sive** \-ˌhī-pər-ˈten-siv\ *also* **an•ti•hy•per•ten•sion** \-ˌhī-pər-ˈten-chən\ *adj* : used or effective against high blood pressure

²**antihypertensive** *n* : an antihypertensive agent (as a drug)

an•ti–id•io•type \ˌan-tī-ˈi-dē-ə-ˌtīp\ *n* : an antibody that binds to the antigen combining site of another antibody either suppressing or enhancing the immune response — **anti–idiotype** *adj* — **an•ti–id•io•typ•ic** \-ˌi-dē-ə-ˈti-pik\ *adj*

¹**an•ti–im•mu•no•glob•u•lin** \ˌan-tē-ˌi-myə-nō-ˈglä-byə-lən, ˌan-ˌtī-, -i-ˌmyü-nō-\ *adj* : acting against specific antibodies ⟨~ antibodies⟩ ⟨~ sera⟩

²**anti–immunoglobulin** *n* : an anti-immunoglobulin agent

an•ti–im•po•tence \-ˈim-pə-tən(t)s\ *adj* : used or effective against sexual impotence

¹**an•ti–in•fec•tive** \-in-ˈfek-tiv\ *adj* : used against or tending to counteract or prevent infection ⟨~ agents⟩

²**anti–infective** *n* : an anti-infective agent

¹**an•ti–in•flam•ma•to•ry** \-in-ˈfla-mə-ˌtōr-ē\ *adj* : reducing or counteracting inflammation

²**anti–inflammatory** *n, pl* **-ries** : a drug (as aspirin or ibuprofen) that reduces inflammation

an•ti–in•flu•en•za \-ˌin-(ˌ)flü-ˈen-zə\ *adj* : ANTIFLU

¹**an•ti–in•su•lin** \-ˈin-sə-lən\ *adj* : tending to counteract the physiological action of insulin

²**anti–insulin** *n* : an anti-insulin substance

an•ti–itch \-ˈich\ *adj* : preventing or alleviating itching : ANTIPRURITIC ⟨~ creams⟩

an•ti•ke•to•gen•ic \-ˈje-nik\ *adj* : tending to prevent or counteract ketosis

an•ti•leu•ke•mic \-lü-ˈkē-mik\ *also* **an•ti•leu•ke•mia** \-mē-ə\ *adj* : counteracting the effects of leukemia

an•ti•leu•ko•tri•ene \-ˌlü-kə-ˈtrī-ˌēn\ *n* : any of various compounds that oppose the action of leukotrienes and are used in the treatment of asthma — **antileukotriene** *adj*

an•ti•lu•et•ic \-lü-ˈe-tik\ *n* : ANTISYPHILITIC

an•ti•lym•pho•cyte globulin \-ˈlim-fə-ˌsīt-\ *n* : serum globulin containing antibodies against lymphocytes that is used similarly to antilymphocyte serum

antilymphocyte serum *n* : a serum containing antibodies against lymphocytes that is used for suppressing graft rejection

an•ti•lym•pho•cyt•ic globulin \-ˌlim-fə-ˈsi-tik-\ *n* : ANTILYMPHOCYTE GLOBULIN

antilymphocytic serum *n* : ANTILYMPHOCYTE SERUM

¹**an•ti•ma•lar•i•al** \-mə-ˈler-ē-əl\ *or* **an•ti•ma•lar•ia** \-ə\ *adj* : serving to prevent, check, or cure malaria

²**antimalarial** *n* : an antimalarial drug

an•ti•man•ic \-ˈman-ik\ *adj* : counteracting or preventing mania and esp. mania associated with bipolar disorder

an•ti•me•tab•o•lite \-mə-ˈta-bə-ˌlīt\ *n* : a substance (as a sulfa drug) that replaces or inhibits the utilization of a metabolite

an•ti•met•a•stat•ic \-ˌme-tə-ˈsta-tik\ *adj* : inhibiting metastasis ⟨~ activity⟩

¹**an•ti•mi•cro•bi•al** \-mī-ˌkrō-bē-əl\ *also* **an•ti•mi•cro•bic** \-ˈkrō-bik\ *adj* : destroying or inhibiting the growth of microorganisms and esp. pathogenic microorganisms

²**antimicrobial** *also* **antimicrobic** *n* : an antimicrobial substance

an•ti•mi•graine \-ˈmī-ˌgrān\ *adj* : used to relieve or prevent the symptoms of migraine headache ⟨~ drugs⟩

¹**an•ti•mi•tot•ic** \-mī-ˈtä-tik\ *adj* : inhibiting or disrupting mitosis ⟨~ agents⟩

²**antimitotic** *n* : an antimitotic substance

an•ti•mo•ny \ˈan-tə-ˌmō-nē\ *n, pl* **-nies** : a usu. silvery-white crystalline metalloid element that is used in medicine as a constituent of antiprotozoal agents (as tartar emetic) — symbol *Sb;* see ELEMENT table

antimonyltartrate — see POTASSIUM ANTIMONYLTARTRATE

antimony potassium tartrate *n* : TARTAR EMETIC

an•ti•mo•til•i•ty \-mō-ˈti-lə-tē\ *adj* : inhibiting or slowing gastrointestinal motility ⟨~ agents to treat diarrhea⟩

anti–Mul•ler•ian hormone \-myü-ˈlir-ē-ən-, -mi-, -mə-\ *or* **anti–Müellerian hormone** *n* : MÜLLERIAN INHIBITING SUBSTANCE — abbr. *AMH*

an•ti•mus•ca•rin•ic \-ˌməs-kə-ˈri-nik\ *adj* : inhibiting muscarinic physiological effects ⟨an ~ agent⟩

an•ti•mu•ta•gen•ic \-ˌmyü-tə-ˈje-nik\ *adj* : reducing the rate of mutation

an•ti•my•cin A \ˌan-ti-ˌmīs-ᵊn-ˈā\ *n* : a crystalline antibiotic $C_{28}H_{40}N_2O_9$ used esp. as a fungicide, insecticide, and miticide — called also *antimycin*

an•ti•my•cot•ic \ˌan-ti-mī-ˈkä-tik, ˌan-ˌtī-\ *adj or n* : ANTIFUNGAL

an•ti–nau•sea \-ˈnȯ-zē-ə, -sē-; -ˈnȯ-zhə, -shə\ *also* **an•ti•nau•se•ant** \-ˈnȯ-zē-ənt, -zhē-, -sē-, -shē-\ *adj* : preventing or counteracting nausea ⟨~ drugs⟩

antinauseant *n* : an anti-nausea agent

[1]**an·ti·neo·plas·tic** \-ˌnē-ə-ˈplas-tik\ *adj* : inhibiting or preventing the growth and spread of neoplasms or malignant cells ⟨~ drugs⟩

[2]**antineoplastic** *n* : an antineoplastic agent

an·ti·neu·rit·ic \-nu̇-ˈri-tik, -nyu̇-\ *adj* : preventing or relieving neuritis

an·ti·neu·tro·phil cytoplasmic antibody \-ˈn(y)ü-trə-ˌfil-\ *also* **an·ti·neu·tro·phil·ic cytoplasmic antibody** \-ˌn(y)ü-trə-ˈfi-lik-\ *n* : any of a group of autoantibodies that bind to cytoplasmic regions of neutrophils and are associated with diseases (as granulomatosis with polyangiitis and polyarteritis nodosa) marked by inflammation of small blood vessels — abbr. *ANCA*

an·ti·no·ci·cep·tive \ˌan-ti-nō-si-ˈsep-tiv, ˌan-ˌtī-\ *adj* : ANALGESIC

an·ti·nu·cle·ar \-ˈnü-klē-ər, -ˈnyü-\ *adj* : being antibodies or autoantibodies that react with components and esp. DNA of cell nuclei and that tend to occur frequently in connective tissue diseases

an·ti·nu·tri·ent \-ˈn(y)ü-trē-ənt\ *n* : a naturally-occurring substance (such as oxalate) found in plant-derived foods that interferes with absorption or proper functioning of nutrients in the body; *also* : a substance (such as refined sugar) that has little nutritive value and typically depletes the body of more nutrients than it provides when metabolized

an·ti–obe·si·ty \-ō-ˈbē-sə-tē\ *adj* : used to treat obesity : promoting the loss of excessive bodily fat

an·ti–on·co·gene \-ˈäŋ-kō-ˌjēn\ *n* : TUMOR SUPRESSOR GENE

an·ti·ox·i·dant \-ˈäk-sə-dənt\ *n* : a substance (as beta-carotene or vitamin C) that inhibits oxidation or reactions promoted by oxygen, peroxides, or free radicals — **antioxidant** *adj*

an·ti·par·a·sit·ic \-ˌpar-ə-ˈsi-tik\ *adj* : acting against parasites

an·ti·par·kin·so·nian \-ˌpär-kən-ˈsō-nē-ən, -nyən\ *also* **an·ti·par·kin·son** \-ˈpär-kən-sən\ *adj* : tending to relieve parkinsonism ⟨~ drugs⟩

[1]**an·ti·pe·ri·od·ic** \-ˌpir-ē-ˈä-dik\ *adj* : preventing periodic returns of disease

[2]**antiperiodic** *n* : an antiperiodic agent

an·ti·peri·stal·sis \-ˌper-ə-ˈstȯl-səs, -ˈstäl-, -ˈstal-\ *n, pl* **-stal·ses** \-ˌsēz\ : reversed peristalsis

an·ti·peri·stal·tic \-tik\ *adj* **1** : opposed to or checking peristaltic motion **2** : relating to antiperistalsis

an·ti·per·spi·rant \-ˈpər-spə-rənt\ *n* : a preparation used to check perspiration

an·ti·phlo·gis·tic \-flə-ˈjis-tik\ *adj or n* : ANTI-INFLAMMATORY

an·ti·phos·pho·lip·id \-ˌfäs-fō-ˈli-pəd\ *adj* : relating to or being an antibody (as anticardiolipin antibody) that acts against phospholipids or proteins that bind to phospholipids and is associated with antiphospholipid syndrome

antiphospholipid syndrome *n* : an autoimmune disorder characterized esp. by the presence of antiphospholipid antibodies and an increased risk of venous and arterial blood clots and recurrent miscarriage — abbr. *APS;* called also *antiphospholipid antibody syndrome, Hughes syndrome*

an·ti·plas·min \-ˈplaz-mən\ *n* : a substance (as an antifibrinolysin) that inhibits the action of plasmin

an·ti·plate·let \-ˈplāt-lət\ *adj* : acting against or destroying blood platelets

an·ti·pneu·mo·coc·cal \-ˌnü-mə-ˈkä-kəl, -ˌnyü-\ *or* **an·ti·pneu·mo·coc·cic** \-ˈkäk-(ˌ)sik\ *or* **an·ti·pneu·mo·coc·cus** \-ˈkä-kəs\ *adj* : destroying or inhibiting pneumococci

an·ti·pro·lif·er·a·tive \-prə-ˈli-fə-ˌrā-tiv\ *adj* : used or tending to inhibit cell growth ⟨~ agents⟩

an·ti·pro·te·ase \-ˈprō-tē-ˌās, -ˌāz\ *n* : a substance that inhibits the enzymatic activity of a protease

an·ti·pro·throm·bin \-(ˌ)prō-ˈthräm-bən\ *n* : a substance that interferes with the conversion of prothrombin to thrombin — compare ANTITHROMBIN, HEPARIN

[1]**an·ti·pro·to·zo·al** \-ˌprō-tə-ˈzō-əl\ *adj* : tending to destroy or inhibit the growth of protozoa

[2]**antiprotozoal** *n* : an antiprotozoal agent

[1]**an·ti·pru·rit·ic** \-prü-ˈri-tik\ *adj* : tending to check or relieve itching

[2]**antipruritic** *n* : an antipruritic agent

an·ti·pseu·do·mo·nal \-ˌsü-də-ˈmōn-ᵊl, -sü-ˈdä-mən-ᵊl\ *adj* : tending to destroy bacteria of the genus *Pseudomonas* ⟨~ activity⟩

[1]**an·ti·psy·chot·ic** \-sī-ˈkä-tik\ *adj* : of, being, or involving the use of an antipsychotic ⟨~ drugs⟩

[2]**antipsychotic** *n* : any of the powerful tranquilizers (as the phenothiazines and butyrophenones) used esp. to treat psychosis and believed to act by blocking dopamine nervous receptors — called also *neuroleptic*

an·ti·py·re·sis \-ˌpī-ˈrē-səs\ *n, pl* **-re·ses** \-ˌsēz\ : treatment of fever by use of antipyretics

[1]**an·ti·py·ret·ic** \-pī-ˈre-tik\ *n* : an antipyretic agent — called also *febrifuge*

[2]**antipyretic** *adj* : preventing, removing, or allaying fever

an·ti·py·rine \-ˈpī-ˌrēn\ *also* **an·ti·py·rin** \-rən\ *n* : an analgesic and antipyretic $C_{11}H_{12}N_2O$ that has been used topically to treat ear pain associated with middle ear infection — called also *phenazone*

[1]**an·ti·ra·chit·ic** \-rə-ˈki-tik\ *adj* : used or tending to prevent the development of rickets ⟨an ~ vitamin⟩

[2]**antirachitic** *n* : an antirachitic agent

an·ti–re·flux \-ˈrē-ˌfləks\ *adj* : used to prevent, control, or treat gastroesophageal reflux or gastroesophageal reflux disease ⟨∼ surgery⟩

an·ti·re·jec·tion \-ri-ˈjek-shən\ *adj* : used or tending to prevent organ transplant rejection ⟨∼ drugs⟩

an·ti·re·sorp·tive \-rē-ˈsȯrp-tiv, -ˈzȯrp-\ *adj* : tending to slow or block the resorption of bone ⟨an ∼ agent⟩

¹an·ti·ret·ro·vi·ral \-ˈre-trō-ˌvī-rəl\ *adj* : acting, used, or effective against retroviruses ⟨∼ drugs⟩ ⟨∼ therapy⟩ — see HIGHLY ACTIVE ANTIRETROVIRAL THERAPY

²antiretroviral *n* : an antiretroviral drug — abbr. *ARV*

¹an·ti·rheu·mat·ic \-rü-ˈma-tik\ *adj* : alleviating or preventing rheumatism

²antirheumatic *n* : an antirheumatic agent

an·ti·schis·to·so·mal \-ˌshis-tə-ˈsō-məl\ *adj* : tending to destroy or inhibit the development and reproduction of schistosomes

an·ti·schizo·phren·ic \-ˌskit-sə-ˈfre-nik\ *or* **an·ti·schizo·phre·nia** \-ˌskit-sə-ˈfrē-nē-ə\ *adj* : tending to relieve or treat the symptoms of schizophrenia

¹an·ti·scor·bu·tic \-skȯr-ˈbyü-tik\ *adj* : counteracting scurvy ⟨the ∼ vitamin is vitamin C⟩

²antiscorbutic *n* : a remedy for scurvy

an·ti·seb·or·rhe·ic \-ˌse-bə-ˈrē-ik\ *adj* : preventing or relieving the symptoms of seborrhea or seborrheic dermatitis ⟨∼ shampoos⟩

an·ti·se·cre·tory \-ˈsē-krə-ˌtōr-ē\ *adj* : tending to inhibit secretion

an·ti·sei·zure \-ˈsē-zhər\ *adj* : preventing or counteracting seizures ⟨∼ drugs⟩

an·ti·sense \ˈan-ˌtī-ˌsens, ˈan-ti-\ *adj* : of, being, relating to, or possessing a sequence of DNA or RNA that is complementary to and pairs with a specific messenger RNA blocking it from being translated into protein and serving to inhibit gene function ⟨∼ RNA⟩ ⟨∼ drug therapy⟩ — compare MISSENSE, NONSENSE

an·ti·sep·sis \ˌan-tə-ˈsep-səs\ *n, pl* **-sep·ses** \-ˌsēz\ : the inhibiting of the growth and multiplication of microorganisms by antiseptic means

¹an·ti·sep·tic \ˌan-tə-ˈsep-tik\ *adj* **1 a** : opposing sepsis, putrefaction, or decay; *esp* : preventing or arresting the growth of microorganisms (as on living tissue) **b** : acting or protecting like an antiseptic **2** : relating to or characterized by the use of antiseptics **3** : free of living microorganisms : scrupulously clean : ASEPTIC — **an·ti·sep·ti·cal·ly** \-ti-k(ə-)lē\ *adv*

²antiseptic *n* : a substance that checks the growth or action of microorganisms esp. in or on living tissue; *also* : GERMICIDE

an·ti·se·rum \ˈan-ti-ˌsir-əm, ˈan-ˌtī-, -ˌser-\ *n* : a serum containing antibodies — called also *immune serum*

an·ti·shock \-ˈshäk\ *adj* : counteracting the effects of bodily shock; *specif* : used to treat hypovolemic shock (as that resulting from hemorrhage) esp. by improving blood flow and pressure in the upper body

an·ti·so·cial \-ˈsō-shəl\ *adj* : hostile or harmful to organized society: as **a** : being or marked by behavior deviating sharply from the social norm **b** : of, relating to, or characterized by an antisocial personality, the antisocial personality disorder, or behavior typical of either

antisocial personality *n* : a personality exhibiting traits typical of the antisocial personality disorder — called also *psychopathic personality*

antisocial personality disorder *n* : a personality disorder that is characterized by antisocial behavior exhibiting pervasive disregard for and violation of the rights, feelings, and safety of others

¹an·ti·spas·mod·ic \-spaz-ˈmä-dik\ *n* : an antispasmodic agent

²antispasmodic *adj* : preventing or relieving spasms or convulsions

an·ti·sperm \-ˈspərm\ *adj* : destroying or inactivating sperm ⟨∼ pills⟩

an·ti·strep·to·coc·cal \-ˌstrep-tə-ˈkä-kəl\ *or* **an·ti·strep·to·coc·cic** \-ˈkä-kik, -ˈkäk-sik\ *adj* : tending to destroy or inhibit the growth and reproduction of streptococci ⟨∼ antibodies⟩

an·ti·strep·to·ki·nase \-ˌstrep-tō-ˈkī-ˌnās, -ˌnāz\ *n* : an antibody that acts against streptokinase — often used before *antibody*

an·ti·strep·to·ly·sin \-ˌstrep-tə-ˈlīs-ᵊn\ *n* : an antibody against a streptolysin produced by an individual injected with a streptolysin-forming streptococcus

an·ti–stroke \-ˈstrōk\ *adj* : used to prevent a stroke or to reduce the neurological damage following a stroke ⟨∼ drugs⟩ ⟨∼ therapy⟩

¹an·ti·syph·i·lit·ic \-ˌsi-fə-ˈli-tik\ *adj* : effective against syphilis ⟨∼ therapy⟩

²antisyphilitic *n* : an antisyphilitic agent

anti–TB \-(ˌ)tē-ˈbē\ *adj* : used to treat tuberculosis : ANTITUBERCULOUS

an·ti·throm·bin \-ˈthräm-bən\ *n* : any of a group of substances in blood that inhibit blood clotting by inactivating thrombin — compare ANTIPROTHROMBIN, HEPARIN

an·ti·throm·bo·gen·ic \-ˌthräm-bə-ˈje-nik\ *adj* : preventing the formation of a blood clot esp. within a blood vessel — **an·ti·throm·bo·ge·nic·i·ty** \-jə-ˈni-sə-tē\ *n*

an·ti·throm·bo·plas·tin \-ˌthräm-bə-ˈplas-tən\ *n* : an anticoagulant substance that counteracts the effects of thromboplastin

¹an·ti·throm·bot·ic \-thräm-ˈbä-tik\ *adj* : used against or tending to prevent thrombosis ⟨∼ agents⟩ ⟨∼ therapy⟩

²antithrombotic *n* : an antithrombotic agent

an·ti·thy·mo·cyte globulin \-ˈthī-mə-ˌsīt-\ *n* : a mixture of usu. IgG antibodies against human T cells that is administered by intravenous injection esp. to suppress immune system function (as to prevent rejection in kidney transplant)

an·ti·thy·roid \-ˈthī-ˌrȯid\ *adj* : able to counteract excessive thyroid activity

an·ti·tox·ic \-ˈtäk-sik\ *adj* **1** : counteracting toxins **2** : being or containing antitoxins ⟨~ serum⟩

an·ti·tox·in \ˌan-ti-ˈtäk-sən\ *n* : an antibody that is capable of neutralizing the specific toxin (as a specific causative agent of disease) that stimulated its production in the body and is produced in animals for medical purposes by injection of a toxin or toxoid with the resulting serum being used to counteract the toxin in other individuals; *also* : an antiserum containing antitoxins

an·ti·trag·i·cus \ˌan-ti-ˈtra-jə-kəs\ *n, pl* **-i·ci** \-jə-ˌsī, -ˌsē\ : a small muscle arising from the outer part of the antitragus and inserted into the antihelix

an·ti·tra·gus \-ˈtrā-gəs\ *n, pl* **-gi** \-ˌjī, -ˌgī\ : a prominence on the lower posterior portion of the concha of the external ear opposite the tragus

an·ti·try·pano·som·al \-tri-ˌpa-nə-ˈsō-məl\ *also* **an·ti·try·pano·some** \-tri-ˈpa-nə-ˌsōm\ *adj* : TRYPANOCIDAL

an·ti·tryp·sin \ˈan-ti-ˌtrip-sən, ˌan-ˌtī-\ *n* : a substance that inhibits the action of trypsin — see ALPHA-1-ANTITRYPSIN — **an·ti·tryp·tic** \-ˌtrip-tik\ *adj*

an·ti·tu·ber·cu·lous \ˌan-ti-tu̇-ˈbər-kyə-ləs, ˌan-ˌtī-, -tyu̇-\ *or* **an·ti·tu·ber·cu·lo·sis** \-ˌbər-kyə-ˈlō-səs\ *also* **an·ti·tu·ber·cu·lar** \-ˈbər-kyə-lər\ *adj* : used or effective against tuberculosis

an·ti·tu·mor \ˈan-ti-ˌtü-mər, ˈan-ˌtī-, -ˌtyü-\ *also* **an·ti·tu·mor·al** \-mə-rəl\ *adj* : ANTICANCER ⟨~ agents⟩

[1]**an·ti·tus·sive** \ˌan-ti-ˈtə-siv, ˌan-ˌtī-\ *adj* : tending to prevent or suppress coughing ⟨~ action⟩

[2]**antitussive** *n* : a cough suppressant

an·ti·ty·phoid \-ˈtī-ˌfȯid, -tī-ˈfȯid\ *adj* : used to prevent or treat typhoid fever ⟨an ~ vaccine⟩

an·ti·ul·cer \-ˈəl-sər\ *adj* : tending to prevent or heal ulcers ⟨~ drugs⟩

an·ti·ven·in \-ˈve-nən\ *n* : an antitoxin to a venom; *also* : an antiserum containing such an antitoxin

An·ti·vert \ˈan-ti-ˌvərt, -ˌtī-\ *trademark* — used for a preparation of the hydrochloride of meclizine

[1]**an·ti·vi·ral** \ˌan-ti-ˈvī-rəl, ˌan-ˌtī-\ *also* **an·ti·vi·rus** \-ˈvī-rəs\ *adj* : acting, effective, or directed against viruses

[2]**antiviral** *n* : an antiviral agent

an·ti·vi·ta·min \ˈan-ti-ˌvī-tə-mən, ˈan-ˌtī-\ *n* : a substance that makes a vitamin metabolically ineffective

An·ton's syndrome \ˈan-ˌtänz-\ *also* **Anton syndrome** *n* : a rare disorder in which blindness associated with damage to the cerebral cortex esp. of the occipital lobes is accompanied by denial of visual loss by the patient

An·ton \ˈän-ˌtōn\, **Gabriel (1858–1933),** German neuropsychiatrist.

antr- *or* **antro-** *comb form* : antrum ⟨*antro*stomy⟩

an·tral \ˈan-trəl\ *adj* : of or relating to an antrum ⟨~ gastritis⟩

an·trec·to·my \an-ˈtrek-tə-mē\ *n, pl* **-mies** : surgical removal of the lower portion of the stomach

an·tros·to·my \an-ˈträs-tə-mē\ *n, pl* **-mies** : the operation of opening an antrum (as for drainage); *also* : the opening made in such an operation

an·trot·o·my \-ˈträ-tə-mē\ *n, pl* **-mies** : incision of an antrum; *also* : ANTROSTOMY

an·trum \ˈan-trəm\ *n, pl* **an·tra** \-trə\ : a cavity within a bone (as the maxilla) or hollow organ (as the stomach)

antrum of High·more \-ˈhī-ˌmōr\ *n* : MAXILLARY SINUS

Highmore, Nathaniel (1613–1685), British surgeon.

anu·cle·ate \(ˌ)ā-ˈnü-klē-ət, -ˈnyü-\ *also* **anu·cle·at·ed** \-klē-ˌā-təd\ *adj* : lacking a cell nucleus

anulus *var of* ANNULUS

an·uria \ə-ˈnu̇r-ē-ə, a-, -ˈnyu̇r-\ *n* : absence of or defective urine excretion — **an·uric** \-ˈnu̇r-ik, -ˈnyu̇r-\ *adj*

anus \ˈā-nəs\ *n, pl* **anus·es** *or* **ani** \ˈā-(ˌ)nī\ : the posterior opening of the digestive tract

an·vil \ˈan-vəl\ *n* : INCUS

anx·i·ety \aŋ-ˈzī-ə-tē\ *n, pl* **-eties** **1 a** (1) : apprehensive uneasiness or nervousness usu. over an impending or anticipated ill : a state of being anxious (2) : an abnormal and overwhelming sense of apprehension and fear often marked by physical signs (as tension, sweating, and increased pulse rate), by doubt concerning the reality and nature of the threat, and by self-doubt about one's capacity to cope with it **b** : mentally distressing concern or interest ⟨a child's illness can be a source of ~ for a parent⟩ **2** : a cause of anxiety

anxiety disorder *n* : any of various disorders (as panic disorder, obsessive-compulsive disorder, or generalized anxiety disorder) in which anxiety is a predominant feature — called also *anxiety neurosis, anxiety state*

anxiety reaction *n* : reaction to a feared situation or object in which various manifestations of anxiety are prominent

anxiety state *n* **1** : ANXIETY DISORDER **2** : an episode of usu. intense anxiety : a temporary condition during which a person experiences significant levels of anxiety

an·xi·o·gen·ic \ˌaŋ-zē-ō-ˈje-nik, ˌaŋ(k)-sē-\ *adj* : producing anxiety ⟨~ agents⟩ — **anxiogenic** *n*

[1]**anx·io·lyt·ic** \ˌaŋ-zē-ō-ˈli-tik, ˌaŋ-sē-\ *n* : a drug that relieves anxiety

[2]**anxiolytic** *adj* : relieving anxiety

anx·ious \ˈaŋk-shəs\ *adj* **1** : characterized by extreme uneasiness of mind or brooding fear about some contingency **2** : characterized by, resulting from, or causing anxiety

AOB *abbr* alcohol on breath

AOM *abbr* acute otitis media

A1c \ˌā-ˌwən-ˈsē\ *n* : HEMOGLOBIN A1C

aort- *or* **aorto-** *comb form* **1** : aorta ⟨*aort*itis⟩ **2** : aortic and ⟨*aorto*coronary⟩

aor·ta \ā-ˈȯr-tə\ *n, pl* **-tas** *or* **-tae** \-tē\ : the large arterial trunk that carries blood from the heart to be distributed by branch arteries through the body

aor·tic \ā-ˈȯr-tik\ *also* **aor·tal** \-ˈȯrt-ᵊl\ *adj* : of, relating to, or affecting an aorta ⟨an ∼ aneurysm⟩

aortic arch *n* : ARCH OF THE AORTA

aortic dissection *n* : a pathological splitting of the aortic media

aortic hiatus *n* : an opening in the diaphragm through which the aorta passes

aortic incompetence *n* : AORTIC REGURGITATION

aortic insufficiency *n* : AORTIC REGURGITATION

aor·tico·pul·mo·nary \ā-ˌȯr-tə-kō-ˈpu̇l-mə-ˌner-ē, -ˈpəl-\ *adj* : AORTOPULMONARY

aor·tico·re·nal \-ˈrēn-ᵊl\ *adj* : relating to or situated near the aorta and the kidney

aortic regurgitation *n* : leakage of blood from the aorta back into the left ventricle during diastole because of failure of an aortic valve to close properly — called also *aortic incompetence, aortic insufficiency*

aortic sinus *n* : SINUS OF VALSALVA

aortic stenosis *n* : narrowing of the orifice of the aortic valve (as from calcium deposition or congenital heart defect) that is marked esp. by fainting, chest pain, fatigue, shortness of breath, and heart palpitations

aortic valve *n* : the semilunar valve separating the aorta from the left ventricle that prevents blood from flowing back into the left ventricle

aor·ti·tis \ˌā-ˌȯr-ˈtī-təs\ *n* : inflammation of the aorta

aor·to·cor·o·nary \ˌā-ˌȯr-tō-ˈkȯr-ə-ˌner-ē, -ˈkär-\ *adj* : of, relating to, or joining the aorta and the coronary arteries ⟨∼ bypass surgery⟩

aor·to·fem·o·ral \-ˈfe-mə-rəl\ *adj* : of, relating to, or joining the abdominal aorta and the femoral arteries ⟨an ∼ bypass graft⟩

aor·to·gram \ā-ˈȯr-tə-ˌgram\ *n* : an X-ray picture of the aorta made by arteriography

aor·tog·ra·phy \ˌā-ˌȯr-ˈtä-grə-fē\ *n, pl* **-phies** : arteriography of the aorta — **aor·to·graph·ic** \(ˌ)ā-ˌȯr-tə-ˈgra-fik\ *adj*

aor·to·il·i·ac \ˌā-ˌȯr-tō-ˈi-lē-ˌak\ *adj* : of, relating to, or joining the abdominal aorta and the iliac arteries

aor·to·pul·mo·nary \ˌā-ˌȯr-tō-ˈpu̇l-mə-ˌner-ē, -ˈpəl-\ *adj* : of, relating to, or joining the aorta and the pulmonary artery ⟨an ∼ shunt⟩

aortopulmonary window *n* : a congenital circulatory defect in which there is direct communication between the aorta and the pulmonary artery — called also *aortopulmonary fenestration*

aor·to·sub·cla·vi·an \-ˌsəb-ˈklā-vē-ən\ *adj* : relating to or joining the aorta and the subclavian arteries

AOTA *abbr* American Occupational Therapy Association

ap- — see APO-

APA *abbr* **1** American Psychiatric Association **2** American Psychological Association

APAP *abbr* acetaminophen — used esp. when combined with a prescription drug ⟨hydrocodone/*APAP*⟩

apar·a·lyt·ic \ˌā-ˌpar-ə-ˈli-tik\ *adj* : not characterized by paralysis

ap·a·thet·ic \ˌa-pə-ˈthe-tik\ *adj* : having or showing little or no feeling or emotion — **ap·a·thet·i·cal·ly** \-ti-k(ə-)lē\ *adv*

ap·a·thy \ˈa-pə-thē\ *n, pl* **-thies** : lack of feeling or emotion

ap·a·tite \ˈa-pə-ˌtīt\ *n* : any of a group of calcium phosphate minerals comprising the chief constituent of bones and teeth; *specif* : calcium phosphate fluoride $Ca_5F(PO_4)_3$

APC \ˌā-ˌpē-ˈsē\ *n* : a tumor suppressor gene that in a defective form tends to be associated with a high risk of colorectal cancer

APC *abbr* **1** antigen-presenting cell **2** aspirin, phenacetin, and caffeine

ape·ri·ent \ə-ˈpir-ē-ənt\ *adj* : gently causing the bowels to move : LAXATIVE — **aperient** *n*

ape·ri·od·ic \ˌā-ˌpir-ē-ˈä-dik\ *adj* : of irregular occurrence

aperi·stal·sis \ˌā-ˌper-ə-ˈstȯl-səs, -ˈstäl-, -ˈstal-\ *n, pl* **-stal·ses** \-ˌsēz\ : absence of peristalsis

Apert syndrome \ä-ˈper-\ *also* **Apert's syndrome** *n* : a rare congenital condition in which premature closure of the cranial sutures results in malformation of the skull with characteristic facial features (as widely spaced eyes and a prominent forehead) and fusion and webbing of the toes and fingers — see ACROCEPHALOSYNDACTYLY

Apert, Eugène Charles (1868–1940), French pediatrician.

apex \ˈā-ˌpeks\ *n, pl* **apex·es** *or* **api·ces** \ˈā-pə-ˌsēz\ : a narrowed or pointed end of an anatomical structure: as **a** : the narrow somewhat conical upper part of a lung extending into the root **b** : the lower pointed end of the heart situated in humans opposite the space between the cartilages of the fifth and sixth ribs on the left side **c** : the extremity of the root of a tooth

apex·car·di·og·ra·phy \ˌā-ˌpeks-ˌkär-dē-ˈä-grə-fē\ *n, pl* **-phies** : a procedure for measuring the beat in the apex region of the heart by recording movements in the nearby wall of the chest

Ap•gar score \ˈap-ˌgär-\ *n* : an index used to evaluate the condition of a newborn infant based on a rating of 0, 1, or 2 for each of the five characteristics of color, heart rate, response to stimulation of the sole of the foot, muscle tone, and respiration with 10 being a perfect score

Apgar, Virginia (1909–1974), American physician.

aph- — see APO-

apha•gia \ə-ˈfā-jə, a-, -jē-ə\ *n* : loss of the ability to swallow

apha•kia \ə-ˈfā-kē-ə, a-\ *n* : absence of the crystalline lens of the eye; *also* : the resulting anomalous state of refraction

[1]**apha•kic** \ə-ˈfā-kik, a-\ *adj* : of, relating to, or affected with aphakia

[2]**aphakic** *n* : an individual who has had the lens of an eye removed

apha•sia \ə-ˈfā-zhə, -zhē-ə\ *n* : loss or impairment of the power to use or comprehend words usu. resulting from brain damage — see MOTOR APHASIA; compare ANARTHRIA

[1]**apha•sic** \ə-ˈfā-zik\ *adj* : of, relating to, or affected with aphasia

[2]**aphasic** *or* **apha•si•ac** \ə-ˈfā-zē-ˌak, -zhē-\ *n* : an individual affected with aphasia

apha•si•ol•o•gy \ə-ˈfā-zē-ˈä-lə-jē, -zhē-\ *n, pl* **-gies** : the study of aphasia — **apha•si•ol•o•gist** \-jist\ *n*

aphe•re•sis \ä-fə-ˈrē-səs\ *n, pl* **-re•ses** \-ˌsēz\ : withdrawal of blood from a donor's body, removal of one or more components (as plasma or white blood cells) from the blood, and transfusion of the remaining blood back into the donor — called also *pheresis;* see LEUKAPHERESIS, PLASMAPHERESIS, PLATELETPHERESIS

apho•nia \(ˌ)ā-ˈfō-nē-ə\ *n* : loss of voice and of all but whispered speech — **apho•nic** \-ˈfä-nik, -ˈfō-\ *adj*

aphos•pho•ro•sis \ˌā-ˌfäs-fə-ˈrō-səs\ *n, pl* **-ro•ses** \-ˌsēz\ : a deficiency disease esp. of cattle caused by inadequate intake of dietary phosphorus

[1]**aph•ro•di•si•ac** \ˌa-frə-ˈdē-zē-ˌak, -ˈdi-\ *also* **aph•ro•di•si•a•cal** \ˌa-frə-də-ˈzī-ə-kəl, -ˈsī-\ *adj* : exciting sexual desire

[2]**aphrodisiac** *n* : an aphrodisiac agent

aph•tha \ˈaf-thə\ *also* **ap•tha** \ˈap-\ *n, pl* **aph•thae** *also* **ap•thae** \-ˌthē\ : a blister or ulcer on a mucous membrane (as of the mouth or lip) — **aph•thous** \-thəs\ *adj*

aph•thoid \ˈaf-ˌthȯid\ *adj* : resembling thrush ⟨~ ulcers⟩

aphthous fever *n* : FOOT-AND-MOUTH DISEASE

aphthous stomatitis *n* : a very common disorder of the oral mucosa that is characterized by the formation of canker sores on movable mucous membranes and that has a multiple etiology but is not caused by the virus causing herpes simplex

apic- *or* **apici-** *or* **apico-** *comb form* : apex : tip esp. of an organ ⟨*apic*ectomy⟩

api•cal \ˈā-pi-kəl, ˈa-\ *adj* : of, relating to, or situated at an apex — **api•cal•ly** \-k(ə-)lē\ *adv*

apical foramen *n* : the opening of the pulp canal in the root of a tooth

apic•ec•to•my \ˌā-pə-ˈsek-tə-mē\ *n, pl* **-mies** : surgical removal of an anatomical apex (as of the root of a tooth)

apices *pl of* APEX

api•ci•tis \ˌā-pə-ˈsī-təs, ˌa-pə-\ *n, pl* **-ci•tes** \-ˈsī-ˌtēz\ : inflammation of the apex of an organ or anatomical part (as the lung or the root of a tooth): as **a** : inflammation and infection of the apex of the petrous portion of the temporal bone **b** : PATELLAR TENDINITIS

api•co•ec•to•my \ˌā-pi-(ˌ)kō-ˈek-tə-mē, ˌa-\ *n, pl* **-mies** : excision of the root tip of a tooth

api•ther•a•py \ˌā-pi-ˈther-ə-pē, ˌa-\ *n* : the use of substances produced by honeybees (such as venom or honey) to treat various medical conditions

apix•a•ban \ə-ˈpik-sə-ˌban\ *n* : an anticoagulant drug $C_{25}H_{25}N_5O_4$ that inhibits the activated form of factor X and is used to prevent or treat thromboembolic disease (as deep vein thrombosis) — see ELIQUIS

apla•sia \(ˌ)ā-ˈplā-zhə, -zhē-ə, ə-\ *n* : incomplete or faulty development of an organ or part — **aplas•tic** \-ˈplas-tik\ *adj*

aplastic anemia *n* : anemia that results from defective functioning of the bone marrow, is characterized esp. by headache, fatigue, paleness, fever, recurrent infections, bruising or rashes, and rapid or irregular heartbeat, and is often of unknown cause but may occur as a congenital or inherited condition (as in Fanconi's anemia) or be caused by exposure to toxic agents (as chemicals) or infection with pathogens (as hepatitis virus) — called also *hypoplastic anemia*

ap•nea \ˈap-nē-ə, ap-ˈnē \ *n* **1** : transient cessation of respiration; *esp* : SLEEP APNEA **2** : ASPHYXIA — **ap•ne•ic** \ap-ˈnē-ik\ *adj*

ap•neu•sis \ap-ˈnü-səs, -ˈnyü-\ *n, pl* **ap•neu•ses** \-ˌsēz\ : sustained tonic contraction of the respiratory muscles resulting in prolonged inspiration — **ap•neus•tic** \-ˈnü-stik, -ˈnyü-\ *adj*

ap•noea \ap-ˈnē-ə, ˈap-nē-\ *chiefly Brit var of* APNEA

apo \ˈa-ˌpō\ *n, often cap* : APOLIPOPROTEIN

apo- *or* **ap-** *or* **aph-** *prefix* : formed from : related to ⟨*apo*morphine⟩

apo•crine \ˈa-pə-krən, -ˌkrīn, -ˌkrēn\ *adj* : producing a fluid secretion by pinching off one end of the secreting cells which then reform and repeat the process; *also* : produced by an apocrine gland — compare ECCRINE, HOLOCRINE, MEROCRINE

apo•en•zyme \ˌa-pō-ˈen-ˌzīm\ *n* : a protein that forms an active enzyme system by combination with a coenzyme and determines the specificity of this system for a substrate

ap•o•fer•ri•tin \ˌa-pə-ˈfer-ət-ᵊn\ *n* : a protein capable of storing iron in bodily cells esp. of the liver

apo•li•po•pro•tein \ˌa-pə-ˌlī-pō-ˈprō-ˌtēn, -ˌli-\ *n* : any of the proteins that combine with a lipid (as cholesterol) to form a lipoprotein and are grouped into several classes designated by letters (as A or B) with specific class members typically identified with a number ⟨∼ B is a major component of LDL⟩ — called also *apo*

apo•mor•phine \ˌa-pə-ˈmȯr-ˌfēn\ *n* : a morphine derivative that is a dopamine agonist and is injected subcutaneously in the form of its hydrochloride $C_{17}H_{17}NO_2 \cdot HCl \cdot {}^1/_2H_2O$ to treat immobility associated with advanced Parkinson's disease

apo•neu•ro•sis \ˌa-pə-nu̇-ˈrō-səs, -nyu̇-\ *n, pl* **-ro•ses** \-ˌsēz\ : any of the broad flat sheets of dense fibrous collagenous connective tissue that cover, invest, and form the terminations and attachments of various muscles — **apo•neu•rot•ic** \-ˈrä-tik\ *adj*

aponeurotica — see GALEA APONEUROTICA

ap•o•phe•nia \ˌa-pə-ˈfē-nē-ə\ *n* : the tendency to perceive a connection or meaningful pattern between unrelated or random things (as objects or ideas) — compare PAREIDOLIA

apoph•y•sis \ə-ˈpä-fə-səs\ *n, pl* **-y•ses** \-ˌsēz\ : an expanded or projecting part esp. of an organism — **apoph•y•se•al** \-ˌpä-fə-ˈsē-əl\ *adj*

apoph•y•si•tis \ə-ˌpä-fə-ˈsī-təs\ *n* : inflammation of a bony outgrowth and esp. the area of active growth at the end of bone (as of the heel or shin) where a muscle or tendon attaches ⟨calcaneal ∼⟩

ap•o•plec•tic \ˌa-pə-ˈplek-tik\ *adj* **1** : of, relating to, or causing stroke **2** : affected with, inclined to, or showing symptoms of stroke — **ap•o•plec•ti•cal•ly** \-ti-k(ə-)lē\ *adv*

ap•o•plexy \ˈa-pə-ˌplek-sē\ *n, pl* **-plex•ies** **1** : STROKE **2** : copious hemorrhage into a cavity or into the substance of an organ ⟨abdominal ∼⟩

apo•pro•tein \ˌa-pə-ˈprō-ˌtēn\ *n* : a protein that combines with a prosthetic group to form a conjugated protein

ap•o•pto•sis \ˌa-pə-ˈtō-sis\ *n, pl* **-pto•ses** \-ˌsēz\ : a genetically directed process of cell self-destruction that is marked by the fragmentation of nuclear DNA and is a normal physiological process eliminating DNA-damaged, superfluous, or unwanted cells — called also *cell suicide, programmed cell death* — **ap•o•pto•tic** \-ˈtä-tik\ *adj*

ap•o•tem•no•phil•ia \ˌa-pə-ˌtem-nō-ˈfi-lē-ə, -ˈfē-\ *n* : an overwhelming or obsessive desire to have one or more healthy body parts and esp. a limb removed by amputation

apothecaries' measure *n* : a system of liquid units of measure used in compounding medical prescriptions that include the gallon, pint, fluid ounce, fluid dram, and minim

apothecaries' weight *n* : a system of weights used chiefly by pharmacists in compounding medical prescriptions that include the pound of 12 ounces, the dram of 60 grains, and the scruple

apoth•e•cary \ə-ˈpä-thə-ˌker-ē\ *n, pl* **-car•ies** **1** : a person who prepares and sells drugs or compounds for medicinal purposes : DRUGGIST, PHARMACIST **2** : PHARMACY 2a

ap•pa•ra•tus \ˌa-pə-ˈra-təs, -ˈrā-\ *n, pl* **-tus•es** *or* **-tus** : a group of anatomical or cytological parts functioning together — see GOLGI APPARATUS

append- *or* **appendo-** *or* **appendic-** *or* **appendico-** *comb form* : vermiform appendix ⟨*append*ectomy⟩

ap•pend•age \ə-ˈpen-dij\ *n* : a subordinate or derivative body part; *esp* : a limb or analogous part

ap•pen•dec•to•my \ˌa-pən-ˈdek-tə-mē\ *n, pl* **-mies** : surgical removal of the vermiform appendix

ap•pen•di•ceal \ə-ˌpen-də-ˈsē-əl\ *also* **ap•pen•di•cal** \ə-ˈpen-di-kəl\ *adj* : of, relating to, or involving the vermiform appendix ⟨∼ inflammation⟩

ap•pen•di•cec•to•my \ə-ˌpen-də-ˈsek-tə-mē\ *n, pl* **-mies** *Brit* : APPENDECTOMY

ap•pen•di•ces epi•ploi•cae \ə-ˈpen-də-ˌsēz-ˌe-pi-ˈplȯi-sē\ *n pl* : small peritoneal pouches filled with fat that are situated along the large intestine

ap•pen•di•ci•tis \ə-ˌpen-də-ˈsī-təs\ *n* : inflammation of the vermiform appendix

ap•pen•dic•u•lar \ˌa-pən-ˈdi-kyə-lər\ *adj* : of or relating to an appendage: **a** : of or relating to a limb or limbs ⟨the ∼ skeleton⟩ **b** : APPENDICEAL

ap•pen•dix \ə-ˈpen-diks\ *n, pl* **-dix•es** *or* **-di•ces** \-də-ˌsēz\ : a bodily outgrowth or process; *specif* : VERMIFORM APPENDIX

ap•per•ceive \ˌa-pər-ˈsēv\ *vb* **-ceived; -ceiv•ing** : to have apperception of

ap•per•cep•tion \ˌa-pər-ˈsep-shən\ *n* : mental perception; *esp* : the process of understanding something perceived in terms of previous experience — compare ASSIMILATION 3 — **ap•per•cep•tive** \-ˈsep-tiv\ *adj*

ap•pe•stat \ˈa-pə-ˌstat\ *n* : a hypothetical region in the hypothalamus that is thought to regulate appetite

ap•pe•tite \ˈa-pə-ˌtīt\ *n* : any of the instinctive desires necessary to keep up organic life; *esp* : the desire to eat — **ap•pe•ti•tive** \-ˌtī-tiv\ *adj*

ap•pla•na•tion \ˌa-plə-ˈnā-shən\ *n* : abnormal flattening of a convex surface (as of the cornea of the eye)

applanation tonometer *n* : an ophthalmologic instrument used to determine pressure by measuring the force necessary to flatten an area of the cornea with a small disk

ap·pli·ance \ə-ˈplī-əns\ *n* : an instrument or device designed for a particular use ⟨prosthetic ~*s*⟩

ap·pli·ca·tion \ˌa-plə-ˈkā-shən\ *n* **1** : an act of applying **2** : a medicated or protective layer or material

ap·pli·ca·tor \ˈa-plə-ˌkā-tər\ *n* : one that applies; *specif* : a device for applying a substance (as medicine)

applied behavior analysis *also* **applied behavioral analysis** *n* : psychological therapy that uses techniques (as operant conditioning) developed from the objective analysis of observable behavior to make changes to socially significant behaviors that are abnormal or harmful — abbr. *ABA*

applied kinesiology *n* : a diagnostic system that uses manual testing of the functional integrity of muscles to identify illness in other parts of the body — **applied kinesiologist** *n*

ap·ply \ə-ˈplī\ *vb* **ap·plied; ap·ply·ing** : to lay or spread on

ap·po·si·tion \ˌa-pə-ˈzi-shən\ *n* **1** : the placing of things in juxtaposition or proximity; *specif* : deposition of successive layers upon those already present — compare ACCRETION **2** : the state of being in juxtaposition or proximity (as in the drawing together of cut edges of tissue in healing) — **ap·pose** \a-ˈpōz\ *vb* — **ap·po·si·tion·al** \ˌa-pə-ˈzi-shə-nəl\ *adj*

ap·proach \ə-ˈprōch\ *n* : the surgical procedure by which access is gained to a bodily part

approach–approach conflict *n* : psychological conflict that results when a choice must be made between two desirable alternatives — compare APPROACH-AVOIDANCE CONFLICT, AVOIDANCE-AVOIDANCE CONFLICT

approach–avoidance conflict *n* : psychological conflict that results when a goal is both desirable and undesirable — compare APPROACH-APPROACH CONFLICT, AVOIDANCE-AVOIDANCE CONFLICT

ap·prox·i·mate \ə-ˈpräk-sə-ˌmāt\ *vb* **-mat·ed; -mat·ing** : to bring together ⟨~ cut edges of tissue⟩

aprax·ia \(ˌ)ā-ˈprak-sē-ə\ *n* : loss or impairment of the ability to execute complex coordinated movements without muscular or sensory impairment — **aprac·tic** \-ˈprak-tik\ *or* **aprax·ic** \-ˈprak-sik\ *adj*

aprep·i·tant \ə-ˈpre-pə-tənt\ *n* : an antiemetic drug $C_{23}H_{21}F_7N_4O_3$ taken orally to prevent nausea and vomiting associated with cancer chemotherapy or surgery — see EMEND

apro·ti·nin \ā-ˈprō-tə-nin\ *n* : a polypeptide used to reduce blood loss and preserve platelet function during heart surgery but now withdrawn from use due to safety concerns

APS *abbr* antiphospholipid syndrome; antiphospholipid antibody syndrome

APSAC \ˈap-ˌsak\ *n* : ANISTREPLASE

aptha *var of* APHTHA

ap·ti·tude \ˈap-tə-ˌtüd, -ˌtyüd\ *n* : a natural or acquired capacity or ability; *esp* : a tendency, capacity, or inclination to learn or understand

aptitude test *n* : a standardized test designed to predict an individual's ability to learn certain skills

apy·rex·ia \ˌā-ˌpī-ˈrek-sē-ə, ˌa-pə-ˈrek-\ *n* : absence or intermission of fever

aqua \ˈa-kwə, ˈä-\ *n, pl* **aquae** \ˈa-(ˌ)kwē, ˈä-ˌkwī\ *or* **aquas** : WATER; *esp* : an aqueous solution

aqua·gen·ic \ˌä-kwə-ˈje-nik, ˌa-\ *adj* : caused by water and esp. by contact with water ⟨~ urticaria⟩

aq·ue·duct \ˈa-kwə-ˌdəkt\ *n* : a canal or passage in a part or organ

aqueduct of Syl·vi·us \-ˈsil-vē-əs\ *n* : a channel connecting the third and fourth ventricles of the brain — called also *cerebral aqueduct*

Du·bois \dü̅-ˈbwä, dü-, dyü-\, **Jacques (*Latin* Jacobus Sylvius) (1478–1555)**, French anatomist.

[1]**aque·ous** \ˈā-kwē-əs, ˈa-\ *adj* **1 a** : of, relating to, or resembling water ⟨an ~ vapor⟩ **b** : made from, with, or by water ⟨an ~ solution⟩ **2** : of or relating to the aqueous humor

[2]**aqueous** *n* : AQUEOUS HUMOR

aqueous flare *n* : FLARE 3

aqueous humor *n* : a transparent fluid occupying the space between the crystalline lens and the cornea of the eye

Ar *symbol* argon

ara–A \ˌar-ə-ˈā\ *n* : VIDARABINE

arab·i·nose \ə-ˈra-bə-ˌnōs, -ˌnōz\ *n* : a white crystalline sugar $C_5H_{10}O_5$ occurring esp. in vegetable gums

ara·bi·no·side \ˌar-ə-ˈbi-nə-ˌsīd, ə-ˈra-bə-nō-ˌsīd\ *n* : a glycoside that yields arabinose on hydrolysis

Ara–C \ˌar-ə-ˈsē\ *n* : CYTOSINE ARABINOSIDE

ar·a·chi·don·ic acid \ˌar-ə-kə-ˈdä-nik-\ *n* : an unsaturated fatty acid $C_{20}H_{32}O_2$ that occurs in most animal fats, is a precursor of prostaglandins and leukotrienes, and is considered essential in nutrition

arachn- *or* **arachno-** *comb form* : spider ⟨*arachno*dactyly⟩

arach·nid \ə-ˈrak-nəd\ *n* : any of a large class of arthropods (Arachnida) including the spiders and scorpions, mites, and ticks and having a segmented body divided into two regions of which the anterior bears four pairs of legs but no antennae — **arach·nid** *adj*

arach·nid·ism \-nə-ˌdi-zəm\ *n* : poisoning caused by the bite or sting of an arachnid (as a spider, tick, or scorpion); *esp* : a syndrome marked by extreme pain and muscular rigidity due to the bite of a black widow spider

arach•no•dac•ty•ly \ə-ˌrak-nō-ˈdak-tə-lē\ *n, pl* **-lies** : a hereditary condition characterized esp. by excessive length of the fingers and toes
arach•noid \ə-ˈrak-ˌnȯid\ *n* : a thin membrane of the brain and spinal cord that lies between the dura mater and the pia mater — **arachnoid** *also* **arach•noi•dal** \ə-ˌrak-ˈnȯid-ᵊl\ *adj*
arachnoid granulation *n* : any of the small whitish processes that are enlarged villi of the arachnoid membrane of the brain which protrude into the superior sagittal sinus and into depressions in the neighboring bone — called also *arachnoid villus, pacchionian body*
arach•noid•itis \ə-ˌrak-ˌnȯi-ˈdī-təs\ *n* : inflammation of the arachnoid membrane
arach•no•pho•bia \ə-ˌrak-nə-ˈfō-bē-ə\ *n* : pathological fear or loathing of spiders — **arach•no•phobe** \ə-ˈrak-nə-ˌfōb\ *n* — **arach•no•pho•bic** \ə-ˌrak-nə-ˈfō-bik\ *adj or n*
Ara•nesp \ˈar-ə-ˌnesp\ *trademark* — used for a preparation of darbepoetin alfa
ARB *abbr* angiotensin receptor blocker
ar•bor \ˈär-bər\ *n* : a branching anatomical structure resembling a tree
ar•bo•ri•za•tion \ˌär-bə-rə-ˈzā-shən\ *n* : a treelike figure or arrangement of branching parts; *esp* : a treelike part or process (as a dendrite) of a nerve cell
ar•bo•rize \ˈär-bə-ˌrīz\ *vb* **-rized; -riz•ing** : to branch freely and repeatedly
ar•bo•vi•rus \ˌär-bə-ˈvī-rəs\ *n* : any of various RNA viruses (as the causative agents of Japanese B encephalitis, West Nile virus, yellow fever, and dengue) transmitted chiefly by arthropods — **ar•bo•vi•ral** \-rəl\ *adj*
ARC *abbr* **1** AIDS-related complex **2** American Red Cross
ar•cade \är-ˈkād\ *n* **1** : an anatomical structure comprising a series of arches **2** : DENTAL ARCH
arch \ˈärch\ *n* **1** : an anatomical structure that resembles an arch in form or function: as **a** : either of two vaulted portions of the bony structure of the foot that impart elasticity to it **b** : ARCH OF THE AORTA **2** : a fingerprint in which all the ridges run from side to side with no backward turn
arch- *or* **archi-** *prefix* : primitive : original : primary ⟨*arch*enteron⟩
arch•en•ter•on \är-ˈken-tə-ˌrän, -rən\ *n, pl* **-tera** \-tə-rə\ : the cavity of the gastrula of an embryo forming a primitive gut
ar•che•type \ˈär-ki-ˌtīp\ *n* : an inherited idea or mode of thought in the psychology of C. G. Jung that is present in the unconscious of the individual — **ar•che•typ•al** \ˌär-ki-ˈtī-pəl\ *adj*
ar•chi•pal•li•um \ˌär-ki-ˈpa-lē-əm\ *n* : the olfactory part of the cerebral cortex comprising the hippocampus and part of the parahippocampal gyrus — compare NEOPALLIUM
ar•chi•tec•ton•ics \-tek-ˈtä-niks\ *n sing or pl* : the structural arrangement or makeup of an anatomical part or system — **ar•chi•tec•ton•ic** \-nik\ *adj*
ar•chi•tec•ture \ˈär-kə-ˌtek-chər\ *n* : the basic structural form (as of a body part or molecule) — **ar•chi•tec•tur•al** \ˌär-kə-ˈtek-chə-rəl, -ˈtek-shrəl\ *adj* — **ar•chi•tec•tur•al•ly** *adv*
arch of the aorta *n* : the curved transverse part of the aorta that connects the ascending aorta with the descending aorta — called also *aortic arch*
ar•cu•ate \ˈär-kyə-wət, -ˌwāt\ *adj* : curved like a bow
arcuate artery *n* : any of several arteries that curve and arch: as **a** : any of the branches of an interlobar artery of the kidney that form arches over the base of the renal pyramids **b** : a branch of the dorsalis pedis artery of the foot that arches across the top of the middle of the foot and supplies blood esp. to the toes
arcuate ligament — see LATERAL ARCUATE LIGAMENT, MEDIAL ARCUATE LIGAMENT, MEDIAN ARCUATE LIGAMENT
arcuate nucleus *n* : any of several cellular masses in the thalamus, hypothalamus, or medulla oblongata
arcuate popliteal ligament *n* : a triangular ligamentous band in the posterior part of the knee that passes medially downward from the lateral condyle of the femur to the area between the condyles of the tibia and to the head of the fibula — compare OBLIQUE POPLITEAL LIGAMENT
arcuate vein *n* : any of the veins of the kidney that accompany the arcuate arteries, drain blood from the interlobular veins, and empty into the interlobar veins
ar•cus \ˈär-kəs\ *n, pl* **arcus** : an anatomical arch
arcus se•nil•is \-sə-ˈni-ləs\ *n* : a whitish ring-shaped or bow-shaped deposit in the cornea that frequently occurs in old age
ARDS *abbr* acute respiratory distress syndrome; adult respiratory distress syndrome
ar•ea \ˈar-ē-ə\ *n* : a part of the cerebral cortex having a particular function — see ASSOCIATION AREA, MOTOR AREA, SENSORY AREA
area po•stre•ma \-pōs-ˈtrē-mə, -päs-\ *n* : a tongue-shaped structure in the caudal region of the fourth ventricle of the brain
areata — see ALOPECIA AREATA
arec•o•line \ə-ˈre-kə-ˌlēn\ *n* : a toxic parasympathomimetic alkaloid $C_8H_{13}NO_2$ obtained from betel nuts and used as a veterinary anthelmintic
are•flex•ia \ˌā-ri-ˈflek-sē-ə\ *n* : absence of reflexes — **are•flex•ic** \-ˈflek-sik\ *adj*
ar•e•na•vi•rus \ˌar-ə-nə-ˈvī-rəs\ *n* **1** *cap* : a genus of single-stranded RNA vi-

ruses (family *Arenaviridae*) having dense lipid envelope on the virion covered by club-shaped projections and including the Machupo virus, the Junin virus, and the viruses causing lymphocytic choriomeningitis and Lassa fever **2** : any virus of the genus *Arenavirus* or of the family (*Arenaviridae*) to which it belongs

are•o•la \ə-ˈrē-ə-lə\ *n, pl* **-lae** \-ˌlē\ *or* **-las** **1** : the colored ring around the nipple or around a vesicle or pustule **2** : the portion of the iris that borders the pupil of the eye

are•o•lar \-lər\ *adj* **1** : of, relating to, or like an areola **2** : of, relating to, or consisting of areolar tissue

areolar tissue *n* : fibrous connective tissue having the fibers loosely arranged in a net or meshwork

Ar•gas \ˈär-gəs, -ˌgas\ *n* : a genus of ticks (family Argasidae) including the fowl ticks (as *A. persicus*)

argent- *or* **argenti-** *or* **argento-** *comb form* : silver ⟨*argento*phil⟩

ar•gen•taf•fin cell \är-ˈjen-tə-fən-\ *or* **ar•gen•taf•fine cell** \-fən-, -ˌfēn-\ *n* : any of various specialized epithelial cells of the gastrointestinal tract that stain readily with silver salts

ar•gen•to•philic \är-ˌjen-tə-ˈfi-lik\ *also* **ar•gen•to•phil** \-ˈjen-tə-ˌfil\ *or* **ar•gen•to•phile** \-ˌfīl\ *adj* : ARGYROPHILIC

ar•gi•nine \ˈär-jə-ˌnēn\ *n* : a crystalline basic amino acid $C_6H_{14}N_4O_2$ derived from guanidine

arginine vasopressin *n* : vasopressin in which the eighth amino acid residue in its polypeptide chain is an arginine residue — abbr. *AVP*

ar•gon \ˈär-ˌgän\ *n* : a colorless odorless inert gaseous element — symbol *Ar;* see ELEMENT table

Ar•gyll Rob•ert•son pupil \ˈär-gīl-ˈrä-bərt-sən-, är-ˈgīl-\ *n* : a pupil characteristic of neurosyphilis that fails to react to light but still reacts in accommodation to distance

Robertson, Douglas Argyll (1837–1909), British ophthalmologist.

argyr- *or* **argyro-** *comb form* : silver ⟨*argyr*ia⟩

ar•gyr•ia \är-ˈjir-ē-ə\ *n* : dark discoloration of skin caused by overuse of medicinal silver preparations

Ar•gy•rol \ˈär-jə-ˌrȯl, -ˌrōl\ *trademark* — used for a silver-protein compound whose aqueous solution is used as a topical antiseptic

ar•gyr•o•phil•ic \ˌär-jə-(ˌ)rō-ˈfi-lik, -rə-\ *also* **ar•gyr•o•phil** \ˌär-jə-(ˌ)rō-ˌfil, -rə-\ *or* **ar•gyr•o•phile** \-ˌfīl\ *adj* : having an affinity for silver ⟨∼ cells⟩

ari•bo•fla•vin•osis \ˌā-ˌrī-bə-ˌflā-və-ˈnō-səs\ *n, pl* **-oses** \-ˌsēz\ : a deficiency disease due to inadequate intake of riboflavin and characterized by sores on the mouth

Ar•i•cept \ˈar-ə-ˌsept\ *trademark* — used for a preparation of the hydrochloride of donepezil

Arim•i•dex \ə-ˈri-mə-ˌdeks\ *trademark* — used for a preparation of anastrozole

ar•i•pip•ra•zole \ˌa-rə-ˈpi-prə-ˌzōl, -ˌzȯl\ *n* : an antipsychotic drug $C_{23}H_{27}Cl_2N_3O_2$ used in the treatment of schizophrenia, bipolar disorder, major depressive disorder, and irritability associated with autism — see ABILIFY

arith•mo•ma•nia \ə-ˌrith-mō-ˈmā-nē-ə, -nyə\ *n* : an abnormal compulsion to count objects or actions and make mathematical calculations

-ar•i•um \ˈar-ē-əm\ *n suffix, pl* **-ariums** *or* **-ar•ia** \-ē-ə\ : thing or place belonging to or connected with ⟨sanit*arium*⟩

arm \ˈärm\ *n* **1** : a human upper limb; *esp* : the part between the shoulder and the wrist **2 a** : the forelimb of a vertebrate other than a human being **b** : a limb of an invertebrate animal **c** : any of the usu. two parts of a chromosome lateral to the centromere — **armed** \ˈärmd\ *adj*

ar•ma•men•tar•i•um \ˌär-mə-ˌmen-ˈter-ē-əm, -mən-\ *n, pl* **-tar•ia** \-ē-ə\ : the equipment, methods, and pharmaceuticals used in medicine

arm lift *n* : BRACHIOPLASTY

arm•pit \ˈärm-ˌpit\ *n* : the hollow beneath the junction of the arm and shoulder : AXILLA

Ar•nold–Chi•ari malformation \ˈär-nᵊld-kē-ˈär-ē-\ *n* : a congenital abnormality that is a type of Chiari malformation in which the lower surface of the cerebellum and the lower brain stem protrude into the spinal canal through the foramen magnum

Arnold, Julius (1835–1915), German pathologist.

H. Chiari — see CHIARI MALFORMATION

Aro•ma•sin \ə-ˈrō-mə-ˌsin\ *trademark* — used for a preparation of exemestane

aro•ma•tase \ə-ˈrō-mə-ˌtās, -ˌtāz\ *n* : an enzyme or complex of enzymes that promotes the conversion of an androgen into estrogen

aromatase inhibitor *n* : any of a class of drugs (as anastrozole) that suppress the synthesis of estrogen in the body by inhibiting the action of aromatase and are used to treat breast cancer in postmenopausal women

aro•ma•ther•a•py \ə-ˌrō-mə-ˈther-ə-pē\ *n, pl* **-pies** : inhalation or bodily application (as by massage) of fragrant essential oils (as from flowers and fruits) for therapeutic purposes; *broadly* : the use of aroma to enhance a feeling of well-being — **aro•ma•ther•a•pist** \-pist\ *n*

arous•al \ə-ˈrau̇-zəl\ *n* **1 a** : the act of arousing ⟨∼ from sleep⟩ **b** : the state of being aroused; *specif* : responsiveness to stimuli **2** : a state of physiological and psychological excitation caused by sexual contact or other erotic stimulation

arouse \ə-ˈrau̇z\ *vb* **aroused; arousing** **1 a** : to awake from sleep **b** : to rouse or stimulate to action **2** : to excite sexually : to cause sexual arousal in — **arous•able** \ə-ˈrau̇-zə-bəl\ *adj*

ar•rec•tor pi•li muscle \ə-ˈrek-tər-ˈpī-ˌlī-, -ˈpi-lē-\ *n* : one of the small fan-shaped smooth muscles associated with the base of each hair that contract when the body surface is chilled and erect the hairs, compress an oil gland above each muscle, and produce the appearance of goose bumps

[1]**ar•rest** \ə-ˈrest\ *vb* : to bring to a standstill or state of inactivity

[2]**arrest** *n* : the condition of being stopped — see CARDIAC ARREST

ar•rhe•no•blas•to•ma \ˌar-ə-ˌnō-ˌbla-ˈstō-mə, ə-ˌrē-ˌnō-\ *n, pl* **-mas** *also* **-ma•ta** \-mə-tə\ : a sometimes malignant tumor of the ovary that by the secretion of male hormone induces development of secondary male characteristics — compare GYNANDROBLASTOMA

ar•rhyth•mia \ā-ˈrit͟h-mē-ə\ *n* : an alteration in rhythm of the heartbeat either in time or force

ar•rhyth•mic \-mik\ *adj* **1** : lacking rhythm or regularity **2** : of, relating to, characterized by, or resulting from arrhythmia ⟨~ death⟩

ar•rhyth•mo•gen•ic \(ˈ)ā-ˌrit͟h-mə-ˈjenik, (ˈ)a- *also* -ˌrith-\ *adj* : producing or tending to produce cardiac arrhythmia

arrhythmogenic right ventricular dysplasia *n* : a disease of the heart that is characterized by replacement of the muscle of the right ventricle by fatty and fibrous tissue which typically results in arrhythmias and that is often inherited as an autosomal dominant trait

ARRT *abbr* **1** American registered respiratory therapist **2** American Registry of Radiologic Technologists

ars- *comb form* : arsenic ⟨*ars*ine⟩

ar•se•nate \ˈär-sə-nət, -ˌnāt\ *n* : a salt or ester of an arsenic acid

ar•se•nic \ˈär-sə-nik\ *n* **1** : a solid poisonous element that is commonly metallic steel-gray, crystalline, and brittle — symbol *As;* see ELEMENT table **2** : ARSENIC TRIOXIDE

ar•sen•ic acid \är-ˈse-nik-\ *n* : any of three arsenic-containing acids that are analogous to the phosphoric acids

[1]**ar•sen•i•cal** \är-ˈse-ni-kəl\ *adj* : of, relating to, containing, or caused by arsenic ⟨~ poisoning⟩

[2]**arsenical** *n* : a compound or preparation containing arsenic

arsenic trioxide *n* : a poisonous trioxide of arsenic As_2O_3 or As_4O_6 that is used as a rodenticide and weed killer and is used in medicine to treat some forms of leukemia — called also *arsenic*

ar•sen•i•cum album \är-ˈse-ni-kəm-ˈal-bəm\ *n* : a preparation of arsenic trioxide used in homeopathy — called also *arsenicum*

ar•sine \är-ˈsēn, ˈär-ˌ\ *n* : a colorless flammable extremely poisonous gas AsH_3 with an odor like garlic

ars•phen•a•mine \ärs-ˈfe-nə-ˌmēn, -mən\ *n* : a toxic powder $C_{12}Cl_2H_{14}As_2N_2O_2{\cdot}2H_2O$ formerly used in the treatment esp. of syphilis and yaws — called also *salvarsan, six-o-six*

ART *abbr* **1** accredited record technician **2** assisted reproductive technology

ar•te•fact *chiefly Brit var of* ARTIFACT

ar•tem•e•ther \är-ˈte-mə-t͟hər\ *n* : an antimalarial drug $C_{16}H_{26}O_5$ that is a water-insoluble derivative of artemisinin administered by intramuscular injection or taken orally in tablets usu. in combination with lumefantrine — see COARTEM

ar•te•mis•i•nin \ˌär-tə-ˈmi-sᵊn-ən\ *n* : an antimalarial drug $C_{15}H_{22}O_5$ that is obtained from the leaves of a Chinese herb (*Artemisia annua*) or is made synthetically and is typically administered with other antimalarial agents (as mefloquine or amodiaquine) — see ARTEMETHER, ARTESUNATE

arteri- *or* **arterio-** *comb form* **1** : artery ⟨*arterio*graphy⟩ **2** : arterial and ⟨*arterio*venous⟩

ar•te•ria \är-ˈtir-ē-ə\ *n, pl* **-ri•ae** \-ē-ˌē\ : ARTERY

ar•te•ri•al \är-ˈtir-ē-əl\ *adj* **1** : of or relating to an artery **2** : relating to or being the bright red blood present in most arteries that has been oxygenated in lungs or gills — compare VENOUS 3 — **ar•te•ri•al•ly** *adv*

ar•te•rio•gram \är-ˈtir-ē-ə-ˌgram\ *n* : a radiograph of an artery made by arteriography

ar•te•ri•og•ra•phy \är-ˌtir-ē-ˈä-grə-fē\ *n, pl* **-phies** : the radiographic visualization of an artery after injection of a radiopaque substance — **ar•te•ri•o•graph•ic** \-ē-ə-ˈgra-fik\ *adj* — **ar•te•rio•graph•i•cal•ly** \-fi-k(ə-)lē\ *adv*

ar•te•ri•o•la \är-ˌtir-ē-ˈō-lə\ *n, pl* **-lae** \-ˌlē\ : ARTERIOLE

ar•te•ri•ole \är-ˈtir-ē-ˌōl\ *n* : any of the small terminal twigs of an artery that ends in capillaries — **ar•te•ri•o•lar** \-ˌtir-ē-ˈō-ˌlär, -lər\ *adj*

ar•te•rio•li•tis \är-ˌtir-ē-ō-ˈlī-təs\ *n* : inflammation of the arterioles

ar•te•rio•lu•mi•nal \är-ˌtir-ē-ō-ˈlü-mən-ᵊl\ *adj* : relating to or being the small vessels that branch from the arterioles of the heart and empty directly into its lumen

ar•te•ri•op•a•thy \är-ˌtir-ē-ˈä-pə-thē\ *n, pl* **-thies** : a disease of the arteries

ar•te•ri•or•rha•phy \är-ˌtir-ē-ˈór-ə-fē\ *n, pl* **-phies** : a surgical operation of suturing an artery

ar•te•rio•scle•ro•sis \är-ˌtir-ē-ō-sklə-ˈrō-səs\ *n, pl* **-ro•ses** \-ˌsēz\ : a chronic disease characterized by abnormal thickening and hardening of the arterial walls with resulting loss of elasticity — see ATHEROSCLEROSIS

arteriosclerosis ob•lit•e•rans \-ä-ˈbli-tə-ˌranz\ *n* : chronic arteriosclerosis marked by occlusion of arteries and esp. those supplying the extremities

[1]**ar·te·rio·scle·rot·ic** \-ˈrä-tik\ *adj* : of, relating to, or affected with arteriosclerosis

[2]**arteriosclerotic** *n* : an arteriosclerotic individual

arteriosi — see CONUS ARTERIOSUS

ar·te·rio·si·nu·soi·dal \är-ˌtir-ē-ō-ˌsī-nyə-ˈsȯid-ᵊl, -nə-\ *adj* : relating to or being the vessels that connect the arterioles and sinusoids of the heart

ar·te·rio·spasm \är-ˈtir-ē-ō-ˌspa-zəm\ *n* : spasm of an artery — **ar·te·ri·o·spas·tic** \-ˌtir-ē-ō-ˈspas-tik\ *adj*

arteriosum — see LIGAMENTUM ARTERIOSUM

arteriosus — see CONUS ARTERIOSUS, DUCTUS ARTERIOSUS, PATENT DUCTUS ARTERIOSUS

ar·te·ri·ot·o·my \är-ˌtir-ē-ˈä-tə-mē\ *n, pl* **-mies** : the surgical incision of an artery

ar·te·rio·ve·nous \är-ˌtir-ē-ō-ˈvē-nəs\ *adj* : of, relating to, or connecting the arteries and veins ⟨~ anastomoses⟩

ar·ter·i·tis \ˌär-tə-ˈrī-təs\ *n* : arterial inflammation — see GIANT CELL ARTERITIS — **ar·ter·it·ic** \-ˈri-tik\ *adj*

ar·tery \ˈär-tə-rē\ *n, pl* **-ter·ies** : any of the tubular branching muscular- and elastic-walled vessels that carry blood from the heart through the body

ar·tes·u·nate \är-ˈte-zə-ˌnāt\ *n* : an antimalarial drug $C_{19}H_{28}O_8$ that is a water-soluble derivative of artemisinin taken orally or administered by intramuscular or intravenous injection

arthr- *or* **arthro-** *comb form* : joint ⟨*arthr*algia⟩ ⟨*arthro*pathy⟩

ar·thral·gia \är-ˈthral-jə, -jē-ə\ *n* : pain in one or more joints — **ar·thral·gic** \-jik\ *adj*

ar·threc·to·my \är-ˈthrek-tə-mē\ *n, pl* **-mies** : surgical excision of a joint

[1]**ar·thrit·ic** \är-ˈthri-tik\ *adj* : of, relating to, or affected with arthritis — **ar·thrit·i·cal·ly** \-ti-k(ə-)lē\ *adv*

[2]**arthritic** *n* : a person affected with arthritis

ar·thri·tis \är-ˈthrī-təs\ *n, pl* **-thrit·i·des** \-ˈthri-tə-ˌdēz\ : inflammation of joints due to infectious, metabolic, or constitutional causes; *also* : a specific arthritic condition (as gouty arthritis or psoriatic arthritis)

arthritis de·for·mans \-dē-ˈfȯr-ˌmanz\ *n* : a chronic arthritis marked by deformation of affected joints

ar·thro·cen·te·sis \ˌär-(ˌ)thrō-sen-ˈtē-səs\ *n, pl* **-te·ses** \-ˌsēz\ : surgical puncture of a joint esp. for aspiration of fluid

ar·throd·e·sis \är-ˈthrä-də-səs\ *n, pl* **-e·ses** \-ˌsēz\ : the surgical immobilization of a joint so that the bones grow solidly together : artificial ankylosis

ar·thro·dia \är-ˈthrō-dē-ə\ *n, pl* **-di·ae** \-dē-ˌē\ : GLIDING JOINT

ar·thro·dys·pla·sia \ˌär-(ˌ)thrō-dis-ˈplā-zhə, -zhē-ə, -zē-ə\ *n* : abnormal development of a joint

ar·thro·gram \ˈär-thrō-ˌgram\ *n* : a radiograph of a joint made by arthrography

ar·throg·ra·phy \är-ˈthrä-grə-fē\ *n, pl* **-phies** : the radiographic visualization of a joint after the injection of a radiopaque substance — **ar·thro·graph·ic** \ˌär-thrə-ˈgra-fik\ *adj*

ar·thro·gry·po·sis \ˌär-(ˌ)thrō-gri-ˈpō-səs\ *n* **1** : congenital fixation of a joint in an extended or flexed position **2** : any of a group of congenital conditions characterized by reduced mobility of multiple joints due to contractures causing fixation of the joints in extension or flexion — **ar·thro·gry·pot·ic** \ˌär-(ˌ)thrō-gri-ˈpä-tik\ *adj*

arthrogryposis mul·ti·plex con·gen·i·ta \-ˈməl-tə-ˌpleks-kən-ˈje-nə-tə\ *n* : ARTHROGRYPOSIS 2

ar·throl·o·gy \är-ˈthrä-lə-jē\ *n, pl* **-gies** : a science concerned with the study of joints

ar·throp·a·thy \är-ˈthrä-pə-thē\ *n, pl* **-thies** : a disease of a joint — **ar·thro·path·ic** \ˌär-thrə-ˈpa-thik\ *adj*

ar·thro·plas·ty \ˈär-thrə-ˌplas-tē\ *n, pl* **-ties** : plastic surgery of a joint : the operative formation or restoration of a joint

ar·thro·pod \ˈär-thrə-ˌpäd\ *n* : any of a phylum (Arthropoda) of invertebrate animals (as insects or arachnids) that have a segmented body and jointed appendages and usu. a shell of chitin — **arthropod** *adj* — **ar·throp·o·dan** \är-ˈthrä-pəd-ᵊn\ *adj*

ar·thro·scope \ˈär-thrə-ˌskōp\ *n* : an endoscope inserted through an incision near a joint (as the knee) and used to visually examine, diagnose, and treat the interior of a joint

ar·thros·co·py \är-ˈthrä-skə-pē\ *n, pl* **-pies** : a minimally invasive surgical procedure involving visual examination of the interior of a joint with an arthroscope to diagnose or treat various conditions or injuries of a joint esp. to repair or remove damaged or diseased tissue or bone — **ar·thro·scop·ic** \ˌär-thrə-ˈskä-pik\ *adj* — **ar·thro·scop·ic·al·ly** \-pi-k(ə-)lē\ *adv*

ar·thro·sis \är-ˈthrō-səs\ *n, pl* **-thro·ses** \-ˌsēz\ **1** : an articulation or line of juncture between bones **2** : a degenerative disease of a joint

ar·throt·o·my \är-ˈthrä-tə-mē\ *n, pl* **-mies** : incision into a joint

Ar·thus reaction \ˈär-thəs-, ȧr-ˈtües-\ *n* : a hypersensitivity reaction that occurs several hours to days following injection of a vaccine and is marked by the formation of antigen-antibody complexes accompanied by localized inflammation, pain, redness, and sometimes tissue destruction

Arthus, Nicolas Maurice (1862–1945), French bacteriologist and physiologist.

ar·tic·u·lar \är-ˈti-kyə-lər\ *adj* : of or relating to a joint

articular capsule *n* : JOINT CAPSULE

articular cartilage *n* : cartilage that covers the articular surfaces of bones

articular disk *n* : a cartilage interposed between two articular surfaces and partially or completely separating the joint cavity into two compartments

articular process *n* : either of two processes on each side of a vertebra that articulate with adjoining vertebrae: **a** : one on each side of the neural arch that projects upward and articulates with an inferior articular process of the next more cranial vertebra — called also *superior articular process* **b** : one on each side of the neural arch that projects downward and articulates with a superior articular process of the next more caudal vertebra — called also *inferior articular process*

ar·tic·u·late \är-ˈti-kyə-ˌlāt\ *vb* **-lat·ed; -lat·ing** **1** : to unite or be united by means of a joint ⟨bones that ~ with each other⟩ **2** : to arrange (artificial teeth) on an articulator

ar·tic·u·la·tion \är-ˌti-kyə-ˈlā-shən\ *n* **1** : the action or manner in which the parts come together at a joint **2 a** : a joint between bones or cartilages in the vertebrate skeleton that is immovable when the bones are directly united, slightly movable when they are united by an intervening substance, or more or less freely movable when the articular surfaces are covered with smooth cartilage and surrounded by a joint capsule — see AMPHIARTHROSIS, DIARTHROSIS, SYNARTHROSIS **b** : a movable joint between rigid parts of any animal (as between the segments of an insect appendage) **3 a** (1) : the act of properly arranging artificial teeth (2) : an arrangement of artificial teeth **b** : OCCLUSION 2a

ar·tic·u·la·tor \är-ˈti-kyə-ˌlā-tər\ *n* : an apparatus used in dentistry for obtaining correct articulation of artificial teeth

ar·tic·u·la·to·ry \är-ˈti-kyə-lə-ˌtōr-ē\ *adj* : of or relating to articulation

ar·ti·fact \ˈär-tə-ˌfakt\ *n* **1** : a product of artificial character due to usu. extraneous (as human) agency; *specif* : a product or formation in a microscopic preparation of a fixed tissue or cell that is caused by manipulation or reagents and is not indicative of actual structural relationships **2** : an electrocardiographic and electroencephalographic wave that arises from sources other than the heart or brain — **ar·ti·fac·tu·al** \ˌär-tə-ˈfak-chə-wəl, -shə-wəl\ *adj*

ar·ti·fi·cial \ˌär-tə-ˈfi-shəl\ *adj* : humanly contrived often on a natural model ⟨an ~ limb⟩ — **ar·ti·fi·cial·ly** *adv*

artificial insemination *n* : introduction of semen into part of the female reproductive tract (as the cervical opening, uterus, or fallopian tube) by other than natural means — abbr. *AI;* called also *alternative insemination*

artificial kidney *n* : an apparatus designed to do the work of the kidney during temporary stoppage of kidney function — called also *hemodialyzer*

artificial respiration *n* : the process of restoring or initiating breathing by forcing air into and out of the lungs to establish the rhythm of inspiration and expiration — see MOUTH-TO-MOUTH

art therapy *n* : therapy based on engagement in artistic activities (as painting or drawing) as a means of creative expression and symbolic communication esp. in individuals affected with a mental or emotional disorder or cognitive impairment — **art therapist** *n*

ARV *abbr* antiretroviral

ary·ep·i·glot·tic \ˌar-ē-ˌe-pə-ˈglä-tik\ *adj* : relating to or linking the arytenoid cartilage and the epiglottis ⟨~ folds⟩

¹ary·te·noid \ˌar-ə-ˈtē-ˌnȯid, ə-ˈrit-ᵊn-ˌȯid\ *adj* **1** : relating to or being either of two small cartilages to which the vocal cords are attached and which are situated at the upper back part of the larynx **2** : relating to or being either of a pair of small muscles or an unpaired muscle of the larynx

²arytenoid *n* : an arytenoid cartilage or muscle

ary·te·noi·dec·to·my \ˌar-ə-ˌtē-ˌnȯi-ˈdek-tə-mē, ə-ˌrit-ᵊn-ˌȯi-\ *n, pl* **-mies** : surgical excision of an arytenoid cartilage

ary·te·noi·do·pexy \ˌar-ə-tə-ˈnȯi-də-ˌpek-sē, ə-ˌrit-ᵊn-ˈȯid-\ *n, pl* **-pex·ies** : surgical fixation of arytenoid muscles or cartilages

As *symbol* arsenic

AS *abbr* **1** ankylosing spondylitis **2** aortic stenosis **3** arteriosclerosis **4** [Latin *auris sinistra*] left ear — used esp. in audiology and in writing medical prescriptions

ASA *abbr* [*a*cetyl*s*alicylic *a*cid] aspirin

asa·fet·i·da *or* **asa·foet·i·da** \ˌa-sə-ˈfi-tə-dē, -ˈfe-tə-də\ *n* : the fetid gum resin of an Asian plant (*Ferula assa-foetida*) of the carrot family (Umbelliferae) used as an herbal remedy (as in the treatment of asthma, whooping cough, and flatulence)

as·bes·tos \as-ˈbes-təs, az-\ *n* : any of several minerals that readily separate into long flexible fibers, that cause asbestosis and have been implicated as causes of certain cancers, and that have been used esp. formerly as fireproof insulating materials

as·bes·to·sis \ˌas-ˌbes-ˈtō-səs, ˌaz-\ *n, pl* **-to·ses** \-ˌsēz\ : a pneumoconiosis due to asbestos particles that is marked by fibrosis and scarring of lung tissue

as·ca·ri·a·sis \ˌas-kə-ˈrī-ə-səs\ *n, pl* **-a·ses** \-ˌsēz\ : infestation with or disease caused by ascarids

as·car·i·cid·al \ə-ˌskar-ə-ˈsīd-ᵊl\ *adj* : capable of destroying ascarids

as•car•i•cide \ə-ˈskar-ə-ˌsīd\ *n* : an agent destructive of ascarids

as•ca•rid \ˈas-kə-rəd\ *n* : any of a family (Ascaridae) of nematode worms that are usu. parasitic in the intestines of vertebrates — see ASCARIDIA, ASCARIS — **ascarid** *adj*

As•ca•rid•ia \ˌas-kə-ˈri-dē-ə\ *n* : a genus of ascarid nematode worms that include an important intestinal parasite (*A. galli*) of some domestic fowl

as•car•i•di•a•sis \ə-ˌskar-ə-ˈdī-ə-səs\ *n, pl* **-a•ses** : ASCARIASIS

as•car•i•do•sis \ə-ˌskar-ə-ˈdō-səs\ *n, pl* **-do•ses** \-ˌsēz\ : ASCARIASIS

as•ca•ris \ˈas-kə-rəs\ *n* **1** *cap* : a genus of ascarid nematode worms that resemble earthworms in size and superficial appearance and include one (*A. lumbricoides*) parasitic in the human intestine **2** *pl* **as•car•i•des** \ə-ˈskar-ə-ˌdēz\ : ASCARID

As•ca•rops \ˈas-kə-ˌräps\ *n* : a genus of nematode worms (family Spiruridae) including a common stomach worm (*A. strongylina*) of swine

as•cend \ə-ˈsend\ *vb* : to move upward: as **a** : to conduct nerve impulses toward or to the brain **b** : to affect the extremities and esp. the lower limbs first and then the central nervous system

ascending aorta *n* : the part of the aorta from its origin to the beginning of the arch

ascending colon *n* : the part of the large intestine that extends from the cecum to the bend on the right side below the liver — compare DESCENDING COLON, TRANSVERSE COLON

ascending lumbar vein *n* : a longitudinal vein on each side that connects the lumbar veins and is frequently the origin of the azygos vein on the right side and of the hemiazygos vein on the left

ascending palatine artery *n* : PALATINE ARTERY 1a

Asch•heim–Zon•dek test \ˈäsh-ˌhīm-ˈzän-dik-, -ˈtsän-\ *n* : a test formerly used esp. to determine human pregnancy in its early stages on the basis of the effect of a subcutaneous injection of the patient's urine on the ovaries of an immature female mouse

Asch•heim \ˈäsh-ˌhīm\, **Selmor Samuel (1878–1965)**, and **Zon•dek** \ˈtsȯn-ˌdek\, **Bernhard (1891–1966)**, German obstetrician-gynecologists.

Asch•off body \ˈä-ˌshȯf-\ *n* : one of the small nodules in heart muscle typical of rheumatic heart disease; *also* : one of the similar but larger nodules found under the skin esp. in rheumatic fever or polyarthritis — called also *Aschoff nodule*

Aschoff, Karl Albert Ludwig (1866–1942), German pathologist.

as•ci•tes \ə-ˈsī-tēz\ *n, pl* **ascites** : abnormal accumulation of serous fluid in the spaces between tissues and organs in the cavity of the abdomen — **as•cit•ic** \-ˈsi-tik\ *adj*

as•co•my•cete \ˌas-kō-ˈmī-ˌsēt, -ˌmī-ˈsēt\ *n* : any of a group (as class Ascomycetes or subdivision Ascomycotina) of fungi (as yeasts or molds) with spores formed in asci — **as•co•my•ce•tous** \-ˌmī-ˈsē-təs\ *adj*

ascor•bate \ə-ˈskȯr-ˌbāt, -bət\ *n* : a salt of ascorbic acid

ascor•bic acid \ə-ˈskȯr-bik-\ *n* : VITAMIN C

ASCP *abbr* American Society of Clinical Pathologists

as•cus \ˈas-kəs\ *n, pl* **as•ci** \ˈas-ˌkī, -ˌkē; ˈa-ˌsī\ : the membranous oval or tubular spore case of an ascomycete

ASCUS *abbr* atypical squamous cells of undetermined significance

ASCVD *abbr* arteriosclerotic cardiovascular disease

ASD *abbr* autism spectrum disorder

-ase *n suffix* : enzyme ⟨prote*ase*⟩

asep•sis \(ˌ)ā-ˈsep-səs, ə-\ *n, pl* **asep•ses** \-ˌsēz\ **1** : the condition of being aseptic **2** : the methods of producing or maintaining an aseptic condition

asep•tic \-ˈsep-tik\ *adj* **1** : preventing or not involving infection ⟨~ techniques⟩ **2** : free or freed from pathogenic microorganisms ⟨an ~ wound⟩ ⟨an ~ operating room⟩ — **asep•ti•cal•ly** \-ti-k(ə-)lē\ *adv*

aseptic meningitis *n* : meningitis not caused by a bacterial infection that is of the milder type typically caused by any of numerous viruses

aseptic necrosis *n* : AVASCULAR NECROSIS

asex•u•al \(ˌ)ā-ˈsek-shə-wəl\ *adj* **1** : lacking sex or functional sexual organs ⟨~ plants⟩ **2** : produced without sexual action or differentiation ⟨~ spores⟩ **3** : devoid of sexuality ⟨an ~ relationship⟩ — **asex•u•al•ly** *adv*

asexual generation *n* : a generation that reproduces only by asexual processes — used of organisms exhibiting alternation of a sexual and an asexual generation

asexual reproduction *n* : reproduction (as spore formation, fission, or budding) without union of individuals or gametes

ASHD *abbr* arteriosclerotic heart disease

ash•wa•gan•dha \ˌä-shwə-ˈgän-də\ *n* : a preparation usu. of the leaves of an evergreen shrub (*Withania somnifera*) used in herbal medicine esp. as a tonic, anti-inflammatory, and adaptogen

Asian flu *n* : influenza that is caused by a subtype (H2N2) of the orthomyxovirus causing influenza A and that was responsible for about 70,000 deaths in the U.S. in the influenza pandemic of 1957–58 — called also *Asian influenza;* compare HONG KONG FLU, SPANISH FLU

Asian tiger mosquito *n* : a black-and-white striped Asian mosquito of the genus *Aedes* (*A. albopictus*) that transmits the causative viruses of several diseases (as dengue) and has been introduced into the U.S. — called also *tiger mosquito*

Asi•at•ic cholera \ˌā-zhē-ˈa-tik-, -zē-\ *n* : cholera of Asian origin that is produced by virulent strains of the causative vibrio (*Vibrio cholerae*)

As•ma•nex \ˈaz-mə-ˌneks\ *trademark* — used for a preparation of mometasone for oral inhalation

aso•cial \(ˌ)ā-ˈsō-shəl\ *adj* : not social: as **a** : not involving or taking part in social interaction with others **b** : ANTISOCIAL

as•pa•rag•i•nase \ˌas-pə-ˈra-jə-ˌnās, -ˌnāz\ *n* : an enzyme that hydrolyzes asparagine to aspartic acid and ammonia

L–asparaginase — see entry alphabetized in the letter *l*

as•par•a•gine \ə-ˈspar-ə-ˌjēn\ *n* : a white crystalline amino acid $C_4H_8N_2O_3$ that is an amide of aspartic acid

as•par•tame \ˈas-pər-ˌtām, ə-ˈspär-\ *n* : a crystalline compound $C_{14}H_{18}N_2O_5$ that is synthesized from the amino acids phenylalanine and aspartic acid and is used as a low-calorie sweetener — see NUTRASWEET

as•par•tate \-ˌtāt\ *n* : a salt or ester of aspartic acid

aspartate aminotransferase *n* : an enzyme that promotes transfer of an amino group from glutamic acid to oxaloacetic acid and when present in abnormally high levels in the blood is a diagnostic indication of heart attack or liver disease — abbr. *AST;* called also *aspartate transaminase, glutamic-oxaloacetic transaminase*

as•par•tic acid \ə-ˈspär-tik-\ *n* : a crystalline amino acid $C_4H_7NO_4$ that is obtained from many proteins by hydrolysis

as•par•tyl \ə-ˈspär-təl, a-, -ˌtēl\ *n* : the bivalent radical $-OCCH_2CH(NH_2)CO-$ of aspartic acid

as•pect \ˈas-ˌpekt\ *n* : the part of an object (as an organ) in a particular position

aspera — see LINEA ASPERA

As•per•ger's syndrome \ˈäs-ˌpər-gərz-\ *also* **As•per•ger syndrome** \-gər-\ *n* : an autism spectrum disorder that is characterized by impaired social interaction, by repetitive patterns of behavior and restricted interests, by normal language and cognitive development but poor conversational skills and difficulty with nonverbal communication, and often by above average performance in a narrow field against a general background of impaired functioning — called also *Asperger's, Asperger's disorder*

Asperger, Hans (1906–1980), Austrian psychiatrist.

as•per•gil•lin \ˌas-pər-ˈji-lən\ *n* : an antibacterial substance isolated from molds of the genus *Aspergillus*

as•per•gil•lo•sis \ˌas-pər-(ˌ)ji-ˈlō-səs\ *n, pl* **-lo•ses** \-ˌsēz\ : infection with or disease caused by molds of the genus *Aspergillus*

as•per•gil•lus \-ˈji-ləs\ *n* **1** *cap* : a genus of ascomycetous fungi that include many common molds **2** *pl* **-gil•li** \-ˈji-ˌlī, -(ˌ)lē\ : any fungus of the genus *Aspergillus*

asper•mia \(ˈ)ā-ˈspər-mē-ə\ *n* : inability to produce or ejaculate semen — compare AZOOSPERMIA — **asper•mic** \-mik\ *adj*

as•phyx•ia \as-ˈfik-sē-ə, əs-\ *n* : a lack of oxygen or excess of carbon dioxide in the body that is usu. caused by interruption of breathing and that causes unconsciousness — **as•phyx•i•al** \-sē-əl\ *adj*

as•phyx•i•ant \-sē-ənt\ *n* : an agent (as a gas) capable of causing asphyxia

as•phyx•i•ate \-sē-ˌāt\ *vb* **-at•ed; -at•ing 1** : to cause asphyxia in; *also* : to kill or make unconscious by inadequate oxygen, presence of noxious agents, or other obstruction to normal breathing **2** : to become asphyxiated — **as•phyx•i•a•tion** \-ˌfik-sē-ˈā-shən\ *n* — **as•phyx•i•a•tor** \-ˈfik-sē-ˌā-tər\ *n*

[1]**as•pi•rate** \ˈas-pə-ˌrāt\ *vb* **-rat•ed; -rat•ing 1** : to draw by suction **2** : to remove (as blood) by aspiration **3** : to take into the lungs by aspiration

[2]**as•pi•rate** \-rət\ *n* : material removed by aspiration

as•pi•ra•tion \ˌas-pə-ˈrā-shən\ *n* **1** : the act of breathing and esp. of breathing in **2** : the withdrawal of fluid or friable tissue from the body **3** : the taking of foreign matter into the lungs with the respiratory current — **as•pi•ra•tion•al** \-sh(ə-)nəl\ *adj*

as•pi•ra•tor \ˈas-pə-ˌrā-tər\ *n* : an apparatus for producing suction or moving or collecting materials by suction; *esp* : a hollow tubular instrument connected with a partial vacuum and used to remove fluid or tissue or foreign bodies from the body

as•pi•rin \ˈas-prən, -pə-rən\ *n, pl* **aspirin** *or* **aspirins 1** : a white crystalline derivative $C_9H_8O_4$ of salicylic acid used for relief of pain and fever **2** : a tablet of aspirin

asple•nia \(ˌ)ā-ˈsplē-nē-ə\ *n* : absence of the spleen or of normal spleen function or activity — **asplen•ic** \(ˌ)ā-ˈsple-nik\ *adj*

as•say \ˈa-ˌsā, a-ˈsā\ *n* **1** : examination and determination as to characteristics (as weight, measure, or quality) **2** : analysis (as of a drug) to determine the presence, absence, or quantity of one or more components — compare BIOASSAY **3** : a substance to be assayed; *also* : the tabulated result of assaying — **as•say** \a-ˈsā, ˈa-ˌsā\ *vb*

as•sim•i•la•ble \ə-ˈsi-mə-lə-bəl\ *adj* : capable of being assimilated

[1]**as•sim•i•late** \ə-ˈsi-mə-ˌlāt\ *vb* **-lat•ed; -lat•ing 1** : to take in and utilize as nourishment : absorb into the system **2** : to become absorbed or incorporated into the system

²as·sim·i·late \-lət, -ˌlāt\ *n* : something that is assimilated

as·sim·i·la·tion \ə-ˌsi-mə-ˈlā-shən\ *n* **1 a** : an act, process, or instance of assimilating **b** : the state of being assimilated **2** : the incorporation or conversion of nutrients into protoplasm that follows digestion and absorption **3** : the process of receiving new facts or of responding to new situations in conformity with what is already available to consciousness — compare APPERCEPTION

as·sist·ed hatching \ə-ˌsis-təd-\ *n* : a technique for assisting reproduction in cases of infertility that involves manipulating the zona pellucida of a fertilized egg usu. a few days after in vitro fertilization

assisted living *n* : a system of housing and limited care that is designed for senior citizens who need some assistance with daily activities but do not require care in a nursing home

assisted reproductive technology *n* : the use of technology to assist human reproduction in the treatment of infertility; *esp* : a procedure (as in vitro fertilization or gamete intrafallopian transfer) that involves the removal of eggs from an ovary and fertilization by sperm in vitro — abbr. *ART*

assisted suicide *n* : suicide committed by someone with assistance from another person; *esp* : PHYSICIAN-ASSISTED SUICIDE

as·sist·ive \ə-ˈsis-tiv\ *adj* : providing aid or assistance; *specif* : designed or intended to assist a disabled person in performing an activity, task, or function esp. in an independent manner ⟨∼ devices⟩

as·so·ci·a·tion \ə-ˌsō-sē-ˈā-shən, -shē-\ *n* **1** : something linked in memory or imagination with a thing or person **2** : the process of forming mental connections or bonds between sensations, ideas, or memories **3** : the aggregation of chemical species to form (as with hydrogen bonds) loosely bound chemical complexes — compare POLYMERIZATION — **as·so·ci·a·tion·al** \-sh(ə-)nəl\ *adj*

association area *n* : an area of the cerebral cortex that functions in linking and coordinating the sensory and motor areas — called also *association cortex*

association fiber *n* : a nerve fiber connecting different parts of the brain; *esp* : any of the fibers connecting different areas within the cortex of each cerebral hemisphere — compare PROJECTION FIBER

as·so·cia·tive \ə-ˈsō-shē-ˌā-tiv, -sē-; -shə-tiv\ *adj* **1** : of or relating to association esp. of ideas or images ⟨an ∼ symbol⟩ **2 a** : dependent on or characterized by association ⟨an ∼ reaction⟩ **b** : acquired by a process of learning ⟨an ∼ reflex⟩

associative learning *n* : a learning process in which discrete ideas and percepts which are experienced together become linked to one another — compare PAIRED-ASSOCIATE LEARNING

associative neuron *n* : INTERNEURON

as·sort·ment \ə-ˈsȯrt-mənt\ — see INDEPENDENT ASSORTMENT

AST *abbr* aspartate aminotransferase; aspartate transaminase

asta·sia \ə-ˈstā-zhə, -zhē-ə\ *n* : muscular incoordination in standing — compare ABASIA — **astat·ic** \ə-ˈsta-tik\ *adj*

as·ta·tine \ˈas-tə-ˌtēn\ *n* : an unstable radioactive halogen element — symbol *At;* see ELEMENT table

as·tem·i·zole \ə-ˈste-mə-ˌzōl\ *n* : an antihistamine $C_{28}H_{31}FN_4O$ now withdrawn from use because of its link to ventricular arrhythmias and cardiac arrest

as·ter \ˈas-tər\ *n* : a system of microtubules arranged radially about a centriole at either end of the mitotic or meiotic spindle

astere·og·no·sis \(ˌ)ā-ˌster-ē-äg-ˈnō-səs, -ˌstir-\ *n, pl* **-no·ses** \-ˌsēz\ : loss of the ability to recognize the shapes of objects by handling them

as·te·rix·is \ˌas-tə-ˈrik-sis\ *n* : a motor disorder characterized by jerking movements (as of the outstretched hands) and associated with various encephalopathies due esp. to faulty metabolism

asthen- *or* **astheno-** *comb form* : weak ⟨*asthen*opia⟩

as·the·nia \as-ˈthē-nē-ə\ *n* : lack or loss of strength : DEBILITY

as·then·ic \as-ˈthe-nik\ *adj* **1** : of, relating to, or exhibiting asthenia : DEBILITATED **2** : characterized by slender build and slight muscular development : ECTOMORPHIC

as·the·no·pia \ˌas-thə-ˈnō-pē-ə\ *n* : weakness or rapid fatigue of the eyes often accompanied by pain and headache — **as·the·no·pic** \-ˈnä-pik, -ˈnō-\ *adj*

asth·ma \ˈaz-mə\ *n* : a chronic lung disorder that is marked by recurrent episodes of airway obstruction (as from bronchospasm) manifested by labored breathing accompanied by wheezing and coughing and by a sense of constriction in the chest, and that is triggered by hyperreactivity to various stimuli (as allergens or a rapid change in air temperature)

¹asth·mat·ic \az-ˈma-tik\ *adj* : of, relating to, or affected with asthma ⟨an ∼ attack⟩ — **asth·mat·i·cal·ly** \-ti-k(ə-)lē\ *adv*

²asthmatic *n* : a person affected with asthma

asthmaticus — see STATUS ASTHMATICUS

asth·mo·gen·ic \ˌaz-mə-ˈje-nik\ *adj* : causing asthmatic attacks

[1]**as·tig·mat·ic** \ˌas-tig-ˈma-tik\ *adj* : affected with, relating to, or correcting astigmatism 〈~ eyes〉

[2]**astigmatic** *n* : a person affected with astigmatism

astig·ma·tism \ə-ˈstig-mə-ˌti-zəm\ *n* **1** : a defect of an optical system (as a lens) causing rays from a point to fail to meet in a focal point resulting in a blurred and imperfect image **2** : a defect of vision due to astigmatism of the refractive system of the eye and esp. to corneal irregularity — compare EMMETROPIA, MYOPIA

as tol *abbr* as tolerated

astr- *or* **astro-** *comb form* **1** : star : star-shaped 〈*astro*cyte〉 **2** : astrocyte 〈*astro*blastoma〉 〈*astro*glia〉

astragal- *or* **astragalo-** *comb form* : astragalus 〈*astragal*ectomy〉

astrag·a·lec·to·my \ə-ˌstra-gə-ˈlek-tə-mē\ *n, pl* **-mies** : surgical removal of the astragalus

as·trag·a·lus \ə-ˈstra-gə-ləs\ *n, pl* **-li** \-ˌlī, -ˌlē\ **1** : one of the proximal bones of the tarsus of the higher vertebrates — see TALUS 1 **2** : the dried root of an Asian herb (*Astragalus membranaceus* syn. *A. propinquus*) used esp. as an herbal remedy in traditional Chinese medicine; *also* : a preparation or extract of this root

astral ray *n* : one of the microtubules that make up the mitotic or meiotic aster

[1]**as·trin·gent** \ə-ˈstrin-jənt\ *adj* : having the property of drawing together the soft organic tissues 〈~ cosmetic lotions〉: **a** : tending to shrink mucous membranes or raw or exposed tissues : checking discharge (as of serum or mucus) : STYPTIC **b** : tending to pucker the tissues of the mouth 〈~ fruits〉 — **as·trin·gen·cy** \-jən-sē\ *n*

[2]**astringent** *n* : an astringent agent or substance

as·tro·blas·to·ma \ˌas-trə-(ˌ)blas-ˈtō-mə\ *n, pl* **-mas** *also* **-ma·ta** \-mə-tə\ : an astrocytoma of moderate malignancy

as·tro·cyte \ˈas-trə-ˌsīt\ *n* : a star-shaped cell; *esp* : any comparatively large much-branched neuroglial cell — **as·tro·cyt·ic** \ˌas-trə-ˈsi-tik\ *adj*

as·tro·cy·to·ma \ˌas-trə-sī-ˈtō-mə\ *n, pl* **-mas** *also* **-ma·ta** \-mə-tə\ : a nerve-tissue tumor composed of astrocytes

as·tro·glia \as-ˈträ-glē-ə, ˌas-trə-ˈglī-ə\ *n* : glial tissue composed of astrocytes — **as·tro·gli·al** \-əl\ *adj*

as·tro·gli·o·sis \ˌa-strə-ˌglī-ˈō-səs\ *n, pl* **-o·ses** \-ˈō-ˌsēz\ : excessive development of the astroglia : GLIOSIS

as·tro·vi·rus \ˌa-strə-ˈvī-rəs\ *n* : any of a family (*Astroviridae*) of single-stranded RNA viruses that cause gastroenteritis esp. in children

asy·lum \ə-ˈsī-ləm\ *n* : an institution providing care and protection to needy individuals (as the infirm or destitute) and esp. the mentally ill

asym·bo·lia \ˌā-(ˌ)sim-ˈbō-lē-ə\ *n* : loss of the power to understand previously familiar symbols and signs

asym·met·ri·cal \ˌā-sə-ˈme-tri-kəl\ *or* **asym·met·ric** \-trik\ *adj* **1** : not symmetrical **2** *usu asymmetric, of a carbon atom* : bonded to four different atoms or groups — **asym·met·ri·cal·ly** \-tri-k(ə-)lē\ *adv*

asym·me·try \(ˌ)ā-ˈsi-mə-trē\ *n, pl* **-tries** **1** : lack or absence of symmetry: as **a** : lack of proportion between the parts of a thing; *esp* : want of bilateral symmetry 〈~ in brain development〉 **b** : lack of coordination of two parts acting in connection with one another 〈~ of convergence of the eyes〉 **2** : lack of symmetry in spatial arrangement of atoms and groups in a molecule

asymp·tom·at·ic \ˌā-ˌsimp-tə-ˈma-tik\ *adj* : presenting no symptoms of disease 〈an ~ infection〉 — **asymp·tom·at·i·cal·ly** \-ti-k(ə-)lē\ *adv*

asyn·ap·sis \ˌā-sə-ˈnap-səs\ *n, pl* **-ap·ses** \-ˌsēz\ : failure of pairing of homologous chromosomes in meiosis

asyn·clit·ism \(ˌ)ā-ˈsin-klə-ˌti-zəm, -ˈsiŋ-\ *n* : presentation of the fetal head during childbirth with the axis oriented obliquely to the axial planes of the pelvis — **asyn·clit·ic** \(ˈ)ā-(ˈ)sin-ˈkli-tik, -sən-, -(ˈ)siŋ-, -səŋ-\ *adj*

asy·ner·gia \ˌā-sə-ˈnər-jē-ə, -jə\ *or* **asyn·er·gy** \(ˌ)ā-ˈsi-nər-jē\ *n, pl* **-gi·as** *or* **-gies** : lack of coordination (as of muscles) — **asy·ner·gic** \ˌā-sə-ˈnər-jik\ *adj*

asys·to·le \(ˌ)ā-ˈsis-tə-(ˌ)lē\ *n* : a condition of weakening or cessation of systole — **asys·tol·ic** \ˌā-sis-ˈtä-lik\ *adj*

At *symbol* astatine

Ata·brine \ˈa-tə-brən\ *n* : a preparation of quinacrine — formerly a U.S. registered trademark

At·a·cand \ˈa-tə-ˌkand\ *trademark* — used for a preparation of candesartan

Atacand HCT *trademark* — used for a preparation of hydrochlorothiazide and candesartan

[1]**at·a·rac·tic** \ˌa-tə-ˈrak-tik\ *or* **at·a·rax·ic** \-ˈrak-sik\ *adj* : tending to tranquilize 〈~ drugs〉

[2]**ataractic** *or* **ataraxic** *n* : TRANQUILIZER

at·a·rax·ia \ˌa-tə-ˈrak-sē-ə\ *or* **at·a·raxy** \ˈa-tə-ˌrak-sē\ *n, pl* **-rax·ias** *or* **-rax·ies** : calmness untroubled by mental or emotional disquiet

at·a·vism \ˈa-tə-ˌvi-zəm\ *n* **1** : recurrence in an organism of a trait or character typical of an ancestral form and usu. due to genetic recombination **2** : an individual or character manifesting atavism — **at·a·vis·tic** \ˌa-tə-ˈvis-tik\ *adj*

atax·ia \ə-ˈtak-sē-ə, (ˌ)ā-\ *n* : an inability to coordinate voluntary muscular movements that is symptomatic of some disorders of the central nervous system — **atax·ic** \-sik\ *adj*

ataxia–telangiectasia *n* : a genetic disorder that is inherited as a recessive autosomal trait and is marked esp. by progressive pathological changes in the nervous system resulting in loss of motor coordination, telangiectasias esp. on the eye, ears, and cheeks, and immunodeficiency leading to increased susceptibility to cancer esp. of lymphoid tissue

ataxic cerebral palsy *n* : cerebral palsy marked by hypotonic muscles and poor coordination and balance

at•a•zan•a•vir \ˌa-tə-ˈza-nə-ˌvir\ *n* : a protease inhibitor used in the form of its sulfate $C_{38}H_{52}N_6O_7 \cdot H_2SO_4$ in conjunction with other antiretroviral agents to treat HIV infection — see EVOTAZ, REYATAZ

atel- *or* **atelo-** *comb form* : defective ⟨*atel*ectasis⟩

at•el•ec•ta•sis \ˌat-ᵊl-ˈek-tə-səs\ *n, pl* **-ta•ses** \-ˌsēz\ : collapse of the expanded lung; *also* : defective expansion of the pulmonary alveoli at birth — **at•el•ec•tat•ic** \-ek-ˈta-tik\ *adj*

ate•li•o•sis \ə-ˌte-lē-ˈō-səs, -ˌtē-\ *n, pl* **-o•ses** \-ˌsēz\ : incomplete development; *esp* : dwarfism associated with anterior pituitary deficiencies and marked by normal proportions

Atel•via \ə-ˈtel-vē-ə\ *trademark* — used for a preparation of the sodium salt of risedronate

aten•o•lol \ə-ˈte-nə-ˌlȯl, -ˌlōl\ *n* : a beta-blocker $C_{14}H_{22}N_2O_3$ used to treat hypertension — see TENORMIN

ath•er•ec•to•my \ˌa-thə-ˈrek-tə-mē\ *n, pl* **-mies** : removal of atheromatous plaque from within a blood vessel by utilizing a catheter usu. fitted with a cutting blade or grinding burr

athero- *comb form* : atheroma ⟨*athero*genic⟩

ath•ero•gen•e•sis \ˌa-thə-rō-ˈje-nə-səs\ *n, pl* **-e•ses** \-ˌsēz\ : the formation of atheroma

ath•ero•gen•ic \-ˈje-nik\ *adj* : relating to or causing atherogenesis ⟨~ diets⟩ — **ath•ero•ge•nic•i•ty** \-jə-ˈni-sə-tē\ *n*

ath•er•o•ma \ˌa-thə-ˈrō-mə\ *n, pl* **-mas** *also* **-ma•ta** \-mə-tə\ **1** : fatty degeneration of the inner coat of the arteries **2** : an abnormal fatty deposit in an artery — **ath•er•o•ma•tous** \-ˈrō-mə-təs\ *adj*

ath•er•o•ma•to•sis \ˌa-thə-rō-mə-ˈtō-səs\ *n, pl* **-to•ses** \-ˌsēz\ : a disease characterized by atheromatous degeneration of the arteries

ath•ero•scle•ro•sis \ˌa-thə-rō-sklə-ˈrō-səs\ *n, pl* **-ro•ses** \-ˌsēz\ : an arteriosclerosis characterized by atheromatous deposits in and fibrosis of the inner layer of the arteries — **ath•ero•scle•rot•ic** \-sklə-ˈrä-tik\ *adj* — **ath•ero•scle•rot•i•cal•ly** \-i-k(ə-)lē\ *adv*

ath•ero•throm•bo•sis \ˌa-thə-(ˌ)rō-thräm-ˈbō-səs, -thrəm-\ *n, pl* **-bo•ses** \–ˌsēz\ : the formation of a blood clot within an artery as a result of atherosclerosis — **ath•ero•throm•bot•ic** \ˌa-thə-(ˌ)rō-thräm-ˈbä-tik, -thrəm-\ *adj*

[1]**ath•e•toid** \ˈa-thə-ˌtȯid\ *adj* : exhibiting or characteristic of athetosis

[2]**athetoid** *n* : an athetoid individual

athetoid cerebral palsy *n* : cerebral palsy marked by involuntary uncontrolled writhing movements — called also *dyskinetic cerebral palsy*

ath•e•to•sis \ˌa-thə-ˈtō-səs\ *n, pl* **-to•ses** \-ˌsēz\ : a nervous disorder that is marked by continual slow movements esp. of the extremities and is usu. due to a brain lesion

athlete's foot *n* : ringworm of the feet — called also *tinea pedis*

ath•let•ic \ath-ˈle-tik\ *adj* : characterized by heavy frame, large chest, and powerful muscular development : MESOMORPHIC

athletic supporter *n* : a supporter for the genitals worn by boys and men participating in sports or strenuous activities — called also *jockstrap;* see CUP 1

ath•ro•cyte \ˈa-thrə-ˌsīt\ *n* : a cell capable of athrocytosis — **ath•ro•cyt•ic** \ˌa-thrə-ˈsi-tik\ *adj*

ath•ro•cy•to•sis \ˌa-thrə-sī-ˈtō-səs\ *n, pl* **-to•ses** \-ˌsēz\ : the capacity of some cells (as of the proximal convoluted tubule of the kidney) to pick up foreign material and store it in granular form in the cytoplasm

athy•mic \(ˌ)ā-ˈthī-mik\ *adj* : lacking a thymus

At•i•van \ˈat-i-ˌvan\ *trademark* — used for a preparation of lorazepam

At•kins diet \ˈat-kənz-\ *n* : a weight loss program that emphasizes a diet low in carbohydrates along with little restriction on protein, fat, or total caloric intake

Atkins, Robert Coleman (1930–2003), American cardiologist and nutritionist.

ATL *abbr* adult T-cell leukemia

atlant- *or* **atlanto-** *comb form* **1** : atlas ⟨*atlant*al⟩ **2** : atlantal and ⟨*atlanto*-occipital⟩

at•lan•tal \-ˈlant-ᵊl\ *adj* **1** : of or relating to the atlas **2** : ANTERIOR 1, CEPHALIC

at•lan•to•ax•i•al \ət-ˌlan-tō-ˈak-sē-əl, at-\ *adj* : relating to or being anatomical structures that connect the atlas and the axis

at•lan•to–oc•cip•i•tal \-äk-ˈsi-pət-ᵊl\ *adj* : relating to or being structures (as a joint or ligament) joining the atlas and the occipital bone

at•las \ˈat-ləs\ *n* : the first vertebra of the neck

ATLS *trademark* — used for an instruction course for assessing patient condition in the case of trauma

at•mo•sphere \ˈat-mə-ˌsfir\ *n* **1** : the whole mass of air surrounding the earth **2** : a unit of pressure equal to the pressure of the air at sea level or approximately 14.7 pounds per square inch (101,352 pascals) — **at•mo•spher•ic** \ˌat-mə-ˈsfir-ik, -ˈsfer-\ *adj*

atmospheric pressure *n* : the pressure exerted in every direction at any given point by the weight of the atmosphere

at•om \ˈa-təm\ *n* : the smallest particle of an element that can exist either alone or in combination — **atom•ic** \ə-ˈtä-mik\ *adj*

atomic cocktail *n* : a radioactive substance (as iodide of sodium) dissolved in water and administered orally to patients with cancer

atomic number *n* : the number of protons in the nucleus of an element — see ELEMENT table

atomic weight *n* : the average mass of an atom of an element as it occurs in nature — see ELEMENT table

at•om•ize \ˈa-tə-ˌmīz\ *vb* **-ized; -iz•ing** : to convert to minute particles or to a fine spray — **at•om•i•za•tion** \ˌa-tə-mə-ˈzā-shən\ *n*

at•om•iz•er \ˈa-tə-ˌmī-zər\ *n* : an instrument for atomizing usu. a perfume, disinfectant, or medicament

at•om•ox•e•tine \ˌa-tə-ˈmäk-sə-ˌtēn\ *n* : an SNRI taken orally in the form of its hydrochloride $C_{17}H_{21}NO \cdot HCl$ in the treatment of attention deficit disorder — see STRATTERA

aton•ic \(ˌ)ā-ˈtä-nik, (ˌ)a-\ *adj* : characterized by atony ⟨an ∼ bladder⟩

at•o•ny \ˌat-ᵊn-ē\ *or* **ato•nia** \(ˌ)ā-ˈtō-nē-ə\ *n, pl* **-nies** *or* **-ni•as** : lack of physiological tone esp. of a contractile organ

atopic dermatitis *n* : a chronic eczematous skin condition primarily affecting children that is marked esp. by intense itching, inflammation, and xerosis and occurs chiefly in those with a personal or familial history of atopy — abbr. *AD*

at•o•py \ˈa-tə-pē\ *n, pl* **-pies** : a genetic disposition to develop an allergic reaction (as allergic rhinitis, asthma, or atopic dermatitis) and produce elevated levels of IgE upon exposure to an environmental antigen and esp. one inhaled or ingested — **ato•pic** \(ˌ)ā-ˈtä-pik, -ˈtō-\ *adj*

ator•va•stat•in \ə-ˌtȯr-və-ˈsta-tᵊn\ *n* : a statin that is administered orally in the form of its hydrated calcium salt $(C_{33}H_{34}FN_2O_5)_2Ca \cdot 3H_2O$ to lower lipid levels in the blood — see CADUET, LIPITOR

ato•va•quone \ə-ˈtō-və-ˌkwōn\ *n* : an antiprotozoal drug $C_{22}H_{19}O_3Cl$ taken orally esp. to prevent or treat Pneumocystis carinii pneumonia and falciparum malaria — see MALARONE

ATP \ˌā-(ˌ)tē-ˈpē\ *n* : a phosphorylated nucleotide $C_{10}H_{16}N_5O_{13}P_3$ composed of adenosine and three phosphate groups that supplies energy for many biochemical cellular processes by undergoing enzymatic hydrolysis esp. to ADP — called also *adenosine triphosphate*

ATPase \ˌā-(ˌ)tē-ˈpē-ˌās, -ˌāz\ *n* : an enzyme that hydrolyzes ATP; *esp* : one that hydrolyzes ATP to ADP and inorganic phosphate — called also *adenosine triphosphatase*

at•ra•cu•ri•um \ˌa-trə-ˈkyu̇r-ē-əm\ *n* : a muscle relaxant $C_{65}H_{82}N_2O_{18}S_2$ administered intravenously esp. in conjunction with general anesthesia

atrau•mat•ic \(ˈ)ā-trə-ˈma-tik, trȯ-, trau̇-\ *adj* **1** : designed to minimize tissue damage : not causing injury or trauma ⟨∼ sutures⟩ **2** : not resulting from injury or trauma ⟨an ∼ fracture⟩

atre•sia \ə-ˈtrē-zhə\ *n* **1** : absence or closure of a natural passage of the body ⟨∼ of the small intestine⟩ **2** : absence or disappearance of an anatomical part (as an ovarian follicle) by degeneration — **atret•ic** \ə-ˈtre-tik\ *adj*

atri- *or* **atrio-** *comb form* **1** : atrium ⟨*atri*al⟩ **2** : atrial and ⟨*atrio*ventricular⟩

atria *pl of* ATRIUM

atri•al \ˈā-trē-əl\ *adj* : of, relating to, or affecting an atrium ⟨∼ disorders⟩

atrial fibrillation *n* : very rapid uncoordinated contractions of the atria of the heart resulting in a lack of synchronism between heartbeat and pulse beat — abbr. *AF;* called also *A-fib, auricular fibrillation*

atrial flutter *n* : an irregularity of the heartbeat in which the contractions of the atrium exceed in number those of the ventricle — called also *auricular flutter*

atrial natriuretic peptide *n* : a peptide hormone secreted by the cardiac atria that promotes salt and water excretion and lowers blood pressure — called also *atrial natriuretic factor*

atrial septal defect *n* : a congenital defect in the interatrial septum of the heart

atrial septum *n* : INTERATRIAL SEPTUM

atrich•ia \ā-ˈtri-kē-ə, ə-\ *n* : congenital or acquired baldness : ALOPECIA

atrio•ven•tric•u•lar \ˌā-trē-(ˌ)ō-ˌven-ˈtri-kyə-lər\ *adj* **1** : of, relating to, or situated between an atrium and ventricle **2** : of, involving, or being the atrioventricular node

atrioventricular bundle *n* : BUNDLE OF HIS

atrioventricular canal *n* : the canal joining the atrium and ventricle in the tubular embryonic heart

atrioventricular node *n* : a small mass of tissue that is situated in the wall of the right atrium adjacent to the septum between the atria and passes impulses received from the sinoatrial node to the ventricles by way of the bundle of His

atrioventricular valve *n* : a valve between an atrium and ventricle of the heart: **a** : MITRAL VALVE **b** : TRICUSPID VALVE

Atrip•la \ə-ˈtrip-lə\ *trademark* — used for a preparation of efavirenz, emtricitabine, and the fumarate of tenofovir

atri•um \ˈā-trē-əm\ *n, pl* **atria** \-trē-ə\ *also* **atri•ums** : an anatomical cavity or passage; *esp* : a chamber of the heart that receives blood from the veins and forces it into a ventricle or ventricles

At•ro•pa \ˈa-trə-pə\ *n* : a genus of Eurasian and African herbs (as belladonna) of the nightshade family (Solanaceae) that are a source of medicinal alkaloids (as atropine)

atro•phic \(ˌ)ā-ˈtrō-fik, ə-, -ˈträ-\ *adj* : relating to or characterized by atrophy ⟨an ∼ jaw⟩

atrophicans — see ACRODERMATITIS CHRONICA ATROPHICANS

atrophic gastritis *n* : chronic inflammation of the mucous membrane of the stomach leading to atrophy and thinning of parts of the gastric mucosa and often gastric metaplasia

atrophic rhinitis *n* **1** : chronic inflammation of the mucous membrane of the nose resulting in atrophy and sclerosis of the nasal mucosa; *esp* : OZENA **2** : a disease of swine that is characterized by purulent inflammation of the nasal mucosa, atrophy of the nasal conchae, and abnormal swelling of the face

atrophicus — see LICHEN SCLEROSUS ET ATROPHICUS

atrophic vaginitis *n* : inflammation of the vagina with thinning of the epithelial lining that occurs following menopause and is due to a deficiency of estrogen

¹at•ro•phy \ˈa-trə-fē\ *n, pl* **-phies** : decrease in size or wasting away of a body part or tissue; *also* : arrested development or loss of a part or organ incidental to the normal development or life of an animal or plant

²atrophy \ˈa-trə-fē, -ˌfī\ *vb* **-phied; -phy•ing** : to undergo or cause to undergo atrophy

at•ro•pine \ˈa-trə-ˌpēn\ *n* : a racemic mixture of hyoscyamine usu. obtained from belladonna and related plants (family Solanaceae) and used esp. in the form of its hydrated sulfate $(C_{17}H_{23}NO_3)_2 \cdot H_2SO_4 \cdot H_2O$ for its anticholinergic effects (as pupil dilation or relief of smooth muscle spasms)

at•ro•pin•ism \-ˌpē-ˌni-zəm\ *n* : poisoning by atropine

at•ro•pin•i•za•tion \ˌa-trə-ˌpē-nə-ˈzā-shən\ *n* : the act or process of treating with atropine : the condition of being under the influence of atropine — **at•ro•pin•ize** \ˈa-trə-pə-ˌnīz\ *vb*

at•ro•scine \ˈa-trə-ˌsēn, -sən\ *n* : racemic scopolamine

At•ro•vent \ˈa-trō-ˌvent\ *trademark* — used for a preparation of ipratropium bromide for oral inhalation

at•tach•ment \ə-ˈtach-mənt\ *n* **1** : a strong emotional bond that an infant forms with a caregiver (as a mother) esp. when viewed as a basis for normal emotional and social development; *also* : the process by which an infant forms an attachment **2** : the physical connection by which one thing is attached to another — **at•tach** \ə-ˈtach\ *vb*

attachment disorder *n* : a psychological disorder of infancy and early childhood that is characterized by disturbed or developmentally inappropriate patterns of social interaction and is typically associated with inadequate parental care — called also *reactive attachment disorder*

¹at•tack \ə-ˈtak\ *vb* : to begin to affect or to act on injuriously

²attack *n* : a fit of sickness; *esp* : an active episode of a chronic or recurrent disease

at•tempt•er \ə-ˈtem(p)-tər\ *n* : one who attempts suicide

at•tend \ə-ˈtend\ *vb* : to visit with or care for in a professional capacity

¹at•tend•ing \ə-ˈten-diŋ\ *adj* : serving as a physician or surgeon on the staff of a hospital or similar health-care facility and having primary responsibility over the treatment of a patient and often supervising treatment given by interns, residents, and fellows

²attending *n* : an attending physician or surgeon

at•ten•tion \ə-ˈten-chən\ *n* **1** : the act or state of attending : the application of the mind to any object of sense or thought **2 a** : an organismic condition of selective awareness or perceptual receptivity **b** : the process of focusing consciousness to produce greater vividness and clarity of certain of its contents relative to others — **at•ten•tion•al** \-ˈten-chə-nəl\ *adj*

attention deficit disorder *n* : a developmental disorder that is marked esp. by symptoms of inattention (as distractibility, forgetfulness, or disorganization) or by symptoms of hyperactivity and impulsivity (as fidgeting or speaking out of turn) or by symptoms of all three, that is not caused by any serious underlying physical or mental disorder, and that interferes with normal development and daily functioning — abbr. *ADD*

attention deficit hyperactivity disorder *n* : ATTENTION DEFICIT DISORDER — abbr. *ADHD*

at•ten•u•ate \ə-ˈten-yə-ˌwāt\ *vb* **-at•ed; -at•ing** : to reduce the severity of (a disease) or virulence or vitality of (a pathogenic agent) ⟨a procedure to ∼ severe diabetes⟩ ⟨*attenuated* bacilli⟩

at•ten•u•a•tion \ə-ˌten-yə-ˈwā-shən\ *n* : a decrease in the pathogenicity or vitality of a microorganism or in the severity of a disease

at•tic \ˈa-tik\ *n* : the small upper space of the middle ear — called also *epitympanic recess*

at•ti•co•to•my \ˌa-tə-ˈkä-tə-mē\ *n, pl* **-mies** : surgical incision of the tympanic attic

at•ti•tude \ˈa-tə-ˌtüd, -ˌtyüd\ *n* **1** : the arrangement of the parts of the body : POSTURE **2 a** : a mental position with regard to a fact or state **b** : a feeling or emotion toward a fact or state **3** : an organismic state of readiness to respond in a characteristic way to a stimulus (as an object, concept, or situation)

at·ti·tu·di·nal \ˌa-tə-ˈtüd-ᵊn-əl, -ˈtyüd-\ *adj* : relating to, based on, or expressive of personal attitudes or feelings

at·tri·tion \ə-ˈtri-shən\ *n* : the act of rubbing together; *also* : the act of wearing or grinding down by friction ⟨∼ of teeth⟩

atyp·ia \(ˌ)ā-ˈti-pē-ə\ *n* : ATYPISM

atyp·i·cal \(ˌ)ā-ˈti-pi-kəl\ *adj* **1** : not typical : not like the usual or normal type ⟨∼ cells⟩ **2** : relating to or being an antipsychotic drug (as aripiprazole) that tends to produce fewer adverse side effects on movement (as dyskinesia) than previously used antipsychotic drugs (as haloperidol) — **atyp·i·cal·ly** \-pi-k(ə-)lē\ *adv*

atypical pneumonia *n* : PRIMARY ATYPICAL PNEUMONIA

atyp·ism \(ˌ)ā-ˈtī-ˌpi-zəm\ *n* : the condition of being uncharacteristic or lacking uniformity

Au *symbol* [L *aurum*] gold

AU *abbr* [Latin *aures unitas*] both ears — used esp. in audiology and in writing prescriptions

au·di·ble \ˈȯ-də-bəl\ *adj* : heard or capable of being heard — **au·di·bil·i·ty** \ˌȯ-də-ˈbi-lə-tē\ *n* — **au·di·bly** \ˈȯ-də-blē\ *adv*

[1]**au·dile** \ˈȯ-ˌdīl\ *n* : a person whose mental imagery is auditory rather than visual or motor — compare TACTILE, VISUALIZER

[2]**audile** *adj* **1** : of or relating to hearing : AUDITORY **2** : of, relating to, or being an audile

audio- *comb form* **1** : hearing ⟨*audio*logy⟩ **2** : sound ⟨*audio*genic⟩

au·dio·gen·ic \ˌȯ-dē-ō-ˈje-nik\ *adj* : produced by frequencies corresponding to sound waves — used esp. of epileptoid responses ⟨∼ seizures⟩

au·dio·gram \ˈȯ-dē-ō-ˌgram\ *n* : a graphic representation of the relation of vibration frequency and the minimum sound intensity for hearing

au·di·ol·o·gist \ˌȯ-dē-ˈä-lə-jist\ *n* : a specialist in audiology

au·di·ol·o·gy \ˌȯ-dē-ˈä-lə-jē\ *n, pl* **-gies** : a branch of science dealing with hearing; *specif* : therapy of individuals having impaired hearing — **au·di·o·log·i·cal** \-dē-ə-ˈlä-ji-kəl\ *also* **au·di·o·log·ic** \-dē-ə-ˈlä-jik\ *adj*

au·di·om·e·ter \ˌȯ-dē-ˈä-mə-tər\ *n* : an instrument used in measuring the acuity of hearing

au·di·om·e·try \ˌȯ-dē-ˈä-mə-trē\ *n, pl* **-tries** : the testing and measurement of hearing acuity for variations in sound intensity and pitch and for tonal purity — **au·dio·met·ric** \-ō-ˈme-trik\ *adj* — **au·di·om·e·trist** \-ˈä-mə-trist\ *n*

aud·ism \ˈȯ-ˌdi-zəm\ *n* : discrimination or prejudice against individuals who are deaf or hard-of-hearing

au·di·to·ry \ˈȯ-də-ˌtōr-ē\ *adj* **1** : of or relating to hearing **2** : attained, experienced, or produced through or as if through hearing ⟨∼ images⟩ ⟨∼ hallucinations⟩ **3** : marked by great susceptibility to impressions and reactions produced by acoustic stimuli

auditory canal *n* : either of two passages of the ear — called also *acoustic meatus, auditory meatus;* compare EXTERNAL AUDITORY CANAL, INTERNAL AUDITORY CANAL

auditory cortex *n* : a sensory area of the temporal lobe associated with the organ of hearing — called also *auditory area, auditory center*

auditory nerve *n* : either of the eighth pair of cranial nerves connecting the inner ear with the brain, transmitting impulses concerned with hearing and balance, and composed of the cochlear nerve and the vestibular nerve — called also *acoustic nerve, auditory, eighth cranial nerve, vestibulocochlear nerve*

auditory processing disorder *n* : CENTRAL AUDITORY PROCESSING DISORDER

auditory tube *n* : EUSTACHIAN TUBE

Auer·bach's plexus \ˈau̇-ər-ˌbäks-, -ˌbäks-\ *n* : MYENTERIC PLEXUS

Auer·bach \ˈau̇-ər-ˌbäk, -ˌbäk\, **Leopold (1828–1897)**, German anatomist.

aug·ment \ȯg-ˈment, ˈȯg-ˌment\ *vb* : to increase in size, amount, degree, or severity — **aug·men·ta·tion** \ˌȯg-mən-ˈtā-shən, -ˌmen-\ *n*

Aug·men·tin \ȯg-ˈmen-tᵊn\ *trademark* — used for a preparation of amoxicillin and the potassium salt of clavulanic acid

aur- *or* **auri-** *comb form* : ear ⟨*aur*al⟩

au·ra \ˈȯr-ə\ *n, pl* **auras** *also* **au·rae** \-ē\ : a subjective sensation (as of voices or colored lights) experienced at the onset of a neurological condition and esp. an epileptic seizure or migraine

au·ral \ˈȯr-əl\ *adj* : of or relating to the ear or to the sense of hearing — **au·ral·ly** *adv*

au·ran·o·fin \ȯ-ˈra-nə-fən\ *n* : a gold-containing compound $C_{20}H_{34}AuO_9PS$ used in the treatment of rheumatoid arthritis — see RIDAURA

Au·reo·my·cin \ˌȯr-ē-ō-ˈmī-sən\ *trademark* — used for a preparation of the hydrochloride of chlortetracycline

au·ri·cle \ˈȯr-i-kəl\ *n* **1 a** : PINNA **b** : an atrium of the heart **2** : an angular or ear-shaped anatomical lobe or process

au·ric·u·la \ȯ-ˈri-kyu̇-lə\ *n, pl* **-lae** \-ˌlē\ : AURICLE; *esp* : AURICULAR APPENDAGE

au·ric·u·lar \ȯ-ˈri-kyu̇-lər\ *adj* **1** : of, relating to, or using the ear or the sense of hearing **2** : understood or recognized by the sense of hearing **3** : of or relating to an auricle or auricular appendage ⟨∼ fibrillation⟩

auricular appendage *n* : an ear-shaped pouch projecting from each atrium of the heart — called also *auricular appendix*

auricular artery — see POSTERIOR AURICULAR ARTERY

auricular fibrillation *n* : ATRIAL FIBRILLATION

auricular flutter *n* : ATRIAL FLUTTER

au•ric•u•lar•is \ȯ-ˌri-kyu̇-ˈlar-əs, -ˈlär-\ *n, pl* **-lar•es** \-ˌēz\ : any of three muscles attaching the cartilage of the external ear to the skull that assist in moving the scalp and in some individuals the external ear itself and that consist of one that is anterior, one superior, and one posterior in position — called also respectively *auricularis anterior, auricularis superior, auricularis posterior*

auricular vein — see POSTERIOR AURICULAR VEIN

auriculo- *comb form* : of or belonging to an auricle of the heart and ⟨*auriculo*ventricular⟩

au•ric•u•lo•tem•po•ral nerve \ȯ-ˌri-kyu̇-(ˌ)lō-ˈtem-pə-rəl-\ *n* : the branch of the mandibular nerve that supplies sensory fibers to the skin of the external ear and temporal region and autonomic fibers from the otic ganglion to the parotid gland

au•ric•u•lo•ven•tric•u•lar \-ven-ˈtri-kyu̇-lər,-vən-\ *adj* : ATRIOVENTRICULAR

au•ro•thio•glu•cose \ˌȯr-ō-ˌthī-ō-ˈglü-ˌkōs, -ˌkōz\ *n* : GOLD THIOGLUCOSE

aus•cul•ta•tion \ˌȯ-skəl-ˈtā-shən\ *n* : the act of listening to sounds arising within organs (as the lungs or heart) as an aid to diagnosis and treatment — **aus•cul•tate** \ˈȯ-skəl-ˌtāt\ *vb* — **aus•cul•ta•to•ry** \ȯ-ˈskəl-tə-ˌtȯr-ē\ *adj*

Aus•tra•lia antigen \ȯ-ˈstrāl-yə-\ *also* **Aus•tra•lian antigen** \-yən-\ *n* : HEPATITIS B SURFACE ANTIGEN

aut- *or* **auto-** *comb form* : self : same one ⟨*aut*ism⟩: **a** : of, by, affecting, from, or for the same individual ⟨*auto*graft⟩ ⟨*auto*transfusion⟩ **b** : arising or produced within the individual and acting or directed toward or against the individual or the individual's own body, tissues, or molecules ⟨*auto*immunity⟩ ⟨*auto*suggestion⟩

au•ta•coid \ˈȯ-tə-ˌkȯid\ *n* : a physiologically active substance (as serotonin, bradykinin, or angiotensin) that is produced by the body and typically has a localized effect of brief duration

au•tism \ˈȯ-ˌti-zəm\ *n* : a developmental disorder that appears by age three and that is variable in expression but is recognized and diagnosed by impairment of the ability to form normal social relationships, by impairment of the ability to communicate with others, and by stereotyped behavior patterns esp. as exhibited by a preoccupation with repetitive activities of restricted focus rather than with flexible and imaginative ones — called also *autistic disorder*

autism spectrum disorder *n* : any of a group of developmental disorders (as autism and Asperger's syndrome) marked by impairments in the ability to communicate and interact socially and by the presence of repetitive behaviors or restricted interests — abbr. *ASD;* called also *autistic spectrum disorder, pervasive developmental disorder*

au•tist \ˈȯ-ˌtist\ *n* : AUTISTIC

[1]**au•tis•tic** \ȯ-ˈtis-tik\ *adj* : of, relating to, or marked by autism or autism spectrum disorder ⟨~ behavior⟩

[2]**autistic** *n* : a person affected with autism or autism spectrum disorder

autistic disorder *n* : AUSTISM

autistic savant *n* : a person affected with autism who exhibits exceptional skill or brilliance in some limited field (as mathematics or music)

au•to•ag•glu•ti•na•tion \ˌȯ-tō-ə-ˌglüt-ᵊn-ˈā-shən\ *n* : agglutination of red blood cells by cold agglutinins in an individual's own serum usu. at lower than body temperature

au•to•ag•glu•ti•nin \-ə-ˈglüt-ᵊn-ən\ *n* : an antibody that agglutinates the red blood cells of the individual producing it — compare COLD AGGLUTININ

Au•to•an•a•lyz•er \ˌȯ-tō-ˈan-ᵊl-ˌī-zər\ *trademark* — used for an instrument designed for automatic chemical analysis (as of blood glucose level)

au•to•an•ti•body \ˌȯ-(ˌ)tō-ˈan-ti-ˌbä-dē\ *n, pl* **-bod•ies** : an antibody active against a tissue constituent of the individual producing it

au•to•an•ti•gen \ˌȯ-tō-ˈan-ti-jen\ *n* : an antigen that is a normal bodily constituent and against which the immune system produces autoantibodies — **au•to•an•ti•gen•ic** \-ˌan-ti-ˈjen-ik\ *adj*

au•toch•tho•nous \(ˌ)ȯ-ˈtäk-thə-nəs\ *adj* **1 a** : indigenous or endemic to a region ⟨~ malaria⟩ **b** : contracted in the area where reported **2** : originated in that part of the body where found — used chiefly of pathological conditions — **au•toch•tho•nous•ly** *adv*

au•to•clav•able \ˈȯ-tə-ˌklā-və-bəl\ *adj* : able to withstand the action of an autoclave — **au•to•clav•abil•i•ty** \ˌȯ-tə-ˌklā-və-ˈbi-lə-tē\ *n*

au•to•clave \ˈȯ-tō-ˌklāv\ *n* : an apparatus (as for sterilizing) using superheated steam under pressure — **autoclave** *vb*

au•to•crine \ˈȯ-tō-ˌkrin\ *adj* : of, relating to, promoted by, or being a substance secreted by a cell and acting on surface receptors of the same cell ⟨~ action⟩ — compare PARACRINE

au•to•er•o•tism \ˌȯ-tō-ˈer-ə-ˌti-zəm\ *or* **au•to•erot•i•cism** \-i-ˈrä-tə-ˌsi-zəm\ *n* **1** : sexual gratification obtained solely through stimulation by oneself of one's own body **2** : sexual feeling arising without known external stimulation — **au•to•erot•ic** \-i-ˈrä-tik\ *adj* — **au•to•erot•i•cal•ly** \-ti-k(ə-)lē\ *adv*

au•to•gen•ic \ˌȯ-tə-ˈje-nik\ *adj* **1** : AUTOGENOUS **2** : of or relating to any of several relaxation techniques that actively involve the patient (as by meditation or biofeedback) in attempts to control physiological variables (as blood pressure)

au•tog•e•nous \ȯ-ˈtä-jə-nəs\ *adj* **1** : produced independently of external influence or aid : ENDOGENOUS **2** : originating or derived from sources within the same individual ⟨an ~ graft⟩ ⟨~ vaccine⟩

au•to•graft \ˈȯ-tō-ˌgraft\ *n* : a tissue or organ that is transplanted from one part to another part of the same body — **autograft** *vb*

au•to•he•mo•ly•sin \ˌȯ-tō-ˌhē-mə-ˈlīs-ᵊn\ *n* : a hemolysin that acts on the red blood cells of the individual in whose blood it is found

au•to•he•mo•ly•sis \-hi-ˈmä-lə-səs, -ˌhē-mə-ˈlī-səs\ *n, pl* **-ly•ses** \-ˌsēz\ : hemolysis of red blood cells by factors in the serum of the person from whom the blood is taken

au•to•he•mo•ther•a•py \-ˌhē-mō-ˈther-ə-pē\ *n, pl* **-pies** : treatment of disease by modification (as by irradiation) of the patient's own blood or by its introduction (as by intramuscular injection) outside the bloodstream

au•to•hyp•no•sis \ˌȯ-tō-hip-ˈnō-səs\ *n, pl* **-no•ses** \-ˌsēz\ : self-induced and usu. automatic hypnosis — **au•to•hyp•not•ic** \-ˈnä-tik\ *adj*

au•to•im•mune \-i-ˈmyün\ *adj* : of, relating to, or caused by antibodies or T cells that attack molecules, cells, or tissues of the organism producing them ⟨~ diseases⟩

autoimmune hemolytic anemia *n* : anemia caused by the excessive destruction of red blood cells by autoantibodies

autoimmune hepatitis *n* : chronic hepatitis occurring as a result of an immune system attack on cells of the liver

au•to•im•mu•ni•ty \ˌȯ-tō-i-ˈmyü-nə-tē\ *n, pl* **-ties** : a condition in which the body produces an immune response against its own tissue constituents — **au•to•im•mu•ni•za•tion** \-ˌi-myə-nə-ˈzā-shən *also* i-ˌmyü-nə-\ *n* — **au•to•im•mu•nize** \-ˈi-myə-ˌnīz\ *vb*

au•to•in•fec•tion \-in-ˈfek-shən\ *n* : reinfection with larvae produced by parasitic worms already in the body — compare HYPERINFECTION

au•to–in•ject•or \ˌȯ-(ˌ)tō-ˌin-ˈjek-tər\ *n* : a device for injecting oneself with a single dose of a drug that consists of a syringe which is activated when the device is pressed firmly against the body

au•to•in•oc•u•la•tion \-i-ˌnä-kyə-ˈlā-shən\ *n* **1** : inoculation with vaccine prepared from material from one's own body **2** : spread of infection from one part to other parts of the same body — **au•to•in•oc•u•la•ble** \ˌȯ-tō-i-ˈnä-kyə-lə-bəl\ *adj*

au•to•ki•ne•sis \ˌȯ-tō-kə-ˈnē-səs, -kī-\ *n, pl* **-ne•ses** \-ˌsēz\ : spontaneous or voluntary movement

au•tol•o•gous \ȯ-ˈtä-lə-gəs\ *adj* **1** : derived from the same individual ⟨~ grafts⟩ — compare HETEROLOGOUS 1, HOMOLOGOUS 2 **2** : involving one individual as both donor and recipient (as of blood) ⟨~ transfusion⟩

au•tol•y•sate \ȯ-ˈtä-lə-ˌsāt, -ˌzāt\ *also* **au•tol•y•zate** \-ˌzāt\ *n* : a product of autolysis

au•tol•y•sin \-lə-sən\ *n* : a substance that produces autolysis

au•tol•y•sis \-lə-səs\ *n, pl* **-y•ses** \-lə-ˌsēz\ : breakdown of all or part of a cell or tissue by self-produced enzymes — **au•to•lyt•ic** \ˌȯt-ᵊl-ˈi-tik\ *adj* — **au•to•lyze** \ˈȯt-ᵊl-ˌīz\ *vb*

automated external defibrillator *n* : a portable device that attaches to the chest and operates automatically to measure the heart's rhythm to determine if an electric shock is needed — abbr. *AED;* called also *automatic external defibrillator*

au•tom•a•tism \ȯ-ˈtä-mə-ˌti-zəm\ *n* **1** : an automatic action; *esp* : any action performed without the doer's intention or awareness **2** : the power or fact of moving or functioning without conscious control either independently of external stimulation (as in the beating of the heart) or more or less directly under the influence of external stimuli (as in the dilating or contracting of the pupil of the eye)

au•to•nom•ic \ˌȯ-tə-ˈnä-mik\ *adj* **1 a** : acting or occurring involuntarily ⟨~ reflexes⟩ **b** : relating to, affecting, or controlled by the autonomic nervous system ⟨~ ganglia⟩ **2** : having an effect upon tissue supplied by the autonomic nervous system ⟨~ drugs⟩ — **au•to•nom•i•cal•ly** \-mi-k(ə-)lē\ *adv*

autonomic dysreflexia *n* : a disorder of spinal reflex activity occurring in those with spinal cord injury that is characterized by a sudden onset of hypertension, bradycardia, excessive sweating, and headache

autonomic nervous system *n* : a part of the vertebrate nervous system that innervates smooth and cardiac muscle and glandular tissues and governs involuntary actions (as secretion, vasoconstriction, or peristalsis) and that consists of the sympathetic nervous system and the parasympathetic nervous system — compare CENTRAL NERVOUS SYSTEM, PERIPHERAL NERVOUS SYSTEM

au•ton•o•my \ȯ-ˈtä-nə-mē\ *n, pl* **-mies** **1** : the quality or state of being independent, free, and self-directing **2** : independence from the organism as a whole in the capacity of a part for growth, reactivity, or responsiveness — **au•ton•o•mous** \-məs\ *adj* — **au•ton•o•mous•ly** *adv*

au•to•pro•throm•bin \ˌȯ-tō-prō-ˈthräm-bən\ *n* : any of several blood factors formed in the conversion of prothrombin to thrombin: as **a** : FACTOR VII — called also *autoprothrombin I* **b** : FACTOR IX — called also *autoprothrombin II*

[1]**au•top•sy** \ˈȯ-ˌtäp-sē, -təp-\ *n, pl* **-sies** : an examination of the body after

death usu. with such dissection as will expose the vital organs for determining the cause of death or the character and extent of changes produced by disease — called also *necropsy, postmortem, postmortem examination*

²**autopsy** *vb* **-sied; -sy·ing** : to perform an autopsy on

au·to·ra·dio·gram \ˌȯ-tō-ˈrā-dē-ə-ˌgram\ *n* : AUTORADIOGRAPH

au·to·ra·dio·graph \-ˌgraf\ *n* : an image produced on a photographic film or plate by the radiations from a radioactive substance in an object which is in close contact with the emulsion — called also *radioautogram, radioautograph* — **autoradiograph** *vb* — **au·to·ra·dio·graph·ic** \-ˌrā-dē-ə-ˈgra-fik\ *adj* — **au·to·ra·di·og·ra·phy** \-ˌrā-dē-ˈä-grə-fē\ *n*

au·to·re·ac·tive \ˌȯ-tō-rē-ˈak-tiv\ *adj* : produced by an organism and acting against its own cells or tissues ⟨~ T cells⟩ — **au·to·re·ac·tiv·i·ty** \ˌȯ-tō-(ˌ)rē-ˌak-ˈti-və-tē\ *n*

au·to·reg·u·la·tion \ˌȯ-tō-ˌre-gyə-ˈlā-shən\ *n* : the maintenance of relative constancy of a physiological process by a bodily part or system under varying conditions; *esp* : the maintenance of a constant supply of blood to an organ in spite of varying arterial pressure — **au·to·reg·u·late** \-ˈre-gyə-ˌlāt\ *vb* — **au·to·reg·u·la·to·ry** \-ˈre-gyə-lə-ˌtōr-ē\ *adj*

au·to·sen·si·ti·za·tion \ˌȯ-tō-ˌsen-sə-tə-ˈzā-shən\ *n* : AUTOIMMUNIZATION

au·to·some \ˈȯ-tə-ˌsōm\ *n* : a chromosome other than a sex chromosome — **au·to·so·mal** \ˌȯ-tə-ˈsō-məl\ *adj* — **au·to·so·mal·ly** *adv*

au·to·sug·ges·tion \-səg-ˈjes-chən, -jesh-\ *n* : an influencing of one's own attitudes, behavior, or physical condition by mental processes other than conscious thought : SELF-HYPNOSIS — **au·to·sug·gest** \-səg-ˈjest\ *vb*

au·to·ther·a·py \ˈȯ-tō-ˌther-ə-pē\ *n, pl* **-pies** : SELF-TREATMENT

au·to·top·ag·no·sia \ˌȯ-tō-ˌtä-pig-ˈnō-zhə\ *n* : loss of the power to recognize or orient a bodily part due to a brain lesion

autotoxicus — see HORROR AUTOTOXICUS

au·to·trans·fu·sion \-trans-ˈfyü-zhən\ *n* : return of blood lost by or taken from a patient to his or her own circulatory system — **au·to·trans·fuse** \-trans-ˈfyüz\ *vb*

au·to·trans·plant \-ˈtrans-ˌplant\ *n* : AUTOGRAFT — **au·to·trans·plant** \-trans-ˈ\ *vb* — **au·to·trans·plan·ta·tion** \-ˌtrans-ˌplan-ˈtā-shən\ *n*

au·to·troph \ˈȯ-tə-ˌtrōf, -ˌträf\ *n* : an autotrophic organism

au·to·tro·phic \ˌȯ-tə-ˈtrō-fik\ *adj* **1** : needing only carbon dioxide or carbonates as a source of carbon and a simple inorganic nitrogen compound for metabolic synthesis **2** : not requiring a specified exogenous factor for normal metabolism — **au·to·tro·phi·cal·ly** \-fi-k(ə-)lē\ *adv* — **au·to·tro·phy** \ˈȯ-tə-ˌtrō-fē, ȯ-ˈtä-trə-fē\ *n*

au·to·vac·ci·na·tion \ˌȯ-tō-ˌvak-sə-ˈnā-shən\ *n* : vaccination of an individual by material from the individual's own body or with a vaccine prepared from such material

au·tumn cro·cus \ˌȯ-təm-ˈkrō-kəs\ *n* : an herb (*Colchicum autumnale*) of the lily family (Liliaceae) that is the source of medicinal colchicum

¹**aux·il·ia·ry** \ȯg-ˈzil-yə-rē, -ˈzi-lə-rē, -ˈzil-rē\ *adj* : serving to supplement or assist ⟨~ springs in a dental appliance⟩

²**auxiliary** *n* **1** : one who assists or serves another person esp. in dentistry **2** : an organization that assists (as by donations or volunteer services) the work esp. of a hospital

AV *abbr* **1** arteriovenous **2** atrioventricular

Avan·dia \ˌä-ˌvan-ˈdē-ə\ *trademark* — used for a preparation of the maleate of rosiglitazone

Av·a·pro \ˈa-və-ˌprō\ *trademark* — used for a preparation of irbesartan

avas·cu·lar \(ˌ)ā-ˈvas-kyə-lər\ *adj* : having few or no blood vessels ⟨~ tissue⟩ — **avas·cu·lar·i·ty** \-ˌvas-kyə-ˈlar-ə-tē\ *n*

avascular necrosis *n* : necrosis of bone tissue due to impaired or disrupted blood supply (as that caused by traumatic injury or disease) resulting in weakened bone that may flatten and collapse — called also *aseptic necrosis, osteonecrosis*

Avas·tin \ə-ˈva-stən\ *trademark* — used for a preparation of bevacizumab

Aven·tyl \ˈa-vən-ˌtil\ *trademark* — used for a preparation of nortriptyline

aver·sion \ə-ˈvər-zhən, -shən\ *n* **1** : a feeling of repugnance toward something with a desire to avoid or turn from it **2** : a tendency to extinguish a behavior or to avoid a thing or situation and esp. a usu. pleasurable one because it is or has been associated with a noxious stimulus

aversion therapy *n* : therapy intended to suppress an undesirable habit or behavior (as smoking or overeating) by associating the habit or behavior with a noxious or punishing stimulus (as an electric shock)

aver·sive \ə-ˈvər-siv, -ziv\ *adj* : tending to avoid or causing avoidance of a noxious or punishing stimulus ⟨behavior modification by ~ conditioning⟩ — **aver·sive·ly** *adv* — **aver·sive·ness** *n*

avi·an cholera \ˈā-vē-ən-\ *n* : FOWL CHOLERA

avian flu *n* : BIRD FLU

avian influenza *n* : BIRD FLU

avian tuberculosis *n* : tuberculosis of birds usu. caused by a bacterium of the genus *Mycobacterium* (*M. avium*); *also* : infection of mammals (as swine) by the same bacterium

avi•o•pho•bia *also* **avi•a•pho•bia** \ˌā-vē-ə-ˈfō-bē-ə, ˌa-\ *n* : fear of flying : AEROPHOBIA
avir•u•lent \(ˌ)ā-ˈvir-ə-lənt, -ˈvir-yə-\ *adj* : not virulent ⟨an ∼ tubercle bacillus⟩
avis — see CALCAR AVIS
avi•ta•min•osis \ˌā-ˌvī-tə-mə-ˈnō-səs\ *n, pl* **-o•ses** \-ˌsēz\ : disease (as pellagra) resulting from a deficiency of one or more vitamins — called also *hypovitaminosis* — **avi•ta•min•ot•ic** \-mə-ˈnä-tik\ *adj*
A–V node *or* **AV node** \ˌā-ˈvē-\ *n* : ATRIOVENTRICULAR NODE
avo•ben•zone \ˌā-və-ˈben-ˌzōn\ *n* : a chemical compound $C_{20}H_{22}O_3$ that absorbs UVA radiation and is used as an ingredient in sunscreens — see PARSOL
Av•o•dart \ˈav-ō-ˌdärt\ *trademark* — used for a preparation of dutasteride
avoid•ance \ə-ˈvȯid-ᵊns\ *n, often attrib* : the act or practice of keeping away from or withdrawing from something undesirable; *esp* : an anticipatory response undertaken to avoid a noxious stimulus
avoidance–avoidance conflict *n* : psychological conflict that results when a choice must be made between two undesirable alternatives — compare APPROACH-APPROACH CONFLICT, APPROACH-AVOIDANCE CONFLICT
avoid•ant \ə-ˈvȯid-ᵊnt\ *adj* : characterized by turning away or by withdrawal or defensive behavior
avoidant personality disorder *n* : a personality disorder that is characterized by excessive sensitivity to social criticism and rejection, low self-esteem, and social withdrawal despite a desire for acceptance and affection
av•oir•du•pois \ˌa-vər-də-ˈpȯiz, -ˈpwä\ *adj* : expressed in avoirdupois weight ⟨∼ units⟩ ⟨5 ounces ∼⟩
avoirdupois pound *n* : POUND b
avoirdupois weight *n* : a system of weights based on a pound of 16 ounces and an ounce of 437.5 grains (28.350 grams)
avo•li•tion \(ˈ)ā-ˌvō-ˈli-shən, -və-\ *n* : lack of interest or engagement in goal-directed behavior — **avo•li•tion•al** \(ˈ)ā-ˌvō-ˈlish-nəl, -ˈli-shə-nᵊl, -və-\ *adj*
Av•o•nex \ˈa-və-ˌneks\ *trademark* — used for a preparation of a recombinant form of beta interferon
AVP *abbr* arginine vasopressin
avul•sion \ə-ˈvəl-shən\ *n* : a tearing away of a body part accidentally or surgically — **avulse** \ə-ˈvəls\ *vb*
avulsion fracture *n* : the detachment of a bone fragment that results from the pulling away of a ligament, tendon, or joint capsule from its point of attachment on a bone — called also *sprain fracture*
ax- *or* **axo-** *comb form* : axon ⟨*axo*dendritic⟩
axe•nic \(ˌ)ā-ˈze-nik, -ˈzē-\ *adj* : free from other living organisms ⟨an ∼ culture of bacteria⟩ — **axe•ni•cal•ly** \-ni-k(ə-)lē\ *adv*
ax•i•al \ˈak-sē-əl\ *adj* **1** : of, relating to, or having the characteristics of an axis **2** : situated around, in the direction of, on, or along an axis
axial skeleton *n* : the skeleton of the trunk and head
Ax•id \ˈak-sid\ *trademark* — used for a preparation of nizatidine
ax•il•la \ag-ˈzi-lə, ak-ˈsi-\ *n, pl* **-lae** \-(ˌ)lē, -ˌlī\ *or* **-las** : the cavity beneath the junction of the arm or anterior appendage and shoulder or shoulder girdle containing the axillary artery and vein, a part of the brachial plexus of nerves, many lymph nodes, and fat and areolar tissue; *esp* : ARMPIT
ax•il•lary \ˈak-sə-ˌler-ē\ *adj* : of, relating to, or located near the axilla ⟨∼ lymph nodes⟩
axillary artery *n* : the part of the main artery of the arm that lies in the axilla and that is continuous with the subclavian artery above and the brachial artery below
axillary nerve *n* : a large nerve arising from the posterior cord of the brachial plexus and supplying the deltoid and teres minor muscles and the skin of the shoulder
axillary node *n* : any of the lymph nodes of the axilla
axillary vein *n* : the large vein passing through the axilla continuous with the basilic vein below and the subclavian vein above
Ax•i•ron \ˈak-sə-ˌrän\ *trademark* — used for a topical preparation of testosterone
ax•is \ˈak-səs\ *n, pl* **ax•es** \-ˌsēz\ **1 a** : a straight line about which a body or a geometric figure rotates or may be thought of as rotating **b** : a straight line with respect to which a body, organ, or figure is symmetrical **2 a** : the second vertebra of the neck of the higher vertebrates that is prolonged anteriorly within the foramen of the first vertebra and united with the dens which serves as a pivot for the atlas and head to turn upon — called also *epistropheus* **b** : any of various central, fundamental, or axial parts ⟨the cerebrospinal ∼⟩ ⟨the skeletal ∼⟩ **c** : AXILLA
axis cylinder *n* : AXON; *esp* : the axon of a myelinated neuron
axo–ax•on•ic \ˌak-sō-ak-ˈsän-ik\ *also* **axo–ax•o•nal** \-ˈak-sən-ᵊl, -ak-ˈsän-, -ˈsōn-\ *adj* : relating to or being a synapse between an axon of one neuron and an axon of another
axo•den•drit•ic \ˌak-sō-den-ˈdri-tik\ *adj* : relating to or being a nerve synapse between an axon of one neuron and a dendrite of another
axo•lem•ma \ˈak-sə-ˌle-mə\ *n* : the plasma membrane of an axon — **axo•lem•mal** \ˈak-sə-ˌle-məl\ *adj*
ax•on \ˈak-ˌsän\ *also* **ax•one** \-ˌsōn\ *n* : a usu. long and single nerve-cell process

that usu. conducts impulses away from the cell body — **ax•o•nal** \ˈak-sən-ᵊl; ak-ˈsän-, -ˈsōn-\ *adj* — **ax•o•nal•ly** *adv*

ax•on•o•tme•sis \ˌak-sə-nət-ˈmē-səs\ *n, pl* **-me•ses** \-ˌsēz\ : axonal nerve damage that does not completely sever the surrounding endoneurial sheath so that regeneration can take place

axo•plasm \ˈak-sə-ˌpla-zəm\ *n* : the protoplasm of an axon — **axo•plas•mic** \ˌak-sə-ˈplaz-mik\ *adj*

axo•so•mat•ic \ˌak-sō-sō-ˈma-tik\ *adj* : relating to or being a nerve synapse between the cell body of one neuron and an axon of another

aya•hua•sca \ˌī-ə-ˈ(h)wä-skə\ *n* : a hallucinogenic beverage that is prepared from the bark of a South American vine (*Banisteriopsis caapi* of the family Malpighiaceae) typically in a mixture with other psychoactive plants — called also *yage*

Ayer•za's disease \ə-ˈyər-zəz-\ *n* : a complex of symptoms marked esp. by cyanosis, dyspnea, polycythemia, and sclerosis of the pulmonary artery

Ayerza, Abel (1861–1918), Argentinean physician.

Ay•ur•ve•da \ˌī-yər-ˈvā-də\ *n* : the traditional system of medicine of India that seeks to treat and integrate body, mind, and spirit using a holistic approach that emphasizes diet, herbal remedies, exercise, meditation, breathing, and physical therapy — **Ay•ur•ve•dic** \-dik\ *adj*

Ayurvedic medicine *n* : AYURVEDA

az- *or* **azo-** *comb form* : containing nitrogen esp. as an azo group ⟨*azo*sulfamide⟩

aza•ci•ti•dine \ˌa-zə-ˈsi-tə-ˌden, -ˈsī-\ *or* **5–aza•cy•ti•dine** \ˈfīv-\ *also* **azacytidine** *n* : an antineoplastic cytidine analog $C_8H_{12}N_4O_5$ that is administered by subcutaneous injection in the treatment of myelodysplastic syndrome

aza•thi•o•prine \ˌa-zə-ˈthī-ə-ˌprēn\ *n* : a purine antimetabolite $C_9H_7N_7O_2S$ that is used esp. as an immunosuppressant — see IMURAN

az•e•la•ic acid \ˌa-zə-ˌlā-ik-\ *n* : a crystalline acid $C_9H_{16}O_4$ that has antimicrobial properties and is applied topically in the treatment of acne and rosacea

azel•a•stine \ə-ˈze-lə-ˌstēn\ *n* : an antihistamine drug used in the form of its hydrochloride $C_{22}H_{24}ClN_3O{\cdot}HCl$ as a nasal spray to treat rhinitis and as eye drops to treat itching associated with allergic conjunctivitis

az•i•do•thy•mi•dine \ˌa-zi-dō-ˈthī-mə-ˌdēn\ *n* : AZT

azith•ro•my•cin \ə-ˌzith-rō-ˈmī-sᵊn\ *n* : a semisynthetic macrolide antibiotic $C_{38}H_{72}N_2O_{12}$ that is derived from erythromycin and is used esp. as an antibacterial agent — see ZITHROMAX, Z-PAK

Az•ma•cort \ˈaz-mə-ˌkȯrt\ *trademark* — used for a preparation of triamcinolone

azo \ˈā-(ˌ)zō, ˈa-\ *adj* : relating to, containing, or being the group N=N united at both ends to carbon

azo dye *n* : any of numerous dyes containing azo groups

azo•osper•mia \ā-ˌzō-ə-ˈspər-mē-ə, ə-ˌzō-\ *n* : absence of spermatozoa from the seminal fluid — compare ASPERMIA — **azo•osper•mic** \-ˈspər-mik\ *adj*

Azor \ˈā-ˌzȯr\ *trademark* — used for a preparation of amlodipine and olmesartan

azo•sul•fa•mide \ˌā-zō-ˈsəl-fə-ˌmīd\ *n* : a dark red crystalline azo compound $C_{18}H_{14}N_4Na_2O_{10}S_3$ of the sulfa class having antibacterial effect similar to that of sulfanilamide — called also *prontosil*

azot- *or* **azoto-** *comb form* : nitrogen : nitrogenous substance ⟨*azot*uria⟩

azo•te•mia \ˌā-zō-ˈtē-mē-ə\ *n* : an excess of nitrogenous bodies in the blood as a result of kidney insufficiency — compare UREMIA — **azo•te•mic** \-ˈtē-mik\ *adj*

azo•tu•ria \ˌā-zō-ˈtu̇r-ē-ə, -ˈtyu̇r-\ *n* : an abnormal condition of horses characterized by an excess of urea or other nitrogenous substances in the urine and by muscle damage esp. to the hindquarters

AZT \ˌā-(ˌ)zē-ˈtē\ *n* : an antiviral drug $C_{10}H_{13}N_5O_4$ that inhibits replication of some retroviruses (as HIV) and is used to treat AIDS — called also *azidothymidine, ZDV, zidovudine;* see RETROVIR

az•tre•o•nam \ˌaz-ˈtrē-ō-ˌnam\ *n* : a synthetic monobactam antibiotic $C_{13}H_{17}N_5O_8S_2$ used esp. against gram-negative bacteria

azygo- *comb form* : azygos ⟨*azygo*graphy⟩

azy•gog•ra•phy \ˌā-zī-ˈgä-grə-fē\ *n, pl* **-phies** : radiographic visualization of the azygos system of veins after injection of a radiopaque medium

[1]**azy•gos** \ā-ˈzī-gəs\ *n* : an azygos anatomical part

[2]**azy•gos** *also* **azy•gous** \(ˌ)ā-ˈzī-gəs\ *adj* : not being one of a pair ⟨the ~ muscle of the uvula⟩

azygos vein *n* : any of a system of three veins which drain the thoracic wall and much of the abdominal wall and which form a collateral circulation when either the inferior or superior vena cava is obstructed; *esp* : a vein that receives blood from the right half of the thoracic and abdominal walls, ascends along the right side of the vertebral column, and empties into the superior vena cava — compare ACCESSORY HEMIAZYGOS VEIN, HEMIAZYGOS VEIN

B

b *abbr* bicuspid

B \ˈbē\ *n* : the one of the four ABO blood groups characterized by the presence of antigens designated by the letter B and by the presence of antibodies against the antigens present in the A blood group

B *symbol* boron

Ba *symbol* barium

ba·be·sia \bə-ˈbē-zhə, -zhē-ə\ *n* **1** *cap* : a genus of sporozoans (family Babesiidae) parasitic in mammalian red blood cells and transmitted by the bite of a tick **2** *pl* **-sias** *or* **-si·ae** \-zhē-ˌē\ : any sporozoan of the genus *Babesia* or sometimes the family (Babesiidae) to which it belongs — called also *piroplasm*

Babès, Victor (1854–1926), Romanian bacteriologist.

babe·si·a·sis \ˌba-bə-ˈsī-ə-səs\ *n, pl* **-a·ses** \-ˌsēz\ : BABESIOSIS

ba·be·si·o·sis \ˌba-bə-ˈsī-ə-səs, bə-ˌbē-zē-ˈō-səs\ *n, pl* **-o·ses** \-ˌsēz\ : infection with or disease caused by babesias — called also *babesiasis*

Ba·bin·ski reflex \bə-ˈbin-skē-\ *also* **Ba·bin·ski's reflex** \-skēz-\ *n* : a reflex movement in which when the sole is tickled the great toe turns upward instead of downward and which is normal in infancy but indicates damage to the central nervous system (as in the pyramidal tracts) when occurring later in life — called also *Babinski sign, Babinski's sign;* compare PLANTAR REFLEX

Babinski, Joseph–François–Felix (1857–1932), French neurologist.

ba·by \ˈbā-bē\ *n, pl* **babies** : an extremely young child or animal; *esp* : INFANT

baby talk *n* **1** : the imperfect speech or modified forms used by small children learning to talk **2** : the consciously imperfect or altered speech often used by adults in speaking to small children

baby tooth *n* : MILK TOOTH

BAC *abbr* blood alcohol concentration

bacill- *or* **bacilli-** *or* **bacillo-** *comb form* : bacillus ⟨*bacill*osis⟩

ba·cil·la·ry \ˈba-sə-ˌler-ē, bə-ˈsi-lə-rē\ *also* **ba·cil·lar** \bə-ˈsi-lər, ˈba-sə-lər\ *adj* **1** : shaped like a rod; *also* : consisting of small rods **2** : of, relating to, or caused by bacilli ⟨~ meningitis⟩

bacillary angiomatosis *n* : a bacterial disease esp. of the skin, subcutaneous tissue, and mucous membranes that occurs in immunocompromised individuals, is characterized by red or purple elevated lesions or scaly nodules, may spread to involve bone and internal organs, and is caused by either of two bacteria of the genus *Bartonella* (*B. henselae* and *B. quintana*) — called also *epithelioid angiomatosis*

ba·cille Calmette–Guérin \ba-ˈsēl-\ *n* : BACILLUS CALMETTE-GUÉRIN

bac·il·le·mia \ˌba-sə-ˈlē-mē-ə\ *n* : BACTEREMIA

bac·il·lo·sis \ˌba-sə-ˈlō-səs\ *n, pl* **-lo·ses** \-ˌsēz\ : infection with bacilli

bac·il·lu·ria \ˌba-sə-ˈlu̇r-ē-ə, -ˈlyu̇r-\ *n* : the passage of bacilli with the urine — **bac·il·lu·ric** \-ik\ *adj*

ba·cil·lus \bə-ˈsi-ləs\ *n, pl* **-li** \-ˌlī *also* -lē\ **1 a** *cap* : a genus of aerobic rod-shaped gram-positive bacteria (family Bacillaceae) that include many saprophytes and some parasites (as *B. anthracis* of anthrax) **b** : any bacterium of the genus *Bacillus*; *broadly* : a straight rod-shaped bacterium **2** : BACTERIUM; *esp* : a disease-producing bacterium

bacillus Cal·mette–Gué·rin \-ˌkal-ˈmet-(ˌ)gā-ˈra^n, -ˈran\ *n* : an attenuated strain of tubercle bacillus developed by repeated culture on a medium containing bile and used in preparation of tuberculosis vaccines — compare BCG VACCINE

Calmette, Albert Léon Charles (1863–1933), French bacteriologist, and **Guérin, Camille (1872–1961),** French veterinarian.

bac·i·tra·cin \ˌba-sə-ˈtrās-^{ə}n\ *n* : a polypeptide antibiotic isolated from a bacillus (*Bacillus subtilis* or *B. licheniformis*) and usu. used topically esp. against gram-positive bacteria

Tra·cy \ˈtrā-sē\, **Margaret,** American hospital patient.

back \ˈbak\ *n* **1 a** : the rear part of the human body esp. from the neck to the end of the spine **b** : the corresponding part of a lower animal (as a quadruped) **c** : SPINAL COLUMN **2** : the part of the upper surface of the tongue behind the front and lying opposite the soft palate when the tongue is at rest

back·ache \ˈbak-ˌāk\ *n* : a pain in the lower back

back·board \ˈbak-ˌbȯrd\ *n* : a stiff board on which an injured person and esp. one with neck or spinal injuries is placed and immobilized in order to prevent further injury during transport

back·bone \-ˌbōn\ *n* **1** : SPINAL COLUMN, SPINE **2** : the longest chain of atoms or groups of atoms in a usu. long molecule (as a protein)

[1]**back·cross** \ˈbak-ˌkrȯs\ *vb* : to cross (a first-generation hybrid) with one of the parental types

[2]**backcross** *n* : a mating that involves backcrossing; *also* : an individual produced by backcrossing

back·ing \ˈba-kiŋ\ *n* : the metal portion of a dental crown, bridge, or similar structure to which a porcelain or plastic tooth facing is attached

back•rest \ˈbak-ˌrest\ *n* : a rest for the back

back•side \-ˈsīd\ *n* : BUTTOCKS — often used in pl.

bac•lo•fen \ˈba-klō-ˌfen\ *n* : a gamma-aminobutyric acid analog $C_{10}H_{12}ClNO_2$ used as a relaxant of skeletal muscle esp. in treating spasticity (as in multiple sclerosis)

bact *abbr* **1** bacteria; bacterial **2** bacteriological; bacteriology **3** bacterium

bacter- *or* **bacteri-** *or* **bacterio-** *comb form* : bacteria : bacterial ⟨*bacterio*lysis⟩

bac•ter•emia \ˌbak-tə-ˈrē-mē-ə\ *n* : the usu. transient presence of bacteria in the blood — **bac•ter•emic** \-mik\ *adj*

[1]**bacteria** *pl of* BACTERIUM

[2]**bacteria** *n* : BACTERIUM — not usu. used technically

bac•te•ri•al \bak-ˈtir-ē-əl\ *adj* : of, relating to, or caused by bacteria ⟨a ~ chromosome⟩ ⟨~ infection⟩ — **bac•te•ri•al•ly** *adv*

bacterial vag•i•no•sis \-ˌva-jə-ˈnō-səs\ *n* : vaginitis that is marked by a grayish vaginal discharge usu. of foul odor and that is associated with the presence of a bacterium esp. of the genus *Gardnerella* (*G. vaginalis* syn. *Haemophilus vaginalis*) — abbr. *BV;* called also *nonspecific vaginitis*

bac•te•ri•cid•al \bak-ˌtir-ə-ˈsīd-ᵊl\ *also* **bac•te•ri•o•cid•al** \-ˌtir-ē-ə-ˈsīd-\ *adj* : destroying bacteria — **bac•te•ri•cid•al•ly** *adv* — **bac•te•ri•cide** \-ˈtir-ə-ˌsīd\ *n*

bac•te•ri•cid•in \bak-ˌtir-ə-ˈsīd-ᵊn\ *or* **bac•te•ri•o•cid•in** \-ˌtir-ē-ə-ˈsīd-\ *n* : a bactericidal antibody

bac•ter•in \ˈbak-tə-rən\ *n* : a suspension of killed or attenuated bacteria for use as a vaccine

bac•te•rio•cin \bak-ˈtir-ē-ə-sən\ *n* : an antibiotic (as colicin) produced by bacteria

bac•te•ri•ol•o•gist \(ˌ)bak-ˌtir-ē-ˈä-lə-jist\ *n* : a specialist in bacteriology

bac•te•ri•ol•o•gy \(ˌ)bak-ˌtir-ē-ˈä-lə-jē\ *n, pl* **-gies** **1** : a science that deals with bacteria and their relations to medicine, industry, and agriculture **2** : bacterial life and phenomena — **bac•te•ri•o•log•ic** \bak-ˌtir-ē-ə-ˈlä-jik\ *or* **bac•te•ri•o•log•i•cal** \-ˈlä-ji-kəl\ *adj* — **bac•te•ri•o•log•i•cal•ly** \-ji-k(ə-)lē\ *adv*

bac•te•rio•ly•sin \bak-ˌtir-ē-ə-ˈlīs-ᵊn\ *n* : an antibody that acts to destroy a bacterium

bac•te•ri•ol•y•sis \(ˌ)bak-ˌtir-ē-ˈä-lə-səs\ *n, pl* **-y•ses** \-ˌsēz\ : destruction or dissolution of bacterial cells — **bac•te•ri•o•lyt•ic** \bak-ˌtir-ē-ə-ˈli-tik\ *adj*

bac•te•rio•phage \bak-ˈtir-ē-ə-ˌfāj, -ˌfäzh\ *n* : a virus that infects bacteria — called also *phage*

bacteriophage lambda *n* : a bacteriophage (species *Enterobacteria phage λ* of the family *Siphoviridae*) containing double-stranded DNA and that can be integrated as a prophage into the genome of some strains of E. coli and is used as a vector to clone DNA from various organisms — called also *lambda phage, phage lambda*

bac•te•rio•sta•sis \bak-ˌtir-ē-ō-ˈstā-səs\ *n, pl* **-sta•ses** \-ˌsēz\ : inhibition of the growth of bacteria without destruction

bac•te•rio•stat \-ˈtir-ē-ō-ˌstat\ *also* **bac•te•rio•stat•ic** \-ˌtir-ē-ō-ˈsta-tik\ *n* : an agent that causes bacteriostasis

bac•te•rio•stat•ic \-ˌtir-ē-ō-ˈsta-tik\ *adj* : causing bacteriostasis ⟨a ~ agent⟩ — **bac•te•rio•stat•i•cal•ly** \-ti-k(ə-)lē\ *adv*

bac•te•ri•o•ther•a•py \-ˈther-ə-pē\ *n, pl* **-pies** : the treatment of disease by the use of bacteria or their products

bac•te•ri•um \bak-ˈtir-ē-əm\ *n, pl* **-ria** \-ē-ə\ : any of a domain (Bacteria) of prokaryotic round, spiral, or rod-shaped single-celled microorganisms that are often aggregated into colonies or motile by means of flagella, that live in soil, water, organic matter, or the bodies of plants and animals, and that are usu. autotrophic, saprophytic, or parasitic in nutrition, and that are noted for their biochemical effects and pathogenicity; *broadly* : PROKARYOTE

bac•te•ri•uria \bak-ˌtir-ē-ˈu̇r-ē-ə, -ˈyu̇r-\ *n* : the presence of bacteria in the urine — **bac•te•ri•uric** \-ik\ *adj*

bac•te•roi•des \-ˈrȯi-(ˌ)dēz\ *n* **1** *cap* : a genus of gram-negative anaerobic bacteria (family Bacteroidaceae) that typically occur as part of the normal intestinal flora **2** *pl* **-roides** : a bacterium of the genus *Bacteroides* or of a closely related genus

Bac•trim \ˈbak-trim\ *trademark* — used for a preparation of sulfamethoxazole and trimethoprim

Bac•tro•ban \ˈbak-trō-ˌban\ *trademark* — used for a preparation of mupirocin

bac•u•lo•vi•rus \ˌba-kyü-lō-ˈvī-rəs\ *n* : any of a family (*Baculoviridae*) of DNA viruses that infect arthropods and esp. insects and have been used as biological control agents for insect pests and experimentally in recombinant DNA technology

bad cholesterol *n* : LDL

[1]**bag** \ˈbag\ *n* **1** : a pouched or pendulous bodily part or organ; *esp* : UDDER **2** : a puffy or sagging protuberance of flabby skin ⟨~*s* under the eyes⟩

[2]**bag** *vb* **bagged; bag•ging** : to ventilate the lungs of (a patient) using a hand-squeezed bag attached to a face mask

ba•gasse \bə-ˈgas\ *n* : plant residue (as of sugarcane or grapes) left after a product (as juice) has been extracted

bag•as•so•sis \ˌba-gə-ˈsō-səs\ *n, pl* **-so•ses** \-ˌsēz\ : an industrial disease characterized by cough, difficult breathing, chills, fever, and prolonged weakness and caused by the inhalation of the dust of bagasse — called also *bagasse disease*

Bagh•dad boil \ˈbag-ˌdad-\ *n* : ORIENTAL SORE

bag of waters *n* : the double-walled fluid-filled sac that encloses and protects the fetus in the mother's womb and that breaks releasing its fluid during the birth process

Bain•bridge reflex \ˈbān-(ˌ)brij-\ *n* : a homeostatic reflex mechanism that causes acceleration of heartbeat following the stimulation of local muscle spindles when blood pressure in the venae cavae and right atrium is increased

Bainbridge, Francis Arthur (1874–1921), British physiologist.

Ba•ker's cyst \ˈbā-kərz-\ *n* : a swelling behind the knee that is composed of a membrane-lined sac filled with synovial fluid and is associated with certain joint disorders (as arthritis)

Baker, William Morrant (1839–1896), British surgeon.

bak•er's itch \ˌbā-kərz-\ *n* : GROCER'S ITCH

bak•ing soda \ˈbā-kiŋ-\ *n* : SODIUM BICARBONATE

BAL \ˌbē-(ˌ)ā-ˈel\ *n* : DIMERCAPROL

balan- *or* **balano-** *comb form* : glans penis ⟨*balan*itis⟩ ⟨*balano*posthitis⟩

bal•ance \ˈba-ləns\ *n* **1** : an instrument for weighing **2** : mental and emotional steadiness **3** : the relation in physiology between the intake of a particular substance and its excretion — see NITROGEN BALANCE, WATER BALANCE

bal•anced \-lənst\ *adj* **1** : having the physiologically active elements mutually counteracting ⟨a ~ solution⟩ **2** *of a diet or ration* : furnishing all needed nutrients in the amount, form, and proportions needed to support healthy growth and productivity

bal•a•ni•tis \ˌba-lə-ˈnī-təs\ *n* : inflammation of the glans penis

bal•a•no•pos•thi•tis \ˌba-lə-(ˌ)nō-päs-ˈthī-təs\ *n* : inflammation of the glans penis and of the foreskin

bal•an•ti•di•a•sis \ˌba-lən-tə-ˈdī-ə-səs, bə-ˌlan-\ *also* **bal•an•tid•i•o•sis** \ˌba-lən-ˌti-dē-ˈō-səs\ *n, pl* **-a•ses** *also* **-o•ses** \-ˌsēz\ : infection with or disease caused by protozoans of the genus *Balantidium*

bal•an•tid•i•um \ˌba-lən-ˈti-dē-əm\ *n* **1** *cap* : a genus of large parasitic ciliate protozoans (order Heterotricha) including one (*B. coli*) that infests the intestines of some mammals and esp. swine and may cause a chronic ulcerative dysentery in humans **2** *pl* **-ia** \-dē-ə\ : a protozoan of the genus *Balantidium* — **ba•lan•tid•i•al** \-dē-əl\ *adj*

bald \ˈbȯld\ *adj* : lacking all or a significant part of the hair on the head or sometimes on other parts of the body — **bald** *vb*

bald•ness *n* : the state of being bald — see MALE-PATTERN BALDNESS

Bal•kan frame \ˈbȯl-kən-\ *n* : a frame employed in the treatment of fractured bones of the leg or arm that provides overhead weights and pulleys for suspension, traction, and continuous extension of the splinted fractured limb

ball \ˈbȯl\ *n* **1** : a roundish protuberant part of the body: as **a** : the rounded eminence by which the base of the thumb is continuous with the palm of the hand **b** : the rounded broad part of the sole of the human foot between toes and arch and on which the main weight of the body first rests in normal walking **2** : EYEBALL **3** *often vulgar* : TESTIS

ball–and–socket joint *n* : an articulation (as the hip joint) in which the rounded head of one bone fits into a cuplike cavity of the other and admits movement in any direction — called also *enarthrosis*

bal•lism \ˈba-ˌli-zəm\ *or* **bal•lis•mus** \bə-ˈliz-məs\ *n, pl* **-lisms** *or* **-lis•mus•es** : the abnormal swinging jerking movements sometimes seen in chorea

bal•lis•to•car•dio•gram \bə-ˌlis-tō-ˈkär-dē-ə-ˌgram\ *n* : the record made by a ballistocardiograph

bal•lis•to•car•dio•graph \-ˌgraf\ *n* : a device for measuring the amount of blood passing through the heart in a specified time by recording the recoil movements of the body that result from contraction of the heart muscle in ejecting blood from the ventricles — **bal•lis•to•car•dio•graph•ic** \-ˌkär-dē-ə-ˈgra-fik\ *adj* — **bal•lis•to•car•di•og•ra•phy** \-ē-ˈä-grə-fē\ *n*

[1]**bal•loon** \bə-ˈlün\ *n* : a nonporous bag of tough light material that can be inflated (as in a bodily cavity) with air or gas

[2]**balloon** *vb* : to inflate, swell, or puff out like a balloon

balloon angioplasty *n* : dilation of an obstructed artherosclerotic artery by the passage of a balloon catheter through the vessel to the area of disease where inflation of the catheter's tip compresses the plaque against the vessel wall

balloon catheter *n* : a catheter with an inflatable tip which can be expanded (as by air or water) esp. to hold the catheter in place or to expand a partly closed or obstructed bodily passage, opening, or vessel (as a coronary artery) — called also *balloon-tipped catheter;* see BALLOON ANGIOPLASTY, PERCUTANEOUS TRANSLUMINAL ANGIOPLASTY

bal•lotte•ment \bə-ˈlät-mənt\ *n* : a sharp upward pushing against the uterine wall with a finger inserted into the vagina for diagnosing pregnancy by feeling the return impact of the displaced fetus; *also* : a similar procedure for detecting a floating kidney

balm \ˈbäm, ˈbälm, ˈbȧm\ *n* **1** : an aromatic preparation (as a healing ointment) **2** : a soothing restorative agency

balne- or **balneo-** *comb form* : bath : bathing ⟨*balneo*therapy⟩

bal•ne•ol•o•gy \ˌbal-nē-ˈä-lə-jē\ *n, pl* **-gies** : the science of the therapeutic use of baths

bal•neo•ther•a•py \ˌbal-nē-ō-ˈther-ə-pē\ *n, pl* **-pies** : the treatment of disease by baths

bal•sam \ˈbȯl-səm\ *n* **1** : any of several resinous substances used esp. in medicine **2** : BALM 2 — **bal•sam•ic** \bȯl-ˈsa-mik\ *adj*

balsam of Pe•ru \-pə-ˈrü\ *n* : a balsam from a tropical tree (*Myroxylon pereirae*) used esp. as an irritant and to promote wound healing — called also *Peru balsam, Peruvian balsam*

balsam of To•lu \-tə-ˈlü\ *n* : a balsam from a tropical tree (*Myroxylon balsamum*) used esp. as an expectorant and as a flavoring for cough syrups — called also *tolu, tolu balsam*

bam•boo spine \(ˌ)bam-ˈbü-\ *n* : a spinal column in the advanced stage of ankylosing spondylitis esp. as observed in an X-ray with ossification of the vertebrae giving the spine an appearance of a stick of bamboo

Ban•croft•i•an filariasis \ˈban-ˌkrȯf-tē-ən-, ˈbaŋ-\ or **Ban•croft's filariasis** \-ˌkrȯfts-\ *n* : filariasis caused by a slender white filaria of the genus *Wuchereria* (*W. bancrofti*) that is transmitted in larval form by mosquitoes, lives in lymph vessels and lymphoid tissues, and often causes elephantiasis by blocking lymphatic drainage

Ban•croft \ˈban-ˌkrȯft, ˈbaŋ-\, **Joseph (1836–1894),** British physician.

band \ˈband\ *n* **1** : a thin flat encircling strip esp. for binding: as **a** : a strip of cloth used to protect a newborn baby's navel — called also *bellyband* **b** : a thin flat strip of metal that encircles a tooth ⟨orthodontic ~*s*⟩ **2** : a strip separated by some characteristic color or texture or considered apart from what is adjacent: as **a** : a line or streak of differentiated cells **b** : one of the alternating dark and light segments of skeletal muscle fibers **c** : a strip of abnormal tissue either congenital or acquired; *esp* : a strip of connective tissue that causes obstruction of the bowel

[1]**ban•dage** \ˈban-dij\ *n* : a strip of fabric used to cover a wound, hold a dressing in place, immobilize an injured part, or apply pressure — see CAPELINE, ESMARCH BANDAGE, PRESSURE BANDAGE, SPICA, VELPEAU BANDAGE

[2]**bandage** *vb* **ban•daged; ban•dag•ing** : to bind, dress, or cover with a bandage

Band–Aid \ˈban-ˌdād\ *trademark* — used for a small adhesive strip with a gauze pad for covering minor wounds

band cell *n* : a young neutrophil in the stage of development following a metamyelocyte and having an elongated nucleus that has not yet become lobed as in a mature neutrophil — called also *band form, band neutrophil, stab cell*

band keratopathy *n* : the deposition of calcium salts in the superficial layers of the cornea immediately below the epithelium that appears as an opaque grayish-white streak across the central cornea and occurs in hypercalcemia and various chronic inflammatory conditions of the eye

bane•ber•ry \ˈbān-ˌber-ē, -bə-rē, -brē\ *n, pl* **-ber•ries** : the acid poisonous berry of any plant of a genus (*Actaea*) of the buttercup family (Ranunculaceae); *also* : one of these plants

bang *var of* BHANG

Bang's disease \ˈbaŋz-\ *n* : BRUCELLOSIS; *specif* : brucellosis of cattle — called also *Bang's*

Bang \ˈbäŋ\, **Bernhard Lauritz Frederik (1848–1932),** Danish veterinarian.

bank \ˈbaŋk\ *n* : a depot for the collection and storage of a biological product of human origin for medical use ⟨a sperm ~⟩ — see BLOOD BANK

Ban•ti's disease \ˈbän-tēz-\ *n* : a disorder characterized by congestion and great enlargement of the spleen usu. accompanied by anemia, leukopenia, and cirrhosis of the liver — called also *Banti's syndrome*

Ban•ti \ˈbän-tē\, **Guido (1852–1925),** Italian physician.

[1]**bar** \ˈbär\ *n, often attrib* **1** : a piece of metal that connects parts of a removable partial denture **2** : a straight stripe, band, or line much longer than it is wide **3** : the space in front of the molar teeth of a horse in which the bit is placed

[2]**bar** *n* : a unit of pressure equal to 100,000 pascals

bar- or **baro-** *comb form* : weight : pressure ⟨*bar*iatrics⟩ ⟨*baro*trauma⟩

Bá•rá•ny chair \bə-ˈrän-(y)ē-ˌcha(ə)r, -ˌche(ə)r\ *n* : a chair used esp. for demonstrating the effects of circular motion (as on airplane pilots)

Bá•rá•ny \ˈbä-ˌränʸ\, **Robert (1876–1936),** Austrian otologist.

barbae — see SYCOSIS BARBAE

bar•ber's itch \ˌbär-bərz-\ *n* : ringworm of the face and neck

bar•bi•tal \ˈbär-bə-ˌtȯl\ *n* : a crystalline barbiturate $C_8H_{12}N_2O_3$ formerly used as a sedative and hypnotic often in the form of its soluble sodium salt

bar•bi•tone \ˈbär-bə-ˌtōn\ *n, Brit* : BARBITAL

bar•bi•tu•rate \bär-ˈbi-chə-rət\ *n* **1** : a salt or ester of barbituric acid **2** : any of various derivatives of barbituric acid (as phenobarbital) used esp. as sedatives, hypnotics, and antispasmodics

bar•bi•tu•ric acid \ˌbär-bə-ˈtůr-ik, -ˈtyůr-\ *n* : a synthetic crystalline acid $C_4H_4N_2O_3$ that is a derivative of pyrimidine; *also* : any of its acid derivatives of which some are used as hypnotics

bar•bi•tur•ism \bär-ˈbi-chə-ˌri-zəm, ˈbär-bi-\ *n* : a condition characterized by deleterious effects on the mind or body by excess use of barbiturates

bar·bo·tage \ˌbär-bə-ˈtäzh\ *n* : the repeated injection and removal of fluid (as saline or anesthetic solution) from a part of the body ⟨bladder ~⟩

Bar·det–Biedl syndrome \bär-ˈdā-ˈbē-dᵊl-\ *n* : a genetic disorder that is a ciliopathy characterized by obesity, retinal dysfunction and degeneration, learning disabilities, the presence of extra fingers or toes, abnormalities of the kidney, liver, and heart, short stature, and subnormal development of the genital organs and is inherited as an autosomal recessive trait — compare LAURENCE-MOON SYNDROME

Bardet, George Louis (1885–1970), French physician.

Biedl, Artur (1869–1933), German physician.

barefoot doctor *n* : an auxiliary medical worker trained to provide health care in rural areas of China

bar·ia·tri·cian \ˌbar-ē-ə-ˈtri-shən\ *n* : a specialist in bariatrics

bar·iat·rics \ˌbar-ē-ˈa-triks\ *n* : a branch of medicine that deals with the treatment of obesity — **bar·iat·ric** \-trik\ *adj*

bar·i·to·sis \ˌbar-ə-ˈtō-səs\ *n, pl* **-to·ses** \-ˌsēz\ : pneumoconiosis caused by inhalation of dust composed of barium and esp. barium sulfate

bar·i·um \ˈbar-ē-əm\ *n* : a silver-white malleable toxic metallic element — symbol *Ba;* see ELEMENT table

barium chloride *n* : a water-soluble toxic salt $BaCl_2 \cdot 2H_2O$ used as a reagent in analysis

barium enema *n* : a suspension of barium sulfate injected into the lower bowel to render it radiopaque, usu. followed by injection of air to inflate the bowel and increase definition, and used in the radiographic diagnosis of intestinal lesions

barium meal *n* : a solution of barium sulfate that is swallowed by a patient to facilitate fluoroscopic or radiographic diagnosis

barium sulfate *n* : a colorless crystalline insoluble salt $BaSO_4$ used medically chiefly as a radiopaque substance

Bar·low's disease \ˈbär-ˌlōz-\ *also* **Barlow disease** *n* : INFANTILE SCURVY

Barlow, Sir Thomas (1845–1945), British physician.

Barlow's syndrome *also* **Barlow syndrome** *n* : MITRAL VALVE PROLAPSE — called also *Barlow disease, Barlow's disease*

Barlow, John Brereton (1924–2008), South African cardiologist.

baro- — see BAR-

baro·re·cep·tor \ˌbar-ō-ri-ˈsep-tər\ *also* **baro·cep·tor** \-ō-ˈsep-\ *n* : a sensory nerve ending esp. in the walls of large arteries (as the carotid sinus) that is sensitive to changes in blood pressure — called also *pressoreceptor*

baro·re·flex \ˈbar-ō-ˌrē-fleks\ *n* : the reflex mechanism by which baroreceptors regulate blood pressure — called also *baroreceptor reflex*

baro·trau·ma \-ˈtrau̇-mə, -ˈtrȯ-\ *n, pl* **-mas** *also* **-ma·ta** \-mə-tə\ : injury of a part or organ as a result of changes in barometric pressure; *specif* : AERO-OTITIS MEDIA

Barr body \ˈbär-\ *n* : a densely staining inactivated condensed X chromosome that is present in each somatic cell of most female mammals and is used as a test of genetic femaleness (as in a fetus or an athlete) — called also *sex chromatin*

Barr, Murray Llewellyn (1908–1995), Canadian anatomist.

bar·rel chest \ˈbar-əl-\ *n* : the enlarged chest with a rounded cross section and fixed horizontal position of the ribs that occurs in chronic pulmonary emphysema

bar·ren \ˈbar-ən\ *adj* : incapable of producing offspring — used esp. of females — **bar·ren·ness** \-ən-nəs\ *n*

Bar·rett's esophagus \ˈbar-its-\ *n* : metaplasia of the lower esophagus that occurs esp. as a result of chronic gastroesophageal reflux and is associated with an increased risk for esophageal carcinoma — called also *Barrett's epithelium*

Barrett, Norman Rupert (1903–1979), British surgeon.

bar·ri·er \ˈbar-ē-ər\ *n* **1** : something that separates, demarcates, or hinders movement — see BLOOD-BRAIN BARRIER, PLACENTAL BARRIER **2** : a contraceptive device (as a condom or diaphragm) that prevents sperm from entering the uterus

bar·tho·lin·itis \bär-ˌtō-lə-ˈnī-təs\ *n, pl* **-lin·ites** \-ˌtēz\ : inflammation of the Bartholin's glands

Bar·tho·lin's gland \ˈbärt-ᵊl-ənz-, ˈbär-thə-lənz-\ *n* : either of two oval racemose glands lying one to each side of the lower part of the vagina and secreting a lubricating mucus — called also *gland of Bartholin, greater vestibular gland;* compare COWPER'S GLAND

Bar·tho·lin \bär-ˈtu̇-lin\, **Caspar Thomèson (1655–1738),** Danish anatomist.

bar·ton·el·la \ˌbärt-ᵊn-ˈe-lə\ *n* **1** *cap* : a genus of gram-negative bacteria (family Bartonellaceae) that include the causative agent (*B. bacilliformis*) of bartonellosis **2** : any bacterium of the genus *Bartonella*

Bar·ton \ˈbär-ˌtōn\, **Alberto L. (1874–1950),** Peruvian physician.

bar·ton·el·lo·sis \ˌbärt-ᵊn-ˌe-ˈlō-səs\ *n, pl* **-lo·ses** \-ˌsēz\ : a disease that occurs in So. America, is characterized by severe anemia and high fever followed by an eruption like warts on the skin, and is caused by a bacterium of the genus *Bartonella* (*B. bacilliformis*) that invades the red blood cells and is transmitted by sand flies (genus *Phlebotomus*) — called also *Carrión's disease*

Bart·ter syndrome \ˈbär-tər-\ *also* **Bartter's syndrome** *n* : a genetic kidney disorder that is marked esp. by hypokalemia, aldosteronism, hyperreninemia, and hyperplasia of juxtaglomerular cells, includes a life-threatening form evident at birth and a somewhat less severe form with onset during early childhood, and that is inherited as an autosomal recessive trait

Bartter, Frederic Crosby (1914–1983), American physiologist.

ba·sal \ˈbā-səl, -zəl\ *adj* **1** : relating to, situated at, or forming the base **2** : of, relating to, or essential for maintaining the fundamental vital activities of an organism (as respiration, heartbeat, or excretion) ⟨~ diet⟩ **3** : serving as or serving to induce an initial comatose or unconscious state that forms a basis for further anesthetization ⟨~ anesthesia⟩ — **ba·sal·ly** *adv*

basal body temperature *n* : the temperature of the body at rest that is typically measured immediately after waking from sleep

basal cell *n* : one of the innermost cells of the deeper epidermis of the skin

basal cell carcinoma *n* : a skin cancer derived from and preserving the form of the basal cells of the skin

basale — see STRATUM BASALE

basal ganglion *n* : any of four deeply placed masses of gray matter within each cerebral hemisphere comprising the caudate nucleus, the lentiform nucleus, the amygdala, and the claustrum — usu. used in pl.; called also *basal nucleus*

basalia — see STRATUM BASALE

basalis — see DECIDUA BASALIS

basal lamina *n* **1** : the part of the gray matter of the embryonic neural tube from which the motor nerve roots arise **2** : a thin extracellular layer chiefly of collagen, proteoglycans, and glycoproteins (as laminin) that lies adjacent to the basal surface of epithelial cells or surrounds individual muscle, fat, and Schwann cells and that separates these cells from underlying or surrounding connective tissue or adjacent cells — compare RETICULAR LAMINA

basal metabolic rate *n* : the rate at which heat is given off by an organism at complete rest

basal metabolism *n* : the turnover of energy in a fasting and resting organism using energy solely to maintain vital cellular activity, respiration, and circulation as measured by the basal metabolic rate

basal nucleus *n* : BASAL GANGLION

basal plate *n* : an underlying structure: as **a** : the ventral portion of the neural tube **b** : the part of the decidua of a placental mammal that is intimately fused with the placenta

base \ˈbās\ *n, pl* **bas·es** \ˈbā-səz\ **1** : that portion of a bodily organ or part by which it is attached to another more central structure of the organism ⟨the ~ of the thumb⟩ **2 a** : the usu. inactive ingredient of a preparation serving as the vehicle for the active medicinal preparation **b** : the chief active ingredient of a preparation — called also *basis* **3 a** : any of various typically water-soluble and bitter tasting compounds that in solution have a pH greater than 7, are capable of reacting with an acid to form a salt, and are molecules or ions able to take up a proton from an acid or are substances able to give up a pair of electrons to an acid — compare ALKALI **b** : any of the five purine or pyrimidine bases of DNA and RNA that include cytosine, guanine, adenine, thymine, and uracil — **based** \ˈbāst\ *adj*

Ba·se·dow's disease \ˈbä-zə-ˌdōz-\ *n* : GRAVES' DISEASE

Basedow \ˈbä-zə-ˌdō\, **Karl Adolph von (1799–1854)**, German physician.

base·line \ˈbās-ˌlīn\ *n* : a set of critical observations or data used for comparison or a control

base·ment membrane \ˈbā-smənt-\ *n* **1** : a thin supporting layer that separates a layer of epithelial cells from the underlying lamina propria and is composed of the basal lamina and reticular lamina **2** : BASAL LAMINA 2

base pair *n* : one of the pairs of nucleotide bases on complementary strands of nucleic acid that consist of a purine on one strand joined to a pyrimidine on the other strand by hydrogen bonds and that include adenine linked to thymine in DNA or to uracil in RNA and guanine linked to cytosine in both DNA and RNA

base pairing *n* : the pairing of purine and pyrimidine bases linked by hydrogen bonds in two complementary strands of DNA or RNA

base·plate \ˈbās-ˌplāt\ *n* **1** : the portion of an artificial denture in contact with the jaw **2** : the sheet of plastic material used in the making of trial denture plates

base unit *n* : one of a set of simple units in a system of measurement from which other units may be derived

basi- *also* **baso-** *comb form* **1** : of or belonging to the base or lower part of ⟨*basi*cranial⟩ **2** : chemical base ⟨*baso*philic⟩

ba·sic \ˈbā-sik, -zik\ *adj* **1** : of, relating to, or forming the base or essence **2 a** : of, relating to, containing, or having the character of a base **b** : having an alkaline reaction

ba·si·cra·ni·al \ˌbā-si-ˈkrā-nē-əl\ *adj* : of or relating to the base of the skull

ba•sid•io•my•cete \bə-ˌsi-dē-ō-ˈmī-ˌsēt\ *n* : any of a group of higher fungi that include destructive forms (as rusts and smuts) that cause plant disease as well as edible forms (as many mushrooms) — **ba•sid•io•my•ce•tous** \-mī-ˈsē-təs\ *adj*

bas•i•lar \ˈba-zə-lər, -sə- *also* ˈbā-\ *adj* : of, relating to, or situated at the base ⟨~ fractures of the skull⟩

basilar artery *n* : an unpaired artery that is formed by the union of the two vertebral arteries, runs forward within the skull just under the pons, divides into the two posterior cerebral arteries, and supplies the pons, cerebellum, posterior part of the cerebrum, and the inner ear

basilar membrane *n* : a membrane that extends from the margin of the bony shelf of the cochlea to the outer wall and that supports the organ of Corti

basilar process *n* : an anterior median projection of the occipital bone in front of the foramen magnum articulating in front with the body of the sphenoid by the basilar suture

basilic vein *n* : a vein of the upper arm lying along the inner border of the biceps muscle, draining the whole limb, and opening into the axillary vein

¹ba•si•oc•cip•i•tal \ˌbā-sē-äk-ˈsip-ət-ᵊl\ *adj* : relating to or being a bone in the base of the cranium immediately in front of the foramen magnum that is represented in humans by the basilar process of the occipital bone

²basioccipital *n* : the basioccipital bone

ba•si•on \ˈbā-sē-ˌän, -zē-\ *n* : the midpoint of the anterior margin of the foramen magnum

ba•sis \ˈbā-səs\ *n, pl* **ba•ses** \-ˌsēz\ **1** : any of various anatomical parts that function as a foundation **2** : BASE 2b

ba•si•sphe•noid \ˌbā-səs-ˈfē-ˌnȯid\ *also* **ba•si•sphe•noi•dal** \-səs-fi-ˈnȯid-ᵊl\ *adj* : relating to or being the part of the base of the cranium that lies between the basioccipital and the presphenoid bones and that usu. ossifies separately and becomes a part of the sphenoid bone only in the adult — **basisphenoid** *n*

basket cell *n* : any of the cells in the molecular layer of the cerebellum whose axons pass inward and end in a basketlike network around the Purkinje cells

Basle Nom•i•na An•a•tom•i•ca \ˈbä-zəl-ˈnä-mə-nə-ˌa-nə-ˈtä-mi-kə\ *n* : the anatomical nomenclature adopted at the 1895 meeting of the German Anatomical Society at Basel, Switzerland, and superseded by the Nomina Anatomica in 1955 — abbr. *BNA*

baso- — see BASI-

ba•so•lat•er•al \ˌbā-sō-ˈla-tə-rəl\ *adj* : situated below and toward the side : located in or on the base and one or more sides — **ba•so•lat•er•al•ly** *adv*

ba•so•phil \ˈbā-sə-ˌfil, -zə-\ *also* **ba•so•phile** \-ˌfīl\ *n* : a basophilic substance or structure; *esp* : a white blood cell with basophilic granules that is similar in function to a mast cell

ba•so•phil•ia \ˌbā-sə-ˈfi-lē-ə, -zə-\ *n* **1** : tendency to stain with basic dyes **2** : an abnormal condition in which some tissue element has increased basophilia

ba•so•phil•ic \-ˈfi-lik\ *also* **ba•so•phil** \ˈbā-sə-ˌfil, -zə-\ *or* **ba•so•phile** \-ˌfīl\ *adj* : staining readily with or being a basic stain

basophilism — see PITUITARY BASOPHILISM

Bas•sen–Korn•zweig syndrome \ˈba-sᵊn-ˈkȯrn-ˌzwīg-\ *n* : ABETALIPOPROTEINEMIA

Bassen, Frank Albert (1903–2003), American hematologist.

Kornzweig, Abraham Leon (1900–1982), American ophthalmologist.

bath \ˈbath, ˈbȧth\ *n, pl* **baths** \ˈbat͟hz, ˈbaths, ˈbȧt͟hz, ˈbȧths\ **1** : a washing or soaking (as in water) of all or part of the body — see MUD BATH, SITZ BATH **2** : water used for bathing **3** : SPA 1 — usu. used in pl.

bathe \ˈbāt͟h\ *vb* **bathed; bath•ing** **1** : to wash in a liquid (as water) **2** : to apply water or a liquid medicament to

bath salts *n pl* **1** : a crystalline preparation for perfuming and softening bathwater **2** : any of various synthetic illicit stimulant drugs (as MDPV) containing derivatives of cathinone and typically sold as white or brown crystalline powders

ba•tracho•tox•in \bə-ˌtra-kə-ˈtäk-sən, ˌba-trə-kō-\ *n* : a very powerful steroid venom $C_{31}H_{42}N_2O_6$ extracted from the skin of a So. American frog (*Phyllobates aurotaenia*)

Bat•ten disease \ˈba-tᵊn-\ *also* **Batten's disease** *n* : a fatal lipofuscinosis that is characterized by seizures, progressive loss of vision, mental impairment, and paralysis, has an onset during childhood with death typically occurring during the late teens and twenties, and is typically inherited as an autosomal recessive trait; *also* : any of a group of related diseases

Batten, Frederick Eustace (1865–1918), British neurologist and pediatrician.

battered child syndrome *n* : the complex of physical injuries (as fractures, hematomas, and contusions) that results from gross abuse (as by a parent) of a young child

battered woman syndrome *also* **battered woman's syndrome** *n* : the highly variable symptom complex of physical and psychological injuries exhibited by a woman repeatedly abused esp. physically by her mate — called also *battered wife syndrome, battered women's syndrome*

bat•tery \'ba-tə-rē\ *n, pl* **-ter•ies** : a group or series of tests; *esp* : a group of intelligence or personality tests given to a subject as an aid in psychological analysis

battle fatigue *n* : COMBAT FATIGUE — **bat•tle–fa•tigued** *adj*

Bau•hin's valve \'bō-ˌanz-, bō-'aⁿz-\ *n* : ILEOCECAL VALVE

Bauhin, Gaspard *or* **Caspar (1560–1624),** Swiss anatomist and botanist.

BBB *abbr* **1** blood-brain barrier **2** bundle branch block

BC *abbr* board-certified

BCC *abbr* basal cell carcinoma

B cell *n* : any of the lymphocytes that have antigen-binding antibody molecules on the surface, that comprise the antibody-secreting plasma cells when mature, and that differentiate in the bone marrow — called also *B lymphocyte;* compare T CELL

BCG *abbr* bacillus Calmette-Guérin

BCG vaccine \ˌbē-(ˌ)sē-'jē-\ *n* : a vaccine prepared from a living attenuated strain of tubercle bacilli and used to vaccinate human beings against tuberculosis

A. L. C. Calmette and **C. Guérin** — see BACILLUS CALMETTE-GUÉRIN

BCLS *abbr* basic cardiac life support

BCNU \ˌbē-(ˌ)sē-(ˌ)en-'yü\ *n* : CARMUSTINE

B complex *n* : VITAMIN B COMPLEX

b.d. *abbr* [Latin *bis die*] twice a day — used in writing prescriptions

B–DNA \'bē-ˌdē-ˌen-'ā\ *n* : the typical form of double helix DNA in which the chains twist up and to the right around the front of the axis of the helix — compare Z-DNA

BDNF *abbr* brain-derived neurotrophic factor

Be *symbol* beryllium

BE *abbr* board-eligible

bead•ing \'bē-diŋ\ *n* : the beadlike nodules occurring in rickets at the junction of the ribs with their cartilages — called also *rachitic rosary*

Beals syndrome \'bēlz-\ *n* : CONGENITAL CONTRACTURAL ARACHNODACTYLY

Beals, Rodney K. (1931–2008), American orthopedic surgeon.

bear down *vb* : to contract the abdominal muscles and the diaphragm during childbirth

[1]**beat** \'bēt\ *vb* **beat; beat•en** \'bēt-ᵊn\ *or* **beat; beat•ing** : PULSATE, THROB

[2]**beat** *n* : a single stroke or pulsation (as of the heart) ⟨ectopic ~*s*⟩ — see EXTRASYSTOLE

Beau's lines \'bōz-\ *n pl* : transverse grooves or ridges on a fingernail or toenail that occur from a temporary disruption in nail growth (as that resulting from severe illness, malnutrition, or chemotherapy)

Beau \bō\, **Joseph-Honoré-Simon (1806–1865),** French physician.

Beck Depression Inventory \'bek-\ *n* : a standardized psychiatric questionnaire that is used to diagnose and determine the severity of depression

Beck, Aaron Temkin (*b* 1921), American psychiatrist.

Beck•er muscular dystrophy \'be-kər-\ *or* **Beck•er's muscular dystrophy** \-kərz\ *n* : a less severe form of Duchenne muscular dystrophy with later onset and slower progression of the disease that is inherited as an X-linked recessive trait and is characterized by dystrophin of deficient or abnormal molecular weight

Becker, P. E., 20th-century German human geneticist.

Beck•with–Wie•de•mann syndrome \'bek-wəth-'wē-də-mən-\ *n* : an inherited disease present at birth that is characterized esp. by abdominal wall defects (as umbilical hernia), enlarged tongue, hypoglycemia, tumors (as Wilms' tumor) of usu. embryonic origin, and enlargement of internal organs

Beckwith, John Bruce (*b* 1933), American pathologist.

Wie•de•mann \'vē-də-ˌmän\, **Hans Rudolf (1915–2006),** German pediatrician.

bec•lo•meth•a•sone \ˌbe-klə-'me-thə-ˌzōn, -ˌsōn\ *n* : a steroid anti-inflammatory drug administered in the form of its dipropionate $C_{28}H_{37}ClO_7$ as an inhalant to treat asthma and as a nasal spray to treat rhinitis and prevent nasal polyps — see BECONASE AQ, QNASL, QVAR, VANCENASE, VANCERIL

Bec•on•ase AQ \'bek-ə-ˌnās-, -ˌnāz-\ *trademark* — used for a preparation of the dipropionate of beclomethasone administered as a nasal spray

bed \'bed\ *n* **1 a** : a piece of furniture on or in which one may lie and sleep — see HOSPITAL BED **b** : the equipment and services needed to care for one hospitalized patient **2** : a layer of specialized or altered tissue esp. when separating dissimilar structures — see NAIL BED, VASCULAR BED

BED *abbr* binge eating disorder

bed•bug \'bed-ˌbəg\ *n* : a wingless bloodsucking bug (*Cimex lectularius*) sometimes infesting houses and esp. beds and feeding on human blood — called also *chinch*

bed•pan \'bed-ˌpan\ *n* : a shallow vessel used by a bedridden person for urination or defecation

bed rest *n* : confinement of a sick person to bed

bed•rid•den \'bed-ˌrid-ᵊn\ *also* **bed•rid** \-ˌrid\ *adj* : confined to bed (as by illness)

[1]**bed•side** \'bed-ˌsīd\ *n* : a place beside a bed esp. of a bedridden person

[2]**bedside** *adj* **1** : of, relating to, or conducted at the bedside of a bedridden patient ⟨a ~ diagnosis⟩ **2** : suitable for a bedridden person

bedside manner *n* : the manner that a physician assumes toward patients

bed•so•nia \bed-'sō-nē-ə\ *n, pl* **-ni•ae** \-nē-ˌē, -ˌī\ : CHLAMYDIA 2a

Bed·son \ˈbed-sᵊn\, **Sir Samuel Phillips (1886–1969),** English bacteriologist.

bed·sore \ˈbed-ˌsōr\ *n* : an ulceration of tissue deprived of adequate blood supply by prolonged pressure — called also *decubitus, decubitus ulcer, pressure sore;* compare PRESSURE POINT 1

bed–wet·ting \-ˌwe-tiŋ\ *n* : enuresis esp. when occurring in bed during sleep — **bed–wet·ter** \-ˌwe-tər\ *n*

bee \ˈbē\ *n* : HONEYBEE; *broadly* : any of numerous hymenopterous insects (superfamily Apoidea) that differ from the related wasps esp. in the heavier hairier body and in having sucking as well as chewing mouthparts — see AFRICANIZED BEE

beef measles *n, sing or pl* : the infestation of beef muscle by cysticerci of the beef tapeworm which make oval white vesicles giving a measly appearance to beef

beef tapeworm *n* : a tapeworm of the genus *Taenia* (*T. saginata*) that infests the human intestine as an adult, has a cysticercus larva that develops in cattle, and is contracted through ingestion of the larva in raw or rare beef

bees·wax \ˈbēz-ˌwaks\ *n* **1** : WAX 1 **2** : YELLOW WAX

be·hav·ior \bi-ˈhā-vyər\ *n* **1** : the manner of conducting oneself **2 a** : anything that an organism does involving action and response to stimulation **b** : the response of an individual, group, or species to its environment — **be·hav·ior·al** \-vyə-rəl\ *adj* — **be·hav·ior·al·ly** *adv*

behavioral medicine *n* : an interdisciplinary medical science dealing with the psychological and behavioral causes of bodily symptoms and disease

behavioral psychology *also* **behavior psychology** *n* : BEHAVIORISM

behavioral science *n* : a science (as psychology or sociology) that deals with human action and seeks to generalize about human behavior in society — **behavioral scientist** *n*

be·hav·ior·ism \bi-ˈhā-vyə-ˌri-zəm\ *n* : a school of psychology that takes the objective evidence of behavior (as measured responses to stimuli) as the only concern of its research and the only basis of its theory without reference to conscious experience — **be·hav·ior·ist** \-rist\ *n or adj* — **be·hav·ior·is·tic** \-ˌhā-vyə-ˈris-tik\ *adj*

behavior modification *also* **behavioral modification** *n* : BEHAVIOR THERAPY

behavior therapist *or* **behavioral therapist** *n* : a specialist in behavior therapy

behavior therapy *or* **behavioral therapy** *n* : psychotherapy that is concerned with the treatment (as by desensitization or aversion therapy) of observable behaviors and that applies principles of learning to substitute desirable responses and behavior patterns for undesirable ones (such as phobias or obsessions) — compare COGNITIVE BEHAVIORAL THERAPY, COGNITIVE THERAPY

be·hav·iour, be·hav·iour·ism *chiefly Brit var of* BEHAVIOR, BEHAVIORISM

Beh·cet's disease \bə-ˈchets-\ *n* : a rare disease of unknown cause marked by chronic inflammation of blood vessels with symptoms including ulcerative sores esp. of the mouth and genitals, inflammation of the eye, and joint swelling and pain — called also *Behcet's syndrome*

Behçet, Hulusi (1889–1948), Turkish dermatologist.

bej·el \ˈbe-jəl\ *n* : a disease that is endemic chiefly in children of dry hot regions of northern Africa, Asia, and the Middle East, is marked by bone and skin lesions, and is caused by a spirochete of the genus *Treponema* (*T. endemicum*) closely related to the causative agent of syphilis — called also *endemic syphilis*

[1]**belch** \ˈbelch\ *vb* : to expel gas from the stomach suddenly : ERUCT

[2]**belch** *n* : an act or instance of belching : ERUCTATION

bel·la·don·na \ˌbe-lə-ˈdä-nə\ *n* **1** : an Old World poisonous plant of the genus *Atropa* (*A. belladonna*) having a root and leaves that yield atropine — called also *deadly nightshade* **2** : a medicinal preparation (as atropine) extracted from the belladonna and containing anticholinergic alkaloids

bel·lows \ˈbe-(ˌ)lōz\ *n sing or pl* : LUNGS

Bell's palsy *n* : paralysis of the facial nerve producing distortion on one side of the face

Bell, Sir Charles (1774–1842), British anatomist.

bel·ly \ˈbe-lē\ *n, pl* **bellies 1 a** : ABDOMEN 1a **b** : the undersurface of an animal's body **c** : the stomach and its adjuncts **2** : the enlarged fleshy body of a muscle

bel·ly·ache \ˈbe-lē-ˌāk\ *n* : pain in the abdomen and esp. in the stomach : STOMACHACHE

bel·ly·band \-ˌband\ *n* : a band around or across the belly; *esp* : BAND 1a

belly button *n* : the human navel

bel·o·ne·pho·bia \ˌbe-lə-nə-ˈfō-bē-ə\ *n* : AICHMOPHOBIA

Bel·viq \ˌbel-ˈvēk\ *trademark* — used for a preparation of lorcaserin

be·me·gride \ˈbe-mə-ˌgrīd, ˈbē-\ *n* : an analeptic drug $C_{18}H_{13}NO_2$ used esp. to counteract the effects of barbiturates

Ben·a·dryl \ˈbe-nə-ˌdril\ *trademark* — used for a preparation of the hydrochloride of diphenhydramine

ben·a·ze·pril \bən-ˈā-zə-pril\ *n* : an ACE inhibitor used in the form of its hydrochloride $C_{24}H_{28}N_2O_5{\cdot}HCl$ for the treatment of hypertension — see LOTENSIN, LOTREL

Bence–Jones protein \ˈbens-ˈjōnz-\ *n* : a polypeptide composed of one or two antibody light chains that is found esp. in the urine of persons affected with multiple myeloma

Bence–Jones, Henry (1814–1873), British physician.

ben·da·mus·tine \ˌben-də-ˈməs-ˌtēn\ *n* : a derivative of mechlorethamine administered in the form of its hydrochloride $C_{16}H_{21}Cl_2N_3O_2 \cdot HCl$ by intravenous infusion to treat non-Hodgkin lymphoma of B cell origin and chronic lymphocytic leukemia — see TREANDA

Ben·der Gestalt test \ˌben-dər-\ *n* : a test in which the subject copies geometric figures and which is used esp. to assess organic brain damage and degree of nervous system maturation

Bender, Lauretta (1897–1987), American psychiatrist.

ben·dro·flu·me·thi·a·zide \ˌben-drō-ˌflü-mə-ˈthi-ə-ˌzīd\ *n* : a diuretic $C_{15}H_{14}F_3N_3O_4S_2$ taken orally in the treatment of hypertension often in combination with a beta-blocker (as nadolol)

bends \ˈbendz\ *n sing or pl* : DECOMPRESSION SICKNESS; *also* : intense joint pain occurring as a common manifestation of decompression sickness — usu. used with *the* ⟨a case of the ~⟩

Ben·e·dict's solution \ˈbe-nə-ˌdikts-\ *n* : a blue solution that contains sodium carbonate, sodium citrate, and copper sulfate $CuSO_4$ and is used to test for reducing sugars in Benedict's test

Ben·e·dict \ˈbe-nə-ˌdikt\, **Stanley Rossiter (1884–1936),** American chemist.

Benedict's test *n* : a test for the presence of a reducing sugar (as in urine) by heating the solution to be tested with Benedict's solution which yields a red, yellow, or orange precipitate upon warming with a reducing sugar (as glucose or maltose)

Ben·gay \ˌben-ˈgā\ *trademark* — used for a pain-relieving topical preparation containing menthol and often methyl salicylate

Ben·i·car \ˈben-i-ˌkär\ *trademark* — used for a preparation of olmesartan

Benicar HCT *trademark* — used for a preparation of hydrochlorothiazide and olmesartan

be·nign \bi-ˈnīn\ *adj* **1** : of a mild type or character that does not threaten health or life ⟨~ malaria⟩ ⟨a ~ cyst⟩; *esp* : not becoming cancerous ⟨a ~ lung tumor⟩ — compare MALIGNANT 1 **2** : having a good prognosis : responding favorably to treatment ⟨a ~ psychosis⟩ — **be·nig·ni·ty** \bi-ˈnig-nə-tē\ *n*

benign intracranial hypertension *n* : IDIOPATHIC INTRACRANIAL HYPERTENSION

benign paroxysmal positional vertigo *or* **benign positional vertigo** *n* : a condition marked by short recurrent episodes of vertigo and nystagmus brought about by a change in head position — abbr. *BPPV, BPV*

benign prostatic hyperplasia *n* : adenomatous hyperplasia of the periurethral part of the prostate gland that occurs esp. in men over 50 years old and that tends to obstruct urination by constricting the urethra — abbr. *BPH;* called also *benign prostatic hypertrophy*

ben·ny \ˈbe-nē\ *n, pl* **bennies** *slang* : a tablet of amphetamine taken as a stimulant

bent spine syndrome *n* : CAMPTOCORMIA

benz- *or* **benzo-** *comb form* **1** : related to benzene or benzoic acid ⟨*benzo*ate⟩ **2** : containing a benzene ring fused on one side to one side of another ring ⟨*benz*imidazole⟩

benz·al·ko·ni·um chloride \ˌben-zal-ˈkō-nē-əm-\ *n* : a white or yellowish-white mixture of chloride salts used as an antiseptic and germicide — see ZEPHIRAN

ben·za·thine penicillin G \ˈben-zə-ˌthēn-, -thən-\ *also* **benzathine penicillin** *n* : PENICILLIN G BENZATHINE

Ben·ze·drine \ˈben-zə-ˌdrēn\ *n* : a preparation of the sulfate of amphetamine $(C_9H_{13}N)_2 \cdot H_2SO_4$ formerly used in medicine — formerly a U.S. registered trademark

ben·zene \ˈben-ˌzēn, ben-ˈ\ *n* : a colorless volatile flammable toxic liquid aromatic hydrocarbon C_6H_6 used in organic synthesis, as a solvent, and as a motor fuel

benzene hexa·chlor·ide \-ˌhek-sə-ˈklōr-ˌīd\ *n* : a compound $C_6H_6Cl_6$ occurring in several stereoisomeric forms; *esp* : GAMMA BENZENE HEXACHLORIDE — see LINDANE

benzene ring *n* : a ring of six carbon atoms linked by alternate single and double bonds in a plane symmetrical hexagon that occurs in benzene and related compounds

ben·zes·trol \ben-ˈzes-ˌtrȯl, -ˌtrōl\ *n* : a crystalline estrogenic compound $C_{20}H_{26}O_2$

ben·zi·dine \ˈben-zə-ˌdēn\ *n* : a crystalline base $C_{12}H_{12}N_2$ used esp. in making dyes and in a test for blood

benzidine test *n* : a test for blood (as in urine or feces) based on its production of a blue color in a solution containing benzidine

benzilate — see QUINUCLIDINYL BENZILATE

benz·imid·azole \ˌben-ˌzi-mə-ˈda-ˌzōl, ˌben-zə-ˈmi-də-ˌzōl\ *n* : a crystalline base $C_7H_6N_2$ used esp. to inhibit the growth of various viruses, parasitic worms, and fungi; *also* : one of its derivatives

benzo- — see BENZ-

ben·zo·[a]·py·rene \ˌben-zō-ˌā-ˈpīr-ˌēn, -zō-ˌal-fə-, -pī-ˈrēn\ *n* : the yellow crystalline highly carcinogenic isomer of the benzopyrene mixture that is formed esp. in the burning of cigarettes, coal, wood, and gasoline

ben·zo·ate \ˈben-zə-ˌwāt\ *n* : a salt or ester of benzoic acid

ben·zo·caine \ˈben-zə-ˌkān\ *n* : a crystalline ester $C_9H_{11}NO_2$ used as a local anesthetic — called also *ethyl aminobenzoate*

ben·zo·di·az·e·pine \ˌben-zō-dī-ˈa-zə-ˌpēn\ *n* : any of a group of aromatic lipophilic amines (as diazepam and chlordiazepoxide) used esp. as tranquilizers

ben·zo·ic acid \ben-ˈzō-ik-\ *n* : a white crystalline acid $C_6H_6O_2$ used as a preservative of foods and in medicine

ben·zo·in \ˈben-zə-wən, -ˌwēn; -ˌzȯin\ *n* **1** : a yellowish balsamic resin from trees (genus *Styrax* of the family Styracaceae) of southeastern Asia used esp. as an expectorant and topically to relieve skin irritations **2** : a white crystalline hydroxy ketone $C_{14}H_{12}O_2$

ben·zo·mor·phan \ˌben-zō-ˈmȯr-ˌfan\ *n* : any of a group of synthetic compounds including some potent analgesics (as phenazocine or pentazocine)

ben·zo·phe·none \ˌben-zō-fi-ˈnōn, -ˈfē-ˌnōn\ *n* : a colorless crystalline ketone $C_{13}H_{10}O$ used in sunscreens

ben·zo·py·rene \ˌben-zō-ˈpīr-ˌēn, -pī-ˈrēn\ *or* **benz·py·rene** \benz-ˈpīr-ˌēn, ˌbenz-pī-ˈrēn\ *n* : a mixture of two isomeric hydrocarbons $C_{20}H_{12}$ of which one is highly carcinogenic — see BENZO[A]PYRENE

ben·zo·yl peroxide \ˈben-zə-ˌwil-, -ˌzȯil-\ *n* : a white crystalline compound $C_{14}H_{10}O_4$ used in medicine esp. in the treatment of acne — see EPIDUO

benz·pyr·in·i·um bromide \ˌbenz-pə-ˈri-nē-əm-\ *n* : a cholinergic agent $C_{15}H_{17}BrN_2O_2$ that has actions similar to those of neostigmine — called also *benzpyrinium*

benz·tro·pine \benz-ˈtrō-ˌpēn, -pən\ *n* : an anticholinergic drug used in the form of its mesylate $C_{21}H_{25}NO \cdot CH_4O_3S$ esp. to treat symptoms (as tremors or spasms) of Parkinson's disease or similar symptoms caused as side effects of certain drugs

ben·zyl benzoate \ˈben-ˌzēl-, -zəl-\ *n* : a colorless oily ester $C_{14}H_{12}O_2$ used esp. as a scabicide

ben·zyl·pen·i·cil·lin \ˌben-ˌzēl-(ˌ)pe-nə-ˈsi-lən, -zəl-\ *n* : PENICILLIN G

ben·zyl·pi·per·a·zine \ˌben-(ˌ)zēl-pī-ˈper-ə-ˌzēn, -zəl-\ *n* : a synthetic derivative $C_{11}H_{16}N_2$ of piperazine used illicitly as a stimulant — called also *BZP*

beri·beri \ˌber-ē-ˈber-ē\ *n* : a deficiency disease marked by inflammatory or degenerative changes of the nerves, digestive system, and heart and caused by a lack of or inability to assimilate thiamine

berke·li·um \ˈbər-klē-əm\ *n* : a radioactive metallic element — symbol *Bk;* see ELEMENT table

ber·lock dermatitis \ˈbər-ˌläk-\ *n* : a brownish discoloration of the skin that develops on exposure to sunlight after the use of perfume containing certain essential oils

ber·ry aneurysm \ˈber-ē-\ *n* : an aneurysm of a cerebral artery that resembles a berry or sac in shape and typically occurs at an arterial junction in the circle of Willis

Ber·tin's column \ber-ˈtaⁿz-\ *n* : COLUMN OF BERTIN

Ber·tin \ber-taⁿ\, **Exupère Joseph (1712–1781)**, French anatomist.

be·ryl·li·o·sis \bə-ˌri-lē-ˈō-səs\ *also* **ber·yl·lo·sis** \ˌber-ə-ˈlō-\ *n, pl* **-li·o·ses** \-ˌsēz\; *or* **-lo·ses** \-ˌsēz\ : poisoning resulting from exposure to fumes and dusts of beryllium compounds or alloys and occurring chiefly as an acute pneumonitis or as a granulomatosis involving esp. the lungs

be·ryl·li·um \bə-ˈri-lē-əm\ *n* : a steel-gray light strong brittle toxic bivalent metallic element — symbol *Be;* see ELEMENT table

bes·ti·al·i·ty \ˌbes-chē-ˈa-lə-tē, ˌbēs-\ *n, pl* **-ties** : sexual relations between a human being and a lower animal

[1]**be·ta** \ˈbā-tə\ *n* **1** : the second letter of the Greek alphabet — Β or β **2** : BETA PARTICLE **3** : BETA WAVE

[2]**beta** *or* **β-** *adj* **1** : of or relating to one of two or more closely related chemical substances ⟨the *beta* chain of hemoglobin⟩ — used somewhat arbitrarily to specify ordinal relationship or a particular physical form **2** : second in position in the structure of an organic molecule from a particular group or atom; *also* : occurring at or having a structure characterized by such a position ⟨β–substitution⟩ **3** : producing a zone of decolorization when grown on blood media — used of some hemolytic streptococci or of the hemolysis they cause

be·ta–ad·ren·er·gic \-ˌa-drə-ˈnər-jik\ *adj* : of, relating to, or being a beta-receptor ⟨~ blocking action⟩

beta–adrenergic receptor *n* : BETA-RECEPTOR

be·ta–ad·re·no·cep·tor \-ə-ˈdrē-nə-ˌsep-tər\ *also* **be·ta–ad·re·no·re·cep·tor** \-ri-ˌsep-tər\ *n* : BETA-RECEPTOR

be·ta–ag·o·nist \-ˈa-gə-nəst\ *n* : any of various drugs (as albuterol or terbutaline) that combine with and activate a beta-receptor

be·ta–am·y·loid *also* **β–amyloid** \-ˈa-mə-ˌlȯid\ *n* : an amyloid that is derived from amyloid precursor protein and is the primary component of plaques characteristic of Alzheimer's disease — called also *A-beta, amyloid beta, amyloid beta peptide, amyloid beta protein, beta-amyloid peptide, beta-amyloid protein*

be·ta–block·ade \-blä-ˈkād\ *n* : blockade of beta-receptor activity by a beta-blocker

be·ta–block·er \-ˈblä-kər\ *n* : any of a group of drugs (as propranolol) that combine with and block the activity of a beta-receptor to decrease the heart rate and force of contractions and lower high blood pressure and that are used esp. to treat hypertension, angina pectoris, and ventricular and supraventricular arrhythmias

be•ta–block•ing \-ˈblä-kiŋ\ *adj* : blocking or relating to the blocking of beta-receptor activity ⟨~ drugs⟩

be•ta–car•o•tene *or* **β–carotene** \-ˈkar-ə-ˌtēn\ *n* : a reddish-orange pigment that is an isomer of carotene found chiefly in orange, dark green, and dark yellow vegetables and fruits (as carrots and spinach)

beta cell *n* : any of various secretory cells distinguished by their basophilic staining characters: as **a** : a pituitary basophil **b** : an insulin-secreting cell of the islets of Langerhans — compare ALPHA CELL

Be•ta•dine \ˈbā-tə-ˌdīn\ *trademark* — used for a preparation of povidone-iodine

be•ta–en•dor•phin *or* **β–endorphin** \ˌbā-tə-en-ˈdȯr-fən\ *n* : an endorphin of the pituitary gland with much greater analgesic potency than morphine — see BETA-LIPOTROPIN

beta globin *also* **β–glo•bin** \-ˈglō-bən\ *n* : the chain of hemoglobin that is designated beta and that when deficient or defective causes various anemias (as beta-thalassemia or sickle cell anemia) — compare ALPHA GLOBIN

beta globulin *n* : any of several globulins of plasma or serum that have at alkaline pH electrophoretic mobilities intermediate between those of the alpha globulins and gamma globulins

beta hemolysis *n* : a sharply defined clear colorless zone of hemolysis surrounding colonies of certain streptococci on blood agar plates — **be•ta–he•mo•lyt•ic** \ˌbā-tə-ˌhē-mə-ˈli-tik\ *adj*

beta hydroxy acid *also* **beta hydroxy** *n* : SALICYLIC ACID — abbr. *BHA*

be•ta•ine \ˈbē-tə-ˌēn\ *n* : an ammonium salt $C_5H_{11}NO_2$ that is used to treat homocystinuria and is also used in the form of its hydrochloride $C_5H_{11}NO_2 \cdot HCl$ as a source of hydrochloric acid esp. to treat hypochlorhydria

beta interferon *n* : an interferon that is produced esp. by fibroblasts, possesses antiviral activity, and is used in a form obtained from recombinant DNA esp. in the treatment of multiple sclerosis — called also *interferon beta;* see AVONEX, BETASERON

be•ta–lac•tam *or* **β–lactam** \ˌbā-tə-ˈlak-ˌtam\ *n* : any of a large class of antibiotics (as the penicillins and cephalosporins) with a lactam ring

be•ta–lac•ta•mase *also* **β–lactamase** \-ˈlak-tə-ˌmās, -ˌmāz\ *n* : any of various bacterial enzymes that inactivate beta-lactam antibiotics (as penicillin) by hydrolyzing them — compare PENICILLINASE

beta–lipoprotein *or* **β–lipoprotein** *n* : LDL

be•ta–li•po•tro•pin \ˌbā-tə-ˌli-pə-ˈtrō-pən, -ˌlī-\ *n* : a lipotropin of the anterior pituitary that contains beta-endorphin as the terminal sequence of 31 amino acids in its polypeptide chain

be•ta•meth•a•sone \ˌbā-tə-ˈme-thə-ˌzōn, -ˌsōn\ *n* : a potent glucocorticoid $C_{22}H_{29}FO_5$ that is isomeric with dexamethasone and has potent anti-inflammatory activity

beta particle *n* : a high-speed electron emitted from the nucleus of an atom during radioactive decay

be•ta–pleat•ed sheet \-ˈplē-təd\ *n* : BETA-SHEET

beta ray *n* **1** : BETA PARTICLE **2** : a stream of beta particles — called also *beta radiation*

be•ta–re•cep•tor \ˌbā-tə-ri-ˈsep-tər\ *n* : any of a group of receptors that are present on cell surfaces of some effector organs and tissues innervated by the sympathetic nervous system and that mediate certain physiological responses (as vasodilation, relaxation of bronchial and uterine smooth muscle, and increased heart rate) when bound by specific adrenergic agents — called also *beta-adrenergic receptor, beta-adrenoceptor;* compare ALPHA-RECEPTOR

beta rhythm *n* : BETA WAVE

Be•ta•ser•on \ˌbā-tə-ˈsir-ˌän\ *trademark* — used for a preparation of a recombinant form of beta interferon

be•ta–sheet \-ˌshēt\ *n* : the structural arrangement of many proteins in which two or more short regions of the polypeptide chain align adjacently and are stabilized by hydrogen bonds into sheets with a pleated appearance — called also *beta-pleated sheet;* compare ALPHA-HELIX

beta–si•tos•ter•ol *also* **β–sitosterol** \-sī-ˈtäs-tə-ˌrȯl, -ˌrōl\ *n* : a sterol widespread in plant products (as wheat germ, soybeans, and corn oil) that is used in dietary supplements and is held to lower cholesterol levels and relieve symptoms of benign prostatic hyperplasia

beta–thal•as•se•mia *or* **β–thal•as•se•mia** \-ˌthal-ə-ˈsē-mē-ə\ *n* : thalassemia in which the hemoglobin chains designated beta are affected and which comprises Cooley's anemia in the homozygous condition and thalassemia minor in the heterozygous condition — compare ALPHA-THALASSEMIA

beta thalassemia major *or* **β–thalassemia major** *n* : COOLEY'S ANEMIA

beta wave *n* : an electrical rhythm of the brain with a frequency of 13 to 30 cycles per second that is associated with normal conscious waking experience — called also *beta, beta rhythm*

be•tel nut \ˈbē-tᵊl-\ *n* : the astringent seed of an Asian palm (*Areca catechu*) that is a source of arecoline

be•tha•ne•chol \bə-ˈthā-nə-ˌkȯl, -ˈtha-, -ˌkōl\ *n* : a parasympathomimetic agent administered in the form of its chloride $C_7H_{17}ClN_2O_2$ and used esp. to treat gastric and urinary retention — see URECHOLINE

be•tween•brain \bi-ˈtwēn-ˌbrān\ *n* : DIENCEPHALON

Betz cell \ˈbets-\ *n* : a very large pyramidal nerve cell of the motor area of the cerebral cortex

Betz, Vladimir Aleksandrovich (1834–1894), Russian anatomist.

bev•a•ciz•u•mab \ˌbe-və-ˈsi-zu̇-ˌmab\ *n* : a genetically engineered monoclonal antibody administered intravenously to slow or inhibit tumor growth esp. in some metastatic forms of cancer — see AVASTIN

Bex•tra \ˈbek-strə\ *trademark* — used for a preparation of valdecoxib

be•zoar \ˈbē-ˌzōr\ *n* : any of various calculi found in the gastrointestinal organs esp. of ruminants — called also *bezoar stone*

BFP *abbr* **1** *of a pregnancy test* big fat positive — not used technically **2** biological false-positive; biologic false-positive

BGH *or* **bGH** *abbr* bovine growth hormone

Bh *symbol* bohrium

BHA \ˌbē-(ˌ)āch-ˈā\ *n* : a phenolic antioxidant $C_{11}H_{16}O_2$ used esp. to preserve fats and oils in food — called also *butylated hydroxyanisole*

BHA *abbr* beta hydroxy acid

bhang *also* **bang** \ˈbäŋ, ˈbȯŋ, ˈbaŋ\ *n* **1 a** : HEMP 1 **b** : the leaves and flowering tops of uncultivated hemp : CANNABIS — compare MARIJUANA **2** : an intoxicant product obtained from bhang — compare HASHISH

BHC \ˌbē-(ˌ)āch-ˈsē\ *n* : BENZENE HEXACHLORIDE

BHT \ˌbē-(ˌ)āch-ˈtē\ *n* : a phenolic antioxidant $C_{15}H_{24}O$ used esp. to preserve fats and oils in food, cosmetics, and pharmaceuticals — called also *butylated hydroxytoluene*

Bi *symbol* bismuth

[1]**bi-** *prefix* **1 a** : two ⟨*bi*lateral⟩ **b** : into two parts ⟨*bi*furcate⟩ **2** : twice : doubly : on both sides ⟨*bi*convex⟩ **3** : between, involving, or affecting two (specified) symmetrical parts ⟨*bi*labial⟩ **4 a** : containing one (specified) constituent in double the proportion of the other constituent or in double the ordinary proportion ⟨*bi*carbonate⟩ **b** : DI- ⟨*bi*phenyl⟩

[2]**bi-** *or* **bio-** *comb form* : life : living organisms or tissue ⟨*bio*chemistry⟩

bi•al•le•lic \(ˈ)bī-ə-ˈlē-lik, -ˈle-\ *adj* : of, relating to, or affecting both alleles of a gene

bi•ar•tic•u•lar \ˌbī-är-ˈtik-yə-lər\ *adj* : of or relating to two joints

Bi•ax•in \(ˌ)bī-ˈak-sən\ *trademark* — used for a preparation of clarithromycin

bib•li•o•ther•a•py \ˌbi-blē-ō-ˈther-ə-pē\ *n, pl* **-pies** : the use of selected reading materials as therapeutic adjuvants in medicine and in psychiatry; *also* : guidance in the solution of personal problems through directed reading — **bib•li•o•ther•a•peu•tic** \-ther-ə-ˈpyüt-ik\ *adj* — **bib•li•o•ther•a•pist** \-ˈther-ə-pist\ *n*

bi•carb \ˈbī-ˌkärb, bī-ˈ\ *n* : SODIUM BICARBONATE

bi•car•bon•ate \(ˌ)bī-ˈkär-bə-ˌnāt, -nət\ *n* : an acid carbonate

bicarbonate of soda *n* : SODIUM BICARBONATE

bi•ceps \ˈbī-ˌseps\ *n, pl* **biceps** *also* **bicepses** : a muscle having two heads: as **a** : the large flexor muscle of the front of the upper arm **b** : the large flexor muscle of the back of the upper leg

biceps bra•chii \-ˈbrā-kē-ˌē, -ˌī\ *n* : BICEPS a

biceps fe•mo•ris \-ˈfē-mə-rəs, -ˈfe-\ *n* : BICEPS b

biceps flex•or cu•bi•ti \-ˈflek-ˌsȯr-ˈkyü-bə-ˌtī, -tē\ *n* : BICEPS a

biceps reflex *n* : an involuntary contraction of the biceps muscle of the arm produced by tapping its tendon

bi•chlo•ride of mercury \(ˌ)bī-ˈklōr-ˌīd-\ *n* : MERCURIC CHLORIDE

bi•cip•i•tal \(ˌ)bī-ˈsi-pət-ᵊl\ *adj* **1** *of muscles* : having two heads or origins **2** : of or relating to a biceps muscle

bicipital aponeurosis *n* : an aponeurosis given off from the tendon of the biceps of the arm and continuous with the deep fascia of the forearm

bicipital groove *n* : a furrow on the upper part of the humerus occupied by the long head of the biceps — called also *intertubercular groove*

bicipital tuberosity *n* : the rough eminence which is on the anterior inner aspect of the neck of the radius and into which the tendon of the biceps is inserted

BiC•NU \ˈbik-ˌnü\ *trademark* — used for a preparation of carmustine

bi•con•cave \ˌbī-(ˌ)kän-ˈkāv, (ˌ)bī-ˈkän-ˌ\ *adj* : concave on both sides — **bi•con•cav•i•ty** \ˌbī-(ˌ)kän-ˈka-və-tē\ *n*

bi•con•vex \ˌbī-(ˌ)kän-ˈveks, (ˌ)bī-ˈkän-ˌ, ˌbī-kən-ˈ\ *adj* : convex on both sides — **bi•con•vex•i•ty** \ˌbī-kən-ˈvek-sə-tē, -(ˌ)kän-\ *n*

bi•cor•nu•ate \(ˌ)bī-ˈkȯrn-yə-ˌwāt, -wət\ *or* **bi•cor•nate** \-ˈkȯr-ˌnāt, -nət\ *adj* : having two horns or horn-shaped processes ⟨a ∼ uterus⟩

bi•cu•cul•line \bī-ˈkü-kyə-ˌlēn, -lən\ *n* : a convulsant alkaloid $C_{20}H_{17}NO_6$ obtained from plants (family Fumariaceae) and having the capacity to antagonize the action of gamma-aminobutyric acid

[1]**bi•cus•pid** \(ˌ)bī-ˈkəs-pəd\ *adj* : having or ending in two points ⟨∼ teeth⟩

[2]**bicuspid** *n* : either of the two double-pointed teeth that are situated between the canines and the molars on each side of each jaw : PREMOLAR

bicuspid valve *n* : MITRAL VALVE

bi·cy·clic \(ˌ)bī-ˈsī-klik, -ˈsi-\ *adj* : containing two usu. fused rings in the structure of a molecule

bid *abbr* [Latin *bis in die*] twice a day — used in writing prescriptions

bi·det \bi-ˈdā\ *n* : a bathroom fixture used esp. for bathing the external genitals and the anal region

bi·di·rec·tion·al \ˌbī-də-ˈrek-sh(ə-)nəl, -dī-\ *adj* : involving, moving, or taking place in two usu. opposite directions ⟨~ flow⟩ — **bi·di·rec·tion·al·ly** *adv*

bi·fid \ˈbī-ˌfid, -fəd\ *adj* : divided into two equal lobes or parts by a median cleft ⟨repair of a ~ digit⟩

bifida — see SPINA BIFIDA, SPINA BIFIDA OCCULTA

bi·fi·do·bac·te·ri·um \ˌbī-fə-(ˌ)dō-ˌbak-ˈtir-ē-əm\ *n* **1** *cap* : a genus (family Bifidobacteriaceae) of gram-positive, nonmotile, anaerobic bacteria that occur as part of the normal intestinal and vaginal flora of humans **2** *pl* **-ria** : any bacterium of the genus *Bifidobacterium*

[1]**bi·fo·cal** \(ˌ)bī-ˈfō-kəl\ *adj* **1** : having two focal lengths **2** : having one part that corrects for near vision and one for distant vision ⟨a ~ eyeglass lens⟩

[2]**bifocal** *n* **1** : a bifocal glass or lens **2 bifocals** *pl* : eyeglasses with bifocal lenses

bi·func·tion·al \ˌbī-ˈfəŋk-sh(ə-)nəl\ *adj* : having two functions ⟨~ neurons⟩

bi·fur·cate \ˈbī-(ˌ)fər-ˌkāt, bī-ˈfər-\ *vb* **-cat·ed; -cat·ing** : to divide into two branches or parts — **bi·fur·cate** \(ˌ)bī-ˈfər-kət, -ˌkāt; ˈbī-(ˌ)fər-ˌkāt\ *or* **bi·fur·cat·ed** \-ˌkā-təd\ *adj* — **bi·fur·ca·tion** \ˌbī-(ˌ)fər-ˈkā-shən\ *n*

bi·gem·i·ny \bī-ˈje-mə-nē\ *n, pl* **-nies** : the state of having a pulse characterized by two beats close together with a pause following each pair of beats — **bi·gem·i·nal** \-nəl\ *adj*

big·head \ˈbig-ˌhed\ *n* : any of several diseases of animals: as **a** : equine osteoporosis **b** : an acute photosensitization of sheep and goats that follows the ingestion of various plants

big·orex·ia \ˌbi-gə-ˈrek-sē-ə, -shə\ *n* : MUSCLE DYSMORPHIA

big toe *n* : the innermost and largest digit of the foot — called also *great toe*

bi·gua·nide \(ˌ)bī-ˈgwä-ˌnīd, -nəd\ *n* : any of various derivatives of a strong base $C_2H_7N_5$ that includes drugs (as metformin) used in the treatment of type 2 diabetes as well as antiseptic and disinfecting agents (as chlorhexidine) — see PROGUANIL

bi·ki·ni incision \bə-ˈkē-nē-\ *n* : PFANNENSTIEL INCISION — called also *bikini cut*

bi·la·bi·al \(ˌ)bī-ˈlā-bē-əl\ *adj* : of or relating to both lips

bi·lat·er·al \(ˌ)bī-ˈla-tə-rəl, -ˈla-trəl\ *adj* **1** : of, relating to, or affecting the right and left sides of the body or the right and left members of paired organs ⟨~ nephrectomy⟩ **2** : having bilateral symmetry — **bi·lat·er·al·i·ty** \(ˌ)bī-ˌla-tə-ˈra-lə-tē\ *n* — **bi·lat·er·al·ly** *adv*

bilateral symmetry *n* : symmetry in which similar anatomical parts are arranged on opposite sides of a median axis so that one and only one plane can divide the individual into essentially identical halves

bi·lay·er \ˈbī-ˌlā-ər\ *n* : a film or membrane with two molecular layers — **bilayer** *adj*

bil·ber·ry \ˈbil-ˌber-ē\ *n* : the fruit of a Eurasian shrub (*Vaccinium myrtillus*) resembling a blueberry; *also* : the dried fruit or an extract of this fruit used as an herbal remedy

bile \ˈbīl\ *n* : a yellow or greenish viscid alkaline fluid secreted by the liver and passed into the duodenum where it aids esp. in the emulsification and absorption of fats

bile acid *n* : any of several steroid acids (as cholic acid) that occur in bile usu. in the form of sodium salts conjugated with glycine or taurine

bile duct *n* : a duct by which bile passes from the liver or gallbladder to the duodenum

bile fluke *n* : CHINESE LIVER FLUKE

bile pigment *n* : any of several coloring matters (as bilirubin) in bile

bile salt *n* **1** : a salt of bile acid **2 bile salts** *pl* : a dry mixture of the salts of the gall of the ox used as a liver stimulant and as a laxative

bil·har·zia \bil-ˈhär-zē-ə, -ˈhärt-sē-\ *n* **1** : SCHISTOSOME **2** : SCHISTOSOMIASIS — **bil·har·zi·al** \-zē-əl, -sē-\ *adj*

Bil·harz \ˈbil-ˌhärts\, **Theodor Maximillian (1825–1862)**, German anatomist and helminthologist.

bil·har·zi·a·sis \ˌbil-ˌhär-ˈzī-ə-səs, -ˌhärt-ˈsī-\ *n, pl* **-a·ses** \-ˌsēz\ : SCHISTOSOMIASIS

bili- *comb form* **1** : bile ⟨*bili*ary⟩ **2** : derived from bile ⟨*bili*rubin⟩

bil·i·ary \ˈbi-lē-ˌer-ē\ *adj* **1** : of, relating to, or conveying bile **2** : affecting the bile-conveying structures

biliary atresia *n* : a life-threatening congenital condition marked by the absence, underdevelopment, or blockage of the bile ducts and esp. the extrahepatic bile ducts

biliary cirrhosis *n* : chronic progressive liver disease marked by inflammation, obstruction, and damage to the bile ducts resulting in the accumulation of bile in and functional impairment or failure of the liver

biliary dyskinesia *n* : pain or discomfort in the epigastric region resulting from spasm esp. of the sphincter of Oddi following cholecystectomy

biliary fever *n* : piroplasmosis esp. of dogs and horses

biliary tree *n* : the bile ducts and gallbladder — called also *biliary tract*

bil·io·pan·cre·at·ic \ˌbi-lē-ō-ˌpaŋ-krē-ˈa-tik, -ˌpan-\ *adj* : of, relating to, or involving the bile-conveying structures (as the gallbladder) and the pancreas ⟨~ secretions⟩

biliopancreatic diversion *n* : a gastric bypass procedure to treat severe obesity that limits the intestinal area available for breakdown of food by bile and pancreatic digestive enzymes

bil•ious \ˈbil-yəs\ *adj* **1** : of or relating to bile **2** : marked by or affected with disordered liver function and esp. excessive secretion of bile — **bil•ious•ness** *n*

bil•i•ru•bin \ˌbi-li-ˈrü-bən, ˈbi-li-ˌ\ *n* : a reddish-yellow pigment $C_{33}H_{36}N_4O_6$ that is formed by the breakdown of heme, is excreted by liver cells into bile, and occurs in blood and urine in disease states (as cirrhosis or hemolytic anemia) — see JAUNDICE

bil•i•ru•bi•nae•mia \ˌbi-li-ˌrü-bə-ˈnē-mē-ə\ *chiefly Brit var of* BILIRUBINEMIA

bil•i•ru•bi•ne•mia \-ˈnē-mē-ə\ *n* : HYPERBILIRUBINEMIA

bil•i•ru•bin•u•ria \-ˈnu̇r-ē-ə, -nyu̇r-\ *n* : excretion of bilirubin in the urine

bil•i•ver•din \ˌbi-li-ˈvərd-ᵊn, ˈbi-li-ˌ\ *n* : a green pigment $C_{33}H_{34}N_4O_6$ that occurs in bile and is an intermediate in the degradation of hemoglobin heme groups to bilirubin

bi•lobed \(ˌ)bī-ˈlōbd\ *adj* : divided into two lobes ⟨a ~ organ⟩

Bil•tri•cide \ˈbil-trə-ˌsīd\ *trademark* — used for a preparation of praziquantel

bi•man•u•al \(ˌ)bī-ˈman-yə-wəl\ *adj* : done with or requiring the use of both hands ⟨a ~ pelvic examination⟩

bi•mat•o•prost \bi-ˈma-tə-ˌpräst\ *n* : a prostaglandin analog $C_{25}H_{37}NO_4$ used topically to reduce elevated intraocular pressure and promote the growth of longer and thicker lashes — see LATISSE, LUMIGAN

bin- *comb form* : two : two by two : two at a time ⟨*bin*aural⟩

bi•na•ry \ˈbī-nə-rē\ *adj* **1** : compounded or consisting of or marked by two things or parts **2** : composed of two chemical elements, an element and a radical that acts as an element, or two such radicals

binary fission *n* : reproduction of a cell by division into two approximately equal parts

bin•au•ral \(ˌ)bī-ˈnȯr-əl, (ˌ)bi-\ *adj* : of, relating to, or involving two or both ears — **bin•au•ral•ly** *adv*

bind \ˈbīnd\ *vb* **bound** \ˈbau̇nd\; **bind•ing** **1** : to wrap up (an injury) with a cloth : BANDAGE **2** : to take up and hold usu. by chemical forces : combine with ⟨cellulose ~*s* water⟩ **3** : to combine or be taken up esp. by chemical action ⟨an antibody *bound* to a specific antigen⟩ **4** : to make costive : CONSTIPATE

bind•er \ˈbīn-dər\ *n* **1** : a broad bandage applied (as about the chest) for support **2** : a substance (as glucose or acacia) used in pharmacy to hold together the ingredients of a compressed tablet

binding site *n* : a region on a molecule or cell surface where the combining of chemical substances takes place

Bi•net age \bē-ˈnā-, bi-\ *n* : mental age as determined by the Binet-Simon scale
Bi•net \bē-nā\, **Alfred (1857–1911)**, French psychologist, and **Si•mon** \sē-mōⁿ\, **Théodore (1873–1961)**, French physician.

Bi•net–Si•mon scale \bi-ˈnā-sē-ˈmōⁿ-\ *n* : an intelligence test consisting orig. of tasks graded from the level of the average 3-year-old to that of the average 12-year-old but later extended in range — called also *Binet-Simon test, Binet test;* see STANFORD-BINET TEST

¹binge \ˈbinj\ *n* : an act of excessive or compulsive consumption esp. of food or alcoholic beverages

²binge *vb* **binged; binge•ing** *or* **bing•ing** : to go on a binge — **bing•er** \ˈbin-jər\ *n*

binge eating disorder *n* : an eating disorder characterized by recurring episodes of excessive food consumption accompanied by a sense of lack of control but without intervening periods of compensatory behavior (as self-induced vomiting or purging by laxatives) — abbr. *BED*

bin•oc•u•lar \bī-ˈnä-kyə-lər, bə-\ *adj* : of, relating to, using, or adapted to the use of both eyes ⟨a ~ infection⟩ ⟨~ vision⟩ — **bin•oc•u•lar•ly** *adv*

bi•no•mi•al \bī-ˈnō-mē-əl\ *n* : a biological species name consisting of two terms — **binomial** *adj*

binomial nomenclature *n* : a system of nomenclature in which each species of animal or plant receives a name of two terms of which the first identifies the genus to which it belongs and the second the species itself

bin•ovu•lar \(ˌ)bī-ˈnä-vyə-lər, -ˈnō-\ *adj* : BIOVULAR ⟨~ twinning⟩

bi•nu•cle•ate \(ˌ)bī-ˈnü-klē-ət, -ˈnyü-\ *also* **bi•nu•cle•at•ed** \-klē-ˌā-təd\ *adj* : having two nuclei ⟨~ lymphocytes⟩

bio- — see BI-

bio•ab•sorb•able \ˌbī-ō-əb-ˈzȯr-bə-bəl, -ˈsȯr-\ *adj* : capable of being absorbed into living tissue ⟨~ sutures⟩

bio•ac•cu•mu•la•tion \ˌbī-(ˌ)ō-ə-ˌkyü-myə-ˈlā-shən\ *n* : the accumulation of a substance (as a pesticide) in a living organism

bio•ac•tive \ˌbī-ō-ˈak-tiv\ *adj* : having an effect on a living organism — **bio•ac•tiv•i•ty** \-ak-ˈti-və-te\ *n*

bio•ad•he•sive \-ad-ˈhē-siv, -əd-\ *adj* : tending to adhere to or cause adhesion in living tissue ⟨~ gels⟩ — **bioadhesive** *n*

bio•aero•sol \-ˈer-ə-ˌsäl, -ˌsȯl\ *n* : a tiny, airborne particle (as a pollen grain or endotoxin) that is composed of or derived from biological matter

bio•as•say \ˌbī-(ˌ)ō-ˈa-ˌsā, -a-ˈsā\ *n* : determination of the relative strength of a substance (as a drug) by comparing its effect on a test organism with that of a standard preparation — **bio•as•say** \-a-ˈsā, -ˈa-ˌsā\ *vb*

bio•avail•abil•i•ty \ˌbī-(ˌ)ō-ə-ˌvā-lə-ˈbi-lə-tē\ *n, pl* **-ties** : the degree and rate at which a substance (as a drug) is absorbed into a living system or is made available at the site of physiological activity — **bio•avail•able** \-ˈvā-lə-bəl\ *adj*

bio•bank \-ˈbaŋk\ *n* : a storage place for biological samples (as blood or DNA) that may be used esp. for future medical research — called also *biorepository* — **bio•bank•ing** \-ˈbaŋ-kiŋ\ *n*

bio•cat•a•lyst \ˌbī-ō-ˈkat-ᵊl-əst\ *n* : a catalyst and esp. an enzyme of biological origin — **bio•ca•tal•y•sis** \-kə-ˈtal-ə-səs\ *n* — **bio•cat•a•lyt•ic** \-ˌkat-ᵊl-ˈit-ik\ *adj*

bio•chem•i•cal \ˌbī-ō-ˈke-mi-kəl\ *adj* **1** : of or relating to biochemistry **2** : characterized by, produced by, or involving chemical reactions in living organisms ⟨~ abnormalities⟩ ⟨~ processes⟩ — **biochemical** *n* — **bio-chem•i•cal•ly** \-k(ə-)lē\ *adv*

bio•chem•is•try \ˌbī-ō-ˈke-mə-strē\ *n, pl* **-tries** **1** : chemistry that deals with the chemical compounds and processes occurring in organisms **2** : the chemical characteristics and reactions of a particular living organism or biological substance ⟨a change in the patient's ~⟩ — **bio•chem•ist** \-ˈke-mist\ *n*

bio•chip \ˈbī-ō-ˌchip\ *n* : MICROARRAY

bio•cide \ˈbī-ə-ˌsīd\ *n* : a substance (as glutaraldehyde) that is destructive to many different organisms — **bio•cid•al** \ˌbī-ə-ˈsīd-ᵊl\ *adj*

bio•com•pat•i•bil•i•ty \ˌbī-ō-kəm-ˌpa-tə-ˈbi-lə-tē\ *n, pl* **-ties** : the condition of being compatible with living tissue or a living system by not being toxic or injurious and not causing immunological rejection — **bio•com•pat•i•ble** \-kəm-ˈpa-tə-bəl\ *adj*

bio•de•grad•able \ˌbī-(ˌ)ō-di-ˈgrā-də-bəl\ *adj* : capable of being broken down esp. into innocuous products by the action of living things (as microorganisms) — **bio•de•grad•abil•i•ty** \-ˌgrā-də-ˈbi-lə-tē\ *n* — **bio•deg•ra•da•tion** \-ˌde-grə-ˈdā-shən\ *n* — **bio•de•grade** \-di-ˈgrād\ *vb*

bio•elec•tri•cal \-i-ˈlek-tri-kəl\ *also* **bio•elec•tric** \-trik\ *adj* : of or relating to electric phenomena in living organisms ⟨human cortical ~ activity⟩ — **bio•elec•tric•i•ty** \-ˌlek-ˈtri-sə-tē\ *n*

bio•elec•tron•ics \-i-(ˌ)lek-ˈträ-niks\ *n* **1** : a branch of science that deals with electronic control of physiological function **2** : a branch of science that deals with the role of electron transfer in biological processes — **bio•elec•tron•ic** \-nik\ *adj*

bio•en•er•get•ics \-ˌe-nər-ˈje-tiks\ *n* : a system of therapy that combines breathing and body exercises, psychological therapy, and the free expression of impulses and emotions and that is held to increase well-being by releasing blocked physical and psychic energy — **bio•en•er•get•ic** \-tik\ *adj*

bio•en•gi•neer•ing \-ˌen-jə-ˈnir-iŋ\ *n* **1** : biological or medical application of engineering principles or engineering equipment — called also *biomedical engineering* **2** : the application of biological techniques (as genetic recombination) to create modified versions of organisms (as crops); *esp* : GENETIC ENGINEERING — **bio•en•gi•neer** \-ˈnir\ *n or vb*

bio•equiv•a•lence \-i-ˈkwi-və-ləns\ *n* : the property wherein two drugs with identical active ingredients or two different dosage forms (as tablet and oral suspension) of the same drug possess similar bioavailability and produce the same effect at the site of physiological activity — **bio•equiv•a•lent** \-lənt\ *adj*

bio•equiv•a•len•cy \-lən-sē\ *n, pl* **-cies** : BIOEQUIVALENCE

bio•eth•i•cist \-ˈe-thə-sist\ *n* : an expert in bioethics

bio•eth•ics \-ˈe-thiks\ *n* : the discipline dealing with the ethical implications of biological research and applications esp. in medicine — **bio•eth•ic** \-thik\ *n* — **bio•eth•i•cal** \-thi-kəl\ *adj*

bio•feed•back \-ˈfēd-ˌbak\ *n* : the technique of making unconscious or involuntary bodily processes (as heartbeat or brain waves) perceptible to the senses (as by the use of an oscilloscope) in order to manipulate them by conscious mental control

bio•film \ˈbī-ō-ˌfilm\ *n* : a thin usu. resistant layer of microorganisms (as bacteria) that form on and coat various surfaces (as of catheters)

bio•fla•vo•noid \-ˈflā-və-ˌnȯid\ *n* : any of various biologically active flavonoids (as quercetin) derived from plants and found esp. in fruits and vegetables

bio•ge•ner•ic \-jə-ˈner-ik\ *n* : BIOSIMILAR — **biogeneric** *adj*

bio•gen•ic \-ˈje-nik\ *adj* : produced by living organisms ⟨~ amines⟩

bio•haz•ard \ˈbī-ō-ˌha-zərd\ *n* : a biological agent or condition that constitutes a hazard to humans or the environment; *also* : a hazard posed by such an agent or condition — **bio•haz•ard•ous** \ˌbī-ō-ˈha-zər-dəs\ *adj*

bio•iden•ti•cal \ˌbī-ō-ī-ˈden-ti-kəl\ *adj* : having the same molecular structure as a substance produced in the body ⟨~ hormones⟩ — **bioidentical** *n*

bio•in•for•mat•ics \ˌbī-ō-ˌin-fər-ˈma-tiks\ *n* : the collection, classification, storage, and analysis of biochemical and biological information using computers esp. as applied in molecular genetics and genomics — **bio•in•for•mat•ic** \-tik\ *adj*

biol *abbr* biologic; biological; biologist; biology

bi•o•log•ic \ˌbī-ə-ˈlä-jik\ *or* **bi•o•log•i•cal** \-ji-kəl\ *n* : a biological product (as a globulin or antigen) used in the prevention or treatment of disease

biological *also* **biologic** *adj* **1** : of or relating to biology or to life and living processes **2** : used in or produced by applied biology **3** : related by direct genetic relationship rather than by adoption or marriage 〈~ parents〉 — **bi•o•log•i•cal•ly** \-ji-k(ə-)lē\ *adv*

biological clock *n* : an inherent timing mechanism in a living system (as a cell) that is inferred to exist in order to explain various cyclical behaviors and physiological processes

biological control *n* **1** : the reduction in numbers or elimination of pest organisms by interference with their ecology **2** : an agent used in biological control

biological false–positive *also* **biologic false–positive** *n* : a positive serological reaction for syphilis given by blood of a person who does not have syphilis

biological half–life *or* **biologic half–life** *n* : the time that a living body requires to eliminate one half the quantity of an administered substance (as a radioisotope) through its normal channels of elimination

biological warfare *n* : warfare involving the use of biological weapons; *also* : warfare involving the use of herbicides

biological weapon *n* : a harmful biological agent (as a pathogenic microorganism) used as a weapon to cause death or disease

bi•ol•o•gist \bī-ˈä-lə-jist\ *n* : a specialist in biology

bi•ol•o•gy \bī-ˈä-lə-jē\ *n, pl* **-gies** **1** : a branch of science that deals with living organisms and vital processes **2** : the laws and phenomena relating to an organism or group

bio•mag•net•ic \ˌbī-ō-ˌmag-ˈne-tik\ *adj* **1** : of or relating to the generation of magnetic fields by biological tissues 〈~ materials〉 **2** : of, relating to, or utilizing magnetic therapy 〈~ bracelets〉

biomagnetic therapy *n* : MAGNETIC THERAPY

bio•mag•ne•tism \-ˈmag-nə-ˌti-zəm\ *n* **1** : the generation of magnetic fields by living organisms **2** : MAGNETIC THERAPY

bio•mark•er \ˈbī-ō-ˌmär-kər\ *n* : a biological or biologically derived indicator (as a metabolite in the body) of a process, event, or condition (as disease or exposure to a toxin)

bio•ma•te•ri•al \ˌbī-ō-mə-ˈtir-ē-əl\ *n* : material that is suitable for introduction into living tissue esp. as part of a medical device (as an artificial heart valve or joint)

bio•me•chan•ics \ˌbī-ō-mi-ˈka-niks\ *n sing or pl* : the mechanics of biological and esp. musculoskeletal activity (as in locomotion or exercise); *also* : the scientific study of such mechanics — **bio•me•chan•i•cal** \-ni-kəl\ *adj*

bio•med•i•cal \-ˈme-di-kəl\ *adj* **1** : of or relating to biomedicine 〈~ studies〉 **2** : of, relating to, or involving biological, medical, and physical science — **bio•med•i•cal•ly** \-k(ə-)lē\ *adv*

biomedical engineering *n* : BIOENGINEERING 1 — **biomedical engineer** *n*

bio•med•i•cine \-ˈme-də-sən\ *n* : medicine based on the application of the principles of the natural sciences and esp. biology and biochemistry

bio•met•ric \ˌbī-ō-ˈme-trik\ *also* **bio•met•ri•cal** \-tri-kəl\ *adj* **1** : of or relating to biometry 〈~ analysis〉 **2** : utilizing biometrics 〈~ identification〉

bio•met•rics \-ˈme-triks\ *n sing or pl* **1** : BIOMETRY 1 **2** : the measurement and analysis of unique characteristics (as fingerprint or voice patterns) esp. as a means of verifying personal identity

bi•om•e•try \bī-ˈä-mə-trē\ *n, pl* **-tries** **1** : the application of statistical methods to the collection and analysis of biological data **2** : measurement (as by ultrasound) of living tissue or bodily structures — **bio•me•tri•cian** \-me-ˈtri-shən\ *n*

bio•mi•cro•scope \ˌbī-ō-ˈmī-krə-ˌskōp\ *n* : a binocular microscope used for examination of the anterior part of the eye

bio•mi•cros•co•py \-mī-ˈkräs-kə-pē\ *n, pl* **-pies** : the microscopic examination and study of living cells and tissues; *specif* : examination of the living eye with the biomicroscope

bio•mol•e•cule \ˌbī-ō-ˈmä-li-ˌkyül\ *n* : an organic molecule and esp. a macromolecule (as a protein or nucleic acid) in living organisms — **bio•mo•lec•u•lar** \-mə-ˈle-kyə-lər\ *adj*

bi•on•ic \bī-ˈä-nik\ *adj* **1** : of or relating to bionics **2** : having normal biological capability or performance enhanced by or as if by electronic or electrically actuated mechanical devices

bi•on•ics \bī-ˈä-niks\ *n sing or pl* : a science concerned with the application of data about the functioning of biological systems to the solution of engineering problems

[1]**bio•phar•ma•ceu•ti•cal** \ˌbī-ō-ˌfär-mə-ˈsü-ti-kəl\ *adj* : of or relating to biopharmaceutics or biopharmaceuticals

[2]**biopharmaceutical** *n* : a pharmaceutical derived from biological sources and esp. one produced by biotechnology

bio•phar•ma•ceu•tics \ˌbī-ō-ˌfär-mə-ˈsü-tiks\ *n* : the study of the relationships between the physical and chemical properties, dosage, and form of administration of a drug and its activity in the living body

bio•phys•i•cal \-ˈfi-zi-kəl\ *adj* **1** : of or relating to biophysics **2** : involving biological and physical factors or considerations

bio•phys•i•cist \-ˈfi-zə-sist\ *n* : a specialist in biophysics

bio•phys•ics \ˌbī-ō-ˈfi-ziks\ *n* : a branch of science concerned with the application of physical principles and methods to biological problems

bio·poly·mer \ˌbī-ō-ˈpä-lə-mər\ *n* : a polymer (as a protein or polysaccharide) formed in a biological system

bio·pros·the·sis \-präs-ˈthē-səs\ *n, pl* **-the·ses** \-ˌsēz\ : a prosthesis (as a porcine heart valve) consisting of an animal part or containing animal tissue — **bio·pros·thet·ic** \-präs-ˈthet-ik\ *adj*

bi·op·sy \ˈbī-ˌäp-sē\ *n, pl* **-sies** : the removal and examination of tissue, cells, or fluids from the living body — **biopsy** *vb*

bio·psy·chol·o·gy \ˌbī-ō-sī-ˈkä-lə-jē\ *n, pl* **-gies** : PSYCHOBIOLOGY — **bio·psy·cho·log·i·cal** \-ˌsī-kə-ˈlä-ji-kəl\ *adj* — **bio·psy·chol·o·gist** \-sī-ˈkä-lə-jist\ *n*

bio·psy·cho·so·cial \-ˌsī-kō-ˈsō-shəl\ *adj* : of, relating to, or concerned with the biological, psychological, and social aspects of disease

bio·re·ac·tor \-rē-ˈak-tər\ *n* : a device or apparatus in which organisms and esp. bacteria synthesize useful substances (as interferon) or break down harmful ones (as in sewage)

bio·re·pos·i·to·ry \-ri-ˈpä-zə-ˌtȯr-ē\ *n, pl* **-ries** : BIOBANK

bio·rhythm \ˈbī-ō-ˌri-t͟həm\ *n* : an innately determined rhythmic biological process or function (as sleep behavior); *also* : an innate rhythmic determiner of such a process or function — **bio·rhyth·mic** \ˌbī-ō-ˈrit͟h-mik\ *adj*

bio·safe·ty \ˈbī-ō-ˌsāf-tē\ *n, pl* **-ties** : safety with respect to the effects of biological research on humans and the environment

bio·sci·ence \ˈbī-ō-ˌsī-əns\ *n* : BIOLOGY; *also* : LIFE SCIENCE — **bio·sci·en·tist** \ˌbī-ō-ˈsī-ən-tist\ *n*

bio·sen·sor \ˈbī-ō-ˌsen-ˌsȯr, -sər\ *n* : a device and esp. one consisting of a biological component (as an enzyme or bacterium) that aids in the detection of a target substance

bio·sim·i·lar \-ˈsi-mə-lər, -ˈsim-lər\ *n* : a substance of biological origin that is very similar to a previously-approved biologic preparation and is considered interchangeable with it — **biosimilar** *adj* — **bio·sim·i·lar·i·ty** \-ˌsi-mə-ˈler-ə-tē\ *n*

-bi·o·sis \(ˌ)bī-ˈō-səs, bē-\ *n comb form, pl* **-bi·o·ses** \-ˌsēz\ : mode of life ⟨para*biosis*⟩ ⟨sym*biosis*⟩

bio·sta·tis·tics \ˌbī-ō-stə-ˈtis-tiks\ *n* : statistical processes and methods applied to the collection and analysis of biological data — **bio·stat·is·ti·cian** \-ˌsta-tə-ˈsti-shən\ *n*

bio·syn·the·sis \ˌbī-ō-ˈsin-thə-səs\ *n, pl* **-the·ses** : production of a chemical compound by a living organism — **bio·syn·the·size** \-ˈsin-thə-ˌsīz\ *vb* — **bio·syn·thet·ic** \-sin-ˈthe-tik\ *adj* — **bio·syn·thet·i·cal·ly** \-ti-k(ə-)lē\ *adv*

bio·tech \ˈbī-ō-ˌtek\ *n* **1** : BIOTECHNOLOGY 1 **2** : a company that uses biotechnology (as to develop drugs)

bio·tech·ni·cal \ˌbī-ō-ˈtek-ni-kəl\ *adj* : of or relating to biotechnology

bio·tech·nol·o·gy \ˌbī-ō-tek-ˈnä-lə-jē\ *n, pl* **-gies** **1** : the manipulation (as through genetic engineering) of living organisms or their components to produce useful usu. commercial products (as novel pharmaceuticals); *also* : any of various applications of biological science used in such manipulation **2** : ERGONOMICS 1 — **bio·tech·no·log·i·cal** \-ˌtek-nə-ˈlä-ji-kəl\ *adj* — **bio·tech·no·log·i·cal·ly** \-k(ə-)lē\ *adv* — **bio·tech·nol·o·gist** \-tek-ˈnä-lə-jəst\ *n*

bio·te·lem·e·try \-tə-ˈle-mə-trē\ *n, pl* **-tries** : remote detection and measurement of a human or animal condition, activity, or function (as heartbeat or body temperature) — **bio·tel·e·met·ric** \-ˌte-lə-ˈme-trik\ *adj*

bi·ot·ic \bī-ˈä-tik\ *adj* : of or relating to life; *esp* : caused or produced by living beings

-bi·ot·ic \bī-ˈä-tik\ *adj comb form* **1** : relating to life ⟨anti*biotic*⟩ **2** : having a (specified) mode of life ⟨necro*biotic*⟩

bi·o·tin \ˈbī-ə-tən\ *n* : a colorless crystalline growth vitamin $C_{10}H_{16}N_2O_3S$ of the vitamin B complex found esp. in yeast, liver, and egg yolk — called also *vitamin H*

bio·tox·in \ˈbī-ō-ˌtäk-sən\ *n* : a toxic substance of biological origin

bio·trans·for·ma·tion \ˈbī-ō-ˌtrans-fər-ˈmā-shən, -ˌfȯr-\ *n* : the transformation of chemical compounds within a living system

bi·ovu·lar \(ˌ)bī-ˈä-vyə-lər, -ˈō-\ *adj, of fraternal twins* : derived from two ova

bi·pa·ri·etal \ˌbī-pə-ˈrī-ət-ᵊl\ *adj* : of or relating to the parietal bones; *specif* : being a measurement between the most distant opposite points of the two parietal bones

bi·ped \ˈbī-ˌped\ *n* : a two-footed animal — **biped** *or* **bi·ped·al** \(ˌ)bī-ˈped-ᵊl\ *adj*

bi·pen·nate \(ˌ)bī-ˈpe-ˌnāt\ *adj* : having the fibers arranged obliquely and inserting on both sides into a tendon ⟨a ~ muscle⟩

bi·pen·ni·form \-ˈpe-ni-ˌfȯrm\ *adj* : BIPENNATE

bi·per·i·den \bī-ˈper-ə-dən\ *n* : a white crystalline muscle relaxant $C_{21}H_{29}NO$ used esp. to reduce the symptoms (as tremors and muscle rigidity) associated with Parkinson's disease

bi·phe·nyl \(ˌ)bī-ˈfen-ᵊl, -ˈfēn-\ *n* : a white crystalline hydrocarbon $C_6H_5 \cdot C_6H_5$

[1]**bi·po·lar** \(ˌ)bī-ˈpō-lər\ *adj* **1** : involving or being electrodes or leads attached to two different bodily sites (as the arms and legs) for recording the difference in electrical potential between the two sites **2** *of a neuron* : having an efferent and an afferent process **3** : being, characteristic of, or

affected with a bipolar disorder <~ depression> — compare UNIPOLAR

[2]**bipolar** *n* : a person affected with bipolar disorder

bipolar disorder *n* : any of several mood disorders characterized usu. by alternating episodes of depression and mania in which the mania may be of the euphoric or irritable type or both — called also *bipolar affective disorder, bipolar illness, manic depression, manic-depressive illness, manic-depressive psychosis*

bird flu *n* : influenza of birds caused esp. by strains of a subtype (H5N1) of the orthomyxovirus causing influenza A that have produced epidemics in domestic birds esp. in Asia and may mutate and be passed to humans causing mild to fatally severe respiratory illness — called also *avian flu; avian influenza, fowl plague*

bird louse *n* : BITING LOUSE

[1]**birth** \ˈbərth\ *n, often attrib* **1** : the emergence of a new individual from the body of its parent **2** : the act or process of bringing forth young from the womb — **birth** *vb*

[2]**birth** *adj* : BIOLOGICAL 3

birth canal *n* : the channel formed by the cervix, vagina, and vulva through which the fetus passes during birth

birth certificate *n* : a copy of an official record of a person's date and place of birth and parentage

birth control *n* **1** : control of the number of children born esp. by preventing or lessening the frequency of conception : CONTRACEPTION **2** : contraceptive devices or preparations

birth control pill *n* : any of various preparations that usu. contain progestogen and an estrogen, are taken orally esp. on a daily basis, and act as contraceptives typically by preventing ovulation — called also *oral contraceptive, oral contraceptive pill*

birth defect *n* : a physical or biochemical defect (as cleft palate, phenylketonuria, or Down syndrome) that is present at birth and may be inherited or environmentally induced

birthing center *n* : a facility usu. staffed by nurse-midwives that provides a less institutionalized setting than a hospital for women who wish to deliver by natural childbirth

birthing room *n* : a comfortably furnished hospital room where both labor and delivery take place and in which the baby usu. remains during the hospital stay

birth•mark \ˈbərth-ˌmärk\ *n* : an unusual mark or blemish on the skin at birth : NEVUS — **birthmark** *vb*

birth pang *n* : one of the regularly recurrent pains that are characteristic of childbirth — usu. used in pl.

birth•rate \ˈbərth-ˌrāt\ *n* : the ratio between births and individuals in a specified population and time often expressed as number of live births per hundred or per thousand population per year — called also *natality*

birth trauma *n* : physical injury (as cephalhematoma, facial paralysis, or clavicular fracture) sustained by an infant in the process of birth

bis•a•co•dyl \ˌbi-sə-ˈkō-(ˌ)dil\ *n* : a white crystalline laxative $C_{22}H_{19}NO_4$ used orally or as a suppository

[1]**bi•sex•u•al** \(ˌ)bī-ˈsek-shə-wəl\ *adj* **1 a** : possessing characters of both sexes and esp. both male and female reproductive structures : HERMAPHRODITIC **b** : of, relating to, or characterized by a tendency to be sexually attracted toward individuals of both sexes : engaging in sexual activity with partners of either sex **2** : of, relating to, or involving two sexes <~ reproduction> — **bi•sex•u•al•i•ty** \ˌbī-ˌsek-shə-ˈwa-lə-tē\ *n* — **bi•sex•u•al•ly** *adv*

[2]**bisexual** *n* : a bisexual individual

bis•hy•droxy•cou•ma•rin \ˌbis-(ˌ)hī-ˌdräk-sē-ˈkü-mə-rən\ *n* : DICUMAROL

bis•muth \ˈbiz-məth\ *n* : a brittle grayish-white chiefly trivalent metallic element — symbol *Bi;* see ELEMENT table

bismuth sub•car•bon•ate \-ˌsəb-ˈkär-bə-ˌnāt, -nət\ *n* : a white or pale yellowish-white powder used chiefly in treating gastrointestinal disorders, topically as a protective in lotions and ointments, and in cosmetics

bismuth sub•ni•trate \-ˌsəb-ˈnī-ˌtrāt\ *n* : a white powder $Bi_5O(OH)_9(NO_3)_4$ that is used in medicine similarly to bismuth subcarbonate

bismuth sub•sa•lic•y•late \-ˌsəb-sə-ˈli-sə-ˌlāt\ *n* : an antidiarrheal drug $C_7H_5BiO_4$ also used to relieve heartburn, indigestion, and nausea — see PEPTO-BISMOL

bis•o•pro•lol \ˌbi-sō-ˈprō-ˌlȯl\ *n* : a beta-blocker taken orally in the form of its fumarate $(C_{18}H_{31}NO_4)_2{\cdot}C_4H_4O_4$ to treat hypertension — see ZEBETA

bis•phe•nol A \ˌbis-ˈfē-ˌnōl-, -ˌnȯl-\ *n* : a chemical compound $C_{15}H_{16}O_2$ that is a component esp. of hard plastics and epoxy resins — abbr. *BPA*

bis•phos•pho•nate \bis-ˈfäs-fə-ˌnāt\ *n* : any of a group of drugs (as alendronate) that slow the breakdown of bone by osteoclasts

bis•tou•ry \ˈbis-tə-rē\ *n, pl* **-ries** : a small slender straight or curved surgical knife with a sharp or blunt point

bi•sul•fate \bī-ˈsəl-ˌfāt\ *n* : an acid sulfate

bi•tar•trate \bī-ˈtär-ˌtrāt\ *n* : an acid tartrate

[1]**bite** \ˈbīt\ *vb* **bit** \ˈbit\; **bit•ten** \ˈbit-ᵊn\ *also* **bit; bit•ing 1** : to seize esp. with teeth or jaws so as to enter, grip, or wound **2** : to wound, pierce, or sting esp. with a fang or a proboscis

[2]**bite** *n* **1** : the act or manner of biting; *esp* : OCCLUSION 2a **2** : a wound made by biting

bite block *n* : a device used in dentistry for recording the spatial relation of the jaws esp. in respect to the occlusion of the teeth

bi•tem•po•ral \(ˌ)bī-ˈtem-pə-rəl\ *adj* : relating to, involving, or joining the two temporal bones or the areas that they occupy

bite plane *n* : a removable dental appliance used to cover the occlusal surfaces of the teeth so that they cannot be brought into contact

bite plate *n* : a removable usu. plastic dental appliance used in orthodontics and prosthodontics: as **a** : a U-shaped device worn in the upper or lower jaw and used esp. to reposition that jaw or prevent bruxism **b** : RETAINER 2

bite•wing \ˈbīt-ˌwiŋ\ *n* : dental X-ray film designed to show the crowns of the upper and lower teeth simultaneously

biting fly *n* : a dipteran fly (as a mosquito or horsefly) having mouthparts adapted for piercing and biting

biting louse *n* : any of numerous wingless insects (order Mallophaga) parasitic esp. on birds — called also *bird louse*

biting midge *n* : any of a family (Ceratopogonidae) of small dipteran flies including vectors of filarial worms

Bi•tot's spots \bē-ˈtōz-\ *n* : shiny pearly spots of triangular shape occurring on the conjunctiva in severe vitamin A deficiency esp. in children

Bi•tot \bē-ˈtō\, **Pierre A. (1822–1888)**, French physician.

bit•ter \ˈbi-tər\ *adj* : being or inducing the one of the four basic taste sensations that is peculiarly acrid, astringent, or disagreeable — compare SALT, SOUR, SWEET — **bit•ter•ness** *n*

bitter almond *n* : an almond with a bitter taste that contains amygdalin; *also* : a tree (*Prunus dulcis amara*) of the rose family (Rosaceae) producing bitter almonds

bi•uret \ˌbī-yə-ˈret\ *n* : a white crystalline compound $N_3H_5C_2O_2$ formed by heating urea

biuret reaction *n* : a chemical reaction that produces a violet or purple color when biuret or most proteins are exposed to an alkaline solution of copper sulfate and is typically used to indicate the presence of protein in a test sample

biuret test *n* : a test esp. for the presence of proteins using the biuret reaction

[1]**bi•va•lent** \(ˌ)bī-ˈvā-lənt\ *adj* **1** : having two combining sites ⟨a ~ antibody⟩ **2** : associated in pairs in synapsis **3** : conferring immunity to two diseases or two serotypes ⟨a ~ vaccine⟩

[2]**bivalent** *n* : a pair of synaptic chromosomes

bi•valve \ˈbī-ˌvalv\ *vb* **bi•valved; bi•valv•ing** : to split (a cast) along one or two sides (as to relieve pressure)

bi•ven•tric•u•lar \(ˈ)bī-ven-ˈtri-kyə-lər\ *adj* : of, relating to, or affecting both ventricles of the heart ⟨~ hypertrophy⟩

Bk *symbol* berkelium

BK *abbr* below knee

black–and–blue \ˌblak-ən-ˈblü\ *adj* : darkly discolored from blood effused by bruising

black box *adj* : being or containing a warning of a serious or life-threatening side effect (as stroke or suicidal tendencies) that is highlighted by a black border on a label or accompanying informational insert for a prescription drug ⟨*black box* warnings⟩

black cohosh *n* : the root of a woodland herb (*Cimicifuga racemosa* syn. *Actaea recemosa*) used esp. as an herbal remedy to treat menopausal symptoms; *also* : a preparation or extract of this root

black death *n, often cap B&D* : PLAGUE 2; *also* : a severe epidemic of plague and esp. bubonic plague that occurred in Asia and Europe in the 14th century

black disease *n* : a fatal toxemia of sheep associated with simultaneous infection by liver flukes (*Fasciola hepatica*) and an anaerobic toxin-producing clostridium (*Clostridium novyi*)

black eye *n* : a discoloration of the skin around the eye from bruising

black•fly \ˈblak-ˌflī\ *n, pl* **-flies** : any of a family (Simuliidae) and esp. genus *Simulium* of bloodsucking dipteran flies

black hairy tongue *n* : a dark furry or hairy discoloration of the tongue that is due to hyperplasia of the filiform papillae usu. with an overgrowth of microorganisms — called also *blacktongue*

black•head \ˈblak-ˌhed\ *n* **1** : a small plug of sebum blocking the duct of a sebaceous gland esp. on the face — compare MILIUM **2** : a destructive disease of turkeys and related birds caused by a protozoan of the genus *Histomonas* (*H. meleagridis*)

black henbane *n* : HENBANE

black•leg \ˈblak-ˌleg\ *n* : a usu. fatal toxemia esp. of young cattle caused by toxins produced by an anaerobic soil bacterium of the genus *Clostridium* (*C. chauvoei* syn. *C. feseri*)

black–legged tick *n* : either of two ixodid ticks : **a** : DEER TICK **b** : WESTERN BLACK-LEGGED TICK

black lung *n* : pneumoconiosis caused by habitual inhalation of coal dust — called also *black lung disease*

black mold *n* : a greenish-black mold (genus *Stachybotrys* and esp. *S. chartarum*) found esp. on waterlogged cellulose materials (as cardboard)

black•out \ˈblak-ˌau̇t\ *n* : a transient dulling or loss of vision, consciousness, or memory (as from temporary impairment of cerebral circulation or an alcoholic binge) — compare GRAYOUT, REDOUT — **black out** *vb*

black quarter *n* : BLACKLEG

black rat *n* : a rat of the genus *Rattus* (*R. rattus*) that has been the chief vector of bubonic plague

black•tongue \ˈblak-ˌtəng\ *n* **1** : BLACK HAIRY TONGUE **2** : a disease of dogs caused by a deficient diet and analogous to pellagra in humans

black•wa•ter \ˈblak-ˌwȯ-tər, -ˌwä-\ *n* : any of several diseases (as blackwater fever or Texas fever) characterized by dark-colored urine

blackwater fever *n* : a rare febrile complication of repeated malarial attacks that is marked by destruction of blood cells with hemoglobinuria and extensive kidney damage

black widow *n* : a venomous New World spider of the genus *Latrodectus* (*L. mactans*) the female of which is black with an hourglass-shaped red mark on the abdominal underside; *broadly* : any other spider of the genus *Latrodectus*

blad•der \ˈbla-dər\ *n* **1** : a membranous sac in animals that serves as the receptacle of a liquid or contains gas; *esp* : URINARY BLADDER **2** : a vesicle or pouch forming part of an animal body ⟨the ~ of a tapeworm larva⟩

bladder worm *n* : CYSTICERCUS

blade \ˈblād\ *n* **1** : a broad flat body part (as the shoulder blade) **2** : the flat portion of the tongue immediately behind the tip; *also* : this portion together with the tip **3** : a flat working and esp. cutting part of an implement (as a scalpel)

blain \ˈblān\ *n* : an inflammatory swelling or sore

Bla•lock–Taus•sig operation \ˈblā-ˌläk-ˈtaů-sig-\ *n* : surgical correction of the tetralogy of Fallot — called also *blue-baby operation*

Blalock, Alfred (1899–1964), and **Taussig, Helen B. (1898–1986),** American physicians.

blast \ˈblast\ *n* : BLAST CELL

blast- *or* **blasto-** *comb form* : bud : budding : germ ⟨*blasto*disc⟩ ⟨*blas-tu*la⟩

-blast \ˌblast\ *n comb form* : formative unit esp. of living matter : germ : cell layer ⟨epi*blast*⟩

blast cell *n* : an immature cell; *esp* : a usu. large blood cell precursor that is in the earliest stage of development in which it is recognizably committed to development along a particular cell lineage

blast crisis *n* : the terminal stage of chronic myelogenous leukemia that is marked by a significant increase in the proportion of blast cells — called also *blastic crisis*

blas•te•ma \bla-ˈstē-mə\ *n, pl* **-mas** *also* **-ma•ta** \-mə-tə\ : a mass of living substance capable of growth and differentiation

-blas•tic \ˈblas-tik\ *adj comb form* : sprouting or germinating (in a specified way) ⟨hemocyto*blastic*⟩ : having (such or so many) sprouts, buds, or germ layers ⟨meso*blastic*⟩

blas•to•coel *or* **blas•to•coele** \ˈblas-tə-ˌsēl\ *n* : the cavity of a blastula — **blas•to•coe•lic** \ˌblas-tə-ˈsē-lik\ *adj*

blas•to•cyst \ˈblas-tə-ˌsist\ *n* : the modified blastula of a placental mammal

blas•to•derm \-ˌdərm\ *n* : a blastodisc after completion of cleavage and formation of the blastocoel

blas•to•derm•ic vesicle \ˌblas-tə-ˈdər-mik-\ *n* : BLASTOCYST

blas•to•disc *or* **blas•to•disk** \ˈblas-tə-ˌdisk\ *n* : the embryo-forming portion of an egg with discoidal cleavage usu. appearing as a small disc on the upper surface of the yolk mass

blas•to•gen•e•sis \ˌblas-tə-ˈje-nə-səs\ *n, pl* **-e•ses** \-ˌsēz\ : the transformation of lymphocytes into larger cells capable of undergoing mitosis — **blas•to•gen•ic** \-ˈje-nik\ *adj*

blas•to•mere \ˈblas-tə-ˌmir\ *n* : a cell produced during cleavage of a fertilized egg — called also *cleavage cell*

Blas•to•my•ces \ˌblas-tə-ˈmī-ˌsēz\ *n* : a genus of yeastlike fungi that contains the causative agent (*B. dermatitidis*) of North American blastomycosis

blas•to•my•co•sis \-ˌmī-ˈkō-səs\ *n, pl* **-co•ses** \-ˌsēz\ : either of two infectious diseases caused by yeastlike fungi — see NORTH AMERICAN BLASTOMYCOSIS, SOUTH AMERICAN BLASTOMYCOSIS — **blas•to•my•cot•ic** \-ˈkä-tik\ *adj*

blas•to•pore \ˈblas-tə-ˌpō(ə)r, -ˌpȯ(ə)r\ *n* : the opening of the archenteron

blas•tu•la \ˈblas-chə-lə\ *n, pl* **-las** *or* **-lae** \-ˌlē\ : an early metazoan embryo typically having the form of a hollow fluid-filled rounded cavity bounded by a single layer of cells — compare GASTRULA, MORULA — **blas•tu•lar** \-lər\ *adj* — **blas•tu•la•tion** \ˌblas-chə-ˈlā-shən\ *n*

bleb \ˈbleb\ *n* **1** : a small blister — compare BULLA 2 **2** : a vesicular outpocketing of a plasma or nuclear membrane

¹bleed \ˈblēd\ *vb* **bled** \ˈbled\; **bleed•ing** **1** : to emit or lose blood **2** : to escape by oozing or flowing (as from a wound); *also* : to remove or draw blood from

²bleed *n* : the escape of blood from vessels : HEMORRHAGE

bleed•er \ˈblē-dər\ *n* **1** : BLOODLETTER **2** : HEMOPHILIAC **3** : a large blood vessel (as one cut during surgery) that is losing blood **4** : a horse that has experienced exercise-induced pulmonary hemorrhage

bleed•ing *n* : an act, instance, or result of being bled or the process by which something is bled: as **a** : the escape of blood from vessels : HEMORRHAGE **b** : PHLEBOTOMY

bleeding time *n* : a period of time of usu. about two and a half minutes during which a small wound (as a pinprick) continues to bleed

blem•ish \ˈble-mish\ *n* : a mark of physical deformity or injury; *esp* : any small mark on the skin (as a pimple)

blen•nor•rha•gia \ˌble-nə-ˈrā-jē-ə, -jə\ *n* **1** : BLENNORRHEA **2** : GONORRHEA

blennorrhagica — see KERATOSIS BLENNORRHAGICA

blennorrhagicum — see KERATODERMA BLENNORRHAGICUM

blen•nor•rhea \ˌble-nə-ˈrē-ə\ *n* : an excessive secretion and discharge of mucus — **blen•nor•rheal** \-ˈrē-əl\ *adj*

blen•nor•rhoea *chiefly Brit var of* BLENNORRHEA

bleo•my•cin \ˌblē-ə-ˈmīs-ᵊn\ *n* : a mixture of glycoprotein antibiotics derived from a streptomyces (*Streptomyces verticillus*) and used in the form of the sulfates as an antineoplastic agent — see ABVD

blephar- *or* **blepharo-** *comb form* : eyelid ⟨*blepharo*spasm⟩

bleph•a•ri•tis \ˌble-fə-ˈrī-təs\ *n, pl* **-rit•i•des** \-ˈri-tə-ˌdēz\ : inflammation esp. of the margins of the eyelids

bleph•a•ro•con•junc•ti•vi•tis \ˌble-fə-(ˌ)rō-kən-ˌjəŋk-tə-ˈvī-təs\ *n* : inflammation of the eyelid and conjunctiva

bleph•a•ro•plas•ty \ˈble-fə-rō-ˌplas-tē\ *n, pl* **-ties** : plastic surgery on an eyelid esp. to remove fatty or excess tissue

bleph•a•rop•to•sis \ˌble-fə-rəp-ˈtō-səs\ *n, pl* **-to•ses** \-ˌsēz\ : a drooping or abnormal relaxation of the upper eyelid

bleph•a•ro•spasm \ˈble-fə-rō-ˌspa-zəm, -rə-\ *n* : spasmodic winking from involuntary contraction of the orbicularis oculi muscle of the eyelids

bleph•a•rot•o•my \ˌble-fə-ˈrä-tə-mē\ *n, pl* **-mies** : surgical incision of an eyelid

blind \ˈblīnd\ *adj* **1 a** : lacking or deficient in sight; *esp* : having less than 1/10 of normal vision in the more efficient eye when refractive defects are fully corrected by lenses **b** : of or relating to sightless persons ⟨~ care⟩ **2** : designed to prevent participants from having information that could cause bias ⟨a ~ clinical trial⟩ — see DOUBLE-BLIND, SINGLE-BLIND **3** : having but one opening or outlet ⟨the cecum is a ~ pouch⟩ — **blind** *vb* — **blind•ly** *adv* — **blind•ness** *n*

blind gut *n* : the cecum of the large intestine

blind•sight \ˈblīn(d)-ˌsīt\ *n* : the ability of individuals with blindness to detect and respond to visual stimuli — **blind•sight•ed** \-ˌsī-təd\ *adj*

blind spot *n* : the point in the retina where the optic nerve enters that is devoid of rods and cones and is insensitive to light — called also *optic disk*

blind stag•gers \-ˈsta-gərz\ *n sing or pl* : a severe form of selenosis marked esp. by impaired vision and an unsteady gait; *also* : a similar condition not caused by selenium poisoning

blink \ˈbliŋk\ *vb* **1** : to close and open the eye involuntarily **2** : to remove (as tears) from the eye by blinking — **blink** *n*

blis•ter \ˈblis-tər\ *n* **1** : a fluid-filled elevation of the epidermis **2** : an agent that causes blistering — **blister** *vb* — **blis•tery** \-tə-rē\ *adj*

blister pack *n* : a card holding medicinal tablets or capsules that are individually packaged in a clear plastic case sealed to the card — called also *blister card*

¹**bloat** \ˈblōt\ *vb* : to make or become turgid: **a** : to produce edema in **b** : to cause or result in accumulation of gas in the digestive tract of **c** : to cause abdominal distension in

²**bloat** *n* **1** : a flatulent digestive disturbance of domestic animals and esp. cattle **2** : a condition of large dogs marked by distension and usu. life-threatening rotation of the stomach

¹**block** \ˈbläk\ *n, often attrib* **1** : interruption of normal physiological function of a tissue or organ; *esp* : HEART BLOCK **2 a** : BLOCK ANESTHESIA **b** : NERVE BLOCK 1 **3** : interruption of a train of thought by competing thoughts or psychological suppression

²**block** *vb* **1** : to prevent normal functioning of (a bodily element) **2** : to experience or exhibit psychological blocking or blockage **3** : to obstruct the effect of

block•ade \blä-ˈkād\ *n* **1** : interruption of normal physiological function (as transmission of nerve impulses) of a tissue or organ **2** : inhibition of a physiologically active substance (as a hormone) — **blockade** *vb*

block•age \ˈblä-kij\ *n* **1** : the action of blocking or the state of being blocked **2** : internal resistance to understanding a communicated idea, to learning new material, or to adopting a new mode of response because of existing habitual ways of thinking, perceiving, and acting — compare BLOCKING

block anesthesia *n* : local anesthesia (as by injection) produced by interruption of the flow of impulses along a nerve trunk — compare REGIONAL ANESTHESIA

block•er \ˈblä-kər\ *n* : one that blocks — see ALPHA-BLOCKER, BETA-BLOCKER, CALCIUM CHANNEL BLOCKER

block•ing \ˈblä-kiŋ\ *n* : interruption of a trend of associative thought by the arousal of an opposing trend or through the welling up into consciousness of a complex of unpleasant ideas — compare BLOCKAGE 2

blocking antibody *n* : an antibody that combines with an antigen without visible reaction and blocks another antibody from combining with it

blood \ˈbləd\ *n, often attrib* **1** : the fluid that circulates in the heart, arteries, capillaries, and veins of a vertebrate animal carrying nourishment and oxygen to and bringing away waste products from all parts of the body **2** : a fluid of an invertebrate comparable to blood

blood alcohol *n* : the amount of alcohol in the blood

blood bank *n* : a place for storage of or an institution storing blood or plasma; *also* : blood so stored

blood banking *n* : the activity of administering or working in a blood bank

blood–borne \-ˌbȯrn\ *adj* : carried or transmitted by the blood

blood–brain barrier *n* : a barrier created by the modification of brain capillaries (as by reduction in fenestration and formation of tight cell-to-cell contacts) that prevents many substances from leaving the blood and crossing the capillary walls into the brain tissues — abbr. *BBB*

blood cell *n* : a cell or platelet normally present in blood — see RED BLOOD CELL, WHITE BLOOD CELL

blood clot *n* : CLOT

blood count *n* : the determination of the blood cells in a definite volume of blood; *also* : the number of cells so determined — see COMPLETE BLOOD COUNT, DIFFERENTIAL BLOOD COUNT

blood doping *n* : a technique for temporarily improving athletic performance in which oxygen-carrying red blood cells previously withdrawn from an athlete are injected back just before an event

blood fluke *n* : SCHISTOSOME

blood gas *n* : dissolved carbon dioxide and oxygen in blood typically expressed in terms of partial pressure; *also* : a test of usu. arterial blood to measure the partial pressures and concentrations of carbon dioxide and oxygen along with the pH and bicarbonate level

blood group *n* : one of the classes (as A, B, AB, or O) into which individuals or their blood can be separated on the basis of the presence or absence of specific antigens in the blood — called also *blood type*

blood grouping *n* : BLOOD TYPING

blood•less \ˈbləd-ləs\ *adj* : free from or lacking blood ⟨a ∼ surgical field⟩

blood•let•ter \ˈbləd-ˌle-tər\ *n* : a practitioner of phlebotomy

blood•let•ting \-ˌle-tiŋ\ *n* : PHLEBOTOMY

blood•mo•bile \-mō-ˌbēl\ *n* : a motor vehicle staffed and equipped for collecting blood from donors

blood packing *n* : BLOOD DOPING

blood plasma *n* : the pale yellow fluid portion of whole blood that consists of water and its dissolved constituents including proteins (as albumin, fibrinogen, and globulins), electrolytes (as sodium and chloride), glucose, lipids (as cholesterol and triglycerides), metabolic waste products (as urea), amino acids, hormones, and vitamins

blood platelet *n* : PLATELET

blood poisoning *n* : SEPTICEMIA

blood pressure *n* : pressure exerted by the blood upon the walls of the blood vessels and esp. arteries, usu. measured on the radial artery by means of a sphygmomanometer, and expressed in millimeters of mercury either as a fraction having as numerator the maximum pressure that follows systole of the left ventricle of the heart and as denominator the minimum pressure that accompanies cardiac diastole or as a whole number representing the first value only ⟨a *blood pressure* of 120/80⟩ ⟨a *blood pressure* of 120⟩ — abbr. *BP*

blood serum *n* : SERUM a(1)

blood•shot \ˈbləd-ˌshät\ *adj, of an eye* : inflamed to redness

blood•stain \-ˌstān\ *n* : a discoloration caused by blood — **blood•stained** \-ˌstānd\ *adj*

blood•stream \-ˌstrēm\ *n* : the flowing blood in a circulatory system

blood•suck•er \-ˌsə-kər\ *n* : an animal that sucks blood; *esp* : LEECH — **blood•suck•ing** \-kiŋ\ *adj*

blood sugar *n* : the glucose in the blood; *also* : its concentration (as in milligrams per 100 milliliters)

blood test *n* : the analysis of a sample of blood to determine the level of specific components (as glucose or blood cells) which indicate the presence or likely development of a disease or condition or serve to indicate the degree of function of an organ

blood thinner *n* : a drug used to prevent the formation of blood clots by hindering coagulation of the blood — **blood–thinning** *adj*

blood type *n* : BLOOD GROUP

blood typ•ing \-ˌtī-piŋ\ *n* : the action or process of determining an individual's blood group

blood urea nitrogen *n* : BUN

blood vessel *n* : a vessel through which blood circulates in the body

blood work *n* : the diagnostic testing of blood

blood•worm \ˈbləd-ˌwərm\ *n* : any of several nematode worms of the genus *Strongylus* that are parasitic in the large intestine of horses — called also *palisade worm, red worm*

bloody \ˈblə-dē\ *adj* **blood•i•er; -est 1 a** : containing or made up of blood **b** : of or contained in the blood **2 a** : smeared or stained with blood **b** : dripping blood : BLEEDING ⟨a ∼ nose⟩

blot \ˈblät\ *n* : a sheet usu. of a cellulose derivative that contains spots of immobilized macromolecules (as of DNA, RNA, or protein) or their fragments and that is used to identify specific components of the spots by applying a suitable molecular probe (as a complementary nucleic acid or a radioactively labeled antibody) — see NORTHERN BLOT, SOUTHERN BLOT, WESTERN BLOT — **blot** *vb*

blotch \ˈbläch\ *n* : a discolored patch on the skin ⟨a face covered with ~*es*⟩ — **blotch** *vb* — **blotchy** \ˈblä-chē\ *adj*

blow•fish \ˈblō-ˌfish\ *n* : PUFFER FISH

blow•fly \-ˌflī\ *n, pl* **-flies** : any of a family (Calliphoridae) of dipteran flies (as a bluebottle or screwworm)

BLS *abbr* basic life support

blue baby *n* : an infant with a bluish tint usu. from a congenital heart defect marked by mingling of venous and arterial blood

blue–baby operation *n* : BLALOCK-TAUSSIG OPERATION

blue bag *n* : gangrenous mastitis of sheep

blue•bot•tle \ˈblü-ˌbät-ᵊl\ *n* : any of several blowflies (genus *Calliphora*) with iridescent blue bodies

blue comb \ˈblü-ˈkōm\ *n* : an acute infectious disease of domestic turkeys that is caused by a coronavirus (species *Avian coronavirus* of the genus *Gammacoronavirus*)

blue heaven *n, slang* : amobarbital or its sodium derivative in a blue tablet or capsule

blue mold *n* : any of various fungi of the genus *Penicillium* that produce blue or blue-green surface growth

blue nevus *n* : a small blue or bluish-black spot on the skin that is sharply circumscribed, rounded, and flat or slightly raised and is usu. benign but often mistaken for a melanoma

blues \ˈblüz\ *n sing or pl* : low spirits : MELANCHOLY

blue•tongue \ˈblü-ˌtəŋ\ *n* : a serious febrile virus disease esp. of sheep that is caused by a reovirus of the genus *Orbivirus* (species *Bluetongue virus*) transmitted chiefly by biting midges of the genus *Culicoides*

blunt dissection *n* : surgical separation of tissue layers by means of an instrument without a cutting edge or by the fingers

blunt trauma *n* : an injury caused by a blunt object or collision with a blunt surface (as in a car accident) — called also *blunt force trauma*

B lym•pho•cyte \ˈbē-ˈlim-fə-ˌsīt\ *n* : B CELL

BM *abbr* **1** Bachelor of Medicine **2** bowel movement

BMD *abbr* bone mineral density

BMI *abbr* body mass index

BMP *abbr* bone morphogenetic protein

BMR *abbr* basal metabolic rate

BMT *abbr* **1** bachelor of medical technology **2** bone marrow transplant; bone marrow transplantation

BNA *abbr* Basle Nomina Anatomica

BNP *abbr* brain natriuretic peptide; B-type natriuretic peptide

BO *abbr* body odor

board \ˈbōrd\ *n* **1** : a group of persons having supervisory, managerial, investigative, or advisory powers ⟨medical licensing ~*s*⟩ ⟨a ~ of health⟩ **2** : an examination given by an examining board — often used in pl.

board–certified *adj, of a physician* : having graduated from medical school, completed residency, trained under supervision in a specialty, and passed a qualifying exam given by a medical specialty board — abbr. *BC*

board–eligible *adj, of a physician* : eligible to take a qualifying exam given by a medical specialty board after having graduated from medical school, completed residency, and trained under supervision in a specialty — abbr. *BE*

Bo•dan•sky unit \bə-ˈdan-skē-, -ˈdän-\ *n* : a unit that is used as a measure of phosphatase concentration (as in the blood) esp. in the diagnosis of various pathological conditions and that has a normal value for the blood averaging about 7 for children and about 4 for adults

Bodansky, Aaron (1887–1960), American biochemist.

bodi•ly \ˈbäd-ᵊl-ē\ *adj* : of or relating to the body ⟨~ organs⟩

body \ˈbä-dē\ *n, pl* **bod•ies** **1 a** (1) : the material part or nature of a human being (2) : a dead organism : CORPSE **b** : a human being **2 a** : the main part of a plant or animal body esp. as distinguished from limbs and head : TRUNK **b** : the main part of an organ (as the uterus)

body bag *n* : a large zippered bag in which a human corpse is placed esp. for transportation

body build \-ˌbild\ *n* : the distinctive physical makeup of a human being

body cavity *n* : a cavity within an animal body; *specif* : COELOM

body clock *n* : the internal mechanisms that schedule bodily functions and activities — not usu. used technically

body dysmorphic disorder *n* : pathological preoccupation with an imagined or slight physical defect of one's body — called also *body dysmorphia*

body fat *n* : fat contained in adipose tissue; *also* : ADIPOSE TISSUE

body fluid *n* : a fluid or fluid secretion (such as blood, lymph, saliva, semen, or urine) of the body

body heat *n* : heat produced in the body of a living animal by metabolic and physical activity — called also *animal heat*

body image *n* : a subjective picture of one's own physical appearance established both by self-observation and by noting the reactions of others

body louse *n* : a louse feeding primarily on the body; *esp* : a sucking louse of the genus *Pediculus* (*P. humanus humanus* syn. *P. h. corporis*) feeding on the human body and living in clothing — called also *cootie*

body mass index *n* : a measure of body fat that is the ratio of the weight of the body in kilograms to the square of its height in meters ⟨a *body mass index* in adults of 25 to 29.9 is considered an indication of overweight, and 30 or more an indication of obesity⟩ — abbr. *BMI*

body odor *n* : an unpleasant odor from a perspiring or unclean person

body ringworm *n* : TINEA CORPORIS

body stalk *n* : the mesodermal cord that contains the umbilical vessels and that connects a fetus with its chorion

body•work \-ˌwərk\ *n* : therapeutic touching or manipulation of the body by using specialized techniques

Boeck's sarcoid \ˈbeks-\ *n* : SARCOIDOSIS

Boeck \ˈbek\, **Caesar Peter Moeller (1845–1917),** Norwegian dermatologist.

Bohr effect \ˈbōər-\ *n* : the decrease in oxygen affinity of a respiratory pigment (as hemoglobin) in response to decreased blood pH resulting from increased carbon dioxide concentration

Bohr, Christian (1855–1911), Danish physiologist.

bohr•i•um \ˈbōr-ē-əm\ *n* : a short-lived radioactive element that is artificially produced — symbol *Bh;* see ELEMENT table

boil \ˈbȯil\ *n* : a localized swelling and inflammation of the skin resulting from usu. bacterial infection of a hair follicle and adjacent tissue, having a hard central core, and forming pus — called also *furuncle*

boiling point *n* : the temperature at which a liquid boils

bo•lus \ˈbō-ləs\ *n* **1** : a rounded mass: as **a** : a large pill **b** : a soft mass of chewed food **2 a** : a dose of a substance (as a drug) given intravenously **b** : a large dose of a substance given by injection for the purpose of rapidly achieving the needed therapeutic concentration in the bloodstream

bombé — see IRIS BOMBÉ

bom•be•sin \ˈbäm-bə-sin\ *n* : a polypeptide that is found in the brain and gastrointestinal tract and has been shown experimentally to cause the secretion of various substances (as gastrin and cholecystokinin) and to inhibit intestinal motility

bond \ˈbänd\ *n* : an attractive force that holds together atoms, ions, or groups of atoms in a molecule or crystal — usu. represented in formulas by a line or dot — **bond** *vb*

bond•ing *n* **1** : the formation of a close personal relationship (as between a mother and child) esp. through frequent or constant association — see MALE BONDING **2** : a dental technique in which a material and esp. plastic or porcelain is attached to a tooth surface to correct minor defects (as chipped or discolored teeth) esp. for cosmetic purposes

bone \ˈbōn\ *n, often attrib* **1** : one of the hard parts of the skeleton of a vertebrate ⟨the ∼*s* of the arm⟩ **2** : the hard largely calcareous connective tissue of which the adult skeleton of most vertebrates is chiefly composed ⟨cancellous ∼⟩ ⟨compact ∼⟩ — compare CARTILAGE 1

bone density *n* : the amount of mineral content per unit volume of bone; *also* : a measurement of this mineral content used to determine the strength of bone and esp. to detect osteoporosis — called also *bone mineral density*

bone marrow *n* : a soft highly vascular modified connective tissue that occupies the cavities and cancellous part of most bones and occurs in two forms: **a** : one that is whitish or yellowish, consists chiefly of fat cells, and is found esp. in the cavities of long bones — called also *yellow marrow* **b** : one that is reddish, contains little fat, is the chief site of red blood cell and blood granulocyte formation, and occurs in the normal adult in cancellous tissue esp. of certain flat bones — called also *red marrow*

bone morphogenetic protein *n* : any of several proteins that are transforming growth factors involved in inducing bone and cartilage formation; *also* : a recombinant version used esp. in spinal surgery to promote new bone growth — abbr. *BMP*

bone spur *n* : a bony outgrowth : OSTEOPHYTE — called also *bony spur*

Bo•nine \ˈbō-ˌnēn\ *trademark* — used for a preparation of the hydrochloride of meclizine

Bo•ni•va \bō-ˈnē-və\ *trademark* — used for a preparation of ibandronate

bont tick \ˈbänt-\ *n* : a southern African tick of the genus *Amblyomma* (*A. hebraeum*) that attacks livestock, birds, and sometimes humans and transmits heartwater of sheep, goats, and cattle; *broadly* : any African tick of the genus *Amblyomma*

bony *also* **bon•ey** \ˈbō-nē\ *adj* **bon•i•er; -est** : consisting of or resembling bone ⟨∼ prominences of the skull⟩

bony labyrinth *n* : the cavity in the petrous portion of the temporal bone that contains the membranous labyrinth of the inner ear and is divided into the vestibule, cochlea, and semicircular canals — called also *osseous labyrinth*

Bo•oph•i•lus \bō-ˈä-fə-ləs\ *n* : a genus of ticks some of which are pests esp. of cattle and vectors of disease — see CATTLE TICK

boost•er \ˈbü-stər\ *n* : a substance or dose used to renew or increase the effect of a drug or immunizing agent; *esp* : BOOSTER SHOT

booster dose *n* : a supplementary dose of a therapeutic agent designed to increase the effectiveness of one or more previously administered doses; *esp* : BOOSTER SHOT

booster shot *n* : a supplementary dose of an immunizing agent administered as an injection— see BOOSTER, BOOSTER DOSE

bo•rac•ic acid \bə-ˈra-sik-\ *n* : BORIC ACID

bor•bo•ryg•mus \ˌbȯr-bə-ˈrig-məs\ *n, pl* **-mi** \-ˌmī\ : a rumbling sound made by the movement of gas in the intestine — **bor•bo•ryg•mic** \-mik\ *adj*

[1]**bor•der•line** \ˈbȯr-dər-ˌlīn\ *adj* **1** : being in an intermediate position or state : not fully classifiable as one thing or its opposite; *esp* : not quite up to what is usual, standard, or expected ⟨~ intelligence⟩ **2** : exhibiting typical but not altogether conclusive symptoms ⟨a ~ diabetic⟩ **3** : of, relating to, being, or exhibiting a behavior pattern typical or suggestive of borderline personality disorder

[2]**borderline** *n* : a person affected with borderline personality disorder

borderline personality disorder *n* : a disordered behavior pattern that is marked by unstable intense emotions and mood with variable symptoms (as instability in interpersonal relationships and impulsive or unpredictable behavior) and has an onset during adolescence or early adulthood — abbr. *BPD*

Bor•de•tel•la \ˌbȯr-də-ˈte-lə\ *n* : a genus of gram-negative strictly aerobic bacteria including the causative agent (*B. pertussis*) of whooping cough

J.–J.–B.–V. Bordet — see BORDET-GENGOU BACILLUS

Bor•det–Gen•gou bacillus \bȯr-ˈdā-zhäⁿ-ˈgü-\ *n* : a small ovoid bacteria of the genus *Bordetella* (*B. pertussis*) that is the causative agent of whooping cough

Bordet, Jules–Jean–Baptiste–Vincent (1870–1961), Belgian bacteriologist, and **Gengou, Octave (1875–1957),** French bacteriologist.

bore \ˈbōr\ *n* : the internal diameter of a tube (as a hypodermic needle or catheter)

bo•ric acid \ˈbōr-ik-\ *n* : a white crystalline acid H_3BO_3 used esp. as a weak antiseptic — called also *boracic acid*

bor•na•vi•rus \ˌbȯr-nə-ˈvī-rəs\ *n* : a single-stranded RNA virus (family *Bornaviridae*) that chiefly infects the central nervous system of birds and mammals (as dogs and horses)

Born•holm disease \ˈbȯrn-ˌhōlm-\ *n* : EPIDEMIC PLEURODYNIA

bo•ron \ˈbōr-ˌän\ *n* : a trivalent metalloid element found in nature only in combination — symbol *B;* see ELEMENT table

bor•re•lia \bə-ˈre-lē-ə, -ˈrē-\ *n* **1** *cap* : a genus of small spirochetes (family Spirochaetaceae) that are parasites of humans and warm-blooded animals and include the causative agents of relapsing fever in Africa (*B. duttoni*) and Lyme disease in the U.S. (*B. burgdorferi*) **2** : a spirochete of the genus *Borrelia*

bor•rel•i•o•sis \bə-ˌre-lē-ˈō-səs\ *n, pl* **-o•ses** \-ˌsēz\ : infection with or disease caused by a spirochete of the genus *Borrelia; specif* : LYME DISEASE

bor•tez•o•mib \ˌbȯr-ˈte-zō-ˌmib\ *n* : an antineoplastic drug $C_{19}H_{25}BN_4O_4$ administered by injection esp. in the treatment of multiple myeloma — see VELCADE

bos•se•lat•ed \ˈbä-sə-ˌlā-təd, ˈbȯ-\ *adj* : marked or covered with protuberances ⟨a ~ tumor⟩

bot *also* **bott** \ˈbät\ *n* : the larva of a botfly; *esp* : one infesting the horse

bo•tan•i•cal \bə-ˈta-ni-kəl\ *n* : a medicinal preparation derived from a plant : HERBAL REMEDY

bot•fly \ˈbät-ˌflī\ *n, pl* **-flies** : any of various stout dipteran flies (family Oestridae) with larvae parasitic in body cavities or tissues

[1]**Bo•tox** \ˈbō-ˌtäks\ *trademark* — used for a preparation of botulinum toxin type A

[2]**Botox** *vb* : to inject botulinum toxin into (part of the body and usu. part of the face) esp. for cosmetic purposes (as to minimize wrinkles)

bot•ry•oid \ˈbä-trē-ˌȯid\ *adj* : having the form of a bunch of grapes ⟨~ sarcoma⟩

botryoides — see SARCOMA BOTRYOIDES

bot•ry•o•my•co•sis \ˌbä-trē-(ˌ)ō-mī-ˈkō-səs\ *n, pl* **-co•ses** \-ˌsēz\ : a bacterial infection of domestic animals and humans marked by the formation of usu. superficial vascular granulomatous masses, associated esp. with wounds, and sometimes followed by metastatic visceral tumors — **bot•ry•o•my•cot•ic** \-ˈkä-tik\ *adj*

bot•tle \ˈbät-ᵊl\ *n, often attrib* : liquid food usu. consisting of milk and supplements that is fed from a bottle (as to an infant) in place of mother's milk

bottle baby *n* : a baby that is primarily bottle-fed as contrasted with a baby that is primarily breastfed

bot•tle–feed \ˈbät-ᵊl-ˌfēd\ *vb* **-fed; -feed•ing** : to feed (an infant) from a nursing bottle rather than by breast-feeding

bottle jaw *n* : a pendulous edematous condition of the tissues under the lower jaw in cattle and sheep resulting from infestation with bloodsucking gastrointestinal parasites (as of the genus *Haemonchus*)

bot•u•lin \ˈbä-chə-lən\ *n* : BOTULINUM TOXIN

bot•u•li•num \ˌbä-chə-ˈlī-nəm\ *also* **bot•u•li•nus** \-nəs\ *n* : a spore-forming bacterium of the genus *Clostridium*

(*C. botulinum*) that produces botulinum toxin — **bo·tu·li·nal** \-ˈlīn-ᵊl\ *adj*

botulinum toxin *also* **botulinus toxin** *n* : a very powerful neurotoxin that is produced by the botulinum bacterium (*Clostridium botulinum*), acts primarily on the parasympathetic nervous system, and causes botulism; *also* BOTULINUM TOXIN TYPE A

botulinum toxin type A *or* **botulinum toxin A** *n* : a solution of purified botulinum toxin that is used by injection for medical and cosmetic purposes (as to treat blepharospasm, spasmodic torticollis, and severe axillary hyperhidrosis and to minimize wrinkles) — see BOTOX

bot·u·lism \ˈbä-chə-ˌli-zəm\ *n* : acute food poisoning caused by botulinum toxin produced in food by a bacterium of the genus *Clostridium* (*C. botulinum*) and characterized by muscle weakness and paralysis, disturbances of vision, swallowing, and speech, and a high mortality rate

Bou·chard's node \bü-ˈshärz\ *n* : a bony enlargement of the middle joint of a finger that is commonly associated with osteoarthritis — compare HEBERDEN'S NODE

Bouchard, Charles Jacques (1837–1915), French pathologist.

bou·gie \ˈbü-ˌzhē, -ˌjē\ *n* **1** : a tapering cylindrical instrument for introduction into a tubular passage of the body **2** : SUPPOSITORY

bou·gie·nage *or* **bou·gi·nage** \ˌbü-zhē-ˈnäzh\ *n* : the dilation of a tubular cavity (as a constricted esophagus) with a bougie

-boulia — see -BULIA

bound \ˈbau̇nd\ *adj* **1** : made costive : CONSTIPATED **2** : held in chemical or physical combination

bou·ton \bü-ˈtōⁿ\ *n* : a terminal club-shaped enlargement of a nerve fiber at a synapse with another neuron

bou·ton·neuse fever \ˌbü-tȯ-ˈnüz-, -ˈnœ̄z-\ *n* : a tick-borne illness of the Mediterranean region, central Asia, and Africa that is typically marked by mild symptoms (as fever, headache, and red rash) but may in rare cases progress to serious disease and that is caused by a rickettsial bacteria (*Rickettsia conorii*) — called also *Marseilles fever, Mediterranean spotted fever, tick-bite fever;* see TACHE NOIR

Bo·vic·o·la \bō-ˈvi-kə-lə\ *n* : a genus of biting lice (order Mallophaga) including several that infest the hair of domestic mammals

bo·vine \ˈbō-ˌvīn, -ˌvēn\ *n* : an ox (genus *Bos*) or a closely related animal — **bovine** *adj*

bovine growth hormone *n* : BOVINE SOMATOTROPIN; *also* : a genetically engineered form of bovine somatotropin that is injected into cows to stimulate milk production — abbr. *bGH, BGH*

bovine mastitis *n* : inflammation of the udder of a cow resulting from injury or more commonly from bacterial infection

bovine somatotropin *n* : a growth hormone of cows that stimulates milk production; *also* : genetically engineered bovine growth hormone — abbr. *bST, BST*

bovine spongiform encephalopathy *n* : a fatal prion disease of cattle that affects the nervous system, resembles or is identical to scrapie of sheep and goats, and is prob. transmitted by infected tissue in food — abbr. *BSE;* called also *mad cow disease*

bovine viral diarrhea *or* **bovine virus diarrhea** *n* : an infectious disease of cattle that may range from a subclinical or mild infection to a severe illness marked chiefly by fever, diarrhea, anorexia, and ulceration esp. of the mouth and is caused by two flaviviruses of the genus *Pestivirus* (species *Bovine viral diarrhea virus 1* and *Bovine viral diarrhea virus 2*) — see MUCOSAL DISEASE

bovinum — see COR BOVINUM

bow \ˈbō\ *n* : a frame for the lenses of eyeglasses; *also* : the curved sidepiece of the frame passing over the ear

bow·el \ˈbau̇l\ *n* : INTESTINE, GUT; *also* : one of the divisions of the intestines — usu. used in pl. except in medical use ⟨move your ~*s*⟩ ⟨surgery of the involved ~⟩

bowel movement *n* : an act of passing usu. solid waste through the rectum and anus

bowel worm *n* : a common strongylid nematode worm of the genus *Chabertia* (*C. ovina*) infesting the colon of sheep and feeding on blood and tissue

bow·en·oid papulosis \ˈbō-ə-ˌnȯid-\ *n* : a skin condition associated with certain human papillomaviruses (such as HPV-16) that is marked by pigmented lesions in the anogenital area which usu. follow a benign course but may sometimes develop into squamous cell carcinoma

J. T. Bowen — see BOWEN'S DISEASE

Bow·en's disease \ˈbō-ənz-\ *n* : a precancerous lesion of the skin or mucous membranes characterized by small solid elevations covered by thickened horny tissue

Bow·en \ˈbō-ən\, **John Templeton (1857–1941),** American dermatologist.

bow·leg \ˈbō-ˌleg\ *n* : a leg bowed outward at or below the knee — called also *genu varum*

bow·legged \ˈbō-ˌle-gəd, -ˌlegd\ *adj* : having bowlegs

Bow·man's capsule \ˈbō-mənz-\ *n* : a thin membranous double-walled capsule surrounding the glomerulus of a vertebrate nephron — called also *capsule of Bowman, glomerular capsule*

Bow•man \ˈbō-mən\, **Sir William (1816–1892),** British ophthalmologist, anatomist, and physiologist.

Bowman's gland *n* : OLFACTORY GLAND

Bowman's membrane *n* : the thin outer layer of the substantia propria of the cornea immediately underlying the epithelium

box•ing \ˈbäk-siŋ\ *n* : construction of the base of a dental cast by building up the walls of an impression while preserving important landmarks

box jellyfish *n* : SEA WASP

bp *abbr* base pair

BP *abbr* blood pressure

BPA *abbr* bisphenol A

BPD *abbr* borderline personality disorder

BPH *abbr* benign prostatic hyperplasia

BPharm *abbr* bachelor of pharmacy

BPPV *abbr* benign paroxysmal positional vertigo

BPV *abbr* benign positional vertigo

Br *symbol* bromine

[1]**brace** \ˈbrās\ *n, pl* **brac•es** **1** : an appliance that gives support to movable parts (as a joint), to weak muscles, or to strained ligaments (as of the lower back) **2 braces** *pl* : an orthodontic appliance usu. of metallic wire that is used esp. to exert pressure to straighten misaligned teeth and that is not removable by the patient

[2]**brace** *vb* **braced; brac•ing** : to furnish or support with a brace

brachi- *or* **brachio-** *comb form* **1** : arm ⟨*brachio*radialis⟩ **2** : brachial and ⟨*brachio*cephalic artery⟩

bra•chi•al \ˈbrā-kē-əl\ *adj* : of or relating to the arm

brachial artery *n* : the chief artery of the upper arm that is a direct continuation of the axillary artery and divides into the radial and ulnar arteries just below the elbow — see DEEP BRACHIAL ARTERY

bra•chi•alis \ˌbrā-kē-ˈa-ləs, -ˈā-, -ˈä-\ *n* : a flexor that lies in front of the lower part of the humerus whence it arises and is inserted into the ulna

brachial plexus *n* : a complex network of nerves that is formed chiefly by the lower four cervical nerves and the first thoracic nerve and supplies nerves to the chest, shoulder, and arm

brachial vein *n* : one of a pair of veins accompanying the brachial artery and uniting with each other and with the basilic vein to form the axillary vein

brachii — see BICEPS BRACHII, TRICEPS BRACHII

bra•chio•ce•phal•ic artery \ˌbrā-kē-(ˌ)ō-sə-ˈfa-lik-\ *n* : a short artery that arises from the arch of the aorta and divides into the carotid and subclavian arteries of the right side — called also *innominate artery*

brachiocephalicus — see TRUNCUS BRACHIOCEPHALICUS

brachiocephalic vein *n* : either of two large veins that occur one on each side of the neck, receive blood from the head and neck, are formed by the union of the internal jugular and the subclavian veins, and unite to form the superior vena cava — called also *innominate vein*

bra•chio•plas•ty \ˈbrā-kē-ō-ˌpla-stē\ *n, pl* **-ties** : plastic surgery that removes excess skin and fat from the undersurface of the upper arm chiefly for cosmetic purposes to reduce sagging — called also *arm lift*

bra•chio•ra•di•alis \ˌbrā-kē-ō-ˌrā-dē-ˈa-ləs, -ˈā-, -ˈä-\ *n, pl* **-ales** \-ˌlēz\ : a flexor of the radial side of the forearm arising from the lateral supracondylar ridge of the humerus and inserted into the styloid process of the radius

bra•chi•um \ˈbrā-kē-əm\ *n, pl* **-chia** \-kē-ə\ : the upper segment of the arm extending from the shoulder to the elbow

brachium con•junc•ti•vum \-ˌkän-(ˌ)jəŋk-ˈtī-vəm\ *n* : CEREBELLAR PEDUNCLE a

brachium pon•tis \-ˈpän-təs\ *n* : CEREBELLAR PEDUNCLE b

brachy- *comb form* : short ⟨*brachy*cephalic⟩ ⟨*brachy*dactylous⟩

brachy•ce•phal•ic \ˌbra-ki-sə-ˈfa-lik\ *adj* : short-headed or broad-headed with a cephalic index of over 80 — **brachy•ceph•a•ly** \-ˈse-fə-lē\ *n*

brachy•dac•ty•lous \ˌbra-ki-ˈdak-tə-ləs\ *adj* : having abnormally short digits — **brachy•dac•ty•ly** \-lē\ *n*

brachy•ther•a•py \-ˈther-ə-pē\ *n, pl* **-pies** : radiotherapy in which the source of radiation is placed (as by implantation) in or close to the area being treated

Brad•ford frame \ˈbrad-fərd-\ *n* : a frame used to support a patient with disease or fractures of the spine, hip, or pelvis

Bradford, Edward Hickling (1848–1926), American orthopedist.

brady- *comb form* : slow ⟨*brady*cardia⟩

bra•dy•car•dia \ˌbrā-di-ˈkär-dē-ə *also* ˌbra-\ *n* : relatively slow heart action whether physiological or pathological — compare TACHYCARDIA

bra•dy•ki•ne•sia \-kī-ˈnē-zhē-ə, -zhə, -zē-ə\ *n* : extreme slowness of movements and reflexes (as that caused by Parkinson's disease or antipsychotic drugs)

bra•dy•ki•nin \-ˈkī-nən\ *n* : a kinin that is formed locally in injured tissue, acts in vasodilation of small arterioles, and is considered to play a part in inflammatory processes

bra•dy•phre•nia \-ˈfrē-nē-ə\ *n* : slowed cognitive functioning

bra•dy•pnea \ˌbrā-dəp-ˈnē-ə, ˌbra-\ *n* : abnormally slow breathing

bra•dy•pnoea *chiefly Brit var of* BRADYPNEA

braille \ˈbrāl\ *n, often cap* : a system of writing for the blind that uses characters made up of raised dots — **braille** *vb*

Braille \ˈbrī, ˈbrāl\, **Louis (1809–1852)**, French inventor and teacher.

brain \ˈbrān\ *n* : the portion of the vertebrate central nervous system enclosed in the skull and continuous with the spinal cord through the foramen magnum that is composed of neurons and supporting and nutritive structures (as glia) and that integrates sensory information from inside and outside the body in controlling autonomic function (as heartbeat and respiration), in coordinating and directing correlated motor responses, and in the process of learning

brain attack *n* : STROKE

brain·case \-ˌkās\ *n* : the part of the skull that encloses the brain — see CRANIUM

brain death *n* : final cessation of activity in the central nervous system esp. as indicated by a flat electroencephalogram for a predetermined length of time — **brain–dead** *adj*

brain–derived neurotrophic factor *n* : a neuropeptide that regulates the growth, survival, and differentiation of neurons

brain fog *n* : a usu. temporary state of diminished mental capacity marked by inability to concentrate or to think or reason clearly

brain natriuretic peptide *n* : B-TYPE NATRIURETIC PEPTIDE

brain stem *n* : the part of the brain composed of the midbrain, pons, and medulla oblongata and connecting the spinal cord with the forebrain and cerebrum

brain vesicle *n* : any of the divisions into which the developing embryonic brain of vertebrates is marked off by incomplete transverse constrictions

brain·wash·ing \ˈbrān-ˌwȯ-shiŋ, -ˌwä-\ *n* : a forcible indoctrination to induce someone to give up basic political, social, or religious beliefs and attitudes and to accept contrasting regimented ideas — **brain·wash** *vb*

brain wave *n* **1** : rhythmic fluctuations of voltage between parts of the brain resulting in the flow of an electric current **2** : a current produced by brain waves — compare ALPHA WAVE, BETA WAVE

bran \ˈbran\ *n* : the edible broken seed coats of cereal grain separated from the flour or meal by sifting

branch \ˈbranch\ *n* : something that extends from or enters into a main body or source ⟨a ~ of an artery⟩ — **branch** *vb* — **branched** \ˈbrancht\ *adj*

bran·chi·al \ˈbran-kē-əl\ *adj* : of or relating to the parts of the body derived from the embryonic branchial arches and clefts

branchial arch *n* : one of a series of bony or cartilaginous arches that develop in the walls of the mouth cavity and pharynx of a vertebrate embryo and correspond to the gill arches of fishes and amphibians — called also *pharyngeal arch, visceral arch*

branchial cleft *n* : one of the open or potentially open clefts that occur on each side of the neck region of a vertebrate embryo between the branchial arches and correspond to the gill slits of fishes and amphibians — called also *pharyngeal cleft*

brash \ˈbrash\ *n* : WATER BRASH

Brax·ton–Hicks contractions \ˈbrak-stən-ˈhiks-\ *n pl* : relatively painless nonrhythmic contractions of the uterus that occur during pregnancy with increasing frequency over time but are not associated with labor

Hicks, John Braxton (1823–1897), British gynecologist.

braxy \ˈbrak-sē\ *n, pl* **brax·ies** : a malignant edema of sheep that involves gastrointestinal invasion by a bacterium of the genus *Clostridium* (*C. septicum*)

BRCA \ˌbē-ˌär-ˌsē-ˈā\ *n* : either of two tumor suppressor genes that in mutated form tend to be associated with an increased risk of certain cancers and esp. breast and ovarian cancers

[1]**break** \ˈbrāk\ *vb* **broke** \ˈbrōk\; **bro·ken** \ˈbrō-kən\; **break·ing** **1 a** : to snap into pieces : FRACTURE ⟨~ a bone⟩ **b** : to fracture the bone of (a bodily part) ⟨the blow *broke* her arm⟩ **c** : to dislocate or dislocate and fracture a bone of (the neck or back) **2 a** : to cause an open wound in : RUPTURE ⟨~ the skin⟩ **b** : to rupture the surface of and permit flowing out or effusing ⟨~ an artery⟩ **3** : to fail in health or strength — often used with *down* **4** : to suffer complete or marked loss of resistance, composure, resolution, morale, or command of a situation — often used with *down*

[2]**break** *n* **1** : an act or action of breaking : FRACTURE **2** : a condition produced by breaking ⟨the ~ in his leg⟩

break·bone fever \ˈbrāk-ˌbōn-\ *n* : DENGUE

[1]**break·down** \ˈbrāk-ˌdau̇n\ *n* **1** : a failure to function **2** : a physical, mental, or nervous collapse **3** : the process of decomposing ⟨~ of food during digestion⟩ — **break down** *vb*

[2]**breakdown** *adj* : obtained or resulting from disintegration or decomposition of a substance

break·out \ˈbrā-ˌkau̇t\ *n* : an eruption or inflammation of the skin

break out *vb* **1** : to become affected with a skin eruption **2** *of a disease* : to manifest itself by skin eruptions **3** : to become covered with ⟨*break out* in a sweat⟩

break·through bleeding \ˌbrāk-ˌthrü-\ *n* : an abnormal flow of blood from the uterus that occurs between menstrual periods esp. due to irregular sloughing of the endometrium in women on contraceptive hormones

breakthrough pain *n* : a transient usu. severe episode of pain occurring in individuals being treated for chronic pain

breast \ˈbrest\ *n* **1** : either of the pair of mammary glands extending from the front of the chest in pubescent and adult females; *also* : either of the analogous but rudimentary organs of the male chest esp. when enlarged **2** : the fore or ventral part of the body between the neck and the abdomen

breast·bone \ˈbrest-ˌbōn\ *n* : STERNUM

breast·feed \ˈbrest-ˌfēd\ *or* **breast–feed** *vb* **1** : to feed (a baby) from a mother's breast rather than from a nursing bottle **2** *of a baby* : to feed oneself by sucking milk from a mother's breast — **breast·feed·er** *or* **breast–feeder** *n*

breast lift *n* : plastic surgery to elevate, firm, and often reshape a sagging breast — called also *mastopexy*

breath \ˈbreth\ *n* **1 a** : the faculty of breathing **b** : an act or an instance of breathing or inhaling <recovering her ~ after the race> **2 a** : air inhaled and exhaled in breathing <bad ~> **b** : something (as moisture on a cold surface) produced by breath or breathing — **out of breath** : breathing very rapidly (as from strenuous exercise)

Breath·a·ly·zer \ˈbre-thə-ˌlī-zər\ *trademark* — used for a device that is used to determine the alcohol content of a breath sample

breathe \ˈbrēth\ *vb* **breathed; breath·ing 1** : to draw air into and expel it from the lungs : RESPIRE; *broadly* : to take in oxygen and give out carbon dioxide through natural processes **2** : to inhale and exhale freely

breath·er \ˈbrē-thər\ *n* : one that breathes usu. in a specified way — see MOUTH BREATHER

breathing machine *n* : a device that assists breathing (as by keeping the air passages open) or maintains artificial respiration

breathing tube *n* : ENDOTRACHEAL TUBE

breath·less \ˈbreth-ləs\ *adj* **1** : panting or gasping for breath **2** : suffering from dyspnea

breath test *n* : a test to detect the presence of one or more substances in a person's exhaled breath — **breath testing** *n*

breech \ˈbrēch\ *n* **1** : the hind end of the body : BUTTOCKS **2** : BREECH PRESENTATION; *also* : a fetus that is presented at the uterine cervix buttocks or legs first

breech delivery *n* : delivery of a fetus by breech presentation — called also *breech birth*

breech presentation *n* : presentation of the fetus in which the buttocks or legs are the first parts to appear at the uterine cervix

breg·ma \ˈbreg-mə\ *n, pl* **-ma·ta** \-mə-tə\ : the point of junction of the coronal and sagittal sutures of the skull — **breg·mat·ic** \breg-ˈma-tik\ *adj*

bre·tyl·i·um \brə-ˈti-lē-əm\ *n* : an antiarrhythmic drug administered by injection in the form of its tosylate $C_{18}H_{24}BrNO_3S$ to treat ventricular fibrillation and tachycardia

brev·e·tox·in \ˌbre-və-ˈtäk-sən\ *n* : any of several neurotoxic substances produced by a dinoflagellate (esp. *Karenia brevis*) found in red tides that in humans may cause respiratory symptoms when inhaled and neurotoxic shellfish poisoning when ingested

brevis — see ABDUCTOR POLLICIS BREVIS, ADDUCTOR BREVIS, EXTENSOR CARPI RADIALIS BREVIS, EXTENSOR DIGITORUM BREVIS, EXTENSOR HALLUCIS BREVIS, EXTENSOR POLLICIS BREVIS, FLEXOR DIGITI MINIMI BREVIS, FLEXOR DIGITORUM BREVIS, FLEXOR HALLUCIS BREVIS, FLEXOR POLLICIS BREVIS, PALMARIS BREVIS, PERONEUS BREVIS

brewer's yeast *n* : the dried pulverized cells of a yeast of the genus *Saccharomyces* (*S. cerevisiae*) used as a source of B-complex vitamins

bridge \ˈbrij\ *n* **1 a** : the upper bony part of the nose **b** : the curved part of a pair of glasses that rests upon this part of the nose **2 a** : PONS **b** : a strand of protoplasm extending between two cells **c** : a partial denture held in place by anchorage to adjacent teeth

bridge·work \-ˌwərk\ *n* : dental bridges; *also* : prosthodontics concerned with their construction

bright·ness \ˈbrīt-nəs\ *n* : the one of the three psychological dimensions of color perception by which visual stimuli are ordered continuously from light to dark and which is correlated with light intensity — compare HUE, SATURATION

Bright's disease \ˈbrīts-\ *n* : any of several kidney diseases marked esp. by albumin in the urine

Bright \ˈbrīt\, **Richard (1789–1858),** British internist and pathologist.

Brill's disease \ˈbrilz-\ *n* : an acute infectious disease milder than epidemic typhus but caused by the same rickettsia

Brill \ˈbril\, **Nathan Edwin (1860–1925),** American physician.

bri·mo·ni·dine \bri-ˈmō-nə-ˌdēn\ *n* : an alpha-blocker $C_{11}H_{10}BrN_5 \cdot C_4H_6O_6$ used in a topical ophthalmic solution to reduce intraocular pressure or in a topical gel to reduce redness associated with rosacea — see ALPHAGAN, COMBIGAN, MIRVASO

bring up *vb* : VOMIT

Bris·delle \briz-ˈdel\ *trademark* — used for a preparation of the mesylate of paroxetine

British an·ti–lew·is·ite \-ˌan-tē-ˈlü-ə-ˌsīt, -ˌan-ˌtī-\ *n* : DIMERCAPROL

W. L. Lewis — see LEWISITE

brit•tle \ˈbrit-ᵊl\ *adj* : affected with or being a form of type 1 diabetes characterized by large and unpredictable fluctuations in blood glucose level ⟨∼ diabetes⟩

brittle bone disease *n* : OSTEOGENESIS IMPERFECTA — called also *brittle bones*

broach \ˈbrōch\ *n* : a fine tapered flexible instrument used in dentistry to remove dental pulp and to dress a root canal

broad bean *n* : the large flat edible seed of an Old World upright vetch (*Vicia faba*); *also* : the plant itself — called also *fava bean;* see FAVISM

broad ligament *n* : either of the two lateral ligaments of the uterus composed of a double sheet of peritoneum and bearing the ovary suspended from the dorsal surface

broad–spectrum *adj* **1** : effective against a wide range of organisms (as insects or bacteria) ⟨∼ antibiotics⟩ — compare NARROW-SPECTRUM **2** : absorbing or blocking both UVA and UVB rays ⟨∼ sunscreen⟩

Bro•ca's aphasia \ˈbrō-ˌkəz-\ *n* : MOTOR APHASIA

Bro•ca \brō-ˈkä\, **Pierre–Paul (1824–1880),** French surgeon and anthropologist.

Broca's area *n* : a brain center associated with the motor control of speech and usu. located in the left but sometimes in the right inferior frontal gyrus — called also *Broca's convolution, Broca's gyrus, convolution of Broca*

Brod•mann area \ˈbräd-mən-\ *or* **Brod•mann's area** \-mənz-\ *n* : one of the several structurally distinguishable and presumably functionally distinct regions into which the cortex of each cerebral hemisphere can be divided

Brod•mann \ˈbrōt-ˌmän, ˈbräd-mən\, **Korbinian (1868–1918),** German neurologist.

broke *past of* BREAK

bro•ken \ˈbrō-kən\ *adj* : having undergone or been subjected to fracture

brom- *or* **bromo-** *comb form* **1** : bromine ⟨*brom*ide⟩ **2** *now usu* *bromo-* : containing bromine in place of hydrogen — in names of organic compounds ⟨*bromo*uracil⟩

bro•me•lain *also* **bro•me•lin** \ˈbrō-mə-lən\ *n* : a protease obtained from the juice of the pineapple (*Ananas comosus* of the family Bromeliaceae)

brom•hi•dro•sis \ˌbrō-mə-ˈdrō-səs *also* ˌbrōm-hə-\ *also* **bro•mi•dro•sis** \ˌbrō-mə-\ *n, pl* **-dro•ses** \-ˌsēz\ : foul-smelling sweat

bro•mide \ˈbrō-ˌmīd\ *n* **1** : a binary compound of bromine with another element or a radical including some (as potassium bromide) used as sedatives **2** : a dose of bromide taken usu. as a sedative

bro•mine \ˈbrō-ˌmēn\ *n* : a nonmetallic element that is normally a red corrosive toxic liquid — symbol *Br;* see ELEMENT table

bro•mism \ˈbrō-ˌmi-zəm\ *n* : an abnormal state due to excessive or prolonged use of bromides

bro•mo \ˈbrō-(ˌ)mō\ *n, pl* **bromos** : a dose of a proprietary effervescent mixture used as a headache remedy, sedative, and antacid; *also* : such a proprietary product

bro•mo•crip•tine \ˌbrō-mō-ˈkrip-ˌtēn\ *n* : a polypeptide alkaloid $C_{32}H_{40}BrN_5O_5$ that is a derivative of ergot and mimics the activity of dopamine in selectively inhibiting prolactin secretion

bro•mo•de•oxy•ur•i•dine \ˌbrō-mō-ˌdē-ˌäk-sē-ˈyu̇r-ə-ˌdēn, -dən\ *or* **5–bro•mo•de•oxy•ur•i•dine** \ˈfīv-\ *n* : a mutagenic analog $C_9H_{11}O_5NBr$ of thymidine that induces chromosomal breakage esp. in heterochromatic regions — abbr. *BUdR*

bro•mo•der•ma \ˈbrō-mə-ˌdər-mə\ *n* : a skin eruption caused by a hypersensitive reaction to the ingestion of bromides

bro•mo•ura•cil \ˌbrō-mō-ˈyu̇r-ə-ˌsil, -səl\ *n* : a mutagenic uracil derivative $C_4H_3N_2O_2Br$ that is an analog of thymine and pairs readily with adenine and sometimes with guanine

brom•phen•ir•a•mine \ˌbrōm-fen-ˈir-ə-ˌmēn\ *n* : an H_1 antagonist used in the form of its maleate $C_{16}H_{19}BrN_2 \cdot C_4H_4O_4$ as an antihistamine

bronch- *or* **broncho-** *comb form* : bronchial tube : bronchial ⟨*bronch*itis⟩

bronchi *pl of* BRONCHUS

bronchi- *or* **bronchio-** *comb form* : bronchial tubes ⟨*bronchi*ectasis⟩

bron•chi•al \ˈbräŋ-kē-əl\ *adj* : of or relating to the bronchi or their ramifications in the lungs — **bron•chi•al•ly** *adv*

bronchial artery *n* : any branch of the descending aorta or first intercostal artery that accompanies the bronchi

bronchial asthma *n* : asthma resulting from spasmodic contraction of bronchial muscles

bronchial pneumonia *n* : BRONCHOPNEUMONIA

bronchial tree *n* : the bronchi together with their branches

bronchial tube *n* : a primary bronchus; *also* : any of its branches

bronchial vein *n* : any vein accompanying the bronchi and their branches and emptying into the azygos and superior intercostal veins

bron•chi•ec•ta•sis \ˌbräŋ-kē-ˈek-tə-səs\ *also* **bron•chi•ec•ta•sia** \-ek-ˈtā-zhə, -zhē-ə\ *n, pl* **-ta•ses** \-ˌsēz\ *also* **-ta•sias** \-zhəz, -zhē-əz\ : a chronic inflammatory or degenerative condition of one or more bronchi or bronchioles marked by dilatation and loss of elasticity of the walls — **bron·chi·ec·tat·ic** \-ek-ˈta-tik\ *adj*

bron·chi·o·al·ve·o·lar \ˌbräŋ-kē-ō-al-ˈvē-ə-lər\ *adj* : BRONCHOALVEOLAR

bron·chio·gen·ic \ˌbräŋ-kē-ō-ˈje-nik\ *adj* : BRONCHOGENIC

bron·chi·ole \ˈbräŋ-kē-ˌōl\ *n* : a minute thin-walled branch of a bronchus — **bron·chi·o·lar** \ˌbräŋ-kē-ˈō-lər\ *adj*

bron·chi·ol·itis \ˌbräŋ-kē-ō-ˈlī-təs\ *n* : inflammation of the bronchioles

bronchiolitis ob·lit·er·ans \-ə-ˈbli-tə-ˌranz\ *n* : progressive obstruction of the bronchioles due to inflammation and fibrosis

bron·chi·o·lus \bräŋ-ˈkī-ə-ləs\ *n, pl* **-o·li** \-ˌlī\ : BRONCHIOLE

bron·chi·tis \brän-ˈkī-təs, bräŋ-\ *n* : acute or chronic inflammation of the bronchial tubes; *also* : a disease marked by this — **bron·chit·ic** \-ˈki-tik\ *adj*

broncho- — see BRONCH-

bron·cho·al·ve·o·lar \ˌbräŋ-kō-al-ˈvē-ə-lər\ *adj* : of, relating to, or involving the bronchioles and alveoli of the lungs ⟨~ lavage⟩ ⟨~ carcinoma⟩

bron·cho·con·stric·tion \-kən-ˈstrik-shən\ *n* : constriction of the bronchial air passages — **bron·cho·con·stric·tive** \-tiv\ *adj*

bron·cho·con·stric·tor \-ˈstrik-tər\ *adj* : causing or involving bronchoconstriction — **bronchoconstrictor** *n*

bron·cho·di·la·ta·tion \-ˌdi-lə-ˈtā-shən, -ˌdī-\ *n* : BRONCHODILATION

bron·cho·di·la·tion \-dī-ˈlā-shən\ *n* : expansion of the bronchial air passages

bron·cho·di·la·tor \-dī-ˈlā-tər, -ˈdī-ˌlā-\ *also* **bron·cho·di·la·to·ry** \-dī-ˈlā-tə-rē\ *adj* : causing or involving bronchodilation ⟨~ activity⟩ ⟨~ drugs⟩ — **bronchodilator** *n*

bron·cho·gen·ic \ˌbräŋ-kə-ˈje-nik\ *adj* : of, relating to, or arising in or by way of the air passages of the lungs ⟨~ carcinoma⟩

bron·cho·gram \ˈbräŋ-kə-ˌgram, -kō-\ *n* : a radiograph of the bronchial tree after injection of a radiopaque substance

bron·chog·ra·phy \brän-ˈkä-grə-fē, bräŋ-\ *n, pl* **-phies** : the radiographic visualization of the bronchi and their branches after injection of a radiopaque substance — **bron·cho·graph·ic** \ˌbräŋ-kə-ˈgra-fik\ *adj*

bron·choph·o·ny \bräŋ-ˈkä-fə-nē\ *n, pl* **-nies** : the sound of the voice heard through the stethoscope over a healthy bronchus and over other portions of the chest in cases of consolidation of the lung tissue — compare PECTORILOQUY

bron·cho·plas·ty \ˈbräŋ-kə-ˌplas-tē\ *n, pl* **-ties** : surgical repair and reconstruction of a bronchus — **bron·cho·plas·tic** \ˌbräŋ-kə-ˈplas-tik\ *adj*

bron·cho·pleu·ral \ˌbräŋ-kō-ˈplu̇r-əl\ *adj* : joining a bronchus and the pleural cavity ⟨a ~ fistula⟩

bron·cho·pneu·mo·nia \ˌbräŋ-(ˌ)kō-nu̇-ˈmō-nyə, -nyu̇-\ *n* : pneumonia involving many relatively small areas of lung tissue — called also *bronchial pneumonia* — **bron·cho·pneu·mon·ic** \-ˈmä-nik\ *adj*

bron·cho·pul·mo·nary \ˌbräŋ-kō-ˈpu̇l-mə-ˌner-ē, -ˈpəl-\ *adj* : of, relating to, or affecting the bronchi and the lungs

bronchopulmonary dysplasia *n* : a chronic lung condition that is caused by tissue damage to the lungs and usu. occurs in immature infants who have received mechanical ventilation and supplemental oxygen as treatment for respiratory distress syndrome

bron·cho·scope \ˈbräŋ-kə-ˌskōp\ *n* : a usu. flexible endoscope for inspecting or passing instruments into the bronchi — **bron·cho·scop·ic** \ˌbräŋ-kə-ˈskä-pik\ *adj* — **bron·chos·co·pist** \brän-ˈkäs-kə-pist\ *n* — **bron·chos·co·py** \brän-ˈkäs-kə-pē\ *n*

bron·cho·spasm \ˈbräŋ-kə-ˌspa-zəm\ *n* : constriction of the air passages of the lung (as in asthma) by spasmodic contraction of the bronchial muscles — **bron·cho·spas·tic** \ˌbräŋ-kə-ˈspas-tik\ *adj*

bron·cho·spi·rom·e·try \ˌbräŋ-kō-spī-ˈrä-mə-trē\ *n, pl* **-tries** : independent measurement of the vital capacity of each lung by means of a spirometer in direct continuity with one of the primary bronchi — **bron·cho·spi·rom·e·ter** \-ˈrä-mə-tər\ *n*

bron·cho·ste·no·sis \ˌbräŋ-kō-stə-ˈnō-səs\ *n, pl* **-no·ses** \-ˌsēz\ : stenosis of a bronchus

bron·chus \ˈbräŋ-kəs\ *n, pl* **bron·chi** \ˈbräŋ-ˌkī, -ˌkē\ : either of the two primary divisions of the trachea that lead respectively into the right and the left lung; *broadly* : BRONCHIAL TUBE

brow \ˈbrau̇\ *n* **1** : EYEBROW **2** : either of the lateral prominences of the forehead **3** : FOREHEAD

brow bone *n* : the bony prominence above each eye formed by part of the supraorbital ridge; *also* : the skin overlying this bony prominence

brown alga *n* : any of a division (Phaeophyta) of variable mostly marine algae with chlorophyll masked by brown pigment

brown dog tick *n* : a widely distributed reddish-brown tick of the genus *Rhipicephalus* (*R. sanguineus*) that occurs esp. on dogs and that transmits canine babesiosis

brown fat *n* : a mammalian heat-producing tissue occurring esp. in human newborn infants — called also *brown adipose tissue*

brown lung disease *n* : BYSSINOSIS

brown rat *n* : a common domestic rat of the genus *Rattus* (*R. norvegicus*) that has been introduced worldwide — called also *Norway rat*

brown recluse spider *n* : a venomous spider of the genus *Loxosceles* (*L. reclusa*) esp. of the southern and central U.S. that produces a dangerous cytotoxin — called also *brown recluse*

brown snake *n* : any of several Australian venomous elapid snakes (genus *Pseudonaja* syn. *Demansia*); *esp* : a widely distributed brownish or blackish snake (*P. textilis*)

brow ridge \ˈbrau̇-ˌrij\ *n* : SUPRAORBITAL RIDGE

BRP *abbr* bathroom privileges

bru·cel·la \brü-ˈse-lə\ *n* **1** *cap* : a genus of nonmotile capsulated bacteria (family Brucellaceae) that cause disease in humans and domestic animals **2** *pl* **-cel·lae** \-ˈse-(ˌ)lē\ *or* **-cel·las** : any bacterium of the genus *Brucella*

Bruce \ˈbrüs\, **Sir David (1855–1931),** British bacteriologist.

bru·cel·lo·sis \ˌbrü-sə-ˈlō-səs\ *n, pl* **-lo·ses** \-ˌsēz\ **1** : a disease of domestic animals that is caused by bacteria of the genus *Brucella* (*B. melitensis* of goats, *B. suis* of swine and rarely cattle, *B. abortus* of cattle and rarely swine, and *B. canis* of dogs) and is marked esp. by abortion — see BANG'S DISEASE **2** : an acute or chronic disease of humans that is acquired esp. through direct contact with animals or animal products (as unpasteurized milk) infected with bacteria of the genus *Brucella* and is marked chiefly by fever, fatigue, joint and muscle pain, loss of appetite, and swelling of internal organs (as the liver or heart) — called also *Malta fever, Mediterranean fever, undulant fever*

Bruch's membrane \ˈbru̇ks-, ˈbrüks-\ *n* : the inner membrane of the retina separating the pigmented layer of the retina from the choroid of the eye

Bruch, Karl Wilhelm Ludwig (1819–1884), German anatomist.

bru·cine \ˈbrü-ˌsēn\ *n* : a poisonous alkaloid $C_{23}H_{26}N_2O_4$ found with strychnine esp. in nux vomica

Bruce \ˈbrüs\, **James (1730–1794),** British explorer.

Brud·zin·ski sign \brü-ˈjin-skē-, brüd-ˈzin-\ *or* **Brud·zin·ski's sign** \-skēz-\ *n* : any of several symptoms of meningeal irritation occurring esp. in meningitis; *esp* : involuntary bending of the knees and hips of a supine patient caused by lifting the head of the patient so that the chin moves towards the chest

Brudzinski, Josef (1874–1917), Polish physician.

Bru·ga·da syndrome \brü-ˈgä-də-\ *n* : an inherited life-threatening cardiac disorder of abnormal heart rhythm

Brugada, Pedro (*b* 1952) and **Josep (*b* 1958),** Spanish cardiologists.

¹bruise \ˈbrüz\ *vb* **bruised; bruis·ing 1** : to inflict a bruise on : CONTUSE **2** : WOUND, INJURE; *esp* : to inflict psychological hurt on **3** : to become bruised

²bruise *n* **1** : an injury transmitted through unbroken skin to underlying tissue causing rupture of small blood vessels and escape of blood into the tissue with resulting discoloration : CONTUSION **2** : an injury esp. to the feelings

bruit \ˈbrü-ē\ *n* : any of several generally abnormal sounds heard on auscultation

Brun·ner's gland \ˈbru̇-nərz-\ *n* : any of the compound racemose glands in the submucous layer of the duodenum that secrete alkaline mucus and a potent proteolytic enzyme — called also *gland of Brunner*

Brun·ner \ˈbru̇-nər\, **Johann Conrad (1653–1727),** Swiss anatomist.

brush border *n* : a stria of microvilli on the plasma membrane of an epithelial cell (as in a kidney tubule) that is specialized for absorption

brux·ism \ˈbrək-ˌsi-zəm\ *n* : the habit of unconsciously gritting or grinding the teeth esp. in situations of stress or during sleep — **brux** \ˈbrəks\ *vb*

BS *abbr* **1** bowel sounds **2** breath sounds

BSE *abbr* **1** bovine spongiform encephalopathy **2** breast self-exam; breast self-examination

BSN *abbr* bachelor of science in nursing

BST *abbr* **1** blood serological test **2** *also* **bST** bovine somatotropin

B–type natriuretic peptide \ˈbē-ˌtīp-\ *n* : a peptide hormone secreted mainly by myocytes of the cardiac ventricles in response to stretching of heart muscle with elevated levels in the blood indicative of heart failure — abbr. *BNP;* called also *brain natriuretic peptide*

bubble boy disease *n* : SEVERE COMBINED IMMUNODEFICIENCY

bu·bo \ˈbü-(ˌ)bō, ˈbyü-\ *n, pl* **buboes** : an inflammatory swelling of a lymph node esp. in the groin — **bu·bon·ic** \bü-ˈbä-nik, byü-\ *adj*

bubonic plague *n* : plague caused by a bacterium of the genus *Yersinia* (*Y. pestis* syn. *Pasteurella pestis*) and characterized esp. by the formation of buboes — compare PNEUMONIC PLAGUE

buc·cal \ˈbə-kəl\ *adj* **1** : of, relating to, near, involving, or supplying a cheek ⟨the ~ surface of a tooth⟩ **2** : of, relating to, involving, or lying in the mouth — **buc·cal·ly** *adv*

buccal gland *n* : any of the small racemose mucous glands in the mucous membrane lining the cheeks

buc·ci·na·tor \ˈbək-sə-ˌnā-tər\ *n* : a thin broad muscle forming the wall of the cheek and serving to compress the cheek against the teeth — called also *buccinator muscle*

bucco- *comb form* : buccal and ⟨*bucco*lingual⟩

buc·co·lin·gual \ˌbə-kō-ˈliŋ-gwəl, -gyə-wəl\ *adj* **1** : relating to or affecting the cheek and the tongue **2** : of or relating to the buccal and lingual aspects of a tooth ⟨the ∼ width of a molar⟩ — **buc·co·lin·gual·ly** *adv*

buc·co·pha·ryn·geal \-ˌfar-ən-ˈjē-əl, -fə-ˈrin-jəl, -jē-əl\ *adj* : relating to or near the cheek and the pharynx

bucket handle *adj* : being an injury of internal body tissue that resembles the shape of the curved handle of a bucket ⟨a *bucket handle* fracture⟩

buck·thorn \ˈbək-ˌthȯrn\ *n* : any of a genus (*Rhamnus* of the family Rhamnaceae) of shrubs and trees some of which yield purgative principles in their bark or sap

buck·tooth \-ˈtüth\ *n, pl* **buck·teeth** : a large projecting front tooth — **buck–toothed** \-ˌtütht\ *adj*

[1]**bud** \ˈbəd\ *n* **1 a** : an asexual reproductive structure **b** : a primordium having potentialities for growth and development into a definitive structure ⟨an embryonic limb ∼⟩ **2** : an anatomical structure (as a tactile corpuscle) resembling a bud

[2]**bud** *vb* **bud·ded; bud·ding** : to reproduce asexually esp. by the pinching off of a small part of the parent

bu·des·o·nide \ˌbyü-ˈde-sō-ˌnīd\ *n* : an anti-inflammatory glucocorticoid $C_{25}H_{34}O_6$ used esp. to treat asthma, allergic rhinitis, nasal polyps, Crohn's disease, and ulcerative colitis — see ENTOCORT, PULMICORT, RHINOCORT AQUA, SYMBICORT, UCERIS

BUdR *abbr* bromodeoxyuridine

Buer·ger's disease \ˈbər-gərz-, ˈbu̇r-\ *n* : thromboangiitis of the small arteries and veins of the extremities and esp. the feet resulting in occlusion, ischemia, and gangrene — called also *thromboangiitis obliterans*

Buer·ger \ˈbər-gər, ˈbu̇r-\, **Leo (1879–1943),** American pathologist.

buffalo hump *n* : an excess deposit of fat localized on the back of the neck that is caused esp. by excess cortisol in the body (as in Cushing's syndrome)

[1]**buff·er** \ˈbə-fər\ *n* : a substance or mixture of substances (as bicarbonates) that in solution tends to stabilize the hydrogen-ion concentration by neutralizing within limits both acids and bases

[2]**buffer** *vb* : to treat (as a solution or its acidity) with a buffer; *also* : to prepare (aspirin) with an antacid

buffy coat \ˈbə-fē-\ *n* : the superficial layer of yellowish or buff coagulated plasma from which the red corpuscles have settled out in slowly coagulated blood

bu·fo·ten·ine \ˌbyü-fə-ˈte-ˌnēn, -nən\ *or* **bu·fo·ten·in** \-nən\ *n* : a toxic hallucinogenic alkaloid $C_{12}H_{16}N_2O$ that is obtained esp. from poisonous secretions of toads (order Anura and esp. family Bufonidae) and from some mushrooms and has hypertensive and vasoconstrictor activity

bug \ˈbəg\ *n* **1 a** : an insect or other creeping or crawling invertebrate animal (as a spider) — not used technically **b** : any of several insects (as the bedbug or cockroach) commonly considered obnoxious **c** : any of an order (Hemiptera and esp. its suborder Heteroptera) of insects that have sucking mouthparts and forewings thickened at the base **2 a** : a microorganism (as a bacterium or virus) esp. when causing illness or disease **b** : an often unspecified or nonspecific sickness presumed to be caused by such a microorganism ⟨a stomach ∼⟩

building–related illness *n* : a clinically diagnosable disease or condition (as Legionnaires' disease or an allergic reaction) caused by a microorganism or substance demonstrably present in a building

bulb \ˈbəlb\ *n* **1** : a rounded dilation or expansion of something cylindrical ⟨the ∼ of a thermometer⟩; *esp* : a rounded or pear-shaped enlargement on a small base ⟨the ∼ of an eyedropper⟩ **2** : a rounded part: as **a** : a rounded enlargement of one end of a part — see BULB OF THE PENIS, BULB OF THE VESTIBULE, END BULB, OLFACTORY BULB **b** : MEDULLA OBLONGATA; *broadly* : the hindbrain exclusive of the cerebellum

bulb- *or* **bulbo-** *comb form* **1** : bulb ⟨*bulb*ar⟩ **2** : bulbar and ⟨*bulbo*spinal⟩

bul·bar \ˈbəl-bər, -ˌbär\ *adj* : of or relating to a bulb; *specif* : involving the medulla oblongata

bulbar paralysis *n* : destruction of nerve centers of the medulla oblongata and paralysis of the parts innervated from the medulla with interruption of their functions (as swallowing or speech)

bulbi — see PHTHISIS BULBI

bul·bo·cav·er·no·sus \ˌbəl-(ˌ)bō-ˌka-vər-ˈnō-səs\ *n, pl* **-no·si** \-ˌsī\ : a muscle that in the male surrounds and compresses the bulb of the penis and the bulbar portion of the urethra and in the female serves to compress the vagina — see SPHINCTER VAGINAE

bulb of the penis *n* : the proximal expanded part of the corpus cavernosum of the male urethra

bulb of the vestibule *n* : a structure in the female vulva that is homologous to the bulb of the penis and the adjoining corpus spongiosum in the male and that consists of an elongated mass of erectile tissue on each side of the vaginal opening united anteriorly to the contralateral mass by a narrow median band passing along the lower surface of the clitoris

bul·bo·spi·nal \ˌbəl-bō-ˈspīn-ᵊl\ *adj* : of, relating to, or connecting the medulla oblongata and the spinal cord

bul·bo·spon·gi·o·sus muscle \ˌbəl-(ˌ)bō-ˌspən-jē-ˈō-səs-\ *n* : BULBOCAVERNOSUS

bul·bo·ure·thral gland \-yu̇-ˈrē-thrəl-\ *n* : COWPER'S GLAND

bul·bous \ˈbəl-bəs\ *adj* : resembling a bulb esp. in roundness or the gross enlargement of a part

bul·bus \ˈbəl-bəs\ *n, pl* **bul·bi** \-ˌbī, -ˌbē\ : a bulb-shaped anatomical part

-bulia *also* **-boulia** *n comb form* : condition of having (such) will ⟨a*bulia*⟩

-bulic *adj comb form* : of, relating to, or characterized by a (specified) state of will ⟨a*bulic*⟩

bu·lim·a·rex·ia \bü-ˌli-mə-ˈrek-sē-ə, byü-, -ˌlē-\ *n* **1** : BULIMIA 2 **2** : an eating disorder in which symptoms of both bulimia and anorexia nervosa are present — **bu·lim·a·rex·ic** \-sik\ *n or adj*

bu·lim·ia \bü-ˈli-mē-ə, byü-, -ˈlē-\ *n* **1** : an abnormal and constant craving for food **2** : a serious eating disorder that occurs chiefly in females, is characterized by compulsive overeating usu. followed by self-induced vomiting or laxative or diuretic abuse, and is often accompanied by guilt and depression

bulimia ner·vo·sa \-(ˌ)nər-ˈvō-sə, -zə\ *n* : BULIMIA 2

[1]**bu·lim·ic** \-mik\ *adj* : of, relating to, or affected with bulimia ⟨∼ patients⟩

[2]**bulimic** *n* : a person affected with bulimia

bulk \ˈbəlk\ *n* : material (as indigestible fibrous residues of food) that forms a mass in the intestine; *esp* : FIBER 2

bul·la \ˈbu̇-lə\ *n, pl* **bul·lae** \ˈbu̇-ˌlē, -ˌlī\ **1** : a hollow thin-walled rounded bony prominence **2** : a large vesicle or blister — compare BLEB

bull·nose \ˈbu̇l-ˌnōz\ *n* : a necrobacillosis arising in facial wounds of swine

bullosa — see EPIDERMOLYSIS BULLOSA

bul·lous \ˈbu̇-ləs\ *adj* : resembling or characterized by bullae : VESICULAR

bullous pemphigoid *n* : a chronic skin disease that is characterized by the formation of numerous hard blisters usu. over a widespread area and typically affects older individuals

bu·met·a·nide \byü-ˈme-tə-ˌnīd\ *n* : a diuretic $C_{17}H_{20}N_2O_5S$ used in the treatment of edema — see BUMEX

Bu·mex \ˈbyü-ˌmeks\ *trademark* — used for a preparation of bumetanide

BUN \ˌbē-(ˌ)yü-ˈen\ *n* : the concentration of nitrogen in the form of urea in the blood

Bu·na·vail \ˈbyü-nə-ˌvāl\ *trademark* — used for a film containing buprenorphine and naloxone that is placed on the inside of the cheek

bun·dle \ˈbənd-ᵊl\ *n* : a small band of mostly parallel fibers (as of nerve or muscle) : FASCICULUS, TRACT

bundle branch *n* : either of the parts of the bundle of His passing respectively to the right and left ventricles

bundle branch block *n* : heart block due to a lesion in one of the bundle branches

bundle of His \-ˈhis\ *n* : a slender bundle of modified cardiac muscle that passes from the atrioventricular node in the right atrium to the right and left ventricles by way of the septum and that maintains the normal sequence of the heartbeat — called also *atrioventricular bundle, His bundle*

His, Wilhelm (1863–1934), German physician.

bun·ga·ro·tox·in \ˈbəŋ-gə-rō-ˌtäk-sən\ *n* : a potent neurotoxin obtained from the venom of an Asian elapid snake (genus *Bungarus*)

bun·ion \ˈbən-yən\ *n* : an inflamed swelling of the small fluid-filled sac on the first joint of the big toe accompanied by enlargement and protrusion of the joint

bun·io·nec·to·my \ˌbən-yə-ˈnek-tə-mē\ *n, pl* **-mies** : surgery to remove all or part of a bunion that involves removing soft tissue and bone and may also involve realigning the toe joint

Bu·nos·to·mum \byü-ˈnäs-tə-məm\ *n* : a genus of nematode worms including the hookworms of sheep and cattle

bun·ya·vi·rus \ˈbən-yə-ˌvī-rəs\ *n* : any of a family (*Bunyaviridae*) of single-stranded RNA viruses that are usu. transmitted by the bite of an arthropod (as a mosquito or tick) or in the bodily secretions of rodents and that include the hantaviruses and the causative agents of Rift Valley fever, sandfly fever, and some forms of encephalitis (as La Crosse encephalitis) and hemorrhagic fever

Bun·ya·vi·rus \ˈbən-yə-ˌvī-rəs\ *n, syn of* ORTHOBUNYAVIRUS

buph·thal·mos \büf-ˈthal-məs, byüf-, ˌbəf-, -ˌmäs\ *also* **buph·thal·mia** \-mē-ə\ *n, pl* **-mos·es** *also* **-mias** : marked enlargement of the eye that is usu. congenital and attended by symptoms of glaucoma

bu·piv·a·caine \byü-ˈpi-və-ˌkān\ *n* : a local anesthetic $C_{18}H_{28}N_2O$ that is like lidocaine in its action but is longer acting

Bu·pre·nex \ˈbyü-prə-ˌneks\ *trademark* — used for a preparation of buprenorphine administered by injection

bu·pre·nor·phine \ˌbyü-prə-ˈnȯr-ˌfēn\ *n* : a narcotic analgesic that is used in the form of its hydrochloride $C_{29}H_{41}NO_4·HCl$ to control moderate to severe pain and to treat opioid dependence — see BUNAVAIL, BUPRENEX, BUTRANS, SUBUTEX, SUBOXONE, ZUBSOLV

bu·pro·pi·on \byü-ˈprō-pē-ˌän\ *n* : a drug used in the form of its hydrochloride $C_{13}H_{18}ClNO·HCl$ as an antidepressant and as an aid to stop smoking — see WELLBUTRIN, ZYBAN

bur \ˈbər\ *n* **1** *usu* **burr** : a small surgical cutting tool (as for making an opening in bone) **2** : a bit used on a dental drill

bur·den \ˈbər-dən\ *n* : LOAD 1

Burk·hol·de·ria \ˌbərk-hōl-ˈder-ē-ə\ *n* : a genus of bacteria (family Burkholderiaceae) formerly placed in the genus *Pseudomonas* and including the causative agents of glanders (*B. mallei*) and melioidosis (*B. pseudomallei*)

Burkholder, Walter Hagemeyer (1891–1983), American botanist.

Bur·kitt's lymphoma \ˈbər-kəts-\ *also* **Burkitt lymphoma** \-kət-\ *n* : a non-Hodgkin lymphoma of B cell origin that occurs esp. in children of central Africa and is associated with Epstein-Barr virus

Bur·kitt \ˈbər-kət\, **Denis Parsons (1911–1993),** British surgeon.

Burkitt's tumor *also* **Burkitt tumor** *n* : BURKITT'S LYMPHOMA

[1]**burn** \ˈbərn\ *vb* **burned** \ˈbərnd, ˈbərnt\ *or* **burnt** \ˈbərnt\; **burn·ing 1** : to produce or undergo discomfort or pain ⟨iodine ~*s* so⟩; *also* : to injure or damage by exposure to fire, heat, or radiation ⟨~*ed* his hand⟩ **2** : to become reddened or irritated by or as if by exposure to sun or wind ⟨she ~*s* easily⟩ **3** : to break down and use as a source of energy ⟨~ calories⟩

[2]**burn** *n* **1** : bodily injury resulting from exposure to heat, caustics, electricity, or some radiations, marked by varying degrees of skin destruction and hyperemia often with the formation of watery blisters and in severe cases by charring of the tissues, and classified according to the extent and degree of the injury — see FIRST-DEGREE BURN, SECOND-DEGREE BURN, THIRD-DEGREE BURN **2** : an abrasion having the appearance of a burn ⟨friction ~*s*⟩ **3** : a burning sensation

burn center *or* **burn unit** *n* : a specialized facility usu. affiliated with a hospital that provides advanced care and treatment for patients with severe burn — called also *burns center, burns unit*

burn·er \ˈbər-nər\ *n* : STINGER 2

[1]**burn·ing** \ˈbər-niŋ\ *adj* **1** : affecting with or as if with heat ⟨a ~ fever⟩ **2** : resembling that produced by a burn ⟨a ~ sensation⟩

[2]**burning** *n* : a sensation of being on fire or excessively heated ⟨gastric ~⟩

burning mouth syndrome *n* : a chronic burning sensation of the oral mucous membranes esp. of the tongue that chiefly affects postmenopausal women and is of unknown cause

burn·out \ˈbərn-ˌau̇t\ *n* **1 a** : exhaustion of physical or emotional strength usu. as a result of prolonged stress or frustration **b** : a person affected with burnout **2** : a person showing the effects of drug abuse

Bu·row's solution \ˈbü-(ˌ)rōz-\ *n* : a solution of the acetate of aluminum used as an antiseptic and astringent

Bu·row \ˈbü-(ˌ)rō\, **Karl August von (1809–1874),** German military surgeon and anatomist.

[1]**burp** \ˈbərp\ *n* : BELCH

[2]**burp** *vb* **1** : BELCH **2** : to help (a baby) expel gas from the stomach esp. by patting or rubbing the back

burr *var of* BUR

bur·row \ˈbər-(ˌ)ō\ *n* : a passage or gallery formed in or under the skin by the wandering of a parasite (as the mite of scabies) — **burrow** *vb*

bur·sa \ˈbər-sə\ *n, pl* **bur·sas** \-səz\ *or* **bur·sae** \-ˌsē, -ˌsī\ : a bodily pouch or sac: as **a** : a small serous sac between a tendon and a bone **b** : BURSA OF FABRICIUS — **bur·sal** \-səl\ *adj*

bursa of Fa·bri·cius \-fə-ˈbri-shəs, -shē-əs\ *n* : a blind glandular sac that opens into the cloaca of birds and functions in B cell production

Fabricius, Johann Christian (1745–1808), Danish entomologist.

bur·sec·to·my \(ˌ)bər-ˈsek-tə-mē\ *n, pl* **-mies** : the excision of a bursa (as of the hip or shoulder joint)

bur·si·tis \(ˌ)bər-ˈsī-təs\ *n* : inflammation of a bursa (as of the shoulder or elbow)

bush·mas·ter \ˈbu̇sh-ˌmas-tər\ *n* : a tropical American pit viper (*Lachesis mutus*)

Bu·Spar \ˈbyü-ˌspär\ *trademark* — used for a preparation of the hydrochloride of buspirone

bu·spi·rone \byü-ˈspī-ˌrōn\ *n* : a mild antianxiety tranquilizer that is used in the form of its hydrochloride $C_{21}H_{31}N_5O_2 \cdot HCl$ and does not induce significant tolerance or psychological dependence — see BUSPAR

bu·sul·fan \byü-ˈsəl-fən\ *n* : an antineoplastic agent $C_6H_{14}O_6S_2$ used in the treatment of chronic myelogenous leukemia — see MYLERAN

bu·ta·bar·bi·tal \ˌbyü-tə-ˈbär-bə-ˌtal\ *n* : a synthetic barbiturate used esp. in the form of its sodium salt $C_{10}H_{15}N_2NaO_3$ as a sedative and sleep aid

bu·ta·caine \ˈbyü-tə-ˌkān\ *n* : a local anesthetic that is applied in the form of its sulfate $(C_{18}H_{30}N_2O_2)_2 \cdot H_2SO_4$ to mucous membranes

Bu·ta·zol·i·din \ˌbyü-tə-ˈzä-lə-dən\ *n* : a preparation of phenylbutazone — formerly a U.S. registered trademark

bute \ˈbyüt\ *n* : PHENYLBUTAZONE

bu·tor·pha·nol \ˌbyü-ˈtȯr-fə-ˌnȯl\ *n* : a synthetic opioid drug administered in the form of its tartrate $C_{21}H_{29}NO_2 \cdot C_4H_6O_6$ as a nasal spray or by injection esp. for the relief of pain — see STADOL

butoxide — see PIPERONYL BUTOXIDE

Bu·trans \ˈbyü-ˌtranz\ *trademark* — used for a transdermal patch containing buprenorphine

[1]**but·ter·fly** \ˈbə-tər-ˌflī\ *n, pl* **-flies** **1** *pl* : a feeling of hollowness or queasiness caused esp. by emotional or nervous tension or anxious anticipation **2** : BUTTERFLY BANDAGE

[2]**butterfly** *adj* : affecting the part of the face including the cheeks and the bridge of the nose ⟨the typical ∼ lesion of lupus erythematosus⟩

butterfly bandage *n* : an adhesive bandage with wing-shaped extensions used esp. to close small cuts and incisions

butterfly needle *n* : a short needle that has plastic tabs on either side which aid esp. in manipulating and stabilizing the needle during insertion

but·tock \ˈbə-tək\ *n* **1** : the back of a hip that forms one of the fleshy parts on which a person sits **2 buttocks** *pl* : the seat of the body; *also* : the corresponding part of a quadruped : RUMP

but·ton \ˈbət-ᵊn\ *n* : something that resembles a small knob or disk: as **a** : the terminal segment of a rattlesnake's rattle **b** : COTYLEDON 1

bu·tyl·at·ed hy·droxy·an·i·sole \ˈbyüt-ᵊl-ˌā-təd-ˌhī-ˌdräk-sē-ˈa-nə-ˌsōl\ *n* : BHA

butylated hy·droxy·tol·u·ene \-(ˌ)hī-ˌdräk-sē-ˈtäl-yə-ˌwēn\ *n* : BHT

bu·tyl nitrite \ˈbyüt-ᵊl-\ *n* : a colorless pungent liquid $C_4H_9NO_2$ inhaled illicitly for its stimulating effects which are similar to those of amyl nitrite — called also *isobutyl nitrite;* compare POPPER

bu·tyr·ic acid \byü-ˈtir-ik-\ *n* : either of two isomeric fatty acids $C_4H_8O_2$; *esp* : one of unpleasant odor found in rancid butter and in perspiration

bu·ty·ro·phe·none \ˌbyü-tə-(ˌ)rō-fə-ˈnōn\ *n* : any of a class of antipsychotic drugs (as haloperidol) used esp. in the treatment of schizophrenia

bu·tyr·yl·cho·lin·es·ter·ase \ˌbyüt-ə-rəl-ˌkō-lə-ˈnes-tə-ˌrās, -ˌrāz\ *n* : an enzyme related to acetylcholinesterase that promotes the hydroysis of choline esters — called also *cholinesterase, pseudocholinesterase*

BV *abbr* bacterial vaginosis

B vitamin *n* : any vitamin of the vitamin B complex

Bx *abbr* [by analogy with *Rx*] biopsy

by·pass \ˈbī-ˌpas\ *n* : a surgically established shunt; *also* : a surgical procedure for the establishment of a shunt — see CORONARY BYPASS, GASTRIC BYPASS, JEJUNOILEAL BYPASS — **bypass** *vb*

bys·si·no·sis \ˌbi-sə-ˈnō-səs\ *n, pl* **-no·ses** \-ˌsēz\ : an occupational respiratory disease associated with inhalation of cotton, flax, or hemp dust and characterized initially by chest tightness, shortness of breath, and cough, and eventually by irreversible lung disease — called also *brown lung, brown lung disease*

Bys·tol·ic \bis-ˈtä-lik\ *trademark* — used for a preparation of nebivolol

BZ \ˌbē-ˈzē\ *n* : a gas $C_{21}H_{23}NO_3$ that when breathed produces incapacitating physical and mental effects — called also *quinuclidinyl benzilate*

BZP \ˌbē-ˌzē-ˈpē\ *n* : BENZYLPIPERAZINE

C

c *abbr* **1** canine **2** centimeter **3** curie **4** *or* c̄ [Latin *cum*] with — used in writing prescriptions
C *abbr* **1** Celsius **2** centigrade **3** cervical — used esp. with a number from 1 to 7 to indicate a vertebra or segment of the spinal cord **4** cocaine **5** [Latin *congius*] gallon **6** cytosine
C *symbol* carbon
Ca *symbol* calcium
CA *abbr* chronological age
CABG \ˈka-bij\ *abbr* coronary artery bypass graft
cacao butter *var of* COCOA BUTTER
ca•chec•tic \kə-ˈkek-tik, ka-\ *adj* : relating to or affected by cachexia
ca•chet \ka-ˈshā\ *n* : a medicinal preparation for swallowing consisting of a case usu. of rice-flour paste containing an unpleasant-tasting medicine
ca•chex•ia \kə-ˈkek-sē-ə, ka-\ *n* : general physical wasting and malnutrition usu. associated with chronic disease
cac•o•dyl•ic acid \ˌka-kə-ˈdi-lik-\ *n* : a toxic crystalline compound of arsenic $C_2H_7AsO_2$ used esp. as an herbicide
ca•cos•mia \kə-ˈkäs-mē-ə, ka-,-ˈkäz-\ *n* : a hallucination of a disagreeable odor
CAD *abbr* coronary artery disease
ca•dav•er \kə-ˈda-vər\ *n* : a dead body; *specif* : one intended for dissection — **ca•dav•er•ic** \-və-rik\ *adj*
ca•dav•er•ous \kə-ˈda-və-rəs\ *adj* **1** : of or relating to a corpse **2** *of a complexion* : being pallid or livid like a corpse
cade oil *n* : JUNIPER TAR
cad•mi•um \ˈkad-mē-əm\ *n* : a bluish-white malleable ductile toxic bivalent metallic element — symbol *Cd;* see ELEMENT table
cadmium sulfide *n* : a yellow-brown poisonous salt CdS used esp. in the treatment of seborrheic dermatitis of the scalp
ca•du•ceus \kə-ˈdü-sē-əs, -ˈdyü-, -shəs\ *n, pl* **-cei** \-sē-ˌī\ : a medical insignia bearing a representation of a staff with two entwined snakes and two wings at the top that is sometimes used to symbolize a physician but is often considered to be an erroneous representation— compare STAFF OF AESCULAPIUS
Cad•u•et \ˈka-dü-ˌet\ *trademark* — used for a preparation of amlodipine and atorvastatin
caec- *or* **caeci-** *or* **caeco-** *chiefly Brit var of* CEC-
cae•cal, cae•cum *chiefly Brit var of* CECAL, CECUM
caesarean *also* **caesarian** *var of* CESAREAN
cae•si•um *chiefly Brit var of* CESIUM
ca•fé au lait spot \ka-ˈfā-ō-ˈlā-\ *n* : any of the medium brown spots usu. on the trunk, pelvis, and creases of the elbow and knees that are often numerous in neurofibromatosis — usu. used in pl.
caf•feine \ka-ˈfēn,ˈka-ˌ\ *n* : a bitter alkaloid $C_8H_{10}N_4O_2$ found esp. in coffee and tea and used medicinally as a stimulant and diuretic — **caf•fein•ic** \ka-ˈfē-nik\ *adj*
caf•fein•ism \-ˌni-zəm\ *n* : a condition caused by the ingestion of excessive caffeine and marked by restlessness, irritability, insomnia, diuresis, tremors, and tachycardia
CAH *abbr* congenital adrenal hyperplasia
-caine *n comb form* : synthetic alkaloid anesthetic ⟨pro*caine*⟩ ⟨lido*caine*⟩
cais•son disease \ˈkā-ˌsän-, ˈkās-ᵊn-\ *n* : DECOMPRESSION SICKNESS
caj•e•put•ol *or* **caj•u•put•ol** \ˈka-jə-pə-ˌtȯl, -ˌtōl\ *n* : EUCALYPTOL
caked breast \ˈkākt-\ *n* : a localized hardening in one or more segments of a lactating breast caused by accumulation of blood in dilated veins and milk in obstructed ducts
cal *abbr* small calorie
Cal *abbr* large calorie
Cal•a•bar swelling \ˈka-lə-ˌbär-\ *n* : a transient subcutaneous swelling marking the migratory course through the tissues of the adult filarial eye worm of the genus *Loa* (*L. loa*)
cal•a•mine \ˈka-lə-ˌmīn, -mən\ *n* : a mixture of zinc oxide or zinc carbonate with a small amount of ferric oxide that is used in lotions, liniments, and ointments
Cal•an \ˈka-ˌlän\ *trademark* — used for a preparation of the hydrochloride of verapamil
cal•ca•ne•al \kal-ˈkā-nē-əl\ *adj* **1** : relating to the heel **2** : relating to the calcaneus
calcaneal tendon *n* : ACHILLES TENDON
calcaneo- *comb form* : calcaneal and ⟨*calcaneo*cuboid⟩
cal•ca•neo•cu•boid \(ˌ)kal-ˌkā-nē-ō-ˈkyü-ˌbȯid\ *adj* : of or relating to the calcaneus and the cuboid bone
calcaneonavicular — see PLANTAR CALCANEONAVICULAR LIGAMENT
cal•ca•ne•um \kal-ˈkā-nē-əm\ *n, pl* **-nea** \-nē-ə\ : CALCANEUS
cal•ca•ne•us \-nē-əs\ *n, pl* **-nei** \-nē-ˌī\ : a tarsal bone that in humans is the large bone of the heel — called also *heel bone, os calcis*
cal•car \ˈkal-ˌkär\ *n, pl* **cal•car•ia** \kal-ˈkar-ē-ə\ : a small anatomical prominence or projection
calcar avis \-ˈā-vəs, -ˈä-\ *n, pl* **calcaria avi•um** \-vē-əm\ : a curved ridge on the medial wall of the posterior horn of each lateral ventricle of the brain opposite the calcarine sulcus

cal·car·e·ous \kal-ˈkar-ē-əs\ *adj* : resembling, consisting of, or containing calcium carbonate; *also* : containing calcium

cal·ca·rine sulcus \ˈkal-kə-ˌrīn-\ *n* : a sulcus in the mesial surface of the occipital lobe of the cerebrum — called also *calcarine fissure*

cal·cif·er·ol \kal-ˈsi-fə-ˌrȯl, -ˌrōl\ *n* : an alcohol $C_{28}H_{43}OH$ usu. prepared by irradiation of ergosterol and used as a dietary supplement in nutrition and medicinally esp. in the control of rickets — called also *ergocalciferol, viosterol, vitamin D, vitamin D₂;* see DRISDOL

cal·cif·ic \kal-ˈsi-fik\ *adj* : involving or caused by calcification ⟨~ lesions⟩

cal·ci·fi·ca·tion \ˌkal-sə-fə-ˈkā-shən\ *n* **1** : impregnation with calcareous matter: as **a** : deposition of calcium salts within the matrix of cartilage often as the preliminary step in the formation of bone **b** : abnormal deposition of calcium salts within soft tissue often causing thickening or hardening **2** : a calcified structure or part; *also* : an abnormal deposit of calcium salts ⟨arterial ~⟩ — **cal·ci·fy** \ˈkal-sə-ˌfī\ *vb*

cal·ci·no·sis \ˌkal-sə-ˈnō-səs\ *n, pl* **-no·ses** \-ˌsēz\ : the abnormal deposition of calcium salts in a part or tissue of the body

cal·ci·po·tri·ene \ˌkal-sə-(ˌ)pō-ˈtrī-ˌēn\ *n* : a drug $C_{27}H_{40}O_3$ that is a synthetic analog of vitamin D_3 used topically to treat psoriasis

calcis — see OS CALCIS

cal·ci·to·nin \ˌkal-sə-ˈtō-nən\ *n* **1** : a polypeptide hormone esp. from the thyroid gland that tends to lower the level of calcium in the blood plasma — called also *thyrocalcitonin* **2** : a synthetic or recombinant form of calcitonin used to treat Paget's disease of bone and postmenopausal osteoporosis

cal·ci·tri·ol \ˌkal-sə-ˈtrī-ˌȯl, -ˌōl\ *n* : a physiologically active metabolic derivative $C_{27}H_{44}O_3$ of cholecalciferol that is synthesized in the liver and kidney and stimulates the intestinal absorption of calcium — called also *1,25-dihydroxycholecalciferol*

cal·ci·um \ˈkal-sē-əm\ *n, often attrib* : a silver-white bivalent metal that is an essential constituent of most plants and animals — symbol *Ca;* see ELEMENT table

calcium blocker *n* : CALCIUM CHANNEL BLOCKER

calcium carbonate *n* : a calcium salt $CaCO_3$ that is found in limestone, chalk, and bones and that is used in pharmaceuticals as an antacid and to supplement bodily calcium stores

calcium channel blocker *n* : any of a class of drugs (as verapamil) that prevent or slow the influx of calcium ions into smooth muscle cells esp. of the heart and that are used to treat some forms of angina pectoris and some cardiac arrhythmias — called also *calcium blocker*

calcium chloride *n* : a white salt $CaCl_2$ used in medicine as a source of calcium and as a diuretic

calcium citrate *n* : a white, odorless powder $C_{12}H_{10}Ca_3O_{14}$ used esp. as a calcium dietary supplement

calcium gluconate *n* : a white powdery salt $C_{12}H_{22}CaO_{14}$ used to supplement bodily calcium stores

calcium hydroxide *n* : a strong alkali $Ca(OH)_2$ — see SODA LIME

calcium lactate *n* : a white crystalline salt $C_6H_{10}CaO_6 \cdot 5H_2O$ used chiefly in medicine as a source of calcium and in foods (as in baking powder)

calcium levulinate *n* : a white powdery salt $C_{10}H_{14}CaO_6 \cdot H_2O$ used in medicine as a source of calcium

calcium oxalate *n* : an insoluble crystalline salt $CaC_2O_4 \cdot H_2O$ that is sometimes excreted in urine or retained in the form of urinary calculi

calcium pantothenate *n* : a white powdery salt $C_{18}H_{32}CaN_2O_{10}$ made synthetically and used as a source of pantothenic acid

calcium phosphate *n* : any of various phosphates of calcium: as **a** : the phosphate $CaHPO_4$ used in pharmaceutical preparations and animal feeds **b** : a naturally occurring phosphate $Ca_5(F,Cl,OH,{}^1/_2CO_3)(PO_4)_3$ that contains other elements or radicals and is the chief constituent of bones and teeth

calcium propionate *n* : a mold-inhibiting salt $C_6H_{10}CaO_4$ used chiefly as a food preservative

calcium stearate *n* : a white powder consisting essentially of calcium salts of stearic acid and palmitic acid and used as a conditioning agent in food and pharmaceuticals

calcium sulfate *n* : a white calcium salt $CaSO_4$ used esp. as a diluent in tablets and in plaster of paris

cal·co·sphe·rite \ˌkal-kō-ˈsfir-ˌīt\ *n* : a granular or laminated deposit of calcium salts in the body

cal·cu·lo·sis \ˌkal-kyə-ˈlō-səs\ *n, pl* **-lo·ses** \-ˌsēz\ : the formation of or the condition of having a calculus or calculi

cal·cu·lous \ˈkal-kyə-ləs\ *adj* : caused or characterized by a calculus or calculi ⟨~ disease⟩

cal·cu·lus \-ləs\ *n, pl* **-li** \-ˌlī, -ˌlē\; *also* **-lus·es** **1** : a concretion usu. of mineral salts around organic material found esp. in hollow organs or ducts **2** : a concretion on teeth : TARTAR

Cald·well–Luc operation \ˈkȯld-ˌwel-ˈlük-, ˈkäld-, -ˈlu̇k-\ *n* : surgery esp. for clearing a blocked or infected maxillary sinus that involves entering the sinus through the mouth by way of an incision into the canine fossa above a canine tooth, cleaning the sinus, and creating a new and enlarged opening for drainage through the nose — called also *Caldwell-Luc procedure*

Caldwell, George Walter (1866–1946), American surgeon.

Luc \lu̇̄k\, **Henri (1855–1925),** French laryngologist.

calf \ˈkaf, ˈkȧf\ *n, pl* **calves** \ˈkavz, ˈkȧvz\ : the fleshy back part of the leg below the knee

calf bone *n* : FIBULA

calf diphtheria *n* : an infectious disease of the mouth and pharynx of calves and young cattle associated with the presence of a bacterium of the genus *Fusobacterium* (*F. necrophorum*) and usu. resulting in pneumonia or septicemia if untreated

cal•i•ber \ˈka-lə-bər\ *n* : the diameter of a round body; *esp* : the internal diameter of a hollow cylinder

cal•i•bre *chiefly Brit var of* CALIBER

caliceal *var of* CALYCEAL

cal•i•ci•vi•rus \kə-ˈli-sə-ˌvī-rəs\ *n* : any of a family (*Caliciviridae*) of single-stranded RNA viruses that include the Norwalk virus and the causative virus of vesicular exanthema — see HEPATITIS E

cal•i•for•ni•um \ˌka-lə-ˈfȯr-nē-əm\ *n* : an artificially prepared radioactive element — symbol *Cf;* see ELEMENT table

cal•i•per \ˈka-lə-pər\ *n* : any of various measuring instruments having two usu. adjustable arms, legs, or jaws used esp. to measure diameter or thickness — usu. used in pl.

cal•is•then•ics \ˌka-ləs-ˈthe-niks\ *n sing or pl* : systematic rhythmic bodily exercises performed usu. without apparatus — **cal•is•then•ic** \-nik\ *adj*

calix *var of* CALYX

cal•li•per *chiefly Brit var of* CALIPER

cal•lis•then•ics *Brit var of* CALISTHENICS

cal•lo•sal \ka-ˈlō-səl\ *adj* : of, relating to, or adjoining the corpus callosum

cal•los•i•ty \ka-ˈlä-sə-tē\ *n, pl* **-ties** : the quality or state of being callous; *esp* : marked or abnormal hardness and thickness (as of the skin)

callosum — see CORPUS CALLOSUM

cal•lous \ˈka-ləs\ *adj* **1** : being hardened and thickened **2** : having calluses

cal•loused *or* **cal•lused** \ˈka-ləst\ *adj* : CALLOUS 2 ⟨~ hands⟩

cal•lus \ˈka-ləs\ *n* **1** : a thickening of or a hard thickened area on skin **2** : a mass of exudate and connective tissue that forms around a break in a bone and is converted into bone in the healing of the break

calm•ant \ˈkä-mənt, ˈkälm-\ *n* : SEDATIVE

calm•ative \ˈkä-mə-tiv, ˈkäl-mə-\ *n or adj* : SEDATIVE

cal•mod•u•lin \ˌkal-ˈmä-jə-lən\ *n* : a calcium-binding protein that regulates cellular metabolic processes (as muscle-fiber contraction) by modifying the activity of specific calcium-dependent enzymes

cal•o•mel \ˈka-lə-məl, -ˌmel\ *n* : a white tasteless compound Hg_2Cl_2 used esp. as a fungicide and insecticide and formerly in medicine as a purgative — called also *mercurous chloride*

cal•or \ˈka-ˌlȯr\ *n* : bodily heat that is a sign of inflammation

calori- *comb form* : heat ⟨*calori*genic⟩ ⟨*calori*meter⟩

ca•lo•ric \kə-ˈlōr-ik, -ˈlär-; ˈka-lə-rik\ *adj* **1** : of or relating to heat **2** : of or relating to calories — **ca•lo•ri•cal•ly** \kə-ˈlōr-i-k(ə-)lē, -ˈlär-\ *adv*

cal•o•rie *also* **cal•o•ry** \ˈka-lə-rē\ *n, pl* **-ries** **1 a** : the amount of heat required at a pressure of one atmosphere to raise the temperature of one gram of water one degree Celsius that is equal to about 4.19 joules — abbr. *cal;* called also *gram calorie, small calorie* **b** : the amount of heat required to raise the temperature of one kilogram of water one degree Celsius that is equal to 1000 gram calories — abbr. *Cal;* called also *kilocalorie, kilogram calorie, large calorie* **2 a** : a unit equivalent to the large calorie expressing heat-producing or energy-producing value in food when oxidized in the body **b** : an amount of food having an energy-producing value of one large calorie

cal•o•rif•ic \ˌka-lə-ˈri-fik\ *adj* **1** : CALORIC **2** : of or relating to the production of heat

ca•lor•i•gen•ic \kə-ˌlōr-ə-ˈje-nik, -ˌlär-; ˌka-lə-rə-\ *adj* : generating heat or energy ⟨~ foodstuffs⟩

cal•o•rim•e•ter \ˌka-lə-ˈri-mə-tər\ *n* : any of several apparatuses for measuring quantities of absorbed or evolved heat or for determining specific heats — **ca•lo•ri•met•ric** \ˌka-lə-rə-ˈme-trik; kə-ˌlōr-ə-, -ˌlär-\ *adj* — **ca•lo•ri•met•ri•cal•ly** \-tri-k(ə-)lē\ *adv* — **cal•o•rim•e•try** \ˌka-lə-ˈri-mə-trē\ *n*

cal•va \ˈkal-və\ *n, pl* **calvas** *or* **cal•vae** \-ˌvē, -ˌvī\ : the upper part of the human cranium

cal•var•ia \kal-ˈvar-ē-ə\ *n, pl* **-i•ae** \-ē-ˌē, -ē-ˌī\ : CALVARIUM

cal•var•i•um \-ē-əm\ *n, pl* **-ia** \-ē-ə\ : an incomplete skull; *esp* : the portion of a skull including the braincase and excluding the lower jaw or lower jaw and facial portion — **cal•var•i•al** \-ē-əl\ *adj*

calves *pl of* CALF

cal•vi•ti•es \kal-ˈvi-shē-ˌēz, -(ˌ)shēz\ *n, pl* **calvities** : the condition of being bald : BALDNESS

calx \ˈkalks\ *n, pl* **cal•ces** \ˈkal-ˌsēz\ : HEEL

ca•ly•ce•al *or* **ca•li•ce•al** \ˌka-lə-ˈsē-əl, ˌkā-\ *adj* : of or relating to a calyx

calyces *pl of* CALYX

ca•lyx *also* **ca•lix** \ˈkā-liks, ˈka-\ *n, pl* **ca•lyx•es** *or* **ca•ly•ces** \ˈkā-lə-ˌsēz, ˈka-\ : a cuplike division of the renal pelvis surrounding one or more renal papillae

CAM *abbr* complementary and alternative medicine

cam·i·sole \ˈka-mə-ˌsōl\ *n* : a long-sleeved straitjacket

cAMP *abbr* cyclic AMP

cam·phor \ˈkam-fər\ *n* : a gummy volatile aromatic crystalline compound $C_{10}H_{16}O$ obtained esp. from the wood and bark of an evergreen tree (*Cinnamomum camphora*) of the laurel family (Lauraceae) and used esp. as a liniment and mild topical analgesic and as an insect repellent

cam·phor·at·ed \ˈkam-fə-ˌrā-təd\ *adj* : impregnated or treated with camphor

cam·phor·ic acid \kam-ˈfȯr-ik-, -ˈfär-\ *n* : the dextrorotatory form of a white crystalline acid $C_{10}H_{16}O_2$ that is used in pharmaceuticals

cam·pim·e·ter \kam-ˈpi-mə-tər\ *n* : an instrument for testing indirect or peripheral visual perception of form and color — **cam·pim·e·try** \-trē\ *n*

camp·to·cor·mia \ˌkam-tə-ˈkȯr-mē-ə\ *n* : abnormal forward bending of the trunk during standing or walking that resolves in the supine position and may be of neurological, muscular, or psychological origin — called also *bent spine syndrome*

camp·to·dac·ty·ly \ˌkam-tə-ˈdak-tə-lē\ *n, pl* **-lies** : permanent flexion of one or more finger joints

camp·to·the·cin \ˌkamp-tə-ˈthē-sən\ *n* : an alkaloid $C_{20}H_{16}N_2O_4$ from the wood of a Chinese tree (*Camptotheca acuminata* of the family Nyssaceae) that has shown some antileukemic and antitumor activity; *also* : a semisynthetic or synthetic derivative of this

cam·py·lo·bac·ter \ˈkam-pə-lō-ˌbak-tər\ *n* **1** *cap* : a genus of slender spirally curved rod bacteria (family Spirillaceae) including some forms pathogenic for domestic animals or humans — HELICOBACTER **2** : any bacterium of the genus *Campylobacter*

cam·py·lo·bac·te·ri·o·sis \ˌkam-pi-lō-bak-ˌtir-ē-ˈō-səs, kam-ˌpi-lə-\ *n, pl* **-o·ses** \-ˌsēz\ : illness caused by infection with bacteria of the genus *Campylobacter* (as *C. jejuni*) that is marked esp. by diarrhea, abdominal pain, fever, nausea, vomiting, and fatigue and that may become life-threatening in immunocompromised individuals

CA–MRSA *abbr* community-acquired MRSA

can·a·gli·flo·zin \ˌka-nə-glə-ˈflō-zən\ *n* : a drug $C_{24}H_{25}FO_5S{\cdot}\frac{1}{2}H_2O$ that lowers blood sugar by reducing the reabsorption of glucose from the kidneys and is taken orally to treat type 2 diabetes — see INVOKAMET, INVOKANA

ca·nal \kə-ˈnal\ *n* : a tubular anatomical passage or channel : DUCT

can·a·lic·u·lus \ˌkan-ᵊl-ˈi-kyə-ləs\ *n, pl* **-li** \-ˌlī, -ˌlē\ : a minute canal in a bodily structure — **can·a·lic·u·lar** \-lər\ *adj*

ca·na·lis \kə-ˈna-ləs, -ˈnä-\ *n, pl* **ca·na·les** \-ˈna-(ˌ)lēz, -ˈnä-(ˌ)lās\ : CANAL

ca·na·li·za·tion \ˌkan-ᵊl-ə-ˈzā-shən\ *n* **1** : surgical formation of holes or canals for drainage without tubes **2** : natural formation of new channels in tissue (as formation of new blood vessels through a blood clot) **3** : establishment of new pathways in the central nervous system by repeated passage of nerve impulses

can·a·lize \ˈkan-ᵊl-ˌīz\ *vb* **-lized; -liz·ing** **1** : to drain (a wound) by forming channels without the use of tubes **2** : to develop new channels (as new capillaries in a blood clot)

canal of Schlemm \-ˈshlem\ *n* : a circular canal lying in the substance of the sclerocorneal junction of the eye and draining the aqueous humor from the anterior chamber into the veins draining the eyeball — called also *Schlemm's canal, sinus venosus sclerae*

Schlemm, Friedrich S. (1795–1858), German anatomist.

Can·a·van disease \ˈka-nə-ˌvan-\ *also* **Can·a·van's disease** \-ˌvanz-\ *n* : a rare usu. fatal demyelinating disease of infancy that is caused by an enzyme deficiency inherited as an autosomal recessive trait and that typically affects individuals of eastern European Jewish ancestry

Canavan, Myrtelle May (1879–1953), American pathologist.

can·cel·lous \kan-ˈse-ləs, ˈkan-sə-\ *adj* : having a porous structure made up of intersecting plates and bars that form small cavities or cells ⟨~ bone⟩ — compare COMPACT

can·cer \ˈkan-sər\ *n* **1** : a malignant tumor of potentially unlimited growth that expands locally by invasion and systemically by metastasis **2** : an abnormal state marked by a cancer — **can·cer·ous** \-sə-rəs\ *adj*

cancer eye *n* : a malignant squamous cell epithelioma of cattle

can·cer·i·ci·dal *or* **can·cer·o·ci·dal** \ˌkan-sə-rə-ˈsīd-ᵊl\ *adj* : destructive of cancer cells

can·cer·i·za·tion \-ˈzā-shən\ *n* : transformation into cancer or from a normal to a cancerous state

can·cer·o·gen·ic \-ˈje-nik, -rō-\ *or* **can·cer·i·gen·ic** \-rə-\ *adj* : CARCINOGENIC

can·cer·ol·o·gy \ˌkan-sə-ˈrä-lə-jē\ *n, pl* **-gies** : the study of cancer — **can·cer·ol·o·gist** \-jist\ *n*

can·cer·pho·bia \ˌkan-sər-ˈfō-bē-ə\ *or* **can·cer·o·pho·bia** \-sər-ō-ˈfō-\ *n* : an abnormal dread of cancer

can·crum oris \ˌkaŋ-krəm-ˈōr-əs, -ˈär-\ *n, pl* **can·cra oris** \-krə-\ : noma of the oral tissues — called also *gangrenous stomatitis*

can·de·la \kan-ˈdē-lə, -ˈde-\ *n* : a unit of luminous intensity in the International System of Units — called also *candle*

can·de·sar·tan \ˌkan-də-ˈsär-ˌtan\ *n* : an antihypertensive drug $C_{33}H_{34}N_6O_6$ that is taken orally and blocks the action of angiotensin II — see ATACAND, ATACAND HCT

can·di·ci·din \ˌkan-də-ˈsīd-ᵊn\ *n* : an antibiotic obtained from a streptomyces (*Streptomyces griseus*) and active against some fungi of the genus *Candida*

can·di·da \ˈkan-də-də\ *n* **1** *cap* : a genus of parasitic fungi that resemble yeasts and occur esp. in the mouth, vagina, and intestinal tract where they are usu. benign but can become pathogenic **2** : any fungus of the genus *Candida; esp* : one (*C. albicans*) causing thrush **3** : infection with fungi of the genus *Candida* : CANDIDIASIS — **can·di·dal** \-dəd-ᵊl\ *adj*

can·di·de·mia \ˌkan-də-ˈdē-mē-ə\ *n* : infection of the bloodstream with fungi of the genus *Candida* (as *C. albicans* or *C. parapsilosis*)

can·di·di·a·sis \ˌkan-də-ˈdī-ə-səs\ *n, pl* **-a·ses** \-ˌsēz\ : infection with or disease caused by a fungus of the genus *Candida* — called also *monilia, moniliasis*

can·dle \ˈkand-ᵊl\ *n* : CANDELA

candy striper *n* : a volunteer nurse's aide

ca·nic·o·la fever \kə-ˈni-kə-lə-\ *n* : a disease of humans and dogs marked by gastroenteritis and mild jaundice and caused by a spirochete of the genus *Leptospira* (*L. canicola*)

[1]**ca·nine** \ˈkā-ˌnīn\ *n* **1** : a conical pointed tooth; *esp* : one situated between the lateral incisor and the first premolar **2** : a canine mammal : DOG

[2]**canine** *adj* : of or relating to dogs or to the family (Canidae) to which they belong

canine distemper *n* : DISTEMPER 1

canine fossa *n* : a depression external to and somewhat above the prominence on the surface of the superior maxillary bone caused by the socket of the canine tooth

ca·ni·nus \kā-ˈnī-nəs, kə-\ *n, pl* **ca·ni·ni** \-ˈnī-ˌnī\ : LEVATOR ANGULI ORIS

ca·ni·ti·es \kə-ˈni-shē-ˌēz\ *n* : grayness or whiteness of the hair

can·ker \ˈkaŋ-kər\ *n* **1 a** : an erosive or spreading sore **b** : CANKER SORE **2 a** : a chronic inflammation of the ear in dogs, cats, or rabbits; *esp* : a localized form of mange **b** : a chronic inflammation of the hooves of horses — **can·kered** \-kərd\ *adj*

canker sore *n* : a painful shallow ulceration of the oral mucous membranes that has a grayish-white base surrounded by a reddish inflamed area and is characteristic of aphthous stomatitis

can·na·bi·noid \ˈka-nə-bə-ˌnȯid, kə-ˈna-\ *n* : any of various chemical constituents (as THC) of cannabis or marijuana

can·na·bis \ˈka-nə-bəs\ *n* **1 a** *cap* : a genus of annual herbs (family Moraceae) that have leaves with three to seven leaflets and female flowers in spikes along the erect stems and that include the hemp (*C. sativa*) **b** : HEMP 1 **2** : any of the preparations (as marijuana or hashish) or chemicals (as THC) that are derived from the hemp and are psychoactive

cannabis in·di·ca \-ˈin-di-kə\ *n, pl* **can·na·bes in·di·cae** \ˈka-nə-ˌbēz-ˈin-də-ˌsē, -ˌbās-ˈin-di-ˌkī\ : cannabis of a variety obtained in India

can·na·bism \ˈka-nə-ˌbi-zəm\ *n* **1** : habituation to the use of cannabis **2** : chronic poisoning from excessive smoking or chewing of cannabis

can·non \ˈka-nən\ *n* : the part of the leg in which the cannon bone is found

cannon bone *n* : a bone in hoofed mammals that supports the leg from the hock joint to the fetlock

can·nu·la *also* **can·u·la** \ˈkan-yə-lə\ *n, pl* **-las** *or* **-lae** \-ˌlē, -ˌlī\ : a small tube for insertion into a body cavity, duct, or vessel

can·nu·late \-ˌlāt\ *vb* **-lat·ed; -lat·ing** : to insert a cannula into — **can·nu·la·tion** \ˌkan-yə-ˈlā-shən\ *n*

can·nu·lize \ˈkan-yə-ˌlīz\ *vb* **-lized; -liz·ing** : CANNULATE — **can·nu·li·za·tion** \ˌkan-yə-lə-ˈzā-shən\ *n*

ca·no·la \kə-ˈnō-lə\ *n* **1** : a rape plant (*Brassica napus*) of the mustard family of an improved variety with seeds that are low in erucic acid and are the source of canola oil **2** : CANOLA OIL

canola oil *n* : an edible vegetable oil obtained from the seeds of canola that is high in monounsaturated fatty acids

can·thar·i·din \kan-ˈthar-əd-ᵊn\ *n* : a bitter crystalline compound $C_{10}H_{12}O_4$ that is the active blister-producing ingredient of cantharides

can·tha·ris \ˈkan-thə-rəs\ *n, pl* **can·thar·i·des** \kan-ˈthar-ə-ˌdēz\ **1** : SPANISH FLY 1 **2** *cantharides* : a preparation of dried beetles and esp. Spanish flies that contains cantharidin and is used in medicine as a blister-producing agent and formerly as an aphrodisiac — used with a sing. or pl. verb; called also *Spanish fly*

can·tha·xan·thin \ˌkan-thə-ˈzan-ˌthin\ *n* : a carotenoid $C_{40}H_{52}O_2$ used esp. as a color additive in food

can·thus \ˈkan-thəs\ *n, pl* **can·thi** \ˈkan-ˌthī, -ˌthē\ : either of the angles formed by the meeting of the upper and lower eyelids

[1]**cap** \ˈkap\ *n, often attrib* **1** : something that serves as a cover or protection esp. for a tip, knob, or end (as of a tooth) **2** : PATELLA, KNEECAP **3** *Brit* : CERVICAL CAP

[2]**cap** *vb* **capped; cap·ping** **1** : to invest (a student nurse) with a cap as an indication of completion of a probationary period of study **2** : to cover (a

diseased or exposed part of a tooth) with a protective substance

cap *abbr* capsule

ca·pac·i·ta·tion \kə-ˌpa-sə-ˈtā-shən\ *n* : the change undergone by sperm in the female reproductive tract that enables them to penetrate and fertilize an egg — **ca·pac·i·tate** \-ˌtāt\ *vb*

ca·pac·i·ty \kə-ˈpa-sə-tē, -ˈpas-tē\ *n, pl* **-ties** **1** : a measure of content : VOLUME — see VITAL CAPACITY **2** : legal qualification, competency, power, or fitness

CAPD *abbr* **1** central auditory processing disorder **2** continuous ambulatory peritoneal dialysis

cap·e·ci·ta·bine \ˌkap-ə-ˈsīt-ə-ˌbēn\ *n* : an antineoplastic drug $C_{15}H_{22}FN_3O_6$ used to treat metastatic breast cancer and cancers of the colon and rectum — see XELODA

cap·e·line \ˈka-pə-ˌlēn, -lən\ *n* : a cup-shaped bandage for the head, the shoulder, or the stump of an amputated limb

Cap·gras syndrome \ˌkap-ˈgrä-\ *n* : a delusional condition characterized by the false belief that known individuals (as family members) have been replaced by doubles or impostors

Capgras, Jean-Marie Joseph (1873–1950), French psychiatrist.

cap·il·lar·ia \ˌka-pə-ˈlar-ē-ə\ *n* **1** *cap* : a genus of slender white nematode worms (family Trichuridae) that include serious pathogens of the digestive tract of fowls and some parasites of mammals including one (*C. hepatica*) which is common in rodents and occas. invades the human liver sometimes with fatal results **2** : a nematode worm of the genus *Capillaria* — **cap·il·lar·id** \-ˈlar-əd, kə-ˈpi-lə-rəd\ *n*

ca·pil·la·ri·a·sis \kə-ˌpi-lə-ˈrī-ə-səs\ *also* **cap·il·lar·i·o·sis** \ˌka-pə-ˌler-ē-ˈō-səs\ *n, pl* **-a·ses** \-ˈrī-ə-ˌsēz\ *also* **-o·ses** \-ˈō-ˌsēz\ : infestation with or disease caused by nematode worms of the genus *Capillaria*

cap·il·lar·o·scope \ˌka-pə-ˈlar-ə-ˌskōp\ *n* : a microscope that permits visual examination of the living capillaries in nail beds, skin, and conjunctiva — **cap·il·la·ros·co·py** \ˌka-pə-lə-ˈräs-kə-pē\ *n*

[1]**cap·il·lary** \ˈka-pə-ˌler-ē\ *adj* **1 a** : resembling a hair esp. in slender elongated form **b** : having a very small bore ⟨a ~ tube⟩ **2** : of or relating to capillaries

[2]**capillary** *n, pl* **-lar·ies** **1** : a minute thin-walled vessel of the body; *esp* : any of the smallest blood vessels connecting arterioles with venules and forming networks throughout the body **2** : a capillary tube

capillary bed *n* : the whole system of capillaries of a body, part, or organ

capita *pl of* CAPUT

capitate *n* : the largest bone of the wrist that is situated between the hamate and the trapezoid in the distal row of carpal bones and that articulates with the third metacarpal

cap·i·tat·ed \ˈka-pə-ˌtā-təd\ *adj* : of, relating to, participating in, or being a health-care system in which a medical provider is given a set fee per patient (as by an HMO) regardless of the treatment required

cap·i·ta·tion \ˌka-pə-ˈtā-shən\ *n* **1** : a fixed per capita payment made periodically to a medical service provider (as a physician) by a managed care group (as an HMO) in return for medical care provided to enrolled individuals **2** : a capitated health-care system

cap·i·ta·tum \ˌka-pə-ˈtā-təm, -ˈtä-\ *n, pl* **cap·i·ta·ta** \-tə\ : CAPITATE

cap·i·tel·lum \ˌka-pə-ˈte-ləm\ *n, pl* **-tel·la** \-lə\ : a knoblike protuberance esp. at the end of a bone (as the humerus)

capitis — see LONGISSIMUS CAPITIS, LONGUS CAPITIS, OBLIQUUS CAPITIS INFERIOR, OBLIQUUS CAPITIS SUPERIOR, PEDICULOSIS CAPITIS, RECTUS CAPITIS POSTERIOR MAJOR, RECTUS CAPITIS POSTERIOR MINOR, SEMISPINALIS CAPITIS, SPINALIS CAPITIS, SPLENIUS CAPITIS, TINEA CAPITIS

ca·pit·u·lum \kə-ˈpi-chə-ləm\ *n, pl* **-la** \-lə\ : a rounded protuberance of an anatomical part — **ca·pit·u·lar** \-lər, -ˌlär\ *adj*

cap·let \ˈka-plət\ *n* : a capsule-shaped medicinal tablet

-capnia *n comb form* : carbon dioxide in the blood ⟨hyper*capnia*⟩

cap·no·gram \ˈkap-nō-ˌgram\ *n* : the waveform tracing produced by a capnograph

cap·no·graph \ˈkap-nō-ˌgraf\ *n* : a monitoring device that measures the concentration of carbon dioxide in exhaled air and displays a numerical readout and waveform tracing — **cap·no·graph·ic** \ˌkap-nō-ˈgra-fik\ *adj* — **cap·nog·ra·phy** \kap-ˈnä-grə-fē\ *n*

cap·nom·e·ter \kap-ˈnä-mə-tər\ *n* : a monitoring device that measures and numerically displays the concentration of carbon dioxide in exhaled air — **cap·nom·e·try** \-trē\ *n*

Cap·o·ten \ˈka-pō-ˌten\ *trademark* — used for a preparation of captopril

cap·re·o·my·cin \ˌka-prē-ō-ˈmīs-ᵊn\ *n* : an antibiotic obtained from a bacterium of the genus *Streptomyces* (*S. capreolus*) that is administered by injection to treat tuberculosis

ca·pro·ic acid \kə-ˈprō-ik-\ *n* : a liquid fatty acid $C_6H_{12}O_2$ that is found as a glycerol ester in fats and oils and is used in pharmaceuticals and flavors

cap·ry·late \ˈka-prə-ˌlāt\ *n* : a salt or ester of caprylic acid — see SODIUM CAPRYLATE

ca·pryl·ic acid \kə-ˈpri-lik-\ *n* : a fatty acid $C_8H_{16}O_2$ of rancid odor occurring in fats and oils

cap·sa·i·cin \kap-ˈsā-ə-sən\ *n* : a colorless irritant substance $C_{18}H_{27}NO_3$ obtained from various capsicums and used in topical creams for its analgesic properties — see ZOSTRIX

cap·si·cum \ˈkap-si-kəm\ *n* **1** : any of a genus (*Capsicum*) of tropical plants of the nightshade family (Solanaceae) that are widely cultivated for their many-seeded usu. fleshy-walled berries **2** : the dried ripe fruit of some capsicums (as *C. frutescens*) used as a gastric and intestinal stimulant

cap·sid \ˈkap-səd\ *n* : the protein shell of a virus particle that surrounds its nucleic acid

cap·so·mer \ˈkap-sə-mər\ *or* **cap·so·mere** \ˈkap-sə-ˌmir\ *n* : one of the subunits making up a viral capsid

capsul- *or* **capsuli-** *or* **capsulo-** *comb form* : capsule ⟨*capsul*itis⟩

cap·su·la \ˈkap-sə-lə\ *n, pl* **cap·su·lae** \-ˌlē, -ˌlī\ : CAPSULE

cap·su·lar \ˈkap-sə-lər\ *adj* : of, relating to, affecting, or resembling a capsule

capsular contracture *n* : shrinking and tightening of the mass of scar tissue around a breast implant that may result in pain and in unnatural firmness and distortion of the breast

capsularis — see DECIDUA CAPSULARIS

cap·su·lat·ed \-ˌlā-təd\ *also* **cap·su·late** \-ˌlāt, -lət\ *adj* : enclosed in a capsule

cap·su·la·tion \ˌkap-sə-ˈlā-shən\ *n* : enclosure in a capsule

cap·sule \ˈkap-səl, -(ˌ)sül\ *n* **1 a** : a membrane or saclike structure enclosing a part or organ ⟨the ~ of the kidney⟩ **b** : either of two layers or laminae of white matter in the cerebrum: (1) : a layer that consists largely of fibers passing to and from the cerebral cortex and that lies internal to the lentiform nucleus — called also *internal capsule* (2) : one that lies between the lentiform nucleus and the claustrum — called also *external capsule* **2** : a shell usu. of gelatin for packaging something (as a drug or vitamins); *also* : a usu. medicinal or nutritional preparation for oral use consisting of the shell and its contents **3** : a viscous or gelatinous often polysaccharide envelope surrounding certain microscopic organisms (as the pneumococcus)

cap·su·lec·to·my \ˌkap-sə-ˈlek-tə-mē\ *n, pl* **-mies** : excision of a capsule (as of a joint, kidney, or lens)

capsule endoscopy *n* : visualization of the interior of the digestive tract by means of a wireless camera encased in a pill-sized capsule that is swallowed — **capsule endoscope** *n*

capsule of Bow·man \-ˈbō-mən\ *n* : BOWMAN'S CAPSULE

capsule of Te·non \-tə-ˈnōⁿ\ *n* : TENON'S CAPSULE

cap·su·li·tis \ˌkap-sə-ˈlī-təs\ *n* : inflammation of a capsule (as that of the crystalline lens)

cap·su·lor·rha·phy \ˌkap-sə-ˈlȯr-ə-fē\ *n, pl* **-phies** : suture of a cut or wounded capsule (as of the knee joint)

cap·su·lot·o·my \-ˈlä-tə-mē\ *n, pl* **-mies** : incision of a capsule esp. of the crystalline lens (as in cataract surgery)

cap·to·pril \ˈkap-tə-ˌpril\ *n* : an antihypertensive drug $C_9H_{15}NO_3S$ that is an ACE inhibitor — see CAPOTEN

ca·put \ˈkä-ˌpu̇t, -pət; ˈka-pət\ *n, pl* **ca·pi·ta** \ˈkä-pə-ˌtä, ˈka-pə-tə\ **1** : a knoblike protuberance (as of a bone or muscle) **2** : CAPUT SUCCEDANEUM

caput suc·ce·da·ne·um \-ˌsək-sə-ˈdā-nē-əm\ *n, pl* **capita suc·ce·da·nea** \-ə\ : an edematous swelling formed upon the presenting part of the scalp of a newborn infant as a result of trauma sustained during delivery

Car·a·fate \ˈkar-ə-ˌfāt\ *trademark* — used for a preparation of sucralfate

ca·ra·te \kə-ˈrä-tē\ *n* : PINTA

carb \ˈkärb\ *or* **car·bo** \ˈkär-ˌbō\ *n* : CARBOHYDRATE; *also* : a high-carbohydrate food — usu. used in pl.

car·ba·chol \ˈkär-bə-ˌkȯl, -ˌkōl\ *n* : a synthetic parasympathomimetic drug $C_6H_{15}ClN_2O_2$ that is used topically to treat glaucoma

car·ba·mate \ˈkär-bə-ˌmāt, kär-ˈba-ˌmāt\ *n* : a salt or ester of carbamic acid — see URETHANE

car·ba·maz·e·pine \ˌkär-bə-ˈma-zə-ˌpēn\ *n* : a tricyclic anticonvulsant and analgesic $C_{15}H_{12}N_2O$ used in the treatment of trigeminal neuralgia and epilepsy — see TEGRETOL

car·bam·ic acid \(ˌ)kär-ˈba-mik-\ *n* : an acid CH_3NO_2 known in the form of salts and esters

carb·ami·no·he·mo·glo·bin \ˌkär-bə-ˌmē-(ˌ)nō-ˈhē-mə-ˌglō-bən\ *n* : a compound of hemoglobin with carbon dioxide

car·ba·pen·em \ˌkär-bə-ˈpe-nəm\ *n* : any of a class of broad-spectrum beta-lactam antibiotics (as imipenem)

carbapenem–resistant Enterobacteriaceae *n pl* : CRE

car·bar·sone \kär-ˈbär-ˌsōn\ *n* : a white powder $C_7H_9N_2O_4As$ used esp. in treating intestinal amebiasis

car·ba·zole \ˈkär-bə-ˌzōl\ *n* : a crystalline slightly basic cyclic compound $C_{12}H_9N$ used in testing for carbohydrates (as sugars)

car·ben·i·cil·lin \ˌkär-ˌbe-nə-ˈsi-lən\ *n* : a broad-spectrum semisynthetic penicillin $C_{17}H_{18}N_2O_6S$ that is used esp. against gram-negative bacteria (as pseudomonas)

carb·he·mo·glo·bin \(ˌ)kärb-ˈhē-mə-ˌglō-bən\ *or* **car·bo·hemo·glo·bin** \ˌkär-bō-\ *n* : CARBAMINOHEMOGLOBIN

car·bi·do·pa \ˌkär-bə-ˈdō-pə\ *n* : a drug $C_{10}H_{14}N_2O_4{\cdot}H_2O$ that is typically administered with L-dopa in the treatment of Parkinson's disease to increase the amount of L-dopa available for transport to the brain — see DUOPA,

LODOSYN, PARCOPA, RYTARY, SINEMET, STALEVO

carbo *var of* CARB

car•bo•hy•drase \ˌkär-bō-ˈhī-ˌdrās, -bə-, -ˌdrāz\ *n* : any of a group of enzymes (as amylase) that promote hydrolysis or synthesis of a carbohydrate (as a disaccharide)

car•bo•hy•drate \-ˌdrāt, -drət\ *n* : any of various neutral compounds of carbon, hydrogen, and oxygen (as sugars, starches, and celluloses) most of which are formed by green plants and which constitute a major class of animal foods

car•bol•fuch•sin paint \ˈkär-(ˌ)bäl-ˈfyük-sən-, -(ˌ)bȯl-\ *n* : a solution containing boric acid, phenol, resorcinol, and fuchsin in acetone, alcohol, and water that is applied externally in the treatment of fungal infections of the skin — called also *Castellani's paint*

car•bol•ic \kär-ˈbä-lik\ *n* : PHENOL 1

carbolic acid *n* : PHENOL 1

car•bo–load \ˈkär-ˌbō-ˈlōd\ *vb* : to consume foods high in carbohydrates esp. in preparation for an activity (as distance running) requiring long-lasting energy and endurance

car•bo•my•cin \ˌkär-bə-ˈmīs-ᵊn\ *n* : a colorless crystalline basic macrolide antibiotic $C_{42}H_{67}NO_{16}$ produced by a bacterium of the genus *Streptomyces* (*S. halstedii*) and active against gram-positive bacteria

car•bon \ˈkär-bən\ *n, often attrib* : a nonmetallic element found native (as in diamonds and graphite) or as a constituent of coal, petroleum, asphalt, limestone, and organic compounds or obtained artificially (as in activated charcoal) — symbol *C;* see ELEMENT table

car•bon•ate \ˈkär-bə-ˌnāt, -nət\ *n* : a salt or ester of carbonic acid

carbon dioxide *n* : a heavy colorless gas CO_2 that does not support combustion, dissolves in water to form carbonic acid and is formed esp. in animal respiration and in the decay or combustion of animal and vegetable matter

carbon 14 *n* : a heavy radioactive isotope of carbon of mass number 14 used esp. in tracer studies

car•bon•ic acid \kär-ˈbä-nik-\ *n* : a weak acid H_2CO_3 known only in solution that reacts with bases to form carbonates

carbonic an•hy•drase \an-ˈhī-ˌdrās, -ˌdrāz\ *n* : a zinc-containing enzyme that occurs in living tissues (as red blood cells) and aids carbon-dioxide transport from the tissues and its release from the blood in the lungs by catalyzing the reversible hydration of carbon dioxide to carbonic acid

carbon monoxide *n* : a colorless odorless very toxic gas CO that is formed as a product of the incomplete combustion of carbon

carbon tetrachloride *n* : a colorless nonflammable toxic carcinogenic liquid CCl_4 that has an odor resembling that of chloroform and is used as a solvent and a refrigerant

car•bo•plat•in \ˈkär-bō-ˌpla-tᵊn\ *n* : a platinum-containing antineoplastic drug $C_6H_{12}N_2O_4Pt$ that is an analog of cisplatin with somewhat reduced toxicity and that is used in the treatment of various cancers

car•boxy•he•mo•glo•bin \(ˌ)kär-ˌbäk-sē-ˈhē-mə-ˌglō-bən\ *n* : a very stable combination of hemoglobin and carbon monoxide formed in the blood when carbon monoxide is inhaled with resulting loss of ability of the blood to combine with oxygen

car•box•yl \kär-ˈbäk-səl\ *n* : a monovalent group –COOH typical of organic acids — called also *carboxyl group* — **car•box•yl•ic** \ˌkär-(ˌ)bäk-ˈsi-lik\ *adj*

car•box•yl•ase \kär-ˈbäk-sə-ˌlās, -ˌlāz\ *n* : an enzyme that catalyzes decarboxylation or carboxylation

car•box•yl•ate \-ˌlāt, -lət\ *n* : a salt or ester of a carboxylic acid — **car•box•yl•ate** \-ˌlāt\ *vb* — **car•box•yl•ation** \(ˌ)kär-ˌbäk-sə-ˈlā-shen\ *n*

carboxylic acid *n* : an organic acid (as an acetic acid) containing one or more carboxyl groups

car•boxy•meth•yl•cel•lu•lose \(ˌ)kär-ˌbäk-sē-ˌme-thəl-ˈsel-yə-ˌlōs, -ˌlōz\ *n* : a derivative of cellulose that in the form of its sodium salt is used as a bulk laxative in medicine

car•boxy•pep•ti•dase \-ˈpep-tə-ˌdās, -ˌdāz\ *n* : an enzyme that hydrolyzes peptides and esp. polypeptides by splitting off sequentially the amino acids at the end of the peptide chain which contain free carboxyl groups

car•bun•cle \ˈkär-ˌbəŋ-kəl\ *n* : a painful local purulent inflammation of the skin and deeper tissues with multiple openings for the discharge of pus and usu. necrosis and sloughing of dead tissue — **car•bun•cu•lar** \kär-ˈbəŋ-kyə-lər\ *adj*

car•bun•cu•lo•sis \kär-ˌbəŋ-kyə-ˈlō-səs\ *n, pl* **-lo•ses** \-ˌsēz\ : a condition marked by the formation of many carbuncles simultaneously or in rapid succession

carcin- *or* **carcino-** *comb form* : tumor : cancer ⟨*carcino*genic⟩

car•ci•no•em•bry•on•ic antigen \ˌkärs-ᵊn-ō-ˌem-brē-ˈä-nik-\ *n* : a glycoprotein present in fetal gut tissues during the first two trimesters of pregnancy and in peripheral blood of patients with some forms of cancer (as of the digestive system) — abbr. *CEA*

car•cin•o•gen \kär-ˈsi-nə-jən, ˈkärs-ᵊn-ə-ˌjen\ *n* : a substance or agent causing cancer

car•ci•no•gen•e•sis \ˌkärs-ᵊn-ō-ˈje-nə-səs\ *n, pl* **-e•ses** \-ˌsēz\ : the production of cancer

car•ci•no•gen•ic \ˌkärs-ᵊn-ō-ˈje-nik\ *adj* : producing or tending to produce cancer ⟨~ compounds⟩ — **car·ci·no·gen·i·cal·ly** \-ni-k(ə-)lē\ *adv* — **car·ci·no·ge·nic·i·ty** \-jə-ˈni-sə-tē\ *n*

car·ci·noid \ˈkärs-ᵊn-ˌȯid\ *n* : a benign or malignant tumor arising esp. from the mucosa of the gastrointestinal tract (as in the stomach or appendix)

carcinoid syndrome *n* : a syndrome that is caused by vasoactive substances secreted by carcinoid tumors and is characterized by flushing, cyanosis, abdominal cramps, diarrhea, and valvular heart disease

car·ci·no·ma \ˌkärs-ᵊn-ˈō-mə\ *n, pl* **-mas** *also* **-ma·ta** \-mə-tə\ : a malignant tumor of epithelial origin — compare SARCOMA — **car·ci·no·ma·tous** \-mə-təs\ *adj*

carcinoma in situ *n* : carcinoma in the stage of development when the cancer cells are still within their site of origin (as the mouth or uterine cervix)

car·ci·no·ma·to·sis \-ˌō-mə-ˈtō-səs\ *n, pl* **-to·ses** \-ˌsēz\ : a condition in which multiple carcinomas develop simultaneously usu. after dissemination from a primary source

car·ci·no·sar·co·ma \ˈkärs-ᵊn-ō-(ˌ)sär-ˈkō-mə\ *n, pl* **-mas** *also* **-ma·ta** \-mə-tə\ : a malignant tumor combining elements of carcinoma and sarcoma

car·ci·no·stat·ic \ˌkär-sə-nō-ˈsta-tik\ *adj* : capable of inhibiting the growth of malignant tumors

cardi- *or* **cardio-** *comb form* : heart : cardiac : cardiac and ⟨*cardio*gram⟩

car·dia \ˈkär-dē-ə\ *n, pl* **car·di·ae** \-ˌē\ *or* **cardias** **1** : the opening of the esophagus into the stomach **2** : the part of the stomach adjoining the cardia

¹-car·dia \ˈkär-dē-ə\ *n comb form* : heart action or location (of a specified type) ⟨tachy*cardia*⟩

²-cardia *pl of* -CARDIUM

¹car·di·ac \ˈkär-dē-ˌak\ *adj* **1 a** : of, relating to, situated near, or acting on the heart **b** : of or relating to the cardia of the stomach **2** : of, relating to, or affected with heart disease

²cardiac *n* : a person with heart disease

cardiac arrest *n* : abrupt temporary or permanent cessation of the heartbeat (as from ventricular fibrillation or asystole) — called also *sudden cardiac arrest*

cardiac asthma *n* : asthma due to heart disease (as heart failure) that occurs in paroxysms usu. at night and is characterized by difficult wheezing respiration, pallor, and anxiety — called also *paroxysmal dyspnea*

cardiac catheterization *n* : a medical procedure in which a catheter is inserted through an artery or vein (as of the arm or leg) and passed into the heart for diagnosis and treatment of heart conditions — **cardiac catheter** *n*

cardiac cycle *n* : the complete sequence of events in the heart from the beginning of one beat to the beginning of the following beat : a complete heartbeat including systole and diastole

cardiac failure *n* : HEART FAILURE

cardiac gland *n* : any of the branched tubular mucus-secreting glands of the cardia of the stomach; *also* : one of the similar glands of the esophagus

cardiac glycoside *n* : a glycoside (as digitoxin) that acts on the heart to increase the force and rate of myocardial contraction

cardiac index *n* : a measure of cardiac output per square meter of body surface area

cardiac massage *n* : the manual application of rhythmic pressure on the heart esp. to resuscitate a person experiencing cardiac arrest — called also *heart massage*

cardiac muscle *n* : the principal muscle tissue of the vertebrate heart that is made up of elongated striated fibers joined at usu. branched ends by intercalated disks and that is synchronized to function in contraction esp. by electrical signals of extrinsic origin passing through gap junctions in the intercalated disks — compare SMOOTH MUSCLE, STRIATED MUSCLE

cardiac nerve *n* : any of the three nerves connecting the cervical ganglia of the sympathetic nervous system with the cardiac plexus

cardiac neurosis *n* : NEUROCIRCULATORY ASTHENIA

cardiac output *n* : the volume of blood ejected from the left side of the heart in one minute — called also *minute volume*

cardiac plexus *n* : a nerve plexus of the autonomic nervous system supplying the heart and neighboring structures and situated near the heart and the arch and ascending part of the aorta

cardiac reserve *n* : the difference between the rate at which a heart pumps blood at a particular time and its maximum capacity for pumping blood

cardiac sphincter *n* : the somewhat thickened muscular ring surrounding the opening between the esophagus and the stomach

cardiac tamponade *n* : mechanical compression of the heart by large amounts of fluid or blood within the pericardial space that limits the normal range of motion and function of the heart

cardiac valve *n* : HEART VALVE

cardiac vein *n* : any of the veins returning the blood from the tissues of the heart that open into the right atrium either directly or through the coronary sinus

car·di·al·gia \ˌkär-dē-ˈal-jə, -jē-ə\ *n* **1** : HEARTBURN **2** : pain in the heart

car·di·ec·to·my \ˌkär-dē-ˈek-tə-mē\ *n, pl* **-mies** : excision of the cardiac portion of the stomach

cardinal vein *n* : any of four longitudinal veins of the vertebrate embryo running anteriorly and posteriorly along each side of the spinal column with the pair on each side meeting at and discharging blood to the heart through a large venous sinus — called also *cardinal sinus, Cuvierian vein*

[1]**car·dio** \ˈkär-dē-ō\ *adj* : CARDIOVASCULAR 2 ⟨~ exercises⟩

[2]**cardio** *n* : cardiovascular exercise

cardio- — see CARDI-

car·dio·ac·cel·er·a·tor \ˌkär-dē-(ˌ)ō-ik-ˈse-lə-ˌrā-tər, -ak-\ *adj* : speeding up the action of the heart — **car·dio·ac·cel·er·a·tion** \-ˌse-lə-ˈrā-shən\ *n*

car·dio·ac·tive \-ˈak-tiv\ *adj* : having an influence on the heart ⟨~ drugs⟩

car·dio·cir·cu·la·to·ry \-ˈsər-kyə-lə-ˌtōr-ē\ *adj* : of or relating to the heart and circulatory system ⟨~ failure⟩

car·dio·dy·nam·ics \-dī-ˈna-miks\ *n sing or pl* : the dynamics of the heart's action in pumping blood — **car·dio·dy·nam·ic** \-mik\ *adj*

car·dio·gen·ic \ˈ-je-nik\ *adj* : originating in the heart : caused by a cardiac condition ⟨~ pulmonary edema⟩

cardiogenic shock *n* : shock resulting from failure of the heart to pump an adequate amount of blood as a result of heart disease and esp. heart attack

car·dio·gram \ˈkär-dē-ə-ˌgram\ *n* : the curve or tracing made by a cardiograph

car·dio·graph \ˌ-graf\ *n* : an instrument that registers graphically movements of the heart — **car·dio·graph·ic** \ˌkär-dē-ə-ˈgra-fik\ *adj* — **car·di·og·ra·phy** \ˌkär-dē-ˈä-grə-fē\ *n*

car·dio·in·hib·i·to·ry \ˌkär-dē-(ˌ)ō-in-ˈhi-bə-ˌtōr-ē\ *adj* : interfering with or slowing the normal sequence of events in the cardiac cycle ⟨the ~ center of the medulla⟩

car·dio·lip·in \ˌkär-dē-ō-ˈli-pən\ *n* : a phospholipid used in combination with lecithin and cholesterol as an antigen in diagnostic blood tests for syphilis

car·di·ol·o·gy \ˌkär-dē-ˈä-lə-jē\ *n, pl* **-gies** : the study of the heart and its action and diseases — **car·di·o·log·i·cal** \-ə-ˈlä-ji-kəl\ *adj* — **car·di·ol·o·gist** \-ˈä-lə-jist\ *n*

car·dio·meg·a·ly \ˌkär-dē-ō-ˈme-gə-lē\ *n, pl* **-lies** : enlargement of the heart

car·dio·myo·cyte \ˌkär-dē-ō-ˈmī-ə-ˌsīt\ *n* : a muscle cell of the heart

car·dio·my·op·a·thy \ˈkär-dē-ō-(ˌ)mī-ˈä-pə-thē\ *n, pl* **-thies** : any structural or functional disease of heart muscle that is marked esp. by enlargement of the heart, by hypertrophy of cardiac muscle, or by rigidity and loss of flexibility of the heart walls and that may be idiopathic or attributable to a specific cause (as heart valve disease, untreated high blood pressure, or viral infection)

car·di·op·a·thy \ˌkär-dē-ˈä-pə-thē\ *n, pl* **-thies** : any disease of the heart

car·dio·plas·ty \ˈkär-dē-ō-ˌplas-tē\ *n, pl* **-ties** : surgical repair of the gastric cardiac sphincter — called also *esophagogastroplasty*

car·dio·ple·gia \ˌkär-dē-ō-ˈplē-jə, -jē-ə\ *n* : temporary cardiac arrest induced (as by drugs) during heart surgery — **car·dio·ple·gic** \-jik\ *adj*

car·dio·pro·tec·tive \ˌkär-dē-ō-prə-ˈtek-tiv\ *adj* : serving to protect the heart esp. from heart disease ⟨~ drugs⟩ — **car·dio·pro·tec·tion** \-prə-ˈtek-shən\ *n*

car·dio·pul·mo·nary \ˌkär-dē-ō-ˈpu̇l-mə-ˌner-ē, -ˈpəl-\ *adj* : of or relating to the heart and lungs ⟨a ~ bypass⟩

cardiopulmonary resuscitation *n* : a procedure designed to restore normal breathing after cardiac arrest that includes the clearance of air passages to the lungs, the mouth-to-mouth method of artificial respiration, and cardiac massage by the exertion of pressure on the chest — abbr. *CPR*

car·dio·re·nal \-ˈrēn-ᵊl\ *adj* : of or relating to the heart and the kidneys

car·dio·re·spi·ra·to·ry \ˌkär-dē-ō-ˈres-pə-rə-ˌtōr-ē, -ri-ˈspī-rə-\ *adj* : of or relating to the heart and the respiratory system : CARDIOPULMONARY

car·dio·scle·ro·sis \ˌkär-dē-(ˌ)ō-sklə-ˈrō-səs\ *n, pl* **-ro·ses** \-ˌsēz\ : induration of the heart caused by formation of fibrous tissue in the cardiac muscle

car·dio·spasm \ˈkär-dē-ō-ˌspa-zəm\ *n* : failure of the cardiac sphincter to relax during swallowing with resultant esophageal obstruction

car·dio·ta·chom·e·ter \ˌkär-dē-(ˌ)ō-ta-ˈkä-mə-tər\ *n* : a device for prolonged graphic recording of the heartbeat

car·dio·tho·ra·cic \-thə-ˈra-sik\ *adj* : relating to, involving, or specializing in the heart and chest ⟨~ surgery⟩

car·di·ot·o·my \ˌkär-dē-ˈä-tə-mē\ *n, pl* **-mies 1** : surgical incision of the heart **2** : surgical incision of the stomach cardia

[1]**car·dio·ton·ic** \ˌkär-dē-ō-ˈtä-nik\ *adj* : tending to increase the tonus of heart muscle ⟨~ steroids⟩

[2]**cardiotonic** *n* : a cardiotonic substance

car·dio·tox·ic \-ˈtäk-sik\ *adj* : having a toxic effect on the heart — **car·dio·tox·ic·i·ty** \-täk-ˈsi-sə-tē\ *n*

[1]**car·dio·vas·cu·lar** \-ˈvas-kyə-lər\ *adj* **1** : of, relating to, or involving the heart and blood vessels ⟨~ disease⟩ **2** : used, designed, or performed to cause a temporary increase in heart rate ⟨a ~ workout⟩

[2]**cardiovascular** *n* : a substance (as a drug) that affects the heart or blood vessels

car·dio·ver·sion \-ˈvər-zhən, -shən\ *n* : application of an electric shock in order to restore normal heartbeat

car·dio·ver·ter \ˈkär-dē-ō-ˌvər-tər\ *n* : a device for the administration of an electric shock in cardioversion

car·di·tis \kär-ˈdī-təs\ *n, pl* **car·dit·i·des** \-ˈdi-tə-ˌdēz\ : inflammation of the heart muscle : MYOCARDITIS

-car·di·um \ˈkär-dē-əm\ *n comb form, pl* **-car·dia** \-ē-ə\ : heart ⟨epi*cardium*⟩

Car·di·zem \ˈkär-də-ˌzem\ *trademark* — used for a preparation of the hydrochloride of diltiazem

Car·dura \kär-ˈdu̇r-ə\ *trademark* — used for a preparation of the mesylate of doxazosin

care \ˈker, ˈkar\ *n* : responsibility for or attention to health, well-being, and safety — see ACUTE CARE, HEALTH CARE, INTENSIVE CARE, PRIMARY CARE, TERTIARY CARE — **care** *vb*

care·giv·er \-ˌgi-vər\ *n* : a person who provides direct care (as for children, elderly people, or the chronically ill) — **care·giv·ing** \-ˌgi-viŋ\ *n*

car·ies \ˈkar-ēz, ˈker-\ *n, pl* **caries** : a progressive destruction of bone or tooth; *esp* : tooth decay

ca·ri·na \kə-ˈrī-nə, -ˈrē-\ *n, pl* **carinas** *or* **ca·ri·nae** \-ˈrī-ˌnē, -ˈrē-ˌnī\ : any of various keel-shaped anatomical structures, ridges, or processes

carinii — see PNEUMOCYSTIS CARINII PNEUMONIA

cario- *comb form* : caries ⟨*cario*genic⟩

car·io·gen·ic \ˌkar-ē-ō-ˈje-nik\ *adj* : producing or promoting the development of tooth decay ⟨~ foods⟩

car·io·stat·ic \-ˈsta-tik\ *adj* : tending to inhibit the formation of dental caries

car·i·ous \ˈkar-ē-əs, ˈker-\ *adj* : affected with caries ⟨~ teeth⟩

ca·ri·so·pro·dol \kə-ˌrī-sə-ˈprō-ˌdȯl, -zə-, -ˌdōl\ *n* : a drug $C_{12}H_{24}N_2O_4$ related to meprobamate that is used to relax muscle and relieve pain — see SOMA

[1]**car·mi·na·tive** \kär-ˈmi-nə-tiv, ˈkär-mə-ˌnā-\ *adj* : expelling gas from the stomach or intestines so as to relieve flatulence or abdominal pain or distension

[2]**carminative** *n* : a carminative agent

car·mus·tine \ˈkär-mə-ˌstēn\ *n* : a nitrosourea $C_5H_9Cl_2N_3O_2$ used as an antineoplastic drug (as in the treatment of brain tumors) — called also *BCNU;* see BICNU

car·ni·tine \ˈkär-nə-ˌtēn\ *n* : a quaternary ammonium compound $C_7H_{15}NO_3$ present esp. in muscle and involved in the transfer of fatty acids across mitochondrial membranes

car·o·ten·ae·mia *chiefly Brit var of* CAROTENEMIA

car·o·tene \ˈkar-ə-ˌtēn\ *n* : any of several orange or red hydrocarbon pigments (as $C_{40}H_{56}$) that occur in plants and in the fatty tissues of plant-eating animals and are convertible to vitamin A — see BETA-CAROTENE

car·o·ten·emia \ˌkar-ə-tə-ˈnē-mē-ə\ *n* : a yellowing of the skin resembling jaundice that is associated with increased levels of carotene in the blood

ca·rot·enoid \kə-ˈrät-ᵊn-ˌȯid\ *n* : any of various usu. yellow to red pigments (as carotenes) found widely in plants and animals — **carotenoid** *adj*

caroticum — see GLOMUS CAROTICUM

ca·rot·id \kə-ˈrä-təd\ *adj* : of, situated near, or involving a carotid artery

carotid artery *n* : either of the two main arteries that supply blood to the head of which the left in humans arises from the arch of the aorta and the right by bifurcation of the brachiocephalic artery — called also *carotid;* see COMMON CAROTID ARTERY, EXTERNAL CAROTID ARTERY, INTERNAL CAROTID ARTERY

carotid body *n* : a small body of vascular tissue that adjoins the carotid sinus, functions as a chemoreceptor sensitive to change in the oxygen content of blood, and mediates reflex changes in respiratory activity — called also *carotid gland, glomus caroticum*

carotid canal *n* : the canal by which the internal carotid artery enters the skull — called also *carotid foramen*

carotid plexus *n* : a network of nerves of the sympathetic nervous system surrounding the internal carotid artery

carotid sinus *n* : a small but richly innervated arterial enlargement that is located near the point in the neck where the common carotid artery divides into the internal and the external carotid arteries and that functions in the regulation of heart rate and blood pressure

carotid triangle *n* : a space in each lateral half of the neck that is bounded in back by the sternocleidomastoid muscle, below by the omohyoid muscle, and above by the stylohyoid and digastric muscles

carp- *or* **carpo-** *comb form* **1** : carpus ⟨*carp*ectomy⟩ **2** : carpal and ⟨*carpo*metacarpal⟩

[1]**car·pal** \ˈkär-pəl\ *adj* : relating to the carpus

[2]**carpal** *n* : a carpal element : CARPALE

car·pa·le \kär-ˈpa-(ˌ)lē, -ˈpā-, -ˈpä-\ *n, pl* **-lia** \-lē-ə\ : a carpal bone; *esp* : one of the distal series articulating with the metacarpals

carpal tunnel *n* : a passage between the flexor retinaculum of the hand and the carpal bones that is sometimes a site of compression of the median nerve

carpal tunnel syndrome *n* : a condition caused by compression of the median nerve in the carpal tunnel and characterized esp. by weakness, pain, and disturbances of sensation in the hand and fingers

car·pec·to·my \kär-ˈpek-tə-mē\ *n, pl* **-mies** : excision of a carpal bone

carpi — see EXTENSOR CARPI RADIALIS BREVIS, EXTENSOR CARPI RADIALIS LONGUS, EXTENSOR CARPI ULNARIS,

FLEXOR CARPI RADIALIS, FLEXOR CARPI ULNARIS

carpo- — see CARP-

car•po•meta•car•pal \ˌkär-pō-ˈme-tə-ˌkär-pəl\ *adj* : relating to, situated between, or joining a carpus and metacarpus ⟨a ~ joint⟩

car•po•ped•al spasm \ˌkär-pə-ˈped-ᵊl-, -ˈpēd-\ *n* : a spasmodic contraction of the muscles of the hands, feet, or esp. the wrists and ankles (as that occurring in alkalosis and tetany)

car•pus \ˈkär-pəs\ *n, pl* **car•pi** \-ˌpī, -ˌpē\ **1** : WRIST **2** : the group of bones supporting the wrist comprising in humans a proximal row which contains the scaphoid, lunate, triquetrum, and pisiform that articulate with the radius and a distal row which contains the trapezium, trapezoid, capitate, and hamate that articulate with the metacarpals

car•riage \ˈkar-ij\ *n* : the condition of harboring a pathogen within the body

car•ri•er \ˈkar-ē-ər\ *n* **1 a** : a person, animal, or plant that harbors and transmits the causative agent of an infectious disease; *esp* : one that carries the causative agent systemically but is asymptomatic or immune to it ⟨a ~ of typhoid fever⟩ — compare RESERVOIR 2, VECTOR 1 **b** : an individual possessing a specified gene and capable of transmitting it to offspring but not expressing or only weakly expressing its phenotype; *esp* : one that is heterozygous for a recessive factor **2** : a vehicle serving esp. as a diluent (as for a drug)

Car•ri•ón's disease \ˌkar-ē-ˈōnz-\ *n* : BARTONELLOSIS

Carrión, Daniel A. (1850–1885), Peruvian medical student.

car•ry \ˈkar-ē\ *vb* **1** : to harbor (a pathogen) within the body **2** : to possess a specified gene; *specif* : to possess one copy of a specified recessive gene and be capable of transmitting it to offspring

car•sick \ˈkär-ˌsik\ *adj* : affected with motion sickness esp. in an automobile — **car sickness** *n*

car•ti•lage \ˈkärt-ᵊl-ij, ˈkärt-lij\ *n* **1** : a usu. translucent somewhat elastic tissue that composes most of the skeleton of vertebrate embryos and except for a small number of structures (as some joints, respiratory passages, and the external ear) is replaced by bone during ossification in the higher vertebrates **2** : a part or structure composed of cartilage

car•ti•lag•i•nous \ˌkärt-ᵊl-ˈa-jə-nəs\ *adj* : composed of, relating to, or resembling cartilage

car•un•cle \ˈkar-əŋ-kəl, kə-ˈrəŋ-\ *n* : a small fleshy growth; *specif* : a reddish growth situated at the urethral meatus in women and causing pain and bleeding — see LACRIMAL CARUNCLE

ca•run•cu•la \kə-ˈrəŋ-kyə-lə\ *n, pl* **-lae** \-ˌlē, -ˌlī\ : CARUNCLE

car•ve•dil•ol \ˈkär-və-ˌdil-ˌȯl\ *n* : a beta-blocker $C_{24}H_{26}N_2O_4$ that is used to treat congestive heart failure and hypertension and to manage patients with left ventricular dysfunction following heart attack — see COREG

cary- *or* **caryo-** — see KARY-

ca•san•thra•nol \kə-ˈsan-thrə-ˌnȯl\ *n* : a mixture of glycosides extracted from cascara sagrada and having laxative properties

cas•cade \(ˌ)kas-ˈkād\ *n* : a molecular, biochemical, or physiological process occurring in a succession of stages each of which is closely related to or depends on the output of the previous stage ⟨an enzymatic ~⟩

cas•cara sa•gra•da \kas-ˈkar-ə-sə-ˈgrä-də, -ˈkär-; ˈkas-kə-rə-\ *n* : the dried bark of a buckthorn (*Rhamnus purshiana*) used as a mild laxative — called also *cascara*

case \ˈkās\ *n* **1** : the circumstances and situation of a particular person or group **2 a** : an instance of disease or injury ⟨90 ~*s* of flu⟩ **b** : PATIENT 1

ca•se•ation \ˌkā-sē-ˈā-shən\ *n* : necrosis with conversion of damaged tissue into a soft cheesy substance — **ca•se•ate** \ˈkā-sē-ˌāt\ *vb*

case•book \ˈkās-ˌbu̇k\ *n* : a book containing medical records of illustrative cases that is used for reference and instruction

case history *n* : a record of an individual's personal or family history and environment for use in analysis or instructive illustration

ca•sein \kā-ˈsēn, ˈkā-sē-ən\ *n* : any of several phosphoproteins of milk

case•load \ˈkās-ˌlōd\ *n* : the number of cases handled (as by a clinic) in a particular period

caseosa — see VERNIX CASEOSA

ca•se•ous \ˈkā-sē-əs\ *adj* : marked by caseation

caseous lymphadenitis *n* : a chronic infectious disease of sheep and goats characterized by caseation esp. of the lymph glands that is caused by a bacterium of the genus *Corynebacterium* (*C. pseudotuberculosis*) — called also *pseudotuberculosis*

case•work \ˈkās-ˌwərk\ *n* : social work involving direct consideration of the problems, needs, and adjustments of the individual case (as a person or family in need of psychiatric aid) — **case•work•er** \-ˌwər-kər\ *n*

cas•sette *also* **ca•sette** \kə-ˈset, ka-\ *n* : a lightproof magazine for holding the intensifying screens and film in X-ray photography

cast \ˈkast\ *n* **1** : a slight strabismus **2** : a rigid casing (as of fiberglass or of gauze impregnated with plaster of paris) used for immobilizing a usu. diseased or broken part **3** : a mass of plastic matter formed in cavities of diseased organs (as the kidneys) and discharged from the body

Cas·tel·la·ni's paint \ˌkas-tə-ˈlä-nēz-\ *n* : CARBOLFUCHSIN PAINT
Cas·tel·la·ni \ˌkäs-tə-ˈlä-nē\, **Aldo (1878–1971),** Italian physician.

Cas·tle·man's disease \ˈkas-əl-mənz-\ *or* **Castleman disease** *n* : a disorder that is characterized by enlargement of the lymph nodes due to benign overgrowth of lymphoid tissue and is marked esp. by fever, weight loss, and fatigue — called also *angiofollicular lymph node hyperplasia, giant lymph node hyperplasia*
Castleman, Benjamin (1906–1982), American pathologist.

cas·tor bean \ˈkas-tər-\ *n* : the very poisonous seed of the castor-oil plant; *also* : CASTOR-OIL PLANT

castor oil *n* : a pale viscous fatty oil from castor beans used esp. as a cathartic

castor–oil plant *n* : a tropical Old World herb (*Ricinus communis*) of the spurge family (Euphorbiaceae) bearing oil-rich castor beans that are a source of castor oil

[1]**cas·trate** \ˈkas-ˌtrāt\ *vb* **cas·trat·ed; cas·trat·ing 1 a** : to deprive of the testes : GELD **b** : to deprive of the ovaries : SPAY **2** : to render impotent or deprive of vitality esp. by psychological means — **cas·trat·er** *or* **cas·tra·tor** \-ˈtrā-tər\ *n*

[2]**castrate** *n* : a castrated individual

cas·tra·tion \kas-ˈtrā-shən\ *n* **1** : the removal of testes or ovaries **2** : CHEMICAL CASTRATION

castration complex *n, in Freudian psychoanalytic theory* : a child's fear of genital injury at the hands of the parent of the same sex as punishment for unconscious guilt over oedipal strivings; *broadly* : the often unconscious fear or feeling of bodily injury or loss of power at the hands of authority

ca·su·al·ty \ˈka-zhəl-tē, ˈka-zhə-wəl-\ *n, pl* **-ties 1** : a serious or fatal accident **2** : a military person lost through death, wounds, injury, sickness, internment, or capture or through being missing in action **3 a** : injury or death from accident **b** : one injured or killed (as by accident)

CAT *abbr* computed axial tomography; computerized axial tomography

cata- *or* **cat-** *or* **cath-** *prefix* : down ⟨*cata*mnesis⟩ ⟨*cata*plexy⟩

ca·tab·o·lism \kə-ˈta-bə-ˌli-zəm\ *n* : destructive metabolism involving the release of energy and resulting in the breakdown of complex materials within the organism — compare ANABOLISM — **cat·a·bol·ic** \ˌka-tə-ˈbä-lik\ *adj* — **cat·a·bol·i·cal·ly** \-li-k(ə-)lē\ *adv*

ca·tab·o·lite \-ˌlīt\ *n* : a product of catabolism

ca·tab·o·lize \-ˌlīz\ *vb* **-lized; -liz·ing** : to subject to or undergo catabolism

cat·a·gen \ˈka-tə-ˌjen\ *n* : a short transition phase of the hair growth cycle in which hair growth ends and the resting phase begins

cat·a·lase \ˈkat-ᵊl-ˌās, -ˌāz\ *n* : an enzyme that consists of a protein complex with hematin groups and catalyzes the decomposition of hydrogen peroxide into water and oxygen

cat·a·lep·sy \ˈkat-ᵊl-ˌep-sē\ *n, pl* **-sies** : a trancelike state of consciousness (as that occurring in catatonic schizophrenia) that is marked by a loss of voluntary motion and a fixed posture in which the limbs remain in whatever position they are placed — compare WAXY FLEXIBILITY

[1]**cat·a·lep·tic** \ˌkat-ᵊl-ˈep-tik\ *adj* : of, having the characteristics of, or affected with catalepsy ⟨a ~ state⟩

[2]**cataleptic** *n* : one affected with catalepsy

ca·tal·y·sis \kə-ˈta-lə-səs\ *n, pl* **-y·ses** \-ˌsēz\ : a change and esp. increase in the rate of a chemical reaction induced by a catalyst — **cat·a·lyt·ic** \ˈkat-ᵊl-ˈi-tik\ *adj* — **cat·a·lyt·i·cal·ly** \-ti-k(ə-)lē\ *adv*

cat·a·lyst \ˈka-tᵊl-əst\ *n* : a substance (as an enzyme) that enables a chemical reaction to proceed at a usu. faster rate or under different conditions (as at a lower temperature) than otherwise possible

cat·a·lyze \ˈkat-ᵊl-ˌīz\ *vb* **-lyzed; -lyz·ing** : to bring about the catalysis of (a chemical reaction) — **cat·a·lyz·er** *n*

cata·me·nia \ˌka-tə-ˈmē-nē-ə\ *n pl* : MENSES

cata·me·ni·al \-nē-əl\ *adj* : relating to or associated with menstruation ⟨~ pneumothorax⟩

cat·am·ne·sis \ˌkat-ˌam-ˈnē-səs\ *n, pl* **-ne·ses** \-ˌsēz\ : the follow-up medical history of a patient — **cat·am·nes·tic** \-ˈnes-tik\ *adj*

cat·a·plasm \ˈka-tə-ˌpla-zəm\ *n* : POULTICE

cat·a·plexy \ˈka-tə-ˌplek-sē\ *n, pl* **-plex·ies** \-sēz\ : sudden loss of muscle power with retention of clear consciousness following a strong emotional stimulus (as shock or anger)

cat·a·ract \ˈka-tə-ˌrakt\ *n* : a clouding of the lens of the eye or its surrounding transparent membrane that obstructs the passage of light

cat·a·ract·ous \ˈka-tə-ˌrak-təs\ *adj* : of, relating to, or affected with an eye cataract

ca·tarrh \kə-ˈtär\ *n* : inflammation of a mucous membrane in humans or animals; *esp* : one chronically affecting the human nose and air passages — **ca·tarrh·al** \-əl\ *adj*

catarrhal fever *n* : MALIGNANT CATARRHAL FEVER

cata·to·nia \ˌka-tə-ˈtō-nē-ə\ *n* : a marked psychomotor disturbance that may involve stupor or mutism, negativism, rigidity, purposeless excitement, echolalia, echopraxia, and inappropriate or bizarre posturing and is associated with various medical conditions (as schizophrenia, Wilson's disease, or meningoencephalitis)

[1]**cata·ton·ic** \ˌka-tə-ˈtä-nik\ *adj* : of, relating to, marked by, or affected with catatonia ⟨~ schizophrenia⟩ — **cata·ton·i·cal·ly** \-ni-k(ə-)lē\ *adv*

[2]**catatonic** *n* : a catatonic person

catch·ment area \ˈkach-mənt-\ *n* : the geographical area served by an institution

cat cry syndrome *or* **cat's cry syndrome** *n* : CRI DU CHAT SYNDROME

cat distemper *n* : PANLEUKOPENIA

cat·e·chol·amine \ˌka-tə-ˈkō-lə-ˌmēn, -ˈkȯ-\ *n* : any of various amines (as epinephrine, norepinephrine, and dopamine) that function as hormones or neurotransmitters or both

cat·e·chol·amin·er·gic \-ˌkō-lə-mē-ˈnər-jik\ *adj* : involving, liberating, or mediated by catecholamine ⟨~ transmission in the nervous system⟩

cat fever *n* : PANLEUKOPENIA

cat flea *n* : a common flea of the genus *Ctenocephalides* (*C. felis*) that breeds chiefly on cats, dogs, and rats

cat·gut \ˈkat-ˌgət\ *n* : a tough cord made usu. from sheep intestines and used for sutures in closing wounds

[1]**cath** \ˈkath\ *n* : CATHETERIZATION; *esp* : CARDIAC CATHETERIZATION

[2]**cath** *vb* : to insert a catheter into : subject to catheterization

cath *abbr* **1** cathartic **2** catheter

cath- — see CATA-

ca·thar·sis \kə-ˈthär-səs\ *n, pl* **ca·thar·ses** \-ˌsēz\ **1** : PURGATION **2** : elimination of a complex by bringing it to consciousness and affording it expression

[1]**ca·thar·tic** \kə-ˈthär-tik\ *adj* : of, relating to, or producing catharsis

[2]**cathartic** *n* : a cathartic medicine : PURGATIVE

ca·thect \kə-ˈthekt, ka-\ *vb* : to invest with mental or emotional energy

ca·thec·tic \kə-ˈthek-tik, ka-\ *adj* : of, relating to, or invested with mental or emotional energy

cath·e·ter \ˈka-thə-tər, ˈkath-tər\ *n* : a tubular medical device for insertion into canals, vessels, passageways, or body cavities for diagnostic or therapeutic purposes (as to permit injection or withdrawal of fluids or to keep a passage open)

cath·e·ter·i·za·tion \ˌka-thə-tə-rə-ˈzā-shən, ˌkath-tə-rə-\ *n* : the use of or insertion of a catheter (as in or into the bladder, trachea, or heart) — **cath·e·ter·ize** \ˈka-thə-tə-ˌrīz, ˈkath-tə-\ *vb*

cath·e·ter·ized *adj* : obtained by catheterization ⟨~ urine specimens⟩

ca·thex·is \kə-ˈthek-səs, ka-\ *n, pl* **ca·thex·es** \-ˌsēz\ : investment of mental or emotional energy in a person, object, or idea

cath·i·none \ˈka-thə-ˌnōn\ *n* : an alkaloid $C_9H_{11}NO$ found in the leaves of a tropical shrub and possessing properties similar to those of amphetamine; *also* : a derivative of this alkaloid — see BATH SALTS 2

cath·ode–ray oscilloscope \ˈka-ˌthōd-\ *n* : OSCILLOSCOPE

cathode–ray tube *n* : a vacuum tube in which a beam of electrons is projected on a fluorescent screen to produce a luminous spot

cat·ion \ˈkat-ˌī-ən, ˈka-(ˌ)tī-ən\ *n* : the ion in an electrolyte that migrates to the cathode; *also* : a positively charged ion — **cat·ion·ic** \ˌkat-(ˌ)ī-ˈä-nik, ˌka-(ˌ)tī-\ *adj* — **cat·ion·i·cal·ly** *adv*

cat louse *n* : a biting louse (*Felicola subrostratus* of the family Trichodectidae) common on cats esp. in warm regions

CAT scan \ˈkat-\ *n* : CT SCAN — **CAT scanning** *n*

CAT scanner *n* : CT SCANNER

cat scratch disease *n* : an illness that is characterized by chills, slight fever, and swelling of the lymph glands and is usu. caused by a gram-negative bacterium of the genus *Bartonella* (*B. henselae* syn. *Rochalimaea henselae*) transmitted esp. by a cat scratch — called also *cat scratch fever*

cat tapeworm *n* : a tapeworm of the genus *Taenia* (*T. taeniaeformis*) occurring in cats

cattle grub *n* : either of two warble flies of the genus *Hypoderma* esp. in the larval stage: **a** : COMMON CATTLE GRUB **b** : NORTHERN CATTLE GRUB

cattle louse *n* : a louse (as *Haematopinus eurysternus* or *Linognathus vituli*) infesting cattle

cattle tick *n* : either of two ixodid ticks of the genus *Boophilus* (*B. annulatus* and *B. microplus*) that infest cattle and transmit the protozoan which causes Texas fever

cau·dad \ˈkȯ-ˌdad\ *adv* : toward the tail or posterior end

cau·da equi·na \ˈkau̇-də-ē-ˈkwē-nə, ˈkȯ-də-, -ˈkwī-\ *n, pl* **caudae equi·nae** \ˈkau̇-ˌdī-ē-ˈkwē-ˌnī, ˈkȯ-ˌdē-ē-ˈkwī-ˌnē\ : the roots of the spinal nerves that extend beyond the termination of the spinal cord at the first lumbar vertebra in the form of a bundle of filaments within the spinal canal resembling a horse's tail

cauda equina syndrome *n* : a group of symptoms that are caused by compression of the cauda equina and include pain in the lower back and legs, weakness and numbness in the groin, buttocks and legs, and impaired functioning of the bladder and bowel

cau·dal \ˈkȯd-ᵊl\ *adj* **1** : of, relating to, or being a tail **2** : situated in or directed toward the hind part of the body — **cau·dal·ly** *adv*

caudal anesthesia *n* : loss of pain sensation below the umbilicus produced by injection of an anesthetic into the caudal portion of the spinal canal — called also *caudal analgesia*

cau·date lobe \ˈkȯ-ˌdāt-\ *n* : a lobe of the liver bounded on the right by the inferior vena cava, on the left by the fissure of the ductus venosus, and connected with the right lobe by a narrow prolongation

caudate nucleus *n* : the one of the four basal ganglia in each cerebral hemisphere that comprises a mass of gray matter in the corpus striatum, forms part of the floor of the lateral ventricle, and is separated from the lentiform nucleus by the internal capsule — called also *caudate*

caul \ˈkȯl\ *n* **1** : GREATER OMENTUM **2** : the inner embryonic membrane esp. when covering the head at birth

cauliflower ear *n* : an ear deformed from injury and excessive growth of reparative tissue

cau•sal•gia \kȯ-ˈzal-jə, -ˈsal-, -jē-ə\ *n* : a constant usu. burning pain that results from injury to a peripheral nerve and is often considered a type of complex regional pain syndrome — **cau•sal•gic** \-jik\ *adj*

¹**caus•tic** \ˈkȯ-stik\ *adj* : capable of destroying or eating away organic tissue by chemical action

²**caustic** *n* : a caustic agent : as **a** : a substance that burns or destroys organic tissue by chemical action : ESCHAROTIC **b** : a strong corrosive alkali (as sodium hydroxide)

cau•ter•ize \ˈkȯ-tə-ˌrīz\ *vb* **-ized; -iz•ing** : to sear with a cautery or caustic — **cau•ter•i•za•tion** \ˌkȯ-tə-rə-ˈzā-shən\ *n*

cau•tery \ˈkȯ-tə-rē\ *n, pl* **-ter•ies** **1** : the act or effect of cauterizing : CAUTERIZATION **2** : a substance or medical device used to burn, sear, or destroy tissue

¹**ca•va** \ˈkä-və, ˈkā-\ *n, pl* **ca•vae** \ˈkä-ˌvē, -ˌvī; ˈkā-ˌvē\ : VENA CAVA — **ca•val** \-vəl\ *adj*

²**cava** *pl of* CAVUM

cavernosum, cavernosa — see CORPUS CAVERNOSUM

cav•ern•ous \ˈka-vər-nəs\ *adj* **1** : having caverns or cavities **2** *of tissue* : composed largely of vascular sinuses and capable of dilating with blood to bring about the erection of a body part

cavernous sinus *n* : either of a pair of large venous sinuses situated in a groove at the side of the body of the sphenoid bone in the cranial cavity and opening behind into the petrosal sinuses

cav•i•tary \ˈka-və-ˌter-ē\ *adj* : of, relating to, or characterized by bodily cavitation ⟨~ lesions⟩

cav•i•ta•tion \ˌka-və-ˈtā-shən\ *n* **1** : the formation of cavities in an organ or tissue esp. in disease **2** : a cavity formed by cavitation — **cav•i•tate** \ˈka-və-ˌtāt\ *vb*

cav•i•ty \ˈka-və-tē\ *n, pl* **-ties** **1** : an unfilled space within a mass **2** : an area of decay in a tooth : CARIES

ca•vum \ˈkä-vəm, ˈkā-\ *n, pl* **ca•va** \-və\ : an anatomical recess or hollow

cavus — see PES CAVUS

Cb *symbol* columbium

CB *abbr* [Latin *Chirurgiae Baccalaureus*] bachelor of surgery

CBC *abbr* complete blood count

CBT *abbr* cognitive behavioral therapy

CBW *abbr* chemical and biological warfare

cc *abbr* cubic centimeter

CC *abbr* **1** chief complaint **2** current complaint

CCK *abbr* cholecystokinin

CCU *abbr* **1** cardiac care unit **2** coronary care unit **3** critical care unit

Cd *symbol* cadmium

CD *abbr* cluster of differentiation — used with a number to denote any of numerous antigenic proteins on the surface of white blood cells (as T cells or B cells); see CD8, CD4

CDC *abbr* Centers for Disease Control and Prevention

CD8 \ˌsē-(ˌ)dē-ˈāt\ *n, often attrib* : a glycoprotein found esp. on the surface of cytotoxic T cells that usu. functions to facilitate recognition by cytotoxic T cell receptors of antigens complexed with molecules of a class that are found on the surface of most nucleated cells and are the product of genes of the major histocompatibility complex

CD4 \ˌsē-(ˌ)dē-ˈfōr\ *n, often attrib* : a large glycoprotein that is found esp. on the surface of helper T cells, that is the receptor for HIV, and that usu. functions to facilitate recognition by helper T cells of antigens complexed with molecules of a class that are found on the surface of antigen-presenting cells and are the product of genes of the major histocompatibility complex

C. diff \ˈsē-ˈdif\ *n, pl* **C. diff** : a rod-shaped spore-producing bacterium (*Clostridium difficile*) that occurs widely in soil and water and sometimes in the intestine and may produce a toxin causing intestinal illness esp. in those receiving antibiotic therapy

cDNA \ˌsē-(ˌ)dē-(ˌ)en-ˈā\ *n* : a DNA that is complementary to a given RNA which serves as a template for synthesis of the DNA in the presence of a reverse transcriptase — called also *complementary DNA*

Ce *symbol* cerium

CEA *abbr* carcinoembryonic antigen

cec- *or* **ceci-** *or* **ceco-** *comb form* : cecum ⟨*cec*itis⟩ ⟨*ceco*stomy⟩

ce•cal \ˈsē-kəl\ *adj* : of or like a cecum — **ce•cal•ly** *adv*

ce•ci•tis \sē-ˈsī-təs\ *n* : inflammation of the cecum

Ce•clor \ˈsē-klȯr\ *trademark* — used for a preparation of cefaclor

ce•co•pexy \ˈsē-kə-ˌpek-sē\ *n, pl* **-pex•ies** : a surgical operation to fix the cecum to the abdominal wall

ce•cos•to•my \sē-ˈkäs-tə-mē\ *n, pl* **-mies** : the surgical formation of an opening into the cecum to serve as an artificial anus

ce•cum \ˈsē-kəm\ *n, pl* **ce•ca** \-kə\ : the blind pouch at the beginning of the large intestine into which the ileum opens from one side and which is continuous with the colon

cef•a•clor \ˈse-fə-klȯr\ *n* : a semisynthetic cephalosporin antibiotic $C_{15}H_{14}ClN_3O_4S·H_2O$ that is administered orally to treat bacterial infections— see CECLOR

ce•faz•o•lin \si-ˈfa-zə-lən\ *n* : a semisynthetic cephalosporin antibiotic administered parenterally in the form of its sodium salt $C_{14}H_{13}N_8NaO_4S_3$

ce•fix•ime \ˌse-ˈfiks-ˌēm\ *n* : a semisynthetic broad-spectrum cephalosporin antibiotic $C_{16}H_{15}N_5O_7S_2$

ce•fo•tax•ime \ˌse-fə-ˈtak-ˌsēm\ *n* : a semisynthetic cephalosporin antibiotic that is administered parenterally in the form of its sodium salt $C_{16}H_{16}N_5NaO_7S_2$

ce•fox•i•tin \si-ˈfäk-sə-tən\ *n* : a semisynthetic cephamycin antibiotic administered parenterally in the form of its sodium salt $C_{16}H_{16}N_3NaO_7S_2$

cef•taz•i•dime \sef-ˈtaz-ə-ˌdēm\ *n* : a semisynthetic cephalosporin antibiotic that is administered parenterally in the form of its hydrate $C_{22}H_{22}N_6O_7S_2·5H_2O$

Cef•tin \ˈsef-tin\ *trademark* — used for a preparation of an ester of cefuroxime

cef•tri•ax•one \ˌsef-ˌtrī-ˈak-ˌsōn\ *n* : a semisynthetic cephalosporin antibiotic that is administered parenterally in the form of its hydrated disodium salt $C_{18}H_{16}N_8Na_2O_7S_3·3\frac{1}{2}H_2O$

ce•fur•o•xime \si-ˈfyu̇r-ə-ˌzēm\ *n* : a semisynthetic cephalosporin antibiotic that is administered parenterally in the form of its sodium salt $C_{16}H_{15}N_4NaO_8S$ or orally as an ester derivative $C_{20}H_{22}N_4O_{10}S$ — see CEFTIN

-cele *n comb form* : tumor : hernia ⟨cysto*cele*⟩

-cele — see -COELE

Cel•e•brex \ˈse-lə-ˌbreks\ *trademark* — used for a preparation of celecoxib

cel•e•cox•ib \ˌse-lə-ˈkäk-sib\ *n* : an NSAID $C_{17}H_{14}F_3N_3O_2S$ that is a COX-2 inhibitor administered orally esp. to relieve the pain and inflammation of osteoarthritis and rheumatoid arthritis — see CELEBREX

Ce•lexa \sə-ˈlek-sə\ *trademark* — used for a preparation of the hydrobromide of citalopram

celi- *or* **celio-** *comb form* : belly : abdomen ⟨*celio*scopy⟩ ⟨*celio*tomy⟩

[1]**ce•li•ac** \ˈsē-lē-ˌak\ *adj* **1** : of or relating to the abdominal cavity **2** : belonging to or prescribed for celiac disease ⟨the ~ syndrome⟩ ⟨a ~ diet⟩

[2]**celiac** *n* : a celiac part (as a nerve)

celiac artery *n* : a short thick artery arising from the aorta just below the diaphragm and dividing almost immediately into the gastric, hepatic, and splenic arteries — called also *celiac axis, truncus celiacus*

celiac disease *n* : a chronic hereditary intestinal disorder in which an inability to absorb the gliadin portion of gluten results in the gliadin triggering an immune response that damages the intestinal mucosa — called also *celiac sprue, gluten-sensitive enteropathy, nontropical sprue, sprue*

celiac ganglion *n* : either of a pair of collateral sympathetic ganglia that are the largest of the autonomic nervous system and lie one on each side of the celiac artery near the adrenal gland on the same side

celiac plexus *n* : a nerve plexus that is situated in the abdomen behind the stomach and in front of the aorta and the crura of the diaphragm, surrounds the celiac artery and the root of the superior mesenteric artery, contains several ganglia of which the most important are the celiac ganglia, and distributes nerve fibers to all the abdominal viscera — called also *solar plexus*

celiac sprue *n* : CELIAC DISEASE

celiacus — see TRUNCUS CELIACUS

ce•li•os•co•py \ˌsē-lē-ˈäs-kə-pē\ *n, pl* **-pies** : examination of the abdominal cavity by surgical insertion of an endoscope through the abdominal wall

ce•li•ot•o•my \ˌsē-lē-ˈä-tə-mē\ *n, pl* **-mies** : surgical incision of the abdomen

cell \ˈsel\ *n* : a small usu. microscopic mass of protoplasm bounded externally by a semipermeable membrane, usu. including one or more nuclei and various nonliving products, capable alone or interacting with other cells of performing all the fundamental functions of life, and forming the smallest structural unit of living matter capable of functioning independently

cell body *n* : the nucleus-containing central part of a neuron exclusive of its axons and dendrites that is the major structural element of the gray matter of the brain and spinal cord, the ganglia, and the retina — called also *perikaryon, soma*

cell count *n* : a count of cells esp. of the blood or other body fluid in a standard volume (as a cubic millimeter)

cell cycle *n* : the complete series of events from one cell division to the next — see G_1 PHASE, G_2 PHASE, M PHASE, S PHASE

cell division *n* : the process by which cells multiply involving both nuclear and cytoplasmic division — compare MEIOSIS, MITOSIS

celled \ˈseld\ *adj* : having (such or so many) cells — used in combination ⟨single-*celled* organisms⟩

cell line *n* : a cell culture selected for uniformity from a cell population derived from a usu. homogeneous tissue source (as an organ) ⟨a *cell line* derived from a malignant tumor⟩

cell–me·di·at·ed \ˈsel-ˈmē-dē-ˌā-təd\ *adj* : relating to or being the part of immunity or the immune response that is mediated primarily by T cells and esp. cytotoxic T cells rather than by antibodies secreted by B cells ⟨~ immunity⟩ — compare HUMORAL 2

cell membrane *n* : a membrane of a cell; *esp* : PLASMA MEMBRANE

cell of Ley·dig \-ˈlī-dig\ *n* : LEYDIG CELL

cell sap *n* **1** : the liquid contents of a plant cell vacuole **2** : CYTOSOL

cell suicide *n* : APOPTOSIS

cel·lu·lar \ˈsel-yə-lər\ *adj* **1** : of, relating to, or consisting of cells **2** : CELL-MEDIATED ⟨~ immunity⟩ — **cel·lu·lar·i·ty** \ˌsel-yə-ˈlar-ə-tē\ *n*

cellular respiration *n* : any of various energy-yielding oxidative reactions in living matter that typically involve transfer of oxygen and production of carbon dioxide and water as end products

cel·lu·lite \ˈsel-yə-ˌlīt, -ˌlēt\ *n* : deposits of subcutaneous fat within fibrous connective tissue (as in the thighs, hips, and buttocks) that give a puckered and dimpled appearance to the skin surface

cel·lu·li·tis \ˌsel-yə-ˈlī-təs\ *n* : diffuse and esp. subcutaneous inflammation of connective tissue

cel·lu·lose \ˈsel-yə-ˌlōs, -ˌlōz\ *n* : a polysaccharide $(C_6H_{10}O_5)_x$ of glucose units that constitutes the chief part of the cell walls of plants — **cel·lu·los·ic** \ˌsel-yə-ˈlō-sik, -zik\ *adj*

cellulose acetate phthal·ate \-ˈta-ˌlāt\ *n* : a derivative of cellulose used as a coating for enteric tablets

cell wall *n* : the usu. rigid nonliving permeable wall that surrounds a plasma membrane

Cel·sius \ˈsel-sē-əs, -shəs\ *adj* : relating to or having a scale for measuring temperature on which the interval between the triple point and the boiling point of water is divided into 99.99 degrees with 0.01° being the triple point and 100.00° the boiling point — abbr. *C;* compare CENTIGRADE

Celsius, Anders (1701–1744), Swedish astronomer.

ce·ment \si-ˈment\ *n* **1** : CEMENTUM **2** : a plastic composition made esp. of zinc or silica for filling dental cavities

ce·men·ta·tion \ˌsē-ˌmen-ˈtā-shən\ *n* : the act or process of attaching (as a dental restoration to a natural tooth) by means of cement

ce·ment·i·cle \si-ˈmen-ti-kəl\ *n* : a calcified body formed in the periodontal ligament of a tooth

ce·mento·enam·el \si-ˌmen-tō-i-ˈna-məl\ *adj* : of, relating to, or joining the cementum and enamel of a tooth

ce·men·to·ma \ˌsē-ˌmen-ˈtō-mə\ *n, pl* **-mas** *also* **-ma·ta** \-mə-tə\ : a tumor resembling cementum in structure

ce·men·tum \si-ˈmen-təm\ *n* : a specialized external bony layer covering the dentin of the part of a tooth normally within the gum — called also *cement;* compare DENTIN, ENAMEL

cen·sor \ˈsen-sər\ *n* : a hypothetical psychic agency that represses unacceptable notions before they reach consciousness

cen·sor·ship \ˈsen-sər-ˌship\ *n* : exclusion from consciousness by the psychic censor

Cen·ta·ny \ˈsen-tə-nē\ *trademark* — used for a preparation of mupirocin

cen·ter \ˈsen-tər\ *n* : a group of nerve cells having a common function — called also *nerve center*

cen·te·sis \sen-ˈtē-səs\ *n, pl* **cen·te·ses** \-ˌsēz\ : surgical puncture (as of a tumor or membrane) — usu. used in compounds ⟨para*centesis*⟩

cen·ti·grade \ˈsen-tə-ˌgrād, ˈsän-\ *adj* : relating to, conforming to, or having a thermometer scale on which the interval between the freezing and boiling points of water is divided into 100 degrees with 0° representing the freezing point and 100° the boiling point ⟨10° ~⟩ — abbr. *C;* compare CELSIUS

cen·ti·gram \-ˌgram\ *n* : a unit of mass and weight equal to 1/100 gram

cen·ti·li·ter \-ˌlē-tər\ *n* : a unit of liquid capacity equal to 1/100 liter

cen·ti·me·ter \-ˌmē-tər\ *n* : a unit of length equal to 1/100 meter

centimeter–gram–second *adj* : CGS

cen·ti·pede \ˈsen-tə-pēd\ *n* : any of a class (Chilopoda) of long flattened many-segmented predaceous arthropods with each segment bearing one pair of legs of which the foremost pair is modified into poison fangs

centra *pl of* CENTRUM

cen·tral \ˈsen-trəl\ *adj* **1** : of or concerning the centrum of a vertebra **2 a** : of, relating to, or comprising the brain and spinal cord **b** : originating within or caused by factors originating in the central nervous system ⟨~ precocious puberty⟩ **3** : affecting or involving the trunk of the body and esp. the abdomen ⟨~ adiposity⟩ — **cen·tral·ly** *adv*

central artery *n* : a branch of the ophthalmic artery or the lacrimal artery that enters the substance of the optic nerve and supplies the retina

central artery of the retina *n* : a branch of the ophthalmic artery that passes to the retina in the middle of the optic nerve and branches to form the arterioles of the retina — called also *central retinal artery*

central auditory processing disorder *n* : a disorder that is marked by a deficit in the way the brain receives, differentiates, analyzes, and interprets auditory information (as speech) and that is not attributable to impairments in peripheral hearing or intellect — abbr. *CAPD*

central canal *n* : a minute canal running through the gray matter of the whole length of the spinal cord and continuous anteriorly with the ventricles of the brain

central deafness *n* : hearing loss or impairment resulting from defects in the central nervous system (as in the auditory cortex) rather than in the ear itself or the auditory nerve — compare CONDUCTION DEAFNESS, NERVE DEAFNESS

central diabetes insipidus *n* : diabetes insipidus caused by insufficient production of vasopressin and resulting from damage to the pituitary gland or hypothalamus

centralis — see FOVEA CENTRALIS

central line *n* : an IV line that is inserted into a large vein (as the superior vena cava) typically in the neck or near the heart for therapeutic or diagnostic purposes

central lobe *n* : INSULA

central nervous system *n* : the part of the nervous system which in vertebrates consists of the brain and spinal cord, to which sensory impulses are transmitted and from which motor impulses pass out, and which supervises and coordinates the activity of the entire nervous system — compare AUTONOMIC NERVOUS SYSTEM, PERIPHERAL NERVOUS SYSTEM

central pontine myelinolysis *n* : demyelination that occurs in the pons and is associated with malnutrition, alcoholism, liver disease, or hyponatremia

central retinal artery *n* : CENTRAL ARTERY OF THE RETINA

central retinal vein *n* : CENTRAL VEIN OF THE RETINA

central sleep apnea *n* : sleep apnea that is caused by a disturbance in the brain's respiratory center — compare OBSTRUCTIVE SLEEP APNEA

central sulcus *n* : the sulcus separating the frontal lobe of the cerebral cortex from the parietal lobe — called also *fissure of Rolando, Rolandic fissure*

central tendon *n* : a 3-lobed aponeurosis located near the central portion of the diaphragm caudal to the pericardium and composed of intersecting planes of collagenous fibers

central vein *n* : any of the veins in the lobules of the liver that occur one in each lobule running from the apex to the base, receive blood from the sinusoids, and empty into the sublobular veins — called also *intralobular vein*

central vein of the retina *n* : a vein that is formed by union of the veins draining the retina, passes with the central artery of the retina in the optic nerve, and empties into the superior ophthalmic vein — called also *central retinal vein*

central venous pressure *n* : the venous pressure of the right atrium of the heart obtained by inserting a catheter into a vein (as the subclavian vein) and advancing it to the right atrium through the superior vena cava — abbr. *CVP*

cen•tre *chiefly Brit var of* CENTER

cen•tric \ˈsen-trik\ *adj* **1** : of or relating to a nerve center **2** *of dental occlusion* : involving spatial relationships such that all teeth of both jaws meet in a normal manner and forces exerted by the lower on the upper jaw are perfectly distributed in the dental arch

cen•trif•u•gal \sen-ˈtri-fyə-gəl, -fi-\ *adj* : passing outward (as from a nerve center to a muscle or gland) : EFFERENT — **cen•trif•u•gal•ly** *adv*

cen•trif•u•ga•tion \ˌsen-trə-fyu̇-ˈgā-shən\ *n* : the process of centrifuging

[1]**cen•tri•fuge** \ˈsen-trə-ˌfyüj\ *n* : a machine using centrifugal force for separating substances of different densities, for removing moisture, or for simulating gravitational effects

[2]**centrifuge** *vb* **-fuged; -fug•ing** : to subject to centrifugal action esp. in a centrifuge

cen•tri•lob•u•lar \ˌsen-trə-ˈlä-byə-lər\ *adj* : relating to or affecting the center of a lobule ⟨~ necrosis in the liver⟩; *also* : affecting the central parts of the lobules containing clusters of branching functional and anatomical units of the lung ⟨~ emphysema⟩

cen•tri•ole \ˈsen-trē-ˌōl\ *n* : one of a pair of cellular organelles that occur esp. in animals, are found near the nucleus, function in the formation of the spindle apparatus during cell division, and consist of a cylinder with nine microtubules arranged peripherally in a circle

cen•trip•e•tal \sen-ˈtri-pət-ᵊl\ *adj* : passing inward (as from a sense organ to the brain or spinal cord) : AFFERENT — **cen•trip•e•tal•ly** *adv*

cen•tro•mere \ˈsen-trə-ˌmir\ *n* : the point or region on a chromosome to which the spindle attaches during mitosis and meiosis — called also *kinetochore* — **cen•tro•mer•ic** \ˌsen-trə-ˈmer-ik, -ˈmir-\ *adj*

cen•tro•some \ˈsen-trə-ˌsōm\ *n* : the centriole-containing region of clear cytoplasm adjacent to the cell nucleus

cen•trum \ˈsen-trəm\ *n, pl* **centrums** *or* **cen•tra** \-trə\ **1** : the center esp. of an anatomical part **2** : the body of a vertebra ventral to the neural arch

Cen•tru•roi•des \ˌsen-trə-ˈrȯi-(ˌ)dēz\ *n* : a genus of scorpions containing the only U.S. forms dangerous to humans

cephal- *or* **cephalo-** *comb form* **1** : head ⟨*cephal*algia⟩ ⟨*cephalo*metry⟩ **2** : cephalic and ⟨*cephalo*pelvic⟩

ceph•a•lad \ˈse-fə-ˌlad\ *adv* : toward the head or anterior end of the body

ceph•a•lal•gia \ˌse-fə-ˈlal-jə, -jē-ə\ *n* : HEADACHE

ceph•a•lex•in \ˌse-fə-ˈlek-sən\ *n* : a semisynthetic cephalosporin $C_{16}H_{17}N_3O_4S$ with a spectrum of antibiotic activity similar to the penicillins that is often administered in the form of its hydrochloride $C_{16}H_{17}N_3O_4S \cdot HCl$ or hydrate $C_{16}H_{17}N_3O_4S \cdot H_2O$ — see KEFLEX

ce•phal•gia \se-ˈfal-jə, -jē-ə\ *n* : HEADACHE

ceph•al•he•ma•to•ma \ˌse-fəl-ˌhē-mə-ˈtō-mə\ *or* **ceph•a•lo•he•ma•to•ma** \ˌsef-ə-lō-ˌhē-mə-ˈtō-mə\ *n, pl* **-mas** *also* **-ma•ta** \-mə-tə\ : a usu. benign swelling formed from a hemorrhage beneath the periosteum of the skull and occurring esp. over one or both of the parietal bones in newborn infants as a result of trauma sustained during delivery

-cephali *pl of* -CEPHALUS

ce•phal•ic \sə-ˈfa-lik\ *adj* **1** : of or relating to the head **2** : directed toward or situated on or in or near the head — **ce•phal•i•cal•ly** \-li-k(ə-)lē\ *adv*

cephalic flexure *n* : the middle of the three anterior flexures of an embryo in which the front part of the brain bends downward in an angle of 90 degrees

cephalic index *n* : the ratio multiplied by 100 of the maximum breadth of the head to its maximum length — compare CRANIAL INDEX

cephalic vein *n* : any of various superficial veins of the arm; *specif* : a large vein of the upper arm lying along the outer edge of the biceps muscle and emptying into the axillary vein

ceph•a•lin \ˈke-fə-lən, ˈse-\ *n* : PHOSPHATIDYLETHANOLAMINE

cephalo- — see CEPHAL-

ceph•a•lo•cau•dal \ˌse-fə-lō-ˈkȯd-ᵊl\ *adj* : proceeding or occurring in the long axis of the body esp. in the direction from head to tail — **ceph•a•lo•cau•dal•ly** *adv*

ceph•a•lom•e•ter \ˌse-fə-ˈlä-mə-tər\ *n* : an instrument for measuring the head

ceph•a•lom•e•try \ˌse-fə-ˈlä-mə-trē\ *n, pl* **-tries** : the science of measuring the head in living individuals — **ceph•a•lo•met•ric** \-lō-ˈme-trik\ *adj*

ceph•a•lo•pel•vic disproportion \ˌse-fə-lō-ˈpel-vik-\ *n* : a condition in which a maternal pelvis is small in relation to the size of the fetal head

ceph•a•lor•i•dine \ˌse-fə-ˈlȯr-ə-ˌdēn, -ˈlär-\ *n* : a semisynthetic broad-spectrum antibiotic $C_{19}H_{17}N_3O_4S_2$ derived from cephalosporin

ceph•a•lo•spo•rin \ˌse-fə-lə-ˈspōr-ən\ *n* : any of several beta-lactam antibiotics produced by an imperfect fungus (genus *Acremonium*) or made semisynthetically

ceph•a•lo•thin \ˈse-fə-lə-(ˌ)thin\ *n* : a semisynthetic broad-spectrum antibiotic $C_{16}H_{15}N_2NaO_6S_2$ that is an analog of a cephalosporin and is effective against penicillin-resistant staphylococci

ceph•a•lo•tho•ra•cop•a•gus \ˌse-fə-ˌlō-ˌthōr-ə-ˈkä-pə-gəs\ *n, pl* **-a•gi** \-ˌgī, -ˌgē\ : teratological twin fetuses joined at the head, neck, and thorax

-cephalus *n comb form, pl* **-cephali** : cephalic abnormality (of a specified type) ⟨hydro*cephalus*⟩

ceph•a•my•cin \ˌse-fə-ˈmī-sᵊn\ *n* : any of several beta-lactam antibiotics produced by bacteria of the genus *Streptomyces* or made semisynthetically

cer•amide \ˈsir-ə-ˌmīd\ *n* : any of a group of lipids formed by linking a fatty acid to sphingosine

cer•amide tri•hexo•si•dase \ˌsir-ə-ˌmīd-ˌtrī-ˌhek-sə-ˈsī-ˌdās, -ˌdāz\ *n* : an enzyme that breaks down ceramide trihexoside and is deficient in individuals affected with Fabry disease

cer•amide tri•hexo•side \-(ˌ)trī-ˈhek-sə-ˌsīd\ *n* : a lipid that accumulates in body tissues of individuals affected with Fabry disease

ce•rate \ˈsir-ˌāt\ *n* : an unctuous preparation for external use consisting of wax or resin mixed with oil, lard, and medicinal ingredients

cer•a•to•hy•al \ˌser-ə-(ˌ)tō-ˈhī-əl\ *or* **cer•a•to•hy•oid** \-ˈhī-ˌȯid\ *n* : the smaller inner projection of the two lateral projections on each side of the human hyoid bone — called also *lesser cornu;* compare THYROHYAL

cer•car•ia \(ˌ)sər-ˈkar-ē-ə, -ˈker-\ *n, pl* **-i•ae** \-ē-ˌē\ : a usu. tadpole-shaped larval trematode worm that develops in a molluscan host from a redia — **cer•car•i•al** \-əl\ *adj*

cer•clage \ser-ˈkläzh, (ˌ)sər-\ *n* : any of several procedures for increasing tissue resistance in a functionally incompetent uterine cervix that usu. involve reinforcement with an inert substance esp. in the form of sutures near the internal opening

ce•rea flex•i•bil•i•tas \ˌsir-ē-ə-ˌflek-sə-ˈbi-lə-ˌtas, -ˌtäs\ *n* : the capacity (as in catalepsy) to maintain the limbs or other bodily parts in whatever position they have been placed

cerebell- *or* **cerebelli-** *or* **cerebello-** *comb form* : cerebellum ⟨*cerebell*itis⟩

cerebella *pl of* CEREBELLUM

cer•e•bel•lar \ˌser-ə-ˈbe-lər\ *adj* **1** : of, relating to, or affecting the cerebellum ⟨~ neurons⟩ **2** : caused by disease of the cerebellum ⟨~ ataxia⟩

cerebellar artery *n* : any of several branches of the basilar and vertebral arteries that supply the cerebellum

cerebellaris — see PEDUNCULUS CEREBELLARIS INFERIOR, PEDUNCULUS CEREBELLARIS MEDIUS, PEDUNCULUS CEREBELLARIS SUPERIOR

cerebellar peduncle *n* : any of three large bands of nerve fibers that join each hemisphere of the cerebellum with the parts of the brain below and in front: **a** : one connecting the cerebellum with the midbrain — called also *brachium conjunctivum, pedunculus cerebellaris superior, superior cerebellar peduncle* **b** : one connecting the cerebellum with the pons —

called also *brachium pontis, middle cerebellar peduncle, middle peduncle, pedunculus cerebellaris medius* **c** : one that connects the cerebellum with the medulla oblongata and the spinal cord — called also *inferior cerebellar peduncle, pedunculus cerebellaris inferior, restiform body*

cerebelli — see FALX CEREBELLI, TENTORIUM CEREBELLI

cer•e•bel•li•tis \ˌser-ə-bə-ˈlī-təs, -be-\ *n* : inflammation of the cerebellum

cer•e•bel•lo•pon•tine angle \ˌser-ə-ˌbe-lō-ˌpän-ˌtēn-, -ˌtīn-\ *n* : a region of the brain at the junction of the pons and cerebellum that is a frequent site of tumor formation

cer•e•bel•lum \ˌser-ə-ˈbe-ləm\ *n, pl* **-bellums** *or* **-bel•la** \-lə\ : a large dorsally projecting part of the brain concerned esp. with the coordination of muscles and the maintenance of bodily equilibrium, situated between the brain stem and the back of the cerebrum and formed in humans of two lateral lobes and a median lobe

cerebr- *or* **cerebro-** *comb form* **1** : brain : cerebrum ⟨*cerebr*ation⟩ **2** : cerebral and ⟨*cerebro*spinal⟩

cerebra *pl of* CEREBRUM

ce•re•bral \sə-ˈrē-brəl, ˈser-ə-\ *adj* **1** : of or relating to the brain or the intellect **2** : of, relating to, or being the cerebrum ⟨~ blood flow⟩

cerebral accident *n* : STROKE

cerebral aqueduct *n* : AQUEDUCT OF SYLVIUS

cerebral artery *n* : any of the arteries supplying the cerebral cortex: **a** : an artery that arises from the internal carotid artery, forms the anterior portion of the circle of Willis where it is linked to the artery on the opposite side by the anterior communicating artery, and passes on to supply the medial surfaces of the cerebrum — called also *anterior cerebral artery* **b** : an artery that arises from the internal carotid artery, passes along the lateral fissure, and supplies the lateral surfaces of the cerebral cortex — called also *middle cerebral artery* **c** : an artery that arises by the terminal forking of the basilar artery where it forms the posterior portion of the circle of Willis and passes on to supply the lower surfaces of the temporal and occipital lobes — called also *posterior cerebral artery*

cerebral cortex *n* : the convoluted surface layer of gray matter of the cerebrum that functions chiefly in coordination of sensory and motor information — called also *pallium;* see NEOCORTEX

cerebral dominance *n* : dominance in development and functioning of one of the cerebral hemispheres

cerebral edema *n* : the accumulation of fluid in and resultant swelling of the brain (as that caused by trauma, a tumor, lack of oxygen at high altitudes, or exposure to a toxin)

cerebral hemisphere *n* : either of the two hollow convoluted lateral halves of the cerebrum

cerebral hemorrhage *n* : bleeding from a ruptured blood vessel in the brain and esp. in the cerebrum that is often life-threatening and is marked by sudden headache, nausea, impaired consciousness, and neurological dysfunction — called also *intracerebral hemorrhage*

cerebral palsy *n* : a disability resulting from damage to the brain before, during, or shortly after birth and outwardly manifested by muscular incoordination and speech disturbances — see ATAXIC CEREBRAL PALSY, ATHETOID CEREBRAL PALSY, SPASTIC CEREBRAL PALSY — **cerebral palsied** *adj*

cerebral peduncle *n* : either of two large bundles of nerve fibers passing from the pons forward and outward to form the main connection between the cerebral hemispheres and the spinal cord

cerebral vein *n* : any of various veins that drain the surface and inner tissues of the cerebral hemispheres — see GALEN'S VEIN, GREAT CEREBRAL VEIN

cer•e•brate \ˈser-ə-ˌbrāt\ *vb* **-brat•ed; -brat•ing** : to use the mind — **cer•e•bra•tion** \ˌser-ə-ˈbrā-shən\ *n*

cerebri — see CRURA CEREBRI, FALX CEREBRI, HYPOPHYSIS CEREBRI, PSEUDOTUMOR CEREBRI

cerebro- — see CEREBR-

ce•re•bro•side \sə-ˈrē-brə-ˌsīd, ˈser-ə-\ *n* : any of various lipids composed of ceramide and a monosaccharide and found esp. in the myelin sheath of nerves

ce•re•bro•spi•nal \sə-ˌrē-brō-ˈspīn-ᵊl, ˌser-ə-\ *adj* : of or relating to the brain and spinal cord or to these together with the cranial and spinal nerves that innervate voluntary muscles

cerebrospinal fluid *n* : a liquid that is comparable to serum but contains less dissolved material, that is secreted from the blood into the lateral ventricles of the brain, and that serves chiefly to maintain uniform pressure within the brain and spinal cord — called also *spinal fluid*

cerebrospinal meningitis *n* : inflammation of the meninges of both brain and spinal cord; *specif* : an infectious epidemic and often fatal meningitis caused by the meningococcus — called also *cerebrospinal fever*

ce•re•bro•vas•cu•lar \sə-ˌrē-brō-ˈvas-kyə-lər, ˌser-ə-\ *adj* : of or involving the cerebrum and the blood vessels supplying it ⟨~ disease⟩

cerebrovascular accident *n* : STROKE

ce•re•brum \sə-ˈrē-brəm, ˈser-ə-\ *n, pl* **-brums** *or* **-bra** \-brə\ : the expanded anterior portion of the brain that overlies the rest of the brain, consists of cerebral hemispheres and connecting structures, and is considered to be the seat of conscious mental processes : TELENCEPHALON

cer•e•sin \ˈser-ə-sən\ *n* : a white or yellow hard brittle wax

Cer•e•zyme \ˈser-ə-ˌzīm\ *trademark* — used for a preparation of imiglucerase

ce•ri•um \ˈsir-ē-əm\ *n* : a malleable ductile metallic element — symbol *Ce;* see ELEMENT table

ce•roid \ˈsir-ˌȯid\ *n* : a yellow to brown pigment similar to lipofuscin that accumulates in the body esp. in diseased states

cert *abbr* certificate; certification; certified; certify

cer•ti•fy \ˈsər-tə-ˌfī\ *vb* **-fied; -fy•ing** : to designate as having met the requirements to practice medicine or a particular medical specialty — **cer•ti•fi•able** \ˈsər-tə-ˌfī-ə-bəl, ˌsər-tə-ˈfī-\ *adj* — **cer•ti•fi•ably** \-blē\ *adv* — **cer•ti•fi•ca•tion** \-fə-ˈkā-shən\ *n*

cer•to•liz•u•mab peg•ol \ˌsər-tə-ˈliz-yü-ˌmab-ˈpeg-ˌȯl\ *n* : a monoclonal antibody fragment that inhibits the activity of tumor necrosis factor and is administered by subcutaneous injection to treat Crohn's disease, rheumatoid arthritis, psoriatic arthritis, and ankylosing arthritis — see CIMZIA

cerulea — see PHLEGMASIA CERULEA DOLENS

ceruleus, cerulei — see LOCUS COERULEUS

ce•ru•lo•plas•min \sə-ˌrü-lō-ˈplaz-mən\ *n* : a blue copper-binding serum oxidase that appears to catalyze the conversion of ferrous iron in tissues to ferric iron and is deficient in Wilson's disease

ce•ru•men \sə-ˈrü-mən\ *n* : EARWAX

ce•ru•mi•nous gland \sə-ˈrü-mə-nəs-\ *n* : one of the modified sweat glands of the ear that produce earwax

Cer•va•rix \ˈsər-və-ˌriks\ *trademark* — used for a vaccine against some types of human papillomavirus

cervic- *or* **cervici-** *or* **cervico-** *comb form* **1** : neck : cervix of an organ ⟨*cervic*itis⟩ **2** : cervical and ⟨*cervico*thoracic⟩ ⟨*cervico*vaginal⟩

cer•vi•cal \ˈsər-vi-kəl\ *adj* : of or relating to a neck or cervix ⟨~ cancer⟩

cervical canal *n* : the passage through the cervix uteri

cervical cap *n* : a usu. rubber or plastic contraceptive device in the form of a thimble-shaped molded cap that fits snugly over the uterine cervix and blocks sperm from entering the uterus — called also *Dutch cap*

cervical dystonia *n* : an often painful condition characterized by involuntary contraction of the neck muscles that causes the head to tilt or turn sideways, forward, or backward or jerk abnormally — called also *spasmodic torticollis*

cervical flexure *n* : a ventral bend in the neural tube of the embryo marking the point of transition from brain to spinal cord

cervical ganglion *n* : any of three sympathetic ganglia on each side of the neck

cervicalis — see ANSA CERVICALIS

cervical nerve *n* : one of the spinal nerves of the cervical region of which there are eight on each side in most mammals including humans

cervical plexus *n* : a plexus formed by the anterior divisions of the four upper cervical nerves

cervical plug *n* : a mass of tenacious secretion by glands of the uterine cervix present during pregnancy and tending to close the uterine orifice

cervical rib *n* : a supernumerary rib sometimes found in the neck above the usual first rib

cervical vertebra *n* : any of the seven vertebrae of the neck

cer•vi•cec•to•my \ˌsər-və-ˈsek-tə-mē\ *n, pl* **-mies** : surgical excision of the uterine cervix — called also *trachelectomy*

cervici- *or* **cervico-** — see CERVIC-

cervicis — see ILIOCOSTALIS CERVICIS, LONGISSIMUS CERVICIS, SEMISPINALIS CERVICIS, SPINALIS CERVICIS, SPLENIUS CERVICIS, TRANSVERSALIS CERVICIS

cer•vi•ci•tis \ˌsər-və-ˈsī-təs\ *n* : inflammation of the uterine cervix

cer•vi•co•fa•cial \ˌsər-və-kō-ˈfā-shəl\ *adj* : of, relating to, or affecting the neck and face ⟨~ actinomycosis⟩

cervicofacial nerve \ˌsər-və-(ˌ)kō-ˈfā-shəl-\ *n* : a branch of the facial nerve supplying the lower part of the face and upper part of the neck

cer•vi•co•tho•rac•ic \ˌsər-vi-(ˌ)kō-thə-ˈra-sik, -thȯ-\ *adj* : of or relating to the neck and thorax

cer•vi•co•vag•i•nal \-ˈva-jən-ᵊl\ *adj* : of or relating to the uterine cervix and the vagina ⟨~ flora⟩ ⟨~ carcinoma⟩

cer•vix \ˈsər-viks\ *n, pl* **cer•vi•ces** \-və-ˌsēz, ˌsər-ˈvī-(ˌ)sēz\ *or* **cervixes** **1** : NECK 1a; *esp* : the back part of the neck **2** : a constricted portion of an organ or part: as **a** : the narrow lower or outer end of the uterus **b** : the constricted cementoenamel junction on a tooth

cervix ute•ri \-ˈyü-tə-ˌrī\ *n* : CERVIX 2a

¹ce•sar•e•an *or* **cae•sar•e•an** *also* **ce•sar•i•an** *or* **cae•sar•i•an** \si-ˈzar-ē-ən\ *adj* : of, relating to, or being a cesarean section ⟨a ~ birth⟩

²cesarean *or* **caesarean** *also* **cesarian** *or* **caesarian** *n, sometimes cap* : CESAREAN SECTION

Cae•sar \ˈsē-zər\, **Gaius Julius (100–44 BC)**, Roman general and statesman.

cesarean section *n* : a surgical procedure involving incision of the walls of the abdomen and uterus for delivery of offspring

ce•si•um \'sē-zē-əm\ *n* : a silver-white soft ductile element — symbol *Cs;* see ELEMENT table

ces•tode \'ses-ˌtōd\ *n* : TAPEWORM — **cestode** *adj*

ce•tir•i•zine \se-'tir-ə-ˌzēn\ *n* : an H_1 antagonist administered orally in the form of its dihydrochloride $C_{21}H_{25}ClN_2O_3·2HCl$ as an antihistamine to treat allergic rhinitis and chronic hives — see ZYRTEC

cet•ri•mide \'se-trə-ˌmīd\ *n* : a mixture of bromides of ammonium used esp. as a detergent and antiseptic

ce•tux•i•mab \sə-'tək-sə-ˌmab\ *n* : an antineoplastic drug used to treat colorectal cancer and some forms of head and neck cancer — see ERBITUX

ce•tyl alcohol \'sēt-ᵊl-\ *n* : a waxy crystalline alcohol $C_{16}H_{34}O$ used in pharmaceutical and cosmetic preparations

ce•tyl•py•ri•din•i•um chloride \ˌsēt-ᵊl-ˌpī-rə-'di-nē-əm-\ *n* : a white powder consisting of a quaternary ammonium salt $C_{21}H_{38}ClN·H_2O$ and used as a detergent and antiseptic

Cf *symbol* californium

CF *abbr* cystic fibrosis

CFS *abbr* chronic fatigue syndrome

CG *abbr* chorionic gonadotropin

cGMP *abbr* cyclic GMP; cyclic guanosine monophosphate

cgs *adj, often cap C&G&S* : of, relating to, or being a system of units based on the centimeter as the unit of length, the gram as the unit of mass, and the second as the unit of time

Cha•ber•tia \shə-'ber-tē-ə, -'bər-\ *n* : a genus of strongylid nematode worms including one (*C. ovina*) that infests the colon esp. of sheep

Cha•bert \shȧ-'ber\, **Philibert (1737–1814)**, French veterinarian.

chafe \'chāf\ *n* : injury caused by friction — **chafe** *vb*

Cha•gas disease \'shä-gəs-\ *or* **Cha•gas' disease** \'shäg-əs-(əz-)\ *n* : a tropical American disease that is caused by a trypanosome (*Trypanosoma cruzi*) transmitted by blood-sucking insects and that has an acute form marked by usu. mild symptoms (as fever, fatigue, and swelling at the infection site) and which may sometimes progress years later to a chronic form marked esp. by cardiac and gastrointestinal complications — called also *American trypanosomiasis*

Chagas, Carlos Ribeiro Justiniano (1879–1934), Brazilian physician.

cha•go•ma \shə-'gō-mə\ *n, pl* **-mas** *or* **-ma•ta** \-tə\ : a swelling resembling a tumor that appears at the site of infection in Chagas disease

chain \'chān\ *n* : a number of atoms or chemical groups connected by chemical bonds ⟨a carbon ~⟩

κ–chain *var of* KAPPA CHAIN

chain reflex *n* : a series of responses each serving as a stimulus that evokes the next response

chair•side \'char-ˌsīd\ *adj* : relating to, performed in the vicinity of, or assisting in the work done on a patient in a dentist's chair ⟨a dental ~ assistant⟩

chair time *n* : the amount of time that a patient spends in the chair of a health care provider (as a dentist or optometrist) for examination or treatment

cha•la•sia \kə-'lā-zhə, ka-\ *n* : the relaxation of a ring of muscle (as the cardiac sphincter of the esophagus) surrounding a bodily opening

cha•la•zi•on \kə-'lā-zē-ən, -ˌän\ *n, pl* **-zia** \-zē-ə\ : a small circumscribed tumor of the eyelid formed by retention of secretions of the meibomian gland

chal•i•co•sis \ˌka-li-'kō-səs\ *n, pl* **-co•ses** \-ˌsēz\ : a pulmonary disorder occurring among stone cutters that is caused by inhalation of stone dust

chalk \'chȯk\ *n* : a soft limestone sometimes used medicinally as a source of calcium carbonate — see PRECIPITATED CHALK, PREPARED CHALK — **chalky** \'chȯ-kē\ *adj*

chal•lenge \'cha-lənj\ *n* : the process of provoking or testing physiological activity by exposure to a specific substance; *esp* : a test of immunity by exposure to an antigen after immunization against it — **challenge** *vb*

chal•lenged *adj* : having a physical or mental disability or impairment

cha•lone \'kā-ˌlōn, 'ka-\ *n* : a substance that inhibits mitosis in the specific tissue which secretes it

cham•ber \'chām-bər\ *n* : an enclosed space within the body of an animal — see ANTERIOR CHAMBER, POSTERIOR CHAMBER, PULP CHAMBER, VITREOUS CHAMBER

chamber pot *n* : a bedroom vessel for urination and defecation

chan•cre \'shaŋ-kər\ *n* : a primary sore or ulcer at the site of entry of a pathogen (as in tularemia); *esp* : the initial lesion of syphilis

chan•croid \'shaŋ-ˌkrȯid\ *n* : a venereal disease caused by a bacterium of the genus *Haemophilus* (*H. ducreyi*) and characterized by chancres that unlike those of syphilis lack firm indurated margins — called also *soft chancre;* see DUCREY'S BACILLUS

change of life *n* **1** : MENOPAUSE 1a(2) **2** : ANDROPAUSE

chan•nel \'chan-ᵊl\ *n* **1** : a usu. tubular enclosed passage **2** : a passage created in a selectively permeable membrane by a conformational change in membrane proteins; *also* : the proteins of such a passage — see ION CHANNEL

chan•ne•lop•a•thy \ˌcha-nə-'lä-pə-thē\ *n, pl* **-thies** : a disorder (as epilepsy, cystic fibrosis, and myotonia) caused by the malfunction of an ion channel

Chan•tix \'chan-ˌtiks\ *trademark* — used for a preparation of the tartrate of varenicline

chap \ˈchap\ *n* : a crack in or a sore roughening of the skin caused by exposure to wind or cold — **chap** *vb*

Chap Stick \ˈchap-ˌstik\ *trademark* — used for a lip balm in stick form

char•ac•ter \ˈkar-ik-tər\ *n* **1** : one of the attributes or features that make up and distinguish the individual **2** : the detectable expression of the action of a gene or group of genes **3** : the complex of mental and ethical traits marking and often individualizing a person, group, or nation

[1]**char•ac•ter•is•tic** \ˌkar-ik-tə-ˈris-tik\ *adj* : serving to reveal and distinguish the individual character — **char•ac•ter•is•ti•cal•ly** \-ti-k(ə-)lē\ *adv*

[2]**characteristic** *n* : a distinguishing trait, quality, or property

cha•ras \ˈchär-əs\ *n* : HASHISH

char•coal \ˈchär-ˌkōl\ *n* : a dark or black porous carbon prepared from vegetable or animal substances — see ACTIVATED CHARCOAL

Char•cot joint \(ˌ)shär-ˈkō-\ *also* **Char•cot's joint** \-ˈkōz-\ *n* : a degenerative joint condition affecting esp. the foot or ankle that is marked by bone fragmentation, swelling, redness, pain, and joint deformity and typically occurs following loss of nerve sensation (as in diabetes and spina bifida) — called also *Charcot arthropathy, Charcot disease, Charcot neuroarthropathy, neuroarthropathy, neuropathic arthropathy*

Char•cot \shär-ˈkō\, **Jean–Martin (1825–1893),** French neurologist.

Char•cot–Ley•den crystals \ˌshär-ˌkō-ˈlī-dᵊn-\ *n pl* : minute colorless crystals found in bodily tissues or discharges (as of sputum or feces) that are released from eosinophils and are indicative of an inflammatory response esp. to parasitic infections or allergic states

Leyden, Ernst Viktor von (1832–1910), German physician.

Char•cot–Ma•rie–Tooth disease \(ˌ)shär-ˈkō-mə-ˈrē-ˈtüth-\ *n* : an inherited neurological disorder affecting the peripheral nerves that is marked esp. by progressive muscular weakness in the foot and lower leg and later the forearms and hands and typically has an onset during adolescence or early adulthood — called also *peroneal muscular atrophy*

P. Marie — see MARIE-STRÜMPELL DISEASE

Tooth, Howard Henry (1856–1925), British physician.

charge nurse \ˈchärj-\ *n* : a nurse who is in charge of a health-care unit (as a hospital ward or emergency room)

char•la•tan \ˈshär-lə-tən\ *n* : QUACK

char•ley horse \ˈchär-lē-ˌhȯrs\ *n* : a muscular pain, cramping, or stiffness esp. of the quadriceps that results from a strain or bruise

chart \ˈchärt\ *n* : a record of medical information for a patient

CHD *abbr* coronary heart disease

check•bite \ˈchek-ˌbīt\ *n* **1 a** : an act of biting into a sheet of material (as wax) to record the relation between the opposing surfaces of upper and lower teeth **b** : the record obtained **2** : the material for checkbites

check ligament *n* **1** : ALAR LIGAMENT **2** : either of two expansions of the sheaths of rectus muscles of the eye each of which prob. restrains the activity of the muscle with which it is associated

check•up \ˈchek-ˌəp\ *n* : EXAMINATION; *esp* : a general physical examination

Che•diak–Hi•ga•shi syndrome \shād-ˈyäk-hē-ˈgä-shē-\ *n* : a genetic disorder inherited as an autosomal recessive trait and characterized by partial albinism, abnormal granules in the white blood cells, and marked susceptibility to bacterial infections

Che•diak \shād-ˈyäk\, **Moises (*fl* 1952),** French physician.

Hi•ga•shi \hē-ˈgä-shē\, **Ototaka (*fl* 1954),** Japanese physician.

cheek \ˈchēk\ *n* **1** : the fleshy side of the face below the eye and above and to the side of the mouth; *broadly* : the lateral aspect of the head **2** : BUTTOCK 1

cheek•bone \ˈchēk-ˌbōn\ *n* : the prominence below the eye that is formed by the zygomatic bone; *also* : ZYGOMATIC BONE

cheek tooth *n* : any of the molar or premolar teeth

cheese skipper *n* : the larva of a dipteran fly (*Piophila casei*) that lives in cheese and cured meats and is a cause of intestinal myiasis

cheesy \ˈchē-zē\ *adj* **chees•i•er; -est** : resembling cheese in consistency ⟨~ lesions⟩ ⟨a ~ discharge⟩

cheil- *or* **cheilo-** *also* **chil-** *or* **chilo-** *comb form* : lip ⟨*cheil*itis⟩ ⟨*cheilo*plasty⟩

chei•li•tis \kī-ˈlī-təs\ *n* : inflammation of the lip

chei•lo•plas•ty \ˈkī-lō-ˌplas-tē\ *n, pl* **-ties** : plastic surgery to repair lip defects

chei•los•chi•sis \kī-ˈläs-kə-səs\ *n, pl* **-chi•ses** \-ˌsēz\ : CLEFT LIP

chei•lo•sis \kī-ˈlō-səs\ *n, pl* **-lo•ses** \-ˌsēz\ : an abnormal condition of the lips characterized by scaling of the surface and by the formation of fissures in the corners of the mouth

cheir- *or* **cheiro-** — see CHIR-

chei•ro•pom•pho•lyx \ˌkī-rō-ˈpäm-fə-ˌliks\ *n* : a skin disease characterized by itching vesicles or blebs occurring in groups on the hands or feet

che•late \ˈkē-ˌlāt\ *n* : a compound having a ring structure that usu. contains a metal ion held by coordinate bonds — **chelate** *adj or vb* — **che•la•tion** \kē-ˈlā-shən\ *n*

che•lat•ing agent \ˈkē-ˌlā-tiŋ-\ *n* : CHELATOR

che·la·tion therapy \kē-ˈlā-shən-\ *n* : the use of a chelator (as EDTA) to bind with a metal in the body to form a chelate so that the metal loses its toxic effect or physiological activity

che·la·tor \ˈkē-ˌlā-tər\ *n* : any of various compounds that combine with metals to form chelates and include some used medically to treat metal poisoning (as by lead)

chem *abbr* chemical; chemist; chemistry

chem- *or* **chemo-** *also* **chemi-** *comb form* : chemical : chemistry ⟨*chemo*therapy⟩

[1]**chem·i·cal** \ˈke-mi-kəl\ *adj* **1** : of, relating to, used in, or produced by chemistry **2** : acting or operated or produced by chemicals — **chem·i·cal·ly** \-mi-k(ə-)lē\ *adv*

[2]**chemical** *n* **1** : a substance obtained by a chemical process or used for producing a chemical effect **2** : DRUG 2

chemical castration *n* : the administration of a drug (as medroxyprogesterone acetate) to bring about a marked decrease in the body's production of androgens and esp. testosterone

chemical dependence *n* : addiction to or dependence on drugs — **chemically dependent** *adv*

chemical dependency *n* : CHEMICAL DEPENDENCE

chemical peel *n* : a cosmetic procedure for the removal of facial blemishes and wrinkles involving the application of a caustic chemical and esp. an acid to the skin

chemical warfare *n* : warfare using incendiary mixtures, smokes, or irritant, burning, poisonous, or asphyxiating gases

chem·ist \ˈke-məst\ *n* **1** : one trained in chemistry **2** *Brit* : PHARMACIST

chem·is·try \ˈke-mə-strē\ *n, pl* **-tries** **1** : a science that deals with the composition, structure, and properties of substances and of the transformations that they undergo **2 a** : the composition and chemical properties of a substance ⟨the ~ of hemoglobin⟩ **b** : chemical processes and phenomena (as of an organism) ⟨blood ~⟩

chemist's shop *n, Brit* : a place where medicines are sold

chemo \ˈkē-ˌmō\ *n* : CHEMOTHERAPY

chemo- — see CHEM-

chemo brain *n* : impaired cognition (as memory loss or lack of concentration) that has been observed in patients who have received chemotherapy

che·mo·dec·to·ma \ˌkē-mō-ˈdek-tə-mə, ˌke-\ *n, pl* **-mas** *also* **-ma·ta** \-mə-tə\ : a tumor that affects tissue (as of the carotid body) populated with chemoreceptors

che·mo·em·bo·li·za·tion \-ˌem-bə-lə-ˈzā-shən\ *n* : a technique for treating cancer that involves the use of a catheter to administer high doses of chemotherapeutic agents into a blood vessel supplying the tumor along with an obstructing material (as particles of gelatin sponge) which blocks the tumor's blood supply and prevents the dissipation of the chemotherapeutic agents

che·mo·nu·cle·ol·y·sis \-ˌnü-klē-ˈä-lə-səs, -ˌnyü-\ *n, pl* **-y·ses** \-ˌsēz\ : treatment of a slipped disk by the injection of chymopapain to dissolve the displaced nucleus pulposus

che·mo·pal·li·dec·to·my \-ˌpa-lə-ˈdek-tə-mē\ *n, pl* **-mies** : destruction of the globus pallidus by the injection of a chemical agent esp. formerly for the relief of parkinsonian tremors

che·mo·pho·bia \-ˈfō-bē-ə\ *n* : abnormal or excessive fear of chemicals

che·mo·pre·ven·tion \-pri-ˈven-chən\ *n* : the use of chemical agents to prevent the development of cancer — **che·mo·pre·ven·tive** \-tiv\ *adj*

che·mo·pro·phy·lax·is \-ˌprō-fə-ˈlak-səs, -ˌprä-\ *n, pl* **-lax·es** \-ˌsēz\ : the prevention of infectious disease by the use of chemical agents — **che·mo·pro·phy·lac·tic** \-ˈlak-tik\ *adj*

che·mo·ra·di·a·tion \-ˌrā-dē-ˈā-shən\ *n* : CHEMORADIOTHERAPY

che·mo·ra·dio·ther·a·py \-ˌrā-dē-ō-ˈther-ə-pē\ *n* : treatment that combines chemotherapy and radiotherapy

che·mo·re·cep·tion \-ri-ˈsep-shən\ *n* : the physiological reception of chemical stimuli — **che·mo·re·cep·tive** \-tiv\ *adj*

che·mo·re·cep·tor \-ri-ˈsep-tər\ *n* : a sense organ (as a taste bud) responding to chemical stimuli

chemoreceptor trigger zone *n* : an area in or near the area postrema of the brain with receptors that stimulate the reticular formation to induce vomiting

che·mo·re·flex \ˌkē-mō-ˈrē-ˌfleks *also* ˌke-\ *n* : a physiological reflex initiated by a chemical stimulus or in a chemoreceptor — **chemoreflex** *adj*

che·mo·re·sis·tance \-ri-ˈzis-təns\ *n* : the quality or state of being resistant to a chemical (as a drug) — **che·mo·re·sis·tant** \-tənt\ *adj*

che·mo·sen·si·tiv·i·ty \-ˌsen-sə-ˈti-və-tē\ *n, pl* **-ties** : susceptibility to the action of a chemical agent (as a therapeutic drug) ⟨~ of cancer cells⟩ — **che·mo·sen·si·tive** \-ˈsen-sə-tiv\ *adj*

che·mo·sis \kə-ˈmō-səs\ *n, pl* **-mo·ses** \-ˌsēz\ : swelling of the conjunctival tissue around the cornea

che·mo·sur·gery \ˌkə-mō-ˈsər-jə-rē\ *n, pl* **-ger·ies** : removal by chemical means of diseased or unwanted tissue — **che·mo·sur·gi·cal** \-ˈsər-ji-kəl\ *adj*

che·mo·tac·tic \-ˈtak-tik\ *adj* : involving, inducing, or exhibiting chemotaxis — **che·mo·tac·ti·cal·ly** \-ti-k(ə-)lē\ *adv*

che·mo·tax·is \-ˈtak-səs\ *n, pl* **-tax·es** \-ˌsēz\ : orientation or movement of an organism or cell in relation to chemical agents

[1]**che•mo•ther•a•peu•tic** \-ˌther-ə-ˈpyü-tik\ *adj* : of, relating to, or used in chemotherapy — **che•mo•ther•a•peu•ti•cal•ly** \-ti-k(ə-)lē\ *adv*

[2]**chemotherapeutic** *n* : an agent used in chemotherapy

che•mo•ther•a•py \-ˈther-ə-pē\ *n, pl* **-pies** : the therapeutic use of chemical agents to treat disease; *esp* : the administration of one or more cytotoxic drugs to destroy or inhibit the growth of malignant cells in the treatment of cancer — **che•mo•ther•a•pist** \-pist\ *n*

che•mot•ic \ki-ˈmä-tik\ *adj* : marked by or affected with chemosis

che•no•de•oxy•cho•lic acid \ˌkē-(ˌ)nō-ˌdē-ˌäk-si-ˈkō-lik-, -ˈkä-\ *n* : a bile acid $C_{24}H_{40}O_4$ that facilitates fat absorption and cholesterol excretion

che•no•di•ol \ˌkē-nō-ˈdī-ˌȯl, -ˌōl\ *n* : CHENODEOXYCHOLIC ACID

cher•ub•ism \ˈcher-ü-ˌbi-zəm\ *n* : a hereditary condition characterized by swelling of the jawbones and esp. in young children by a characteristic facies marked by protuberant cheeks and upturned eyes

chest \ˈchest\ *n* **1** : MEDICINE CHEST **2** : the part of the body enclosed by the ribs and sternum

chesty \ˈches-tē\ *adj, chiefly Brit, of a cough* : accompanied by the raising of phlegm

Cheyne–Stokes respiration \ˈchān-ˈstōks-\ *n* : cyclic breathing marked by a gradual increase in the rapidity of respiration followed by a gradual decrease and total cessation for from 5 to 50 seconds and found esp. in advanced kidney and heart disease, asthma, and increased intracranial pressure — called also *Cheyne-Stokes breathing*

Cheyne \ˈchān, ˈchā-nē\, **John (1777–1836),** British physician.

Stokes \ˈstōks\, **William (1804–1878),** British physician.

CHF *abbr* congestive heart failure

Chi•ari–From•mel syndrome \kē-ˈär-ē-ˈfrȯ-məl-, -ˈfrä-\ *n* : a condition usu. occurring postpartum and marked by amenorrhea, galactorrhea, obesity, and atrophy of the uterus and ovaries

Chiari, Johann Baptist (1817–1854), German surgeon.

Frommel, Richard Julius Ernst (1854–1912), German gynecologist.

Chi•ari malformation \kē-ˈär-ē-\ *n* : a congenital abnormality of the hindbrain in which the cerebellum and often parts of the brain stem protrude into the spinal canal through the foramen magnum

Chiari, Hans (1851–1916), Austrian pathologist.

chi•asm \ˈkī-ˌa-zəm, ˈkē-\ *n* : CHIASMA 1

chi•as•ma \kī-ˈaz-mə, kē-\ *n, pl* **-ma•ta** \-mə-tə\ **1** : an anatomical intersection or decussation — see OPTIC CHIASMA **2** : a cross-shaped configuration of paired chromatids visible in the diplotene of meiotic prophase and considered the cytological equivalent of genetic crossing-over — **chi•as•mat•ic** \ˌkī-əz-ˈma-tik, ˌkē-\ *adj*

chiasmatic groove *n* : a narrow transverse groove that lies near the front of the superior surface of the body of the sphenoid bone, is continuous with the optic foramen, and houses the optic chiasma

chicken mite *n* : a small mite of the genus *Dermanyssus* (*D. gallinae*) that infests poultry esp. in warm regions

chicken pox *n* : an acute contagious disease esp. of children that is marked by low-grade fever and formation of vesicles and is caused by a herpesvirus of the genus *Varicellovirus* (species *Human herpesvirus 3*) — called also *varicella;* see SHINGLES

chief cell *n* **1** : one of the cells that line the lumen of the fundic glands of the stomach; *esp* : a small cell with granular cytoplasm that secretes pepsin — compare PARIETAL CELL **2** : one of the secretory cells of the parathyroid glands

chig•ger \ˈchi-gər, ˈji-\ *n* **1** : CHIGOE 1 **2** : a six-legged usu. red or orange mite larva (family Trombiculidae) that feeds on skin cells and causes intensely itchy reddish welts; *also* : the adult mite of this larva

chi•goe \ˈchi-(ˌ)gō, ˈchē-\ *n* **1** : a tropical flea belonging to the genus *Tunga* (*T. penetrans*) of which the gravid female burrows under the skin esp. of the feet causing itching, irritation, and often inflammation — called also *chigger, sand flea* **2** : CHIGGER 2

chi kung \ˈchē-ˈkůŋ\ *n, often cap C&K* : QIGONG

chik•un•gun•ya \ˌchi-kən-ˈgůn-yə\ *n* : a febrile disease that resembles dengue, occurs esp. in parts of Africa, India, and southeastern Asia, and is caused by a togavirus of the genus *Alphavirus* (species *Chikungunya virus*) transmitted by mosquitoes esp. of the genus *Aedes* — called also *chikungunya fever*

chil- *or* **chilo-** — see CHEIL-

chil•blain \ˈchil-ˌblān\ *n* : an inflammatory swelling or sore caused by exposure (as of the feet or hands) to cold — called also *pernio*

child \ˈchīld\ *n, pl* **chil•dren** \ˈchil-drən, -dərn\ **1** : an unborn or recently born person **2** : a young person esp. between infancy and youth — **with child** : PREGNANT

child•bear•ing \ˈchīld-ˌbar-iŋ\ *n* : the act of bringing forth children : CHILDBIRTH — **childbearing** *adj*

child•bed \-ˌbed\ *n* : the condition of a woman in childbirth

childbed fever *n* : PUERPERAL FEVER

child•birth \-ˌbərth\ *n* : the act or process of giving birth to a baby : PARTURITION

child guidance *n* : the clinical study and treatment of the behavioral and emotional problems of children by a staff of specialists

child•hood \ˈchīld-ˌhu̇d\ *n* : the state or period of being a child

childhood absence epilepsy *n* : epilepsy that typically begins between the ages of four and eight and is marked by the frequent, daily occurrence of absence seizures

child psychiatry *n* : psychiatry applied to the treatment of children

child psychology *n* : the study of the psychological characteristics of infants and children and the application of general psychological principles to infancy and childhood

[1]**chill** \ˈchil\ *n* **1** : a sensation of cold accompanied by shivering **2** : a disagreeable sensation of coldness

[2]**chill** *vb* **1 a** : to make or become cold **b** : to shiver or quake with or as if with cold **2** : to become affected with a chill

chill factor *n* : WINDCHILL

chi•mae•ra *chiefly Brit var of* CHIMERA

chi•me•ra \kī-ˈmir-ə, kə-\ *n* : an individual, organ, or part containing tissue with two or more genetically distinct groups of cells — **chi•me•ric** \-ˈmir-ik, -ˈmer-\ *adj* — **chi•me•rism** \-ˈmir-ˌi-zəm, kə-; ˈkī-mə-ˌri-\ *n*

chin \ˈchin\ *n* : the lower portion of the face lying below the lower lip and including the prominence of the lower jaw — called also *mentum* — **chin•less** \-ləs\ *adj*

Chi•na white \ˈchī-nə-ˈ(h)wīt\ *n, often cap W, slang* **1** : a pure potent form of heroin originating in southeastern Asia **2** : an illicit analog of the analgesic fentanyl that resembles heroin in its physical appearance and physiological effects

chin•bone \ˈchin-ˌbōn\ *n* : JAW 1b; *esp* : the median anterior part of the bone of the lower jaw

chinch \ˈchinch\ *n* : BEDBUG

Chinese liver fluke *n* : a destructive Asian liver fluke of the genus *Clonorchis* (*C. sinensis*) that is a serious human parasite invading the liver following consumption of raw infected fish and causing clonorchiasis

Chinese restaurant syndrome *n* : a group of symptoms (as chest pain, headache, and facial flushing) that is held to affect susceptible persons eating food and esp. Chinese food heavily seasoned with monosodium glutamate

chip \ˈchip\ *n* : MICROARRAY

chip–blow•er \ˈchip-ˌblō-ər\ *n* : a dental instrument used to blow drilling debris from a cavity being prepared for filling

chir- *or* **chiro-** *also* **cheir-** *or* **cheiro-** *comb form* : hand ⟨*chiro*practic⟩

chi•rop•o•dy \kə-ˈrä-pə-dē, shə-, kī-\ *n, pl* **-dies** : PODIATRY — **chi•ro•po•di•al** \ˌkī-rə-ˈpō-dē-əl\ *adj* — **chi•rop•o•dist** \kə-ˈrä-pə-dist, shə-, kī-\ *n*

chi•ro•prac•tic \ˈkī-rə-ˌprak-tik\ *n* : a system of therapy which holds that disease results from a lack of normal nerve function and which employs manipulation and specific adjustment of body structures (as the spinal column) — **chiropractic** *adj* — **chi•ro•prac•tor** \-tər\ *n*

chis•el \ˈchi-zəl\ *n* : a metal tool with a cutting edge at the end of a blade; *esp* : one used in dentistry

chi•tin \ˈkīt-ᵊn\ *n* : a horny polysaccharide that forms part of the hard outer integument esp. of insects, arachnids, and crustaceans — **chi•tin•ous** \ˈkīt-ᵊn-əs\ *adj*

chla•myd•ia \klə-ˈmi-dē-ə\ *n* **1** *cap* : a genus of coccoid to spherical gram-negative intracellular bacteria (family Chlamydiaceae) including one (*C. trachomatis*) that causes or is associated with various diseases of the eye and genitourinary tract including trachoma, lymphogranuloma venereum, cervicitis, and some forms of nongonococcal urethritis **2** *pl* **-iae** *also* **-ias** **a** : a bacterium of the genus *Chlamydia* **b** : an infection or disease caused by chlamydiae — **chla•myd•ial** \-əl\ *adj*

chla•myd•i•o•sis \klə-ˌmi-dē-ˈō-səs\ *n, pl* **-o•ses** \-ˌsēz\ : an infection or disease (as psittacosis or feline pneumonitis) caused by bacteria of the genus *Chlamydia*

chlo•as•ma \klō-ˈaz-mə\ *n, pl* **-ma•ta** \-mə-tə\ : irregular brownish or blackish spots esp. on the face that occur sometimes in pregnancy and in disorders of or functional changes in the uterus and ovaries

chlor- *or* **chloro-** *comb form* **1** : green ⟨*chlor*osis⟩ **2** : chlorine : containing or caused by chlorine ⟨*chlor*acne⟩

chloracetophenone *var of* CHLOROACETOPHENONE

chlor•ac•ne \(ˌ)klōr-ˈak-nē\ *n* : a skin eruption resembling acne and resulting from exposure to chlorine or its compounds

chlo•ral \ˈklōr-əl\ *n* : CHLORAL HYDRATE

chloral hydrate *n* : a bitter white crystalline drug $C_2H_3Cl_3O_2$ used as a hypnotic and sedative

chlo•ral•ose \ˈklōr-ə-ˌlōs, -ˌlōz\ *n* : a bitter crystalline compound $C_8H_{11}Cl_3O_6$ used esp. to anesthetize animals

chlo•ram•bu•cil \klōr-ˈam-byə-ˌsil\ *n* : an anticancer drug $C_{14}H_{19}Cl_2NO_2$ used esp. to treat leukemias, multiple myeloma, and some lymphomas

chlo•ra•mine \ˈklōr-ə-ˌmēn\ *n* : any of various organic compounds containing nitrogen and chlorine; *esp* : CHLORAMINE-T

chloramine–T \-ˈtē\ *n* : a white or faintly yellow crystalline compound

$C_7H_7ClNNaO_2S{\cdot}3H_2O$ used as an antiseptic (as in treating wounds)

chlor·am·phen·i·col \ˌklōr-ˌam-ˈfe-ni-kȯl, -ˌkōl\ *n* : a broad-spectrum antibiotic $C_{11}H_{12}Cl_2N_2O_5$ isolated from cultures of a soil actinomycete of the genus *Streptomyces* (*S. venezuelae*) or prepared synthetically

chlor·bu·tol \ˈklȯr-byə-ˌtȯl\ *n, chiefly Brit* : CHLOROBUTANOL

chlor·cy·cli·zine \klȯr-ˈsī-klə-ˌzēn\ *n* : a cyclic antihistamine administered in the form of its hydrochloride $C_{18}H_{21}ClN_2{\cdot}HCl$

chlor·dane \ˈklȯr-ˌdān\ *n* : a viscous volatile liquid insecticide $C_{10}H_6Cl_8$ formerly used in the U.S.

chlor·di·az·epox·ide \ˌklōr-dī-ˌa-zə-ˈpäk-ˌsīd\ *n* : a benzodiazepine structurally and pharmacologically related to diazepam and used in the form of its hydrochloride $C_{16}H_{14}ClN_3O{\cdot}HCl$ esp. as a tranquilizer and to treat the withdrawal symptoms of alcoholism — see LIBRIUM

chlor·hex·i·dine \klōr-ˈhek-sə-ˌdīn, -ˌdēn\ *n* : an antibacterial compound $C_{22}H_{30}Cl_2N_{10}$ used as a local antiseptic (as in mouthwash) and disinfectant esp. in the form of its hydrochloride, gluconate, or acetate

chlo·ride \ˈklōr-ˌīd\ *n* : a compound of chlorine with another element or radical; *esp* : a salt or ester of hydrochloric acid

chloride shift *n* : the passage of chloride ions from the plasma into the red blood cells when carbon dioxide enters the plasma from the tissues and their return to the plasma when the carbon dioxide is discharged in the lungs that is a major factor both in maintenance of blood pH and in transport of carbon dioxide

chlo·ri·nate \ˈklōr-ə-ˌnāt\ *vb* **-nat·ed; -nat·ing** : to treat or cause to combine with chlorine or a chlorine compound — **chlo·ri·na·tion** \ˌklōr-ə-ˈnā-shən\ *n*

chlo·rine \ˈklōr-ˌēn, -ən\ *n* : a halogen element that is isolated as a heavy greenish-yellow gas of pungent odor and is used esp. as a bleach, oxidizing agent, and disinfectant in water purification — symbol *Cl;* see ELEMENT table

chlor·mer·o·drin \klōr-ˈmer-ə-drən\ *n* : a mercurial compound $C_5H_{11}ClHgN_2O_2$ formerly used esp. as a diuretic

chloro- — see CHLOR-

chlo·ro·ace·to·phe·none \ˌklōr-ō-ˌa-sə-(ˌ)tō-fə-ˈnōn, -ə-ˌsē-\ *or* **chlor·ace·to·phe·none** \ˌklōr-ˌa-, ˌklōr-ə-ˌsē\ *n* : a chlorine-containing compound C_8H_7ClO used esp. as a tear gas

chlo·ro·az·o·din \ˌklōr-ō-ˈa-zəd-ᵊn\ *n* : a yellow crystalline compound $C_2H_4Cl_2N_6$ used in solution as a surgical antiseptic

chlo·ro·bu·ta·nol \-ˈbyüt-ᵊn-ˌȯl, -ōl\ *n* : a white crystalline alcohol $C_4H_7Cl_3O$ that is used as a local anesthetic, sedative, and preservative

chlo·ro·cre·sol \-ˈkrē-ˌsȯl, -ˌsōl\ *n* : a chlorine derivative C_7H_7ClO of cresol used as an antiseptic and preservative

[1]**chlo·ro·form** \ˈklōr-ə-ˌfȯrm\ *n* : a colorless volatile heavy toxic liquid $CHCl_3$ with an ether odor used esp. as a solvent — called also *trichloromethane*

[2]**chloroform** *vb* : to treat with chloroform esp. so as to produce anesthesia or death

chlo·ro·gua·nide \ˌklōr-o-ˈgwä-ˌnīd, -nəd\ *n* : PROGUANIL

chlo·ro·leu·ke·mia \-lü-ˈkē-mē-ə\ *n* : CHLOROMA

chlo·ro·ma \klə-ˈrō-mə\ *n, pl* **-mas** *also* **-ma·ta** \-mə-tə\ : a leukemic condition marked by the formation of usu. green-colored tumors composed of myeloid tissue; *also* : one of these tumors

Chlo·ro·my·ce·tin \ˌklōr-ō-mī-ˈsēt-ᵊn\ *n* : a preparation of chloramphenicol — formerly a U.S. registered trademark

chlo·ro·phyll \ˈklōr-ə-ˌfil, -fəl\ *n* **1** : the green photosynthetic coloring matter of plants **2** : a waxy green chlorophyll-containing substance extracted from green plants and used as a coloring agent or deodorant

chlo·ro·pic·rin \ˌklōr-ə-ˈpik-rən\ *n* : a heavy colorless liquid CCl_3NO_2 that causes tears and vomiting and is used esp. as a soil fumigant

chlo·ro·pro·caine \ˌklōr-ō-ˈprō-ˌkān\ *n* : a local anesthetic administered by injection in the form of its hydrochloride $C_{13}H_{19}ClN_2O_2{\cdot}HCl$ — see NESACAINE

chlo·ro·quine \ˈklōr-ə-ˌkwēn\ *n* : an antimalarial drug administered in the form of its diphosphate $C_{18}H_{26}ClN_3{\cdot}2H_3PO_4$ or hydrochloride $C_{18}H_{26}ClN_3{\cdot}HCl$

chlo·ro·sis \klə-ˈrō-səs\ *n, pl* **-ro·ses** \-ˌsēz\ : an iron-deficiency anemia esp. of adolescent girls that may impart a greenish tint to the skin — called also *greensickness* — **chlo·rot·ic** \-ˈrä-tik\ *adj*

chlo·ro·thi·a·zide \ˌklōr-ə-ˈthī-ə-ˌzīd, -zəd\ *n* : a thiazide diuretic $C_7H_6ClN_3O_4S_2$ that is taken orally or is administered in the form of its sodium salt $C_7H_5ClN_3NaO_4S_2$ by intravenous injection esp. in the treatment of edema and hypertension — see DIURIL

chlo·ro·tri·an·i·sene \-ˌtrī-ˈa-nə-ˌsēn\ *n* : a synthetic estrogen $C_{23}H_{21}ClO_3$ used esp. formerly to treat menopausal symptoms

chlor·phen·e·sin carbamate \(ˌ)klōr-ˈfe-nə-sin-\ *n* : a drug $C_{10}H_{12}ClNO_4$ used as a skeletal muscle relaxant

chlor·phen·ir·amine \(ˌ)klōr-fen-ˈir-ə-ˌmēn\ *n* : an antihistamine that is usu. administered in the form of its maleate $C_{16}H_{19}ClN_2{\cdot}C_4H_4O_4$ — see ACTIFED

chlor·prom·a·zine \klōr-ˈprä-mə-ˌzēn\ *n* : a phenothiazine derivative that has antipsychotic, sedative, and antiemetic properties and is used in the form of its hydrochloride $C_{17}H_{19}ClN_2S{\cdot}HCl$ esp. to manage the symptoms of psychotic disorders (as in schizophrenia) — see LARGACTIL, THORAZINE

chlor·prop·amide \-ˈprä-pə-ˌmīd, -ˈprō-\ *n* : a sulfonylurea drug $C_{10}H_{13}ClN_2O_3S$ used orally to reduce blood sugar in the treatment of type 2 diabetes

chlor·tet·ra·cy·cline \ˌklōr-ˌte-trə-ˈsī-ˌklēn\ *n* : a broad-spectrum antibiotic $C_{22}H_{23}ClN_2O_8$ produced by a soil actinomycete of the genus *Streptomyces* (*S. aureofaciens*) and sometimes used in animal feeds to stimulate growth — see AUREOMYCIN

chlor·thal·i·done \klōr-ˈtha-lə-ˌdōn\ *n* : a diuretic sulfonamide $C_{14}H_{11}ClN_2O_4S$ used esp. in the treatment of edema and hypertension — see HYGROTON

cho·a·na \ˈkō-ə-nə\ *n, pl* **-nae** \-ˌnē\ : either of the pair of posterior apertures of the nasal cavity that open into the nasopharynx — called also *posterior naris* — **cho·a·nal** \-nəl\ *adj*

Cho·a·no·tae·nia \ˌkō-ə-(ˌ)nō-ˈtē-nē-ə\ *n* : a genus of tapeworms including one (*C. infundibulum*) which is an intestinal parasite of birds

[1]**choke** \ˈchōk\ *vb* **choked; chok·ing 1** : to keep from breathing in a normal way by compressing or obstructing the windpipe or by poisoning or adulterating available air **2** : to have the windpipe blocked entirely or partly

[2]**choke** *n* **1** : the act of choking **2 chokes** *pl* : pulmonary manifestations of decompression sickness including shortness of breath, chest pain, and cough — used with *the*

choked disk *n* : PAPILLEDEMA

chol- *or* **chole** *or* **cholo-** *comb form* : bile : gall ⟨*chol*ate⟩ ⟨*cholo*rrhea⟩

cho·lae·mia *chiefly Brit var of* CHOLEMIA

cho·la·gogue \ˈkä-lə-ˌgäg, ˈkō-\ *n* : an agent that promotes an increased flow of bile — **cho·la·gog·ic** \ˌkä-lə-ˈgä-jik, ˌkō-\ *adj*

chol·an·gio·car·ci·noma \kə-ˌlan-jē-ə-ˌkär-sᵊn-ˈō-mə\ *n* : a usu. slow-growing malignant tumor of the bile duct that arises from biliary epithelium and is typically an adenocarcinoma

chol·an·gio·gram \kə-ˈlan-jē-ə-ˌgram, kō-\ *n* : a radiograph of the bile ducts made after the ingestion or injection of a radiopaque substance

chol·an·gi·og·ra·phy \kə-ˌlan-jē-ˈä-grə-fē, (ˌ)kō-\ *n, pl* **-phies** : radiographic visualization of the bile ducts after ingestion or injection of a radiopaque substance — **chol·an·gio·graph·ic** \-jē-ə-ˈgra-fik\ *adj*

chol·an·gi·o·li·tis \-ə-ˈlī-təs, (ˌ)kō-\ *n, pl* **-lit·i·des** \-ˈli-tə-ˌdēz\ : inflammation of bile capillaries — **chol·an·gi·o·lit·ic** \-ˈli-tik\ *adj*

cholangiopancreatography — see ENDOSCOPIC RETROGRADE CHOLANGIOPANCREATOGRAPHY

chol·an·gi·tis \ˌkō-ˌlan-ˈjī-təs\ *n, pl* **-git·i·des** \-ˈji-tə-ˌdēz\ : inflammation of one or more bile ducts

cho·late \ˈkō-ˌlāt\ *n* : a salt or ester of cholic acid

cho·le·cal·cif·er·ol \ˌkō-lə-(ˌ)kal-ˈsi-fə-ˌrȯl, -ˌrōl\ *n* : a sterol $C_{27}H_{43}OH$ that is a natural form of vitamin D found esp. in fish, egg yolks, and fish-liver oils and is formed in the skin on exposure to sunlight or ultraviolet rays — called also *vitamin D, vitamin* D_3

cho·le·cys·tec·to·my \ˌkō-lə-(ˌ)sis-ˈtek-tə-mē\ *n, pl* **-mies** : surgical excision of the gallbladder — **cho·le·cys·tec·to·mized** \-ˌmīzd\ *adj*

cho·le·cys·ti·tis \-(ˌ)sis-ˈtī-təs\ *n, pl* **-tit·i·des** \-ˈti-tə-ˌdēz\ : inflammation of the gallbladder

cho·le·cys·to·en·ter·os·to·my \-ˌsis-tō-ˌen-tə-ˈräs-tə-mē\ *n, pl* **-mies** : surgical union of and creation of a passage between the gallbladder and the intestine

cho·le·cys·to·gram \-ˈsis-tə-ˌgram\ *n* : a radiograph of the gallbladder made after ingestion or injection of a radiopaque substance

cho·le·cys·tog·ra·phy \-(ˌ)sis-ˈtä-grə-fē\ *n, pl* **-phies** : the radiographic visualization of the gallbladder after ingestion or injection of a radiopaque substance — **cho·le·cys·to·graph·ic** \-ˌsis-tə-ˈgra-fik\ *adj*

cho·le·cys·to·ki·net·ic \-ˌsis-tə-kə-ˈne-tik, -kī-\ *adj* : tending to cause the gallbladder to contract and discharge bile

cho·le·cys·to·ki·nin \-ˌsis-tə-ˈkī-nən\ *n* : a hormone secreted esp. by the duodenal mucosa that regulates the emptying of the gallbladder and secretion of enzymes by the pancreas and that has been found in the brain — called also *cholecystokinin-pancreozymin, pancreozymin*

cho·le·cys·tor·rha·phy \-(ˌ)sis-ˈtȯr-ə-fē\ *n, pl* **-phies** : repair of the gallbladder by suturing

cho·le·cys·tos·to·my \-(ˌ)sis-ˈtäs-tə-mē\ *n, pl* **-mies** : surgical incision of the gallbladder usu. to effect drainage

cho·le·cys·tot·o·my \-ˈtä-tə-mē\ *n, pl* **-mies** : surgical incision of the gallbladder esp. for exploration or to remove a gallstone

cho·le·doch·al \ˈkō-lə-ˌdä-kəl, kə-ˈle-də-kəl\ *adj* : relating to, being, or occurring in the common bile duct

cho·le·do·chi·tis \kə-ˌle-də-ˈkī-təs, ˌkō-lə-\ *n* : inflammation of the common bile duct

cho·led·o·cho·je·ju·nos·to·my \kə-ˌle-də-(ˌ)kō-ji-(ˌ)jü-ˈnäs-tə-mē\ *n, pl* **-mies** : surgical creation of a passage uniting the common bile duct and the jejunum

cho·led·o·cho·li·thi·a·sis \-li-ˈthī-ə-səs\ *n, pl* **-a·ses** \-ˌsēz\ : a condition marked by presence of calculi in the gallbladder and common bile duct

cho•led•o•cho•li•thot•o•my \-li-ˈthä-tə-mē\ *n, pl* **-mies** : surgical incision of the common bile duct for removal of a gallstone

cho•led•o•chor•rha•phy \kə-ˌle-də-ˈkȯr-ə-fē\ *n, pl* **-rha•phies** : surgical union of the separated ends of the common bile duct by suturing

cho•led•o•chos•to•my \-ˈkäs-tə-mē\ *n, pl* **-mies** : surgical incision of the common bile duct usu. to effect drainage

cho•led•o•chot•o•my \-ˈkä-tə-mē\ *n, pl* **-mies** : surgical incision of the common bile duct

cho•led•o•chus \kə-ˈle-də-kəs\ *n, pl* **-o•chi** \-ˌkī, -ˌkē\ : COMMON BILE DUCT

cho•le•glo•bin \ˈkō-lə-ˌglō-bən, ˈkä-\ *n* : a green pigment that occurs in bile and is formed by breakdown of hemoglobin

cho•le•lith \ˈkō-li-ˌlith, ˈkä-\ *n* : GALLSTONE

cho•le•li•thi•a•sis \ˌkō-li-li-ˈthī-ə-səs\ *n, pl* **-a•ses** \-ˌsēz\ : production of gallstones; *also* : the resulting abnormal condition

cho•le•mia \kō-ˈlē-mē-ə\ *n* : the presence of excess bile in the blood usu. indicative of liver disease — **cho•le•mic** \-mik\ *adj*

cho•le•poi•e•sis \ˌkō-lə-ˌpȯi-ˈē-səs, ˌkä-\ *n, pl* **-e•ses** \-ˌsēz\ : production of bile — **cho•le•poi•et•ic** \-ˈe-tik\ *adj*

chol•era \ˈkä-lə-rə\ *n* : any of several diseases of humans and domestic animals usu. marked by severe gastrointestinal symptoms: as **a** : an acute diarrheal disease caused by an enterotoxin produced by a comma-shaped gram-negative bacillus of the genus *Vibrio* (*V. cholerae* syn. *V. comma*) when it is present in large numbers in the proximal part of the human small intestine — see ASIATIC CHOLERA **b** : FOWL CHOLERA **c** : HOG CHOLERA — **chol•e•ra•ic** \ˌkä-lə-ˈrā-ik\ *adj*

cholera mor•bus \-ˈmȯr-bəs\ *n* : a gastrointestinal disturbance characterized by abdominal pain, diarrhea, and sometimes vomiting — not used technically

cho•le•re•sis \ˌkō-lə-ˈrē-səs, ˌkä-\ *n, pl* **-re•ses** \-ˌsēz\ : the flow of bile from the liver esp. when increased above a previous or normal level

[1]**cho•le•ret•ic** \ˌkō-lə-ˈre-tik, ˌkä-\ *adj* : promoting bile secretion by the liver ⟨~ action of bile salts⟩

[2]**choleretic** *n* : a choleretic agent

cho•le•scin•tig•ra•phy \ˌkō-lə-sin-ˈti-grə-fē\ *n, pl* **-phies** : scintigraphy of the biliary system

cho•le•sta•sis \ˌkō-lə-ˈstā-səs, ˌkä-\ *n, pl* **-sta•ses** \-ˈstā-ˌsēz\ : a checking or failure of bile flow — **cho•le•stat•ic** \-ˈsta-tik\ *adj*

cho•les•te•a•to•ma \kə-ˌles-tē-ə-ˈtō-mə, ˌkō-lə-ˌstē-, ˌkä-lə-\ *n, pl* **-mas** *also* **-ma•ta** \-mə-tə\ **1** : an epidermoid cyst usu. in the brain appearing as a compact shiny flaky mass **2** : a tumor usu. growing in a confined space (as the middle ear) and frequently constituting a sequel to chronic otitis media — **cho•les•te•a•to•ma•tous** \-mə-təs\ *adj*

cho•les•ter•ol \kə-ˈles-tə-ˌrōl, -ˌrȯl\ *n* : a steroid alcohol $C_{27}H_{45}OH$ present in animal cells and body fluids that regulates membrane fluidity, functions as a precursor molecule in various metabolic pathways, and as a constituent of LDL may cause atherosclerosis — **cho•les•ter•ic** \kə-ˈles-tə-rik; ˌkō-lə-ˈster-ik, ˌkä-\ *adj*

cho•les•ter•ol•ae•mia *also* **cho•les•te•rae•mia** *chiefly Brit var of* CHOLESTEROLEMIA

cho•les•ter•ol•emia \kə-ˌles-tə-rə-ˈlē-mē-ə\ *also* **cho•les•ter•emia** \-ˈrē-mē-ə\ *n* : the presence of cholesterol in the blood

cho•les•ter•ol•osis \kə-ˌles-tə-rə-ˈlō-səs\ *or* **cho•les•ter•o•sis** \kə-ˌles-tə-ˈrō-səs\ *n, pl* **-o•ses** \-ˌsēz\ : abnormal deposition of cholesterol (as in blood vessels or the gallbladder)

cho•le•styr•amine \kō-ˈles-tir-ə-ˌmēn\ *n* : a strongly basic synthetic resin used esp. to lower cholesterol levels

cho•lic acid \ˈkō-lik-\ *n* : a crystalline bile acid $C_{24}H_{40}O_5$

cho•line \ˈkō-ˌlēn\ *n* : a basic compound $C_5H_{14}NO$ that is found in various foods (as egg yolks and legumes) or is synthesized in the liver, is a precursor of acetylcholine, and is essential to liver function

choline ace•tyl•trans•fer•ase \-ə-ˌsē-tᵊl-ˈtrans-fər-ˌās\ *n* : an enzyme that catalyzes the synthesis of acetylcholine from acetyl coenzyme A and choline

cho•lin•er•gic \ˌkō-lə-ˈnər-jik\ *adj* **1** *of autonomic nerve fibers* : liberating, activated by, or involving acetylcholine — compare ADRENERGIC 1, NORADRENERGIC **2** : resembling acetylcholine esp. in physiologic action — **cho•lin•er•gi•cal•ly** \-ji-k(ə-)lē\ *adv*

cho•lin•es•ter•ase \ˌkō-lə-ˈnes-tə-ˌrās, -ˌrāz\ *n* **1** : an enzyme that occurs chiefly at neuromuscular junctions and promotes the hydrolysis of acetylcholine at postsynaptic receptors : ACETYLCHOLINESTERASE **2** : BUTYRYLCHOLINESTERASE

[1]**cho•li•no•lyt•ic** \ˌkō-lə-nō-ˈli-tik\ *adj* : interfering with the action of acetylcholine or cholinergic agents

[2]**cholinolytic** *n* : a cholinolytic substance

[1]**cho•li•no•mi•met•ic** \ˌkō-lə-nō-mə-ˈme-tik, ˌkä-, -mī-\ *adj* : resembling acetylcholine or simulating its physiologic action

[2]**cholinomimetic** *n* : a cholinomimetic substance

cholo- — see CHOL-

cho•lor•rhea \ˌkä-lə-ˈrē-ə, ˌkō-\ *n* : excessive secretion of bile

cho•lor•rhoea *chiefly Brit var of* CHOLORRHEA

chol•uria \kō-ˈlu̇r-ē-ə, kōl-ˈyu̇r-\ *n* : presence of bile in urine

chondr- *or* **chondri-** *or* **chondro-** *comb form* : cartilage ⟨*chondro*clast⟩

chon•dral \ˈkän-drəl\ *adj* : of or relating to cartilage

chon•dri•tis \kän-ˈdrī-təs\ *n* : inflammation of cartilage

chon•dro•blast \ˈkän-drə-ˌblast, -drō-\ *n* : a cell that produces cartilage — **chon•dro•blas•tic** \ˌkän-drə-ˈblas-tik, -drō-\ *adj*

chon•dro•cal•ci•no•sis \ˌkän-drō-ˌkal-sə-ˈnō-səs\ *n, pl* **-no•ses** \-ˈnō-ˌsēz\ : the abnormal deposition of calcium salts in cartilage (as of joints)

chon•dro•clast \ˈkän-drə-ˌklast, -drō-\ *n* : a cell that absorbs cartilage

chon•dro•cos•tal \ˌkän-drə-ˈkäst-ᵊl, -drō-\ *adj* : of or relating to the costal cartilages and the ribs

chon•dro•cyte \ˈkän-drə-ˌsīt, -drō-\ *n* : a cartilage cell

chon•dro•dys•pla•sia \ˌkän-drə-dis-ˈplā-zhə, -drō-, -zhē-ə\ *n* : a hereditary skeletal disorder characterized by the formation of exostoses at the epiphyses and resulting in arrested development and deformity — called also *dyschondroplasia*

chon•dro•dys•tro•phia \-dis-ˈtrō-fē-ə\ *n* : ACHONDROPLASIA

chon•dro•dys•tro•phy \-ˈdis-trə-fē\ *n, pl* **-phies** : ACHONDROPLASIA — **chon•dro•dys•tro•phic** \-dis-ˈtrō-fik\ *adj*

chon•dro•gen•e•sis \-ˈje-nə-səs\ *n, pl* **-e•ses** \-ˌsēz\ : the development of cartilage — **chon•dro•gen•ic** \-ˈje-nik\ *adj*

chon•droid \ˈkän-ˌdrȯid\ *adj* : resembling cartilage

chon•droi•tin \kän-ˈdrȯit-ᵊn, -ˈdrō-ət-ᵊn\ *n* : any of several glycosaminoglycans occurring in sulfated form in various tissues (as cartilage and tendons)

chon•drol•o•gy \kän-ˈdrä-lə-jē\ *n, pl* **-gies** : a branch of anatomy concerned with cartilage

chon•dro•ma \kän-ˈdrō-mə\ *n, pl* **-mas** \-məz\ *also* **-ma•ta** \-mə-tə\ : a benign tumor containing the structural elements of cartilage — **chon•dro•ma•tous** \(ˈ)kän-ˈdrä-mə-təs, -ˈdrō-\ *adj*

chon•dro•ma•la•cia \ˌkän-drō-mə-ˈlā-shə, -shē-ə\ *n* : abnormal softness of cartilage

chondromalacia patellae *or* **chondromalacia patella** *n* : pain over the front of the knee with softening of the articular cartilage of the patella — see RUNNER'S KNEE

chon•dro–os•teo•dys•tro•phy \-ˌäs-tē-ō-ˈdis-trə-fē\ *n, pl* **-phies** : any of several mucopolysaccharidoses (as Hurler syndrome) characterized esp. by disorders of bone and cartilage

chon•dro•phyte \ˈkän-drō-ˌfīt\ *n* : an outgrowth or spur of cartilage

chon•dro•sar•co•ma \ˌkän-drō-sär-ˈkō-mə\ *n, pl* **-mas** *also* **-ma•ta** \-mə-tə\ : a sarcoma containing cartilage cells

chon•dro•ster•nal \ˌkän-drō-ˈstərn-ᵊl\ *adj* : of or relating to the costal cartilages and sternum

Cho•part's joint \(ˌ)shō-ˈpärz-\ *n* : the tarsal joint that comprises the talonavicular and calcaneocuboid articulations

Cho•part \shō-pȧr\, **François (1743–1795)**, French surgeon.

chor•da ten•din•ea \ˈkȯr-də-ˌten-ˈdi-nē-ə\ *n, pl* **chor•dae ten•din•e•ae** \-nē-ˌē\ : any of the delicate tendinous cords that are attached to the edges of the atrioventricular valves of the heart and to the papillary muscles and serve to prevent the valves from being pushed into the atrium during the ventricular contraction

chorda tym•pa•ni \-ˈtim-pə-ˌnī\ *n* : a branch of the facial nerve that traverses the middle ear cavity and the infratemporal fossa and supplies autonomic fibers to the sublingual and submandibular glands and sensory fibers to the anterior part of the tongue

chor•dee \ˈkȯr-ˌdē, -ˌdā, ˌkȯr-ˈ\ *n* : painful erection of the penis often with a downward curvature that may be present in a congenital condition (as hypospadias) or accompany gonorrhea

chor•do•ma \kȯr-ˈdō-mə\ *n, pl* **-mas** *also* **-ma•ta** \-mə-tə\ : a malignant tumor that is derived from remnants of the embryonic notochord and occurs along the spine

chordotomy *var of* CORDOTOMY

cho•rea \kə-ˈrē-ə\ *n* : a movement disorder marked by involuntary spasmodic movements esp. of the limbs and facial muscles and typically symptomatic of neurological dysfunction (as that associated with a neurodegenerative disease) — see HUNTINGTON'S DISEASE, SYDENHAM'S CHOREA — **cho•re•at•ic** \ˌkōr-ē-ˈa-tik\ *adj* — **cho•re•ic** \kə-ˈrē-ik\ *adj*

cho•re•i•form \kə-ˈrē-ə-ˌfȯrm\ *adj* : resembling chorea ⟨~ convulsions⟩

cho•reo•ath•e•to•sis \-ˌa-thə-ˈtō-səs\ *n, pl* **-to•ses** \-ˌsēz\ : a nervous disturbance marked by the involuntary movements characteristic of chorea and athetosis

cho•rio•al•lan•to•is \ˌkōr-ē-ō-ə-ˈlan-tə-wəs\ *n, pl* **-to•ides** \-ō-ˌa-lən-ˈtō-ə-ˌdēz, -ˌlan-\ : a vascular fetal membrane composed of the fused chorion and adjacent wall of the allantois — called also *chorioallantoic membrane* — **cho•rio•al•lan•to•ic** \-ˌa-lən-ˈtō-ik\ *adj*

cho•rio•am•ni•o•ni•tis \-ˌam-nē-ō-ˈnī-təs\ *n* : inflammation of the fetal membranes

cho•rio•an•gi•o•ma \-ˌan-jē-ˈō-mə\ *n, pl* **-mas** *also* **-ma•ta** \-mət-ə\ : a benign vascular tumor of the chorion

cho•rio•cap•il•lar•is \-ˌka-pə-ˈlar-əs\ *n* : the inner of the two vascular layers of the choroid of the eye that is composed largely of capillaries

cho•rio•car•ci•no•ma \-ˌkärs-ᵊn-ˈō-mə\ *n, pl* **-mas** *also* **-ma•ta** \-mə-tə\ : a malignant tumor derived from trophoblastic tissue that develops typically in the uterus following pregnancy, miscarriage, or abortion esp. when associated with a hydatidiform mole or rarely in the testes or ovaries chiefly as a component of a mixed germ-cell tumor

cho•rio•ep•i•the•li•o•ma \-ˌe-pə-ˌthē-lē-ˈō-mə\ *n, pl* **-mas** *also* **-ma•ta** \-mə-tə\ : CHORIOCARCINOMA

cho•ri•o•ma \ˌkōr-ē-ˈō-mə\ *n, pl* **-mas** *also* **-ma•ta** \-mə-tə\ : a tumor formed of chorionic tissue

cho•rio•men•in•gi•tis \ˌkōr-ē-(ˌ)ō-ˌme-nən-ˈjī-təs\ *n, pl* **-git•i•des** \-ˈji-tə-ˌdēz\ : cerebral meningitis; *specif* : LYMPHOCYTIC CHORIOMENINGITIS

cho•ri•on \ˈkōr-ē-ˌän\ *n* : the highly vascular outer embryonic membrane that is associated with the allantois in the formation of the placenta

cho•ri•on•ep•i•the•li•o•ma \ˌkōr-ē-ˌä-ˌne-pə-ˌthē-lē-ˈō-mə\ *n, pl* **-mas** *also* **-ma•ta** \-mə-tə\ : CHORIOCARCINOMA

chorion fron•do•sum \-frən-ˈdō-səm\ *n* : the part of the chorion that has persistent villi and that with the decidua basalis forms the placenta — see CHORIONIC VILLUS SAMPLING

cho•ri•on•ic \ˌkōr-ē-ˈä-nik\ *adj* **1** : of, relating to, or being part of the chorion ⟨~ villi⟩ **2** : secreted or produced by chorionic or a related tissue (as in the placenta or a choriocarcinoma)

chorionic so•ma•to•mam•mo•tro•pin \-ˌsō-mə-tə-ˌma-mə-ˈtrō-pᵊn\ *n* : PLACENTAL LACTOGEN

chorionic villus sampling *also* **chorionic villi sampling** *n* : biopsy of the chorion frondosum through the abdominal wall or by way of the vagina and uterine cervix at 10 to 12 weeks of gestation to obtain fetal cells for the prenatal diagnosis of chromosomal abnormalities — abbr. *CVS*

chorion lae•ve \-ˈlē-və\ *n* : the smooth part of the chorion that lacks villi

Cho•ri•op•tes \ˌkōr-ē-ˈäp-ˌtēz\ *n* : a genus of small parasitic mites infesting domestic animals — **cho•ri•op•tic** \-ˈäp-tik\ *adj*

chorioptic mange *n* : mange caused by mites of the genus *Chorioptes* that usu. attack only the surface of the skin — compare DEMODECTIC MANGE, SARCOPTIC MANGE

cho•rio•ret•i•nal \ˌkōr-ē-ō-ˈret-ᵊn-əl\ *adj* : of, relating to, or affecting the choroid and the retina of the eye

cho•rio•ret•i•ni•tis \-ˌret-ᵊn-ˈī-təs\ *also* **cho•roi•do•ret•i•ni•tis** \kə-ˌrȯi-dō-\ *n, pl* **-nit•i•des** \-ˈi-tə-ˌdēz\ : inflammation of the retina and choroid of the eye

cho•roid \ˈkōr-ˌȯid\ *n* : a vascular membrane containing large branched pigment cells that lies between the retina and the sclera of the eye — called also *choroid coat* — **choroid** *or* **cho•roi•dal** \kə-ˈrȯid-ᵊl\ *adj*

choroidea — see TELA CHOROIDEA

cho•roi•de•re•mia \ˌkōr-ˌȯi-də-ˈrē-mē-ə\ *n* : progressive degeneration of the choroid that is an X-linked trait chiefly affecting males and that is characterized by night blindness, constriction of the visual field, and eventual blindness

cho•roid•itis \ˌkōr-ˌȯi-ˈdī-təs\ *also* **cho•ri•oid•itis** \ˌkōr-ē-ȯi-\ *n* : inflammation of the choroid of the eye

cho•roi•do•iri•tis \kə-ˌrȯi-dō-ī-ˈrī-təs\ *n* : inflammation of the choroid and the iris of the eye

cho•roid•op•a•thy \ˌkōr-ˌȯi-ˈdä-pə-thē\ *n, pl* **-thies** : a diseased condition affecting the choroid of the eye

choroid plexus *n* : a highly vascular portion of the pia mater that projects into the ventricles of the brain and secretes cerebrospinal fluid

Christ•mas disease \ˈkris-məs-\ *n* : HEMOPHILIA B

Christmas, Stephen, British child patient.

Christmas factor *n* : FACTOR IX

chrom•aes•the•sia *chiefly Brit var of* CHROMESTHESIA

chro•maf•fin \ˈkrō-mə-fən\ *adj* : staining deeply with chromium salts

chro•maf•fi•no•ma \ˌkrō-mə-fə-ˈnō-mə, krō-ˌma-\ *n, pl* **-mas** *also* **-ma•ta** \-mə-tə\ : a tumor containing chromaffin cells; *esp* : PHEOCHROMOCYTOMA

chro•ma•phil \ˈkrō-mə-ˌfil\ *adj* : CHROMAFFIN ⟨~ tissue⟩

chromat- *or* **chromato-** *comb form* **1** : color ⟨*chromat*id⟩ **2** : chromatin ⟨*chromato*lysis⟩

chro•mat•ic \krō-ˈma-tik\ *adj* **1** : of, relating to, or characterized by color or color phenomena or sensations ⟨~ stimuli⟩ **2** : capable of being colored by staining agents ⟨~ substances⟩

chromatic vision *n* **1** : normal color vision in which the colors of the spectrum are distinguished and evaluated **2** : CHROMATOPSIA

chro•ma•tid \ˈkrō-mə-təd\ *n* : one of the usu. paired and parallel strands of a duplicated chromosome joined by a single centromere — see CHROMONEMA

chro•ma•tin \ˈkrō-mə-tən\ *n* : a complex of a nucleic acid with basic proteins (as histone) in eukaryotic cells that is usu. dispersed in the interphase nucleus and condensed into chromosomes in mitosis and meiosis — **chro•ma•tin•ic** \ˌkrō-mə-ˈti-nik\ *adj*

chro•ma•tism \ˈkrō-mə-ˌti-zəm\ *n* : CHROMESTHESIA

chromato- — see CHROMAT-

chro•mato•gram \krō-ˈma-tə-ˌgram, krə-\ *n* **1** : the pattern formed on the adsorbent medium by the layers of components separated by chromatography **2** : a time-based graphic record of a chromatographic separation

chro•mato•graph \krō-ˈma-tə-ˌgraf, krə-\ *n* : an instrument for producing chromatograms — **chromatograph** *vb*

chro•ma•tog•ra•phy \ˌkrō-mə-ˈtä-grə-fē\ *n, pl* **-phies** : a process in which a chemical mixture carried by a liquid or gas is separated into components as a result of differential distribution of the solutes as they flow around or over a stationary liquid or solid phase — **chro•mato•graph•ic** \krō-ˌma-tə-ˈgra-fik, krə-\ *adj* — **chro•mato•graph•i•cal•ly** \-fi-k(ə-)lē\ *adv*

chro•ma•tol•y•sis \ˌkrō-mə-ˈtä-lə-səs\ *n, pl* **-y•ses** \-ˌsēz\ : the dispersal of Nissl substance in the cell body of a neuron resulting from axonal stress (as that induced by injury or neurodegenerative disease) — **chro•ma•to•lyt•ic** \krō-ˌmat-ᵊl-ˈi-tik, krə-\ *adj*

chro•mato•phore \krō-ˈma-tə-ˌfōr, krə-\ *n* : a pigment-bearing cell esp. in the skin

chro•ma•top•sia \ˌkrō-mə-ˈtäp-sē-ə\ *n* : a disturbance of vision in which colorless objects appear colored

chro•ma•to•sis \ˌkrō-mə-ˈtō-səs\ *n, pl* **-to•ses** \-ˌsēz\ : PIGMENTATION; *specif* : deposit of pigment in a normally unpigmented area or excessive pigmentation in a normally pigmented site

chrom•es•the•sia \ˌkrō-mes-ˈthē-zhə, -zhē-ə\ *n* : synesthesia in which color is perceived in response to stimuli (as words or numbers) that contain no element of color — called also *chromatism*

chro•mi•dro•sis \ˌkrō-mə-ˈdrō-səs\ *also* **chrom•hi•dro•sis** \ˌkrōm-(h)ə-\ *n, pl* **-dro•ses** \-ˌsēz\ : secretion of colored sweat

chro•mi•um \ˈkrō-mē-əm\ *n* : a blue-white metallic element found naturally only in combination — symbol *Cr;* see ELEMENT table

chromium picolinate *n* : a biologically active chromium salt $C_{18}H_{12}CrN_3O_6$ that is used as a dietary supplement

chro•mo•blas•to•my•co•sis \ˌkrō-mə-ˌblas-tə-ˌmī-ˈkō-səs\ *n, pl* **-co•ses** \-ˌsēz\ : a chronic infection of skin and subcutaneous tissues that is caused by pigmented fungi (as *Fonsecaea pedrosoi*, *Phialophora verrucosa*, and *Cladophialophora carrionii*) and is marked by the formation of usu. warty, nodular, or scaly lesions esp. on the legs or feet — called also *chromomycosis*

chro•mo•en•dos•co•py \ˌkrō-mō-en-ˈdä-skə-pē\ *also* **chro•mos•co•py** \krō-ˈmä-skə-pē\ *n, pl* **-pies** : a technique involving the application of stains or dyes to tissues esp. of the esophagus and gastrointestinal tract during endoscopic examination to facilitate detection and identification of abnormal cell growth — **chro•mo•en•do•scop•ic** \ˌkrō-mō-ˌen-də-ˈskä-pik\ *also* **chro•mo•scop•ic** \ˌkrō-mə-ˈskä-pik\ *adj*

¹**chro•mo•mere** \ˈkrō-mə-ˌmir\ *n* : the highly refractile portion of a blood platelet — compare HYALOMERE

²**chromomere** *n* : one of the small bead-shaped and heavily staining concentrations of chromatin that are linearly arranged along the chromosome — **chro•mo•mer•ic** \ˌkrō-mə-ˈmer-ik, -ˈmir-\ *adj*

chro•mo•my•co•sis \ˌkrō-mə-ˌmī-ˈkō-səs\ *n, pl* **-co•ses** \-ˌsēz\ : CHROMOBLASTOMYCOSIS

chro•mo•ne•ma \ˌkrō-mə-ˈnē-mə\ *n, pl* **-ne•ma•ta** \-ˈnē-mə-tə\ : the coiled filamentous core of a chromatid — **chro•mo•ne•mat•ic** \-ni-ˈma-tik\ *adj*

chro•mo•nych•ia \ˌkrō-mə-ˈni-kē-ə\ *n* : discoloration or abnormal pigmentation of the fingernails or toenails or the underlying tissue

chro•mo•phil \ˈkrō-mə-ˌfil\ *adj* : staining readily with dyes

¹**chro•mo•phobe** \ˈkrō-mə-ˌfōb\ *adj* : not readily absorbing stains : difficult to stain ⟨~ tumors⟩

²**chromophobe** *n* : a chromophobe cell esp. of the pituitary gland

chro•mo•pro•tein \ˌkro-mə-ˈprō-ˌtēn\ *n* : any of various proteins (as hemoglobins or carotenoids) having a pigment as a prosthetic group

chro•mo•some \ˈkrō-mə-ˌsōm, -ˌzōm\ *n* : any of the rod-shaped or threadlike DNA-containing structures of cellular organisms that are located in the nucleus of eukaryotes, are usu. ring-shaped in prokaryotes (as bacteria), and contain most or all of the genes of the organism; *also* : the genetic material of a virus — **chro•mo•som•al** \ˌkrō-mə-ˈsō-məl, -ˈzō-\ *adj* — **chro•mo•som•al•ly** *adv*

chromosome complement *n* : the entire group of chromosomes in a nucleus

chromosome number *n* : the usu. constant number of chromosomes characteristic of a particular kind of animal or plant

chron•ax•ie *or* **chron•axy** \ˈkrō-ˌnak-sē, ˈkrä-\ *n, pl* **-ax•ies** : the minimum time required for excitation of a structure (as a nerve cell) by a constant electric current of twice the threshold voltage

¹**chron•ic** \ˈkrä-nik\ *also* **chron•i•cal** \-ni-kəl\ *adj* **1 a** : marked by long duration, by frequent recurrence over a long time, and often by slowly progressing seriousness : not acute ⟨~ indigestion⟩ **b** : suffering from a disease or ailment of long duration or frequent recurrence ⟨a ~ arthritic⟩ **2 a** : having a slow progressive course of indefinite duration — used esp. of degenerative invasive diseases, some infections, psychoses, and inflammations ⟨~ heart disease⟩ ⟨~ arthritis⟩; compare ACUTE 2b **b** : infected with a disease-causing agent (as a virus) and remaining infectious over a long period of time but not necessarily ex-

pressing symptoms <~ carriers> — **chron•i•cal•ly** \-ni-k(ə-)lē\ *adv* — **chro•nic•i•ty** \krä-ˈni-sə-tē, krō-\ *n*

²**chronic** *n* : one that suffers from a chronic disease

chronica — see ACRODERMATITIS CHRONICA ATROPHICANS

chronic alcoholism *n* : ALCOHOLISM 2b

chronic care *adj* : providing or concerned with long-term medical care lasting usu. more than 90 days esp. for individuals with chronic physical or mental impairment — **chronic care** *n*

chronic fatigue syndrome *n* : a disorder of uncertain cause that is characterized by persistent profound fatigue usu. accompanied by impairment in short-term memory or concentration, sore throat, tender lymph nodes, muscle or joint pain, and headache unrelated to any preexisting medical condition and that typically has an onset at about 30 years of age — abbr. *CFS;* called also *myalgic encephalomyelitis*

chronic granulocytic leukemia *n* : CHRONIC MYELOGENOUS LEUKEMIA

chronic granulomatous disease *n* : an immune system disorder that is marked by recurrent often serious infections (as of the skin or lungs) and excessive granuloma formation, results from the inability of white blood cells to destroy certain bacteria and fungi, and is inherited as an X-linked or autosomal trait

chronic lymphocytic leukemia *n* : lymphocytic leukemia that is marked by an abnormal increase in the number of mature lymphocytes and esp. B cells, that is characterized by slow onset and progression, and that occurs esp. in older adults — abbr. *CLL;* compare ACUTE LYMPHOCYTIC LEUKEMIA

chronic myelogenous leukemia *n* : myelogenous leukemia that is marked by an abnormal increase in granulocytes esp. in bone marrow and blood, occurs esp. in adults, and is associated with the presence of the Philadelphia chromosome — abbr. *CML;* called also *chronic myelocytic leukemia, chronic myeloid leukemia, chronic granulocytic leukemia;* compare ACUTE MYELOGENOUS LEUKEMIA

chronic obstructive pulmonary disease *n* : pulmonary disease (as emphysema or chronic bronchitis) that is characterized by chronic typically irreversible airway obstruction resulting in a slowed rate of exhalation — called also *chronic obstructive lung disease, COPD*

chronic traumatic encephalopathy *n* : a progressive neurological disease that is found esp. in athletes who have experienced repetitive usu. minor injury (as concussion) to the brain and is characterized by cognitive deficits (as short-term memory loss), depression, behavioral and personality changes, speech and gait abnormalities, parkinsonism, and dementia — abbr. *CTE;* called also *dementia pugilistica, punch-drunk syndrome*

chronicum — see ERYTHEMA CHRONICUM MIGRANS

chronicus — see LICHEN SIMPLEX CHRONICUS

chronic venous insufficiency *n* : inability of the veins of the legs to return blood to the heart that is chiefly due to absence of or damage to venous valves (as from deep vein thrombosis or phlebitis) resulting in the pooling of blood in the lower legs and that is marked by edema, pain, reddened or discolored skin, varicose veins, eczema, and ulceration of the legs — called also *postphlebitic syndrome*

chro•no•bi•ol•o•gy \ˌkrä-nə-bī-ˈä-lə-jē, ˌkrō-\ *n, pl* **-gies** : the study of biological rhythms — **chro•no•bi•o•log•ic** \-ˌbī-ə-ˈlä-jik\ *or* **chro•no•bi•o•log•i•cal** \-ji-kəl\ *adj* — **chro•no•bi•ol•o•gist** \-bī-ˈä-lə-jist\ *n*

chro•no•log•i•cal age \ˌkrän-ᵊl-ˈä-ji-kəl-, ˌkrōn-\ *n* : the age of a person as measured from birth to a given date

chro•no•ther•a•peu•tics \-ˌther-ə-ˈpyüt-iks\ *n* : CHRONOTHERAPY 2 — **chro•no•ther•a•peu•tic** \-ˈpyüt-ik\ *adj*

chro•no•ther•a•py \ˌkrä-nə-ˈther-ə-pē, ˌkrō-\ *n, pl* **-pies** **1** : treatment of a sleep disorder (as insomnia) by changing sleeping and waking times in an attempt to reset the patient's biological clock **2** : the administration of medication or treatment in coordination with the body's circadian rhythms to maximize effectiveness and minimize side effects

chro•no•trop•ic \-ˈträ-pik\ *adj* : influencing the rate esp. of the heartbeat

chro•not•ro•pism \krə-ˈnä-trə-ˌpi-zəm\ *n* : interference with the rate of the heartbeat

chro•no•type \ˈkrō-nə-ˌtīp\ *n* : the internal circadian rhythm or body clock of a person that influences the cycle of sleep

chrys•a•ro•bin \ˌkri-sə-ˈrō-bən\ *n* : a brownish to orange-yellow powder that is obtained from the wood of a Brazilian leguminous tree (*Andira araroba*) and is used to treat skin diseases

chry•si•a•sis \krə-ˈsī-ə-səs\ *n, pl* **-a•ses** \-ˌsēz\ : a grayish-purple to grayish-blue pigmentation of the skin and whites of the eyes due to deposition of gold particles in the tissues

Chrys•ops \ˈkri-ˌsäps\ *n* : a genus of horseflies (family Tabanidae) including the deerflies and mango flies

chryso•ther•a•py \ˌkri-sə-ˈther-ə-pē\ *n, pl* **-pies** : treatment (as of rheumatoid arthritis) by injection of gold salts

Churg–Strauss syndrome \ˈchərg-ˈstraus-\ *n* : a rare progressive inflammatory disease affecting esp. the lungs and skin and usu. beginning with asthma, allergic rhinitis, nasal polyps, and sinusitis followed by eosinophilia and eventually systemic inflammation of blood vessels — called also *allergic granulomatosis;* see ANTINEUTROPHIL CYTOPLASMIC ANTIBODY

Churg, Jacob (1910–2005), and **Strauss, Lotte (1913–1985),** American pathologists.

Chvos·tek's sign \ˈvȯs-ˌteks-, ˈkvȯs-\ *or* **Chvos·tek sign** \-ˌtek-\ *n* : a twitch of the facial muscles following gentle tapping over the facial nerve in front of the ear that indicates hyperirritability of the facial nerve

Chvostek, Franz (1835–1884), Austrian surgeon.

chyl- *or* **chyli-** *or* **chylo-** *comb form* : chyle ⟨*chyl*uria⟩ ⟨*chylo*thorax⟩

chyle \ˈkīl\ *n* : lymph that is milky from emulsified fats, is characteristically present in the lacteals, and is most apparent during intestinal absorption of fats

chyli — see CISTERNA CHYLI

-chylia *n comb form* : condition of having (such) chyle ⟨a*chylia*⟩

chy·lo·mi·cron \ˌkī-lō-ˈmī-ˌkrän\ *n* : a lipoprotein rich in triglyceride and common in the blood during fat digestion and assimilation

chy·lo·mi·cro·nae·mia *chiefly Brit var of* CHYLOMICRONEMIA

chy·lo·mi·cro·ne·mia \-ˌmī-krə-ˈnē-mē-ə\ *n* : an excessive number of chylomicrons in the blood

chy·lo·tho·rax \-ˈthōr-ˌaks\ *n, pl* **-rax·es** *or* **-ra·ces** \-ˈthōr-ə-ˌsēz\ : an effusion of chyle or chylous fluid into the thoracic cavity

chy·lous \ˈkī-ləs\ *adj* : consisting of or like chyle ⟨~ ascites⟩

chyl·uria \kī-ˈlu̇r-ē-ə, kīl-ˈyu̇r-\ *n* : the presence of chyle in the urine as a result of organic disease (as of the kidney) or of mechanical lymphatic esp. parasitic obstruction

chyme \ˈkīm\ *n* : the semifluid mass of partly digested food expelled by the stomach into the duodenum — **chy·mous** \ˈkī-məs\ *adj*

chy·mo·pa·pa·in \ˌkī-mō-pə-ˈpā-ən, -ˈpī-ən\ *n* : a proteolytic enzyme from the latex of the papaya that is used in meat tenderizer and has been used medically in chemonucleolysis

chy·mo·tryp·sin \ˌkī-mō-ˈtrip-sən\ *n* : a protease that hydrolyzes peptide bonds and is formed in the intestine from chymotrypsinogen — **chy·mo·tryp·tic** \-ˈtrip-tik\ *adj*

chy·mo·tryp·sin·o·gen \-ˌtrip-ˈsi-nə-jən\ *n* : a zymogen that is secreted by the pancreas and is converted by trypsin to chymotrypsin

Ci·al·is \sē-ˈa-ləs\ *trademark* — used for a preparation of tadalafil

ci·ca·trix \ˈsi-kə-ˌtriks, sə-ˈkā-triks\ *n, pl* **ci·ca·tri·ces** \ˌsi-kə-ˈtrī-(ˌ)sēz, sə-ˈkā-trə-ˌsēz\ : a scar resulting from formation and contraction of fibrous tissue in a flesh wound — **cic·a·tri·cial** \ˌsi-kə-ˈtri-shəl\ *adj*

cic·a·tri·zant \ˌsi-kə-ˈtrīz-ᵊnt\ *adj* : promoting the healing of a wound or the formation of a cicatrix

cic·a·tri·za·tion \ˌsi-kə-trə-ˈzā-shən\ *n* : scar formation at the site of a healing wound — **cic·a·trize** \ˈsi-kə-ˌtrīz\ *vb*

ci·cles·o·nide \sī-ˈkle-sə-ˌnīd\ *n* : a corticosteroid drug $C_{32}H_{44}O_7$ that is used as an inhalational aerosol to treat asthma and as a nasal spray or aerosol to treat allergic rhinitis — see ALVESCO, OMNARIS, ZETONNA

Ci·clo·dan \ˌsī-klə-ˌdan\ *trademark* — used for a preparation of ciclopirox

ci·clo·pir·ox \ˌsī-klō-ˈpir-ˌäks\ *n* : a synthetic, topical, antifungal agent $C_{12}H_{17}NO_2$ or its derivative $C_{12}H_{17}NO_2 \cdot C_2H_7NO$ (ciclopirox ol·a·mine \-ˈä-lə-ˌmēn\) used to treat fungal infections of the skin, scalp, and nails — see CICLODAN, LOPROX, PENLAC

CICU *abbr* coronary intensive care unit; cardiovascular intensive care unit; coronary intensive care unit

cic·u·tox·in \ˌsi-kyə-ˈtäk-sən, ˈsi-kyə-ˌ\ *n* : an amorphous poisonous principle $C_{19}H_{26}O_3$ in water hemlock, spotted cowbane, and related plants

ci·dof·o·vir \sī-ˈdä-fə-ˌvir\ *n* : an antiviral agent $C_8H_{14}N_3O_6P \cdot 2H_2O$ administered intravenously esp. to treat cytomegalovirus infection of the eye — see VISTIDE

cigarette drain *n* : a cigarette-shaped gauze wick enclosed in rubber dam tissue or rubber tubing for draining wounds — called also *Penrose drain*

ci·gua·tera \ˌsē-gwə-ˈter-ə, ˌsi-\ *n* : poisoning caused by the ingestion of various normally edible tropical fish in whose flesh a toxic substance has accumulated

ci·gua·tox·in \ˈsē-gwə-ˌtäk-sən, ˈsi-\ *n* : a potent neurotoxin that is produced by a marine dinoflagellate (*Gambierdiscus toxicus*) and causes ciguatera poisoning in those who eat fish in which toxic levels of it have become concentrated; *also* : any of several related neurotoxins causing ciguatera

ci·la·stat·in \ˌsī-lə-ˈsta-tᵊn\ *n* : a drug $C_{16}H_{25}N_2O_5SNa$ administered intravenously in combination with the antibiotic imipenem to increase its effectiveness — called also *cilastatin sodium*

cilia *pl of* CILIUM

ciliaris — see ORBICULUS CILIARIS, ZONULA CILIARIS

cil·i·ary \ˈsi-lē-ˌer-ē\ *adj* **1** : of or relating to cilia **2** : of, relating to, or being the annular suspension of the lens of the eye

ciliary artery *n* : any of several arteries that arise from the ophthalmic artery or its branches and supply various parts of the eye — see LONG POSTERIOR CILIARY ARTERY, SHORT POSTERIOR CILIARY ARTERY

ciliary body *n* : a vascular structure encircling the inner surface of the eye behind the iris that secretes the aqueous humor and contains the ciliary muscle and ciliary processes

ciliary ganglion *n* : a small autonomic ganglion on the nasociliary branch of the ophthalmic nerve receiving preganglionic fibers from the oculomotor nerve and sending postganglionic fibers to the ciliary muscle and to the sphincter pupillae

ciliary muscle *n* : a circular band of smooth muscle fibers situated in the ciliary body and serving as the chief agent in accommodation when it contracts by drawing the ciliary processes centripetally and relaxing the suspensory ligament of the lens so that the lens is permitted to become more convex

ciliary nerve — see LONG CILIARY NERVE, SHORT CILIARY NERVE

ciliary process *n* : any of the vascular folds on the inner surface of the ciliary body producing the aqueous humor and between which pass the suspensory zonular fibers joining the ciliary muscle to the lens — see PARS PLICATA

ciliary ring *n* : PARS PLANA

cil•i•ate \ˈsi-lē-ət, -ˌāt\ *n* : any of a phylum or subphylum (Ciliophora) of ciliated protozoans

cil•i•at•ed \ˈsi-lē-ˌā-təd\ *or* **ciliate** *adj* : provided with cilia

cil•i•op•a•thy \ˌsi-lē-ˈä-pə-thē\ *n, pl* **-thies** : any of a group of genetic disorders (as polycystic kidney disease or retinitis pigmentosa) that are caused by the abnormal formation or function of cellular cilia

cil•io•ret•i•nal \ˌsi-lē-ō-ˈret-ᵊn-əl\ *adj* : of, relating to, or supplying the part of the eye including the ciliary body and the retina

cil•i•um \ˈsi-lē-əm\ *n, pl* **cil•ia** \-ə\ **1** : EYELASH **2** : a minute short hairlike process that projects from the surface of most eukaryotic cells, is composed chiefly of microtubules, in unicellular organisms functions chiefly in locomotion, and in higher forms serves esp. in the movement of fluids and particles (as the passage of mucus and dust from the lungs) and in sensory reception — see CILIOPATHY

ci•met•i•dine \sī-ˈme-tə-ˌdēn\ *n* : an H_2 antagonist $C_{10}H_{16}N_6S$ that is used to inhibit gastric acid secretion in conditions in which such secretion produces duodenal or gastric ulcers or erosive lesions — see TAGAMET

Ci•mex \ˈsī-ˌmeks\ *n* : a genus of bloodsucking bugs (family Cimicidae) that includes the common bedbug

Cim•zia \ˈsim-zē-ə\ *trademark* — used for a preparation of certolizumab pegol

cin- *or* **cino-** — see KIN-

cin•a•cal•cet \ˌsin-ə-ˈkal-ˌset\ *n* : a drug $C_{22}H_{22}F_3NHCl$ sometimes used to treat hyperparathyroidism or hypercalcemia — see SENSIPAR

cin•cho•caine \ˈsiŋ-kə-ˌkān, ˈsin-\ *n, chiefly Brit* : DIBUCAINE

cin•cho•na \siŋ-ˈkō-nə, sin-ˈchō-\ *n* : the dried bark of any of several trees (genus *Cinchona* of the family Rubiaceae and esp. *C. ledgeriana* and *C. succirubra*) containing alkaloids (as quinine) used esp. formerly as a specific in malaria, an antipyretic in other fevers, and a tonic and stomachic — called also *cinchona bark*

Chin•chón \chin-ˈchōn\, **Countess of (Doña Francisca Henriquez de Ribera),** Spanish noblewoman.

cin•cho•nism \ˈsiŋ-kə-ˌni-zəm, ˈsin-chə-\ *n* : a disorder due to excessive or prolonged use of cinchona or its alkaloids and marked by temporary deafness, ringing in the ears, headache, dizziness, and rash

cine•an•gio•car•di•og•ra•phy \ˌsi-nē-ˌan-jē-ō-ˌkär-dē-ˈä-grə-fē\ *n, pl* **-phies** : motion-picture photography of a fluoroscopic screen recording passage of a contrasting medium through the chambers of the heart and large blood vessels — **cine•an•gio•car•dio•graph•ic** \-ˌkär-dē-ə-ˈgra-fik\ *adj*

cine•an•gi•og•ra•phy \-ˌan-jē-ˈä-grə-fē\ *n, pl* **-phies** : motion-picture photography of a fluorescent screen recording passage of a contrasting medium through the blood vessels — **cine•an•gio•graph•ic** \-jē-ə-ˈgra-fik\ *adj*

cine•flu•o•rog•ra•phy \-ˌflu̇r-ˈä-grə-fē\ *n, pl* **-phies** : the process of making motion pictures of images of objects by means of X-rays with the aid of a fluorescent screen (as for revealing the motions of organs in the body) — compare CINERADIOGRAPHY — **cine•flu•o•ro•graph•ic** \-ˌflu̇r-ə-ˈgra-fik\ *adj*

cin•e•ole \ˈsi-nē-ˌōl\ *n* : EUCALYPTOL

cin•e•plas•ty \ˈsi-nə-ˌplas-tē\ *also* **ki•ne•plasty** \ˈki-nə-, ˈkī-\ *n, pl* **-ties** **1** : surgical fitting of a lever to a muscle in an amputation stump to facilitate the operation of an artificial hand **2** : surgical isolation of a loop of muscle of chest or arm, covering it with skin, and attaching to it a prosthetic device to be operated by contraction of the muscle in the loop — **cin•e•plas•tic** \ˌsi-nə-ˈplas-tik\ *also* **ki•ne•plas•tic** \ˌki-nə-, ˌkī-\ *adj*

cine•ra•di•og•ra•phy \ˌsi-nē-ˌrā-dē-ˈä-grə-fē\ *n, pl* **-phies** : the process of making radiographs of moving objects (as the heart or joints) in sufficiently rapid sequence so that the radiographs or copies made from them may be projected as motion pictures — compare CINEFLUOROGRAPHY — **cine•ra•dio•graph•ic** \-ˌrā-dē-ō-ˈgra-fik\ *adj*

ci•ne•rea \sə-ˈnir-ē-ə\ *n* : the gray matter of nerve tissue

cinereum — see TUBER CINEREUM

cine•roent•gen•og•ra•phy \ˌsi-nē-ˌrent-gən-ˈä-grə-fē\ *n, pl* **-phies** : CINERADIOGRAPHY

cin•gu•late gyrus \ˈsiŋ-gyə-lət-, -ˌlāt-\ *n* : a medial gyrus of each cerebral hemisphere that partly surrounds the corpus callosum

cin•gu•lot•o•my \ˌsiŋ-gyə-ˈlä-tə-mē\ *n, pl* **-mies** : surgical destruction of all or part (as the cingulum) of the cingulate gyrus

cin•gu•lum \ˈsiŋ-gyə-ləm\ *n, pl* **cin•gu•la** \-lə\ **1** : a ridge about the base of the crown of a tooth **2** : a tract of association fibers lying within the cingulate gyrus and connecting the callosal and hippocampal convolutions of the brain

cin•na•mon \ˈsi-nə-mən\ *n, often attrib* : an aromatic spice prepared from the dried inner bark of an Asian tree (esp. *Cinnamomum zeylanicum*) of the laurel family (Lauraceae); *also* : the bark

cino- — see KIN-

Cip•ro \ˈsi-prō\ *trademark* — used for a preparation of ciprofloxacin

cip•ro•flox•a•cin \sip-rə-ˈfläk-sə-sən\ *n* : a fluoroquinolone $C_{17}H_{18}FN_3O_3$ that is often administered in the form of its hydrochloride $C_{17}H_{18}FN_3O_3{\cdot}HCl$ and is effective esp. against gram-negative bacteria — see CIPRO

cir•ca•di•an \(ˌ)sər-ˈka-dē-ən, -ˈkā-; ˌsər-kə-ˈdī-ən, -ˈdē-\ *adj* : being, having, characterized by, or occurring in approximately 24-hour periods or cycles (as of biological activity or function) ⟨~ rhythms in behavior⟩

cir•ci•nate \ˈsərs-ᵊn-ˌāt\ *adj, of lesions* : having a sharply circumscribed and somewhat circular margin

circle of Wil•lis \-ˈwi-ləs\ *n* : a complete ring of arteries at the base of the brain that is formed by the cerebral and communicating arteries and is a site of aneurysms

Willis, Thomas (1621–1675), British physician.

circling disease *n* : listeriosis of sheep or cattle

cir•cu•lar \ˈsər-kyə-lər\ *adj* : MANIC-DEPRESSIVE; *esp* : BIPOLAR 3

circulares — see PLICAE CIRCULARES

circular sinus *n* : a circular venous channel around the pituitary gland formed by the cavernous and intercavernous sinuses

cir•cu•late \ˈsər-kyə-ˌlāt\ *vb* **-lat•ed; -lat•ing** : to flow or be propelled naturally through a closed system of channels (as blood vessels)

circulating nurse *n* : a registered nurse who makes preparations for an operation and continually monitors patient and staff during its course and who works outside the sterile field in which the operation takes place

cir•cu•la•tion \ˌsər-kyə-ˈlā-shən\ *n* : the movement of blood through the vessels of the body that is induced by the pumping action of the heart and serves to distribute nutrients and oxygen to and remove waste products from all parts of the body — see PULMONARY CIRCULATION, SYSTEMIC CIRCULATION

cir•cu•la•to•ry \ˈsər-kyə-lə-ˌtōr-ē\ *adj* : of or relating to circulation or the circulatory system ⟨~ failure⟩

circulatory system *n* : the system of blood, blood vessels, lymphatics, and heart concerned with the circulation of the blood and lymph

cir•cu•lus \ˈsər-kyə-ləs\ *n, pl* **-li** \-ˌlī\ : an anatomical circle or ring esp. of veins or arteries

cir•cum•cise \ˈsər-kəm-ˌsīz\ *vb* **-cised; -cis•ing** : to cut off the foreskin of (a male) or the prepuce or clitoris and labia minora of (a female) — **cir•cum•cis•er** *n*

cir•cum•ci•sion \ˌsər-kəm-ˈsi-zhən\ *n* **1 a** : the act of circumcising; *esp* : the cutting off of the foreskin of males that is practiced as a religious rite by Jews and Muslims and by others as a social custom or for potential health benefits (as improved hygiene) **b** : FEMALE GENITAL MUTILATION **2** : the condition of being circumcised

cir•cum•cor•ne•al \ˌsir-kəm-ˈkȯr-nē-əl\ *adj* : surrounding the cornea ⟨~ redness⟩

circumcorneal injection *n* : enlargement of the ciliary and conjunctival blood vessels near the margin of the cornea with reduction in size peripherally

cir•cum•duc•tion \ˌsər-kəm-ˈdək-shən\ *n* : movement of a limb or extremity so that the distal end describes a circle while the proximal end remains fixed — **cir•cum•duct** \-ˈdəkt\ *vb*

cir•cum•flex \ˈsər-kəm-ˌfleks\ *adj, of nerves and blood vessels* : bending around

circumflex artery *n* : any of several paired curving arteries: as **a** : either of two arteries that branch from the deep femoral artery or from the femoral artery itself: (1) : LATERAL FEMORAL CIRCUMFLEX ARTERY (2) : MEDIAL FEMORAL CIRCUMFLEX ARTERY **b** : either of two branches of the axillary artery that wind around the neck of the humerus: (1) ANTERIOR HUMERAL CIRCUMFLEX ARTERY (2) : POSTERIOR HUMERAL CIRCUMFLEX ARTERY **c** : CIRCUMFLEX ILIAC ARTERY **d** : a branch of the subscapular artery supplying the muscles of the shoulder

circumflex iliac artery *n* : either of two arteries arching anteriorly near the inguinal ligament: **a** : an artery lying internal to the iliac crest and arising from the external iliac artery **b** : a more superficially located artery that is a branch of the femoral artery

circumflex nerve *n* : AXILLARY NERVE

cir•cum•oral \ˌsər-kəm-ˈōr-əl, -ˈär-\ *adj* : surrounding the mouth ⟨~ pallor⟩

cir•cum•scribed \'sər-kəm-ˌskrībd\ *adj* : confined to a limited area ⟨~ patches of hair loss⟩
cir•cum•stan•ti•al•i•ty \ˌsər-kəm-ˌstan-chē-'a-lə-tē\ *n, pl* **-ties** : a conversational pattern (as in some manic states) exhibiting excessive attention to irrelevant and digressive details
cir•cum•val•late \ˌsər-kəm-'va-ˌlāt, -lət\ *adj* : enclosed by a ridge of tissue
circumvallate papilla *n* : any of the usu. 8 to 12 large papillae near the back of the tongue each of which is surrounded with a marginal sulcus and supplied with taste buds responsive esp. to bitter flavors — called also *vallate papilla*
cir•rho•sis \sə-'rō-səs\ *n, pl* **-rho•ses** \-ˌsēz\ : widespread disruption of normal liver structure by fibrosis and the formation of regenerative nodules that is caused by any of various chronic progressive conditions affecting the liver (as long-term alcohol abuse or hepatitis) — see BILIARY CIRRHOSIS
[1]**cir•rhot•ic** \sə-'rä-tik\ *adj* : of, relating to, caused by, or affected with cirrhosis ⟨~ degeneration⟩ ⟨a ~ liver⟩
[2]**cirrhotic** *n* : an individual affected with cirrhosis
cirs- *or* **cirso-** *comb form* : swollen vein : varix ⟨*cirs*oid⟩
cir•soid \'sər-ˌsȯid\ *adj* : resembling a dilated tortuous vein ⟨~ aneurysms⟩
CIS *abbr* carcinoma in situ
cis•plat•in \'sis-'plat-ᵊn\ *n* : a platinum-containing antineoplastic drug $Cl_2H_6N_2Pt$ used esp. as a palliative therapy in testicular and ovarian tumors and in advanced bladder cancer — see PLATINOL
cis–platinum \-'plat-ᵊn-əm\ *n* : CISPLATIN
13–cis–retinoic acid *n* : ISOTRETINOIN
cis•ter•na \sis-'tər-nə\ *n, pl* **-nae** \-ˌnē\ : a fluid-containing sac or cavity in an organism: as **a** : CISTERNA MAGNA **b** : CISTERNA CHYLI
cisterna chy•li \-'kī-ˌlī\ *n, pl* **cisternae chyli** : a dilated lymph channel usu. opposite the first and second lumbar vertebrae and marking the beginning of the thoracic duct
cis•ter•nal \(ˌ)sis-'tərn-ᵊl\ *adj* : of or relating to a cisterna and esp. the cisterna magna — **cis•ter•nal•ly** *adv*
cisterna mag•na \-'mag-nə\ *n, pl* **cisternae mag•nae** \-ˌnē\ : a large subarachnoid space between the caudal part of the cerebellum and the medulla oblongata
cis•ter•nog•ra•phy \ˌsis-(ˌ)tər-'nä-grə-fē\ *n, pl* **-phies** : radiographic visualization of the subarachnoid spaces containing cerebrospinal fluid following injection of an opaque contrast medium
cis•tron \'sis-ˌträn\ *n* : a segment of DNA that is equivalent to a gene and that specifies a single functional unit (as a protein or enzyme) — **cis•tron•ic** \sis-'trä-nik\ *adj*
ci•tal•o•pram \sī-'ta-lə-ˌpram\ *n* : a drug that functions as an SSRI and is administered orally in the form of its hydrobromide $C_{20}H_{21}FN_2O{\cdot}HBr$ to treat depression and anxiety — see CELEXA
cit•rate \'si-ˌtrāt\ *n* : a salt or ester of citric acid
cit•rat•ed \'si-ˌtrā-təd\ *adj* : treated with a citrate esp. of sodium or potassium to prevent coagulation ⟨~ blood⟩
cit•ric acid \'si-trik-\ *n* : a sour organic acid $C_6H_8O_7$ occurring in cellular metabolism, obtained esp. from lemon and lime juices or by fermentation of sugars, and used as a flavoring
citric acid cycle *n* : KREBS CYCLE
ci•tri•nin \si-'trī-nən\ *n* : a toxic antibiotic $C_{13}H_{14}O_5$ that is produced esp. by two molds of the genus *Penicillium* (*P. citrinum*) and the genus *Aspergillus* (*A. niveus*) and is effective against some gram-positive bacteria
ci•trov•o•rum factor \sə-'trä-və-rəm-\ *n* : LEUCOVORIN
cit•rul•lin•ae•mia *chiefly Brit var of* CITRULLINEMIA
cit•rul•line \'si-trə-ˌlēn; si-'trə-ˌlēn, -lən\ *n* : a crystalline amino acid $C_6H_{13}N_3O_3$ formed esp. as an intermediate in the conversion of ornithine to arginine in the living system
cit•rul•lin•emia \ˌsi-trə-lə-'nē-mē-ə, si-ˌtrə-lə-'nē-\ *n* : an inherited disorder of amino acid metabolism that is marked by excess amounts of citrulline in the blood and urine and typically by hyperammonemia and is inherited as an autosomal recessive trait
cit•rus \'si-trəs\ *n, often attrib* : an acidic fruit (as an orange or lemon) with a usu. thick rind and pulpy flesh that is borne by a shrub or tree (*Citrus* and related genera of the family Rutaceae) grown in warm regions
CJD *abbr* Creutzfeldt-Jakob disease
CK *abbr* creatine kinase
cl *abbr* centiliter
Cl *symbol* chlorine
CLA *abbr* certified laboratory assistant
clair•voy•ance \klar-'vȯi-əns, kler-\ *n* : the power or faculty of discerning objects or matters not present to the senses — **clair•voy•ant** \-ənt\ *adj or n*
clam•my \'kla-mē\ *adj* **clam•mi•er; -est** : being moist and sticky ⟨~ hands⟩
clamp \'klamp\ *n* : any of various instruments or appliances having parts brought together for holding or compressing something; *esp* : an instrument used to hold, compress, or crush vessels and hollow organs and to aid in surgical excision of parts ⟨an arterial ~⟩ — **clamp** *vb*
clang association *n* : association of words based on their similar sound rather than meaning

clap \ˈklap\ *n* : GONORRHEA — often used with *the*

Clar·i·nex \ˈklar-ə-ˌneks\ *trademark* — used for a preparation of desloratadine

cla·rith·ro·my·cin \klə-ˌrith-rə-ˈmī-sᵊn\ *n* : a semisynthetic macrolide antibiotic $C_{38}H_{69}NO_{13}$ used esp. in the treatment of various mild to moderate bacterial infections — see BIAXIN

Clar·i·tin \ˈklar-ə-ˌtin\ *trademark* — used for a preparation of loratadine

clasp \ˈklasp\ *n* : a device designed to encircle a tooth to hold a denture in place

class \ˈklas\ *n* : a major category in biological taxonomy ranking above the order and below the phylum

clas·sic \ˈkla-sik\ *or* **clas·si·cal** \-si-kəl\ *adj* : standard or recognized esp. because of great frequency or consistency of occurrence ⟨the ~ symptoms of a disease⟩

classical conditioning *n* : conditioning in which the conditioned stimulus (as the sound of a bell) is paired with and precedes the unconditioned stimulus (as the sight of food) until the conditioned stimulus alone is sufficient to elicit the response (as salivation in a dog) — compare OPERANT CONDITIONING

clau·di·ca·tion \ˌklȯ-də-ˈkā-shən\ *n* **1** : the quality or state of being lame **2** : INTERMITTENT CLAUDICATION

claus·tro·phobe \ˈklȯ-strə-ˌfōb\ *n* : one affected with claustrophobia

claus·tro·pho·bia \ˌklȯ-strə-ˈfō-bē-ə\ *n* : abnormal dread of being in closed or narrow spaces

[1]**claus·tro·pho·bic** \ˌklȯ-strə-ˈfō-bik\ *adj* **1** : suffering from or inclined to claustrophobia **2** : inducing or suggesting claustrophobia — **claus·tro·pho·bi·cal·ly** \-bi-k(ə-)lē\ *adv*

[2]**claustrophobic** *n* : CLAUSTROPHOBE

claus·trum \ˈklȯ-strəm, ˈklau̇-\ *n, pl* **claus·tra** \-strə\ : the one of the four basal ganglia in each cerebral hemisphere that consists of a thin lamina of gray matter between the lentiform nucleus and the insula

clav·i·cle \ˈkla-vi-kəl\ *n* : a bone of the shoulder girdle that links the scapula and sternum, is situated just above the first rib on either side of the neck, and has the form of a narrow elongated S — called also *collarbone* — **cla·vic·u·lar** \kla-ˈvi-kyə-lər, klə-\ *adj*

clavicular notch *n* : a notch on each side of the upper part of the manubrium that is the site of articulation with a clavicle

cla·vic·u·lec·to·my \kla-ˌvi-kyə-ˈlek-tə-mē, klə-\ *n, pl* **-mies** : surgical removal of all or part of a clavicle

clav·u·lan·ic acid \ˌklav-yə-ˌla-nik-\ *n* : a beta-lactam antibiotic $C_8H_9NO_5$ produced by a bacterium of the genus *Streptomyces* (*S. clavuligerus*) — see AUGMENTIN

cla·vus \ˈklā-vəs, ˈklä-\ *n, pl* **cla·vi** \ˈklā-ˌvī, ˈklä-ˌvē\ : CORN

claw foot *n* : a deformity of the foot characterized by an exaggerated curvature of the longitudinal arch

claw hand *n* : a deformity of the hand characterized by extreme extension of the wrist and the first phalanges and extreme flexion of the other phalanges

claw toe *n* : HAMMERTOE

[1]**clean** \ˈklēn\ *adj* **1 a** : free from dirt or pollution **b** : free from disease or infectious agents **2** : free from drug addiction

[2]**clean** *vb* **1** : to brush (the teeth) with a cleanser (as a dentifrice) **2** : to perform dental prophylaxis on (the teeth)

[1]**clear** \ˈklir\ *adj* **1** *of the skin or complexion* : good in texture and color and without blemish or discoloration **2** : free from abnormal sounds on auscultation

[2]**clear** *vb* : to rid (the throat) of phlegm or of something that makes the voice indistinct or husky

clear·ance \ˈklir-əns\ *n* : the volume of blood or plasma that could be freed of a specified constituent in a specified time (usu. one minute) by excretion of the constituent into the urine through the kidneys — called also *renal clearance*

cleav·age \ˈklē-vij\ *n* **1** : the series of synchronized mitotic cell divisions of the fertilized egg that results in the formation of the blastomeres and changes the single-celled zygote into a multicellular embryo; *also* : one of these cell divisions **2** : the splitting of a molecule into simpler molecules — **cleave** \ˈklēv\ *vb*

cleavage cell *n* : BLASTOMERE

cleft \ˈkleft\ *n* **1** : a usu. abnormal fissure or opening esp. when resulting from failure of parts to fuse during embryonic development **2** : a usu. V-shaped indented formation : a hollow between ridges or protuberances **3** : SYNAPTIC CLEFT

cleft lip *n* : a birth defect characterized by one or more clefts in the upper lip resulting from failure of the embryonic parts of the lip to unite — called also *cheiloschisis*

cleft palate *n* : congenital fissure of the roof of the mouth produced by failure of the two maxillae to unite during embryonic development and often associated with cleft lip

cleid- *or* **cleido-** *comb form* : clavicular : clavicular and ⟨*cleido*cranial⟩

clei·do·cra·ni·al dysplasia \ˌklī-dō-ˈkrā-nē-əl-\ *n* : a rare condition inherited as an autosomal dominant trait and characterized esp. by partial or complete absence of the clavicles, defective ossification of the skull, and faulty occlusion due to missing, misplaced, or extra teeth — called also *cleidocranial dysostosis*

clem•as•tine \'kle-mə-ˌstēn\ *n* : an antihistamine administered in the form of its fumarate $C_{21}H_{26}ClNO{\cdot}C_4H_4O_4$

clen•bu•te•rol \klen-'byü-tə-ˌrȯl, -ˌrōl\ *n* : a bronchodilator $C_{12}H_{18}Cl_2N_2O{\cdot}HCl$ approved in the U.S. only for veterinary use but sometimes used illicitly by athletes to enhance performance

cle•oid \'klē-ˌȯid\ *n* : a dental excavator with a claw-shaped working point

clerk \'klərk\ *n* : a third- or fourth-year medical student undergoing clinical training in a clerkship — **clerk** *vb*

clerk•ship \'klərk-ˌship\ *n* : a course of clinical medical training in a specialty that usu. lasts a minimum of several weeks and takes place during the third or fourth year of medical school

click \'klik\ *n* : a short sharp sound heard in auscultation and associated with various heart abnormalities

cli•mac•ter•ic \klī-'mak-tə-rik, ˌklī-ˌmak-'ter-ik\ *n* **1** : MENOPAUSE 1a(2) **2** : ANDROPAUSE — **climacteric** *adj*

cli•mac•te•ri•um \ˌklī-ˌmak-'tir-ē-əm\ *n, pl* **-ria** \-ē-ə\ : the bodily and mental changes occurring during the latter part of middle age; *specif* : menopause and the bodily and psychological changes that accompany it

cli•mac•tic \klī-'mak-tik\ *adj* : of, relating to, or constituting a climax

cli•ma•to•ther•a•py \ˌklī-mə-tō-'ther-ə-pē\ *n, pl* **-pies** : treatment of disease by means of residence in a suitable climate

cli•max \'klī-ˌmaks\ *n* **1** : the highest or most intense point **2** : ORGASM **3 a** : MENOPAUSE 1a(2) **b** : ANDROPAUSE

clin *abbr* clinical

clin•da•my•cin \ˌklin-də-'mī-sən\ *n* : an antibiotic $C_{18}H_{33}ClN_2O_5S$ derived from and used similarly to lincomycin

clin•ic \'kli-nik\ *n* **1 a** : a session or class of medical instruction in a hospital held at the bedside of patients serving as case studies **b** : a group of selected patients presented with discussion before doctors for purposes of instruction **2 a** : an institution connected with a hospital or medical school where diagnosis and treatment are made available to outpatients **b** : a form of group practice in which several physicians (as specialists) work in cooperative association

clin•i•cal \'kli-ni-kəl\ *adj* : of, relating to, or conducted in or as if in a clinic: as **a** : involving or concerned with the direct observation of living patients ⟨a full-time ~ practice⟩ **b** : of, relating to, based on, or characterized by observable or diagnosable symptoms of disease ⟨~ tuberculosis⟩ ⟨the ~ presentation of Lyme disease⟩ **c** : applying objective or standardized methods (as interviews and personality tests) to the description, evaluation, and modification of human behavior ⟨~ psychology⟩ — **clin•i•cal•ly** \-k(ə-)lē\ *adv*

clinical crown *n* : the part of a tooth that projects above the gums

clinical depression *n* : depression of sufficient severity to be brought to the attention of a physician and to require treatment; *specif* : MAJOR DEPRESSIVE DISORDER

clinical thermometer *n* : a thermometer for measuring body temperature that has a constriction in the tube above the bulb preventing movement of the column of liquid downward once it has reached its maxium temperature so that it continues to indicate the maximum temperature until the liquid is shaken back down into the bulb — called also *fever thermometer*

clinical trial *n* : a scientifically controlled study of the safety and effectiveness of a therapeutic agent (as a drug or vaccine) using consenting human subjects

cli•ni•cian \kli-'ni-shən\ *n* : one qualified in the clinical practice of medicine, psychiatry, or psychology

clinico- *comb form* : clinical : clinical and ⟨*clinico*pathologic⟩

clin•i•co•path•o•log•ic \'kli-ni-(ˌ)kō-ˌpa-thə-'lä-jik\ *or* **clin•i•co•path•o•log•i•cal** \-'lä-ji-kəl\ *adj* : relating to or concerned both with the signs and symptoms directly observable by the physician and with the results of laboratory examination ⟨a ~ study of the patient⟩ — **clin•i•co•path•o•log•i•cal•ly** \-ji-k(ə-)lē\ *adv*

cli•no•dac•ty•ly \ˌklī-nō-'dak-tə-lē\ *n, pl* **-ty•lies** : a deformity of the hand marked by deviation or deflection of the fingers

cli•noid process \'klī-ˌnȯid-\ *n* : any of several processes of the sphenoid bone

clip \'klip\ *n* : a device used to arrest bleeding from vessels or tissues during operations

clitorid- *or* **clitorido-** *comb form* : clitoris ⟨*clitorid*ectomy⟩

clit•o•ri•dec•to•my \ˌkli-tə-rə-'dek-tə-mē\ *also* **clit•o•rec•to•my** \-'rek-tə-mē\ *n, pl* **-mies** : excision of all or part of the clitoris

clitoridis — see PREPUTIUM CLITORIDIS

cli•to•ris \'kli-tə-rəs, kli-'tȯr-əs\ *n, pl* **cli•to•ris•es** *also* **cli•to•ri•des** \kli-'tȯr-ə-ˌdēz\ : a small erectile female organ at the anterior junction of the labia minora that develops from the same embryonic mass of tissue as the penis and is responsive to sexual stimulation — **cli•to•ral** \'kli-tə-rəl\ *also* **cli•tor•ic** \kli-'tȯr-ik, -'tär-\ *adj*

cli•vus \'klī-vəs\ *n, pl* **cli•vi** \-ˌvī\ : the smooth sloping surface on the upper posterior part of the body of the sphenoid bone supporting the pons and the basilar artery

CLL *abbr* chronic lymphocytic leukemia

clo·aca \klō-ˈā-kə\ *n, pl* **-acae** \-ˌkē, -ˌsē\ **1** : the terminal part of the embryonic hindgut of a mammal before it divides into rectum, bladder, and genital precursors **2** : a passage in a bone leading to a cavity containing a sequestrum — **clo·acal** \-kəl\ *adj*

cloacal membrane *n* : a plate of fused embryonic ectoderm and endoderm closing the fetal anus

clo·be·ta·sol \klō-ˈbā-tə-ˌsōl\ *n* : a potent synthetic corticosteroid that is used topically in the form of its propionate $C_{25}H_{32}ClFO_5$ esp. to treat inflammatory skin conditions — called also *clobetasol propionate*

clock \ˈkläk\ *n* : BIOLOGICAL CLOCK

clo·faz·i·mine \klō-ˈfā-zə-ˌmēn\ *n* : a reddish-brown powdered dye $C_{27}H_{22}Cl_2N_4$ that is used esp. to treat lepromatous leprosy

clo·fi·brate \klō-ˈfī-ˌbrāt, -ˈfi-\ *n* : a synthetic drug $C_{12}H_{15}ClO_3$ used esp. to lower abnormally high concentrations of fats and cholesterol in the blood

Clo·mid \ˈklō-mid\ *trademark* — used for a preparation of the citrate of clomiphene

clo·mi·phene \ˈklä-mə-ˌfēn, ˈklō-\ *n* : a synthetic drug used in the form of its citrate $C_{26}H_{28}ClNO·C_6H_8O_7$ to induce ovulation — see CLOMID

clo·mip·ra·mine \klō-ˈmi-prə-ˌmēn\ *n* : a tricyclic antidepressant used in the form of its hydrochloride $C_{19}H_{23}ClN_2·HCl$ to treat obsessive-compulsive disorder — see ANAFRANIL

clo·naz·e·pam \(ˌ)klō-ˈna-zə-ˌpam\ *n* : a benzodiazepine $C_{15}H_{10}ClN_3O_3$ used esp. to prevent and control seizures and to reduce anxiety

clone \ˈklōn\ *n* **1** : the aggregate of genetically identical cells or organisms asexually produced by a single progenitor cell or organism **2** : an individual grown from a single somatic cell or cell nucleus and genetically identical to it **3** : a group of replicas of all or part of a macromolecule and esp. DNA — **clon·al** \ˈklōn-ᵊl\ *adj* — **clon·al·ly** *adv* — **clone** *vb*

clon·ic \ˈklä-nik\ *adj* : exhibiting, relating to, or involving clonus ⟨~ contraction⟩ ⟨~ spasm⟩ — **clo·nic·i·ty** \klō-ˈni-sə-tē, klä-\ *n*

clo·ni·dine \ˈklä-nə-ˌdēn, ˈklō-, -ˌdīn\ *n* : an antihypertensive drug used in the form of its hydrochloride $C_9H_9Cl_2N_3·HCl$ esp. to treat essential hypertension, to prevent migraine headache, and to diminish opiate withdrawal symptoms

clo·nor·chi·a·sis \ˌklō-nȯr-ˈkī-ə-səs\ *n, pl* **-a·ses** \-ˌsēz\ : infestation with or disease caused by the Chinese liver fluke (*Clonorchis sinensis*) that invades bile ducts of the liver after ingestion in uncooked fish and when present in numbers causes severe systemic reactions including edema, liver enlargement, and diarrhea

Clo·nor·chis \klō-ˈnȯr-kəs\ *n* : a genus of trematode worms (family Opisthorchiidae) that includes the Chinese liver fluke (*C. sinensis*)

clo·nus \ˈklō-nəs\ *n* : a series of alternating contractions and partial relaxations of a muscle that in some diseases of the central nervous system occurs in the form of convulsive spasms — compare TONUS 2

clo·pid·o·grel \klō-ˈpi-də-ˌgrel\ *n* : an antithrombotic agent that is administered in the form of its bisulfate $C_{16}H_{16}ClNO_2S·H_2SO_4$ and inhibits ADP-induced aggregation of platelets — see PLAVIX

clor·az·e·pate \ˌklȯr-ˈa-zə-ˌpāt\ *n* : a benzodiazepine $C_{16}H_{10}ClKN_2O_3·KOH$ taken orally to treat anxiety, partial seizures, and acute alcohol withdrawal — called also *clorazepate dipotassium;* see TRANXENE

closed \ˈklōzd\ *adj* **1 a** : covered by unbroken skin ⟨a ~ fracture⟩ **b** : not penetrating the skull ⟨a ~ head injury⟩ **2** : not discharging pathogenic organisms to the outside ⟨~ tuberculosis⟩ — compare OPEN 1c

closed–angle glaucoma *n* : ANGLE-CLOSURE GLAUCOMA

closed reduction *n* : the reduction of a displaced part (as a fractured bone) by manipulation without incision — compare OPEN REDUCTION

clos·trid·i·um \kläs-ˈtri-dē-əm\ *n* **1** *cap* : a genus of saprophytic mostly anaerobic bacteria (family Clostridiaceae) that are commonly found in soil and in the intestinal tracts of humans and animals and that include important pathogens — see BLACKLEG, BOTULISM, C. DIFF, GAS GANGRENE, TETANUS BACILLUS; compare LIMBERNECK **2** *pl* **clos·trid·ia** \-dē-ə\ **a** : any bacterium of the genus *Clostridium* **b** : a spindle-shaped or ovoid bacterial cell; *esp* : one swollen at the center by an endospore — **clos·trid·i·al** \-dē-əl\ *adj*

clo·sure \ˈklō-zhər\ *n* **1 a** : an act of closing up or condition of being closed up **b** : a drawing together of edges or parts to form a united integument **2** : the perception of incomplete figures or situations as though complete by ignoring the missing parts or by compensating for them by projection based on past experience **3** : an often comforting or satisfying sense of finality

[1]**clot** \ˈklät\ *n* : a coagulated mass produced by clotting of blood

[2]**clot** *vb* **clot·ted; clot·ting** : to undergo a sequence of reactions that results in conversion of fluid blood into a coagulum and that involves shedding of blood, release of thromboplastin, inactivation of heparin, conversion of prothrombin to thrombin, interaction of thrombin with fibrinogen to form an insoluble fibrin network, and con-

traction of the network to squeeze out excess fluid : COAGULATE

clot–bust·er \ˈklät-ˌbəs-tər\ *n* : a drug (as streptokinase or tissue plasminogen activator) used to dissolve blood clots — **clot–bust·ing** \-tiŋ\ *adj*

clot retraction *n* : the process by which a blood clot becomes smaller and draws the edges of a broken blood vessel together and which involves the shortening of fibrin threads and the squeezing out of excess serum

clo·tri·ma·zole \klō-ˈtrī-mə-ˌzōl, -ˌzȯl\ *n* : an antifungal agent $C_{22}H_{17}ClN_2$ used to treat candida infections, tinea, and ringworm — see LOTRIMIN

clotting factor *n* : any of several plasma components (as fibrinogen, prothrombin, and thromboplastin) that are involved in the clotting of blood — called also *coagulation factor;* see FACTOR VIII, PLASMA THROMBOPLASTIN ANTECEDENT, TRANSGLUTAMINASE; compare FACTOR V, FACTOR VII, FACTOR IX, FACTOR X, FACTOR XII, FACTOR XIII

clove oil \ˈklōv-\ *n* : a colorless to pale yellow essential oil that is obtained from the dried aromatic flower buds of a tropical tree (*Syzygium aromaticum*) of the myrtle family (Myrtaceae) and is a source of eugenol, has a powerful germicidal action, and is used topically to relieve toothache

cloverleaf skull *n* : a birth defect in which some or all of the usu. separate bones of the skull have grown together resulting in a 3-lobed skull with associated deformities of the features and skeleton

clox·a·cil·lin \ˌkläk-sə-ˈsi-lən\ *n* : a semisynthetic oral penicillin $C_{19}H_{17}ClN_3NaO_5S$ effective esp. against staphylococci which secrete beta-lactamase — see TEGOPEN

clo·za·pine \ˈklō-zə-ˌpēn\ *n* : an antipsychotic drug $C_{18}H_{19}ClN_4$ with serious side effects that is used in the management of severe schizophrenia — see CLOZARIL

Clo·za·ril \ˈklō-zə-ril\ *trademark* — used for a preparation of clozapine

clubbed \ˈkləbd\ *adj* **1** : having a bulbous enlargement of the tip with convex overhanging nail ⟨a ~ finger⟩ **2** : affected with clubfoot — **club·bing** \ˈklə-biŋ\ *n*

club·foot \ˈkləb-ˌfu̇t\ *n, pl* **club·feet** \-ˌfēt\ **1** : any of numerous congenital deformities of the foot in which it is twisted out of position or shape — called also *talipes;* compare TALIPES EQUINOVARUS, TALIPES EQUINUS, TALIPES VALGUS, TALIPES VARUS **2** : a foot affected with clubfoot — **club·foot·ed** \-ˌfu̇-təd\ *adj*

club·hand \-ˌhand\ *n* **1** : a congenital deformity in which the hand is short and distorted **2** : a hand affected with clubhand

clump \ˈkləmp\ *n* : a clustered mass of particles (as cells) — compare AGGLUTINATION — **clump** *vb*

clus·ter \ˈklə-stər\ *n* : a larger than expected number of cases of disease occurring in a particular locality, group of people, or period of time

cluster headache *n* : a headache that is characterized by severe unilateral pain in the eye or temple, affects primarily men, and tends to recur in a series of attacks

clut·ter·ing \ˈklə-tə-riŋ\ *n* : a speech defect in which phonetic units are dropped, condensed, or otherwise distorted as a result of overly rapid agitated utterance

Clut·ton's joints \ˈklət-ᵊnz-\ *n pl* : symmetrical hydrarthrosis esp. of the knees or elbows that occurs in congenital syphilis

Clut·ton \ˈklət-ᵊn\, **Henry Hugh (1850–1909)**, British surgeon.

cly·sis \ˈklī-səs\ *n, pl* **cly·ses** \-ˌsēz\ : the introduction of large amounts of fluid into the body usu. by parenteral injection to replace that lost (as from hemorrhage or in dysentery or burns), to provide nutrients, or to maintain blood pressure — see HYPODERMOCLYSIS, PROCTOCLYSIS

clys·ter \ˈklis-tər\ *n* : ENEMA

cm *abbr* centimeter

Cm *symbol* curium

CMA *abbr* certified medical assistant

CMHC *abbr* Community Mental Health Center

CML *abbr* chronic myelogenous leukemia; chronic myeloid leukemia

CMV *abbr* cytomegalovirus

Cn *symbol* copernicium

CNA *abbr* certified nurse aide; certified nurse assistant; certified nurse's aide; certified nurse's assistant

cne·mi·al \ˈnē-mē-əl\ *adj* : relating to the shin or shinbone

cni·dar·i·an \nī-ˈdar-ē-ən\ *n* : COELENTERATE — **cnidarian** *adj*

CNM *abbr* certified nurse-midwife

CNS *abbr* central nervous system

Co *symbol* cobalt

c/o *abbr* complains of

co·ad·min·is·tra·tion \ˌkō-əd-ˌmi-nə-ˈstrā-shən\ *n* : the administration of two or more drugs together — **co·ad·min·is·ter** \-ˈmi-nə-stər\ *vb*

co·ag·u·lant \kō-ˈa-gyə-lənt\ *n* : something that produces coagulation

co·ag·u·lase \kō-ˈa-gyə-ˌlās, -ˌlāz\ *n* : any of several enzymes that cause coagulation (as of blood)

¹co·ag·u·late \kō-ˈa-gyə-ˌlāt\ *vb* **-lat·ed; -lat·ing** **1** : to become or cause to become viscous or thickened into a coherent mass : CLOT **2** : to subject to coagulation — **co·ag·u·la·bil·i·ty** \kō-ˌa-gyə-lə-ˈbi-lə-tē\ *n* — **co·ag·u·la·ble** \-ˈa-gyə-lə-bəl\ *adj*

²co·ag·u·late \-lət, -ˌlāt\ *n* : COAGULUM

co·ag·u·la·tion \kō-ˌa-gyə-ˈlā-shən\ *n* **1 a** : a change to a viscous, jellylike, or solid state; *esp* : a change from a liquid to a thickened curdlike state not by evaporation but by chemical reaction **b** : the process by which such change of state takes place consisting of the alteration of a soluble substance (as protein) into an insoluble form or of the flocculation or separation of colloidal or suspended matter **2** : a substance or body formed by coagulation : COAGULUM **3** : disruption of tissue by physical means (as by application of an electric current) so that denaturation and clumping of protein occur

coagulation factor *n* : CLOTTING FACTOR

coagulation time *n* : the time required by shed blood to clot that is a measure of the normality of the blood

co•ag•u•lop•a•thy \kō-ˌa-gyə-ˈlä-pə-thē\ *n, pl* **-thies** : a disease or condition affecting the blood's ability to coagulate

co•ag•u•lum \kō-ˈa-gyə-ləm\ *n, pl* **-u•la** \-lə\ *or* **-u•lums** : a coagulated mass or substance : CLOT

coal tar *n* : tar obtained by distillation of bituminous coal and used in the treatment of some skin diseases by direct local application to the skin

co•apt \kō-ˈapt\ *vb* : to close or fasten together : cause to adhere — **co•ap•ta•tion** \(ˌ)kō-ˌap-ˈtā-shən\ *n*

co•arct \kō-ˈärkt\ *vb* : to cause (the aorta) to become narrow or (the heart) to constrict

co•arc•ta•tion \(ˌ)kō-ˌärk-ˈtā-shən\ *n* : a stricture or narrowing esp. of a canal or vessel (as the aorta)

coarse \ˈkōrs\ *adj* **1** : visible to the naked eye or by means of a compound microscope **2** *of a tremor* : of wide excursion **3** : harsh, raucous, or rough in tone — used of some sounds heard in auscultation in pathological states of the chest ⟨~ rales⟩

Co•ar•tem \kō-ˈär-ˌtem\ *trademark* — used for a preparation of artemether and lumefantrine

coat \ˈkōt\ *n* **1** : the external growth on an animal **2** : a layer of one substance covering or lining another; *esp* : one covering or lining an organ

coat•ed \ˈkō-təd\ *adj, of the tongue* : covered with a whitish or yellowish deposit of desquamated cells, bacteria, and debris

Coats' disease \ˈkōts, ˈkōt-səz-\ *also* **Coats disease** *or* **Coat's disease** \ˈkōts-\ *n* : a chronic progressive disease of the eye that is caused by the accumulation of fluid and blood debris beneath the retina, is typically marked by a whitish mass in the pupil of one eye, and may lead to retinal detachment and blindness if untreated

Coats \ˈkōts\, **George (1876–1915)**, British ophthalmologist.

co•bal•a•min \kō-ˈba-lə-mən\ *n* : VITAMIN B_{12}

co•balt \ˈkō-ˌbȯlt\ *n* : a tough lustrous silver-white magnetic metallic element — symbol *Co;* see ELEMENT table

cobalt 60 *n* : a heavy radioactive isotope of cobalt having the mass number 60 and used as a source of gamma rays esp. in place of radium (as in the treatment of cancer and in radiography) — called also *radiocobalt*

co•bic•i•stat \kō-ˈbik-i-ˌstat\ *n* : a drug $C_{40}H_{53}N_7O_5S_2$ administered chiefly in conjunction with atazanavir or darunavir to improve their effectiveness in the treatment of HIV infection — see EVOTAZ, PREZCOBIX, STRIBILD, TYBOST

co•bra \ˈkō-brə\ *n* **1** : any of several venomous Asian and African elapid snakes (genera *Naja* and *Ophiophagus*) **2** : RINGHALS **3** : MAMBA

COC *abbr* combination oral contraceptive; combined oral contraceptive

co•ca \ˈkō-kə\ *n* **1** : any of several So. American shrubs (genus *Erythroxylon* of the family Erythroxylaceae); *esp* : one (*E. coca*) that is the primary source of cocaine **2** : dried leaves of a coca (as *Erythroxylon coca*) containing alkaloids including cocaine

co•caine \kō-ˈkān, ˈkō-ˌ\ *n* : a bitter crystalline alkaloid $C_{17}H_{21}NO_4$ obtained from coca leaves that is used medically esp. in the form of its hydrochloride $C_{17}H_{21}NO_4 \cdot HCl$ as a topical anesthetic and illicitly for its euphoric effects and that may result in a compulsive psychological need

co•cain•ize \kō-ˈkā-ˌnīz\ *vb* **-ized; -iz•ing** : to treat or anesthetize with cocaine — **co•cain•i•za•tion** \-ˌkā-nə-ˈzā-shən\ *n*

co•car•cin•o•gen \ˌkō-kär-ˈsi-nə-jən, kō-ˈkärs-ᵊn-ə-ˌjen\ *n* : an agent that aggravates the carcinogenic effects of another substance — **co•car•cin•o•gen•ic** \ˌkō-ˌkärs-ᵊn-ō-ˈje-nik\ *adj*

coc•cal \ˈkä-kəl\ *adj* : of or relating to a coccus

[1]**coc•ci** \ˈkäk-sē\ *n* : COCCIDIOIDOMYCOSIS

[2]**coc•ci** \ˈkäk-ˌ(s)ī *also* -(ˌ)(s)ē\ *pl of* COCCUS

coc•cid•ia \käk-ˈsi-dē-ə\ *n pl* : sporozoans of an order (Coccidia) parasitic in the digestive epithelium of vertebrates — **coc•cid•ian** \-dē-ən\ *adj or n*

Coc•cid•i•oi•des \käk-ˌsi-dē-ˈȯi-ˌdēz\ *n* : a genus of ascomycetous fungi (family Onygenaceae) esp. of dry warm soils that cause coccidioidomycosis

coc•cid•i•oi•din \-ˈȯid-ᵊn, -ˈȯi-ˌdin\ *n* : an antigen prepared from a fungus of the genus *Coccidioides* (*C. immitis*) and used to detect skin sensitivity to and, by inference, infection with this organism

coc•cid•i•oi•do•my•co•sis \-ˌȯi-dō-(ˌ)mī-ˈkō-səs\ *n, pl* **-co•ses** \-ˌsēz\ : a disease that is caused by inhalation of spores from either of two fungi (*Coccidioides immitis* and *C. posadasii*) found in dry soils of the southwestern U.S. and that may be asymptomatic or present as a mild to serious flu-like illness which sometimes spreads beyond the lungs causing painful lesions, swollen joints, or meningitis — called also *cocci, San Joaquin fever, San Joaquin valley fever, valley fever*

coc·cid·io·my·co·sis \(ˌ)käk-ˌsi-dē-ō-(ˌ)mī-ˈkō-səs\ *n, pl* **-co·ses** \-ˌsēz\ : COCCIDIOIDOMYCOSIS

coc·cid·i·o·sis \(ˌ)käk-ˌsi-dē-ˈō-səs\ *n, pl* **-o·ses** \-ˌsēz\ : infestation with or disease caused by coccidia

coc·cid·io·stat \(ˌ)käk-ˈsi-dē-ō-ˌstat\ *n* : a chemical agent added to animal feed that inhibits the growth of pathogenic coccidia so that disease is minimized and the host develops immunity

coc·co·ba·cil·lus \ˌkä-(ˌ)kō-bə-ˈsi-ləs\ *n, pl* **-li** \-ˌlī, -ˌlē\ : a very short bacillus esp. of the genus *Pasteurella* — **coc·co·ba·cil·la·ry** \-ˈba-sə-ˌler-ē, -bə-ˈsi-lə-rē\ *adj*

coc·coid \ˈkä-ˌkȯid\ *adj* : of, related to, or resembling a coccus — **coccoid** *n*

coc·cus \ˈkä-kəs\ *n, pl* **coc·ci** \ˈkä-ˌkī, -ˌkē; ˈkäk-ˌsī, -ˌsē\ : a spherical bacterium

coccyg- *or* **coccygo-** *comb form* : coccyx ⟨*coccyg*ectomy⟩

coc·cy·geal \käk-ˈsi-jəl, -jē-əl\ *adj* : of, relating to, or affecting the coccyx

coccygeal body *n* : GLOMUS COCCYGEUM

coccygeal gland *n* : GLOMUS COCCYGEUM

coccygeal nerve *n* : either of the 31st or lowest pair of spinal nerves

coc·cy·gec·to·my \ˌkäk-sə-ˈjek-tə-mē\ *n, pl* **-mies** : the surgical removal of the coccyx

coccygeum — see GLOMUS COCCYGEUM

coc·cyg·e·us \käk-ˈsi-jē-əs\ *n, pl* **coc·cyg·ei** \-jē-ˌī\ : a muscle arising from the ischium and sacrospinous ligament and inserted into the coccyx and sacrum — called also *coccygeus muscle, ischiococcygeus*

coc·cy·go·dyn·ia \ˌkäk-sə-(ˌ)gō-ˈdi-nē-ə\ *n* : pain in the coccyx and adjacent regions

coc·cyx \ˈkäk-siks\ *n, pl* **coc·cy·ges** \-sə-ˌjēz\ *also* **coc·cyx·es** \-sik-səz\ : a small bone that articulates with the sacrum and that usu. consists of four fused vertebrae which form the terminus of the spinal column

co·chle·a \ˈkō-klē-ə, ˈkä-\ *n, pl* **co·chle·as** *or* **co·chle·ae** \-ē, -ī\ : a division of the bony labyrinth of the inner ear coiled into the form of a snail shell and consisting of a spiral canal in the petrous part of the temporal bone in which lies a smaller membranous spiral passage that communicates with the saccule at the base of the spiral, ends blindly near its apex, and contains the organ of Corti — **co·chle·ar** \-ər\ *adj*

cochlear canal *n* : COCHLEAR DUCT

cochlear duct *n* : the spirally arranged canal in the bony canal of the cochlea that contains the organ of Corti, is triangular in cross section, and is bounded by the vestibular membrane above, by the periosteum lined wall of the cochlea laterally, and by the basilar membrane below — called also *cochlear canal, scala media*

cochlear implant *n* : an electronic prosthetic device that enables individuals with sensorineural hearing loss to recognize some sounds and consists of an external microphone and speech processor and one or more electrodes implanted in the cochlea — **cochlear implantation** *n*

cochlear microphonic *n* : an electrical potential arising in the cochlea when the mechanical energy of a sound stimulus is transformed to electrical energy as the action potential of the transmitting nerve — called also *microphonic*

cochlear nerve *n* : a branch of the auditory nerve that arises in the spiral ganglion of the cochlea and conducts sensory stimuli from the organ of hearing to the brain — called also *cochlear, cochlear branch, cochlear division*

cochlear nucleus *n* : the nucleus of the cochlear nerve situated in the caudal part of the pons and consisting of dorsal and ventral parts which are continuous and lie on the dorsal and lateral aspects of the inferior cerebellar peduncle

co·chleo·ves·tib·u·lar \ˌkō-klē-(ˌ)ō-ve-ˈsti-byə-lər, ˌkä-\ *adj* : relating to or affecting the cochlea and vestibule of the ear ⟨~ disorders⟩

Coch·lio·my·ia \ˌkä-klē-ə-ˈmī-ə\ *n* : a genus of No. American blowflies that includes the screwworms (*C. hominivorax* and *C. macellaria*)

Cock·ayne syndrome \kä-ˈkān-\ *also* **Cockayne's syndrome** *n* : a rare disease that is inherited as an autosomal recessive trait, is marked esp. by growth and developmental failure, photosensitivity, and premature aging, and that is either present at birth or has an onset during infancy or childhood

Cockayne, Edward Alfred (1880–1956), British physician.

cock·roach \ˈkäk-ˌrōch\ *n* : any of an order (Blattodea) of chiefly nocturnal insects including some that are domestic pests — see AMERICAN COCKROACH, GERMAN COCKROACH

cock·tail \ˈkäk-ˌtāl\ *n* : a mixture of agents usu. in solution that is taken or used esp. for medical treatment or diagnosis

cocoa butter *or* **cacao butter** *n* : a pale vegetable fat obtained from cacao beans that is used in the manufacture of chocolate candy, in cosmetics as an emollient, and in pharmacy for making suppositories — called also *theobroma oil*

co·con·scious \(ˌ)kō-ˈkän-chəs\ *n* : mental processes outside the main stream of consciousness but sometimes available to it — **coconscious** *adj*

co·con·scious·ness *n* : COCONSCIOUS

[1]**code** \ˈkōd\ *n* **1** : GENETIC CODE **2** : CODE BLUE

[2]**code** *vb* **cod•ed; cod•ing 1 :** to specify the genetic code ⟨a gene that ~*s* for a protein⟩ **2 :** to experience cardiac arrest or respiratory failure ⟨the patient *coded* a second time⟩

code blue *n, often cap C&B* : a declaration of or a state of medical emergency and call for medical personnel and equipment to attempt to resuscitate a patient esp. when in cardiac arrest or respiratory distress or failure; *also* : the attempt to resuscitate the patient

co•deine \ˈkō-ˌdēn, ˈkō-dē-ən\ *n* : a morphine derivative that is found in opium, is weaker in action than morphine, and is used chiefly in the form of its sulfate $(C_{18}H_{21}NO_3)_2 \cdot H_2SO_4$ or phosphate $C_{18}H_{21}NO_3 \cdot H_3PO_4$ esp. as a pain reliever and cough suppressant

co•de•pen•dence \ˌkō-di-ˈpen-dəns\ *n* : CODEPENDENCY

co•de•pen•den•cy \-dən-sē\ *n, pl* **-cies** : a psychological condition or a relationship in which a person with low self-esteem and need for approval has an unhealthy attachment to and tries to satisfy the needs of another person who is often controlling or manipulative and who may have an addictive or emotionally unstable personality; *broadly* : dependence on the needs of or control by another

[1]**co•de•pen•dent** \-dənt\ *n* : a codependent person

[2]**codependent** *adj* : participating in or exhibiting codependency

co•dex \ˈkō-ˌdeks\ *n, pl* **co•di•ces** \ˈkō-də-ˌsēz, ˈkä-\ : an official or standard collection of drug formulas and descriptions

cod–liver oil *n* : a pale yellow fatty oil obtained from the liver of the cod (*Gadus morhua* of the family Gadidae) and related fishes and used in medicine chiefly as a source of vitamins A and D

co•dom•i•nant \(ˌ)kō-ˈdä-mə-nənt\ *adj* : being fully expressed in the heterozygous condition — **codominant** *n*

co•don \ˈkō-ˌdän\ *n* : a specific sequence of three consecutive nucleotides that is part of the genetic code and that specifies a particular amino acid in a protein or starts or stops protein synthesis — called also *triplet*

co•ef•fi•cient \ˌkō-ə-ˈfi-shənt\ *n* : a number that serves as a measure of some property or characteristic (as of a substance, device, or process)

-coele *or* **-coel** *also* **-cele** *n comb form* : cavity : chamber ⟨blasto*coel*⟩

coe•len•ter•ate \si-ˈlen-tə-ˌrāt, -rət\ *n* : any of a phylum (Cnidaria syn. Coelenterata) of invertebrate animals including the jellyfishes, corals, and sea anemones — called also *cnidarian* — **coelenterate** *adj*

coeli- *or* **coelio-** *chiefly Brit var of* CELI-

coe•li•ac, coe•li•os•co•py, coe•li•ot•o•my *chiefly Brit var of* CELIAC, CELIOSCOPY, CELIOTOMY

coe•lom \ˈsē-ləm\ *n, pl* **coeloms** *or* **coe•lo•ma•ta** \si-ˈlō-mə-tə\ : the usu. epithelium-lined metazoancavity between the body wall and digestive tract — **coe•lo•mate** \ˈsē-lə-ˌmāt\ *adj or n* — **coe•lo•mic** \si-ˈlä-mik, -ˈlō-\ *adj*

coe•nu•ro•sis \ˌsēn-yə-ˈrō-səs, ˌsen-\ *or* **coe•nu•ri•a•sis** \-ˈrī-ə-səs\ *n, pl* **-o•ses** \-ˌsēz\ *or* **-a•ses** \-ˌsēz\ : infestation with or disease caused by coenuri

coe•nu•rus \sə-ˈnu̇r-əs, sē-, -ˈnyur-\ *n, pl* **-nu•ri** \-ˈnu̇r-ˌī, -ˈnyu̇r-\ : a complex tapeworm larva growing interstitially in vertebrate tissues and consisting of a large fluid-filled sac from the inner wall of which numerous scolices develop — see GID

co•en•zyme \(ˌ)kō-ˈen-ˌzīm\ *n* : a thermostable nonprotein compound that forms the active portion of an enzyme system after combination with an apoenzyme — **co•en•zy•mat•ic** \-ˌen-zə-ˈma-tik, -(ˌ)zī-\ *adj* — **co•en•zy•mat•i•cal•ly** \-ti-k(ə-)lē\ *adv*

coenzyme A *n* : a coenzyme $C_{21}H_{36}N_7O_{16}P_3S$ that occurs in all living cells and is essential to the metabolism of carbohydrates, fats, and some amino acids

coenzyme Q *n* : UBIQUINONE

coenzyme Q10 *n* : a ubiquinone $C_{59}H_{90}O_4$ of humans and most other mammals that possesses antioxidant properties — abbr. *CoQ10*

coeruleus, coerulei — see LOCUS COERULEUS

co•fac•tor \ˈkō-ˌfak-tər\ *n* **1 :** a substance that acts with another substance to bring about certain effects; *esp* : COENZYME **2 :** something (as a diet or virus) that acts with or aids another factor in causing disease

cogener *var of* CONGENER

Cog•gins test \ˈkä-gənz-\ *n* : a serological immunodiffusion test for the diagnosis of equine infectious anemia esp. in horses by the presence of antibodies to the causative virus — called also *Coggins* — **Coggins test** *vb*

Coggins, Leroy (1932–2014), American veterinary virologist.

Cog•nex \ˈkäg-ˌneks\ *trademark* — used for a preparation of tacrine

cog•ni•tion \käg-ˈni-shən\ *n* : cognitive mental processes; *also* : a product of these processes

cog•ni•tive \ˈkäg-nə-tiv\ *adj* : of, relating to, or being conscious intellectual activity (as thinking, reasoning, remembering, imagining, or learning words) — **cog•ni•tive•ly** *adv*

cognitive behavioral therapy *also* **cognitive behavior therapy** *n* : psychotherapy that combines cognitive therapy with behavior therapy to substitute desirable patterns of thinking, emotional response, and behavior for undesirable ones — abbr. *CBT*

cognitive dissonance *n* : psychological conflict resulting from simultaneously held incongruous beliefs and attitudes

cognitive psychology *n* : a branch of psychology concerned with cognition esp. with respect to the internal events occurring between sensory stimulation and the overt expression of behavior — compare BEHAVIORISM — **cognitive psychologist** *n*

cognitive science *n* : an interdisciplinary science that draws on many fields (as psychology, artificial intelligence, linguistics, and philosophy) in developing theories about human perception, thinking, and learning — **cognitive scientist** *n*

cognitive therapy *n* : psychotherapy that emphasizes the substitution of desirable patterns of thinking for maladaptive or faulty ones; *esp* : COGNITIVE BEHAVIORAL THERAPY — abbr. *CT;* compare BEHAVIOR THERAPY

cogwheel rigidity *n* : muscular rigidity in which passive movement of the limbs (as during a physical examination) elicits ratchet-like start-and-stop movements through the range of motion of a joint (as of the elbow) and that occurs esp. in individuals affected with Parkinson's disease — called also *cogwheeling*

co•he•sion \kō-ˈhē-zhən\ *n* **1** : the act or process of sticking together tightly **2** : the molecular attraction by which the particles of a body are united throughout the mass — **co•he•sive** \kō-ˈhē-siv, -ziv\ *adj* — **co•he•sive•ly** *adv* — **co•he•sive•ness** *n*

co•hort \ˈkō-ˌhȯrt\ *n* : a group of individuals having a statistical factor (as age or risk) in common

coil \ˈkȯi(ə)l\ *n* : INTRAUTERINE DEVICE

co•in•fec•tion \ˌkō-in-ˈfek-shən\ *n* : concurrent infection of a cell or organism with two microorganisms — **co•in•fect** \-ˈfekt\ *vb*

coin lesion *n* : a round well-circumscribed nodule in a lung that is seen in an X-ray photograph as a shadow the size and shape of a coin

coital exanthema *n* : EQUINE COITAL EXANTHEMA

co•ition \kō-ˈi-shən\ *n* : COITUS — **co•ition•al** \-ˈish-nəl, -ˈi-shən-ᵊl\ *adj*

co•itus \ˈkō-ə-təs, kō-ˈē-; ˈkȯi-təs\ *n* : physical union of male and female genitalia accompanied by rhythmic movements : SEXUAL INTERCOURSE 1 — compare ORGASM — **co•ital** \-ət-ᵊl, -ˈēt-\ *adj* — **co•ital•ly** \-ᵊl-ē\ *adv*

coitus in•ter•rup•tus \-ˌin-tə-ˈrəp-təs\ *n* : coitus in which the penis is withdrawn prior to ejaculation to prevent the deposit of sperm in the vagina

coitus res•er•va•tus \-ˌre-zər-ˈvā-təs\ *n* : prolonged coitus in which ejaculation of sperm is deliberately withheld

col- *or* **coli-** *or* **colo-** *comb form* **1** : colon ⟨*col*itis⟩ **2** : colon bacillus ⟨*coli*form⟩

cola *pl of* COLON

Co•lace \kō-ˈlās\ *trademark* — used for a preparation of the sodium salt of docusate

col•chi•cine \ˈkäl-chə-ˌsēn, ˈkäl-kə-\ *n* : a poisonous alkaloid $C_{22}H_{25}NO_6$ that inhibits mitosis, is extracted from the corms or seeds of the autumn crocus, and is used in the treatment of gout and acute attacks of gouty arthritis

col•chi•cum \-kəm\ *n* : the dried corm or dried ripe seeds of the autumn crocus containing the alkaloid colchicine

[1]**cold** \ˈkōld\ *adj* **1 a** : having or being a temperature that is noticeably lower than body temperature and esp. that is uncomfortable for humans **b** : having a relatively low temperature or one that is lower than normal or expected **c** : receptive to the sensation of coldness : stimulated by cold **2** : marked by the loss of normal body heat ⟨~ hands⟩ **3** : DEAD **4** : exhibiting little or no radioactivity — **cold•ness** *n*

[2]**cold** *n* **1** : bodily sensation produced by loss or lack of heat **2** : a bodily disorder popularly associated with chilling: **a** *in humans* : COMMON COLD **b** *in domestic animals* : CORYZA

COLD *abbr* chronic obstructive lung disease

cold agglutinin *n* : any of several agglutinins sometimes present in the blood (as of patients with primary atypical pneumonia) that at low temperatures agglutinate compatible as well as incompatible red blood cells, including the patient's own — compare AUTOAGGLUTININ

cold–blood•ed \ˈkōld-ˈblə-dəd\ *adj* : having a body temperature not internally regulated but approximating that of the environment : POIKILOTHERMIC — **cold–blood•ed•ness** *n*

cold cream *n* : a soothing and cleansing cosmetic basically consisting of a perfumed emulsion of a bland vegetable oil or heavy mineral oil

cold pack *n* : a sheet or blanket wrung out of cold water, wrapped around the patient's body, and covered with dry blankets — compare HOT PACK

cold sore *n* : a vesicular lesion that typically occurs in or around the mouth, that initially causes pain, burning, or itching before bursting and crusting over, and that is caused by a herpes simplex virus — called also *fever blister*

cold sweat *n* : perspiration accompanied by feelings of chill or cold and usu. induced or accompanied by dread, fear, or shock

cold turkey *n* : abrupt complete cessation of the use of an addictive drug; *also* : the symptoms experienced by one undergoing withdrawal from a drug — **cold–turkey** *adv or vb*

col•ec•to•my \kə-ˈlek-tə-mē, kō-\ *n, pl* **-mies** : excision of a portion or all of the colon

co•le•sev•e•lam \ˌkō-lə-ˈsev-ə-ˌlam\ *n* : a drug that is taken orally to lower LDL levels in the treatment of hyperlipidemia and to control levels of blood sugar in the treatment of type 2 diabetes — see WELCHOL

co·les·ti·pol \kə-ˈles-tə-ˌpōl\ *n* : a drug that binds to bile acids and is used esp. to lower LDL levels in the treatment of hypercholesterolemia

co·li \ˈkō-ˌlī\ *adj* : of or relating to bacteria normally inhabiting the intestine or colon and esp. to species of the genus *Escherichia* (as *E. coli*) — **coli** *n*

coli- — see COL-

co·li·ba·cil·lo·sis \ˌkō-lə-ˌba-sə-ˈlō-səs\ *n, pl* **-lo·ses** \-ˌsēz\ : infection with or disease caused by colon bacilli (esp. E. coli)

[1]**col·ic** \ˈkä-lik\ *n* **1** : an attack of acute abdominal pain localized in a hollow organ and often caused by spasm, obstruction, or twisting **2** : a condition marked by recurrent episodes of prolonged and uncontrollable crying and irritability in an otherwise healthy infant that is of unknown cause and usu. subsides after three to four months of age

[2]**colic** *adj* : of or relating to colic : COLICKY ⟨~ crying⟩

[3]**co·lic** \ˈkō-lik, ˈkä-\ *adj* : of or relating to the colon

colic artery *n* : any of three arteries that branch from the mesenteric arteries and supply the large intestine

co·li·cin \ˈkō-lə-sən\ *also* **co·li·cine** \-ˌsēn\ *n* : any of various antibacterial proteins that are produced by strains of intestinal bacteria (as E. coli) and that often act to inhibit macromolecular synthesis in related strains

col·icky \ˈkä-li-kē\ *adj* **1** : relating to or associated with colic ⟨~ pain⟩ **2** : suffering from colic ⟨~ babies⟩

co·li·form \ˈkō-lə-ˌfȯrm, ˈkä-\ *adj* : of, relating to, or being gram-negative rod-shaped bacteria (as E. coli) normally present in the intestine — **coliform** *n*

co·li·phage \ˈkō-lə-ˌfāj, -ˌfäzh\ *n* : a bacteriophage active against colon bacilli

co·lis·tin \kə-ˈlis-tən, kō-\ *n* : a polymyxin produced by a bacterium of the genus *Bacillus* (*B. polymyxa* var. *colistinus*)

co·li·tis \kō-ˈlī-təs, kə-\ *n* : inflammation of the colon — see ULCERATIVE COLITIS

colla *pl of* COLLUM

col·la·gen \ˈkä-lə-jən\ *n* : an insoluble fibrous protein of vertebrates that is the chief constituent of the fibrils of connective tissue (as in skin and tendons) and of the organic substance of bones and yields gelatin and glue on prolonged heating with water — **col·lag·e·nous** \kə-ˈla-jə-nəs\ *adj*

col·la·ge·nase \kə-ˈla-jə-ˌnās, ˈkä-lə-, -ˌnāz\ *n* : any of a group of proteolytic enzymes that decompose collagen and gelatin

collagen disease *n* : CONNECTIVE TISSUE DISEASE

col·la·gen·o·lyt·ic \ˌkä-lə-jə-nə-ˈli-tik, -ˌje-\ *adj* : relating to or having the capacity to break down collagen

col·la·ge·no·sis \ˌkä-lə-jə-ˈnō-səs\ *n, pl* **-no·ses** \-ˌsēz\ : CONNECTIVE TISSUE DISEASE

collagen vascular disease *n* : CONNECTIVE TISSUE DISEASE

[1]**col·lapse** \kə-ˈlaps\ *vb* **col·lapsed; col·laps·ing** **1** : to fall or shrink together abruptly and completely : fall into a jumbled or flattened mass through the force of external pressure ⟨a blood vessel that *collapsed*⟩ **2** : to break down in vital energy, stamina, or self-control through exhaustion or disease; *esp* : to fall helpless or unconscious — **col·laps·ibil·i·ty** \-ˌlap-sə-ˈbi-lə-tē\ *n* — **col·laps·ible** \-ˈlap-sə-bəl\ *adj*

[2]**collapse** *n* **1** : a breakdown in vital energy, strength, or stamina : complete sudden enervation **2** : a state of extreme prostration and physical depression resulting from circulatory failure, great loss of body fluids, or heart disease and occurring terminally in diseases such as cholera, typhoid fever, and pneumonia **3** : an airless state of a lung of spontaneous origin or induced surgically — see ATELECTASIS **4** : an abnormal falling together of the walls of an organ

col·lar \ˈkä-lər\ *n* : a protective or supportive device (as a brace or cast) worn around the neck

col·lar·bone \ˈkä-lər-ˌbōn\ *n* : CLAVICLE

[1]**col·lat·er·al** \kə-ˈla-tə-rəl, -trəl\ *adj* **1** : relating to or being branches of a bodily part ⟨~ sprouting of nerves⟩ **2** : relating to or being part of the collateral circulation ⟨~ blood flow⟩

[2]**collateral** *n* **1** : a branch esp. of a blood vessel, nerve, or the axon of a nerve cell **2** : a bodily part that is lateral in position

collateral circulation *n* : circulation of blood established through enlargement of minor vessels and anastomosis of vessels with those of adjacent parts when a major vein or artery is functionally impaired (as by obstruction); *also* : the modified vessels through which such circulation occurs

collateral ligament *n* : any of various ligaments on one or the other side of a hinge joint (as the knee, elbow, or the joints between the phalanges of the toes and fingers): as **a** : LATERAL COLLATERAL LIGAMENT **b** : MEDIAL COLLATERAL LIGAMENT **c** : RADIAL COLLATERAL LIGAMENT **d** : ULNAR COLLATERAL LIGAMENT

collateral sulcus *n* : a sulcus of the tentorial surface of the cerebrum lying below and external to the calcarine sulcus and causing an elevation on the floor of the lateral ventricle between the hippocampi — called also *collateral fissure*

collecting duct *n* : any of several ducts that receive urine from the nephrons and discharge it into the pelvis of the kidney — called also *collecting tubule*

collecting tubule *n* **1** : COLLECTING DUCT **2** : a tubule that connects the distal convoluted tubule of the nephron with the collecting ducts — called also *connecting tubule*

collective unconscious *n* : the genetically determined part of the unconscious in the psychoanalytic theory of C. G. Jung

Col•les' fracture \ˈkä-ləs-, -ˌlēz-\ *n* : a fracture of the lower end of the radius with backward displacement of the lower fragment and radial deviation of the hand at the wrist that produces a characteristic deformity — compare SMITH FRACTURE

Col•les \ˈkä-ləs\, **Abraham (1773–1843),** British surgeon.

col•lic•u•lus \kə-ˈli-kyə-ləs\ *n, pl* **-u•li** \-ˌlī, -ˌlē\ : an anatomical prominence; *esp* : any of the four prominences constituting the corpora quadrigemina — see INFERIOR COLLICULUS, SUPERIOR COLLICULUS

col•li•ma•tor \ˈkä-lə-ˌmā-tər\ *n* : a device for obtaining a beam of radiation (as X-rays) of limited cross section

col•li•qua•tion \ˌkä-lə-ˈkwā-zhən, -shən\ *n* : the breakdown and liquefaction of tissue — **col•li•qua•tive** \ˈkä-li-ˌkwā-tiv, kə-ˈli-kwə-\ *adj*

col•lo•di•on \kə-ˈlō-dē-ən\ *n* : a viscous solution of pyroxylin used as a coating for wounds

col•loid \ˈkä-ˌlȯid\ *n* **1** : a gelatinous or mucinous substance found in tissues in disease or normally (as in the thyroid) **2 a** : a substance that consists of particles dispersed throughout another substance which are too small for resolution with an ordinary light microscope but are incapable of passing through a semipermeable membrane **b** : a mixture (as smoke) consisting of a colloid together with the medium in which it is dispersed — **col•loi•dal** \kə-ˈlȯid-ᵊl, kä-\ *adj* — **col•loi•dal•ly** *adv*

colloidal silver *n* : a preparation consisting of silver particles suspended in liquid that is sometimes used as a dietary supplement

col•lum \ˈkä-ləm\ *n, pl* **col•la** \-lə\ : an anatomical neck or neckline part or process

col•lu•to•ri•um \ˌkä-lə-ˈtōr-ē-əm\ *n, pl* **-to•ria** \-ē-ə\ : MOUTHWASH

col•lyr•i•um \kə-ˈlir-ē-əm\ *n, pl* **-ia** \-ē-ə\ *or* **-i•ums** : an eye lotion : EYEWASH

colo- — see COL-

col•o•bo•ma \ˌkä-lə-ˈbō-mə\ *n, pl* **-mas** *also* **-ma•ta** \-mə-tə\ : a fissure of the eye usu. of congenital origin

co•lon \ˈkō-lən\ *n, pl* **colons** *or* **co•la** \-lə\ : the part of the large intestine that extends from the cecum to the rectum

colon bacillus *n* : any of several bacilli esp. of the genus *Escherichia* that are normally commensal in vertebrate intestines; *esp* : E. COLI

[1]**co•lon•ic** \kō-ˈlä-nik, kə-\ *adj* : of or relating to the colon

[2]**colonic** *n* : ENEMA — see HIGH COLONIC

colonic irrigation *n* : ENEMA

col•o•nize \ˈkä-lə-ˌnīz\ *vb* **-nized; -niz•ing** : to establish a colony in or on — **col•o•ni•za•tion** \ˌkä-lə-nə-ˈzā-shən\ *n*

co•lo•nog•ra•phy \ˌkō-lə-ˈnä-grə-fē\ *n, pl* **-phies** : noninvasive visualization of the interior of the colon by means of computed tomography or magnetic resonance imaging; *esp* : CT COLONOGRAPHY — called also *virtual colonography, virtual colonoscopy*

co•lon•o•scope \kō-ˈlä-nə-ˌskōp\ *n* : a flexible endoscope for inspecting and passing instruments into the colon (as to obtain tissue for biopsy)

co•lo•nos•co•py \ˌkō-lə-ˈnäs-kə-pē, ˌkä-\ *n, pl* **-pies** : endoscopic examination of the colon — **co•lon•o•scop•ic** \kō-ˌlä-nə-ˈskä-pik\ *adj*

col•o•ny \ˈkä-lə-nē\ *n, pl* **-nies** : a circumscribed mass of microorganisms usu. growing in or on a solid medium

colony–stimulating factor *n* : any of several glycoproteins that promote the differentiation of stem cells esp. into blood granulocytes and macrophages and that stimulate their proliferation into colonies in culture

co•lo•proc•tos•to•my \ˌkō-lə-ˌpräk-ˈtäs-tə-mē, ˌkä-\ *n, pl* **-mies** : surgical formation of an artificial passage between the colon and the rectum

col•or \ˈkə-lər\ *n, often attrib* **1 a** : a phenomenon of light (as red, brown, pink, or gray) or visual perception that enables one to differentiate otherwise identical objects **b** : the aspect of objects and light sources that may be described in terms of hue, lightness, and saturation for objects and hue, brightness, and saturation for light sources **c** : a hue as contrasted with black, white, or gray **2** : complexion tint; *esp* : the tint characteristic of good health

Colorado tick fever *n* : a mild disease of the western U.S. and western Canada that is characterized by the absence of a rash, intermittent fever, malaise, headaches, and myalgia and is caused by a reovirus (species *Colorado tick fever virus* of the genus *Coltivirus*) transmitted by the Rocky Mountain wood tick

col•or–blind \-ˌblīnd\ *adj* : affected with partial or total inability to distinguish one or more chromatic colors — **color blindness** *n*

co•lo•rec•tal \ˌkō-lə-ˈrekt-ᵊl, ˌkä-\ *adj* : relating to or affecting the colon and the rectum ⟨∼ cancer⟩ ⟨∼ surgery⟩

co•lo•rec•tum \-ˈrek-təm\ *n* : the colon and the rectum

col•or•im•e•ter \ˌkə-lə-ˈri-mə-tər\ *n* : any of various instruments used to objectively determine the color of a solution — **col•or•i•met•ric** \ˌkə-lə-rə-ˈme-trik\ *adj* — **col•or•i•met•ri•cal•ly** \-tri-k(ə-)lē\ *adv* — **col•or•im•e•try** \ˌkə-lə-ˈri-mə-trē\ *n*

color index *n* : a figure that represents the ratio of the amount of hemoglobin to the number of red cells in a given volume of blood and that is a measure of the normality of the hemoglobin content of the individual cells

color vision *n* : perception of and ability to distinguish colors

co•los•to•mize \kə-ˈläs-tə-ˌmīz\ *vb* **-mized; -miz•ing** : to perform a colostomy on

co•los•to•my \kə-ˈläs-tə-mē\ *n, pl* **-mies** : surgical formation of an artificial anus by connecting the colon to an opening in the abdominal wall

colostomy bag *n* : a container kept constantly in position to receive feces discharged through a colostomy

co•los•trum \kə-ˈläs-trəm\ *n* : milk secreted for a few days after childbirth and characterized esp. by high protein and antibody content — **co•los•tral** \-trəl\ *adj*

col•our *chiefly Brit var of* COLOR

colp- *or* **colpo-** *comb form* : vagina ⟨*colp*itis⟩ ⟨*colpo*scope⟩

col•pec•to•my \käl-ˈpek-tə-mē\ *n, pl* **-to•mies** : VAGINECTOMY

col•pi•tis \käl-ˈpī-təs\ *n* : VAGINITIS 1

col•po•cen•te•sis \ˌkäl-(ˌ)pō-sen-ˈtē-səs\ *n, pl* **-te•ses** \-ˌsēz\ : surgical puncture of the vagina

col•po•clei•sis \ˌkäl-pō-ˈklī-səs\ *n, pl* **-clei•ses** \-ˌsēz\ : the suturing of posterior and anterior walls of the vagina to prevent uterine prolapse

col•po•per•i•ne•or•rha•phy \ˌkäl-pō-ˌper-ə-(ˌ)nē-ˈȯr-ə-fē\ *n, pl* **-phies** : the suturing of an injury to the vagina and the perineum

col•po•pexy \ˈkäl-pə-ˌpek-sē\ *n, pl* **-pex•ies** : fixation of the vagina by suturing it to the adjacent abdominal wall

col•por•rha•phy \käl-ˈpȯr-ə-fē\ *n, pl* **-phies** : surgical repair of the vaginal wall

-colpos *n comb form* : vaginal disorder (of a specified type) ⟨hemato*colpos*⟩

col•po•scope \ˈkäl-pə-ˌskōp\ *n* : an instrument designed to facilitate visual inspection of the vagina — **col•po•scop•ic** \ˌkäl-pə-ˈskä-pik\ *adj* — **col•po•scop•i•cal•ly** \-pi-k(ə-)lē\ *adv* — **col•pos•co•py** \käl-ˈpäs-kə-pē\ *n*

col•pot•o•my \käl-ˈpä-tə-mē\ *n, pl* **-mies** : surgical incision of the vagina

co•lum•bi•um \kə-ˈləm-bē-əm\ *n* : NIOBIUM

col•u•mel•la \ˌkä-lə-ˈme-lə, ˌkäl-yə-\ *n, pl* **-mel•lae** \-ˈme-(ˌ)lē, -ˌlī\ : any of various anatomical parts likened to a column: **a** : the bony central axis of the cochlea **b** : the lower part of the nasal septum — **col•u•mel•lar** \-lər\ *adj*

col•umn \ˈkä-ləm\ *n* : a longitudinal subdivision of the spinal cord that resembles a column or pillar: as **a** : any of the principal longitudinal subdivisions of gray matter or white matter in each lateral half of the spinal cord — see DORSAL HORN, GRAY COLUMN, LATERAL COLUMN 1, VENTRAL HORN; compare FUNICULUS a **b** : any of a number of smaller bundles of spinal nerve fibers : FASCICULUS

co•lum•nar \kə-ˈləm-nər\ *adj* : of, relating to, being, or composed of tall narrow somewhat cylindrical epithelial cells ⟨~ epithelium⟩

column of Ber•tin \-ber-ˈtaⁿ\ *n* : any of the masses of cortical tissue extending between the sides of the renal pyramids of the kidney as far as the renal pelvis — called also *Bertin's column, renal column*

E. J. Bertin — see BERTIN'S COLUMN

column of Bur•dach \-ˈbər-dək, -ˈbu̇r-, -ˌdäk\ *n* : FASCICULUS CUNEATUS

Bur•dach \ˈbu̇r-däk\, **Karl Friedrich (1776–1847)**, German anatomist.

co•ma \ˈkō-mə\ *n* : a state of profound unconsciousness caused by disease, injury, or poison

co•ma•tose \ˈkō-mə-ˌtōs, ˈkä-\ *adj* : of, resembling, or affected with coma ⟨a ~ patient⟩ ⟨a ~ condition⟩

combat fatigue *n* : a post-traumatic stress disorder occurring under wartime conditions (as combat) that cause intense stress — called also *battle fatigue, shell shock, war neurosis*

Com•bi•gan \ˈkäm-bi-gən\ *trademark* — used for an ophthalmic solution containing brimonidine and timolol

combination therapy *n* : the use of two or more therapies and esp. drugs to treat a disease or condition

Com•bi•vent \ˈkäm-bə-ˌvent\ *trademark* — used for a preparation of ipratropium bromide and the sulfate of albuterol for oral inhalation

com•e•do \ˈkä-mə-ˌdō\ *n, pl* **com•e•do•nes** \ˌkä-mə-ˈdō-(ˌ)nēz\ : BLACKHEAD 1

com•e•do•car•ci•no•ma \ˌkä-mə-ˌdō-ˌkärs-ᵊn-ˈō-mə\ *n, pl* **-mas** *also* **-ma•ta** \-mə-tə\ : a breast cancer that arises in the larger ducts and is characterized by slow growth, late metastasis, and the accumulation of solid plugs of atypical and degenerating cells in the ducts

com•e•do•gen•ic \ˌkä-mə-də-ˈje-nik\ *adj* : tending to clog pores esp. by the formation of blackheads ⟨~ cosmetics⟩

come to *vb* : to recover consciousness

comfort care *n* : PALLIATIVE CARE

comitans — see VENA COMITANS

com•men•sal•ism \kə-ˈmen-sə-ˌli-zəm\ *n* : a relation between two kinds of organisms in which one obtains food or other benefits from the other without damaging or benefiting it — **com•men•sal** \-səl\ *adj or n* — **com•men•sal•ly** *adv*

com•mi•nut•ed \ˌkä-mə-ˈnü-təd, -ˈnyü-\ *adj* : being a fracture in which the bone is splintered or crushed into numerous pieces

com•mis•su•ra \ˌkä-mə-ˈshu̇r-ə\ *n, pl* **-rae** \-ˈshu̇r-ē\ : COMMISSURE

com•mis•sure \ˈkä-mə-ˌshu̇r\ *n* **1** : a point or line of union or junction between two anatomical parts (as the lips at their angles or adjacent heart valves) **2** : a connecting band of nerve tissue in the brain or spinal cord — see ANTERIOR COMMISSURE, CORPUS CALLOSUM, GRAY COMMISSURE, HABENULAR COMMISSURE, HIPPOCAMPAL COMMISSURE, POSTERIOR COMMISSURE — **com•mis•su•ral** \ˌkä-mə-ˈshu̇r-əl\ *adj*

com•mis•sur•ot•o•my \ˌkä-mə-ˌshu̇r-ˈä-tə-mē, -shə-ˈrä-\ *n, pl* **-mies** : the operation of cutting through a band of muscle or nerve fibers; *specif* : separation of the flaps of a mitral valve to relieve mitral stenosis : VALVULOTOMY

com•mit \kə-ˈmit\ *vb* **com•mit•ted; com•mit•ting** : to place in a prison or mental institution — **com•mit•ment** \kə-ˈmit-mənt\ *n* — **com•mit•ta•ble** \-ˈmi-tə-bəl\ *adj*

com•mon \ˈkä-mən\ *adj* : formed of or dividing into two or more branches ⟨the ~ facial vein⟩ ⟨~ iliac vessels⟩

common bile duct *n* : the duct formed by the union of the hepatic and cystic ducts and opening into the duodenum

common carotid artery *n* : the part of either carotid artery between its point of origin and its division into the internal and external carotid arteries — called also *common carotid*

common cattle grub *n* : a cattle grub of the genus *Hypoderma* (*H. lineatum*) whose larva is particularly destructive to cattle : HEEL FLY

common cold *n* : an acute contagious disease of the upper respiratory tract that is marked by inflammation of the mucous membranes of the nose, throat, eyes, and eustachian tubes with a watery then purulent discharge and is caused by any of several viruses (as a rhinovirus or an adenovirus)

common iliac artery *n* : ILIAC ARTERY 1

common iliac vein *n* : ILIAC VEIN a

common interosseous artery *n* : a short thick artery that arises from the ulnar artery near the proximal end of the radius and that divides into anterior and posterior branches which pass down the forearm toward the wrist

common peroneal nerve *n* : the smaller of the branches into which the sciatic nerve divides passing outward and downward from the popliteal space and to the neck of the fibula where it divides into the deep peroneal nerve and the superficial peroneal nerve — called also *lateral popliteal nerve, peroneal nerve*

com•mo•tio \kə-ˈmō-shē-ō\ *n* : CONCUSSION

commotio cor•dis \-ˈkȯr-dəs\ *n* : concussion of the heart that is caused by a blow to the chest over the region of the heart by a blunt object which does not penetrate the body and that usu. results in ventricular fibrillation leading to sudden cardiac death if treatment by defibrillation is not immediately given

com•mu•ni•ca•ble \kə-ˈmyü-ni-kə-bəl\ *adj* : capable of being transmitted from person to person, animal to animal, animal to human, or human to animal : TRANSMISSIBLE — **com•mu•ni•ca•bil•i•ty** \-ˌmyü-ni-kə-ˈbi-lə-tē\ *n*

communicable disease *n* : an infectious disease transmissible (as from person to person) by direct contact with an affected individual or the individual's discharges or by indirect means (as by a vector) — compare CONTAGIOUS DISEASE

communicans — see RAMUS COMMUNICANS, WHITE RAMUS COMMUNICANS

communicantes — see RAMUS COMMUNICANS

com•mu•ni•cate \kə-ˈmyü-nə-ˌkāt\ *vb* **-cat•ed; -cat•ing** : to cause to pass from one to another ⟨some diseases are easily *communicated*⟩

communicating artery *n* : any of three arteries in the brain that form parts of the circle of Willis: **a** : one connecting the anterior cerebral arteries — called also *anterior communicating artery* **b** : either of two arteries that occur one on each side of the circle of Willis and connect an internal carotid artery with a posterior cerebral artery — called also *posterior communicating artery*

com•mu•ni•ca•tion \kə-ˌmyü-nə-ˈkā-shən\ *n* **1** : the act or process of transmitting information (as about ideas, attitudes, emotions, or objective behavior) **2** : information communicated **3** : a connection between bodily parts ⟨an artificial ~ between the esophagus and the stomach⟩

communis — see EXTENSOR DIGITORUM COMMUNIS

community–acquired *adj, of an infection* : acquired or arising in the general population : not acquired or arising in a hospital ⟨~ pneumonia⟩

co•mor•bid \kō-ˈmȯr-bəd\ *adj* : existing simultaneously with and usu. independently of another medical condition ⟨bipolar disorder with ~ substance abuse⟩

co•mor•bid•i•ty \kō-mȯr-ˈbi-də-tē\ *n* **1** : a comorbid condition **2** : the occurrence of comorbid conditions : occurrence as a comorbid condition

com•pact \kəm-ˈpakt, käm-ˈ, ˈkäm-ˌ\ *adj* : having a dense structure without small cavities or cells ⟨~ bone⟩ — compare CANCELLOUS

compacta — see PARS COMPACTA

compactum — see STRATUM COMPACTUM

com•par•a•tive \kəm-ˈpar-ə-tiv\ *adj* : characterized by the systematic comparison of phenomena and esp. of likenesses and dissimilarities ⟨~ anatomy⟩

com•part•ment syndrome \kəm-ˈpärt-mənt-\ *n* : a painful condition resulting from the expansion or overgrowth of enclosed tissue (as of a leg muscle) within its anatomical enclosure (as a muscular sheath) producing pressure that interferes with circulation and adversely affects the function and health of the tissue itself — called also *com•part•men•tal syndrome* \kəm-ˌpärt-ˈmen-tᵊl-\

com•pat•i•ble \kəm-ˈpa-tə-bəl\ *adj* **1** : capable of existing together in a satisfactory relationship (as marriage) **2** : capable of being used in transfusion or grafting without immunological reaction (as agglutination or tissue rejection) **3** *of medications* : capable of being administered jointly without interacting to produce deleterious effects or impairing their respective actions — **com•pat•i•bil•i•ty** \-ˌpa-tə-ˈbi-lə-tē\ *n*

Com•pa•zine \ˈkäm-pə-ˌzēn\ *trademark* — used for a preparation of prochlorperazine

com•pen•sate \ˈkäm-pən-ˌsāt, -ˌpen-\ *vb* **-sat•ed; -sat•ing 1** : to subject to or remedy by physiological compensation **2** : to undergo, experience, or engage in psychological or physiological compensation

com•pen•sat•ed *adj* : buffered so that there is no change in the pH of the blood ⟨~ acidosis⟩ — compare UNCOMPENSATED

com•pen•sa•tion \ˌkäm-pən-ˈsā-shən, -ˌpen-\ *n* **1** : correction of an organic defect by excessive development or by increased functioning of another organ or unimpaired parts of the same organ ⟨cardiac ~⟩ — see DECOMPENSATION **2** : a psychological mechanism by which feelings of inferiority, frustration, or failure in one field are counterbalanced by achievement in another

com•pen•sa•to•ry \kəm-ˈpen-sə-ˌtōr-ē\ *adj* : making up for a loss; *esp* : serving as psychological or physiological compensation

com•pe•tence \ˈkäm-pə-təns\ *n* : the quality or state of being functionally adequate ⟨immune system ~⟩

com•pe•ten•cy \-tən-sē\ *n, pl* **-cies** : COMPETENCE

com•pe•tent \ˈkäm-pə-tənt\ *adj* : having the capacity to function or develop in a particular way

com•pet•i•tive \kəm-ˈpe-tə-tiv\ *adj* : depending for effectiveness on the relative concentration of two or more substances ⟨~ protein binding⟩

com•plain \kəm-ˈplān\ *vb* : to speak of one's illness or symptoms

com•plaint \kəm-ˈplānt\ *n* : a bodily ailment or disease

com•ple•ment \ˈkäm-plə-mənt\ *n* **1** : a group or set (as of chromosomes) that is typical of the complete organism or one of its parts — see CHROMOSOME COMPLEMENT **2** : the thermolabile group of proteins in normal blood serum and plasma that in combination with antibodies causes the destruction esp. of particulate antigens

com•ple•men•tar•i•ty \ˌkäm-plə-(ˌ)men-ˈtar-ə-tē, -mən-\ *n, pl* **-ties** : correspondence in reverse of part of one molecule to part of another: as **a** : the arrangement of chemical groups and electric charges that enables a combining group of an antibody to combine with a specific determinant group of an antigen or hapten **b** : the correspondence between strands or nucleotides of DNA or sometimes RNA that permits their precise pairing

com•ple•men•ta•ry \ˌkäm-plə-ˈmen-tə-rē, -trē\ *adj* : characterized by molecular complementarity; *esp* : characterized by the capacity for precise pairing of purine and pyrimidine bases between strands of DNA and sometimes RNA such that the structure of one strand determines the other — **com•ple•men•ta•ri•ly** \-ˈmen-trə-lē, -(ˌ)men-ˈter-ə-lē, -ˈmen-tə-rə-lē\ *adv* — **com•ple•men•ta•ri•ness** \-ˈmen-tə-rē-nəs, -ˈmen-trē-\ *n*

complementary DNA *n* : CDNA

complementary medicine *n* : any of the practices (as acupuncture) of alternative medicine accepted and utilized by mainstream medical practitioners; *also* : ALTERNATIVE MEDICINE

complement fixation *n* : the process of binding serum complement to the product formed by the union of an antibody and the antigen for which it is specific

complement fixation test *n* : a diagnostic test for the presence of a particular antibody in the serum of a patient that involves inactivation of the complement in the serum, addition of measured amounts of the antigen for which the antibody is specific and of foreign complement, and detection of the presence or absence of complement fixation by the addition of a suitable indicator system — see WASSERMAN TEST

Com•plera \kəm-ˈpler-ə\ *trademark* — used for a preparation of emtricitabine, rilpivirine, and the fumarate of tenofovir

com•plete \kəm-ˈplēt\ *adj* **1** *of a bone fracture* : characterized by a break passing entirely across the bone — compare INCOMPLETE 1 **2** *of a protein* : containing all essential amino acids — compare INCOMPLETE 2

complete blood count *n* : a blood count that includes separate counts for red and white blood cells — called also *complete blood cell count;* compare DIFFERENTIAL BLOOD COUNT

[1]**com•plex** \käm-ˈpleks, kəm-ˈ, ˈkäm-ˌ\ *adj* : formed by the union of simpler chemical substances ⟨~ proteins⟩

[2]**com•plex** \ˈkäm-ˌpleks\ *n* **1** : a group of repressed memories, desires, and ideas that exert a dominant influence on the personality and behavior ⟨a guilt ~⟩ — see CASTRATION COMPLEX, ELECTRA COMPLEX, INFERIORITY COMPLEX, OEDIPUS COMPLEX, PERSECUTION COMPLEX, SUPERIORITY COMPLEX **2** : a group of chromosomes arranged or behaving in a particular way — see GENE COMPLEX **3** : a chemical association of two or more species (as ions or molecules) joined usu. by weak electrostatic bonds rather than covalent bonds **4** : the sum of the factors (as symptoms and lesions) characterizing a disease ⟨primary tuberculous ~⟩

[3]**com•plex** \käm-ˈpleks, kəm-ˈ, ˈkäm-ˌ\ *vb* : to form or cause to form into a complex ⟨RNA ~*ed* with protein⟩

com•plex•ion \kəm-ˈplek-shən\ *n* : the hue or appearance of the skin and esp. of the face ⟨a dark ~⟩ — **com•plex•ioned** \-shənd\ *adj*

complex regional pain syndrome *n* : a condition of chronic severe often burning pain usu. of part or all of one or more extremities that typically occurs following an injury, is often accompanied by swelling, skin discoloration, allodynia, abnormal sweating, and impaired motor function in the affected area, and is of unknown pathogenesis — abbr. *CRPS;* see CAUSALGIA, REFLEX SYMPATHETIC DYSTROPHY

com•plex•us \kəm-ˈplek-səs, käm-\ *n* : SEMISPINALIS CAPITIS — called also *complexus muscle*

com•pli•ance \kəm-ˈplī-əns\ *n* **1** : the ability or process of yielding to changes in pressure without disruption of structure or function ⟨pulmonary ~⟩ **2** : the process of complying with a regimen of treatment

com•pli•cate \ˈkäm-plə-ˌkāt\ *vb* **-cat•ed; -cat•ing** : to cause to be more complex or severe ⟨a virus disease *complicated* by bacterial infection⟩

com•pli•cat•ed *adj, of a bone fracture* : characterized by injury to nearby parts

com•pli•ca•tion \ˌkäm-plə-ˈkā-shən\ *n* : a secondary disease or condition that develops in the course of a primary disease or condition and arises either as a result of it or from independent causes

com•pos men•tis \ˌkäm-pəs-ˈmen-təs\ *adj* : of sound mind, memory, and understanding

[1]**com•pound** \käm-ˈpau̇nd, kəm-ˈ, ˈkäm-ˌ\ *vb* : to form by combining parts ⟨~ a medicine⟩

[2]**com•pound** \ˈkäm-ˌpau̇nd, käm-ˈ, kəm-ˈ\ *adj* : composed of or resulting from union of separate elements, ingredients, or parts ⟨~ glands⟩

[3]**com•pound** \ˈkäm-ˌpau̇nd\ *n* : something formed by a union of elements or parts; *specif* : a distinct substance formed by chemical union of two or more ingredients in definite proportion by weight

compound benzoin tincture *n* : FRIAR'S BALSAM

compound fracture *n* : a bone fracture resulting in an open wound through which bone fragments usu. protrude — compare SIMPLE FRACTURE

compound microscope *n* : a microscope consisting of an objective and an eyepiece mounted in a telescoping tube

[1]**com•press** \kəm-ˈpres\ *vb* : to press or squeeze together ⟨a ~*ed* nerve⟩

[2]**com•press** \ˈkäm-ˌpres\ *n* **1** : a covering consisting usu. of a folded cloth that is applied and held firmly by the aid of a bandage over a wound dressing to prevent oozing **2** : a folded wet or dry cloth applied firmly to a part (as to allay inflammation)

compressed–air illness *n* : DECOMPRESSION SICKNESS

com•pres•sion \kəm-ˈpre-shən\ *n* : the act, process, or result of compressing esp. when involving a compressing force on a bodily part ⟨~ of a nerve⟩

compression fracture *n* : fracture (as of a vertebra) caused by compression of one bone against another

[1]**com•pro•mise** \ˈkäm-prə-ˌmīz\ *vb* **-mised; -mis•ing** : to cause the impairment of ⟨a *compromised* immune system⟩

[2]**compromise** *n* : the condition of having been compromised : IMPAIRMENT ⟨cardiovascular ~⟩

com•pul•sion \kəm-ˈpəl-shən\ *n* : an irresistible persistent impulse to perform an act (as excessive hand washing); *also* : the act itself — compare OBSESSION, PHOBIA

[1]**com•pul•sive** \-siv\ *adj* : of, relating to, caused by, or suggestive of psychological compulsion or obsession ⟨~ behavior⟩ ⟨~ hoarding⟩ ⟨a ~ gambler⟩ — **com•pul•sive•ly** *adv* — **com•pul•sive•ness** *n* — **com•pul•siv•i•ty** \kəm-ˌpəl-ˈsi-və-tē, ˌkäm-\ *n*

[2]**compulsive** *n* : one who is subject to a psychological compulsion

com•put•ed axial tomography \kəm-ˈpyü-təd-\ *n* : COMPUTED TOMOGRAPHY — abbr. *CAT*

computed tomographic *adj* : using, produced by, or obtained by computed tomography

computed tomographic colonography *n* : CT COLONOGRAPHY — called also *computerized tomographic colonography, computed tomography colonography* — abbr. *CTC*

computed tomography *n* : a method of producing a three-dimensional image of an internal body structure by computerized combination of two-dimensional cross-sectional X-ray images made along an axis — abbr. *CT;* see CT SCAN, CT COLONOGRAPHY

com·pu·ter·ized axial tomography \kəm-ˈpyü-tə-ˌrīzd-\ *n* : COMPUTED TOMOGRAPHY — abbr. *CAT*

computerized tomography *n* : COMPUTED TOMOGRAPHY — abbr. *CT*

Com·tan \ˈkäm-ˌtan\ *trademark* — used for a preparation of entacapone

co·na·tion \kō-ˈnā-shən\ *n* : an inclination (as an instinct or a craving) to act purposefully : IMPULSE 2 — **co·na·tive** \ˈkō-nə-tiv, -ˌnā-; ˈkä-\ *adj*

conc *abbr* concentrated; concentration

con·ca·nav·a·lin \ˌkän-kə-ˈna-və-lən\ *n* : either of two crystalline globulins occurring esp. in the seeds of a tropical American leguminous plant (*Canavalia ensiformis*); *esp* : one that is a potent hemagglutinin

con·ceive \kən-ˈsēv\ *vb* **con·ceived; con·ceiv·ing** : to become pregnant

con·cen·trate \ˈkän-sən-ˌtrāt, -ˌsen-\ *vb* **-trat·ed; -trat·ing 1 a** : to bring or direct toward a common center or objective **b** : to accumulate (a toxic substance) in bodily tissues ⟨fish ~ mercury⟩ **2** : to make less dilute **3** : to fix one's powers, efforts, or attention on one thing

con·cen·tra·tion \ˌkän-sən-ˈtrā-shən, -ˌsen-\ *n* **1** : the act or action of concentrating: as **a** : a directing of the attention or of the mental faculties toward a single object **b** : an increasing of strength (as of a solute) by partial or total removal of diluents **2** : a crude active principle of a vegetable esp. for pharmaceutical use in the form of a powder or resin **3** : the relative content of a component (as dissolved or dispersed material) of a solution, mixture, or dispersion that may be expressed in percentage by weight or by volume, in parts per million, or in grams per liter

con·cep·tion \kən-ˈsep-shən\ *n* **1 a** : the process of becoming pregnant involving fertilization or implantation or both **b** : EMBRYO, FETUS **2 a** : the capacity, function, or process of forming or understanding ideas or abstractions or their symbols **b** : a general idea

con·cep·tive \kən-ˈsep-tiv\ *adj* : capable of or relating to conceiving

con·cep·tus \kən-ˈsep-təs\ *n* : a fertilized egg, embryo, or fetus

Con·cer·ta \kän-ˈsər-tə\ *trademark* — used for a preparation of the hydrochloride of methylphenidate

conch \ˈkäŋk, ˈkänch, ˈkȯŋk\ *n, pl* **conchs** \ˈkäŋks, ˈkȯŋks\ *or* **conch·es** \ˈkän-chəz\ : CONCHA 1

con·cha \ˈkäŋ-kə, ˈkȯŋ-\ *n, pl* **con·chae** \-ˌkē, -ˌkī\ **1** : the largest and deepest concavity of the external ear **2** : NASAL CONCHA — **con·chal** \-kəl\ *adj*

con·cor·dant \kən-ˈkȯrd-ᵊnt\ *adj, of twins* : similar with respect to one or more particular characters — compare DISCORDANT — **con·cor·dance** \-ᵊn(t)s\ *n*

con·cre·ment \ˈkäŋ-krə-mənt, ˈkän-\ *n* : CONCRETION

con·cre·tion \kän-ˈkrē-shən, kən-\ *n* : a hard usu. inorganic mass (as a tophus) formed esp. from mineral salts in a living body

con·cuss \kən-ˈkəs\ *vb* : to affect with concussion

con·cus·sion \kən-ˈkə-shən\ *n* **1** : a hard blow or collision **2** : a condition resulting from the effects of a hard blow; *esp* : a jarring injury of the brain resulting in disturbance of cerebral function — **con·cus·sive** \-ˈkə-siv\ *adj*

con·den·sa·tion \ˌkän-ˌden-ˈsā-shən, -dən-\ *n* **1** : the act or process of condensing: as **a** : a chemical reaction involving union between molecules often with elimination of a simple molecule (as water) **b** : the conversion of a substance (as water) from the vapor state to a denser liquid or solid state **2** : representation of several apparently discrete ideas by a single symbol esp. in dreams **3** : an abnormal hardening of an organ or tissue ⟨connective tissue ~*s*⟩

con·dense \kən-ˈdens\ *vb* **con·densed; con·dens·ing** : to make denser or more compact; *esp* : to subject to or undergo condensation — **condensed** *adj*

[1]**con·di·tion** \kən-ˈdi-shən\ *n* **1** : something essential to the appearance or occurrence of something else; *esp* : an environmental requirement **2 a** : a usu. defective state of health ⟨a serious heart ~⟩ **b** : a state of physical fitness

[2]**condition** *vb* **con·di·tioned; con·di·tion·ing** : to cause to undergo a change so that an act or response previously associated with one stimulus becomes associated with another — **con·di·tion·able** \kən-ˈdi-sh(ə-)nə-bəl\ *adj*

con·di·tion·al \kən-ˈdish-nəl, -ˈdi-shən-ᵊl\ *adj* **1** : CONDITIONED ⟨~ reflex⟩ **2** : eliciting a conditional response ⟨a ~ stimulus⟩ — **con·di·tion·al·ly** \-ˈdish-nə-lē, -ˈdi-shən-ᵊl-ē\ *adv*

con·di·tioned *adj* : determined or established by conditioning

con·di·tion·ing *n* **1** : the process of training to become physically fit by a regimen of exercise, diet, and rest; *also* : the resulting state of physical fitness **2** : a simple form of learning involving the formation, strengthening, or weakening of an association between a stimulus and a response — see CLASSICAL CONDITIONING, OPERANT CONDITIONING

con·dom \ˈkän-dəm\ *n* **1** : a sheath commonly of rubber worn over the penis (as to prevent conception or venereal infection during sexual intercourse) — called also *sheath* **2** : a device inserted into the vagina that is similar in form and function to a condom

con•duct \kən-ˈdəkt, ˈkän-ˌdəkt\ *vb* **1** : to act as a medium for conveying **2** : to have the quality of transmitting something — **con•duc•tance** \kən-ˈdək-təns\ *n*

con•duc•tion \kən-ˈdək-shən\ *n* **1** : transmission through or by means of something (as a conductor) **2** : the transmission of excitation through living tissue and esp. nervous tissue

conduction deafness *n* : hearing loss or impairment resulting from interference with the transmission of sound waves to the organ of Corti — called also *conductive deafness, transmission deafness;* compare CENTRAL DEAFNESS, NERVE DEAFNESS

con•duc•tive \-ˈdək-tiv\ *adj* **1** : having the power to conduct **2** : caused by failure in the mechanisms for sound transmission in the external or middle ear ⟨~ hearing loss⟩ — **con•duc•tiv•i•ty** \ˌkän-ˌdək-ˈti-və-tē, kən-\ *n*

con•duc•tor \kən-ˈdək-tər\ *n* **1** : a material or object capable of transmitting electricity, heat or sound **2** : a bodily part (as a nerve fiber) that transmits excitation

condyl- *or* **condylo-** *comb form* : joint : condyle ⟨*condyl*ectomy⟩

con•dy•lar•thro•sis \ˌkän-də-lär-ˈthrō-səs\ *n, pl* **-thro•ses** \-ˌsēz\ : articulation by means of a condyle

con•dyle \ˈkän-ˌdīl, ˈkänd-ᵊl\ *n* : an articular prominence of a bone — used chiefly of such as occur in pairs resembling a pair of knuckles (as those of the occipital bone for articulation with the atlas, those at the distal end of the humerus and femur, and those of the lower jaw); see LATERAL CONDYLE, MEDIAL CONDYLE — **con•dy•lar** \ˈkän-də-lər\ *adj* — **con•dy•loid** \ˈkän-də-ˌlȯid\ *adj*

con•dyl•ec•to•my \ˌkän-ˌdī-ˈlek-tə-mē, ˌkänd-ᵊl-ˈek-\ *n, pl* **-mies** : surgical removal of a condyle

con•dy•loid joint \ˈkän-də-ˌlȯid-\ *n* : an articulation in which an ovoid head is received into an elliptical cavity permitting all movements except axial rotation

condyloid process *n* : the rounded process by which the ramus of the mandible articulates with the temporal bone — called also *condylar process*

con•dy•lo•ma \ˌkän-də-ˈlō-mə\ *n, pl* **-ma•ta** \-mə-tə\ *also* **-mas** : GENITAL WART — **con•dy•lo•ma•tous** \-mə-təs\ *adj*

condyloma acu•mi•na•tum \-ə-ˌkyü-mə-ˈnā-təm\ *n, pl* **condylomata acu•mi•na•ta** \-ˈnā-tə\ : GENITAL WART

condyloma la•tum \-ˈlā-təm\ *n, pl* **condylomata la•ta** \-tə\ : a highly infectious flattened often hypertrophic papule of secondary syphilis that forms in moist areas of skin and at mucocutaneous junctions

cone \ˈkōn\ *n* **1** : any of the conical photosensitive receptor cells of the retina that function in color vision — compare ROD 1 **2** : any of a family (Conidae) of tropical marine gastropod mollusks that include a few highly poisonous forms **3** : a cusp of a tooth esp. in the upper jaw

cone•nose \ˈkōn-ˌnōz\ *n* : any of various large bloodsucking bugs esp. of the genus *Triatoma* including some capable of inflicting painful bites — called also *kissing bug*

con•fab•u•la•tion \kən-ˌfa-byə-ˈlā-shən, ˌkän-\ *n* : a filling in of gaps in memory through the creation of false memories by an individual who is affected with a memory disorder and is unaware that the fabricated memories are inaccurate and false — **con•fab•u•late** \kən-ˈfa-byə-ˌlāt\ *vb*

con•fec•tion \kən-ˈfek-shən\ *n* : a medicinal preparation usu. made with sugar, syrup, or honey — called also *electuary*

con•fine \kən-ˈfīn\ *vb* **con•fined; con•fin•ing** : to keep from leaving accustomed quarters (as one's room or bed) under pressure of infirmity, childbirth, or detention

con•fined \kən-ˈfīnd\ *adj* : undergoing childbirth

con•fine•ment \kən-ˈfīn-mənt\ *n* : an act of confining : the state of being confined; *esp* : LYING-IN

con•flict \ˈkän-ˌflikt\ *n* : mental struggle resulting from incompatible or opposing needs, drives, wishes, or external or internal demands — **con•flict•ful** \ˈkän-ˌflikt-fəl\ *adj* — **con•flic•tu•al** \kän-ˈflik-chə-wəl, kən-\ *adj*

con•flict•ed \kən-ˈflik-təd\ *adj* : having or expressing emotional conflict ⟨~ about one's sexual identity⟩

con•flu•ence of sinuses \ˈkän-ˌflü-ənts-, kən-ˈflü-\ *n* : the junction of several of the sinuses of the dura mater in the internal occipital region — called also *confluence of the sinuses*

con•flu•ent \ˈkän-ˌflü-ənt, kən-ˈ\ *adj* **1** : flowing or coming together; *also* : run together ⟨~ pustules⟩ **2** : characterized by confluent lesions ⟨~ smallpox⟩ — compare DISCRETE

con•for•ma•tion \ˌkän-(ˌ)fȯr-ˈmā-shən, -fər-\ *n* : any of the spatial arrangements of a molecule that can be obtained by rotation of the atoms about a single bond — **con•for•ma•tion•al** \-shnəl, -shən-ᵊl\ *adj* — **con•for•ma•tion•al•ly** *adv*

con•form•er \kən-ˈfȯr-mər\ *n* : a mold (as of plastic) used to prevent collapse or closing of a cavity, vessel, or opening during surgical repair

con•fu•sion \kən-ˈfyü-zhən\ *n* : disturbance of consciousness characterized by inability to engage in orderly thought or by lack of power to distinguish, choose, or act decisively —

con•fused \-ˈfyüzd\ *adj* — **con•fu•sion•al** \-zhnəl, -zhən-ᵊl\ *adj*

con•geal \kən-ˈjēl\ *vb* **1** : to change from a fluid to a solid state by or as if by cold **2** : to make viscid or curdled : COAGULATE

con•ge•ner \ˈkän-jə-nər, kən-ˈjē-\ *also* **co•ge•ner** \ˈkō-ˌjē-nər\ *n* **1** : a member of the same taxonomic genus as another plant or animal **2** : a chemical substance related to another — **con•ge•ner•ic** \ˌkän-jə-ˈner-ik\ *adj*

congenita — see AMYOTONIA CONGENITA, ARTHROGRYPOSIS MULTIPLEX CONGENITA, MYOTONIA CONGENITA, OSTEOGENESIS IMPERFECTA CONGENITA

con•gen•i•tal \kän-ˈje-nət-ᵊl\ *adj* **1** : existing at or dating from birth ⟨~ deafness⟩ **2** : acquired during development in the uterus and not through heredity ⟨~ syphilis⟩ — compare ACQUIRED 1, FAMILIAL, HEREDITARY — **con•gen•i•tal•ly** *adv*

congenital adrenal hyperplasia *n* : any of several hereditary disorders that are marked by inadequate synthesis of cortisol and often aldosterone, are typically marked by excessive androgen production, virilization of female external genitalia, and hypertension, and are inherited as an autosomal recessive trait — abbr. *CAH*

congenital con•trac•tur•al arachnodactyly \-kən-ˈtrak-chə-rəl-, -kän-\ *n* : a disorder that is similar to or a variant of Marfan syndrome, is inherited as a dominant autosomal trait, and is characterized esp. by arachnodactyly, joint contracture, and scoliosis — called also *Beals syndrome*

congenital megacolon *n* : HIRSCHSPRUNG'S DISEASE

con•gest•ed \kən-ˈjes-təd\ *adj* : containing an excessive accumulation of blood or mucus ⟨~ lungs⟩

con•ges•tion \kən-ˈjes-chən, -ˈjesh-\ *n* : an excessive accumulation esp. of blood or mucus ⟨nasal ~⟩ ⟨vascular ~⟩ — **con•ges•tive** \-ˈjes-tiv\ *adj*

congestive heart failure *n* : heart failure in which the heart is unable to maintain adequate circulation of blood in the tissues of the body or to pump out the venous blood returned to it by the venous circulation

con•glu•ti•nate \kən-ˈglüt-ᵊn-ˌāt, kän-\ *vb* **-nat•ed; -nat•ing** : to unite or become united by or as if by a glutinous substance ⟨blood platelets ~ in blood clotting⟩ — **con•glu•ti•na•tion** \-ˌglüt-ᵊn-ˈā-shən\ *n*

Congo red \ˈkäŋ-(ˌ)gō-\ *n* : an azo dye $C_{32}H_{22}N_6Na_2O_6S_2$ used in a number of diagnostic tests and esp. for the detection of amyloidosis

coni *pl of* CONUS

con•iza•tion \ˌkō-nə-ˈzā-shən, ˌkä-\ *n* : the electrosurgical excision of a cone of tissue from a diseased uterine cervix

con•joined \kən-ˈjȯind\ *adj* : of, relating to, or being conjoined twins

conjoined twins *n pl* : twins that are physically united at some part or parts of their bodies at birth

con•ju•ga•ta \ˌkän-jə-ˈgā-tə\ *n, pl* **-ga•tae** \-ˈgā-ˌtē\ : CONJUGATE DIAMETER

[1]**con•ju•gate** \ˈkän-ji-gət, -jə-ˌgāt\ *adj* **1** : functioning or operating simultaneously as if joined **2** *of an acid or base* : related by the difference of a proton — **con•ju•gate•ly** *adv*

[2]**con•ju•gate** \-jə-ˌgāt\ *vb* **-gat•ed; -gat•ing 1** : to unite (as with the elimination of water) so that the product is easily broken down (as by hydrolysis) into the original compounds **2** : to pair and fuse in conjugation **3** : to pair in synapsis

[3]**con•ju•gate** \-ji-gət, -jə-ˌgāt\ *n* : a chemical compound formed by the union of two compounds or united with another compound — **con•ju•gat•ed** \ˈkän-jə-ˌgā-təd\ *adj*

conjugated estrogen *n* : a mixture of estrogens and esp. of estrone and equilin for oral administration in the form of the sodium salts of their sulfate esters — usu. used in pl. with a sing. or pl. verb; see PREMARIN, PREMPRO

conjugate diameter *n* : the anteroposterior diameter of the human pelvis measured from the sacral promontory to the pubic symphysis — called also *conjugata, true conjugate*

conjugated protein *n* : a compound of a protein with a nonprotein ⟨hemoglobin is a *conjugated protein* of heme and globin⟩

conjugate vaccine *n* : a vaccine containing bacterial capsular polysaccharide joined to a protein to enhance immunogenicity; *esp* : one that is used to immunize infants and children against invasive disease caused by Hib bacteria

con•ju•ga•tion \ˌkän-jə-ˈgā-shən\ *n* **1** : the act of conjugating : the state of being conjugated **2 a** : temporary cytoplasmic union with exchange of nuclear material that is the usual sexual process in ciliated protozoans **b** : the one-way transfer of DNA between bacteria in cellular contact — **con•ju•ga•tion•al** \-shnəl, -shən-ᵊl\ *adj*

con•junc•ti•va \ˌkän-ˌjəŋk-ˈtī-və, kən-\ *n, pl* **-vas** *or* **-vae** \-(ˌ)vē\ : the mucous membrane that lines the inner surface of the eyelids and is continued over the forepart of the eyeball — **con•junc•ti•val** \-vəl\ *adj*

con•junc•ti•vi•tis \kən-ˌjəŋk-ti-ˈvī-təs\ *n* : inflammation of the conjunctiva that is typically marked by pinkness or redness of the sclera and by itching, burning, irritation, discharge, or excessive tearing of the eye and that is typically caused by pathogenic microorganisms (as bacteria or viruses), allergens, or irritants — see PINK EYE

con•junc•tivo•plas•ty \kən-ˈjəŋk-ti-(ˌ)vō-ˌplas-tē\ *n, pl* **-plas•ties** : plastic repair of a defect in the conjunctiva

con•junc•tivo•rhi•nos•to•my \kən-ˌjəŋk-ti-(ˌ)vō-ˌrī-ˈnäs-tə-mē\ *n, pl* **-to•mies** : surgical creation of a passage through the conjunctiva to the nasal cavity

conjunctivum — see BRACHIUM CONJUNCTIVUM

connecting tubule *n* : COLLECTING TUBULE 2

connective tissue *n* : a tissue of mesodermal origin that consists of various cells (as fibroblasts and macrophages) and interlacing protein fibers (as of collagen) embedded in a chiefly carbohydrate ground substance, that supports, ensheathes, and binds together other tissues, and that includes loose and dense forms (as adipose tissue, tendons, ligaments, and aponeuroses) and specialized forms (as cartilage and bone)

connective tissue disease *n* : any of various diseases or abnormal states (as scleroderma, systemic lupus erythematosus, polyarteritis nodosa, and dermatomyositis) characterized by inflammatory or degenerative changes in connective tissue — called also *collagen disease, collagenosis, collagen vascular disease*

con•nec•tor \kə-ˈnek-tər\ *n* : a part of a partial denture which joins its components

conniventes — see VALVULAE CONNIVENTES

Conn's syndrome \ˈkänz-\ *n* : PRIMARY ALDOSTERONISM

Conn, Jerome W. (1907–1994), American physician.

con•san•guine \kän-ˈsaŋ-gwən, kən-\ *adj* : CONSANGUINEOUS

con•san•guin•e•ous \ˌkän-ˌsan-ˈgwi-nē-əs, -ˌsaŋ-\ *adj* : of the same blood or origin; *specif* : relating to or involving persons (as first cousins) that are relatively closely related ⟨~ marriages⟩ — **con•san•guin•i•ty** \-nə-tē\ *n*

con•science \ˈkän-chəns\ *n* : the part of the superego in psychoanalysis that transmits commands and admonitions to the ego

[1]**con•scious** \ˈkän-chəs\ *adj* **1** : capable of or marked by thought, will, design, or perception : relating to, being, or being part of consciousness ⟨the ~ mind⟩ **2** : having mental faculties undulled by sleep, faintness, or stupor — **con•scious•ly** *adv*

[2]**conscious** *n* : CONSCIOUSNESS 3

con•scious•ness \-nəs\ *n* **1** : the totality in psychology of sensations, perceptions, ideas, attitudes, and feelings of which an individual or a group is aware at any given time or within a given time span **2** : waking life (as that to which one returns after sleep, trance, or fever) in which one's normal mental powers are present **3** : the upper part of mental life of which the person is aware as contrasted with unconscious processes

conscious sedation *n* : an induced state of sedation characterized by a minimally depressed consciousness such that the patient is able to continuously and independently maintain a patent airway, retain protective reflexes, and remain responsive to verbal commands and physical stimulation — compare DEEP SEDATION

con•sen•su•al \kən-ˈsen-chə-wəl\ *adj* **1** : existing or made by mutual consent ⟨~ sexual behavior⟩ **2** : relating to or being the constrictive pupillary response of an eye that is covered when the other eye is exposed to light — **con•sen•su•al•ly** *adv*

con•ser•va•tive \kən-ˈsər-və-tiv\ *adj* : designed to preserve parts or restore or preserve function ⟨~ surgery⟩ — compare AGGRESSIVE 2, RADICAL — **con•ser•va•tive•ly** *adv*

con•serve \kən-ˈsərv\ *vb* **con•served; con•serv•ing** : to maintain (a quantity) constant during a process of chemical, physical, or evolutionary change

con•sol•i•da•tion \kən-ˌsä-lə-ˈdā-shən\ *n* : the process by which an infected lung passes from an aerated collapsible condition to one of airless solid consistency through the accumulation of exudate in the alveoli and adjoining ducts; *also* : tissue that has undergone consolidation

con•spe•cif•ic \ˌkän-spi-ˈsi-fik\ *adj* : of the same species — **conspecific** *n*

constant region *n* : the part of the polypeptide chain of a light or heavy chain of an antibody that ends in a free carboxyl group –COOH and that is relatively constant in its sequence of amino-acid residues from one antibody to another — called also *constant domain;* compare VARIABLE REGION

con•stel•la•tion \ˌkän-stə-ˈlā-shən\ *n* : a set of ideas, conditions, symptoms, or traits that fall into or appear to fall into a pattern

con•sti•pa•tion \ˌkän-stə-ˈpā-shən\ *n* : abnormally delayed or infrequent passage of usu. dry hardened feces — **con•sti•pate** \ˈkän-stə-ˌpāt\ *vb* — **con•sti•pat•ed** \-ˌpā-təd\ *adj*

con•sti•tu•tion \ˌkän-stə-ˈtü-shən, -ˈtyü-\ *n* : the physical makeup of the individual comprising inherited qualities modified by environment — **con•sti•tu•tion•al** \-shnəl, -shən-ᵊl\ *adj*

con•sti•tu•tion•al \-shnəl, -shən-ᵊl\ *n* : a walk taken for one's health

con•strict \kən-ˈstrikt\ *vb* **1** : to make narrow or draw together **2** : to subject (as a body part) to compression ⟨~ a nerve⟩ — **con•stric•tion** \-ˈstrik-shən\ *n* — **con•stric•tive** \-ˈstrik-tiv\ *adj*

con•stric•tor \-ˈstrik-tər\ *n* : a muscle that contracts a cavity or orifice or compresses an organ — see INFERIOR CONSTRICTOR, MIDDLE CONSTRICTOR, SUPERIOR CONSTRICTOR

constrictor pha·ryn·gis inferior \-fə-ˈrin-jəs-\ *n* : INFERIOR CONSTRICTOR

constrictor pharyngis me·di·us \-ˈmē-dē-əs\ *n* : MIDDLE CONSTRICTOR

constrictor pharyngis superior *n* : SUPERIOR CONSTRICTOR

con·struct \ˈkän-ˌstrəkt\ *n* : something constructed esp. by mental synthesis ⟨form a ~ of a physical object⟩

con·sult \kən-ˈsəlt\ *vb* : to ask the advice or opinion of ⟨~ a doctor⟩

con·sul·tant \kən-ˈsəlt-ᵊnt\ *n* : one (as a physician, surgeon, or psychologist) called in for professional advice or services

con·sul·ta·tion \ˌkän-səl-ˈtā-shən\ *n* : a deliberation between physicians on a case or its treatment — **con·sul·ta·tive** \kən-ˈsəl-tə-tiv, ˈkän-səl-ˌtā-tiv\ *adj*

con·sult·ing \kən-ˈsəl-tiŋ\ *adj* **1** : serving as a consultant ⟨a ~ physician⟩ **2** : of or relating to consultation or a consultant ⟨a ~ room⟩

con·sum·ma·to·ry \kən-ˈsə-mə-ˌtōr-ē\ *adj* : of, relating to, or being a response or act (as eating or copulating) that terminates a period of usu. goal-directed behavior

con·sump·tion \kən-ˈsəmp-shən\ *n* **1** : a progressive wasting away of the body esp. from pulmonary tuberculosis **2** : TUBERCULOSIS

[1]**con·sump·tive** \-ˈsəmp-tiv\ *adj* : of, relating to, or affected with consumption ⟨a ~ cough⟩

[2]**consumptive** *n* : a person affected with consumption

[1]**con·tact** \ˈkän-ˌtakt\ *n* **1** : union or junction of body surfaces ⟨sexual ~⟩ **2** : direct experience through the senses **3** : CONTACT LENS

[2]**contact** *adj* : caused or transmitted by direct or indirect contact (as with an allergen or a contagious disease)

contact dermatitis *n* : inflammation of the skin caused by direct contact with an irritant or allergen — see ALLERGIC CONTACT DERMATITIS, IRRITANT CONTACT DERMATITIS

contact lens *n* : a thin lens designed to fit over the cornea and usu. worn to correct defects in vision

con·ta·gion \kən-ˈtā-jən\ *n* **1** : the transmission of a disease by direct or indirect contact **2** : CONTAGIOUS DISEASE **3** : a disease-producing agent (as a virus)

contagiosa — see IMPETIGO CONTAGIOSA, MOLLUSCUM CONTAGIOSUM

contagiosum — see MOLLUSCUM CONTAGIOSUM

con·ta·gious \-jəs\ *adj* **1** : communicable by contact — compare INFECTIOUS 2 **2** : bearing contagion **3** : used for contagious diseases ⟨a ~ ward⟩ — **con·ta·gious·ly** *adv* — **con·tagious·ness** *n*

contagious disease *n* : an infectious disease communicable by contact with one who has it, with a bodily discharge of such a patient, or with an object touched by such a patient or by bodily discharges — compare COMMUNICABLE DISEASE

con·ta·gium \kən-ˈtā-jəm, -jē-əm\ *n, pl* **-gia** \-jə, -jē-ə\ : a virus or living organism capable of causing a communicable disease

con·tam·i·nant \kən-ˈta-mə-nənt\ *n* : something that contaminates

con·tam·i·nate \kən-ˈta-mə-ˌnāt\ *vb* **-nat·ed; -nat·ing** **1** : to soil, stain, or infect by contact or association ⟨bacteria *contaminated* the wound⟩ **2** : to make unfit for use by the introduction of unwholesome or undesirable elements ⟨water *contaminated* by sewage⟩ — **con·tam·i·na·tion** \kən-ˌta-mə-ˈnā-shən\ *n*

con·tent \ˈkän-ˌtent\ *n* : the subject matter or symbolic significance of something — see LATENT CONTENT, MANIFEST CONTENT

con·ti·nence \ˈkänt-ᵊn-əns\ *n* **1** : self-restraint in refraining from sexual intercourse **2** : the ability to retain a bodily discharge voluntarily ⟨fecal ~⟩ — **con·ti·nent** \-ənt\ *adj* — **con·ti·nent·ly** *adv*

continuous positive airway pressure *n* : a technique for relieving breathing problems (as those associated with sleep apnea or congestive heart failure) by pumping a steady flow of air through the nose to prevent the narrowing or collapse of air passages or to help the lungs to expand — abbr. *CPAP*

con·tra·cep·tion \ˌkän-trə-ˈsep-shən\ *n* : deliberate prevention of conception or impregnation — **con·tra·cep·tive** \-ˈsep-tiv\ *adj or n*

contraceptive pill *n* : BIRTH CONTROL PILL

con·tract \kən-ˈtrakt, ˈkän-ˌtrakt\ *vb* **1** : to become affected with ⟨~ pneumonia⟩ **2** : to draw together so as to become diminished in size **3** *of a muscle or muscle fiber* : to undergo contraction; *esp* : to shorten and thicken

con·trac·tile \kən-ˈtrakt-ᵊl, -ˈtrak-ˌtīl\ *adj* : having or concerned with the power or property of contracting

con·trac·til·i·ty \ˌkän-ˌtrak-ˈti-lə-tē\ *n, pl* **-ties** : the capability or quality of shrinking or contracting; *esp* : the power of muscle fibers of shortening into a more compact form

con·trac·tion \kən-ˈtrak-shən\ *n* **1** : the action or process of contracting : the state of being contracted **2** : the action of a functioning muscle or muscle fiber in which force is generated accompanied esp. by shortening and thickening of the muscle or muscle fiber or sometimes by its lengthening; *esp* : the shortening and thickening of a functioning muscle or muscle fiber **3** : one of usu. a series of rhythmic tightening actions of the uterine muscles (as during labor)

con·trac·tor \ˈkän-ˌtrak-tər, kən-ˈ\ *n* : something (as a muscle) that contracts or shortens

con·trac·ture \kən-ˈtrak-chər\ *n* : a permanent shortening (as of muscle, tendon, or scar tissue) producing deformity or distortion — see DUPUYTREN'S CONTRACTURE

con·tra·in·di·ca·tion \ˌkän-trə-ˌin-də-ˈkā-shən\ *n* : something (as a symptom or condition) that makes a particular treatment or procedure inadvisable — **con·tra·in·di·cate** \-ˈin-də-ˌkāt\ *vb*

con·tra·lat·er·al \-ˈla-tə-rəl, -ˈla-trəl\ *adj* : occurring on, affecting, or acting in conjunction with a part on the opposite side of the body — compare IPSILATERAL

contrast bath *n* : a therapeutic immersion of a part of the body (as an extremity) alternately in hot and cold water

contrast medium *n* : a substance comparatively opaque to X-rays that is introduced into the body to contrast an internal part with its surrounding tissue in radiographic visualization — called also *contrast agent, contrast material*

con·tre·coup \ˈkōn-trə-ˌkü, ˈkän-\ *n* : injury (as when the brain strikes the skull) occurring on the side of an organ opposite to the side on which a blow or impact is received — compare COUP

¹con·trol \kən-ˈtrōl\ *vb* **con·trolled; con·trol·ling** **1** : to incorporate suitable controls in ⟨a *controlled* experiment⟩ **2** : to reduce the incidence or severity of esp. to innocuous levels ⟨~ outbreaks of cholera⟩

²control *n* **1** : an act or instance of controlling something ⟨~ of acute intermittent porphyria⟩ **2** : one that is used in controlling something: as **a** : an experiment in which the subjects are treated as in a parallel experiment except for omission of the procedure or agent under test and which is used as a standard of comparison in judging experimental effects — called also *control experiment* **b** : one (as an organism) that is part of a control

con·trolled \kən-ˈtrōld\ *adj* : regulated by law with regard to possession and use ⟨~ drugs⟩

controlled hypotension *n* : low blood pressure induced and maintained to reduce blood loss or to provide a bloodless field during surgery

controlled–release *adj* : designed to slowly release a drug in the body in a prolonged controlled fashion; *also* : SUSTAINED-RELEASE

con·tu·sion \kən-ˈtü-zhən, -ˈtyü-\ *n* : injury to tissue usu. without laceration : BRUISE 1 — **con·tuse** \-ˈtüz, -ˈtyüz\ *vb*

co·nus \ˈkō-nəs\ *n, pl* **co·ni** \-ˌnī, -(ˌ)nē\ : CONUS ARTERIOSUS

conus ar·te·ri·o·sus \-är-ˌtir-ē-ˈō-səs\ *n, pl* **co·ni ar·te·ri·o·si** \-ˌnī-är-ˌtir-ē-ˈō-ˌsī, -(ˌ)nē-\ : a conical prolongation of the right ventricle from which the pulmonary arteries emerge

conus med·ul·lar·is \-ˌmed-ᵊl-ˈer-əs, -ˌme-jə-ˈler-\ *n* : a tapering lower part of the spinal cord at the level of the first lumbar segment

con·va·les·cence \ˌkän-və-ˈles-ᵊns\ *n* **1** : gradual recovery of health and strength after disease **2** : the time between the subsidence of a disease and complete restoration to health — **con·va·lesce** \ˌkän-və-ˈles\ *vb*

¹con·va·les·cent \ˌkän-və-ˈles-ᵊnt\ *adj* **1** : recovering from sickness or debility : partially restored to health or strength **2** : of, for, or relating to convalescence or convalescents ⟨a ~ ward⟩

²convalescent *n* : one recovering from sickness

convalescent home *n* : an institution for the care of convalescing patients

con·ver·gence \kən-ˈvər-jəns\ *n* **1** : movement of the two eyes so coordinated that the images of a single point fall on corresponding points of the two retinas **2** : overlapping synaptic innervation of a single cell by more than one nerve fiber — compare DIVERGENCE 2 — **con·verge** \-ˈvərj\ *vb* — **con·ver·gent** \-ˈvər-jənt\ *adj*

convergent thinking *n* : thinking that weighs alternatives within an existing construct or model in solving a problem or answering a question to find one best solution and that is measured by IQ tests — compare DIVERGENT THINKING

con·ver·sion \kən-ˈvər-zhən, -shən\ *n* : the transformation of an unconscious mental conflict into a symbolically equivalent bodily symptom

conversion disorder *n* : a psychiatric disorder in which bodily symptoms (as paralysis of the limbs) appear without physical basis and that is typically associated with psychological stress or conflict — called also *conversion hysteria, conversion reaction*

con·vo·lut·ed \ˈkän-və-ˌlü-təd\ *adj* : folded in curved or tortuous windings; *specif* : having convolutions

convoluted tubule *n* **1** : PROXIMAL CONVOLUTED TUBULE **2** : DISTAL CONVOLUTED TUBULE

con·vo·lu·tion \ˌkän-və-ˈlü-shən\ *n* : any of the irregular ridges on the surface of the brain and esp. of the cerebrum — called also *gyrus;* compare SULCUS

convolution of Broca *n* : BROCA'S AREA

¹con·vul·sant \kən-ˈvəl-sənt\ *adj* : causing convulsions : CONVULSIVE

²convulsant *n* : an agent and esp. a drug that produces convulsions

con·vulse \kən-ˈvəls\ *vb* **con·vulsed; con·vuls·ing** **1** : to shake or agitate violently; *esp* : to shake or cause to shake with or as if with irregular spasms **2** : to become affected with convulsions

con•vul•sion \kən-ˈvəl-shən\ *n* **1** : an abnormal violent and involuntary contraction or series of contractions of the muscles — often used in pl. **2** : SEIZURE 1 — **con•vul•sive** \-siv\ *adj* — **con•vul•sive•ly** *adv*

convulsive therapy *n* : SHOCK THERAPY

Coo•ley's anemia \ˈkü-lēz-\ *n* : a disorder of hemoglobin synthesis that is the most severe form of beta-thalassemia, is inherited as an autosomal recessive trait, is marked by severe anemia, the presence of microcytes, enlargement of the liver and spleen, bone deformities, and poor growth rate, and occurs esp. in individuals of Mediterranean ancestry — called also *beta-thalassemia major, Cooley's disease, thalassemia major*

Coo•ley \ˈkü-lē\, **Thomas Benton (1871–1945)**, American pediatrician.

Coo•mas•sie blue \kü-ˈma-sē-, -ˈmä-\ *n* : a bright blue acid dye used as a biological stain esp. for proteins in gel electrophoresis

Coombs test \ˈkümz-\ *n* : an agglutination test used to detect proteins and esp. antibodies on the surface of red blood cells

Coombs, Robert Royston Amos (1921–2005), British immunologist.

Coo•pe•ria \kü-ˈpir-ē-ə\ *n* : a genus of small reddish-brown nematode worms (family Trichostrongylidae) including several infesting the small intestine of sheep, goats, and cattle

Curtice, Cooper (1856–1939), American veterinarian.

coordinate bond *n* : a covalent bond that consists of a pair of electrons supplied by only one of the two atoms it joins

co•or•di•na•tion \(ˌ)kō-ˌȯrd-ᵊn-ˈā-shən\ *n* **1** : the act or action of bringing into a common action, movement, or condition **2** : the harmonious functioning of parts (as muscle and nerves) for most effective results — **co•or•di•nate** \kō-ˈȯrd-ᵊn-ˌāt\ *vb* — **co•or•di•nat•ed** \-ˌā-təd\ *adj*

coo•tie \ˈkü-tē\ *n* : BODY LOUSE

Co•pax•one \kō-ˈpak-ˌsōn\ *trademark* — used for a preparation of glatiramer

co–pay \ˈkō-ˈpā\ *n* : CO-PAYMENT

co–pay•ment \(ˌ)kō-ˈpā-mənt\ *n* : a relatively small fixed fee that a health insurer (as an HMO) requires the patient to pay upon incurring a medical expense (as for a routine office visit, surgical procedure, or prescription drug) covered by the health insurer

COPD \ˌsē-ˌō-ˌpē-ˈdē\ *n* : CHRONIC OBSTRUCTIVE PULMONARY DISEASE

cope \ˈkōp\ *vb* **coped; cop•ing** : to deal with and attempt to overcome problems and difficulties — usu. used with *with* ⟨helping children ~ with grief⟩

COPE *abbr* chronic obstructive pulmonary emphysema

co•per•nic•i•um \ˌkō-pər-ˈni-sē-əm\ *n* : a short-lived radioactive element that is artificially produced — symbol *Cn;* see ELEMENT table

cop•per \ˈkä-pər\ *n, often attrib* : a common reddish metallic element that is ductile and malleable — symbol *Cu;* see ELEMENT table

cop•per•head \ˈkä-pər-ˌhed\ *n* : a pit viper (*Agkistrodon contortrix*) of the eastern and central U.S. that usu. has a copper-colored head and often a reddish-brown hourglass pattern on the body and is capable of inflicting a very painful but rarely fatal bite

copper sulfate *n* : a sulfate of copper; *esp* : a blue hydrous crystalline compound $CuSO_4 \cdot 5H_2O$ used as an algicide and fungicide and formerly in solution as an emetic

copr- *or* **copro-** *comb form* **1** : dung : feces ⟨*copro*phagy⟩ **2** : obscenity ⟨*copro*lalia⟩

cop•ro•an•ti•body \ˌkä-prō-ˈan-ti-ˌbä-dē\ *n, pl* **-bod•ies** : an antibody whose presence in the intestinal tract can be demonstrated by examination of an extract of the feces

cop•ro•la•lia \ˌkä-prə-ˈlā-lē-ə\ *n* **1** : obsessive or uncontrollable use of obscene language **2** : the use of obscene language as sexual gratification — **cop•ro•la•lic** \-ˈla-lik\ *adj*

cop•ro•pha•gia \ˌkä-prə-ˈfā-jə, -jē-ə\ *n* : COPROPHAGY

co•proph•a•gy \kə-ˈprä-fə-jē\ *n, pl* **-gies** : the eating of feces that is normal behavior among many animals — **co•proph•a•gous** \-gəs\ *adj*

cop•ro•phil•ia \ˌkä-prə-ˈfi-lē-ə\ *n* : marked interest in excrement; *esp* : the use of feces or filth for sexual excitement — **cop•ro•phil•i•ac** \-ˌak\ *n*

cop•ro•por•phy•rin \ˌkä-prə-ˈpȯr-fə-rən\ *n* : any of four isomeric porphyrins $C_{36}H_{38}N_4O_8$ of which types I and III are found in feces and urine esp. in certain pathological conditions

cop•u•late \ˈkä-pyə-ˌlāt\ *vb* **-lat•ed; -lat•ing** : to engage in sexual intercourse — **cop•u•la•tion** \ˌkä-pyə-ˈlā-shən\ *n* — **cop•u•la•to•ry** \ˈkä-pyə-lə-ˌtōr-ē\ *adj*

CoQ10 *abbr* coenzyme Q10

coraco- *comb form* : coracoid and ⟨*coraco*humeral⟩

cor•a•co•acro•mi•al \ˌkȯr-ə-(ˌ)kō-ə-ˈkrō-mē-əl\ *adj* : relating to or connecting the acromion and the coracoid process

cor•a•co•bra•chi•a•lis \ˌkȯr-ə-(ˌ)kō-ˌbrā-kē-ˈā-ləs\ *n, pl* **-a•les** \-ˌlēz\ : a muscle extending between the coracoid process and the middle of the medial surface of the humerus — called also *coracobrachialis muscle*

cor•a•co•cla•vic•u•lar ligament \-klə-ˌvi-kyə-lər-, -kla-\ *n* : a ligament that joins the clavicle and the coracoid process of the scapula

cor·a·co·hu·mer·al \-ˈhyü-mə-rəl\ *adj* : relating to or connecting the coracoid process and the humerus

[1]**cor·a·coid** \ˈkȯr-ə-ˌkȯid, ˈkär-\ *adj* : of, relating to, or being a process of the scapula in most mammals or a well-developed cartilage bone of many lower vertebrates that extends from the scapula to or toward the sternum

[2]**coracoid** *n* : a coracoid bone or process

coracoid process *n* : a process of the scapula in most mammals representing the remnant of the coracoid bone of lower vertebrates that has become fused with the scapula and in humans is situated on its superior border and serves for the attachment of various muscles

coral snake \ˈkȯr-əl-, ˈkär-\ *n* : any of several venomous chiefly tropical New World elapid snakes of the genus *Micrurus* that are brilliantly banded in red, black, and yellow or white and include two (*M. fulvius* and *M. euryxanthus*) ranging northward into the southern U.S.

cor bo·vi·num \ˈkȯr-bō-ˈvī-nəm\ *n* : a greatly enlarged heart

cord \ˈkȯrd\ *n* : a slender flexible anatomical structure (as a nerve) — see SPERMATIC CORD, SPINAL CORD, UMBILICAL CORD, VOCAL CORD 1

cord blood *n* : blood from the umbilical cord of a fetus or newborn

cor·dec·to·my \kȯr-ˈdek-tə-mē\ *n, pl* **-mies** : surgical removal of one or more vocal cords

cordia pulmonalia *pl of* COR PULMONALE

cordis — see VENAE CORDIS MINIMAE

cor·do·cen·te·sis \ˌkȯr-dō-sen-ˈtē-səs\ *n* : the withdrawal of a sample of fetal blood from the umbilical cord by transabdominal insertion of a needle guided by ultrasound

cor·dot·o·my *or* **chor·dot·o·my** \kȯr-ˈdä-tə-mē\ *n, pl* **-mies** : surgical division of a tract of the spinal cord for relief of severe intractable pain

core \ˈkōr\ *n* : the central part of a body, mass, or part

core biopsy *n* : a biopsy in which a cylindrical sample of tissue is obtained (as from a kidney or breast) by a hollow needle

Co·reg \ˈkȯr-ˌeg\ *trademark* — used for a preparation of carvedilol

co·re·pres·sor \ˌkō-ri-ˈpres-ər\ *n* : a substance that activates a particular genetic repressor by combining with it

core temperature *n* : the temperature deep within a living body (as in the viscera)

Co·ri cycle \ˈkōr-ē-\ *n* : the cycle in carbohydrate metabolism consisting of the conversion of glycogen to lactic acid in muscle, diffusion of the lactic acid into the bloodstream which carries it to the liver where it is converted into glycogen, and the breakdown of liver glycogen to glucose which is transported to muscle by the bloodstream and reconverted into glycogen

Cori, Carl Ferdinand (1896–1984), and Gerty Theresa (1896–1957), American biochemists.

co·ri·um \ˈkōr-ē-əm\ *n, pl* **co·ria** \-ē-ə\ : DERMIS

corn \ˈkȯrn\ *n* : a local hardening and thickening of epidermis (as on a toe)

corne- *or* **corneo-** *comb form* : cornea : corneal and ⟨*corneo*scleral⟩

cor·nea \ˈkȯr-nē-ə\ *n* : the transparent part of the coat of the eyeball that covers the iris and pupil and admits light to the interior — **cor·ne·al** \-əl\ *adj*

cor·neo·scler·al \ˌkȯr-nē-ə-ˈskler-əl\ *adj* : of, relating to, or affecting both the cornea and the sclera

cor·ne·um \ˈkȯr-nē-əm\ *n, pl* **cor·nea** \-nē-ə\ : STRATUM CORNEUM

cor·nic·u·late cartilage \kȯr-ˈni-kyə-lət-\ *n* : either of two small nodules of yellow elastic cartilage articulating with the apex of the arytenoid

cor·ni·fi·ca·tion \ˌkȯr-nə-fə-ˈkā-shən\ *n* **1** : conversion into horn or a horny substance or tissue : KERATINIZATION **2** : the cytological changes that occur in the vaginal epithelium esp. of rodents in response to stimulation by estrogen — **cor·ni·fy** \ˈkȯr-nə-fī\ *vb*

corn oil *n* : a yellow fatty oil obtained from the germ of corn kernels

cor·nu \ˈkȯr-(ˌ)nü, -(ˌ)nyü\ *n, pl* **cor·nua** \-nü-ə, -nyü-\ : a horn-shaped anatomical structure (as either of the lateral divisions of a bicornuate uterus or one of the lateral processes of the hyoid bone) — **cor·nu·al** \-nü-əl, -nyü-\ *adj*

co·ro·na \kə-ˈrō-nə\ *n* : the upper portion of a bodily part

co·ro·nal \ˈkȯr-ən-ᵊl, ˈkär-; kə-ˈrōn-\ *adj* **1** : of, relating to, or being a corona **2** : lying in the direction of the coronal suture **3** : of or relating to the frontal plane that passes through the long axis of the body

coronal suture *n* : a suture extending across the skull between the parietal and frontal bones — called also *frontoparietal suture*

co·ro·na ra·di·a·ta \kə-ˈrō-nə-ˌrā-dē-ˈā-tə, -ˈä-\ *n, pl* **co·ro·nae ra·di·a·tae** \-(ˌ)nē-ˌrā-dē-ˈā-(ˌ)tē, -ˈä-\ **1** : the zone of small follicular cells immediately surrounding the ovum in the graafian follicle and accompanying the ovum on its discharge from the follicle **2** : a large mass of myelinated nerve fibers radiating from the internal capsule to the cerebral cortex

[1]**cor·o·nary** \ˈkȯr-ə-ˌner-ē, ˈkär-\ *adj* **1** : of, relating to, affecting, or being the coronary arteries or veins of the heart ⟨~ sclerosis⟩; *broadly* : of or relating to the heart **2** : of, relating to, or affected with coronary artery disease ⟨a ~ care unit⟩

[2]**coronary** *n, pl* **-nar·ies** **1 a** : CORONARY ARTERY **b** : CORONARY VEIN **2**

: CORONARY THROMBOSIS; *broadly* : HEART ATTACK

coronary artery *n* : either of two arteries that arise one from the left and one from the right side of the aorta immediately above the semilunar valves and supply the tissues of the heart itself

coronary artery bypass *n* : a surgical procedure performed to shunt blood around a narrowing or blockage in the coronary artery that usu. involves grafting one end of a segment of blood vessel (as the saphenous vein) removed from another part of the body into the aorta and the other end of the segment into the coronary artery beyond the obstructed area to allow for increased blood flow — called also *coronary artery bypass graft, coronary artery bypass grafting, coronary bypass, coronary bypass graft, coronary bypass grafting*

coronary artery bypass graft *or* **coronary artery bypass grafting** *n* : CORONARY ARTERY BYPASS — abbr. *CABG*

coronary artery disease *n* : CORONARY HEART DISEASE

coronary band *n* : a thickened band of extremely vascular tissue that lies at the upper border of the wall of the hoof of the horse and related animals and that plays an important part in the secretion of the horny walls — called also *coronary cushion*

coronary bypass *n* : CORONARY ARTERY BYPASS

coronary bypass graft *or* **coronary bypass grafting** *n* : CORONARY ARTERY BYPASS

coronary disease *n* : CORONARY HEART DISEASE

coronary failure *n* : heart failure in which the heart muscle is deprived of the blood necessary to meet its functional needs as a result of narrowing or blocking of one or more of the coronary arteries — compare CONGESTIVE HEART FAILURE

coronary heart disease *n* : a condition and esp. one caused by atherosclerosis that reduces the blood flow through the coronary arteries to the heart muscle and typically results in chest pain or heart damage — called also *coronary artery disease, coronary disease*

coronary insufficiency *n* : cardiac insufficiency of relatively mild degree — compare ANGINA PECTORIS, HEART ATTACK, HEART FAILURE 1

coronary ligament *n* **1** : the folds of peritoneum connecting the posterior surface of the liver and the diaphragm **2** : a part of the joint capsule of the knee connecting each meniscus with the margin of the head of the tibia

coronary occlusion *n* : the partial or complete blocking (as by a thrombus or by sclerosis) of a coronary artery

coronary plexus *n* : one of two nerve plexuses that are extensions of the cardiac plexus along the coronary arteries

coronary sinus *n* : a venous channel that is derived from the sinus venosus, is continuous with the largest of the cardiac veins, receives most of the blood from the walls of the heart, and empties into the right atrium

coronary thrombosis *n* : the blocking of a coronary artery of the heart by a thrombus

coronary vein *n* **1 a** : any of several veins that drain the tissues of the heart and empty into the coronary sinus **b** : CARDIAC VEIN — not used technically **2** : a vein draining the lesser curvature of the stomach and emptying into the portal vein

co•ro•na•vi•rus \kə-ˈrō-nə-ˌvī-rəs\ *n* : any of a family (*Coronaviridae*) of single-stranded RNA viruses that infect birds and many mammals including humans and that include the causative agents of blue comb, feline infectious peritonitis, MERS, and SARS — abbr. *CoV*

cor•o•ner \ˈkȯr-ə-nər, ˈkär-\ *n* : a usu. elected public officer who is typically not required to have specific medical qualifications and whose principal duty is to inquire by an inquest into the cause of any death which there is reason to suppose is not due to natural causes — see MEDICAL EXAMINER 1

cor•o•net \ˌkȯr-ə-ˈnet, ˌkär-\ *n* : the lower part of a horse's pastern where the horn terminates in skin

cor•o•noid•ec•to•my \ˌkȯr-ə-ˌnȯi-ˈdek-tə-mē\ *n, pl* **-mies** : surgical removal of the mandibular coronoid process

cor•o•noid fossa \ˈkȯr-ə-ˌnȯid-\ *n* : a depression of the humerus into which the coronoid process fits when the arm is flexed — compare OLECRANON FOSSA

coronoid process *n* **1** : the anterior process of the superior border of the ramus of the mandible **2** : a flared process of the lower anterior part of the upper articular surface of the ulna fitting into the coronoid fossa when the arm is flexed

corpora *pl of* CORPUS

cor•po•ral \ˈkȯr-pə-rəl, -prəl\ *adj* : of, relating to, or affecting the body ⟨~ injury⟩

cor•po•ra quad•ri•gem•i•na \ˌkȯr-pə-rə-ˌkwä-drə-ˈje-mə-nə, ˌkȯr-prə-\ *n pl* : two pairs of colliculi on the dorsal surface of the midbrain composed of white matter externally and gray matter within, the superior pair containing correlation centers for optic reflexes and the inferior pair containing correlation centers for auditory reflexes

cor•po•re•al \kȯr-ˈpōr-ē-əl\ *adj* : having, consisting of, or relating to a physical material body

corporis — see PEDICULOSIS CORPORIS, TINEA CORPORIS

corpse \ˈkȯrps\ *n* : a dead body esp. of a human being

corps•man \ˈkōr-mən, ˈkōrz-\ *n, pl* **corps•men** \-mən\ : a military enlisted person trained to give first aid and minor medical treatment

cor pul•mo•na•le \ˌkȯr-ˌpu̇l-mə-ˈnä-lē, -ˌpəl-, -ˈna-\ *n, pl* **cor•dia pul•mo•na•lia** \ˈkȯr-dē-ə-ˌpu̇l-mə-ˈnä-lē-ə, -ˌpəl-, -ˈna-\ : disease of the heart characterized by hypertrophy and dilatation of the right ventricle and secondary to disease of the lungs or their blood vessels

cor•pus \ˈkȯr-pəs\ *n, pl* **cor•po•ra** \-pə-rə, -prə\ **1** : the human or animal body esp. when dead **2** : the main part or body of a bodily structure or organ

corpus al•bi•cans \-ˈal-bə-ˌkanz\ *n, pl* **corpora al•bi•can•tia** \-ˌal-bə-ˈkan-chē-ə\ **1** : MAMMILLARY BODY **2** : the white fibrous scar that remains in the ovary after resorption of the corpus luteum and replaces a discharged graafian follicle

corpus cal•lo•sum \-ka-ˈlō-səm\ *n, pl* **corpora cal•lo•sa** \-sə\ : the great band of commissural fibers uniting the cerebral hemispheres

corpus ca•ver•no•sum \-ˌka-vər-ˈnō-səm\ *n, pl* **corpora ca•ver•no•sa** \-sə\ : a mass of erectile tissue with large interspaces capable of being distended with blood; *esp* : one of those that form the bulk of the body of the penis or of the clitoris

cor•pus•cle \ˈkȯr-(ˌ)pə-səl\ *n* **1** : a living cell; *esp* : one (as a red or white blood cell or a cell in cartilage or bone) not aggregated into continuous tissues **2** : any of various small circumscribed multicellular bodies — usu. used with a qualifying term ⟨Malpighian ~*s*⟩ — **cor•pus•cu•lar** \kȯr-ˈpəs-kyə-lər\ *adj*

corpuscle of Krause *n* : KRAUSE'S CORPUSCLE

corpus he•mor•rhag•i•cum \-ˌhe-mə-ˈra-ji-kəm\ *n* : a ruptured graafian follicle containing a blood clot that is absorbed as the cells lining the follicle form the corpus luteum

corpus lu•te•um \-ˈlü-tē-əm, -lü-ˈtē-əm\ *n, pl* **corpora lu•tea** \-ə\ : a yellowish mass of progesterone-secreting endocrine tissue that consists of pale secretory cells derived from granulosa cells, that forms immediately after ovulation from the ruptured graafian follicle in the mammalian ovary, and that regresses rather quickly if the ovum is not fertilized but persists throughout the ensuing pregnancy if it is fertilized

corpus spon•gi•o•sum \-ˌspən-jē-ˈō-səm, -ˌspän-\ *n* : the median longitudinal column of erectile tissue of the penis that contains the urethra and is ventral to the two corpora cavernosa

corpus stri•a•tum \-ˌstrī-ˈā-təm\ *n, pl* **corpora stri•a•ta** \-ˈā-tə\ : either of a pair of masses of nerve tissue which lie beneath and external to the anterior cornua of the lateral ventricles of the brain and form part of their floor and each of which contains a caudate nucleus and a lentiform nucleus separated by sheets of white matter to give the mass a striated appearance in section

corpus ute•ri \-ˈyü-tə-ˌrī\ *n* : the main body of the uterus above the constriction behind the cervix and below the openings of the fallopian tubes

[1]**cor•rec•tive** \kə-ˈrek-tiv\ *adj* : intended to correct ⟨~ lenses⟩ ⟨~ surgery⟩ — **cor•rec•tive•ly** *adv*

[2]**corrective** *n* : a medication that removes undesirable or unpleasant side effects of other medication

corresponding points *n pl* : points on the retinas of the two eyes which when simultaneously stimulated normally produce a single visual impression

Cor•ri•gan's pulse \ˌkȯr-i-gənz-\ *or* **Corrigan pulse** *n* : a pulse characterized by a sharp rise to full expansion followed by immediate collapse that is seen in aortic insufficiency — called also *water-hammer pulse*

Cor•ri•gan \ˈkȯr-i-gən\, **Sir Dominic John (1802–1880)**, British pathologist.

cor•rode \kə-ˈrōd\ *vb* **cor•rod•ed; cor•rod•ing** : to eat or be eaten away gradually (as by chemical action) — **cor•ro•sion** \kə-ˈrō-zhən\ *n*

[1]**cor•ro•sive** \-ˈrō-siv, -ziv\ *adj* : tending or having the power to corrode ⟨~ acids⟩ — **cor•ro•sive•ness** *n*

[2]**corrosive** *n* : a substance that corrodes : CAUSTIC

corrosive sublimate *n* : MERCURIC CHLORIDE

cor•ru•ga•tor \ˈkȯr-ə-ˌgā-tər\ *n* : a muscle that contracts the skin into wrinkles; *esp* : one that draws the eyebrows together and wrinkles the brow in frowning

cor•tex \ˈkȯr-ˌteks\ *n, pl* **cor•ti•ces** \ˈkȯr-tə-ˌsēz\ *or* **cor•tex•es** : the outer or superficial part of an organ or body structure (as the kidney, adrenal gland, or a hair); *esp* : CEREBRAL CORTEX

cor•ti•cal \ˈkȯr-ti-kəl\ *adj* **1** : of, relating to, or consisting of cortex ⟨~ tissue⟩ **2** : involving or resulting from the action or condition of the cerebral cortex ⟨~ blindness⟩ — **cor•ti•cal•ly** *adv*

cortico- *comb form* **1** : cortex ⟨*cortico*tropic⟩ **2** : cortical and ⟨*cortico*spinal⟩

cor•ti•co•ad•re•nal \ˌkȯr-ti-kō-ə-ˈdrēn-ᵊl\ *adj* : of or relating to the cortex of the adrenal gland ⟨~ insufficiency⟩

cor•ti•co•bul•bar \-ˈbəl-bər, -ˌbär\ *adj* : relating to or connecting the cerebral cortex and the medulla oblongata

cor•ti•coid \ˈkȯr-ti-ˌkȯid\ *n* : CORTICOSTEROID — **corticoid** *adj*

cor•ti•co•pon•tine \ˌkȯr-ti-kō-ˈpän-ˌtīn\ *adj* : relating to or connecting the cerebral cortex and the pons

cor•ti•co•pon•to•cer•e•bel•lar \-ˌpän-tō-ˌser-ə-ˈbe-lər\ *adj* : of, relating to, or being a tract of nerve fibers or a path for nerve impulses that passes from the cerebral cortex through the internal capsule to the pons to the white matter and cortex of the cerebellum

cor·ti·co·spi·nal \-ˈspīn-ᵊl\ *adj* : of or relating to the cerebral cortex and spinal cord or to the corticospinal tract

corticospinal tract *n* : any of four columns of motor fibers of which two run on each side of the spinal cord and which are continuations of the pyramids of the medulla oblongata: **a** : LATERAL CORTICOSPINAL TRACT **b** : VENTRAL CORTICOSPINAL TRACT

cor·ti·co·ste·roid \ˌkȯr-ti-kō-ˈstir-ˌȯid, -ˈster-\ *n* : any of various adrenal-cortex steroids (as corticosterone, cortisone, and aldosterone) that are divided on the basis of their major biological activity into glucocorticoids and mineralocorticoids

cor·ti·co·ste·rone \ˌkȯr-tə-ˈkäs-tə-ˌrōn, -kō-stə-ˈ; ˌkȯr-ti-kō-ˈstir-ˌōn, -ˈster-\ *n* : a colorless crystalline corticosteroid $C_{21}H_{30}O_4$ of the adrenal cortex that is important in protein and carbohydrate metabolism

cor·ti·co·tro·pic \ˌkȯr-ti-kō-ˈtrō-pik\ *also* **cor·ti·co·tro·phic** \-fik\ *adj* : influencing or stimulating the adrenal cortex ⟨∼ cells⟩

cor·ti·co·tro·pin \-ˈtrō-pən\ *also* **cor·ti·co·tro·phin** \-fən\ *n* : ACTH; *also* : a preparation of ACTH that is used esp. in the treatment of rheumatoid arthritis and rheumatic fever

corticotropin–releasing factor *also* **corticotrophin–releasing factor** *n* : a substance secreted by the median eminence of the hypothalamus that regulates the release of ACTH by the anterior lobe of the pituitary gland

corticotropin–releasing hormone *also* **corticotrophin–releasing hormone** *n* : CORTICOTROPIN-RELEASING FACTOR

cor·tin \ˈkȯrt-ᵊn\ *n* : the active principle of the adrenal cortex now known to consist of several hormones

cor·ti·sol \ˈkȯrt-ə-ˌsȯl, -ˌzȯl, -ˌsōl, -ˌzōl\ *n* : a glucocorticoid $C_{21}H_{30}O_5$ produced by the adrenal cortex upon stimulation by ACTH that mediates various metabolic processes (as gluconeogenesis), has anti-inflammatory and immunosuppressive properties, and whose levels in the blood may become elevated in response to physical or psychological stress — called also *hydrocortisone*

cor·ti·sone \-ˌsōn, -ˌzōn\ *n* : a glucocorticoid $C_{21}H_{28}O_5$ that is produced naturally in small amounts by the adrenal cortex and is used in the form of its synthetic acetate $C_{23}H_{30}O_6$ esp. as replacement therapy for deficient adrenocortical secretion and as an anti-inflammatory agent (as for rheumatoid arthritis) — compare 11-DEHYDROCORTICOSTERONE

cor·y·ne·bac·te·ri·um \ˌkȯr-ə-(ˌ)nē-bak-ˈtir-ē-əm\ *n* **1** *cap* : a genus of usu. gram-positive nonmotile bacteria that occur as irregular or branching rods and include the causative agents of diphtheria and caseous lymphadenitis **2** *pl* **-ria** \-ē-ə\ : any bacterium of the genus *Corynebacterium*

co·ryne·form \kə-ˈri-nə-ˌfȯrm\ *adj* : being or resembling bacteria of the genus *Corynebacterium*

co·ry·za \kə-ˈrī-zə\ *n* : an acute inflammatory contagious disease involving the upper respiratory tract: **a** : COMMON COLD **b** : any of several diseases of domestic animals; *esp* : INFECTIOUS CORYZA — **co·ry·zal** \-zəl\ *adj*

cos·me·ceu·ti·cal \ˌkäz-mə-ˈsü-ti-kəl\ *n* : a preparation (as of benzoyl peroxide or retinol) having both cosmetic and pharmaceutical properties

cos·me·sis \käz-ˈmē-səs\ *n, pl* **-me·ses** \-ˌsēz\ **1** : preservation, restoration, or enhancement of physical appearance **2** : the outer aesthetic covering (as of silicone) of a limb prosthesis

[1]**cos·met·ic** \käz-ˈme-tik\ *n* : a cosmetic preparation for external use

[2]**cosmetic** *adj* **1** : of, relating to, or making for beauty esp. of the complexion ⟨∼ salves⟩ **2** : correcting defects esp. of the face ⟨∼ surgery⟩ — **cos·met·i·cal·ly** *adv*

cos·mid \ˈkäz-məd\ *n* : a plasmid into which a short nucleotide sequence of a bacteriophage has been inserted to create a vector capable of cloning large segments of DNA

cost- *or* **costi-** *or* **costo-** *comb form* : rib : costal and ⟨*costo*chondral⟩

cos·ta \ˈkäs-tə\ *n, pl* **cos·tae** \-(ˌ)tē, -ˌtī\ : RIB

cos·tal \ˈkäst-ᵊl\ *adj* : of, relating to, involving, or situated near a rib

costal breathing *n* : inspiration and expiration produced chiefly by movements of the ribs

costal cartilage *n* : any of the cartilages that connect the distal ends of the ribs with the sternum and by their elasticity permit movement of the chest in respiration

costarum — see LEVATORES COSTARUM

cos·tive \ˈkäs-tiv, ˈkȯs-\ *adj* **1** : affected with constipation **2** : causing constipation — **cos·tive·ness** *n*

cos·to·cer·vi·cal trunk \ˌkäs-tə-ˈsər-və-kəl-, -tō-\ *n* : a branch of the subclavian artery that divides to supply the first or first two intercostal spaces and the deep structures of the neck — see INTERCOSTAL ARTERY b

cos·to·chon·dral \-ˈkän-drəl\ *adj* : relating to or joining a rib and costal cartilage ⟨a ∼ junction⟩

cos·to·chon·dri·tis \-kän-ˈdrī-təs\ *n* : TIETZE'S SYNDROME

cos·to·di·a·phrag·mat·ic \ˌkäs-tə-ˌdī-ə-frə-ˈma-tik, ˌkäs-tō-, -frəg-, -ˌfrag-\ *adj* : relating to or involving the ribs and diaphragm

cos·to·phren·ic \ˌkäs-tə-ˈfre-nik, -tō-\ *adj* : of or relating to the ribs and the diaphragm

cos·to·trans·verse \ˌkäs-tə-trans-ˈvərs, -tō-, -tranz-, -ˈtrans-ˌ, -ˈtranz-ˌ\ *adj* : relating to or connecting a rib and the transverse process of a vertebra ⟨a ~ joint⟩

cos·to·trans·ver·sec·to·my \-ˌtrans-(ˌ)vər-ˈsek-tə-mē, -ˌtranz-\ *n, pl* **-mies** : surgical excision of part of a rib and the transverse process of the adjoining vertebra

cos·to·ver·te·bral \-(ˌ)vər-ˈtē-brəl, -ˈvər-tə-\ *adj* : of or relating to a rib and its adjoining vertebra ⟨~ pain⟩

[1]**cot** \ˈkät\ *n* : a protective cover for a finger — called also *fingerstall*

[2]**cot** *n* : a wheeled stretcher for hospital, mortuary, or ambulance service

COTA *abbr* certified occupational therapy assistant

cot death *n, chiefly Brit* : SUDDEN INFANT DEATH SYNDROME

co·throm·bo·plas·tin \(ˌ)kō-ˌthräm-bō-ˈplas-tən\ *n* : FACTOR VII

co·tin·ine \ˈkō-tᵊn-ˌēn, -ˌīn\ *n* : an alkaloid $C_{10}H_{12}N_2O$ that is the principal metabolite of nicotine and is widely used as an indicator of recent exposure to nicotine

co–tri·mox·a·zole \ˌkō-ˌtrī-ˈmäk-sə-ˌzōl\ *n* : a bactericidal combination of trimethoprim and sulfamethoxazole in the ratio of one to five used esp. for chronic urinary tract infections

cot·ton·mouth \ˈkät-ᵊn-ˌmau̇th\ *n* : WATER MOCCASIN

cottonmouth moccasin *n* : WATER MOCCASIN

cot·y·le·don \ˌkät-ᵊl-ˈēd-ᵊn\ *n* : a lobule of a mammalian placenta — **cot·y·le·don·ary** \-ˈēd-ᵊn-ˌer-ē\ *adj*

[1]**couch** \ˈkau̇ch\ *vb* : to treat (a cataract or a person who has a cataract) by displacing the lens of the eye into the vitreous humor

[2]**couch** *n* : an article of furniture used (as by a patient undergoing psychoanalysis) for sitting or reclining — **on the couch** : receiving psychiatric treatment

[1]**cough** \ˈkȯf\ *vb* **1** : to expel air from the lungs suddenly with a sharp short noise usu. in a series of efforts **2** : to expel by coughing — often used with *up* ⟨~ up mucus⟩

[2]**cough** *n* **1** : a condition marked by repeated frequent coughing ⟨he has a bad ~⟩ **2** : a sudden sharp-sounding expulsion of air from the lungs acting as a protective mechanism to clear the air passages or as a symptom of pulmonary disturbance

cough drop *n* : a lozenge used to relieve coughing

cough syrup *n* : any of various sweet usu. medicated liquids used to relieve coughing

cou·lomb \ˈkü-ˌläm, -ˌlōm, kü-ˈ\ *n* : the practical mks unit of electric charge equal to the quantity of electricity transferred by a current of one ampere in one second

Coulomb, Charles–Augustin de (1736–1806), French physicist.

Cou·ma·din \ˈkü-mə-dən\ *trademark* — used for a preparation of the sodium salt of warfarin

cou·ma·phos \ˈkü-mə-ˌfäs\ *n* : an organophosphorus systemic insecticide $C_{14}H_{16}ClO_5PS$ administered esp. to cattle and poultry as a feed additive

cou·ma·rin \ˈkü-mə-rən\ *n* : a toxic white crystalline lactone $C_9H_6O_2$ found in plants or made synthetically and used as the parent compound in anticoagulant agents (as warfarin); *also* : a derivative of this compound

coun·sel·ing \ˈkau̇n-s(ə-)liŋ\ *n* : professional guidance of the individual by utilizing psychological methods

coun·sel·or *or* **coun·sel·lor** \ˈkau̇n-s(ə-)lər\ *n* : a person engaged in counseling

[1]**count** \ˈkau̇nt\ *vb* : to indicate or name by units or groups so as to find the total number of units involved

[2]**count** *n* : the total number of individual things in a given unit or sample (as of blood) obtained by counting all or a subsample of them

[1]**count·er** \ˈkau̇n-tər\ *n* : a level surface over which transactions are conducted or food is served or on which goods are displayed or work is conducted — **over the counter** : without a prescription ⟨drugs available *over the counter*⟩

[2]**counter** *n* : a device for indicating a number or amount — see GEIGER COUNTER

coun·ter·act \ˌkau̇n-tər-ˈakt\ *vb* : to make ineffective or restrain or neutralize the usu. ill effects of by an opposite force — **coun·ter·ac·tion** \-ˈak-shən\ *n*

coun·ter·con·di·tion·ing \-kən-ˈdi-shə-niŋ\ *n* : conditioning in order to replace an undesirable response (as fear) to a stimulus (as an engagement in public speaking) by a favorable one

coun·ter·cur·rent \ˌkau̇n-tər-ˈkər-ənt, -ˈkə-rənt\ *adj* **1** : flowing in an opposite direction **2** : involving flow of materials in opposite directions

coun·ter·elec·tro·pho·re·sis \-i-ˌlek-trə-fə-ˈrē-səs\ *n, pl* **-re·ses** \-ˌsēz\ : an electrophoretic method of testing blood esp. for hepatitis antigens

coun·ter·im·mu·no·elec·tro·pho·re·sis \-ˌim-yə-nō-i-ˌlek-trō-fə-ˈrē-səs\ *n, pl* **-re·ses** : COUNTERELECTROPHORESIS

coun·ter·ir·ri·tant \-ˈir-ə-tənt\ *n* : an agent applied locally to produce superficial inflammation with the object of reducing inflammation in deeper adjacent structures — **counterirritant** *adj*

coun·ter·ir·ri·ta·tion \-ˌtā-shən\ *n* : the reaction produced by treatment with a counterirritant; *also* : the treatment itself

coun·ter·pho·bic \-ˌfō-bik\ *adj* : relating to or characterized by a preference for or the seeking out of a situation that is feared ⟨~ reaction patterns⟩

coun·ter·pul·sa·tion \-ˌpəl-ˈsā-shən\ *n* : a technique for reducing the work load on the heart by lowering systemic blood pressure just before or during expulsion of blood from the ventricle and by raising blood pressure during diastole — see INTRA-AORTIC BALLOON COUNTERPULSATION

coun·ter·shock \-ˌshäk\ *n* : therapeutic electric shock applied to a heart for the purpose of altering a disturbed rhythm

coun·ter·stain \-ˌstān\ *n* : a stain used to color parts of a microscopy specimen not affected by another stain; *esp* : a cytoplasmic stain used to contrast with or enhance a nuclear stain — **counterstain** *vb*

coun·ter·trac·tion \ˈkau̇n-tər-ˌtrak-shən\ *n* : a traction opposed to another traction used in reducing fractures

coun·ter·trans·fer·ence \ˌkau̇n-tər-trans-ˈfər-əns, -ˈtrans-(ˌ)\ *n* **1** : psychological transference esp. by a psychotherapist during the course of treatment; *esp* : the psychotherapist's reactions to the patient's transference **2** : the complex of feelings of a psychotherapist toward the patient

coup \ˈkü\ *n* : injury occurring on the side of an organ (as the brain) on which a blow or impact is received — compare CONTRECOUP

couples counseling *n* : COUPLES THERAPY — **couples counselor** *n*

couples therapy *n* : usu. short-term counseling designed to help couples understand and resolve problems, dissatisfaction, and conflict in their relationship : MARRIAGE COUNSELING — **couples therapist** *n*

course \ˈkōrs\ *n* **1** : the series of events or stages comprising a natural process **2** : a series of doses or medications administered over a designated period

cou·vade \kü-ˈväd\ *n* **1** : a custom in some cultures in which when a child is born the father takes to bed as if bearing the child **2** : COUVADE SYNDROME

couvade syndrome *n* : a phenomenon in which a male experiences symptoms of pregnancy (as nausea or weight gain) during the time his partner or another woman he is particularly close to is pregnant

Cou·ve·laire uterus \ˌkü-və-ˈler-\ *n* : a pregnant uterus in which the placenta has detached prematurely with extravasation of blood into the uterine musculature

Couvelaire, Alexandre (1873–1948), French obstetrician.

CoV *abbr* coronavirus

co·va·lent bond \(ˌ)kō-ˈvā-lənt-\ *n* : a chemical bond formed between atoms by the sharing of electrons

cover glass *n* : a piece of very thin glass or plastic used to cover material on a microscope slide

cov·er·slip \ˈkə-vər-ˌslip\ *n* : COVER GLASS

cow·hage *also* **cow·age** \ˈkau̇-ij\ *n* : a tropical leguminous woody vine (*Mucuna pruriens*) with crooked pods covered with barbed hairs that cause severe itching; *also* : these hairs formerly used as a vermifuge

Cow·per's gland \ˈkau̇-pərz-, ˈkü-, ˈku̇-\ *n* : either of two small glands of which one lies on each side of the male urethra below the prostate gland and discharges a secretion into the semen — called also *bulbourethral gland;* compare BARTHOLIN'S GLAND

Cow·per \ˈkau̇-pər, ˈkü-, ˈku̇-\, **William (1666–1709),** British anatomist.

cow·pox \ˈkau̇-ˌpäks\ *n* : a mild eruptive disease of the cow that is caused by a poxvirus of the genus *Orthopoxvirus* (species *Cowpox virus*) and that when communicated to humans protects against smallpox — called also *variola vaccinia*

COX \ˈkäks\ *n* : CYCLOOXYGENASE — see COX-1, COX-2

cox- *or* **coxo-** *comb form* : hip : thigh : of the hip and ⟨*coxo*femoral⟩

coxa \ˈkäk-sə\ *n, pl* **cox·ae** \-ˌsē, -ˌsī\ : HIP JOINT, HIP

coxa vara \ˈkäk-sə-ˈvar-ə\ *n* : a deformed hip joint in which the neck of the femur is bent downward

Cox·i·el·la \ˌkäk-sē-ˈe-lə\ *n* : a genus of small pleomorphic gram-negative bacteria occurring intercellularly in ticks and intracellularly in the cytoplasm of vertebrates and including the causative organism (*C. burnetii*) of Q fever

Cox \ˈkäks\, **Herald Rea (1907–1986),** American bacteriologist.

coxo·fem·o·ral \ˌkäk-sō-ˈfe-mə-rəl\ *adj* : of or relating to the hip and thigh

COX–1 \ˈkäks-ˈwən\ *n* : the isoform of cyclooxygenase that is expressed in most tissues of the body and is not involved in producing the pain and inflammation of arthritis

Cox·sack·ie·vi·rus \(ˌ)käk-ˌsa-kē-ˈvī-rəs\ *or* **Cox·sack·ie virus** *n* : any of numerous serotypes of three viruses of the genus *Enterovirus* (species *Human enterovirus A, Human enterovirus B*, and *Human enterovirus C*) associated with mild to serious illness (as sore throat, diarrhea, conjunctivitis, meningitis, hepatitis, and epidemic pleurodynia)

COX–2 \ˈkäks-ˈtü\ *n* **1** : the isoform of cyclooxygenase that is expressed esp. in the brain and kidneys and at sites of inflammation **2** : COX-2 INHIBITOR

COX–2 inhibitor *n* : any of a class of NSAID drugs (as celecoxib) that selectively block the isoform COX-2 but not the isoform COX-1 of cyclooxygenase and that are used chiefly to relieve the pain and inflammation of arthritis while minimizing gastrointestinal side effects — called also *COX-2 blocker*

Co·zaar \ˈkō-ˌzär\ *trademark* — used for a preparation of the potassium salt of losartan

CP *abbr* **1** cerebral palsy **2** chest pain

CPAP *abbr* continuous positive airway pressure

CPB *abbr* competitive protein binding

C–pep·tide \ˈsē-ˈpep-ˌtīd\ *n* : a protein fragment 35 amino-acid residues long produced by enzymatic cleavage of proinsulin in the formation of insulin

CPK *abbr* creatine phosphokinase

CPR *abbr* cardiopulmonary resuscitation

Cr *symbol* chromium

CR *abbr* **1** conditioned response **2** controlled-release

crab louse *n* : PUBIC LOUSE

crabs \ˈkrabz\ *n pl* : infestation with pubic lice

crack \ˈkrak\ *n, often attrib* : a potent form of cocaine that is obtained by treating the hydrochloride of cocaine with sodium bicarbonate to create small chips used illicitly usu. for smoking

crack baby *n* : an infant subjected to prolonged exposure to crack cocaine in the mother's womb

cra·dle \ˈkrād-ᵊl\ *n* : a frame to keep the bedding from contact with an injured part of the body

cradle cap *n* : a seborrheic condition in infants that usu. affects the scalp and is characterized by greasy gray or dark brown adherent scaly crusts

¹cramp \ˈkramp\ *n* **1** : a painful involuntary spasmodic contraction of a muscle ⟨a ~ in the leg⟩ **2** : a temporary paralysis of muscles from overuse — see WRITER'S CRAMP **3 a** : sharp abdominal pain — usu. used in pl. **b** : persistent and often intense though dull lower abdominal pain associated with dysmenorrhea — usu. used in pl.

²cramp *vb* : to affect with or be affected with a cramp or cramps

crani- *or* **cranio-** *comb form* **1** : cranium ⟨*cranio*synostosis⟩ **2** : cranial and ⟨*cranio*sacral⟩

-crania *n comb form* : condition of the skull or head ⟨hemi*crania*⟩

cra·ni·ad \ˈkrā-nē-ˌad\ *adv* : toward the head or anterior end

cra·ni·al \ˈkrā-nē-əl\ *adj* **1** : of or relating to the skull or cranium **2** : CEPHALIC — **cra·ni·al·ly** *adv*

cranial arteritis *n* : GIANT CELL ARTERITIS

cranial fossa *n* : any of the three large depressions in the posterior, middle, and anterior aspects of the floor of the cranial cavity

cranial index *n* : the ratio multiplied by 100 of the maximum breadth of the bare skull to its maximum length from front to back — compare CEPHALIC INDEX

cranial nerve *n* : any of the 12 paired nerves that arise from the lower surface of the brain with one of each pair on each side and pass through openings in the skull to the periphery of the body — see ABDUCENS NERVE, ACCESSORY NERVE, AUDITORY NERVE, FACIAL NERVE, GLOSSOPHARYNGEAL NERVE, HYPOGLOSSAL NERVE, OCULOMOTOR NERVE, OLFACTORY NERVE, OPTIC NERVE, TRIGEMINAL NERVE, TROCHLEAR NERVE, VAGUS NERVE

cra·ni·ec·to·my \ˌkrā-nē-ˈek-tə-mē\ *n, pl* **-mies** : the surgical removal of a portion of the skull

cra·nio·ce·re·bral \ˌkrā-nē-ō-sə-ˈrē-brəl, -ˈser-ə-\ *adj* : involving both cranium and brain ⟨~ injury⟩

cra·nio·fa·cial \ˌkrā-nē-ō-ˈfā-shəl\ *adj* : of, relating to, or involving both the cranium and the face

craniofacial dysostosis *n* : CROUZON SYNDROME

cra·ni·ol·o·gy \ˌkrā-nē-ˈä-lə-jē\ *n, pl* **-gies** : a science dealing with variations in size, shape, and proportions of the human skull

cra·ni·om·e·try \-ˈä-mə-trē\ *n, pl* **-tries** : a science dealing with cranial measurement

cra·ni·op·a·gus \ˌkrā-nē-ˈä-pə-gəs\ *n, pl* **-a·gi** \-pə-ˌjē, -ˌjī\ : a pair of twins joined at the heads

cra·nio·pha·ryn·geal \ˌkrā-nē-ō-ˌfar-ən-ˈjē-əl, -fə-ˈrin-jəl, -jē-əl\ *adj* : relating to or connecting the cavity of the skull and the pharynx

cra·nio·pha·ryn·gi·o·ma \-ˌfar-ən-jē-ˈō-mə, -fə-ˌrin-jē-ˈō-mə\ *n, pl* **-mas** *also* **-ma·ta** \-mə-tə\ : a tumor of the brain near the pituitary gland that develops esp. in children or young adults from epithelium derived from the embryonic craniopharyngeal canal and that is often associated with increased intracranial pressure

cra·nio·plas·ty \ˈkrā-nē-(ˌ)ō-ˌplas-tē\ *n, pl* **-ties** : the surgical correction of skull defects

cra·nio·ra·chis·chi·sis \ˌkrā-nē-(ˌ)ō-rə-ˈkis-kə-səs\ *n, pl* **-chi·ses** \-ˌsēz\ : a congenital fissure of the skull and spine

cra·nio·sa·cral \ˌkrā-nē-ō-ˈsa-krəl, -ˈsā-\ *adj* **1** : of or relating to the cranium and the sacrum **2** : PARASYMPATHETIC

craniosacral therapy *n* : a system of gentle touch designed to enhance the functioning of the membranes, tissues, fluids, and bones surrounding or associated with the brain and spinal cord — **craniosacral therapist** *n*

cra·ni·os·chi·sis \ˌkrā-nē-ˈäs-kə-səs\ *n, pl* **-chi·ses** \-ˌsēz\ : a congenital fissure of the skull

cra·nio·ste·no·sis \ˌkrā-nē-(ˌ)ō-stə-ˈnō-səs\ *n, pl* **-no·ses** \-ˌsēz\ : malformation of the skull caused by premature closure of the cranial sutures

cra·nio·syn·os·to·sis \-ˌsi-ˌnäs-ˈtō-səs\ *n, pl* **-to·ses** \-ˌsēz\ : the premature closure during infancy of the fibrous joints of the skull

cra·nio·ta·bes \ˌkrā-nē-ə-ˈtā-(ˌ)bēz\ *n, pl* **craniotabes** : a thinning and softening of the infantile skull in spots usu. due to rickets or syphilis

cra·ni·ot·o·my \ˌkrā-nē-ˈä-tə-mē\ *n, pl* **-mies** **1** : the operation of cutting or crushing the fetal head to effect delivery **2** : surgical opening of the skull

cra•ni•um \ˈkrā-nē-əm\ *n, pl* **-ni•ums** *or* **-nia** \-nē-ə\ : SKULL; *specif* : BRAINCASE
crank \ˈkraŋk\ *n* : CRYSTAL METH; *specif* : an impure form of crystal meth
crash diet \ˈkrash-\ *n* : a diet intended to help a person lose a large amount of weight in a short period of time typically by reducing the amount of food consumed to minimal levels — **crash dieter** *n* — **crash dieting** *n*
cra•ter \ˈkrā-tər\ *n* : an eroded lesion of a wall or surface ⟨ulcer ∼*s*⟩
cra•ter•i•za•tion \ˌkrā-tər-ə-ˈzā-shən\ *n* : surgical excision of a crater-shaped piece of bone
craz•ing \ˈkrāz-iŋ\ *n* : the formation of minute cracks (as in the enamel of a tooth)
cra•zy \ˈkrā-zē\ *adj* **craz•i•er; -est** : marked by a severely disordered state of mind — not used technically — **cra•zi•ly** \-zə-lē\ *adv* — **cra•zi•ness** \-zē-nəs\ *n*
crazy bone *n* : FUNNY BONE
CRD *abbr* chronic respiratory disease
CRE \ˌsē-ˌär-ˈē\ *n, pl* **CRE** [*c*arbapenem-*r*esistant *E*nterobacteriaceae] : any enterobacterium that is resistant to most antibiotics including carbapenems and may cause severe infections (as of the blood or urinary tract) esp. in hospitalized patients
C–re•ac•tive protein \ˈsē-rē-ˈak-tiv-\ *n* : a protein produced by the liver that is normally present in trace amounts in the blood serum but is elevated during episodes of acute inflammation
cream \ˈkrēm\ *n* **1** : the yellowish part of milk containing from 18 to about 40 percent butterfat **2** : something having the consistency of cream; *esp* : a usu. emulsified medicinal or cosmetic preparation — **creamy** \ˈkrē-mē\ *adj*
crease \ˈkrēs\ *n* : a line or mark made by or as if by folding a pliable substance (as the skin) — **crease** *vb*
cre•atine \ˈkrē-ə-ˌtēn, -ət-ᵊn\ *n* : a nitrogenous substance $C_4H_9N_3O_2$ found esp. in vertebrate muscles either free or as phosphocreatine
creatine kinase *n* : any of three isoenzymes found esp. in skeletal and myocardial muscle and the brain that catalyze the transfer of a high-energy phosphate group from phosphocreatine to ADP with the formation of ATP and creatine and typically occur in elevated levels in the blood following injury to brain or muscle tissue
creatine phosphate *n* : PHOSPHOCREATINE
creatine phosphokinase *n* : CREATINE KINASE
cre•at•i•nine \krē-ˈat-ᵊn-ˌēn, -ᵊn-ən\ *n* : a white crystalline strongly basic compound $C_4H_7N_3O$ formed from creatine and found esp. in muscle, blood, and urine
cre•a•tin•uria \ˌkrē-ə-tə-ˈnu̇r-ē-ə, -ˈnyu̇r-\ *n* : the presence of creatine in urine; *esp* : an increased or abnormal amount in the urine
creeping eruption *n* : a human skin disorder that is characterized by a red line of eruption which fades at one end as it progresses at the other and that is usu. caused by insect or worm larvae and esp. those of the dog hookworm burrowing in the deeper layers of the skin — called also *larval migrans, larva migrans*
cre•mas•ter \krē-ˈmas-tər, krə-\ *n* : a thin muscle consisting of loops of fibers derived from the internal oblique muscle and descending upon the spermatic cord to surround and suspend the testicle — called also *cremaster muscle* — **cre•mas•ter•ic** \ˌkrē-mə-ˈster-ik\ *adj*
crème \ˈkrem, ˈkrēm\ *n, pl* **crèmes** \ˈkrem, ˈkremz, ˈkrēmz\ : CREAM 2
cre•nat•ed \ˈkrē-ˌnā-təd\ *also* **cre•nate** \-ˌnāt\ *adj* : having the margin or surface cut into rounded scallops ⟨∼ red blood cells⟩
cre•na•tion \kri-ˈnā-shən\ *n* : shrinkage of red blood cells resulting in crenated margins
cre•o•sote \ˈkrē-ə-ˌsōt\ *n* **1** : an oily liquid mixture of phenolic compounds obtained by the distillation of wood tar and used esp. as a disinfectant and as an expectorant in chronic bronchitis **2** : a brownish oily liquid consisting chiefly of aromatic hydrocarbons obtained by distillation of coal tar and used esp. as a wood preservative
crep•i•tant rale \ˈkre-pə-tənt-\ *n* : a peculiar crackling sound audible with inspiration in pneumonia and other lung diseases
crep•i•ta•tion \ˌkre-pə-ˈtā-shən\ *n* : a grating or crackling sound or sensation (as that produced by the fractured ends of a bone moving against each other) ⟨∼ in the arthritic knee⟩
crep•i•tus \ˈkre-pə-təs\ *n, pl* **crepitus** : CREPITATION
crescent of Gian•nuz•zi *or* **crescent of Gia•nuz•zi** \-jə-ˈnüt-sē\ *n* : DEMILUNE
G. Giannuzzi — see DEMILUNE OF GIANNUZZI
cre•sol \ˈkrē-ˌsȯl, -ˌsōl\ *n* : any of three poisonous colorless crystalline or liquid isomeric phenols C_7H_8O that are used as disinfectants, in making phenolic resins, and in organic synthesis — see METACRESOL
crest \ˈkrest\ *n* : a ridge esp. on a bone ⟨the ∼ of the tibia⟩ — see OCCIPITAL CREST
Cres•tor \ˈkre-ˌstȯr\ *trademark* — used for the calcium salt of rosuvastatin
cre•tin \ˈkrēt-ᵊn\ *n, often offensive* : one affected with cretinism — **cre•tin•ous** \-ᵊn-əs\ *adj*
cre•tin•ism \-ᵊn-ˌi-zəm\ *n* : a usu. congenital condition marked by physical stunting and intellectual disability and caused by severe thyroid deficiency

Creutz•feldt–Ja•kob disease *also* **Creutz•feld–Ja•cob disease** \ˈkrȯits-ˌfelt-ˈyä-(ˌ)kōb-, -(ˌ)kōp-\ *n* : a rare progressive fatal prion disease marked by development of porous brain tissue, premature dementia in middle age, and gradual loss of muscular coordination — abbr. *CJD;* called also *Jakob-Creutzfeldt disease;* see VARIANT CREUTZFELDT-JAKOB DISEASE

Creutzfeldt, Hans Gerhard (1885–1964), and **Jakob, Alfons Maria (1884–1931),** German psychiatrists.

crev•ice \ˈkre-vəs\ *n* : a narrow fissure or cleft — see GINGIVAL CREVICE

cre•vic•u•lar \krə-ˈvi-kyə-lər\ *adj* : of, relating to, or involving a crevice and esp. the gingival crevice

crib death *n* : SUDDEN INFANT DEATH SYNDROME

crib•ri•form plate \ˈkri-brə-ˌfȯrm-\ *n* **1** : the horizontal plate of the ethmoid bone perforated with numerous foramina for the passage of the olfactory nerve filaments from the nasal cavity — called also *lamina cribrosa* **2** : LAMINA DURA

cribrosa — see LAMINA CRIBROSA

crick \ˈkrik\ *n* : a painful spasmodic condition of muscles (as of the neck or back) — **crick** *vb*

crico- *comb form* **1** : cricoid cartilage and ⟨*crico*thyroid⟩ **2** : of the cricoid cartilage and ⟨*crico*pharyngeal⟩

cri•co•ar•y•te•noid \ˌkrī-kō-ˌar-ə-ˈtē-ˌnȯid, -kō-ə-ˈrit-ᵊn-ˌȯid\ *n* **1** : a muscle of the larynx that arises from the upper margin of the arch of the cricoid cartilage, inserts into the front of the process of the arytenoid cartilage, and helps to narrow the opening of the vocal cords — called also *lateral cricoarytenoid* **2** : a muscle of the larynx that arises from the posterior surface of the lamina of the cricoid cartilage, inserts into the posterior of the process of the arytenoid cartilage, and widens the opening of the vocal cords — called also *posterior cricoarytenoid*

cri•coid cartilage \ˈkrī-ˌkȯid-\ *n* : a cartilage of the larynx which articulates with the lower cornua of the thyroid cartilage and with which the arytenoid cartilages articulate — called also *cricoid*

cri•co•pha•ryn•geal \ˌkrī-kō-ˌfar-ən-ˈjē-əl, -fə-ˈrin-jəl, -jē-əl\ *adj* : of or relating to the cricoid cartilage and the pharynx

¹cri•co•thy•roid \-ˈthī-ˌrȯid\ *adj* : relating to or connecting the cricoid cartilage and the thyroid cartilage

²cricothyroid *n* : a triangular muscle of the larynx that is attached to the cricoid and thyroid cartilages and is the principal tensor of the vocal cords — called also *cricothyroid muscle*

cri•co•thy•roi•de•us \ˌkrī-kō-thī-ˈrȯi-dē-əs\ *n, pl* **-dei** \-dē-ˌī\ : CRICOTHYROID

cricothyroid membrane *n* : a membrane of yellow elastic tissue that is attached below to the cricoid cartilage, in front to the thyroid cartilage, and in back to the arytenoid cartilages and that forms the vocal ligaments with its thickened upper margins

cri•co•thy•roi•dot•o•my \ˌkrī-kō-ˌthī-ˌrȯi-ˈdä-tə-mē\ *n, pl* **-mies** : tracheotomy by incision through the skin and cricothyroid membrane esp. as an emergency procedure for relief of an obstructed airway

cri du chat syndrome \ˌkrē-dü-ˈshä-, -də-\ *n* : an inherited condition characterized by a mewing cry, intellectual disability, physical anomalies, and the absence of part of a chromosome — called also *cat cry syndrome*

¹crip•ple \ˈkri-pəl\ *n, sometimes offensive* : an individual having a physical disability and esp. a physically impaired leg or foot

²cripple *vb* **crip•pled; crip•pling** \-p(ə-)liŋ\ : to deprive of the use of a limb and esp. a leg ⟨*crippled* by arthritis⟩

crip•pler \-p(ə-)lər\ *n* : a disease that results in physical disability

cri•sis \ˈkrī-səs\ *n, pl* **cri•ses** \-ˌsēz\ **1** : the turning point for better or worse in an acute disease or fever; *esp* : a sudden turn for the better (as sudden abatement in severity of symptoms or abrupt drop in temperature) — compare LYSIS 1 **2** : a paroxysmal attack of pain, distress, or disordered function ⟨tabetic ~⟩ ⟨cardiac ~⟩ **3** : an emotionally significant event or radical change of status in a person's life **4** : a psychological or social condition characterized by unusual instability caused by excessive stress and either endangering or felt to endanger the continuity of an individual or group; *esp* : such a social condition requiring the transformation of cultural patterns and values

crisis center *n* : a facility run usu. by nonprofessionals who counsel those who telephone for help in a personal crisis

cris•ta \ˈkris-tə\ *n, pl* **cris•tae** \-ˌtē, -ˌtī\ **1** : one of the areas of specialized sensory epithelium in the ampullae of the semicircular canals of the ear serving as end organs for the vestibular sense **2** : an elevation of the surface of a bone for the attachment of a muscle or tendon **3** : any of the inwardly projecting folds of the inner membrane of a mitochondrion

crista am•pul•lar•is \-ˌam-p(y)ü-ˈlar-əs\ *n* : CRISTA 1

crista gal•li \-ˈga-lē, -ˈgȯ-\ *n* : an upright process on the anterior portion of the cribriform plate to which the anterior part of the falx cerebri is attached

crit•i•cal \ˈkri-ti-kəl\ *adj* **1** : relating to, indicating, or being the stage of a disease at which an abrupt change for better or worse may be anticipated with reasonable certainty ⟨the ~ phase of a fever⟩ **2** : being or relating to an illness or condition involving danger of death ⟨~ care⟩ ⟨a ~ head injury⟩ — **crit·i·cal·ly** \-k(ə-)lē\ *adv*

Crix·i·van \ˈkrik-sə-ˌvan\ *trademark* — used for a preparation of the sulfate of indinavir

CRNA *abbr* certified registered nurse anesthetist

crock \ˈkräk\ *n, slang* : a complaining medical patient whose illness is largely imaginary or psychosomatic

Crohn's disease \ˈkrōnz-\ *also* **Crohn disease** \ˈkrōn-\ *n* : chronic ileitis that typically involves the distal portion of the ileum, often spreads to the colon, and is characterized by diarrhea, cramping, and loss of appetite and weight with local abscesses and scarring — called also *regional enteritis, regional ileitis*

Crohn \ˈkrōn\, **Burrill Bernard (1884–1983),** American physician.

cromoglycate — see DISODIUM CROMOGLYCATE, SODIUM CROMOGLYCATE

cro·mo·lyn \ˈkrō-mə-lən\ *n* : a drug $C_{23}H_{14}Na_2O_{11}$ that inhibits the release of histamine from mast cells and is used as an inhalant to prevent the onset of bronchial asthma attacks, as a nasal spray to treat allergic rhinitis, as eye drops to treat allergic conjunctivitis, keratitis, or keratoconjunctivitis, and as an oral solution to treat mastocytosis — called also *cromolyn sodium, disodium cromoglycate, sodium cromoglycate*

[1]**cross** \ˈkrȯs\ *n* **1** : an act of crossing dissimilar individuals **2** : a crossbred individual or kind

[2]**cross** *vb* : to interbreed or cause (an animal or plant) to interbreed with one of a different kind : HYBRIDIZE

[3]**cross** *adj* : CROSSBRED, HYBRID

cross·bred \ˈkrȯs-ˈbred\ *adj* : produced by crossbreeding : HYBRID — **cross·bred** \-ˌbred\ *n*

[1]**cross·breed** \ˈkrȯs-ˌbrēd, -ˈbrēd\ *vb* **-bred** \-ˌbred, -ˈbred\; **-breed·ing** : HYBRIDIZE, CROSS; *esp* : to cross (two varieties or breeds) within the same species

[2]**cross·breed** \-ˌbrēd\ *n* : HYBRID

cross·bridge \ˈkrȯs-ˌbrij\ *n* : the globular head of a myosin molecule that projects from a myosin filament in muscle and in the sliding filament hypothesis of muscle contraction is held to attach temporarily to an adjacent actin filament and draw it into the A band of a sarcomere between the myosin filaments

crossed \ˈkrȯst\ *adj* : forming a decussation ⟨a ~ tract of nerve fibers⟩

cross–eye \ˈkrȯs-ˌī\ *n* **1** : strabismus in which the eye turns inward toward the nose — called also *esotropia;* compare WALLEYE 2a **2 cross–eyes** \-ˈīz\ *pl* : eyes affected with cross-eye — **cross–eyed** \-ˈīd\ *adj*

cross·ing–over \ˌkrȯ-siŋ-ˈō-vər\ *n* : an interchange of genes or segments between homologous chromosomes

cross–link \ˈkrȯs-ˌliŋk\ *n* : a crosswise connecting part (as an atom) that connects parallel chains in a complex chemical molecule (as a protein) — **cross–link** *vb*

cross·match·ing \ˈkrȯs-ˈma-chiŋ\ *or* **cross·match** \-ˈmach\ *n* : the testing of the compatibility of the bloods of a transfusion donor and a recipient by mixing the serum of each with the red cells of the other to determine the absence of agglutination reactions — **crossmatch** *vb*

[1]**cross·over** \ˈkrȯs-ˌō-vər\ *n* **1** : an instance or product of genetic crossing-over **2** : a crossover interchange in an experiment

[2]**crossover** *adj* : involving or using interchange of the control group and the experimental group during the course of an experiment

cross–re·ac·tion \ˌkrȯs-rē-ˈak-shən\ *n* : reaction of one antigen with antibodies developed against another antigen — **cross–re·act** \-ˈakt\ *vb* — **cross–re·ac·tive** \-rē-ˈak-tiv\ *adj* — **cross–re·ac·tiv·i·ty** \-(ˌ)rē-ˌak-ˈti-və-tē\ *n*

cross–re·sis·tance \ˌkrȯs-ri-ˈzis-tən(t)s\ *n* : tolerance (as of a bacteria or malignant cell) to a usu. toxic substance (as an antibiotic or chemotherapy drug) that is acquired not as a result of direct exposure but by exposure to a related substance

cross section *n* : a cutting or piece of something cut off at right angles to an axis; *also* : a representation of such a cutting — **cross–sec·tion·al** \ˌkrȯs-ˈsek-shə-nəl\ *adj*

cross–tol·er·ance \ˈkrȯs-ˈtä-lə-rəns\ *n* : tolerance or resistance to a drug that develops through continued use of another drug with similar pharmacological action

cro·ta·lar·ia \ˌkrō-tə-ˈlar-ē-ə, ˌkrä-\ *n* **1** *cap* : a genus of leguminous plants including some containing toxic alkaloids **2** : any plant of the genus *Crotalaria* — called also *rattlebox*

Cro·ta·lus \ˈkrōt-ᵊl-əs, ˈkrät-\ *n* : a genus of American pit vipers including many of the rattlesnakes

crotch \ˈkräch\ *n* : an angle formed by the parting of two legs, branches, or members

-crotic *adj comb form* : having (such) a heartbeat or pulse ⟨di*crotic*⟩

-crotism *n comb form* : condition of having (such) a heartbeat or pulse ⟨di*crotism*⟩

Cro·ton bug \ˈkrōt-ᵊn-\ *n* : GERMAN COCKROACH

cro·ton oil \ˈkrōt-ᵊn-\ *n* : a viscid irritating oil from an Asian plant (*Croton tiglium* of the family Euphorbiaceae) that has been used in folk medicine as a cathartic

croup \ˈkrüp\ *n* : inflammation, edema, and subsequent obstruction of the larynx, trachea, and bronchi esp. of infants and young children that is typically caused by a parainfluenza virus and is marked by episodes of difficult breathing and low-pitched cough resembling the bark of a seal — **croup·ous** \ˈkrü-pəs\ *adj* — **croupy** \-pē\ *adj*

Crou·zon syndrome \ˌkrü-ˈzän-\ *also* **Crou·zon's syndrome** \-ˈzänz-\ *n* : a craniofacial disorder that is inherited as an autosomal dominant trait and is characterized by malformation of the skull due to premature ossification and closure of the sutures — called also *craniofacial dysostosis, Crouzon's disease*

Crouzon, Octave (1874–1938), French neurologist.

[1]**crown** \ˈkrau̇n\ *n* **1** : the topmost part of the skull or head **2** : the part of a tooth external to the gum or an artificial substitute for this

[2]**crown** *vb* **1** : to put an artificial crown on (a tooth) **2** *in childbirth* : to appear at the vaginal opening — used of the first part (as the crown of the head) of the infant to appear

crow's–foot \ˈkrōz-ˌfu̇t\ *n, pl* **crow's–feet** \-ˌfēt\ : a wrinkle extending from the outer corner of the eye — usu. used in pl.

CRPS *abbr* complex regional pain syndrome

CRT \ˌsē-(ˌ)är-ˈtē\ *n, pl* **CRTs** *or* **CRT's** : CATHODE-RAY TUBE; *also* : a display device incorporating a cathode-ray tube

CRTT *abbr* certified respiratory therapy technician

cru·ci·ate \ˈkrü-shē-ˌāt\ *adj* : shaped like a cross

cruciate ligament *n* : any of several more or less cross-shaped ligaments: as **a** : either of two ligaments in the knee joint which cross each other from femur to tibia: (1) : ANTERIOR CRUCIATE LIGAMENT (2) : POSTERIOR CRUCIATE LIGAMENT **b** : a complex ligament made up of the transverse ligament of the atlas and vertical fibrocartilage extending from the dens to the border of the foramen magnum

crude protein *n* : the approximate amount of protein in foods that is calculated from the determined nitrogen content and that may contain an appreciable error if the nitrogen is derived from nonprotein material or from a protein of unusual composition

crura *pl of* CRUS

cru·ra ce·re·bri \ˌkru̇r-ə-ˈser-ə-ˌbrī, -ˈker-ə-ˌbrē\ *n pl* : CRUS 2c

crura for·ni·cis \-ˈfȯr-nə-ˌsis, -nə-ˌkis\ *n pl* : CRUS 2e

cru·ral \ˈkru̇r-əl\ *adj* : of or relating to the thigh or leg; *specif* : FEMORAL

cruris — see TINEA CRURIS

crus \ˈkrüs, ˈkrəs\ *n, pl* **cru·ra** \ˈkru̇r-ə\ **1** : the lower or hind limb esp. between the knee and the ankle or tarsus : SHANK **2** : any of various anatomical parts likened to a leg or to a pair of legs: as **a** : either of the diverging proximal ends of the corpora cavernosa **b** : the tendinous attachments of the diaphragm to the bodies of the lumbar vertebrae forming the sides of the aortic opening — often used in pl. **c** *pl* : the peduncles of the cerebrum — called also *crura cerebri* **d** *pl* : the peduncles of the cerebellum **e** *pl* : the posterior pillars of the fornix — called also *crura fornicis* **f** (1) : a long bony process of the incus that articulates with the stapes; *also* : a shorter one projecting from the body of the incus perpendicular to this (2) : either of the two bony processes forming the sides of the arch of the stapes

crush syndrome *n* : the physical responses to severe crushing injury of muscle tissue involving esp. shock and partial or complete renal failure; *also* : the renal failure associated with such responses

crust \ˈkrəst\ *n* **1** : SCAB 2 **2** : an encrusting deposit of serum, cellular debris, and bacteria present over or about lesions in some skin diseases (as impetigo or eczema) — **crust** *vb*

crutch \ˈkrəch\ *n* **1** : a support typically fitting under the armpit for use as an aid in walking **2** : the crotch esp. of an animal

cry- *or* **cryo-** *comb form* : cold : freezing ⟨*cryo*surgery⟩

cryo·ab·la·tion \ˌkrī-ō-a-ˈblā-shən\ *n* : the destruction of tissue by freezing — **cryo·ab·late** \-a-ˈblāt\ *vb*

cryo·bi·ol·o·gy \ˌkrī-ō-bī-ˈä-lə-jē\ *n, pl* **-gies** : the study of the effects of extremely low temperature on living organisms and cells — **cryo·bi·o·log·i·cal** \-ˌbī-ə-ˈlä-ji-kəl\ *adj* — **cryo·bi·ol·o·gist** \ˌkrī-ō-bī-ˈä-lə-jist\ *n*

cryo·cau·tery \-ˈkȯ-tə-rē\ *n, pl* **-ter·ies** : destruction of tissue by use of extreme cold

cryo·ex·trac·tion \-ik-ˈstrak-shən\ *n* : extraction of a cataract through use of a cryoprobe whose refrigerated tip adheres to and freezes tissue of the lens permitting its removal

cryo·ex·trac·tor \-ik-ˈstrak-tər, -ˈek-ˌ\ *n* : a cryoprobe used for removal of cataracts

cryo·fi·brin·o·gen \-fī-ˈbri-nə-jən\ *n* : an abnormal fibrinogen that precipitates upon cooling to 4°C (39°F) and redissolves at 37°C (98.6°F) and is sometimes associated with vasculitis

cryo·gen·ic \ˌkrī-ə-ˈje-nik\ *adj* **1 a** : of or relating to the production of very low temperatures **b** : being or relating to very low temperatures **2** : requiring or involving the use of a cryogenic temperature ⟨∼ surgery⟩ — **cryo·gen·i·cal·ly** \-ni-k(ə-)lē\ *adv*

cryo·gen·ics \-niks\ *n* : a branch of physics that deals with the production and effects of very low temperatures

cryo·glob·u·lin \ˌkrī-ō-ˈglä-byə-lən\ *n* : any of several proteins similar to gamma globulins (as in molecular weight) that precipitate usu. in the cold from blood serum esp. in pathological conditions (as multiple myeloma)

cryo•glob•u•lin•emia \-ˌglä-byə-lə-ˈnē-mē-ə\ *n* : the condition of having abnormal quantities of cryoglobulins in the blood

cry•on•ics \krī-ˈä-niks\ *n* : the practice of freezing the body of a person who has died from a disease in hopes of restoring life at some future time when a cure for the disease has been developed — **cry•on•ic** \-nik\ *adj*

cryo•pexy \ˈkrī-ə-ˌpek-sē\ *n, pl* **-pex•ies** : cryosurgery for fixation of the retina in retinal detachment or for repair of a retinal tear or hole

cryo•pre•cip•i•tate \ˌkrī-ō-prə-ˈsi-pə-tət, -ˌtāt\ *n* : a precipitate that is formed by cooling a solution — **cryo•pre•cip•i•ta•tion** \-ˌsi-pə-ˈtā-shən\ *n*

cryo•pres•er•va•tion \-ˌpre-zər-ˈvā-shən\ *n* : preservation (as of sperm or eggs) by subjection to extremely low temperatures — **cryo•pre•serve** \-pri-ˈzərv\ *vb*

cryo•probe \ˈkrī-ə-ˌprōb\ *n* : a blunt chilled instrument used to freeze tissues in cryosurgery

cryo•pro•tec•tive \ˌkrī-ō-prə-ˈtek-tiv\ *adj* : serving to protect against the deleterious effects of subjection to freezing temperatures ⟨a ~ agent⟩ — **cryo•pro•tec•tant** \-tənt\ *n or adj*

cryo•stat \ˈkrī-ə-ˌstat\ *n* : an apparatus for maintaining a constant low temperature esp. below 0°C; *esp* : one containing a microtome for obtaining sections of frozen tissue — **cryo•stat•ic** \ˌkrī-ə-ˈsta-tik\ *adj*

cryo•sur•gery \ˌkrī-ō-ˈsərj-rē, -ˈsər-jə-rē\ *n, pl* **-ger•ies** : surgery in which diseased or abnormal tissue (as a tumor or wart) is destroyed or removed by freezing (as by the use of liquid nitrogen) — **cryo•sur•geon** \-ˈsər-jən\ *n* — **cryo•sur•gi•cal** \-ˈsər-ji-kəl\ *adj*

cryo•ther•a•py \-ˈther-ə-pē\ *n, pl* **-pies** : the therapeutic use of cold; *esp* : CRYOSURGERY

crypt \ˈkript\ *n* **1** : an anatomical pit or depression **2** : a simple tubular gland (as a crypt of Lieberkühn)

crypt- *or* **crypto-** *comb form* : hidden : covered ⟨*crypto*genic⟩

crypt•ec•to•my \krip-ˈtek-tə-mē\ *n, pl* **-mies** : surgical removal or destruction of a crypt

cryp•tic \ˈkrip-tik\ *adj* : not recognized ⟨a ~ infection⟩

cryp•ti•tis \krip-ˈtī-təs\ *n* : inflammation of a crypt (as an anal crypt)

cryp•to \ˈkrip-(ˌ)tō\ *n* : CRYPTOSPORIDIUM 2; *also* : CRYPTOSPORIDIOSIS

cryp•to•coc•co•sis \ˌkrip-tə-(ˌ)kä-ˈkō-səs\ *n, pl* **-co•ses** \-(ˌ)sēz\ : an infectious disease that is caused by a fungus of the genus *Cryptococcus* (*C. neoformans*) and is characterized by the production of nodular lesions or abscesses in the subcutaneous tissues, joints, and esp. the lungs, brain, and meninges — called also *torulosis*

cryp•to•coc•cus \-ˈkä-kəs\ *n* **1** *cap* : a genus of imperfect fungi that resemble yeasts and include a few serious pathogens **2** *pl* **-coc•ci** \-ˈkäk-ˌsī, -ˌsē; -ˈkä-ˌkī, -ˌkē\ : any fungus of the genus *Cryptococcus* — **cryp•to•coc•cal** \-ˈkä-kəl\ *adj*

crypt of Lie•ber•kühn \-ˈlē-bər-ˌkün, -ˌkyün, -ˌkue̅n-\ *n* : any of the tubular glands of the intestinal mucous membrane — called also *intestinal gland*

Lieberkühn, Johannes Nathanael (1711–1756), German anatomist.

crypt of Mor•ga•gni \-mȯr-ˈgän-yē\ *n* : any of the pouched cavities of the rectal mucosa immediately above the anorectal junction, intervening between vertical folds of the rectal mucosa

Morgagni, Giovanni Battista (1682–1771), Italian anatomist and pathologist.

cryp•to•ge•net•ic \ˌkrip-tō-jə-ˈne-tik\ *adj* : CRYPTOGENIC

cryp•to•gen•ic \ˌkrip-tə-ˈje-nik\ *adj* : of obscure or unknown origin

crypt•or•chid \krip-ˈtȯr-kəd\ *n* : one affected with cryptorchidism — compare MONORCHID — **cryptorchid** *adj*

crypt•or•chi•dism \-kə-ˌdi-zəm\ *also* **crypt•or•chism** \-ˌki-zəm\ *n* : a condition in which one or both testes fail to descend normally — compare MONORCHIDISM

cryp•to•spo•rid•i•o•sis \ˌkrip-tō-spȯr-ˌi-dē-ˈō-səs\ *n, pl* **-o•ses** \-ˌsēz\ : a disease caused by cryptosporidia

cryp•to•spo•rid•i•um \ˌkrip-tō-spȯr-ˈi-dē-əm\ *n* **1** *cap* : a genus of coccidian protozoans parasitic in the gut of many vertebrates including humans and sometimes causing diarrhea esp. in individuals who are immunocompromised (as in AIDS) **2** *pl* **-rid•ia** \-dē-ə\ : any protozoan of the genus *Cryptosporidium*

cryp•to•xan•thin \ˌkrip-tə-ˈzan-thən\ *n* : a carotenoid alcohol $C_{40}H_{55}OH$ that occurs in many plants, in blood serum, and in some animal products (as butter and egg yolk) and that is a precursor of vitamin A

cryp•to•zo•ite \-ˈzō-ˌīt\ *n* : a malaria parasite that develops in tissue cells and gives rise to the forms that invade blood cells

crys•tal \ˈkrist-ᵊl\ *n* **1** : a body that is formed by the solidification of a chemical element, a compound, or a mixture and has a regularly repeating internal arrangement of its atoms and often external plane faces **2** : CRYSTAL METH; *broadly* : methamphetamine in any form when used illicitly — **crystal** *adj* — **crys•tal•line** \ˈkris-tə-lən, -ˌlīn, -ˌlēn\ *adj*

crys•tal•lin \ˈkris-tə-lən\ *n* : either of two globulins in the crystalline lens

crystallina — see MILIARIA CRYSTALLINA
crystalline lens *n* : the lens of the eye
crys•tal•lize *also* **crys•tal•ize** \ˈkris-tə-ˌlīz\ *vb* **-lized** *also* **-ized; -liz•ing** *also* **-iz•ing** : to cause to form crystals or assume crystalline form — **crys•tal•liz•able** \-ˌkris-tə-ˈlī-zə-bəl\ *adj* — **crys•tal•li•za•tion** \ˌkris-tə-lə-ˈzā-shən\ *n*
crys•tal•lu•ria \ˌkris-tə-ˈlu̇r-ē-ə, -təl-ˈyu̇r-\ *n* : the presence of crystals in the urine indicating renal irritation
crystal meth *n* : methamphetamine in the form of crystals of its hydrochloride salt $C_{10}H_{15}N{\cdot}HCl$ when used illicitly for smoking, snorting, or injecting — called also *crank, crystal, crystal methamphetamine, ice*
cs *abbr* conditioned stimulus
Cs *symbol* cesium
CS \ˌsē-ˈes\ *n* : a potent lacrimatory and nausea-producing gas $C_{10}H_5ClN_2$ used in riot control and chemical warfare
C–sec•tion \ˈsē-ˌsek-shən\ *n* : CESAREAN SECTION
CSF \ˌsē-(ˌ)es-ˈef\ *n* : COLONY-STIMULATING FACTOR
CSF *abbr* cerebrospinal fluid
CT *abbr* **1** cognitive therapy **2** computed tomography; computerized tomography
CTC *abbr* computed tomographic colonography; computed tomography colonography; computerized tomographic colonography; CT colonography
CT colonography *n* : a noninvasive medical imaging technique that uses computed tomography to visualize the interior of the colon and rectum esp. to screen for polyps or cancerous growths; *also* : a procedure utilizing CT colonography — abbr. *CTC;* called also *colonography, computed tomographic colonography*
CTD *abbr* cumulative trauma disorder
CTE *abbr* chronic traumatic encephalopathy
Cteno•ce•phal•i•des \ˌte-nō-sə-ˈfa-lə-ˌdēz\ *n* : a genus of fleas (family Pulicidae) including the dog flea (*C. canis*) and cat flea (*C. felis*)
CTL \ˌsē-(ˌ)tē-ˈel\ *n* : CYTOTOXIC T LYMPHOCYTE
CTS *abbr* carpal tunnel syndrome
CT scan \ˈsē-ˈtē-\ *n* : a cross-sectional three-dimensional image of an internal body part produced by computed tomography chiefly for diagnostic purposes — called also *CAT scan* — **CT scanning** *n*
CT scanner *n* : a medical instrument consisting of X-ray and computing equipment and used for computed tomography — called also *CAT scanner*
Cu *symbol* copper
[1]**cu•bi•tal** \ˈkyü-bət-ᵊl\ *adj* : of or relating to a cubitus
[2]**cubital** *n* : CUBITUS
cubiti — see BICEPS FLEXOR CUBITI
cu•bi•tus \ˈkyü-bə-təs\ *n, pl* **cu•bi•ti** \-ˌtī\ **1** : FOREARM, ANTEBRACHIUM **2** : ULNA
cubitus valgus *n* : a condition of the arm in which the forearm deviates away from the midline of the body when extended
cubitus varus *n* : a condition of the arm in which the forearm deviates toward the midline of the body when extended
[1]**cu•boid** \ˈkyü-ˌbȯid\ *adj* **1** : relating to or being the cuboid ⟨the ~ bone⟩ **2** : shaped approximately like a cube
[2]**cuboid** *n* : the outermost bone in the distal row of tarsal bones of the foot that supports the fourth and fifth metatarsals
cu•boi•dal \kyü-ˈbȯid-ᵊl\ *adj* **1** : CUBOID 2 **2** : composed of nearly cubical elements ⟨~ epithelium⟩
cud \ˈkəd\ *n* : food brought up into the mouth by a ruminating animal from its first stomach to be chewed again
cue \ˈkyü\ *n* : a minor stimulus acting as an indication of the nature of the perceived object or situation
cuff \ˈkəf\ *n* **1** : an inflatable band that is wrapped around an extremity to control the flow of blood through the part when recording blood pressure with a sphygmomanometer **2** : an anatomical structure shaped like a cuff; *esp* : ROTATOR CUFF
cuffed \ˈkəft\ *adj* : provided with an often inflatable encircling part ⟨a ~ endotracheal tube⟩
cui•rass \kwi-ˈras, kyu̇-\ *n* **1** : a plaster cast for the trunk and neck **2** : a respirator that covers the chest or the chest and abdomen and provides artificial respiration by means of an electric pump
cul–de–sac \ˌkəl-di-ˈsak, ˌku̇l-\ *n, pl* **culs–de–sac** *same or* ˌkəlz-, ˌku̇lz-\ *also* **cul–de–sacs** \-ˈsaks\ **1** : a blind diverticulum or pouch; *also* : the closed end of such a pouch **2** : POUCH OF DOUGLAS
cul–de–sac of Douglas *n* : POUCH OF DOUGLAS
culdo- *comb form* : pouch of Douglas ⟨*culdo*scopy⟩
cul•do•cen•te•sis \ˌkəl-dō-ˌsen-ˈtē-səs, ˌku̇l-\ *n, pl* **-te•ses** \-ˌsēz\ : removal of material from the pouch of Douglas by means of puncture of the vaginal wall
cul•dos•co•py \ˌkəl-ˈdäs-kə-pē, ˌku̇l-\ *n, pl* **-pies** : a technique for endoscopic visualization and minor operative procedures on the female pelvic organs in which the instrument is introduced through a puncture in the wall of the pouch of Douglas — **cul•do•scop•ic** \ˌkəl-də-ˈskä-pik, ˌku̇l-\ *adj*
cul•dot•o•my \ˌkəl-ˈdä-tə-mē, ˌku̇l-\ *n, pl* **-mies** : surgical incision of the pouch of Douglas
cu•lex \ˈkyü-ˌleks\ *n* **1** *cap* : a large cosmopolitan genus of mosquitoes

(family Culicidae) that includes the common house mosquito (*C. pipiens*) of Europe and No. America, a widespread tropical mosquito (*C. quinquefasciatus* syn. *C. fatigans*) which transmits some filarial worms parasitic in humans, and other mosquitoes which act as vectors of viral encephalitides **2** : a mosquito of the genus *Culex* — **cu·li·cine** \ˈkyü-lə-ˌsīn\ *adj or n*

cu·li·cide \ˈkyü-lə-ˌsīd\ *n* : an insecticide that destroys mosquitoes

Cu·li·coi·des \ˌkyü-lə-ˈkȯi-ˌdēz\ *n* : a genus of bloodsucking midges (family Ceratopogonidae) of which some are intermediate hosts of filarial parasites

cul·men \ˈkəl-mən\ *n* : a lobe of the cerebellum lying in the superior vermis just in front of the primary fissure

cul·ti·vate \ˈkəl-tə-ˌvāt\ *vb* **-vat·ed; -vat·ing** : CULTURE 1

cul·ti·va·tion \ˌkəl-tə-ˈvā-shən\ *n* : CULTURE 2

[1]**cul·ture** \ˈkəl-chər\ *n* **1 a** : the integrated pattern of human behavior that includes thought, speech, action, and artifacts and depends upon the human capacity for learning and transmitting knowledge to succeeding generations **b** : the customary beliefs, social forms, and material traits of a racial, religious, or social group **2 a** : the act or process of growing living material (as bacteria or viruses) in prepared nutrient media **b** : a product of cultivation in nutrient media — **cul·tur·al** \ˈkəl-chə-rəl\ *adj* — **cul·tur·al·ly** *adv*

[2]**culture** *vb* **cul·tured; cul·tur·ing** **1** : to grow (as microorganisms or tissues) in a prepared medium **2** : to start a culture from; *also* : to make a culture of ⟨~ milk⟩

culture shock *n* : a sense of confusion and uncertainty sometimes with feelings of anxiety that may affect people exposed to an alien culture or environment without adequate preparation

cu·mu·la·tive \ˈkyü-myə-lə-tiv, -ˌlā-\ *adj* : increasing in effect by successive doses (as of a drug or poison) — **cu·mu·la·tive·ly** *adv*

cumulative trauma disorder *n* : REPETITIVE STRAIN INJURY

cu·mu·lus \ˈkyü-myə-ləs\ *n, pl* **cu·mu·li** \-ˌlī, -ˌlē\ : the projecting mass of granulosa cells that bears the developing ovum in a graafian follicle — called also *discus proligerus*

cumulus ooph·o·rus \-ō-ˈä-fə-rəs\ *n* : CUMULUS

cu·ne·ate fasciculus \ˈkyü-nē-ˌāt-, -ət-\ *n, pl* **cuneate fasciculi** : FASCICULUS CUNEATUS

cuneate nucleus *n* : NUCLEUS CUNEATUS

cuneatus — see FASCICULUS CUNEATUS, NUCLEUS CUNEATUS

[1]**cu·ne·i·form** \kyu̇-ˈnē-ə-ˌfȯrm, ˈkyü-; ˈkyü-nə-\ *adj* **1** : of, relating to, or being a cuneiform bone or cartilage **2** *of a human skull* : wedge-shaped as viewed from above

[2]**cuneiform** *n* : a cuneiform bone or cartilage

cuneiform bone *n* **1** : any of three small bones of the tarsus situated between the navicular and the first three metatarsals: **a** : one on the medial side of the foot that is just proximal to the first metatarsal bone and is the largest of the three bones — called also *medial cuneiform, medial cuneiform bone* **b** : one that is situated between the other two bones proximal to the second metatarsal bone and is the smallest of the three bones — called also *intermediate cuneiform, intermediate cuneiform bone* **c** : one that is situated proximal to the third metatarsal bone and that lies between the intermediate cuneiform bone and the cuboid — called also *lateral cuneiform bone* **2** : TRIQUETRAL BONE

cuneiform cartilage *n* : either of a pair of rods of yellow elastic cartilage of which each lies on one side of the larynx in an aryepiglottic fold just below the arytenoid cartilage

cu·ne·us \ˈkyü-nē-əs\ *n, pl* **cu·nei** \-nē-ˌī\ : a convolution of the mesial surface of the occipital lobe of the brain above the calcarine sulcus that forms a part of the visual cortex

cun·ni·lin·gus \ˌkə-ni-ˈliŋ-gəs\ *also* **cun·ni·linc·tus** \-ˈliŋk-təs\ *n* : oral stimulation of the vulva or clitoris

[1]**cup** \ˈkəp\ *n* **1** : an athletic supporter reinforced for providing extra protection to the wearer in certain strenuous sports (as hockey or football) **2** : a cap of metal or plastic shaped like the femoral head and used in plastic reconstruction of the hip joint

[2]**cup** *vb* **cupped; cup·ping** **1** : to treat by cupping **2** : to undergo or perform cupping

cup·ping *n* : a technique formerly employed for drawing blood to the surface of the body by application of a glass vessel from which air had been evacuated by heat to form a partial vacuum

cu·pu·la \ˈkyü-pyu̇-lə, -pu̇-\ *n, pl* **cu·pu·lae** \-ˌlē\ **1** : the bony apex of the cochlea **2** : the peak of the pleural sac covering the apex of the lung

cur·able \ˈkyu̇r-ə-bəl\ *adj* : capable of being cured

cu·ra·re *also* **cu·ra·ri** \kyu̇-ˈrär-ē, ku̇-\ *n* : a dried aqueous extract esp. of a vine (as *Strychnos toxifera* of the family Loganiaceae or *Chondodendron tomentosum* of the family Menispermaceae) that produces muscle relaxation and is used in arrow poisons by So. American Indians — compare TUBOCURARINE

cu·ra·ri·form \kyu̇-ˈrär-ə-ˌfȯrm, ku̇-\ *adj* : producing or characterized by the muscular relaxation typical of curare ⟨~ drugs⟩

cu·ra·rize \-ˈrär-ˌīz\ *vb* **-rized; -riz·ing** : to treat with curare — **cu·ra·ri·za·tion** \-ˌrär-ə-ˈzā-shən\ *n*

cu·ra·tive \ˈkyu̇r-ə-tiv\ *adj* : relating to or used in the cure of diseases — **curative** *n* — **cu·ra·tive·ly** *adv*

curb \ˈkərb\ *n* : a swelling of the lower part of the hock of a horse that is due to ligament strain or rupture and usu. causes lameness

cur·cu·min \ˈkər-kyə-mən\ *n* : an orange-yellow crystalline compound $C_{21}H_{20}O_6$ that constitutes the chief coloring principle of turmeric

¹**cure** \ˈkyu̇r\ *n* **1** : recovery from a disease ⟨his ~ was complete⟩; *also* : remission of signs or symptoms of a disease esp. during a prolonged period of observation ⟨a clinical ~⟩ **2** : a drug, treatment, regimen, or other agency that cures a disease **3** : a course or period of treatment; *esp* : one designed to interrupt an addiction or compulsive habit or to improve general health **4** : SPA

²**cure** *vb* **cured; cur·ing** **1 a** : to make or become healthy, sound, or normal again ⟨~ a patient of his illness⟩ **b** : to bring about recovery from ⟨~ a disease⟩ **2** : to take a cure (as at a spa) — **cur·er** *n*

cu·ret·tage \ˌkyu̇r-ə-ˈtäzh\ *n* : a surgical scraping or cleaning by means of a curette

¹**cu·rette** *also* **cu·ret** \kyu̇-ˈret\ *n* : a surgical instrument that has a scoop, loop, or ring at its tip and is used in performing curettage

²**curette** *also* **curet** *vb* **cu·rett·ed; cu·rett·ing** : to perform curettage on — **cu·rette·ment** \kyu̇-ˈret-mənt\ *n*

cu·rie \ˈkyu̇r-(ˌ)ē, kyu̇-ˈrē\ *n* **1** : a unit quantity of any radioactive nuclide in which 3.7×10^{10} disintegrations occur per second **2** : a unit of radioactivity equal to 3.7×10^{10} disintegrations per second

Curie, Pierre (1859–1906), and **Marie Słodowska (1867–1934),** French chemists and physicists.

cu·ri·um \ˈkyu̇r-ē-əm\ *n* : a metallic radioactive trivalent element produced artificially — symbol *Cm;* see ELEMENT table

Cur·ling's ulcer \ˈkər-liŋz-\ *n* : acute gastroduodenal ulceration following severe skin burns

Cur·ling \ˈkər-liŋ\, **Thomas Blizard (1811–1888),** British surgeon.

cur·rent \ˈkər-ənt\ *n* : a flow of electric charge; *also* : the rate of such flow

cur·va·ture \ˈkər-və-ˌchu̇r, -chər, -ˌtyu̇r\ *n* **1** : an abnormal curving (as of the spine) — see KYPHOSIS, SCOLIOSIS **2** : a curved surface of an organ (as the stomach) — see GREATER CURVATURE, LESSER CURVATURE

cush·ing·oid \ˈku̇-shiŋ-ˌȯid\ *adj, often cap* : resembling Cushing's disease esp. in facies or habitus

Cush·ing's disease \ˈku̇-shiŋz-\ *n* : Cushing's syndrome esp. when caused by excessive production of ACTH by the pituitary gland

Cush·ing, Harvey Williams (1869–1939), American neurosurgeon.

Cushing's syndrome *n* : an abnormal condition that is caused by excess corticosteroids and esp. cortisol due either to hyperfunction of the adrenal gland or to prolonged use of corticosteroid medications and is characterized esp. by moon face with plethora, truncal obesity, fatigue, hypertension, muscle weakness, and easy bruising — called also *adrenogenital syndrome;* compare CUSHING'S DISEASE, HYPERADRENOCORTICISM

cush·ion \ˈku̇-shən\ *n* **1** : a bodily part resembling a pad **2** : a medical procedure or drug that eases discomfort without necessarily affecting the basic condition of the patient

cusp \ˈkəsp\ *n* **1** : a point on the grinding surface of a tooth **2** : a fold or flap of a cardiac valve — **cus·pal** \ˈkəs-pəl\ *adj*

cus·pid \ˈkəs-pəd\ *n* : a canine tooth

cus·to·di·al \ˌkəs-ˈtō-dē-əl\ *adj* **1** : relating to, providing, or being protective care or services for basic needs ⟨~ care⟩ **2** : having sole or primary custody of a child ⟨~ parents⟩

¹**cut** \ˈkət\ *vb* **cut; cut·ting** **1 a** : to penetrate with or as if with an edged instrument **b** : to cut or operate on in surgery: as (1) : to subject (a domestic animal) to castration (2) : to perform lithotomy on **c** : to experience the emergence of (a tooth) through the gum **2** : to function as or in the manner of an edged tool ⟨a knife that ~*s* well⟩ **3** : to subject to trimming or paring ⟨~ one's nails⟩

²**cut** *n* **1 a** : an opening made with an edged instrument **b** : a wound made by something sharp **2** : a stroke or blow with the edge of a sharp implement (as a knife)

cu·ta·ne·ous \kyu̇-ˈtā-nē-əs\ *adj* : of, relating to, or affecting the skin ⟨a ~ infection⟩ — **cu·ta·ne·ous·ly** *adv*

cutaneous T–cell lymphoma *n* : any of several non-Hodgkin lymphomas (as mycosis fungoides or Sezary syndrome) that are marked by clusters of malignant helper T cells in the epidermis causing skin lesions and eruptions which typically progress to tumors and may spread to lymph nodes and internal organs

cut·down \ˈkət-ˌdau̇n\ *n* : incision of a superficial blood vessel (as a vein) to facilitate insertion of a catheter (as for administration of fluids)

Cu·te·re·bra \ˌkyü-tə-ˈrē-brə, kyu̇-ˈter-ə-brə\ *n* : a genus of botflies (family Cuterebridae) with larvae that form tumors under the skin of small mammals (as rodents and rabbits)

cu·ti·cle \ˈkyü-ti-kəl\ *n* **1 a** : the outermost layer of integument composed of epidermis **b** : the outermost membranous layer of a hair consisting of cornified epithelial cells **2** : dead or horny epidermis (as that surrounding the base and sides of a fingernail or toenail) — **cu·tic·u·lar** \kyu̇-ˈti-kyə-lər\ *adj*

cu·ti·re·ac·tion \ˌkyü-ti-rē-ˈak-shən, ˈkyü-ti-rē-ˌ\ *n* : a local inflammatory reaction of the skin that occurs in certain infectious diseases following the application to or injection into the skin of a preparation of organisms producing the disease

cu·tis \ˈkyü-təs\ *n, pl* **cu·tes** \-ˌtēz\ *or* **cu·tis·es** : DERMIS

Cu·vie·ri·an vein \(ˌ)kyü-ˈvir-ē-ən-, ˌkyü-vē-ˈir-\ *n* : CARDINAL VEIN

Cu·vier \ˈkü-vē-ˌā, ˈkyü-; kūē-ˈvyā\, **Georges** (*orig.* **Jean–Léopold–Nicolas–Frédéric**) **(1769–1832),** French naturalist.

CVA *abbr* cerebrovascular accident

CVD *abbr* cardiovascular disease

CVP *abbr* central venous pressure

CVS *abbr* chorionic villus sampling

cyan- *or* **cyano-** *comb form* **1** : blue ⟨*cyan*osis⟩ **2** : cyanide ⟨*cyano*genetic⟩

cy·a·nide \ˈsī-ə-ˌnīd, -nəd\ *n* : any of several compounds (as potassium cyanide) that contain the monovalent group –CN, react with and inactivate respiratory enzymes, and are rapidly lethal producing drowsiness, tachycardia, coma, and finally death

cy·a·no·ac·ry·late \ˌsī-ə-nō-ˈa-krə-ˌlāt, sī-ˌa-nō-\ *n* : any of several liquid acrylate monomers used as adhesives in medicine on living tissue to close wounds in surgery

cy·a·no·co·bal·a·min \-kō-ˈba-lə-mən\ *also* **cy·a·no·co·bal·a·mine** \-ˌmēn\ *n* : VITAMIN B_{12}

cy·a·no·gen·ic \ˌsī-ə-nō-ˈjen-ik, sī-ˌa-nō-\ *also* **cy·a·no·ge·net·ic** \-jə-ˈnet-ik\ *adj* : capable of producing cyanide (as hydrogen cyanide) ⟨~ glycosides⟩ — **cy·a·no·gen·e·sis** \-ˈje-nə-səs\ *n*

cy·a·no·met·he·mo·glo·bin \ˌsī-ə-ˌnō-(ˌ)met-ˈhē-mə-ˌglō-bən\ *or* **cy·an·met·he·mo·glo·bin** \ˌsī-ˌan-(ˌ)met-, ˌsī-ən-\ *n* : a bright red crystalline compound formed by the action of hydrogen cyanide on methemoglobin in the cold or on oxyhemoglobin at body temperature

cy·a·nosed \ˈsī-ə-ˌnōst, -ˌnōzd\ *adj* : affected with cyanosis

cy·a·no·sis \ˌsī-ə-ˈnō-səs\ *n, pl* **-no·ses** \-ˌsēz\ : a bluish or purplish discoloration (as of skin) due to deficient oxygenation of the blood — **cy·a·not·ic** \-ˈnä-tik\ *adj*

cycl- *or* **cyclo-** *comb form* **1** : ciliary body (of the eye) ⟨*cycl*itis⟩ ⟨*cyclo*dialysis⟩ **2** : containing a ring of atoms — in names of organic compounds ⟨*cyclo*hexane⟩

cy·cla·mate \ˈsī-klə-ˌmāt, -mət\ *n* : an artificially prepared salt of sodium or calcium used esp. formerly as a sweetener but now largely discontinued because of the possibly harmful effects of its metabolic breakdown product cyclohexylamine

cy·clan·de·late \ˌsī-ˈkland-ᵊl-ˌāt\ *n* : an antispasmodic drug $C_{17}H_{24}O_3$ used esp. formerly as a vasodilator

cy·claz·o·cine \sī-ˈkla-zə-ˌsēn, -sən\ *n* : an analgesic drug $C_{18}H_{25}NO$ that inhibits the effect of morphine and related addictive drugs and is used in the treatment of drug addiction

[1]**cy·cle** \ˈsī-kəl\ *n* : a recurring series of events: as **a** (1) : a series of stages through which an organism tends to pass once in a fixed order; *also* : a series of stages through which a population of organisms tends to pass more or less together — see LIFE CYCLE (2) : a series of physiological, biochemical, or psychological stages that recur in the same individual — see CARDIAC CYCLE, MENSTRUAL CYCLE, KREBS CYCLE **b** : one complete performance of a vibration, electric oscillation, current alternation, or other periodic process — **cy·clic** \ˈsī-klik, ˈsi-\ *or* **cy·cli·cal** \ˈsī-kli-kəl, ˈsi-\ *adj* — **cy·cli·cal·ly** *also* **cy·clic·ly** *adv*

[2]**cycle** *vb* **cycled; cycling** : to undergo the estrous cycle

cy·clec·to·my \sī-ˈklek-tə-mē, si-\ *n, pl* **-mies** : surgical removal of part of the ciliary muscle or body

cyclic adenosine monophosphate *n* : CYCLIC AMP

cyclic AMP *n* : a cyclic mononucleotide of adenosine that is formed from ATP and is responsible for the intracellular mediation of hormonal effects on various cellular processes — abbr. *cAMP*

cyclic GMP \-ˌjē-(ˌ)em-ˈpē\ *n* : a cyclic mononucleotide of guanosine that acts similarly to cyclic AMP as a second messenger in response to hormones

cyclic guanosine monophosphate *n* : CYCLIC GMP

cy·clic·i·ty \sī-ˈkli-sə-tē, si-\ *n, pl* **-ties** : the quality or state of being cyclic

cy·clin \ˈsī-klən, ˈsi-\ *n* : any of a group of proteins active in controlling the cell cycle and in initiating DNA synthesis

cy·cli·tis \sə-ˈklī-təs, sī-\ *n* : inflammation of the ciliary body

cy·cli·zine \ˈsī-klə-ˌzēn\ *n* : an antiemetic drug used esp. in the form of its hydrochloride $C_{18}H_{22}N_2 \cdot HCl$ in the treatment of motion sickness — see MAREZINE

cyclo- — see CYCL-

cy·clo·ben·za·prine \ˌsī-klō-ˈben-zə-ˌprēn\ *n* : a skeletal muscle relaxant used in the form of its hydrochloride $C_{20}H_{21}N \cdot HCl$ to relieve muscle spasms and pain — see AMRIX, FEXMID, FLEXERIL

cy·clo·di·al·y·sis \ˌsī-klō-dī-ˈa-lə-səs\ *n, pl* **-y·ses** \-ˌsēz\ : surgical detachment of the ciliary body from the sclera to reduce tension in the eyeball in some cases of glaucoma

cy·clo·dia·ther·my \-ˈdī-ə-ˌthər-mē\ *n, pl* **-mies** : partial or complete destruction of the ciliary body by diathermy to relieve some conditions (as glaucoma) characterized by increased tension within the eyeball

Cy•clo•gyl \ˈsī-klō-ˌgil\ *trademark* — used for a preparation of the hydrochloride of cyclopentolate

cy•clo•hex•ane \ˌsī-klō-ˈhek-ˌsān\ *n* : a pungent hydrocarbon C_6H_{12} found in petroleum or made synthetically

cy•clo•hex•yl•a•mine \-hek-ˈsi-lə-ˌmēn\ *n* : a colorless liquid amine $C_6H_{11}NH_2$ of cyclohexane that is believed to be harmful as a metabolic breakdown product of cyclamate

[1]**cy•cloid** \ˈsī-ˌklȯid\ *n* : a cycloid individual

[2]**cycloid** *adj* : relating to, having, or being a personality characterized by alternating high and low moods — compare CYCLOTHYMIC

cy•clo•ox•y•gen•ase \ˌsī-klō-ˈäk-si-jə-ˌnās, -äk-ˈsi-jə-, -ˌnāz\ *n* : an enzyme that catalyzes the conversion of arachidonic acid to prostaglandins, is inactivated by aspirin and other NSAIDs, and has two isoforms — see COX-1, COX-2

cy•clo•pen•to•late \ˌsī-klō-ˈpen-tə-ˌlāt, ˌsi-\ *n* : an anticholinergic drug used esp. in the form of its hydrochloride $C_{17}H_{25}NO_3{\cdot}HCl$ to dilate the pupil of the eye for ophthalmologic examination — see CYCLOGYL

cy•clo•phos•pha•mide \-ˈfäs-fə-ˌmīd\ *n* : an immunosuppressive and antineoplastic drug $C_7H_{15}Cl_2N_2O_2P$ used in the treatment of lymphomas and some leukemias — see CYTOXAN

cy•clo•pia \sī-ˈklō-pē-ə\ *n* : a developmental anomaly characterized by the presence of a single median eye

cy•clo•ple•gia \ˌsī-klō-ˈplē-jə, ˌsi-, -jē-ə\ *n* : paralysis of the ciliary muscle of the eye

[1]**cy•clo•ple•gic** \-ˈplē-jik\ *adj* : producing, involving, or characterized by cycloplegia ⟨~ agents⟩ ⟨~ refraction⟩

[2]**cycloplegic** *n* : a cycloplegic agent

cy•clo•pro•pane \-ˈprō-ˌpān\ *n* : a flammable gaseous saturated cyclic hydrocarbon C_3H_6 sometimes used as a general anesthetic

cy•clops \ˈsī-ˌkläps\ *n, pl* **cy•clo•pes** \sī-ˈklō-(ˌ)pēz\ : an individual or fetus abnormal in having a single eye or the usual two orbits fused

cy•clo•ser•ine \ˌsī-klō-ˈser-ˌēn, ˌsi-\ *n* : a broad-spectrum antibiotic $C_3H_6N_2O_2$ produced by an actinomycete of the genus *Streptomyces* (*S. orchidaceus*) and used esp. in the treatment of tuberculosis

cy•clo•spora \ˌsī-klō-ˈspȯr-ə\ *n* **1** *cap* : a genus of coccidian protozoans including one (*C. cayetanensis*) causing diarrhea in humans **2** : a protozoan of the genus *Cyclospora*

cy•clo•spo•ri•a•sis \ˌsī-klō-spə-ˈrī-ə-səs\ *n, pl* **-a•ses** \-ˌsēz\ : infection with or disease caused by a cyclospora

cy•clo•spor•in \ˌsī-klə-ˈspȯr-ᵊn\ *n* : any of a group of polypeptides with immunosuppressive properties obtained as metabolites from various fungi or prepared synthetically; *esp* : CYCLOSPORINE

cy•clo•spor•ine \ˌsī-klə-ˈspȯr-ᵊn, -ˌēn\ *n* : a cyclosporin $C_{62}H_{111}N_{11}O_{12}$ that is obtained from a fungus (*Beauveria nivea* syn. *Tolypocladium inflatum*) and is used as an immunosuppressant esp. to prevent rejection of transplanted organs and to treat rheumatoid arthritis and psoriasis — see NEORAL, RESTASIS, SANDIMMUNE

cyclosporine A *or* **cyclosporin A** *n* : CYCLOSPORINE

cy•clo•thyme \ˈsī-klə-ˌthīm\ *n* : a cyclothymic individual

cy•clo•thy•mia \ˌsī-klə-ˈthī-mē-ə\ *n* : a cyclothymic mood disorder

[1]**cy•clo•thy•mic** \-ˈthī-mik\ *adj* : relating to, having, or being a mood disorder characterized by alternating short episodes of depression and hypomania in a form less severe than that of bipolar disorder — compare CYCLOID

[2]**cyclothymic** *n* : a cyclothymic individual

cy•clo•tome \ˈsī-klə-ˌtōm\ *n* : a knife used in cyclotomy

cy•clot•o•my \sī-ˈklä-tə-mē\ *n, pl* **-mies** : incision or division of the ciliary body

cy•clo•tro•pia \ˌsī-klə-ˈtrō-pē-ə\ *n* : squint in which the eye rolls outward or inward around its front-to-back axis

cy•e•sis \sī-ˈē-səs\ *n, pl* **cy•e•ses** \-ˌsēz\ : PREGNANCY

cyl•in•droid \ˈsi-lən-ˌdrȯid, sə-ˈlin-\ *n* : a spurious or mucous urinary cast that resembles a hyaline cast but has one tapered, stringy, twisted end

cyl•in•dro•ma \ˌsi-lən-ˈdrō-mə\ *n, pl* **-mas** *also* **-ma•ta** \mə-tə\ : a tumor characterized by cylindrical masses consisting of epithelial cells and hyalinized stroma: **a** : a malignant tumor esp. of the respiratory tract or salivary glands **b** : a benign tumor of the skin and esp. the scalp

cyl•in•dru•ria \ˌsi-lən-ˈdru̇r-ē-ə\ *n* : the presence of casts in the urine

Cym•bal•ta \sim-ˈbȯl-tə\ *trademark* — used for a preparation of duloxetine

cy•no•pho•bia \-ˈfō-bē-ə\ *n* : a morbid fear of dogs

cy•pro•hep•ta•dine \ˌsī-prō-ˈhep-tə-ˌdēn\ *n* : a drug used orally in the form of its hydrochloride $C_{21}H_{21}N{\cdot}HCl$ esp. as an antihistamine to treat allergy symptoms (as sneezing and runny nose)

cy•prot•er•one \sī-ˈprä-tə-ˌrōn\ *n* : a synthetic steroid used in the form of its acetate $C_{24}H_{29}ClO_4$ to inhibit the action and secretion of testosterone

cyst \ˈsist\ *n* **1** : a closed sac having a distinct membrane and developing abnormally in a body cavity or structure **2** : a body resembling a cyst: as **a** : a capsule formed about a minute organism going into a resting or spore stage; *also* : this capsule with its contents **b** : a resistant cover about a parasite produced by the parasite or the host — compare HYDATID 2a

cyst- *or* **cysti-** *or* **cysto-** *comb form* **1** : bladder ⟨*cyst*itis⟩ ⟨*cysto*plasty⟩ **2** : cyst ⟨*cysto*gastrostomy⟩

-cyst \ˌsist\ *n comb form* : bladder : sac ⟨blasto*cyst*⟩

cyst•ad•e•no•ma \ˌsis-ˌtad-ᵊn-ˈō-mə\ *n, pl* **-mas** *also* **-ma•ta** \-mə-tə\ : an adenoma marked by a cystic structure — **cyst•ad•e•no•ma•tous** \-mə-təs\ *adj*

cys•te•amine \sis-ˈtē-ə-mən\ *n* : a cysteine derivative used in the form of its bitartrate $C_2H_7NS·C_4H_6O_6$ to treat cystinosis and esp. formerly as an antidote for acetaminophen overdose

cys•tec•to•my \sis-ˈtek-tə-mē\ *n, pl* **-mies** **1** : the surgical excision of a cyst ⟨ovarian ~⟩ **2** : the removal of all or a portion of the urinary bladder

cys•teine \ˈsis-tə-ˌēn\ *n* : a sulfur-containing amino acid $C_3H_7NO_2S$ occurring in many proteins and glutathione and readily oxidizable to cystine

cysti- — see CYST-

cys•tic \ˈsis-tik\ *adj* **1** : relating to, composed of, or containing cysts ⟨a ~ tumor⟩ **2** : of or relating to the urinary bladder or the gallbladder **3** : enclosed in a cyst ⟨a ~ worm larva⟩

cystica — see OSTEITIS FIBROSA CYSTICA, OSTEITIS FIBROSA CYSTICA GENERALISTA

cystic duct *n* : the duct from the gallbladder that unites with the hepatic duct to form the common bile duct

cys•ti•cer•coid \ˌsis-tə-ˈsər-ˌkȯid\ *n* : a tapeworm larva having an invaginated scolex and solid hind part

cys•ti•cer•co•sis \-(ˌ)sər-ˈkō-səs\ *n, pl* **-co•ses** \-ˌsēz\ : infestation with or disease caused by cysticerci

cys•ti•cer•cus \-ˈsər-kəs\ *n, pl* **-cer•ci** \-ˈsər-ˌsī, -ˌkī\ : a tapeworm larva that consists of a fluid-filled sac containing an invaginated scolex, is situated in the tissues of an intermediate host, and is capable of developing into an adult tapeworm when eaten by a suitable definitive host — called also *bladder worm, measle* — **cys•ti•cer•cal** \-ˈsər-kəl\ *adj*

cystic fibrosis *n* : a common hereditary disease esp. in Caucasian populations that appears usu. in early childhood, is inherited as an autosomal recessive trait, involves functional disorder of the exocrine glands, and is marked esp. by faulty digestion due to a deficiency of pancreatic enzymes, by difficulty in breathing due to mucus accumulation in airways, and by excessive loss of salt in the sweat — called also *fibrocystic disease of the pancreas, mucoviscidosis*

cys•tine \ˈsis-ˌtēn\ *n* : a crystalline amino acid $C_6H_{12}N_2O_4S_2$ that is widespread in proteins (as keratins) and is a major metabolic sulfur source

cys•ti•no•sis \ˌsis-tə-ˈnō-səs\ *n, pl* **-no•ses** \-ˌsēz\ : a recessive autosomally inherited disease characterized esp. by cystinuria and deposits of cystine throughout the body — **cys•ti•not•ic** \-ˈnä-tik\ *adj*

cys•tin•uria \ˌsis-tə-ˈnu̇r-ē-ə, -ˈnyu̇r-\ *n* : a metabolic defect that is characterized by excretion of excessive amounts of cystine in the urine and sometimes by the formation of calculi in the urinary tract and is inherited as an autosomal recessive trait — **cys•tin•uric** \-ˈnu̇r-ik, -ˈnyu̇r-\ *adj*

cys•ti•tis \sis-ˈtī-təs\ *n, pl* **cys•tit•i•des** \-ˈti-tə-ˌdēz\ : inflammation of the urinary bladder — **cys•tit•ic** \(ˈ)sis-ˈti-tik\ *adj*

cysto- — see CYST-

cys•to•cele \ˈsis-tə-ˌsēl\ *n* : hernia of a bladder and esp. the urinary bladder : vesical hernia

cys•to•gas•tros•to•my \ˌsis-tō-(ˌ)gas-ˈträs-tə-mē\ *n, pl* **-mies** : creation of a surgical opening between the stomach and a nearby cyst for drainage

cys•to•gram \ˈsis-tə-ˌgram\ *n* : a radiograph made by cystography

cys•tog•ra•phy \sis-ˈtä-grə-fē\ *n, pl* **-phies** : X-ray photography of the urinary bladder after injection of a contrast medium — **cys•to•graph•ic** \-tə-ˈgra-fik\ *adj*

cys•toid \ˈsis-ˌtȯid\ *adj* : resembling a bladder

cys•to•lith \ˈsis-tə-ˌlith\ *n* : a urinary calculus

cys•to•li•thi•a•sis \ˌsis-tō-li-ˈthī-ə-səs\ *n, pl* **-a•ses** \-ˌsēz\ : the presence of calculi in the urinary bladder

cys•to•li•thot•o•my \-li-ˈthä-tə-mē\ *n, pl* **-mies** : surgical removal of a calculus from the urinary bladder

cys•tom•e•ter \sis-ˈtä-mə-tər\ *n* : an instrument designed to measure pressure within the urinary bladder in relation to its capacity — **cys•to•met•ric** \ˌsis-tə-ˈme-trik\ *adj* — **cys•tom•e•try** \sis-ˈtä-mə-trē\ *n*

cys•to•met•ro•gram \ˌsis-tə-ˈme-trə-ˌgram, -ˈmē-\ *n* : a graphic recording of a cystometric measurement

cys•to•me•trog•ra•phy \-mə-ˈträ-grə-fē\ *n, pl* **-phies** : the process of making a cystometrogram

cys•to•plas•ty \ˈsis-tə-ˌplas-tē\ *n, pl* **-ties** : a plastic surgery on the urinary bladder

cys•to•py•eli•tis \ˌsis-tə-ˌpī-ə-ˈlī-təs\ *n* : inflammation of the urinary bladder and of the pelvis of one or both kidneys

cys•tor•rha•phy \sis-ˈtōr-ə-fē\ *n, pl* **-phies** : suture of a wound, injury, or rupture in the urinary bladder

cys•to•sar•co•ma phyl•lo•des \ˌsis-tō-ˌsär-ˈkō-mə-fi-ˈlō-ˌdēz\ *n* : a slow-growing tumor of the breast that resembles a fibroadenoma

cys•to•scope \ˈsis-tə-ˌskōp\ *n* : a rigid endoscope for inspecting and passing instruments into the urethra and bladder — **cys•to•scop•ic** \ˌsis-tə-ˈskä-pik\ *adj* — **cys•tos•co•pist** \sis-ˈtäs-kə-pist\ *n*

cys•tos•co•py \sis-ˈtäs-kə-pē\ *n, pl* **-pies** : the use of a cystoscope to examine the bladder
cys•tos•to•my \sis-ˈtäs-tə-mē\ *n, pl* **-mies** : formation of an opening into the urinary bladder by surgical incision
cys•tot•o•my \sis-ˈtä-tə-mē\ *n, pl* **-mies** : surgical incision of the urinary bladder
cys•to•ure•ter•itis \ˌsis-tō-ˌyu̇r-ə-tə-ˈrī-təs\ *n* : combined inflammation of the urinary bladder and ureters
cys•to•ure•thro•cele \ˌsis-tō-yu̇-ˈrē-thrə-ˌsēl\ *n* : herniation of the neck of the female bladder and associated urethra into the vagina
cys•to•ure•thro•gram \-yu̇-ˈrē-thrə-ˌgram\ *n* : an X-ray photograph of the urinary bladder and urethra made after injection of these organs with a contrast medium — **cys•to•ure•throg•ra•phy** \-ˌyu̇r-i-ˈthrä-grə-fē\ *n*
cys•to•ure•thro•scope \ˌsis-tō-yu̇-ˈrē-thrə-ˌskōp\ *n* : an instrument used for the examination of the posterior urethra and bladder — **cys•to•ure•thros•co•py** \-ˌyu̇r-i-ˈthräs-kə-pē\ *n*
cyt- *or* **cyto-** *comb form* **1** : cell ⟨*cyto*logy⟩ **2** : cytoplasm ⟨*cyto*kinesis⟩
cyt•ar•a•bine \sī-ˈtar-ə-ˌbēn\ *n* : CYTOSINE ARABINOSIDE
-cyte \ˌsīt\ *n comb form* : cell ⟨leuko*cyte*⟩
cy•ti•dine \ˈsi-tə-ˌdēn\ *n* : a nucleoside containing cytosine
cy•to•ar•chi•tec•ton•ics \ˌsī-tō-ˌär-kə-(ˌ)tek-ˈtä-niks\ *n sing or pl* : CYTOARCHITECTURE — **cy•to•ar•chi•tec•ton•ic** \-nik\ *adj*
cy•to•ar•chi•tec•ture \ˌsī-tō-ˈär-kə-ˌtek-chər\ *n* : the cellular makeup of a bodily tissue or structure — **cy•to•ar•chi•tec•tur•al** \-ˌär-kə-ˈtek-chə-rəl\ *adj* — **cy•to•ar•chi•tec•tur•al•ly** *adv*
cy•to•chem•is•try \-ˈke-mə-strē\ *n, pl* **-tries** **1** : microscopic biochemistry **2** : the chemistry of cells — **cy•to•chem•i•cal** \-ˈke-mi-kəl\ *adj* — **cy•to•chem•i•cal•ly** \-mi-k(ə-)lē\ *adv* — **cy•to•chem•ist** \-ˈke-mist\ *n*
cy•to•chrome \ˈsī-tə-ˌkrōm\ *n* : any of several intracellular hemoprotein respiratory pigments that are enzymes functioning in electron transport as carriers of electrons
cytochrome c *n, often italicized third c* : the most abundant and stable of the cytochromes
cytochrome oxidase *n* : an iron-porphyrin enzyme important in cell respiration because of its ability to catalyze the oxidation of reduced cytochrome c in the presence of oxygen
cy•to•cid•al \ˌsī-tə-ˈsīd-ᵊl\ *adj* : killing or tending to kill individual cells ⟨~ RNA viruses⟩
cy•to•di•ag•no•sis \ˌsī-tō-ˌdī-ig-ˈnō-səs, -əg-\ *n, pl* **-no•ses** \-ˌsēz\ : diagnosis based upon the examination of cells found in the tissues or fluids of the body — **cy•to•di•ag•nos•tic** \-ˈnäs-tik\ *adj*
cy•to•dif•fer•en•ti•a•tion \ˌsī-tō-ˌdi-fə-ˌren-chē-ˈā-shən\ *n* : the development of specialized cells (as muscle, blood, or nerve cells) from undifferentiated precursors
cy•to•ge•net•ics \-jə-ˈne-tiks\ *n sing or pl* : a branch of biology that deals with the study of heredity and variation by the methods of both cytology and genetics — **cy•to•ge•net•ic** \-jə-ˈne-tik\ *or* **cy•to•ge•net•i•cal** \-ti-kəl\ *adj* — **cy•to•ge•net•i•cal•ly** \-ti-k(ə-)lē\ *adv* — **cy•to•ge•net•i•cist** \-ˈne-tə-sist\ *n*
cy•toid body \ˈsī-ˌtȯid-\ *n* : one of the white globular masses resembling cells that are found in the retina in some abnormal conditions
cy•to•ker•a•tin \ˌsī-tō-ˈker-ə-tᵊn\ *n* : any of a class of fibrous proteins that are intermediate filaments of the cytoplasm of epithelial cells and are sometimes used as markers to identify malignancies of epithelial origin
cy•to•kine \ˈsī-tə-ˌkīn\ *n* : any of a class of immunoregulatory substances (as lymphokines) that are secreted by cells of the immune system
cy•to•ki•ne•sis \ˌsī-tō-kə-ˈnē-səs, -kī-\ *n, pl* **-ne•ses** \-ˌsēz\ **1** : the cytoplasmic changes accompanying mitosis **2** : cleavage of the cytoplasm into daughter cells following nuclear division — compare KARYOKINESIS — **cy•to•ki•net•ic** \-ˈne-tik\ *adj*
cytol *abbr* cytological; cytology
cy•tol•o•gy \sī-ˈtä-lə-jē\ *n, pl* **-gies** **1 a** : a branch of biology dealing with the structure, function, multiplication, pathology, and life history of cells **b** : the cellular aspects of a process or structure **2** : the microscopic examination of cells obtained from the body (as by scraping) for diagnostic purposes : EXFOLIATIVE CYTOLOGY — called also *cytopathology* — **cy•to•log•i•cal** \ˌsīt-ᵊl-ˈä-ji-kəl\ *or* **cy•to•log•ic** \-ˈä-jik\ *adj* — **cy•to•log•i•cal•ly** \-ji-k(ə-)lē\ *adv* — **cy•tol•o•gist** \sī-ˈtä-lə-jist\ *n*
cy•to•ly•sin \ˌsīt-ᵊl-ˈīs-ᵊn\ *n* : a substance (as an antibody that lyses bacteria) producing cytolysis
cy•tol•y•sis \sī-ˈtä-lə-səs\ *n, pl* **-y•ses** \-ˌsēz\ : the usu. pathologic dissolution or disintegration of cells — **cy•to•lyt•ic** \ˌsīt-ᵊl-ˈi-tik\ *adj*
cytolytic T cell *n* : CYTOTOXIC T CELL
cytolytic T lymphocyte *n* : CYTOTOXIC T CELL
cy•to•me•gal•ic \ˌsī-tō-mi-ˈga-lik\ *adj* : characterized by or causing the formation of enlarged cells
cytomegalic inclusion disease *n* : a severe disease esp. of newborns that is caused by a cytomegalovirus and usu. affects the salivary glands, brain, kidneys, liver, and lungs — called also *inclusion disease*
cy•to•meg•a•lo•vi•rus \ˌsī-tə-ˌme-gə-lō-ˈvī-rəs\ *n* **1** : a herpesvirus (species *Human herpesvirus 5* of the genus *Cytomegalovirus*) that is transmitted chiefly in infected body fluids and secretions and that in healthy indi-

viduals causes an infection that is asymptomatic or is accompanied by mild symptoms (as fever or fatigue) but in immunocompromised individuals and newborns may cause an infection marked by serious symptoms (as pneumonia, retinitis, or seizures) **2** : infection with or disease caused by the cytomegalovirus — abbr. *CMV*

cy·tom·e·ter \sī-ˈtä-mə-tər\ *n* : an apparatus for counting and measuring cells

cy·tom·e·try \sī-ˈtä-mə-trē\ *n, pl* **-tries** : a technical specialty concerned with the counting of cells and esp. blood cells — see FLOW CYTOMETRY — **cy·to·met·ric** \ˌsī-tə-ˈme-trik\ *adj*

cy·to·mor·phol·o·gy \ˌsī-tə-mȯr-ˈfä-lə-jē\ *n, pl* **-gies** : the morphology of cells — **cy·to·mor·pho·log·i·cal** \-ˌmȯr-fə-ˈlä-ji-kəl\ *adj*

cy·to·path·ic \ˌsī-tə-ˈpa-thik\ *adj* : of, relating to, characterized by, or producing pathological changes in cells

cy·to·patho·gen·ic \-ˌpa-thə-ˈje-nik\ *adj* : causing or involving pathological changes in cells — **cy·to·patho·ge·nic·i·ty** \-jə-ˈni-sə-tē\ *n*

cy·to·pa·thol·o·gy \-pə-ˈthä-lə-jē, -pa-\ *n, pl* **-gies** **1** : a branch of pathology that deals with manifestations of disease at the cellular level **2** : CYTOLOGY 2 — **cy·to·patho·log·ic** \-ˌpa-thə-ˈlä-jik\ *also* **cy·to·patho·log·i·cal** \-ji-kəl\ *adj* — **cy·to·pa·thol·o·gist** \-pə-ˈthä-lə-jist, -pa-\ *n*

cy·to·pe·nia \-ˈpē-nē-ə\ *n* : a deficiency of cellular elements of the blood; *esp* : deficiency of a specific element (as granulocytes in granulocytopenia) — **cy·to·pe·nic** \-ˈpē-nik\ *adj*

cy·to·phil·ic \ˌsī-tə-ˈfi-lik\ *adj* : having an affinity for cells

cy·to·pho·tom·e·ter \ˌsī-tō-fō-ˈtä-mə-tər\ *n* : a photometer for use in cytophotometry

cy·to·pho·tom·e·try \-(ˌ)fō-ˈtä-mə-trē\ *n, pl* **-tries** : photometry applied to the study of the cell or its constituents — **cy·to·pho·to·met·ric** \-ˌfō-tə-ˈme-trik\ *adj* — **cy·to·pho·to·met·ri·cal·ly** \-tri-k(ə-)lē\ *adv*

cy·to·phys·i·ol·o·gy \-ˌfi-zē-ˈä-lə-jē\ *n, pl* **-gies** : the physiology of cells — **cy·to·phys·i·o·log·i·cal** \-zē-ə-ˈlä-ji-kəl\ *adj*

cy·to·pi·pette \ˌsī-tō-pī-ˈpet\ *n* : a pipette with a bulb that contains a fluid which is released into the vagina and then sucked back with a sample of cells for a vaginal smear

cy·to·plasm \ˈsī-tə-ˌpla-zəm\ *n* : the organized complex of inorganic and organic substances external to the nuclear membrane of a cell and including the cytosol and membrane-bound organelles (as mitochondria) — **cy·to·plas·mic** \ˌsī-tə-ˈplaz-mik\ *adj* — **cy·to·plas·mi·cal·ly** \-mi-k(ə-)lē\ *adv*

cy·to·sine \ˈsī-tə-ˌsēn\ *n* : a pyrimidine base $C_4H_5N_3O$ that codes genetic information in the polynucleotide chain of DNA or RNA — compare ADENINE, GUANINE, THYMINE, URACIL

cytosine arabinoside *n* : a cytotoxic antineoplastic agent $C_9H_{13}N_3O_5$ that is a synthetic isomer of the naturally occurring nucleoside of cytosine and arabinose and is used esp. in the treatment of acute myelogenous leukemia in adults — called also *Ara-C*

cy·to·skel·e·ton \ˌsī-tō-ˈske-lət-ᵊn\ *n* : the network of protein filaments and microtubules in the cytoplasm that controls cell shape, maintains intracellular organization, and is involved in cell movement — **cy·to·skel·e·tal** \-ᵊl\ *adj*

cy·to·sol \ˈsī-tə-ˌsäl, -ˌsȯl\ *n* : the fluid portion of the cytoplasm exclusive of organelles and membranes — called also *hyaloplasm, ground substance* — **cy·to·sol·ic** \ˌsī-tə-ˈsä-lik, -ˈsȯ-\ *adj*

¹**cy·to·stat·ic** \ˌsī-tə-ˈsta-tik\ *adj* : tending to retard cellular activity and multiplication ⟨~ treatment of tumors⟩ — **cy·to·stat·i·cal·ly** \-ti-k(ə-)lē\ *adv*

²**cytostatic** *n* : a cytostatic agent

cy·to·tech·ni·cian \ˌsī-tə-(ˌ)tek-ˈni-shən\ *n* : CYTOTECHNOLOGIST

cy·to·tech·nol·o·gist \-ˈnä-lə-jist\ *n* : a medical technician trained in cytotechnology

cy·to·tech·nol·o·gy \-ˈnä-lə-jē\ *n, pl* **-gies** : a specialty in medical technology concerned with the identification of cells and cellular abnormalities (as in cancer)

cy·to·tox·ic \ˌsī-tə-ˈtäk-sik\ *adj* : toxic to cells ⟨~ lymphocytes⟩ ⟨~ drugs⟩ — **cy·to·tox·ic·i·ty** \-(ˌ)täk-ˈsi-sə-tē\ *n*

cytotoxic T cell *n* : a T cell that usu. bears CD8 molecular markers on its surface and that functions in cell-mediated immunity by destroying a cell (as one infected with a virus) having a specific antigenic molecule on its surface — called also *CTL, cytolytic T cell, cytolytic T lymphocyte, killer T cell, killer T lymphocyte;* compare HELPER T CELL, SUPPRESSOR T CELL

cy·to·tox·in \-ˈtäk-sən\ *n* : a substance (as a toxin or antibody) having a toxic effect on cells

cy·to·tro·pho·blast \ˌsī-tə-ˈtrō-fə-ˌblast\ *n* : the inner cellular layer of the trophoblast of an embryonic placenta-forming mammal that gives rise to the plasmodial syncytiotrophoblast covering the placental villi — **cy·to·tro·pho·blas·tic** \-ˌtrō-fə-ˈblas-tik\ *adj*

Cy·tox·an \sī-ˈtäk-sən\ *trademark* — used for a preparation of cyclophosphamide

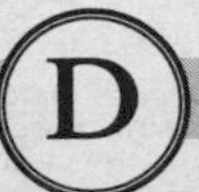

d *abbr* **1** died **2** diopter **3** disease

d- \ˌdē, ˈdē\ *prefix* **1** : dextrorotatory — usu. printed in italic ⟨*d*-tartaric acid⟩ **2** : having a similar configuration at a selected carbon atom to the configuration of dextrorotatory glyceraldehyde — usu. printed as a small capital ⟨D-fructose⟩

2,4–D — see entry alphabetized as TWO,FOUR-D in the letter *t*

da·big·a·tran \də-ˈbig-ə-ˌtran, ˌdab-ə-ˈga-\ *n* : an anticoagulant drug $C_{34}H_{41}N_7O_5 \cdot CH_4O_3S$ that inhibits the action of thrombin and is used orally to reduce the risk of stroke and treat or prevent deep vein thrombosis and pulmonary embolism — called also *dabigatran etexilate, dabigatran etexilate mesylate;* see PRADAXA

da·car·ba·zine \dä-ˈkär-bə-ˌzēn\ *n* : an antineoplastic agent $C_6H_{10}N_6O$ used to treat esp. metastatic malignant melanoma, tumors of adult soft tissue, and Hodgkin's lymphoma — see ABVD

dacry- *or* **dacryo-** *comb form* : lacrimal ⟨*dacryo*cystitis⟩

dac·ryo·ad·e·nec·to·my \ˌda-krē-(ˌ)ō-ˌad-ᵊn-ˈek-tə-mē\ *n, pl* **-mies** : excision of a lacrimal gland

dac·ry·o·cyst \ˈda-krē-ə-ˌsist\ *n* : LACRIMAL SAC

dac·ryo·cys·tec·to·my \ˌda-krē-(ˌ)ō-sis-ˈtek-tə-mē\ *n, pl* **-mies** : excision of a lacrimal sac

dac·ryo·cys·ti·tis \-sis-ˈtī-təs\ *n* : inflammation of the lacrimal sac

dac·ry·o·cys·tog·ra·phy \-sis-ˈtä-grə-fē\ *n, pl* **-phies** : radiographic visualization of the lacrimal sacs and associated structures after injection of a contrast medium

dac·ryo·cys·to·rhi·nos·to·my \-ˌsis-tə-ˌrī-ˈnäs-tə-mē\ *n, pl* **-mies** : surgical creation of a passage for drainage between the lacrimal sac and the nasal cavity

dac·ryo·cys·tos·to·my \-sis-ˈtäs-tə-mē\ *n, pl* **-mies** : an operation on a lacrimal sac to form a new opening (as for drainage)

dac·ryo·cys·tot·o·my \-sis-ˈtä-tə-mē\ *n, pl* **-mies** : incision (as for drainage) of a lacrimal sac

dac·ryo·lith \ˈda-krē-ə-ˌlith\ *n* : a concretion formed in a lacrimal passage

dac·ryo·ste·no·sis \ˌda-krē-(ˌ)ō-sti-ˈnō-səs\ *n, pl* **-o·ses** \-ˌsēz\ : a narrowing of the lacrimal duct

dac·ti·no·my·cin \ˌdak-tə-nō-ˈmīs-ᵊn\ *n* : a toxic antineoplastic drug $C_{62}H_{86}N_{12}O_{16}$ of the actinomycin group — called also *actinomycin D*

dactyl- *or* **dactylo-** *comb form* : finger : toe : digit ⟨*dactylo*logy⟩

-dac·tyl·ia *n comb form* : -DACTYLY ⟨*adactylia*⟩

-dac·tyl·ism *n comb form* : -DACTYLY ⟨oligo*dactylism*⟩

dac·ty·lol·o·gy \ˌdak-tə-ˈlä-lə-jē\ *n, pl* **-gies** : FINGER SPELLING

-dac·ty·lous *adj comb form* : having (such or so many) fingers or toes ⟨brachy*dactylous*⟩

-dac·ty·ly *n comb form, pl* **-lies** : condition of having (such or so many) fingers or toes ⟨poly*dactyly*⟩

dag·ga \ˈda-gə, ˈdä-\ *n, chiefly SoAfr* : MARIJUANA

DAH *abbr* disordered action of the heart

Dal·mane \ˈdal-ˌmān\ *n* : a preparation of the hydrochloride of flurazepam — formerly a U.S. registered trademark

Dal·ton·ism \ˈdȯlt-ᵊn-ˌi-zəm\ *n* : red-green color blindness occurring as a recessive sex-linked genetic trait; *broadly* : any form of color blindness

Dalton, John (1766–1844), British chemist and physicist.

¹dam \ˈdam\ *n* : a female parent — used esp. of a domestic animal

²dam *n* : RUBBER DAM — see DENTAL DAM

dam *abbr* dekameter

damp \ˈdamp\ *n* : a noxious or stifling gas or vapor; *esp* : one occurring in coal mines — usu. used in pl.; see BLACK DAMP, FIREDAMP

da·na·zol \ˈdä-nə-ˌzōl, ˈda-, -ˌzȯl\ *n* : a synthetic androgenic derivative $C_{22}H_{27}NO_2$ of ethisterone that suppresses hormone secretion by the adenohypophysis and is used esp. in the treatment of endometriosis

D&C *n* : DILATION AND CURETTAGE

D&E *n* : DILATION AND EVACUATION

dan·der \ˈdan-dər\ *n* : DANDRUFF; *specif* : minute scales from hair, feathers, or skin that may act as allergens

dan·druff \ˈdan-drəf\ *n* : scaly white or grayish flakes of dead skin cells esp. of the scalp; *also* : the condition marked by excessive shedding of such flakes and usu. accompanied by itching — **dan·druffy** \-drə-fē\ *adj*

D&X *n* : DILATION AND EXTRACTION

dan·dy fever \ˈdan-dē-\ *n* : DENGUE

Dane particle \ˈdān-\ *n* : a spherical particle found in the serum in hepatitis B that is the virion of the causative virus

Dane, David Maurice Surrey (1923–1998), British pathologist.

dap·a·gli·flo·zin \ˌda-pə-glə-ˈflō-zən\ *n* : a drug $C_{21}H_{25}ClO_6 \cdot C_3H_8O_2 \cdot H_2O$ that lowers blood sugar by reducing the reabsorption of glucose from the kidneys and is taken orally to treat type 2 diabetes — see FARXIGA

dap·sone \ˈdap-ˌsōn, -ˌzōn\ *n* : an antimicrobial agent $C_{12}H_{12}N_2O_2S$ used orally to treat leprosy and dermatitis herpetiformis and topically to treat acne vulgaris — called also *diaminodiphenyl sulfone;* see ACZONE

Dar•a•prim \ˈder-ə-ˌprim\ *trademark* — used for a preparation of pyrimethamine

dar•be•poe•tin al•fa \ˌdär-bə-ˈpō-ə-tən-ˈal-fə, -ˈpȯi-tən-\ *n* : a glycoprotein that is similar to human erythropoietin, stimulates the production of red blood cells, and is administered by injection esp. to treat anemia (as that associated with chemotherapy) — see ARANESP

Da•rier's disease \dar-ˈyāz-\ *n* : a genetically determined skin condition characterized by patches of keratotic papules — called also *keratosis follicularis*

Da•rier \dȧr-ˈyā\, **Jean Ferdinand (1856–1938)**, French dermatologist.

dark adaptation *n* : the phenomena including dilation of the pupil, increase in retinal sensitivity, shift of the region of maximum luminosity toward the blue, and regeneration of rhodopsin by which the eye adapts to conditions of reduced illumination — compare LIGHT ADAPTATION — **dark–adapted** *adj*

dark field *n* : the dark area that serves as the background for objects viewed in an ultramicroscope — **dark–field** *adj*

dark–field microscope *n* : ULTRAMICROSCOPE — **dark–field microscopy** *n*

darm•stadt•i•um \ˌdärm-ˈsta-tē-əm\ *n* : a short-lived radioactive element that is artificially produced — symbol *Ds;* see ELEMENT table

dar•tos \ˈdär-ˌtäs, -təs\ *n* : a thin layer of vascular contractile tissue that contains smooth muscle fibers but no fat and is situated beneath the skin of the scrotum or beneath that of the labia majora

da•ru•na•vir \də-ˈrü-nə-ˌvir\ *n* : a protease inhibitor $C_{27}H_{37}N_3O_7S{\cdot}C_2H_5OH$ taken orally in conjunction with other antiretroviral agents in the treatment of HIV infection — see PREZCOBIX, PREZISTA

Dar•vo•cet–N \ˈdär-vō-ˌset-ˈen\ *trademark* — used for a preparation of the napsylate of propoxyphene in combination with acetaminophen

Dar•von \ˈdär-ˌvän\ *trademark* — used for a preparation of the hydrochloride of propoxyphene

Darwin's tubercle *n* : the slight projection occas. present on the edge of the external human ear and assumed by some scientists to represent the pointed part of the ear of quadrupeds

Dar•win \ˈdär-wən\, **Charles Robert (1809–1882)**, British naturalist.

DASH \ˈdash\ *n* [*d*ietary *a*pproaches to *s*top *h*ypertension] : a diet that is designed to lower blood pressure and emphasizes the consumption of fruit, vegetables, grains, and low-fat or nonfat dairy products

da•ta \ˈdā-tə, ˈda-, ˈdä-\ *n sing or pl* : factual information (as measurements or statistics) used as a basis for reasoning, discussion, or calculation

date rape *n* : rape committed by the victim's date; *broadly* : ACQUAINTANCE RAPE

date rape drug *n* : a drug (as GHB) given surreptitiously (as in a drink) to induce an unconscious or sedated state in a potential date rape victim

da•tu•ra \də-ˈtu̇r-ə, -ˈtyu̇r-\ *n* **1** *cap* : a genus of strong-scented herbs, shrubs, and trees (family Solanaceae) related to the potato and tomato and including some used as sources of medicinal alkaloids (as stramonium from jimsonweed) or in folk rites or illicitly for their poisonous, narcotic, or hallucinogenic properties **2** : any plant of the genus *Datura*

dau *abbr* daughter

[1]**daugh•ter** \ˈdȯ-tər\ *n* **1 a** : a human female having the relation of child to a parent **b** : a female offspring of an animal **2** : an atomic species that is the immediate product of the radioactive decay of a given element

[2]**daughter** *adj* **1** : having the characteristics or relationship of a daughter **2** : belonging to the first generation of offspring, organelles, or molecules produced by reproduction, division, or replication ⟨a ~ cell⟩ ⟨~ chromosomes⟩ ⟨~ DNA molecules⟩

dau•no•my•cin \ˌdȯ-nə-ˈmīs-ᵊn, ˌdau̇-\ *n* : DAUNORUBICIN

dau•no•ru•bi•cin \-ˈrü-bə-sən\ *n* : an antibiotic that is a nitrogenous glycoside used in the form of its hydrochloride $C_{27}H_{29}NO_{10}{\cdot}HCl$ esp. in the treatment of some leukemias

dawn phenomenon *n* : a rise in the level of glucose in the blood plasma that occurs in early morning before breakfast and that may progress to hyperglycemia in diabetics — compare SOMOGYI EFFECT

day•dream \ˈdā-ˌdrēm\ *n* : a visionary creation of the imagination experienced while awake; *esp* : a gratifying reverie usu. of wish fulfillment — **daydream** *vb* — **day•dream•er** *n*

day•mare \ˈdā-ˌmar\ *n* : a nightmarish fantasy experienced while awake

Day•pro *trademark* — used for a preparation of oxaprozin

Db *symbol* dubnium

DBCP \ˌdē-(ˌ)bē-(ˌ)sē-ˈpē\ *n* : an agricultural pesticide $C_3H_5Br_2Cl$ that is a suspected carcinogen and cause of sterility in human males — called also *dibromochloropropane*

DBP *abbr* diastolic blood pressure

DBS *abbr* deep brain stimulation

DC *abbr* doctor of chiropractic

DCIS *abbr* ductal carcinoma in situ

DD *abbr* developmentally disabled

DDAVP \ˌdē-ˌdē-ˌā-ˌvē-ˈpē\ *trademark* — used for a preparation of the acetate of desmopressin

ddC \ˌdē-(ˌ)dē-ˈsē\ *n, often all cap* : a synthetic nucleoside analog $C_9H_{13}N_3O_3$ that inhibits replication of retroviruses and is used in the treatment

of advanced HIV infection — called also *dideoxycytidine, zalcitabine*
DDD \-ˈdē\ *n* : an insecticide $C_{14}H_{10}Cl_4$ closely related chemically and similar in properties to DDT
DDE \-ˈē\ *n* : a persistent organochlorine $C_{15}H_8Cl_4$ that is produced by the metabolic breakdown of DDT
ddI \-ˈī\ *n, often all cap* : a synthetic nucleoside analog $C_{10}H_{12}N_4O_3$ having properties and uses similar to those of ddC — called also *didanosine, dideoxyinosine;* see VIDEX
DDS *abbr* doctor of dental surgery
DDT \ˌdēd-(ˌ)ē-ˈtē\ *n* : a colorless odorless water-insoluble crystalline insecticide $C_{14}H_9Cl_5$ that tends to accumulate in ecosystems and has toxic effects on many vertebrates
DDVP \ˌdē-(ˌ)dē-(ˌ)vē-ˈpē\ *n* : DICHLORVOS
[1]**dead** \ˈded\ *adj* **1** : deprived of life : having died **2** : lacking power to move, feel, or respond : NUMB
[2]**dead** *n, pl* **dead** : one that is dead — usu. used collectively
dead·ly \ˈded-lē\ *adj* **dead·li·er; -est** : likely to cause or capable of causing death ⟨a ∼ disease⟩ ⟨a ∼ poison⟩ — **dead·li·ness** \-nəs\ *n*
deadly nightshade *n* : BELLADONNA 1
dead space *n* **1** : space in the respiratory system in which air does not undergo significant gaseous exchange — see ANATOMICAL DEAD SPACE, PHYSIOLOGICAL DEAD SPACE **2** : a space (as that in the chest following excision of a lung) left in the body as the result of a surgical procedure
deaf \ˈdef\ *adj* : lacking or deficient in the sense of hearing — **deaf·ness** *n*
deaf–aid \ˈdef-ˌād\ *n, chiefly Brit* : HEARING AID
deaf·en \ˈde-fən\ *vb* **deaf·ened; deaf·en·ing 1** : to make deaf **2** : to cause deafness or stun one with noise — **deaf·en·ing·ly** \-f(ə-)niŋ-lē\ *adv*
de·af·fer·en·ta·tion \ˌdē-ˌa-fə-ˌren-ˈtā-shən\ *n* : the freeing of a motor nerve from sensory components by severing the dorsal root central to the dorsal ganglion
[1]**deaf–mute** \ˈdef-ˈmyüt\ *adj, often offensive* : lacking the sense of hearing and the ability to speak — **deaf–mute·ness** *n, sometimes offensive* — **deaf–mut·ism** \-ˈmyü-ˌti-zəm\ *n, sometimes offensive*
[2]**deaf–mute** *n, often offensive* : a deaf person who cannot speak
de·am·i·nase \(ˌ)dē-ˈa-mə-ˌnās, -ˌnāz\ *also* **des·am·i·nase** \(ˌ)des-\ *n* : an enzyme that hydrolyzes amino compounds (as amino acids) with removal of the amino group
de·am·i·nate \-ˌnāt\ *vb* **-nat·ed; -nat·ing** : to remove the amino group from (a compound) — **de·am·i·na·tion** \(ˌ)dē-ˌa-mə-ˈnā-shən\ *n*
de·a·nol \ˈdē-ə-ˌnȯl\ *n* : DMAE
death \ˈdeth\ *n* **1** : the irreversible cessation of all vital functions esp. as indicated by permanent stoppage of the heart, respiration, and brain activity : the end of life — see BRAIN DEATH **2** : the cause or occasion of loss of life ⟨drinking was the ∼ of him⟩ **3** : the state of being dead
death·bed \ˈdeth-ˌbed\ *n* **1** : the bed in which a person dies **2** : the last hours of life — **on one's deathbed** : near the point of death
death cap *n* : a very poisonous mushroom of the genus *Amanita* (*A. phalloides*) of deciduous woods of No. America and Europe that varies in color from pure white to olive or yellow and has a prominent cup at the base of the stem — called also *death cup;* see THIOCTIC ACID
death instinct *n* : an innate and unconscious tendency toward self-destruction postulated in psychoanalytic theory to explain aggressive and destructive behavior not satisfactorily explained by the pleasure principle — called also *Thanatos;* compare EROS
death rate *n* : a measure of the number of deaths in a specified population during a particular time period
death rattle *n* : a rattling or gurgling sound produced by air passing through mucus in the lungs and air passages of a dying person
death wish *n* : the conscious or unconscious desire for the death of another or of oneself
de·bil·i·tate \di-ˈbi-lə-ˌtāt\ *vb* **-tat·ed; -tat·ing** : to impair the strength of ⟨a body *debilitated* by disease⟩ — **de·bil·i·ta·tion** \-ˌbi-lə-ˈtā-shən\ *n*
de·bil·i·ty \di-ˈbi-lə-tē\ *n, pl* **-ties** : the quality or state of being weak, feeble, or infirm; *esp* : physical weakness
de·bride·ment \di-ˈbrēd-mənt, dā-, -ˌmänt, -ˌmäⁿ\ *n* : the usu. surgical removal of lacerated, devitalized, or contaminated tissue — **de·bride** \də-ˈbrēd, dā-\ *vb*
de·bris \də-ˈbrē, dā-ˈ, ˈdā-ˌ\ *n, pl* **de·bris** : organic waste from dead or damaged tissue
de·bris·o·quin \di-ˈbri-sō-ˌkwin\ *or* **de·bris·o·quine** \-ˌkwīn\ *n* : an antihypertensive drug used esp. in the form of its sulfate $(C_{10}H_{13}N_3)_2 \cdot H_2SO_4$
de·bulk \dē-ˈbəlk\ *vb* : to remove all or most of the substance of (a tumor or lesion)
dec *abbr* deceased
Dec·a·dron \ˈde-kə-ˌdrän\ *trademark* — used for a preparation of dexamethasone
de·cal·ci·fi·ca·tion \(ˌ)dē-ˌkal-sə-fə-ˈkā-shən\ *n* : the removal or loss of calcium or calcium compounds (as from bones) — **de·cal·ci·fy** \-ˈkal-sə-ˌfī\ *vb*
deca·me·tho·ni·um \ˌde-kə-mə-ˈthō-nē-əm\ *n* : a synthetic ion used in the form of either its bromide $C_{16}H_{38}Br_2N_2$ or iodide salts $C_{16}H_{38}I_2N_2$ as a skeletal muscle relaxant

de·cap·i·tate \di-ˈka-pə-ˌtāt\ *vb* **-tat·ed; -tat·ing** : to cut off the head of — **de·cap·i·ta·tion** \-ˌka-pə-ˈtā-shən\ *n*

de·cap·su·late \(ˌ)dē-ˈkap-sə-ˌlāt\ *vb* **-lat·ed; -lat·ing** : to remove the capsule from ‹~ a kidney› — **de·cap·su·la·tion** \-ˌkap-sə-ˈlā-shən\ *n*

de·car·box·yl·ase \ˌdē-kär-ˈbäk-sə-ˌlās, -ˌlāz\ *n* : any of a group of enzymes that accelerate decarboxylation esp. of amino acids

de·car·box·yl·ate \-sə-ˌlāt\ *vb* **-lat·ed; -lat·ing** : to remove carboxyl from — **de·car·box·yl·ation** \-ˌbäk-sə-ˈlā-shən\ *n*

de·cay \di-ˈkā\ *n* **1 a** : ROT 1; *specif* : aerobic decomposition of proteins chiefly by bacteria **b** : the product of decay **2 a** : spontaneous decrease in the number of radioactive atoms in radioactive material **b** : spontaneous disintegration (as of an atom or a nuclear particle) — **decay** *vb*

de·ceased \di-ˈsēst\ *adj* : no longer living; *esp* : recently dead — used of persons

deceased *n, pl* **deceased** : a dead person

de·cer·e·brate \(ˌ)dē-ˈser-ə-brət, -ˌbrāt; ˌdē-sə-ˈrē-brət\ *adj* : having the cerebrum removed or made inactive; *also* : characteristic of decerebration ‹~ rigidity›

de·cer·e·bra·tion \(ˈ)dē-ˌser-ə-ˈbrā-shən\ *n* : loss of cerebral function (as from disease or surgical cutting of the brain stem); *also* : removal of the cerebrum (as by surgery) — **de·cer·e·brate** \(ˈ)dē-ˈser-ə-ˌbrāt\ *vb*

deci·bel \ˈde-sə-ˌbel, -bəl\ *n* : a unit for expressing the relative intensity of sounds on a scale from zero for the average least perceptible sound to about 130 for the average pain level

de·cid·ua \di-ˈsi-jə-wə\ *n, pl* **-uae**\-ˌwē\ **1** : the part of the mucous membrane lining the uterus that undergoes special modifications in preparation for and during pregnancy and is cast off at childbirth, being made up of a part lining the uterus, a part enveloping the embryo, and a part participating with the chorion in the formation of the placenta — see DECIDUA BASALIS, DECIDUA CAPSULARIS, DECIDUA PARIETALIS **2** : the part of the mucous membrane of the uterus cast off in the ordinary process of menstruation — **de·cid·u·al** \-wəl\ *adj*

decidua ba·sa·lis \-bə-ˈsā-ləs\ *n* : the part of the endometrium in the pregnant human female that participates with the chorion in the formation of the placenta

decidua cap·su·lar·is \-ˌkap-sə-ˈlar-əs\ *n* : the part of the decidua in the pregnant human female that envelops the embryo

decidua pa·ri·etal·is \-pə-ˌrī-ə-ˈta-ləs\ *n* : the part of the decidua in the pregnant human female lining the uterus

decidua pla·cen·tal·is \-ˌplā-sən-ˈta-ləs, -sen-\ *n* : DECIDUA BASALIS

decidua re·flexa \-ri-ˈflek-sə\ *n* : DECIDUA CAPSULARIS

decidua ser·o·ti·na \-ˌser-ə-ˈtē-nə, -ˈtī-\ *n* : DECIDUA BASALIS

de·cid·u·ate \di-ˈsi-jə-wət\ *adj* : having the fetal and maternal tissues firmly interlocked so that a layer of maternal tissue is torn away at childbirth and forms a part of the afterbirth

decidua ve·ra \-ˈvir-ə, -ˈver-\ *n* : DECIDUA PARIETALIS

de·cid·u·oma \di-ˌsi-jə-ˈwō-mə\ *n, pl* **-ma·ta** \-mə-tə\ *also* **-mas** **1** : a mass of tissue formed in the uterus following pregnancy that contains remnants of chorionic or decidual tissue **2** : decidual tissue induced in the uterus (as by trauma) in the absence of pregnancy

de·cid·u·ous \di-ˈsi-jə-wəs\ *adj* **1** : falling off or shed at a certain stage in the life cycle **2** : having deciduous parts ‹a ~ dentition›

deciduous tooth *n* : MILK TOOTH

deci·gram \ˈde-sə-ˌgram\ *n* : a metric unit of mass and weight equal to $^1/_{10}$ gram

deci·li·ter \ˈde-sə-ˌlē-tər\ *n* : a metric unit of capacity equal to $^1/_{10}$ liter

deci·me·ter \ˈde-sə-ˌmē-tər\ *n* : a metric unit of length equal to $^1/_{10}$ meter

de·clar·a·tive \di-ˈklar-ə-tiv\ *adj* : being or comprising memory characterized by the conscious recall of facts and events — compare PROCEDURAL

de·claw \(ˌ)dē-ˈklȯ\ *vb* : to remove the claws of (a cat) usu. with the nail matrix and all or part of the last bone of the toe

de·cline \di-ˈklīn, ˈdē-ˌklīn\ *n* **1** : a gradual physical or mental sinking and wasting away **2** : the period during which the end of life is approaching **3** : a wasting disease; *esp* : pulmonary tuberculosis — **de·cline** \di-ˈklīn\ *vb*

de·clive \di-ˈklīv\ *n* : a part of the monticulus of the cerebellum that is dorsal to the culmen

de·clot \(ˌ)dē-ˈklät\ *vb* **de·clot·ted; de·clot·ting** : to remove blood clots from

de·coc·tion \di-ˈkäk-shən\ *n* **1** : the act or process of boiling usu. in water so as to extract the flavor or active principle — compare INFUSION 2a **2** : an extract or liquid preparation obtained by decoction esp. of a medicinal plant — **de·coct** \-ˈkäkt\ *vb*

de·col·or·ize \(ˌ)dē-ˈkə-lə-ˌrīz\ *vb* **-or·ized; -or·iz·ing** : to remove color from — **de·col·or·iza·tion** \-ˌkə-lə-rə-ˈzā-shən\ *n*

de·com·pen·sa·tion \(ˌ)dē-ˌkäm-pən-ˈsā-shən, -pen-\ *n* : loss of physiological compensation or psychological balance; *esp* : inability of the heart to maintain adequate circulation — **de·com·pen·sate** \-ˈkäm-pən-ˌsāt, -ˌpen-\ *vb* — **de·com·pen·sa·to·ry** \ˌdē-kəm-ˈpen-sə-ˌtōr-ē\ *adj*

de·com·pose \ˌdē-kəm-ˈpōz\ *vb* **-posed; -pos·ing** **1** : to separate into constituent parts or elements or into simpler compounds **2** : to undergo chemical breakdown : DECAY, ROT — **de•com•pos•able** \-ˈpō-zə-bəl\ *adj* — **de•com•po•si•tion** \(ˌ)dē-ˌkäm-pə-ˈzi-shən\ *n*

de•com•pres•sion \ˌdē-kəm-ˈpre-shən\ *n* **1 a** : the decrease of ambient air pressure experienced in an air lock on return to atmospheric pressure after a period of breathing compressed air (as in a diving apparatus or caisson) or experienced in ascent to a great altitude without a pressure suit or pressurized cabin **b** : the decrease of water pressure experienced by a diver when ascending rapidly **2** : an operation or technique used to relieve pressure upon an organ (as in fractures of the skull or spine) or within a hollow organ (as in intestinal obstruction) — **de•com•press** \-ˈpres\ *vb*

decompression chamber *n* **1** : a chamber in which excessive pressure can be reduced gradually to atmospheric pressure **2** : a chamber in which an individual can be gradually subjected to decreased atmospheric pressure (as in simulating conditions at high altitudes)

decompression sickness *n* : a sometimes fatal condition that is caused by the release of gas bubbles typically of nitrogen as it leaves its dissolved form throughout the body upon a rapid decrease in barometric pressure (as that experienced by the rapid ascent of a diver from a deep dive) and is marked chiefly by joint pain which may be accompanied by various symptoms (as fatigue, shortness of breath, numbness, or confusion) — called also *bends, caisson disease, decompression illness, decompression syndrome;* see AEROEMBOLISM, CHOKE 2

de•com•pres•sive \ˌdē-kəm-ˈpre-siv\ *adj* : tending to relieve or reduce pressure ⟨~ lumbar laminectomy⟩

de•con•di•tion \ˌdē-kən-ˈdi-shən\ *vb* **1** : to cause to lose physical fitness **2** : to cause extinction of (a conditioned response)

de•con•di•tion•ing \-ˈdi-shə-niŋ\ *n* : a decrease in the responsiveness of heart muscle that sometimes occurs after long periods of weightlessness and may be marked by decrease in blood volume and pooling of the blood in the legs upon return to normal conditions

[1]**de•con•ges•tant** \ˌdē-kən-ˈjes-tənt\ *n* : an agent that relieves congestion (as of mucous membranes)

[2]**decongestant** *adj* : relieving or tending to relieve congestion

de•con•ges•tion \-ˈjes-chən\ *n* : the process of relieving congestion — **de•con•ges•tive** \-ˈjes-tiv\ *adj*

de•con•tam•i•nate \ˌdē-kən-ˈta-mə-ˌnāt\ *vb* **-nat•ed; -nat•ing** : to rid of contamination (as radioactive material) — **de•con•tam•i•na•tion** \-ˌta-mə-ˈnā-shən\ *n*

[1]**de•cor•ti•cate** \(ˌ)dē-ˈkȯr-tə-ˌkāt\ *vb* **-cat•ed; -cat•ing** : to remove all or part of the cortex from (as the brain)

[2]**de•cor•ti•cate** \-ˌkāt, -kət\ *adj* : lacking a cortex and esp. the cerebral cortex

de•cor•ti•ca•tion \-ˌkȯr-ti-ˈkā-shən\ *n* : the surgical removal of the cortex of an organ, an enveloping membrane, or a constrictive fibrinous covering ⟨the ~ of a lung⟩

de•cu•bi•tal \di-ˈkyü-bət-ᵊl\ *adj* **1** : relating to or resulting from lying down ⟨a ~ sore⟩ **2** : relating to or resembling a decubitus

de•cu•bi•tus \-bə-təs\ *n, pl* **-bi•ti** \-ˌtī, -ˌtē\ **1** : a position assumed in lying down ⟨the dorsal ~⟩ **2 a** : ULCER **b** : BEDSORE **3** : prolonged lying down (as in bed)

decubitus ulcer *n* : BEDSORE

de•cus•sa•tion \ˌdē-(ˌ)kə-ˈsā-shən\ *n* **1** : the action of intersecting or crossing (as of nerve fibers) esp. in the form of an X — see PYRAMIDAL DECUSSATION **2 a** : a band of nerve fibers that connects unlike centers on opposite sides of the nervous system **b** : a crossed tract of nerve fibers passing between centers on opposite sides of the central nervous system : COMMISSURE — **de•cus•sate** \ˈde-kə-ˌsāt, di-ˈkə-ˌsāt\ *vb*

decussation of pyramids *n* : PYRAMIDAL DECUSSATION

de•dif•fer•en•ti•a•tion \(ˌ)dē-ˌdi-fə-ˌren-chē-ˈā-shən\ *n* : reversion of specialized structures (as cells) to a more generalized or primitive condition often as a preliminary to major change — **de•dif•fer•en•ti•ate** \-ˈren-chē-ˌāt\ *vb*

deep \ˈdēp\ *adj* **1** : extending well inward from an outer surface ⟨a ~ gash⟩ **b** (1) : not located superficially within the body or one of its parts ⟨~ veins⟩ (2) : resulting from or involving stimulation of deep structures ⟨~ pain⟩ ⟨~ reflexes⟩ **2** : being below the level of the conscious ⟨~ neuroses⟩ — **deep•ly** *adv*

deep brachial artery *n* : the largest branch of the brachial artery in the upper part of the arm

deep brain stimulation *n* : a procedure for the treatment of neurological disorders (as Parkinson's disease) in which electrical stimulation is delivered to specific areas of the brain by one or more electrodes implanted in the brain and attached by a wire to a device which generates electrical pulses and is usu. implanted in the upper chest — abbr. *DBS*

deep external pudendal artery *n* : EXTERNAL PUDENDAL ARTERY b

deep facial vein *n* : a tributary of the facial vein draining part of the pterygoid plexus and nearby structures

deep fascia *n* : a firm fascia that ensheathes and binds together muscles and other internal structures — compare SUPERFICIAL FASCIA

deep femoral artery *n* : the large deep branch of the femoral artery formed where it divides about two inches (five centimeters) below the inguinal ligament

deep inguinal ring *n* : the internal opening of the inguinal canal — called also *internal inguinal ring;* compare SUPERFICIAL INGUINAL RING, INGUINAL RING

deep palmar arch *n* : PALMAR ARCH a

deep peroneal nerve *n* : a nerve that arises as a branch of the common peroneal nerve and that innervates or gives off branches innervating the muscles of the anterior part of the leg, the extensor digitorum brevis of the foot, and the skin between the big toe and the second toe — compare SUPERFICIAL PERONEAL NERVE

deep petrosal nerve *n* : a sympathetic nerve that originates in the carotid plexus, passes through the cartilage of the Eustachian tube, joins with the greater petrosal nerve to form the Vidian nerve, and as part of this nerve is distributed to the mucous membranes of the nasal cavity and palate

deep sedation *n* : an induced state of sedation characterized by depressed consciousness such that the patient is unable to continuously and independently maintain a patent airway and experiences a partial loss of protective reflexes and ability to respond to verbal commands or physical stimulation — compare CONSCIOUS SEDATION

deep temporal artery *n* : TEMPORAL ARTERY 1

deep temporal nerve *n* : either of two motor branches of the mandibular nerve on each side of the body that are distributed to the temporalis

deep temporal vein *n* : TEMPORAL VEIN b

deep vein thrombosis *n* : a condition marked by the formation of a thrombus within a deep vein (as of the leg or pelvis) that may be asymptomatic or be accompanied by symptoms (as swelling and pain) and that is potentially life threatening if dislodgment of the thrombus results in pulmonary embolism — abbr. *DVT*

deer·fly \ˈdir-ˌflī\ *n* : any of numerous small horseflies esp. of the genus *Chrysops* that include important vectors of tularemia

deer tick *n* : a tick of the genus *Ixodes* (*I. scapularis* syn. *I. dammini*) that transmits the bacterium causing Lyme disease

deet \ˈdēt\ *n, often all cap* : a colorless oily liquid insect and tick repellent $C_{12}H_{17}NO$

def·e·cate \ˈde-fi-ˌkāt\ *vb* **-cat·ed; -cat·ing** **1** : to discharge from the anus **2** : to discharge feces from the bowels — **def·e·ca·tion** \ˌde-fi-ˈkā-shən\ *n*

de·fect \ˈdē-ˌfekt, di-ˈ\ *n* : a lack or deficiency of something necessary for adequacy in form or function

[1]**de·fec·tive** \di-ˈfek-tiv\ *adj* : falling below the norm in structure or in mental or physical function ⟨~ eyesight⟩ — **de·fec·tive·ness** \-nəs\ *n*

[2]**defective** *n* : a person who is subnormal physically or mentally

de·fem·i·nize \(ˌ)dē-ˈfe-mə-ˌnīz\ *vb* **-nized; -niz·ing** : to divest of feminine qualities or physical characteristics : MASCULINIZE — **de·fem·i·ni·za·tion** \-ˌfe-mə-nə-ˈzā-shən\ *n*

de·fense \di-ˈfens\ *n* : a means or method of protecting the physical or functional integrity of body or mind ⟨a ~ against anxiety⟩

defense mechanism *n* : an often unconscious mental process (as repression, projection, or sublimation) that makes possible compromise solutions to personal problems

de·fen·sive \di-ˈfen-siv, ˈdē-ˌ\ *adj* **1** : serving to defend or protect (as the ego) **2** : devoted to resisting or preventing aggression or attack ⟨~ behavior⟩ — **de·fen·sive·ly** *adv* — **de·fen·sive·ness** *n*

defensive medicine *n* : the practice of ordering medical tests, procedures, or consultations of doubtful clinical value in order to protect the prescribing physician from malpractice suits

deferens — see DUCTUS DEFERENS, VAS DEFERENS

deferentes — see DUCTUS DEFERENS

deferentia — see VAS DEFERENS

de·fer·ox·amine \ˌdē-fə-ˈräk-sə-ˌmēn\ *n* : a chelator that is used in the form of its mesylate $C_{25}H_{48}N_6O_8 \cdot CH_4O_3S$ as an antidote to iron poisoning or overload

de·fer·ves·cence \ˌdē-(ˌ)fər-ˈves-ᵊns, ˌde-fər-\ *n* : the subsidence of a fever

de·fi·bril·la·tion \(ˌ)dē-ˌfi-brə-ˈlā-shən, -ˌfī-\ *n* : restoration of the rhythm of a fibrillating heart — **de·fi·bril·late** \(ˈ)dē-ˈfi-brə-ˌlāt, -ˈfī-\ *vb*

de·fi·bril·la·tor \-ˈfi-brə-ˌlā-tər, -ˈfī-\ *n* : an electronic device used to defibrillate a heart by applying an electric shock to it

de·fi·brin·ate \-ˈfi-brə-ˌnāt, -ˈfī-\ *vb* **-at·ed; -at·ing** : to remove fibrin from (blood) — **de·fi·brin·ation** \-ˌfi-brə-ˈnā-shən, -ˌfī-\ *n*

de·fi·cien·cy \di-ˈfi-shən-sē\ *n, pl* **-cies** **1** : a shortage of substances (as vitamins) necessary to health **2** : DELETION

deficiency anemia *n* : NUTRITIONAL ANEMIA

deficiency disease *n* : a disease (as scurvy) caused by a lack of essential dietary elements and esp. a vitamin or mineral

[1]**de·fi·cient** \di-ˈfi-shənt\ *adj* **1** : lacking in some necessary quality or element ⟨a ~ diet⟩ **2** : not up to a normal standard or complement ⟨~ strength⟩

[2]**deficient** *n* : one that is deficient

de·fi·cit \ˈde-fə-sət\ *n* : a deficiency of a substance ⟨a potassium ~⟩; *also* : a lack or impairment of a functional capacity ⟨cognitive ∼*s*⟩

de•fin•i•tive \di-ˈfi-nə-tiv\ *adj* : fully differentiated or developed

definitive host *n* : the host in which the sexual reproduction of a parasite takes place — compare INTERMEDIATE HOST 1

de•flo•ra•tion \ˌde-flə-ˈrā-shən, ˌdē-\ *n* : rupture of the hymen — **de•flo•rate** \ˈde-flə-ˌrāt, ˈdē-\ *vb*

de•flu•vi•um \dē-ˈflü-vē-əm\ *n* : the pathological loss of a part (as hair or nails)

de•fo•cus \(ˌ)dē-ˈfō-kəs\ *vb* **de•fo•cused; de•fo•cus•ing** : to cause to be out of focus ⟨∼*ed* his eye⟩ ⟨a ∼*ed* image⟩

deformans — see ARTHRITIS DEFORMANS, DYSTONIA MUSCULORUM DEFORMANS, OSTEITIS DEFORMANS

de•formed \di-ˈfȯrmd, dē-\ *adj* : misshapen esp. in body or limbs — **de•for•ma•tion** \ˌdē-ˌfȯr-ˈmā-shən, ˌde-fər-\ *n*

de•for•mi•ty \di-ˈfȯr-mə-tē\ *n, pl* **-ties** **1** : the state of being deformed **2** : a physical blemish or distortion

deg *abbr* degree

de•gen•er•a•cy \di-ˈje-nə-rə-sē\ *n, pl* **-cies** **1** : sexual perversion **2** : the coding of an amino acid by more than one codon of the genetic code

¹de•gen•er•ate \-rət\ *adj* **1 a** : having deteriorated progressively (as in the process of evolution) esp. through loss of structure and function **b** : having sunk to a lower and usu. corrupt and vicious state **2** : having more than one codon representing an amino acid; *also* : being such a codon

²degenerate *n* : one that is degenerate

de•gen•er•a•tion \di-ˌje-nə-ˈrā-shən, ˌdē-\ *n* **1** : progressive deterioration of physical characters from a level representing the norm of earlier generations or forms **2** : deterioration of a tissue or an organ in which its function is diminished or its structure impaired — **de•gen•er•ate** \-ˈje-nə-ˌrāt\ *vb* — **de•gen•er•a•tive** \di-ˈje-nə-ˌrā-tiv, -rə-\ *adj*

degenerative arthritis *n* : OSTEOARTHRITIS

degenerative disease *n* : a disease (as arteriosclerosis or osteoarthritis) characterized by progressive degenerative changes in tissue

degenerative joint disease *n* : OSTEOARTHRITIS

de•germ \(ˌ)dē-ˈjərm\ *vb* : to remove germs from (as the skin)

de•glu•ti•tion \ˌdē-ˌglü-ˈti-shən, ˌde-\ *n* : the act, power, or process of swallowing

deg•ra•da•tion \ˌde-grə-ˈdā-shən\ *n* : change of a chemical compound to a less complex compound — **deg•ra•da•tive** \ˈde-grə-ˌdā-tiv\ *adj*

de•grade \di-ˈgrād\ *vb* **1** : to reduce the complexity of (a chemical compound) by splitting off one or more groups or larger components : DECOMPOSE **2** : to undergo chemical degradation — **de•grad•able** \-ˈgrā-də-bəl\ *adj*

de•gran•u•la•tion \(ˌ)dē-ˌgran-yə-ˈlā-shən\ *n* : the process by which cytoplasmic granules (as of mast cells) release their contents — **de•gran•u•late** \-ˈgran-yə-ˌlāt\ *vb*

de•gree \di-ˈgrē\ *n* **1** : a measure of damage to tissue caused by injury or disease — see FIRST-DEGREE BURN, SECOND-DEGREE BURN, THIRD-DEGREE BURN **2** : one of the divisions or intervals marked on a scale of a measuring instrument; *specif* : any of various units for measuring temperature

de•his•cence \di-ˈhis-ᵊns\ *n* : the parting of the sutured lips of a surgical wound — **de•hisce** \-ˈhis\ *vb*

de•hu•mid•i•fy \ˌdē-hyü-ˈmi-də-ˌfī, ˌdē-yü-\ *vb* **-fied; -fy•ing** : to remove moisture from (as air) — **de•hu•mid•i•fi•ca•tion** \-ˌmi-də-fə-ˈkā-shən\ *n* — **de•hu•mid•i•fi•er** \-ˈmi-də-ˌfī-ər\ *n*

de•hy•drate \(ˌ)dē-ˈhī-ˌdrāt\ *vb* **-drat•ed; -drat•ing** **1** : to remove bound water or hydrogen and oxygen from (a chemical compound) in the proportion in which they form water **2** : to remove water from (as foods) **3** : to lose water or body fluids — **de•hy•dra•tor** \-ˌdrā-tər\ *n*

de•hy•dra•tion \ˌdē-hī-ˈdrā-shən\ *n* : the process of dehydrating; *esp* : an abnormal depletion of body fluids

de•hy•dro•ascor•bic acid \(ˌ)dē-ˌhī-drō-ə-ˈskȯr-bik-\ *n* : a crystalline oxidation product $C_6H_6O_6$ of vitamin C

7–de•hy•dro•cho•les•ter•ol \ˈse-vən-(ˌ)dē-ˌhī-drō-kə-ˈles-tə-ˌrȯl, -ˌrōl\ *n* : a crystalline steroid alcohol $C_{27}H_{43}OH$ that occurs (as in the skin) in humans and that yields vitamin D_3 on irradiation with ultraviolet light

24–dehydrocholesterol \ˌtwen-tē-ˈfōr-\ *n* : DESMOSTEROL

de•hy•dro•cho•lic acid \(ˈ)dē-ˌhī-drə-ˈkō-lik-\ *n* : a colorless crystalline acid $C_{24}H_{34}O_5$ used often in the form of its sodium salt $C_{24}H_{33}NaO_5$ esp. as a laxative and choleretic

11–de•hy•dro•cor•ti•co•ste•rone \i-ˈle-vən-(ˌ)dē-ˌhī-drō-ˌkȯr-tə-ˈkäs-tə-ˌrōn, -ˌkō-stə-ˈrōn, -kō-ˈstir-ˌōn\ *n* : a steroid $C_{21}H_{28}O_4$ extracted from the adrenal cortex and also made synthetically — compare CORTISONE

de•hy•dro•epi•an•dros•ter•one \(ˌ)dē-ˌhī-drō-ˌe-pē-an-ˈdräs-tə-ˌrōn\ *n* : an androgenic ketosteroid $C_{19}H_{28}O_2$ that is secreted by the adrenal cortex and is an intermediate in the biosynthesis of testosterone — abbr. *DHA, DHEA*

de•hy•dro•ge•nase \ˌdē-(ˌ)hī-ˈdrä-jə-ˌnās, -ˈhī-drə-jə-, -ˌnāz\ *n* : an enzyme that accelerates the removal of hydrogen from metabolites and its transfer to other substances — see ALCOHOL DEHYDROGENASE

de·hy·dro·ge·nate \ˌdē-(ˌ)hī-ˈdrä-jə-ˌnāt, -ˈhī-drə-jə-\ *vb* **-nat·ed; -nat·ing** : to remove hydrogen from — **de·hy·dro·ge·na·tion** \ˌdē-(ˌ)hī-ˌdrä-jə-ˈnā-shən, -ˌhī-drə-jə-\ *n*

de·hy·dro·ge·nize \(ˌ)dē-ˈhī-drə-jə-ˌnīz\ *vb* **-ized; -iz·ing** : DEHYDROGENATE

de·in·sti·tu·tion·al·iza·tion \(ˌ)dē-ˌin-stə-ˌtü-shə-nə-lə-ˈzā-shən, -ˌtyü-\ *n* : the release of institutionalized individuals from institutional care (as in a psychiatric hospital) to care in the community — **de·in·sti·tu·tion·al·ize**\-ˈtü-shə-nə-ˌlīz, -ˈtyü-\ *vb*

de·ion·ize \(ˌ)dē-ˈī-ə-ˌnīz\ *vb* **-ized; -iz·ing** : to remove ions from ⟨~ water⟩ — **de·ion·iza·tion** \-ˌī-ə-nə-ˈzā-shən\ *n* — **de·ion·iz·er** \-ˈī-ə-ˌnī-zər\ *n*

Dei·ters' nucleus \ˈdī-tərz-\ *n* : LATERAL VESTIBULAR NUCLEUS

dé·jà vu \ˌdā-ˌzhä-ˈvü\ *n* : PARAMNESIA b

delayed hypersensitivity *n* : hypersensitivity (as in a tuberculin test) in which the typical symptoms of inflammation and induration appear in an individual previously exposed to an antigen after an interval of 12 to 48 hours following a subsequent exposure

delayed–release *adj* : designed to delay release of a drug in the body (as through the use of enteric coatings) usu. until it passes through the stomach into the small intestine

delayed–stress disorder *n* : POST-TRAUMATIC STRESS DISORDER

delayed–stress syndrome *n* : POST-TRAUMATIC STRESS DISORDER

de·lead \(ˌ)dē-ˈled\ *vb* : to remove lead from ⟨~ a chemical⟩

del·e·te·ri·ous \ˌde-lə-ˈtir-ē-əs\ *adj* : harmful often in a subtle or an unexpected way ⟨~ genes⟩

de·le·tion \di-ˈlē-shən\ *n* **1** : the absence of a section of genetic material from a gene or chromosome **2** : the mutational process that results in a deletion

de·lin·quen·cy \di-ˈliŋ-kwən-sē, -ˈlin-\ *n, pl* **-cies** : conduct that is out of accord with accepted behavior or the law; *esp* : JUVENILE DELINQUENCY

[1]**de·lin·quent** \-kwənt\ *n* : a delinquent person; *specif* : one whose behavior has been labeled juvenile delinquency

[2]**delinquent** *adj* **1** : offending by neglect or violation of duty or of law **2** : of, relating to, or characteristic of delinquents : marked by delinquency ⟨~ behavior⟩ — **de·lin·quent·ly** *adv*

de·lir·i·um \di-ˈlir-ē-əm\ *n* : a mental disturbance characterized by confusion, disordered speech, and hallucinations — **de·lir·i·ous** \-ē-əs\ *adj* — **de·lir·i·ous·ly** *adv*

delirium tre·mens \-ˈtrē-mənz, -ˈtre-\ *n* : a violent delirium with tremors that is induced by excessive and prolonged use of alcoholic liquors — called also *d.t.'s* /ˌdē-ˈtēz/

de·liv·er \di-ˈli-vər\ *vb* **de·liv·ered; de·liv·er·ing** **1 a** : to assist (a parturient female) in giving birth ⟨she was *~ed* of a fine boy⟩ **b** : to aid in the birth of ⟨~ a child with forceps⟩ **2** : to give birth to ⟨she *~ed* a healthy girl⟩

de·liv·ery \di-ˈli-və-rē\ *n, pl* **-er·ies** **1** : the act of giving birth : the expulsion or extraction of a fetus and its membranes : PARTURITION **2** : the procedure of assisting birth of the fetus and expulsion of the placenta by manual, instrumental, or surgical means

delivery room *n* : a hospital room esp. equipped for the delivery of pregnant women

de·louse \(ˌ)dē-ˈlau̇s, -ˈlau̇z\ *vb* **de·loused; de·lous·ing** : to remove lice from

del·phin·i·um \del-ˈfin-ē-əm\ *n* **1** *cap* : a genus of perennial herbs of the buttercup family (Ranunculaceae) including several esp. of the western U.S. that are toxic to grazing animals and esp. cattle **2** : any plant of the genus *Delphinium*

delt \ˈdelt\ *n* : DELTOID — usu. used in pl.

[1]**del·ta** \ˈdel-tə\ *n* **1** : the fourth letter of the Greek alphabet — symbol Δ or δ **2** : DELTA WAVE

[2]**delta** *or* **δ-** *adj* : of or relating to one of four or more closely related chemical substances ⟨the *delta* chain of fetal hemoglobin⟩ — used somewhat arbitrarily to specify ordinal relationship or a particular physical form

delta agent *n* : HEPATITIS D VIRUS

delta hepatitis *n* : HEPATITIS D

delta–9–tet·ra·hy·dro·can·nab·i·nol \ˈdel-tə-ˈnīn-ˌte-trə-ˌhī-drə-kə-ˈna-bə-ˌnȯl, -ˌnōl\ *n* : THC a

delta–9–THC \-ˌtē-āch-ˈsē\ *n* : THC a

delta virus *n* : HEPATITIS D VIRUS

delta wave *n* : a high amplitude electrical rhythm of the brain with a frequency of less than 6 cycles per second that occurs esp. in deep sleep, in infancy, and in many diseased conditions of the brain — called also *delta, delta rhythm*

[1]**del·toid** \ˈdel-ˌtȯid\ *n* : a large triangular muscle that covers the shoulder joint, serves to raise the arm laterally, arises from the upper anterior part of the outer third of the clavicle and from the acromion and spine of the scapula, and is inserted into the outer side of the middle of the shaft of the humerus — called also *deltoid muscle;* see DELTOID TUBEROSITY

[2]**deltoid** *adj* : relating to, associated with, or supplying the deltoid

del·toi·de·us \del-ˈtȯi-dē-əs\ *n, pl* **-dei** \-dē-ˌē, -ˌī\ : DELTOID

deltoid ligament *n* : a strong radiating ligament of the inner aspect of the ankle that binds the base of the tibia to the bones of the foot

deltoid tuberosity *n* : a rough triangular bump on the outer side of the middle of the humerus that is the site of insertion of the deltoid

delts \ˈdelts\ *pl of* DELT

de•lude \di-ˈlüd\ *vb* **de•lud•ed; de•lud•ing** : to mislead the mind or judgment of

de•lu•sion \di-ˈlü-zhən\ *n* **1 a** : the act of deluding : the state of being deluded **b** : an abnormal mental state characterized by the occurrence of psychotic delusions **2** : a false belief regarding the self or persons or objects outside the self that persists despite the facts and occurs in some psychotic states — **de•lu•sion•al** \di-ˈlü-zhən-ᵊl\ *adj*

delusion of reference *n* : IDEA OF REFERENCE

de•mas•cu•lin•ize \(ˌ)dē-ˈmas-kyə-lə-ˌnīz, di-\ *vb* **-ized; -iz•ing** : to remove the masculine character or qualities of — **de•mas•cu•lin•iza•tion** \-ˌmas-kyə-lə-nə-ˈzā-shən, -ˌni-ˈ\ *n*

dem•e•car•i•um \ˌde-mi-ˈkar-ē-əm, -ˈker-\ *n* : a long-acting cholinesterase-inhibiting ammonium compound that is used as the bromide $C_{32}H_{52}Br_2N_4O_4$ in an ophthalmic solution esp. in the treatment of glaucoma and esotropia

de•mec•lo•cy•cline \ˌde-mə-klō-ˈsī-ˌklēn\ *n* : a broad-spectrum tetracycline antibiotic produced by an actinomycete of the genus *Streptomyces* (*S. aureofaciens*) and used esp. in the form of its hydrochloride $C_{21}H_{21}ClN_2O_8 \cdot HCl$

de•ment•ed \di-ˈmen-təd\ *adj* : suffering from or exhibiting cognitive dementia

de•men•tia \di-ˈmen-chə\ *n* : a usu. progressive condition (as Alzheimer's disease) marked by the development of multiple cognitive deficits (as memory impairment, aphasia, and inability to plan and initiate complex behavior) — **de•men•tial** \-chəl\ *adj*

dementia par•a•lyt•i•ca \-ˌpar-ə-ˈli-ti-kə\ *n, pl* **de•men•ti•ae par•a•lyt•i•cae** \di-ˈmen-chē-ˌē-ˌpar-ə-ˈli-ti-ˌsē\ : GENERAL PARESIS

dementia prae•cox \-ˈprē-ˌkäks\ *n* : SCHIZOPHRENIA

dementia pu•gi•lis•ti•ca \-ˌpyü-jə-ˈli-stə-kə\ *n* : CHRONIC TRAUMATIC ENCEPHALOPATHY

de•ment•ing \di-ˈmen-tiŋ\ *adj* : causing or characterized by dementia

Dem•er•ol \ˈde-mə-ˌrȯl, -ˌrōl\ *trademark* — used for meperidine

demi•lune \ˈde-mē-ˌlün\ *n* : one of the small crescentic groups of granular deeply staining zymogen-secreting cells lying between the clearer mucus-producing cells and the basement membrane in the alveoli of mixed salivary glands — called also *crescent of Giannuzzi*

demilune of Gian•nuz•zi *also* **demilune of Gia•nuz•zi** \-jä-ˈnüt-sē\ *n* : DEMILUNE

Giannuzzi, Giuseppe (1839–1876), Italian anatomist.

de•min•er•al•iza•tion \(ˌ)dē-ˌmi-nə-rə-lə-ˈzā-shən\ *n* **1** : loss of minerals (as salts of calcium) from the body esp. in disease **2** : the process of removing mineral matter or salts (as from water) — **de•min•er•al•ize** \-ˈmi-nə-rə-ˌlīz\ *vb*

dem•o•dec•tic mange \ˌde-mə-ˈdek-tik-\ *n* : mange caused by mites of the genus *Demodex* that burrow in the hair follicles esp. of dogs — compare CHORIOPTIC MANGE, SARCOPTIC MANGE

de•mo•dex \ˈde-mə-ˌdeks, ˈdē-\ *n* **1** *cap* : a genus (family Demodicidae) of minute mites that live in the hair follicles esp. about the face of humans and various furred mammals and in the latter often cause demodectic mange **2** : any mite of the genus *Demodex* : FOLLICLE MITE

dem•o•di•co•sis \ˌde-mō-də-ˈkō-səs\ *n, pl* **-co•ses** \-ˌsēz\ : DEMODECTIC MANGE

de•mog•ra•phy \di-ˈmä-grə-fē\ *n, pl* **-phies** : the statistical study of human populations esp. with reference to size and density, distribution, and vital statistics — **de•mog•ra•pher** \-fər\ *n* — **de•mo•graph•ic** \ˌde-mə-ˈgra-fik, ˌdē-\ *adj* — **de•mo•graph•i•cal•ly** \-fi-k(ə-)lē\ *adv*

¹de•mul•cent \di-ˈməl-sᵊnt\ *adj* : tending to soothe or soften

²demulcent *n* : a usu. mucilaginous or oily substance that can soothe or protect an abraded mucous membrane

de•my•elin•at•ing \(ˌ)dē-ˈmī-ə-lə-ˌnā-tiŋ\ *adj* : causing or characterized by the loss or destruction of myelin

de•my•eli•na•tion \-ˌmī-ə-lə-ˈnā-shən\ *n* : the state resulting from the loss or destruction of myelin; *also* : the process of such loss or destruction

de•my•elin•iza•tion \-lə-nə-ˈzā-shən\ *n* : DEMYELINATION

de•na•tur•ant \(ˌ)dē-ˈnā-chər-ənt\ *n* : a denaturing agent

de•na•ture \-ˈnā-chər\ *vb* **de•na•tured; de•na•tur•ing** **1** : to make (alcohol) unfit for drinking (as by adding an obnoxious substance) without impairing usefulness for other purposes **2** : to modify the molecular structure of (as a protein or DNA) esp. by heat, acid, alkali, or ultraviolet radiation so as to destroy or diminish some of the original properties and esp. the specific biological activity — **de•na•tur•ation** \-ˌnā-chə-ˈrā-shən\ *n*

den•drite \ˈden-ˌdrīt\ *n* : any of the usu. branching protoplasmic processes that conduct impulses toward the body of a nerve cell — **den•drit•ic** \den-ˈdri-tik\ *adj*

dendritic cell *n* : any of various antigen-presenting cells with long irregular processes

den•dro•den•drit•ic \ˌden-drō-ˌden-ˈdri-tik\ *adj* : relating to or being a nerve synapse between a dendrite of one cell and a dendrite of another

de·ner·vate \ˈdē-(ˌ)nər-ˌvāt\ *vb* **-vat·ed; -vat·ing** : to deprive of a nerve supply (as by cutting a nerve) — **de·ner·va·tion** \ˌdē-(ˌ)nər-ˈvā-shən\ *n*

den·gue \ˈdeŋ-gē, -ˌgā\ *n* : an acute infectious disease that is characterized by headache, severe joint pain, and a rash and that is caused by a virus of the genus *Flavivirus* (species *Dengue virus*) transmitted by mosquitoes of the genus *Aedes* — called also *breakbone fever, dandy fever, dengue fever*

dengue hemorrhagic fever *n* : dengue marked by hemorrhagic symptoms (as hemorrhagic lesions of the skin and thrombocytopenia) — called also *hemorrhagic dengue*

de·ni·al \di-ˈnī-əl\ *n* : a psychological defense mechanism in which confrontation with a personal problem or with reality is avoided by denying the existence of the problem or reality

den·i·da·tion \ˌde-nə-ˈdā-shən\ *n* : the sloughing of the endometrium of the uterus esp. during menstruation

de·ni·trog·e·nate \(ˌ)dē-ˌnī-ˈträ-jə-ˌnāt\ *vb* **-nat·ed; -nat·ing** : to reduce the stored nitrogen in the body of by forced breathing of pure oxygen for a period of time esp. as a measure designed to prevent development of decompression sickness — **de·ni·trog·e·na·tion** \-ˌträ-jə-ˈnā-shən\ *n*

den·o·su·mab \ˌden-ˈō-sə-ˌmab\ *n* : a drug that reduces bone resorption and increases bone mass and is administered by injection to prevent fractures associated with osteoporosis and malignant bone tumors and to treat hypercalcemia associated with various cancers — see PROLIA, XGEVA

dens \ˈdenz\ *n, pl* **den·tes** \ˈden-ˌtēz\ : a toothlike process that projects from the anterior end of the centrum of the axis in the spinal column and serves as a pivot on which the atlas rotates — called also *odontoid process*

densa — see MACULA DENSA

den·si·tom·e·ter \ˌden-sə-ˈtä-mə-tər\ *n* : an instrument for determining optical, photographic, or mass density ⟨an X-ray bone ~⟩ — **den·si·to·met·ric** \ˌden-sə-tə-ˈme-trik\ *adj* — **den·si·tom·e·try** \ˌden-sə-ˈtä-mə-trē\ *n*

den·si·ty \ˈden-sə-tē\ *n, pl* **-ties** **1** : the quantity per unit volume, unit area, or unit length: as **a** : the mass of a substance per unit volume **b** : the distribution of a quantity (as mass, electricity, or energy) per unit usu. of space **c** : the average number of individuals or units per space unit **2** : the degree of opacity of a translucent medium

dent- *or* **denti-** *or* **dento-** *comb form* **1** : tooth : teeth ⟨*dent*al⟩ **2** : dental and ⟨*dento*facial⟩

den·tal \ˈdent-ᵊl\ *adj* **1** : relating to, specializing in, or used in dentistry **2** : relating to or used on the teeth ⟨~ paste⟩ — **den·tal·ly** *adv*

dental arch *n* : the curve of the row of teeth in each jaw — called also *arcade*

dental dam *n* : a rubber dam used in dentistry

dental floss *n* : a thread used to clean between the teeth

dental formula *n* : an abridged expression for the number and kind of teeth of mammals in which the kind of teeth are represented by *i* (incisor), *c* (canine), *pm* (premolar) or *b* (bicuspid), and *m* (molar) and the number in each jaw is written like a fraction with the figures above the horizontal line showing the number in the upper jaw and those below the number in the lower jaw and with a dash separating the figures representing the teeth on each side of the jaw ⟨the *dental formula* of a human adult is

$$i\,\frac{2\text{–}2}{2\text{–}2},\ c\,\frac{1\text{–}1}{1\text{–}1},\ b \text{ or } pm\,\frac{2\text{–}2}{2\text{–}2},$$

$$m\,\frac{3\text{–}3}{3\text{–}3} = 32\rangle$$

dental hygienist *n* : one who assists a dentist esp. in cleaning teeth

dental lamina *n* : a linear zone of epithelial cells of the covering of each embryonic jaw that gives rise to the enamel organs of the teeth — called also *dental ridge*

dental nerve — see INFERIOR ALVEOLAR NERVE

dental papilla *n* : the mass of mesenchyme that gives rise to the dentin and the pulp of the tooth

dental plate *n* : DENTURE 2

dental pulp *n* : the highly vascular sensitive tissue occupying the central cavity of a tooth

dental surgeon *n* : DENTIST; *esp* : one engaging in oral surgery

dental technician *n* : a technician who makes dental appliances

den·tate \ˈden-ˌtāt\ *adj* : having teeth or pointed conical projections ⟨the ~ border of the retina⟩

dentate gyrus *n* : a narrow strip of cortex associated with the hippocampal sulcus that continues forward to the uncus

dentate nucleus *n* : a large laminar nucleus of gray matter forming an incomplete capsule within the white matter of each cerebellar hemisphere

dentes *pl of* DENS

denti- — see DENT-

den·ti·cle \ˈden-ti-kəl\ *n* : PULP STONE

den·tic·u·late ligament \den-ˈti-kyə-lət-\ *n* : a band of fibrous pia mater extending along the spinal cord on each side between the dorsal and ventral roots

den·ti·frice \ˈden-tə-frəs\ *n* : a powder, paste, or liquid for cleaning the teeth

den·tig·er·ous cyst \den-ˈti-jə-rəs-\ *n* : an epithelial cyst containing fluid and one or more imperfect teeth

den·tin \ˈdent-ᵊn\ *or* **den·tine** \ˈden-ˌtēn, den-ˈtēn\ *n* : a calcareous material similar to bone but harder and denser that composes the principal mass of a tooth and is formed by the odontoblasts — compare CEMENTUM, ENAMEL — **den·tin·al** \ˈdent-ᵊn-əl; ˈden-ˌtēn-ᵊl, den-ˈ\ *adj*

dentinal tubule *n* : one of the minute parallel tubules of the dentin of a tooth that communicate with the dental pulp

den·tino·enam·el \den-ˌtē-nō-i-ˈna-məl\ *adj* : relating to or connecting the dentin and enamel of a tooth ⟨the ~ junction⟩

den·tino·gen·e·sis \den-ˌtē-nə-ˈje-nə-səs\ *n, pl* **-e·ses** \-ˌsēz\ : the formation of dentin

dentinogenesis im·per·fec·ta \-ˌim-pər-ˈfek-tə\ *n* : a disorder of tooth development inherited as an autosomal dominant trait and characterized by relatively soft enamel that makes the teeth abnormally vulnerable to fracture, abrasion, and wear

den·tist \ˈden-tist\ *n* : a licensed practitioner who is skilled in the prevention, diagnosis, and treatment of diseases, injuries, and malformations of the teeth, jaws, and mouth and who makes and inserts false teeth — **den·tist·ry** \ˈden-tə-strē\ *n*

den·ti·tion \den-ˈti-shən\ *n* **1** : the development and cutting of teeth **2** : the character of a set of teeth esp. with regard to their number, kind, and arrangement **3** : TEETH

dento- — see DENT-

den·to·al·ve·o·lar \ˌden-tō-al-ˈvē-ə-lər\ *adj* : of, relating to, or involving the teeth and their sockets ⟨~ structures⟩

den·to·fa·cial \ˌden-tə-ˈfā-shəl\ *adj* : of or relating to the dentition and face

den·to·gin·gi·val \ˌden-tō-ˈjin-jə-vəl\ *adj* : of, relating to, or connecting the teeth and the gums ⟨the ~ junction⟩

den·tu·lous \ˈden-chə-ləs\ *adj* : having teeth

den·ture \ˈden-chər\ *n* **1** : a set of teeth **2** : an artificial replacement for one or more teeth; *esp* : a set of false teeth

den·tur·ist \-chə-rist\ *n* : a dental technician who makes, fits, and repairs dentures directly for the public

de·nu·da·tion \ˌdē-nü-ˈdā-shən, ˌde-, -nyü-\ *n* : the act or process of removing surface layers (as of skin) or an outer covering (as of myelin); *also* : the condition that results from this — **de·nude** \di-ˈnüd, -ˈnyüd\ *vb*

¹**de·odor·ant** \dē-ˈō-də-rənt\ *adj* : destroying or masking offensive odors

²**deodorant** *n* : any of various preparations or solutions (as a soap or disinfectant) that destroy or mask unpleasant odors; *esp* : a cosmetic that neutralizes perspiration odors

de·odor·ize \dē-ˈō-də-ˌrīz\ *vb* **-ized; -iz·ing** : to eliminate or prevent the offensive odor of — **de·odor·iza·tion** \-ˌō-də-rə-ˈzā-shən\ *n* — **de·odor·iz·er** *n*

de·oxy \(ˌ)dē-ˈäk-sē\ *also* **des·oxy** \(ˌ)dez-\ *adj* : containing less oxygen per molecule than the compound from which it is derived — usu. used in combination ⟨*deoxy*ribonucleic acid⟩

de·oxy·cho·late \(ˌ)dē-ˌäk-sē-ˈkō-ˌlāt\ *n* : a salt or ester of deoxycholic acid

de·oxy·cho·lic acid \-ˈkō-lik-\ *n* : a crystalline acid $C_{24}H_{40}O_4$ found esp. in bile

deoxycorticosterone *var of* DESOXYCORTICOSTERONE

de·oxy·cor·tone *chiefly Brit var of* DESOXYCORTONE

de·ox·y·gen·ate \(ˌ)dē-ˈäk-si-jə-ˌnāt, ˌdē-äk-ˈsi-jə-\ *vb* **-at·ed; -at·ing** : to remove oxygen from — **de·ox·y·gen·ation** \-ˌäk-si-jə-ˈnā-shən, ˌdē-äk-ˌsi-jə-\ *n*

de·ox·y·gen·at·ed *adj* : having the hemoglobin in the reduced state

de·oxy·ri·bo·nu·cle·ase \(ˌ)dē-ˈäk-si-ˌrī-bō-ˈnü-klē-ˌās, -ˈnyü-, -ˌāz\ *n* : an enzyme that hydrolyzes DNA to nucleotides — called also *DNase*

de·oxy·ri·bo·nu·cle·ic acid \(ˌ)dē-ˌäk-si-ˌrī-bō-nu̇-ˈklē-ik-, -nyu̇-, -ˈklā-\ *also* **des·oxy·ri·bo·nu·cle·ic acid** \(ˌ)des-\ *n* : DNA

de·oxy·ri·bo·nu·cle·o·tide \-ˈnü-klē-ə-ˌtīd, -ˈnyü-\ *n* : a nucleotide that contains deoxyribose and is a constituent of DNA

de·oxy·ri·bose \(ˌ)dē-ˌäk-si-ˈrī-ˌbōs, -ˌbōz\ *n* : a pentose sugar $C_5H_{10}O_4$ that is a structural element of DNA

Dep·a·kene \ˈde-pə-ˌkēn\ *trademark* — used for a preparation of valproic acid

Dep·a·kote \ˈde-pə-ˌkōt\ *trademark* — used for a preparation of divalproex sodium

de·pen·dence \di-ˈpen-dəns\ *n* **1** : the quality or state of being dependent upon or unduly subject to the influence of another **2 a** : drug addiction **b** : HABITUATION 2b

de·pen·den·cy \-dən-sē\ *n, pl* **-cies** : DEPENDENCE

de·pen·dent \di-ˈpen-dənt\ *adj* **1** : unable to exist, sustain oneself, or act appropriately or normally without the assistance or direction of another **2** : affected with a drug dependence **3 a** : occurring under the influence of gravity ⟨~ drainage⟩ **b** : affecting the lower part of the body and esp. the legs ⟨~ edema⟩ — **de·pen·dent·ly** *adv*

dependent lividity *n* : LIVOR MORTIS

de·per·son·al·iza·tion \(ˌ)dē-ˌpər-sə-nə-lə-ˈzā-shən\ *n* : the act or process of causing or the state resulting from loss of the sense of personal identity; *esp* : a psychopathological syndrome characterized by loss of identity and feelings of unreality or strangeness about one's own behavior — **de·per·son·al·ize** \(ˈ)dē-ˈpər-sə-nə-ˌlīz\ *vb*

de·phos·phor·y·la·tion \(ˌ)dē-ˌfäs-ˌfȯr-ə-ˈlā-shən\ *n* : the process of removing phosphate groups from an organic compound (as ATP) by hydrolysis; *also* : the resulting state — **de·phos·phor·y·late** \-fäs-ˈfȯr-ə-ˌlāt\ *vb*

de·pig·men·ta·tion \(ˌ)dē-ˌpig-mən-ˈtā-shən, -ˌmen-\ *n* : loss of normal pigmentation — **de·pig·ment·ed** \-ˈpig-mən-təd, -ˌmen-\ *adj* — **de·pig·ment·ing** \-tiŋ\ *adj*

dep·i·la·tion \ˌde-pə-ˈlā-shən\ *n* : the removal of hair, wool, or bristles by chemical or mechanical methods — **dep·i·late** \ˈde-pə-ˌlāt\ *vb*

[1]**de·pil·a·to·ry** \di-ˈpi-lə-ˌtōr-ē\ *adj* : having the power to remove hair

[2]**depilatory** *n* : a cosmetic for the temporary removal of undesired hair

de·plete \di-ˈplēt\ *vb* **de·plet·ed; de·plet·ing** : to empty of a principal substance ⟨tissues *depleted* of vitamins⟩

de·ple·tion \di-ˈplē-shən\ *n* : the act or process of depleting or the state of being depleted: as **a** : the reduction or loss of blood, body fluids, chemical constituents, or stored materials from the body (as by hemorrhage or malnutrition) **b** : a debilitated state caused by excessive loss of body fluids or other constituents

de·po·lar·iza·tion \(ˌ)dē-ˌpō-lə-rə-ˈzā-shən\ *n* : loss of polarization; *esp* : loss of the difference in charge between the inside and outside of the plasma membrane of a muscle or nerve cell due to a change in permeability and migration of sodium ions to the interior — **de·po·lar·ize** \-ˈpō-lə-ˌrīz\ *vb*

Depo–Pro·vera \ˈde-pō-prō-ˈver-ə\ *trademark* — used for a preparation of medroxyprogesterone acetate administered by intramuscular injection

de·pos·it \də-ˈpä-zət\ *n* : matter laid down or accumulated by a normal or abnormal process — **deposit** *vb*

[1]**de·pot** \ˈde-(ˌ)pō, ˈdē-\ *n* : a bodily location where a substance is stored usu. for later utilization ⟨fat ∼*s*⟩

[2]**depot** *adj* : being in storage ⟨∼ fat⟩; *also* : acting over a prolonged period ⟨∼ insulin⟩

dep·re·nyl \ˈdep-rə-ˌnil\ *n* : a monoamine oxidase inhibitor $C_{13}H_{17}N$; *esp* : SELEGILINE

de·press \di-ˈpres\ *vb* **1** : to diminish the activity, strength, or yield of **2** : to lower in spirit or mood

[1]**de·pres·sant** \-ᵊnt\ *adj* : tending to depress; *esp* : lowering or tending to lower functional or vital activity ⟨a drug with a ∼ effect on heart rate⟩

[2]**depressant** *n* : one that depresses; *specif* : an agent that reduces bodily functional activity or an instinctive desire (as appetite)

de·pressed \di-ˈprest\ *adj* **1** : low in spirits; *specif* : affected by psychological depression ⟨a severely ∼ patient⟩ **2** : having the central part lower than the margin ⟨a ∼ pustule⟩

depressed fracture *n* : a fracture esp. of the skull in which the fragment is depressed below the normal surface

de·pres·sion \di-ˈpre-shən\ *n* **1** : a displacement downward or inward ⟨∼ of the jaw⟩ **2** : an act of depressing or a state of being depressed: as **a** (1) : a state of feeling sad (2) : a mood disorder marked esp. by sadness, inactivity, difficulty with thinking and concentration, a significant increase or decrease in appetite and time spent sleeping, feelings of dejection and hopelessness, and sometimes suicidal thoughts or an attempt to commit suicide **b** : a reduction in functional activity, amount, quality, or force ⟨∼ of autonomic function⟩

[1]**de·pres·sive** \di-ˈpre-siv\ *adj* **1** : tending to depress **2** : of, relating to, marked by, or affected by psychological depression ⟨∼ symptoms⟩

[2]**depressive** *n* : one who is affected with or prone to psychological depression

depressive disorder *n* : any of several mood disorders and esp. dysthymia and major depressive disorder that are characterized by prolonged or recurring symptoms of psychological depression without manic episodes

de·pres·sor \di-ˈpre-sər\ *n* : one that depresses: as **a** : a muscle that draws down a part — compare LEVATOR **b** : a device for pressing a part down or aside — see TONGUE DEPRESSOR **c** : a nerve or nerve fiber that decreases the activity or the tone of the organ or part it innervates

depressor sep·ti \-ˈsep-ˌtī\ *n* : a small muscle of each side of the upper lip that is inserted into the nasal septum and wing of the nose on each side and constricts the nasal opening by drawing the wing downward

de·pri·va·tion \ˌde-prə-ˈvā-shən, ˌdē-ˌprī-\ *n* : the act or process of removing or the condition resulting from removal of something normally present and usu. essential for mental or physical well-being ⟨sleep ∼⟩ ⟨sensory ∼⟩ — **de·prive** \di-ˈprīv\ *vb*

de·pro·gram \(ˌ)dē-ˈprō-ˌgram\ *vb* **-grammed** *also* **-gramed; -gram·ming** *also* **-gram·ing** : to dissuade or try to dissuade from strongly held convictions (as of a religious nature) or a firmly established or innate behavior pattern

de·pro·tein·ate \(ˌ)dē-ˈprō-ˌtē-ˌnāt, -ˈprō-tē-ə-ˌnāt\ *vb* **-at·ed; -at·ing** : DEPROTEINIZE — **de·pro·tein·ation** \(ˌ)dē-ˌprō-ˌtē-ˈnā-shən, -ˌprō-tē-ə-\ *n*

de·pro·tein·i·za·tion \(ˌ)dē-ˌprō-ˌtē-nə-ˈzā-shən, -ˌprō-tē-ə-nə-\ *n* : the process of removing protein

de·pro·tein·ize \(ˌ)dē-ˈprō-ˌtē-ˌnīz, -ˈprō-tē-ə-ˌnīz\ *vb* **-ized; -iz·ing** : to subject to deproteinization

depth \ˈdepth\ *n, pl* **depths** **1** : the distance between upper and lower or between dorsal and ventral points of a body **2** : the quality of a state of consciousness, a bodily state, or a physiological function of being intense or complete ⟨the ~ of anesthesia⟩

depth perception *n* : the ability to judge the distance of objects and the spatial relationship of objects at different distances

depth psychology *n* : PSYCHOANALYSIS; *also* : psychology concerned esp. with the unconscious mind

de·Quer·vain's disease \də-(ˌ)kər-ˈvaⁿz-\ *n* : inflammation of tendons and their sheaths at the styloid process of the radius that often causes pain in the thumb side of the wrist

Quer·vain \ker-ˈvaⁿ\, **Fritz de (1868–1940),** Swiss physician.

de·range·ment \di-ˈrānj-mənt\ *n* : a disturbance of normal bodily functioning or operation — **de·range** \di-ˈrānj\ *vb*

de·re·al·iza·tion \(ˌ)dē-ˌrē-ə-lə-ˈzā-shən\ *n* : a feeling of altered reality that occurs often in schizophrenia and in some drug reactions

de·re·press \ˌdē-ri-ˈpres\ *vb* : to activate (a gene or enzyme) by releasing from a blocked state — **de·re·pres·sion** \-ˈpre-shən\ *n*

[1]**de·riv·a·tive** \di-ˈri-və-tiv\ *adj* **1** : formed by derivation **2** : made up of or marked by derived elements

[2]**derivative** *n* **1** : something that is obtained from, grows out of, or results from an earlier or more fundamental state or condition **2** : a chemical substance related structurally to another substance and theoretically derivable from it **b** : a substance that can be made from another substance

de·rive \di-ˈrīv\ *vb* **de·rived; de·riv·ing** : to take, receive, or obtain, esp. from a specified source; *specif* : to obtain (a chemical substance) actually or theoretically from a parent substance — **der·i·va·tion** \ˌder-ə-ˈvā-shən\ *n*

derm- *or* **derma-** *or* **dermo-** *comb form* : skin ⟨*derm*al⟩ ⟨*dermo*pathy⟩

-derm \ˌdərm\ *n comb form* : skin : covering ⟨ecto*derm*⟩

-der·ma \ˈdər-mə\ *n comb form, pl* **-dermas** *or* **-der·ma·ta** \-mə-tə\ : skin or skin ailment of a (specified) type ⟨sclero*derma*⟩

derm·abra·sion \ˌdər-mə-ˈbrā-zhən\ *n* : surgical removal of skin blemishes or imperfections (as scars or tattoos) by abrasion

Der·ma·cen·tor \ˈdər-mə-ˌsen-tər\ *n* : a large widely distributed genus of ornate ixodid ticks including several vectors of important diseases (as Rocky Mountain spotted fever)

der·mal \ˈdər-məl\ *adj* **1** : of or relating to skin and esp. to the dermis : CUTANEOUS **2** : EPIDERMAL

Der·ma·nys·sus \ˌdər-mə-ˈni-səs\ *n* : a genus (family Dermanyssidae) of blood-sucking mites that are parasitic on birds — see CHICKEN MITE

dermat- *or* **dermato-** *comb form* : skin ⟨*dermat*itis⟩ ⟨*dermato*logy⟩

der·ma·ti·tis \ˌdər-mə-ˈtī-təs\ *n, pl* **-ti·tis·es** *or* **-tit·i·des** \-ˈti-tə-ˌdēz\ : inflammation of the skin — **der·ma·tit·ic** \-ˈti-tik\ *adj*

dermatitis her·pe·ti·for·mis \-ˌhər-pə-tə-ˈfȯr-məs\ *n* : chronic dermatitis characterized by eruption of itching papules, vesicles, and lesions resembling hives typically in clusters

Der·ma·to·bia \ˌdər-mə-ˈtō-bē-ə\ *n* : a genus of botflies including one (*D. hominis*) whose larvae live under the skin of domestic mammals and sometimes of humans in tropical America

der·ma·to·fi·bro·ma \ˌdər-mə-tō-fī-ˈbrō-mə\ *n, pl* **-mas** *also* **-ma·ta** \-mə-tə\ : a benign chiefly fibroblastic nodule of the skin found esp. on the extremities of adults

der·ma·to·fi·bro·sar·co·ma \-ˌfī-brō-sär-ˈkō-mə\ *n, pl* **-mas** *also* **-ma·ta** \-mə-tə\ : a fibrosarcoma affecting the skin

dermatofibrosarcoma pro·tu·ber·ans \-prō-ˈtü-bə-rənz, -ˈtyü-\ *n* : a dermal fibroblastic tumor composed of firm nodular masses that usu. do not metastasize

der·ma·to·glyph·ics \ˌdər-mə-tə-ˈgli-fiks\ *n* **1** : skin patterns; *esp* : patterns of the specialized skin of the inferior surfaces of the hands and feet **2** : the science of the study of skin patterns — **der·ma·to·glyph·ic** \-fik\ *adj*

der·ma·to·graph·ia \-ˈgra-fē-ə\ *n* : DERMOGRAPHISM

der·ma·to·graph·ism \-ˈgra-ˌfi-zəm\ *n* : DERMOGRAPHISM

der·ma·to·log·ic \ˌdər-mət-ᵊl-ˈä-jik\ *or* **der·ma·to·log·i·cal** \-ji-kəl\ *adj* : of or relating to dermatology

der·ma·to·log·i·cal \-ji-kəl\ *n* : a medicinal agent for application to the skin

der·ma·tol·o·gy \ˌdər-mə-ˈtä-lə-jē\ *n, pl* **-gies** : a branch of medicine dealing with the skin, its structure, functions, and diseases — **der·ma·tol·o·gist** \-mə-ˈtä-lə-jist\ *n*

der·ma·tome \ˈdər-mə-ˌtōm\ *n* **1** : an instrument for cutting skin for use in grafting **2** : the lateral wall of a somite from which the dermis is produced — **der·ma·to·mal** \ˌdər-mə-ˈtō-məl\ *or* **der·ma·to·mic** \-mik\ *adj*

der·ma·to·my·co·sis \ˌdər-mə-tō-ˌmī-ˈkō-səs, (ˌ)dər-ma-\ *n, pl* **-co·ses** \-ˌsēz\ : a disease (as ringworm) of the skin caused by infection with a fungus

der·ma·to·my·o·si·tis \-ˌmī-ə-ˈsī-təs\ *n, pl* **-si·tis·es** *or* **-sit·i·des** \-ˈsi-tə-ˌdēz\ : polymyositis that is accompanied by involvement of the skin and that is marked esp. by reddish erythematous eruptions, by periorbital edema, and by violet-colored erythema of the eyelids and region over the upper eyelids — abbr. *DM*

der•ma•to•pa•thol•o•gy \-pə-ˈthä-lə-jē, -pa-\ *n, pl* **-gies** : pathology of the skin — **der•ma•to•pa•thol•o•gist** \-jist\ *n*

Der•ma•toph•a•goi•des \ˌdər-mə-ˌtä-fə-ˈgȯi-(ˌ)dēz\ *n* : a genus of mites (family Pyroglyphidae) including several that scavenge shed flakes of human skin and dander and cause allergy — see HOUSE DUST MITE

der•ma•to•phyte \(ˌ)dər-ˈma-tə-ˌfīt, ˈdər-mə-tə-\ *n* : a fungus parasitic upon the skin or skin derivatives (as hair or nails) — compare DERMATOMYCOSIS — **der•ma•to•phy•tic** \(ˌ)dər-ˌma-tə-ˈfi-tik, ˌdər-mə-\ *adj*

der•ma•to•phy•tid \(ˌ)dər-ˌma-tə-ˈfī-təd, ˌdər-mə-\ *n* : a skin eruption associated with a fungus infection; *esp* : one considered to be due to allergic reaction

der•ma•to•phy•to•sis \-fī-ˈtō-səs\ *n, pl* **-to•ses** \-ˌsēz\ : a disease (as athlete's foot) of the skin or skin derivatives that is caused by a dermatophyte

der•ma•to•plas•ty \(ˌ)dər-ˈma-tə-ˌplas-tē, ˈdər-mə-\ *n, pl* **-ties** : plastic surgery of the skin

der•ma•to•sis \ˌdər-mə-ˈtō-səs\ *n, pl* **-to•ses** \-ˌsēz\ : a disease of the skin

-der•ma•tous \ˈdər-mə-təs\ *adj comb form* : having a (specified) type of skin ⟨sclero*dermatous*⟩

-der•mia \ˈdər-mē-ə\ *n comb form* : skin or skin ailment of a (specified) type ⟨kerato*dermia*⟩

der•mis \ˈdər-məs\ *n* : the vascular thick layer of the skin lying below the epidermis and above the superficial fascia that contains fibroblasts, macrophages, mast cells, B cells, and sensory nerve endings and has an extracellular matrix composed of proteoglycans and glycoproteins embedded with collagen and elastin fibers — called also *corium, cutis*

-der•mis \ˈdər-məs\ *n comb form* : layer of skin or tissue ⟨epi*dermis*⟩

dermo- — see DERM-

der•mo•graph•ia \ˌdər-mə-ˈgra-fē-ə\ *n* : DERMOGRAPHISM

der•mog•ra•phism \(ˌ)dər-ˈmä-grə-ˌfi-zəm\ *n* : a condition in which pressure or friction on the skin gives rise to a transient raised usu. reddish mark so that a line traced on the skin becomes visible — called also *dermatographia, dermatographism*

der•moid \ˈdər-ˌmȯid\ *also* **der•moi•dal** \(ˌ)dər-ˈmȯid-ᵊl\ *adj* **1** : made up of cutaneous elements and esp. ectodermal derivatives ⟨a ~ tumor⟩ **2** : resembling skin

dermoid cyst *n* : a cystic tumor often of the ovary that contains skin and skin derivatives (as hair or teeth) — called also *dermoid*

der•mo•ne•crot•ic \ˌdər-mō-ni-ˈkrä-tik\ *adj* : relating to or causing necrosis of the skin ⟨a ~ toxin⟩

der•mop•a•thy \(ˌ)dər-ˈmä-pə-thē\ *n, pl* **-thies** : a disease of the skin

DES \ˌdē-(ˌ)ē-ˈes\ *n* : DIETHYLSTILBESTROL

desaminase *var of* DEAMINASE

des•ce•met•o•cele \ˌde-sə-ˈme-tə-ˌsēl\ *n* : protrusion of Descemet's membrane through the cornea

Des•ce•met's membrane \ˌde-sə-ˈmāz-, ˌdes-ˈmāz-\ *n* : a transparent highly elastic apparently structureless membrane that covers the inner surface of the cornea and is lined with endothelium — called also *membrane of Descemet, posterior elastic lamina*

Des•ce•met \des-ˈmā\, **Jean (1732–1810),** French physician.

descending *adj* **1** : moving or directed downward **2** : being a nerve, nerve fiber, or nerve tract that carries nerve impulses in a direction away from the central nervous system : EFFERENT, MOTOR

descending aorta *n* : the part of the aorta from the arch to its bifurcation into the two common iliac arteries that passes downward in the thoracic and abdominal cavities

descending colon *n* : the part of the large intestine on the left side that extends from the bend below the spleen to the sigmoid colon — compare ASCENDING COLON, TRANSVERSE COLON

de•scen•sus \di-ˈsen-səs\ *n* : the process of descending or prolapsing

de•sen•si•tize \(ˌ)dē-ˈsen-sə-ˌtīz\ *vb* **-tized; -tiz•ing 1** : to make (a sensitized or hypersensitive individual) insensitive or nonreactive to a sensitizing agent **2** : to extinguish an emotional response (as of fear or anxiety) to stimuli which formerly induced it : make emotionally insensitive — **de•sen•si•ti•za•tion** \-ˌsen-sə-tə-ˈzā-shən\ *n*

de•sen•si•tiz•er \-ˈsen-sə-ˌtī-zər\ *n* : a desensitizing agent; *esp* : a drug that reduces sensitivity to pain

de•ser•pi•dine \di-ˈsər-pə-ˌdēn\ *n* : an alkaloid $C_{32}H_{38}N_2O_8$ that is obtained from a tropical plant (*Rauvolfia canescens*) and is used esp. as an antihypertensive

de•sex \(ˌ)dē-ˈseks\ *vb* : CASTRATE, SPAY

[1]**des•ic•cant** \ˈde-si-kənt\ *adj* : tending to dry or desiccate

[2]**desiccant** *n* : a drying agent (as calcium chloride)

des•ic•cate \ˈde-si-ˌkāt\ *vb* **-cat•ed; -cat•ing** : to dry up or cause to dry up : deprive or exhaust of moisture; *esp* : to dry thoroughly

des•ic•ca•tion \ˌde-si-ˈkā-shən\ *n* : the act or process of desiccating or the state of being or becoming desiccated; *esp* : a complete or nearly complete deprivation of moisture or of water not chemically combined : DEHYDRATION

designer drug *n* **1** : a synthetic version of a controlled substance (as heroin) that is produced with a slightly altered molecular structure to avoid classification as an illicit drug **2** : a synthetic therapeutic agent designed to have a highly selective mode of action so that effectiveness is maximized and side effects are minimized compared with existing therapies

de·si·pra·mine \ˌde-zə-ˈpra-mən, də-ˈzi-prə-ˌmēn\ *n* : a tricyclic antidepressant administered in the form of its hydrochloride $C_{18}H_{22}N_2{\cdot}HCl$ esp. in the treatment of endogenous depressions (as bipolar disorder) — see NORPRAMIN, PERTOFRANE

-de·sis \də-səs\ *n comb form, pl* **-de·ses** \-ˌsēz\ : binding or fixation ⟨arthro*desis*⟩

des·lo·rat·a·dine \ˌdez-lə-ˈra-tə-ˌdēn, -ˌdīn\ *n* : a long-acting H_1 antagonist $C_{19}H_{19}ClN_2$ that is used to treat seasonal and perennial allergic rhinitis and chronic hives — see CLARINEX

desm- *or* **desmo-** *comb form* : connective tissue ⟨*desmo*plasia⟩

des·meth·yl·imip·ra·mine \ˌdes-ˌme-thəl-im-ˈi-prə-ˌmēn\ *n* : DESIPRAMINE

des·moid \ˈdez-ˌmȯid\ *n* : a dense benign connective-tissue tumor

des·mo·pla·sia \ˌdez-mə-ˈplā-zhə, -zhē-ə\ *n* : formation of fibrous connective tissue by proliferation of fibroblasts

des·mo·plas·tic \-ˈplas-tik\ *adj* : characterized by the formation of fibrous tissue ⟨~ fibromas⟩

des·mo·pres·sin \ˌdes-mō-ˈpre-sᵊn\ *n* : a synthetic hormone that is used in the form of its hydrated acetate salt $C_{46}H_{64}N_{14}O_{12}S_2{\cdot}C_2H_4O_2{\cdot}3H_2O$ for its antidiuretic effect and for its effect of increasing certain clotting factors — see DDAVP

des·mo·some \ˈdez-mə-ˌsōm\ *n* : a specialized local thickening of the plasma membrane of an epithelial cell that serves to anchor contiguous cells together — **des·mo·som·al** \-ˌsō-məl\ *adj*

des·mos·ter·ol \dez-ˈmä-stə-ˌrȯl, -ˌrōl\ *n* : a precursor $C_{27}H_{43}OH$ of cholesterol that tends to accumulate in blood serum when cholesterol synthesis is inhibited — called also *24-dehydrocholesterol*

deso·ges·trel \ˌdes-ə-ˈjes-trəl\ *n* : a synthetic progestogen $C_{22}H_{30}O$ used in birth control pills in combination with ethinyl estradiol

desoxy *var of* DEOXY

des·oxy·cor·ti·co·ste·rone \(ˌ)dez-ˌäk-si-ˌkȯr-ti-ˈkäs-tə-ˌrōn, -ˌkō-stə-ˈrōn\ *or* **de·oxy·cor·ti·co·ste·rone** \(ˌ)dē-\ *n* : a steroid hormone $C_{21}H_{30}O_3$ of the adrenal cortex

des·oxy·cor·tone \(ˌ)dez-ˌäk-si-ˈkȯr-ˌtōn\ *n* : DESOXYCORTICOSTERONE

desoxyribonucleic acid *var of* DEOXYRIBONUCLEIC ACID

des·qua·mate \ˈdes-kwə-ˌmāt\ *vb* **-mat·ed; -mat·ing** : to peel off in the form of scales : scale off ⟨*desquamated* epithelial cells⟩ — **des·qua·ma·tion** \ˌdes-kwə-ˈmā-shən\ *n* — **des·qua·ma·tive** \ˈdes-kwə-ˌmā-tiv, di-ˈskwa-mə-\ *adj*

destroying angel *n* : any of several very poisonous white mushrooms of the genus *Amanita* (as *A. verna or A. virosa*); *also* : a death cap (*A. phalloides*) whether white or colored

des·ven·la·fax·ine \des-ˌven-lə-ˈfak-ˌsēn\ *n* : a drug that functions as an SNRI and is administered orally chiefly in the form of its succinate $C_{16}H_{25}NO_2{\cdot}C_4H_6O_4{\cdot}H_2O$ or fumarate $C_{16}H_{25}NO_2{\cdot}C_4H_4O_4$ esp. to treat depression — see PRISTIQ

detached retina *n* : RETINAL DETACHMENT

detachment of the retina *n* : RETINAL DETACHMENT

detail man *n* : a representative of a drug manufacturer who introduces new drugs esp. to physicians and pharmacists — called also *detailer*

¹de·ter·gent \di-ˈtər-jənt\ *adj* : having a cleansing action

²detergent *n* : a cleansing agent (as a soap)

de·te·ri·o·rate \di-ˈtir-ē-ə-ˌrāt\ *vb* **-rat·ed; -rat·ing** : to become impaired in quality, functioning, or condition : DEGENERATE — **de·te·ri·o·ra·tion** \di-ˌtir-ē-ə-ˈrā-shən\ *n*

de·ter·mi·nant \di-ˈtər-mə-nənt\ *n* **1** : GENE **2** : EPITOPE

de·ter·mi·nate \di-ˈtər-mə-nət\ *adj* : relating to, being, or undergoing determinate cleavage ⟨a ~ egg⟩

determinate cleavage *n* : cleavage of an egg in which each division irreversibly separates portions of the zygote with specific potencies for further development — compare INDETERMINATE CLEAVAGE

de·ter·min·er \-ˈtər-mə-nər\ *n* : GENE

de·tick \(ˌ)dē-ˈtik\ *vb* : to remove ticks from ⟨~ dogs⟩

¹de·tox \(ˌ)dē-ˈtäks\ *vb* **1** : to subject oneself to or to undergo detoxification : DETOXIFY 2 **2** : to remove a harmful or intoxicating substance from : DETOXIFY 1

²de·tox \ˈdē-ˌtäks\ *n, often attrib* **1 a** : detoxification from an intoxicating or addictive substance ⟨a ~ clinic⟩ **b** : a detox program or facility **2** : a regimen or treatment to remove toxins and impurities from the body

de·tox·i·cant \(ˌ)dē-ˈtäk-si-kənt\ *n* : a detoxicating agent

de·tox·i·cate \-ˈtäk-sə-ˌkāt\ *vb* **-cat·ed; -cat·ing** : DETOXIFY — **de·tox·i·ca·tion** \-ˌtäk-sə-ˈkā-shən\ *n*

de·tox·i·fy \-ˈtäk-sə-ˌfī\ *vb* **-fied; -fy·ing 1 a** : to remove a poison or toxin or the effect of such from **b** : to render (a harmful substance) harmless **2** : to free (as a drug user or an alcoholic) from an intoxicating or an addictive substance in the body or from dependence on or addiction to such a substance — **de·tox·i·fi·ca·tion** \-ˌtäk-sə-fə-ˈkā-shən\ *n*

Det•rol \ˈdet-ˌrōl\ *trademark* — used for a preparation of tolterodine

de•tru•sor \di-ˈtrü-zər, -sər\ *n* : the outer largely longitudinally arranged musculature of the bladder wall — called also *detrusor muscle*

detrusor uri•nae \-yə-ˈrī-(ˌ)nē\ *n* : the external longitudinal musculature of the urinary bladder

de•tu•mes•cence \ˌdē-tü-ˈmes-ᵊns, -tyü-\ *n* : subsidence or diminution of swelling or erection — **de•tu•mes•cent** \-ᵊnt\ *adj*

deu•ter•anom•a•lous \ˌdü-tə-rə-ˈnä-mə-ləs, ˌdyü-\ *adj* : exhibiting partial loss of green color vision so that an increased intensity of this color is required in a mixture of red and green to match a given yellow

deu•ter•anom•a•ly \-mə-lē\ *n, pl* **-lies** : the condition of being deuteranomalous — compare PROTANOMALY, TRICHROMATISM

deu•ter•an•ope \ˈdü-tə-rə-ˌnōp, ˈdyü-\ *n* : an individual affected with deuteranopia

deu•ter•an•opia \ˌdü-tə-rə-ˈnō-pē-ə, ˌdyü-\ *n* : color blindness marked by usu. complete loss of ability to distinguish colors — **deu•ter•an•opic** \-ˈnō-pik, -ˈnä-\ *adj*

deux — see FOLIE À DEUX

de•vas•cu•lar•iza•tion \(ˌ)dē-ˌvas-kyə-lə-rə-ˈzā-shən\ *n* : loss of the blood supply to a bodily part due to destruction or obstruction of blood vessels — **de•vas•cu•lar•ized** \-ˈvas-kyə-lə-ˌrīzd\ *adj*

de•vel•op \di-ˈve-ləp\ *vb* **1 a** : to make active or promote the growth of ⟨~*ed* her muscles by weight lifting⟩ **b** : to go through a process of natural growth, differentiation, or evolution by successive stages **2** : to become infected or affected by ⟨~*ed* tuberculosis⟩ **3** : to acquire secondary sex characteristics

de•vel•op•ment \di-ˈve-ləp-mənt\ *n* **1** : the action or process of developing: as **a** : the process of growth and differentiation by which the potentialities of a zygote, spore, or embryo are realized **b** : the gradual advance through evolutionary stages : EVOLUTION **2** : the state of being developed — **de•vel•op•men•tal** \-ˌve-ləp-ˈment-ᵊl\ *adj* — **de•vel•op•men•tal•ly** *adv*

developmental disability *n* : any of various conditions (as autism spectrum disorder, cerebral palsy, or intellectual disability) that are marked by delayed development or functional limitations esp. in learning, language, communication, cognition, behavior, socialization, or mobility — **developmentally disabled** *adj*

developmental quotient *n* : a number expressing the development of a child determined by dividing the age of the group into which test scores place the child by the child's chronological age and multiplying by 100

de•vi•ance \ˈdē-vē-əns\ *n* : deviant quality, state, or behavior

[1]**de•vi•ant** \-ənt\ *adj* : deviating esp. from some accepted norm : characterized by deviation (as from a standard of conduct) ⟨socially ~ behavior⟩

[2]**deviant** *n* : something that deviates from a norm; *esp* : a person who differs markedly (as in social adjustment or sexual behavior) from what is considered normal for a group

[1]**de•vi•ate** \ˈdē-vē-ət, -vē-ˌāt\ *adj* : characterized by or given to significant departure from the behavioral norms of a particular society

[2]**deviate** *n* : one that deviates from a norm; *esp* : a person who differs markedly from a group norm

de•vi•at•ed septum \ˌdē-vē-ˌā-təd-\ *n* : deviation of the nasal septum from its normal position that results from a developmental abnormality or trauma

de•vi•a•tion \ˌdē-vē-ˈā-shən\ *n* : an act or instance of diverging (as in growth or behavior) from an established way or in a new direction

de•vi•tal•iza•tion \(ˌ)dē-ˌvīt-ᵊl-ə-ˈzā-shən\ *n* : destruction and usu. removal of the pulp from a tooth — **de•vi•tal•ize** \-ˈvīt-ᵊl-ˌīz\ *vb*

dew•claw \ˈdü-ˌklȯ, ˈdyü-\ *n* : a vestigial digit not reaching to the ground on the foot of a mammal; *also* : a claw or hoof terminating such a digit — **dew•clawed** \-ˌklȯd\ *adj*

de•worm \(ˌ)dē-ˈwərm\ *vb* : to rid (as a dog) of worms : WORM

de•worm•er \-ˈwər-mər\ *n* : WORMER

dex \ˈdeks\ *n* : the sulfate of dextroamphetamine

DEXA *abbr* dual-energy X-ray absorptiometry

dexa•meth•a•sone \ˌdek-sə-ˈme-thə-ˌsōn, -ˌzōn\ *n* : a synthetic glucocorticoid $C_{22}H_{29}FO_5$ also used in the form of its acetate $C_{24}H_{31}FO_6$ or sodium phosphate $C_{22}H_{28}FNa_2O_8P$ esp. as an anti-inflammatory and anti-allergy agent — see DECADRON

Dex•e•drine \ˈdek-sə-ˌdrēn, -drən\ *trademark* — used for a preparation of the sulfate of dextroamphetamine

dex•fen•flur•a•mine \ˌdeks-ˈfen-flu̇r-ə-ˌmēn\ *n* : the dextrorotatory form of fenfluramine formerly used in the form of its hydrochloride to treat obesity but no longer used due to its association with heart disease affecting the heart valves — see FEN-PHEN 1

dex•ies \ˈdek-sēz\ *n pl, slang* : tablets or capsules of the sulfate of dextroamphetamine

Dex•i•lant \ˈdek-sə-ˌlant\ *trademark* — used for a preparation of dexlansoprazole

dex•lan•so•pra•zole \ˌdeks-ˌlan-ˈsō-prə-ˌzōl\ *n* : a drug $C_{16}H_{14}F_3N_3O_2S$ that acts as a proton pump inhibitor and is used to treat heartburn and promote healing of erosive esophagitis — see DEXILANT

dex•meth•yl•phen•i•date \ˌdeks-ˌmeth-əl-ˈfen-ə-ˌdāt\ *n* : a mild stimulant of the central nervous system $C_{14}H_{19}NO_2 \cdot HCl$ used orally to treat attention deficit disorder — see FOCALIN

dextr- *or* **dextro-** *comb form* **1** : right : on or toward the right ⟨*dextro*cardia⟩ **2** *usu dextro-* : dextrorotatory ⟨*dextro*amphetamine⟩

[1]**dex•tral** \ˈdek-strəl\ *adj* : of or relating to the right; *esp* : RIGHT-HANDED — **dex•tral•ly** *adv*

[2]**dextral** *n* : a person exhibiting dominance of the right hand and eye

dex•tral•i•ty \dek-ˈstra-lə-tē\ *n, pl* **-ties** : the quality or state of having the right side or some parts (as the hand or eye) different from and usu. more efficient than the left or corresponding parts; *also* : RIGHT-HANDEDNESS

dex•tran \ˈdek-ˌstran, -strən\ *n* : any of numerous biopolymers $(C_6H_{10}O_5)_n$ of variable molecular weight that are produced by bacteria (genus *Leuconostoc*), are found in dental plaque, and are used esp. after suitable chemical modification as blood plasma substitutes and as pharmaceutical agents

dex•tran•ase \-strə-ˌnās, -ˌnāz\ *n* : a hydrolase that prevents tooth decay by breaking down dextran and eliminating plaque

dex•trin \ˈdek-strən\ *n* : any of various soluble gummy polysaccharides $(C_6H_{10}O_5)_n$ obtained from starch by the action of heat, acids, or enzymes

dex•tro \ˈdek-(ˌ)strō\ *adj* : DEXTROROTATORY

dex•tro•am•phet•amine \ˌdek-(ˌ)strō-am-ˈfe-tə-ˌmēn, -mən\ *n* : a stimulant drug consisting of dextrorotatory amphetamine that is usu. used in the form of its sulfate $(C_9H_{13}N)_2 \cdot H_2SO_4$ to treat narcolepsy and attention deficit disorder and is a common drug of abuse — see ADDERALL, DEXEDRINE

dex•tro•car•dia \ˌdek-strō-ˈkär-dē-ə\ *n* : an abnormal condition in which the heart is situated on the right side and the great blood vessels of the right and left sides are reversed — **dex•tro•car•di•al** \-dē-əl\ *adj*

dex•tro•me•thor•phan \ˌdek-strō-mi-ˈthȯr-ˌfan\ *n* : a cough suppressant that is widely used esp. in the form of its hydrobromide $C_{18}H_{25}NO \cdot HBr$ in over-the-counter cough and cold preparations — abbr. *DXM*

dex•tro•pro•poxy•phene \ˌdek-strə-prō-ˈpäk-sə-ˌfēn\ *n* : PROPOXYPHENE

dex•tro•ro•ta•to•ry \-ˈrō-tə-ˌtȯr-ē\ *also* **dex•tro•ro•ta•ry** \-ˈrō-tə-rē\ *adj* : turning clockwise or toward the right; *esp* : rotating the plane of polarization of light toward the right ⟨∼ crystals⟩ — compare LEVOROTATORY

dex•trose \ˈdek-ˌstrōs, -ˌstrōz\ *n* : dextrorotatory glucose — called also *grape sugar*

d4T \ˌdē-ˌfȯr-ˈtē\ *n* : STAVUDINE

DFP \ˌdē-(ˌ)ef-ˈpē\ *n* : ISOFLUROPHATE

DHA *abbr* **1** dehydroepiandrosterone **2** dihydroxyacetone **3** docosahexaenoic acid

DHEA *abbr* dehydroepiandrosterone

DHPG \ˌdē-(ˌ)āch-(ˌ)pē-ˈjē\ *n* : GANCICLOVIR

DHT *abbr* dihydrotestosterone

di- *comb form* **1** : twice : twofold : double ⟨*di*zygotic⟩ **2** : containing two atoms, radicals, or groups ⟨*di*oxide⟩

di•a•be•si•ty \ˌdī-ə-ˈbē-sə-tē\ *n* : obesity associated with diabetes : the state of being very overweight or obese and of having type 2 diabetes

Di•a•ßeta \ˌdī-ə-ˈbā-tə\ *trademark* — used for a preparation of glyburide

di•a•be•tes \ˌdī-ə-ˈbē-tēz, -təs\ *n, pl* **diabetes** : any of various abnormal conditions characterized by the secretion and excretion of excessive amounts of urine; *esp* : DIABETES MELLITUS

diabetes in•sip•i•dus \-in-ˈsi-pə-dəs\ *n* : a disorder that is caused by insufficient secretion of vasopressin by the pituitary gland or by a failure of the kidneys to respond to circulating vasopressin and that is characterized by intense thirst and by the excretion of large amounts of urine — see CENTRAL DIABETES INSIPIDUS, NEPHROGENIC DIABETES INSIPIDUS

diabetes mel•li•tus \-ˈme-lə-təs\ *n* : a variable disorder of carbohydrate metabolism caused by a combination of hereditary and environmental factors and usu. characterized by inadequate secretion or utilization of insulin, by excessive urine production, by excessive amounts of sugar in the blood and urine, and by thirst, hunger, and loss of weight — see TYPE 1 DIABETES, TYPE 2 DIABETES

[1]**di•a•bet•ic** \ˌdī-ə-ˈbe-tik\ *adj* **1** : of or relating to diabetes or diabetics **2** : affected with diabetes **3** : occurring in or caused by diabetes ⟨∼ coma⟩ **4** : suitable for diabetics ⟨∼ food⟩

[2]**diabetic** *n* : a person affected with diabetes

diabeticorum — see NECROBIOSIS LIPOIDICA DIABETICORUM

di•a•be•to•gen•ic \ˌdī-ə-ˌbē-tə-ˈje-nik\ *adj* : producing diabetes ⟨∼ drugs⟩

di•a•be•tol•o•gist \ˌdī-ə-bə-ˈtä-lə-jist\ *n* : a specialist in diabetes

di•ace•tic acid \ˌdī-ə-ˌsēt-ik-\ *n* : ACETOACETIC ACID

di•ace•tyl•mor•phine \ˌdī-ə-ˌsēt-ᵊl-ˈmȯr-ˌfēn, dī-ˌa-sət-ᵊl-\ *n* : HEROIN

di•ag•nose \ˈdī-ig-ˌnōs, -ˌnōz, ˌdī-ig-ˈ, -əg-\ *vb* **-nosed; -nos•ing** **1** : to recognize (as a disease) by signs and symptoms **2** : to diagnose a disease or condition in ⟨*diagnosed* the patient⟩ — **di·ag·nos·able** *also* **di·ag·nose·able** \ˌdī-ig-ˈnō-sə-bəl, -əg-, -zə-\ *adj*

di·ag·no·sis \ˌdī-ig-ˈnō-səs, -əg-\ *n, pl* **-no·ses** \-ˌsēz\ **1** : the art or act of identifying a disease from its signs and symptoms **2** : the decision reached by diagnosis

diagnosis related group *n* : DRG

[1]**di·ag·nos·tic** \-ˈnäs-tik\ *also* **di·ag·nos·ti·cal** \-ti-kəl\ *adj* **1** : of, relating to, or used in diagnosis **2** : using the methods of or yielding a diagnosis — **di·ag·nos·ti·cal·ly** \-ti-k(ə-)lē\ *adv*

[2]**diagnostic** *n* : the art or practice of diagnosis — often used in pl.

di·ag·nos·ti·cian \-(ˌ)näs-ˈti-shən\ *n* : a specialist in medical diagnostics

dia·ki·ne·sis \ˌdī-ə-kə-ˈnē-səs, -(ˌ)kī-\ *n, pl* **-ne·ses** \-ˌsēz\ : the final stage of the meiotic prophase marked by contraction of each chromosome pair — **dia·ki·net·ic** \-ˈne-tik\ *adj*

di·al·y·sance \dī-ˈa-lə-səns\ *n* : blood volume in milliliters per unit time cleared of a substance by dialysis

di·al·y·sate \dī-ˈa-lə-ˌzāt, -ˌsāt\ *also* **di·al·y·zate** \-ˌzāt\ *n* **1** : the material that passes through the membrane in dialysis **2** : the liquid into which material passes by way of the membrane in dialysis

di·al·y·sis \dī-ˈa-lə-səs\ *n, pl* **-y·ses** \-ˌsēz\ **1** : the separation of substances in solution by means of their unequal diffusion through semipermeable membranes; *esp* : such a separation of colloids from soluble substances **2** : either of two medical procedures to remove wastes or toxins from the blood and adjust fluid and electrolyte imbalances by utilizing rates at which substances diffuse through a semipermeable membrane: **a** : the process of removing blood from an artery (as of a kidney patient), purifying it by dialysis, adding vital substances, and returning it to a vein — called also *hemodialysis* **b** : a procedure performed in the peritoneal cavity in which the peritoneum acts as the semipermeable membrane — called also *peritoneal dialysis* — **di·a·lyt·ic** \ˌdī-ə-ˈli-tik\ *adj*

dialysis dementia *n* : a neurological syndrome that occurs in some long-term dialysis patients, is associated with aluminum intoxication (as from aluminum-containing compounds in the dialysis fluid), and is marked esp. by motor and speech disturbance (as dysarthria and myoclonus), progressive dementia, and seizures

di·a·lyze \ˈdī-ə-ˌlīz\ *vb* **-lyzed; -lyz·ing** **1** : to subject to or undergo dialysis **2** : to separate or obtain by dialysis — **di·a·lyz·abil·i·ty** \ˌdī-ə-ˌlī-zə-ˈbi-lə-tē\ *n* — **di·a·lyz·able** \-ˈlī-zə-bəl\ *adj*

di·a·lyz·er \-ˌlī-zər\ *n* : an apparatus in which dialysis is carried out consisting essentially of one or more containers for liquids separated into compartments by membranes

di·am·e·ter \dī-ˈa-mə-tər\ *n* **1** : a unit of magnification of a magnifying device equal to the number of times the linear dimensions of the object are increased **2** : one of the maximal breadths of a part of the body ⟨the transverse ~ of the inlet of the pelvis⟩

di·ami·no·di·phe·nyl sul·fone \ˌdī-ə-ˌmē-(ˌ)nō-ˌdī-ˈfen-ᵊl-ˈsəl-ˌfōn, -ˈfēn-\ *n* : DAPSONE

di·a·mond·back rattlesnake \ˈdī-mənd-ˌbak-, ˈdī-ə-\ *n* : either of two large and deadly rattlesnakes of the genus *Crotalus* (*C. adamanteus* of the southeastern U.S. and *C. atrox* of the south central and southwestern U.S. and Mexico) — called also *diamondback, diamondback rattler*

dia·mor·phine \ˌdī-ə-ˈmȯr-ˌfēn\ *n* : HEROIN

di·a·pe·de·sis \ˌdī-ə-pə-ˈdē-səs\ *n, pl* **-de·ses** \-ˌsēz\ : the passage of blood cells through capillary walls into the tissues — **di·a·pe·det·ic** \-ˈde-tik\ *adj*

[1]**di·a·per** \ˈdī-pər, ˈdī-ə-\ *n* : a basic garment esp. for infants consisting of a folded cloth or other absorbent material drawn up between the legs and fastened about the waist

[2]**diaper** *vb* **di·a·pered; di·a·per·ing** : to put on or change the diaper of (an infant)

diaper rash *n* : skin irritation of the diaper-covered area and usu. the buttocks of an infant esp. from exposure to feces and urinary ammonia

di·a·pho·re·sis \ˌdī-ə-fə-ˈrē-səs, (ˌ)dī-ˌa-fə-\ *n, pl* **-re·ses** \-ˌsēz\ : PERSPIRATION; *esp* : profuse perspiration artificially induced

[1]**di·a·pho·ret·ic** \-ˈre-tik\ *adj* **1** : having the power to increase sweating **2** : perspiring profusely : SWEATY

[2]**diaphoretic** *n* : an agent capable of inducing sweating

di·a·phragm \ˈdī-ə-ˌfram\ *n* **1** : a body partition of muscle and connective tissue; *specif* : the partition separating the chest and abdominal cavities in mammals — compare PELVIC DIAPHRAGM, UROGENITAL DIAPHRAGM **2** : a device that limits the aperture of a lens or optical system **3** : a molded cap usu. of thin rubber fitted over the uterine cervix to act as a mechanical contraceptive barrier

di·a·phrag·ma sel·lae \dī-ə-ˈfrag-mə-ˈse-ˌlī, -ˌlē\ *n, pl* : a small horizontal fold of the dura mater that roofs over the sella turcica and contains a small opening for passage of the infundibulum

di·a·phrag·mat·ic \ˌdī-ə-frə-ˈma-tik, -ˌfrag-\ *adj* : of, involving, or resembling a diaphragm ⟨~ hernia⟩

di·aph·y·se·al \dī-ˌa-fə-ˈsē-əl, -ˈzē-\ *or* **di·a·phys·i·al** \ˌdī-ə-ˈfi-zē-əl\ *adj* : of, relating to, or involving a diaphysis

di·a·phy·sec·to·my \ˌdī-ə-fə-ˈzek-tə-mē, -ˈsek-\ *n, pl* **-mies** : surgical excision of all or part of a diaphysis (as of the femur)

di·aph·y·sis \dī-ˈa-fə-səs\ *n, pl* **-y·ses** \-ˌsēz\ : the shaft of a long bone — compare EPIPHYSIS 1

di·ar·rhea \ˌdī-ə-ˈrē-ə\ *n* : abnormally frequent intestinal evacuations with more or less fluid stools

di·ar·rhe·al \-ˈrē-əl\ *adj* : of, relating to, or marked by diarrhea ⟨a ~ disease⟩

diarrheal shellfish poisoning *n* : shellfish poisoning that is marked by diarrhea, nausea, vomiting, and abdominal pain and is caused by toxins produced by dinoflagellates (as of the genera *Dinophysis* and *Prorocentrum*) and consumed in contaminated shellfish

di·ar·rhe·ic \-ˈrē-ik\ *adj* **1** : affected with diarrhea ⟨~ patients⟩ **2** : DIARRHEAL ⟨~ illness⟩

di·ar·rhet·ic \-ˈre-tik\ *adj* : DIARRHEAL

di·ar·rhoea, di·ar·rhoe·al, di·ar·rhoe·ic, di·ar·rhoet·ic *chiefly Brit var of* DIARRHEA, DIARRHEAL, DIARRHEIC, DIARRHETIC

di·ar·thro·sis \ˌdī-är-ˈthrō-səs\ *n, pl* **-thro·ses** \-ˌsēz\ **1** : articulation that permits free movement **2** : a freely movable joint — called also *synovial joint* — **di·ar·thro·di·al** \ˌdī-ˌär-ˈthrō-dē-əl\ *adj*

di·a·stase \ˈdī-ə-ˌstās, -ˌstāz\ *n* **1** : AMYLASE; *esp* : a mixture of amylases from malt **2** : ENZYME

di·as·ta·sis \dī-ˈas-tə-səs\ *n, pl* **-ta·ses** \-ˌsēz\ **1** : an abnormal separation of parts normally joined together **2** : the rest phase of cardiac diastole occurring between filling of the ventricle and the start of atrial contraction

di·a·stat·ic \ˌdī-ə-ˈsta-tik\ *adj* : relating to or having the properties of diastase; *esp* : converting starch into sugar

di·a·ste·ma \ˌdī-ə-ˈstē-mə\ *n, pl* **-mas** *or* **-ma·ta** \-mə-tə\ : a space between teeth in a jaw

di·a·ste·ma·to·my·e·lia \ˌdī-ə-ˌstē-mə-tō-mī-ˈē-lē-ə, -ˌste-\ *n* : congenital division of all or part of the spinal cord

di·as·to·le \dī-ˈas-tə-(ˌ)lē\ *n* : the passive rhythmical expansion or dilation of the cavities of the heart during which they fill with blood — compare SYSTOLE — **di·a·stol·ic** \ˌdī-ə-ˈstä-lik\ *adj*

diastolic blood pressure *n* : the lowest arterial blood pressure of a cardiac cycle occurring during diastole of the heart — called also *diastolic pressure;* compare SYSTOLIC BLOOD PRESSURE

di·a·stroph·ic dwarfism \ˌdī-ə-ˈsträ-fik-\ *n* : an inherited dysplasia affecting bones and joints and characterized esp. by clubfoot, deformities of the digits of the hand, malformed pinnae, and cleft palate

dia·ther·my \ˈdī-ə-ˌthər-mē\ *n, pl* **-mies** : the generation of heat in tissue by electric currents for medical or surgical purposes — see ELECTROCOAGULATION — **dia·ther·mic** \ˌdī-ə-ˈthər-mik\ *adj*

di·ath·e·sis \dī-ˈa-thə-səs\ *n, pl* **-e·ses** \-ˌsēz\ : a constitutional predisposition toward a particular state or condition and esp. one that is abnormal or diseased

di·a·tom \ˈdī-ə-ˌtäm\ *n* : any of a class (Bacillariophyceae) of planktonic one-celled or colonial algae with skeletons of silica

dia·tri·zo·ate \ˌdī-ə-ˌtrī-ˈzō-ˌāt\ *n* : either of two salts of the acid $C_{11}H_9I_3N_2O_4$ administered in solution as a radiopaque medium for various forms of radiographic diagnosis — see HYPAQUE

di·az·e·pam \dī-ˈa-zə-ˌpam\ *n* : a synthetic tranquilizer $C_{16}H_{13}ClN_2O$ used esp. to relieve anxiety and tension and as a muscle relaxant — see VALIUM

Di·az·i·non \dī-ˈa-zə-ˌnän\ *trademark* — used for an organophosphate insecticide $C_{12}H_{21}N_2O_3PS$ that is a cholinesterase inhibitor dangerous to humans if ingested

di·az·ox·ide \ˌdī-ˌa-ˈzäk-ˌsīd\ *n* : a drug $C_8H_7ClN_2O_2S$ used in the treatment of hypoglycemia and in the emergency treatment of hypertension

di·benz·an·thra·cene *or* **1,2:5,6–di·benz·an·thra·cene** \(ˌ)wən-ˌtü-ˌfīv-ˌsiks-)dī-ˌben-ˈzan-thrə-ˌsēn\ *n* : a carcinogenic cyclic hydrocarbon $C_{22}H_{14}$ found in trace amounts in coal tar

di·ben·zo·fu·ran \ˈdī-ˌben-zō-ˈfyu̇-ˌran, -fyə-ˈran\ *n* : a highly toxic chemical compound $C_{12}H_8O$ that is used in chemical synthesis and as an insecticide and is a hazardous pollutant in its chlorinated form

di·bro·mo·chlo·ro·pro·pane \(ˌ)dī-ˌbrō-mō-ˌklōr-ō-ˈprō-ˌpān\ *n* : DBCP

di·bu·caine \dī-ˈbyü-ˌkān, ˈdī-ˌ\ *n* : a local anesthetic $C_{20}H_{29}N_3O_2$ used for temporary relief of pain and itching esp. from burns, sunburn, insect bites, or hemorrhoids — called also *cinchocaine*

dibucaine number *n* : a number expressing the percentage by which cholinesterase activity in a serum sample is inhibited by dibucaine

DIC *abbr* disseminated intravascular coagulation

di·cen·tric \(ˌ)dī-ˈsen-trik\ *adj* : having two centromeres ⟨a ~ chromosome⟩ — **dicentric** *n*

dich- *or* **dicho-** *comb form* : apart : separate ⟨*dich*otic⟩

di·chlo·ra·mine–T \ˌdī-ˌklōr-ə-ˌmēn-ˈtē\ *n* : a yellow crystalline compound

$C_7H_7Cl_2NO_2S$ used esp. formerly as an antiseptic

***p*–dichlorobenzene** *var of* PARADICHLOROBENZENE

2,4–di•chlo•ro•phen•oxy•ace•tic acid *also* **di•chlo•ro•phen•oxy•ace•tic acid** \(ˌ)tü-ˌfōr-)ˌdī-ˌklōr-ō-(ˌ)phe-ˌnäk-sē-ə-ˈsē-tik-\ *n* : 2,4-D

di•chlor•vos \(ˌ)dī-ˈklōr-ˌväs, -vəs\ *n* : an organophosphorus insecticide and anthelmintic $C_4H_7Cl_2O_4P$ used esp. in veterinary medicine — called also *DDVP*

dich•otic \(ˌ)dī-ˈkō-tik\ *adj* : relating to or involving the presentation of a stimulus to one ear that differs in some respect (as pitch, loudness, frequency, or energy) from a stimulus presented to the other ear ⟨~ listening⟩ — **dich•oti•cal•ly** \-ti-k(ə-)lē\ *adv*

di•chot•o•my \dī-ˈkä-tə-mē\ *n, pl* **-mies** : a division or forking into branches; *esp* : repeated bifurcation — **di•chot•o•mous** \dī-ˈkä-tə-məs\ *adj*

di•chro•mat \ˈdī-krō-ˌmat, (ˌ)dī-ˈ\ *n* : one affected with dichromatism

di•chro•ma•tism \dī-ˈkrō-mə-ˌti-zəm\ *n* : partial color blindness in which only two colors are perceptible — **di•chro•mat•ic** \ˌdī-krō-ˈma-tik\ *adj*

Dick test \ˈdik-\ *n* : a test to determine susceptibility or immunity to scarlet fever by an injection of scarlet fever toxin

Dick, George Frederick (1881–1967), and **Gladys Henry (1881–1963),** American physicians.

di•clo•fe•nac \dī-ˈklō-fə-ˌnak\ *n* : a nonsteroidal anti-inflammatory drug used in the form of its sodium salt $C_{14}H_{10}Cl_2NNaO_2$ or potassium salt $C_{14}H_{10}Cl_2KNaO_2$ esp. to treat the symptoms of rheumatoid arthritis, osteoarthritis, and ankylosing spondylitis — see VOLTAREN

di•clox•a•cil•lin \(ˌ)dī-ˌkläk-sə-ˈsi-lən\ *n* : a semisynthetic penicillin used in the form of its sodium salt $C_{19}H_{16}Cl_2N_3NaO_5S·H_2O$ esp. against beta-lactamase producing staphylococci

di•cou•ma•rin \(ˌ)dī-ˈkü-mə-rən\ *n* : DICUMAROL

Di•cro•coe•li•um \ˌdī-krə-ˈsē-lē-əm\ *n* : a genus (family Dicrocoeliidae) of small digenetic trematodes infesting the livers of ruminants or occas. other mammals including humans — see LANCET FLUKE

di•crot•ic \(ˌ)dī-ˈkrä-tik\ *adj* **1** *of the pulse* : having a double beat (as in certain febrile states in which the heart is overactive and the arterial walls are lacking in tone) — compare MONOCROTIC **2** : being or relating to the second part of the arterial pulse occurring during diastole of the heart or of an arterial pressure recording made during the same period — **di•cro•tism** \ˈdī-krə-ˌti-zəm\ *n*

dicrotic notch *n* : a secondary upstroke in the descending part of a pulse tracing corresponding to the transient increase in aortic pressure upon closure of the aortic valve

Dic•ty•o•cau•lus \ˌdik-tē-ə-ˈkȯ-ləs\ *n* : a genus (family Metastrongylidae) of lungworms infesting various mammals (as sheep and horses)

dic•tyo•some \ˈdik-tē-ə-ˌsōm\ *n* : GOLGI APPARATUS

di•cu•ma•rol *or* **di•cou•ma•rol** \dī-ˈkü-mə-ˌrȯl, -ˈkyü-, -ˌrōl\ *n* : an anticoagulant $C_{19}H_{12}O_6$ that acts similarly to warfarin and is used esp. in preventing and treating thromboembolic disease

di•cy•clo•mine \(ˌ)dī-ˈsī-klə-ˌmēn, -ˈsi-\ *n* : an anticholinergic drug used in the form of its hydrochloride $C_{19}H_{35}NO_2·HCl$ for its antispasmodic effect on smooth muscle in gastrointestinal functional disorders

di•dan•o•sine \dī-ˈda-nə-ˌsēn\ *n* : DDI

di•de•oxy•cy•ti•dine \ˌdī-(ˌ)dē-ˌäk-sē-ˈsi-tə-dēn, -ˈsī-\ *n* : DDC

di•de•oxy•ino•sine \-ˈi-nə-ˌsēn, -ˈī-, -sən\ *n* : DDI

die \ˈdī\ *vb* **died; dy•ing** \ˈdī-iŋ\ **1** : to suffer total and irreversible loss of the bodily attributes and functions that constitute life **2** : to suffer or face the pains of death

diel•drin \ˈdēl-drən\ *n* : a white crystalline persistent chlorinated hydrocarbon insecticide $C_{12}H_8Cl_6O$

Diels \ˈdēls\, **Otto Paul Hermann (1876–1954),** and **Al•der** \ˈȯl-dər\, **Kurt (1902–1958),** German chemists.

di•en•ceph•a•lon \ˌdī-ən-ˈse-fə-ˌlän, ˌdī-(ˌ)en-, -lən\ *n* : the posterior subdivision of the forebrain — called also *betweenbrain* — **di•en•ce•phal•ic** \-sə-ˈfa-lik\ *adj*

die•ner \ˈdē-nər\ *n* : a laboratory helper esp. in a medical school

di•en•es•trol \ˌdī-ə-ˈnes-ˌtrȯl, -ˌtrōl\ *n* : a white crystalline estrogenic compound $C_{18}H_{18}O_2$ structurally related to diethylstilbestrol and used topically to treat atrophic vaginitis and kraurosis vulvae

di•en•oes•trol \ˌdī-ə-ˈnēs-ˌtrȯl, -ˌtrōl\ *chiefly Brit var of* DIENESTROL

Di•ent•amoe•ba \ˌdī-ˌen-tə-ˈmē-bə\ *n* : a genus of amoebic protozoans parasitic in the intestines of humans and monkeys that include one (*D. fragilis*) known to cause abdominal pain, anorexia, and loose stools in humans

di•es•trus \(ˌ)dī-ˈes-trəs\ *n* : a period of sexual quiescence that intervenes between two periods of estrus — **di•es•trous** \-trəs\ *adj*

¹di•et \ˈdī-ət\ *n* **1** : food and drink regularly provided or consumed **2** : habitual nourishment **3** : the kind and amount of food prescribed for a person or animal for a special reason **4** : a regimen of eating and drinking sparingly so as to reduce one's weight

²diet *vb* : to eat or cause to eat less or according to a prescribed rule

³diet *adj* **1 :** reduced in calories or without calories ⟨a ~ soft drink⟩ **2 :** promoting weight loss ⟨~ pills⟩

¹di•etary \ˈdī-ə-ˌter-ē\ *n, pl* **di•etar•ies :** the kinds and amounts of food available to or eaten by an individual, group, or population

²dietary *adj* **:** of or relating to a diet or to the rules of a diet ⟨~ habits⟩ — **di•etari•ly** \ˌdī-ə-ˈter-ə-lē\ *adv*

dietary fiber *n* **:** FIBER 2

Dietary Reference Intake *n* **:** a set of guidelines for the daily intake of nutrients (as vitamins, protein, and fats) and other food components (as fiber) — abbr. *DRI*

dietary supplement *n* **:** a product taken orally that contains one or more ingredients (as vitamins or herbs) that are intended to supplement one's diet and are not considered food

di•et•er \ˈdī-ə-tər\ *n* **:** one that diets; *esp* **:** a person that consumes a reduced allowance of food in order to lose weight

di•etet•ic \ˌdī-ə-ˈte-tik\ *adj* **1 :** of or relating to diet **2 :** adapted (as by the elimination of salt or sugar) for use in special diets — **di•etet•i•cal•ly** \-ti-k(ə-)lē\ *adv*

di•etet•ics \-ˈte-tiks\ *n, sing or pl* **:** the science or art of applying the principles of nutrition to feeding

diethylamide — see LYSERGIC ACID DIETHYLAMIDE

di•eth•yl•car•bam•azine \ˌdī-ˌe-thəl-kär-ˈba-mə-ˌzēn, -zən\ *n* **:** an anthelmintic derived from piperazine and administered in the form of its crystalline citrate $C_{10}H_{21}N_3O·C_6H_8O_7$ esp. to control filariasis in humans and roundworms in dogs and cats

di•eth•yl ether \(ˌ)dī-ˈe-thəl-\ *n* **:** ETHER 1

di•eth•yl•pro•pi•on \(ˌ)dī-ˌe-thəl-ˈprō-pē-ˌän\ *n* **:** a sympathomimetic amine related structurally to amphetamine and used esp. in the form of its hydrochloride $C_{13}H_{19}NO·HCl$ as an appetite suppressant to promote weight loss — see TENUATE

di•eth•yl•stil•bes•trol \-stil-ˈbes-ˌtrȯl, -ˌtrōl\ *n* **:** a synthetic estrogen $C_{18}H_{20}O_2$ used formerly to prevent miscarriage or premature delivery but was discontinued in the U.S. in the 1970s due to its association with serious side effects (as reproductive tract abnormalities) in offspring exposed while developing in the uterus — called also *DES, stilbestrol*

di•eth•yl•stil•boes•trol \-ˈbēs-ˌtrȯl, -ˌtrōl\ *chiefly Brit var of* DIETHYLSTILBESTROL

di•eti•tian *or* **di•eti•cian** \ˌdī-ə-ˈti-shən\ *n* **:** a specialist in dietetics

Die•tl's crisis \ˈdēt-ᵊlz-\ *n* **:** an attack of violent pain in the kidney region accompanied by chills, nausea, vomiting, and collapse that is caused by the formation of kinks in the ureter and is usu. associated with a floating kidney

Dietl \ˈdēt-ᵊl\, **Josef (1804–1878),** Polish physician.

diet pill *n* **:** a pill and esp. one containing amphetamine prescribed esp. formerly to promote weight loss by increasing metabolism or depressing appetite

differential blood count *n* **:** a blood count which includes separate counts for each kind of white blood cell — compare COMPLETE BLOOD COUNT

differential cell count *n* **:** a count of cells that includes a separate count for each type of cell; *esp* **:** DIFFERENTIAL BLOOD COUNT

differential diagnosis *n* **:** the distinguishing of a disease or condition from others presenting similar symptoms

dif•fer•en•ti•ate \ˌdi-fə-ˈren-chē-ˌāt\ *vb* **-at•ed; -at•ing 1 :** to constitute a difference that distinguishes **2 a :** to cause differentiation of in the course of development **b :** to undergo differentiation **3 :** to sense, recognize, or give expression to a difference (as in stimuli) **4 :** to cause differentiation in (a specimen for microscopic examination) by staining

dif•fer•en•ti•a•tion \-ˌren-chē-ˈā-shən\ *n* **1 a :** the act or process of differentiating **b :** the enhancement of microscopically visible differences between tissue or cell parts by partial selective decolorization or removal of excess stain **2 a :** modification of different parts of the body for performance of particular functions **b :** the sum of the developmental processes whereby apparently unspecialized cells, tissues, and structures attain their adult form and function

differently abled *adj* **:** DISABLED, CHALLENGED

Dif•fe•rin \ˈdi-fə-rən\ *trademark* — used for a preparation of adapalene

dif•flu•ent \ˈdi-(ˌ)flü-ənt\ *adj* **:** soft like mush ⟨a ~ spleen⟩

dif•fu•sate \di-ˈfyü-ˌzāt\ *n* **:** DIALYSATE

¹dif•fuse \di-ˈfyüs\ *adj* **:** not concentrated or localized ⟨~ sclerosis⟩

²dif•fuse \di-ˈfyüz\ *vb* **dif•fused; dif•fus•ing 1 :** to subject to or undergo diffusion **2 :** to break up and distribute (incident light) by reflection (as from a rough surface) — **dif•fus•ible** \di-ˌfyü-zə-bəl\ *adj* — **dif•fus•ibil•i•ty** \-ˌfyü-zə-ˈbi-lə-tē\ *n*

dif•fu•sion \di-ˈfyü-zhən\ *n* **1 :** the process whereby particles of liquids, gases, or solids intermingle as the result of their spontaneous movement caused by thermal agitation and in dissolved substances move from a region of higher to one of lower concentration **2 a :** reflection of light by a rough reflecting surface **b :** transmission of light through a translucent material — **dif•fu•sion•al** \-ˈfyü-zhə-nəl\ *adj*

Di•flu•can \dī-ˈflük-ˌän\ *trademark* — used for a preparation of fluconazole

di·flu·ni·sal \(ˌ)dī-ˈflü-nə-ˌsal\ *n* : a nonsteroidal anti-inflammatory drug $C_{13}H_8F_2O_3$ related to aspirin that is used to relieve mild to moderately severe pain — see DOLOBID

di·flu·pred·nate \ˌdī-flü-ˈpred-ˌnāt\ *n* : a corticosteroid $C_{27}H_{34}F_2O_7$ used in an emulsion applied as eye drops to treat uveitis of the iris and ciliary body and inflammation and pain associated with ocular surgery — see DUREZOL

di·gas·tric muscle \(ˌ)dī-ˈgas-trik-\ *n* : either of a pair of muscles that extend from the anterior inferior margin of the mandible to the temporal bone and serve to depress the lower jaw and raise the hyoid bone esp. during swallowing — called also *digastric*

di·gas·tri·cus \-tri-kəs\ *n* : DIGASTRIC MUSCLE

di·ge·net·ic \ˌdī-jə-ˈne-tik\ *adj* : of or relating to a subclass (Digenea) of trematode worms in which sexual reproduction as an internal parasite of a vertebrate alternates with asexual reproduction in a mollusk and which include a number of parasites (as the Chinese liver fluke) of humans

Di·George syndrome \də-ˈjȯrj-\ *also* **Di·George's syndrome** \-ˈjȯr-jəz-\ *n* : a rare congenital disease that is characterized esp. by absent or underdeveloped thymus and parathyroid glands, heart defects, immunodeficiency, hypocalcemia, and characteristic facial features (as wide-set eyes and small jaws)

Di George, Angelo Mario (1921–2009), American endocrinologist and pediatrician.

¹di·gest \ˈdī-ˌjest\ *n* : a product of digestion

²di·gest \dī-ˈjest, də-\ *vb* **1** : to convert (food) into absorbable form **2 a** : to soften, decompose, or break down by heat and moisture or chemicals **b** : to extract soluble ingredients from by warming with a liquid — **di·ges·ter** \-ˈjes-tər\ *n*

di·ges·tant \-ˈjes-tənt\ *n* : a substance that digests or aids in digestion

di·gest·ibil·i·ty \-ˌjes-tə-ˈbi-lə-tē\ *n, pl* **-ties** **1** : the fitness of something for digestion **2** : the percentage of a foodstuff taken into the digestive tract that is absorbed into the body

di·gest·ible \-ˈjes-tə-bəl\ *adj* : capable of being digested

di·ges·tion \-ˈjes-chən\ *n* : the action, process, or power of digesting; *esp* : the process of making food absorbable by mechanically and enzymatically breaking it down into simpler chemical compounds in the digestive tract

¹di·ges·tive \-ˈjes-tiv\ *n* **1** : something that aids digestion esp. of food **2** : a substance which promotes suppuration

²digestive *adj* **1** : relating to or functioning in digestion ⟨~ processes⟩ **2** : having the power to cause or promote digestion ⟨~ enzymes⟩

digestive gland *n* : a gland secreting digestive enzymes

digestive system *n* : the bodily system concerned with the ingestion, digestion, and absorption of food and the discharge of residual wastes and consisting of the digestive tract and accessory glands (as the salivary glands and the pancreas) that secrete digestive enzymes — called also *alimentary system*

digestive tract *n* : the tubular passage typically extending from mouth to anus or cloaca that functions in digestion and absorption of food and elimination of residual waste and that in most mammals includes the mouth, pharynx, esophagus, stomach, intestine, and anus — called also *alimentary canal, alimentary tract*

dig·i·lan·id \ˌdi-jə-ˈla-nəd\ *or* **dig·i·lan·ide** \-ˌnīd, -nəd\ *n* : LANATOSIDE

digilanid A *or* **digilanide A** *n* : LANATOSIDE a

digilanid B *or* **digilanide B** *n* : LANATOSIDE b

digilanid C *or* **digilanide C** *n* : LANATOSIDE c

dig·it \ˈdi-jət\ *n* : any of the divisions (as a finger or toe) in which the limbs of amphibians and all higher vertebrates terminate and which in humans are five in number on each limb

dig·i·tal \ˈdi-jət-ᵊl\ *adj* **1** : of, relating to, or supplying one or more fingers or toes ⟨a ~ branch of an artery⟩ **2** : done with a finger ⟨a ~ rectal examination⟩ — **dig·i·tal·ly** *adv*

dig·i·tal·in \ˌdi-jə-ˈta-lən, -ˈtā-\ *n* **1** : a white crystalline steroid glycoside $C_{36}H_{56}O_{14}$ obtained from seeds esp. of a common European foxglove (*Digitalis purpurea*) **2** : a mixture of the glycosides of digitalis leaves or seeds

dig·i·tal·is \-ləs\ *n* **1 a** *cap* : a genus of Eurasian herbs (family Scrophulariaceae) that have stalks of showy bell-shaped flowers **b** : FOXGLOVE **2** : the dried leaf of a common European foxglove (*D. purpurea*) that contains physiologically active glycosides, that is a powerful cardiac stimulant and a diuretic, and that is used in standardized powdered form esp. in the treatment of congestive heart failure and in the management of atrial fibrillation, atrial flutter, and paroxysmal tachycardia of the atria; *broadly* : any of various glycosides (as digoxin or digitoxin) that are constituents of digitalis or are derived from a related foxglove (*D. lanata*)

dig·i·ta·li·za·tion \ˌdi-jət-ᵊl-ə-ˈzā-shən\ *n* : the administration of digitalis (as in heart disease) until the desired physiological adjustment is attained; *also* : the bodily state so produced — **dig·i·ta·lize** \ˈdi-jət-ᵊl-ˌīz\ *vb*

digital nerve *n* **1** : any of several branches of the median nerve and the ulnar nerve supplying the fingers and thumb **2** : any of several branches of the medial plantar nerve supplying the toes

Dig•i•tek \ˈdi-jə-ˌtek\ *trademark* — used for a preparation of digoxin

digiti — see ABDUCTOR DIGITI MINIMI, EXTENSOR DIGITI MINIMI, EXTENSOR DIGITI QUINTI PROPRIUS, FLEXOR DIGITI MINIMI BREVIS, OPPONENS DIGITI MINIMI

digitorum — see EXTENSOR DIGITORUM BREVIS, EXTENSOR DIGITORUM COMMUNIS, EXTENSOR DIGITORUM LONGUS, FLEXOR DIGITORUM BREVIS, FLEXOR DIGITORUM LONGUS, FLEXOR DIGITORUM PROFUNDUS, FLEXOR DIGITORUM SUPERFICIALIS

dig•i•tox•in \ˌdi-jə-ˈtäk-sən\ *n* : a poisonous glycoside $C_{41}H_{64}O_{13}$ that is the most active constituent of digitalis; *also* : a mixture of digitalis glycosides consisting chiefly of digitoxin

di•glyc•er•ide \dī-ˈgli-sə-ˌrīd\ *n* : an ester of glycerol that contains two ester groups and involves one or two acids

di•gox•in \di-ˈjäk-sən, -ˈgäk-\ *n* : a poisonous cardiotonic glycoside $C_{41}H_{64}O_{14}$ obtained from the leaves of a foxglove (*Digitalis lanata*) and used similarly to digitalis — see DIGITEK, LANOXIN

di•hy•dro•chlo•ride \(ˌ)dī-ˌhī-drə-ˈklōr-ˌīd\ *n* : a chemical compound with two molecules of hydrochloric acid

di•hy•dro•co•de•inone \-kō-ˈdē-ə-ˌnōn\ *n* : HYDROCODONE

di•hy•dro•er•got•a•mine \-ˌhī-drō-ˌər-ˈgä-tə-ˌmēn\ *n* : a hydrogenated derivative of ergotamine that is used in the form of its mesylate $C_{33}H_{37}N_5O_5 \cdot CH_4O_3S$ in the treatment of migraine

di•hy•dro•fo•late reductase \-ˈfō-ˌlāt\ *n* : an enzyme that is essential for DNA and protein synthesis

di•hy•dro•mor•phi•none \-ˈmȯr-fə-ˌnōn\ *n* : HYDROMORPHONE

di•hy•dro•strep•to•my•cin \-ˌstrep-tə-ˈmīs-ᵊn\ *n* : a toxic antibiotic $C_{21}H_{41}N_7O_{12}$ formerly used but abandoned because of its tendency to impair hearing

di•hy•dro•tachy•ste•rol \-ˌta-ki-ˈster-ˌȯl, -ˈstir-, -ˌōl\ *n* : an alcohol $C_{28}H_{45}OH$ used in the treatment of hypocalcemia

di•hy•dro•tes•tos•ter•one \-te-ˈstäs-tə-ˌrōn\ *n* : a biologically active metabolite $C_{19}H_{30}O_2$ of testosterone having similar androgenic activity — abbr. *DHT*

di•hy•dro•the•elin \-ˈthē-ə-lən\ *n* : ESTRADIOL

di•hy•droxy•ac•e•tone \ˌdī-hī-ˌdräk-sē-ˈa-sə-ˌtōn\ *n* : a glyceraldehyde isomer $C_3H_6O_3$ that is used esp. to stain the skin to simulate a tan

1,25–di•hy•droxy•cho•le•cal•cif•er•ol \ˌwən-ˌtwen-tē-ˌfīv-ˌdī-hī-ˌdräk-sē-ˌkō-lə-(ˌ)kal-ˈsi-fə-ˌrȯl, -ˌrōl\ *n* : CALCITRIOL

di•hy•droxy•phe•nyl•al•a•nine \ˌdī-hī-ˌdräk-sē-ˌfen-ᵊl-ˈa-lə-ˌnēn, -ˌfēn-\ *n* **1** *or* **3,4–dihydroxyphenylalanine** \ˌthrē-ˌfōr-\ : DOPA **2** *or* **L–3,4–dihydroxyphenylalanine** \ˌel-\ *or* **L dihydroxyphenylalanine** : L-DOPA

di•io•do•hy•droxy•quin \ˌdī-ˌī-ə-ˌdō-hī-ˈdräk-si-kwən\ *n* : IODOQUINOL

di•io•do•hy•droxy•quin•o•line \-hī-ˌdräk-si-ˈkwin-ᵊl-ˌēn\ *n* : IODOQUINOL

di•io•do•ty•ro•sine \-ˈtī-rə-ˌsēn\ *n* : a compound $C_9H_9I_2NO_3$ of tyrosine and iodine that is produced in the thyroid gland from monoiodotyrosine and that combines with monoiodotyrosine to form triiodothyronine

di•iso•pro•pyl flu•o•ro•phos•phate \ˌdī-ˌī-sə-ˈprō-pəl-ˌflu̇r-ō-ˈfäs-ˌfāt\ *n* : ISOFLUROPHATE

di•lac•er•a•tion \(ˌ)dī-ˌla-sə-ˈrā-shən\ *n* : injury (as partial fracture) to a developing tooth that results in a curve in the long axis as development continues — **di•lac•er•at•ed** \(ˌ)dī-ˈla-sə-ˌrā-təd\ *adj*

Di•lan•tin \dī-ˈlant-ᵊn, də-\ *trademark* — used for a preparation of phenytoin

di•la•ta•tion \ˌdi-lə-ˈtā-shən, ˌdī-\ *n* **1** : the condition of being stretched beyond normal dimensions esp. as a result of overwork or disease or of abnormal relaxation **2** : DILATION 2

di•la•ta•tor \ˈdi-lə-ˌtā-tər, ˈdī-\ *n* : DILATOR b

di•late \dī-ˈlāt, ˈdī-ˌ\ *vb* **di•lat•ed; di•lat•ing** **1** : to enlarge, stretch, or cause to expand **2** : to become expanded or swollen

di•la•tion \dī-ˈlā-shən\ *n* **1** : the state of being dilated : DILATATION **2** : the action of stretching or enlarging an organ or part of the body

dilation and curettage *n* : a medical procedure in which the uterine cervix is dilated and a curette is inserted into the uterus to scrape away the endometrium (as for the diagnosis or treatment of abnormal bleeding or for surgical abortion during the early part of the second trimester of pregnancy) — called also *D&C*

dilation and evacuation *n* : a surgical abortion that is typically performed midway during the second trimester of pregnancy and in which the uterine cervix is dilated and fetal tissue is removed using surgical instruments (as a forceps and curette) and suction — called also *D&E*

dilation and extraction *n* : a surgical abortion that is typically performed during the third trimester or later part of the second trimester of pregnancy and in which the death of the fetus is induced after it has passed partway through the dilated cervix — called also *D&X, partial-birth abortion*

di•la•tor \(ˌ)dī-ˈlā-tər, də-\ *n* : one that dilates: as **a** : an instrument for expanding a tube, duct, or cavity ⟨a urethral ~〉 **b** : a muscle that dilates a part **c** : a drug (as a vasodilator) causing dilation

Di·lau·did \(ˌ)dī-ˈlȯ-did\ *trademark* — used for a preparation of hydromorphone

dil·do \ˈdil-(ˌ)dō\ *n, pl* **dildos** *also* **dildoes** : an object resembling a penis used for sexual stimulation

dil·ti·a·zem \dil-ˈtī-ə-(ˌ)zem\ *n* : a calcium channel blocker used esp. in the form of its hydrochloride $C_{22}H_{26}N_2O_4S·HCl$ as a coronary vasodilator — see CARDIZEM

[1]**dil·u·ent** \ˈdil-yə-wənt\ *n* : a diluting agent (as the vehicle in a medicinal preparation)

[2]**diluent** *adj* : making thinner or less concentrated by admixture

[1]**di·lute** \dī-ˈlüt, də-\ *vb* **di·lut·ed; di·lut·ing** : to make thinner or more liquid by admixture — **di·lut·er** *also* **di·lut·or** \-ˈlü-tər\ *n*

[2]**dilute** *adj* : of relatively low strength or concentration

di·lu·tion \dī-ˈlü-shən, də-\ *n* **1** : the action of diluting : the state of being diluted **2** : something (as a solution) that is diluted

di·men·hy·dri·nate \ˌdī-ˌmen-ˈhī-drə-ˌnāt\ *n* : an antihistamine $C_{24}H_{28}ClN_5O_3$ used esp. to prevent nausea (as in motion sickness)

di·mer \ˈdī-mər\ *n* : a polymer formed from two molecules of a monomer — **di·mer·ic** \(ˌ)dī-ˈmer-ik\ *adj*

di·mer·cap·rol \ˌdī-(ˌ)mər-ˈka-ˌprȯl, -ˌprōl\ *n* : a colorless viscous oily compound $C_3H_8OS_2$ with an offensive odor used in treating arsenic, mercury, and gold poisoning — called also *BAL, British anti-lewisite*

di·meth·yl·ami·no·eth·a·nol \(ˈ)dī-ˈme-thə-lə-ˌmē-nō-ˈe-thə-ˌnȯl, -nōl\ *n* : DMAE

di·meth·yl fumarate \(ˈ)dī-ˈme-thəl-\ *n* : a drug $C_6H_8O_4$ taken by mouth in the treatment of relapsing multiple sclerosis — see TECFIDERA

di·meth·yl·ni·tros·amine \(ˌ)dī-ˌme-thəl-(ˌ)nī-ˈtrō-sə-ˌmēn\ *n* : a carcinogenic nitrosamine $C_2H_6N_2O$ that occurs esp. in tobacco smoke — called also *nitrosodimethylamine*

dimethyl sul·fox·ide \-səl-ˈfäk-sīd\ *n* : an anti-inflammatory agent $(CH_3)_2SO$ used in the treatment of interstitial cystitis — called also *DMSO*

di·meth·yl·tryp·ta·mine \-ˈtrip-tə-ˌmēn\ *n* : a hallucinogenic drug $C_{12}H_{16}N_2$ that is chemically similar to but shorter acting than psilocybin — called also *DMT*

dim·ple \ˈdim-pəl\ *n* : a slight natural indentation or hollow in the surface of some part of the human body (as on a cheek or the chin) — **dimple** *vb*

dinitrate — see ISOSORBIDE DINITRATE

di·ni·tro·phe·nol \ˌdī-ˌnī-trō-ˈfē-ˌnōl, -fi-ˈ\ *n* : any of six isomeric compounds $C_6H_4N_2O_5$ some of whose derivatives are pesticides; *esp* : a highly toxic compound formerly used in weight control

di·no·fla·gel·late \ˌdī-nō-ˈfla-jə-lət, -ˌlāt, -flə-ˈje-lət\ *n* : any of an order (Dinoflagellata) of chiefly marine planktonic plantlike unicellular protists of which some cause red tide

Di·oc·to·phy·ma \(ˌ)dī-ˌäk-tə-ˈfī-mə\ *n* : a genus (family Dioctophymidae) of nematode worms including a single species (*D. renale*) which is a destructive parasite of the kidney of dogs, minks, and sometimes humans

di·oes·trus *chiefly Brit var of* DIESTRUS

di·op·ter \dī-ˈäp-tər, ˈdī-ˌäp-\ *n* : a unit of measurement of the refractive power of a lens equal to the reciprocal of the focal length in meters

di·op·tric \(ˌ)dī-ˈäp-trik\ *adj* **1** : producing or serving in refraction of a beam of light : REFRACTIVE; *specif* : assisting vision by refracting and focusing light **2** : produced by means of refraction

Di·o·van \ˈdī-ə-ˌvan\ *trademark* — used for a preparation of valsartan

di·ox·ide \(ˌ)dī-ˈäk-ˌsīd\ *n* : an oxide (as carbon dioxide) containing two atoms of oxygen in a molecule

di·ox·in \(ˌ)dī-ˈäk-sən\ *n* : any of several persistent toxic hydrocarbons that occur esp. as by-products of various industrial processes and waste incineration; *esp* : TCDD — see AGENT ORANGE

di·oxy·ben·zone \(ˌ)dī-ˌäk-sē-ˈben-ˌzōn, -ben-ˈ\ *n* : a sunscreen $C_{14}H_{12}O_4$ that absorbs UVB and some UVA radiation

dip \ˈdip\ *n* : a liquid preparation of an insecticide, parasiticide, or fungicide which is applied to animals by immersing them in it — **dip** *vb*

di·pep·ti·dase \dī-ˈpep-tə-ˌdās, -ˌdāz\ *n* : any of various enzymes that hydrolyze dipeptides but not polypeptides

di·pep·tide \(ˌ)dī-ˈpep-ˌtīd\ *n* : a peptide that yields two molecules of amino acid on hydrolysis

di·pha·sic \(ˌ)dī-ˈfā-zik\ *adj* : having two phases: as **a** : exhibiting a stage of stimulation followed by a stage of depression or vice versa 〈the ~ action of certain drugs〉 **b** : relating to or being a record of a nerve impulse that is negative and positive — compare MONOPHASIC 1, POLYPHASIC 1

di·phen·hy·dra·mine \ˌdī-ˌfen-ˈhī-drə-ˌmēn\ *n* : an antihistamine used esp. in the form of its hydrochloride $C_{17}H_{21}NO·HCl$ to treat allergy symptoms and motion sickness and to induce sleep — see BENADRYL

di·phen·oxy·late \ˌdī-ˌfen-ˈäk-sə-ˌlāt\ *n* : an antidiarrheal agent used in the form of its hydrochloride $C_{30}H_{32}N_2O_2·HCl$ in combination with the sulfate of atropine — see LOMOTIL

di·phe·nyl·hy·dan·to·in \(ˌ)dī-ˌfen-ᵊl-hī-ˈdan-tə-wən, -ˌfēn-\ *n* : PHENYTOIN

di·phos·phate \(ˌ)dī-ˈfäs-ˌfāt\ *n* : a phosphate containing two phosphate groups

2,3–di·phos·pho·glyc·er·ate *also* **di·phos·pho·glyc·er·ate** \(ˌtü-ˌthrē-)ˌdī-ˌfäs-fō-ˈgli-sə-ˌrāt\ *n* : a phosphate that occurs in human red blood cells and facilitates release of oxygen by decreasing the oxygen affinity of hemoglobin

di·phos·pho·nate \(ˌ)dī-ˈfäs-fə-ˌnāt\ *n* : BISPHOSPHONATE

di·phos·pho·pyr·i·dine nucleotide \-ˌpir-ə-ˌdēn-\ *n* : NAD

diph·the·ria \dif-ˈthir-ē-ə, dip-\ *n* : an acute febrile contagious disease marked by the formation of a false membrane esp. in the throat and caused by a bacterium of the genus *Corynebacterium* (*C. diphtheriae*) which produces a toxin causing inflammation of the heart and nervous system — **diph·the·ri·al** \-ē-əl\ *adj*

diph·the·rit·ic \ˌdif-thə-ˈri-tik, ˌdip-\ *adj* : relating to, produced in, or affected with diphtheria; *also* : resembling diphtheria esp. in the formation of a false membrane ⟨~ dysentery⟩

[1]**diph·the·roid** \ˈdif-thə-ˌrȯid\ *adj* : resembling diphtheria

[2]**diphtheroid** *n* : a bacterium (esp. genus *Corynebacterium*) that resembles the bacterium of diphtheria but does not produce diphtheria toxin

di·phyl·lo·both·ri·a·sis \(ˌ)dī-ˌfi-lō-bä-ˈthrī-ə-səs\ *n, pl* **-a·ses** \-ˌsēz\ : infestation with or disease caused by the fish tapeworm

Di·phyl·lo·both·ri·um \-ˈbä-thrē-əm\ *n* : a genus of tapeworms (family Diphyllobothriidae) that includes the fish tapeworm (*D. latum*) of humans

dipl- *or* **diplo-** *comb form* : double : twofold ⟨*diplo*coccus⟩ ⟨*dipl*opia⟩

dip·la·cu·sis \ˌdi-plə-ˈkyü-səs\ *n, pl* **-cu·ses** \-ˌsēz\ : the hearing of a single tone as if it were two tones of different pitch

di·ple·gia \dī-ˈplē-jə, -jē-ə\ *n* : paralysis of corresponding parts (as the legs) on both sides of the body

dip·lo·coc·cus \ˌdi-plō-ˈkä-kəs\ *n, pl* **-coc·ci** \-ˈkä-ˌkī, -kē; ˈkäk-ˌsī, -sē\ : any of various encapsulated bacteria (as the pneumococcus) that usu. occur in pairs and that were formerly grouped in a single taxon (genus *Diplococcus*) but are now all assigned to other genera — **di·plo·coc·cal** \-kəl\ *adj*

dip·loe \ˈdi-plə-ˌwē\ *n* : cancellous bony tissue between the external and internal layers of the skull — **di·plo·ic** \də-ˈplō-ik, dī-\ *adj*

diploic vein *n* : any of several veins situated in channels in the diploe

[1]**dip·loid** \ˈdi-ˌplȯid\ *adj* : having the basic chromosome number doubled — **dip·loi·dy** \-ˌplȯi-dē\ *n*

[2]**diploid** *n* : a single cell, individual, or generation characterized by the diploid chromosome number

dip·lo·mate \ˈdi-plə-ˌmāt\ *n* : a physician qualified to practice in a medical specialty by advanced training and experience in the specialty followed by passing an intensive examination by a national board of senior specialists

dip·lo·pia \di-ˈplō-pē-ə\ *n* : a disorder of vision in which two images of a single object are seen (as from unequal action of the eye muscles) — called also *double vision* — **dip·lo·pic** \-ˈplō-pik, -ˈplä-\ *adj*

dip·lo·tene \ˈdi-plə-ˌtēn\ *n* : a stage of meiotic prophase which follows the pachytene and during which the paired homologous chromosomes begin to separate and chiasmata become visible — **diplotene** *adj*

di·pole \ˈdī-ˌpōl\ *n* **1** : a pair of equal and opposite electric charges or magnetic poles of opposite sign separated by a small distance **2** : a body or system (as a molecule) having such charges — **di·po·lar** \-ˌpō-lər, -ˈpō-\ *adj*

di·po·tas·sium \ˌdī-pə-ˈta-sē-əm\ *adj* : containing two atoms of potassium in a molecule

di·pro·pi·o·nate \(ˌ)dī-ˈprō-pē-ə-ˌnāt\ *n* : an ester containing two propionate groups

dip·so·gen·ic \ˌdip-sə-ˈje-nik, -sō-\ *adj* : producing thirst ⟨~ diabetes insipidus⟩

dip·so·ma·nia \ˌdip-sə-ˈmā-nē-ə, -nyə\ *n* : an uncontrollable craving for alcoholic liquors — **dip·so·ma·ni·ac** \-nē-ˌak\ *n* — **dip·so·ma·ni·a·cal** \ˌdip-sō-mə-ˈnī-ə-kəl\ *adj*

dip·stick \ˈdip-ˌstik\ *n* : a chemically sensitive strip of paper used to identify one or more constituents (as glucose or protein) of urine by immersion

dip·ter·an \ˈdip-tə-rən\ *adj* : of, relating to, or being a fly (sense 2a) — **dipteran** *n* — **dip·ter·ous** \-rəs\ *adj*

Di·py·lid·i·um \ˌdī-ˌpī-ˈli-dē-əm, -pə-\ *n* : a genus of taenioid tapeworms including the dog tapeworm (*D. caninum*)

di·pyr·i·dam·ole \(ˌ)dī-ˌpir-ə-ˈda-ˌmȯl, -ˌmōl\ *n* : a drug $C_{24}H_{40}N_8O_4$ used chiefly to prevent blood clot formation — see AGGRENOX, PERSANTINE

di·rec·tive \də-ˈrek-tiv, dī-\ *adj* : of or relating to psychotherapy in which the therapist introduces information, content, or attitudes not previously expressed by the client

di·rec·tor \də-ˈrek-tər, dī-\ *n* : an instrument grooved to guide and limit the motion of a surgical knife

direct pyramidal tract *n* : VENTRAL CORTICOSPINAL TRACT

Di·ro·fi·lar·ia \ˌdī-(ˌ)rō-fə-ˈlar-ē-ə\ *n* : a genus of filarial worms that includes the heartworm (*D. immitis*) — **di·ro·fi·lar·i·al** \-ē-əl\ *adj*

di•ro•fil•a•ri•a•sis \-ˌfi-lə-ˈrī-ə-səs\ *n, pl* **-a•ses** \-ˌsēz\ : infestation with filarial worms of the genus *Dirofilaria* and esp. with the heartworm (*D. immitis*)

dirty \ˈdər-tē\ *adj* **dirt•i•er; -est** : contaminated with infecting organisms

dis•abil•i•ty \ˌdi-sə-ˈbi-lə-tē\ *n, pl* **-ties** **1** : a physical, mental, cognitive, or developmental condition that impairs, interferes with, or limits a person's ability to engage in certain tasks or actions; *also* : impaired function or ability **2 a** (1) : an impairment (as a chronic medical condition or injury) that prevents one from engaging in gainful employment (2) : an impairment (as spina bifida) that results in serious functional limitations for a minor **b** : a program providing financial support to one affected with disability

dis•able \di-ˈsā-bəl, -ˈzā-\ *vb* **dis•abled; dis•abling** : to impair physically or mentally : to cause disability in

dis•abled *adj* **1** : incapacitated by illness or injury **2** : impaired or limited by a physical, mental, cognitive, or developmental condition : affected by disability

dis•able•ment \-mənt\ *n* : the act of becoming disabled; *also* : the state of being disabled

di•sac•cha•ri•dase \(ˌ)dī-ˈsa-kə-rə-ˌdās, -ˌdāz\ *n* : an enzyme (as maltase) that hydrolyzes disaccharides

di•sac•cha•ride \(ˌ)dī-ˈsa-kə-ˌrīd\ *n* : any of a class of sugars (as sucrose) that on hydrolysis yields two monosaccharide molecules

dis•ar•tic•u•la•tion \ˌdi-sär-ˌti-kyə-ˈlā-shən\ *n* : separation or amputation of a body part at a joint ⟨∼ of the shoulder⟩ — **dis•ar•tic•u•late** \-ˈti-kyə-ˌlāt\ *vb*

disc, discectomy *var of* DISK, DISKECTOMY

disc- *or* **disci-** *or* **disco-** *comb form* : disk ⟨*disci*form⟩

[1]**dis•charge** \dis-ˈchärj, ˈdis-ˌ\ *vb* **discharged; dis•charg•ing** **1** : to release from confinement, custody, or care ⟨∼ a patient from the hospital⟩ **2 a** : to give outlet to or emit ⟨a boil *discharging* pus⟩ **b** : to release or give expression to (as a pent-up emotion)

[2]**dis•charge** \ˈdis-ˌchärj, dis-ˈ\ *n* **1** : the act of relieving of something ⟨∼ of a repressed impulse⟩ **2** : release from confinement, custody, or care **3** : something that is emitted or evacuated ⟨a purulent ∼⟩

disci *pl of* DISCUS

dis•ci•form \ˈdi-sə-ˌfȯrm\ *adj* : round or oval in shape

dis•cis•sion \də-ˈsi-shən, -zhən\ *n* : an incision (as in treating cataract) of the capsule of the lens of the eye

dis•clos•ing \dis-ˈklō-ziŋ\ *adj* : being or using an agent (as a tablet or liquid) that contains a usu. red dye that adheres to and stains dental plaque

dis•co•gen•ic \ˌdi-skə-ˈje-nik\ *also* **dis•ko•gen•ic** *adj* : originating in an intervertebral disk : produced by factors (as herniation) occurring in an intervertebral disk ⟨∼ pain⟩

discogram, discography *var of* DISKOGRAM, DISKOGRAPHY

[1]**dis•coid** \ˈdis-ˌkȯid\ *adj* **1** : resembling a disk : being flat and circular **2** : characterized by macules ⟨∼ lupus erythematosus⟩

[2]**discoid** *n* : an instrument with a disk-shaped blade used in dentistry for carving

dis•coi•dal \dis-ˈkȯid-ᵊl\ *adj* : of, resembling, or producing a disk; *esp* : having the villi restricted to one or more disklike areas

dis•cop•a•thy \dis-ˈkä-pə-thē\ *n, pl* **-thies** : any disease affecting an intervertebral disk

dis•cor•dant \dis-ˈkȯrd-ᵊnt\ *adj, of twins* : dissimilar with respect to one or more particular characters — compare CONCORDANT — **dis•cor•dance** \-ᵊns\ *n*

dis•crete \dis-ˈkrēt, ˈdis-ˌ\ *adj* : characterized by distinct unconnected lesions ⟨∼ smallpox⟩ — compare CONFLUENT 2

dis•crim•i•nate \dis-ˈkri-mə-ˌnāt\ *vb* **-nat•ed; -nat•ing** : to respond selectively to (a stimulus)

dis•crim•i•na•tion \dis-ˌkri-mə-ˈnā-shən\ *n* : the process by which two stimuli differing in some aspect are responded to differently

dis•cus \ˈdis-kəs\ *n, pl* **dis•ci** \-ˌkī, -kē\ : any of various rounded and flattened anatomical structures

discus pro•lig•er•us \-prō-ˈli-jə-rəs\ *n* : CUMULUS

dis•ease \di-ˈzēz\ *n* : an impairment of the normal state of the living body or one of its parts that interrupts or modifies the performance of the vital functions and is a response to environmental factors (as malnutrition), to specific infective agents (as viruses), to inherent defects of the organism (as genetic anomalies), or to combinations of these factors : SICKNESS, ILLNESS — **dis•eased** \-ˈzēzd\ *adj*

dis•equi•lib•ri•um \(ˌ)di-ˌsē-kwə-ˈli-brē-əm, -ˌse-\ *n, pl* **-ri•ums** *or* **-ria** : loss or lack of equilibrium

disfunction *var of* DYSFUNCTION

dis•har•mo•ny \(ˌ)dis-ˈhär-mə-nē\ *n, pl* **-nies** : lack of harmony — see OCCLUSAL DISHARMONY

dish•pan hands \ˈdish-ˌpan-\ *n sing or pl* : irritant contact dermatitis of the hands that is marked by dry, red, and scaly skin and results from repeated exposure to cleaning materials (as detergents) typically used in housework

dis•in•fect \ˌdis-ᵊn-ˈfekt\ *vb* : to free from infection esp. by destroying harmful microorganisms — **dis•in•fec•tion** \-ˈfek-shən\ *n*

[1]**dis•in•fec•tant** \-ˈfek-tənt\ *n* : a chemical that destroys vegetative forms of

harmful microorganisms (as bacteria and fungi) esp. on inanimate objects but that may be less effective in destroying spores

[2]**disinfectant** *adj* : serving or tending to disinfect : suitable for use in disinfecting

dis•in•fest \ˌdis-ᵊn-ˈfest\ *vb* : to rid of small animal pests (as insects or rodents) — **dis•in•fes•ta•tion** \(ˌ)dis-ˌin-ˌfes-ˈtā-shən\ *n*

dis•in•fes•tant \ˌdis-ᵊn-ˈfes-tənt\ *n* : a disinfesting agent

dis•in•hib•it \ˌdis-in-ˈhi-bət\ *vb* : to cause the loss or reduction of an inhibition ⟨~ of a reflex⟩ — **dis•in•hi•bi•tion** \(ˌ)dis-ˌin-hə-ˈbi-shən, -ˌsi-nə-\ *n*

dis•in•hib•i•to•ry \-in-ˈhi-bə-ˌtōr-ē\ *adj* : tending to overcome psychological inhibition ⟨~ drugs⟩

dis•in•ter \ˌdis-in-ˈtər\ *vb* : to take out of the grave or tomb — **dis•in•ter•ment** \-mənt\ *n*

dis•junc•tion \dis-ˈjəŋk-shən\ *n* : the separation of chromosomes or chromatids during anaphase of mitosis or meiosis

disk *or* **disc** \ˈdisk\ *n* : any of various rounded or flattened anatomical structures: as **a** : a mammalian blood cell **b** : BLIND SPOT **c** : INTERVERTEBRAL DISK — see SLIPPED DISK

disk•ec•to•my *also* **disc•ec•to•my** \dis-ˈkek-tə-mē\ *n, pl* **-mies** : surgical removal of an intervertebral disk

disk•o•gram *also* **disc•o•gram** \ˈdis-kə-ˌgram\ *n* : a radiograph of an intervertebral disk made after injection of a radiopaque substance

dis•kog•ra•phy *also* **dis•cog•ra•phy** \dis-ˈkä-grə-fē\ *n, pl* **-phies** : the process of making a diskogram

dis•lo•cate \ˈdis-lō-ˌkāt, -lə-; (ˌ)dis-ˈlō-ˌkāt\ *vb* **-cat•ed; -cat•ing** : to put (a body part) out of order by displacing a bone from its normal connections with another bone ⟨he *dislocated* his shoulder⟩; *also* : to displace (a bone) from normal connections with another bone ⟨the humerus was *dislocated* in the fall⟩

dis•lo•ca•tion \ˌdis-(ˌ)lō-ˈkā-shən, -lə-\ *n* : displacement of one or more bones at a joint : LUXATION

dismutase — see SUPEROXIDE DISMUTASE

di•so•di•um \(ˌ)dī-ˈsō-dē-əm\ *adj* : containing two atoms of sodium in a molecule

disodium cromoglycate \-ˌkrō-mō-ˈglī-ˌkāt\ *n* : CROMOLYN

disodium ed•e•tate \-ˈe-də-ˌtāt\ *n* : a disodium salt $C_{10}H_{14}N_2Na_2O_8{\cdot}2H_2O$ of EDTA that has an affinity for calcium and is used to treat hypercalcemia and pathological calcification

di•so•mic \dī-ˈsō-mik\ *adj* : having one or more chromosomes present in two copies ⟨the ~ state is normal in humans⟩ — **di•so•my** \-mē\ *n*

di•so•pyr•a•mide \ˌdī-(ˌ)sō-ˈpir-ə-ˌmīd\ *n* : a cardiac depressant used in the form of its phosphate $C_{21}H_{29}N_3O{\cdot}H_3PO_4$ to treat life-threatening ventricular arrhythmias

[1]**dis•or•der** \(ˌ)di-ˈsȯr-dər, -ˈzȯr-\ *vb* **dis•or•dered; dis•or•der•ing** : to disturb the regular or normal functions of

[2]**disorder** *n* : an abnormal physical or mental condition : AILMENT

dis•or•dered *adj* **1** : not functioning in a normal orderly healthy way ⟨~ bodily functions⟩ **2** : mentally unbalanced

dis•or•ga•ni•za•tion \(ˌ)di-ˌsȯr-gə-nə-ˈzā-shən\ *n* : psychopathological inconsistency in personality, mental functions, or overt behavior — **dis•or•ga•nize** \(ˌ)di-ˈsȯr-gə-ˌnīz\ *vb*

dis•ori•ent \(ˌ)di-ˈsōr-ē-ˌent\ *vb* : to produce a state of disorientation in : DISORIENTATE

dis•ori•en•ta•tion \(ˌ)di-ˌsōr-ē-ən-ˈtā-shən, -ˌen-\ *n* : a usu. transient state of confusion esp. as to time, place, or identity often as a result of disease or drugs — **dis•ori•en•tate** \-ˈsōr-ē-ən-ˌtāt, -ˌen-\ *vb*

dis•par•i•ty \di-ˈspar-ə-tē\ *n, pl* **-ties** : the state of being different or dissimilar (as in the sensory information received) — see RETINAL DISPARITY

dis•pen•sa•ry \di-ˈspen-sə-rē\ *n, pl* **-ries** : a place where medicine or medical or dental treatment is dispensed

dis•pen•sa•to•ry \di-ˈspen-sə-ˌtōr-ē\ *n, pl* **-ries 1** : a book or medicinal formulary containing a systematic description of the drugs and preparations used in medicine **2** : DISPENSARY

dis•pense \dis-ˈpens\ *vb* **dis•pensed; dis•pens•ing 1** : to put up (a prescription or medicine) **2** : to prepare and distribute (medication) — **dis•pen•sa•tion** \ˌdis-pən-ˈsā-shən, -pen-\ *n*

dispensing optician *n, Brit* : a person qualified and licensed to fit and supply eyeglasses

dis•place•ment \di-ˈsplā-smənt\ *n* **1** : the act or process of removing something from its usual or proper place or the state resulting from this : DISLOCATION ⟨the ~ of a knee joint⟩ **2** : the quantity in which or the degree to which something is displaced **3 a** : the direction of an emotion or impulse away from its original object (as an idea or person) to something that is more acceptable **b** : SUBLIMATION **c** : the substitution of another form of behavior for what is usual or expected esp. when the usual response is nonadaptive — **dis•place** \-ˈsplās\ *vb*

dis•pro•por•tion \ˌdis-prə-ˈpōr-shən\ *n* : absence of symmetry or the proper dimensional relationship — see CEPHALOPELVIC DISPROPORTION

dis•rup•tive \dis-ˈrəp-tiv\ *adj* : characterized by psychologically disorganized behavior ⟨a confused and ~ patient in the manic phase⟩

dissecans — see OSTEOCHONDRITIS DISSECANS

dis•sect \di-ˈsekt, dī-; ˈdī-ˌ\ *vb* **1** : to cut so as to separate into pieces or to expose the several parts of (as an animal or a cadaver) for scientific examination; *specif* : to separate or follow along natural lines of cleavage (as through connective tissue) **2** : to make a medical dissection — **dis•sec•tor** \-ˈsek-tər, -ˌsek-\ *n*

dis•sec•tion \di-ˈsek-shən, dī-; ˈdī-ˌ\ *n* **1** : the act or process of dissecting or separating: as **a** : the surgical removal along natural lines of cleavage of tissues which are or might become diseased **b** : the digital separation of tissues (as in heart-valve operations) **c** : a pathological splitting or separation of tissue — see AORTIC DISSECTION **2 a** : something (as a part or the whole of an animal) that has been dissected **b** : an anatomical specimen prepared in this way

dis•sem•i•nat•ed \di-ˈse-mə-ˌnā-təd\ *adj* : widely dispersed in a tissue, organ, or the entire body — see ACUTE DISSEMINATED ENCEPHALOMYELITIS — **dis•sem•i•na•tion** \-ˌse-mə-ˈnā-shən\ *n*

disseminated intravascular coagulation *n* : an acute or chronic thrombotic and hemorrhagic disorder that arises secondary to various disease states (as acute promyelocytic leukemia, abruptio placentae, or major trauma) and is marked by uncontrolled systemic coagulation resulting in thrombosis which in acute cases typically leads to generalized bleeding due to depletion of clotting factors and increased fibrinolysis — abbr. *DIC*

dis•so•ci•a•tion \(ˌ)di-ˌsō-sē-ˈā-shən, -shē-\ *n* **1** : the process by which a chemical combination breaks up into simpler constituents **2** : the separation of whole segments of the personality (as in multiple personality disorder) or of discrete mental processes (as in the schizophrenias) from the mainstream of consciousness or of behavior — **dis•so•ci•ate** \-ˈsō-sē-ˌāt, -shē-\ *vb* — **dis•so•cia•tive** \(ˌ)di-ˈsō-shē-ˌā-tiv, -sē-, -shə-tiv\ *adj*

dissociative identity disorder *n* : MULTIPLE PERSONALITY DISORDER

dis•so•lu•tion \ˌdi-sə-ˈlü-shən\ *n* : the act or process of dissolving

dis•solve \di-ˈzälv, -ˈzölv\ *vb* **dis•solved; dis•solv•ing** **1** : to pass or cause to pass into solution **2** : to cause to melt or liquefy **3** : to become fluid — **dis•solv•er** *n*

dis•so•nance \ˈdi-sə-nəns\ *n* : inconsistency between the beliefs one holds or between one's actions and one's beliefs — see COGNITIVE DISSONANCE

dist- — see DISTO-

dis•tal \ˈdist-ᵊl\ *adj* **1** : situated away from the point of attachment or origin or a central point: as **a** : located away from the center of the body ⟨the ~ end of a bone⟩ — compare PROXIMAL 1a **b** : located away from the mesial plane of the body — compare MESIAL 2 **c** : of, relating to, or being the surface of a tooth that is next to the following tooth counting from the middle of the front of the upper or lower jaw or that faces the back of the mouth in the case of the last tooth on each side — compare MESIAL 3, PROXIMAL 1b **2** : physical or social rather than sensory — compare PROXIMAL 2 — **dis•tal•ly** *adv*

distal convoluted tubule *n* : the convoluted portion of the nephron lying between the loop of Henle and the nonsecretory part of the nephron and concerned esp. with the concentration of urine — called also *convoluted tubule, distal tubule*

distalis — see PARS DISTALIS

distal radioulnar joint *n* : a pivot joint between the lower end of the ulna and the ulnar notch on the lower end of the radius that permits rotation of the distal end of the radius around the longitudinal axis of the ulna — called also *inferior radioulnar joint*

dis•tem•per \dis-ˈtem-pər\ *n* **1** : a highly contagious virus disease esp. of dogs that is marked by fever, leukopenia, and respiratory, gastrointestinal, and neurological symptoms and that is caused by a paramyxovirus of the genus *Morbillivirus* (species *Canine distemper virus*) — called also *canine distemper* **2** : STRANGLES **3** : PANLEUKOPENIA

dis•tend \di-ˈstend\ *vb* : to enlarge or stretch out (as from internal pressure)

dis•ten•si•ble \-ˈsten-sə-bəl\ *adj* : capable of being distended, extended, or dilated ⟨~ blood vessels⟩ — **dis•ten•si•bil•i•ty** \-ˌsten-sə-ˈbi-lə-tē\ *n*

dis•ten•sion *or* **dis•ten•tion** \di-ˈsten-chən\ *n* : the act of distending or the state of being distended esp. unduly or abnormally

disto- *also* **dist-** *or* **disti-** *comb form* : distal ⟨*disto*buccal⟩

dis•to•buc•cal \ˌdis-tō-ˈbə-kəl\ *adj* : relating to or located on the distal and buccal surfaces of a molar or premolar — **dis•to•buc•cal•ly** *adv*

dis•to•lin•gual \-ˈliŋ-gwəl, -gyə-wəl\ *adj* : relating to or situated on the distal and lingual surfaces of a tooth

di•sto•ma•to•sis \ˌdī-ˌstō-mə-ˈtō-səs\ *n, pl* **-to•ses** \-ˌsēz\ : infestation with or disease (as liver rot) caused by digenetic trematode worms

di•sto•mi•a•sis \ˌdī-stō-ˈmī-ə-səs\ *n, pl* **-a•ses** \-ˌsēz\ : DISTOMATOSIS

dis•tor•tion \di-ˈstȯr-shən\ *n* **1** : the censorship of unacceptable unconscious impulses so that they are unrecognizable to the ego in the manifest content of a dream **2** : a lack of correspondence of size or intensity in an image resulting from defects in an optical system

dis•tract•i•bil•i•ty \di-ˌstrak-tə-ˈbi-lə-tē\ *n, pl* **-ties** : a condition in which the attention of the mind is easily distracted by small and irrelevant stimuli — **dis•tract•ible** \-ˈstrak-tə-bəl\ *adj*

dis•trac•tion \di-ˈstrak-shən\ *n* **1 a** : diversion of the attention **b** : mental confusion **2** : excessive separation (as from improper traction) of fracture fragments — **dis•tract** \di-ˈstrakt\ *vb*

dis•tress \di-ˈstres\ *n* : pain or suffering affecting the body, a bodily part, or the mind ⟨gastric ~⟩ ⟨respiratory ~⟩

dis•tri•bu•tion \ˌdis-trə-ˈbyü-shən\ *n* : the pattern of branching and termination of a ramifying anatomical structure (as a nerve or artery)

district nurse *n, Brit* : a qualified nurse who is employed by a local authority to visit and treat patients in their own homes — compare VISITING NURSE

dis•turbed \di-ˈstərbd\ *adj* : showing symptoms of emotional or mental illness ⟨~ children⟩ — **dis•tur•bance** \-ˈstər-bəns\ *n*

di•sul•fi•ram \dī-ˈsəl-fə-ˌram\ *n* : a compound $C_{10}H_{20}N_2S_4$ that causes a severe physiological reaction to alcohol and is used esp. in the treatment of alcoholism — called also *tetraethylthiuram disulfide;* see ANTABUSE

di•sul•phi•ram *chiefly Brit var of* DISULFIRAM

di•thra•nol \ˈdī-thrə-ˌnȯl, ˈdi-, -ˌnōl\ *n, chiefly Brit* : ANTHRALIN

di•ure•sis \ˌdī-yə-ˈrē-səs\ *n, pl* **di•ure•ses** \-ˌsēz\ : an increased excretion of urine

[1]**di•uret•ic** \ˌdī-yə-ˈre-tik\ *adj* : tending to increase the excretion of urine — **di•uret•i•cal•ly** \-ti-k(ə-)lē\ *adv*

[2]**diuretic** *n* : an agent that increases the excretion of urine

Di•ur•il \ˈdī-yu̇r-il\ *trademark* — used for a preparation of chlorothiazide

di•ur•nal \dī-ˈərn-ᵊl\ *adj* **1** : having a daily cycle ⟨~ rhythms⟩ **2** : of, relating to, or occurring in the daytime ⟨~ activity⟩ — **di•ur•nal•ly** *adv*

di•val•pro•ex sodium \ˌdī-ˈval-prō-eks-\ *n* : a combination of valproate and valproic acid that is used esp. to treat manic episodes of bipolar disorder and absence seizures of epilepsy — called also *divalproex;* see DEPAKOTE

di•ver•gence \də-ˈvər-jəns, dī-\ *n* **1** : a drawing apart **2** : dissemination of the effect of activity of a single nerve cell through multiple synaptic connections — compare CONVERGENCE 2 — **di•verge** \-ˈvərj\ *vb* — **di•ver•gent** \-ˈvər-jənt\ *adj*

divergent thinking *n* : creative thinking that may follow many lines of thought and tends to generate new and original solutions to problems — compare CONVERGENT THINKING

diverticula *pl of* DIVERTICULUM

di•ver•tic•u•lar \ˌdī-vər-ˈti-kyə-lər\ *adj* : consisting of or resembling a diverticulum

diverticular disease *n* : a disorder characterized by diverticulosis or diverticulitis

di•ver•tic•u•lec•to•my \ˌdī-vər-ˌti-kyə-ˈlek-tə-mē\ *n, pl* **-mies** : the surgical removal of a diverticulum

di•ver•tic•u•li•tis \-ˈlī-təs\ *n* : inflammation or infection of a diverticulum of the colon that is marked by abdominal pain or tenderness often accompanied by fever, chills, and cramping

di•ver•ti•cu•lop•exy \-ˈlä-pək-sē\ *n, pl* **-ex•ies** : surgical obliteration or fixation of a diverticulum

di•ver•tic•u•lo•sis \-ˈlō-səs\ *n, pl* **-lo•ses** \-ˌsēz\ : an intestinal disorder characterized by the presence of many diverticula in the colon that is typically symptomless but may be marked by symptoms (as bleeding or constipation)

di•ver•tic•u•lum \ˌdī-vər-ˈti-kyə-ləm\ *n, pl* **-la** \-lə\ **1** : an abnormal pouch or sac opening from a hollow organ (as the colon or bladder) **2** : a blind tube or sac branching off from a cavity or canal of the body

di•vide \də-ˈvīd\ *vb* **di•vid•ed; di•vid•ing** **1** : to separate into two or more parts ⟨~ a nerve surgically⟩ **2** : to undergo replication, multiplication, fission, or separation into parts ⟨actively *dividing* cells⟩

di•vi•sion \də-ˈvi-zhən\ *n* **1** : the act or process of dividing : the state of being divided — see CELL DIVISION **2** : a group of organisms forming part of a larger group; *specif* : a primary category of the plant kingdom that is typically equivalent to a phylum — **di•vi•sion•al** \-ˈvi-zhə-nəl\ *adj*

di•zy•got•ic \ˌdī-zī-ˈgä-tik\ *also* **di•zy•gous** \(ˌ)dī-ˈzī-gəs\ *adj, of twins* : FRATERNAL

diz•zi•ness \ˈdi-zē-nəs\ *n* : the condition of being dizzy; *esp* : a sensation of unsteadiness accompanied by a feeling of movement within the head

diz•zy \ˈdi-zē\ *adj* **diz•zi•er; -est** **1** : having a whirling sensation in the head with a tendency to fall **2** : mentally confused — **diz•zi•ly** \ˈdi-zə-lē\ *adv*

DJD *abbr* degenerative joint disease

DKA *abbr* diabetic ketoacidosis

DM *abbr* **1** dermatomyositis **2** diabetes mellitus **3** diastolic murmur **4** [Latin *dystrophia myotonica*] myotonic dystrophy

DMAE \ˌdē-ˌem-ˌā-ˈē\ *n* : a choline analog $C_4H_{11}NO$ used esp. as a dietary supplement and skin toner — called also *deanol, dimethylaminoethanol*

DMD *abbr* **1** [Latin *dentariae medicinae doctor*] doctor of dental medicine **2** Duchenne muscular dystrophy; Duchenne's muscular dystrophy

DMF *abbr* decayed, missing, and filled teeth

DMSO \ˌdē-(ˌ)em-(ˌ)es-ˈō\ *n* : DIMETHYL SULFOXIDE

DMT \ˌdē-(ˌ)em-ˈtē\ *n* : DIMETHYLTRYPTAMINE

DNA \ˌdē-(ˌ)en-ˈā\ *n* : any of various nucleic acids that are usu. the molecular basis of heredity, are localized esp. in cell nuclei, and are constructed of a double helix held together by hydrogen bonds between purine and pyrimidine bases which project inward from two chains containing alternate links of deoxyribose and phosphate — called also *deoxyribonucleic acid;* see RECOMBINANT DNA

DNA fingerprint *n* : the base-pair pattern in an individual's DNA obtained by DNA fingerprinting — called also *genetic fingerprint*

DNA fingerprinting *n* : a technique that involves extracting and identifying the base-pair pattern of an individual's DNA — called also *DNA typing, genetic fingerprinting*

DNA methylation *n* : the enzymatically controlled methylation of a nucleotide base (as cytosine) in a molecule of DNA that plays a role in suppressing gene expression

DNA polymerase *n* : any of several polymerases that promote replication or repair of DNA usu. using single-stranded DNA as a template

DNAR *abbr* do not attempt resuscitation

DN·ase \(ˌ)dē-ˈen-ˌās, -ˌāz\ *also* **DNA·ase** \(ˌ)dē-ˌen-ˈā-ˌās, -ˌāz\ *n* : DEOXYRIBONUCLEASE

DNA virus *n* : a virus whose genome consists of DNA

DNR *abbr* do not resuscitate

DO *abbr* doctor of osteopathic medicine; doctor of osteopathy

DOA *abbr* dead on arrival

DOB *abbr* date of birth

do·bu·ta·mine \dō-ˈbyü-tə-ˌmēn\ *n* : a drug administered intravenously in the form of its hydrochloride $C_{18}H_{23}NO_3 \cdot HCl$ esp. to increase cardiac output and lower wedge pressure in heart failure and after cardiopulmonary bypass surgery

doc \ˈdäk\ *n* : DOCTOR — used chiefly as a familiar term of address

do·ce·tax·el \ˌdō-sə-ˈtak-səl\ *n* : a semisynthetic antineoplastic drug $C_{43}H_{53}NO_{14} \cdot 3H_2O$ administered intravenously to treat various cancers (as of the lung or breast) and derived from the needles of a European yew tree (*Taxus baccata*) — see TAXOTERE

do·co·sa·hex·a·e·no·ic acid \ˌdō-kō-sə-ˌhek-sə-ˌē-ˌnō-ik-\ *n* : an omega-3 fatty acid $C_{22}H_{32}O_2$ found esp. in fish of cold waters — abbr. *DHA*

¹doc·tor \ˈdäk-tər\ *n* **1 a** : a person who has earned one of the highest academic degrees (as a PhD) conferred by a university **b** : a person awarded an honorary doctorate by a college or university **2** : a person skilled or specializing in healing arts; *esp* : one (as a physician, dentist, or veterinarian) who holds an advanced degree and is licensed to practice

²doctor *vb* **doc·tored; doc·tor·ing 1 a** : to give medical treatment to **b** : to practice medicine **2** : CASTRATE, SPAY

doc·u·sate \ˈdä-kyu̇-ˌsāt\ *n* : any of several laxative salts and esp. the sodium salt $C_{20}H_{37}NaO_7S$ used to soften stools in the treatment or prevention of constipation

dog flea \ˈdȯg-\ *n* : a flea of the genus *Ctenocephalides* (*C. canis*) that feeds chiefly on dogs and cats

dog tapeworm *n* : a tapeworm of the genus *Dipylidium* (*D. caninum*) occurring in dogs and cats and sometimes in humans

dog tick *n* : any of several ticks infesting dogs and commonly other animals; *esp* : AMERICAN DOG TICK

dolens — see PHLEGMASIA ALBA DOLENS, PHLEGMASIA CERULEA DOLENS

dolicho- *comb form* : long ⟨*dolicho*cephalic⟩

dol·i·cho·ce·phal·ic \ˌdä-li-kō-sə-ˈfa-lik\ *adj* : having a relatively long head with a cephalic index of less than 75 — **dol·i·cho·ceph·a·ly** \-ˈse-fə-lē\ *n*

Do·lo·bid \ˈdō-lə-ˌbid\ *trademark* — used for a preparation of diflunisal

do·lor \ˈdō-lər, ˈdä-\ *n* : mental suffering or anguish

DOM \ˌdē-(ˌ)ō-ˈem\ *n* : STP

do·main \dō-ˈmān\ *n* **1** : any of the three-dimensional subunits of a protein that together make up its tertiary structure **2** : the highest taxonomic category in biological classification ranking above the kingdom

dome \ˈdōm\ *n* : a rounded-arch element in the wave tracing in an electroencephalogram

do·mi·cil·i·ary \ˌdä-mə-ˈsi-lē-ˌer-ē, ˌdō-\ *adj* **1** : provided or attended in the home rather than in an institution ⟨~ midwifery⟩ **2** : providing, constituting, or provided by an institution for chronically ill or permanently disabled persons requiring minimal medical attention ⟨~ care⟩

dom·i·nance \ˈdä-mə-nəns\ *n* : the fact or state of being dominant: as **a** : the property of one of a pair of alleles or traits that suppresses expression of the other in the heterozygous condition **b** : functional asymmetry between a pair of bodily structures (as the right and left hands)

¹dom·i·nant \-nənt\ *adj* **1** : exerting forcefulness or having dominance in a social hierarchy **2** : being the one of a pair of bodily structures that is the more effective or predominant in action ⟨the ~ eye⟩ **3** : of, relating to, or exerting genetic dominance — **dom·i·nant·ly** *adv*

²dominant *n* **1** : a dominant genetic character or factor **2** : a dominant individual in a social hierarchy

do·mo·ic acid \də-ˈmō-ik-\ *n* : a neurotoxin $C_{15}H_{21}NO_6$ that is produced chiefly by marine diatoms (as *Pseudo-nitzschia pungens*) and has caused amnesic shellfish poisoning in people who have consumed contaminated fish or shellfish

DOMS *abbr* delayed onset muscle soreness

do·nee \dō-ˈnē\ *n* : a recipient of biological material (as blood or a graft)

don·ep·e·zil \ˌdä-ˈne-pə-zil\ *n* : a drug taken orally in the form of its hydrochloride $C_{24}H_{29}NO_3{\cdot}HCl$ to treat dementia associated with Alzheimer's disease— see ARICEPT, NAMZARIC

dong quai \ˈdäŋ-ˈkwī, ˈdȯŋ-\ *n* : the root of an Asian plant (*Angelica sinensis*) used esp. in traditional Chinese medicine as a tonic, analgesic, antispasmodic, and laxative

Don Juan·ism \ˈdän-ˈhwä-ˌni-zəm, -ˈwä-\ *n* : male sexual promiscuity

do·nor \ˈdō-nər, -ˌnȯr\ *n* **1** : one used as a source of biological material (as blood or an organ) **2** : a compound capable of giving up a part (as an atom) for combination with an acceptor

Don·o·van body \ˈdä-nə-vən-, ˈdə-\ *n* : an encapsulated gram-negative bacterium of the genus *Klebsiella* (*K. granulomatis*) that is the causative agent of granuloma inguinale — compare LEISHMAN-DONOVAN BODY

C. Donovan — see LEISHMAN-DONOVAN BODY

don·o·va·no·sis \ˌdä-nə-və-ˈnō-səs\ *n* : GRANULOMA INGUINALE

do·pa \ˈdō-pə, -(ˌ)pä\ *n* : an amino acid $C_9H_{11}NO_4$ that in the levorotatory form is found in the broad bean and is used in the treatment of Parkinson's disease

L–dopa — see entry alphabetized in the letter *l*

do·pa·mine \ˈdō-pə-ˌmēn\ *n* : a monoamine $C_8H_{11}NO_2$ that is a decarboxylated form of dopa and occurs esp. as a neurotransmitter in the brain and as an intermediate in the biosynthesis of epinephrine — see INTROPIN

do·pa·mi·ner·gic \ˌdō-pə-ˌmē-ˈnər-jik\ *adj* : liberating, activated by, or involving dopamine or related substances ⟨~ activity⟩ ⟨~ neurons⟩

dope \ˈdōp\ *n* **1** : a preparation of an illicit, habit-forming, or narcotic drug (as heroin or marijuana) **2** : a preparation given to a racehorse to help or hinder its performance — **dope** *vb*

dop·ing \ˈdō-piŋ\ *n* : the use of a substance (as an anabolic steroid or erythropoietin) or technique (as blood doping) to improve athletic performance and that is typically banned in many competitive sports

Dopp·ler \ˈdä-plər\ *adj* **1** : of, relating to, or utilizing a shift in frequency in accordance with the Doppler effect **2** : of, relating to, using, or produced by Doppler ultrasound ⟨~ images⟩ ⟨~ echocardiography⟩

Doppler, Christian Johann (1803–1853), Austrian physicist and mathematician.

Doppler effect *n* : a change in the frequency with which waves (as sound or light) from a given source reach an observer when the source and the observer are in motion with respect to each other so that the frequency increases or decreases according to the speed at which the distance is decreasing or increasing

Doppler ultrasound *n* : ultrasound that utilizes the Doppler effect to measure movement or flow in the body and esp. blood flow — called also *Doppler ultrasonography*

dors- — see DORSO-

dorsa *pl of* DORSUM

¹dor·sal \ˈdȯr-səl\ *adj* **1** : being or located near, on, or toward the upper surface of an animal (as a quadruped) opposite the lower or ventral surface **2** : being or located near, on, or toward the back or posterior part of the human body — **dor·sal·ly** \-sə-lē\ *adv*

²dorsal *n* : a dorsally located part; *esp* : a thoracic vertebra

dorsal horn *n* : a longitudinal subdivision of gray matter in the dorsal part of each lateral half of the spinal cord that receives terminals from some afferent fibers of the dorsal roots of the spinal nerves — called also *dorsal column, posterior column, posterior gray column, posterior horn;* compare LATERAL COLUMN 1, VENTRAL HORN

dorsal interosseus *n* **1** : any of four small muscles of the hand that act to draw the fingers away from the long axis of the middle finger, flex the fingers at the metacarpophalangeal joints, and extend their distal two phalanges **2** : any of four small muscles of the foot that act to draw the toes away from the long axis of the second toe, flex their proximal phalanges, and extend the distal phalanges

dorsalis — see INTEROSSEUS DORSALIS, SACROCOCCYGEUS DORSALIS, TABES DORSALIS

dor·sa·lis pe·dis artery \dȯr-ˈsa-ləs-ˈpe-dəs-, -ˈsā-, -ˈsä-, -ˈpē-\ *n* : an artery of the upper surface of the foot that is a direct continuation of the anterior tibial artery — called also *dorsalis pedis*

dorsal lip *n* : the margin of the fold of blastula wall that delineates the dorsal limit of the blastopore

dorsal mesogastrium *n* : MESOGASTRIUM 2

dorsal root *n* : the one of the two roots of a spinal nerve that passes posteriorly to the spinal cord separating the posterior and lateral funiculi and that consists of sensory fibers — called also *posterior root;* compare VENTRAL ROOT

dorsal root ganglion *n* : SPINAL GANGLION

dorsal spinocerebellar tract *n* : SPINOCEREBELLAR TRACT a

dorsi — see ILIOCOSTALIS DORSI, LATISSIMUS DORSI, LONGISSIMUS DORSI

dor•si•flex•ion \ˌdȯr-sə-ˈflek-shən\ *n* : flexion in a dorsal direction; *esp* : flexion of the foot in an upward direction — compare PLANTAR FLEXION — **dor•si•flex** \ˈdȯr-sə-ˌfleks\ *vb*

dor•si•flex•or \ˈdȯr-sə-ˌflek-sər\ *n* : a muscle causing flexion in a dorsal direction

dorso- *or* **dorsi-** *also* **dors-** *comb form* **1** : dorsal ⟨*dorsi*flexion⟩ **2** : dorsal and ⟨*dorso*lateral⟩

dor•so•lat•er•al \ˌdȯr-sō-ˈla-tə-rəl, -ˈla-trəl\ *adj* : of, relating to, or involving both the back and the sides ⟨the ~ prefrontal cortex⟩ — **dor•so•lat•er•al•ly** *adv*

dorsolateral tract *n* : a slender column of white matter between the dorsal gray column and the periphery of the spinal cord — called also *tract of Lissauer*

dor•so•lum•bar \ˌdȯr-sō-ˈləm-bər\ *adj* : of or involving structures in the region occupied by the dorsal and lumbar vertebrae ⟨the ~ spine⟩

dor•so•me•di•al \-ˈmē-dē-əl\ *adj* : located toward the back and near the midline ⟨the ~ hypothalamus⟩

dor•so•ven•tral \-ˈven-trəl\ *adj* : relating to, involving, or extending along the axis joining the dorsal and ventral sides — **dor•so•ven•tral•ly** *adv*

dor•sum \ˈdȯr-səm\ *n, pl* **dor•sa** \-sə\ **1** : the upper surface of an appendage or part **2** : BACK; *esp* : the entire dorsal surface of an animal

dos•age \ˈdō-sij\ *n* **1 a** : the addition of an ingredient or the application of an agent in a measured dose **b** : the presence and relative representation or strength of a factor or agent (as a gene) **2 a** : DOSE 1 **b** (1) : the giving of a dose (2) : regulation or determination of doses

[1]**dose** \ˈdōs\ *n* **1 a** : the measured quantity of a therapeutic agent to be taken at one time **b** : the quantity of radiation administered or absorbed **2** : a gonorrheal infection

[2]**dose** *vb* **dosed; dos•ing** **1** : to divide (as a medicine) into doses **2** : to give a dose to; *esp* : to give medicine to **3** : to take medicine **4** : to treat with an application or agent

dose–response *adj* : of, relating to, or graphing the pattern of physiological response to varied dosage (as of a drug or toxic substance)

do•sim•e•ter \dō-ˈsi-mə-tər\ *n* : a device for measuring doses of radiations (as X-rays) — **do•si•met•ric** \ˌdō-sə-ˈme-trik\ *adj* — **do•sim•e•try** \dō-ˈsi-mə-trē\ *n*

double bind *n* : a psychological predicament in which a person receives from a single source conflicting messages that allow no appropriate response to be made

dou•ble–blind \ˌdə-bəl-ˈblīnd\ *adj* : of, relating to, or being an experimental procedure in which neither the subjects nor the experimenters know which subjects are in the test and control groups during the actual course of the experiments — compare OPEN-LABEL, SINGLE-BLIND

double bond *n* : a chemical bond in which two pairs of electrons are shared by two atoms in a molecule and which is usu. represented in chemical formulas by two lines

double chin *n* : a fleshy or fatty fold under the chin — **dou•ble–chinned** \-ˈchind\ *adj*

double helix *n* : the structural arrangement of DNA in space that consists of paired polynucleotide strands stabilized by chemical bonds between the chains linking purine and pyrimidine bases — compare ALPHA-HELIX, WATSON-CRICK MODEL — **dou•ble–he•li•cal** \-ˈhe-li-kəl, -ˈhē-\ *adj*

dou•ble–joint•ed \ˌdə-bəl-ˈjȯin-təd\ *adj* : having a joint that permits an exceptional degree of freedom of motion of the parts joined

double pneumonia *n* : pneumonia affecting both lungs

double vision *n* : DIPLOPIA

douche \ˈdüsh\ *n* **1 a** : a jet or current of liquid (as a cleansing solution) directed against or into a bodily part or cavity (as the vagina) **b** : an act of cleansing with a douche **2** : a device for giving douches — **douche** *vb*

Doug•las bag \ˈdə-gləs-\ *n* : an inflatable bag used to collect expired air for the determination of oxygen consumption and basal metabolic rate

Douglas, Claude Gordon (1882–1963), British physiologist.

Douglas's cul–de–sac \ˈdə-glə-səz-\ *n* : POUCH OF DOUGLAS

Douglas's pouch *n* : POUCH OF DOUGLAS

dou•la \ˈdü-lə\ *n* : a woman experienced in childbirth who provides advice, information, emotional support, and physical comfort to a mother before, during, and just after childbirth

douloureux — see TIC DOULOUREUX

dow•a•ger's hump \ˈdau̇-i-jərz-\ *n* : an abnormal outward curvature of the upper back with round shoulders and stooped posture caused esp. by bone loss and anterior compression of the vertebrae in osteoporosis

down•er \ˈdau̇-nər\ *n* : a depressant drug; *esp* : BARBITURATE

down•stream \ˈdau̇n-ˈstrēm\ *adv or adj* **1** : in the same direction along a molecule of DNA or RNA as that in which transcription and translation take place and toward the end having a hydroxyl group attached to the position labeled 3′ in the terminal nucleotide — compare UPSTREAM 1 **2** : toward the end of or following a series of cellular processes — compare UPSTREAM 2

Down syndrome \ˈdau̇n-\ *or* **Down's syndrome** \ˈdau̇nz-\ *n* : a congenital condition characterized esp. by developmental delays, usu. mild to moderate impairment in cognitive functioning, short stature, relatively small head, upward slanting eyes usu. with epicanthal folds, flattened nasal bridge, broad hands with short fingers, decreased muscle tone, and by trisomy of the human chromosome numbered 21 — called also *Down, Down's, trisomy 21*

Down \ˈdau̇n\, **John Langdon Haydon (1828–1896)**, British physician.

dox·a·zo·sin \ˌdäk-ˈsā-zō-sin\ *n* : an alpha-blocker used in the form of its mesylate $C_{23}H_{25}N_5O_5{\cdot}CH_4O_3S$ to relieve urethral obstruction in benign prostatic hyperplasia and to treat hypertension — see CARDURA

dox·e·pin \ˈdäk-sə-ˌpin, -pən\ *n* : a tricyclic antidepressant administered as the hydrochloride $C_9H_{21}NO{\cdot}HCl$ — see SINEQUAN

doxo·ru·bi·cin \ˌdäk-sə-ˈrü-bə-sən\ *n* : an antibiotic with broad antitumor activity that is obtained from a bacterium of the genus *Streptomyces* (*S. peucetius*) and is used in the form of its hydrochloride $C_{27}H_{29}NO_{11}{\cdot}HCl$ — see ABVD, ADRIAMYCIN

doxy·cy·cline \ˌdäk-sə-ˈsī-ˌklēn\ *n* : a broad-spectrum tetracycline antibiotic $C_{22}H_{24}N_2O_8$ used orally to treat various bacterial infections

dox·yl·amine \däk-ˈsi-lə-ˌmēn, -mən\ *n* : an antihistamine usu. used in the form of its succinate $C_{17}H_{22}N_2O{\cdot}C_4H_6O_4$ to treat respiratory symptoms of the common cold and allergies, to induce sleep in the treatment of insomnia, and combined with pyridoxine hydrochloride to control nausea and vomiting during pregnancy

DP *abbr* doctor of podiatry

DPH *abbr* **1** department of public health **2** doctor of public health

DPM *abbr* doctor of podiatric medicine

DPT *abbr* diphtheria-pertussis-tetanus (vaccine)

dr *abbr* dram

Dr *abbr* doctor

drac·on·ti·a·sis \ˌdra-ˌkän-ˈtī-ə-səs\ *n, pl* **-a·ses** \-ˌsēz\ : DRACUNCULIASIS

dra·cun·cu·li·a·sis \drə-ˌkəŋ-kyə-ˈlī-ə-səs\ *n, pl* **-a·ses** \-ˌsēz\ : infestation with or disease caused by the guinea worm — called also *Guinea worm disease*

dra·cun·cu·lo·sis \-ˈlō-səs\ *n, pl* **-lo·ses** \-ˌsēz\ : DRACUNCULIASIS

Dra·cun·cu·lus \drə-ˈkəŋ-kyə-ləs\ *n* : a genus (family Dracunculidae) of greatly elongated nematode worms including the Guinea worm

draft \ˈdraft, ˈdráft\ *n* **1** : a portion (as of medicine) poured out or mixed for drinking : DOSE **2** : a current of air in a closed-in space — **drafty** \ˈdraf-tē, ˈdráf-\ *adj*

[1]**drain** \ˈdrān\ *vb* **1** : to draw off (liquid) gradually or completely ⟨~ pus from an abscess⟩ **2** : to carry away or give passage to a bodily fluid or a discharge from ⟨~ an abscess⟩

[2]**drain** *n* : a tube or cylinder usu. of absorbent material for drainage of a wound — see CIGARETTE DRAIN

drain·age \ˈdrā-nij\ *n* : the act or process of drawing off fluids from a cavity or wound by means of suction or gravity

Draize test \ˈdrāz-\ *n* : a test that is used as a criterion for harmfulness of chemicals to the human eye and that involves dropping the test substance into one eye of rabbits without anesthesia with the other eye used as a control — called also *Draize eye test*

Draize, John H. (1900–1992), American pharmacologist.

dram \ˈdram\ *n* **1** : either of two units of weight: **a** : an avoirdupois unit equal to 1.772 grams or 27.344 grains **b** : a unit of apothecaries' weight equal to 3.888 grams or 60 grains **2** : FLUID DRAM

Dram·amine \ˈdra-mə-ˌmēn\ *trademark* — used for a preparation of dimenhydrinate

drape \ˈdrāp\ *n* : a sterile covering used in an operating room — usu. used in pl. — **drape** *vb*

dras·tic \ˈdras-tik\ *adj* : acting rapidly or violently — used chiefly of purgatives — **dras·ti·cal·ly** \-ti-k(ə-)lē\ *adv*

draught *chiefly Brit var of* DRAFT

draw \ˈdrȯ\ *vb* **drew** \ˈdrü\; **drawn** \ˈdrȯn\; **draw·ing** **1** : INHALE **2 a** : to localize in or cause to move toward a surface — used in the phrase *draw to a head* ⟨using a poultice to ~ inflammation to a head⟩ **b** : to cause local congestion : induce blood or other body fluid to localize at a particular point

draw·sheet \ˈdrȯ-ˌshēt\ *n* : a narrow sheet used chiefly in hospitals and stretched across the bed lengthwise often over a rubber sheet underneath the patient's trunk

DRE *abbr* digital rectal exam; digital rectal examination

dream \ˈdrēm\ *n, often attrib* : a series of thoughts, images, or emotions occurring during sleep and esp. during REM sleep — **dream** *vb*

drench \ˈdrench\ *n* : a large dose of medicine mixed with liquid and put down the throat of an animal

dress \ˈdres\ *vb* : to apply dressings or medicaments to

dress·ing *n* : a covering (as of ointment or gauze) applied to a lesion

Dress·ler's syndrome \ˈdre-slərz-\ *n* : pericarditis after heart attack or open-heart surgery that is often recurrent and is typically accompanied by fever, chest pain, difficulty in breathing, pleurisy, and pericardial and pleural effusions

Dressler, William (1890–1969), American cardiologist.

DRG \ˌdē-(ˌ)är-ˈjē\ *n* : any of the payment categories that are used to classify patients and esp. Medicare patients for the purpose of reimbursing hospitals for each case in a given category with a fixed fee regardless of the actual costs incurred — called also *diagnosis related group*

DRI *abbr* Dietary Reference Intake

drier *comparative of* DRY

driest *superlative of* DRY

drift \ˈdrift\ *n* **1** : movement of a tooth in the dental arch **2** : GENETIC DRIFT — **drift** *vb*

drill *n* : an instrument with an edged or pointed end for making holes in hard substances (as teeth) by revolving — **drill** *vb*

Drink•er respirator \ˈdriŋ-kər-\ *n* : IRON LUNG

Drinker, Philip (1894–1972), American industrial hygienist.

drip \ˈdrip\ *n* **1 a** : a falling in drops — see POSTNASAL DRIP **b** : liquid that falls, overflows, or is extruded in drops **2** : a device for the administration of a fluid at a slow rate esp. into a vein; *also* : a material so administered ⟨a glucose ~⟩ — see GRAVITY DRIP — **drip** *vb*

Dris•dol \ˈdris-ˌdȯl, -ˌdōl\ *trademark* — used for a preparation of calciferol

drive \ˈdrīv\ *n* : an urgent, basic, or instinctual need : a motivating physiological condition of the organism ⟨a sexual ~⟩

dro•nab•i•nol \ˌdrō-ˈna-bə-ˌnȯl\ *n* : a synthetic delta-9-tetrahydrocannabinol used to control nausea caused by chemotherapy and to stimulate appetite in cases of AIDS-induced anorexia — see MARINOL

drool \ˈdrül\ *vb* **1** : to secrete saliva in anticipation of food **2** : to let saliva or some other substance flow from the mouth — **drool** *n*

[1]**drop** \ˈdräp\ *n* **1 a** : the quantity of fluid that falls in one spherical mass **b drops** *pl* : a dose of medicine measured by drops ⟨eye ~*s*⟩ **2** : the smallest practical unit of liquid measure that varies in size according to the specific gravity and viscosity of the liquid and to the conditions under which it is formed

[2]**drop** *vb* **dropped; drop•ping 1** : to fall in drops **2** *of an animal* : to give birth to ⟨lambs *dropped* in June⟩ **3** : to take (a drug) orally ⟨~ acid⟩

dro•per•i•dol \drō-ˈper-ə-ˌdȯl\ *n* : a butyrophenone tranquilizer $C_{22}H_{22}FN_3O_2$ used esp. as a sedative, antiemetic, and antipsychotic

drop foot *n* : FOOT DROP

drop•let \ˈdräp-lət\ *n* : a tiny drop (as of a liquid)

droplet infection *n* : infection transmitted by airborne droplets of saliva or sputum containing infectious organisms

drop•per \ˈdrä-pər\ *n* : a short glass tube fitted with a rubber bulb and used to measure liquids by drops — called also *eyedropper, medicine dropper* — **drop•per•ful** \-ˌfu̇l\ *n*

drop•si•cal \ˈdräp-si-kəl\ *adj* : relating to or affected with edema

drop•sy \ˈdräp-sē\ *n, pl* **drop•sies** : EDEMA

dros•pir•e•none \drō-ˈspir-ə-ˌnōn\ *n* : a synthetic progestogen $C_{24}H_{30}O_3$ that is an analog of spironolactone and is used in birth control pills in combination with ethinyl estradiol — see YAZ

drown \ˈdrau̇n\ *vb* **drowned** \ˈdrau̇nd\; **drown•ing** \ˈdrau̇-niŋ\ **1** : to suffocate in water or some other liquid **2** : to suffocate because of excess of body fluid that interferes with the passage of oxygen from the lungs to the body tissues (as in pulmonary edema)

DrPH *abbr* doctor of public health

[1]**drug** \ˈdrəg\ *n* **1 a** : a substance used as a medication or in the preparation of medication **b** *according to the Food, Drug, and Cosmetic Act* (1) : a substance recognized in an official pharmacopoeia or formulary (2) : a substance intended for use in the diagnosis, cure, mitigation, treatment, or prevention of disease (3) : a substance other than food intended to affect the structure or function of the body (4) : a substance intended for use as a component of a medicine but not a device or a component, part, or accessory of a device **2** : something and often an illicit substance that causes addiction, habituation, or a marked change in consciousness

[2]**drug** *vb* **drugged; drug•ging 1** : to affect with a drug; *esp* : to stupefy by a narcotic drug **2** : to administer a drug to **3** : to take drugs for narcotic effect

drug•gist \ˈdrə-gist\ *n* : one who sells or dispenses drugs and medicines: as **a** : PHARMACIST **b** : a person who owns or manages a drugstore

drug•mak•er \ˈdrəg-ˌmā-kər\ *n* : a company that manufactures pharmaceuticals

drug•store \-ˌstōr\ *n* : a retail store where medicines and miscellaneous articles (as food, cosmetics, and film) are sold — called also *pharmacy*

drum \ˈdrəm\ *n* : TYMPANIC MEMBRANE

drum•head \-ˌhed\ *n* : TYMPANIC MEMBRANE

drum•stick \-ˌstik\ *n* : a small projection from the cell nucleus that occurs esp. in neutrophils of the normal human female and is comprised of an inactivated condensed X chromosome

druse \ˈdrüz, ˈdrü-zə\ *n, pl* **dru•sen** \ˈdrü-zən\ : one of the small yellowish deposits of cellular debris that accumulate between the pigmented epithelial layer of the retina and the inner collagenous layer of the choroid

dry \ˈdrī\ *adj* **dri•er** \ˈdrī-ər\; **dri•est** \-əst\ **1** : marked by the absence or scantiness of secretions, effusions, or other forms of moisture **2** *of a cough* : not accompanied by the raising of mucus or phlegm

dry eye *n* : a condition associated with inadequate tear production and marked by redness of the conjunctiva and by itching and burning of the eye — called also *dry eye syndrome, keratoconjunctivitis sicca*

dry gangrene *n* : gangrene that develops in the presence of arterial obstruction, is sharply localized, and is characterized by dryness of the dead tissue which is distinguishable from adjacent tissue by a line of inflammation

dry heaves *n pl* : repeated involuntary retching unaccompanied by vomit

dry mouth *n* : XEROSTOMIA

dry out *vb* : to undergo an extended period of withdrawal from alcohol or drug use esp. at a special clinic : DETOXIFY

dry socket *n* : a tooth socket in which after tooth extraction a blood clot fails to form or disintegrates without undergoing organization; *also* : a condition that is marked by the occurrence of such a socket or sockets and that is usu. accompanied by neuralgic pain but without suppuration

Ds *symbol* darmstadtium

DSC *abbr* doctor of surgical chiropody

DSM *abbr* Diagnostic and Statistical Manual of Mental Disorders

DTaP *abbr* diphtheria, tetanus, acellular pertussis (vaccine)

DTP *abbr* diphtheria, tetanus, pertussis (vaccine)

d.t.'s \ˌdē-ˈtēz\ *n, pl often cap D&T* : DELIRIUM TREMENS

dual–energy X–ray absorptiometry *n* : absorptiometry in which the density or mass of a material (as bone) is measured by comparing the material's absorption of X-rays of two different energies and which is used esp. for determining the mineral content and density of bone — abbr. *DEXA, DXA*

DUB *abbr* dysfunctional uterine bleeding

dub•ni•um \ˈdüb-nē-əm\ *n* : a short-lived radioactive element that is artificially produced — symbol *Db;* see ELEMENT table

Du•chenne \dü-ˈshen, də-\ *also* **Du•chenne's** \-ˈshenz\ *adj* : relating to or being Duchenne muscular dystrophy

Du•chenne \dūē-ˈshen\, **Guillaume–Benjamin–Amand (1806–1875)**, French neurologist.

Duchenne dystrophy *also* **Duchenne's dystrophy** *n* : DUCHENNE MUSCULAR DYSTROPHY

Duchenne muscular dystrophy *also* **Duchenne's muscular dystrophy** *n* : a severe progressive form of muscular dystrophy of males that appears in early childhood, affects the muscles of the legs before those of the arms, is inherited as an X-linked recessive trait, is characterized by complete absence of the protein dystrophin, and usu. has a fatal outcome by age 20 — abbr. *DMD;* see BECKER MUSCULAR DYSTROPHY

Du•crey's bacillus \dü-ˈkrāz-\ *n* : a gram-negative bacillus of the genus *Haemophilus* (*H. ducreyi*) that is the causative agent of chancroid

Du•crey \dü-ˈkrā\, **Augusto (1860–1940)**, Italian dermatologist.

duct \ˈdəkt\ *n* : a bodily tube or vessel esp. when carrying the secretion of a gland

duc•tal \ˈdək-tᵊl\ *adj* : of or belonging to a duct : made up of ducts

ductal carcinoma in situ *n* : any of a histologically variable group of precancerous growths or early carcinomas of the lactiferous ducts that have the potential of becoming invasive and spreading to other tissues — abbr. *DCIS*

duc•tion \ˈdək-shən\ *n* : a turning or rotating movement of the eye

duct•less \ˈdəkt-ləs\ *adj* : being without a duct

ductless gland *n* : ENDOCRINE GLAND

duct of Bel•li•ni \-be-ˈlē-nē\ *n* : any of the large excretory ducts of the uriniferous tubules of the kidney that open on the free surface of the papillae

Bellini, Lorenzo (1643–1704), Italian anatomist and physiologist.

duct of Gart•ner \-ˈgärt-nər\ *n* : GARTNER'S DUCT

duct of Ri•vi•nus \-rə-ˈvē-nəs\ *n* : any of several small inconstant efferent ducts of the sublingual gland

Rivinus, Augustus Quirinus (1652–1723), German anatomist and botanist.

duct of San•to•ri•ni \-ˌsan-tə-ˈrē-nē, -ˌsän-\ *n* : ACCESSORY PANCREATIC DUCT

Santorini, Giovanni Domenico (1681–1737), Italian anatomist.

duct of Wir•sung \-ˈvir-(ˌ)zúŋ, -zəŋ\ *n* : PANCREATIC DUCT a

Wirsung, Johann Georg (1589–1643), German anatomist.

duct•ule \ˈdək-(ˌ)tyül\ *n* : a small duct

duc•tu•li ef•fe•ren•tes \ˈdək-tyù-ˌlī-ˌef-ə-ˈren-(ˌ)tēz, -tù-, -(ˌ)lē-\ *n pl* : a group of ducts that convey sperm from the testis to the epididymis

duc•tu•lus \ˈdək-tyù-ləs, -tù-\ *n, pl* **-li** \-ˌlī, -(ˌ)lē\ : DUCTULE

duc•tus \ˈdək-təs\ *n, pl* **ductus** : DUCT

ductus ar•te•ri•o•sus \-är-ˌtir-ē-ˈō-səs\ *n* : a short broad vessel in the fetus that connects the pulmonary artery with the aorta and conducts most of the blood directly from the right ventricle to the aorta bypassing the lungs

duc·tus de·fer·ens \-ˈde-fə-ˌrenz, -rənz\ *n, pl* **ductus de·fer·en·tes** \-ˌde-fə-ˈren-tēz\ : VAS DEFERENS

ductus re·uni·ens \-rē-ˈyü-nē-ˌenz, -ˈü-\ *n* : a passage in the ear that connects the cochlea and the saccule

ductus ve·no·sus \-vi-ˈnō-səs\ *n* : a vein passing through the liver and connecting the left umbilical vein with the inferior vena cava of the fetus, losing its circulatory function after birth, and persisting as the ligamentum venosum of the liver

Duf·fy \ˈdə-fē\ *adj* : relating to, characteristic of, or being a system of blood groups determined by the presence or absence of any of several antigens in red blood cells ⟨~ blood typing⟩

Duffy, Richard (1906–1956), British hemophiliac.

Dührs·sen's incisions \ˈdu̅e̅r-sənz-\ *n pl* : a set of three incisions in the cervix of the uterus to facilitate delivery if dilation is inadequate

Dührs·sen \ˈdu̅e̅r-sən\, **Alfred (1862–1933)**, German obstetrician-gynecologist.

Du·lera \dü-ˈler-ə\ *trademark* — used for a preparation of formoterol and mometasone for oral inhalation

dull \ˈdəl\ *adj* **1** : mentally slow or stupid **2** : slow in perception or sensibility **3** : lacking sharpness or edge or point ⟨a ~ scalpel⟩ **4** : lacking in force, intensity, or acuteness ⟨a ~ pain⟩ — **dull** *vb* — **dull·ness** *or* **dul·ness** \ˈdəl-nəs\ *n* — **dul·ly** *adv*

du·lox·e·tine \dü-ˈläk-sə-ˌtēn\ *n* : a drug that functions as an SNRI and is taken orally in the form of its hydrochloride $C_{18}H_{19}NOS{\cdot}HCl$ esp. to treat depression, anxiety, and chronic pain (as that associated with fibromyalgia) — see CYMBALTA

dumb \ˈdəm\ *adj, often offensive* : lacking the ability to speak

dumb rabies *n* : PARALYTIC RABIES

dum·dum fever \ˈdəm-ˌdəm-\ *n* : KALA-AZAR

[1]**dum·my** \ˈdə-mē\ *n, pl* **dummies** : PLACEBO

[2]**dummy** *adj* : being a placebo ⟨a ~ pill⟩

dump·ing syndrome \ˈdəm-piŋ-\ *n* : a condition characterized by weakness, dizziness, flushing and warmth, nausea, and palpitation immediately or shortly after eating and produced by abnormally rapid emptying of the stomach esp. in persons who have had part of the stomach removed

duoden- *or* **duodeno-** *comb form* **1** : duodenum ⟨*duoden*itis⟩ **2** : duodenal and ⟨*duodeno*jejunal⟩

du·o·de·nal ulcer \ˌdü-ə-ˈdēn-ᵊl-, ˌdyü-; dü-ˈäd-ᵊn-əl-, dyü-\ *n* : a peptic ulcer situated in the duodenum

du·o·de·ni·tis \dü-ˌäd-ᵊn-ˈī-təs, dyü-\ *n* : inflammation of the duodenum

du·o·de·no·cho·led·o·chot·o·my \dü-ˌäd-ᵊn-ō-kə-ˌle-də-ˈkä-tə-mē, dyü-\ *n, pl* **-mies** : choledochotomy performed by approach through the duodenum by incision

du·o·de·nog·ra·phy \dü-ˌäd-ᵊn-ˈä-grə-fē, dyü-\ *n, pl* **-phies** : radiographic visualization of the duodenum with a contrast medium

du·o·de·no·je·ju·nal \dü-ˌäd-ᵊn-ō-ji-ˈjün-ᵊl, dyü-\ *adj* : of, relating to, or joining the duodenum and the jejunum

du·o·de·no·je·ju·nos·to·my \-ji-jü-ˈnäs-tə-mē\ *n, pl* **-mies** : a surgical operation that joins part of the duodenum and the jejunum with creation of an artificial opening between them

du·o·de·no·scope \ˌd(y)ü-ə-ˈdē-nə-ˌskōp\ *n* : a long flexible endoscope that is inserted through the mouth and is used to visually examine and pass instruments into the duodenum — **du·o·de·nos·co·py** \ˌd(y)ü-ə-də-ˈnä-skə-pē\ *n*

du·o·de·not·o·my \dü-ˌäd-ᵊn-ˈä-tə-mē, dyü-\ *n, pl* **-mies** : incision of the duodenum

du·o·de·num \ˌdü-ə-ˈdē-nəm, ˌdyü-; dü-ˈäd-ᵊn-əm, dyü-\ *n, pl* **-de·na** \-ˈdē-nə, -ᵊn-ə\ *or* **-de·nums** : the first, shortest, and widest part of the small intestine that in humans is about 10 inches (25 centimeters) long and that extends from the pylorus to the undersurface of the liver where it descends for a variable distance and receives the bile and pancreatic ducts and then bends to the left and finally upward to join the jejunum near the second lumbar vertebra — **du·o·de·nal** \-ˈden-ᵊl, -ᵊn-əl\ *adj*

Du·o·pa \dü-ˈō-pə\ *trademark* — used for a liquid suspension containing carbidopa and L-dopa that is administered by infusion pump

du·plex \ˈdü-ˌpleks, ˈdyü-\ *n* : a molecule having two complementary polynucleotide strands of DNA or of DNA and RNA — **duplex** *adj*

du·pli·cate \ˈdü-pli-ˌkāt, ˈdyü-\ *vb* **-cat·ed; -cat·ing** : to become duplicate : REPLICATE

du·pli·ca·tion \ˌdü-pli-ˈkā-shən, ˌdyü-\ *n* **1** : the act or process of duplicating : the quality or state of being duplicated **2** : a part of a chromosome in which the genetic material is repeated; *also* : the process of forming a duplication

Du·puy·tren's contracture \də-ˌpwē-ˈtraⁿz-, -ˈpwē-trənz-\ *n* : a condition marked by fibrosis with shortening and thickening of the palmar aponeurosis resulting in flexion contracture of the fingers into the palm of the hand

Du·puy·tren \də-pwē-ˈtraⁿ\, **Guillaume (1777–1835)**, French surgeon.

dura — see LAMINA DURA

du·ral \'du̇r-əl, 'dyu̇r-\ *adj* : of or relating to the dura mater

dural sinus *n* : SINUS OF THE DURA MATER

du·ra ma·ter \'du̇r-ə-ˌmā-tər, 'dyu̇r-, -ˌmä-\ *n* : the tough fibrous membrane lined with endothelium on the inner surface that envelops the brain and spinal cord external to the arachnoid and pia mater, that in the cranium closely lines the bone and contains numerous blood vessels and venous sinuses, and that in the spinal cord is separated from the bone by a considerable space and contains no venous sinuses — called also *dura*

Dur·e·zol \'du̇r-ə-ˌzȯl, -ˌzōl\ *trademark* — used for an ophthalmic preparation containing difluprednate

dust cell *n* : a pulmonary macrophage that takes up and eliminates foreign particles introduced into the lung alveoli with inspired air

dust·ing powder \'dəs-tiŋ-\ *n* : a powder used on the skin or on wounds esp. for allaying irritation or absorbing moisture

dust mite *n* : any of various mites (esp. family Pyroglyphidae) commonly found in dust; *esp* : HOUSE DUST MITE

du·tas·te·ride \dü-'tas-tə-ˌrīd\ *n* : a synthetic drug $C_{27}H_{30}F_6N_2O_2$ that inhibits 5-alpha-reductase and is used to treat benign prostatic hyperplasia — see AVODART

Dutch cap *n* : CERVICAL CAP

DV *abbr* daily value

DVM *abbr* doctor of veterinary medicine

DVT *abbr* deep vein thrombosis

[1]**dwarf** \'dwȯrf\ *n, pl* **dwarfs** \'dwȯrfs\ *also* **dwarves** \'dwȯrvz\ *often attrib* **1** : a person of unusually small stature; *esp* : a person whose height does not exceed 4 feet 10 inches (1.47 meters) and is typically less than 4 feet 5 inches (1.35 meters) **2** : an animal much below normal size

[2]**dwarf** *vb* : to restrict the growth of

dwarf·ism \'dwȯr-ˌfi-zəm\ *n* : a condition of stunted growth; *esp* : a condition (as achondroplasia) marked by unusually small size or short stature

Dx *or* **DX** *abbr* **1** diagnosis **2** diagnostic

DXA *abbr* dual-energy X-ray absorptiometry

DXM *abbr* dextromethorphan

Dy *symbol* dysprosium

dy·ad \'dī-ˌad, -əd\ *n* : a meiotic chromosome after separation of the two homologous members of a tetrad

Dy·a·zide \'dī-ə-ˌzīd\ *trademark* — used for a preparation of hydrochlorothiazide and triamterene

dy·dro·ges·ter·one \ˌdī-drō-'jes-tə-ˌrōn\ *n* : a synthetic progestational agent $C_{21}H_{28}O_2$ — called also *isopregnenone*

dying *pres part of* DIE

-dynamia *n comb form* : strength : condition of having (such) strength ⟨*adynamia*⟩

dy·nam·ic \dī-'na-mik\ *also* **dy·nam·i·cal** \-mi-kəl\ *adj* **1 a** : of or relating to physical force or energy **b** : of or relating to dynamics **2** : FUNCTIONAL 1b ⟨a ~ disease⟩ — **dy·nam·i·cal·ly** \-mi-k(ə-)lē\ *adv*

dy·nam·ics \dī-'na-miks\ *n sing or pl* **1** : a branch of mechanics that deals with forces and their relation primarily to the motion but sometimes also to the equilibrium of bodies **2** : PSYCHODYNAMICS **3** : the pattern of change or growth of an object or phenomenon ⟨personality ~⟩

dy·na·mom·e·ter \ˌdī-nə-'mä-mə-tər\ *n* : an instrument for measuring the force of muscular contraction esp. of the hand

dyne \'dīn\ *n* : the unit of force in the cgs system equal to the force that would give a free mass of one gram an acceleration of one centimeter per second per second

dy·nein \'dī-ˌnēn, -ˌnē-ən\ *n* : an ATPase that regulates that movement of cellular organelles and structures (as cilia and chromosomes) by controlling the motion of microtubules

dy·nor·phin \dī-'nȯr-fən\ *n* : any of a group of potent opioid peptides found in the mammalian central nervous system

dy·phyl·line \dī-'fi-ˌlēn\ *n* : a theophylline derivative $C_{10}H_{14}N_4O_4$ used as a diuretic and for its bronchodilator and peripheral vasodilator effects

dys- *prefix* **1** : abnormal ⟨*dys*plasia⟩ **2** : difficult ⟨*dys*pnea⟩ **3** : impaired ⟨*dys*function⟩

dys·aes·the·sia *chiefly Brit var of* DYSESTHESIA

dys·ar·thria \dis-'är-thrē-ə\ *n* : difficulty in articulating words due to disease of the central nervous system — compare DYSPHASIA — **dys·ar·thric** \-thrik\ *adj*

dys·ar·thro·sis \ˌdis-ˌär-'thrō-səs\ *n, pl* **-thro·ses** \-ˌsēz\ **1** : a condition of reduced joint motion due to deformity, dislocation, or disease **2** : DYSARTHRIA

dys·au·to·no·mia \ˌdis-ˌȯ-tə-'nō-mē-ə\ *n* : a disorder of the autonomic nervous system that causes disturbances in all or some autonomic functions and may result from the course of a disease (as diabetes) or from injury or poisoning; *esp* : FAMILIAL DYSAUTONOMIA — **dys·au·to·nom·ic** \-'nä-mik\ *adj*

dys·ba·rism \'dis-bə-ˌri-zəm\ *n* : the complex of symptoms (as the bends or headache) that accompanies exposure to excessively low or rapidly changing environmental air pressure

dys·cal·cu·lia \ˌdis-ˌkal-'kyü-lē-ə\ *n* : impairment of mathematical ability due to an organic condition of the brain

dys·che·zia \dis-'kē-zē-ə, -'ke-, -zhə, -zhē-ə\ *n* : constipation associated with a defective reflex for defecation

dys·chon·dro·pla·sia \dis-ˌkän-drō-'plā-zhə, -zhē-ə\ *n* : CHONDRODYSPLASIA

dys·cra·sia \dis-ˈkrā-zhə, -zhē-ə\ *n* : an abnormal condition of the body; *esp* : an imbalance of components of the blood — see PLASMA CELL DYSCRASIA

dys·di·ad·o·cho·ki·ne·sia *or* **dys·di·ad·o·ko·ki·ne·sia** \ˌdis-ˌdī-ˌa-də-ˌkō-kī-ˈnē-zhə, -zhē-ə\ *n* : impairment of the ability to make movements exhibiting a rapid change of motion that is caused by cerebellar dysfunction

dys·en·ter·ic \ˌdis-ᵊn-ˈter-ik\ *adj* : of or relating to dysentery

dys·en·tery \ˈdis-ᵊn-ˌter-ē\ *n, pl* **-ter·ies** **1** : a disease characterized by severe diarrhea with passage of mucus and blood and usu. caused by infection **2** : DIARRHEA

dys·es·the·sia \ˌdi-ses-ˈthē-zhə, -zhē-ə\ *n* : impairment of sensitivity esp. to touch — **dys·es·thet·ic** \-ˈthe-tik\ *adj*

dys·func·tion *also* **dis·func·tion** \(ˈ)dis-ˈfəŋk-shən\ *n* : impaired or abnormal functioning (as of an organ of the body) — **dys·func·tion·al** \-shnəl, -shən-ᵊl\ *adj* — **dys·func·tion·ing** \-shə-niŋ\ *n*

dysfunctional uterine bleeding *n* : abnormal uterine bleeding that is not associated with a physical lesion (as a tumor), inflammation, or pregnancy — abbr. *DUB*

dys·gam·ma·glob·u·li·ne·mia \ˌdis-ˌga-mə-ˌglä-byə-lə-ˈnē-mē-ə\ *n* : a disorder involving abnormality in structure or frequency of gamma globulins — compare AGAMMAGLOBULINEMIA

dys·gen·e·sis \(ˌ)dis-ˈje-nə-səs\ *n, pl* **-e·ses** \-ˌsēz\ : defective development esp. of the gonads (as in Klinefelter's syndrome or Turner's syndrome)

dys·ger·mi·no·ma \dis-ˌjər-mə-ˈnō-mə\ *n, pl* **-mas** *also* **-ma·ta** \-mə-tə\ : a germinoma of the ovary

dys·geu·sia \(ˌ)dis-ˈgü-zē-ə, -ˈgyü-, -zhə, -zhē-ə\ *n* : dysfunction of the sense of taste

dys·graph·ia \(ˌ)dis-ˈgra-fē-ə\ *n* : impairment of handwriting ability marked esp. by very poor or illegible writing

dys·hi·dro·sis \ˌdis-ˌhī-ˈdrō-səs, -hə-\ *n, pl* **-dro·ses** \-ˌsēz\ : POMPHOLYX

dys·kary·o·sis \ˌdis-kar-ē-ˈō-səs\ *n, pl* **-o·ses** \-ˌsēz\ *or* **-o·sis·es** : abnormality esp. of exfoliated cells (as from the uterine cervix) that affects the nucleus but not the cytoplasm

dys·ker·a·to·sis \ˌdis-ˌker-ə-ˈtō-səs\ *n, pl* **-to·ses** \-ˌsēz\ : faulty development of the epidermis with abnormal keratinization — **dys·ker·a·tot·ic** \-ˈtä-tik\ *adj*

dys·ki·ne·sia \ˌdis-kə-ˈnē-zhə, -kī-, -zhē-ə\ *n* : impairment of voluntary movements resulting in fragmented or jerky motions (as in Parkinson's disease) — see TARDIVE DYSKINESIA — **dys·ki·net·ic** \-ˈne-tik\ *adj*

dyskinetic cerebral palsy *n* : ATHETOID CEREBRAL PALSY

dys·lec·tic \dis-ˈlek-tik\ *adj or n* : DYSLEXIC

dys·lex·ia \dis-ˈlek-sē-ə\ *n* : a variable often familial learning disability that involves difficulties in acquiring and processing language and is typically manifested by a lack of proficiency in reading, spelling, and writing

[1]**dys·lex·ic** \-ˈlek-sik\ *adj* : affected with dyslexia

[2]**dyslexic** *n* : a person affected with dyslexia

dys·lip·id·emia \dis-ˌli-pə-ˈdē-mē-ə\ *n* : a condition marked by abnormal concentrations of lipids or lipoproteins in the blood — **dys·lip·id·emic** \-mik\ *adj*

dys·men·or·rhea \(ˌ)dis-ˌme-nə-ˈrē-ə\ *n* : painful menstruation — **dys·men·or·rhe·ic** \-ˈrē-ik\ *adj*

dys·met·ria \dis-ˈme-trē-ə\ *n* : impaired ability to estimate distance in muscular action

dys·mor·phia \-ˈmȯr-fē-ə\ *n* **1** : DYSMORPHISM ⟨craniofacial ~⟩ **2** : BODY DYSMORPHIC DISORDER

dys·mor·phic \-ˈmȯr-fik\ *adj* : characterized by or having an anatomical malformation

dys·mor·phism \-ˈmȯr-ˌfi-zəm\ *n* : an anatomical malformation

dys·mor·phol·o·gy \-mȯr-ˈfä-lə-jē\ *n* : a branch of clinical medicine concerned with human teratology — **dys·mor·phol·o·gist** \-jist\ *n*

dys·os·mia \di-ˈsäz-mē-ə, -ˈsäs-\ *n* : dysfunction of the sense of smell

dys·os·to·sis \ˌdi-ˌsäs-ˈtō-səs\ *n, pl* **-to·ses** \-ˌsēz\ : defective formation of bone — **dys·os·tot·ic** \-ˈtä-tik\ *adj*

dys·pa·reu·nia \ˌdis-pə-ˈrü-nē-ə, -nyə\ *n* : difficult or painful sexual intercourse

dys·pep·sia \dis-ˈpep-shə, -sē-ə\ *n* : INDIGESTION

[1]**dys·pep·tic** \-ˈpep-tik\ *adj* : relating to or having dyspepsia

[2]**dyspeptic** *n* : a person having dyspepsia

dys·pha·gia \dis-ˈfā-jə, -jē-ə\ *n* : difficulty in swallowing — **dys·phag·ic** \-ˈfa-jik\ *adj*

dys·pha·sia \dis-ˈfā-zhə, -zhē-ə\ *n* : loss of or deficiency in the power to use or understand language as a result of injury to or disease of the brain — compare DYSARTHRIA

[1]**dys·pha·sic** \-ˈfā-zik\ *adj* : relating to or affected with dysphasia

[2]**dysphasic** *n* : a dysphasic person

dys·pho·nia \dis-ˈfō-nē-ə\ *n* : defective use of the voice

dys·pho·ria \dis-ˈfōr-ē-ə\ *n* : a state of feeling unwell or unhappy — compare EUPHORIA — **dys·phor·ic** \-ˈfȯr-ik, -ˈfär-\ *adj*

dys·pla·sia \dis-ˈplā-zhə, -zhē-ə\ *n* : abnormal growth or development (as of organs or cells); *broadly* : abnormal anatomic structure due to such growth — **dys·plas·tic** \-ˈplas-tik\ *adj*

dys·pnea \ˈdis-nē-ə, ˈdisp-\ *n* : difficult or labored respiration — compare EUPNEA — **dys·pne·ic** \-nē-ik\ *adj*

dys·pnoea *chiefly Brit var of* DYSPNEA

dys•prax•ia \dis-ˈprak-sē-ə, -ˈprak-shə, -shē-ə\ *n* : impairment of the ability to perform coordinated movements — **dys•prax•ic** \-sik\ *adj*

dys•pro•si•um \dis-ˈprō-zē-əm, -zhəm, -zhē-əm\ *n* : an element that forms highly magnetic compounds — symbol *Dy;* see ELEMENT table

dys•pro•tein•ae•mia *chiefly Brit var of* DYSPROTEINEMIA

dys•pro•tein•emia \ˌdis-ˌprōt-ᵊn-ˈē-mē-ə, -ˌprō-ˌtē-ˈnē-, -ˌprō-tē-ə-ˈnē-\ *n* : any abnormality of the protein content of the blood — **dys•pro•tein•emic** \-mik\ *adj*

dys•ra•phism \dis-ˈrā-ˌfi-zəm\ *n* : incomplete fusion of parts; *esp* : defective closure of the neural tube ⟨spinal ~⟩

dys•re•flex•ia \ˌdis-rē-ˈflek-sē-ə\ *n* : abnormal physiological reflexes in response to stimuli; *esp* : AUTONOMIC DYSREFLEXIA

dys•reg•u•la•tion \ˌdis-ˌre-gyə-ˈlā-shən\ *n* : impairment of regulatory mechanisms (as those governing metabolism or organ function) — **dys•reg•u•lat•ed** \-ˈre-gyə-ˌlā-təd\ *adj*

dys•rhyth•mia \dis-ˈrith-mē-ə\ *n* **1** : an abnormal rhythm; *esp* : a disordered rhythm exhibited in a record of electrical activity of the brain or heart **2** : JET LAG — **dys•rhyth•mic** \-mik\ *adj*

dys•sy•ner•gia \ˌdis-sə-ˈnər-jə, -jē-ə\ *n* : DYSKINESIA — **dys•sy•ner•gic** \-ˈnər-jik\ *adj*

dys•thy•mia \dis-ˈthī-mē-ə\ *n* : a mood disorder characterized by chronic mildly depressed or irritable mood often accompanied by other symptoms (as eating and sleeping disturbances, and poor self-esteem) — **dys•thy•mic** \-mik\ *adj or n*

dysthymic disorder *n* : DYSTHYMIA

dys•to•cia \dis-ˈtō-shə, -shē-ə\ *or* **dys•to•kia** \-ˈtō-kē-ə\ *n* : slow or difficult labor or delivery

dys•to•nia \dis-ˈtō-nē-ə\ *n* : a state of disordered tonicity of tissues (as of muscle) — **dys•ton•ic** \-ˈtä-nik\ *adj*

dystonia mus•cu•lo•rum de•for•mans \-ˌməs-kyə-ˈlȯr-əm-di-ˈfȯr-ˌmanz\ *n* : a rare inherited neurological disorder characterized by progressive muscular spasticity causing severe involuntary contortions esp. of the trunk and limbs — called also *torsion dystonia*

dys•tro•phic \dis-ˈtrō-fik\ *adj* **1** : relating to or caused by faulty nutrition **2** : relating to or affected with a dystrophy ⟨~ muscles⟩ **3 a** : occurring at sites of damaged or necrotic tissue ⟨~ calcification⟩ **b** : characterized by disordered growth ⟨~ nails⟩

dystrophica — see MYOTONIA DYSTROPHICA

dystrophic epidermolysis bullosa *n* : any of several inherited forms of epidermolysis bullosa that are marked esp. by blister formation between the basement membrane and lamina propria

dys•tro•phin \ˈdis-trə-ˌfin\ *n* : a protein that is absent in Duchenne muscular dystrophy and deficient or of abnormal molecular weight in Becker muscular dystrophy

dys•tro•phy \ˈdis-trə-fē\ *n, pl* **-phies** **1** : a condition produced by faulty nutrition **2** : any myogenic atrophy; *esp* : MUSCULAR DYSTROPHY

dys•uria \dis-ˈyu̇r-ē-ə\ *n* : difficult or painful discharge of urine — **dys•uric** \-ˈyu̇r-ik\ *adj*

E

e- *prefix* : missing : absent ⟨*e*dentulous⟩
EAE *abbr* experimental allergic encephalomyelitis
ear \ˈir\ *n* **1** : the vertebrate organ of hearing and equilibrium consisting in most mammals of a sound-collecting outer ear separated by the tympanic membrane from a sound-transmitting middle ear that in turn is separated from a sensory inner ear by membranous fenestrae **2 a** : the external ear of humans and most mammals **b** : a human earlobe — **eared** \ˈird\ *adj*
ear·ache \ˈir-ˌāk\ *n* : an ache or pain in the ear — called also *otalgia*
ear canal *n* : the tubular passage of the outer ear leading to the tympanic membrane
ear·drum \-ˌdrəm\ *n* : TYMPANIC MEMBRANE
ear·lobe \ˈir-ˌlōb\ *n* : the pendent part of the ear esp. of humans
ear mange *n* : canker of the ear esp. in cats and dogs that is caused by mites; *esp* : OTODECTIC MANGE
ear mite *n* : any of various mites attacking the ears of mammals
ear·mold \ˈir-ˌmōld\ *n* : a device that fits within the outer ear, is connected by way of a tube to a hearing aid worn behind the ear, and serves esp. to channel the amplified sound from the hearing aid to the ear canal
ear pick *n* : a device for removing wax or foreign bodies from the ear
ear·piece \ˈir-ˌpēs\ *n* **1** : a part of an instrument (as a stethoscope) that is inserted into the outer opening of the ear **2** : one of the two sidepieces that support eyeglasses by passing over or behind the ears
ear·plug \-ˌpləg\ *n* : a device of pliable material for insertion into the outer opening of the ear (as to keep out water or deaden sound)
ear tick *n* : any of several ticks infesting the ears of mammals; *esp* : SPINOSE EAR TICK
ear·wax \ˈir-ˌwaks\ *n* : the yellow waxy secretion from the glands of the external ear — called also *cerumen*
east coast fever *n* : an acute fatal febrile disease of cattle that occurs in Africa and is caused by a protozoan of the genus *Theileria* (*T. parva*) transmitted by ticks esp. of the genera *Rhipicephalus* and *Hyalomma*
eastern equine encephalitis *also* **eastern equine encephalomyelitis** *n* : EQUINE ENCEPHALITIS a — abbr. *EEE;* called also *triple E*
eating disorder *n* : any of several psychological disorders (as anorexia nervosa or bulimia) characterized by serious disturbances of eating behavior
Ea·ton agent \ˈēt-ᵊn-\ *n* : a bacterium of the genus *Mycoplasma* (*M. pneumoniae*) that is the causative agent of primary atypical pneumonia
Eaton, Monroe Davis (1904–1989), American microbiologist.
Eaton–Lambert syndrome *n* : LAMBERT-EATON SYNDROME
Ebo·la \i-ˈbō-lə, ē-\ *n* **1** : EBOLA VIRUS **2** : the hemorrhagic fever caused by the Ebola virus — called also *Ebola fever*
Ebola virus *n* : any of several filoviruses (esp. species *Zaire ebolavirus* of the genus *Ebolavirus*) of African origin that cause an often fatal hemorrhagic fever
eb·ur·nat·ed \ˈe-bər-ˌnā-təd, ˈē-\ *adj* : hard and dense like ivory ⟨~ cartilage⟩ ⟨~ bone⟩ — **eb·ur·na·tion** \ˌe-bər-ˈnā-shən, ˌē-\ *n*
EBV *abbr* Epstein-Barr virus
EB virus \ˌē-ˈbē-\ *n* : EPSTEIN-BARR VIRUS
ec- *prefix* : out of : outside of : outside ⟨*ec*crine⟩
eccentric hypertrophy *n* : hypertrophy of the wall of a hollow organ and esp. the heart with dilatation of its cavity
ec·chon·dro·ma \ˌe-kən-ˈdrō-mə\ *n, pl* **-ma·ta** \-mə-tə\ *also* **-mas** : a cartilaginous tumor projecting from bone or cartilage
ec·chy·mo·sis \ˌe-kə-ˈmō-səs\ *n, pl* **-mo·ses** \-ˌsēz\ : the escape of blood into the tissues from ruptured blood vessels marked by a livid black-and-blue or purple spot or area; *also* : the discoloration so caused — **ec·chy·mosed** \ˈe-kə-ˌmōzd, -ˌmōst\ *adj* — **ec·chy·mot·ic** \-ˈmä-tik\ *adj*
ec·crine \ˈe-krən, -ˌkrīn, -ˌkrēn\ *adj* : of, relating to, having, or being eccrine glands — compare APOCRINE, HOLOCRINE, MEROCRINE
eccrine gland *n* : any of the rather small sweat glands that produce a fluid secretion without removing cytoplasm from the secreting cells and that are restricted to the human skin — called also *eccrine sweat gland*
ECG *abbr* electrocardiogram
Echid·noph·a·ga \ˌek-(ˌ)id-ˈnä-fə-gə\ *n* : a genus of fleas (family Pulicidae) including the sticktight flea (*E. gallinacea*)
ech·i·na·cea \ˌe-ki-ˈnā-sē-ə, -shə\ *n* : the dried root or other part of any of three herbs (*Echinacea angustifolia*, *E. pallida*, and *E. purpurea*) that are used chiefly in dietary supplements and herbal remedies and that are held to stimulate the immune system; *also* : any of these herbs
echi·no·coc·co·sis \i-ˌkī-nə-kä-ˈkō-səs\ *n, pl* **-co·ses** \-ˌsēz\ : infestation with or disease caused by a tapeworm of the

genus *Echinococcus; esp* : HYDATID DISEASE
echi•no•coc•cus \-nə-ˈkä-kəs\ *n* **1** *cap* : a genus of taeniid tapeworms (as *E. granulosus* and *E. multilocularis*) that alternate a minute adult living as a harmless commensal in the intestine of dogs and other carnivores with a hydatid larva invading tissues esp. of the liver of mammals (as cattle, sheep, swine, and humans) and acting as a serious often fatal pathogen — see HYDATID DISEASE **2** *pl* **-coc•ci** \-ˈkä-ˌkī, -ˌkē; -ˈkäk-ˌsī, -ˌsē\ : any tapeworm of the genus *Echinococcus; also* : HYDATID 1
echo *abbr* — echocardiogram; echocardiography
echo•car•dio•gram \ˌe-kō-ˈkär-dē-ə-ˌgram\ *n* : a visual record made by echocardiography; *also* : the procedure for producing such a record
echo•car•di•og•ra•phy \-ˌkär-dē-ˈä-grə-fē\ *n, pl* **-phies** : the use of ultrasound to examine and measure the structure and functioning of the heart and to diagnose abnormalities and disease — **echo•car•di•og•raph•er** \-grə-fər\ *n* — **echo•car•dio•graph•ic** \-dē-ə-ˈgra-fik\ *adj*
echo•en•ceph•a•lo•gram \ˌe-kō-in-ˈse-fə-lə-ˌgram\ *n* : a visual record obtained by echoencephalography
echo•en•ceph•a•log•ra•phy \-in-ˌse-fə-ˈlä-grə-fē\ *n, pl* **-phies** : the use of ultrasound to examine and measure internal structures (as the ventricles) of the skull and to diagnose abnormalities and disease — **echo•en•ceph•alo•graph•ic** \-fə-lə-ˈgra-fik\ *adj*
echo•gen•ic \ˌe-kə-ˈje-nik\ *adj* : reflecting ultrasound waves — **echo•ge•nic•i•ty** \-jə-ˈni-sə-tē\ *n*
echo•gram \ˈe-kō-ˌgram\ *n* : SONOGRAM
echo•graph \-ˌgraf\ *n* : an instrument used for echography
echog•ra•phy \i-ˈkä-grə-fē\ *n, pl* **-phies** : ULTRASOUND 2 — **echo•graph•ic** \ˌe-kō-ˈgra-fik\ *adj* — **echo•graph•i•cal•ly** \-fi-k(ə-)lē\ *adv*
echo•la•lia \ˌe-kō-ˈlā-lē-ə\ *n* : the often pathological repetition of what is said by other people as if echoing them — **echo•lal•ic** \-ˈla-lik\ *adj*
echo•prax•ia \ˌe-kō-ˈprak-sē-ə\ *n* : pathological repetition of the actions of other people as if echoing them
echo•thi•o•phate iodide \-ˈthī-ə-ˌfāt-\ *n* : a long-acting anticholinesterase $C_9H_{23}INO_3PS$ used esp. to reduce intraocular pressure in the treatment of glaucoma — called also *echothiophate*
echo•vi•rus \ˈe-kō-ˌvī-rəs\ *n* : any of numerous serotypes of a picornavirus of the genus *Enterovirus* (species *Human enterovirus B*) that are found in the gastrointestinal tract and are sometimes associated with respiratory ailments and meningitis
ec•lamp•sia \i-ˈklamp-sē-ə, e-\ *n* : a convulsive state : an attack of convulsions: as **a** : convulsions or coma late in pregnancy in an individual affected with preeclampsia **b** : a condition comparable to milk fever of cows occurring in domestic animals (as dogs and cats) — **ec•lamp•tic** \-tik\ *adj*
ECLS *abbr* extracorporeal life support
ECMO \ˈek-(ˌ)mō\ *n* : EXTRACORPOREAL MEMBRANE OXYGENATION
E. coli \ˌē-ˈkō-ˌlī\ *n, pl* **E. coli** *also* **E. colis** : a straight rod-shaped gram-negative bacterium (*Escherichia coli* of the family Enterobacteriaceae) occurring in various strains that may live as harmless inhabitants of the human lower intestine or may produce a toxin causing intestinal illness marked esp. by diarrhea
e–col•lar \ˈē-ˌkä-lər\ *n* : ELIZABETHAN COLLAR
ecol•o•gy \i-ˈkä-lə-jē, e-\ *n, pl* **-gies** **1** : a branch of science concerned with the interrelationship of organisms and their environments **2** : the totality or pattern of relations between organisms and their environment **3** : HUMAN ECOLOGY — **eco•log•i•cal** \ˌē-kə-ˈlä-ji-kəl, ˌe-\ *also* **eco•log•ic** \-jik\ *adj* — **eco•log•i•cal•ly** \-ji-k(ə-)lē\ *adv* — **ecol•o•gist** \i-ˈkä-lə-jist, e-\ *n*
eco•sys•tem \ˈē-kō-ˌsis-təm, ˈe-\ *n* : the complex of a community and its environment functioning as an ecological unit in nature
écra•seur \ā-krä-ˈzər, ˌē-\ *n* : a surgical instrument used to encircle and sever a projecting mass of tissue
ec•sta•sy \ˈek-stə-sē\ *n, pl* **-sies** **1** : a trance state in which intense absorption is accompanied by loss of sense perception and voluntary control **2** *often cap* : a synthetic amphetamine analog $C_{11}H_{15}NO_2$ used illicitly for its mood-enhancing and hallucinogenic properties — called also *MDMA, methylene dioxymethamphetamine* — **ec•stat•ic** \ek-ˈsta-tik\ *adj*
ECT *abbr* electroconvulsive therapy
ec•ta•sia \ek-ˈtā-zhē-ə, -zhə\ *n* : the expansion of a hollow or tubular organ — **ec•tat•ic** \ek-ˈta-tik\ *adj*
ec•ta•sis \ˈek-tə-səs\ *n, pl* **-ta•ses** \-ˌsēz\ : ECTASIA
ec•thy•ma \ek-ˈthī-mə\ *n* **1** : a cutaneous eruption marked by large flat pustules that have a hardened base surrounded by inflammation and occur esp. on the lower legs **2** : sore mouth of sheep — **ec•thy•ma•tous** \ek-ˈthi-mə-təs, -ˈthī-\ *adj*
ecto- *also* **ect-** *comb form* : outside : external ⟨*ecto*derm⟩
ec•to•derm \-ˌdərm\ *n* **1** : the outermost of the three primary germ layers of an embryo **2** : a tissue (as neural tissue) derived from ectoderm — **ec•to•der•mal** \ˌek-tə-ˈdər-məl\ *adj*
ec•to•en•zyme \ˌek-tō-ˈen-ˌzīm\ *n* : an enzyme acting outside the cell

ec•to•mor•phic \ˌek-tə-ˈmȯr-fik\ *adj* : having a light lean body build — compare ENDOMORPHIC, MESOMORPHIC — **ec•to•morph** \ˈek-tə-ˌmȯrf\ *n* — **ec•to•mor•phy** \ˈek-tə-ˌmȯr-fē\ *n*

-ec•to•my \ˈek-tə-mē\ *n comb form, pl* **-ec•to•mies** : surgical removal ⟨appen*dectomy*⟩

ec•to•par•a•site \ˌek-tō-ˈpar-ə-ˌsīt\ *n* : a parasite that lives on the exterior of its host — compare ENDOPARASITE — **ec•to•par•a•sit•ic** \-ˌpar-ə-ˈsi-tik\ *adj*

ec•to•pia \ek-ˈtō-pē-ə\ *n* : an abnormal congenital or acquired position of an organ or part ⟨∼ of the heart⟩

ec•top•ic \ek-ˈtä-pik\ *adj* **1** : occurring in an abnormal position ⟨an ∼ kidney⟩ **2** : originating in an area of the heart other than the sinoatrial node ⟨∼ beats⟩; *also* : initiating ectopic heartbeats ⟨an ∼ pacemaker⟩ — **ec•top•i•cal•ly** \-pi-k(ə-)lē\ *adv*

ectopic pregnancy *n* : gestation elsewhere than in the uterus (as in a fallopian tube or in the peritoneal cavity) — called also *ectopic gestation, extrauterine pregnancy*

ec•to•pla•cen•ta \ˌek-tō-plə-ˈsen-tə\ *n* : TROPHOBLAST — **ec•to•pla•cen•tal** \-ˈsent-ᵊl\ *adj*

ec•to•plasm \ˈek-tə-ˌpla-zəm\ *n* : the outer relatively rigid granule-free layer of the cytoplasm — compare ENDOPLASM

ec•to•py \ˈek-tə-pē\ *n, pl* **-pies** : ECTOPIA

ectro- *comb form* : congenitally absent — usu. indicating absence of a particular limb or part ⟨*ectro*dactyly⟩

ec•tro•dac•ty•ly \-ˈdak-tə-lē\ *n, pl* **-lies** : congenital complete or partial absence of one or more digits

ec•tro•me•lia \ˌek-trō-ˈmē-lē-ə\ *n* **1** : congenital absence or imperfection of one or more limbs **2** : MOUSEPOX

ec•tro•pi•on \ek-ˈtrō-pē-ˌän, -ən\ *n* : an abnormal turning out of a part (as an eyelid)

ec•ze•ma \ig-ˈzē-mə, ˈeg-zə-mə, ˈek-sə-\ *n* : an inflammatory condition of the skin characterized by redness, itching, and oozing vesicular lesions which become scaly, crusted, or hardened — **ec•zem•a•tous** \ig-ˈze-mə-təs\ *adj*

ec•ze•ma•toid \ig-ˈzē-mə-ˌtȯid, -ˈze-\ *adj* : resembling eczema

ED *abbr* **1** effective dose **2** emergency department **3** erectile dysfunction

EDB *abbr* ethylene dibromide

ede•ma \i-ˈdē-mə\ *n, pl* **-mas** *also* **-ma•ta** \-mə-tə\ : an abnormal excess accumulation of serous fluid in connective tissue or in a serous cavity — called also *dropsy* — **edem•a•tous** \-ˈde-mə-təs\ *adj*

eden•tu•lous \(ˌ)ē-ˈden-chə-ləs\ *adj* : TOOTHLESS ⟨an ∼ upper jaw⟩

edetate — see DISODIUM EDETATE

Ed•ing•er–West•phal nucleus \ˌe-diŋ-ər-ˈwest-ˌfäl-, -ˌfōl-\ *n* : the lateral portion of the group of nerve cells lying ventral to the aqueduct of Sylvius which give rise to autonomic fibers of the oculomotor nerve

Ed•ing•er \ˈe-diŋ-ər\, **Ludwig (1855–1918)**, German neurologist.

West•phal \ˈwest-ˌfäl, -ˌfōl\, **Carl Friedrich Otto (1833–1890)**, German neurologist.

EDR *abbr* electrodermal response

ed•ro•pho•ni•um \ˌe-drə-ˈfō-nē-əm\ *n* : an anticholinesterase $C_{10}H_{16}ClNO$ used esp. to stimulate skeletal muscle and in the diagnosis of myasthenia gravis — called also *edrophonium chloride;* see TENSILON

EDTA \ˌē-(ˌ)dē-(ˌ)tē-ˈā\ *n* : a white crystalline acid $C_{10}H_{16}N_2O_8$ used in medicine as an anticoagulant and as a chelator in the treatment of lead poisoning — called also *ethylenediaminetetraacetic acid*

ed•u•ca•ble \ˈe-jə-kə-bəl\ *adj* : affected with mild intellectual disability and capable of developing academic, social, and occupational skills within the capabilities of one with a mental age between 9 and 12 years — compare TRAINABLE

Edu•rant \ˈē-də-rənt\ *trademark* — used for a preparation of rilpivirine

Ed•wards syndrome \ˈed-wərdz-\ *n* : TRISOMY 18

Edwards, John Hilton (1928–2007), British geneticist.

EEE *abbr* eastern equine encephalitis; eastern equine encephalomyelitis

EEG *abbr* electroencephalogram; electroencephalograph

EENT *abbr* eye, ear, nose, and throat

ef•a•vi•renz \ˌef-ə-ˈvī-ˌrenz\ *n* : a reverse transcriptase inhibitor $C_{14}H_9ClF_3NO_2$ taken orally with other antiretroviral agents in the treatment of HIV infection — see ATRIPLA, SUSTIVA

ef•face•ment \i-ˈfās-mənt, e-\ *n* : the thinning or obliteration of tissue or narrowing of an internal anatomical space; *esp* : the shortening and thinning of the uterine cervix during labor so that only the external orifice remains — **ef•face** \-ˈfās\ *vb*

ef•fect \i-ˈfekt\ *n* : something that is produced by an agent or cause

ef•fec•tive \i-ˈfek-tiv\ *adj* : producing a decided, decisive, claimed, or desired effect — **ef•fec•tive•ness** *n*

ef•fec•tor \i-ˈfek-tər, -ˌtȯr\ *n* **1** : a bodily organ (as a gland or muscle) that becomes active in response to stimulation **2** : a substance (as an inducer or corepressor) that activates, controls, or inactivates a process or action (as protein synthesis)

[1]**ef•fer•ent** \ˈe-fə-rənt; ˈe-ˌfer-ənt, ˈē-ˌfer-\ *adj* : conducting outward from a part or organ; *specif* : conveying nerve impulses to an effector ⟨∼ neurons⟩ — compare AFFERENT

[2]**efferent** *n* : an efferent part (as a blood vessel or nerve fiber)

efferentes — see DUCTULI EFFERENTES

efferentia — see VASA EFFERENTIA

Ef•fex•or \ə-ˈfek-ˌsȯr\ *trademark* — used for a preparation of the hydrochloride of venlafaxine

Ef•fi•ent \ˈef-ē-ənt\ *trademark* — used for a preparation of prasugrel

ef•fleu•rage \ˌe-flə-ˈräzh, -(ˌ)flü-\ *n* : a light stroking movement used in massage

effort syndrome *n* : NEUROCIRCULATORY ASTHENIA

ef•fuse \i-ˈfyüs, e-\ *adj* : spread out flat without definite form

ef•fu•sion \i-ˈfyü-zhən, e-\ *n* **1** : the escape of a fluid from anatomical vessels by rupture or exudation **2** : the fluid that escapes by extravasation — see PLEURAL EFFUSION

ef•i•na•con•a•zole \ˌef-i-nə-ˈkä-nə-ˌzōl\ *n* : a topical antifungal agent $C_{18}H_{22}F_2N_4O$ used to treat toenail fungus — see JUBLIA

eges•tion \i-ˈjes-chən\ *n* : the act or process of discharging undigested or waste material from a cell or organism; *specif* : DEFECATION — **egest** \i-ˈjest\ *vb*

EGF *abbr* epidermal growth factor

egg \ˈeg, ˈāg\ *n* **1** : the hard-shelled reproductive body produced by a bird and esp. by the common domestic chicken (*Gallus gallus*) **2** : an animal reproductive body consisting of an ovum together with its nutritive and protective envelopes and having the capacity to develop into a new individual capable of independent existence **3** : OVUM

egg cell *n* : OVUM

ego \ˈē-(ˌ)gō\ *n, pl* **egos** **1** : the self esp. as contrasted with another self or the world **2** : the one of the three divisions of the psyche in psychoanalytic theory that serves as the organized conscious mediator between the person and reality esp. by functioning both in the perception of and adaptation to reality — compare [1]ID, SUPEREGO

[1]**ego•cen•tric** \ˌē-gō-ˈsen-trik\ *adj* **1** : limited in outlook or concern to one's own activities or needs **2** : being self-centered or selfish — **ego•cen•tri•cal•ly** \-tri-k(ə-)lē\ *adv* — **ego•cen•tric•i•ty** \ˌē-gō-(ˌ)sen-ˈtris-ət-ē, -sən-\ *n* — **ego•cen•trism** \-ˈsen-ˌtri-zəm\ *n*

[2]**egocentric** *n* : an egocentric person

ego–defense *n* : DEFENSE MECHANISM

ego–dys•ton•ic \-dis-ˈtä-nik\ *adj* : incompatible with or unacceptable to the ego — compare EGO-SYNTONIC

ego ideal *n* : the positive standards, ideals, and ambitions that according to psychoanalytic theory are assimilated from the superego

ego–involvement *n* : an involvement of one's self-esteem in the performance of a task or in an object — **ego–involve** *vb*

ego•ism \ˈē-gə-ˌwi-zəm\ *n* **1 a** : a doctrine that individual self-interest is the actual motive of all conscious action **b** : a doctrine that individual self-interest is the valid end of all actions **2** : excessive concern for oneself without exaggerated feelings of self-importance — compare EGOTISM — **ego•ist** \-wist\ *n* — **ego•is•tic** \ˌē-gə-ˈwis-tik\ *also* **ego•is•ti•cal** \-ti-kəl\ *adj* — **ego•is•ti•cal•ly** \-ti-k(ə-)lē\ *adv*

ego•ma•nia \ˌē-gō-ˈmā-nē-ə, -nyə\ *n* : the quality or state of being extremely egocentric — **ego•ma•ni•ac** \-nē-ˌak\ *n* — **ego•ma•ni•a•cal** \-mə-ˈnī-ə-kəl\ *adj* — **ego•ma•ni•a•cal•ly** \-k(ə-)lē\ *adv*

egoph•o•ny \ē-ˈgä-fə-nē\ *n, pl* **-nies** : a modification of the voice resembling bleating heard on auscultation of the chest in some diseases (as in pleurisy with effusion)

ego–syn•ton•ic \ˌē-gō-sin-ˈtä-nik\ *adj* : compatible with or acceptable to the ego — compare EGO-DYSTONIC

ego•tism \ˈē-gə-ˌti-zəm\ *n* : an exaggerated sense of self-importance — compare EGOISM 2 — **ego•tist** \-tist\ *n* — **ego•tis•tic** \ˌē-gə-ˈtis-tik\ *or* **ego•tis•ti•cal** \-ˈtis-ti-kəl\ *adj* — **ego•tis•ti•cal•ly** \-ˈtis-ti-k(ə-)lē\ *adv*

Eh•lers–Dan•los syndrome \ˈā-lərz-ˈdan-(ˌ)läs-\ *n* : a rare inherited disorder of connective tissue characterized esp. by extremely flexible joints, elastic skin, and excessive bruising

Eh•lers \ˈā-(ˌ)lerz\, **Edvard L. (1863–1937)**, Danish dermatologist.

Dan•los \dän-lō\, **Henri–Alexandre (1844–1912)**, French dermatologist.

Ehr•lich•ia \er-ˈli-kē-ə\ *n* : a genus of gram-negative nonmotile bacteria that are transmitted chiefly by tick bites, are intracellular parasites esp. of white blood cells (as monocytes and granulocytes), and include some (as *E. equi* and *E. phagocytophila*) that are now typically placed in the genus *Anaplasma*

Ehr•lich \ˈār-ˌlik\, **Paul (1854–1915)**, German chemist and bacteriologist.

ehr•lich•i•o•sis \er-ˌlik-ē-ˈō-sis\ *n, pl* **-o•ses** \-ˌsēz\ : infection with or a disease caused by bacteria of the genus *Ehrlichia; also* : ANAPLASMOSIS b — see HUMAN MONOCYTIC EHRLICHIOSIS

EIA *abbr* **1** enzyme immunoassay **2** equine infectious anemia **3** exercise-induced asthma

ei•co•sa•noid \ī-ˈkō-sə-ˌnȯid\ *n* : any of a class of compounds (as the prostaglandins and leukotrienes) derived from polyunsaturated fatty acids and involved in cellular activity

ei•co•sa•pen•ta•e•no•ic acid \ˌī-kō-sə-ˌpen-tə-ē-ˌnō-ik-\ *n* : an omega-3 fatty acid $C_{20}H_{30}O_2$ found esp. in the oil of cold-water fish (as mackerel and herring) — abbr. *EPA*

ei•det•ic \ī-ˈde-tik\ *adj* : marked by or involving extraordinarily accurate and vivid recall esp. of visual images — **ei•det•i•cal•ly** \-ti-k(ə-)lē\ *adv*

eighth cranial nerve *n* : AUDITORY NERVE

eighth nerve *n* : AUDITORY NERVE

ei·ko·nom·e·ter \ˌī-kə-ˈnä-mə-tər\ *n* : a device to detect aniseikonia or to test stereoscopic vision

Ei·me·ria \ī-ˈmir-ē-ə\ *n* : a genus of coccidian protozoans that invade the visceral epithelia and esp. the intestinal wall of many vertebrates and include serious pathogens

Ei·mer \ˈī-mər\, **Theodor Gustav Heinrich (1843–1898),** German zoologist.

ein·stei·ni·um \īn-ˈstī-nē-əm\ *n* : a radioactive element produced artificially — symbol *Es;* see ELEMENT table

Ein·stein \ˈīn-ˌstīn, -ˌshtīn\, **Albert (1879–1955),** German physicist.

Ei·sen·meng·er complex \ˈī-zən-ˌmeŋ-ər-\ *or* **Ei·sen·meng·er's complex** \-ərz-\ *n* : the combination of a congenital defect in the septum between the ventricles of the heart with its early complications (as left to right blood flow through the defect and increased blood pressure in the pulmonary arteries)

Eisenmenger, Victor (1864–1932), German physician.

Eisenmenger syndrome *or* **Eisenmenger's syndrome** *n* : the septal defect of Eisenmenger complex with its later complications (as right to left blood flow through the septal defect and marked hypertrophy of the right ventricle) that are essentially surgically irreversible

[1]**ejac·u·late** \i-ˈja-kyə-ˌlāt\ *vb* **-lat·ed; -lat·ing** : to eject from a living body; *specif* : to eject (semen) in orgasm — **ejac·u·la·tor** \-ˌlā-tər\ *n*

[2]**ejac·u·late** \-lət\ *n* : the semen released by one ejaculation

ejac·u·la·tion \i-ˌja-kyə-ˈlā-shən\ *n* : the act or process of ejaculating; *specif* : the sudden or spontaneous discharging of a fluid (as semen in orgasm) from a duct — see PREMATURE EJACULATION

ejac·u·la·tio prae·cox \-ˈlā-shē-ō-ˈprē-ˌkäks\ *n* : PREMATURE EJACULATION

ejac·u·la·to·ry \i-ˈja-kyə-lə-ˌtōr-ē\ *adj* : of, relating to, or functioning in physiological ejaculation ⟨~ vessels⟩

ejaculatory duct *n* : either of the paired ducts in the human male that are formed by the junction of the duct from the seminal vesicle with the vas deferens, pass through the prostate, and open into or close to the prostatic utricle

ejection fraction *n* : the ratio of the volume of blood the heart empties during systole to the volume of blood in the heart at the end of diastole expressed as a percentage usu. between 50 and 80 percent

ejec·tor \i-ˈjek-tər\ *n* : something that ejects — see SALIVA EJECTOR

EKG \ˌē-(ˌ)kā-ˈjē\ *n* **1** : ELECTROCARDIOGRAM **2** : ELECTROCARDIOGRAPH

el·a·pid \ˈe-lə-pəd\ *n* : any of a family (Elapidae) of venomous snakes with hollow fangs that include the cobras and mambas, the coral snakes of the New World, and the majority of Australian snakes — **elapid** *adj*

elast- *or* **elasto-** *comb form* : elasticity ⟨*elast*osis⟩

elas·tase \i-ˈlas-ˌtās, -ˌtāz\ *n* : an enzyme esp. of pancreatic juice that digests elastin

[1]**elas·tic** \i-ˈlas-tik\ *adj* : capable of being easily stretched or expanded and resuming former shape — **elas·ti·cal·ly** \-ti-k(ə-)lē\ *adv* — **elas·tic·i·ty** \i-ˌlas-ˈtis-ə-tē\ *n*

[2]**elastic** *n* **1 a** : easily stretched rubber usu. prepared in cords, strings, or bands **b** : a band of elastic used esp. in orthodontics; *also* : one placed around a tooth at the gum line in effecting its nonsurgical removal **2 a** : an elastic fabric usu. made of yarns containing rubber **b** : something made from this fabric

elastic cartilage *n* : a yellowish flexible cartilage having the matrix infiltrated in all directions by a network of elastic fibers and occurring chiefly in the external ear, eustachian tube, and some cartilages of the larynx and epiglottis

elastic fiber *n* : a thick very elastic smooth yellowish anastomosing fiber of connective tissue that contains elastin

elastic stocking *n* : a stocking woven or knitted with an elastic material and used (as in the treatment of varicose veins) to provide support for the leg

elastic tissue *n* : tissue consisting chiefly of elastic fibers that is found esp. in some ligaments and tendons

elasticum — see PSEUDOXANTHOMA ELASTICUM

elas·tin \i-ˈlas-tən\ *n* : a protein that is similar to collagen and is the chief constituent of elastic fibers

elas·to·sis \i-ˌlas-ˈtō-səs\ *n, pl* **-to·ses** \-ˌsēz\ : a condition marked by thickening and degeneration of elastic fibers and loss of elasticity in connective tissue esp. of the skin (as due to prolonged sun exposure)

El·a·vil \ˈe-lə-ˌvil\ *trademark* — used for a preparation of amitriptyline

el·bow \ˈel-ˌbō\ *n* : the joint between the human forearm and the upper arm that supports the outer curve of the arm when bent — called also *elbow joint*

el·der·care \ˈel-dər-ˌker\ *n* : the care of older persons and esp. the care of an older parent by a son or daughter

elec·tive \i-ˈlek-tiv\ *adj* : beneficial to the patient but not essential for survival ⟨~ vascular surgery⟩

elective mutism *n* : SELECTIVE MUTISM

Elec·tra complex \i-ˈlek-trə-\ *n* : the Oedipus complex when it occurs in a female

electrical potential *or* **electric potential** *n* : the potential energy measured in volts of a unit of positive charge in an electric field

electric eel *n* : a large eel-shaped South American fish (*Electrophorus electricus* of the family Electrophoridae) that can deliver a severe shock of electricity

electric ray *n* : any of various round-bodied short-tailed rays (family Torpedinidae) of warm seas capable of delivering a shock of electricity

electric scalpel *n* : a needlelike surgical instrument using high-frequency oscillations in the form of a tiny electric arc to cut through tissue while at the same time sterilizing the edges of the wound and sealing blood vessels — called also *electric knife, radio knife*

electric shock *n* **1** : SHOCK 3 **2** : ELECTROCONVULSIVE THERAPY

electric shock therapy *n* : ELECTROCONVULSIVE THERAPY

electric shock treatment *n* : ELECTROCONVULSIVE THERAPY

elec•tro•car•dio•gram \-ˈkär-dē-ə-ˌgram\ *n* : the tracing made by an electrocardiograph; *also* : the procedure for producing an electrocardiogram

elec•tro•car•dio•graph \-ˌgraf\ *n* : an instrument for recording the changes of electrical potential occurring during the heartbeat used esp. in diagnosing abnormalities of heart action — **elec•tro•car•dio•graph•ic** \-ˌkär-dē-ə-ˈgra-fik\ *adj* — **elec•tro•car•dio•graph•i•cal•ly** \-fi-k(ə-)lē\ *adv* — **elec•tro•car•di•og•ra•phy** \-dē-ˈä-grə-fē\ *n*

elec•tro•cau•tery \-ˈkȯ-tə-rē\ *n, pl* **-ter•ies 1** : a cautery operated by an electric current **2** : the cauterization of tissue by means of an electrocautery

elec•tro•co•ag•u•la•tion \-kō-ˌa-gyə-ˈlā-shən\ *n* : the surgical coagulation of tissue by diathermy — **elec•tro•co•ag•u•late** \-kō-ˈa-gyə-ˌlāt\ *vb*

elec•tro•con•vul•sive \i-ˌlek-trō-kən-ˈvəl-siv\ *adj* : of, relating to, or involving a convulsive response to a shock of electricity

electroconvulsive therapy *n* : the treatment of mental illness and esp. depression by the application of electric current to the head of a usu. anesthetized patient that induces unconsciousness and convulsive seizures in the brain — abbr. *ECT;* called also *electric shock, electric shock therapy, electroshock therapy*

elec•tro•cor•ti•cal \-ˈkȯr-ti-kəl\ *adj* : of, relating to, or being electrical activity occurring in the cerebral cortex

elec•tro•cor•ti•co•gram \-ˈkȯr-ti-kə-ˌgram\ *n* : an electroencephalogram made with the electrodes in direct contact with the brain

elec•tro•cor•ti•cog•ra•phy \-ˌkȯr-ti-ˈkä-grə-fē\ *n, pl* **-phies** : the process of recording electrical activity in the brain by placing electrodes in direct contact with the cerebral cortex — **elec•tro•cor•ti•co•graph•ic** \-kə-ˈgra-fik\ *adj* — **elec•tro•cor•ti•co•graph•i•cal•ly** \-fi-k(ə-)lē\ *adv*

elec•troc•u•lo•gram \i-ˌlek-ˈträ-kyə-lə-ˌgram\ *n* : a recording of the moving eye

elec•tro•cute \i-ˈlek-trə-ˌkyüt\ *vb* **-cut•ed; -cut•ing 1** : to execute (a criminal) by electricity **2** : to kill by a shock of electricity — **elec•tro•cu•tion** \-ˌlek-trə-ˈkyü-shən\ *n*

elec•trode \i-ˈlek-ˌtrōd\ *n* : a conductor used to establish electrical contact with a nonmetallic part of a circuit

elec•tro•der•mal \i-ˌlek-trō-ˈdər-məl\ *adj* : of or relating to electrical activity in or electrical properties of the skin

elec•tro•des•ic•ca•tion \-ˌde-si-ˈkā-shən\ *n* : the drying of tissue by a high-frequency electric current applied with a needle-shaped electrode — called also *fulguration* — **elec•tro•des•ic•cate** \-ˈde-si-ˌkāt\ *vb*

elec•tro•di•ag•no•sis \-ˌdī-ig-ˈnō-səs\ *n, pl* **-no•ses** \-ˌsēz\ : diagnosis based on electrodiagnostic methods

elec•tro•di•ag•nos•tic \-ˌdī-ig-ˈnäs-tik\ *adj* : involving or obtained by the recording of responses to electrical stimulation or of spontaneous electrical activity (as in electromyography) for purposes of diagnosing a pathological condition — **elec•tro•di•ag•nos•ti•cal•ly** \-ti-k(ə-)lē\ *adv*

elec•tro•di•al•y•sis \i-ˌlek-trō-dī-ˈa-lə-səs\ *n, pl* **-y•ses** \-ˌsēz\ : dialysis accelerated by an electromotive force applied to electrodes adjacent to the membranes — **elec•tro•di•a•lyt•ic** \-ˌdī-ə-ˈli-tik\ *adj*

elec•tro•en•ceph•a•lo•gram \-in-ˈse-fə-lə-ˌgram\ *n* : the tracing of brain waves made by an electroencephalograph

elec•tro•en•ceph•a•lo•graph \-ˌgraf\ *n* : an apparatus for detecting and recording brain waves — called also *encephalograph* — **elec•tro•en•ceph•a•lo•graph•ic** \-ˌse-fə-lə-ˈgra-fik\ *adj* — **elec•tro•en•ceph•a•lo•graph•i•cal•ly** \-fi-k(ə-)lē\ *adv* — **elec•tro•en•ceph•a•log•ra•phy** \-ˈlä-grə-fē\ *n*

elec•tro•en•ceph•a•log•ra•pher \-in-ˌse-fə-ˈlä-grə-fər\ *n* : a person who specializes in electroencephalography

elec•tro•gen•ic \-ˈje-nik\ *adj* : of or relating to the production of electrical activity in living tissue — **elec•tro•gen•e•sis** \i-ˌlek-trə-ˈje-nə-səs\ *n*

elec•tro•gram \i-ˈlek-trə-ˌgram\ *n* : a tracing of the electrical potentials of a tissue (as the brain or heart) made by means of electrodes placed directly in the tissue instead of on the surface of the body

elec•tro•graph•ic \i-ˌlek-trə-ˈgra-fik\ *adj* : relating to, involving, or produced by the use of electrodes implanted directly in living tissue <~ stimulation of the brain> — **elec•tro•graph•i•cal•ly** \-fi-k(ə-)lē\ *adv*

elec•tro•ky•mo•graph \-ˈkī-mə-ˌgraf\ *n* : an instrument for recording graphically the motion of the heart as seen in silhouette on a fluoroscopic screen — **elec·tro·ky·mog·ra·phy** \-kī-ˈmä-grə-fē\ *n*

elec·trol·o·gist \i-ˌlek-ˈträ-lə-jist\ *n* : a person who removes hair by means of an electric current applied to the body with a needle-shaped electrode

elec·trol·o·gy \i-ˌlek-ˈträl-ə-jē\ *n* : ELECTROLYSIS 2

elec·trol·y·sis \-ˈträ-lə-səs\ *n, pl* **-y·ses** \-ˌsēz\ **1 a** : the process of producing chemical changes by passage of an electric current through an electrolyte **b** : subjection to this action **2** : the destruction of hair roots by an electrologist by means of an electric current applied to the body with a needle-shaped electrode

elec·tro·lyte \i-ˈlek-trə-ˌlīt\ *n* **1** : a nonmetallic electric conductor in which current is carried by the movement of ions **2 a** : a substance (as an acid or salt) that when dissolved in a suitable solvent (as water) or when fused becomes an ionic conductor **b** : any of the ions (as of sodium, potassium, or calcium) that in a biological fluid regulate or affect most metabolic processes (as the flow of nutrients into and waste products out of cells)

elec·tro·lyt·ic \i-ˌlek-trə-ˈli-tik\ *adj* : of or relating to electrolysis or an electrolyte; *also* : involving or produced by electrolysis — **elec·tro·lyt·i·cal·ly** \-ti-k(ə-)lē\ *adv*

elec·tro·mag·net·ic \-mag-ˈne-tik\ *adj* : of, relating to, or produced by electromagnetism

electromagnetic field *n* : a field (as around a high voltage power line) that possesses a definite amount of electromagnetic energy

electromagnetic radiation *n* : a series of electromagnetic waves

electromagnetic spectrum *n* : the entire range of wavelengths or frequencies of electromagnetic radiation extending from gamma rays to the longest radio waves

electromagnetic wave *n* : one of the waves propagated by simultaneous periodic variations of electric and magnetic field intensity and including radio waves, infrared, visible light, ultraviolet, X-rays, and gamma rays

elec·tro·mag·ne·tism \i-ˌlek-trō-ˈmag-nə-ˌti-zəm\ *n* **1** : magnetism developed by a current of electricity **2** : physics dealing with the relations between electricity and magnetism

elec·tro·mo·tive force \i-ˌlek-trō-ˈmō-tiv-, -trə-\ *n* : something that moves or tends to move electricity : the amount of energy derived from an electrical source per unit quantity of electricity passing through the source (as a cell or generator)

elec·tro·myo·gram \i-ˌlek-trō-ˈmī-ə-ˌgram\ *n* : a tracing made with an electromyograph

elec·tro·myo·graph \-ˌgraf\ *n* : an instrument that converts the electrical activity associated with functioning skeletal muscle into a visual record or into sound and has been used to diagnose neuromuscular disorders and in biofeedback training — **elec·tro·myo·graph·ic** \-ˌmī-ə-ˈgra-fik\ *adj* — **elec·tro·myo·graph·i·cal·ly** \-fi-k(ə-)lē\ *adv* — **elec·tro·my·og·ra·phy** \-mī-ˈä-grə-fē\ *n*

elec·tron \i-ˈlek-ˌträn\ *n* : an elementary particle consisting of a charge of negative electricity equal to about 1.602×10^{-19} coulomb and having a mass when at rest of about 9.109534×10^{-28} gram

elec·tro·nar·co·sis \i-ˌlek-trō-när-ˈkō-səs\ *n, pl* **-co·ses** \-ˌsēz\ : unconsciousness induced by passing a weak electric current through the brain

elec·tron·ic \i-ˌlek-ˈträ-nik\ *adj* : of or relating to electrons or electronics — **elec·tron·i·cal·ly** \-ni-k(ə-)lē\ *adv*

elec·tron·ics \i-ˌlek-ˈträ-niks\ *n* **1** : the physics of electrons and electronic devices **2** : electronic devices or equipment

electron micrograph *n* : a micrograph made with an electron microscope

electron microscope *n* : an electron-optical instrument in which a beam of electrons is used to produce an enlarged image of a minute object — **electron microscopist** *n* — **electron microscopy** *n*

electron transport *n* : the sequential transfer of electrons esp. by cytochromes in cellular respiration from an oxidizable substrate to molecular oxygen by a series of oxidation-reduction reactions

elec·tro·nys·tag·mog·ra·phy \i-ˌlek-trō-ˌnis-ˌtag-ˈmä-grə-fē\ *n, pl* **-phies** : the use of electrooculography to study nystagmus — **elec·tro·nys·tag·mo·graph·ic** \-(ˌ)nis-ˌtag-mə-ˈgra-fik\ *adj*

elec·tro·oc·u·lo·gram \-ˈä-kyə-lə-ˌgram\ *n* : a record of the standing voltage between the front and back of the eye that is correlated with eyeball movement (as in REM sleep) and obtained by electrodes suitably placed on the skin near the eye

elec·tro·oc·u·log·ra·phy \-ˌä-kyə-ˈlä-grə-fē\ *n, pl* **-phies** : the preparation and study of electrooculograms — **elec·tro·oc·u·lo·graph·ic** \-lə-ˈgra-fik\ *adj*

elec·tro·phe·ro·gram \-trə-ˈfir-ə-ˌgram, -ˈfer-\ *n* : ELECTROPHORETOGRAM

elec·tro·pho·re·sis \-trə-fə-ˈrē-səs\ *n, pl* **-re·ses** \-ˌsēz\ : the movement of suspended particles through a fluid or gel under the action of an electromotive force applied to electrodes in contact with the suspension — **elec·tro·pho·rese** \-ˈrēs, -ˈrēz\ *vb* — **elec·tro·pho·ret·ic** \-ˈre-tik\ *adj* — **elec·tro·pho·ret·i·cal·ly** \-ti-k(ə-)lē\ *adv*

elec·tro·pho·reto·gram \-fə-ˈre-tə-ˌgram\ *n* : a record that consists of the separated components of a mixture (as of proteins) produced by electrophoresis in a supporting medium

elec•tro•phren•ic \i-ˌlek-trə-ˈfre-nik\ *adj* : relating to or induced by electrical stimulation of the phrenic nerve

elec•tro•phys•i•ol•o•gy \i-ˌlek-trō-ˌfi-zē-ˈä-lə-jē\ *n, pl* **-gies** **1** : physiology that is concerned with the electrical aspects of physiological phenomena **2** : electrical phenomena associated with a physiological process (as the function of a body or bodily part) — **elec•tro•phys•i•o•log•i•cal** \-ə-ˈlä-ji-kəl\ *also* **elec•tro•phys•i•o•log•ic** \-jik\ *adj* — **elec•tro•phys•i•o•log•i•cal•ly** \-ji-k(ə-)lē\ *adv* — **elec•tro•phys•i•ol•o•gist** \-ˈä-lə-jist\ *n*

elec•tro•re•sec•tion \-rē-ˈsek-shən\ *n* : resection by electrosurgical means

elec•tro•ret•i•no•gram \-ˈret-ᵊn-ə-ˌgram\ *n* : a graphic record of electrical activity of the retina

elec•tro•ret•i•no•graph \-ˌgraf\ *n* : an instrument for recording electrical activity in the retina — **elec•tro•ret•i•no•graph•ic** \-ˌret-ᵊn-ə-ˈgra-fik\ *adj* — **elec•tro•ret•i•nog•ra•phy** \-ᵊn-ˈä-grə-fē\ *n*

elec•tro•shock \i-ˈlek-trō-ˌshäk\ *n* **1** : SHOCK 3 **2** : ELECTROCONVULSIVE THERAPY

electroshock therapy *n* : ELECTROCONVULSIVE THERAPY

elec•tro•sleep \-ˌslēp\ *n* : profound relaxation or a state of unconsciousness induced by the passage of a very low voltage electric current through the brain

elec•tro•stat•ic \i-ˌlek-trə-ˈsta-tik\ *adj* : of or relating to stationary electric charges or to the study of the forces of attraction and repulsion acting between such charges

elec•tro•stim•u•la•tion \i-ˌlek-trō-ˌstim-yə-ˈlā-shən\ *n* : shocks of electricity administered in nonconvulsive doses

elec•tro•sur•gery \-ˈsər-jə-rē\ *n, pl* **-ger•ies** : surgery by means of diathermy — **elec•tro•sur•gi•cal** \-ji-kəl\ *adj*

elec•tro•ther•a•py \-ˈther-ə-pē\ *n, pl* **-pies** : treatment of disease by means of electricity (as in diathermy)

elec•tro•tome \i-ˈlek-trə-ˌtōm\ *n* : an electric cutting instrument used in electrosurgery

elec•tro•ton•ic \i-ˌlek-trə-ˈtä-nik\ *adj* **1** : of, induced by, relating to, or constituting electrotonus ⟨the ~ condition of a nerve⟩ **2** : of, relating to, or being the spread of electrical activity through living tissue or cells in the absence of repeated action potentials — **elec•tro•ton•i•cal•ly** \-ni-k(ə-)lē\ *adv*

elec•trot•o•nus \i-ˌlek-ˈträt-ᵊn-əs\ *n* : the altered sensitivity of a nerve when a constant current of electricity passes through any part of it

elec•tu•ary \i-ˈlek-chə-ˌwer-ē\ *n, pl* **-ar•ies** : CONFECTION; *esp* : a medicated paste prepared with a sweet (as honey) and used in veterinary practice

el•e•doi•sin \ˌe-lə-ˈdȯis-ᵊn\ *n* : a small protein $C_{54}H_{85}N_{13}O_{15}S$ from the salivary glands of several octopuses (genus *Eledone*) that is a powerful vasodilator and hypotensive agent

el•e•ment \ˈe-lə-mənt\ *n* **1** : any of more than 100 fundamental substances that consist of atoms of only one kind and that singly or in combination constitute all matter **2** : one of the basic constituent units (as a cell or fiber) of a tissue

☞ The ELEMENT table is on page 234

el•e•men•tal \ˌe-lə-ˈment-ᵊl\ *adj* : of, relating to, or being an element; *specif* : existing as an uncombined chemical element

elementary body *n* : an infectious particle of any of several microorganisms; *esp* : a chlamydial cell of an extracellular infectious form that attaches to receptors on the membrane of the host cell and is taken up by endocytosis — compare RETICULATE BODY

elementary particle *n* : any of the subatomic units of matter and energy (as the electron, neutrino, proton, or photon) that do not appear to be made up of other smaller particles

el•e•phan•ti•a•sis \ˌe-lə-fən-ˈtī-ə-səs, -ˌfan-\ *n, pl* **-a•ses** \-ˌsēz\ : enlargement and thickening of tissues; *specif* : the enormous enlargement of a limb or the scrotum caused by obstruction of lymphatics by filarial worms of the genus *Wuchereria* (*W. bancrofti*) or a related genus (*Brugia malayi*)

el•e•trip•tan \ˌe-lə-ˈtrip-ˌtan\ *n* : a triptan taken orally in the form of its hydrobromide $C_{22}H_{26}N_2O_2S·HBr$ to treat migraine attacks — see RELPAX

el•e•vat•ed \ˈe-lə-ˌvā-təd\ *adj* : increased esp. abnormally ⟨an ~ pulse rate⟩ ⟨~ temperature⟩

el•e•va•tion \ˌe-lə-ˈvā-shən\ *n* **1** : a swelling esp. on the skin **2** : a usu. abnormal increase (as in degree or amount) ⟨an ~ of temperature⟩

el•e•va•tor \ˈe-lə-ˌvā-tər\ *n* **1** : a dental instrument that is used for removing teeth or the roots of teeth which cannot be gripped with a forceps **2** : a surgical instrument for raising a depressed part (as a bone) or for separating contiguous parts

eleventh cranial nerve *n* : ACCESSORY NERVE

El•i•gard \ˈel-ə-ˌgärd\ *trademark* — used for a preparation of the acetate of leuprolide

elim•i•nate \iˈli-mə-ˌnāt\ *vb* **-nat•ed; -nat•ing** : to expel (as waste) from the living body

elim•i•na•tion \i-ˌli-mə-ˈnā-shən\ *n* **1** : the act of discharging or excreting waste products or foreign substances from the body **2** **eliminations** *pl* : bodily discharges (as urine and feces)

El•i•quis \ˈe-lə-kwəs\ *trademark* — used for a preparation of apixaban

ELISA \ē-ˈlī-sə, -zə\ *n* : ENZYME-LINKED IMMUNOSORBENT ASSAY

elix•ir \i-ˈlik-sər\ *n* : a sweetened liquid usu. containing alcohol that is used in medication either for its medicinal ingredients or as a flavoring

CHEMICAL ELEMENTS

ELEMENT NAME	SYMBOL & ATOMIC NUMBER	ATOMIC WEIGHT[1]	ELEMENT NAME	SYMBOL & ATOMIC NUMBER	ATOMIC WEIGHT[1]
actinium	(Ac = 89)	227.0277	manganese	(Mn = 25)	54.93805
aluminum	(Al = 13)	26.98154	meitnerium	(Mt = 109)	(268)
americium	(Am = 95)	(243)	mendelevium	(Md = 101)	(258)
antimony	(Sb = 51)	121.760	mercury	(Hg = 80)	200.59
argon	(Ar = 18)	39.948	molybdenum	(Mo = 42)	95.94
arsenic	(As = 33)	74.92160	neodymium	(Nd = 60)	144.24
astatine	(At = 85)	(210)	neon	(Ne = 10)	20.180
barium	(Ba = 56)	137.33	neptunium	(Np = 93)	(237)
berkelium	(Bk = 97)	(247)	nickel	(Ni = 28)	58.6934
beryllium	(Be = 4)	9.012182	niobium	(Nb = 41)	92.90638
bismuth	(Bi = 83)	208.98038	nitrogen	(N = 7)	14.0067
bohrium	(Bh = 107)	(264)	nobelium	(No = 102)	(259)
boron	(B = 5)	10.81	osmium	(Os = 76)	190.23
bromine	(Br = 35)	79.904	oxygen	(O = 8)	15.9994
cadmium	(Cd = 48)	112.41	palladium	(Pd = 46)	106.42
calcium	(Ca = 20)	40.078	phosphorus	(P = 15)	30.973761
californium	(Cf = 98)	(251)	platinum	(Pt = 78)	195.078
carbon	(C = 6)	12.011	plutonium	(Pu = 94)	(244)
cerium	(Ce = 58)	140.116	polonium	(Po = 84)	(209)
cesium	(Cs = 55)	132.90545	potassium	(K = 19)	39.0983
chlorine	(Cl = 17)	35.453	praseodymium	(Pr = 59)	140.90765
chromium	(Cr = 24)	51.996	promethium	(Pm = 61)	(145)
cobalt	(Co = 27)	58.93320	protactinium	(Pa = 91)	(231)
copernicium	(Cn = 112)	(285)	radium	(Ra = 88)	(226)
copper	(Cu = 29)	63.546	radon	(Rn = 86)	(222)
curium	(Cm = 96)	(247)	rhenium	(Re = 75)	186.207
darmstadtium	(Ds = 110)	(269)	rhodium	(Rh = 45)	102.90550
dubnium	(Db = 105)	(262)	roentgenium	(Rg = 111)	(280)
dysprosium	(Dy = 66)	162.50	rubidium	(Rb = 37)	85.4678
einsteinium	(Es = 99)	(252)	ruthenium	(Ru = 44)	101.07
erbium	(Er = 68)	167.259	rutherfordium	(Rf = 104)	(261)
europium	(Eu = 63)	151.964	samarium	(Sm = 62)	150.36
fermium	(Fm = 100)	(257)	scandium	(Sc = 21)	44.95591
flerovium	(Fl = 114)	(289)	seaborgium	(Sg = 106)	(266)
fluorine	(F = 9)	18.998403	selenium	(Se = 34)	78.96
francium	(Fr = 87)	(223)	silicon	(Si = 14)	28.0855
gadolinium	(Gd = 64)	157.25	silver	(Ag = 47)	107.8682
gallium	(Ga = 31)	69.723	sodium	(Na = 11)	22.989770
germanium	(Ge = 32)	72.64	strontium	(Sr = 38)	87.62
gold	(Au = 79)	196.96655	sulfur	(S = 16)	32.07
hafnium	(Hf = 72)	178.49	tantalum	(Ta = 73)	180.9479
hassium	(Hs = 108)	(277)	technetium	(Tc = 43)	(98)
helium	(He = 2)	4.002602	tellurium	(Te = 52)	127.60
holmium	(Ho = 67)	164.93032	terbium	(Tb = 65)	158.92534
hydrogen	(H = 1)	1.0079	thallium	(Tl = 81)	204.3833
indium	(In = 49)	114.818	thorium	(Th = 90)	232.0381
iodine	(I = 53)	126.90447	thulium	(Tm = 69)	168.93421
iridium	(Ir = 77)	192.217	tin	(Sn = 50)	118.71
iron	(Fe = 26)	55.845	titanium	(Ti = 22)	47.867
krypton	(Kr = 36)	83.80	tungsten	(W = 74)	183.84
lanthanum	(La = 57)	138.9055	uranium	(U = 92)	(238)
lawrencium	(Lr = 103)	(262)	vanadium	(V = 23)	50.9415
lead	(Pb = 82)	207.2	xenon	(Xe = 54)	131.29
lithium	(Li = 3)	6.941	ytterbium	(Yb = 70)	173.04
livermorium	(Lv = 116)	(293)	yttrium	(Y = 39)	88.90585
lutetium	(Lu = 71)	174.967	zinc	(Zn = 30)	65.39
magnesium	(Mg = 12)	24.305	zirconium	(Zr = 40)	91.224

[1]Weights are based on the naturally occurring isotope compositions and scaled to $^{12}C = 12$. For elements lacking stable isotopes, the mass number of the most stable nuclide is shown in parentheses.

Eliz·a·be·than collar \i-ˌli-zə-ˈbē-thən-\ *n* : a typically cone-shaped device of stiff material (as plastic) placed about the neck of an animal and usu. a cat or dog to prevent it from licking, biting, or scratching a wound or injury or to stop obsessive licking or grooming — called also *e-collar*
el·lip·to·cyte \i-ˈlip-tə-ˌsīt\ *n* : an elliptical red blood cell
el·lip·to·cy·to·sis \i-ˌlip-tə-ˌsī-ˈtō-səs\ *n, pl* **-to·ses** \-ˌsēz\ : a human hereditary trait manifested by the presence in the blood of red blood cells which are oval in shape with rounded ends
El·o·con \ˈe-lə-ˌkän\ *trademark* — used for a topical preparation of mometasone
el·u·ant *or* **el·u·ent** \ˈel-yə-wənt\ *n* : a solvent used in eluting
el·u·ate \ˈel-yə-wət, -ˌwāt\ *n* : the washings obtained by eluting
elute \ē-ˈlüt\ *vb* **elut·ed; elut·ing** : to wash out or extract; *specif* : to remove (adsorbed material) from an adsorbent by means of a solvent
el·vi·teg·ra·vir \ˌel-ˌvī-ˈteg-rə-ˌvir\ *n* : an antiretroviral drug $C_{23}H_{23}ClFNO_5$ used in conjunction with ritonavir and a protease inhibitor in the treatment of HIV infection — see STRIBILD, VITEKTA
EM *abbr* **1** electromagnetic **2** electron microscope; electron microscopy **3** emergency medicine
ema·ci·ate \i-ˈmā-shē-ˌāt\ *vb* **-at·ed; -at·ing** **1** : to cause to lose flesh so as to become very thin **2** : to waste away physically — **ema·ci·a·tion** \-ˌmā-shē-ˈā-shən, -sē-\ *n*
emas·cu·late \i-ˈmas-kyə-ˌlāt\ *vb* **-lat·ed; -lat·ing** : to deprive of virility or procreative power : CASTRATE — **emas·cu·la·tion** \-ˌmas-kyə-ˈlā-shən\ *n*
em·balm \im-ˈbäm, -ˈbälm\ *vb* : to treat (a dead body) so as to protect from decay — **em·balm·er** *n*
em·bar·rass \im-ˈbar-əs\ *vb* : to impair the activity of (a bodily function) or the function of (a bodily part)
em·bar·rass·ment \im-ˈbar-əs-mənt\ *n* : difficulty in functioning as a result of disease <respiratory ~>
em·bed *also* **im·bed** \im-ˈbed\ *vb* **em·bed·ded** *also* **im·bed·ded; em·bed·ding** *also* **im·bed·ding** : to prepare (a microscopy specimen) for sectioning by infiltrating with and enclosing in a supporting substance — **em·bed·ment** \-ˈbed-mənt\ *n*
embol- *comb form* : embolus <*embolectomy*>
em·bo·lec·to·my \ˌem-bə-ˈlek-tə-mē\ *n, pl* **-mies** : surgical removal of an embolus
emboli *pl of* EMBOLUS
em·bol·ic \em-ˈbä-lik, im-\ *adj* : of or relating to an embolus or embolism
em·bo·lism \ˈem-bə-ˌli-zəm\ *n* **1** : the sudden obstruction of a blood vessel by an embolus **2** : EMBOLUS
em·bo·li·za·tion \ˌem-bə-lə-ˈzā-shən\ *n* **1** : the process by which or state in which a blood vessel or organ is obstructed by the lodgment of a material mass (as an embolus) <pulmonary ~> <~ of a thrombus> **2** : an operation in which pellets are introduced into the circulatory system in order to induce embolization in specific abnormal blood vessels
em·bo·lize \ˈem-bə-ˌlīz\ *vb* **-lized; -liz·ing** **1** *of an embolus* : to lodge in and obstruct (as a blood vessel or organ) **2** : to break up into emboli or become an embolus
em·bo·lo·ther·a·py \ˌem-bə-lō-ˈther-ə-pē\ *n* : the intentional blockage of an artery with an object (as a balloon inserted by a catheter) to control or prevent hemorrhaging
em·bo·lus \ˈem-bə-ləs\ *n, pl* **-li** \-ˌlī\ : an abnormal particle (as an air bubble) circulating in the blood — compare THROMBUS
em·bra·sure \im-ˈbrā-zhər\ *n* : the sloped valley between adjacent teeth
em·bro·ca·tion \ˌem-brə-ˈkā-shən\ *n* : LINIMENT
embry- *or* **embryo-** *comb form* : embryo <*embry*oma> <*embryo*genesis>
em·bryo \ˈem-brē-ˌō\ *n, pl* **em·bry·os** : an animal in the early stages of growth and differentiation that are characterized by cleavage, the laying down of fundamental tissues, and the formation of primitive organs and organ systems; *esp* : the developing human individual from the time of implantation to the end of the eighth week after conception — compare FETUS
em·bryo·gen·e·sis \ˌem-brē-ō-ˈje-nə-səs\ *n, pl* **-e·ses** \-ˌsēz\ : the formation and development of the embryo — **em·bryo·ge·net·ic** \-jə-ˈne-tik\ *adj*
em·bry·og·e·ny \ˌem-brē-ˈä-jə-nē\ *n, pl* **-nies** : EMBRYOGENESIS — **em·bryo·gen·ic** \-brē-ō-ˈje-nik\ *adj*
em·bry·ol·o·gist \ˌem-brē-ˈä-lə-jist\ *n* : a specialist in embryology
em·bry·ol·o·gy \-jē\ *n, pl* **-gies** **1** : a branch of biology dealing with embryos and their development **2** : the features and phenomena exhibited in the formation and development of an embryo — **em·bry·o·log·i·cal** \-brē-ə-ˈlä-ji-kəl\ *also* **em·bry·o·log·ic** \-jik\ *adj* — **em·bry·o·log·i·cal·ly** \-ji-k(ə-)lē\ *adv*
em·bry·o·ma \ˌem-brē-ˈō-mə\ *n, pl* **-mas** *also* **-ma·ta** \-mə-tə\ : a tumor derived from embryonic structures : TERATOMA
embryon- *or* **embryoni-** *comb form* : embryo <*embryon*ic>
em·bry·o·nal \em-ˈbrī-ən-ᵊl\ *adj* : EMBRYONIC 1
embryonal carcinoma *n* : a highly malignant cancer of the testis
em·bry·o·nate \ˈem-brē-ə-ˌnāt\ *vb* **-nat·ed; -nat·ing** *of an egg or zygote* : to produce or differentiate into an embryo

em·bry·o·nat·ed *adj* : having an embryo

em·bry·on·ic \ˌem-brē-ˈä-nik\ *adj* **1** : of or relating to an embryo **2** : being in an early stage of development — **em·bry·on·i·cal·ly** \-ni-k(ə-)lē\ *adv*

embryonic disk *or* **embryonic disc** *n* **1 a** : BLASTODISC **b** : BLASTODERM **2** : the part of the inner cell mass of a blastocyst from which the embryo of a placental mammal develops

embryonic membrane *n* : a structure (as the amnion) that derives from the fertilized ovum but does not form a part of the embryo

em·bry·op·a·thy \ˌem-brē-ˈä-pə-thē\ *n, pl* **-thies** : a developmental abnormality of an embryo or fetus esp. when caused by maternal disease or drug exposure ⟨diabetic ~⟩ ⟨warfarin ~⟩

em·bryo·tox·ic·i·ty \ˌem-brē-ō-ˌtäk-ˈsi-sə-tē\ *n, pl* **-ties** : the state of being toxic to embryos — **em·bryo·tox·ic** \-ˈtäk-sik\ *adj*

embryo transfer *n* : the final procedure of the in vitro fertilization process that involves transfer of one or more embryos into the uterine cavity typically by using a catheter inserted through the uterine cervix

Emend \i-ˈmend\ *trademark* — used for a preparation of aprepitant

emer·gence \i-ˈmər-jəns\ *n* : a recovering of consciousness (as from anesthesia)

emer·gen·cy \i-ˈmər-jən-sē\ *n, pl* **-cies** : an unforeseen combination of circumstances or the resulting state that calls for immediate action: as **a** : a sudden bodily alteration (as a ruptured appendix) such as is likely to require immediate medical attention **b** : a usu. distressing event or condition that can often be anticipated or prepared for but seldom exactly foreseen

emergency medical technician *n* : EMT

emergency medicine *n* : a medical specialty concerned with the care and treatment of acutely ill or injured patients who need immediate medical attention

emergency room *n* : a hospital room or area staffed and equipped for the reception and treatment of persons with conditions (as illness or trauma) requiring immediate medical care

emer·gent \i-ˈmər-jənt\ *adj* : calling for prompt or urgent action

eme·sis \ˈe-mə-səs, i-ˈmē-\ *n, pl* **eme·ses** \-ˌsēz\ : VOMITING

[1]**emet·ic** \i-ˈme-tik\ *n* : an agent that induces vomiting

[2]**emetic** *adj* : having the capacity to induce vomiting

em·e·tine \ˈe-mə-ˌtēn\ *n* : an amorphous alkaloid $C_{29}H_{40}N_2O_4$ extracted from ipecac root and used as an emetic and expectorant

em·e·to·gen·ic \ˌem-ə-tō-ˈjen-ik\ *adj* : causing nausea and vomiting : EMETIC

EMF *abbr* **1** electromagnetic field **2** electromotive force

EMG *abbr* electromyogram; electromyograph; electromyography

-emia \ˈē-mē-ə\ *or* **-he·mia** \ˈhē-\ *n comb form* **1** : condition of having (such) blood ⟨leuk*emia*⟩ ⟨septic*emia*⟩ **2** : condition of having (a specified thing) in the blood ⟨ur*emia*⟩

Em·i·nase \ˈe-mi-ˌnās, -ˌnāz\ *trademark* — used for a preparation of anistreplase

em·i·nence \ˈe-mə-nəns\ *n* : a protuberance or projection on a bodily part and esp. a bone

emissary vein *n* : any of the veins that pass through apertures in the skull and connect the venous sinuses of the dura mater with veins external to the skull

emis·sion \ē-ˈmi-shən\ *n* **1** : a discharge of fluid from a living body; *esp* : EJACULATE — see NOCTURNAL EMISSION **2** : substances and esp. pollutants discharged into the air (as by a smokestack or an automobile engine)

em·men·a·gogue \ə-ˈme-nə-ˌgäg, e-\ *n* : an agent that promotes the menstrual discharge

em·me·tro·pia \ˌe-mə-ˈtrō-pē-ə\ *n* : the normal refractive condition of the eye in which with accommodation relaxed parallel rays of light are all brought accurately to a focus upon the retina — compare ASTIGMATISM, MYOPIA — **em·me·trop·ic** \-ˈträ-pik, -ˈtrō-\ *adj*

[1]**emol·lient** \i-ˈmäl-yənt\ *adj* : making soft or supple; *also* : soothing esp. to the skin or mucous membrane

[2]**emollient** *n* : an emollient agent

emo·tion \i-ˈmō-shən\ *n* : a conscious mental reaction (as anger or fear) subjectively experienced as strong feeling usu. directed toward a specific object and typically accompanied by physiological and behavioral changes in the body — **emo·tion·al** \-shə-nəl\ *adj* — **emo·tion·al·i·ty** \-ˌmō-shə-ˈna-lə-tē\ *n* — **emo·tion·al·ly** *adv*

em·pa·thy \ˈem-pə-thē\ *n, pl* **-thies** : the action of understanding, being aware of, being sensitive to, and vicariously experiencing the feelings, thoughts, and experience of another of either the past or present without having the feelings, thoughts, and experience fully communicated in an objectively explicit manner; *also* : the capacity for empathy — **em·path·ic** \em-ˈpa-thik, im-\ *adj* — **em·path·i·cal·ly** *adv* — **em·pa·thize** \ˈem-pə-ˌthīz\ *vb*

em·phy·se·ma \ˌem-fə-ˈzē-mə, -ˈsē-\ *n* : a condition characterized by air-filled expansions like blisters in interstitial or subcutaneous tissues; *specif* : a condition of the lung that is marked by distension and eventual rupture of the alveoli with progressive loss of pulmonary elasticity, that is accompanied by shortness of breath with or without cough, and that may lead to impairment of heart action —

em·phy·se·ma·tous \-ˈze-mə-təs, -ˈse-, -ˈzē-, -ˈsē-\ *adj* — **em·phy·se·mic** \-ˈzē-mik, -ˈsē-\ *adj*

em·pir·ic \im-ˈpir-ik, em-\ *n* : EMPIRICIST

em·pir·i·cal \-i-kəl\ *or* **em·pir·ic** \-ik\ *adj* **1** : originating in or based on observation or experiment **2** : capable of being verified or disproved by observation or experiment ⟨~ laws⟩ — **em·pir·i·cal·ly** \-i-k(ə-)lē\ *adv*

empirical formula *n* : a chemical formula showing the simplest ratio of elements in a compound rather than the total number of atoms in the molecule ⟨CH_2O is the *empirical formula* for glucose⟩

em·pir·i·cism \im-ˈpir-ə-ˌsi-zəm, em-\ *n* **1 a** : a former school of medical practice founded on experience without the aid of science or theory **b** : QUACKERY **2** : the practice of relying on observation and experiment esp. in the natural sciences

em·pir·i·cist \-sist\ *n* : one who relies on observation and experiment

empty sella syndrome *n* : a condition in which the subarachnoid space extends into the sella turcica causing it to become filled with cerebrospinal fluid and the pituitary gland is compressed but usu. functions normally

em·py·ema \ˌem-ˌpī-ˈē-mə\ *n, pl* **-ema·ta** \-mə-tə\ *also* **-emas** : the presence of pus in a bodily cavity (as the pleural cavity) — called also *pyothorax* — **em·py·emic** \-mik\ *adj*

EMS *abbr* **1** emergency medical service; emergency medical services **2** eosinophilia-myalgia syndrome

EMT \ˌē-(ˌ)em-ˈtē\ *n* : a specially trained medical technician licensed to provide basic emergency services (as cardiopulmonary resuscitation) before and during transportation to a hospital — called also *emergency medical technician;* compare PARAMEDIC 2

em·tri·cit·a·bine \ˌem-trə-ˈsī-tə-ˌbēn\ *n* : a synthetic reverse transcriptase inhibitor $C_8H_{10}FN_3O_3S$ typically used with other antiretroviral agents to treat HIV infection — see ATRIPLA, COMPLERA, EMTRIVA, STRIBILD, TRUVADA

Em·tri·va \ˈem-trə-və\ *trademark* — used for a preparation of emtricitabine

emul·si·fi·er \i-ˈməl-sə-ˌfī-ər\ *n* : a surface-active agent (as a soap) promoting the formation and stabilization of an emulsion

emul·si·fy \-ˌfī\ *vb* **-fied; -fy·ing** : to disperse (as an oil) in an emulsion; *also* : to convert (two or more mutually insoluble liquids) into an emulsion — **emul·si·fi·ca·tion** \-ˌməl-sə-fə-ˈkā-shən\ *n*

emul·sion \i-ˈməl-shən\ *n* **1 a** : a mixture of mutually insoluble liquids in which one is dispersed throughout the other usu. in droplets of larger than colloidal size **b** : the state of such a mixture **2** : SUSPENSION 2

en·abler \i-ˈnā-b(ə-)lər\ *n* : one who enables another to persist in self-destructive behavior (as substance abuse) by providing excuses or by helping that individual avoid the consequences of such behavior

enal·a·pril \e-ˈna-lə-ˌpril\ *n* : an antihypertensive drug that is an ACE inhibitor administered orally in the form of its maleate $C_{20}H_{28}N_2O_5{\cdot}C_4H_4O_4$ — see VASOTEC

enal·a·pril·at \e-ˈna-lə-ˌpri-lət\ *n* : the metabolically active form $C_{18}H_{24}N_2O_5{\cdot}2H_2O$ of enalapril administered intravenously — see VASOTEC

enam·el \in-ˈa-məl\ *n* : the hard calcareous substance that forms a thin layer partly covering the teeth and consists of minute prisms secreted by ameloblasts, arranged at right angles to the surface, and bound together by a cement substance — compare CEMENTUM, DENTIN

enamel organ *n* : an ectodermal ingrowth from the dental lamina that encloses the anterior part of the developing dental papilla and the cells of the inner enamel layer adjacent to the papilla and differentiates into columnar ameloblasts which lay down the enamel rods of the tooth

enamel rod *n* : one of the elongated prismatic bodies making up the enamel of a tooth — called also *enamel prism*

enanthate — see TESTOSTERONE ENANTHATE

en·an·them \i-ˈnan-thəm\ *or* **en·an·the·ma** \ˌen-ˌan-ˈthē-mə\ *n, pl* **-thems** *or* **-the·ma·ta** \-mə-tə\ : an eruption on a mucous surface

en·an·tio·mer \i-ˈnan-tē-ə-mər\ *n* : either of a pair of chemical compounds whose molecular structures have a mirror-image relationship to each other — **en·an·tio·mer·ic** \-ˌnan-tē-ə-ˈmer-ik\ *adj* — **en·an·tio·mer·i·cal·ly** \-i-k(ə-)lē\ *adv*

en·an·tio·morph \i-ˈnan-tē-ə-ˌmȯrf\ *n* : ENANTIOMER

en·ar·thro·sis \ˌe-ˌnar-ˈthrō-səs\ *n, pl* **-thro·ses** \-ˌsēz\ : BALL-AND-SOCKET JOINT

En·brel \ˈen-ˌbrel\ *trademark* — used for a preparation of etanercept

en·cap·su·late \in-ˈkap-sə-ˌlāt\ *vb* **-lat·ed; -lat·ing** : to encase or become encased in or as if in a capsule — **en·cap·su·la·tion** \-ˌkap-sə-ˈlā-shən\ *n*

en·cap·su·lat·ed *adj* : surrounded by a gelatinous or membranous envelope

en·ceinte \äⁿ-ˈsant\ *adj* : PREGNANT

encephal- *or* **encephalo-** *comb form* **1** : brain ⟨*encephal*itis⟩ ⟨*encephalo*cele⟩ **2** : of, relating to, or affecting the brain and ⟨*encephalo*myelitis⟩

-encephali *pl of* -ENCEPHALUS

en·ceph·a·li·tis \in-ˌse-fə-ˈlī-təs\ *n, pl* **-lit·i·des** \-ˈli-tə-ˌdēz\ : inflammation of the brain that is caused esp. by infection with a virus (as herpes simplex or West Nile virus) and is characterized by mild to severe symptoms (as fever, headache, confusion, seizures, or coma) or may be asymptomatic — **en•ceph•a•lit•ic** \-ˈli-tik\ *adj*

encephalitis le•thar•gi•ca \-li-ˈthär-ji-kə, -le-\ *n* : epidemic virus encephalitis in which somnolence is marked

en•ceph•a•lit•o•gen \in-ˌse-fə-ˈli-tə-jən, -ˌjen\ *n* : an encephalitogenic agent (as a virus)

en•ceph•a•lit•o•gen•ic \in-ˌse-fə-ˌli-tə-ˈje-nik\ *adj* : tending to cause encephalitis ⟨an ∼ strain of a virus⟩

en•ceph•a•lo•cele \in-ˈse-fə-lō-ˌsēl\ *n* : hernia of the brain that is either congenital or due to trauma

en•ceph•a•lo•gram \in-ˈse-fə-lə-ˌgram\ *n* : an X-ray picture of the brain made by encephalography

en•ceph•a•lo•graph \-ˌgraf\ *n* **1** : ENCEPHALOGRAM **2** : ELECTROENCEPHALOGRAPH

en•ceph•a•log•ra•phy \in-ˌse-fə-ˈlä-grə-fē\ *n, pl* **-phies** : radiography of the brain after the cerebrospinal fluid has been replaced by a gas (as air) — **en•ceph•a•lo•graph•ic** \-lə-ˈgra-fik\ *adj* — **en•ceph•a•lo•graph•i•cal•ly** \-fi-k(ə)lē\ *adv*

en•ceph•a•lo•ma•la•cia \in-ˌse-fə-lō-mə-ˈlā-shē-ə, -shə\ *n* : softening of the brain due to degenerative changes in nervous tissue

en•ceph•a•lo•my•eli•tis \in-ˌse-fə-lō-ˌmī-ə-ˈlī-təs\ *n, pl* **-elit•i•des** \-ə-ˈli-tə-ˌdēz\ : concurrent inflammation of the brain and spinal cord — see ACUTE DISSEMINATED ENCEPHALOMYELITIS, ALLERGIC ENCEPHALOMYELITIS, EQUINE ENCEPHALOMYELITIS — **en•ceph•a•lo•my•elit•ic** \-ə-ˈli-tik\ *adj*

en•ceph•a•lo•my•elop•a•thy \-ˌmī-ə-ˈlä-pə-thē\ *n, pl* **-thies** : any disease that affects the brain and spinal cord

en•ceph•a•lo•myo•car•di•tis \-ˌmī-ə-kär-ˈdī-təs\ *n* : an acute febrile virus disease that is caused by a picornavirus (genus *Cardiovirus*) and is marked by degeneration and inflammation of skeletal and cardiac muscle and lesions of the central nervous system

en•ceph•a•lop•a•thy \in-ˌse-fə-ˈlä-pə-thē\ *n, pl* **-thies** : a disease of the brain; *esp* : one involving alterations of brain structure — **en•ceph•a•lo•path•ic** \-lə-ˈpa-thik\ *adj*

-en•ceph•a•lus \in-ˈse-fə-ləs\ *n comb form, pl* **-en•ceph•a•li** \-ˌlī, -ˌlē\ **1** : fetus having (such) a brain ⟨ini*encephalus*⟩ **2** : condition of having (such) a brain ⟨hydr*encephalus*⟩

-en•ceph•a•ly \in-ˈse-fə-lē\ *n comb form, pl* **-en•ceph•a•lies** \in-ˈse-fə-lēz\ : condition of having (such) a brain ⟨micr*encephaly*⟩

en•chon•dral \(ˌ)en-ˈkän-drəl, (ˌ)eŋ-\ *adj* : ENDOCHONDRAL

en•chon•dro•ma \ˌen-ˌkän-ˈdrō-mə, ˌeŋ-\ *n, pl* **-mas** *also* **-ma•ta** \-mə-tə\ : a tumor consisting of cartilaginous tissue; *esp* : one arising where cartilage does not normally exist

en•code \in-ˈkōd, en-\ *vb* : to specify the genetic code for

en•cop•re•sis \ˌen-ˌkä-ˈprē-səs, -kə-\ *n, pl* **-re•ses** \-ˌsēz\ : involuntary passage of feces

encounter group *n* : a usu. unstructured group that seeks to develop the capacity of the individual to express feelings and to form emotional ties by unrestrained confrontation of individuals — compare T-GROUP

encrustation *var of* INCRUSTATION

en•cyst \in-ˈsist, en-\ *vb* : to enclose in or become enclosed in a cyst ⟨an ∼*ed* tumor⟩ — **en•cyst•ment** *n*

end- *or* **endo-** *comb form* **1** : within : inside ⟨*end*aural⟩ ⟨*endo*skeleton⟩ **2** : taking in ⟨*endo*cytosis⟩

end•ar•ter•ec•to•my \ˌen-ˌdär-tə-ˈrek-tə-mē\ *n, pl* **-mies** : surgical removal of the inner layer of an artery when thickened and atheromatous or occluded (as by intimal plaques)

end•ar•te•ri•tis \ˌen-ˌdär-tə-ˈrī-təs\ *n* : inflammation of the intima of one or more arteries

endarteritis ob•lit•er•ans \-ə-ˈbli-tə-ˌranz, -rənz\ *n* : endarteritis in which the intimal tissue plugs the lumen of an affected artery — called also *obliterating endarteritis*

end artery *n* : a terminal artery (as a coronary artery) supplying all or most of the blood to a body part

end•au•ral \(ˌ)en-ˈdȯr-əl\ *adj* : performed or applied within the ear

end•brain \ˈend-ˌbrān\ *n* : TELENCEPHALON

end brush *n* : END PLATE

end bud *n* : TAIL BUD

end bulb *n* : a bulbous termination of a sensory nerve fiber (as in the skin)

end–di•a•stol•ic \ˌen-ˌdī-ə-ˈstä-lik\ *adj* : relating to or occurring in the moment immediately preceding contraction of the heart ⟨∼ pressure⟩

[1]**en•dem•ic** \en-ˈde-mik, in-\ *adj* : restricted or peculiar to a locality or region ⟨∼ diseases⟩ — compare EPIDEMIC 1, SPORADIC — **en•dem•i•cal•ly** \-mi-k(ə-)lē\ *adv*

[2]**endemic** *n* **1** : an endemic disease or an instance of its occurrence **2** : an endemic organism

en•de•mic•i•ty \ˌen-ˌde-ˈmi-sə-tē, -də-\ *n, pl* **-ties** : the quality or state of being endemic

endemic syphilis *n* : BEJEL

endemic typhus *n* : MURINE TYPHUS

en•de•mism \ˈen-də-ˌmi-zəm\ *n* : ENDEMICITY

end foot *n, pl* **end feet** : BOUTON

en•do \ˈen-(ˌ)dō\ *n* : ENDOMETRIOSIS

endo- — see END-

en•do•ab•dom•i•nal \ˌen-dō-ab-ˈdä-mən-ᵊl\ *adj* : relating to or occurring in the interior of the abdomen

en•do•an•eu•rys•mor•rha•phy \ˌen-dō-ˌan-yə-ˌriz-ˈmȯr-ə-fē\ *n, pl* **-phies** : a surgical treatment of aneurysm that

involves opening its sac and collapsing, folding, and suturing its walls
en·do·bron·chi·al \ˌen-dō-ˈbräŋ-kē-əl\ *adj* : located within a bronchus ⟨~ tumors⟩ — **en·do·bron·chi·al·ly** *adv*
en·do·car·di·al \-ˈkär-dē-əl\ *adj* **1** : situated within the heart **2** : of or relating to the endocardium ⟨~ biopsy⟩
endocardial fibroelastosis *n* : a condition usu. associated with congestive heart failure and enlargement of the heart that is characterized by conversion of the endocardium to fibroelastic tissue
en·do·car·di·tis \-ˌkär-ˈdī-təs\ *n* : inflammation of the lining of the heart and its valves
en·do·car·di·um \-ˈkär-dē-əm\ *n, pl* **-dia** \-dē-ə\ : a thin serous membrane lining the cavities of the heart
en·do·cer·vi·cal \ˈsər-vi-kəl\ *adj* : of, relating to, or affecting the endocervix
en·do·cer·vi·ci·tis \-ˌsər-və-ˈsī-təs\ *n* : inflammation of the lining of the uterine cervix
en·do·cer·vix \-ˈsər-viks\ *n, pl* **-vi·ces** \-və-ˌsēz\ : the epithelial and glandular lining of the uterine cervix
en·do·chon·dral \ˌen-də-ˈkän-drəl\ *adj* : relating to, formed by, or being ossification that takes place from centers arising in cartilage and involves deposition of lime salts in the cartilage matrix followed by secondary absorption and replacement by true bony tissue
¹**en·do·crine** \ˈen-də-krən, -ˌkrīn, -ˌkrēn\ *adj* **1** : secreting internally; *specif* : producing secretions that are distributed in the body by way of the bloodstream **2** : of, relating to, affecting, or resembling an endocrine gland or secretion
²**endocrine** *n* **1** : HORMONE **2** : ENDOCRINE GLAND
endocrine gland *n* : a gland (as the thyroid or the pituitary) that produces an endocrine secretion — called also *ductless gland, gland of internal secretion*
endocrine system *n* : the glands and parts of glands that produce endocrine secretions, help to integrate and control bodily metabolic activity, and include esp. the pituitary, thyroid, parathyroids, adrenals, islets of Langerhans, ovaries, and testes
endocrine therapy *n* : HORMONE THERAPY b
en·do·cri·no·log·ic \ˌen-də-ˌkrin-ᵊl-ˈä-jik, -ˌkrīn-, -ˌkrēn-\ *or* **en·do·cri·no·log·i·cal** \-ji-kəl\ *adj* : involving or relating to the endocrine glands or secretions or to endocrinology
en·do·cri·nol·o·gy \ˌen-də-kri-ˈnä-lə-jē, -ˌkrī-\ *n, pl* **-gies** : a science dealing with the endocrine glands — **en·do·cri·nol·o·gist** \-jist\ *n*
en·do·cri·nop·a·thy \-krə-ˈnä-pə-thē, -ˌkrī-, -ˌkrē-\ *n, pl* **-thies** : a disease marked by dysfunction of an endocrine gland — **en·do·crin·o·path·ic** \-ˌkri-nə-ˈpa-thik, -ˌkrī-, -ˌkrē-\ *adj*
en·do·cyt·ic \-ˈsi-tik\ *adj* : of or relating to endocytosis : ENDOCYTOTIC
en·do·cy·to·sis \-sī-ˈtō-səs\ *n, pl* **-to·ses** \-ˌsēz\ : incorporation of substances into a cell by phagocytosis or pinocytosis — **en·do·cy·tose** \-ˈsī-ˌtōs, -ˌtōz\ *vb* — **en·do·cy·tot·ic** \-sī-ˈtä-tik\ *adj*
en·do·derm \ˈen-də-ˌdərm\ *n* : the innermost of the three primary germ layers of an embryo that is the source of the epithelium of the digestive tract and its derivatives and of the lower respiratory tract; *also* : a tissue that is derived from this germ layer — **en·do·der·mal** \ˌen-də-ˈdər-məl\ *adj*
end·odon·tia \ˌen-də-ˈdän-chē-ə, -chə\ *n* : ENDODONTICS
end·odon·tics \-ˈdän-tiks\ *n* : a branch of dentistry concerned with diseases of the pulp — **end·odon·tic** \-tik\ *adj* — **end·odon·ti·cal·ly** \-ti-k(ə-)lē\ *adv*
end·odon·tist \-tist\ *n* : a specialist in endodontics
en·do·en·zyme \ˌen-dō-ˈen-ˌzīm\ *n* : an enzyme that functions inside the cell — compare EXOENZYME
en·dog·e·nous \en-ˈdä-jə-nəs\ *also* **en·do·gen·ic** \ˌen-də-ˈje-nik\ *adj* **1** : caused by factors within the body or mind or arising from internal structural or functional causes ⟨~ malnutrition⟩ ⟨~ depression⟩ **2** : relating to or produced by metabolic synthesis in the body ⟨~ opioids⟩ — compare EXOGENOUS — **en·dog·e·nous·ly** *adv*
en·do·lymph \ˈen-də-ˌlimf\ *n* : the watery fluid in the membranous labyrinth of the ear — **en·do·lym·phat·ic** \ˌen-də-lim-ˈfa-tik\ *adj*
en·do·me·ninx \ˌen-də-ˈmē-nis, -ˈme-\ *n, pl* **-nin·ges** \-mə-ˈnin-(ˌ)jēz\ : the layer of embryonic mesoderm from which the arachnoid coat and pia mater of the brain develop
en·do·me·tri·al \ˌen-də-ˈmē-trē-əl\ *adj* : of, belonging to, or consisting of endometrium
en·do·me·tri·o·ma \-ˌmē-trē-ˈō-mə\ *n, pl* **-mas** *also* **-ma·ta** \-mə-tə\ **1** : a tumor containing endometrial tissue **2** : ENDOMETRIOSIS — used chiefly of isolated foci of endometrium outside the uterus
en·do·me·tri·osis \ˌen-dō-ˌmē-trē-ˈō-səs\ *n, pl* **-oses** \-ˌsēz\ : the presence and growth of functioning endometrial tissue in places other than the uterus that often results in severe pain and infertility — see ADENOMYOSIS — **en·do·me·tri·ot·ic** \-ˈä-tik\ *adj*
en·do·me·tri·tis \-mə-ˈtrī-təs\ *n* : inflammation of the endometrium
en·do·me·tri·um \-ˈmē-trē-əm\ *n, pl* **-tria** \-trē-ə\ : the mucous membrane lining the uterus
en·do·morph \ˈen-də-ˌmȯrf\ *n* : an endomorphic individual
en·do·mor·phic \ˌen-də-ˈmȯr-fik\ *adj* : having a heavy rounded body build often with a marked tendency

to become overweight — compare ECTOMORPHIC, MESOMORPHIC — **en·do·mor·phy** \ˈen-də-ˌmȯr-fē\ *n*

en·do·myo·car·di·al \ˌen-dō-ˌmī-ə-ˈkär-dē-əl\ *adj* : of, relating to, or affecting the endocardium and the myocardium ⟨~ fibrosis⟩ — **en·do·myo·car·di·um** \-dē-əm\ *n*

en·do·my·si·um \ˌen-də-ˈmi-zē-əm, -zhē-əm, -zhəm\ *n, pl* **-sia** \-zē-ə, -zhē-ə, -zhə\ : the delicate connective tissue surrounding the individual muscular fibers — compare EPIMYSIUM — **en·do·my·si·al** \-zē-əl, -zhē-əl, -zhəl\ *adj*

en·do·neu·ri·um \ˌen-dō-ˈnu̇r-ē-əm, -ˈnyu̇r-\ *n, pl* **-ria** \-ē-ə\ : the delicate connective tissue network holding together the individual fibers of a nerve trunk — **en·do·neu·ri·al** \-ē-əl\ *adj*

en·do·nu·cle·ase \-ˈnü-klē-ˌās, -ˈnyü-, -ˌāz\ *n* : an enzyme that breaks down a nucleotide chain into two or more shorter chains by breaking the internal phosphodiester bonds — compare EXONUCLEASE

en·do·nu·cleo·lyt·ic \-ˌnü-klē-ō-ˈli-tik, -ˌnyü-\ *adj* : breaking a nucleotide chain into two parts at an internal point ⟨~ nicks⟩

en·do·par·a·site \-ˈpar-ə-ˌsīt\ *n* : a parasite that lives in the internal organs or tissues of its host — compare ECTOPARASITE — **en·do·par·a·sit·ic** \-ˌpar-ə-ˈsi-tik\ *adj* — **en·do·par·a·sit·ism** \-ˈpar-ə-ˌsī-ˌti-zəm, -sə-\ *n*

en·do·pep·ti·dase \-ˈpep-tə-ˌdās, -ˌdāz\ *n* : any of a group of enzymes that hydrolyze peptide bonds within the long chains of protein molecules : PROTEASE — compare EXOPEPTIDASE

en·do·per·ox·ide \-pə-ˈräk-ˌsīd\ *n* : any of various biosynthetic intermediates in the formation of prostaglandins

en·do·phle·bi·tis \ˌen-dō-fli-ˈbī-təs\ *n, pl* **-bi·tis·es** *or* **-bit·i·des** \-ˈbi-tə-ˌdēz\ : inflammation of the intima of a vein

en·doph·thal·mi·tis \ˌen-ˌdäf-thal-ˈmī-təs\ *n* : inflammation that affects the interior of the eyeball

en·do·phyt·ic \ˌen-dō-ˈfi-tik\ *adj* : tending to grow inward into tissues in fingerlike projections from a superficial site of origin — used of tumors; compare EXOPHYTIC

en·do·plasm \ˈen-də-ˌpla-zəm\ *n* : the inner relatively fluid part of the cytoplasm — compare ECTOPLASM — **en·do·plas·mic** \ˌen-də-ˈplaz-mik\ *adj*

endoplasmic reticulum *n* : a system of interconnected vesicular and lamellar cytoplasmic membranes that functions esp. in the transport of materials within the cell and that is studded with ribosomes in some places

en·do·pros·the·sis \ˌen-dō-präs-ˈthē-səs\ *n, pl* **-the·ses** \-ˌsēz\ : an artificial device to replace a missing bodily part that is placed inside the body

end organ *n* : a structure forming the peripheral end of a path of nerve conduction and consisting of an effector or a receptor with its associated nerve terminations

en·dor·phin \en-ˈdȯr-fən\ *n* : any of a group of endogenous peptides (as enkephalin and dynorphin) that are found esp. in the brain and produce some of the same effects (as pain relief) as those of opiates; *specif* : BETA-ENDORPHIN

β–endorphin *var of* BETA-ENDORPHIN

en·do·scope \ˈen-də-ˌskōp\ *n* : an illuminated usu. fiber-optic flexible or rigid tubular instrument for visualizing the interior of a hollow organ (as the bladder or esophagus) and that typically has one or more channels to enable passage of instruments (as forceps or scissors) — **en·dos·co·py** \en-ˈdäs-kə-pē\ *n*

en·do·scop·ic \ˌen-də-ˈskä-pik\ *adj* : of, relating to, or performed by means of an endoscope or endoscopy — **en·do·scop·i·cal·ly** \-pi-k(ə-)lē\ *adv*

endoscopic retrograde chol·an·gio·pan·cre·atog·ra·phy \-kə-ˌlan-jē-ə-ˌpaŋ-krē-ə-ˈtäg-rə-fē\ *n* : radiographic visualization of the pancreatic and biliary ducts by means of endoscopic injection of a contrast medium through the ampulla of Vater — abbr. *ERCP*

en·dos·co·pist \en-ˈdäs-kə-pist\ *n* : a person trained in the use of the endoscope

en·do·skel·e·ton \ˌen-dō-ˈskel-ət-ᵊn\ *n* : an internal skeleton or supporting framework in an animal — **en·do·skel·e·tal** \-ət-ᵊl\ *adj*

en·do·spore \-ˌspōr\ *n* : an asexual spore developed within the cell esp. in bacteria

en·do·stat·in \ˌen-də-ˈsta-tᵊn\ *n* : a polypeptide that is found esp. in epithelial basement membrane and inhibits angiogenesis, tumor growth, and endothelial cell proliferation

end·os·te·al \en-ˈdäs-tē-əl\ *adj* **1** : of or relating to the endosteum **2** : located within bone or cartilage — **end·os·te·al·ly** *adv*

end·os·te·um \en-ˈdäs-tē-əm\ *n, pl* **-tea** \-ə\ : the layer of vascular connective tissue lining the medullary cavities of bone

endotheli- *or* **endothelio-** *comb form* : endothelium ⟨*endothelio*ma⟩

en·do·the·li·al \ˌen-də-ˈthē-lē-əl\ *adj* : of, relating to, or produced from endothelium

en·do·the·lin \ˌen-dō-ˈthē-lin\ *n* : any of several polypeptides that play a role in regulating vasomotor activity, cell proliferation, and the production of hormones, and that have been implicated in the development of vascular disease

en·do·the·li·o·ma \-ˌthē-lē-ˈō-mə\ *n, pl* **-mas** *also* **-ma·ta** \-mə-tə\ : a tumor developing from endothelial tissue

en·do·the·li·um \ˌen-də-ˈthē-lē-əm\ *n, pl* **-lia** \-ə\ : an epithelium of mesoblastic origin composed of a single layer of thin flattened cells that lines internal body cavities (as the serous cavities or the interior of the heart)

en•do•tox•emia \ˌen-dō-täk-ˈsē-mē-ə\ *n* : the presence of endotoxins in the blood

en•do•tox•in \ˌen-dō-ˈtäk-sən\ *n* : a toxin of internal origin; *specif* : a poisonous substance present in bacteria but separable from the cell body only on its disintegration — compare EXOTOXIN — **en•do•tox•ic** \-sik\ *adj*

en•do•tra•che•al \-ˈtrā-kē-əl\ *adj* **1** : placed within the trachea **2** : applied or effected through the trachea ⟨~ anesthesia⟩ ⟨~ intubation⟩

endotracheal tube *n* : a small usu. plastic tube inserted into the trachea through the mouth or nose to maintain an unobstructed passageway esp. to deliver oxygen or anesthesia to the lungs — called also *breathing tube*

end plate *n* : a complex terminal arborization of the axon of a motor neuron that contacts with a muscle fiber — called also *end brush*

end–stage \ˈend-ˌstāj\ *adj* : being or occurring in the final stages of a terminal disease or condition ⟨~ liver failure⟩

end–stage renal disease *n* : the final stage of kidney failure that is marked by the complete or nearly complete irreversible loss of renal function — called also *end-stage kidney disease, end-stage kidney failure, end-stage renal failure*

end–tid•al \ˈend-ˌtī-dᵊl\ *adj* : of or relating to the last portion of expired tidal air ⟨~ carbon dioxide concentrations⟩

en•e•ma \ˈe-nə-mə\ *n, pl* **enemas** *also* **ene•ma•ta** \ˌe-nə-ˈmä-tə, ˈe-nə-mə-tə\ : the injection of liquid into the rectum and colon by way of the anus (as for cleansing); *also* : the liquid so injected

en•er•get•ics \-tiks\ *n* : the total energy relations and transformations of a physical, chemical, or biological system

en•er•giz•er \ˈe-nər-ˌjī-zər\ *n* : ANTIDEPRESSANT

en•er•gy \ˈe-nər-jē\ *n, pl* **-gies** **1** : PSYCHIC ENERGY **2** : the capacity for doing work

en•er•vate \ˈe-nər-ˌvāt\ *vb* **-vat•ed; -vat•ing** : to lessen the vitality or strength of — **en•er•va•tion** \ˌe-nər-ˈvā-shən\ *n*

en•flur•ane \en-ˈflu̇r-ˌān\ *n* : a liquid inhalational general anesthetic $C_3H_2ClF_5O$ prepared from methanol

en•gage•ment \in-ˈgāj-mənt\ *n* : the phase of childbirth in which the fetal head passes into the cavity of the true pelvis

en•gi•neer \ˌen-jə-ˈnir\ *vb* : to modify or produce by genetic engineering

en•gorge \in-ˈgȯrj\ *vb* **en•gorged; en•gorg•ing** **1** : to fill with blood to the point of congestion ⟨the gastric mucosa was greatly *engorged*⟩ **2** : to suck blood to the limit of body capacity ⟨a tick *engorging* on its host⟩ — **en•gorge•ment** *n*

en•graft \in-ˈgraft\ *vb* : GRAFT — **en•graft•ment** *n*

en•gram *also* **en•gramme** \ˈen-ˌgram\ *n* : a hypothetical change in neural tissue postulated in order to account for persistence of memory : MEMORY TRACE

en•hanc•er \in-ˈhan-sər, en-\ *n* : a nucleotide sequence that increases the rate of genetic transcription by increasing the activity of the nearest promoter on the same DNA molecule

en•keph•a•lin \in-ˈke-fə-lən, -(ˌ)lin\ *n* : either of two pentapeptide endorphins: **a** : LEUCINE-ENKEPHALIN **b** : METHIONINE-ENKEPHALIN

en•keph•a•lin•er•gic \-ˌke-fə-lə-ˈnər-jik\ *adj* : liberating or activated by enkephalins ⟨~ neurons⟩

eno•lase \ˈē-nə-ˌlās, -ˌlāz\ *n* : an enzyme that is found esp. in muscle and is important in the metabolism of carbohydrates

en•oph•thal•mos \ˌe-ˌnäf-ˈthal-məs, -ˌnäp-, -ˌmäs\ *also* **en•oph•thal•mus** \-məs\ *n* : a sinking of the eyeball into the orbital cavity

en•os•to•sis \ˌe-ˌnäs-ˈtō-səs\ *n, pl* **-to•ses** \-ˌsēz\ : a bony tumor arising within a bone

Eno•vid \e-ˈnō-vid\ *n* : a preparation of norethynodrel and mestranol — formerly a U.S. registered trademark

enox•a•par•in \i-ˌnäk-sə-ˈper-ən\ *n* : heparin of low molecular weight that is administered in the form of its sodium salt by subcutaneous injection esp. to treat deep vein thrombosis and pulmonary embolism — see LOVENOX

en•sheathe \in-ˈshēth\ *vb* : to cover with or as if with a sheath

ensiform cartilage *n* : XIPHOID PROCESS

ensiform process *n* : XIPHOID PROCESS

ENT \ˌē-ˌen-ˈtē\ *n* : OTOLARYNGOLOGIST

ENT *abbr* ear, nose, and throat

ent- *or* **ento-** *comb form* : inner : within ⟨*ent*optic⟩ ⟨*ento*derm⟩

en•tac•a•pone \en-ˈtak-ə-ˌpōn\ *n* : a drug $C_{14}H_{15}N_3O_5$ that inhibits the breakdown of L-dopa and is used in conjunction with L-dopa and carbidopa in the treatment of Parkinson's disease — see COMTAN, STALEVO

ent•am•e•bi•a•sis *or* **ent•am•oe•bi•a•sis** \ˌen-ˌta-mi-ˈbī-ə-səs\ *n, pl* **-a•ses** \-ˌsēz\ : infection with or disease caused by an entamoeba

ent•amoe•ba \ˌen-tə-ˈmē-bə\ *n* **1** *cap* : a genus of amoeboid protozoans (order Amoebida) that are parasitic in the vertebrate digestive tract and esp. in the intestines and that include the causative agent (*E. histolytica*) of amebic dysentery **2** *also* **ent•ame•ba** *pl* **-bas** *or* **-bae** \-bē\ : any protozoan of the genus *Entamoeba* — **ent•amoe•bic** *also* **ent•ame•bic** \-bik\ *adj*

enter- *or* **entero-** *comb form* **1** : intestine ⟨*enter*itis⟩ **2** : intestinal and ⟨*entero*hepatic⟩

en·ter·al \ˈen-tə-rəl\ *adj* : ENTERIC — **en·ter·al·ly** *adv*

en·ter·ec·to·my \ˌen-tə-ˈrek-tə-mē\ *n, pl* **-mies** : the surgical removal of a portion of the intestine

en·ter·ic \en-ˈter-ik, in-\ *adj* **1** : of, relating to, or affecting the intestines ⟨~ diseases⟩; *broadly* : ALIMENTARY **2** : being or possessing a coating designed to pass through the stomach unaltered and disintegrate in the intestines ⟨~ aspirin⟩

enteric fever *n* : TYPHOID FEVER; *also* : PARATYPHOID

entericus — see SUCCUS ENTERICUS

en·ter·i·tis \ˌen-tə-ˈrī-təs\ *n, pl* **en·ter·it·i·des** \-ˈri-tə-ˌdēz\ *or* **en·ter·i·tis·es** **1** : inflammation of the intestines and esp. of the human ileum **2** : a disease of domestic animals (as panleukopenia of cats) marked by enteritis and diarrhea

En·tero·bac·ter \ˈen-tə-rō-ˌbak-tər\ *n* : a genus of enterobacteria that are widely distributed in nature (as in feces, soil, or water) and include some that may be pathogenic

en·tero·bac·te·ri·um \ˌen-tə-rō-bak-ˈtir-ē-əm\ *n, pl* **-ria** \-ē-ə\ : any of a family (Enterobacteriaceae) of gram-negative rod-shaped bacteria (as E. coli or salmonella) that ferment glucose and include some serious pathogens — **en·tero·bac·te·ri·al** \-ē-əl\ *adj*

en·tero·bi·a·sis \-ˈbī-ə-səs\ *n, pl* **-a·ses** \-ˌsēz\ : infestation with or disease caused by pinworms of the genus *Enterobius* that occurs esp. in children

En·te·ro·bi·us \ˌen-tə-ˈrō-bē-əs\ *n* : a genus of small nematode worms (family Oxyuridae) that includes the common pinworm (*E. vermicularis*) of the human intestine

en·ter·o·cele \ˈen-tə-rō-ˌsēl\ *n* : a hernia containing a portion of the intestines

en·tero·chro·maf·fin \ˌen-tə-rō-ˈkrō-mə-fən\ *adj* : of, relating to, or being epithelial cells of the intestinal mucosa that stain esp. with chromium salts and usu. contain serotonin

en·tero·coc·cus \ˌen-tə-rō-ˈkä-kəs\ *n* **1** *cap* : a genus of gram-positive bacteria that resemble streptococci and were formerly classified with them **2** *pl* **-coc·ci** \-ˈkäk-ˌsī, -ˌsē; -ˈkä-ˌkī, -ˌkē\ : any bacterium of the genus *Enterococcus; esp* : one (*E. faecalis*) normally present in the intestine — **en·tero·coc·cal** \-ˈkä-kəl\ *adj*

en·tero·co·li·tis \ˌen-tə-rō-kə-ˈlī-təs\ *n* : enteritis affecting both the large and small intestine

en·tero·en·te·ros·to·my \-ˌen-tə-ˈräs-tə-mē\ *n, pl* **-mies** : surgical anastomosis of two parts of the intestine with creation of an opening between them

en·tero·gas·tric reflex \-ˌgas-trik-\ *n* : reflex inhibition of the emptying of the stomach's contents through the pylorus that occurs when the duodenum is stimulated by the presence of irritants, is overloaded, or is obstructed

en·tero·gas·trone \-ˈgas-ˌtrōn\ *n* : a hormone that is produced by the duodenal mucosa and inhibits gastric motility and secretion

en·tero·he·pat·ic \-hi-ˈpa-tik\ *adj* : of or involving the intestine and the liver

en·tero·hep·a·ti·tis \-ˌhe-pə-ˈtī-təs\ *n* : BLACKHEAD 2

en·tero·ki·nase \-ˈkī-ˌnās, -ˌnāz\ *n* : an enzyme that activates trypsinogen by converting it to trypsin

en·ter·o·lith \ˈen-tə-rō-ˌlith\ *n* : a calculus occurring in the intestine

enteropathica — see ACRODERMATITIS ENTEROPATHICA

en·tero·patho·gen·ic \ˌen-tə-rō-ˌpa-thə-ˈje-nik\ *adj* : tending to produce disease in the intestinal tract ⟨~ bacteria⟩ — **en·tero·patho·gen** \-ˈpa-thə-jən\ *n*

en·ter·op·a·thy \ˌen-tə-ˈrä-pə-thē\ *n, pl* **-thies** : a disease of the intestinal tract

en·ter·os·to·my \ˌen-tə-ˈräs-tə-mē\ *n, pl* **-mies** : a surgical formation of an opening into the intestine through the abdominal wall — **en·ter·os·to·mal** \-tə-məl\ *adj*

en·te·rot·o·my \ˌen-tə-ˈrä-tə-mē\ *n, pl* **-mies** : incision into the intestines

en·tero·tox·emia \ˌen-tə-rō-ˌtäk-ˈsē-mē-ə\ *n* : a disease (as pulpy kidney disease of lambs) attributed to absorption of a toxin from the intestine — called also *overeating disease*

en·tero·toxi·gen·ic \-ˌtäk-sə-ˈje-nik\ *adj* : producing enterotoxin

en·tero·tox·in \-ˈtäk-sən\ *n* : a toxin that is produced by microorganisms (as some staphylococci) and causes gastrointestinal symptoms

en·tero·vi·rus \-ˈvī-rəs\ *n* **1** *cap* : a genus of picornaviruses that typically occur in the gastrointestinal tract but may infect other tissues (as nerve and muscle) and that include the polioviruses, Coxsackieviruses, and echoviruses **2** : any virus of the genus *Enterovirus* — **en·tero·vi·ral** \-rəl\ *adj*

ento- — see ENT-

En·to·cort \ˈen-tō-ˌkȯrt\ *trademark* — used for a preparation of budesonide taken by mouth

en·to·derm \ˈen-tə-ˌdərm\ *n* : ENDODERM

en·to·mo·pho·bia \ˌen-tə-mō-ˈfō-bē-ə\ *n* : fear of insects

ent·op·tic \(ˌ)en-ˈtäp-tik\ *adj* : lying or originating within the eyeball — used esp. of visual sensations due to the shadows of retinal blood vessels or of opaque particles in the vitreous body falling upon the retina

en·to·rhi·nal \ˌen-tə-ˈrī-nᵊl\ *adj* : of, relating to, or being the part of the cerebral cortex in the medial temporal lobe that serves as the main cortical input to the hippocampus

en·trap·ment \in-ˈtrap-mənt\ *n* : chronic compression of a peripheral nerve (as the median nerve or ulnar nerve) usu. between ligamentous and bony surfaces that is marked by pain, numbness, tingling, or weakness

en·tro·pi·on \en-ˈtrō-pē-ˌän, -ən\ *n* : the inversion or turning inward of the border of the eyelid against the eyeball

[1]**enu·cle·ate** \(ˌ)ē-ˈnü-klē-ˌāt, -ˈnyü-\ *vb* **-at·ed; -at·ing 1** : to deprive of a nucleus **2** : to remove without cutting into ⟨~ the eyeball⟩ — **enu·cle·ation** \(ˌ)ē-ˌnü-klē-ˈā-shən, -ˌnyü-\ *n*

[2]**enu·cle·ate** \-klē-ət, -ˌāt\ *adj* : lacking a nucleus ⟨~ cells⟩

en·ure·sis \ˌen-yu̇-ˈrē-səs\ *n, pl* **-ure·ses** \-ˌsēz\ : an involuntary discharge of urine : incontinence of urine — **en·uret·ic** \-ˈre-tik\ *adj or n*

en·ve·lope \ˈen-və-ˌlōp, ˈän-\ *n* : a natural enclosing covering (as a membrane or integument)

en·ven·om·ation \in-ˌve-nə-ˈmā-shən\ *n* : an act or instance of impregnating with a venom (as of a snake or spider); *also* : ENVENOMIZATION — **en·ven·om·ate** \-ˈve-nə-ˌmāt\ *vb*

en·ven·om·iza·tion \-mə-ˈzā-shən\ *n* : a poisoning caused by a bite or sting

en·vi·ron·ment \in-ˈvī-rən-mənt, -ˈvī-ərn-\ *n* **1** : the complex of physical, chemical, and biotic factors (as climate, soil, and living things) that act upon an organism or an ecological community and ultimately determine its form and survival **2** : the aggregate of social and cultural conditions that influence the life of an individual or community — **en·vi·ron·men·tal** \-ˌvī-rən-ˈment-ᵊl, -ˌvī-ərn-\ *adj* — **en·vi·ron·men·tal·ly** *adv*

[1]**en·zo·ot·ic** \ˌen-zə-ˈwä-tik\ *adj, of animal diseases* : peculiar to or constantly present in a locality — **en·zo·ot·i·cal·ly** \-ti-k(ə-)lē\ *adv*

[2]**enzootic** *n* : an enzootic disease

en·zy·mat·ic \ˌen-zə-ˈma-tik\ *also* **en·zy·mic** \en-ˈzī-mik\ *adj* : of, relating to, or produced by an enzyme — **en·zy·mat·i·cal·ly** \-ti-k(ə-)lē\ *also* **en·zy·mi·cal·ly** \en-ˈzī-mi-k(ə-)lē\ *adv*

en·zyme \ˈen-ˌzīm\ *n* : any of numerous complex proteins that are produced by living cells and catalyze specific biochemical reactions at body temperatures

enzyme immunoassay *n* : an immunoassay (as an enzyme-linked immunosorbent assay) in which an enzyme bound to an antigen or antibody functions as a label — abbr. *EIA*

enzyme–linked immunosorbent assay *n* : a quantitative in vitro test for an antibody or antigen in which the test material is adsorbed on a surface and exposed to a complex of an enzyme linked to an antibody specific for the antigen or an enzyme linked to an anti-immunoglobulin specific for the antibody followed by reaction of the enzyme with a substrate to yield a colored product corresponding to the concentration of the test material — called also *ELISA*

en·zy·mol·o·gy \ˌen-ˌzī-ˈmä-lə-jē, -zə-\ *n, pl* **-gies** : a branch of biochemistry dealing with enzymes, their nature, activity, and significance — **en·zy·mo·log·i·cal** \-mə-ˈlä-ji-kəl\ *adj* — **en·zy·mol·o·gist** \ˌen-ˌzī-ˈmä-lə-jist\ *n*

EOG *abbr* electrooculogram

EOM *abbr* **1** external oblique muscle **2** external otitis media **3** extraocular movement; extraocular muscle

eon·ism \ˈē-ə-ˌni-zəm\ *n* : TRANSVESTISM

Éon de Beau·mont \ā-ō^{n}-də-bō-mō^{n}\, **Charles (1728–1810),** French chevalier and adventurer.

eo·sin \ˈē-ə-sən\ *also* **eo·sine** \-sən, -ˌsēn\ *n* : a red fluorescent dye $C_{20}H_8Br_4O_5$; *also* : its red to brown sodium or potassium salt used esp. as a biological stain

eo·sin·o·pe·nia \ˌē-ə-ˌsi-nə-ˈpē-nē-ə, -nyə\ *n* : an abnormal decrease in the number of eosinophils in the blood — **eo·sin·o·pe·nic** \-ˈpē-nik\ *adj*

[1]**eo·sin·o·phil** \ˌē-ə-ˈsi-nə-ˌfil\ *also* **eo·sin·o·phile** \-ˌfīl\ *adj* : EOSINOPHILIC 1

[2]**eosinophil** *also* **eosinophile** *n* : a white blood cell or other granulocyte with cytoplasmic inclusions readily stained by eosin

eo·sin·o·phil·ia \-ˌsi-nə-ˈfi-lē-ə\ *n* : abnormal increase in the number of eosinophils in the blood that is characteristic of allergic states and various parasitic infections

eosinophilia–myalgia syndrome *n* : eosinophilia with severe myalgia that occurred esp. in 1989 and 1990 in individuals who made extensive use of L-tryptophan containing a toxic contaminant — abbr. *EMS;* called also *eosinophilia-myalgia*

eo·sin·o·phil·ic \-ˌsi-nə-ˈfi-lik\ *adj* **1** : staining readily with eosin **2** : of, relating to, or characterized by eosinophilia

eosinophilic granuloma *n* : a disease of adolescents and young adults marked by the formation of granulomas in bone and the presence in them of macrophages and eosinophilic cells with secondary deposition of cholesterol

ep- — see EPI-

EPA *abbr* eicosapentaenoic acid

ep·ar·te·ri·al \ˌe-pär-ˈtir-ē-əl\ *adj* : situated above an artery; *specif* : of or relating to the first branch of the right bronchus

ependym- *or* **ependymo-** *comb form* : ependyma ⟨*ependym*itis⟩

ep·en·dy·ma \e-ˈpen-də-mə\ *n* : an epithelial membrane lining the ventricles of the brain and the canal of the spinal cord — **ep·en·dy·mal** \(ˌ)e-ˈpen-də-məl\ *adj*

ep·en·dy·mi·tis \ˌe-ˌpen-də-ˈmī-təs\ *n, pl* **-mit·i·des** \-ˈmi-tə-ˌdēz\ : inflammation of the ependyma

ep•en•dy•mo•ma \(ˌ)e-ˌpen-də-ˈmō-mə\ *n, pl* **-mas** *also* **-ma•ta** \-mə-tə\ : a glioma arising in or near the ependyma

ep•eryth•ro•zo•on \ˌe-pə-ˌrith-rə-ˈzō-ˌän\ *n* **1** *cap* : a genus of bacteria (family Anaplasmataceae) comprising blood parasites of vertebrates **2** *pl* **-zoa** \-ˈzō-ə\ : a bacterium of the genus *Eperythrozoon*

ep•eryth•ro•zo•on•o•sis \-ˌzō-ə-ˈnō-səs\ *n, pl* **-o•ses** \-ˌsēz\ : infection with or disease caused by bacteria of the genus *Eperythrozoon*

ephed•ra \i-ˈfe-drə, ˈe-fə-drə\ *n* **1 a** *cap* : a genus of shrubs (family Gnetaceae) of dry regions **b** : any plant of the genus *Ephedra* **2** : an extract of any of several Asian ephedras (esp. *E. sinica*) that contains ephedrine and related alkaloids, was formerly used as a dietary supplement to promote weight loss and increase energy, and was banned in 2004 due to adverse side effects — called also *ma huang*

ephed•rine \i-ˈfe-drən\ *n* : a crystalline alkaloid $C_{10}H_{15}NO$ extracted from a Chinese ephedra (*Ephedra sinica*) or synthesized that has the physiological action of epinephrine and is usu. used in the form of its hydrochloride or sulfate as a bronchodilator, nasal decongestant, and vasopressor — see PSEUDOEPHEDRINE

ephe•lis \i-ˈfē-ləs\ *n, pl* **-li•des** \-ˈfē-lə-ˌdēz, -ˈfe-\ : FRECKLE

ephem•er•al \i-ˈfe-mə-rəl\ *adj* : lasting a very short time

epi- *or* **ep-** *prefix* : upon ⟨*epi*cranial⟩ : besides ⟨*epi*phenomenon⟩ : attached to ⟨*epi*didymis⟩ : outer ⟨*epi*blast⟩

epi•an•dros•ter•one \ˌe-pē-ˌan-ˈdräs-tə-ˌrōn\ *n* : an androsterone derivative $C_{19}H_{30}O_2$ that occurs in normal human urine

epi•blast \ˈe-pə-ˌblast\ *n* : the outer layer of the blastoderm : ECTODERM — **epi•blas•tic** \ˌe-pə-ˈblas-tik\ *adj*

epi•can•thal fold \ˌe-pə-ˈkan-thəl-\ *n* : a prolongation of a fold of the skin of the upper eyelid over the inner angle or both angles of the eye — called also *epicanthic fold*

epi•can•thus \-ˈkan-thəs\ *n* : EPICANTHAL FOLD

epi•car•di•um \ˌe-pi-ˈkär-dē-əm\ *n, pl* **-dia** \-ə\ : the visceral part of the pericardium that closely envelops the heart — called also *visceral pericardium;* compare PARIETAL PERICARDIUM — **epi•car•di•al** \-dē-əl\ *adj*

epi•con•dyle \ˌe-pi-ˈkän-ˌdīl, -dəl\ *n* : any of several prominences on the distal part of a long bone serving for the attachment of muscles and ligaments: **a** : one on the outer aspect of the distal part of the humerus or proximal to the lateral condyle of the femur — called also *lateral epicondyle* **b** : a larger and more prominent one on the inner aspect of the distal part of the humerus or proximal to the medial condyle of the femur — called also *medial epicondyle;* see EPITROCHLEA — **epi•con•dy•lar** \-də-lər\ *adj*

epi•con•dy•li•tis \-ˌkän-ˌdī-ˈlī-təs, -də-\ *n* : inflammation of an epicondyle or of adjacent tissues — compare TENNIS ELBOW

epi•cra•ni•al \-ˈkrā-nē-əl\ *adj* : situated on the cranium

epicranial aponeurosis *n* : GALEA APONEUROTICA

epi•cra•ni•um \-ˈkrā-nē-əm\ *n, pl* **-nia** \-nē-ə\ : the structures covering the vertebrate cranium

epi•cra•ni•us \ˌe-pə-ˈkrā-nē-əs\ *n, pl* **-cra•nii** \-nē-ˌī\ : OCCIPITOFRONTALIS

ep•i•crit•ic \-ˈkri-tik\ *adj* : of, relating to, being, or mediating cutaneous sensory reception that is marked by accurate discrimination between small degrees of sensation — compare PROTOPATHIC

[1]**ep•i•dem•ic** \ˌe-pə-ˈde-mik\ *also* **ep•i•dem•i•cal** \-mi-kəl\ *adj* **1** : affecting or tending to affect an atypically large number of individuals within a population, community, or region at the same time ⟨typhoid was ~⟩ — compare ENDEMIC, SPORADIC **2** : of, relating to, or constituting an epidemic — **ep•i•dem•i•cal•ly** \-mi-k(ə-)lē\ *adv*

[2]**epidemic** *n* : an outbreak of epidemic disease

epidemic hemorrhagic fever *n* : KOREAN HEMORRHAGIC FEVER

ep•i•de•mic•i•ty \ˌe-pə-ˌde-ˈmi-sə-tē, -də-\ *n, pl* **-ties** : the quality or state of being epidemic; *specif* : the relative ability to spread from one host to others ⟨~ of typhoid bacteria⟩

epidemic keratoconjunctivitis *n* : an infectious often epidemic disease that is caused by an adenovirus of the genus *Mastadenovirus* (esp. species *Human adenovirus B* and *Human adenovirus D*) and is marked by pain, by redness and swelling of the conjunctiva, by edema of the tissues around the eye, and by tenderness of the adjacent lymph nodes

epidemic parotitis *n* : MUMPS

epidemic pleurodynia *n* : an acute epidemic form of pleurisy characterized by sudden onset with fever, headache, and acute diaphragmatic pain and caused by various Coxsackieviruses (esp. serotypes of species *Human enterovirus B* of the genus *Enterovirus*)

epidemic typhus *n* : TYPHUS a

ep•i•de•mi•ol•o•gist \ˌe-pə-ˌdē-mē-ˈä-lə-jist, -ˌde-\ *n* : a specialist in epidemiology

ep•i•de•mi•ol•o•gy \-jē\ *n, pl* **-gies** **1** : a branch of medical science that deals with the incidence, distribution, and control of disease in a population **2** : the sum of the factors controlling the presence or absence of a disease or pathogen — **ep•i•de•mi•o•log•i•cal** \-ə-ˈläj-i-kəl\ *also* **ep•i•de•mi•o•log•ic** \-jik\ *adj* — **ep•i•de•mi•o•log•i•cal•ly** \-ji-k(ə-)lē\ *adv*

ep•i•derm \ˈe-pə-ˌdərm\ *n* : EPIDERMIS

epiderm- *or* **epidermo-** *comb form* : epidermis ⟨*epidermitis*⟩

epi·der·mal \ˌe-pə-ˈdər-məl\ *adj* : of, relating to, or arising from the epidermis

epidermal growth factor *n* : a polypeptide hormone that stimulates cell proliferation esp. of epithelial cells by binding to receptor proteins on the cell surface — abbr. *EGF*

epidermal necrolysis *n* : TOXIC EPIDERMAL NECROLYSIS

epi·der·mic \ˌe-pə-ˈdər-mik\ *adj* : EPIDERMAL

epi·der·mis \-məs\ *n* : the outer epithelial layer of the external integument of the animal body that is derived from the embryonic epiblast; *specif* : the outer nonsensitive and nonvascular layer of the skin that overlies the dermis

epi·der·mi·tis \-(ˌ)dər-ˈmī-təs\ *n, pl* **-mi·tis·es** *or* **-mit·i·des** \-ˈmi-tə-ˌdēz\ : inflammation of the epidermis

epidermo- — see EPIDERM-

epi·der·moid \-ˈdər-ˌmȯid\ *adj* : resembling epidermis or epidermal cells : made up of elements like those of epidermis ⟨~ cancer of the lung⟩

epidermoid cyst *n* : a cystic tumor containing epidermal or similar tissue — called also *epidermoid;* see CHOLESTEATOMA

ep·i·der·mol·y·sis \ˌep-ə-(ˌ)dər-ˈmä-lə-səs\ *n, pl* **-y·ses** \-ˌsēz\ : a state of detachment or loosening of the epidermis

epidermolysis bul·lo·sa \-bə-ˈlō-sə\ *n* : any of a group of inherited disorders (as dystrophic epidermolysis bullosa and junctional epidermolysis bullosa) of variable severity marked esp. by the formation of large fluid-filled blisters which develop chiefly in response to minor mechanical trauma

epidermolysis bullosa ac·qui·si·ta \-ˌa-kwə-ˈsī-tə\ *n* : an autoimmune skin disorder similar to epidermolysis bullosa that occurs in adults and is usu. associated with another disorder (as Crohn's disease or diabetes)

epidermolysis bullosa sim·plex \-ˈsim-ˌpleks\ *n* : any of several forms of epidermolysis bullosa that are marked by blister formation within the epidermis sometimes accompanied by thickening of the skin and that are chiefly inherited as an autosomal dominant trait

Ep·i·der·moph·y·ton \-(ˌ)dər-ˈmä-fə-ˌtän\ *n* : a genus of fungi that comprises dermatophytes causing disease (as athlete's foot and tinea cruris), that now usu. includes a single species (*E. floccosums* syns. *E. inguinale* and *E. cruris*), and that is sometimes considered a synonym of *Trichophyton*

ep·i·der·moph·y·to·sis \-ˌmä-fə-ˈtō-səs\ *n, pl* **-to·ses** \-ˌsēz\ : a disease (as athlete's foot) of the skin or nails caused by a dermatophyte

epididym- *or* **epididymo-** *comb form* **1** : epididymis ⟨*epididym*ectomy⟩ **2** : epididymis and ⟨*epididymo*-orchitis⟩

ep·i·did·y·mec·to·my \-ˌdi-də-ˈmek-tə-mē\ *n, pl* **-mies** : excision of the epididymis

ep·i·did·y·mis \-ˈdi-də-məs\ *n, pl* **-mi·des** \-mə-ˌdēz\ : a system of ductules that emerges posteriorly from the testis, holds sperm during maturation, and forms a tangled mass before uniting into a single coiled duct which comprises the highly convoluted body and tail of the system and is continuous with the vas deferens — see VASA EFFERENTIA — **ep·i·did·y·mal** \-məl\ *adj*

ep·i·did·y·mi·tis \-ˌdi-də-ˈmī-təs\ *n* : inflammation of the epididymis

ep·i·did·y·mo–or·chi·tis \-ˌdi-də-ˌmō-ȯr-ˈkī-təs\ *n* : combined inflammation of the epididymis and testis

ep·i·did·y·mo·vas·os·to·my \-va-ˈsäs-tə-mē\ *n, pl* **-mies** : surgical severing of the vas deferens with anastomosis of the distal part to the epididymis esp. to circumvent an obstruction

Ep·i·duo \ˈep-i-ˌdü-ō\ *trademark* — used for a preparation containing adapalene and benzoyl peroxide

[1]**epi·du·ral** \ˌep-i-ˈdu̇r-əl, -ˈdyu̇r-\ *adj* : situated upon or administered or placed outside the dura mater ⟨~ injections⟩ — **epi·du·ral·ly** *adv*

[2]**epidural** *n* : an injection of an anesthetic to produce epidural anesthesia

epidural anesthesia *n* : anesthesia produced by injection of a local anesthetic into the peridural space of the spinal cord beneath the ligamentum flavum — called also *peridural anesthesia*

epi·gas·tric \ˌe-pə-ˈgas-trik\ *adj* **1** : lying upon or over the stomach **2 a** : of or relating to the anterior walls of the abdomen ⟨~ veins⟩ **b** : of or relating to the abdominal region lying between the hypochondriac regions and above the umbilical region

epigastric artery *n* : any of the three arteries supplying the anterior walls of the abdomen

epi·gas·tri·um \ˌe-pə-ˈgas-trē-əm\ *n, pl* **-tria** \-trē-ə\ : the epigastric region

epi·glot·tic \ˌe-pə-ˈglä-tik\ *or* **epi·glot·tal** \-ˈglät-ᵊl\ *adj* : of, relating to, or produced with the aid of the epiglottis

epi·glot·ti·dec·to·my \-ˌglä-tə-ˈdek-tə-mē\ *n, pl* **-mies** : excision of all or part of the epiglottis

epi·glot·tis \-ˈglä-təs\ *n* : a thin lamella of yellow elastic cartilage that ordinarily projects upward behind the tongue and just in front of the glottis and that with the arytenoid cartilages serves to cover the glottis during the act of swallowing

ep·i·glot·ti·tis \-glä-ˈtī-təs\ *n* : inflammation of the epiglottis

epi·ker·a·to·pha·kia \ˌe-pə-ˌker-ə-tə-ˈfā-kē-ə\ *n* : the grafting of human corneal tissue to a recipient in order to correct a refractive defect (as nearsightedness or astigmatism)

ep•i•la•tion \-ˈlā-shən\ *n* : the loss or removal of hair

ep•i•lep•sy \ˈe-pə-ˌlep-sē\ *n, pl* **-sies** : any of various disorders marked by abnormal electrical discharges in the brain and typically manifested by sudden brief episodes of altered or diminished consciousness, involuntary movements, or convulsions — see GRAND MAL 1, PETIT MAL 1; ABSENCE EPILEPSY, FOCAL EPILEPSY, JACKSONIAN EPILEPSY, MYOCLONIC EPILEPSY, TEMPORAL LOBE EPILEPSY

epilept- *or* **epilepti-** *or* **epilepto-** *comb form* : epilepsy ⟨*epilepti*form⟩

ep•i•lep•tic \ˌe-pə-ˈlep-tik\ *adj* : relating to, affected with, or having the characteristics of epilepsy — **epileptic** *n* — **ep•i•lep•ti•cal•ly** \-ti-k(ə-)lē\ *adv*

epilepticus — see STATUS EPILEPTICUS

ep•i•lep•ti•form \-ˈlep-tə-ˌfȯrm\ *adj* : resembling that of epilepsy ⟨an ~ seizure⟩

ep•i•lep•to•gen•ic \-ˌlep-tə-ˈje-nik\ *adj* : inducing or tending to induce epilepsy ⟨an ~ drug⟩

ep•i•lep•toid \-ˈlep-ˌtȯid\ *adj* **1** : EPILEPTIFORM **2** : exhibiting symptoms resembling those of epilepsy

ep•i•loia \ˌe-pə-ˈlȯi-ə\ *n* : TUBEROUS SCLEROSIS

epi•my•si•um \ˌe-pə-ˈmizh-ē-əm, -zē-\ *n, pl* **-sia** \-zhē-ə, -zē-ə\ : the external connective-tissue sheath of a muscle — compare ENDOMYSIUM

epi•neph•rine *also* **epi•neph•rin** \ˌe-pə-ˈne-frən\ *n* : a crystalline sympathomimetic hormone $C_9H_{13}NO_3$ that is the principal blood-pressure-raising hormone secreted by the adrenal medulla, is prepared from adrenal extracts or made synthetically, and is used medicinally to stimulate the heart during cardiac arrest and to treat life-threatening allergic reactions — called also *adrenaline*

[1]**epi•neu•ral** \ˌe-pə-ˈnu̇r-əl, -ˈnyu̇r-\ *adj* : arising from the neural arch of a vertebra

[2]**epineural** *n* : a spine or process arising from the neural arch of a vertebra

epi•neu•ri•um \ˌe-pə-ˈnu̇r-ē-əm, -ˈnyu̇r-\ *n* : the external connective-tissue sheath of a nerve trunk

Epi•Pen \ˈe-pē-ˌpen\ *trademark* — used for a preparation of epinephrine administered by auto-injector

epi•phe•nom•e•non \ˌe-pi-fə-ˈnä-mə-ˌnän, -nən\ *n* : an accidental or accessory event or process occurring in the course of a disease but not necessarily related to that disease

epiph•o•ra \i-ˈpi-fə-rə\ *n* : a watering of the eyes due to excessive secretion of tears or to obstruction of the lacrimal passages

epiph•y•se•al \i-ˌpi-fə-ˈsē-əl\ *also* **ep•i•phys•i•al** \ˌe-pə-ˈfi-zē-əl\ *adj* : of or relating to an epiphysis

epiphyseal line *n* : the line marking the site of an ossified epiphyseal plate

epiphyseal plate *n* : the cartilage that unites an epiphysis with the shaft of a long bone and is the site where the bone grows in length : GROWTH PLATE — called also *epiphyseal cartilage*

epiph•y•si•od•e•sis \i-ˌpi-fə-sē-ˈä-də-səs, ˌe-pə-ˌfi-zē-\ *n, pl* **-e•ses** \-ˌsēz\ : the surgical reattachment of a separated epiphysis to the shaft of its bone

epiph•y•sis \i-ˈpi-fə-səs\ *n, pl* **-y•ses** \-ˌsēz\ **1** : a part or process of a bone that ossifies separately and later becomes ankylosed to the main part of the bone; *esp* : the usu. rounded end of a long bone — compare DIAPHYSIS **2** : PINEAL GLAND

epiph•y•si•tis \i-ˌpi-fə-ˈsī-təs\ *n* : inflammation of an epiphysis

epi•plo•ec•to•my \ˌe-pə-plō-ˈek-tə-mē\ *n, pl* **-mies** : OMENTECTOMY

ep•i•plo•ic \ˌe-pə-ˈplō-ik\ *adj* : of or associated with an omentum : OMENTAL

epiploicae — see APPENDICES EPIPLOICAE

epiploic foramen *n* : the only opening between the omental bursa and the general peritoneal sac — called also *foramen of Winslow*

ep•i•plo•on \ˌe-pə-ˈplō-ˌän\ *n, pl* **-ploa** \-ˈplō-ə\ : OMENTUM; *specif* : GREATER OMENTUM

epi•pter•ic \ˌep-ip-ˈter-ik\ *adj* : relating to or being a small Wormian bone sometimes present in the human skull between the parietal and the greater wing of the sphenoid

epi•sclera \ˌe-pə-ˈskler-ə\ *n* : the layer of connective tissue between the conjunctiva and the sclera of the eye

epi•scler•al \-ˈskler-əl\ *adj* **1** : situated upon the sclerotic coat of the eye **2** : of or relating to the episclera

epi•scle•ri•tis \-sklə-ˈrī-təs\ *n* : inflammation of the superficial layers of the sclera

episio- *comb form* **1** : vulva ⟨*episio*tomy⟩ **2** : vulva and ⟨*episio*perineorrhaphy⟩

epi•sio•per•i•ne•or•rha•phy \i-ˌpi-zē-ō-ˌper-ə-nē-ˈȯr-ə-fē, -ˌpē-\ *n, pl* **-phies** : surgical repair of the vulva and perineum by suturing

epi•si•or•rha•phy \-zē-ˈȯr-ə-fē\ *n, pl* **-phies** : surgical repair of injury to the vulva by suturing

epi•si•ot•o•my \i-ˌpi-zē-ˈä-tə-mē, -ˌpē-\ *n, pl* **-mies** : surgical enlargement of the vulval orifice for obstetrical purposes during childbirth

ep•i•sode \ˈe-pə-ˌsōd, -ˌzōd\ *n* : an event that is distinctive and separate although part of a larger series; *esp* : an occurrence of a usu. recurrent pathological abnormal condition — **ep•i•sod•ic** \ˌe-pə-ˈsä-dik, -ˈzä-\ *adj* — **ep•i•sod•i•cal•ly** \-di-k(ə-)lē\ *adv*

episodic memory *n* : long-term memory of a specific event that was personally experienced at a particular time or place in the past — compare SEMANTIC MEMORY

epi•some \'e-pə-ˌsōm, -ˌzōm\ *n* : a genetic determinant (as the DNA of some bacteriophages) that can replicate either autonomously in bacterial cytoplasm or as an integral part of their chromosomes — compare PLASMID — **epi•som•al** \ˌe-pə-'sō-məl, -'zō-\ *adj* — **epi•som•al•ly** \-mə-lē\ *adv*

ep•i•spa•di•as \ˌe-pə-'spā-dē-əs\ *n* : a congenital defect in which the urethra opens upon the upper surface of the penis

epis•ta•sis \i-'pis-tə-səs\ *n, pl* **-ta•ses** \-ˌsēz\ **1 a** : suppression of a secretion or discharge **b** : a scum on the surface of urine **2** : suppression of the effect of a gene by a nonallelic gene — **epi•stat•ic** \ˌe-pə-'sta-tik\ *adj*

ep•i•stax•is \ˌe-pə-'stak-səs\ *n, pl* **-stax•es** \-ˌsēz\ : NOSEBLEED

ep•i•stro•phe•us \ˌe-pə-'strō-fē-əs\ *n* : AXIS 2a

epi•thal•a•mus \ˌe-pə-'tha-lə-məs\ *n, pl* **-mi** \-ˌmī\ : a dorsal segment of the diencephalon containing the habenula and the pineal gland

epithel- *or* **epitheli-** *or* **epithelio-** *comb form* : epithelium ⟨*epitheli*oma⟩

ep•i•the•li•al \ˌe-pə-'thē-lē-əl\ *adj* : of or relating to epithelium ⟨~ cells⟩

ep•i•the•li•oid \-'thē-lē-ˌȯid\ *adj* : resembling epithelium

epithelioid angiomatosis *n* : BACILLARY ANGIOMATOSIS

ep•i•the•li•o•ma \-ˌthē-lē-'ō-mə\ *n, pl* **-mas** *also* **-ma•ta** \-mə-tə\ : a tumor derived from epithelial tissue

ep•i•the•li•um \ˌe-pə-'thē-lē-əm\ *n, pl* **-lia** \-lē-ə\ : a membranous cellular tissue that covers a free surface or lines a tube or cavity of an animal body and serves esp. to enclose and protect the other parts of the body, to produce secretions and excretions, and to function in assimilation

ep•i•the•li•za•tion \ˌe-pə-ˌthē-lə-'zā-shən\ *or* **ep•i•the•lial•i•za•tion** \-ˌthē-lē-ə-lə-\ *n* : the process of becoming covered with or converted to epithelium — **ep•i•the•lize** \ˌe-pə-'thē-ˌlīz\ *or* **ep•i•the•li•al•ize** \-'thē-lē-ə-ˌlīz\ *vb*

ep•i•thet \'e-pə-ˌthet, -thət\ *n* : the part of a scientific name identifying the species, variety, or other subunit within a genus — see SPECIFIC EPITHET

epi•tope \'e-pə-ˌtōp\ *n* : a molecular region on the surface of an antigen capable of eliciting an immune response and of combining with the specific antibody produced by such a response — called also *determinant, antigenic determinant*

epi•troch•lea \ˌe-pi-'trä-klē-ə\ *n* : the medial epicondyle at the distal end of the humerus — **epi•troch•le•ar** \-klē-ər\ *adj*

epi•tym•pan•ic \-tim-'pa-nik\ *adj* : situated above the tympanic membrane

epitympanic recess *n* : ATTIC

epi•tym•pa•num \-'tim-pə-nəm\ *n* : the upper portion of the middle ear — compare HYPOTYMPANUM

Ep•i•vir \'e-pə-ˌvir\ *trademark* — used for a preparation of lamivudine

epi•zo•ot•ic \ˌe-pə-zō-'wä-tik\ *n* : an outbreak of disease affecting many animals of one kind at the same time; *also* : the disease itself — **epizootic** *adj*

epizootic lymphangitis *n* : a chronic contagious inflammation chiefly affecting the superficial lymphatics and lymph nodes of horses, mules, and donkeys and caused by a fungus of the genus *Histoplasma* (*H. farciminosum*)

epi•zo•ot•i•ol•o•gy \ˌe-pə-zō-ˌwä-tē-'ä-lə-jē\ *also* **epi•zo•otol•o•gy** \-ˌzō-ə-'tä-lə-jē\ *n, pl* **-gies** **1** : a science that deals with the character, ecology, and causes of outbreaks of animal diseases **2** : the sum of the factors controlling the occurrence of a disease or pathogen of animals — **epi•zo•oti•o•log•i•cal** \-zō-ˌwō-tē-ə-'lä-ji-kəl, -ˌwä-\ *also* **epi•zo•oti•o•log•ic** \-jik\ *adj*

EPO *abbr* erythropoietin

epo•e•tin \i-'pō-ə-tən\ *n* : a glycoprotein produced by recombinant DNA technology that is identical to human erythropoietin and is administered by injection esp. to treat anemia or to reduce the need of some surgery-related blood transfusions — see EPOGEN, MIRCERA, PROCRIT

Ep•o•gen \'e-pə-jən\ *trademark* — used for a preparation of epoetin

ep•o•nych•i•um \ˌe-pə-'ni-kē-əm\ *n* : the horny band of epidermis that extends over the proximal edge of a nail : CUTICLE

ep•onym \'e-pə-ˌnim\ *n* **1** : the person for whom something (as a disease) is or is believed to be named **2** : a name (as of a drug or a disease) based on or derived from the name of a person — **epon•y•mous** \i-'pä-nə-məs, e-\ *adj*

ep•ooph•o•ron \ˌe-pō-'ä-fə-ˌrän\ *n* : a rudimentary organ homologous with the male epididymis that lies in the broad ligament of the uterus — called also *organ of Rosenmüller, parovarium*

Ep•som salts \'ep-səm-\ *or* **Epsom salt** *n* : a bitter white crystalline salt $MgSO_4 \cdot 7H_2O$ that is a hydrated magnesium sulfate with cathartic properties

Ep•stein–Barr virus \'ep-ˌstīn-'bär-\ *n* : a herpesvirus (species *Human herpesvirus 4* of the genus *Lymphocryptovirus*) that causes infectious mononucleosis and is associated with Burkitt's lymphoma and nasopharyngeal carcinoma — abbr. *EBV;* called also *EB virus*

Epstein, Michael Anthony (*b* **1921**), and **Barr, Yvonne M.** (*b* **1932**), British virologists.

Ep•stein's pearls \'ep-ˌstīnz-, -ˌstēnz-\ *n pl* : temporary small white cysts that occur along the midline of the hard palate of many newborn infants

Epstein, Alois (1849–1918), Czech pediatrician.

epu•lis \ə-ˈpyü-ləs\ *n, pl* **epu•li•des** \-lə-ˌdēz\ : a tumor or tumorous growth of the gum

Eq•ua•nil \ˈe-kwə-ˌnil\ *trademark* — used for a preparation of meprobamate

equa•tion•al \i-ˈkwā-zhə-nəl\ *adj* : dividing into two equal parts — used esp. of the mitotic cell division usu. following reduction in meiosis — **equa•tion•al•ly** *adv*

equa•tor \i-ˈkwā-tər, ˈē-ˌ\ *n* **1** : a circle dividing the surface of a body into two usu. equal and symmetrical parts esp. at the place of greatest width ⟨the ~ of the lens of the eye⟩ **2** : EQUATORIAL PLANE — **equa•to•ri•al** \ˌē-kwə-ˈtōr-ē-əl, ˌe-\ *adj*

equatorial plane *n* : the plane perpendicular to the spindle of a dividing cell and midway between the poles

equatorial plate *n* **1** : METAPHASE PLATE **2** : EQUATORIAL PLANE

equi•an•al•ge•sic \ˌē-kwi-ˌan-ᵊl-ˈjē-zik, ˌe-, -sik\ *adj* : producing the same degree of analgesia

equi•len•in \ˌe-kwə-ˈle-nən, ə-ˈkwi-lə-nən\ *n* : a weakly estrogenic steroid hormone $C_{18}H_{18}O_2$ obtained from the urine of pregnant mares

equi•lib•ri•um \ˌē-kwə-ˈli-brē-əm, ˌe-\ *n, pl* **-ri•ums** *or* **-ria** \-brē-ə\ **1** : a state of balance between opposing forces or actions that is either static (as in a body acted on by forces whose resultant is zero) or dynamic (as in a reversible chemical reaction when the velocities in both directions are equal) **2** : a state of intellectual or emotional balance

eq•ui•lin \ˈe-kwə-lən\ *n* : an estrogenic steroid $C_{18}H_{20}O_2$ obtained from the urine of pregnant mares

equina — see CAUDA EQUINA

equine \ˈē-ˌkwīn, ˈe-\ *n* : any of a family (Equidae) of hoofed mammals that include the horses, asses and zebras — **equine** *adj*

equine babesiosis *n* : EQUINE PIROPLASMOSIS

equine coital exanthema *n* : a highly contagious disease of horses that is caused by a herpesvirus of the genus *Varicellovirus* (species *Equid herpesvirus 3*) transmitted chiefly by copulation — called also *coital exanthema*

equine encephalitis *n* : any of three virus diseases chiefly of equines and humans in various parts of No. and So. America that are transmitted esp. by mosquitoes, are characterized in humans by flu-like symptoms which often progress to encephalitis and sometimes to coma and death, and are caused by three togaviruses of the genus *Alphavirus* (species *Eastern equine encephalitis virus, Western equine encephalitis virus*, and *Venezuelan equine encephalitis virus*): **a** : one that occurs in the eastern U.S. and Canada — called also *eastern equine encephalitis, eastern equine encephalomyelitis* **b** : one that occurs in the western U.S. and Canada — called also *western equine encephalitis, western equine encephalomyelitis* **c** : one that occurs from northern So. America to Mexico — called also *Venezuelan equine encephalitis, Venezuelan equine encephalomyelitis*

equine encephalomyelitis *n* : EQUINE ENCEPHALITIS

equine infectious anemia *n* : a serious sometimes fatal disease of horses that is caused by a retrovirus of the genus *Lentivirus* (species *Equine infectious anemia virus*) and is marked by intermittent fever, depression, weakness, edema and anemia — called also *swamp fever*

equine piroplasmosis *n* : a tick-borne disease that affects horses and related equines, is caused by two protozoans of the genus *Babesia* (*B. caballi* and *B. equi*), and is characterized esp. by fever, anemia, weakness, and icterus — called also *equine babesiosis*

equinovarus — see TALIPES EQUINOVARUS

equinus — see TALIPES EQUINUS

equi•po•tent \ˌē-kwə-ˈpōt-ᵊnt, ˌe-\ *adj* : having equal effects or capacities

Er *symbol* erbium

ER *abbr* **1** emergency room **2** extended-release

Erax•is \i-ˈrak-səs\ *trademark* — used for a preparation of anidulafungin

Er•bi•tux \ˈər-bə-ˌtəks\ *trademark* — used for a preparation of cetuximab

er•bi•um \ˈər-bē-əm\ *n* : a metallic element that occurs with yttrium — symbol *Er;* see ELEMENT table

Erb's palsy \ˈerbz-, ˈerps-\ *n* : paralysis affecting the muscles of the upper arm and shoulder that is caused by an injury during birth to the upper part of the brachial plexus

Erb, Wilhelm Heinrich (1840–1921), German neurologist.

ERCP *abbr* endoscopic retrograde cholangiopancreatography

erect \i-ˈrekt\ *adj* **1** : standing up or out from the body ⟨~ hairs⟩ **2** : being in a state of physiological erection

erec•tile \i-ˈrekt-ᵊl, -ˈrek-ˌtīl\ *adj* : capable of being raised to an erect or elevated position; *esp* : CAVERNOUS 2 — **erec•til•i•ty** \-ˌrek-ˈti-lə-tē\ *n*

erectile dysfunction *n* : chronic inability to achieve or maintain an erection satisfactory for sexual intercourse : IMPOTENCE 2 — abbr. *ED*

erec•tion \i-ˈrek-shən\ *n* **1** : the state marked by firm turgid form and erect or elevated position of a previously flaccid bodily part containing cavernous tissue when that tissue becomes dilated with blood **2** : an occurrence of erection in the penis or clitoris

erec•tor \i-ˈrek-tər\ *n* : a muscle that raises or keeps a part erect

erector spi·nae \-ˈspī-ˌnē\ *n* : SACROSPINALIS

erep·sin \i-ˈrep-sən\ *n* : a proteolytic fraction obtained esp. from the intestinal juice

er·e·thism \ˈer-ə-ˌthi-zəm\ *n* : abnormal irritability or responsiveness to stimulation

erg \ˈərg\ *n* : a cgs unit of work equal to the work done by a force of one dyne acting through a distance of one centimeter

ERG *abbr* electroretinogram

erg- *or* **ergo-** *comb form* : work <*ergo*meter>

-er·gic \ˈər-jik\ *adj comb form* **1** : allergic <hyper*ergic*> **2** : exhibiting or stimulating activity esp. of (such) a neurotransmitter substance <adren*ergic*> <dopamin*ergic*>

ergo- *comb form* : ergot <*ergo*sterol>

er·go·cal·cif·er·ol \ˌər-(ˌ)gō-kal-ˈsi-fə-ˌrōl, -ˌrōl\ *n* : CALCIFEROL

er·go·loid mesylates \ˈər-gə-ˌlȯid-\ *n sing or pl* : a combination of equal amounts of three ergot alkaloids used with varying success in the treatment of cognitive decline and dementia esp. in elderly patients — see HYDERGINE

er·gom·e·ter \(ˌ)ər-ˈgä-mə-tər\ *n* : an apparatus for measuring the work performed (as by a person exercising); *also* : an exercise machine equipped with an ergometer — **er·go·met·ric** \ˌər-gə-ˈme-trik\ *adj*

er·go·met·rine \ˌər-gə-ˈme-ˌtrēn, -trən\ *n* : ERGONOVINE

er·go·nom·ics \ˌər-gə-ˈnä-miks\ *n sing or pl* **1** : an applied science concerned with designing and arranging things people use so that the people and things interact most efficiently and safely — called also *biotechnology, human engineering, human factors, human factors engineering* **2** : the design characteristics of an object resulting esp. from the application of the science of ergonomics — **er·go·nom·ic** \-mik\ *adj* — **er·go·nom·i·cal·ly** \-mi-k(ə-)lē\ *adv* — **er·gon·o·mist** \(ˌ)ər-ˈgä-nə-mist\ *n*

er·go·no·vine \ˌər-gə-ˈnō-ˌvēn, -vən\ *n* : an alkaloid $C_{19}H_{23}N_3O_2$ that is derived from ergot and is used esp. in the form of its maleate $C_{19}H_{23}N_3O_2·C_4H_4O_4$ to prevent or treat postpartum bleeding

er·gos·ter·ol \(ˌ)ər-ˈgäs-tə-ˌrȯl, -ˌrōl\ *n* : a steroid alcohol $C_{28}H_{44}O$ that occurs esp. in yeast, molds, and ergot and is converted by ultraviolet irradiation ultimately into vitamin D_2

er·got \ˈər-gət, -ˌgät\ *n* **1** : the black or dark purple sclerotium of fungi of an ascomycetous genus (*Claviceps*); *also* : any fungus of this genus **2 a** : the dried sclerotial bodies of an ergot fungus grown on rye and containing several ergot alkaloids **b** : ERGOT ALKALOID

ergot alkaloid *n* : any of a group of alkaloids found in ergot or produced synthetically that include some (as ergonovine and ergotamine) noted esp. for their contractile effect on smooth muscle (as of the uterus or blood vessels)

er·got·a·mine \(ˌ)ər-ˈgä-tə-ˌmēn\ *n* : an alkaloid that is derived from ergot and is used chiefly in the form of its tartrate $(C_{33}H_{35}N_5O_5)_2·C_4H_6O_6$ esp. in treating migraine

er·got·ism \ˈər-gə-ˌti-zəm\ *n* : a toxic condition produced by eating grain, grain products (as rye bread), or grasses infected with ergot fungus or by chronic excessive use of an ergot drug

er·got·ized \-ˌtīzd\ *adj* : infected with ergot; *also* : poisoned by ergot

erigens, erigentes — see NERVUS ERIGENS

er·i·o·dic·ty·on \ˌer-ē-ə-ˈdik-tē-ˌän\ *n* : the dried leaves of yerba santa used as a flavoring in medicine

erode \i-ˈrōd\ *vb* **erod·ed; erod·ing 1** : to eat into or away by slow destruction of substance <acids that ~ the teeth> <bone *eroded* by cancer> **2** : to remove with an abrasive

erog·e·nous \i-ˈrä-jə-nəs\ *adj* **1** : producing sexual excitement or libidinal gratification when stimulated : sexually sensitive **2** : of, relating to, or arousing sexual feelings — **er·o·ge·ne·ity** \ˌer-ə-jə-ˈnē-ə-tē\ *n*

Eros \ˈer-ˌäs, ˈir-\ *n* : the sum of life-preserving instincts that are manifested as impulses to gratify basic needs (as sex), as sublimated impulses motivated by the same needs, and as impulses to protect and preserve the body and mind — compare DEATH INSTINCT

ero·sion \i-ˈrō-zhən\ *n* **1 a** : the superficial destruction of a surface area of tissue (as mucous membrane) by inflammation, ulceration, or trauma <~ of the uterine cervix> **b** : progressive loss of the hard substance of a tooth **2** : an instance or product of erosion

ero·sive \i-ˈrō-siv, -ziv\ *adj* : tending to erode or to induce erosion <~ lesions>; *also* : caused or marked by erosion <~ osteoarthritis> <~ esophagitis>

erot·ic \i-ˈrä-tik\ *also* **erot·i·cal** \i-ˈrä-ti-kəl\ *adj* **1** : of, devoted to, or tending to arouse sexual love or desire **2** : strongly marked or affected by sexual desire — **erot·i·cal·ly** \-ti-k(ə-)lē\ *adv*

erot·i·cism \i-ˈrä-tə-ˌsi-zəm\ *n* **1** : a state of sexual arousal or anticipation **2** : insistent sexual impulse or desire

erot·i·cize \-ˌsīz\ *vb* **-cized; -ciz·ing** : to make erotic — **erot·i·ci·za·tion** \i-ˌrä-tə-sə-ˈzā-shən\ *n*

er·o·tism \ˈer-ə-ˌti-zəm\ *n* : EROTICISM

er·o·tize \ˈer-ə-ˌtīz\ *vb* **-tized; -tiz·ing** : to invest with erotic significance or sexual feeling — **er·o·ti·za·tion** \ˌer-ə-tə-ˈzā-shən\ *n*

eroto- *comb form* : sexual desire ⟨*erotomania*⟩
ero•to•gen•ic \i-ˌrō-tə-ˈje-nik, -ˌrä-\ *adj* : EROGENOUS
ero•to•ma•nia \-ˈmā-nē-ə\ *n* **1** : excessive sexual desire **2** : a psychological disorder marked by the delusional belief that one is the object of another person's love or sexual desire — **ero•to•ma•ni•ac** \-ˈmā-nē-ˌak\ *n*
ero•to•pho•bia \-ˈfō-bē-ə\ *n* : a morbid aversion to sexual love or desire
ERT *abbr* estrogen replacement therapy
eru•cic acid \i-ˈrü-sik-\ *n* : a crystalline fatty acid $C_{22}H_{42}O_2$ found in the form of glycerides esp. in an oil obtained from the seeds of the rape plant (*Brassica napus* of the mustard family)
eruct \i-ˈrəkt\ *vb* : BELCH
eruc•ta•tion \i-ˌrək-ˈtā-shən, ˌē-\ *n* : an act or instance of belching
erupt \i-ˈrəpt\ *vb* **1** *of a tooth* : to emerge through the gum **2** : to break out (as with a skin eruption) — **erup•tive** \-ˈrəp-tiv\ *adj*
erup•tion \i-ˈrəp-shən\ *n* **1** : an act, process, or instance of erupting; *specif* : the breaking out of an exanthem or enanthem on the skin or mucous membrane (as in measles) **2** : something produced by an act or process of erupting: as **a** : the condition of the skin or mucous membrane caused by erupting **b** : one of the lesions (as a pustule) constituting this condition
er•y•sip•e•las \ˌer-ə-ˈsi-pə-ləs, ˌir-\ *n* **1** : an acute febrile disease that is associated with intense often vesicular and edematous local inflammation of the skin and subcutaneous tissues and that is caused by a hemolytic streptococcus **2** : SWINE ERYSIPELAS — used esp. when the disease affects hosts other than swine
er•y•sip•e•loid \ˌer-ə-ˈsi-pə-ˌlȯid, ˌir-\ *n* : an acute dermatitis resembling erysipelas that is caused by the bacterium of the genus *Erysipelothrix* (*E. rhusiopathiae*) that causes swine erysipelas, is typically marked by usu. painful reddish-purple lesions esp. on the hands, and that is contracted by direct contact with infected animal flesh — **erysipeloid** *adj*
er•y•sip•e•lo•thrix \ˌer-ə-ˈsi-pə-lō-ˌthriks\ *n* **1** *cap* : a genus of gram-positive, rod-shaped bacteria (family Erysipelotrichaceae) including one (*E. rhusiopathiae*) that is the causative agent of swine erysipelas, an arthritis of lambs, and human erysipeloid **2** : a bacterium of the genus *Erysipelothrix*
er•y•the•ma \ˌer-ə-ˈthē-mə\ *n* : abnormal redness of the skin due to capillary congestion (as in inflammation) — **er•y•the•mal** \-məl\ *adj*
erythema chron•i•cum mi•grans \-ˈkrä-nə-kəm-ˈmī-grənz\ *n* : ERYTHEMA MIGRANS
erythema in•fec•ti•o•sum \-in-ˌfek-shē-ˈō-səm\ *n* : FIFTH DISEASE
erythema mi•grans \-ˈmī-grənz\ *n* : a spreading annular erythematous skin lesion that is an early symptom of Lyme disease and that develops at the site of the bite of a tick (as the deer tick) infected with the causative spirochete
erythema mul•ti•for•me \-ˌməl-tə-ˈfȯr-mē\ *n* : a skin disease characterized by papular or vesicular lesions and reddening or discoloration of the skin often in concentric zones about the lesions
erythema no•do•sum \-nō-ˈdō-səm\ *n* : a skin condition characterized by small tender reddened nodules under the skin (as over the shin bones) often accompanied by fever and transitory arthritic pains
erythematosus — see LUPUS ERYTHEMATOSUS, LUPUS ERYTHEMATOSUS CELL, PEMPHIGUS ERYTHEMATOSUS, SYSTEMIC LUPUS ERYTHEMATOSUS
er•y•them•a•tous \ˌer-ə-ˈthe-mə-təs, -ˈthē-\ *adj* : relating to or marked by erythema
er•y•thor•bate \ˌer-ə-ˈthȯr-ˌbāt\ *n* : a salt of erythorbic acid that is used in foods as an antioxidant
er•y•thor•bic acid \ˌer-ə-ˈthȯr-bik-\ *n* : a stereoisomer of vitamin C
erythr- *or* **erythro-** *comb form* **1** : red ⟨*erythrocyte*⟩ **2** : erythrocyte ⟨*erythroid*⟩
er•y•thrae•mia *chiefly Brit var of* ERYTHREMIA
er•y•thras•ma \ˌer-ə-ˈthraz-mə\ *n* : a chronic contagious dermatitis that affects warm moist areas of the body (as the armpit and groin) and is caused by a bacterium of the genus *Corynebacterium* (*C. minutissimum*)
eryth•re•de•ma \i-ˌri-thrə-ˈdē-mə\ *n* : ACRODYNIA
er•y•thre•mia \ˌer-ə-ˈthrē-mē-ə\ *n* : POLYCYTHEMIA VERA
er•y•thrism \ˈer-ə-ˌthri-zəm\ *n* : a condition marked by exceptional prevalence of red pigmentation (as in skin or hair) — **er•y•thris•tic** \ˌer-ə-ˈthris-tik\ *also* **er•y•thris•mal** \-ˈthriz-məl\ *adj*
eryth•ri•tyl tet•ra•ni•trate \i-ˈri-thrə-ˌtil-ˌte-trə-ˈnī-ˌtrāt\ *n* : a vasodilator $C_4H_{10}N_4O_{12}$ used to prevent angina pectoris — called also *erythritol tetranitrate*
erythro- — see ERYTHR-
eryth•ro•blast \i-ˈri-thrə-ˌblast\ *n* : a polychromatic nucleated cell of red marrow that synthesizes hemoglobin and that is an intermediate in the initial stage of red blood cell formation; *broadly* : a cell ancestral to red blood cells — compare NORMOBLAST — **eryth•ro•blas•tic** \-ˌri-thrə-ˈblas-tik\ *adj*
eryth•ro•blas•to•pe•nia \i-ˌri-thrə-ˌblas-tə-ˈpē-nē-ə\ *n* : a deficiency in bone-marrow erythroblasts
eryth•ro•blas•to•sis \-ˌblas-ˈtō-səs\ *n, pl* **-to•ses** \-ˌsēz\ : abnormal presence of erythroblasts in the circulating blood; *esp* : ERYTHROBLASTOSIS FETALIS

erythroblastosis fe•ta•lis \-fi-ˈta-ləs\ *n* : a hemolytic disease of the fetus and newborn that is characterized by an increase in circulating erythroblasts and by jaundice and that occurs when the immune system of an Rh-negative mother produces antibodies to an antigen in the blood of an Rh-positive fetus — called also *hemolytic disease of the newborn, Rh disease*

eryth•ro•blas•tot•ic \i-ˌri-thrə-blas-ˈtä-tik\ *adj* : of, relating to, or affected by erythroblastosis ⟨an ~ infant⟩

Eryth•ro•cin \i-ˈrith-rə-sən\ *trademark* — used for a preparation of erythromycin

eryth•ro•cyte \i-ˈri-thrə-ˌsīt\ *n* : RED BLOOD CELL — **eryth•ro•cyt•ic** \-ˌri-thrə-ˈsi-tik\ *adj*

eryth•ro•cy•to•pe•nia \i-ˌri-thrə-ˌsī-tə-ˈpē-nē-ə\ *n* : deficiency of red blood cells

eryth•ro•cy•tor•rhex•is \-ˈrek-səs\ *n, pl* **-rhex•es** \-ˈrek-ˌsēz\ : rupture of a red blood cell

eryth•ro•cy•to•sis \i-ˌri-thrə-ˌsī-ˈtō-səs\ *n, pl* **-to•ses** \-ˈtō-ˌsēz\ : an increase in the number of circulating red blood cells esp. resulting from a known stimulus (as hypoxia)

eryth•ro•der•ma \-ˈdər-mə\ *n, pl* **-mas** \-məz\ *or* **-ma•ta** \-mə-tə\ : ERYTHEMA

eryth•ro•der•mia \-ˈdər-mē-ə\ *n* : ERYTHEMA

eryth•ro•gen•ic \-ˈje-nik\ *adj* **1** : producing red blood cells : ERYTHROPOIETIC **2** : inducing reddening of the skin

ery•throid \i-ˈri-ˌthrȯid, ˈer-ə-\ *adj* : relating to erythrocytes or their precursors

eryth•ro•leu•ke•mia \i-ˌri-thrə-lü-ˈkē-mē-ə\ *n* : a malignant disorder that is marked by proliferation of erythroblastic and myeloblastic tissue and in later stages by leukemia — **eryth•ro•leu•ke•mic** \-mik\ *adj*

eryth•ro•mel•al•gia \-mə-ˈlal-jə\ *n* : a state of excessive dilation of the superficial blood vessels usu. of the feet accompanied by hyperemia, increased skin temperature, and burning pain

eryth•ro•my•cin \i-ˌri-thrə-ˈmīs-ᵊn\ *n* : a broad-spectrum antibiotic $C_{37}H_{67}NO_{13}$ that resembles penicillin in activity, is produced by a bacterium (*Saccharopolyspora erythraea* syn. *Streptomyces erythreus*), and is used to treat bacterial infections or sometimes infections caused by other microbes (as amoebas)

eryth•ro•phago•cy•to•sis \i-ˈri-thrə-ˌfa-gə-sə-ˈtō-səs, -ˌsī-\ *n, pl* **-to•ses** \-ˈtō-ˌsēz\ : phagocytosis of red blood cells esp. by macrophages

eryth•ro•pla•sia \-ˈplā-zhə, -zhē-ə\ *n* : a reddened patch with a velvety surface on the oral or genital mucosa that is considered to be a precancerous lesion

eryth•ro•poi•e•sis \i-ˌri-thrō-pȯi-ˈē-səs\ *n, pl* **-e•ses** \-ˌsēz\ : the production of red blood cells (as from the bone marrow) — **eryth•ro•poi•et•ic** \-ˈe-tik\ *adj*

erythropoietic protoporphyria *n* : a rare porphyria usu. appearing in young children and marked by excessive protoporphyrin in red blood cells, blood plasma, and feces and by skin lesions resulting from photosensitivity

eryth•ro•poi•e•tin \-ˈpȯi-ət-ᵊn\ *n* : a hormonal substance that is formed esp. in the kidney and stimulates red blood cell formation — abbr. *EPO;* see EPOGEN

eryth•ro•sine \i-ˈri-thrə-sən, -ˌsēn\ *also* **eryth•ro•sin** \-sən\ *n* : a brick-red powdered xanthene dye $C_{20}H_6I_4Na_2O_5$ that is used as a biological stain and in dentistry as an agent to disclose plaque on teeth — called also *erythrosine sodium*

Es *symbol* einsteinium

ESB *abbr* electrical stimulation of the brain

es•cape \i-ˈskāp\ *n* **1** : evasion of something undesirable ⟨~ from pain and suffering⟩ **2** : distraction or relief from routine or reality; *esp* : mental distraction or relief by flight into idealizing fantasy or fiction — **escape** *vb* — **escape** *adj*

escape mechanism *n* : a mode of behavior or thinking adopted to evade unpleasant facts or responsibilities : DEFENSE MECHANISM

es•cap•ism \i-ˈskā-ˌpi-zəm\ *n* : habitual diversion of the mind to purely imaginative activity or entertainment as an escape from reality or routine — **es•cap•ist** \-pist\ *adj or n*

es•char \ˈes-ˌkär\ *n* : a scab formed esp. after a burn

[1]**es•cha•rot•ic** \ˌes-kə-ˈrä-tik\ *adj* : producing an eschar

[2]**escharotic** *n* : an escharotic agent (as a drug)

Esch•e•rich•ia \ˌe-shə-ˈri-kē-ə\ *n* : a genus of aerobic gram-negative rod-shaped bacteria (family Enterobacteriaceae) that include occas. pathogenic forms (as some strains of *E. coli*) normally present in the human intestine and other forms which typically occur in soil and water

Esch•e•rich \ˈe-shə-rik\, **Theodor (1857–1911)**, German pediatrician.

es•ci•tal•o•pram \ˌe-sə-ˈta-lə-ˌpram\ *n* : a drug that functions as an SSRI and is administered orally in the form of its oxalate $C_{20}H_{21}FN_2O \cdot C_2H_2O_4$ to treat depression and anxiety — see LEXAPRO

es•cutch•eon \i-ˈskə-chən\ *n* : the configuration of adult pubic hair

es•er•ine \ˈe-sə-ˌrēn\ *n* : PHYSOSTIGMINE

Es•march bandage \ˈes-ˌmärk, ˈez-\ *or* **Es•march's bandage** \-ˌmärks-\ *n* : a tight rubber bandage for driving the blood out of a limb

Esmarch, Johannes Friedrich August von (1823–1908), German surgeon.

eso- *prefix* : inner ⟨*eso*tropia⟩

es•omep•ra•zole \ˌe-sō-ˈme-prə-ˌzōl\ *n* : an isomer of omeprazole that is administered in the form of its magnesium salt $(C_{17}H_{18}N_3O_3S)_2Mg$ esp. in the treatment of erosive esophagitis, gastroesophageal reflux disease, and duodenal ulcer — see NEXIUM

esophag- *or* **esophago-** *comb form* **1** : esophagus ⟨*esophag*ectomy⟩ ⟨*esophago*plasty⟩ **2** : esophagus and ⟨*esophago*gastrectomy⟩

esoph•a•ge•al \i-ˌsä-fə-ˈjē-əl\ *adj* : of or relating to the esophagus

esophageal artery *n* : any of several arteries that arise from the front of the aorta, anastomose along the esophagus, and terminate by anastomosis with adjacent arteries

esophageal gland *n* : one of the racemose glands in the walls of the esophagus that in humans are small and serve principally to lubricate the food

esophageal hiatus *n* : the aperture in the diaphragm that gives passage to the esophagus — see HIATAL HERNIA

esophageal plexus *n* : a nerve plexus formed by the branches of the vagus nerve which surround and supply the esophagus

esophageal speech *n* : a method of speaking which is used by individuals whose larynx has been removed and in which phonation is achieved by expelling swallowed air from the esophagus

esoph•a•gec•to•my \i-ˌsä-fə-ˈjek-tə-mē\ *n, pl* **-mies** : excision of part of the esophagus

esophagi *pl of* ESOPHAGUS

esoph•a•gi•tis \i-ˌsä-fə-ˈjī-təs, -ˈgī, (ˌ)ē-\ *n* : inflammation of the esophagus

esophago- — see ESOPHAG-

esoph•a•go•gas•trec•to•my \i-ˌsä-fə-gō-ˌgas-ˈtrek-tə-mē\ *n, pl* **-mies** : excision of part of the esophagus (esp. the lower third) and the stomach

esoph•a•go•gas•tric \-ˈgas-trik\ *adj* : of, relating to, involving, or affecting the esophagus and the stomach

esoph•a•go•gas•tro•plas•ty \-ˈga-strə-ˌpla-stē\ *n, pl* **-ties** : CARDIOPLASTY

esoph•a•go•gas•tros•co•py \-ˌgas-ˈträs-kə-pē\ *n, pl* **-pies** : examination of the interior of the esophagus and stomach by means of an endoscope

esoph•a•go•gas•tros•to•my \-ˌgas-ˈträs-tə-mē\ *n, pl* **-mies** : the surgical formation of an artificial communication between the esophagus and the stomach

esoph•a•go•je•ju•nos•to•my \-ˌje-jə-ˈnäs-tə-mē\ *n, pl* **-mies** : the surgical formation of an artificial communication between the esophagus and the jejunum

esoph•a•go•my•ot•o•my \-mī-ˈä-tə-mē\ *n, pl* **-mies** : incision through the musculature of the esophagus and esp. the distal part (as for the relief of esophageal achalasia)

esoph•a•go•plas•ty \i-ˈsä-fə-gə-ˌplas-tē\ *n, pl* **-ties** : plastic surgery for the repair or reconstruction of the esophagus

esoph•a•go•scope \-ˌskōp\ *n* : an endoscope for inspecting the interior of the esophagus

esoph•a•gos•co•py \i-ˌsä-fə-ˈgäs-kə-pē\ *n, pl* **-pies** : examination of the esophagus by means of an esophagoscope — **esoph•a•go•scop•ic** \i-ˌsä-fə-gə-ˈskä-pik\ *adj*

esophagostomiasis *var of* OESOPHAGOSTOMIASIS

esoph•a•gos•to•my \i-ˌsä-fə-ˈgäs-tə-mē\ *n, pl* **-mies** : surgical creation of an artificial opening into the esophagus

esoph•a•got•o•my \-ˈgä-tə-mē\ *n, pl* **-mies** : incision of the esophagus (as for the removal of an obstruction or the relief of esophageal achalasia)

esoph•a•gus \i-ˈsä-fə-gəs\ *n, pl* **-gi** \-ˌgī, -ˌjī\ : a muscular tube that in adult humans is about nine inches (23 centimeters) long and passes from the pharynx down the neck between the trachea and the spinal column and behind the left bronchus where it pierces the diaphragm slightly to the left of the middle line and joins the cardiac end of the stomach

es•o•pho•ria \ˌe-sə-ˈfōr-ē-ə, *sometimes* ˌē-\ *n* : squint in which the eyes tend to turn inward toward the nose

es•o•tro•pia \ˌe-sə-ˈtrō-pē-ə, ˌē-\ *n* : CROSS-EYE 1 — **es•o•trop•ic** \-ˈträ-pik\ *adj*

ESP \ˌē-(ˌ)es-ˈpē\ *n* : EXTRASENSORY PERCEPTION

es•pun•dia \is-ˈpün-dē-ə, -ˈpu̇n-\ *n* : mucocutaneous leishmaniasis of the mouth, pharynx, and nose that is prevalent in Central and So. America — compare UTA

ESR *abbr* erythrocyte sedimentation rate

ESRD *abbr* end-stage renal disease

es•sen•tial \i-ˈsen-chəl\ *adj* **1** : being a substance that is not synthesized by the body in a quantity sufficient for normal health and growth and that must be obtained from the diet ⟨~ fatty acids⟩ — compare NONESSENTIAL **2** : having no obvious or known cause : IDIOPATHIC ⟨~ disease⟩

essential amino acid *n* : any of various alpha-amino acids that are required for normal health and growth, are either not manufactured in the body or manufactured in insufficient quantities, are usu. supplied by dietary protein, and in humans include histidine, isoleucine, leucine, lysine, methionine, phenylalanine, threonine, tryptophan, and valine

essential hypertension *n* : a common form of hypertension that occurs in the absence of any evident cause, is marked by elevated peripheral vascular resistance, and has multiple risk factors (as family history of hypertension, obesity, and sedentary lifestyle) — called also *idiopathic hypertension, primary hypertension;* see MALIGNANT HYPERTENSION

essential oil *n* : any of a large class of volatile oils of vegetable origin that give plants their characteristic odors and are used esp. in perfumes, flavorings, and pharmaceutical preparations — called also *volatile oil*

essential thrombocythemia *n* : THROMBOCYTHEMIA

essential tremor *n* : a common usu. familial disorder of movement characterized by involuntary rhythmic trembling of the hands usu. with nodding of the head and tremulousness of the voice

EST *abbr* electroshock therapy

es•ter \ˈes-tər\ *n* : any of a class of often fragrant compounds that can be represented by the formula RCOOR′ and that are usu. formed by the reaction between an acid and an alcohol usu. with elimination of water

es•ter•ase \ˈes-tə-ˌrās, -ˌrāz\ *n* : an enzyme that accelerates the hydrolysis or synthesis of esters

es•ter•i•fy \e-ˈster-ə-ˌfī\ *vb* **-fied; -fy•ing** : to convert into an ester — **es•ter•i•fi•ca•tion** \e-ˌster-ə-fə-ˈkā-shən\ *n*

estr- *or* **estro-** *comb form* : estrus ⟨*es*trogen⟩

Es•trace \ˈe-ˌstrās\ *trademark* — used for a preparation of estradiol

Es•tra•derm \ˈe-strə-dərm\ *trademark* — used for a preparation of estradiol

es•tra•di•ol \ˌes-trə-ˈdī-ˌȯl, -ˌōl\ *n* : a natural estrogenic hormone $C_{18}H_{24}O_2$ secreted chiefly by the ovaries that is the most potent of the naturally occurring estrogens and is administered in its natural or semisynthetic esterified form esp. to treat menopausal symptoms — called also *dihydrotheelin;* see ESTRACE, ESTRADERM, ESTRING

es•tral cycle \ˈes-trəl-\ *n* : ESTROUS CYCLE

es•trin \ˈes-trən\ *n* : an estrogenic hormone; *esp* : ESTRONE

Es•tring \ˈes-triŋ\ *trademark* — used for a flexible ring containing estradiol that is inserted into the upper part of the vagina

es•tri•ol \ˈes-ˌtrī-ˌȯl, e-ˈstrī-, -ˌōl\ *n* : a relatively weak natural estrogenic hormone $C_{18}H_{24}O_3$ that is found in the body chiefly as a metabolite of estradiol, is the main estrogen secreted by the placenta during pregnancy, and is the estrogen typically found in the urine of pregnant women

estro- — see ESTR-

es•tro•gen \ˈes-trə-jən\ *n* : any of various natural steroids (as estradiol) that are formed from androgen precursors, are secreted chiefly by the ovaries, placenta, adipose tissue, and testes, and stimulate the development of female secondary sex characteristics and promote the growth and maintenance of the female reproductive system; *also* : any of various synthetic or semisynthetic steroids (as ethinyl estradiol) that mimic the physiological effect of natural estrogens — **es•tro•gen–like** \-ˌlīk\ *adj*

es•tro•gen•ic \ˌes-trə-ˈje-nik\ *adj* **1** : promoting estrus **2** : of, relating to, caused by, or being an estrogen — **es•tro•gen•i•cal•ly** \-ni-k(ə-)lē\ *adv* — **es•tro•gen•ic•i•ty** \-jə-ˈni-sə-tē\ *n*

estrogen replacement therapy *n* : the administration of estrogen esp. to treat menopausal symptoms and prevent postmenopausal osteoporosis — abbr. *ERT*

es•trone \ˈes-ˌtrōn\ *n* : a natural estrogenic hormone that is a ketone $C_{18}H_{22}O_2$ found in the body chiefly as a metabolite of estradiol, is also secreted esp. by the ovaries, and is used to treat various conditions relating to estrogen deficiency (as ovarian failure and menopausal symptoms)

es•trous \ˈes-trəs\ *adj* **1** : of, relating to, or characteristic of estrus **2** : being in heat

estrous cycle *n* : the correlated phenomena of the endocrine and generative systems of a female mammal from the beginning of one period of estrus to the beginning of the next — called also *estral cycle, estrus cycle*

es•tru•al \ˈes-trə-wəl\ *adj* : ESTROUS

es•trus \ˈes-trəs\ *n* : a regularly recurrent state of sexual excitability during which the female of most mammals will accept the male and is capable of conceiving : HEAT; *also* : a single occurrence of this state

es•zo•pic•lone \ˌes-zō-ˈpi-ˌklōn\ *n* : a sedative and hypnotic drug $C_{17}H_{17}ClN_6O_3$ used to treat insomnia — see LUNESTA

etan•er•cept \i-ˈtan-ər-ˌsept\ *n* : a drug produced by recombinant DNA technology that binds to and blocks the action of tumor necrosis factor and is administered by injection to treat various inflammatory diseases (as psoriatic arthritis and ankylosing spondylitis) — see ENBREL

eth•a•cryn•ic acid \ˌe-thə-ˈkri-nik-\ *n* : a potent synthetic diuretic $C_{13}H_{12}Cl_2O_4$ used esp. to treat edema

eth•am•bu•tol \e-ˈtham-byu̇-ˌtȯl, -ˌtōl\ *n* : a synthetic drug used in the form of its dihydrochloride $C_{10}H_{24}N_2O_2 \cdot 2HCl$ esp. in the treatment of tuberculosis — see MYAMBUTOL

etha•mi•van \e-ˈtha-mə-ˌvan, ˌe-thə-ˈmī-vən\ *n* : a central nervous stimulant $C_{12}H_{17}NO_3$ used esp. formerly as a respiratory stimulant

eth·a·nol \ˈe-thə-ˌnȯl, -ˌnōl\ *n* : a colorless volatile flammable liquid C_2H_5OH that is the intoxicating agent in liquors and is also used as a solvent — called also *ethyl alcohol, grain alcohol;* see ALCOHOL 1

eth·chlor·vy·nol \eth-ˈklȯr-və-ˌnȯl, -ˌnōl\ *n* : a hypnotic and sedative drug C_7H_9ClO used esp. to treat insomnia — see PLACIDYL

eth·ene \ˈe-ˌthēn\ *n* : ETHYLENE

ether \ˈē-thər\ *n* **1** : a light volatile flammable liquid $C_4H_{10}O$ used esp. formerly as an anesthetic — called also *diethyl ether, ethyl ether* **2** : any of various organic compounds characterized by an oxygen atom attached to two carbon atoms

ether·ize \ˈē-thə-ˌrīz\ *vb* **-ized; -iz·ing** : to treat or anesthetize with ether

¹eth·i·cal \ˈe-thi-kəl\ *also* **eth·ic** \-thik\ *adj* **1** : conforming to accepted professional standards of conduct **2** *of a drug* : restricted to sale only on a doctor's prescription — **eth·i·cal·ly** \-thi-k(ə-)lē\ *adv*

²ethical *n* : an ethical drug

eth·ics \ˈe-thiks\ *n sing or pl* : the principles of conduct governing an individual or a group 〈medical ∼〉

ethid·ium bromide \e-ˈthi-dē-əm-\ *n* : a biological dye $C_{21}H_{20}BrN_3$ that is used esp. to stain nucleic acids

ethi·nyl estradiol *or* **ethy·nyl·es·tra·di·ol** \ˈe-thə-nil-ˌes-trə-ˈdī-ˌȯl, -ˌōl\ *n* : a potent synthetic estrogen $C_{20}H_{24}O_2$ used in combination (as with norgestrel or norethindrone) as a birth control pill or alone in the treatment of menopausal symptoms or female hypogonadism or in the palliative treatment of prostate or breast cancer — see LOESTRIN, MINASTRIN, NUVARING, ORTHO EVRA, ORTHO-NOVUM, ORTHO TRI-CYCLEN, SEASONALE, SEASONIQUE, YASMIN, YAZ

eth·i·on·amide \ˌe-thē-ˈä-nə-ˌmīd\ *n* : a compound $C_8H_{10}N_2S$ used against mycobacteria (as in tuberculosis)

ethi·o·nine \e-ˈthī-ə-ˌnēn\ *n* : an amino acid $C_6H_{13}NO_2S$ that is biologically antagonistic to methionine

ethis·ter·one \i-ˈthis-tə-ˌrōn\ *n* : a synthetic female sex hormone $C_{21}H_{28}O_2$ administered in cases of progesterone deficiency — called also *anhydrohydroxyprogesterone*

ethmo- *comb form* : ethmoid and 〈*ethmo*maxillary〉

¹eth·moid \ˈeth-ˌmȯid\ *or* **eth·moi·dal** \eth-ˈmȯid-ᵊl\ *adj* : of, relating to, adjoining, or being one or more bones of the walls and septum of the nasal cavity

²ethmoid *n* : ETHMOID BONE

ethmoidal air cells *n pl* : the cavities in the lateral masses of the ethmoid bone that communicate with the nasal cavity

ethmoid bone *n* : a light spongy cubical bone forming much of the walls of the nasal cavity and part of those of the orbits

eth·moid·ec·to·my \ˌeth-ˌmȯi-ˈdek-tə-mē\ *n, pl* **-mies** : excision of all or some of the ethmoidal air cells or part of the ethmoid bone

eth·moid·itis \-ˈdī-təs\ *n* : inflammation of the ethmoid bone or its sinuses

ethmoid sinus *also* **ethmoidal sinus** *n* : either of two sinuses each of which is situated in a lateral part of the ethmoid bone alongside the nose and consists of ethmoidal air cells

eth·mo·max·il·lary \ˌeth-(ˌ)mō-ˈmak-sə-ˌler-ē\ *adj* : of or relating to the ethmoid and maxillary bones

eth·no·med·i·cine \ˌeth-nō-ˈme-də-sən\ *n* : the comparative study of how different cultures view disease and how they treat or prevent it; *also* : the medical beliefs and practices of indigenous cultures — **eth·no·med·i·cal** \-ˈme-di-kəl\ *adj*

etho·sux·i·mide \ˌe-(ˌ)thō-ˈsək-sə-ˌmīd, -məd\ *n* : an anticonvulsant drug $C_7H_{11}NO_2$ used to treat epilepsy

eth·o·to·in \ˌe-thə-ˈtō-ən\ *n* : an anticonvulsant drug $C_{11}H_{12}N_2O_2$ used to treat epilepsy — see PEGANONE

eth·yl \ˈe-thəl\ *n* : a monovalent hydrocarbon radical C_2H_5

ethyl alcohol *n* : ETHANOL

ethyl aminobenzoate *n* : BENZOCAINE

ethyl bromide *n* : a volatile liquid compound C_2H_5Br used as an inhalation anesthetic

ethyl carbamate *n* : URETHANE

ethyl chloride *n* : a pungent flammable gaseous or volatile liquid C_2H_5Cl used esp. as a topical anesthetic

eth·yl·ene \ˈe-thə-ˌlēn\ *n* : a colorless flammable gaseous unsaturated hydrocarbon C_2H_4 used in medicine as a general inhalation anesthetic and occurring in plants where it functions esp. as a natural growth regulator that promotes the ripening of fruit — called also *ethene*

ethylene bromide *n* : ETHYLENE DIBROMIDE

eth·yl·ene·di·amine \ˌe-thə-ˌlēn-ˈdī-ə-ˌmēn, -dī-ˈa-mən\ *n* : a colorless volatile liquid base $C_2H_8N_2$ used in medicine to stabilize aminophylline when used in injections

eth·yl·ene·di·amine·tetra·ac·e·tate \ˌe-thə-ˌlēn-ˌdī-ə-ˌmen-ˌte-trə-ˈa-sə-ˌtāt, -dī-ˌa-mən-\ *n* : a salt of EDTA

eth·yl·ene·di·amine·tetra·ace·tic acid \-ə-ˈsē-tik-\ *n* : EDTA

ethylene di·bro·mide \-dī-ˈbrō-ˌmīd\ *n* : a colorless toxic liquid compound $C_2H_4Br_2$ that has been shown by experiments with laboratory animals to be strongly carcinogenic and that was formerly used in the U.S. as an agricultural pesticide — abbr. *EDB;* called also *ethylene bromide*

ethylene glycol *n* : a thick liquid alcohol $C_2H_6O_2$ used esp. as an antifreeze

ethylene oxide *n* : a colorless flammable toxic gaseous or liquid compound

C_2H_4O used in fumigation and sterilization (as of medical instruments)

eth·yl·es·tren·ol \ˌe-thəl-ˈes-trə-ˌnȯl, -ˌnōl\ *n* : an anabolic steroid $C_{20}H_{32}O$ having androgenic activity

ethyl ether *n* : ETHER 1

eth·yl·mor·phine \ˌe-thəl-ˈmȯr-ˌfēn\ *n* : a synthetic toxic alkaloid used esp. in the form of its hydrochloride $C_{19}H_{23}NO_3 \cdot HCl$ similarly to morphine and codeine

eth·y·no·di·ol diacetate \ˌe-thi-nō-ˈdī-ˌōl, -ˌȯl-\ *n* : a synthetic progestogen $C_{24}H_{32}O_4$ used esp. in birth control pills usu. in combination with an estrogen

ethynylestradiol *var of* ETHINYL ESTRADIOL

et·i·dro·nate \ˌē-tə-ˈdrō-ˌnāt, ˌe-\ *n* : a white disodium bisphosphonate salt $C_2H_6Na_2O_7P_2$ that inhibits the formation, growth, and dissolution of hydroxyapatite crystals — called also *etidronate disodium*

etio- *comb form* : cause ⟨*etio*logic⟩

etio·chol·an·ol·one \ˌē-tē-ō-ˌkō-ˈla-nə-ˌlōn, ˌe-\ *n* : a testosterone metabolite $C_{19}H_{30}O_2$ that occurs in urine

eti·o·log·ic \ˌē-tē-ə-ˈlä-jik\ *or* **eti·o·log·i·cal** \-ji-kəl\ *adj* **1** : of, relating to, or based on etiology ⟨~ investigations⟩ **2** : causing or contributing to the cause of a disease or condition — **eti·o·log·i·cal·ly** \-ji-k(ə-)lē\ *adv*

eti·ol·o·gy \ˌē-tē-ˈä-lə-jē\ *n, pl* **-gies 1** : the cause or causes of a disease or abnormal condition **2** : a branch of medical science dealing with the causes and origin of diseases

etio·patho·gen·e·sis \ˌē-tē-ō-ˌpa-thə-ˈje-nə-səs, ˌe-\ *n, pl* **-e·ses** \-ˌsēz\ : the cause and development of a disease or abnormal condition

et·o·no·ges·trel \ˌet-ə-nō-ˈjes-trəl\ *n* : a synthetic progestin $C_{22}H_{28}O_2$ used alone or in combination with an estrogen to prevent pregnancy — see NEXPLANON, NUVARING

eto·po·side \ˌē-tə-ˈpō-ˌsīd, ˌe-\ *n* : a drug $C_{29}H_{32}O_{13}$ used to treat various neoplastic diseases (as carcinoma of the lungs, acute myelogenous leukemia, and Ewing's sarcoma)

etor·phine \ē-ˈtȯr-ˌfēn, i-\ *n* : a synthetic narcotic drug $C_{25}H_{33}NO_4$ related to morphine but with more potent analgesic properties

etret·i·nate \i-ˈtre-tᵊn-ˌāt\ *n* : a retinoid drug $C_{23}H_{30}O_3$ used esp. to treat severe psoriasis that has been withdrawn from use in the U.S. for its tendency to cause birth defects

eu- *comb form* **1** : good : normal ⟨*eu*thyroid⟩ **2** : true ⟨*eu*globulin⟩

Eu *symbol* europium

eu·ca·lyp·tol *also* **eu·ca·lyp·tole** \ˌyü-kə-ˈlip-ˌtōl, -ˌtȯl\ *n* : a liquid $C_{10}H_{18}O$ with an odor of camphor that occurs in many essential oils (as of eucalyptus) and is used esp. as an expectorant — called also *cajeputol, cineole*

eu·ca·lyp·tus oil \ˌyü-kə-ˈlip-təs-\ *n* : any of various essential oils obtained from the leaves of an Australian tree (genus *Eucalyptus* and esp. *E. globulus*) of the myrtle family (Myrtaceae) and used in pharmaceutical preparations (as antiseptics or cough drops)

euc·at·ro·pine \yü-ˈka-trə-ˌpēn\ *n* : a synthetic alkaloid used in the form of its white crystalline hydrochloride $C_{17}H_{25}NO_3 \cdot HCl$ as a mydriatic

eu·chro·ma·tin \(ˌ)yü-ˈkrō-mə-tən\ *n* : the genetically active portion of chromatin that is largely composed of genes — **eu·chro·mat·ic** \ˌyü-krō-ˈma-tik\ *adj*

eu·ge·nol \ˈyü-jə-ˌnȯl, -ˌnōl\ *n* : an aromatic liquid phenol $C_{10}H_{12}O_2$ found esp. in clove oil and used in dentistry as an analgesic

eu·glob·u·lin \yü-ˈglä-byə-lən\ *n* : a simple protein that does not dissolve in pure water

eu·gly·ce·mia \ˌyü-ˌglī-ˈsē-mē-ə\ *n* : a normal level of sugar in the blood

eu·kary·ote *also* **eu·cary·ote** \(ˌ)yü-ˈkar-ē-ˌōt, -ē-ət\ *n* : an organism composed of one or more cells containing visibly evident nuclei and organelles — compare PROKARYOTE — **eu·kary·ot·ic** *also* **eu·cary·ot·ic** \-ˌkar-ē-ˈä-tik\ *adj*

eu·nuch \ˈyü-nək, -nik\ *n* : a man or boy deprived of the testes or external genitals — **eu·nuch·ism** \-nə-ˌki-zəm, -ni-\ *n*

eu·nuch·oid·ism \ˈyü-nə-ˌkȯi-ˌdi-zəm\ *n* : a state marked by deficiency of sexual development, by persistence of prepubertal characteristics, and often by the presence of characteristics typical of the opposite sex — **eu·nuch·oid** \ˈyü-nə-ˌkȯid\ *adj*

eu·pep·sia \yu̇-ˈpep-shə, -sē-ə\ *n* : good digestion — **eu·pep·tic** \-ˈpep-tik\ *adj*

eu·phen·ics \yu̇-ˈfe-niks\ *n* : the amelioration of the deleterious phenotypic effects of a genetic disorder (as phenylketonuria) that involves treatment (as a change in diet) that alters the environment but not the genetic makeup of an individual

eu·pho·ria \yu̇-ˈfōr-ē-ə\ *n* : a feeling of well-being or elation; *esp* : one that is groundless, disproportionate to its cause, or inappropriate to one's life situation — compare DYSPHORIA — **eu·phor·ic** \-ˈfōr-ik, -ˈfär-\ *adj* — **eu·phor·i·cal·ly** \-i-k(ə-)lē\ *adv*

¹eu·pho·ri·ant \yu̇-ˈfōr-ē-ənt\ *n* : a drug that tends to induce euphoria

²euphoriant *adj* : tending to induce euphoria ⟨a ~ drug⟩

eu·phor·i·gen·ic \yu̇-ˌfōr-ə-ˈje-nik\ *adj* : tending to cause euphoria

eup·nea \yu̇p-ˈnē-ə\ *n* : normal respiration — compare DYSPNEA — **eup·ne·ic** \-ˈnē-ik\ *adj*

eup·noea *chiefly Brit var of* EUPNEA

eu·ro·pi·um \yu̇-ˈrō-pē-əm\ *n* : a bivalent and trivalent metallic element — symbol *Eu;* see ELEMENT table
-e·us \ē-əs\ *n comb form, pl* **-ei** \ē-ˌī\ *also* **-e·us·es** \ē-ə-səz\ : muscle that constitutes, has the form of, or joins a (specified) part, thing, or structure ⟨glut*eus*⟩ ⟨rhomboid*eus*⟩
eu·sta·chian tube \yu̇-ˈstā-shən-, -shē-ən-, -kē-ən-\ *n, often cap E* : a bony and cartilaginous tube connecting the middle ear with the nasopharynx and equalizing air pressure on both sides of the tympanic membrane — called also *auditory tube, pharyngotympanic tube*
Eu·sta·chio \āü-ˈstäk-yō\, **Bartolomeo (*ca* 1520–1574),** Italian anatomist.
eu·stress \ˈyü-ˌstres\ *n* : a positive form of stress having a beneficial effect on health, motivation, performance, and emotional well-being
eu·tha·na·sia \ˌyü-thə-ˈnā-zhə, -zhē-ə\ *n* : the act or practice of causing or permitting the death of terminally ill or hopelessly sick or injured individuals in a relatively painless way for reasons of mercy
eu·than·ize \ˈyü-thə-ˌnīz\ *also* **eu·than·a·tize** \yu̇-ˈtha-nə-ˌtīz\ *vb* **-nized** *also* **-tized; -niz·ing** *also* **-tiz·ing** : to subject to euthanasia
eu·then·ics \yu̇-ˈthe-niks\ *n sing or pl* : a science that deals with development of human well-being by improvement of living conditions — **eu·the·nist** \yu̇-ˈthe-nist, ˈyü-thə-\ *n*
eu·thy·mia \yü-ˈthī-mē-ə\ *n* : a normal tranquil mental state or mood; *specif* : a stable mental state or mood in those affected with bipolar disorder that is not manic or depressive — **eu·thy·mic** \-mik\ *adj*
eu·thy·roid \(ˌ)yü-ˈthī-ˌrȯid\ *adj* : characterized by normal thyroid function — **eu·thy·roid·ism** \-ˌrȯi-ˌdi-zəm\ *n*
euvolaemia *chiefly Brit var of* EUVOLEMIA
eu·vo·le·mia \ˌyü-vō-ˈlē-mē-ə\ *n* : NORMOVOLEMIA — **eu·vo·le·mic** \-mik\ *adj*
evac·u·ant \i-ˈva-kyə-wənt\ *n* : an emetic, diuretic, or purgative agent — **evacuant** *adj*
evac·u·ate \i-ˈva-kyə-ˌwāt\ *vb* **-at·ed; -at·ing** **1** : to remove the contents of ⟨∼ an abscess⟩ **2** : to discharge (as urine or feces) from the body as waste : VOID — **evac·u·a·tive** \-ˌwā-tiv\ *adj*
evac·u·a·tion \i-ˌva-kyə-ˈwā-shən\ *n* **1** : the act or process of evacuating **2** : something evacuated or discharged
evag·i·na·tion \i-ˌva-jə-ˈnā-shən\ *n* **1** : a process of turning outward or inside out ⟨∼ of a cell membrane⟩ **2** : a part or structure that is produced by evagination — **evag·i·nate** \i-ˈva-jə-ˌnāt\ *vb*
ev·a·nes·cent \ˌe-və-ˈnes-ᵊnt\ *adj* : tending to disappear quickly : of relatively short duration ⟨an ∼ rash⟩
Ev·ans blue \ˈe-vənz-\ *n* : a dye $C_{34}H_{24}N_6Na_4O_{14}S_4$ that on injection into the bloodstream combines with serum albumin and is used to determine blood volume colorimetrically
Evans, Herbert McLean (1882–1971), American anatomist and physiologist.
event \i-ˈvent\ *n* : an adverse or damaging medical occurrence ⟨a heart attack or other cardiac ∼⟩
even·tra·tion \ˌē-ˌven-ˈtrā-shən\ *n* : protrusion of abdominal organs through the abdominal wall
ev·e·ro·li·mus \ˌe-və-ˈrō-lə-məs\ *n* : an immunosuppressive drug $C_{53}H_{83}NO_{14}$ used esp. to prevent rejection of transplanted organs and to treat some advanced forms of cancer — see AFINITOR, ZORTRESS
ever·sion \i-ˈvər-zhən, -shən\ *n* **1** : the act of turning inside out : the state of being turned inside out ⟨∼ of the eyelid⟩ **2** : the condition (as of the foot) of being turned or rotated outward — compare INVERSION 1b
evert \i-ˈvərt\ *vb* : to turn outward ⟨∼ the foot⟩; *also* : to turn inside out
evis·cer·ate \i-ˈvi-sə-ˌrāt\ *vb* **-at·ed; -at·ing** **1 a** : to remove the viscera of **b** : to remove an organ from (a patient) or the contents of (an organ) **2** : to protrude through a surgical incision or suffer protrusion of a part through an incision — **evis·cer·a·tion** \i-ˌvi-sə-ˈrā-shən\ *n*
Evis·ta \ē-ˈvi-stə\ *trademark* — used for a preparation of raloxifene
evo·ca·tion \ˌē-vō-ˈkā-shən, ˌe-\ *n* : INDUCTION 2b
evo·ca·tor \ˈē-vō-ˌkā-tər, ˈe-\ *n* : the specific chemical constituent responsible for the physiological effects of an organizer
evoked potential \ē-ˈvōkt-\ *n* : an electrical response esp. in the cerebral cortex as recorded following stimulation of a peripheral sense receptor
evo·lu·tion \ˌe-və-ˈlü-shən, ˌē-\ *n* **1** : a process of change in a certain direction **2 a** : the historical development of a biological group (as a race or species) : PHYLOGENY **b** : a theory that the various types of animals and plants have their origin in other preexisting types and that the distinguishable differences are due to modifications in successive generations — **evo·lu·tion·ary** \-shə-ˌner-ē\ *adj*
evolve \i-ˈvälv, -ˈvȯlv\ *vb* **evolved; evolv·ing** : to produce or develop by natural evolutionary processes
Evo·taz \ˈē-vō-ˌtaz\ *trademark* — used for a preparation of atazanavir and cobicistat
evul·sion \i-ˈvəl-shən\ *n* **1** : the act of extracting forcibly : EXTRACTION ⟨∼

of a tooth> **2** : AVULSION <~ of the biceps tendon> — **evulse** \i-ˈvəls\ *vb*

Ev•zio \ˈev-zē-(ˌ)ō\ *trademark* — used for a preparation of the hydrochloride of naloxone administered by injection

Ew•ing's sarcoma \ˈyü-iŋz-\ *n* : a malignant bone tumor esp. of a long bone or the pelvis — called also *Ewing's tumor*

Ewing, James (1866–1943), American pathologist.

ex- — see EXO-

ex•ac•er•bate \ig-ˈza-sər-ˌbāt\ *vb* **-bat•ed; -bat•ing** : to cause (a disease or its symptoms) to become more severe — **ex•ac•er•ba•tion** \-ˌza-sər-ˈbā-shən\ *n*

ex•al•ta•tion \ˌeg-ˌzȯl-ˈtā-shən, ˌek-ˌsȯl-\ *n* **1** : marked or excessive intensification of a mental state or of the activity of a bodily part or function **2** : an abnormal sense of personal well-being, power, or importance : a delusional euphoria

ex•am \ig-ˈzam\ *n* : EXAMINATION

ex•am•i•na•tion \ig-ˌza-mə-ˈnā-shən\ *n* : the act or process of inspecting or testing for evidence of disease or abnormality — see PHYSICAL EXAMINATION — **ex•am•ine** \ig-ˈza-mən\ *vb*

ex•am•in•ee \ig-ˌza-mə-ˈnē\ *n* : a person who is examined

ex•am•in•er \ig-ˈza-mə-nər\ *n* : one that examines — see MEDICAL EXAMINER

ex•an•them \eg-ˈzan-thəm, ˈek-ˌsan-ˌthem\ *or* **ex•an•the•ma** \ˌeg-ˌzan-ˈthē-mə\ *n, pl* **-thems** *also* **-them•a•ta** \ˌeg-ˌzan-ˈthe-mə-tə\ *or* **-themas** : an eruptive disease (as measles) or its symptomatic eruption — **ex•an•them•a•tous** \ˌeg-ˌzan-ˈthe-mə-təs\ *or* **ex•an•the•mat•ic** \-ˌzan-thə-ˈma-tik\ *adj*

exanthema su•bi•tum *or* **exanthem subitum** \-sə-ˈbī-təm\ *n* : ROSEOLA INFANTUM

ex•ca•va•tion \ˌek-skə-ˈvā-shən\ *n* **1** : the action or process of forming or undergoing formation of a cavity or hole **2** : a cavity formed by or as if by cutting, digging, or scooping — **ex•ca•vate** \ˈek-skə-ˌvāt\ *vb*

ex•ca•va•tor \ˈek-skə-ˌvā-tər\ *n* : an instrument used to open bodily cavities (as in the teeth) or remove material from them

excavatum — see PECTUS EXCAVATUM

ex•ce•men•to•sis \ˌeks-si-ˌmen-ˈtō-səs\ *n, pl* **-to•ses** \-ˌsēz\ *or* **-to•sis•es** : abnormal outgrowth of the cementum of the root of a tooth

ex•change transfusion \iks-ˈchānj-\ *n* : simultaneous withdrawal of the recipient's blood and transfusion with the donor's blood esp. in the treatment of erythroblastosis

ex•ci•mer laser \ˈek-si-ˌmər-\ *n* : a laser that uses a compound of a halogen and a noble gas to generate radiation usu. in the ultraviolet region of the spectrum — called also *excimer*

ex•cip•i•ent \ik-ˈsi-pē-ənt\ *n* : a usu. inert substance (as starch) that forms a vehicle (as for a drug)

ex•ci•sion \ik-ˈsi-zhən\ *n* : surgical removal or resection (as of a diseased part) — **ex•cise** \-ˈsīz\ *vb* — **ex•ci•sion•al** \-ˈsi-zhə-nəl\ *adj*

ex•cit•able \ik-ˈsī-tə-bəl\ *adj, of living tissue or an organism* : capable of being activated by and reacting to stimuli : exhibiting irritability — **ex•cit•abil•i•ty** \-ˌsī-tə-ˈbi-lə-tē\ *n*

ex•ci•tant \ik-ˈsīt-ᵊnt, ˈek-sə-tənt\ *n* : an agent that arouses or augments physiological activity (as of the nervous system) — **excitant** *adj*

ex•ci•ta•tion \ˌek-ˌsī-ˈtā-shən, -sə-\ *n* : EXCITEMENT: as **a** : the disturbed or altered condition resulting from arousal of activity (as by neural or electrical stimulation) in an individual organ or tissue **b** : the arousing of such activity

ex•cit•ato•ry \ik-ˈsī-tə-ˌtōr-ē\ *adj* **1** : tending to induce excitation (as of a neuron) **2** : exhibiting, resulting from, related to, or produced by excitement or excitation

ex•cite \ik-ˈsīt\ *vb* **ex•cit•ed; ex•cit•ing** : to increase the activity of (as a living organism) : STIMULATE

ex•cite•ment \-ˈsīt-mənt\ *n* **1** : the act of exciting **2** : the state of being excited: as **a** : aroused, augmented, or abnormal activity of an organism or functioning of an organ or part **b** : extreme motor hyperactivity (as in catatonic schizophrenia or bipolar disorder)

ex•ci•to•tox•ic \ik-ˌsī-tə-ˈtäk-sik\ *adj* : being, involving, or resulting from the action of an agent that binds to a nerve cell receptor, stimulates the cell, and damages it or causes its death <~ neuronal death> — **ex•ci•to•tox•ic•i•ty** \-(ˌ)täk-ˈsi-sə-tē\ *n*

ex•ci•to•tox•in \ik-ˈsī-tə-ˌtäk-sən\ *n* : an excitotoxic agent

ex•co•ri•a•tion \(ˌ)ek-ˌskōr-ē-ˈā-shən\ *n* **1** : the act of abrading or wearing off the skin **2** : a raw irritated lesion (as of the skin or a mucosal surface) — **ex•co•ri•ate** \ek-ˈskōr-ē-āt\ *vb*

ex•cre•ment \ˈek-skrə-mənt\ *n* : waste matter discharged from the body; *esp* : FECES — **ex•cre•men•tal** \ˌek-skrə-ˈment-ᵊl\ *adj*

ex•cres•cence \ik-ˈskres-ᵊns\ *n* : an outgrowth or enlargement: as **a** : a natural and normal appendage or development **b** : an abnormal outgrowth — **ex•cres•cent** \ik-ˈskres-ᵊnt\ *adj*

ex•cre•ta \ik-ˈskrē-tə\ *n pl* : waste matter (as feces) eliminated or discharged from the body — compare EXCRETION 2 — **ex•cre•tal** \-ˈskrē-təl\ *adj*

ex•crete \ik-ˈskrēt\ *vb* **ex•cret•ed; ex•cret•ing** : to separate and eliminate or discharge (waste) from the blood, tissues, or organs or from the active protoplasm

ex•cret•er \-ˈskrē-tər\ *n* : one that excretes something and esp. an atypical bodily product (as a pathogenic microorganism)

ex•cre•tion \ik-ˈskrē-shən\ *n* **1** : the act or process of excreting **2 a** : something excreted; *esp* : a metabolic waste product (as urea or carbon dioxide) that is eliminated from the body and is distinguished from waste materials (as feces) that have merely passed into or through the digestive tract without being incorporated into the body proper **b** : waste material (as feces) discharged from the body : EXCREMENT — not used technically

ex•cre•to•ry \ˈek-skrə-ˌtōr-ē\ *adj* : of, relating to, or functioning in excretion ⟨∼ ducts⟩

ex•cur•sion \ik-ˈskər-zhən\ *n* **1** : a movement outward and back or from a mean position or axis **2** : one complete movement of expansion and contraction of the lungs and their membranes (as in breathing)

ex•cyst \ˌeks-ˈsist\ *vb* : to emerge from a cyst — **ex•cys•ta•tion** \ˌeks-ˌsis-ˈtā-shən\ *n* — **ex•cyst•ment** \ˌeks-ˈsist-mənt\ *n*

Ex•e•lon \ˈek-sə-ˌlän\ *trademark* — used for a transdermal patch containing rivastigmine or an oral preparation of the tartrate of rivastigmine

exe•mes•tane \ˌek-sə-ˈmes-ˌtān\ *n* : a steroidal aromatase inhibitor $C_{20}H_{24}O_2$ administered orally to treat advanced breast cancer in postmenopausal women — see AROMASIN

ex•en•ter•a•tion \ig-ˌzen-tə-ˈrā-shən\ *n* : surgical removal of the contents of a bodily cavity (as the orbit or pelvis) — **ex•en•ter•ate** \ig-ˈzen-tə-ˌrāt\ *vb*

ex•er•cise \ˈek-sər-ˌsīz\ *n* **1** : regular or repeated use of a faculty or bodily organ **2** : bodily exertion for the sake of developing and maintaining physical fitness — **exercise** *vb*

ex•er•cis•er \ˈek-sər-ˌsī-zər\ *n* **1** : one that exercises **2** : an apparatus for use in physical exercise

ex•er•e•sis \ig-ˈzer-ə-səs\ *n, pl* **-e•ses** \-ˌsēz\ : surgical removal of a part or organ (as a nerve)

ex•er•tion•al \ig-ˈzər-shə-nəl\ *adj* : precipitated by physical exertion but usu. relieved by rest ⟨∼ dyspnea⟩

ex•flag•el•la•tion \(ˌ)eks-ˌfla-jə-ˈlā-shən\ *n* : the formation of microgametes in sporozoans (as the malaria parasite) by extrusion of nuclear material into peripheral processes resembling flagella

ex•fo•liant \(ˌ)eks-ˈfō-lē-ənt\ *n* : a mechanical or chemical agent (as an abrasive skin wash or salicylic acid) that is applied to the skin to remove dead cells from the surface — called also *exfoliator*

ex•fo•li•ate \(ˌ)eks-ˈfō-lē-ˌāt\ *vb* **-at•ed; -at•ing** **1** : to cast or come off in scales or laminae **2** : to remove the surface of in scales or laminae **3** : to shed (teeth) by exfoliation

ex•fo•li•a•tion \(ˌ)eks-ˌfō-lē-ˈā-shən\ *n* : the action or process of exfoliating: as **a** : the peeling of the horny layer of the skin **b** : the shedding of surface components **c** : the shedding of a superficial layer of bone or of a tooth or part of a tooth — **ex•fo•li•a•tive** \eks-ˈfō-lē-ˌā-tiv\ *adj*

exfoliative cytology *n* : the microscopic study of cells shed or obtained from the body esp. for diagnostic purposes (as in determining the presence of a cancerous condition)

ex•fo•li•a•tor \(ˌ)eks-ˈfō-lē-ˌā-tər\ *n* : EXFOLIANT

Ex•forge \ˈeks-ˌfȯrj\ *trademark* — used for a preparation of amlodipine and valsartan

ex•ha•la•tion \ˌeks-hə-ˈlā-shən, ˌek-sə-ˈ\ *n* **1** : the action of forcing air out of the lungs **2** : something (as the breath) that is exhaled or given off — **ex•hale** \eks-ˈhāl, ek-ˈsāl\ *vb*

ex•haust \ig-ˈzȯst\ *vb* **1 a** : to draw off or let out completely **b** : to empty by drawing off the contents; *specif* : to create a vacuum in **2 a** : to use up : consume completely **b** : to tire extremely or completely **3** : to extract completely with a solvent

ex•haus•tion \ig-ˈzȯs-chən\ *n* **1** : the act or process of exhausting : the state of being exhausted **2** : neurosis following overstrain or overexertion esp. in military combat

ex•hi•bi•tion•ism \ˌek-sə-ˈbi-shə-ni-zəm\ *n* **1 a** : a perversion marked by a tendency to indecent exposure **b** : an act of such exposure **2** : the act or practice of behaving so as to attract attention to oneself — **ex•hi•bi•tion•ist** \-nist\ *n* — **ex•hi•bi•tion•is•tic** \-ˌbish-ə-ˈnis-tik\ *also* **exhibitionist** *adj*

ex•hume \ig-ˈzüm, igz-ˈyüm; iks-ˈhyüm, -ˈyüm\ *vb* **ex•humed; ex•hum•ing** : DISINTER — **ex•hu•ma•tion** \ˌeks-hyü-ˈmā-shən, ˌeks-yü-; ˌegz-yü-, ˌeg-zü-\ *n*

ex•i•tus \ˈek-sə-təs\ *n, pl* **exitus** : DEATH; *esp* : fatal termination of a disease

exo- *or* **ex-** *comb form* : outside : outer ⟨*exo*enzyme⟩

exo•crine \ˈek-sə-krən, -ˌkrīn, -ˌkrēn\ *adj* : producing, being, or relating to a secretion that is released outside its source ⟨∼ insufficiency⟩

exocrine gland *n* : a gland (as a salivary gland) that releases a secretion external to or at the surface of an organ by means of a canal or duct — called also *gland of external secretion*

exo•cri•nol•o•gy \ˌek-sə-kri-ˈnä-lə-jē, -ˌkrī-, -ˌkrē-\ *n, pl* **-gies** : the study of external secretions (as pheromones) that serve an integrative function

exo·cy·to·sis \ˌek-sō-sī-ˈtō-səs\ *n, pl* **-to·ses** \-ˌsēz\ : the release of cellular substances (as secretory products) contained in cell vesicles by fusion of the vesicular membrane with the plasma membrane and subsequent release of the contents to the exterior of the cell — **exo·cy·tot·ic** \-ˈtä-tik\ *adj*

ex·odon·tia \ˌek-sə-ˈdän-chə, -chē-ə\ *n* : a branch of dentistry that deals with the extraction of teeth — **ex·odon·tist** \-ˈdän-tist\ *n*

exo·en·zyme \ˌek-sō-ˈen-ˌzīm\ *n* : an extracellular enzyme

exo·eryth·ro·cyt·ic \ˌek-sō-i-ˌri-thrə-ˈsi-tik\ *adj* : occurring outside the red blood cells — used of stages of malaria parasites

ex·og·e·nous \ek-ˈsä-jə-nəs\ *also* **ex·o·gen·ic** \ˌek-sō-ˈje-nik\ *adj* **1** : growing from or on the outside **2** : caused by factors (as food or a traumatic event) or an agent (as a disease-producing organism) from outside the organism or system ⟨~ obesity⟩ **3** : introduced from or produced outside the organism or system; *specif* : not synthesized within the organism or system — compare ENDOGENOUS — **ex·og·e·nous·ly** *adv*

ex·om·pha·los \ek-ˈsäm-fə-ləs\ *n* : UMBILICAL HERNIA; *also* : OMPHALOCELE

ex·on \ˈek-ˌsän\ *n* : a polynucleotide sequence in a nucleic acid that codes information for protein synthesis and that is copied and spliced together with other such sequences to form messenger RNA — compare INTRON — **ex·on·ic** \ek-ˈsä-nik\ *adj*

exo·nu·cle·ase \ˌek-sō-ˈnü-klē-ˌās, -ˈnyü-, -ˌāz\ *n* : an enzyme that breaks down a nucleic acid by removing nucleotides one by one from the end of a chain — compare ENDONUCLEASE

exo·nu·cleo·lyt·ic \ˌek-sō-ˌnü-klē-ə-ˈli-tik, -ˌnyü-\ *adj* : breaking a nucleotide chain into two parts at a point adjacent to one of its ends

exo·pep·ti·dase \-ˈpep-tə-ˌdās, -ˌdāz\ *n* : any of a group of enzymes that hydrolyze peptide bonds formed by the terminal amino acids of peptide chains : PEPTIDASE — compare ENDOPEPTIDASE

ex·o·pho·ria \ˌek-sə-ˈfōr-ē-ə\ *n* : latent strabismus in which the visual axes tend outward toward the temple — compare HETEROPHORIA

ex·oph·thal·mia \ˌek-ˌsäf-ˈthal-mē-ə\ *n* : EXOPHTHALMOS

ex·oph·thal·mic goiter \ˌek-säf-ˈthal-mik-\ *n* : GRAVES' DISEASE

ex·oph·thal·mos *also* **ex·oph·thal·mus** \ˌek-säf-ˈthal-məs, -səf-\ *n* : abnormal protrusion of the eyeball — **exophthalmic** *adj*

exo·phyt·ic \ˌek-sō-ˈfi-tik\ *adj* : tending to grow outward beyond the surface epithelium from which it originates — used of tumors; compare ENDOPHYTIC

ex·os·tec·to·my \ˌek-(ˌ)säs-ˈtek-tə-mē\ *n, pl* **-mies** : excision of an exostosis

ex·os·to·sis \ˌek-(ˌ)säs-ˈtō-səs\ *n, pl* **-to·ses** \-ˌsēz\ : a spur or bony outgrowth from a bone or the root of a tooth — **ex·os·tot·ic** \-ˈtä-tik\ *adj*

exo·tox·in \ˌek-sō-ˈtäk-sən\ *n* : a soluble poisonous substance produced during growth of a microorganism and released into the surrounding medium — compare ENDOTOXIN

exo·tro·pia \ˌek-sə-ˈtrō-pē-ə\ *n* : WALLEYE 2a

ex·pand·er \ik-ˈspan-dər\ *n* : any of several colloidal substances (as dextran) of high molecular weight used as a blood or plasma substitute for increasing the blood volume — called also *extender*

ex·pect \ik-ˈspekt\ *vb* : to be pregnant : await the birth of one's child — used in progressive tenses ⟨she's ~*ing* next month⟩

ex·pec·tan·cy \-ˈspek-tən-sē\ *n, pl* **-cies** : the expected amount (as of the number of years of life) based on statistical probability — see LIFE EXPECTANCY

ex·pec·tant \-ˈspek-tənt\ *adj* : expecting the birth of a child ⟨~ mothers⟩

ex·pec·to·rant \ik-ˈspek-tə-rənt\ *n* : an agent that promotes the discharge or expulsion of mucus from the respiratory tract; *broadly* : ANTITUSSIVE — **expectorant** *adj*

ex·pec·to·rate \-ˌrāt\ *vb* **-rat·ed; -rat·ing** **1** : to eject matter from the throat or lungs by coughing or hawking and spitting **2** : SPIT

ex·pec·to·ra·tion \ik-ˌspek-tə-ˈrā-shən\ *n* **1** : the act or an instance of expectorating **2** : expectorated matter

ex·per·i·ment \ik-ˈsper-ə-mənt, -ˈspir-\ *n* **1** : a procedure carried out under controlled conditions in order to discover an unknown effect or law, to test or establish a hypothesis, or to illustrate a known law **2** : the process of testing — **experiment** *vb* — **ex·per·i·men·ta·tion** \ik-ˌsper-ə-mən-ˈtā-shən, -ˌspir-, -ˌmen-\ *n* — **ex·per·i·ment·er** \-ˈsper-ə-ˌmen-tər, -ˈspir-\ *n*

ex·per·i·men·tal \ik-ˌsper-ə-ˈment-ᵊl, -ˌspir-\ *adj* **1** : of, relating to, or based on experience or experiment **2** : founded on or derived from experiment **3** *of a disease* : intentionally produced esp. in laboratory animals for the purpose of study ⟨~ diabetes⟩ — **ex·per·i·men·tal·ly** *adv*

experimental allergic encephalomyelitis *n* : an inflammatory autoimmune disease that has been induced in laboratory animals and esp. mice and is used as an animal model in studying multiple sclerosis in humans — abbr. *EAE;* called also *experimental autoimmune encephalomyelitis*

ex·pi·ra·tion \ˌek-spə-ˈrā-shən\ *n* **1 a** : the act or process of releasing air from the lungs through the nose or mouth **b** : the escape of carbon dioxide from the body protoplasm (as through the blood and lungs or by diffusion) **2** : something produced by breathing out

ex·pi·ra·to·ry \ik-ˈspī-rə-ˌtōr-ē, ek-; ˈek-spə-rə-\ *adj* : of, relating to, or employed in the expiration of air from the lungs ⟨~ muscles⟩

expiratory reserve volume *n* : the additional amount of air that can be expired from the lungs by determined effort after normal expiration — compare INSPIRATORY RESERVE VOLUME

ex·pire \ik-ˈspīr, ek-\ *vb* **ex·pired; ex·pir·ing 1** : to breathe one's last breath : DIE **2 a** : to breathe out from or as if from the lungs **b** : to emit the breath

ex·plant \ˈek-ˌsplant\ *n* : living tissue removed from an organism and placed in a medium for tissue culture — **ex·plant** \(ˌ)ek-ˈsplant\ *vb* — **ex·plan·ta·tion** \ˌek-ˌsplan-ˈtā-shən\ *n*

ex·plor·ato·ry \ik-ˈsplōr-ə-ˌtōr-ē\ *adj* : of, relating to, or being exploration ⟨~ surgery⟩

ex·plore \ik-ˈsplōr\ *vb* **ex·plored; ex·plor·ing** : to examine (as by surgery) esp. for diagnostic purposes — **ex·plo·ra·tion** \ˌek-splə-ˈrā-shən\ *n*

ex·plor·er \ik-ˈsplōr-ər\ *n* : an instrument for exploring cavities esp. in teeth : PROBE 1

ex·pose \ik-ˈspōz\ *vb* **ex·posed; ex·pos·ing 1** : to subject to risk from a harmful action or condition ⟨children *exposed* to measles⟩ **2** : to lay open to view: as **a** : to engage in indecent exposure of (oneself) **b** : to reveal (a bodily part) esp. by dissection

ex·po·sure \ik-ˈspō-zhər\ *n* **1** : the fact or condition of being exposed: as **a** : the condition of being unprotected esp. from severe weather **b** : the condition of being subject to some detrimental effect or harmful condition ⟨~ to bronchial irritants⟩ ⟨~ to the flu⟩ **2** : the act or an instance of exposing — see INDECENT EXPOSURE

exposure therapy *n* : psychotherapy that involves repeated real, visualized, or simulated exposure to or confrontation with a feared situation or object or a traumatic event or memory in order to achieve habituation and that is used esp. in the treatment of post-traumatic stress disorder, anxiety disorder, or phobias

ex·press \ik-ˈspres, ek-\ *vb* **1** : to make known or exhibit by an expression **2** : to force out by pressure ⟨~ breast milk by electric pump⟩ **3** : to cause (a gene) to manifest its effects in the phenotype

ex·pres·sion \ik-ˈspre-shən\ *n* **1 a** : something that manifests, represents, reflects, embodies, or symbolizes something else ⟨the first clinical ~ of a disease⟩ **b** (1) : the detectable effect of a gene; *also* : the sum of the processes (as transcription and translation) by which a gene is manifested in the phenotype (2) : EXPRESSIVITY **2** : facial aspect or vocal intonation as indicative of feeling

ex·pres·siv·i·ty \ˌek-ˌspre-ˈsi-və-tē\ *n, pl* **-ties** : the relative capacity of a gene to affect the phenotype — compare PENETRANCE

ex·pul·sive \ik-ˈspəl-siv\ *adj* : serving to expel ⟨~ efforts during labor⟩

ex·qui·site \ik-ˈskwi-zət\ *adj* : existing in an extreme degree : ACUTE ⟨~ pain⟩ — **ex·qui·site·ly** \-lē\ *adv*

ex·san·gui·na·tion \(ˌ)eks-ˌsaŋ-gwə-ˈnā-shən\ *n* : the action or process of draining or losing blood — **ex·san·gui·nate** \eks-ˈsaŋ-gwə-ˌnāt\ *vb*

ex·sic·co·sis \ˌek-si-ˈkō-səs\ *n, pl* **-co·ses** \-ˌsēz\ : insufficient intake of fluids; *also* : the resulting condition of bodily dehydration

ex·stro·phy \ˈek-strə-fē\ *n, pl* **-phies** : eversion of a part or organ; *specif* : a congenital malformation of the bladder in which the normally internal mucosa of the organ lies exposed on the abdominal wall

ex·tend \ik-ˈstend\ *vb* : to straighten out (as an arm or leg)

extended family *n* : a family that includes in one household near relatives in addition to a nuclear family

extended–release *adj* : designed to slowly release a drug in the body over an extended period of time esp. to reduce dosing frequency

ex·tend·er \ik-ˈsten-dər\ *n* **1** : a substance added to a product esp. in the capacity of a diluent, adulterant, or modifier **2** : EXPANDER

ex·ten·si·bil·i·ty \ik-ˌsten-sə-ˈbi-lə-tē\ *n, pl* **-ties** : the capability of being stretched ⟨~ of muscle⟩ — **ex·ten·si·ble** \ik-ˈsten-sə-bəl\ *adj*

ex·ten·sion \ik-ˈsten-chən\ *n* **1** : the stretching of a fractured or dislocated limb so as to restore it to its natural position **2** : an unbending movement around a joint in a limb (as the knee or elbow) that increases the angle between the bones of the limb at the joint — compare FLEXION 1

ex·ten·sor \ik-ˈsten-sər, -ˌsȯr\ *n* : a muscle serving to extend a bodily part (as a limb) — called also *extensor muscle;* compare FLEXOR

extensor car·pi ra·di·al·is brev·is \-ˈkär-ˌpī-ˌrā-dē-ˈā-ləs-ˈbre-vəs, -ˈkär-ˌpē-\ *n* : a short muscle on the radial side of the back of the forearm that extends and may abduct the hand

extensor carpi radialis lon·gus \-ˈlȯŋ-gəs\ *n* : a long muscle on the radial side of the back of the forearm that extends and abducts the hand

extensor carpi ul·nar·is \-ˌəl-ˈnar-əs\ *n* : a muscle on the ulnar side of the back of the forearm that extends and adducts the hand

extensor dig·i·ti min·i·mi \-ˈdi-jə-ˌtī-ˈmi-nə-ˌmī, -ˈdi-jə-ˌtē-ˈmi-nə-ˌmē\ *n* : a slender muscle on the medial side of the extensor digitorum communis that extends the little finger

extensor digiti quin·ti pro·pri·us \-ˈkwin-ˌtī-ˈprō-prē-əs, -ˈkwin-ˌtē-\ *n* : EXTENSOR DIGITI MINIMI

extensor dig·i·to·rum brev·is \-ˌdi-jə-ˈtōr-əm-ˈbre-vəs\ *n* : a muscle on the dorsum of the foot that extends the toes

extensor digitorum com·mu·nis \-kə-ˈmyü-nəs, -ˈkä-myə-\ *n* : a muscle on the back of the forearm that extends the fingers and wrist

extensor digitorum lon·gus \-ˈlȯŋ-gəs\ *n* : a pennate muscle on the lateral part of the front of the leg that extends the four small toes and dorsally flexes and pronates the foot

extensor hal·lu·cis brev·is \-ˈha-lü-səs-ˈbre-vəs, -lyü-, -ˈha-lə-kəs-\ *n* : the part of the extensor digitorum brevis that extends the big toe

extensor hallucis lon·gus \-ˈlȯŋ-gəs\ *n* : a long thin muscle situated on the shin that extends the big toe and dorsiflexes and supinates the foot

extensor in·di·cis \-ˈin-də-səs, -də-kəs\ *n* : a thin muscle that arises from the ulna in the more distal part of the forearm and extends the index finger

extensor indicis pro·pri·us \-ˈprō-prē-əs\ *n* : EXTENSOR INDICIS

extensor pol·li·cis brev·is \-ˈpä-lə-səs-ˈbre-vəs, -lə-kəs-\ *n* : a muscle that arises from the dorsal surface of the radius, extends the first phalanx of the thumb, and adducts the hand

extensor pollicis lon·gus \-ˈlȯŋ-gəs\ *n* : a muscle that arises dorsolaterally from the middle part of the ulna, extends the second phalanx of the thumb, and abducts the hand

extensor ret·i·nac·u·lum \-ˌret-ᵊn-ˈa-kyə-ləm\ *n* **1** : either of two fibrous bands of fascia crossing the front of the ankle: **a** : a lower band that is attached laterally to the superior aspect of the calcaneus and passes medially to divide in the shape of a Y and that passes over or both over and under the tendons of the extensor muscles at the ankle — called also *inferior extensor retinaculum* **b** : an upper band passing over and binding down the tendons of the tibialis anterior, extensor hallucis longus, extensor digitorum longus, and peroneus tertius just above the ankle joint — called also *superior extensor retinaculum, transverse crural ligament* **2** : a fibrous band of fascia crossing the back of the wrist and binding down the tendons of the extensor muscles

ex·te·ri·or·ize \ek-ˈstir-ē-ə-ˌrīz\ *vb* **-ized; -iz·ing 1** : EXTERNALIZE **2** : to bring out of the body (as for surgery) ⟨the section of perforated colon was *exteriorized*⟩ — **ex·te·ri·or·iza·tion** \-ˌstir-ē-ə-rə-ˈzā-shən\ *n*

ex·tern *also* **ex·terne** \ˈek-ˌstərn\ *n* : a nonresident doctor or medical student at a hospital — **ex·tern·ship** \-ˌship\ *n*

externa — see MUSCULARIS EXTERNA, OTITIS EXTERNA, THECA EXTERNA

ex·ter·nal \ek-ˈstərn-ᵊl\ *adj* **1** : capable of being perceived outwardly : BODILY ⟨∼ signs of a disease⟩ **2 a** : situated at, on, or near the outside ⟨an ∼ muscle⟩ **b** : directed toward the outside : having an outside object ⟨∼ perception⟩ **c** : used by applying to the outside ⟨an ∼ lotion⟩ **3 a** (1) : situated near or toward the surface of the body; *also* : situated away from the mesial plane ⟨the ∼ condyle of the humerus⟩ (2) : arising or acting from outside : having an outside origin ⟨∼ stimuli⟩ **b** : of, relating to, or consisting of something outside the mind : having existence independent of the mind ⟨∼ reality⟩ — **ex·ter·nal·ly** *adv*

external anal sphincter *n* : ANAL SPHINCTER a

external auditory canal *n* : the auditory canal leading from the opening of the external ear to the eardrum — called also *external acoustic meatus, external auditory meatus*

external capsule *n* : CAPSULE 1b (2)

external carotid artery *n* : the outer branch of the carotid artery that supplies the face, tongue, and external parts of the head — called also *external carotid*

external ear *n* : the parts of the ear that are external to the eardrum; *also* : PINNA

external iliac artery *n* : ILIAC ARTERY 2

external iliac node *n* : any of the lymph nodes grouped around the external iliac artery and the external iliac vein — compare INTERNAL ILIAC NODE

external iliac vein *n* : ILIAC VEIN b

external inguinal ring *n* : SUPERFICIAL INGUINAL RING

external intercostal muscle *n* : INTERCOSTAL MUSCLE a — called also *external intercostal*

ex·ter·nal·ize \ek-ˈstərn-ᵊl-ˌīz\ *vb* **-ized; -iz·ing 1 a** : to transform from a mental image into an apparently real object (as in hallucinations) : attribute (a mental image) to external causation **b** : to invent an explanation for by attributing to causes outside the self : RATIONALIZE, PROJECT **2** : to direct outward socially ⟨*externalized* anger⟩ — **ex·ter·nal·iza·tion** \-ˌstərn-ᵊl-ə-ˈzā-shən\ *n*

external jugular vein *n* : JUGULAR VEIN b — called also *external jugular*

external malleolus *n* : MALLEOLUS a

external maxillary artery *n* : FACIAL ARTERY

external oblique *n* : OBLIQUE a (1) — called also *external oblique muscle*

external occipital crest *n* : OCCIPITAL CREST a

external occipital protuberance *n* : OCCIPITAL PROTUBERANCE a

external os *n* : the opening of the uterine cervix into the vagina

external otitis media *n* : OTITIS EXTERNA — abbr. *EOM*
external pterygoid muscle *n* : PTERYGOID MUSCLE a
external pudendal artery *n* : either of two branches of the femoral artery: **a** : one that is distributed to the skin of the lower abdomen, to the penis and scrotum in the male, and to one of the labia majora in the female — called also *superficial external pudendal artery* **b** : one that follows a deeper course, that is distributed to the medial aspect of the thigh, to the skin of the scrotum and perineum in the male, and to one of the labia majora in the female — called also *deep external pudendal artery*
external respiration *n* : exchange of gases between the external environment and the lungs or between the alveoli of the lungs and the blood — compare INTERNAL RESPIRATION
externe *var of* EXTERN
externus — see OBLIQUUS EXTERNUS ABDOMINIS, OBTURATOR EXTERNUS, SPHINCTER ANI EXTERNUS
ex·tero·cep·tive \ˌek-stə-rō-ˈsep-tiv\ *adj* : activated by, relating to, or being stimuli received by an organism from outside
ex·tero·cep·tor \-ˈsep-tər\ *n* : a sense receptor (as of touch, smell, vision, or hearing) excited by exteroceptive stimuli — compare INTEROCEPTOR
ex·tinc·tion \ik-ˈstiŋk-shən\ *n* : the process of eliminating or reducing a conditioned response by not reinforcing it
ex·tin·guish \ik-ˈstiŋ-gwish\ *vb* : to cause extinction of (a conditioned response)
ex·tir·pa·tion \ˌek-stər-ˈpā-shən\ *n* : complete excision or surgical destruction of a body part — **ex·tir·pate** \ˈek-stər-ˌpāt\ *vb*
extra- *prefix* : outside : beyond ⟨*extrauterine*⟩
ex·tra·cap·su·lar \ˌek-strə-ˈkap-sə-lər, -syu̇-lər\ *adj* **1** : situated outside a capsule **2** *of a cataract operation* : involving removal of the front part of the capsule and the central part of the lens — compare INTRACAPSULAR 2
ex·tra·cel·lu·lar \-ˈsel-yə-lər\ *adj* : situated or occurring outside a cell or the cells of the body ⟨~ digestion⟩ ⟨~ enzymes⟩ — **ex·tra·cel·lu·lar·ly** *adv*
ex·tra·chro·mo·som·al \-ˌkrō-mə-ˈsō-məl, -ˈzō-\ *adj* : situated or controlled by factors outside the chromosome ⟨~ inheritance⟩ ⟨~ DNA⟩
ex·tra·cor·po·re·al \-kȯr-ˈpōr-ē-əl\ *adj* : occurring or based outside the living body ⟨heart surgery employing ~ circulation⟩ — **ex·tra·cor·po·re·al·ly** *adv*
extracorporeal life support *n* : life support used when a patient is experiencing cardiac or pulmonary failure unresponsive to conventional therapies (as mechanical ventilation) that typically involves the continuous extracorporeal oxygenation of blood pumped from the body; *esp* : EXTRACORPOREAL MEMBRANE OXYGENATION — abbr. *ECLS*
extracorporeal membrane oxygenation *n* : treatment providing respiratory and circulatory support for a patient that involves pumping blood from the body and through a membrane oxygenator to exchange carbon dioxide for oxygen and a heat exchanger to cool or warm the blood before returning it to the body — called also *ECMO*
ex·tra·cra·ni·al \-ˈkrā-nē-əl\ *adj* : situated or occurring outside the cranium
[1]**ex·tract** \ik-ˈstrakt\ *vb* **1** : to pull or take out forcibly ⟨~*ed* a wisdom tooth⟩ **2** : to separate the medicinally-active components of a plant or animal tissue by the use of solvents — **ex·trac·tion** \-ˈstrak-shən\ *n*
[2]**ex·tract** \ˈek-ˌstrakt\ *n* : something prepared by extracting; *esp* : a medicinally-active pharmaceutical solution
[1]**ex·trac·tive** \ik-ˈstrak-tiv, ˈek-ˌ\ *adj* : of, relating to, or involving the process of extracting
[2]**extractive** *n* : EXTRACT
ex·tra·du·ral \ˌek-strə-ˈdu̇r-əl, -dyu̇r-\ *adj* : situated or occurring outside the dura mater but within the skull ⟨an ~ hemorrhage⟩
ex·tra·em·bry·on·ic \-ˌem-brē-ˈä-nik\ *adj* : situated outside the embryo proper; *esp* : developed from the zygote but not part of the embryo ⟨~ membranes⟩
extraembryonic coelom *n* : the space between the chorion and amnion which in early stages is continuous with the coelom of the embryo proper
ex·tra·fu·sal \ˌek-strə-ˈfyü-zəl\ *adj* : situated outside a striated muscle spindle ⟨~ muscle fibers⟩ — compare INTRAFUSAL
ex·tra·gen·i·tal \-ˈje-nə-tᵊl\ *adj* : situated or originating outside the genital region or organs
ex·tra·he·pat·ic \-hi-ˈpa-tik\ *adj* : situated or originating outside the liver
ex·tra·in·tes·ti·nal \-in-ˈtes-tə-nəl\ *adj* : situated or occurring outside the intestines ⟨~ infections⟩
ex·tra·mac·u·lar \-ˈma-kyə-lər\ *adj* : relating to or being the part of the retina other than the macula
ex·tra·med·ul·lary \-ˈmed-ᵊl-ˌer-ē, -ˈme-jə-ˌler-ē, -mə-ˈdə-lə-rē\ *adj* **1** : situated or occurring outside the spinal cord or the medulla oblongata **2** : located or taking place outside the bone marrow
ex·tra·mi·to·chon·dri·al \-ˌmī-tə-ˈkän-drē-əl\ *adj* : situated or occurring in the cell outside the mitochondria
ex·tra·nu·cle·ar \-ˈnü-klē-ər, -ˈnyü-\ *adj* : situated in or affecting the parts of a cell external to the nucleus : CYTOPLASMIC

ex•tra•oc•u•lar \-ˈä-kyə-lər\ *adj* : occurring or situated outside the eyeball; *also* : involving or relating to the extraocular muscles

extraocular muscle *n* : any of six small voluntary muscles that pass between the eyeball and the orbit and control the movement and stabilization of the eyeball in relation to the orbit — abbr. *EOM;* see OBLIQUE b, RECTUS 2

ex•tra•or•al \-ˈōr-əl, -ˈär-\ *adj* : situated or occurring outside the mouth

ex•tra•peri•to•ne•al \-ˌper-ət-ᵊn-ˈē-əl\ *adj* : located or taking place outside the peritoneal cavity ⟨~ spaces⟩

ex•tra•pi•tu•itary \-pə-ˈtü-ə-ˌter-ē, -ˈtyü-\ *adj* : situated or arising outside the pituitary gland ⟨~ tissue⟩

ex•tra•pla•cen•tal \-plə-ˈsent-ᵊl\ *adj* : being outside of or independent of the placenta

ex•tra•pul•mo•nary \-ˈpu̇l-mə-ˌner-ē, -ˈpəl-\ *adj* : situated or occurring outside the lungs ⟨~ tuberculosis⟩

ex•tra•py•ra•mi•dal \-pə-ˈra-məd-ᵊl, -ˌpir-ə-ˈmid-ᵊl\ *adj* : situated outside of and esp. involving descending nerve tracts other than the pyramidal tracts ⟨~ brain lesions⟩

ex•tra•re•nal \-ˈrēn-ᵊl\ *adj* : situated or occurring outside the kidneys

ex•tra•ret•i•nal \-ˈre-tə-nəl\ *adj* : situated or occurring outside the retina

ex•tra•sen•so•ry \ˌek-strə-ˈsen-sə-rē\ *adj* : residing beyond or outside the ordinary senses

extrasensory perception *n* : perception (as in telepathy, clairvoyance, and precognition) that involves awareness of information about events external to the self not gained through the senses and not deducible from previous experience — called also *ESP*

ex•tra•sys•to•le \-ˈsis-tə-(ˌ)lē\ *n* : a prematurely occurring beat of one of the chambers of the heart that leads to momentary arrhythmia but leaves the fundamental rhythm unchanged — called also *premature beat* — **ex•tra•sys•tol•ic** \-sis-ˈtä-lik\ *adj*

ex•tra•uter•ine \-ˈyü-tə-rən, -ˌrīn\ *adj* : situated or occurring outside the uterus

extrauterine pregnancy *n* : ECTOPIC PREGNANCY

ex•trav•a•sate \ik-ˈstra-və-ˌsāt, -ˌzāt\ *vb* **-sat•ed; -sat•ing** : to force out, cause to escape, or pass by infiltration or effusion from a proper vessel or channel (as a blood vessel) into surrounding tissue

ex•trav•a•sa•tion \ik-ˌstra-və-ˈzā-shən, -ˈsā-\ *n* **1** : the action of extravasating **2 a** : an extravasated fluid (as blood) ⟨~*s* from the nose and mouth⟩ **b** : a deposit formed by extravasation

ex•tra•vas•cu•lar \ˌek-strə-ˈvas-kyə-lər\ *adj* : not occurring or contained in body vessels ⟨~ pulmonary fluid⟩ — **ex•tra•vas•cu•lar•ly** *adv*

ex•tra•ven•tric•u•lar \-ven-ˈtri-kyə lər, -vən-\ *adj* : located or taking place outside a ventricle ⟨~ lesions⟩

extraversion, extravert *var of* EXTROVERSION, EXTROVERT

ex•trem•i•ty \ik-ˈstre-mə-tē\ *n, pl* **-ties 1** : the farthest or most remote part, section, or point **2** : a limb of the body; *esp* : a hand or foot

ex•trin•sic \ek-ˈstrin-zik, -sik\ *adj* **1** : originating or due to causes or factors from or on the outside of a body, organ, or part **2** : originating outside a part and acting on the part as a whole — used esp. of certain muscles; compare INTRINSIC 2 — **ex•trin•si•cal•ly** \-zi-k(ə-)lē, -si-\ *adv*

extrinsic factor *n* : VITAMIN B_{12}

extro- *prefix* : outside : outward ⟨*extro*vert⟩ — compare INTRO-

ex•tro•ver•sion *or* **ex•tra•ver•sion** \ˌek-strə-ˈvər-zhən, -shən\ *n* : the act, state, or habit of being predominantly concerned with and obtaining gratification from what is outside the self — compare INTROVERSION

ex•tro•vert *also* **ex•tra•vert** \ˈek-strə-ˌvərt\ *n* : one whose attention and interests are directed wholly or predominantly toward what is outside the self : one characterized by extroversion; *broadly* : a gregarious and unreserved person — compare INTROVERT — **extrovert** *also* **extravert** *adj* — **ex•tro•vert•ed** *also* **ex•tra•vert•ed** \-ˌver-təd\ *adj*

ex•trude \ik-ˈstrüd\ *vb* **ex•trud•ed; ex•trud•ing** : to force, press, or push out; *also* : to become extruded ⟨blood *extruding* through arteries⟩ — **ex•tru•sion** \ik-ˈstrü-zhən\ *n*

ex•tu•ba•tion \ˌek-ˌstü-ˈbā-shən, -ˌstyü-\ *n* : the removal of a tube esp. from the larynx after intubation — **ex•tu•bate** \ek-ˈstü-ˌbāt, -ˈstyü-, ˈek-ˌstü-, -ˌstyü-\ *vb*

ex•u•ber•ant \ig-ˈzü-bə-rənt\ *adj* : characterized by extreme proliferation ⟨~ granulation tissue⟩

ex•u•date \ˈek-su̇-ˌdāt, -syu̇-, -shu̇-\ *n* : exuded matter; *esp* : the material composed of serum, fibrin, and white blood cells that escapes from blood vessels into a superficial lesion or area of inflammation

ex•u•da•tion \ˌek-su̇-ˈdā-shən, -syu̇-, -shu̇-\ *n* **1** : the process of exuding **2** : EXUDATE — **ex•u•da•tive** \ig-ˈzü-də-tiv; ˈek-su̇-ˌdā-tiv, -syu̇-, -shu̇-\ *adj*

ex•ude \ig-ˈzüd\ *vb* **ex•ud•ed; ex•ud•ing 1** : to ooze or cause to ooze out **2** : to undergo diffusion

eye \ˈī\ *n* **1** : a nearly spherical hollow organ that is lined with a sensitive retina, is lodged in a bony orbit in the skull, is the vertebrate organ of sight, and is normally paired **2** : all the visible structures within and surrounding the orbit and including eyelids, eyelashes, and eyebrows **3** : the faculty of seeing with eyes

eye·ball \ˈī-ˌbȯl\ *n* : the more or less globular capsule of the vertebrate eye formed by the sclera and cornea together with their contained structures

eye bank *n* : a storage place for human corneas from the newly dead for transplanting to the eyes of those blind through corneal defects

eye·brow \ˈī-ˌbrau̇\ *n* : the ridge over the eye or hair growing on it — called also *brow*

eye chart *n* : a chart that is read at a fixed distance for purposes of testing sight; *esp* : one with rows of letters or objects of decreasing size

eye contact *n* : visual contact with another person's eyes

eye·cup \ˈī-ˌkəp\ *n* **1** : a small oval cup with a rim curved to fit the orbit of the eye used for applying liquid remedies to the eyes **2** : OPTIC CUP

eyed \ˈīd\ *adj* : having an eye or eyes esp. of a specified kind or number — often used in combination <a blue-*eyed* patient>

eyed·ness \ˈīd-nəs\ *n* : preference for the use of one eye instead of the other

eye doctor *n* : a specialist (as an optometrist or ophthalmologist) in the examination, treatment, or care of the eyes

eye·drop·per \ˈī-ˌdrä-pər\ *n* : DROPPER

eye drops *n pl* : a medicated solution for the eyes that is applied in drops — **eye–drop** \-ˌdräp\ *adj*

eye·glass \ˈī-ˌglas\ *n* **1 a** : a lens worn to aid vision; *specif* : MONOCLE **b eye·glass·es** *pl* : GLASSES, SPECTACLES **2** : EYECUP 1

eye gnat *n* : any of several small dipteran flies (genus *Hippelates* of the family Chloropidae and esp. *H. pusio*) including some that are held to be vectors of pink eye and yaws — called also *eye fly*

eye·ground \ˈī-ˌgrau̇nd\ *n* : the fundus of the eye; *esp* : the retina as viewed through an ophthalmoscope

eye·lash \ˈī-ˌlash\ *n* **1** : the fringe of hair edging the eyelid — usu. used in pl. **2** : a single hair of the eyelashes

eye·lid \ˈī-ˌlid\ *n* : either of the movable lids of skin and muscle that can be closed over the eyeball — called also *palpebra*

eye·sight \ˈī-ˌsīt\ *n* : SIGHT 2

eye socket *n* : ORBIT

eye·strain \ˈī-ˌstrān\ *n* : weariness or a strained state of the eye

eye·tooth \ˈī-ˌtüth\ *n, pl* **eye·teeth** \-ˌtēth\ : a canine tooth of the upper jaw

eye·wash \ˈī-ˌwȯsh, -ˌwäsh\ *n* : an eye lotion

eye·wear \ˈī-ˌwar, -ˌwer\ *n* : corrective or protective devices (as glasses or contact lenses) for the eyes

eye worm *n* **1** : an African filarial worm of the genus *Loa* (*L. loa*) that migrates through the eyeball and subcutaneous tissues of humans — compare CALABAR SWELLING **2** : any member of the nematode genus *Thelazia* living in the tear duct and beneath the eyelid of dogs, cats, sheep, humans, and other mammals and sometimes causing blindness **3** : either of two nematode worms of the genus *Oxyspirura* (*O. mansoni* and *O. petrowi*) living beneath the nictitating membrane of the eyes of birds

ezet·i·mibe \e-ˈze-tə-ˌmib\ *n* : a drug $C_{24}H_{21}F_2NO_3$ that lowers the amount of cholesterol in the blood by selectively inhibiting its absorption in the intestine — see VYTORIN, ZETIA

F

f *symbol* focal length
F *abbr* Fahrenheit
F *symbol* fluorine
Fab \ˈfab\ *n* : a fragment of an antibody that contains one antigen-binding site, one complete light chain, and part of one heavy chain — called also *Fab fragment*
fab·ri·ca·tion \ˌfa-bri-ˈkā-shən\ *n* : CONFABULATION
Fa·bry disease \ˈfä-brē-\ *or* **Fabry's disease** \-brēz-\ *n* : a disorder of lipid metabolism that is inherited as an X-linked recessive trait and is characterized by skin lesions esp. on the lower trunk, severe pain in the extremities, corneal opacities, and vascular disease affecting the kidneys, heart, or brain
Fabry, Johannes (1860–1930), German dermatologist.
FACC *abbr* Fellow of the American College of Cardiology
FACD *abbr* Fellow of the American College of Dentists
face \ˈfās\ *n, often attrib* : the front part of the head including the chin, mouth, nose, cheeks, eyes, and usu. the forehead
face·bow \ˈfās-ˌbō\ *n* : a device used in dentistry to determine the positional relationships of the maxillae to the temporomandibular joints of a patient
face fly *n* : a European fly of the genus *Musca* (*M. autumnalis*) that is widely established in No. America and causes distress in livestock by clustering about the face
face·lift \ˈfās-ˌlift\ *n* : plastic surgery on the face and neck to remove defects and imperfections (as wrinkles) typical of aging — called also *rhytidectomy* — **face–lift** *vb*
face–lifting \-ˌlif-tiŋ\ *n* : FACELIFT
fac·et \ˈfa-sət\ *n* : a smooth flat or nearly flat circumscribed anatomical surface (as of a bone) — **fac·et·ed** *or* **fac·et·ted** \ˈfa-sə-təd\ *adj*
fac·et·ec·to·my \ˌfa-sə-ˈtek-tə-mē\ *n, pl* **-mies** : excision of a facet esp. of a vertebra
[1]**fa·cial** \ˈfā-shəl\ *adj* **1** : of, relating to, or affecting the face ⟨~ neuralgia⟩ **2** : concerned with or used in improving the appearance of the face **3** : relating to or being the buccal and labial surface of a tooth — **fa·cial·ly** \-shə-lē\ *adv*
[2]**facial** *n* : a treatment to improve the appearance of the face
facial artery *n* : an artery that arises from the external carotid artery and gives off branches supplying the neck and face — called also *external maxillary artery;* compare MAXILLARY ARTERY
facial bone *n* : any of the 14 bones of the facial region of the human skull that do not take part in forming the braincase
facial canal *n* : a passage in the petrous part of the temporal bone that transmits various branches of the facial nerve
facial colliculus *n* : a medial eminence on the floor of the fourth ventricle of the brain produced by the nucleus of the abducens nerve and the flexure of the facial nerve around it
facial nerve *n* : either of the seventh pair of cranial nerves that supply motor fibers esp. to the muscles of the face and jaw and sensory and parasympathetic fibers to the tongue, palate, and fauces — called also *seventh cranial nerve, seventh nerve*
facial vein *n* : a vein that arises as the angular vein, drains the superficial structures of the face, and empties into the internal jugular vein — called also *anterior facial vein;* see DEEP FACIAL VEIN, POSTERIOR FACIAL VEIN
-fa·cient \ˈfā-shənt\ *adj comb form* : making : causing ⟨aborti*facient*⟩
fa·cies \ˈfā-ˌshēz, -shē-ˌēz\ *n, pl* **facies** **1** : an appearance and expression of the face characteristic of a particular condition esp. when abnormal ⟨adenoid ~⟩ **2** : an anatomical surface
fa·cil·i·ta·tion \fə-ˌsi-lə-ˈtā-shən\ *n* **1** : the lowering of the threshold for reflex conduction along a particular neural pathway **2** : the increasing of the ease or intensity of a response by repeated stimulation — **fa·cil·i·tate** \-ˈsi-lə-ˌtāt\ *vb* — **fa·cil·i·ta·to·ry** \-ˈsi-lə-tə-ˌtōr-ē\ *adj*
fac·ing \ˈfā-siŋ\ *n* : a front of porcelain or plastic used in dental crowns and bridgework to face the metal replacement and simulate the natural tooth
facio- *comb form* : facial and ⟨*facio*scapulohumeral⟩
fa·cio·scap·u·lo·hu·mer·al \ˌfā-shē-ō-ˌska-pyə-lō-ˈhyü-mə-rəl\ *adj* : relating to or affecting the muscles of the face, scapula, and arm
FACOG *abbr* Fellow of the American College of Obstetricians and Gynecologists
FACP *abbr* Fellow of the American College of Physicians
FACR *abbr* Fellow of the American College of Radiology
FACS *abbr* Fellow of the American College of Surgeons
F–ac·tin \ˈef-ˌak-tən\ *n* : a fibrous actin polymerized in the form of a double helix that is produced in the presence of a metal cation (as of calcium) and ATP — compare G-ACTIN

fac·ti·tious \fak-ˈti-shəs\ *adj* : not produced by natural means

factitious disorder *n* : a psychological disorder (as Munchausen syndrome) in which someone intentionally produces or feigns symptoms of a disease or injury to convince others medical treatment is needed; *also* : a similar condition (as Munchausen syndrome by proxy) in which a caregiver (as a parent) intentionally produces symptoms of disease or injury in the person being cared for

fac·tor \ˈfak-tər\ *n* **1 a** : something that actively contributes to the production of a result **b** : a substance that functions in or promotes the function of a particular physiological process or bodily system **2** : GENE — **fac·to·ri·al** \fak-ˈtōr-ē-əl\ *adj*

factor VIII \-ˈāt\ *n* : a glycoprotein clotting factor of blood plasma that is essential for blood clotting and is absent or inactive in hemophilia — called also *antihemophilic factor, thromboplastinogen*

factor XI \-i-ˈle-vən\ *n* : PLASMA THROMBOPLASTIN ANTECEDENT

factor V \-ˈfīv\ *n* : a globulin clotting factor produced esp. in the liver that circulates in an inactive form in blood plasma and that in its activated form combines with factor X to accelerate the conversion of prothrombin to thrombin — called also *accelerator globulin, labile factor, proaccelerin*

factor V Lei·den \-ˈlī-dᵊn\ *n* **1** : a point mutation producing an abnormal version of factor V resistant to inactivation **2** : a genetic disorder caused by factor V Leiden that is marked by an increased risk of abnormal blood clot formation leading esp. to deep vein thrombosis or pulmonary embolism and is inherited as an autosomal dominant trait — called also *factor V Leiden thrombophilia*

factor IX \-ˈnīn\ *n* : a clotting factor that activates factor VIII and whose absence is associated with hemophilia B — called also *autoprothrombin II, Christmas factor*

factor VII \-ˈse-vən\ *n* : a clotting factor formed in the kidney under the influence of vitamin K that may be deficient due to a hereditary disorder or to a vitamin K deficiency — called also *autoprothrombin I, cothromboplastin, proconvertin, stable factor*

factor X \-ˈten\ *n* : a clotting factor that is produced esp. in the liver under the influence of vitamin K and in its activated form converts prothrombin to thrombin in a reaction dependent on calcium ions and phospholipids and accelerated by factor V — called also *Stuart-Prower factor*

factor XIII \-ˌthərt-ˈtēn\ *n* : a clotting factor catalyzed by thrombin during the final stage of clot formation to an active form which cross-links strands of fibrin resulting in a stable insoluble clot — called also *fibrinase;* see TRANSGLUTAMINASE

factor XII \-ˈtwelv\ *n* : a clotting factor that facilitates blood coagulation but whose deficiency tends not to promote hemorrhage — called also *Hageman factor*

facts of life *n pl* : the fundamental physiological processes and behavior involved in sex and reproduction

fac·ul·ta·tive \ˈfa-kəl-ˌtā-tiv\ *adj* **1** : taking place under some conditions but not under others ⟨~ parasitism⟩ **2** : exhibiting an indicated lifestyle under some environmental conditions but not under others ⟨~ anaerobes⟩ — **fac·ul·ta·tive·ly** *adv*

FAD \ˌef-(ˌ)ā-ˈdē\ *n* : FLAVIN ADENINE DINUCLEOTIDE

fae·cal, fae·ca·lith, fae·cal·oid, fae·ces *chiefly Brit var of* FECAL, FECALITH, FECALOID, FECES

fag·o·py·rism \ˌfa-gō-ˈpī-ˌri-zəm\ *n* : a photosensitization esp. of swine and sheep that is due to eating large quantities of buckwheat (esp. *Fagopyrum esculentum*)

Fahr·en·heit \ˈfar-ən-ˌhīt\ *adj* : relating or conforming to a thermometric scale on which under standard atmospheric pressure the boiling point of water is at 212 degrees above the zero of the scale and the freezing point is at 32 degrees above zero — abbr. *F*

Fahrenheit, Daniel Gabriel (1686–1736), German physicist.

fail \ˈfāl\ *vb* **1** : to weaken or lose strength **2** : to stop functioning normally ⟨the patient's heart ~*ed*⟩

fail·ure \ˈfāl-yər\ *n* : a state of inability to perform a vital function ⟨respiratory ~⟩ — see HEART FAILURE

¹faint \ˈfānt\ *adj* : weak, dizzy, and likely to faint — **faint·ness** \-nəs\ *n*

²faint *vb* : to lose consciousness because of a temporary decrease in the blood supply to the brain

³faint *n* : the physiological action of fainting; *also* : the resulting condition : SYNCOPE

faith healing *n* : a method of treating diseases by prayer and exercise of faith in God — **faith healer** *n*

falces *pl of* FALX

falciform ligament *n* : an anteroposterior fold of peritoneum attached to the under surface of the diaphragm and sheath of the rectus muscle and along a line on the anterior and upper surfaces of the liver extending back from the notch on the anterior margin

fal·cip·a·rum malaria \fal-ˈsi-pə-rəm-, fȯl-\ *n* : severe malaria caused by a parasite of the genus *Plasmodium* (*P. falciparum*) and marked by irregular recurrence of paroxysms and usu. prolonged or continuous fever — called also *malignant malaria, malignant tertian malaria;* compare VIVAX MALARIA

fallen arch *n* : FLATFOOT

falling sickness *n* : EPILEPSY

fal·lo·pian tube \fə-ˈlō-pē-ən-\ *n, often cap F* : either of the pair of tubes that carry the eggs from the ovary to the uterus — called also *uterine tube*

Fal·lop·pio \fäl-ˈlȯp-yō\ *or* **Fal·lop·pia** \-ˈlȯp-yä\, **Gabriele** (*Latin* **Gabriel Fal·lo·pi·us** \fə-ˈlō-pē-əs\) **(1523–1562)**, Italian anatomist.

Fallot's tetralogy \(ˌ)fa-ˈlōz-\ *n* : TETRALOGY OF FALLOT

fall·out \ˈfȯ-ˌlau̇t\ *n* **1** : the often radioactive particles stirred up by or resulting from a nuclear explosion and descending through the atmosphere; *also* : other polluting particles (as volcanic ash) descending likewise **2** : descent (as of fallout) through the atmosphere

false \ˈfȯls\ *adj* **fals·er; fals·est** **1** : not corresponding to truth or reality **2** : artificially made ⟨a set of ∼ teeth⟩

false cowpox *n* : PSEUDOCOWPOX

false joint *n* : PSEUDARTHROSIS

false labor *n* : pains resembling those of normal labor but occurring at irregular intervals and without dilation of the cervix

false membrane *n* : a fibrinous deposit with enmeshed necrotic cells formed esp. in croup and diphtheria — called also *pseudomembrane*

false mo·rel \-mȯ-ˈrel\ *n* : any fungus of the genus *Gyromitra*

false–negative *adj* : relating to or being an individual or a test result that is erroneously classified in a negative category (as of diagnosis) because of imperfect testing methods or procedures — compare FALSE-POSITIVE — **false negative** *n*

false neurotransmitter *n* : a biological amine that can be stored in presynaptic vesicles but that has little or no effect on postsynaptic receptors when released into the synaptic cleft — called also *false transmitter*

false pelvis *n* : the upper broader portion of the pelvic cavity — called also *false pelvic cavity;* compare TRUE PELVIS

false–positive *adj* : relating to or being an individual or a test result that is erroneously classified in a positive category (as of diagnosis) because of imperfect testing methods or procedures — compare FALSE-NEGATIVE — **false positive** *n*

false pregnancy *n* : PSEUDOCYESIS, PSEUDOPREGNANCY

false rib *n* : a rib whose cartilages unite indirectly or not at all with the sternum — compare FLOATING RIB

false vocal cords *n pl* : the upper pair of vocal cords that are not directly concerned with speech production — called also *superior vocal cords, ventricular folds, vestibular folds*

falx \ˈfalks, ˈfȯlks\ *n, pl* **fal·ces** \ˈfal-ˌsēz, ˈfȯl-\ : a sickle-shaped part or structure: as **a** : FALX CEREBRI **b** : FALX CEREBELLI

falx ce·re·bel·li \-ˌser-ə-ˈbe-ˌlī\ *n* : the smaller of the two folds of dura mater separating the hemispheres of the brain that lies between the lateral lobes of the cerebellum

falx cer·e·bri \-ˈser-ə-ˌbrī\ *n* : the larger of the two folds of dura mater separating the hemispheres of the brain that lies between the cerebral hemispheres and contains the sagittal sinuses

FAMA *abbr* Fellow of the American Medical Association

fam·ci·clo·vir \ˌfam-ˈsī-klō-ˌvir\ *n* : a precursor $C_{14}H_{19}N_5O_4$ of penciclovir that is administered orally esp. to treat shingles and herpes genitalis — see FAMVIR

fa·mil·ial \fə-ˈmil-yəl\ *adj* : tending to occur in more members of a family than expected by chance alone ⟨a ∼ disorder⟩ — compare ACQUIRED 1, CONGENITAL 2, HEREDITARY

familial adenomatous polyposis *n* : a disease of the large intestine that is inherited as an autosomal dominant trait and is marked by the formation esp. in the colon and rectum of numerous adenomatous polyps which typically become malignant if left untreated — abbr. *FAP;* called also *adenomatous polyposis coli, familial polyposis*

familial dysautonomia *n* : a disorder of the autonomic nervous system that is inherited as an autosomal recessive trait, typically affects individuals of eastern European Jewish ancestry, and is characterized esp. by lack of tears, difficulty in swallowing, orthostatic hypotension, poor thermoregulation, episodic vomiting, excessive sweating, and sensory deficits (as of pain) — called also *Riley-Day syndrome*

familial hypercholesterolemia *n* : a disorder of lipid metabolism that is inherited as an autosomal dominant trait and is marked by elevated levels of LDL in the blood plasma resulting esp. in xanthomas, atherosclerosis, and an increased risk of heart attack and coronary artery disease

familial polyposis *n* : any of several inherited diseases (as Gardner's syndrome) that are characterized esp. by the formation of polyps in the gastrointestinal tract; *esp* : FAMILIAL ADENOMATOUS POLYPOSIS

fam·i·ly \ˈfam-lē, ˈfa-mə-\ *n, pl* **-lies** **1** : the basic unit in society traditionally consisting of two parents rearing their children; *also* : any of various social units differing from but regarded as equivalent to the traditional family ⟨a single-parent ∼⟩ **2** : a group of related plants or animals forming a category ranking above a genus and below an order and usu. comprising several to many genera — **family** *adj*

family doctor *n* **1 :** a doctor regularly consulted by a family **2 :** FAMILY PHYSICIAN

family physician *n* **1 :** FAMILY DOCTOR 1 **2 :** a doctor specialized in family practice

family planning *n* **:** planning intended to determine the number and spacing of one's children through effective methods of birth control

family practice *n* **:** a medical practice or specialty which provides continuing general medical care for the individual and family — called also *family medicine*

family practitioner *n* **1 :** FAMILY DOCTOR 1 **2 :** FAMILY PHYSICIAN 2

fa•mo•ti•dine \fə-ˈmō-tə-ˌdīn\ *n* **:** an H_2 antagonist $C_8H_{15}N_7O_2S_3$ used to inhibit gastric acid secretion (as in the treatment of gastric and duodenal ulcers and gastroesophageal reflux disease) — see PEPCID

Fam•vir \ˈfam-ˌvir\ *trademark* — used for a preparation of famciclovir

Fan•co•ni's anemia \fän-ˈkō-nēz-, fan-\ *n* **:** aplastic anemia that is inherited as an autosomal recessive trait and is characterized by progressive pancytopenia, hypoplastic bone marrow, skeletal anomalies (as short stature), microcephaly, hypogonadism, and a predisposition to leukemia

Fanconi, Guido (1892–1979), Swiss pediatrician.

Fanconi syndrome *also* **Fanconi's syndrome** *n* **:** a disorder of reabsorption in the proximal convoluted tubules of the kidney marked esp. by the presence of glucose, amino acids, and phosphates in the urine

fang \ˈfaŋ\ *n* **1 :** a long sharp tooth: as **a :** one by which an animal's prey is seized and held or torn **b :** one of the long hollow or grooved and often erectile teeth of a venomous snake **2 :** the root of a tooth or one of the processes or prongs into which a root divides — **fanged** \ˈfaŋd\ *adj*

fan•go \ˈfaŋ-(ˌ)gō, ˈfäŋ-\ *n* **:** a clay mud from hot springs at Battaglio, Italy, that is applied externally in the therapeutic treatment of certain medical conditions (as rheumatism)

fan•ta•size \ˈfan-tə-ˌsīz\ *vb* **-sized; -siz•ing 1 :** to indulge in fantasy **2 :** to portray in the mind by fantasy

[1]**fan•ta•sy** *also* **phan•ta•sy** \ˈfan-tə-sē, -zē\ *n, pl* **-sies :** the power or process of creating esp. unrealistic or improbable mental images in response to psychological need; *also* **:** a mental image or a series of mental images (as a daydream) so created

[2]**fantasy** *also* **phantasy** *vb* **-sied; -sy•ing :** FANTASIZE

FAP *abbr* familial adenomatous polyposis

FAPA *abbr* Fellow of the American Psychological Association

fa•rad•ic \fə-ˈra-dik, far-ˈa-\ *also* **far•a•da•ic** \far-ə-ˈdā-ik\ *adj* **:** of or relating to an asymmetric alternating current of electricity ⟨~ muscle stimulation⟩

Far•a•day \ˈfar-ə-ˌdā\, **Michael (1791–1867),** British physicist and chemist.

far•a•dism \ˈfar-ə-ˌdi-zəm\ *n* **:** the application of a faradic current of electricity (as for therapeutic purposes)

far•cy \ˈfär-sē\ *n, pl* **far•cies :** GLANDERS; *esp* **:** cutaneous glanders

farmer's lung *n* **:** an acute pulmonary disorder that is characterized by sudden onset, fever, cough, expectoration, and breathlessness and that results from the inhalation of dust from moldy hay or straw

far point *n* **:** the point farthest from the eye at which an object is accurately focused on the retina when the accommodation is completely relaxed — compare NEAR POINT

far•sight•ed \ˈfär-ˌsī-təd\ *adj* **1 :** seeing or able to see to a great distance **2 :** affected with hyperopia — **far•sight•ed•ly** *adv*

far•sight•ed•ness *n* **1 :** the quality or state of being farsighted **2 :** HYPEROPIA

Far•xi•ga \fär-ˈsē-gə\ *trademark* — used for a preparation of dapagliflozin

FAS *abbr* fetal alcohol syndrome

fasc *abbr* fasciculus

fas•cia \ˈfa-shə, ˈfā-, -shē-ə\ *n, pl* **-ci•ae** \-shē-ˌē\ *or* **-cias :** a sheet of connective tissue (as an aponeurosis) covering or binding together body structures; *also* **:** tissue occurring in such a sheet — see DEEP FASCIA, SUPERFICIAL FASCIA — **fas•cial** \-shəl, -shē-əl\ *adj*

fasciae — see TENSOR FASCIAE LATAE

fascia la•ta \-ˈlä-tə, -ˈlā-\ *n, pl* **fasciae la•tae** \-ˈlä-tē, -ˈlā-\ **:** the deep fascia that forms a complete sheath for the thigh

fas•ci•cle \ˈfa-si-kəl\ *n* **:** a small bundle; *esp* **:** FASCICULUS

fasciculata — see ZONA FASCICULATA

fas•cic•u•la•tion \fə-ˌsi-kyə-ˈlā-shən, fa-\ *n* **:** muscular twitching involving the simultaneous contraction of contiguous groups of muscle fibers

fas•cic•u•lus \fə-ˈsi-kyə-ləs, fa-\ *n, pl* **-li** \-ˌlī\ **:** a slender bundle of fibers: **a :** a bundle of skeletal muscle cells bound together by fasciae and forming one of the constituent elements of a muscle **b :** a bundle of nerve fibers that follow the same course but do not necessarily have like functional connections **c :** TRACT 2

fasciculus cu•ne•atus \-ˌkyü-nē-ˈā-təs\ *n* **:** either of a pair of nerve tracts of the posterior funiculus of the spinal cord that are situated on opposite sides of the posterior median septum lateral to the fasciculus gracilis and that carry nerve fibers from the upper part of the body — called also *column of Burdach, cuneate fasciculus*

fasciculus grac•i•lis \-ˈgra-sə-ləs\ *n* **:** either of a pair of nerve tracts of the posterior funiculus of the spinal cord that carry nerve fibers from the lower part of the body — called also *gracile fasciculus*

fas·ci·ec·to·my \ˌfa-shē-ˈek-tə-mē, -sē-\ *n, pl* **-mies** : surgical excision of strips of fascia

fas·ci·i·tis \ˌfa-shē-ˈī-təs,-sē-\ *also* **fas·ci·tis** \fa-ˈshī-təs, -ˈsī-\ *n* : inflammation of a fascia (as from injury)

Fas·ci·o·la \fə-ˈsē-ə-lə, -ˈsī-\ *n* : a genus of digenetic trematode worms (family Fasciolidae) including common liver flukes of various mammals

fa·sci·o·li·a·sis \fə-ˌsē-ə-ˈlī-ə-səs, -ˌsī-\ *n, pl* **-a·ses** \-ˌsēz\ : infestation with or disease caused by liver flukes of the genus *Fasciola* (*F. hepatica* or *F. gigantica*)

fas·ci·o·li·cide \fə-ˈsē-ə-lə-ˌsīd, fa-\ *n* : an agent that destroys liver flukes of the genus *Fasciola*

Fas·ci·o·loi·des \fə-ˌsē-ə-ˈlȯi-(ˌ)dēz, -ˌsī-\ *n* : a genus of trematode worms (family Fasciolidae) including the giant liver flukes of ruminant mammals

fas·ci·o·lop·si·a·sis \-ˌläp-ˈsī-ə-səs\ *n, pl* **-a·ses** \-ˌsēz\ : infestation with or disease caused by an intestinal fluke of the genus *Fasciolopsis* (*F. buski*)

Fas·ci·o·lop·sis \-ˈläp-səs\ *n* : a genus of trematode worms (family Fasciolidae) that includes an intestinal parasite (*F. buski*) esp. of humans and swine in much of eastern Asia

fas·ci·ot·o·my \ˌfa-shē-ˈä-tə-mē\ *n, pl* **-mies** : surgical incision of a fascia

¹fast \ˈfast\ *adj* : resistant to change (as from destructive action) — used chiefly of organisms and in combination with the agent resisted <acid-*fast* bacteria>

²fast *vb* **1 a** : to abstain from food **b** : to eat sparingly or abstain from some foods **2** : to deny food to <the patient was ~*ed* before treatment>

³fast *n* **1** : the practice of fasting **2** : a time of fasting

fas·tig·ial nucleus \fa-ˈsti-jē-əl-\ *n* : a nucleus lying near the midline in the roof of the fourth ventricle of the brain

fas·tig·i·um \fa-ˈsti-jē-əm\ *n* : the period at which the symptoms of a disease are most pronounced

fast·ing \ˈfas-tiŋ\ *adj* : of or taken from a fasting subject <~ blood sugar levels>; *also* : occurring from or caused by fasting <~ hyperglycemia>

fast–twitch \ˈfast-ˌtwich\ *adj* : of, relating to, or being muscle fiber that contracts quickly esp. during brief high-intensity physical activity requiring strength — compare SLOW-TWITCH

¹fat \ˈfat\ *adj* **fat·ter; fat·test** : fleshy with superfluous flabby tissue that is not muscle : OBESE — **fat·ness** *n*

²fat *n* **1** : animal tissue consisting chiefly of cells distended with greasy or oily matter — see BROWN FAT **2 a** : oily or greasy matter making up the bulk of adipose tissue **b** : any of numerous compounds of carbon, hydrogen, and oxygen that are glycerides of fatty acids, are the chief constituents of plant and animal fat, are a major class of energy-rich food, and are soluble in organic solvents but not in water **c** : a solid or semisolid fat as distinguished from an oil **3** : the condition of fatness : OBESITY

fa·tal \ˈfāt-ᵊl\ *adj* : causing death — **fa·tal·ly** *adv*

fatal familial insomnia *n* : a rare fatal prion disease that is inherited as an autosomal dominant trait, that is marked by progressive neurodegenerative changes esp. in the thalamus, and that tends to follow a clinical course exhibiting disturbances of the sleep cycle, intractable insomnia, motor disturbances (as ataxia and myoclonus), dysautonomia, dementia, coma, and death

fa·tal·i·ty \fā-ˈta-lə-tē, fə-\ *n, pl* **-ties** **1** : the quality or state of causing death or destruction : DEADLINESS **2 a** : death resulting from a disaster **b** : one who suffers such a death

fat cell *n* : a fat-containing cell of adipose tissue — called also *adipocyte*

fat de·pot \-ˈde-(ˌ)pō, -ˈdē-\ *n* : ADIPOSE TISSUE

fat farm *n* : a health spa that specializes in weight reduction

father figure *n* : one often of particular power or influence who serves as an emotional substitute for a father

father image *n* : an idealization of one's father often projected onto someone to whom one looks for guidance and protection

fa·ti·ga·bil·i·ty *also* **fa·ti·gua·bil·i·ty** \fə-ˌtē-gə-ˈbi-lə-tē, ˌfa-ti-\ *n, pl* **-ties** : susceptibility to fatigue

fa·tigue \fə-ˈtēg\ *n* **1** : weariness or exhaustion from labor, exertion, or stress **2** : the temporary loss of power to respond induced in a sensory receptor or motor end organ by continued stimulation — **fatigue** *vb*

fat pad *n* : a flattened mass of fatty tissue

fat–sol·u·ble \ˈfat-ˌsäl-yə-bəl\ *adj* : soluble in fats or fat solvents

fat·ty \ˈfa-tē\ *adj* **fat·ti·er; -est** **1 a** : unduly stout **b** : marked by an abnormal deposit of fat **2** : derived from or chemically related to fat — **fat·ti·ness** *n*

fatty acid *n* **1** : any of numerous saturated acids $C_nH_{2n+1}COOH$ (as acetic acid) containing a single carboxyl group and including many that occur naturally usu. in the form of esters in fats, waxes, and essential oils **2** : any of the saturated or unsaturated acids (as palmitic acid) with a single carboxyl group and usu. an even number of carbon atoms that occur naturally in the form of glycerides in fats and fatty oils

fatty degeneration *n* : a process of tissue degeneration marked by the deposition of fat globules in the cells — called also *steatosis*

fatty infiltration *n* : infiltration of the tissue of an organ with excess amounts of fat

fatty liver *n* **1** : an abnormal condition of the liver that is marked by excess lipid accumulation in the hepatocytes, has various causes (as obesity, malnutrition, excessive alcohol consumption, diabetes, and toxins) and is often asymptomatic and benign but may progress to fibrosis and liver failure **2** : a liver affected with fatty liver

fatty oil *n* : a fat that is liquid at ordinary temperatures — called also *fixed oil*

fau•ces \ˈfȯ-ˌsēz\ *n sing or pl* : the narrow passage from the mouth to the pharynx situated between the soft palate and the base of the tongue — called also *isthmus of the fauces* — **fau•cial** \ˈfȯ-shəl\ *adj*

fau•na \ˈfȯn-ə, ˈfän-\ *n, pl* **faunas** *also* **fau•nae** \-ˌē, -ˌī\ : animal life; *esp* : the animals characteristic of a region, period, or special environment — compare FLORA 1 — **fau•nal** \-ᵊl\ *adj* — **fau•nal•ly** \-ᵊl-ē\ *adv*

fa•va bean \ˈfä-və-\ *n* : BROAD BEAN

fa•vism \ˈfä-ˌvi-zəm, ˈfā-\ *n* : a condition esp. of males of Mediterranean descent that is marked by the development of hemolytic anemia upon consumption of broad beans or inhalation of broad bean pollen and is caused by a usu. inherited deficiency of glucose-6-phosphate

fa•vus \ˈfā-vəs\ *n* : a contagious skin disease of humans and many domestic animals and fowls that is caused by a fungus (as *Trichophyton schoenleinii*) — **fa•vic** \-vik\ *adj*

FDA *abbr* Food and Drug Administration

Fe *symbol* iron

febri- *comb form* : fever ⟨*febri*fuge⟩

feb•ri•fuge \ˈfe-brə-ˌfyüj\ *n or adj* : ANTIPYRETIC

fe•brile \ˈfe-ˌbrīl, ˈfē-\ *adj* : marked or caused by fever : FEVERISH

fe•bux•o•stat \fə-ˈbək-sə-ˌstat\ *n* : a drug $C_{16}H_{16}N_2O_3S$ taken orally to treat high levels of uric acid associated with gout — see ULORIC

fe•cal \ˈfē-kəl\ *adj* : of, relating to, or constituting feces — **fe•cal•ly** *adv*

fe•ca•lith \ˈfē-kə-ˌlith\ *n* : a concretion of dry compact feces formed in the intestine or vermiform appendix

fe•cal•oid \-kə-ˌlȯid\ *adj* : resembling dung

fe•ces \ˈfē-(ˌ)sēz\ *n pl* : bodily waste discharged through the anus : EXCREMENT

Fech•ner's law \ˈfek-nərz-, ˈfek-\ *n* : WEBER-FECHNER LAW

fec•u•lent \ˈfe-kyə-lənt\ *adj* : foul with impurities : FECAL

fe•cund \ˈfe-kənd, ˈfē-\ *adj* **1** : characterized by having produced many offspring **2** : capable of producing : not sterile or barren — **fe•cun•di•ty** \fi-ˈkən-də-tē, fe-\ *n*

fe•cun•date \ˈfe-kən-ˌdāt, ˈfē-\ *vb* **-dat•ed; -dat•ing** : IMPREGNATE — **fe•cun•da•tion** \ˌfe-kən-ˈdā-shən, ˌfē-\ *n*

feed•back \ˈfēd-ˌbak\ *n* **1** : the partial reversion of the effects of a process to its source or to a preceding stage **2** : the return to a point of origin of evaluative or corrective information about an action or process; *also* : the information so transmitted

feedback inhibition *n* : inhibition of an enzyme controlling an early stage of a series of biochemical reactions by the end product when it reaches a critical concentration

feed•ing tube \ˈfē-diŋ-\ *n* : a flexible tube passed into the stomach (as by way of the nasal passages or through a surgical opening in the abdominal wall) for introducing fluids and liquid food into the stomach

fee–for–service *n, often attrib* : separate payment to a health-care provider for each medical service rendered to a patient ⟨a ~ health plan⟩

feel•ing \ˈfē-liŋ\ *n* **1** : the one of the basic physical senses of which the skin contains the chief end organs and of which the sensations of touch and temperature are characteristic : TOUCH; *also* : a sensation experienced through this sense **2** : an emotional state or reaction **3** : the overall quality of one's awareness esp. as measured along a pleasantness-unpleasantness continuum

fee splitting *n* : payment by a medical specialist (as a surgeon) of a part of the specialist's fee to the physician who made the referral — **fee splitter** *n*

feet *pl of* FOOT

Feh•ling's solution \ˈfā-liŋz-\ *or* **Fehling solution** \-liŋ-\ *n* : a blue solution of Rochelle salt and copper sulfate used as an oxidizing agent in a test for sugars and aldehydes in which the precipitation of a red oxide of copper indicates a positive result

Fehling, Hermann von (1812–1885), German chemist.

fel•ba•mate \ˈfel-bə-ˌmāt\ *n* : an anticonvulsant drug $C_{11}H_{14}N_2O_4$ used to treat severe epilepsy or epilepsy that is unresponsive to other drugs

Fel•den•krais \ˈfel-dən-ˌkrīs\ *trademark* — used for a system of aided body movements intended to increase bodily awareness and ease tension

fe•line \ˈfē-ˌlīn\ *adj* : of, relating to, or affecting cats or the cat family (Felidae) — **feline** *n*

feline distemper *n* : PANLEUKOPENIA

feline enteritis *n* : PANLEUKOPENIA

feline infectious anemia *n* : a contagious disease of cats characterized by weakness, lethargy, loss of appetite, and hemolytic anemia and caused by a bacterial parasite of red blood cells belonging to the genus *Mycoplasma* (*M. haemofelis*)

feline infectious peritonitis *n* : a usu. fatal infectious disease of cats caused by a coronavirus (species *Alphacoronavirus 1* of the genus *Alphacoronavirus*) and marked esp. by fever, weight and appetite loss, and ascites with a thick yellow fluid

feline leukemia *n* : a disease of cats caused by the feline leukemia virus, characterized by leukemia and lymphoma, and often resulting in death

feline leukemia virus *n* : a retrovirus (species *Feline leukemia virus* of the genus *Gammaretrovirus*) that is widespread in cat populations, is usu. transmitted by direct contact, and is associated with or causes malignant lymphoma, feline leukemia, anemia, glomerulonephritis, and immunosuppression — abbr. *FeLV*

feline panleukopenia *n* : PANLEUKOPENIA

feline pneumonitis *n* : an infectious disease of the eyes and upper respiratory tract of cats that is caused by a bacterium (*Chlamydia psittaci* syn. *Chlamydophila psittaci*) and is marked esp. by conjunctivitis and rhinitis

fel•late \ˈfe-ˌlāt, fə-ˈlāt\ *vb* **fel•lat•ed; fel•lat•ing** : to perform fellatio on someone — **fel•la•tor** \-ˌla-tər, -ˈlā-\ *n*

fel•la•tio \fə-ˈlā-shē-ˌō, fe-, -ˈlä-tē-\ *also* **fel•la•tion** \-ˈlā-shən\ *n, pl* **-tios** *also* **-tions** : oral stimulation of the penis

fellea — see VESICA FELLEA

fel•low \ˈfe-(ˌ)lō\ *n* : a young physician who has completed training as an intern and resident and is granted a stipend and position allowing further study or research in a specialty

fe•lo•di•pine \fə-ˈlō-də-ˌpēn\ *n* : a calcium channel blocker $C_{18}H_{19}Cl_2NO_4$ used esp. in the treatment of hypertension

fel•on \ˈfe-lən\ *n* : a painful abscess of the deep tissues of the palmar surface of the fingertip that is typically caused by infection of a bacterium (as *Staphylococcus aureus*) and is marked by swelling and pain — compare PARONYCHIA, WHITLOW 1

Fel•ty syndrome \ˈfel-tē-\ *or* **Felty's syndrome** \-tēz-\ *n* : a condition characterized esp. by rheumatoid arthritis, neutropenia, and splenomegaly

Felty, Augustus Roi (1895–1964), American physician.

FeLV *abbr* feline leukemia virus

fe•male \ˈfē-ˌmāl\ *n* : an individual that bears young or produces eggs as distinguished from one that produces sperm; *esp* : a woman or girl as distinguished from a man or boy — **female** *adj* — **fe•male•ness** *n*

female genital mutilation *n* : a procedure performed esp. as a cultural rite that includes total or partial excision of the female external genitalia and esp. the clitoris and labia minora and is now outlawed in many nations including the U.S. — abbr. *FGM;* called also *female circumcision*

female hormone *n* : a sex hormone (as an estrogen) primarily produced and functioning in the female

Fem•a•ra \ˈfe-mə-rə\ *trademark* — used for a preparation of letrozole

fem•i•nize \ˈfe-mə-ˌnīz\ *vb* **-nized; -niz•ing** : to cause (a male or castrate) to take on feminine characters (as by implantation of ovaries or administration of estrogenic substances) — **fem•i•ni•za•tion** \ˌfe-mə-nə-ˈzā-shən\ *n*

femora *pl of* FEMUR

fem•o•ral \ˈfe-mə-rəl\ *adj* : of or relating to the femur or thigh

femoral artery *n* : the chief artery of the thigh that lies in the anterior part of the thigh — see DEEP FEMORAL ARTERY

femoral canal *n* : the space that is situated between the femoral vein and the inner wall of the femoral sheath

femoral nerve *n* : the largest branch of the lumbar plexus that supplies extensor muscles of the thigh and skin areas on the front of the thigh and medial surface of the leg and foot and that sends articular branches to the hip and knee joints

femoral ring *n* : the oval upper opening of the femoral canal often the seat of a hernia

femoral sheath *n* : the fascial sheath investing the femoral vessels

femoral triangle *n* : an area in the upper anterior part of the thigh bounded by the inguinal ligament, the sartorius, and the adductor longus — called also *femoral trigone, Scarpa's triangle*

femoral vein *n* : the chief vein of the thigh that is a continuation of the popliteal vein and continues above the inguinal ligament as the external iliac vein

femoris — see BICEPS FEMORIS, PROFUNDA FEMORIS, PROFUNDA FEMORIS ARTERY, QUADRATUS FEMORIS, QUADRICEPS FEMORIS, RECTUS FEMORIS

femoro- *comb form* : femoral and ⟨*femoro*popliteal⟩

fem•o•ro•pop•li•te•al \ˌfe-mə-rō-ˌpä-plə-ˈtē-əl, -pä-ˈpli-tē-əl\ *adj* : of, relating to, or connecting the femoral and popliteal arteries ⟨a ~ bypass⟩

fe•mur \ˈfē-mər\ *n, pl* **fe•murs** *or* **fem•o•ra** \ˈfe-mə-rə\ : the proximal bone of the hind or lower limb that is the longest and largest bone in the human body, extends from the hip to the knee, articulates above with the acetabulum, and articulates with the tibia below by a pair of condyles — called also *thigh bone*

fe•nes•tra \fə-ˈnes-trə\ *n, pl* **-trae** \-ˌtrē, -ˌtrī\ **1** : a small anatomical opening (as in a bone): as **a** : OVAL WINDOW **b** : ROUND WINDOW **2 a** : a small opening cut in bone : WINDOW 2 **b** : a small opening in a surgical instrument — **fe·nes·tral** \-trəl\ *adj*

fenestra coch·le·ae \-ˈkä-klē-ˌē, -ˈkō-klē-ˌī\ *n* : ROUND WINDOW

fenestra oval·is \-ˌō-ˈvā-ləs\ *n* : OVAL WINDOW

fenestra ro·tun·da \-ˌrō-ˈtən-də\ *n* : ROUND WINDOW

fen·es·trat·ed \ˈfe-nə-ˌstrā-təd\ *adj* : having one or more openings or pores ⟨~ blood capillaries⟩

fen·es·tra·tion \ˌfe-nə-ˈstrā-shən\ *n* **1 a** : a natural or surgically created opening in a surface **b** : the presence of such openings **2** : a surgical procedure that involves cutting an opening in the bony labyrinth between the inner ear and tympanum to replace natural fenestrae that are not functional (as in otosclerosis)

fenestra ves·ti·bu·li \-ves-ˈti-byə-ˌlī\ *n* : OVAL WINDOW

fen·flur·amine \ˌfen-ˈflu̇r-ə-ˌmēn\ *n* : an anorectic amphetamine derivative $C_{12}H_{16}F_3N$ formerly used in the form of its hydrochloride to treat obesity but no longer used due to its association with heart valve disease — see DEXFENFLURAMINE, FEN-PHEN 1

fen·o·fi·brate \ˌfe-nō-ˈfī-ˌbrāt\ *n* : a lipid-regulating drug $C_{20}H_{21}ClO_4$ used to reduce levels of LDL, triglyceride, and apolipoprotein B and increase levels of HDL — see ANTARA, FENOGLIDE, LIPOFEN, LOFIBRA, TRICOR, TRIGLIDE; compare FENOFIBRIC ACID

fen·o·fi·bric acid \-ˌfī-brik-\ *n* : a lipid-regulating agent $C_{17}H_{15}ClO_4$ that is the active metabolite of fenofibrate often used in the form of its choline salt $C_{22}H_{28}ClNO_5$ similarly to fenofibrate in the treatment of hypercholesterolemia and hypertriglyceridemia — see FIBRICOR, TRILIPIX

Fen·o·glide \ˈfen-ō-ˌglīd\ *trademark* — used for a preparation of fenofibrate

fen·o·pro·fen \ˌfe-nə-ˈprō-fən\ *n* : an anti-inflammatory analgesic used in the form of its hydrated calcium salt $C_{30}H_{26}CaO_6{\cdot}2H_2O$ esp. to treat arthritis

fen–phen \ˈfen-ˌfen\ *n* **1** : a former diet drug combination of phentermine with either fenfluramine or dexfenfluramine that was withdrawn from use due to its association with heart disease — called also *phen-fen* **2** : a former herbal preparation usu. of ephedra and Saint-John's-wort used as an appetite suppressant until ephedra was banned from use in the U.S. — called also *phen-fen*

fen·ta·nyl \ˈfent-ᵊn-ˌil\ *n* : a synthetic opioid narcotic analgesic $C_{22}H_{28}N_2O$ with pharmacological action similar to morphine that is administered esp. in the form of its citrate $C_{22}H_{28}N_2O{\cdot}C_6H_8O_7$ — see ACTIQ

fer·ment \ˈfər-ˌment, (ˌ)fər-ˈ\ *n* : ENZYME; *also* : FERMENTATION

fer·men·ta·tion \ˌfər-mən-ˈtā-shən, -ˌmen-\ *n* : an enzymatically controlled anaerobic breakdown of an energy-rich compound (as a carbohydrate to carbon dioxide and alcohol); *broadly* : an enzymatically controlled transformation of an organic compound — **fer·ment** \(ˌ)fər-ˈment\ *vb* — **fer·men·ta·tive** \(ˌ)fər-ˈmen-tə-tiv\ *adj*

fer·mi·um \ˈfer-mē-əm, ˈfər-\ *n* : a radioactive metallic element artificially produced — symbol *Fm;* see ELEMENT table

fer·ric \ˈfer-ik\ *adj* **1** : of, relating to, or containing iron **2** : being or containing iron usu. with a valence of three

ferric chloride *n* : a salt $FeCl_3$ that is used in medicine in a water solution or tincture usu. as an astringent or styptic

ferric oxide *n* : the red or black oxide of iron Fe_2O_3

ferric py·ro·phos·phate \-ˌpī-rō-ˈfäs-ˌfāt\ *n* : a green or yellowish-green salt $Fe_4(P_2O_7)_3{\cdot}nH_2O$ that is used as a source of iron esp. to fortify food

fer·ri·he·mo·glo·bin \ˌfer-ˌī-ˈhē-mə-ˌglō-bən, ˌfer-i-\ *n* : METHEMOGLOBIN

fer·ri·tin \ˈfer-ət-ᵊn\ *n* : a crystalline iron-containing protein that functions in the storage of iron and is found esp. in the liver and spleen

fer·rous \ˈfer-əs\ *adj* **1** : of, relating to, or containing iron **2** : being or containing iron with a valence of two

ferrous fumarate *n* : a reddish-orange to red-brown powder $C_4H_2FeO_4$ used orally to treat iron-deficiency anemia

ferrous gluconate *n* : a yellowish-gray or pale greenish-yellow powder or granules $C_{12}H_{22}FeO_{14}$ used as a hematinic in the treatment of iron-deficiency anemia

ferrous sulfate *n* : an astringent iron salt obtained usu. in pale green crystalline form $FeSO_4{\cdot}7H_2O$ and used in medicine chiefly for treating iron-deficiency anemia

fer·tile \ˈfərt-ᵊl, ˈfər-ˌtīl\ *adj* **1** : capable of growing or developing ⟨a ~ egg⟩ **2** : developing spores or spore-bearing organs **3 a** : capable of breeding or reproducing **b** *of an estrous cycle* : marked by the production of one or more viable eggs

fer·til·i·ty \(ˌ)fər-ˈti-lə-tē\ *n, pl* **-ties 1** : the quality or state of being fertile **2** : the birthrate of a population — compare MORTALITY 2b

fer·til·i·za·tion \ˌfərt-ᵊl-ə-ˈzā-shən\ *n* : an act or process of making fertile; *specif* : the process of union of two gametes whereby the somatic chromosome number is restored and the development of a new individual is initiated — **fer·til·ize** \ˈfərt-ᵊl-ˌīz\ *vb*

fertilization membrane *n* : a resistant membranous layer in eggs of many animals that forms following fertilization by the thickening and separation of the vitelline membrane from the cell surface and that prevents multiple fertilization

[1]**fes·ter** \ˈfes-tər\ *n* : a suppurating sore : PUSTULE

[2]**fester** *vb* **fes·tered; fes·ter·ing** : to generate pus

fes·ti·nat·ing \ˈfes-tə-ˌnā-tiŋ\ *adj* : being a walking gait (as in Parkinson's disease) characterized by involuntary acceleration — **fes·ti·na·tion** \ˌfes-tə-ˈnā-shən\ *n*

fe·tal \ˈfēt-ᵊl\ *adj* : of, relating to, or being a fetus

fetal alcohol syndrome *n* : a highly variable group of birth defects including intellectual disability, deficient growth, central nervous system dysfunction, and malformations of the skull and face that tend to occur in the offspring of women who consume large amounts of alcohol during pregnancy — abbr. *FAS*

fetal hemoglobin *n* : hemoglobin that consists of two alpha chains and two gamma chains and that predominates in the blood of a newborn and persists in increased proportions in some forms of anemia (as thalassemia) — called also *hemoglobin F*

fetal hydrops *n* : HYDROPS FETALIS

fetalis — see ERYTHROBLASTOSIS FETALIS, HYDROPS FETALIS

fetal position *n* : a position (as of a sleeping person) in which the body lies curled up on one side with the arms and legs drawn up toward the chest and the head bowed forward and which is assumed in some forms of psychological regression

feti- — see FETO-

fe·ti·cide \ˈfē-tə-ˌsīd\ *n* : the action or process of causing the death of a fetus

fe·tish *also* **fe·tich** \ˈfe-tish, ˈfē-\ *n* : an object or bodily part whose real or fantasized presence is psychologically necessary for sexual gratification and that is an object of fixation to the extent that it may interfere with complete sexual expression

fe·tish·ism *also* **fe·tich·ism** \-ti-ˌshi-zəm\ *n* : the pathological displacement of erotic interest and satisfaction to a fetish — **fe·tish·ist** \-shist\ *n* — **fe·tish·is·tic** \ˌfe-ti-ˈshis-tik *also* ˌfē-\ *adj* — **fe·tish·is·ti·cal·ly** \-ti-k(ə-)lē\ *adv*

fet·lock \ˈfet-ˌläk\ *n* **1 a** : a projection bearing a tuft of hair on the back of the leg above the hoof of a horse or similar animal **b** : the tuft of hair itself **2** : the joint of the limb at the fetlock

feto- *or* **feti-** *comb form* : fetus ⟨*feticide*⟩

fe·tol·o·gist \fē-ˈtä-lə-jist\ *n* : a specialist in fetology

fe·tol·o·gy \fē-ˈtä-lə-jē\ *n, pl* **-gies** : a branch of medical science concerned with the study and treatment of the fetus in the uterus

fe·to·pro·tein \ˌfē-tō-ˈprō-ˌtēn, -tē-ən\ *n* : any of several fetal antigens present in the adult in some abnormal conditions; *esp* : ALPHA-FETOPROTEIN

fe·tor he·pat·i·cus \ˈfē-tər-hi-ˈpa-ti-kəs, -ˌtȯr-\ *n* : a characteristically disagreeable odor to the breath that is a sign of liver failure

fe·to·scope \ˈfē-tə-ˌskōp\ *n* **1** : an endoscope for visual examination of the pregnant uterus **2** : a stethoscope for listening to the fetal heartbeat

fe·tos·co·py \fē-ˈtäs-kə-pē\ *n, pl* **-pies** : examination of the pregnant uterus by means of a fetoscope

fe·to·tox·ic \ˌfē-tə-ˈtäk-sik\ *adj* : toxic to fetuses — **fe·to·tox·i·ci·ty** \-täk-ˈsi-sə-tē\ *n*

fe·tus \ˈfē-təs\ *n, pl* **fe·tus·es** : an unborn or unhatched vertebrate esp. after attaining the basic structural plan of its kind; *specif* : a developing human from usu. two months after conception to birth — compare EMBRYO

Feul·gen reaction \ˈfȯil-gən\ *n* : the development of a purple color by DNA in a microscopic preparation stained with a modified Schiff's reagent

Feulgen, Robert Joachim (1884–1955), German biochemist.

[1]**fe·ver** \ˈfē-vər\ *n* **1** : a rise of body temperature above the normal **2** : an abnormal bodily state characterized by increased production of heat, accelerated heart action and pulse, and systemic debility with weakness, loss of appetite, and thirst **3** : any of various diseases of which fever is a prominent symptom — **fe·ver·ish** \-və-rish\ *adj*

[2]**fever** *vb* **fe·vered; fe·ver·ing** : to affect with or be in a fever

fever blister *n* : COLD SORE

fever therapy *n* : a treatment of disease by fever induced by various artificial means

fever thermometer *n* : CLINICAL THERMOMETER

Fex·mid \ˈfek-smid\ *trademark* — used for a preparation of cyclobenzaprine

fex·o·fen·a·dine \ˌfek-sō-ˈfe-nə-ˌdēn\ *n* : a nonsedating H_1 antagonist administered orally in the form of its hydrochloride $C_{32}H_{39}NO_4·HCl$ to relieve symptoms of seasonal allergic rhinitis and chronic hives — called also *fexofenadine hydrochloride;* see ALLEGRA

FFA *abbr* free fatty acids

FGF *abbr* fibroblast growth factor

FGM *abbr* female genital mutilation

fi·ber \ˈfī-bər\ *n* **1 a** : a strand of nerve tissue : AXON, DENDRITE **b** : one of the filaments composing most of the intercellular matrix of connective tissue **c** : one of the elongated contractile cells of muscle tissue **2** : indigestible material in food that stimulates the intestine to peristalsis — called also *bulk, dietary fiber, roughage*

fiber of Mül·ler \-ˈmyü-lər, -ˈmə-\ *n* : MÜLLER CELL

fiber optics *n pl* **1** : thin transparent fibers of glass or plastic that transmit light throughout their length by internal reflections; *also* : a bundle of such fibers used in an instrument (as an endoscope) **2** : the technique of the use of fiber optics — used with a sing. verb — **fi•ber–op•tic** *adj*

fi•ber•scope \ˈfī-bər-ˌskōp\ *n* : a flexible endoscope that utilizes fiber optics to transmit light and is used for visual examination of inaccessible areas (as the stomach)

fiber tract *n* : TRACT 2

fibr- *or* **fibro-** *comb form* **1** : fiber : fibrous tissue ⟨*fibro*genesis⟩ **2** : fibrous and ⟨*fibro*elastic⟩

fi•brate \ˈfī-ˌbrāt, ˈfi-\ *n* : any of a group of triglyceride-lowering drugs (as fenofibrate and gemfibrozil) that are derivatives of clofibrate

fi•bre *chiefly Brit var of* FIBER

Fi•bri•cor \ˈfī-brə-ˌkȯr\ *trademark* — used for a preparation of fenofibric acid

fi•bril \ˈfī-brəl, ˈfi-\ *n* : a small filament or fiber: as **a** : one of the fine threads into which a striated muscle fiber can be longitudinally split **b** : NEUROFIBRIL

fi•bril•la \fī-ˈbri-lə, fi-; ˈfī-bri-lə, ˈfi-\ *n, pl* **fi•bril•lae** \-ˌlē\ : FIBRIL

fi•bril•lar \ˈfi-brə-lər, ˈfī-; fī-ˈbri-, fi-\ *adj* **1** : of or like fibrils or fibers ⟨a ~ network⟩ **2** : of or exhibiting fibrillation ⟨~ twitchings⟩

fi•bril•lary \ˈfī-brə-ˌler-ē, ˈfi-; fī-ˈbri-lə-rē, fi-\ *adj* **1** : of or relating to fibrils or fibers **2** : of, relating to, or marked by fibrillation ⟨~ chorea⟩

fi•bril•la•tion \ˌfi-brə-ˈlā-shən, ˌfī-\ *n* **1** : an act or process of forming fibers or fibrils **2 a** : a muscular twitching involving individual muscle fibers acting without coordination **b** : very rapid irregular contractions of the muscle fibers of the heart resulting in a lack of synchronism between heartbeat and pulse — **fi•bril•late** \ˈfi-brə-ˌlāt, ˈfī-\ *vb*

fi•bril•lin \ˈfī-brə-lin, ˈfi-\ *n* : a large extracellular glycoprotein of connective tissue that is a structural component of microfibrils associated esp. with elastin

fi•bril•lo•gen•e•sis \ˌfi-brə-ˌlō-ˈje-nə-səs, ˌfī-\ *n, pl* **-e•ses** \-ˌsēz\ : the development of fibrils

fi•brin \ˈfī-brən\ *n* : a white insoluble fibrous protein formed from fibrinogen by the action of thrombin esp. in the clotting of blood

fi•brin•ase \-brə-ˌnās, -nāz\ *n* : FACTOR XIII

fi•brin•o•gen \fī-ˈbri-nə-jən\ *n* : a plasma protein that is produced in the liver and is converted into fibrin during blood clot formation

fi•brin•o•gen•o•pe•nia \(ˌ)fī-ˌbri-nə-ˌje-nə-ˈpē-nē-ə, -nyə\ *n* : a deficiency of fibrin or fibrinogen or both in the blood

fi•bri•noid \ˈfi-brə-ˌnȯid, ˈfī-\ *n, often attrib* : a homogeneous material that resembles fibrin and is formed in the walls of blood vessels and in connective tissue in some pathological conditions and normally in the placenta

fi•bri•no•ly•sin \ˌfī-brən-ᵊl-ˈīs-ᵊn\ *n* : any of several proteolytic enzymes that promote the dissolution of blood clots; *esp* : PLASMIN

fi•bri•no•ly•sis \-ˈī-səs, -brə-ˈnä-lə-səs\ *n, pl* **-ly•ses** \-ˌsēz\ : the usu. enzymatic breakdown of fibrin — **fi•bri•no•lyt•ic** \-brən-ᵊl-ˈi-tik\ *adj*

fi•bri•no•pe•nia \ˌfī-brə-nō-ˈpē-nē-ə, -nyə\ *n* : FIBRINOGENOPENIA

fi•bri•no•pep•tide \-ˈpep-ˌtīd\ *n* : any of the polypeptides that are cleaved from fibrinogen by thrombin during blood clot formation

fi•bri•no•pur•u•lent \-ˈpyu̇r-yə-lənt, -ə-lənt\ *adj* : containing, characterized by, or exuding fibrin and pus

fi•bri•nous \ˈfi-brə-nəs, ˈfī-\ *adj* : marked by the presence of fibrin

fibro- — see FIBR-

fi•bro•ad•e•no•ma \ˌfī-(ˌ)brō-ˌad-ᵊn-ˈō-mə\ *n, pl* **-mas** *also* **-ma•ta** \-mə-tə\ : adenoma with a large amount of fibrous tissue

fi•bro•blast \ˈfī-brə-ˌblast, ˈfi-\ *n* : a connective-tissue cell of mesenchymal origin that secretes proteins and esp. molecular collagen from which the extracellular fibrillar matrix of connective tissue forms — **fi•bro•blas•tic** \ˌfī-brə-ˈblas-tik, ˌfi-\ *adj*

fibroblast growth factor *n* : any of several protein growth factors that stimulate the proliferation esp. of endothelial cells and that promote angiogenesis — abbr. *FGF*

fi•bro•car•ti•lage \ˌfī-(ˌ)brō-ˈkärt-ᵊl-ij\ *n* : cartilage in which the matrix except immediately about the cells is largely composed of fibers like those of ordinary connective tissue; *also* : a structure or part composed of such cartilage — **fi•bro•car•ti•lag•i•nous** \-ˌkärt-ᵊl-ˈa-jə-nəs\ *adj*

fi•bro•cys•tic \ˌfī-brə-ˈsis-tik, ˌfi-\ *adj* : characterized by the presence or development of fibrous tissue and cysts

fibrocystic disease of the pancreas *n* : CYSTIC FIBROSIS

fi•bro•cyte \ˈfī-brə-ˌsīt, ˈfi-\ *n* : FIBROBLAST; *specif* : a spindle-shaped cell of fibrous tissue

fi•bro•dys•pla•sia os•sif•i•cans pro•gres•si•va \ˌfī-brō-di-ˈsplā-zh(ē-)ə-ä-ˈsi-fə-ˌkanz-prə-ˈgre-sə-və\ *n* : a rare hereditary disorder that is characterized by progressive ossification of muscle and connective tissue and is inherited as an autosomal recessive trait — called also *stone man syndrome*

fi•bro•elas•tic \ˌfī-(ˌ)brō-i-ˈlas-tik\ *adj* : consisting of both fibrous and elastic elements ⟨~ tissue⟩

fi•bro•elas•to•sis \-ˌlas-ˈtō-səs\ *n, pl* **-to•ses** \-ˌsēz\ : a condition of the body or one of its organs characterized by proliferation of fibroelastic tissue — see ENDOCARDIAL FIBROELASTOSIS

fi•bro•gen•e•sis \ˌfī-brə-ˈje-nə-səs\ *n, pl* **-e•ses** \-ˌsēz\ : the development or proliferation of fibers or fibrous tissue

fi•bro•gen•ic \-ˈje-nik\ *adj* : promoting the development of fibers

[1]**fi•broid** \ˈfī-ˌbrȯid, ˈfi-\ *adj* : resembling, forming, or consisting of fibrous tissue

[2]**fibroid** *n* : a benign tumor esp. of the uterine wall that consists of fibrous and muscular tissue

fi•bro•ma \fī-ˈbrō-mə\ *n, pl* **-mas** *also* **-ma•ta** \-tə\ : a benign tumor consisting mainly of fibrous tissue — **fi•bro•ma•tous** \-təs\ *adj*

fi•bro•ma•toid \fī-ˈbrō-mə-ˌtȯid\ *adj* : resembling a fibroma

fi•bro•ma•to•sis \(ˌ)fī-ˌbrō-mə-ˈtō-səs\ *n, pl* **-to•ses** \-ˌsēz\ : a condition marked by the presence of or a tendency to develop multiple fibromas

fi•bro•my•al•gia \-ˌmī-ˈal-jə, -jē-ə\ *n* : a chronic disorder characterized by widespread pain, tenderness, and stiffness of muscles and associated connective tissue structures that is typically accompanied by fatigue, headache, and sleep disturbances — called also *fibromyalgia syndrome, fibromyositis*

fi•bro•my•o•ma \-ˌmī-ˈō-mə\ *n, pl* **-mas** *also* **-ma•ta** \-mə-tə\ : a mixed tumor containing both fibrous and muscle tissue — **fi•bro•my•o•ma•tous** \-mə-təs\ *adj*

fi•bro•my•o•si•tis \-ˌmī-ə-ˈsī-təs\ *n* : FIBROMYALGIA

fi•bro•myx•o•ma \-mik-ˈsō-mə\ *n, pl* **-mas** *also* **-ma•ta** \-mə-tə\ : a myxoma containing fibrous tissue

fi•bro•nec•tin \ˌfī-brə-ˈnek-tən\ *n* : any of a group of glycoproteins of cell surfaces, blood plasma, and connective tissue that promote cellular adhesion and migration

fi•bro•pla•sia \ˌfī-brə-ˈplā-zhə, -zhē-ə\ *n* : the process of forming fibrous tissue — **fi•bro•plas•tic** \-ˈplas-tik\ *adj*

fibrosa — see OSTEITIS FIBROSA, OSTEITIS FIBROSA CYSTICA, OSTEITIS FIBROSA CYSTICA GENERALISTA, OSTEODYSTROPHIA FIBROSA

fi•bro•sar•co•ma \-sär-ˈkō-mə\ *n, pl* **-mas** *also* **-ma•ta** \-mə-tə\ : a sarcoma of relatively low malignancy consisting chiefly of spindle-shaped cells that tend to form collagenous fibrils

fi•brose \ˈfī-ˌbrōs\ *vb* **-brosed; -bros•ing** : to form fibrous tissue

fi•bro•se•rous \ˌfī-brō-ˈsir-əs\ *adj* : composed of a serous membrane supported by a firm layer of fibrous tissue

fi•bro•sis \fī-ˈbrō-səs\ *n, pl* **-bro•ses** \-ˌsēz\ : a condition marked by increase of interstitial fibrous tissue : fibrous degeneration — **fi•brot•ic** \-ˈbrä-tik\ *adj*

fi•bro•si•tis \ˌfī-brə-ˈsī-təs\ *n* : a rheumatic disorder of fibrous tissue; *esp* : FIBROMYALGIA — **fi•bro•sit•ic** \-ˈsi-tik\ *adj*

fibrosus — see ANNULUS FIBROSUS

fi•brous \ˈfī-brəs\ *adj* **1** : containing, consisting of, or resembling fibers **2** : characterized by fibrosis

fibrous ankylosis *n* : ankylosis due to the growth of fibrous tissue

fib•u•la \ˈfi-byə-lə\ *n, pl* **-lae** \-lē, -ˌlī\ *or* **-las** : the outer or postaxial and usu. the smaller of the two bones of the hind or lower limb below the knee that is the slenderest bone of the human body in proportion to its length and articulates above with the external tuberosity of the tibia and below with the talus — called also *calf bone* — **fib•u•lar** \-lər\ *adj*

fibular collateral ligament *n* : LATERAL COLLATERAL LIGAMENT 1

Fick principle \ˈfik-\ *n* : a generalization in physiology which states that blood flow is proportional to the difference in concentration of a substance (as oxygen) in the blood as it enters and leaves an organ and which is used to determine cardiac output — called also *Fick method*

Fick, Adolf Eugen (1829–1901), German physiologist.

FICS *abbr* Fellow of the International College of Surgeons

field \ˈfēld\ *n* **1** : a complex of forces that serve as causative agents in human behavior **2** : a region of embryonic tissue potentially capable of a particular type of differentiation **3 a** : an area that is perceived or under observation **b** : the site of a surgical operation

field hospital *n* : a military organization of medical personnel with equipment for establishing a temporary hospital in the field

field of vision *n* : VISUAL FIELD

fièvre bou•ton•neuse \ˈfyev-rə-ˌbü-tȯ-ˈnœ̄z\ *n* : BOUTONNEUSE FEVER

fifth cranial nerve *n* : TRIGEMINAL NERVE

fifth disease *n* : an acute eruptive disease esp. of children that is caused by a parvovirus (species *Human parvovirus B19* of the genus *Erythrovirus*), is first manifested by a blotchy red rash on the cheeks followed by a maculopapular rash on the extremities, and is usu. accompanied by fever and malaise — called also *erythema infectiosum*

fifth nerve *n* : TRIGEMINAL NERVE

figure–ground \ˈfi-gyər-ˈgrau̇nd\ *adj* : relating to or being the relationships between the parts of a perceptual field which is perceived as divided into a part consisting of figures having form and standing out from the part comprising the background and being relatively formless

fil•a•ment \ˈfi-lə-mənt\ *n* : a single thread or a thin flexible threadlike object, process, or appendage; *esp* : an elongated thin series of cells attached one to another (as of some bacteria) — **fil·a·men·tous** \ˌfi-lə-ˈmen-təs\ *adj*

fi·lar·ia \fə-ˈlar-ē-ə\ *n, pl* **fi·lar·i·ae** \-ē-ˌē, -ˌī\ : any of numerous slender filamentous nematodes that as adults are parasites in the blood or tissues and as larvae usu. develop in biting insects and that include forms causing elephantiasis, loaiasis, and onchocerciasis in humans and heartworm in dogs — **fi·lar·i·al** \-ē-əl\ *adj* — **fi·lar·i·id** \-ē-əd\ *adj or n*

fil·a·ri·a·sis \ˌfi-lə-ˈrī-ə-səs\ *n, pl* **-a·ses** \-ˌsēz\ : infestation with or disease caused by filariae

fi·lar·i·cide \fə-ˈlar-ə-ˌsīd\ *n* : an agent that is destructive to filariae — **fi·lar·i·cid·al** \-ˌlar-ə-ˈsīd-ᵊl\ *adj*

fi·lar·i·form \-ə-ˌfȯrm\ *adj, of a larval nematode* : resembling a filaria esp. in having a slender elongated form and in possessing a delicate capillary esophagus

fil·gras·tim \fil-ˈgras-təm\ *n* : a recombinant version of granulocyte colony-stimulating factor that is administered by injection esp. to stimulate production of neutrophils following chemotherapy — see NEUPOGEN

fili- *or* **filo-** *comb form* : thread ⟨*fili*form⟩

fil·ial generation \ˈfi-lē-əl-, ˈfil-yəl-\ *n* : a generation in a breeding experiment that is successive to a parental generation — see F_1 GENERATION, F_2 GENERATION

fi·li·form \ˈfi-lə-ˌfȯrm, ˈfī-\ *n* : an extremely slender bougie

filiform papilla *n* : any of numerous minute pointed papillae on the tongue

fil·i·pin \ˈfi-lə-pin\ *n* : an antifungal antibiotic $C_{35}H_{58}O_{11}$ produced by a bacterium of the genus *Streptomyces* (*S. filipinensis*)

fill \ˈfil\ *vb* **1** : to repair the cavities of (teeth) **2** : to supply as directed ⟨~ a prescription⟩

fil·let \ˈfi-lət\ *n* : a band of anatomical fibers; *specif* : LEMNISCUS

fill·ing \ˈfi-liŋ\ *n* **1** : material (as amalgam) used to fill a cavity in a tooth **2** : simple sporadic lymphangitis of the leg of a horse commonly due to overfeeding and insufficient exercise

film \ˈfilm\ *n* **1 a** : a thin skin or membranous covering **b** : an abnormal growth on or in the eye **2** : an exceedingly thin layer : LAMINA

film badge *n* : a small pack of sensitive photographic film worn as a badge for indicating exposure to radiation

filo- — see FILI-

fi·lo·vi·rus \ˈfī-lō-ˌvī-rəs\ *n* : any of a family (*Filoviridae*) of single-stranded chiefly filamentous RNA viruses that infect vertebrates and include the Ebola viruses and the Marburg virus

fil·ter \ˈfil-tər\ *n* **1** : a porous article or mass (as of paper) through which a gas or liquid is passed to separate out matter in suspension **2** : an apparatus containing a filter medium — **filter** *vb*

fil·ter·able \ˈfil-tə-rə-bəl\ *also* **fil·tra·ble** \-trə-bəl\ *adj* : capable of being filtered or of passing through a filter — **fil·ter·abil·i·ty** \ˌfil-tə-rə-ˈbi-lə-tē\ *n*

filterable virus *n* : any of the infectious agents that pass through a fine filter with the filtrate and remain virulent and that include the viruses and various other groups (as the mycoplasmas and rickettsiae) which were orig. considered viruses before their cellular nature was established

filter paper *n* : porous paper used esp. for filtering

fil·trate \ˈfil-ˌtrāt\ *n* : fluid that has passed through a filter

fil·tra·tion \fil-ˈtrā-shən\ *n* **1** : the process of filtering **2** : the process of passing through or as if through a filter; *also* : DIFFUSION

fi·lum ter·mi·na·le \ˈfī-ləm-ˌtər-mə-ˈnā-(ˌ)lē, ˈfē-ləm-ˌter-mə-ˈnä-ˌlā\ *n, pl* **fi·la ter·mi·na·lia** \ˈfī-lə-tər-mə-ˈnā-lē-ə, ˈfē-lə-ˌter-mə-ˈnä-lē-ə\ : the slender threadlike prolongation of the spinal cord below the origin of the lumbar nerves : the last portion of the pia mater

fim·bria \ˈfim-brē-ə\ *n, pl* **-bri·ae** \-brē-ˌē, -ˌī\ **1** : a bordering fringe esp. at the entrance of the fallopian tubes **2** : a band of nerve fibers bordering the hippocampus and joining the fornix — **fim·bri·al** \-brē-əl\ *adj*

fimbriata — see PLICA FIMBRIATA

fim·bri·at·ed \ˈfim-brē-ˌā-təd\ *also* **fim·bri·ate** \-ˌāt\ *adj* : having the edge or extremity fringed or bordered by slender processes

fi·nas·te·ride \fə-ˈnas-tə-ˌrīd\ *n* : a nitrogenous steroid derivative $C_{23}H_{36}N_2O_2$ that is used esp. to treat symptoms of benign prostatic hyperplasia and to increase hair growth in male-pattern baldness — see PROPECIA, PROSCAR

fine needle *n* : a long thin hollow needle with a narrow bore used esp. to obtain samples by fine needle aspiration; *also* : a solid hairlike needle used in acupuncture

fine needle aspiration *n* : the process of obtaining a sample of cells and bits of tissue for examination by applying suction through a fine needle attached to a syringe — abbr. *FNA*

fin·ger \ˈfiŋ-gər\ *n* : any of the five terminating members of the hand : a digit of the forelimb; *esp* : one other than the thumb — **fin·gered** \ˈfiŋ-gərd\ *adj*

finger fracture *n* : valvulotomy of the mitral commissures performed by a finger thrust through the valve

fin·ger·nail \ˈfiŋ-gər-ˌnāl\ *n* : the nail of a finger

fin·ger·print \-ˌprint\ *n* **1** : an ink impression of the lines on the fingertip taken for purpose of identification **2** : the chromatogram or electrophoretogram obtained by cleaving a protein by enzymatic action and subjecting the resulting collection of peptides to two-dimensional chromatography or electrophoresis — compare DNA FINGERPRINTING — **fingerprint** *vb* — **fin·ger·print·ing** *n*

finger spelling *n* : the representation of individual letters and numbers using standardized finger positions

fin·ger·stall \-ˌstȯl\ *n* : COT

finger–stick \-ˌstik\ *adj* : relating to or being a blood test for which blood is obtained by a finger stick

finger stick *n* : an instance of pricking the skin of a finger to obtain blood from a capillary

fin·ger·tip \-ˌtip\ *n* : the tip of a finger

fin·go·li·mod \fiŋ-ˈgō-lə-ˌmäd\ *n* : an immunomodulator drug $C_{19}H_{32}NO_2 \cdot HCl$ used orally in the treatment of relapsing multiple sclerosis — see GILENYA

fire \ˈfīr\ *vb* **fired; fir·ing** : to transmit or cause to transmit a nerve impulse

fire ant *n* : any ant of the genus *Solenopsis; esp* : IMPORTED FIRE ANT

fire·damp \-ˌdamp\ *n* : a combustible mine gas that consists chiefly of methane; *also* : the explosive mixture of this gas with air

first aid *n* : emergency care or treatment given to an ill or injured person before regular medical aid can be obtained

first cranial nerve *n* : OLFACTORY NERVE

first–degree burn *n* : a mild burn characterized by heat, pain, and reddening of the burned surface but not exhibiting blistering or charring of tissues

first intention *n* : the healing of an incised wound by the direct union of skin edges without granulations — compare SECOND INTENTION

first–line \ˈfərst-ˈlīn\ *adj* : being the preferred, standard, or first choice ⟨~ treatment of advanced breast cancer⟩ — compare SECOND-LINE

first messenger *n* : an extracellular substance (as a hormone or neurotransmitter) that binds to a cell-surface receptor and initiates intracellular activity

first polar body *n* : POLAR BODY a

fish–liv·er oil \ˈfish-ˌli-vər-\ *n* : a fatty oil from the livers of various fishes (as cod, halibut, or sharks) used chiefly as a source of vitamin A

fish oil *n* : a fatty oil obtained from oily fish (as herring) that contains large amounts of unsaturated fatty acids and is used as a dietary supplement

fish tapeworm *n* : a large tapeworm of the genus *Diphyllobothrium* (*D. latum*) that as an adult infests the human intestine and goes through its intermediate stages in freshwater fishes from which it is transmitted to humans when raw fish is eaten

fis·sion \ˈfi-shən, -zhən\ *n* **1** : a method of reproduction in which a living cell or body divides into two or more parts each of which grows into a whole new individual **2** : the splitting of an atomic nucleus resulting in the release of large amounts of energy — called also *nuclear fission* — **fis·sion·able** \ˈfi-shə-nə-bəl, -zhə-\ *adj*

fis·sure \ˈfi-shər\ *n* **1** : a natural cleft between body parts or in the substance of an organ: as **a** : any of several clefts separating the lobes of the liver **b** : any of various clefts between bones or parts of bones in the skull **c** : any of the deep clefts of the brain; *esp* : one of those located at points of elevation in the walls of the ventricles — compare SULCUS **d** : ANTERIOR MEDIAN FISSURE; *also* : POSTERIOR MEDIAN SEPTUM **2** : a break or slit in tissue usu. at the junction of skin and mucous membrane ⟨~ of the lip⟩ **3** : a linear developmental imperfection in the enamel of a tooth — **fis·sured** \ˈfi-shərd\ *adj*

fissure of Ro·lan·do \-rō-ˈlan-(ˌ)dō, -ˈlän-\ *n* : CENTRAL SULCUS

Rolando, Luigi (1773–1831), Italian anatomist and physiologist.

fissure of Syl·vi·us \-ˈsil-vē-əs\ *n* : SYLVIAN FISSURE

F. Dubois or **De Le Boë** — see SYLVIAN

fis·tu·la \ˈfis-chə-lə, -tyu̇-lə\ *n, pl* **-las** *or* **-lae** \-ˌlē, -ˌlī\ : an abnormal passage that leads from an abscess or hollow organ to the body surface or from one hollow organ or part to another and that may be surgically created to permit passage of fluids or secretions — **fis·tu·lat·ed** \-ˌlā-təd\ *adj*

fis·tu·lec·to·my \ˌfis-chə-ˈlek-tə-mē, -tyu̇-\ *n, pl* **-mies** : surgical excision of a fistula

fis·tu·li·za·tion \-lə-ˈzā-shən, -ˌlī-\ *n* **1** : the condition of having a fistula **2** : surgical production of an artificial channel

fis·tu·lous \-ləs\ *adj* : of, relating to, or having the form or nature of a fistula

fistulous withers *n sing or pl* : a deep-seated chronic inflammation of the withers of the horse that is prob. associated with infection by bacteria of the genus *Brucella* (esp. *B. abortus*)

¹fit \ˈfit\ *n* **1** : a sudden violent attack of a disease (as epilepsy) esp. when marked by convulsions or unconsciousness : PAROXYSM **2** : a sudden but transient attack of a physical disturbance

²fit *adj* **fit·ter; fit·test** : sound physically and mentally : HEALTHY — **fit·ness** *n*

¹fix \ˈfiks\ *vb* **1 a** : to make firm, stable, or stationary **b (1)** : to change into a stable compound or available form ⟨bacteria that ~ nitrogen⟩ **(2)** : to kill, harden, and preserve for microscopic study **2** : SPAY, CASTRATE

²fix *n* : a shot of a narcotic

fix·at·ed \ˈfik-ˌsā-təd\ *adj* : arrested in development or adjustment; *esp* : arrested at a pregenital level of psychosexual development

fix·a·tion \fik-ˈsā-shən\ *n* **1 a :** the act or an instance of focusing the eyes upon an object **b** (1) : a persistent concentration of libidinal energies upon objects characteristic of psychosexual stages of development preceding the genital stage (2) : an obsessive or unhealthy preoccupation or attachment **2 :** the immobilization of the parts of a fractured bone esp. by the use of various metal attachments — **fix·ate** \ˈfik-ˌsāt\ *vb*

fixation point *n* **:** the point in the visual field that is fixated by the two eyes in normal vision and for each eye is the point that directly stimulates the fovea of the retina

fix·a·tive \ˈfik-sə-tiv\ *n* **:** a substance used to fix living tissue

fix·a·tor \ˈfik-ˌsā-tər\ *n* **:** a muscle that stabilizes or fixes a part of the body to which a muscle in the process of moving another part is attached

fixed idea *n* **:** IDÉE FIXE

fixed oil *n* **:** a nonvolatile oil; *esp* **:** FATTY OIL

fl *abbr* fluid

Fl *symbol* flerovium

flac·cid \ˈfla-səd, ˈflak-\ *adj* **:** not firm or stiff; *also* **:** lacking normal or youthful firmness ⟨∼ muscles⟩ — **flac·cid·i·ty** \fla-ˈsi-də-tē, flak-\ *n*

flaccid paralysis *n* **:** paralysis in which muscle tone is lacking in the affected muscles and in which tendon reflexes are decreased or absent

fla·gel·lant \ˈfla-jə-lənt, flə-ˈje-lənt\ *n* **:** a person who responds sexually to being beaten by or to beating another person — **flagellant** *adj* — **fla·gel·lant·ism** \-lən-ˌti-zəm\ *n*

fla·gel·lar \flə-ˈje-lər, ˈfla-jə-\ *adj* **:** of or relating to a flagellum

[1]**fla·gel·late** \ˈfla-jə-lət, -ˌlāt; flə-ˈje-lət\ *adj* **1 a** *or* **flag·el·lat·ed** \ˈfla-jə-ˌlā-təd\ **:** having flagella **b :** shaped like a flagellum **2 :** of, relating to, or caused by flagellates ⟨∼ diarrhea⟩

[2]**flagellate** *n* **:** a flagellate protozoan or alga

[1]**flag·el·la·tion** \ˌfla-jə-ˈlā-shən\ *n* **:** the practice of a flagellant

[2]**flagellation** *n* **:** the formation or arrangement of flagella

fla·gel·lum \flə-ˈje-ləm\ *n, pl* **-la** \-lə\ *also* **-lums :** a long tapering process that projects singly or in groups from a cell and is the primary organ of motion of many microorganisms

Flag·yl \ˈfla-gəl\ *trademark* — used for a preparation of metronidazole

flail \ˈflāl\ *adj* **:** exhibiting abnormal mobility and loss of response to normal controls — used of body parts (as joints) damaged by paralysis, accident, or surgery ⟨∼ joint⟩

flammeus — see NEVUS FLAMMEUS

flank \ˈflaŋk\ *n* **:** the fleshy part of the side between the ribs and the hip; *broadly* **:** the side of a quadruped

flap \ˈflap\ *n* **:** a piece of tissue partly severed from its place of origin for use in surgical grafting

[1]**flare** \ˈflar\ *vb* **flared; flar·ing :** to break out or intensify rapidly **:** become suddenly worse or more painful — often used with *up*

[2]**flare** *n* **1 :** FLARE-UP **2 :** an area of skin flush resulting from and spreading out from a local center of vascular dilation and hyperemia ⟨urticaria ∼⟩ **3 :** a cloudy or smoky appearance of the fluid of the anterior chamber of the eye that is seen when a beam of light (as from a slit lamp) passes through it and is caused by the presence of floating protein material — called also *aqueous flare*

flare–up \-ˌəp\ *n* **:** a sudden appearance or worsening of the symptoms of a disease or condition ⟨an asthmatic ∼⟩

flash \ˈflash\ *n* **:** RUSH 2 — see HOT FLASH

flat \ˈflat\ *adj* **flat·ter; flat·test 1 :** being or characterized by a horizontal line or tracing without peaks or depressions **2 :** characterized by general impoverishment in the presence of emotion-evoking stimuli — **flat·ness** *n*

flat bone *n* **:** any of various bones (as of the skull, the jaw, the pelvis, or the rib cage) not rounded in cross section

flat·foot \-ˌfu̇t\ *n, pl* **flat·feet** \-ˌfēt\ **1 :** a condition in which the arch of the instep is flattened so that the entire sole rests upon the ground **2 :** a foot affected with flatfoot — **flat–foot·ed** \-ˌfu̇-təd\ *adj*

flat·line \ˈflat-ˌlīn\ *vb* **flat·lined; flat·lin·ing 1 :** to register on an electronic monitor as having no heartbeat or brain waves **:** to experience cessation of heart contractions or brain wave activity as indicated by a flat line on a electrocardiogram or electroencephalogram **2 :** DIE

flat plate *n* **:** a radiograph esp. of the abdomen taken with the subject lying flat

flat·u·lence \ˈfla-chə-ləns\ *n* **:** the quality or state of being flatulent

flat·u·lent \-lənt\ *adj* **1 :** marked by or affected with gases generated in the intestine or stomach **2 :** likely to cause digestive flatulence — **flat·u·lent·ly** *adv*

fla·tus \ˈflā-təs\ *n* **:** gas generated in the stomach or bowels

flat wart *n* **:** a small smooth slightly elevated wart found esp. on the face and back of the hands that occurs chiefly in children and adolescents — called also *plane wart, verruca plana*

flat·worm \ˈflat-ˌwərm\ *n* **:** any of a phylum (Platyhelminthes) of soft-bodied usu. much flattened worms (as the flukes and tapeworms) — called also *platyhelminth*

fla·vin \ˈflā-vən\ *n* **:** any of a class of yellow water-soluble nitrogenous pigments derived from isoalloxazine and occurring in the form of nucleotides as coenzymes of flavoproteins; *esp* : RIBOFLAVIN

flavin adenine di•nu•cle•o•tide \-ˌdī-ˈnü-klē-ō-ˌtīd, -ˈnyü-\ *n* : a coenzyme $C_{27}H_{33}N_9O_{15}P_2$ of some flavoproteins — called also *FAD*

flavin mononucleotide *n* : FMN

fla•vi•vi•rus \ˈflā-vi-ˌvī-rəs\ *n* **1** *cap* : a genus of single-stranded RNA viruses (family *Flaviviridae*) that are transmitted esp. by ticks and mosquitoes and that include the causative agents of dengue, Japanese B encephalitis, Saint Louis encephalitis, West Nile virus, and yellow fever **2** : any virus of the genus *Flavivirus*; *broadly* : any virus of the family (*Flaviviridae*) to which the genus *Flavivirus* belongs and which includes the causative agents of hepatitis C, bovine viral diarrhea, and cholera

fla•vo•bac•te•ri•um \ˌflā-vō-bak-ˈtir-ē-əm\ *n* : a genus of nonmotile aerobic gram-negative usu. rod-shaped bacteria including one (*F. meningosepticum*) that is found as a contaminant in hospitals and is associated with meningitis and septicemia esp. in newborn infants

fla•vo•noid \ˈflā-və-ˌnȯid, ˈfla-\ *n* : any of a group of plant compounds that include pigments occurring esp. in fruits, vegetables, and herbs — see BIOFLAVONOID — **flavonoid** *adj*

fla•vo•pro•tein \ˌflā-vō-ˈprō-ˌtēn, ˌfla-, -ˈprō-tē-ən\ *n* : a dehydrogenase that contains a flavin and often a metal and plays a major role in biological oxidations

flavum — see LIGAMENTUM FLAVUM

flax•seed \ˈflaks-ˌsēd\ *n* : the seed of flax (esp. *Linum usitatissimum*) used esp. as a demulcent and emollient and as a dietary supplement

flea \ˈflē\ *n* : any of an order (Siphonaptera) comprising small wingless bloodsucking insects that have a hard laterally compressed body and legs adapted to leaping and that feed on warm-blooded animals

flea•bite \-ˌbīt\ *n* : the bite of a flea; *also* : the red spot caused by such a bite — **flea–bit•ten** \-ˌbit-ᵊn\ *adj*

flea collar *n* : a collar for animals that contains insecticide for killing fleas

flea•wort \-ˌwərt, -ˌwȯrt\ *n* : any of three Old World plantains of the genus *Plantago* (esp. *P. psyllium*) that are the source of psyllium seed — called also *psyllium*

fle•cai•nide \ˌfle-ˈkā-ˌnīd\ *n* : an antiarrhythmic drug used in the form of its acetate $C_{17}H_{20}F_6N_2O_3 \cdot C_2H_4O_2$ esp. to treat ventricular arrhythmias

fle•ro•vi•um \flə-ˈrō-vē-əm\ *n* : a short-lived radioactive element that is artificially produced — symbol *Fl;* see ELEMENT table

flesh \ˈflesh\ *n* : the soft parts of the body; *esp* : the parts composed chiefly of skeletal muscle as distinguished from visceral structures, bone, and integuments — see PROUD FLESH — **fleshed** \ˈflesht\ *adj* — **fleshy** \ˈfle-shē\ *adj*

flesh–eating disease *n* : NECROTIZING FASCIITIS

flesh fly *n* : any of a family (Sarcophagidae) of dipteran flies some of which cause myiasis

flesh wound *n* : an injury involving penetration of the body musculature without damage to bones or internal organs

Fletch•er•ism \ˈfle-chər-ˌi-zəm\ *n* : the practice of eating in small amounts and only when hungry and of chewing one's food thoroughly — **fletch•er•ize** \-ˌīz\ *vb*

Fletcher, Horace (1849–1919), American dietitian.

flex \ˈfleks\ *vb* **1** : to bend esp. repeatedly **2 a** : to move muscles so as to cause flexion of (a joint) **b** : to move or tense (a muscle) by contraction

Flex•e•ril \ˈflek-sə-ril\ *trademark* — used for a preparation of cyclobenzaprine

flexibilitas — see CEREA FLEXIBILITAS

flex•i•ble \ˈflek-sə-bəl\ *adj* : capable of being flexed : capable of being turned, bowed, or twisted without breaking — **flex•i•bil•i•ty** \ˌflek-sə-ˈbi-lə-tē\ *n*

flex•ion *also* **flec•tion** \ˈflek-shən\ *n* **1** : a bending movement around a joint in a limb (as the knee or elbow) that decreases the angle between the bones of the limb at the joint — compare EXTENSION 2 **2** : a forward raising of the arm or leg by a movement at the shoulder or hip joint

flex•or \ˈflek-sər, -ˌsȯr\ *n* : a muscle serving to bend a body part (as a limb) — called also *flexor muscle;* compare EXTENSOR

flexor car•pi ra•di•al•is \-ˈkär-ˌpī-ˌrā-dē-ˈā-ləs, -ˈkär-ˌpē-\ *n* : a superficial muscle of the palmar side of the forearm that flexes the hand and assists in abducting it

flexor carpi ul•nar•is \-ˌəl-ˈnar-əs\ *n* : a superficial muscle of the ulnar side of the forearm that flexes the hand and assists in adducting it

flexor dig•i•ti min•i•mi brev•is \-ˈdi-jə-ˌtī-ˈmi-nə-ˌmī-ˈbre-vəs, -ˈdi-jə-ˌtē-ˈmi-nə-ˌmē-\ *n* **1** : a muscle of the ulnar side of the palm of the hand that flexes the little finger **2** : a muscle of the sole of the foot that flexes the first proximal phalanx of the little toe

flexor dig•i•to•rum brevis \-ˌdi-jə-ˈtōr-əm-\ *n* : a muscle of the middle part of the sole of the foot that flexes the second phalanx of each of the four small toes

flexor digitorum lon•gus \-ˈlȯŋ-gəs\ *n* : a muscle of the tibial side of the leg that flexes the terminal phalanx of each of the four small toes

flexor digitorum pro•fund•us \-prō-ˈfən-dəs\ *n* : a deep muscle of the ulnar side of the forearm that flexes esp. the terminal phalanges of the four fingers

flexor digitorum su·per·fi·ci·al·is \-ˌsü-pər-ˌfi-shē-ˈā-ləs\ *n* : a superficial muscle of the palmar side of the forearm that flexes esp. the second phalanges of the four fingers

flexor hal·lu·cis brev·is \-ˈha-lü-səs-ˈbre-vəs, -lyü-, -ˈha-lə-kəs-\ *n* : a short muscle of the sole of the foot that flexes the proximal phalanx of the big toe

flexor hallucis longus *n* : a long deep muscle of the fibular side of the leg that flexes esp. the second phalanx of the big toe

flexor muscle *n* : FLEXOR

flexor pol·li·cis brevis \-ˈpä-lə-səs-, -kəs-\ *n* : a short muscle of the palm that flexes and adducts the thumb

flexor pollicis longus *n* : a muscle of the radial side of the forearm that flexes esp. the second phalanx of the thumb

flexor ret·in·ac·u·lum \-ˌret-ᵊn-ˈa-kyə-ləm\ *n* **1** : a fibrous band of fascia on the medial side of the ankle that extends downward from the medial malleolus of the tibia to the calcaneus and that covers over the bony grooves containing the tendons of the flexor muscles, the posterior tibial artery and vein, and the tibial nerve as they pass into the sole of the foot **2** : a fibrous band of fascia on the palm side of the wrist and base of the hand that forms the roof of the carpal tunnel and covers the tendons of the flexor muscles and the median nerve as they pass into the hand — called also *transverse carpal ligament*

flex·ure \ˈflek-shər\ *n* **1** : the quality or state of being flexed : FLEXION **2** : an anatomical turn, bend, or fold; *esp* : one of three sharp bends of the anterior part of the primary axis of the vertebrate embryo that serve to establish the relationship of the parts of the developing brain — see CEPHALIC FLEXURE, HEPATIC FLEXURE, PONTINE FLEXURE, SPLENIC FLEXURE — **flex·ur·al** \-shər-əl\ *adj*

fli·ban·se·rin \fli-ˈban-sə-rən\ *n* : a drug $C_{20}H_{21}F_3N_4O$ that is taken orally to treat hypoactive sexual desire disorder in premenopausal women and that binds to serotonin receptors causing lowered levels of serotonin and increased levels of dopamine and norepinephrine — see ADDYI

flick·er \ˈfli-kər\ *n* : the wavering or fluttering visual sensation produced by intermittent light when the interval between flashes is not small enough to produce complete fusion of the individual impressions

flicker fusion *n* : FUSION b(2)

flight of ideas *n* : a rapid shifting of ideas that is expressed as a disconnected rambling and occurs esp. in the manic phase of bipolar disorder

flight surgeon *n* : a medical officer (as in the U.S. Air Force) specializing in aerospace medicine

float·er \ˈflō-tər\ *n* : a bit of optical debris (as a dead cell or cell fragment) in the vitreous body or lens that may be perceived as a spot before the eye; *also* : a spot in the visual field due to such debris — usu. used in pl.; compare MUSCAE VOLITANTES

float·ing \ˈflōt-iŋ\ *adj* : located out of the normal position or abnormally movable ⟨a ~ kidney⟩

floating rib *n* : any rib in the last two pairs of ribs that have no attachment to the sternum — compare FALSE RIB

floc·cu·lar \ˈflä-kyə-lər\ *adj* : of or relating to a flocculus

floc·cu·late \ˈflä-kyə-ˌlāt\ *vb* **-lat·ed; -lat·ing** : to aggregate or cause to aggregate into a flocculent mass — **floc·cu·la·tion** \ˌflä-kyə-ˈlā-shən\ *n*

floc·cu·la·tion test \ˌflä-kyə-ˈlā-shən-\ *n* : any of various serological tests (as the Mazzini test for syphilis) in which a positive result depends on the combination of an antigen and antibody to produce a flocculent precipitate

floc·cu·lent \-kyə-lənt\ *adj* : made up of loosely aggregated particles ⟨a ~ precipitate⟩

floc·cu·lo·nod·u·lar lobe \ˌflä-kyə-(ˌ)lō-ˈnä-jə-lər-\ *n* : the posterior lobe of the cerebellum that consists of the nodulus and paired lateral flocculi and is concerned with equilibrium

floc·cu·lus \-ləs\ *n, pl* **-li** \-ˌlī, -ˌlē\ : a small irregular lobe on the undersurface of each hemisphere of the cerebellum that is linked with the corresponding side of the nodulus by a peduncle

Flo·max \ˈflō-ˌmaks\ *trademark* — used for a preparation of the hydrochloride of tamsulosin

Flo·nase \ˈflō-ˌnās\ *trademark* — used for a preparation of fluticasone propionate administered as a nasal spray

flood·ing \ˈflə-diŋ\ *n* : exposure therapy in which there is prolonged confrontation with an anxiety-provoking stimulus

floor \ˈflōr\ *n* : the lower inside surface of a hollow anatomical structure ⟨the ~ of the pelvis⟩

flo·ra \ˈflōr-ə\ *n, pl* **floras** *also* **flo·rae** \ˈflōr-ˌē, -ˌī\ **1** : plant life; *esp* : the plant life characteristic of a region, period, or special environment — compare FAUNA **2** : the microorganisms (as bacteria) living in or on the body — **flo·ral** \ˈflōr-əl\ *adj*

flor·id \ˈflȯr-əd, ˈflär-\ *adj* : fully developed : manifesting a complete and typical clinical syndrome ⟨~ hyperplasia⟩ — **flor·id·ly** *adv*

[1]**floss** \ˈfläs, ˈflȯs\ *n* : DENTAL FLOSS

[2]**floss** *vb* : to use dental floss on (one's teeth)

Flo·vent \ˈflō-ˌvent\ *trademark* — used for a preparation of fluticasone propionate administered as an oral inhalant

[1]**flow** \ˈflō\ *vb* **1** : to move with a continual change of place among the constituent particles **2** : MENSTRUATE

²flow *n* **1 :** the quantity that flows in a certain time **2 :** MENSTRUATION

flow cytometry *n* **:** a technique for identifying and sorting cells and their components (as DNA) by staining with a fluorescent dye and detecting the fluorescence usu. by laser beam illumination — **flow cytometer** *n*

flowers of zinc *n pl* **:** zinc oxide esp. as obtained as a light white powder by burning zinc for use in pharmaceutical and cosmetic preparations

flow·me·ter \ˈflō-ˌmē-tər\ *n* **:** an instrument for measuring the velocity of flow of a fluid (as blood) in a tube or pipe

fl oz *abbr* fluid ounce

flu \ˈflü\ *n* **1 :** INFLUENZA **2 :** any of several chiefly viral illnesses marked esp. by respiratory or gastrointestinal symptoms — see INTESTINAL FLU — **flu–like** \-ˌlīk\ *adj*

flu·con·a·zole \flü-ˈkä-nə-ˌzōl\ *n* **:** a triazole antifungal agent $C_{13}H_{12}F_2N_6O$ used to treat cryptococcal meningitis and local or systemic candida infections — see DIFLUCAN

fluc·tu·ant \ˈflək-chə-wənt\ *adj* **:** movable and compressible — used of abnormal body structures (as some abscesses or tumors)

fluc·tu·a·tion \ˌflək-chə-ˈwā-shən\ *n* **:** the wavelike motion of a fluid collected in a natural or artificial cavity of the body observed by palpation or percussion

flu·cy·to·sine \ˌflü-ˈsī-tə-sēn\ *n* **:** an antifungal agent $C_4H_4FN_3O$ used esp. against fungi of the genera *Candida* and *Cryptococcus* (esp. *Cryptococcus neoformans*)

flu·dar·a·bine \flü-ˈdar-ə-ˌbēn\ *n* **:** an antineoplastic agent administered intravenously in the form of its phosphate $C_{10}H_{13}FN_5O_7P$ esp. to treat chronic lymphocytic leukemia

flu·dro·cor·ti·sone \ˌflü-drō-ˈkȯr-tə-ˌsōn, -ˌzōn\ *n* **:** a potent mineralocorticoid drug that possesses some glucocorticoid activity and is administered in the form of its acetate $C_{23}H_{31}FO_6$ to treat adrenocortical insufficiency

flu·id \ˈflü-əd\ *n* **:** a substance (as a liquid or gas) tending to flow or conform to the outline of its container; *specif* **:** one in the body of an animal or plant — see CEREBROSPINAL FLUID, SEMINAL FLUID — **fluid** *adj*

fluid dram *or* **flu·i·dram** \ˌflü-ə-ˈdram\ *n* **:** either of two units of liquid capacity: **a :** a U.S. unit equal to ⅛ U.S. fluid ounce **b :** a British unit equal to ⅛ British fluid ounce

flu·id·ex·tract \ˌflü-əd-ˈek-ˌstrakt\ *n* **:** an alcohol preparation of a vegetable drug containing the active constituents of one gram of the dry drug in each milliliter

fluid ounce *n* **1 :** a U.S. unit of liquid capacity equal to 1/16 pint **2 :** a British unit of liquid capacity equal to 1/20 pint

fluke \ˈflük\ *n* **:** a flattened digenetic trematode worm; *broadly* **:** TREMATODE — see LIVER FLUKE

Flu·Mist \ˈflü-ˌmist\ *trademark* — used for a vaccine against influenza administered as a nasal spray and composed of live attenuated influenza virus

flu·nis·o·lide \flü-ˈni-sə-ˌlīd\ *n* **:** a synthetic glucocorticoid $C_{24}H_{31}FO_6 \cdot \frac{1}{2}H_2O$ administered as an oral inhalant to treat bronchial asthma and as a nasal spray to treat rhinitis

flu·ni·traz·e·pam \ˌflü-nə-ˈtra-zə-ˌpam\ *n* **:** a powerful benzodiazepine drug $C_{16}H_{12}FN_3O_3$ with sedative and sleep-inducing properties that is not licensed for use in the U.S. but is used medically in other countries and that is a frequent illicit drug of abuse — see ROHYPNOL

flu·o·cin·o·lone ac·e·to·nide \ˌflü-ə-ˈsin-əl-ˌōn-ˌa-sə-ˈtō-ˌnīd\ *n* **:** a glucocorticoid steroid $C_{24}H_{30}F_2O_6$ used esp. as an anti-inflammatory agent in the treatment of skin diseases

flu·o·cin·o·nide \-ˈsin-ə-ˌnīd\ *n* **:** a glucocorticoid drug $C_{26}H_{32}F_2O_7$ used topically to treat inflammation and pruritus associated with various skin disorders (as psoriasis)

fluor- *or* **fluoro-** *comb form* **1 :** fluorine ⟨*fluor*osis⟩ **2** *also* **fluori- :** fluorescence ⟨*fluoro*scope⟩

flu·o·res·ce·in \ˌflu̇-ər-ˈe-sē-ən, ˌflōr-\ *n* **:** a dye $C_{20}H_{12}O_5$ with a bright yellow-green fluorescence in alkaline solution that is used as the sodium salt as an aid in diagnosis

flu·o·res·cence \-ˈes-ᵊns\ *n* **:** luminescence that is caused by the absorption of radiation at one wavelength followed by the nearly immediate emission of radiation usu. at a different wavelength and that ceases almost at once when the source of radiation is removed; *also* **:** the radiation emitted — **flu·o·resce** \-ˈes\ *vb* — **flu·o·res·cent** \-ˈes-ᵊnt\ *adj*

fluorescence microscope *n* **:** ULTRAVIOLET MICROSCOPE

flu·o·ri·date \ˈflu̇r-ə-ˌdāt, ˈflōr-\ *vb* **-dat·ed; -dat·ing :** to add a fluoride to (as drinking water) to reduce tooth decay — **flu·o·ri·da·tion** \ˌflu̇r-ə-ˈdā-shən, ˌflōr-\ *n*

flu·o·ride \ˈflu̇-ər-ˌīd\ *n* **1 :** a compound of fluorine usu. with a more electrically positive element or radical **2 :** the monovalent anion of fluorine — **fluoride** *adj*

flu·o·rine \ˈflu̇-ər-ˌēn, ˈflōr-, -ən\ *n* **:** a nonmetallic monovalent halogen element that is normally a pale yellowish flammable irritating toxic gas — symbol *F;* see ELEMENT table

flu·o·rom·e·ter \ˌflu̇-ər-ˈä-mə-tər\ *or* **flu·o·rim·e·ter** \-ˈi-mə-tər\ *n* **:** an instrument for measuring fluorescence and related phenomena (as intensity of radiation) — **flu·o·ro·met·ric** *or*

flu•o•ri•met•ric \ˌflu̇-ər-ə-ˈme-trik, ˌflōr-\ *adj* — **flu•o•rom•e•try** \-ˈä-mə-trē\ *or* **flu•o•rim•e•try** \-ˈi-mə-trē\ *n*

flu•o•ro•pho•tom•e•ter \ˌflu̇-ər-ō-fō-ˈtä-mə-tər, ˌflōr-ō-\ *n* : FLUOROMETER — **flu•o•ro•pho•to•met•ric** \-ˌfō-tə-ˈme-trik\ *adj* — **flu•o•ro•pho•tom•e•try** \-ˌfō-ˈtä-mə-trē\ *n*

flu•o•ro•quin•o•lone \-ˈkwi-nə-ˌlōn\ *n* : any of a group of fluorinated derivatives (as ciprofloxacin and levofloxacin) of quinolone that are used as antibacterial drugs

flu•o•ro•scope \ˈflu̇r-ə-ˌskōp, ˈflōr-\ *n* : an instrument used in medical diagnosis for observing the internal structure of the body by means of X-rays — **fluoroscope** *vb* — **flu•o•ro•scop•ic** \ˌflu̇r-ə-ˈskä-pik, ˌflōr-\ *adj* — **flu•o•ro•scop•i•cal•ly** \-pi-k(ə-)lē\ *adv* — **flu•o•ros•co•pist** \-ˈäs-kə-pist\ *n* — **flu•o•ros•co•py** \-pē\ *n*

flu•o•ro•sis \ˌflu̇-ər-ˈō-səs, ˌflōr-\ *n* : an abnormal condition (as mottled enamel of human teeth) caused by fluorine or its compounds

flu•o•ro•ura•cil \ˌflu̇-ər-ō-ˈyu̇r-ə-ˌsil, -ˌsəl\ *or* **5–flu•o•ro•ura•cil** \ˈfīv-\ *n* : a fluorine-containing pyrimidine base $C_4H_3FN_2O_2$ used to treat some kinds of cancer

flu•ox•e•tine \ˌflü-ˈäk-sə-ˌtēn\ *n* : a drug that functions as an SSRI and is administered in the form of its hydrochloride $C_{17}H_{18}F_3NO{\cdot}HCl$ esp. to treat depression, panic disorder, and obsessive-compulsive disorder — see PROZAC

flu•oxy•mes•te•rone \flə-ˌwäk-sē-ˈme-stə-ˌrōn\ *n* : a synthetic androgen $C_{20}H_{29}FO_3$ used orally esp. in the treatment of testosterone deficiency in males and in the palliative treatment of breast cancer in females

flu•phen•azine \flü-ˈfe-nə-ˌzēn\ *n* : a phenothiazine tranquilizer used esp. in the form of its dihydrochloride $C_{22}H_{26}F_3N_3OS{\cdot}2HCl$ as an antipsychotic agent— see PERMITIL, PROLIXIN

flur•az•e•pam \ˌflu̇r-ˈa-zə-ˌpam\ *n* : a benzodiazepine closely related structurally to diazepam that is used as a hypnotic in the form of its hydrochloride $C_{21}H_{23}ClFN_3O{\cdot}2HCl$ esp. to treat insomnia — see DALMANE

flur•bip•ro•fen \flu̇r-ˈbi-prə-fən\ *n* : a drug $C_{15}H_{13}FO_2$ that is an NSAID used orally esp. to relieve the symptoms of rheumatoid arthritis and osteoarthritis and is applied topically in the form of its hydrated sodium salt $C_{15}H_{12}FNaO_2{\cdot}2H_2O$ to inhibit miosis during and after ocular surgery— see ANSAID

flur•o•thyl \ˈflu̇r-ə-thil\ *n* : a liquid convulsant $C_4H_4F_6O$ that has been used in place of electroconvulsive therapy in the treatment of mental illness

¹flush \ˈfləsh\ *n* : a transitory sensation of extreme heat (as in response to some physiological states)

²flush *vb* **1** : to blush or become suddenly suffused with color due to vasodilation **2** : to cleanse or wash out with or as if with a rush of liquid

flu shot *n* : an influenza vaccine administered by injection

flu•ta•mide \ˈflü-tə-ˌmīd\ *n* : a nonsteroidal antiandrogen $C_{11}H_{11}F_3N_2O_3$ used to treat prostate cancer

flu•tic•a•sone \flü-ˈti-kə-ˌsōn\ *n* : either of two synthetic corticosteroid drugs with anti-inflammatory activity: **a** *or* **fluticasone propionate** : one $C_{25}H_{31}F_3O_5S$ used as a nasal spray to treat allergic rhinitis, as an oral inhalant to treat asthma and chronic obstructive pulmonary disease, and topically as a cream or ointment to treat skin inflammation and itching — see ADVAIR, FLONASE, FLOVENT **b** *or* **fluticasone fur•o•ate** \-ˈfyu̇r-ə-ˌwāt\ : one $C_{27}H_{29}F_3O_6S$ used as a nasal spray to treat allergic rhinitis and as an oral inhalant to treat asthma and chronic obstructive pulmonary disease

flut•ter \ˈflə-tər\ *n* : an abnormal rapid spasmodic and usu. rhythmic motion or contraction of a body part ⟨a serious ventricular ~⟩ — **flutter** *vb*

flu vaccine *n* : INFLUENZA VACCINE

flu•va•stat•in \ˈflü-və-ˈsta-tᵊn\ *n* : a statin taken orally in the form of its sodium salt $C_{24}H_{25}FNNaO_4$ esp. to lower LDL and triglyceride levels and increase HDL levels — see LESCOL

flu•vox•a•mine \flü-ˈväk-sə-ˌmēn\ *n* : a drug that functions as an SSRI and is administered orally in the form of its maleate $C_{15}H_{21}O_2N_2F_3{\cdot}C_4H_4O_4$ esp. to treat depression and obsessive-compulsive disorder — see LUVOX

flux \ˈfləks\ *n* **1** : a flowing or discharge of fluid from the body esp. when excessive or abnormal: as **a** : DIARRHEA **b** : DYSENTERY **2** : the matter discharged in a flux

fly \ˈflī\ *n, pl* **flies** **1** : any of a large order (Diptera) of usu. winged insects (as the housefly or a mosquito) that have the anterior wings functional, the posterior wings modified to function as sensory flight stabilizers, and segmented often headless, eyeless, and legless lavae **2** : a large stout-bodied fly (as a horsefly)

fly aga•ric \-ˈa-gə-rik, -ə-ˈgar-ik\ *n* : a poisonous mushroom of the genus *Amanita* (*A. muscaria*) that usu. has a bright red cap — called also *fly amanita, fly mushroom*

¹fly•blow \ˈflī-ˌblō\ *vb* **-blew; -blown** : to deposit eggs or young larvae of a flesh fly or blowfly in

²flyblow *n* : FLY-STRIKE

fly•blown \-ˌblōn\ *adj* **1** : infested with fly maggots **2** : covered with flyspecks

fly–strike \-ˌstrīk\ *n* : infestation with fly maggots — **fly–struck** \-ˌstrək\ *adj*

Fm *symbol* fermium

FM *abbr* fibromyalgia

FMN \ˌef-(ˌ)em-ˈen\ *n* : a yellow crystalline phosphoric ester $C_{17}H_{21}N_4O_9P$ of riboflavin that is a coenzyme of several flavoprotein enzymes — called also *flavin mononucleotide, riboflavin phosphate*

fMRI *abbr* functional magnetic resonance imaging

FMS *abbr* fibromyalgia syndrome

FNA *abbr* fine needle aspiration

foam \ˈfōm\ *n* : a light frothy mass of fine bubbles formed in or on the surface of a liquid — **foam** *vb*

foam cell *n* : a swollen vacuolated macrophage filled with lipid inclusions that often accumulates along arterial walls and is characteristic of some conditions of disturbed lipid metabolism

foamy virus \ˈfō-mē-\ *n* : any of a genus (*Spumavirus*) of nonpathogenic retroviruses that are sometimes transmitted to humans from nonhuman primates — called also *spumavirus*

FOBT *abbr* fecal occult blood test; fecal occult blood testing

fo•cal \ˈfō-kəl\ *adj* : of, relating to, being, or having a focus — **fo•cal•ly** \-kə-lē\ *adv*

focal epilepsy *n* : epilepsy characterized by partial seizures — called also *partial epilepsy*

Fo•ca•lin \ˈfō-kə-lən\ *trademark* — used for a preparation of dexmethylphenidate

focal infection *n* : a persistent bacterial infection of some organ or region; *esp* : one causing symptoms elsewhere in the body

focal length *n* : the distance of a focus from the surface of a lens or concave mirror — symbol *f*

focal point *n* : FOCUS 1

focal seizure *n* : PARTIAL SEIZURE

fo•cus \ˈfō-kəs\ *n, pl* **fo•ci** \ˈfō-ˌsī, -ˌkī\ *also* **fo•cus•es** **1** : a point at which rays (as of light) converge or from which they diverge or appear to diverge usu. giving rise to an image after reflection by a mirror or refraction by a lens or optical system **2** : a localized area of disease or the chief site of a generalized disease or infection — **focus** *vb*

foe•ti•cide *chiefly Brit var of* FETICIDE

foeto- *or* **foeti-** *chiefly Brit var of* FETO-

foe•tol•o•gy, foe•tus *chiefly Brit var of* FETOLOGY, FETUS

fog \ˈfäg, ˈfȯg\ *vb* **fogged; fog•ging** : to blur (a visual field) with lenses that prevent a sharp focus in order to relax accommodation before testing vision

foil \ˈfȯil\ *n* : very thin sheet metal (as of gold) used esp. in filling teeth

fo•la•cin \ˈfō-lə-sən\ *n* : FOLIC ACID

fo•late \ˈfō-ˌlāt\ *n* : FOLIC ACID; *also* : a salt or ester of folic acid

fold \ˈfōld\ *n* : a margin formed by the doubling upon itself of a flat anatomical structure (as a membrane)

Fo•ley catheter \ˈfō-lē-\ *n* : a catheter with an inflatable balloon tip for retention in the bladder

Foley, Frederic Eugene Basil (1891–1966), American urologist

fo•lic acid \ˈfō-lik-\ *n* : a crystalline vitamin $C_{19}H_{19}N_7O_6$ of the B complex that is used esp. in the treatment of nutritional anemias — called also *folacin, folate, pteroylglutamic acid, vitamin B_c, vitamin M*

folie à deux \fō-ˈlē-(ˌ)ä-ˈdœ̄, -ˈdər\ *n, pl* **folies à deux** *same or* fō-ˈlēz-\ : the presence of the same or similar delusional ideas in two persons closely associated with one another

fo•lin•ic acid \fō-ˈli-nik-\ *n* : LEUCOVORIN

fo•li•um \ˈfo-lē-əm\ *n, pl* **fo•lia** \-lē-ə\ : one of the lamellae of the cerebellar cortex

folk medicine *n* : traditional medicine as practiced esp. by people isolated from modern medical services and usu. involving the use of plant-derived remedies on an empirical basis

fol•li•cle \ˈfä-li-kəl\ *n* **1** : a small anatomical cavity or deep narrow-mouthed depression; *esp* : a small simple or slightly branched gland : CRYPT **2** : a small lymph node **3** : a vesicle in the mammalian ovary that contains a developing egg surrounded by a covering of cells : OVARIAN FOLLICLE; *esp* : GRAAFIAN FOLLICLE — **fol•lic•u•lar** \fə-ˈli-kyə-lər, fä-\ *adj*

follicle mite *n* : any of several minute mites of the genus *Demodex* that are parasitic in the hair follicles

follicle–stimulating hormone *n* : a hormone from an anterior lobe of the pituitary gland that stimulates the growth of the ovum-containing follicles in the ovary and that activates sperm-forming cells

follicularis — see KERATOSIS FOLLICULARIS

folliculi — see LIQUOR FOLLICULI, THECA FOLLICULI

fol•lic•u•lin \fə-ˈli-kyə-lən, fä-\ *n* : ESTROGEN; *esp* : ESTRONE

fol•lic•u•li•tis \fə-ˌli-kyə-ˈlī-təs\ *n* : inflammation of one or more follicles esp. of the hair

fol•li•tro•pin \ˌfä-lə-ˈtrō-pən\ *n* : FOLLICLE-STIMULATING HORMONE

follow–up \ˈfä-lō-ˌəp\ *n* : maintenance of contact with a patient at one or more designated intervals following diagnosis or treatment esp. to examine again or monitor the progress of therapy; *also* : an instance of such contact — **follow–up** *adj* — **follow up** *vb*

fo•men•ta•tion \ˌfō-mən-ˈtā-shən, -ˌmen-\ *n* **1** : the application of hot moist substances to the body to ease pain **2** : the material applied in fomentation : POULTICE

fo•mite \ˈfō-ˌmīt\ *n, pl* **fo•mites** \-ˌmīts, ˈfä-mə-ˌtēz\ : an object (as a dish or doorknob) that may be contaminated with infectious organisms and serve in their transmission

F₁ generation *n* : the first filial generation produced by a cross and consisting of individuals heterozygous for characters in which the parents differ and are homozygous — compare F₂ GENERATION, P₁ GENERATION

fon•ta•nel *or* **fon•ta•nelle** \ˌfänt-ᵊn-ˈel\ *n* : any of the spaces closed by membranous structures between the uncompleted angles of the parietal bones and the neighboring bones of a fetal or young skull

food \ˈfüd\ *n, often attrib* **1** : material consisting essentially of protein, carbohydrate, and fat used in the body of an organism to sustain growth, repair, and vital processes and to furnish energy; *also* : such food together with supplementary substances (as minerals, vitamins, and condiments) **2** : nutriment in solid form

food poisoning *n* **1** : either of two acute gastrointestinal disorders caused by bacteria or their toxic products: **a** : a rapidly developing intoxication marked by nausea, vomiting, prostration, and often severe diarrhea and caused by the presence in food of toxic products produced by bacteria (as some staphylococci) **b** : a less rapidly developing infection esp. with salmonellae that has generally similar symptoms and results from multiplication of bacteria ingested with contaminated food **2** : a gastrointestinal disturbance occurring after consumption of food that is contaminated with chemical residues or food (as some fungi) that is inherently unsuitable for human consumption

food•stuff \ˈfüd-ˌstəf\ *n* : a substance with food value; *esp* : a specific nutrient (as a fat or protein)

foot \ˈfu̇t\ *n, pl* **feet** \ˈfēt\ *also* **foot** **1** : the terminal part of the vertebrate leg upon which an individual stands **2** : a unit equal to ⅓ yard or 12 inches

foot–and–mouth disease *n* : an acute contagious febrile disease esp. of cloven-hoofed animals that is caused by serotypes of a picornavirus (species *Foot-and-mouth disease virus* of the genus *Aphthovirus*) and is marked by ulcerating vesicles in the mouth, about the hoofs, and on the udder and teats — called also *aftosa, aphthous fever, foot-and-mouth, hoof-and-mouth disease;* compare HAND, FOOT AND MOUTH DISEASE

foot•bath \ˈfu̇t-ˌbath\ *n* : a bath for cleansing, warming, or disinfecting the feet

foot drop *n* : an extended position of the foot caused by paralysis of the flexor muscles of the leg

foot•ed \ˈfu̇-təd\ *adj* : having a foot or feet esp. of a specified kind or number — often used in combination ⟨a 4-*footed* animal⟩

foot•plate \ˈfu̇t-ˌplāt\ *n* : the flat oval base of the stapes

foot–pound \-ˈpau̇nd\ *n, pl* **foot–pounds** : a unit of work equal to the work done by a force of one pound acting through a distance of one foot in the direction of the force

foot–pound–second \ˌfu̇t-ˌpau̇nd-ˈse-kənd\ *adj* : being or relating to a system of units based upon the foot as the unit of length, the pound as the unit of weight or mass, and the second as the unit of time — abbr. *fps*

foot rot *n* : a necrobacillosis of tissues of the foot esp. of sheep and cattle

For•a•dil \ˈfór-ə-ˌdil\ *trademark* — used for a preparation of formoterol for oral inhalation

fo•ra•men \fə-ˈrā-mən\ *n, pl* **fo•ram•i•na** \-ˈra-mə-nə\ *or* **fo•ra•mens** \-ˈrā-mənz\ : a small opening, perforation, or orifice : FENESTRA 1 — **fo•ram•i•nal** \fə-ˈra-mən-ᵊl\ *adj*

foramen ce•cum \-ˈsē-kəm\ *n* : a shallow depression in the posterior dorsal midline of the tongue that is the remnant of the more cranial part of the embryonic duct from which the thyroid gland developed

foramen lac•er•um \-ˈla-sər-əm\ *n* : an irregular aperture on the lower surface of the skull bounded by parts of the temporal, sphenoid, and occipital bones that gives passage to the internal carotid artery

foramen mag•num \-ˈmag-nəm\ *n* : the opening in the skull through which the spinal cord passes to become the medulla oblongata

foramen of Lusch•ka \-ˈlu̇sh-kə\ *n* : either of two openings each of which is situated on one side of the fourth ventricle of the brain and communicates with the subarachnoid space

Luschka, Hubert von (1820–1875), German anatomist.

foramen of Ma•gen•die \-mə-ˌzhän-ˈdē\ *n* : a passage through the midline of the roof of the fourth ventricle of the brain that gives passage to the cerebrospinal fluid from the ventricles to the subarachnoid space

Ma•gen•die, François \mȧ-zhaⁿ-dē\ **(1783–1855),** French physiologist.

foramen of Mon•ro \-mən-ˈrō\ *n* : INTERVENTRICULAR FORAMEN

Monro, Alexander (Secundus) (1733–1817), British anatomist.

foramen of Wins•low \-ˈwinz-ˌlō\ *n* : EPIPLOIC FORAMEN

Winsløw, Jacob (*or* **Jacques–Bénigne) (1669–1760),** Danish anatomist.

foramen ova•le \-ō-ˈva-(ˌ)lē, -ˈvā-, -ˈvä-\ *n* **1** : an opening in the septum between the two atria of the heart that is normally present only in the fetus **2** : an oval opening in the greater wing of the sphenoid for passage of the mandibular nerve

foramen ro•tun•dum \-rō-ˈtən-dəm\ *n* : a circular aperture in the anterior and medial part of the greater wing of the sphenoid that gives passage to the maxillary nerve

foramen spin•o•sum \-spi-ˈnō-səm\ *n* : an aperture in the greater wing of the sphenoid that gives passage to the middle meningeal artery

foramina *pl of* FORAMEN

fo•ram•i•not•o•my \fə-ˌram-ə-ˈnät-ə-mē\ *n, pl* **-mies** : a surgical procedure to enlarge the opening through which the root of a spinal nerve passes as it exits the spinal column esp. to relieve symptoms (as numbness or pain) caused by nerve compression

for•ceps \ˈfȯr-səps, -ˌseps\ *n, pl* **forceps** : an instrument for grasping, holding firmly, or exerting traction upon objects esp. for delicate operations

For•dyce's disease \ˈfȯr-ˌdī-səz-\ *also* **For•dyce disease** \ˈfȯr-ˌdīs-\ *n* : a common anomaly of the oral mucosa in which misplaced sebaceous glands form yellowish-white nodules on the lips or the lining of the mouth

Fordyce, John Addison (1858–1925), American dermatologist.

fore- *comb form* **1** : situated at the front : in front ⟨*fore*leg⟩ **2** : front part of (something specified) ⟨*fore*arm⟩

fore•arm \ˈfōr-ˌärm\ *n* : the part of the arm between the elbow and the wrist

fore•brain \-ˌbrān\ *n* : the anterior of the three primary divisions of the developing vertebrate brain or the corresponding part of the adult brain that includes esp. the cerebral hemispheres, the thalamus, and the hypothalamus and that esp. in higher vertebrates is the main control center for sensory and associative information processing, visceral functions, and voluntary motor functions — called also *prosencephalon;* see DIENCEPHALON, TELENCEPHALON

forebrain bundle — see MEDIAL FOREBRAIN BUNDLE

fore•fin•ger \ˈfōr-ˌfiŋ-gər\ *n* : INDEX FINGER

fore•foot \-ˌfu̇t\ *n* **1** : one of the anterior feet esp. of a quadruped **2** : the front part of the human foot

fore•gut \-ˌgət\ *n* : the anterior part of the digestive tract of a vertebrate embryo that develops into the pharynx, esophagus, stomach, and extreme anterior part of the intestine

fore•head \ˈfȯr-əd, ˈfär-; ˈfōr-ˌhed\ *n* : the part of the face above the eyes — called also *brow*

for•eign \ˈfȯr-ən, ˈfär-\ *adj* **1** : occurring in an abnormal situation in the living body and often introduced from outside **2** : not recognized by the immune system as part of the self

fore•leg \ˈfōr-ˌleg\ *n* : a front leg

fore•limb \-ˌlim\ *n* : a limb (as an arm, wing, fin, or leg) situated anteriorly

fo•ren•sic \fə-ˈren-sik, -zik\ *adj* : relating to or dealing with the application of scientific knowledge to legal problems esp. in regard to criminal evidence or intent ⟨a ~ pathologist⟩ ⟨~ medicine⟩ ⟨a ~ psychiatrist⟩

forensic odontology *n* : a branch of forensic medicine dealing with teeth and marks left by teeth (as in identifying remains of a dead person)

fo•ren•sics \-sikz, -zikz\ *n pl but sing or pl in constr* : scientific analysis of physical evidence (as evidence from a crime scene) — called also *forensic science*

fore•play \ˈfōr-ˌplā\ *n* : erotic stimulation preceding sexual intercourse

fore•skin \-ˌskin\ *n* : a retractable fold of skin that covers the glans of the penis — called also *prepuce*

-form \ˌfȯrm\ *adj comb form* : in the form or shape of : resembling ⟨chorei*form*⟩ ⟨epilepti*form*⟩

form•al•de•hyde \fȯr-ˈmal-də-ˌhīd, fər-\ *n* : a colorless pungent irritating gas CH_2O used as a disinfectant and preservative

for•ma•lin \ˈfȯr-mə-lən, -ˌlēn\ *n* : a clear aqueous solution of formaldehyde containing a small amount of methanol

formed element *n* : one of the red blood cells, white blood cells, or blood platelets as contrasted with the fluid portion of the blood

forme fruste \ˌfȯrm-ˈfrüest, -ˈfrüst\ *n, pl* **formes frustes** *same or* -ˈfrüsts\ : an atypical and usu. incomplete manifestation of a disease

for•mic acid \ˈfȯr-mik-\ *n* : a colorless pungent vesicant liquid acid CH_2O_2 found esp. in ants and in many plants

for•mi•ca•tion \ˌfȯr-mə-ˈkā-shən\ *n* : an abnormal sensation resembling that made by insects creeping in or on the skin

for•mot•e•rol \fȯr-ˈmät-ə-ˌrȯl\ *n* : a beta-agonist drug $(C_{19}H_{24}N_2O_4)_2 \cdot C_4H_4O_4 \cdot 2H_2O$ used as an orally inhaled bronchodilator — called also *formoterol fumarate;* see DULERA, FORADIL, PERFOROMIST, SYMBICORT

for•mu•la \ˈfȯr-myə-lə\ *n, pl* **-las** *or* **-lae** \-ˌlē, -ˌlī\ **1 a** : a recipe or prescription giving method and proportions of ingredients for the preparation of some material (as a medicine) **b** : a milk mixture or substitute (as one containing soybean protein) for feeding an infant **2** : a symbolic expression showing the composition or constitution of a chemical substance and consisting of symbols for the elements present and subscripts to indicate the relative or total number of atoms present in a molecule ⟨the ~ for water is H_2O⟩ — see EMPIRICAL FORMULA, MOLECULAR FORMULA, STRUCTURAL FORMULA

for•mu•lary \ˈfȯr-myə-ˌler-ē\ *n, pl* **-laries** **1** : a book containing a list of medicinal substances and formulas **2** : an official list of pharmaceutical drugs designated by a health insurance provider as approved for coverage under the provider's pharmacy plan benefits

for•ni•ca•tion \ˌfȯr-nə-ˈkā-shən\ *n* : consensual sexual intercourse between two persons not married to each other — **for•ni•cate** \ˈfȯr-nə-ˌkāt\ *vb*

fornicis — see CRURA FORNICIS

for•nix \ˈfȯr-niks\ *n, pl* **for•ni•ces** \-nə-ˌsēz\ : an anatomical arch or fold: as **a** : the vault of the cranium **b** : the junction where the conjunctiva lining the eyelid meets the conjunctiva overlying the sclera **c** : a body of nerve fibers lying beneath the corpus callosum and serving to integrate the hippocampus with other parts of the brain **d** : the vaulted upper part of the vagina surrounding the uterine cervix **e** : the fundus of the stomach **f** : the vault of the pharynx

Fos•a•max \ˈfä-sə-ˌmaks\ *trademark* — used for a preparation of alendronate

fos•car•net \fäs-ˈkär-nət\ *n* : a hydrated sodium salt $Na_3CO_5P{\cdot}6H_2O$ administered intravenously in individuals infected with HIV to treat retinitis caused by a cytomegalovirus — called also *foscarnet sodium*

fo•sin•o•pril \fō-ˈsi-nə-ˌpril\ *n* : an ACE inhibitor used orally in the form of its sodium salt $C_{30}H_{45}NNaO_7P$ to treat hypertension and heart failure — called also *fosinopril sodium;* see MONOPRIL

fos•sa \ˈfä-sə\ *n, pl* **fos•sae** \-ˌsē, -ˌsī\ : an anatomical pit, groove, or depression ⟨the temporal ~ of the skull⟩

fossa na•vic•u•lar•is \-nə-ˌvi-kyə-ˈlar-əs\ *n* : a depression between the posterior margin of the vaginal opening and the fourchette

fossa oval•is \-ō-ˈva-ləs, -ˈvā-, -ˈvä-\ *n* **1** : a depression in the septum between the right and left atria that marks the position of the foramen ovale in the fetus **2** : SAPHENOUS OPENING

Fos•sar•ia \fä-ˈsar-ē-ə, fȯ-\ *n* : a genus of small freshwater snails (family Lymnaeidae) including intermediate hosts of liver flukes

¹foun•der \ˈfau̇n-dər\ *vb* **foun•dered; foun•der•ing 1** : to become disabled; *esp* : to go lame **2** : to disable (an animal) esp. by inducing laminitis through excessive feeding

²founder *n* : LAMINITIS

four•chette *or* **four•chet** \fu̇r-ˈshet\ *n* : a small fold of membrane connecting the labia minora in the posterior part of the vulva

fourth cranial nerve *n* : TROCHLEAR NERVE

fourth ventricle *n* : a somewhat rhomboidal ventricle of the posterior part of the brain that connects at the front with the third ventricle through the aqueduct of Sylvius and at the back with the central canal of the spinal cord

fo•vea \ˈfō-vē-ə\ *n, pl* **fo•ve•ae** \-vē-ˌē, -ˌī\ **1** : a small fossa **2** : a small depression in the center of the macula that contains only cones and constitutes the area of maximum visual acuity — **fo•ve•al** \-əl\ *adj*

fovea cen•tra•lis \-sen-ˈtra-ləs, -ˈträ-, -ˈtrā-\ *n* : FOVEA 2

fo•ve•o•la \fō-ˈvē-ə-lə\ *n, pl* **-lae** \-ˌlē, -ˌlī\ *or* **-las** : a small pit; *specif* : one of the pits in the embryonic gastric mucosa from which the gastric glands develop — **fo•ve•o•lar** \-lər\ *adj*

fowl cholera *n* : an acute contagious septicemic disease of birds that is marked by fever, weakness, diarrhea, and petechial hemorrhages in the mucous membranes and is caused by a bacterium of the genus *Pasteurella* (*P. multocida*) — called also *avian cholera*

fowl mite *n* : CHICKEN MITE — see NORTHERN FOWL MITE

fowl pest *n* : NEWCASTLE DISEASE

fowl plague *n* : BIRD FLU

fowl pox *n* : either of two forms of a disease esp. of chickens and turkeys that is caused by a poxvirus (species *Fowlpox virus* of the genus *Avipoxvirus*): **a** : a cutaneous form marked by pustules, warty growths, and scabs esp. on skin lacking feathers **b** : a more serious form occurring as cheesy lesions of the mucous membranes of the mouth, throat, and eyes

fowl tick *n* : any of several ticks of the genus *Argas* (as *A. persicus*) that attack fowl esp. in warm regions causing anemia and transmitting various diseases (as spirochetosis)

fowl typhoid *n* : an infectious disease of poultry characterized by diarrhea, anemia, and prostration and caused by a bacterium of the genus *Salmonella* (*S. gallinarum*)

fox•glove \ˈfäks-ˌgləv\ *n* : any plant of the genus *Digitalis*; *esp* : a common European biennial or perennial (*D. purpurea*) that is a source of digitalis

FP *abbr* **1** family physician; family practitioner **2** family practice

fps *abbr* foot-pound-second

Fr *symbol* francium

FR *abbr* flocculation reaction

frac•tion \ˈfrak-shən\ *n* : one of several portions (as of a distillate) separable by fractionation

frac•tion•al \-shə-nəl\ *adj* : of, relating to, or involving a process for fractionating components of a mixture

frac•tion•ate \-shə-ˌnāt\ *vb* **-at•ed; -at•ing** : to separate (as a mixture) into different portions (as by precipitation) — **frac•tion•a•tion** \-ˈnā-shən\ *n*

frac•ture \ˈfrak-chər, -shər\ *n* **1** : the act or process of breaking or the state of being broken; *specif* : the breaking of hard tissue and esp. bone **2** : the rupture (as by tearing) of soft tissue ⟨kidney ~⟩ — **fracture** *vb*

fracture zone *n* : the area of bone, soft tissue, and blood vessels affected by or surrounding a bone fracture

fragile X syndrome \-ˈeks-\ *n* : an inherited disorder that is associated with an abnormal X chromosome, that is characterized esp. by moderate to severe intellectual disability, by an elongated face and prominent forehead, chin, and ears, and by enlarged testes in males, and that often has limited or no effect in heterozygous females — called also *fragile X*

fra·gil·i·tas os·si·um \frə-ˈji-lə-təs-ˈä-sē-əm\ *n* : OSTEOGENESIS IMPERFECTA

fram·be·sia \fram-ˈbē-zhə, -zhē-ə\ *n* : YAWS

frame \ˈfrām\ *n* **1** : the physical makeup of an animal and esp. a human body : PHYSIQUE **2 a** : a part of a pair of glasses that holds one of the lenses **b** *pl* : that part of a pair of glasses other than the lenses

frame·shift \-ˌshift\ *adj* : relating to, being, or causing a mutation in which a number of nucleotides not divisible by three is inserted or deleted so that some triplet codons are read incorrectly during genetic translation — **frameshift** *n*

fran·ci·um \ˈfran-sē-əm\ *n* : a radioactive element discovered as a disintegration product of actinium and obtained artificially by the bombardment of thorium with protons — symbol *Fr;* see ELEMENT table

frank \ˈfraŋk\ *adj* : clinically evident ⟨~ pus⟩ ⟨~ gout⟩

Frank·fort horizontal plane \ˈfraŋk-fərt-\ *n* : a plane used in craniometry that is determined by the highest point on the upper margin of the opening of each external auditory canal and the low point on the lower margin of the left orbit — called also *Frankfort horizontal, Frankfort plane*

Frank–Star·ling law \ˈfräŋk-ˈstär-liŋ-\ *n* : STARLING'S LAW OF THE HEART

Frank, Otto (1865–1944), German physiologist.

Starling, Ernest Henry (1866–1927), British physiologist.

Frank–Starling law of the heart *n* : STARLING'S LAW OF THE HEART

fra·ter·nal \frə-ˈtərn-ᵊl\ *adj* : derived from two ova : DIZYGOTIC ⟨~ twins⟩

FRCP *abbr* Fellow of the Royal College of Physicians

FRCS *abbr* Fellow of the Royal College of Surgeons

freck·le \ˈfre-kəl\ *n* : any of the small brownish spots in the skin that are due to augmented melanin production and that increase in number and intensity on exposure to sunlight — called also *ephelis;* compare LENTIGO — **freckle** *vb* — **freck·led** \-kəld\ *adj*

free \ˈfrē\ *adj* **fre·er; fre·est 1 a** (1) : not united with, attached to, combined with, or mixed with something else ⟨a ~ surface of a bodily part⟩ (2) : having the bare axon exposed in tissue ⟨a ~ nerve ending⟩ **b** : not chemically combined ⟨~ oxygen⟩ **2** : having all living connections severed before removal to another site ⟨a ~ graft⟩

free association *n* **1 a** : the expression (as by speaking or writing) of the content of consciousness without censorship as an aid in gaining access to unconscious processes esp. in psychoanalysis **b** : the reporting of the first thought that comes to mind in response to a given stimulus (as a word) **2** : an idea or image elicited by free association **3** : a method using free association — **free–as·so·ci·ate** \ˈfrē-ə-ˈsō-shē-ˌāt, -sē-\ *vb*

¹free·base \ˈfrē-ˌbās\ *vb* **-based; -bas·ing** : to prepare or use (cocaine) as freebase — **free·bas·er** \-ˌbā-sər\ *n*

²freebase *n* : a purified solid form of cocaine (as crack) that is obtained by treating the powdered hydrochloride of cocaine with an alkaloid base (as sodium bicarbonate) and that can be smoked or heated to produce vapors for inhalation; *specif* : a form derived from treatment of the hydrochloride of cocaine with ammonia or similar alkaloid solution followed by extraction with a solvent (as ether)

free fall *n* : the condition of unrestrained motion in a gravitational field; *also* : such motion

free–float·ing \ˈfrē-ˈflō-tiŋ\ *adj* : felt as an emotion without apparent cause ⟨~ anxiety⟩

free–liv·ing \-ˈli-viŋ\ *adj* **1** : not fixed to the substrate but capable of motility ⟨a ~ protozoan⟩ **2** : being metabolically independent : neither parasitic nor symbiotic

free radical *n* : an esp. reactive atom or group of atoms that has one or more unpaired electrons; *esp* : one that is produced in the body by natural biological processes or introduced from outside (as in tobacco smoke, toxins, or pollutants) and that can damage cells, proteins, and DNA by altering their chemical structure

free·stand·ing \ˈfrē-ˈstan-diŋ\ *adj* : being independent; *esp* : not part of or affiliated with another organization ⟨a ~ emergency clinic⟩

free–swimming *adj* : able to swim about : not attached ⟨~ larvae⟩

freeze \ˈfrēz\ *vb* **froze** \ˈfrōz\; **fro·zen** \ˈfrōz-ᵊn\; **freez·ing 1** : to harden or cause to harden into a solid (as ice) by loss of heat **2** : to chill or become chilled with cold **3** : to anesthetize (a part) by cold

freeze–dry \ˈfrēz-ˈdrī\ *vb* **freeze–dried; freeze–dry·ing** : to dry and preserve (as food, vaccines, or tissue) in a frozen state under high vacuum — **freeze–dried** *adj*

freeze–etch·ing \-ˈe-chiŋ\ *n* : FREEZE FRACTURE — **freeze–etch** \-ˈech\ *adj* — **freeze–etched** \-ˌecht\ *adj*

freeze fracture *also* **freeze–fracturing** *n* : preparation of a specimen (as of tissue) for electron microscopic examination by freezing, fracturing along natural structural lines, and preparing a replica — **freeze–fracture** *vb*

freezing point *n* : the temperature at which a liquid solidifies

Frei test \ˈfrī-\ *n* : a serological test for the identification of lymphogranuloma venereum — called also *Frei skin test*

Frei, Wilhelm Siegmund (1885–1943), German dermatologist.

frem•i•tus \ˈfre-mə-təs\ *n* : a sensation felt by a hand placed on a part of the body (as the chest) that vibrates during speech

French \ˈfrench\ *n, pl* **French** : a unit of measure equal to one-third millimeter used in measuring the outside diameter of a tubular instrument (as a catheter) inserted into a body cavity

fren•ec•to•my \frə-ˈnek-tə-mē\ *n, pl* **-mies** : excision of a frenulum

fren•u•lum \ˈfren-yə-ləm\ *n, pl* **-la** \-lə\ : a connecting fold of membrane serving to support or restrain a part (as the tongue)

fre•num \ˈfrē-nəm\ *n, pl* **frenums** *or* **fre•na** \-nə\ : FRENULUM

freq *abbr* frequency

fre•quen•cy \ˈfrē-kwən-sē\ *n, pl* **-cies** **1** : the number of individuals in a single class when objects are classified according to variations in a set of one or more specified attributes **2** : the number of repetitions of a periodic process in a unit of time

Freud•ian \ˈfrȯi-dē-ən\ *adj* : of, relating to, or according with the psychoanalytic theories or practices of Freud — **Freudian** *n* — **Freud•ian•ism** \-ə-ˌni-zəm\ *n*

Freud \ˈfrȯid\, **Sigmund (1856–1939),** Austrian neurologist and psychiatrist.

Freudian slip *n* : something said by mistake that is motivated by and reveals some unconscious aspect of the mind

Freund's adjuvant \ˈfrȯindz-\ *n* : any of several oil and water emulsions that contain antigens and are used to stimulate antibody production in experimental animals

Freund \ˈfrȯind\, **Jules Thomas (1890–1960),** American immunologist.

fri•a•ble \ˈfrī-ə-bəl\ *adj* : easily crumbled or pulverized ⟨~ carcinomatous tissue⟩; *also* : marked by erosion and bleeding ⟨a ~ cervix⟩ — **fri•a•bil•i•ty** \ˌfrī-ə-ˈbi-lə-tē\ *n*

friar's balsam *n* : an alcoholic solution containing essentially benzoin, storax, balsam of Tolu, and aloes applied topically to the skin (as to relieve irritation) and after addition to hot water as an inhalant with expectorant activity — called also *compound benzoin tincture*

Fried•man test \ˈfrēd-mən-\ *also* **Friedman's test** *n* : a modification of the Aschheim-Zondek test for pregnancy using rabbits as test animals

Friedman, Maurice Harold (1903–1991), American physiologist.

Fried•reich's ataxia \ˈfrēd-rīks-, ˈfrēt-rīks-\ *n* : a recessive hereditary degenerative disease affecting the spinal column, cerebellum, and medulla, marked by muscular incoordination and twitching, and usu. becoming manifest in the adult

Friedreich \ˈfrēt-rīk\, **Nikolaus (1825–1882),** German neurologist.

Friend virus \ˈfrend\ *n* : a strain of murine leukemia virus that causes erythroleukemia in mice — called also *Friend leukemia virus*

Friend, Charlotte (1921–1987), American microbiologist.

frig•id \ˈfri-jəd\ *adj* **1** : lacking sexual desire : abnormally averse to sexual intercourse — used esp. of women **2** *of a female* : unable to achieve orgasm during sexual intercourse — **fri•gid•i•ty** \fri-ˈji-də-tē\ *n*

fringed tapeworm *n* : a tapeworm of the genus *Thysanosoma* (*T. actinioides*) found in the intestine and bile ducts of ruminants

frog \ˈfrȯg, ˈfräg\ *n* **1** : the triangular elastic horny pad in the middle of the sole of the foot of a horse **2** : a condition in the throat that produces hoarseness ⟨had a ~ in his throat⟩

Fröh•lich's syndrome *or* **Froeh•lich's syndrome** \ˈfrā-liks-, ˈfrœ-liks-\ *also* **Fröhlich syndrome** *n* : ADIPOSOGENITAL DYSTROPHY

Fröhlich \ˈfrœ-lik\, **Alfred (1871–1953),** Austrian pharmacologist and neurologist.

frondosum — see CHORION FRONDOSUM

fron•tal \ˈfrənt-ᵊl\ *adj* **1** : of, relating to, or adjacent to the forehead or the frontal bone **2** : of, relating to, or situated at the front or anteriorly **3** : parallel to the main axis of the body and at right angles to the sagittal plane ⟨a ~ plane⟩ — **fron•tal•ly** *adv*

frontal bone *n* : a bone that forms the forehead and roofs over most of the orbits and nasal cavity and that at birth consists of two halves separated by a suture

frontal eminence *n* : the prominence of the human frontal bone above each supraorbital ridge

frontal gyrus *n* : any of the convolutions of the outer surface of the frontal lobe of the brain — called also *frontal convolution*

fron•ta•lis \ˌfrən-ˈtā-ləs\ *n* : the muscle of the forehead that forms part of the occipitofrontalis — called also *frontalis muscle*

frontal lobe *n* : the anterior division of each cerebral hemisphere having its lower part in the anterior fossa of the skull and bordered behind by the central sulcus

frontal lobotomy *n* : PREFRONTAL LOBOTOMY

frontal nerve *n* : a branch of the ophthalmic nerve supplying the forehead, scalp, and adjoining parts

frontal process *n* **1** : a long plate that is part of the maxillary bone and contributes to the formation of the lateral part of the nose and of the nasal cavity — called also *nasal process* **2** : a process of the zygomatic bone articulating superiorly with the frontal bone, forming part of the orbit anteriorly, and articulating with the sphenoid bone posteriorly

frontal sinus *n* : either of two air spaces lined with mucous membrane each of which lies within the frontal bone above one of the orbits

fronto- *comb form* : frontal bone and ⟨*fronto*parietal⟩

fron•to–oc•cip•i•tal \ˌfrən-tō-äk-ˈsip-ət-ᵊl, ˌfrän-\ *adj* : of or relating to the forehead and occiput

fron•to•pa•ri•etal \-pə-ˈrī-ət-ᵊl\ *adj* : of, relating to, or involving both frontal and parietal bones of the skull

frontoparietal suture *n* : CORONAL SUTURE

fron•to•tem•po•ral \-ˈtem-pə-rəl\ *adj* : of or relating to the frontal and the temporal bones

frontotemporal dementia *n* : any of several degenerative brain diseases (as Pick's disease) that are caused by progressive atrophic changes in the frontal or temporal lobes — abbr. *FTD;* called also *frontotemporal degeneration*

frost•bite \ˈfrȯst-ˌbīt\ *n* : the superficial or deep freezing of the tissues of some part of the body (as the feet or hands); *also* : the damage to tissues caused by freezing — **frostbite** *vb*

frost•nip \ˈfrȯst-ˌnip\ *n* : the reversible freezing of superficial skin layers that is usu. marked by numbness and whiteness of the skin

frot•tage \frȯ-ˈtäzh\ *n* : FROTTEURISM

frot•teur \frȯ-ˈtər\ *n* : one who practices frotteurism

frot•teur•ism \-ˌi-zəm\ *n* : the paraphiliac practice of achieving sexual stimulation or orgasm by touching and rubbing against a person without the person's consent and usu. in a public place — called also *frottage*

froze *past of* FREEZE

frozen *past part of* FREEZE

frozen shoulder *n* : a shoulder affected by severe pain, stiffening, and restricted motion — called also *adhesive capsulitis*

fruc•to•kin•ase \ˌfrək-tō-ˈkī-ˌnās, -ˈki-, -ˌnāz, ˌfrük-\ *n* : a kinase that catalyzes the transfer of phosphate groups to fructose

fruc•tose \ˈfrək-ˌtōs, ˈfrük-, ˈfru̇k-, -ˌtōz\ *n* **1** : a sugar $C_6H_{12}O_6$ sweeter and more soluble than glucose **2** : the very sweet soluble levorotatory D-form of fructose that occurs esp. in fruit juices and honey — called also *levulose*

fruc•tos•uria \ˌfrək-tə-ˈsu̇r-ē-ə\ *n* : the presence of fructose in the urine

fruit•ar•i•an \frü-ˈter-ē-ən\ *n* : one who lives chiefly on fruit

fruiting body *n* : a plant organ specialized for producing spores; *esp* : SPOROPHORE

fruit sugar *n* : FRUCTOSE 2

fru•se•mide \ˈfrü-sə-ˌmīd\ *n, chiefly Brit* : FUROSEMIDE

frus•trat•ed *adj* : filled with a sense of frustration : feeling deep insecurity, discouragement, or dissatisfaction

frus•tra•tion \(ˌ)frəs-ˈtrā-shən\ *n* **1** : a deep chronic sense or state of insecurity and dissatisfaction arising from unresolved problems or unfulfilled needs **2** : something that frustrates — **frus•trate** \ˈfrəs-ˌtrāt\ *vb*

FSH *abbr* follicle-stimulating hormone

ft *abbr* feet; foot

FTD *abbr* frontotemporal dementia

F_2 generation *n* : the generation produced by interbreeding individuals of an F_1 generation and consisting of individuals that exhibit the result of recombination and segregation of genes controlling traits for which stocks of the P_1 generation differ

fuch•sin *or* **fuch•sine** \ˈfyük-sən, -ˌsēn\ *n* : a dye that yields a brilliant bluish-red and is used in carbolfuchsin paint, in Schiff's reagent, and as a biological stain

fu•cose \ˈfyü-ˌkōs, -ˌkōz\ *n* : an aldose sugar that occurs in bound form in the dextrorotatory D-form in various glycosides and in the levorotatory L-form in some brown algae and in mammalian polysaccharides typical of some blood groups

fu•co•si•dase \ˌfyü-ˈkō-sə-ˌdās, -ˌdāz\ *n* : an enzyme existing in stereoisomeric alpha and beta forms that catalyzes the metabolism of fucose

fu•co•si•do•sis \-ˌkō-sə-ˈdō-səs\ *n, pl* **-do•ses** \-ˌsēz\ : a disorder of metabolism inherited as a recessive trait and characterized by progressive neurological degeneration, deficiency of the alpha stereoisomer of fucosidase, and accumulation of fucose-containing carbohydrates

fugax — see AMAUROSIS FUGAX, PROCTALGIA FUGAX

-fuge \ˌfyüj\ *n comb form* : one that drives away ⟨febri*fuge*⟩ ⟨vermi*fuge*⟩

fu•gi•tive \ˈfyü-jə-tiv\ *adj* : tending to be inconstant or transient

fu•gu \ˈfyü-(ˌ)gü, ˈfü-\ *n* : any of various very poisonous puffer fish that contain tetrodotoxin and that are used as food in Japan after the toxin-containing organs are removed

fugue \ˈfyüg\ *n* : a disturbed state of consciousness in which the one affected seems to perform acts in full awareness but upon recovery cannot recollect them

ful•gu•ra•tion \ˌfu̇l-gə-ˈrā-shən, fəl-, -gyə-, -jə-\ *n* : ELECTRODESICCATION

— **ful·gu·rate** \ˈfu̇l-gə-ˌrāt, ˈfəl-, -gyə-, -jə-\ *vb*

full–blown *adj* : fully developed : being in its most extreme or serious form : possessing or exhibiting the characteristic symptoms ⟨a ~ cold⟩

ful·mi·nant \ˈfu̇l-mə-nənt, ˈfəl-\ *adj* : coming on suddenly with great severity ⟨~ hepatitis⟩

ful·mi·nat·ing \-ˌnā-tiŋ\ *adj* : FULMINANT — **ful·mi·na·tion** \ˌfu̇l-mə-ˈnā-shən, ˌfəl-\ *n*

fu·ma·rate \ˈfyü-mə-ˌrāt\ *n* : a salt or ester of fumaric acid

fu·mar·ic acid \fyu̇-ˈmar-ik-\ *n* : a crystalline acid $C_4H_4O_4$ formed from succinic acid as an intermediate in the Krebs cycle

fu·mi·gant \ˈfyü-mi-gənt\ *n* : a substance used in fumigating

fu·mi·gate \ˈfyü-mə-ˌgāt\ *vb* **-gat·ed; -gat·ing** : to apply smoke, vapor, or gas to esp. for the purpose of disinfecting or of destroying pests — **fu·mi·ga·tion** \ˌfyü-mə-ˈgā-shən\ *n* — **fu·mi·ga·tor** \ˈfyü-mə-ˌgā-tər\ *n*

func·tion \ˈfəŋk-shən\ *n* : any of a group of related actions contributing to a larger action; *esp* : the normal and specific contribution of a bodily part to the economy of a living organism — **function** *vb* — **func·tion·less** \-ləs\ *adj*

func·tion·al \ˈfəŋk-shə-nəl\ *adj* **1 a** : of, connected with, or being a function — compare STRUCTURAL 1 **b** : affecting physiological or psychological functions but not organic structure ⟨~ heart disease⟩ ⟨a ~ psychosis⟩ — compare ORGANIC 1b **2** : performing or able to perform a regular function — **func·tion·al·ly** *adv*

functional food *n* : NUTRACEUTICAL

functional genomics *n pl but sing in constr* : a branch of genomics concerned with analyzing the function of genes and the proteins they produce

functional magnetic resonance imaging *n* : magnetic resonance imaging used to detect physical changes (as of blood flow) in the brain resulting from increased neuronal activity (as during performance of a specific cognitive task) — abbr. *fMRI;* called also *functional MRI*

fun·dal \ˈfənd-ᵊl\ *adj* : FUNDIC

fun·da·ment \ˈfən-də-mənt\ *n* **1** : BUTTOCKS **2** : ANUS

fun·dic \ˈfən-dik\ *adj* : of or relating to a fundus

fundic gland *n* : one of the tubular glands of the fundus of the stomach secreting pepsin and mucus — compare CHIEF CELL 1

fun·do·pli·ca·tion \ˌfən-dō-plī-ˈkā-shən\ *n* : a surgical procedure in which the upper portion of the stomach is wrapped around the lower end of the esophagus and sutured in place as a treatment for the reflux of stomach contents into the esophagus — see NISSEN FUNDOPLICATION

fun·dus \ˈfən-dəs\ *n, pl* **fun·di** \-ˌdī, -ˌdē\ : the bottom of or part opposite the aperture of the internal surface of a hollow organ: as **a** : the greater curvature of the stomach **b** : the lower back part of the bladder **c** : the large upper end of the uterus **d** : the part of the eye opposite the pupil

fun·du·scop·ic *also* **fun·do·scop·ic** \ˌfən-də-ˈskä-pik\ *adj* : of, done by, or obtained by ophthalmoscopic examination of the fundus of the eye — **fun·dus·co·py** \ˌfən-ˈdəs-kə-pē\ *also* **fun·dos·co·py** \-ˈdäs-\ *n*

fun·gae·mia *Brit var of* FUNGEMIA

fun·gal \ˈfəŋ-gəl\ *adj* **1** : of, relating to, or having the characteristics of fungi **2** : caused by a fungus ⟨~ infections⟩

fun·gate \ˈfəŋ-ˌgāt\ *vb* **-gat·ed; -gat·ing** : to assume a fungal form or grow rapidly like a fungus — **fun·ga·tion** \ˌfəŋ-ˈgā-shən\ *n*

fun·ge·mia \fən-ˈgē-mē-ə\ *n* : the presence of fungi in the blood

fungi *pl of* FUNGUS

fungi- *comb form* : fungus ⟨*fungi*cide⟩

fun·gi·cid·al \ˌfən-jə-ˈsīd-ᵊl, ˌfəŋ-gə-\ *adj* : destroying fungi; *broadly* : inhibiting the growth of fungi — **fun·gi·cid·al·ly** *adv*

fun·gi·cide \ˈfən-jə-ˌsīd, ˈfəŋ-gə-\ *n* : an agent that destroys fungi or inhibits their growth

fun·gi·form \ˈfən-jə-ˌfȯrm, ˈfəŋ-gə-\ *adj* : shaped like a mushroom

fungiform papilla *n* : any of numerous papillae on the upper surface of the tongue that are flat-topped and noticeably red from the richly vascular stroma and usu. contain taste buds

fun·gi·stat \ˈfən-jə-ˌstat, ˈfəŋ-gə-\ *n* : a fungistatic agent

fun·gi·stat·ic \ˌfən-jə-ˈsta-tik, ˌfəŋ-gə-\ *adj* : capable of inhibiting the growth and reproduction of fungi without destroying them ⟨a ~ agent⟩ — **fun·gi·stat·i·cal·ly** \-ti-k(ə-)lē\ *adv*

Fun·gi·zone \ˈfən-jə-ˌzōn\ *trademark* — used for a preparation of amphotericin B

fun·goid \ˈfəŋ-ˌgȯid\ *adj* : resembling, characteristic of, caused by, or being a fungus ⟨a ~ ulcer⟩ ⟨a ~ growth⟩

fungoides — see MYCOSIS FUNGOIDES

fun·gous \ˈfəŋ-gəs\ *adj* : FUNGAL

fun·gus \ˈfəŋ-gəs\ *n, pl* **fun·gi** \ˈfən-ˌjī, ˈfəŋ-ˌgī\ *also* **fun·gus·es** \ˈfəŋ-gə-səz\ *often attrib* **1** : any of a kingdom (Fungi) of saprophytic and parasitic spore-producing organisms formerly classified as plants that lack chlorophyll and include molds, rusts, mildews, smuts, mushrooms, and yeasts **2** : infection with a fungus

fu·nic·u·li·tis \fyu̇-ˌni-kyə-ˈlī-təs, fə-\ *n* : inflammation of the spermatic cord

fu·nic·u·lus \fyu̇-ˈni-kyə-les, fə-\ *n, pl* **-li** \-ˌlī, -ˌlē\ : any of various bodily structures more or less like a cord in form: as **a** : one of the longitudinal subdivisions of white matter in each lateral half of the spinal cord — see ANTERIOR FUNICULUS, LATERAL FUNICULUS, POSTERIOR FUNICULUS; compare COLUMN a **b** : SPERMATIC CORD

funnel chest *n* : a depression of the anterior wall of the chest produced by a sinking in of the sternum — called also *funnel breast, pectus excavatum*

funny bone *n* : the place at the back of the elbow where the ulnar nerve rests against a prominence of the humerus — called also *crazy bone*

FUO *abbr* fever of undetermined origin

fur \ˈfər\ *n* : a coat of epithelial debris on the tongue

fu·ra·zol·i·done \ˌfyu̇r-ə-ˈzä-lə-ˌdōn\ *n* : an antimicrobial drug $C_8H_7N_3O_5$ used against bacteria and some protozoans esp. in infections of the gastrointestinal tract

furious rabies *n* : the common form of rabies that is characterized by anxiety, spasm of the muscles of the throat and diaphragm, hyperactive or violent behavior, hallucinations, excessive salivation, paralysis, coma, and death — compare PARALYTIC RABIES

fu·ro·se·mide \fyu̇-ˈrō-sə-ˌmīd\ *n* : a powerful diuretic $C_{12}H_{11}ClN_2O_5S$ used esp. to treat edema — called also *frusemide, fursemide;* see LASIX

furred \ˈfərd\ *adj* : having a coating consisting chiefly of mucus and dead epithelial cells ⟨a ~ tongue⟩

fur·row \ˈfər-(ˌ)ō\ *n* **1** : a marked narrow depression or groove **2** : a deep wrinkle

fur·se·mide \ˈfər-sə-ˌmīd\ *n* : FUROSEMIDE

fu·run·cle \ˈfyu̇r-ˌəŋ-kəl\ *n* : BOIL — **fu·run·cu·lar** \fyu̇-ˈrəŋ-kyə-lər\ *adj* — **fu·run·cu·lous** \-ləs\ *adj*

fu·run·cu·lo·sis \fyu̇-ˌrəŋ-kyə-ˈlō-səs\ *n, pl* **-lo·ses** \-ˌsēz\ **1** : the condition of having or tending to develop multiple furuncles **2** : a highly infectious disease of various salmon and trout (genera *Salmo* and *Oncorhynchus*) and their relatives that is caused by a bacterium (*Aeromonas salmonicida* of the family Vibrionaceae)

fuse \ˈfyüz\ *vb* **fused; fus·ing** : to undergo or cause to undergo fusion

fusi- *comb form* : spindle ⟨*fusi*form⟩

fu·si·form \ˈfyü-zə-ˌfȯrm\ *adj* : tapering toward each end ⟨a ~ aneurysm⟩

fu·sion \ˈfyü-zhən\ *n, often attrib* : a union by or as if by melting together: as **a** : a merging of diverse elements into a unified whole; *specif* : the blending of retinal images in binocular vision **b** (1) : a blend of sensations, perceptions, ideas, or attitudes such that the component elements can seldom be identified by introspective analysis (2) : the perception of light from a source that is intermittent above a critical frequency as if the source were continuous — called also *flicker fusion;* compare FLICKER **c** : the surgical immobilization of a joint — see SPINAL FUSION

fu·so·bac·te·ri·um \ˌfyü-zō-bak-ˈtir-ē-əm\ *n* **1** *cap* : a genus of gram-negative anaerobic strictly parasitic rod-shaped bacteria that is placed in either of two families (Bacteroidaceae or Fusobacteriaceae) and includes some pathogens occurring esp. in purulent or gangrenous infections **2** *pl* **-ria** \-ē-ə\ : any bacterium of the genus *Fusobacterium*

fu·so·spi·ro·chet·al \-ˌspī-rə-ˈkēt-ᵊl\ *adj* : of, relating to, or caused by fusobacteria and spirochetes

G

g \ˈjē\ *n, pl* **g's** *or* **gs** \ˈjēz\ : a unit of force equal to the force exerted by gravity on a body at rest and used to indicate the force to which a body is subjected when accelerated

g *abbr* **1** gram **2** gravity

G *abbr* guanine

Ga *symbol* gallium

GABA \ˈga-bə\ *n or abbr* : GAMMA-AMINOBUTYRIC ACID

gab·a·pen·tin \ˈga-bə-ˌpen-tin\ *n* : an anticonvulsant drug $C_9H_{17}NO_2$ that is administered orally in the treatment of partial seizures — see NEURONTIN

G–ac·tin \ˈjē-ˌak-tən\ *n* : a globular monomeric form of actin produced in solutions of low ionic concentration — compare F-ACTIN

GAD *abbr* generalized anxiety disorder

gad·o·lin·i·um \ˌgad-ᵊl-ˈi-nē-əm\ *n* : a magnetic metallic element — symbol *Gd;* see ELEMENT table

gag reflex *n* : reflex contraction of the muscles of the throat caused esp. by stimulation (as by touch) of the pharynx

gal *abbr* gallon

galact- *or* **galacto-** *comb form* **1** : milk ⟨*galactor*rhea⟩ **2** : galactose ⟨*galacto*kinase⟩

ga·lac·to·cele \gə-ˈlak-tə-ˌsēl\ *n* : a cystic tumor esp. of a mammary gland containing milk or a milky fluid

ga·lac·to·ki·nase \gə-ˌlak-tō-ˈkī-nās, -ˈki-, -ˌnāz\ *n* : a kinase that catalyzes the transfer of phosphate groups to galactose

ga·lac·tor·rhea \gə-ˌlak-tə-ˈrē-ə\ *n* : a spontaneous flow of milk from the nipple

ga·lac·tor·rhoea *chiefly Brit var of* GALACTORRHEA

ga·lac·tos·ae·mia *chiefly Brit var of* GALACTOSEMIA

ga·lac·tos·amine \gə-ˌlak-ˈtō-sə-ˌmēn, -zə-\ *n* : an amino derivative $C_6H_{13}O_5N$ of galactose that occurs in cartilage

ga·lac·tose \gə-ˈlak-ˌtōs, -ˌtōz\ *n* : a sugar $C_6H_{12}O_6$ that is less soluble and less sweet than glucose and is known in dextrorotatory, levorotatory, and racemic forms

ga·lac·tos·emia \gə-ˌlak-tə-ˈsē-mē-ə\ *n* : a metabolic disorder inherited as an autosomal recessive trait in which galactose accumulates in the blood due to deficiency of an enzyme catalyzing its conversion to glucose — **ga·lac·tos·emic** \-mik\ *adj*

ga·lac·to·si·dase \gə-ˌlak-ˈtō-sə-ˌdās, -zə-ˌdāz\ *n* : an enzyme (as lactase) that hydrolyzes a galactoside

ga·lac·to·side \gə-ˈlak-tə-ˌsīd\ *n* : a glycoside that yields galactose on hydrolysis

ga·lac·tos·uria \gə-ˌlak-(ˌ)tō-ˈsu̇r-ē-ə, -ˈsyu̇r-\ *n* : the presence of galactose in the urine

gal·a·nin \ˈga-lə-nin\ *n* : a neurotransmitter that plays a role in regulating various physiological functions (as contraction of gastrointestinal muscle and inhibition of insulin)

Gal·ba \ˈgal-bə, ˈgȯl-\ *n* : a genus of freshwater snails (family Lymnaeidae) that include hosts of a liver fluke of the genus *Fasciola* (*F. hepatica*)

ga·lea \ˈgā-lē-a, ˈga-\ *n* : GALEA APONEUROTICA

galea apo·neu·ro·ti·ca \-ˌa-pō-nu̇-ˈrä-ti-kə, -nyu̇-\ *n* : the aponeurosis underlying the scalp and linking the frontalis and occipitalis muscles — called also *epicranial aponeurosis*

ga·len·i·cal \gə-ˈle-ni-kəl\ *n* : a standard medicinal preparation (as an extract or tincture) containing usu. one or more active constituents of a plant — **ga·len·ic** \-nik\ *also* **galenical** *adj*

Ga·len \ˈgā-lən\ **(*ca* 129–*ca* 199),** Greek physician.

Galen's vein *n* **1** : either of a pair of cerebral veins in the roof of the third ventricle that drain the interior of the brain **2** : GREAT CEREBRAL VEIN

[1]**gall** \ˈgȯl\ *n* : BILE; *esp* : bile obtained from an animal and used in medicine

[2]**gall** *n* : a skin sore caused by chronic irritation

[3]**gall** *vb* : to rub and wear away by friction : CHAFE

gal·la·mine tri·eth·io·dide \ˈga-lə-ˌmēn-ˌtrī-ˌe-ˈthī-ə-ˌdīd\ *n* : an iodide salt $C_{30}H_{60}I_3N_3O_3$ that is used to produce muscle relaxation esp. during anesthesia — called also *gallamine*

gal·late \ˈga-ˌlāt, ˈgȯ-\ *n* : a salt or ester of gallic acid — see PROPYL GALLATE

gall·blad·der \ˈgȯl-ˌbla-dər\ *n* : a membranous muscular sac in which bile from the liver is stored

galli — see CRISTA GALLI

gal·lic acid \ˈga-lik-, ˈgȯ-\ *n* : a white crystalline acid $C_7H_6O_5$ found widely in plants or combined in tannins

gal·li·um \ˈga-lē-əm\ *n* : a rare bluish-white metallic element that is used in the form of its hydrated nitrate salt $Ga(NO_3)_3{\cdot}9H_2O$ to treat hypercalcemia caused by certain cancers — symbol *Ga;* see ELEMENT table

gal·lon \ˈga-lən\ *n* **1** : a U.S. unit of liquid capacity equal to four quarts or 231 cubic inches **2** : a British unit of liquid and dry capacity equal to four quarts or 277.42 cubic inches — called also *imperial gallon*

gal·lop \ˈga-ləp\ *n* : GALLOP RHYTHM

galloping *adj, of a disease* : progressing rapidly toward a fatal conclusion

gallop rhythm *n* : an abnormal heart rhythm marked by the occurrence of three distinct sounds in each heartbeat like the sound of a galloping horse — called also *gallop*

gall sickness *n* : ANAPLASMOSIS b

gall•stone \ˈgȯl-ˌstōn\ *n* : a calculus (as of cholesterol) formed in the gallbladder or biliary passages — called also *cholelith*

gal•van•ic \gal-ˈva-nik\ *adj* : of, relating to, involving, or producing a direct current of electricity ⟨~ stimulation of flaccid muscles⟩ — **gal•van•i•cal•ly** \-ni-k(ə-)lē\ *adv*

Gal•va•ni \gäl-ˈvä-nē\, **Luigi (1737–1798),** Italian physician and physicist.

galvanic skin response *n* : a change in the electrical resistance of the skin in response to emotional arousal which increases sympathetic nervous system activity — abbr. *GSR*

gal•va•nism \ˈgal-və-ˌni-zəm\ *n* : the therapeutic use of direct electric current (as to relieve pain)

gal•va•nom•e•ter \ˌgal-və-ˈnä-mə-tər\ *n* : an instrument for detecting or measuring a small electric current

gamet- *or* **gameto-** *comb form* : gamete ⟨*gamet*ic⟩ ⟨*gameto*genesis⟩

gam•ete \ˈga-ˌmēt, ga-ˈmēt\ *n* : a mature male or female germ cell usu. possessing a haploid chromosome set and capable of initiating formation of a new diploid individual by fusion with a gamete of the opposite sex — called also *sex cell* — **ga•met•ic** \gə-ˈme-tik\ *adj* — **ga•met•i•cal•ly** \-ti-k(ə-)lē\ *adv*

gamete in•tra•fal•lo•pi•an transfer \-ˌin-trə-fə-ˈlō-pē-ən-\ *n* : a method of assisting reproduction in cases of infertility in which eggs are obtained from an ovary, mixed with sperm, and inserted into a fallopian tube — abbr. *GIFT;* called also *gamete intrafallopian tube transfer;* compare ZYGOTE INTRAFALLOPIAN TRANSFER

ga•me•to•cide \gə-ˈmē-tə-ˌsīd\ *n* : an agent that destroys the gametocytes of a malaria parasite

ga•me•to•cyte \-ˌsīt\ *n* : a cell (as of a protozoan causing malaria) that divides to produce gametes

gam•e•to•gen•e•sis \ˌga-mə-tə-ˈje-nə-səs, gə-ˌmē-tə-\ *n, pl* **-e•ses** \-ˌsēz\ : the production of gametes — **gam•e•tog•e•nous** \ˌga-mə-ˈtä-jə-nəs\ *adj*

-gam•ic \ˈgam-ik\ *adj comb form* : -GAMOUS ⟨mono*gamic*⟩

[1]**gam•ma** \ˈga-mə\ *n* **1 :** the third letter of the Greek alphabet — symbol Γ or γ **2 :** GAMMA RAY

[2]**gamma** *or* **γ-** *adj* **1 :** of or relating to one of three or more closely related chemical substances ⟨the *gamma* chain of hemoglobin⟩ — used somewhat arbitrarily to specify ordinal relationship or a particular physical form **2** *of streptococci* : producing no hemolysis on blood agar plates

gam•ma–ami•no•bu•tyr•ic acid *also* **γ-ami•no•bu•tyr•ic acid** \ˌga-mə-ə-ˌmē-(ˌ)nō-byü-ˈtir-ik-, ˌga-mə-ˌa-mə-(ˌ)nō-\ *n* : an amino acid $C_4H_9NO_2$ that is a neurotransmitter that induces inhibition of postsynaptic neurons — called also *GABA*

gamma benzene hexa•chlo•ride \-ˌhek-sə-ˈklōr-ˌīd\ *n* : the gamma isomer of benzene hexachloride that comprises the insecticide lindane and is sometimes used in medicine to treat scabies — called also *gamma BHC*

gamma camera *n* : a camera that detects the gamma-ray photons emitted from a radioactive tracer injected into the body and is used esp. in medical diagnostic scanning

gamma globulin *n* **1 a :** a protein fraction of blood rich in antibodies **b** : a sterile solution of gamma globulin from pooled human blood administered esp. for passive immunity against measles, German measles, hepatitis A, or polio **2 :** any of numerous globulins of blood plasma or serum that have less electrophoretic mobility at alkaline pH than serum albumins, alpha globulins, or beta globulins and that include most antibodies

gamma hydroxybutyrate *n* : GHB

gamma interferon *n* : an interferon produced by T cells that regulates the immune response (as by the activation of macrophages and natural killer cells) and is used in a form obtained from recombinant DNA esp. in the control of infections associated with chronic granulomatous disease — called also *interferon gamma*

Gamma Knife *trademark* — used for a medical device that emits a highly focused beam of gamma radiation used in noninvasive surgery

gamma radiation *n* : radiation that is composed of gamma rays and is used in cancer radiotherapy

gamma ray *n* : a photon emitted spontaneously by a radioactive substance; *also* : a high-energy photon — usu. used in pl.

gam•mop•a•thy \ga-ˈmä-pə-thē\ *n, pl* **-thies :** a disorder characterized by a disturbance in the body's synthesis of antibodies

-g•a•mous \gə-məs\ *adj comb form* **1** : characterized by having or practicing (such) a marriage or (such or so many) marriages ⟨mono*gamous*⟩ **2** : having (such) gametes or reproductive organs or (such) a mode of fertilization ⟨hetero*gamous*⟩

-g•a•my \gə-mē\ *n comb form, pl* **g•a•mies 1 :** marriage ⟨mono*gamy*⟩ **2** : possession of (such) gametes or reproductive organs or (such) a mode of fertilization ⟨hetero*gamy*⟩

gan•ci•clo•vir \gan-ˈsī-klə-(ˌ)vir\ *n* : an antiviral drug $C_9H_{13}N_5O_4$ related to acyclovir and used esp. in the treatment of cytomegalovirus retinitis in immunocompromised patients — called also *DHPG*

gangli- *or* **ganglio-** *comb form* : ganglion ⟨*gangli*oma⟩ ⟨*ganglio*neuroma⟩

ganglia *pl of* GANGLION

gan•gli•al \ˈgaŋ-glē-əl\ *adj* : of, relating to, or resembling a ganglion

gan•gli•at•ed cord \ˈgaŋ-glē-ˌā-təd-\ *n* : either of the two main trunks of the sympathetic nervous system of which one lies on each side of the spinal column

gan•gli•o•ma \ˌgaŋ-glē-ˈō-mə\ *n, pl* **-mas** *also* **-ma•ta** \-mə-tə\ : a tumor of a ganglion

gan•gli•on \ˈgaŋ-glē-ən\ *n, pl* **-glia** \-glē-ə\ *also* **-gli•ons** **1** : a small cystic tumor (as on the back of the wrist) containing viscid fluid and connected either with a joint membrane or tendon sheath **2 a** : a mass of nerve tissue containing cell bodies of neurons that is located outside the central nervous system and forms an enlargement upon a nerve or upon two or more nerves at their point of junction or separation **b** : a mass of gray matter within the brain or spinal cord : NUCLEUS 2 — see BASAL GANGLION

gan•gli•on•at•ed \-ə-ˌnā-təd\ *adj* : furnished with ganglia

ganglion cell *n* : a nerve cell having its body outside the central nervous system

gan•gli•on•ec•to•my \ˌgaŋ-glē-ə-ˈnek-tə-mē\ *n, pl* **-mies** : surgical removal of a nerve ganglion

gan•glio•neu•ro•ma \-(ˌ)ō-nu̇-ˈrō-mə, -nyu̇-\ *n, pl* **-mas** *also* **-ma•ta** \-mə-tə\ : a neuroma derived from ganglion cells

gan•gli•on•ic \ˌgaŋ-glē-ˈä-nik\ *adj* : of, relating to, or affecting ganglia or ganglion cells

ganglionic blocking agent *n* : a drug used to produce blockade at a ganglion

gan•gli•on•it•is \ˌgaŋ-glē-ə-ˈnī-təs\ *n* : inflammation of a ganglion

gan•gli•o•side \ˈgaŋ-glē-ə-ˌsīd\ *n* : any of a group of glycolipids that are found esp. in the plasma membrane of cells of the gray matter and have sialic acid, hexoses, and hexosamines in the carbohydrate part and ceramide as the lipid

gan•gli•o•si•do•sis \ˌgaŋ-glē-ˌō-sī-ˈdō-səs\ *n, pl* **-do•ses** \-ˌsēz\ : any of several inherited metabolic diseases (as Tay-Sachs disease) characterized by an enzyme deficiency which causes accumulation of gangliosides in the tissues

gan•go•sa \gaŋ-ˈgō-sə\ *n* : a destructive ulcerative condition believed to be a manifestation of yaws that usu. originates about the soft palate and spreads into the hard palate, nasal structures, and outward to the face — compare GOUNDOU

gan•grene \ˈgaŋ-ˌgrēn, gaŋ-ˈ\ *n* : local death of soft tissues due to loss of blood supply — **gangrene** *vb* — **gan•gre•nous** \ˈgaŋ-grə-nəs\ *adj*

gangrenosum — see PYODERMA GANGRENOSUM

gangrenous stomatitis *n* : CANCRUM ORIS

gan•ja \ˈgän-jə, ˈgan-\ *n* : a potent preparation of marijuana used esp. for smoking; *broadly* : MARIJUANA

Gan•ser syndrome \ˈgän-zər-\ *or* **Gan•ser's syndrome** *n* : a pattern of psychopathological behavior characterized by the giving of approximate answers (as 2 × 2 = about 5)

Ganser, Sigbert Joseph Maria (1853–1931), German psychiatrist.

gapes \ˈgāps\ *n* : a disease of birds and esp. young birds in which gapeworms invade and irritate the trachea

gape•worm \ˈgāp-ˌwərm\ *n* : a nematode worm of the genus *Syngamus* (*S. trachea*) that causes gapes of birds

gap junction *n* : an area of contact between adjacent cells characterized by modification of the cell membranes for intercellular communication or transfer of low molecular-weight substances — **gap–junc•tion•al** \ˈgap-ˈjəŋk-shə-nəl\ *adj*

Gar•da•sil \ˈgär-də-ˌsil\ *trademark* — used for a vaccine against some types of human papillomavirus associated esp. with genital warts and cervical cancer

Gard•ner•el•la \ˌgärd-nə-ˈre-lə\ *n* : a genus of bacteria that includes one (*G. vaginalis* syn. *Haemophilus vaginalis*) often present in the flora of the healthy vagina and present in greatly increased numbers in bacterial vaginosis

Gard•ner \ˈgärd-nər\, **Herman L.** (*fl* **1955–80),** American physician.

Gard•ner's syndrome \ˈgärd-nərz-\ *n* : a familial polyposis marked by numerous adenomatous polyps in the colon which typically become malignant if left untreated, by osteomas (as of the skull or mandible), and by skin tumors, that is inherited as an autosomal dominant trait, and that is sometimes considered a variant form of familial adenomatous polyposis

gar•get \ˈgär-gət\ *n* : mastitis of domestic animals; *esp* : chronic bovine mastitis

[1]**gar•gle** \ˈgär-gəl\ *vb* **gar•gled; gar•gling** **1** : to hold (a liquid) in the mouth or throat and agitate with air from the lungs **2** : to cleanse or disinfect (the oral cavity) by gargling

[2]**gargle** *n* : a liquid used in gargling

gar•goyl•ism \ˈgar-ˌgȯi-ˌli-zəm\ *n* : MUCOPOLYSACCHARIDOSIS; *esp* : HURLER SYNDROME

Gart•ner's duct \ˈgart-nərz-, ˈgert-\ *n* : the remains in the female mammal of a part of the Wolffian duct of the embryo — called also *duct of Gartner*

Gart•ner \ˈgert-nər\, **Hermann Treschow (1785–1827),** Danish surgeon and anatomist.

gas \ˈgas\ *n, pl* **gas•es** *also* **gas•ses** **1** : a fluid (as air) that has neither independent shape nor volume but tends to expand indefinitely **2** : a gaseous product of digestion; *also* : discomfort from this **3** : a gas or gaseous mixture used to produce anesthesia **4** : a substance that can be used to produce a poisonous, asphyxiating, or irritant atmosphere

gas•eous \ˈga-sē-əs, ˈga-shəs\ *adj* : having the form of or being gas; *also* : of or relating to gases

gas gangrene *n* : progressive gangrene marked by impregnation of the dead and dying tissue with gas and caused by one or more toxin-producing bacteria of the genus *Clostridium* (esp. *C. perfringens* syn. *C. welchii*)

gash \ˈgash\ *n* : a deep long cut esp. in flesh — **gash** *vb*

gas mask *n* : a mask connected to a chemical air filter and used to protect the face and lungs from toxic gases; *broadly* : RESPIRATOR 1

gas•se•ri•an ganglion \ga-ˈsir-ē-ən-\ *n, often cap 1st G* : TRIGEMINAL GANGLION

Gas•ser \ˈgä-sər\, **Johann Laurentius (1723–1765),** Austrian anatomist.

Gas•ter•oph•i•lus \ˌgas-tə-ˈrä-fə-ləs\ *n* : a genus of botflies including several (esp. *G. intestinalis* in the U.S.) that infest horses and rarely humans

gastr- *or* **gastro-** *also* **gastri-** *comb form* **1** : stomach ⟨*gastr*itis⟩ **2** : gastric and ⟨*gastro*intestinal⟩

gas•tral \ˈgas-trəl\ *adj* : of or relating to the stomach or digestive tract

gas•tral•gia \ga-ˈstral-jə\ *n* : pain in the stomach or epigastrium esp. of a neuralgic type — **gas•tral•gic** \-jik\ *adj*

gas•trec•to•my \ga-ˈstrek-tə-mē\ *n, pl* **-mies** : surgical removal of all or part of the stomach

gas•tric \ˈgas-trik\ *adj* : of or relating to the stomach

gastrica — see ACHYLIA GASTRICA

gastric artery *n* **1** : a branch of the celiac artery that passes to the cardiac end of the stomach and along the lesser curvature — called also *left gastric artery;* see RIGHT GASTRIC ARTERY **2** : any of several branches of the splenic artery distributed to the greater curvature of the stomach

gastric banding *n* : a laparoscopic surgical procedure for the treatment of severe obesity that involves placing an adjustable band around the upper stomach to create a small pouch which empties into the remaining stomach through a narrow outlet

gastric bypass *n* : a surgical bypass operation performed to restrict food intake and reduce absorption of calories and nutrients in the treatment of severe obesity that typically involves reducing the size of the stomach and reconnecting the smaller stomach to bypass the first portion of the small intestine; *esp* : ROUX-EN-Y GASTRIC BYPASS

gastric gland *n* : any of various glands in the walls of the stomach that secrete gastric juice

gastric juice *n* : a thin watery acid digestive fluid secreted by the glands in the mucous membrane of the stomach and containing 0.2 to 0.4 percent free hydrochloric acid and several enzymes (as pepsin)

gastric pit *n* : any of the numerous depressions in the mucous membrane lining the stomach into which the gastric glands discharge their secretions

gastric ulcer *n* : a peptic ulcer situated in the stomach

gas•trin \ˈgas-trən\ *n* : any of various polypeptide hormones that are secreted by the gastric mucosa and induce secretion of gastric juice

gas•tri•no•ma \ˌgas-trə-ˈnō-mə\ *n, pl* **-mas** *also* **-ma•ta** \-mə-tə\ : a tumor that often involves blood vessels, usu. occurs in the pancreas or the wall of the duodenum, and produces excessive amounts of gastrin — see ZOLLINGER-ELLISON SYNDROME

gas•tri•tis \ga-ˈstrī-təs\ *n* : inflammation esp. of the mucous membrane of the stomach

gastro- — see GASTR-

gas•troc•ne•mi•us \ˌgas-(ˌ)träk-ˈnē-mē-əs, -trək-\ *n, pl* **-mii** \-mē-ˌī\ : the largest and most superficial muscle of the calf of the leg that arises by two heads from the condyles of the femur and has its tendon of insertion incorporated as part of the Achilles tendon — called also *gastrocnemius muscle*

gas•tro•co•lic \ˌgas-trō-ˈkä-lik, -ˈkō-\ *adj* : of, relating to, or uniting the stomach and colon ⟨a ~ fistula⟩

gastrocolic reflex *n* : the occurrence of peristalsis following the entrance of food into the empty stomach

Gas•tro•dis•coi•des \ˌgas-trō-dis-ˈkȯi-(ˌ)dēz\ *n* : a genus of amphistome trematode worms including an intestinal parasite (*G. hominis*) of humans and swine in southeastern Asia

gas•tro•du•o•de•nal \ˌgas-trō-ˌdü-ə-ˈdēn-ᵊl, -ˌdyü-; -dü-ˈäd-ᵊn-əl, -dyü-\ *adj* : of, relating to, or involving both the stomach and the duodenum

gastroduodenal artery *n* : an artery that arises from the hepatic artery and divides to form the right gastroepiploic artery and a branch supplying the duodenum and pancreas

gas•tro•du•o•de•nos•to•my \-ˌdü-ə-(ˌ)dē-ˈnäs-tə-mē, -ˌdyü-; -dü-ˌäd-ᵊn-ˈäs-tə-mē, -dyü-\ *n, pl* **-mies** : surgical formation of a passage between the stomach and the duodenum

gas•tro•en•ter•i•tis \-ˌen-tə-ˈrī-təs\ *n, pl* **-en•ter•it•i•des** \-ˈri-tə-ˌdēz\ : inflammation of the lining membrane of the stomach and the intestines

gas•tro•en•ter•ol•o•gist \-ˌen-tə-ˈrä-lə-jist\ *n* : a specialist in gastroenterology

gas•tro•en•ter•ol•o•gy \-ˌen-tə-ˈrä-lə-jē\ *n, pl* **-gies** : a branch of medicine concerned with the structure, functions, diseases, and pathology of the stomach and intestines — **gas-**

tro·en·ter·o·log·i·cal \-rə-ˈlä-ji-kəl\ *also* **gas·tro·en·ter·o·log·ic** \-ˈlä-jik\ *adj*

gas·tro·en·ter·op·a·thy \-en-tə-ˈrä-pə-thē\ *n, pl* **-thies** : a disease of the stomach and intestines

gas·tro·en·ter·os·to·my \-ˈräs-tə-mē\ *n, pl* **-mies** : the surgical formation of a passage between the stomach and small intestine

gas·tro·ep·i·plo·ic artery \-ˌe-pə-ˈplō-ik\ *n* : either of two arteries forming an anastomosis along the greater curvature of the stomach: **a** : one that is larger, arises as one of the two terminal branches of the gastroduodenal artery, and passes from right to left — called also *right gastroepiploic artery* **b** : one that is smaller, arises as a branch of the splenic artery, and passes from left to right — called also *left gastroepiploic artery*

gas·tro·esoph·a·ge·al \ˌgas-trō-i-ˌsä-fə-ˈjē-əl\ *adj* : of, relating to, or involving the stomach and esophagus

gastroesophageal reflux *n* : backward flow of the gastric contents into the esophagus due to improper functioning of a sphincter at the lower end of the esophagus and resulting esp. in heartburn — called also *acid reflux*

gastroesophageal reflux disease *n* : a highly variable chronic condition that is characterized by periodic episodes of gastroesophageal reflux usu. accompanied by heartburn and that may result in histopathologic changes in the esophagus — called also *GERD*

gas·tro·in·tes·ti·nal \-in-ˈtes-tən-ᵊl\ *adj* : of, relating to, or affecting both stomach and intestine

gastrointestinal tract *n* : the stomach and intestine as a functional unit

gas·tro·je·ju·nal \-ji-ˈjün-ᵊl\ *adj* : of, relating to, or involving both stomach and jejunum ⟨~ lesions⟩

gas·tro·je·ju·nos·to·my \-ji-(ˌ)jü-ˈnäs-tə-mē\ *n, pl* **-mies** : the surgical formation of a passage between the stomach and jejunum : GASTROENTEROSTOMY

gas·tro·lith \ˈga-strə-ˌlith\ *n* : a gastric calculus

gas·tro·pa·re·sis \ˌgas-trō-pə-ˈrē-səs\ *n, pl* **-re·ses** \-ˌsēz\ : partial paralysis of the stomach

gas·trop·a·thy \ga-ˈsträ-pə-thē\ *n, pl* **-thies** : a disease of the stomach

gas·tro·pexy \ˈgas-trə-ˌpek-sē\ *n, pl* **-pex·ies** : a surgical operation in which the stomach is sutured to the abdominal wall

gas·tro·pod \ˈgas-trə-ˌpäd\ *n* : any of a large class (Gastropoda) of mollusks (as snails) with a one-piece shell or none and usu. a distinct head bearing sensory organs — **gastropod** *adj*

gas·tros·chi·sis \ga-ˈsträs-kə-səs\ *n, pl* **-chi·ses** \-ˌsēz\ : congenital fissure of the ventral abdominal wall

gas·tro·scope \ˈgas-trə-ˌskōp\ *n* : an endoscope for inspecting the interior of the stomach — **gas·tro·scop·ic** \ˌgas-trə-ˈskä-pik\ *adj* — **gas·tros·co·pist** \ga-ˈsträs-kə-pist\ *n* — **gas·tros·co·py** \-pē\ *n*

gas·tro·splen·ic ligament \ˌgas-trō-ˈsple-nik-\ *n* : a mesenteric fold passing from the greater curvature of the stomach to the spleen

gas·tros·to·my \ga-ˈsträs-tə-mē\ *n, pl* **-mies 1** : the surgical formation of an opening through the abdominal wall into the stomach **2** : the opening made by gastrostomy

gas·trot·o·my \ga-ˈsträ-tə-mē\ *n, pl* **-mies** : surgical incision into the stomach

gas·tru·la \ˈgas-trə-lə\ *n, pl* **-las** *or* **-lae** \-ˌlē, -ˌlī\ : an early embryo that develops from the blastula and in mammals is formed by the differentiation of the upper layer of the blastodisc into the ectoderm and the lower layer into the endoderm and by the inward migration of cells through the primitive streak to form the mesoderm — compare BLASTULA, MORULA — **gas·tru·lar** \-lər\ *adj*

gas·tru·la·tion \ˌgas-trə-ˈlā-shən\ *n* : the process of becoming or of forming a gastrula — **gas·tru·late** \ˈgas-trə-ˌlāt\ *vb*

gatch bed \ˈgach-\ *n, often cap* : a hospital bed with a frame in three movable sections equipped with mechanical spring parts that permit raising the head end, foot end, or middle as required; *broadly* : HOSPITAL BED

Gatch, Willis Dew (1878–1954), American surgeon.

gate·keep·er \ˈgāt-ˌkē-pər\ *n* : a health-care professional (as a primary care physician) who regulates access esp. to hospitals and specialists

gate·way drug \ˈgāt-ˌwā-\ *n* : a drug (as marijuana) whose use is thought to lead to the use of and dependence on more dangerous addicting substances (as heroin)

gath·er \ˈga-t͟hər\ *vb* **gath·ered; gath·er·ing** : to swell and fill with pus

gathering *n* : a suppurating swelling : ABSCESS

Gau·cher disease \ˌgō-ˈshā-\ *or* **Gau·cher's disease** \-ˈshāz-\ *n* : a rare hereditary disorder of lipid metabolism that is caused by an enzyme deficiency of glucocerebrosidase, is marked by extreme enlargement of the spleen, pigmentation of the skin, bone lesions, and the accumulation of glucocerebroside in cells, and is inherited as an autosomal recessive trait

Gaucher, Philippe Charles Ernest (1854–1918), French physician.

gaul·the·ria oil \gȯl-ˈthir-ē-ə-\ *n* : OIL OF WINTERGREEN

Gaultier \gō-ˈtyā\, **Jean François (1708–1756),** Canadian physician and botanist.

gauze \ˈgȯz\ *n* : a loosely woven cotton surgical dressing

ga•vage \gə-ˈväzh, gä-\ *n* : introduction of material into the stomach by a tube
gave *past of* GIVE
GB \ˌjē-ˈbē\ *n* : SARIN
GB *abbr* gallbladder
GBS *abbr* **1** Group B streptococcal; Group B streptococcus **2** Guillain-Barré syndrome
GC *abbr* gonococcus
G–CSF *abbr* granulocyte colony-stimulating factor
Gd *symbol* gadolinium
Ge *symbol* germanium
GE *abbr* gastroenterology
Gei•ger counter \ˈgī-gər-\ *n* : an instrument for detecting the presence and intensity of radiations (as particles from a radioactive substance) by means of the ionizing effect on an enclosed gas which results in a pulse that is amplified and fed to a device giving a visible or audible indication
Geiger, Hans (Johannes) Wilhelm (1882–1945), and **Müller** \ˈmue-ler\, **Walther (*fl* 1928),** German physicists.
Geiger–Mül•ler counter \-ˈmyü-lər-\ *n* : GEIGER COUNTER
[1]**gel** \ˈjel\ *n* : a colloid in a more solid form than a sol
[2]**gel** *vb* **gelled; gel•ling** : to change into or take on the form of a gel — **gel•able** \ˈje-lə-bəl\ *adj*
gel•ate \ˈje-ˌlāt\ *vb* **gel•at•ed; gel•at•ing** : GEL
gel•a•tin *also* **gel•a•tine** \ˈje-lə-tən\ *n* **1** : glutinous material obtained from animal tissues by boiling; *esp* : a colloidal protein used as a food and in medicine **2 a** : any of various substances (as agar) resembling gelatin **b** : an edible jelly made with gelatin — **ge•lat•i•nous** \jə-ˈlat-ᵊn-əs\ *adj*
gelatinosa — see SUBSTANTIA GELATINOSA
gel•ation \je-ˈlā-shən\ *n* : the formation of a gel from a sol
gel•cap \ˈjel-ˌkap\ *n* : a capsule-shaped tablet coated with gelatin for easy swallowing
geld \ˈgeld\ *vb* : CASTRATE 1a
geld•ing \ˈgel-diŋ\ *n* : a castrated animal; *specif* : a castrated male horse
gel electrophoresis *n* : electrophoresis in which molecules (as proteins and nucleic acids) migrate through a gel and esp. a polyacrylamide gel and separate into bands according to size
ge•mel•lus \jə-ˈme-ləs\ *n, pl* **ge•mel•li** \-ˌlī\ *also* **ge•mel•lus•es** : either of two small muscles of the hip that insert into the tendon of the obturator internus: **a** : a superior one originating chiefly from the outer surface of the ischial spine — called also *gemellus superior* **b** : an inferior one originating chiefly from the ischial tuberosity — called also *gemellus inferior*
gem•fi•bro•zil \jem-ˈfī-brə-(ˌ)zil, -ˈfi-\ *n* : a drug $C_{15}H_{22}O_3$ that regulates blood serum lipids and is used esp. to lower the levels of triglycerides and increase the levels of HDLs in the treatment of hyperlipidemia — see LOPID
gem•i•na•tion \ˌje-mə-ˈnā-shən\ *n* : a doubling, duplication, or repetition; *esp* : a formation of two teeth from a single tooth germ
gen- *or* **geno-** *comb form* : gene ⟨*ge*nome⟩
-gen \jən, ˌjen\ *also* **-gene** \ˌjēn\ *n comb form* **1** : producer ⟨carcino*gen*⟩ **2** : one that is (so) produced ⟨phos*gene*⟩
gen•der \ˈjen-dər\ *n* **1** : SEX 1 **2** : the behavioral, cultural, or psychological traits typically associated with one sex
gender dysphoria *n* : a distressed state in which a person persistently identifies with the gender that is opposite to their biological sex and is typically manifested by a strong desire to hide or rid oneself of physical attributes of the current gender and to live and be treated as a member of the opposite gender — called also *gender identity disorder*
gender identity *n* **1** : the totality of physical and behavioral traits that are designated by a culture as masculine or feminine **2** : a person's internal sense of being male, female, some combination of male and female, or neither male nor female
gender identity disorder *n* : GENDER DYSPHORIA
gene \ˈjēn\ *n* : a specific sequence of nucleotides in DNA or RNA that is located usu. on a chromosome and that is the functional unit of inheritance controlling the transmission and expression of one or more traits by specifying the structure of a particular polypeptide and esp. a protein or controlling the function of other genetic material — called also *determinant, determiner, factor*
gene complex *n* : a group of genes of an individual or of a potentially interbreeding group that constitute an interacting functional unit
gene flow *n* : the passage and establishment of genes typical of one breeding population into the gene pool of another
gene frequency *n* : the ratio of the number of a specified allele in a population to the total of all alleles at its genetic locus
gene mutation *n* : mutation due to fundamental intramolecular reorganization of a gene — see POINT MUTATION
gene pool *n* : the collection of genes of all the individuals in an interbreeding population
genera *pl of* GENUS
gen•er•al \ˈje-nə-rəl, ˈjen-rəl\ *adj* **1** : not confined by specialization or careful limitation ⟨a ~ surgeon⟩ **2** : involving or affecting practically the entire body or organism : not local

general anesthesia *n* : anesthesia affecting the entire body and accompanied by loss of consciousness

general anesthetic *n* : an anesthetic used to produce general anesthesia

general hospital *n* : a hospital in which patients with many different types of ailments are given care

gen•er•al•ist \ˈjen-rə-list, ˈje-nə-rə-\ *n* : one whose skills or interests extend to several different medical fields; *esp* : GENERAL PRACTITIONER

generalista — see OSTEITIS FIBROSA CYSTICA GENERALISTA

gen•er•al•iza•tion \ˌjen-rə-lə-ˈzā-shən, ˌje-nə-rə-\ *n* **1** : the action or process of becoming widespread or diffuse **2** : the process whereby a response is made to a stimulus similar to but not identical with the conditioned stimulus

gen•er•al•ize \ˈjen-rə-ˌlīz, ˈje-nə-rə-\ *vb* **-ized; -iz•ing** : to spread or extend through all of a body part or region or through most of the entire body

generalized anxiety disorder *n* : an anxiety disorder marked by chronic excessive anxiety and worry that is difficult to control, causes distress or impairment in daily functioning, and is accompanied by three or more associated symptoms (as restlessness, irritability, poor concentration, and sleep disturbances) — abbr. *GAD*

generalized seizure *n* : a seizure (as an absence seizure or tonic-clonic seizure) that originates in both cerebral hemispheres — compare PARTIAL SEIZURE

general paresis *n* : neurosyphilis that is characterized by memory loss, muscle weakness, progressive dementia, seizures, and paralysis — called also *dementia paralytica*

general practitioner *n* : a physician or veterinarian whose practice is not limited to a specialty

gen•er•a•tion \ˌje-nə-ˈrā-shən\ *n* **1** : a body of living beings constituting a single step in the line of descent from an ancestor **2** : the average span of time between the birth of parents and that of their offspring **3** : the action or process of producing offspring : PROCREATION

gen•er•a•tive \ˈje-nə-rə-tiv, -ˌrā-\ *adj* : having the power or function of propagating or reproducing

gen•er•a•tiv•i•ty \ˌje-nə-rə-ˈti-və-tē\ *n, pl* **-ties** : a concern for people besides self and family that usu. develops during middle age; *esp* : a need to nurture and guide younger people and contribute to the next generation — used in the psychology of Erik Erikson

[1]**ge•ner•ic** \jə-ˈner-ik\ *adj* **1** : not protected by trademark registration : NONPROPRIETARY **2** : relating to or having the rank of a biological genus — **ge•ner•i•cal•ly** \-i-k(ə-)lē\ *adv*

[2]**generic** *n* : a generic drug — usu. used in pl.

gene–splic•ing \ˈjēn-ˈsplī-siŋ\ *n* : the process of preparing recombinant DNA

gene therapy *n* : the insertion of usu. genetically altered genes into cells esp. to replace defective genes in the treatment of genetic disorders or to provide a specialized disease-fighting function (as destruction of tumor cells)

ge•net•ic \jə-ˈne-tik\ *also* **ge•net•i•cal** \-ti-kəl\ *adj* **1** : of, relating to, or involving genetics **2** : of, relating to, caused by, or controlled by genes ⟨a ~ disease⟩ — compare ACQUIRED 1 — **ge•net•i•cal•ly** \-ti-k(ə-)lē\ *adv*

-ge•net•ic \jə-ˈne-tik\ *adj comb form* : -GENIC ⟨osteo*genetic*⟩

genetic code *n* : the biochemical basis of heredity consisting of codons in DNA and RNA that determine the specific amino acid sequence in proteins and that appear to be uniform for all known forms of life — **genetic coding** *n*

genetic counseling *n* : guidance provided by a medical professional typically to individuals with an increased risk of having a child with a specific genetic disorder and that includes providing information concerning the probability of having a child with the disorder, prenatal diagnostic tests, and available treatment

genetic drift *n* : random changes in gene frequency esp. in small populations when leading to preservation or extinction of particular genes

genetic engineering *n* : the group of applied techniques of genetics and biotechnology used to cut up and join together genetic material and esp. DNA from one or more species of organism and to introduce the result into an organism in order to change one or more of its characteristics — **genetically engineered** *adj* — **genetic engineer** *n*

genetic fingerprint *n* : DNA FINGERPRINT

genetic fingerprinting *n* : DNA FINGERPRINTING

genetic imprinting *n* : GENOMIC IMPRINTING

genetic load *n* : the decrease in fitness of the average individual in a population due to the presence of deleterious genes or genotypes in the gene pool

genetic map *n* : MAP

genetic marker *n* : a readily recognizable genetic trait, gene, DNA segment, or gene product used for identification purposes esp. when closely linked to a trait or to genetic material that is difficult to identify

ge•net•ics \jə-ˈne-tiks\ *n* **1 a** : a branch of biology that deals with the heredity and variation of organisms **b** : a treatise or textbook on genetics **2** : the genetic makeup and phenomena of an organism, type, group, or condition — **ge•net•i•cist** \jə-ˈne-tə-sist\ *n*

ge•ni•al \ji-ˈnī-əl\ *adj* : of or relating to the chin

genial tubercle *n* : MENTAL TUBERCLE

gen•ic \ˈjē-nik, ˈje-\ *adj* : GENETIC 2 — **gen•i•cal•ly** \-nik(ə-)lē\ *adv*

-gen•ic \ˈje-nik, ˈjē-\ *adj comb form* **1** : producing : forming ⟨carcino*genic*⟩ **2** : produced by : formed from ⟨nephro*genic*⟩

ge•nic•u•lar artery \jə-ˈni-kyə-lər-\ *n* : any of several branches of the femoral and popliteal arteries that supply the region of the knee — called also *genicular*

ge•nic•u•late \-lət, -ˌlāt\ *adj* **1** : bent abruptly at an angle like a bent knee **2** : relating to, comprising, or belonging to a geniculate body or geniculate ganglion ⟨∼ cells⟩ ⟨∼ neurons⟩

geniculate body *n* : either of two prominences of the diencephalon that comprise the metathalamus: **a** : LATERAL GENICULATE BODY **b** : MEDIAL GENICULATE BODY

geniculate ganglion *n* : a small reddish ganglion consisting of sensory and sympathetic nerve cells located at the sharp backward bend of the facial nerve

ge•nic•u•lo•cal•ca•rine \jə-ˌni-kyə-(ˌ)lō-ˈkal-kə-ˌrīn\ *adj* : relating to or comprising the optic radiation from the lateral geniculate body and the pulvinar to the occipital lobe

genio- *comb form* : chin and ⟨*genio*glossus⟩

ge•nio•glos•sus \ˌjē-nē-ō-ˈglä-səs, -ˈglȯ-\ *n, pl* **-glos•si** \-ˌsī\ : a fan-shaped muscle that arises from the superior mental spine, inserts on the hyoid bone and into the tongue, and serves to advance and retract and also to depress the tongue

ge•nio•hyo•glos•sus \-ˌhī-ō-ˈglä-səs, -ˈglȯ-\ *n, pl* **-glos•si** \-ˌsī\ : GENIOGLOSSUS

ge•nio•hy•oid \-ˈhī-ˌȯid\ *adj* : of or relating to the chin and hyoid bone

ge•nio•hy•oid•eus \-ˌhī-ˈȯi-dē-əs\ *n, pl* **-oid•ei** \-dē-ˌī\ : GENIOHYOID MUSCLE

geniohyoid muscle *n* : a slender muscle that arises from the inferior mental spine, is inserted on the hyoid bone, and acts to raise the hyoid bone and draw it forward and to retract and depress the lower jaw — called also *geniohyoid*

ge•nis•tein \jə-ˈni-stē-ən\ *n* : an isoflavone $C_{15}H_{10}O_5$ found esp. in soybeans and shown in laboratory experiments to have antitumor activity

gen•i•tal \ˈje-nə-tᵊl\ *adj* **1** : GENERATIVE **2** : of, relating to, or being a sexual organ **3** : of, relating to, or characterized by the stage of psychosexual development in psychoanalytic theory during which oral and anal impulses are subordinated to adaptive interpersonal mechanisms — compare ANAL 2, ORAL 2, PHALLIC 2 — **gen•i•tal•ly** *adv*

genital herpes *n* : herpes simplex of the type affecting the genitals — called also *herpes genitalis, genital herpes simplex*

gen•i•ta•lia \ˌje-nə-ˈtāl-yə\ *n, pl* : the organs of the reproductive system; *esp* : the external genital organs

genitalis — see HERPES GENITALIS

gen•i•tal•i•ty \-ˈta-lə-tē\ *n, pl* **-ties** : possession of full genital sensitivity and capacity to develop orgasmic potency in relation to a sexual partner of the opposite sex

genital ridge *n* : a ridge of embryonic mesoblast developing from the mesonephros and giving rise to the gonad on either side of the body

gen•i•tals \ˈje-nə-tᵊlz\ *n pl* : GENITALIA

genital tubercle *n* : a conical protuberance on the belly wall of an embryo that develops into the penis in the male and the clitoris in the female

genital wart *n* : a wart on the skin or adjoining mucous membrane usu. near the anus and genital organs — called also *condyloma, condyloma acuminatum, venereal wart*

genito- *comb form* : genital and ⟨*genito*urinary⟩

gen•i•to•cru•ral nerve \ˌjə-nə-(ˌ)tō-ˈkru̇r-əl-\ *n* : GENITOFEMORAL NERVE

gen•i•to•fem•o•ral nerve \-ˈfe-mə-rəl-\ *n* : a nerve that arises from the first and second lumbar nerves and is distributed by way of branches to the skin of the scrotum or labia majora and to the upper anterior aspect of the thigh

gen•i•to•uri•nary \-ˈyu̇r-ə-ˌner-ē\ *adj* : of, relating to, affecting, or being the organs of reproduction and urination : UROGENITAL

genitourinary system *n* : GENITOURINARY TRACT

genitourinary tract *n* : the system of organs comprising those concerned with the production and excretion of urine and those concerned with reproduction — called also *genitourinary system, urogenital system, urogenital tract*

geno — see GEN-

ge•no•gram \ˈjē-nə-ˌgram, ˈje-\ *n* : a diagram outlining the behavioral or medical history of a family's members over several generations

ge•nome \ˈjē-ˌnōm\ *n* : one haploid set of chromosomes with the genes they contain; *broadly* : the genetic material of an organism

ge•nom•ic \ji-ˈnō-mik, -ˈnä-\ *adj* : of or relating to a genome or genomics

genomic imprinting *n* : genetic alteration of a gene or its expression that is inferred to take place from the observation that certain genes are expressed differently depending on whether they are inherited from the paternal or maternal parent — called also *genetic imprinting, imprinting*

ge•no•mics \jē-ˈnō-miks\ *n* : a branch of biotechnology concerned with the genetic mapping and DNA sequencing of sets of genes or the complete genomes of selected organisms using high-speed methods, with organizing the results in databases, and with applications of the data (as in medicine) — compare PROTEOMICS

ge•no•tox•ic \ˌjē-nə-ˈtäk-sik\ *adj* : damaging to genetic material — **ge•no•tox•ic•i•ty** \-täk-ˈsi-sə-tē\ *n*

[1]**ge•no•type** \ˈjē-nə-ˌtīp, ˈje-\ *n* : all or part of the genetic constitution of an individual or group — compare PHENOTYPE — **ge•no•typ•ic** \ˌjē-nə-ˈti-pik, ˌje-\ *also* **ge•no•typ•i•cal** \-pi-kəl\ *adj* — **ge•no•typ•i•cal•ly** \-pi-k(ə-)lē\ *adv*

[2]**genotype** *vb* **-typed; -typ•ing** : to determine the genotype of

-g•e•nous \jə-nəs\ *adj comb form* **1** : producing : yielding ⟨ero*genous*⟩ **2** : produced by : arising or originating in ⟨neuro*genous*⟩ ⟨endo*genous*⟩

gen•ta•mi•cin \ˌjen-tə-ˈmīs-ᵊn\ *n* : a broad-spectrum antibiotic mixture that is derived from an actinomycete of the genus *Micromonospora* (*M. purpurea* and *M. echinospora*) and is extensively used in the form of its sulfate in treating infections esp. of the urinary tract

gen•tian violet \ˈjen-chən-\ *n, often cap G&V* : a greenish mixture that contains not less than 96 percent of a pararosaniline derivative and is used esp. as a bactericide, fungicide, and anthelmintic

gen•tis•ic acid \jen-ˈti-sik-, -zik\ *n* : a crystalline acid $C_7H_6O_4$ used medicinally as an analgesic and diaphoretic

ge•nu \ˈjē-ˌnü, ˈjen-yü\ *n, pl* **gen•ua** \ˈjen-yə-wə\ : an abrupt flexure; *esp* : the bend in the anterior part of the corpus callosum — see GENU VALGUM, GENU VARUM

ge•nus \ˈjē-nəs, ˈje-\ *n, pl* **gen•era** \ˈje-nə-rə\ : a category of biological classification ranking between the family and the species, comprising structurally or phylogenetically related species or an isolated species exhibiting unusual differentiation, and being designated by a capitalized singular noun that is Latin or has a Latin form

genu val•gum \-ˈval-gəm\ *n* : KNOCK-KNEE

genu va•rum \-ˈvar-əm\ *n* : BOWLEG

-g•e•ny \jə-nē\ *n comb form, pl* **-g•e•nies** : generation : production ⟨embryo*geny*⟩ ⟨lyso*geny*⟩

geo•med•i•cine \ˌjē-ō-ˈme-də-sən\ *n* : a branch of medicine that deals with geographic factors in disease

ge•o•pha•gia \-ˈfā-jē-ə-, -jə\ *n* : GEOPHAGY

ge•oph•a•gy \jē-ˈä-fə-jē\ *n, pl* **-gies** : the practice of eating earthy substances (as clay) that in humans is performed esp. to augment a scanty or mineral-deficient diet or as part of a cultural tradition — compare PICA

ge•ot•ri•cho•sis \jē-ˌä-trə-ˈkō-səs\ *n* : infection of the bronchi or lungs and sometimes the mouth and intestines by a fungus of the genus *Geotrichum* (*G. candidum*)

Ge•ot•ri•chum \jē-ˈä-tri-kəm\ *n* : a genus of fungi (family Moniliaceae) including one (*G. candidum*) that causes human geotrichosis

GERD \ˈgərd\ *n* : GASTROESOPHAGEAL REFLUX DISEASE

ge•ri•at•ric \ˌjer-ē-ˈa-trik, ˌjir-\ *n* **1 ge•ri•at•rics** \-triks\ *pl* : a branch of medicine that deals with the problems and diseases of old age and aging people — compare GERONTOLOGY **2** : an aged person — **geriatric** *adj*

ger•i•a•tri•cian \ˌjer-ē-ə-ˈtri-shən, ˌjir-\ *n* : a specialist in geriatrics

ge•ri•a•trist \ˌjer-ē-ˈa-trist, ˌjir-; jə-ˈrī-ə-\ *n* : GERIATRICIAN

germ \ˈjərm\ *n* **1** : a small mass of living substance capable of developing into an organism or one of its parts **2** : MICROORGANISM; *esp* : a microorganism causing disease

Ger•man cockroach \ˈjər-mən-\ *n* : a small active winged cockroach (*Blatella germanica*) that is prob. of African origin and is a common household pest in the U.S. — called also *Croton bug*

ger•ma•nin \jər-ˈmā-nən\ *n* : SURAMIN

ger•ma•ni•um \(ˌ)jər-ˈmā-nē-əm\ *n* : a grayish-white hard brittle element — symbol *Ge;* see ELEMENT table

German measles *n sing or pl* : an acute contagious virus disease that is milder than typical measles but is damaging to the fetus when occurring early in pregnancy and that is caused by a togavirus (species *Rubella virus* of the genus *Rubivirus*) — called also *rubella*

germ cell *n* : an egg or sperm cell or one of their antecedent cells

germ•free \ˈjərm-ˌfrē\ *adj* : free of microorganisms : AXENIC

ger•mi•cid•al \ˌjər-mə-ˈsīd-ᵊl\ *adj* : of or relating to a germicide; *also* : destroying germs

ger•mi•cide \ˈjər-mə-ˌsīd\ *n* : an agent that destroys germs

ger•mi•nal \ˈjər-mə-nəl\ *adj* : of, relating to, or having the characteristics of a germ cell or early embryo

germinal cell *n* : an embryonic cell of the early vertebrate nervous system that is the source of neuroblasts and glial cells

germinal center *n* : the lightly staining central proliferative area of a lymphoid follicle

germinal disk *n* **1** : BLASTODISC **2** : the part of the blastoderm that forms the embryo proper of an amniote vertebrate

germinal epithelium *n* : the epithelial covering of the genital ridges and of the gonads derived from them

germinal vesicle *n* : the enlarged nucleus of the egg before completion of meiosis

ger·mi·na·tive layer \ˈjər-mə-ˌnā-tiv-, -nə-\ *n* : the innermost layer of the epidermis from which new tissue is constantly formed

germinativum — see STRATUM GERMINATIVUM

ger·mi·no·ma \ˌjər-mə-ˈnō-mə\ *n, pl* **-mas** : a malignant tumor (as of the testis or pineal gland) originating from undifferentiated embryonic germ cells — see DYSGERMINOMA, SEMINOMA

germ layer *n* : any of the three primary layers of cells differentiated in most embryos during and immediately following gastrulation

germ line *n* : the cellular lineage from which eggs and sperm are derived and in which a cell undergoing mutation can be passed to the next generation

germ·plasm *n* **1** : germ cells and their precursors serving as the bearers of heredity and being fundamentally independent of other cells **2** : the hereditary material of the germ cells : GENES

germ·proof \ˈjərm-ˌprüf\ *adj* : impervious to the penetration or action of germs

germ theory *n* : a theory in medicine: infections, contagious diseases, and various other conditions result from the action of microorganisms

geront- *or* **geronto-** *comb form* : aged one : old age ⟨*geronto*logy⟩

ger·on·tol·o·gist \ˌjer-ən-ˈtä-lə-jist\ *n* : a specialist in gerontology

ger·on·tol·o·gy \-jē\ *n, pl* **-gies** : the comprehensive study of aging and the problems of the aged — compare GERIATRIC 1 — **ge·ron·to·log·i·cal** \jə-ˌränt-ᵊl-ˈä-ji-kəl\ *also* **ge·ron·to·log·ic** \-jik\ *adj*

Gerst·mann's syndrome \ˈgerst-mänz-, ˈgərst-mənz-\ *n* : cerebral dysfunction characterized esp. by finger agnosia, disorientation with respect to right and left, agraphia, and acalculia and caused by a lesion in the dominant cerebral hemisphere

Gerstmann, Josef (1887–1969), Austrian neurologist and psychiatrist.

Gerst·mann–Sträus·sler–Schein·ker syndrome \ˈgerst-män-ˈshtrȯis-lər-ˈshīŋ-kər-\ *n* : any of several rare fatal prion diseases that are inherited as autosomal dominant traits and are marked by progressive cognitive and motor impairment and by the accumulation of amyloid plaques in the brain — called also *Gerstmann-Sträussler-Scheinker disease, Gerstmann-Sträussler syndrome*

Sträussler, Ernst (1872–1959), and **Scheinker, I.,** Austrian physicians.

ge·stalt \gə-ˈstält, -ˈshtält, -ˈstȯlt, -ˈshtȯlt\ *n, pl* **ge·stalt·en** \-ᵊn\ *or* **gestalts** : a structure, arrangement, or pattern of physical, biological, or psychological phenomena so integrated as to constitute a functional unit with properties not derivable by summation of its parts

ge·stalt·ist \gə-ˈstäl-tist, -ˈshtäl-, -ˈstȯl-, -ˈshtȯl-\ *n, often cap* : a specialist in Gestalt psychology

Gestalt psychology *n* : the study of perception and behavior from the standpoint of an individual's response to gestalten with stress on the uniformity of psychological and physiological events and rejection of analysis into discrete events of stimulus, percept, and response — **Gestalt psychologist** *n*

Gestalt therapy *n* : psychotherapy that focuses on gaining self-awareness of emotions, perceptions, and behaviors in the immediate present

ges·ta·tion \je-ˈstā-shən\ *n* **1** : the carrying of young in the uterus from conception to delivery : PREGNANCY **2** : GESTATION PERIOD — **ges·tate** \ˈjes-ˌtāt\ *vb* — **ges·ta·tion·al** \-shə-nəl\ *adj*

gestation period *n* : the length of time during which gestation takes place — called also *gestation*

ges·to·sis \je-ˈstō-səs\ *n, pl* **-to·ses** \-ˌsēz\ : any disorder of pregnancy; *esp* : TOXEMIA OF PREGNANCY

-geu·sia \ˈgü-zē-ə, ˈjü-, -sē-ə, -zhə\ *n comb form* : a (specified) condition of the sense of taste ⟨dys*geusia*⟩

GG *abbr* gamma globulin

GH *abbr* growth hormone

GHB \ˌjē-ˌāch-ˈbē\ *n* : a fatty acid $C_4H_8O_3$ structurally similar to gamma-aminobutyric acid that is a depressant of the central nervous system, is used medically in the form of its sodium salt $C_4H_7NaO_3$ esp. to treat narcolepsy, is used illicitly in the form of one of several salts to produce sedative and euphoric effects, and is sometimes abused by athletes and body builders to stimulate the release of growth hormone although it has not been shown to increase muscle mass — called also *gamma hydroxybutyrate;* see DATE RAPE DRUG

ghost \ˈgōst\ *n* : a structure (as a cell or tissue) that does not stain normally because of degenerative changes; *specif* : a red blood cell that has lost its hemoglobin

ghrel·in \ˈgre-lən\ *n* : a peptide hormone that is secreted primarily by stomach cells and acts to stimulate the appetite and the secretion of growth hormone

GHRH *abbr* growth hormone-releasing hormone

GI *abbr* **1** gastrointestinal **2** glycemic index

giant cell *n* : a large multinucleate often phagocytic cell (as those characteristic of various sarcomas)

giant cell arteritis *n* : arterial inflammation that often involves the temporal arteries and may lead to blindness when the ophthalmic artery and its branches are affected, is characterized by the formation of giant cells, and may be accompanied by fever, malaise, fatigue, anorexia, weight loss, and arthralgia — called also *temporal arteritis*

giant–cell tumor *n* : an osteolytic tumor affecting the metaphyses and epiphyses of long bones that is usu. benign but sometimes malignant — called also *osteoclastoma*

gi•ant•ism \ˈjī-ən-ˌti-zəm\ *n* : GIGANTISM

giant kidney worm *n* : a blood-red nematode worm of the genus *Dioctophyme* (*D. renale*) that sometimes exceeds a yard in length and invades mammalian kidneys esp. of the dog and occas. of humans

giant lymph node hyperplasia *n* : CASTLEMAN'S DISEASE

giant urticaria *n* : ANGIOEDEMA

giant water bug *n* : any of a family (Belostomatidae and esp. genus *Lethocerus*) of very large bugs capable of inflicting a painful bite

giar•dia \jē-ˈär-dē-ə, ˈjär-\ *n* **1** *cap* : a genus of flagellate protozoans inhabiting the intestines of various mammals and including one (*G. lamblia* syn. *G. intestinalis*) that is associated with diarrhea in humans **2** : any flagellate of the genus *Giardia*

Giard \zhē-ˈär\, **Alfred Mathieu (1846–1908)**, French biologist.

giar•di•a•sis \(ˌ)jē-ˌär-ˈdī-ə-səs, ˌjē-ər-, (ˌ)jär-\ *n, pl* **-a•ses** \-ˌsēz\ : infestation with or disease caused by a flagellate protozoan of the genus *Giardia* (esp. *G. lamblia*) that is often characterized by diarrhea — called also *lambliasis*

gid \ˈgid\ *n* : a disease esp. of sheep that is caused by the presence in the brain of the coenurus of a tapeworm of the genus *Taenia* (*T. multiceps*) — called also *sturdy*

Gi•em•sa stain \gē-ˈem-zə-\ *also* **Giemsa's stain** *n* : a stain consisting of a mixture of eosin and a blue dye and used chiefly in differential staining of blood films — called also *Giemsa*

Giemsa, Gustav (1867–1948), German chemist and pharmacist.

GIFT *abbr* gamete intrafallopian transfer; gamete intrafallopian tube transfer

gi•gan•tism \jī-ˈgan-ˌti-zəm, jə-; ˈjī-gən-\ *n* : development to abnormally large size from excessive growth of the long bones accompanied by muscular weakness and sexual impotence and usu. caused by hyperpituitarism before normal ossification is complete — called also *macrosomia;* compare ACROMEGALY

Gi•la monster \ˈhē-lə-\ *n* : a large orange and black venomous lizard of the genus *Heloderma* (*H. suspectum*) of the southwestern U.S.

Gil•bert's syndrome \zhil-ˈberz-\ *n* : an inherited metabolic disorder that is characterized by elevated levels of serum bilirubin caused esp. by defective uptake of bilirubin by the liver — called also *Gilbert's disease*

Gilbert, Augustin–Nicholas (1858–1927), French physician.

Gil•christ's disease \ˈgil-ˌkrists-\ *n* : NORTH AMERICAN BLASTOMYCOSIS

Gilchrist, Thomas Caspar (1862–1927), American dermatologist.

Gi•len•ya \ji-ˈlen-ē-ə\ *trademark* — used for a preparation of fingolimod

[1]**gill** \ˈjil\ *n* : either of two units of capacity: **a** : a British unit equal to ¼ imperial pint or 8.669 cubic inches **b** : a U.S. liquid unit equal to ¼ U.S. liquid pint or 7.218 cubic inches

[2]**gill** \ˈgil\ *n* **1** : an organ (as of a fish) for obtaining oxygen from water **2** : one of the radiating plates forming the undersurface of the cap of a mushroom — **gilled** \ˈgild\ *adj*

gill arch *n* : one of the bony or cartilaginous arches placed one behind the other on each side of the pharynx and supporting the gills of fishes and amphibians; *also* : BRANCHIAL ARCH

gill cleft *n* : GILL SLIT

Gilles de la Tou•rette syndrome \ˈzhēl-də-lä-tü-ˈret-\ *also* **Gilles de la Tourette's syndrome** *n* : TOURETTE'S SYNDROME

gill slit *n* : one of the openings or clefts between the gill arches in vertebrates that breathe by gills through which water taken in at the mouth passes to the exterior and bathes the gills; *also* : BRANCHIAL CLEFT

gin•ger \ˈjin-jər\ *n* : the aromatic rhizome of a tropical herb (*Zingiber officinale*) of the family Zingiberaceae, the ginger family) that is used as a spice and sometimes medicinally (as to relieve nausea); *also* : the plant

gingiv- *or* **gingivo-** *comb form* **1** : gum : gums ⟨*gingiv*itis⟩ **2** : gums and ⟨*gingivo*stomatitis⟩

gin•gi•va \ˈjin-jə-və, jin-ˈjī-\ *n, pl* **-vae** \-ˌvē, -ˌvī\ : GUM — **gin•gi•val** \ˈjin-jə-vəl\ *adj*

gingival crevice *n* : a narrow space between the free margin of the gingival epithelium and the adjacent enamel of a tooth — called also *gingival trough*

gingival papilla *n* : INTERDENTAL PAPILLA

gingival trough *n* : GINGIVAL CREVICE

gin•gi•vec•to•my \ˌjin-jə-ˈvek-tə-mē\ *n, pl* **-mies** : the excision of a portion of the gingiva

gin•gi•vi•tis \ˌjin-jə-ˈvī-təs\ *n* : inflammation of the gums that is often accompanied by tenderness or bleeding

gin•gi•vo•plas•ty \ˈjin-jə-və-ˌplas-tē\ *n, pl* **-ties** : a surgical procedure that involves reshaping the gums for aesthetic or functional purposes

gin•gi•vo•sto•ma•ti•tis \ˌjin-jə-vō-ˌstō-mə-ˈtī-təs\ *n, pl* **-tit•i•des** \-ˈti-tə-ˌdēz\ *or* **-ti•tis•es** : inflammation of the gums and of the mouth

gin•gly•mus \ˈjiŋ-glə-məs, ˈgiŋ-\ *n, pl* **gin•gly•mi** \-ˌmī, -ˌmē\ : a joint (as between the humerus and ulna) allowing motion in one plane only

gin·seng \ˈjin-ˌseŋ, -ˌsiŋ\ *n* : the aromatic root of a Chinese perennial herb (*Panax ginseng* syn. *P. schinseng* of the family Araliaceae, the ginseng family) used in herbal medicine esp. in eastern Asia; *also* : the plant

gir·dle \ˈgərd-ᵊl\ *n* **1** : SHOULDER GIRDLE **2** : PELVIC GIRDLE

GI series \ˌjē-ˈī-\ *n* : GASTROINTESTINAL SERIES

gi·tal·in \ˈji-tə-lən; jə-ˈtā-lən, -ˈta-\ *n* **1** : a crystalline glycoside $C_{35}H_{56}O_{12}$ obtained from digitalis **2** : a water-soluble mixture of glycosides of digitalis used similarly to digitalis

gi·tox·in \jə-ˈtäk-sən\ *n* : a poisonous crystalline steroid glycoside $C_{41}H_{64}O_{14}$ that is obtained from digitalis and from lanatoside B by hydrolysis

give \ˈgiv\ *vb* **gave** \ˈgāv\; **giv·en** \ˈgi-vən\; **giv·ing** **1** : to administer as a medicine **2** : to cause a person to catch by contagion, infection, or exposure — **give birth** : to have a baby ⟨*gave birth* last Tuesday⟩ — **give birth to** : to produce as offspring ⟨*gave birth to* a daughter⟩

gla·bel·la \glə-ˈbe-lə\ *n, pl* **-bel·lae** \-ˈbe-(ˌ)lē, -ˌlī\ : the smooth prominence between the eyebrows — **gla·bel·lar** \-ˈbe-lər\ *adj*

gla·brous \ˈglā-brəs\ *adj* : having or being a smooth hairless surface ⟨~ skin⟩

glacial acetic acid *n* : acetic acid containing usu. less than 1 percent of water

glad·i·o·lus \ˌgla-dē-ˈō-ləs\ *n, pl* **-li** \-(ˌ)lē, -ˌlī\ : the large middle portion of the sternum lying between the upper manubrium and the lower xiphoid process — called also *mesosternum*

glairy \ˈglar-ē\ *adj* **glair·i·er; -est** : having a slimy viscid consistency suggestive of an egg white

gland \ˈgland\ *n* **1** : a cell, group of cells, or organ of endothelial origin that selectively removes materials from the blood, concentrates or alters them, and secretes them for further use in the body or for elimination from the body **2** : any of various animal structures (as a lymph node) suggestive of glands though not secretory in function — **gland·less** *adj*

glan·dered \ˈglan-dərd\ *adj* : affected with glanders

glan·ders \-dərz\ *n sing or pl* : a contagious and destructive disease esp. of horses caused by a bacterium of the genus *Burkholderia* (*B. mallei*) and characterized by caseating nodular lesions esp. of the respiratory mucosae, lungs, and skin

glandes *pl of* GLANS

gland of Bartholin *n* : BARTHOLIN'S GLAND

gland of Bow·man \-ˈbō-mən\ *n* : OLFACTORY GLAND

W. Bowman — see BOWMAN'S CAPSULE

gland of Brunner *n* : BRUNNER'S GLAND

gland of external secretion *n* : EXOCRINE GLAND

gland of internal secretion *n* : ENDOCRINE GLAND

gland of Lit·tré \-lē-ˈtrā\ *n* : any of the urethral glands of the male

Littré, Alexis (1658–1726), French surgeon and anatomist.

gland of Moll \-ˈmōl, -ˈmȯl, -ˈmäl\ *n* : any of the small glands near the free margin of each eyelid regarded as modified sweat glands — called also *Moll's gland*

Moll \ˈmȯl\, **Jacob Antonius (1832–1914),** Dutch ophthalmologist.

gland of Ty·son \-ˈtīs-ᵊn\ *n* : PREPUTIAL GLAND

Tyson, Edward (1650–1708), British anatomist.

glan·du·lar \ˈglan-jə-lər\ *adj* **1** : of, relating to, or involving glands, gland cells, or their products **2** : having the characteristics or function of a gland ⟨~ tissue⟩

glandular fever *n* : INFECTIOUS MONONUCLEOSIS

glan·du·lous \ˈglan-jə-ləs\ *adj* : GLANDULAR

glans \ˈglanz\ *n, pl* **glan·des** \ˈglan-ˌdēz\ **1** : a conical vascular body that forms the extremity of the penis **2** : a conical vascular body that forms the extremity of the clitoris

glans cli·tor·i·dis \-klə-ˈtȯr-ə-(ˌ)dis\ *n* : GLANS 2

glans clitoris *n* : GLANS 2

glans penis *n* : GLANS 1

Glanz·mann thrombasthenia \ˈglän(t)s-mən-\ *n* : a rare blood disorder that is marked by excessive bleeding and bruising associated with abnormal platelet aggregation and adhesion and is inherited as an autosomal recessive trait

Glanzmann, Eduard (1887–1959), Swiss pediatrician.

Gla·se·ri·an fissure \glə-ˈzir-ē-ən-\ *n* : PETROTYMPANIC FISSURE

Gla·ser \ˈglä-zər\, **Johann Heinrich (1629–1675),** Swiss anatomist and surgeon.

Glas·gow Coma Scale \ˈglas-(ˌ)kō-\ *n* : a scale that is used to assess the severity of a brain injury based on how a patient responds to certain standard stimuli (as by opening the eyes or giving a verbal response) and that for a low score (as 3 to 5) indicates a poor chance of recovery and for a high score (as 8 to 15) indicates a good chance of recovery

glass·es \ˈgla-səz\ *n pl* : a device used to correct defects of vision or to protect the eyes that consists typically of a pair of glass or plastic lenses and the frame by which they are held in place — called also *eyeglasses*

glass eye *n* **1** : an artificial eye made of glass **2** : an eye having a pale, whitish, or colorless iris — **glass–eyed** \-ˈīd\ *adj*

gla·tir·a·mer \glə-ˈtir-ə-mər\ *n* : a drug consisting of a mixture of the acetate salts of synthetic peptides that is administered by subcutaneous injection to treat relapsing multiple sclerosis — called also *glatiramer acetate;* see COPAXONE

Glau·ber's salt \ˈglau̇-bərz-\ *also* **Glau·ber salt** \-bər-\ *n* : a colorless crystalline sodium sulfate $Na_2SO_4 \cdot 10H_2O$ used as a cathartic — sometimes used in pl.

Glauber, Johann Rudolf (1604–1670), German physician and chemist.

glau·co·ma \glau̇-ˈkō-mə, glȯ-\ *n* : a disease of the eye marked by increased pressure within the eyeball that can result in damage to the optic disk and gradual loss of vision — **glau·coma·tous** \-ˈkō-mə-təs, -ˈkä-\ *adj*

Glea·son grade \ˈglē-sᵊn-\ *n* **1** : a grade given to each of the two most prevalent patterns of cancer cells in tissue obtained from biopsy of a prostate tumor that is based on a scale of 1 to 5 with 1 to 3 corresponding to well-differentiated cancer cells similar in appearance to normal cells in surrounding tissue and 4 to 5 corresponding to poorly differentiated cancer cells that look abnormal **2** : GLEASON SCORE

Gleason, Donald F. (1920–2008), American pathologist.

Gleason score *n* : a score that is the sum of the two Gleason grades assigned to a prostate tumor and that is based on a scale of 2 to 10 with the lowest numbers indicating a slow-growing tumor unlikely to spread and the highest numbers indicating an aggressive tumor

gleet \ˈglēt\ *n* : a chronic inflammation (as gonorrhea) of a bodily orifice usu. accompanied by an abnormal discharge; *also* : the discharge itself

Glee·vec \ˈglē-ˌvek\ *trademark* — used for a preparation of the mesylate of imatinib

gle·no·hu·mer·al \ˌgle-(ˌ)nō-ˈhyü-mə-rəl, ˌglē-\ *adj* : of, relating to, or connecting the glenoid cavity and the humerus

glen·oid \ˈgle-ˌnȯid, ˈglē-\ *adj* **1** : having the form of a smooth shallow depression — used chiefly of skeletal articulatory sockets **2** : of or relating to the glenoid cavity or glenoid fossa

glenoid cavity *n* : the shallow cavity of the upper part of the scapula by which the humerus articulates with the shoulder girdle

glenoid fossa *n* : the depression in each lateral wall of the skull with which the mandible articulates — called also *mandibular fossa*

glenoid labrum *or* **glen·oid·al labrum** \gli-ˈnȯid-ᵊl-\ *n* : a fibrocartilaginous ligament forming the margin of the glenoid cavity of the shoulder joint that serves to broaden and deepen the cavity and gives attachment to the long head of the biceps brachii — called also *labrum*

gli- *or* **glio-** *comb form* **1** : gliomatous ⟨*glio*blastoma⟩ **2** : neuroglial ⟨*gli*oma⟩

glia \ˈglē-ə, ˈglī-ə\ *n, pl* **glia** : supporting tissue that is intermingled with the essential elements of nervous tissue esp. in the brain, spinal cord, and ganglia and is composed of a network of fine fibrils and of flattened stellate cells with numerous radiating fibrillar processes — see MACROGLIA, MICROGLIA — **gli·al** \-əl\ *adj*

-g·lia \glē-ə\ *n comb form* : made up of a (specified) kind or size of element ⟨oligodendro*glia*⟩

gli·a·din \ˈglī-ə-dən\ *n* : PROLAMIN; *esp* : one obtained by alcoholic extraction of gluten from wheat and rye

gli·ben·cla·mide \glī-ˈben-klə-ˌmīd\ *n* : GLYBURIDE

gliding joint *n* : a diarthrosis in which the articular surfaces glide upon each other without axial motion — called also *arthrodia, plane joint*

gli·mep·i·ride \gli-ˈmep-ə-ˌrīd\ *n* : a sulfonylurea drug $C_{24}H_{34}N_4O_5S$ that functions chiefly in stimulating the release of insulin from pancreatic beta cells and is taken orally to treat type 2 diabetes

glio·blas·to·ma \ˌglī-(ˌ)ō-bla-ˈstō-mə\ *n, pl* **-mas** *also* **-ma·ta** \-mə-tə\ : a malignant rapidly growing astrocytoma of the central nervous system and usu. of a cerebral hemisphere

glioblastoma mul·ti·for·me \-ˌməl-tə-ˈfȯr-mē\ *n* : GLIOBLASTOMA

Glio·cla·di·um \ˌglī-ō-ˈklā-dē-əm\ *n* : a genus of molds resembling those of the genus *Penicillium*

gli·o·ma \glī-ˈō-mə, glē-\ *n, pl* **-mas** *also* **-ma·ta** \-mə-tə\ : a tumor arising from glial cells — **gli·o·ma·tous** \-mə-təs\ *adj*

gli·o·ma·to·sis \glī-ˌō-mə-ˈtō-səs\ *n, pl* **-to·ses** \-ˌsēz\ : a glioma with diffuse proliferation of glial cells or with multiple foci

gli·o·sis \glī-ˈō-səs\ *n, pl* **gli·o·ses** \-ˌsēz\ : excessive development of glia — **gli·ot·ic** \-ˈä-tik\ *adj*

glio·tox·in \ˌglī-ō-ˈtäk-sən\ *n* : a toxic antibiotic $C_{13}H_{14}N_2O_4S_2$ that is produced by various fungi (as of the genera *Gliocladium* and *Aspergillus*)

glip·i·zide \ˈgli-pə-ˌzīd\ *n* : a sulfonylurea $C_{21}H_{27}N_5O_4S$ that lowers blood glucose levels and is used in the control of hyperglycemia associated with type 2 diabetes — see GLUCOTROL

Glis·son's capsule \ˈglis-ᵊnz-\ *n* : an investment of loose connective tissue entering the liver with the portal vessels and sheathing the larger vessels in their course through the organ

Glisson, Francis (1597–1677), British physician and anatomist.

glit·a·zone \ˈglit-ə-ˌzōn\ *n* : THIAZOLIDINEDIONE

Gln *abbr* glutamine
glob•al \ˈglō-bəl\ *adj* : being comprehensive, all-inclusive, or complete ⟨transient ∼ amnesia⟩
globe \ˈglōb\ *n* : EYEBALL
globe•fish \ˈglōb-ˌfish\ *n* : PUFFER FISH
glo•bin \ˈglō-bən\ *n* : a colorless protein obtained by removal of heme from a conjugated protein and esp. hemoglobin
glo•bo•side \ˈglō-bə-ˌsīd\ *n* : a complex glycolipid that occurs in the red blood cells, serum, liver, and spleen of humans and accumulates in tissues in one of the variants of Tay-Sachs disease
glob•u•lar \ˈglä-byə-lər\ *adj* **1 a** : having the shape of a globe or globule **b** : having a compact folded molecular structure ⟨∼ proteins⟩ **2** : having or consisting of globules — **glob•u•lar•ly** \-lē\ *adv*
glob•ule \ˈglä-(ˌ)byül\ *n* : a small globular body or mass (as a drop of fat)
glob•u•lin \ˈglä-byə-lən\ *n* : any of a class of simple proteins (as myosin) that occur widely in plant and animal tissues — see ALPHA GLOBULIN, BETA GLOBULIN, GAMMA GLOBULIN
glo•bus hys•ter•i•cus \ˈglō-bəs-hisˈter-i-kəs\ *n* : the subjective feeling or sensation of a lump or mass in the throat — called also *globus pharyngeus, globus sensation*
globus pal•li•dus \-ˈpa-lə-dəs\ *n* : the median portion of the lentiform nucleus — called also *pallidum*
globus pha•ryn•ge•us \-fə-ˈrin-jē-əs\ *n* : GLOBUS HYSTERICUS
globus sensation *n* : GLOBUS HYSTERICUS
glom•an•gi•o•ma \ˌglō-ˌman-jē-ˈō-ma\ *n, pl* **-mas** *also* **-ma•ta** \-mə-tə\ : GLOMUS TUMOR
glo•mec•to•my \ˌglō-ˈmek-tə-mē\ *n, pl* **-mies** : excision of a glomus (as the carotid body)
glomerul- *or* **glomerulo-** *comb form* : glomerulus of the kidney ⟨*glomerulitis*⟩ ⟨*glomerulonephritis*⟩
glo•mer•u•lar \glə-ˈmer-yə-lər, glō-, -ə-lər\ *adj* : of, relating to, or produced by a glomerulus ⟨∼ nephritis⟩
glomerular capsule *n* : BOWMAN'S CAPSULE
glo•mer•u•li•tis \glə-ˌmer-yə-ˈlī-təs, glō-, -ə-ˈlī-\ *n* : inflammation of the glomeruli of the kidney
glo•mer•u•lo•ne•phri•tis \-ˌmer-yə-lō-ni-ˈfrī-təs, -ə-lō-\ *n, pl* **-phrit•i•des** \-ˈfri-tə-ˌdēz\ : nephritis that involves inflammation of the capillaries of the renal glomeruli, is marked esp. by blood or protein in the urine, and if untreated may lead to kidney failure
glo•mer•u•lop•a•thy \-yə-ˈlä-pə-thē\ *n, pl* **-thies** : a disease (as glomerulonephritis) affecting the renal glomeruli
glo•mer•u•lo•sa \glə-ˌmer-yə-ˈlō-sə, -ə-ˈlō-, -zə\ *n, pl* **-sae** \-ˌsē, -ˌsī, -ˌzē, -ˌzī\ : ZONA GLOMERULOSA
glo•mer•u•lo•scle•ro•sis \-ˌlō-sklə-ˈrō-səs\ *n, pl* **-ro•ses** \-ˌsēz\ : nephrosclerosis involving the renal glomeruli
glo•mer•u•lus \glə-ˈmer-yə-ləs, glō-, -ə-ləs\ *n, pl* **-li** \-ˌlī, -ˌlē\ : a small convoluted or intertwined mass: as **a** : a tuft of capillaries at the point of origin of each nephron that passes a protein-free filtrate to the surrounding Bowman's capsule **b** : a dense entanglement of nerve fibers in the olfactory bulb that contains the primary synapses of the olfactory pathway — called also *olfactory glomerulus*
glo•mus \ˈglō-məs\ *n, pl* **glom•era** \ˈglä-mə-rə\ *also* **glo•mi** \ˈglō-ˌmī, -ˌmē\ : a small arteriovenous anastomosis together with its supporting structures: as **a** : a vascular tuft that suggests a renal glomerulus and that develops from the embryonic aorta in relation to the pronephros **b** : CAROTID BODY **c** : a tuft of the choroid plexus protruding into each lateral ventricle of the brain
glomus ca•rot•i•cum \-kə-ˈrä-ti-kəm\ *n* : CAROTID BODY
glomus coc•cy•ge•um \-käk-ˈsi-jē-əm\ *n* : a small mass of vascular tissue situated near the tip of the coccyx — called also *coccygeal body, coccygeal gland*
glomus jug•u•la•re \-ˌjə-gyə-ˈlar-ē\ *n* : a mass of chemoreceptors in the adventitia of the dilation in the internal jugular vein where it arises from the transverse sinus in the jugular foramen
glomus tumor *n* : a painful benign tumor that develops by hypertrophy of a glomus — called also *glomangioma*
gloss- *or* **glosso-** *comb form* **1** : tongue ⟨*gloss*itis⟩ **2** : language ⟨*glosso*lalia⟩
glos•sal \ˈglä-səl, ˈglȯ-\ *adj* : of or relating to the tongue ⟨a ∼ cyst⟩
-glos•sia \ˈglä-sē-ə, ˈglȯ-\ *n comb form* : condition of having (such) a tongue ⟨micro*glossia*⟩
glos•si•na \glä-ˈsī-nə, glȯ-, -ˈsē-\ *n* **1** *cap* : an African genus of dipteran flies with a long slender sharp proboscis that includes the tsetse flies **2** : any dipteran fly of the genus *Glossina* : TSETSE FLY
glos•si•tis \-ˈsī-təs\ *n* : inflammation of the tongue
glosso- — see GLOSS-
gloss•odyn•ia \ˌglä-sō-ˈdi-nē-ə, ˌglȯ-\ *n* : pain localized in the tongue
glos•so•la•lia \ˌglä-sə-ˈlā-lē-ə, ˌglȯ-\ *n* : profuse and often emotionally charged speech that mimics coherent speech but is usu. unintelligible to the listener and that is uttered in some states of religious ecstasy and in some schizophrenic states
glos•so•pal•a•tine arch \ˌglä-sō-ˈpa-lə-ˌtīn-, ˌglȯ-\ *n* : PALATOGLOSSAL ARCH
glossopalatine nerve *n* : NERVUS INTERMEDIUS

glos·so·pal·a·ti·nus \-ˌpa-lə-ˈtī-nəs\ *n, pl* **-ni** \-ˌnī, -ˌnē\ : PALATOGLOSSUS

glos·sop·a·thy \glä-ˈsä-pə-thē\ *n, pl* **-thies** : a disease of the tongue

glos·so·pha·ryn·geal \ˌglä-sō-fə-ˈrin-jē-əl, ˌglȯ-, -jəl; -ˌfar-ən-ˈjē-əl\ *adj* **1** : of or relating to both tongue and pharynx **2** : of, relating to, or affecting the glossopharyngeal nerve

glossopharyngeal nerve *n* : either of the ninth pair of cranial nerves that are mixed nerves and supply chiefly the pharynx, posterior tongue, and parotid gland with motor and sensory fibers — called also *glossopharyngeal, ninth cranial nerve*

glottidis — see RIMA GLOTTIDIS

glot·tis \ˈglä-təs\ *n, pl* **glot·tis·es** *or* **glot·ti·des** \-tə-ˌdēz\ : the space between one of the true vocal cords and the arytenoid cartilage on one side of the larynx and those on the other side; *also* : the structures that surround this space — compare EPIGLOTTIS

Glu *abbr* glutamic acid

gluc- *or* **gluco-** *comb form* : glucose ⟨*gluco*kinase⟩ ⟨*gluco*neogenesis⟩

glu·ca·gon \ˈglü-kə-ˌgän\ *n* : a protein hormone that is produced esp. by the pancreatic islets of Langerhans and that promotes an increase in the sugar content of the blood by increasing the rate of breakdown of glycogen in the liver — called also *hyperglycemic factor*

glucagon–like peptide *n* : either of two intestinal hormones that are produced in response to the presence of nutrients in the small intestine and includes one that stimulates insulin secretion and inhibits glucagon secretion

glu·can \ˈglü-ˌkan, -kən\ *n* : a polysaccharide (as glycogen) that is a polymer of glucose

glu·co·ce·re·bro·si·dase \ˌglü-kō-ˌser-ə-ˈbrō-sə-ˌdās, -ˌdāz\ *n* : an enzyme that catalyzes the hydrolysis of the glucose part of a glucocerebroside and is deficient in patients affected with Gaucher disease

glu·co·ce·re·bro·side \-ˈser-ə-brə-ˌsīd, -sə-ˈrē-\ *n* : a lipid composed of a ceramide and glucose that accumulates in the tissues of patients affected with Gaucher disease

glu·co·cor·ti·coid \-ˈkȯr-ti-ˌkȯid\ *n* : any of a group of corticosteroids (as cortisol or dexamethasone) that are involved esp. in carbohydrate, protein, and fat metabolism, that tend to increase liver glycogen and blood sugar by increasing gluconeogenesis, that are anti-inflammatory and immunosuppressive, and that are used widely in medicine (as to alleviate the symptoms of rheumatoid arthritis) — compare MINERALOCORTICOID

glu·co·ki·nase \-ˈkī-ˌnās, -ˌnāz\ *n* : a hexokinase found esp. in the liver that catalyzes the phosphorylation of glucose

glu·com·e·ter \glü-ˈkä-mə-tər\ : an instrument for measuring the concentration of glucose in the blood

glu·co·nate \ˈglü-kə-ˌnāt\ *n* : a salt or ester of a crystalline acid $C_6H_{12}O_7$ — see CALCIUM GLUCONATE, FERROUS GLUCONATE

glu·co·neo·gen·e·sis \ˌglü-kə-ˌnē-ə-ˈje-nə-səs\ *n, pl* **-e·ses** \-ˌsēz\ : formation of glucose esp. by the liver and kidney from precursors (as fats and proteins) other than carbohydrates — **glu·co·neo·gen·ic** \-ˈje-nik\ *adj*

Glu·co·phage \ˈglü-kō-ˌfāj\ *trademark* — used for a preparation of the hydrochloride of metformin

glu·cos·amine \glü-ˈkō-sə-ˌmēn, -zə-\ *n* : an amino derivative $C_6H_{13}NO_5$ of glucose that occurs esp. as a constituent of various polysaccharides that are components of structural substances (as cartilage and chitin)

glu·cose \ˈglü-ˌkōs, -ˌkōz\ *n* : a sugar $C_6H_{12}O_6$ known in dextrorotatory, levorotatory, and racemic forms; *esp* : the sweet soluble dextrorotatory form that occurs widely in nature and is the usual form in which carbohydrate is assimilated by animals

glucose–1–phosphate *n* : an ester $C_6H_{13}O_9P$ that reacts in the presence of a phosphorylase with aldoses and ketoses to yield disaccharides or with itself in liver and muscle to yield glycogen and phosphoric acid

glucose phosphate *n* : a phosphate ester of glucose: as **a** : GLUCOSE-1-PHOSPHATE **b** : GLUCOSE-6-PHOSPHATE

glucose–6–phosphate *n* : an ester $C_6H_{13}O_9P$ that is formed from glucose and ATP in the presence of a glucokinase and that is an essential early stage in glucose metabolism

glucose–6–phosphate dehydrogenase *n* : an enzyme found esp. in red blood cells that dehydrogenates glucose-6-phosphate in a glucose degradation pathway alternative to the Krebs cycle

glucose–6–phosphate dehydrogenase deficiency *n* : a hereditary metabolic disorder affecting red blood cells that is controlled by a variable gene on the X chromosome, that is characterized by a deficiency of glucose-6-phosphate dehydrogenase conferring marked susceptibility to hemolytic anemia which may be chronic, episodic, or induced by certain foods (as broad beans) or drugs (as primaquine), and that occurs esp. in individuals of Mediterranean or African descent

glucose tolerance test *n* : a test of the body's ability to metabolize glucose that involves the administration of a measured dose of glucose to the fasting stomach and the determination of glucose levels in the blood and urine at measured intervals thereafter and that is used esp. to detect diabetes mellitus

glu·co·side \ˈglü-kə-ˌsīd\ *n* : GLYCOSIDE; *esp* : a glycoside that yields glucose on hydrosis — **glu·co·sid·ic** \ˌglü-kə-ˈsi-dik\ *adj*

glu·cos·uria \ˌglü-kō-ˈshu̇r-ē-ə, -ˈsyu̇r-\ *n* : GLYCOSURIA

Glu·co·trol \ˈglü-kə-ˌtrōl\ *trademark* — used for a preparation of glipizide

Glu·co·vance \ˈglü-kō-ˌvans\ *trademark* — used for a preparation of glyburide and the hydrochloride of metformin

gluc·uron·ic acid \ˌglü-kyə-ˈrä-nik-\ *n* : a compound $C_6H_{10}O_7$ that occurs esp. as a constituent of glycosaminoglycans (as hyaluronic acid) and combined as a glucuronide

gluc·uron·i·dase \-ˈrä-nə-ˌdās, -ˌdāz\ *n* : an enzyme that hydrolyzes a glucuronide

gluc·uro·nide \glü-ˈkyu̇r-ə-ˌnīd\ *n* : any of various derivatives of glucuronic acid that are formed esp. as combinations with often toxic aromatic hydroxyl compounds (as phenols) and are excreted in the urine

glue–sniffing *n* : the deliberate inhalation of volatile organic solvents from plastic glues that may result in symptoms ranging from mild euphoria to disorientation and coma

glu·ta·mate \ˈglü-tə-ˌmāt\ *n* : a salt or ester of glutamic acid; *esp* : one that functions as an excitatory neurotransmitter — see MONOSODIUM GLUTAMATE

glutamate dehydrogenase *n* : an enzyme present esp. in liver mitochondria and cytosol that catalyzes the oxidation of glutamate to ammonia and α-ketoglutaric acid

glu·ta·ma·ter·gic \ˌglüt-ə-mə-ˈtər-jik\ *adj* : liberating, activated by, or involving glutamate

glu·tam·ic acid \(ˌ)glü-ˈta-mik-\ *n* : a crystalline amino acid $C_5H_9NO_4$ that is widely distributed in plant and animal proteins and acts esp. in the form of a salt or ester as a neurotransmitter which excites postsynaptic neurons — abbr. *Glu*

glutamic–ox·a·lo·ace·tic transaminase \-ˌäk-sə-lō-ə-ˈsē-tik-\ *also* **glutamic–ox·al·ace·tic transaminase** \-ˌäk-sə-lə-ˈsē-tik-\ *n* : ASPARTATE AMINOTRANSFERASE

glutamic–pyruvic transaminase *n* : ALANINE AMINOTRANSFERASE

glu·ta·mine \ˈglü-tə-ˌmēn\ *n* : a crystalline amino acid $C_5H_{10}N_2O_3$ that is found both free and in proteins in plants and animals and that yields glutamic acid and ammonia on hydrolysis — abbr. *Gln*

glu·tar·al·de·hyde \ˌglü-tə-ˈral-də-ˌhīd\ *n* : a compound $C_5H_8O_2$ used esp. as a disinfectant and in fixing biological tissues

glu·tar·ic acid \glü-ˌtar-ik-\ *n* : a crystalline acid $C_5H_8O_4$ used esp. in organic synthesis

glu·ta·thi·one \ˌglü-tə-ˈthī-ˌōn\ *n* : a peptide $C_{10}H_{17}N_3O_6S$ that contains one amino-acid residue each of glutamic acid, cysteine, and glycine, that occurs widely in plant and animal tissues, and that plays an important role in biological oxidation-reduction processes and as a coenzyme

glute \ˈglüt\ *n* : GLUTEUS; *esp* : GLUTEUS MAXIMUS — usu. used in pl.

glu·te·al \ˈglü-tē-əl, glü-ˈtē-\ *adj* : of or relating to the buttocks or the gluteus muscles

gluteal artery *n* : either of two branches of the internal iliac artery that supply the gluteal region: **a** : the largest branch of the internal iliac artery that sends branches esp. to the gluteal muscles — called also *superior gluteal artery* **b** : a branch that is distributed esp. to the buttocks and the backs of the thighs — called also *inferior gluteal artery*

gluteal nerve *n* : either of two nerves arising from the sacral plexus and supplying the gluteal muscles and adjacent parts: **a** : one arising from the posterior part of the fourth and fifth lumbar nerves and from the first sacral nerve and distributed to the gluteus muscles and to the tensor fasciae latae — called also *superior gluteal nerve* **b** : one arising from the posterior part of the fifth lumbar nerve and from the first and second sacral nerves and distributed to the gluteus maximus — called also *inferior gluteal nerve*

gluteal tuberosity *n* : the lateral ridge of the linea aspera of the femur that gives attachment to the gluteus maximus

glu·ten \ˈglüt-ᵊn\ *n* : a gluey protein substance esp. of wheat flour that causes dough to be sticky

gluten–sensitive enteropathy *n* : CELIAC DISEASE

glutes *pl of* GLUTE

glu·teth·i·mide \glü-ˈte-thə-ˌmīd, -məd\ *n* : a sedative-hypnotic drug $C_{13}H_{15}NO_2$ that has pharmacological properties similar to the barbiturates

glu·te·us \ˈglü-tē-əs, glü-ˈtē-\ *n, pl* **glu·tei** \ˈglü-tē-ˌī, -tē-ˌē; glü-ˈtē-ˌī\ : any of three large muscles of the buttocks: **a** : GLUTEUS MAXIMUS **b** : GLUTEUS MEDIUS **c** : GLUTEUS MINIMUS

gluteus max·i·mus \-ˈmak-sə-məs\ *n, pl* **glutei max·i·mi** \-sə-ˌmī\ : the outermost of the three muscles in each buttock that acts to extend and laterally rotate the thigh

gluteus me·di·us \-ˈmē-dē-us\ *n, pl* **glutei me·dii** \-dē-ˌī\ : the middle of the three muscles in each buttock that acts to abduct and medially rotate the thigh

gluteus min·i·mus \-ˈmi-nə-məs\ *n, pl* **glutei min·i·mi** \-ˌmī\ : the innermost of the three muscles in each buttock that acts similarly to the gluteus medius

Gly *abbr* glycine

gly·bur·ide \ˈglī-byə-ˌrīd\ *n* : a sulfonylurea $C_{23}H_{28}ClN_3O_5S$ used similarly to glipizide — called also *glibenclamide;* see DIAβETA, GLUCOVANCE, MICRONASE

glyc- *or* **glyco-** *comb form* : carbohydrate and esp. sugar ⟨*glyco*protein⟩

gly·cae·mia *chiefly Brit var of* GLYCEMIA

gly·can \ˈglī-ˌkan\ *n* : POLYSACCHARIDE

gly·cat·ed hemoglobin \ˈglī-ˌkā-təd\ *n* : HEMOGLOBIN A1C

gly·ce·mia \glī-ˈsē-mē-ə\ *n* : the presence of glucose in the blood — **gly·ce·mic** \-ˈsē-mik\ *adj*

glycemic index *n* : a measure of the rate at which an ingested food causes the level of glucose in the blood to rise; *also* : a ranking of foods according to their glycemic index — abbr. *GI*

glycer- *or* **glycero-** *comb form* **1** : glycerol ⟨*glyceryl*⟩ **2** : related to glycerol or glyceric acid ⟨*glyceral*dehyde⟩

glyc·er·al·de·hyde \ˌgli-sə-ˈral-də-ˌhīd\ *n* : a sweet crystalline compound $C_3H_6O_3$ that is formed as an intermediate in carbohydrate metabolism

gly·cer·ic acid \gli-ˈser-ik-\ *n* : a syrupy acid $C_3H_6O_4$ obtainable by oxidation of glycerol or glyceraldehyde

glyc·er·ide \ˈgli-sə-ˌrīd\ *n* : an ester of glycerol esp. with fatty acids

glyc·er·in *or* **glyc·er·ine** \ˈgli-sə-rən\ *n* : GLYCEROL

glycero- — see GLYCER-

glyc·er·ol \ˈgli-sə-ˌrȯl, -ˌrōl\ *n* : a sweet syrupy hygroscopic alcohol $C_3H_8O_3$ containing three hydroxy groups per molecule, usu. obtained by the saponification of fats, and used as a moistening agent, emollient, and lubricant, and as an emulsifying agent — called also *glycerin*

glyc·er·yl \ˈgli-sə-rəl\ *n* : a radical derived from glycerol by removal of hydroxide; *esp* : a trivalent radical CH_2CHCH_2

glyceryl guai·a·col·ate \-ˈgwī-ə-ˌkō-ˌlāt, -ˈgī-, -kə-\ *n* : GUAIFENESIN

gly·cine \ˈglī-ˌsēn, ˈglīs-ᵊn\ *n* : a sweet nonessential amino acid $C_2H_5NO_2$ that is a neurotransmitter which induces inhibition of postsynaptic neurons, is obtained by hydrolysis of proteins or is prepared synthetically, and is used in the form of its salt as an antacid — abbr. *Gly*

gly·cin·uria \ˌglīs-ᵊn-ˈu̇r-ē-ə, -ˈyu̇r-\ *n* : a kidney disorder characterized by the presence of excessive amounts of glycine in the urine

glyco- — see GLYC-

gly·co·bi·ar·sol \ˌglī-kō-(ˌ)bī-ˈär-ˌsȯl, -ˌsōl\ *n* : an antiprotozoal drug $C_8H_9AsBiNO_6$

gly·co·chol·ic acid \ˌglī-kō-ˈkä-lik-, -ˈkō-\ *n* : a crystalline acid $C_{26}H_{43}NO_6$ that occurs in bile

gly·co·con·ju·gate \ˌglī-kō-ˈkän-ji-gət, -ˌgāt\ *n* : any of a group of compounds (as the glycolipids and glycoproteins) consisting of sugars linked to proteins or lipids

gly·co·gen \ˈglī-kə-jən\ *n* : a white amorphous tasteless polysaccharide $(C_6H_{10}O_5)_x$ that constitutes the principal form in which carbohydrate is stored in animal tissues and esp. in muscle and liver tissue — called also *animal starch*

gly·cog·e·nase \glī-ˈkä-jə-ˌnās, -ˌnāz\ *n* : an enzyme that catalyzes the hydrolysis of glycogen

gly·co·gen·e·sis \ˌglī-kə-ˈje-nə-səs\ *n, pl* **-e·ses** \-ˌsēz\ : the synthesis of glycogen from glucose that occurs chiefly in the liver and skeletal muscle— compare GLYCOGENOLYSIS

gly·co·gen·ic \-ˈje-nik\ *adj* : of, relating to, or involving glycogen or glycogenesis

gly·co·gen·ol·y·sis \ˌglī-kə-jə-ˈnä-lə-səs\ *n, pl* **-y·ses** \-ˌsēz\ : the breakdown of glycogen esp. to glucose in the body — compare GLYCOGENESIS — **gly·co·gen·o·lyt·ic** \-jən-ᵊl-ˈi-tik, -ˌjen-\ *adj*

gly·co·ge·no·sis \ˌglī-kə-jə-ˈnō-səs\ *n, pl* **-no·ses** \-ˌsēz\ : GLYCOGEN STORAGE DISEASE

glycogen storage disease *n* : any of several metabolic disorders (as McArdle's disease or Pompe disease) that are characterized esp. by abnormal deposits of glycogen in tissue, are caused by enzyme deficiencies in glycogen metabolism, and are usu. inherited as an autosomal recessive trait

gly·co·he·mo·glo·bin \-ˈhē-mə-ˌglō-bən\ *n* : HEMOGLOBIN A1C

gly·col·ic acid *also* **gly·col·lic acid** \glī-ˈkä-lik-\ *n* : an alpha hydroxy acid $C_2H_4O_3$ that is used in chemical peels and that is the major toxic metabolite in ethylene glycol poisoning — called also *hydroxyacetic acid*

gly·co·lip·id \ˌglī-kō-ˈli-pəd\ *n* : a lipid (as a ganglioside or a cerebroside) that contains a carbohydrate radical

gly·col·y·sis \glī-ˈkä-lə-səs\ *n, pl* **-y·ses** \-ˌsēz\ : the enzymatic breakdown of a carbohydrate (as glucose) by way of phosphate derivatives with the production of pyruvic or lactic acid and energy stored in high-energy phosphate bonds of ATP — **gly·co·lyt·ic** \ˌglī-kə-ˈli-tik\ *adj* — **gly·co·lyt·i·cal·ly** *adv*

gly·co·pep·tide \ˌglī-kō-ˈpep-ˌtīd\ *n* : GLYCOPROTEIN

gly·co·pro·tein \-ˈprō-ˌtēn, -ˈprō-tē-ən\ *n* : a conjugated protein in which the nonprotein group is a carbohydrate — compare MUCOPROTEIN

gly·co·pyr·ro·late \-ˈpī-rə-ˌlāt\ *n* : a synthetic anticholinergic drug $C_{19}H_{28}BrNO_3$ used in the treatment of gastrointestinal disorders (as peptic ulcer) esp. when associated with hyperacidity, hypermotility, or spasm — see ROBINUL

gly·cos·ami·no·gly·can \ˌglī-kō-sə-ˌmē-nō-ˈglī-ˌkan, -kō-ˌsa-mə-nō-\ *n* : any of various polysaccharides derived from an amino hexose that are constituents of mucoproteins, glycoproteins, and blood-group substances — called also *mucopolysaccharide*

gly·co·side \ˈglī-kə-ˌsīd\ *n* : any of numerous sugar derivatives that contain a nonsugar group attached through an oxygen or nitrogen bond and that on hydrolysis yield a sugar (as glucose) — see CARDIAC GLYCOSIDE — **gly·co·sid·ic** \ˌglī-kə-ˈsi-dik\ *adj* — **gly·co·sid·i·cal·ly** *adv*

gly·co·sphin·go·lip·id \ˌglī-kō-ˌsfiŋ-gō-ˈli-pəd\ *n* : any of various lipids (as a cerebroside or a ganglioside) which are derivatives of ceramides and some of which accumulate in disorders of lipid metabolism (as Tay-Sachs disease)

gly·cos·uria \ˌglī-kō-ˈshu̇r-ē-ə, -ˈsyu̇r-\ *n* : the presence in the urine of abnormal amounts of sugar — called also *glucosuria* — **gly·cos·uric** \-ˈshu̇r-ik, -ˈsyu̇r-\ *adj*

gly·co·syl·at·ed hemoglobin \glī-ˈkō-sə-ˌlā-təd-\ *n* : HEMOGLOBIN A1C

Gly·set \ˈglī-ˌset\ *trademark* — used for a preparation of miglitol

gm *abbr* gram

GM and S *abbr* General Medicine and Surgery

GM–CSF *abbr* granulocyte-macrophage colony-stimulating factor

GN *abbr* graduate nurse

gnat \ˈnat\ *n* : any of various small usu. biting dipteran flies (as a midge or blackfly)

gna·thi·on \ˈnā-thē-ˌän, ˈna-\ *n* : the midpoint of the lower border of the human mandible

gna·thos·to·mi·a·sis \nə-ˌthäs-tə-ˈmī-ə-səs\ *n, pl* **-a·ses** \-ˌsēz\ : infestation with or disease caused by nematode worms (genus *Gnathostoma*) commonly acquired by eating raw fish

-g·na·thous \g-nə-thəs\ *adj comb form* : having (such) a jaw ⟨pro*gnathous*⟩

-g·no·sia \g-ˈnō-zhə\ *n comb form* : -GNOSIS ⟨a*gnosia*⟩ ⟨prosopa*gnosia*⟩

-g·no·sis \g-ˈnō-səs\ *n comb form, pl* **-g·no·ses** \-ˌsēz\ : knowledge : cognition : recognition ⟨stereo*gnosis*⟩

-g·nos·tic \g-ˈnäs-tik\ *adj comb form* : characterized by or relating to (such) knowledge ⟨pharmaco*gnostic*⟩

-g·no·sy \g-nə-sē\ *n comb form, pl* **-g·no·sies** : -GNOSIS ⟨pharmaco*gnosy*⟩

GnRH *abbr* gonadotropin-releasing hormone

goal–directed *adj* : aimed toward a goal or toward completion of a task ⟨~ behavior⟩

goblet cell *n* : a mucus-secreting epithelial cell (as of columnar epithelium) that is distended with secretion or its precursors at the free end

goi·ter \ˈgȯi-tər\ *n* : an enlargement of the thyroid gland that is commonly visible as a swelling of the anterior part of the neck, that often results from insufficient intake of iodine and then is usu. accompanied by hypothyroidism, and that in other cases is associated with hyperthyroidism usu. together with toxic symptoms and exophthalmos — called also *struma* — **goi·trous** \ˈgȯi-trəs\ *also* **goi·ter·ous** \ˈgȯi-tə-rəs\ *adj*

goi·tre *chiefly Brit var of* GOITER

goi·tro·gen \ˈgȯi-trə-jən\ *n* : a substance (as thiourea or thiouracil) that induces goiter formation

goi·tro·gen·ic \ˌgȯi-trə-ˈje-nik\ *also* **goi·ter·o·gen·ic** \ˌgȯi-tə-rō-ˈje-nik\ *adj* : producing or tending to produce goiter ⟨a ~ agent⟩ — **goi·tro·ge·nic·i·ty** \ˌgȯi-trə-jə-ˈni-sə-tē\ *n*

gold \ˈgōld\ *n, often attrib* : a malleable ductile yellow metallic element used in the form of its salts (as gold sodium thiomalate) esp. in the treatment of rheumatoid arthritis — symbol *Au;* see ELEMENT table

golden hour *n* : the hour immediately following traumatic injury in which medical treatment to prevent irreversible internal damage and optimize the chance of survival is most effective

gold sodium thio·ma·late \-ˌthī-ō-ˈma-lāt, -ˈmā-\ *n* : a mixture of two gold salts $C_4H_3AuNa_2O_4S$ and $C_4H_4AuNaO_4S$ injected intramuscularly esp. in the treatment of rheumatoid arthritis — called also *gold thiomalate;* see MYOCHRYSINE

gold sodium thiosulfate *n* : a soluble gold compound $Na_3Au(S_2O_3)_2{\cdot}2H_2O$ administered by intravenous injection in the treatment of rheumatoid arthritis and lupus erythematosus

gold thio·glu·cose \-ˌthī-ō-ˈglu-ˌkōs\ *n* : an organic compound of gold $C_6H_{11}AuO_5S$ injected intramuscularly in the treatment of active rheumatoid arthritis and nondisseminated lupus erythematosus — called also *aurothioglucose*

Gol·gi apparatus \ˈgȯl-(ˌ)jē-\ *n* : a cytoplasmic organelle that consists of a stack of smooth membranous saccules and associated vesicles active in the modification and transport of proteins — called also *Golgi body, Golgi complex*

Golgi, Camillo (1843 *or* **1844–1926),** Italian histologist and pathologist.

Golgi cell *n* : a neuron with short dendrites and with either a long axon or an axon that breaks into processes soon after leaving the cell body

Golgi tendon organ *n* : a spindle-shaped sensory end organ within a tendon that provides information about muscle tension — called also *neurotendinous spindle*

go·lim·u·mab \gō-ˈlim-yü-ˌmab\ *n* : a genetically engineered monoclonal antibody that inhibits the activity of tumor necrosis factor and is administered by subcutaneous injection to treat rheumatoid arthritis, psoriatic arthritis, ankylosing spondylitis, and ulcerative colitis — see SIMPONI

go·mer \ˈgō-mər\ *n, med slang, usu disparaging* : a chronic problem patient who does not respond to treatment

gom·pho·sis \gäm-ˈfō-səs\ *n* : an immovable articulation in which a hard part is received into a bone cavity (as the teeth into the jaws)

go·nad \ˈgō-ˌnad\ *n* : a gamete-producing reproductive gland (as an ovary or testis) — **go·nad·al** \gō-ˈnad-ᵊl\ *adj*

go·nad·o·troph \gō-ˈna-də-ˌtrōf\ *n* : a cell of the adenohypophysis that secretes a gonadotropic hormone (as luteinizing hormone)

go·nad·o·trop·ic \gō-ˌna-də-ˈträ-pik\ *also* **go·nad·o·tro·phic** \-ˈtrō-fik, -ˈträ-\ *adj* : acting on or stimulating the gonads

go·nad·o·tro·pin \-ˈtrō-pən\ *also* **go·nad·o·tro·phin** \-fən\ *n* : a gonadotropic hormone (as follicle-stimulating hormone) — see HUMAN CHORIONIC GONADOTROPIN

gonadotropin–releasing hormone *n* : a hormone produced by the hypothalamus that stimulates the adenohypophysis to release gonadotropins (as luteinizing hormone and follicle-stimulating hormone) — abbr. *GnRH;* called also *luteinizing hormone-releasing hormone*

G_1 phase \ˌjē-ˈwən-\ *n* : the period in the cell cycle from the end of cell division to the beginning of DNA replication — compare G_2 PHASE, M PHASE, S PHASE

goni- *or* **gonio-** *comb form* : corner : angle ⟨*gonio*meter⟩

gonial angle *n* : the angle formed by the junction of the posterior and lower borders of the human lower jaw — called also *angle of the jaw, angle of the mandible*

go·ni·om·e·ter \ˌgō-nē-ˈä-mə-tər\ *n* : an instrument for measuring angles (as of a joint or the skull) — **go·nio·met·ric** \-nē-ə-ˈme-trik\ *adj* — **go·ni·om·e·try** \-nē-ˈä-mə-trē\ *n*

go·nio·punc·ture \ˈgō-nē-ə-ˌpəŋk-chər\ *n* : a surgical operation for congenital glaucoma that involves making a puncture into the sclera with a knife at the site of discharge of aqueous fluid at the periphery of the anterior chamber of the eye

go·ni·o·scope \-ˌskōp\ *n* : an instrument consisting of a contact lens to be fitted over the cornea and an optical system with which the interior of the eye can be viewed — **go·ni·os·co·py** \ˌgō-nē-ˈäs-kə-pē\ *n*

go·ni·ot·o·my \ˌgō-nē-ˈä-tə-mē\ *n, pl* **-mies** : surgical relief of glaucoma used in some congenital types and achieved by opening the canal of Schlemm

go·ni·tis \gō-ˈnī-təs\ *n* : inflammation of the knee

gono·coc·cae·mia *chiefly Brit var of* GONOCOCCEMIA

gono·coc·ce·mia \ˌgä-nə-ˌkäk-ˈsē-mē-ə\ *n* : the presence of gonococci in the blood — **gono·coc·ce·mic** \-ˈsē-mik\ *adj*

gono·coc·cus \ˌgä-nə-ˈkä-kəs\ *n, pl* **-coc·ci** \-ˈkäk-ˌsī, -ˌsē; -ˈkä-ˌkī, -ˌkē\ : a pus-producing bacterium of the genus *Neisseria* (*N. gonorrhoeae*) that causes gonorrhea — **gono·coc·cal** \-ˈkä-kəl\ *adj*

gon·or·rhea \ˌgä-nə-ˈrē-ə\ *n* : a contagious inflammation of the genital mucous membrane caused by the gonococcus — called also *clap* — **gon·or·rhe·al** \-ˈrē-əl\ *adj*

gon·or·rhoea *chiefly Brit var of* GONORRHEA

-g·o·ny \gə-nē\ *n comb form, pl* **-g·o·nies** : manner of generation or reproduction ⟨schizo*gony*⟩

go·ny·au·lax \ˌgō-nē-ˈȯ-ˌlaks\ *n* **1** *cap* : a large genus of phosphorescent marine dinoflagellates that when unusually abundant cause red tide **2** : any dinoflagellate of the genus *Gonyaulax*

good cholesterol *n* : HDL

Good·pas·ture's syndrome \ˈgu̇d-ˌpas-chərz-\ *also* **Good·pas·ture syndrome** \-chər-\ *n* : an autoimmune disorder of unknown cause that is characterized by the presence of circulating antibodies in the blood which attack the basement membrane of the kidney's glomeruli and the lung's alveoli and that is marked initially by coughing, fatigue, difficulty in breathing, and hemoptysis progressing to glomerulonephritis and pulmonary hemorrhages

Goodpasture, Ernest William (1886–1960), American pathologist.

goose bumps *n pl* : a roughness of the skin produced by erection of its papillae esp. from cold, fear, or a sudden feeling of excitement — called also *goose pimples*

goose·flesh \-ˌflesh\ *n* : GOOSE BUMPS

gork \ˈgȯrk\ *n, med slang, usu disparaging* : a terminal patient whose brain is nonfunctional and the rest of whose body can be kept functioning only by the extensive use of mechanical devices and nutrient solutions — **gorked** \ˈgȯrkt\ *adj, med slang*

goun·dou \ˈgün-(ˌ)dü\ *n* : a tumorous swelling of the nose often considered a late lesion of yaws — compare GANGOSA

gout \ˈgau̇t\ *n* : a metabolic disease marked by a painful inflammation of the joints, deposits of urates in and around the joints, and usu. an excessive amount of uric acid in the blood — **gouty** \ˈgau̇-tē\ *adj*

gouty arthritis *n* : arthritis associated with gout and caused by the deposition of urate crystals in the articular cartilage of joints

GP *abbr* general practitioner

G_1 phase, G_2 phase — see entries alphabetized as G ONE PHASE, G TWO PHASE

gp120 \ˌjē-ˌpē-ˌwən-ˈtwen-tē\ *n* : a glycoprotein that protrudes from the outer surface of the HIV virion and that must bind to a CD4 receptor on a T cell bearing such receptors before infection of the cell can occur

G protein \ˈjē-\ *n* : any of a class of cell membrane proteins that are coupled to cell surface receptors and upon stimulation of the receptor by a molecule (as a hormone) bind to GTP to form an active complex which mediates an intracellular event

gr *abbr* **1** grain **2** gram **3** gravity

graaf·ian follicle \ˈgrä-fē-ən-, ˈgra-\ *n, often cap G* : a mature follicle in a mammalian ovary that contains a liquid-filled cavity and that ruptures during ovulation to release an egg — called also *vesicular ovarian follicle*

de Graaf \də-ˈgräf\, **Reinier (1641–1673),** Dutch physician and anatomist.

grac·ile fasciculus \ˈgra-səl-, -ˌsīl-\ *n, pl* **gracile fasciculi** : FASCICULUS GRACILIS

grac·i·lis \ˈgra-sə-ləs\ *n* : the most superficial muscle of the inside of the thigh that acts to adduct the thigh and to flex the leg at the knee and assist in rotating it medially

grade \ˈgrād\ *n* : a degree of severity of a disease or abnormal condition ⟨a ~ III carcinoma⟩

gra·di·ent echo \ˈgrā-dē-ənt-ˈe-kō\ *n* : a signal that is detected in a nuclear magnetic resonance spectrometer that is analogous to a spin echo but is produced by varying the external magnetic field following application of a single radio-frequency pulse rather than by application of a series of radio-frequency pulses — usu. used attributively ⟨*gradient-echo* magnetic resonance imaging⟩; called also *gradient-recalled echo*

graduate nurse *n* : a person who has completed the regular course of study and practical hospital training in nursing school — abbr. *GN;* called also *trained nurse*

Graf·en·berg spot \ˈgra-fən-bərg-\ *n* : G-SPOT

Gräf·en·berg \ˈgre-fən-ˌberk\, **Ernst (1881–1957),** American (German-born) gynecologist.

¹graft \ˈgraft\ *vb* : to implant (living tissue) surgically

²graft *n* **1** : the act of grafting **2** : something grafted; *specif* : living tissue used in grafting

graft–versus–host *adj* : of, relating to, or caused by graft-versus-host disease

graft–versus–host disease *n* : a bodily condition that results when T cells from a usu. allogeneic tissue or organ transplant and esp. a bone marrow transplant react immunologically against the recipient's antigens attacking cells and tissues (as of the skin and liver) and that may be fatal — abbr. *GVHD;* called also *graft-versus-host reaction*

grain \ˈgrān\ *n* : a unit of avoirdupois, Troy, and apothecaries' weight equal to 0.0648 gram or 0.002286 avoirdupois ounce or 0.002083 Troy ounce — abbr. *gr*

grain alcohol *n* : ETHANOL

grain itch *n* : an itching rash caused by the bite of a mite of the genus *Pyemotes* (*P. ventricosus*) that occurs chiefly on grain, straw, or straw products — compare GROCER'S ITCH

gram \ˈgram\ *n* : a metric unit of mass equal to $^1/_{1000}$ kilogram and nearly equal to the mass of one cubic centimeter of water at its maximum density — abbr. *g*

-gram \ˌgram\ *n comb form* : drawing : writing : record ⟨cardio*gram*⟩

gram calorie *n* : CALORIE 1a

gram·i·ci·din \ˌgra-mə-ˈsīd-ᵊn\ *n* : an antibacterial mixture produced by a soil bacterium of the genus *Bacillus* (*B. brevis*) and used topically against gram-positive bacteria in local infections esp. of the eye

gramme *chiefly Brit var of* GRAM

gram–negative *adj* : not holding the purple dye when stained by Gram's stain — used chiefly of bacteria

gram–positive *adj* : holding the purple dye when stained by Gram's stain — used chiefly of bacteria

Gram's solution \ˈgramz-\ *n* : a watery solution of iodine and the iodide of potassium used in staining bacteria by Gram's stain

Gram \ˈgräm\, **Hans Christian Joachim (1853–1938),** Danish physician.

Gram's stain *or* **Gram stain** \ˈgram-\ *n* **1** : a method for the differential staining of bacteria by treatment with Gram's solution after staining with a triphenylmethane dye — called also *Gram's method* **2** : the chemicals used in Gram's stain

gram–variable *adj* : staining irregularly or inconsistently by Gram's stain

gran·di·ose \ˈgran-dē-ˌōs, ˌgran-dē-ˈ\ *adj* : characterized by affectation of grandeur or splendor or by absurd exaggeration ⟨~ delusions⟩ — **gran·di·os·i·ty** \ˌgran-dē-ˈäs-ət-ē\ *n*

grand mal \ˈgrän-ˈmäl, ˈgräⁿ-, ˈgrand-, -ˈmal\ *n* **1** *or* **grand mal epilepsy** : severe epilepsy characterized by tonic-clonic seizures : tonic-clonic epilepsy **2** *or* **grand mal seizure** : a tonic-clonic seizure

grand rounds *n pl* : rounds involving the formal presentation by an expert of a clinical issue sometimes in the presence of selected patients

granul- *or* **granuli-** *or* **granulo-** *comb form* : granule ⟨*granulo*cyte⟩

gran·u·lar \ˈgran-yə-lər\ *adj* **1 a** : consisting of or containing granules : having a grainy appearance **b** : having granules with an affinity for specific biological stains ⟨~ cytoplasm⟩ **2** : having or marked by granulations

⟨∼ tissue⟩ — **gran•u•lar•i•ty** \ˌgran-yə-ˈlar-ə-tē\ *n*
granular conjunctivitis *n* : TRACHOMA
gran•u•late \ˈgran-yə-ˌlāt\ *vb* **-lat•ed; -lat•ing** **1** : to form or crystallize (as sugar) into grains or granules **2** : to form granulations ⟨a *granulating* wound⟩
gran•u•la•tion \ˌgran-yə-ˈlā-shən\ *n* **1** : the act or process of granulating : the condition of being granulated **2 a** (1) : a minute mass of tissue projecting from the surface of an organ (as on the eyelids in trachoma) (2) : one of the minute red granules made up of loops of newly formed capillaries that form on a raw surface (as of a wound) and that with fibroblasts are the active agents in the process of healing — see GRANULATION TISSUE **b** : the act or process of forming such elevations or granules
granulation tissue *n* : tissue made up of granulations that temporarily replaces lost tissue in a wound
gran•ule \ˈgran-(ˌ)yül\ *n* : a little grain or small particle; *esp* : one of a number of particles forming a larger unit
granule cell *n* : one of the small neurons of the cortex of the cerebellum and cerebrum
granuli- — see GRANUL-
granulo- — see GRANUL-
gran•u•lo•cyte \ˈgran-yə-lō-ˌsīt\ *n* : any of a group of white blood cells (as an eosinophil or neutrophil) with granule-containing cytoplasm and a usu. lobed nucleus — compare AGRANULOCYTE — **gran•u•lo•cyt•ic** \ˌgran-yə-lō-ˈsi-tik\ *adj*
granulocyte colony–stimulating factor *n* : a colony-stimulating factor that acts to promote the maturation of precursor cells into granulocytes — abbr. *G-CSF*
granulocyte–macrophage colony–stimulating factor *n* : a colony-stimulating factor that promotes the differentiation of bone marrow stem cells, stimulates the maturation of precursor cells into granulocytes and macrophages, and activates mature macrophages — abbr. *GM-CSF*
granulocytic leukemia *n* : MYELOGENOUS LEUKEMIA
gran•u•lo•cy•to•pe•nia \ˌgran-yə-lō-ˌsī-tə-ˈpē-nē-ə\ *n* : deficiency of blood granulocytes; *esp* : AGRANULOCYTOSIS — **gran•u•lo•cy•to•pe•nic** \-ˈpē-nik\ *adj*
gran•u•lo•cy•to•poi•e•sis \-ˌsī-tə-pȯi-ˈē-səs\ *n, pl* **-e•ses** \-ˌsēz\ : GRANULOPOIESIS
gran•u•lo•cy•to•sis \ˌgran-yə-lō-ˌsī-ˈtō-səs\ *n, pl* **-to•ses** \-ˌsēz\ : an increase in the number of blood granulocytes — compare LYMPHOCYTOSIS, MONOCYTOSIS
gran•u•lo•ma \ˌgran-yə-ˈlō-mə\ *n, pl* **-mas** *also* **-ma•ta** \-mə-tə\ : a mass or nodule of chronically inflamed tissue with granulations that is usu. associated with an infective process
granuloma an•nu•la•re \-ˌa-nyü-ˈlar-ē\ *n* : a benign chronic rash of unknown cause marked by one or more flat spreading ringlike spots with lighter centers esp. on the feet, legs, hands, or fingers
granuloma in•gui•na•le \-ˌiŋ-gwə-ˈna-lē, -ˈnä-, -ˈnā-\ *n* : a sexually transmitted disease characterized by ulceration and formation of granulations on the genitalia and in the groin area and caused by a bacterium of the genus *Klebsiella* (*K. granulomatis* syn. *Calymmatobacterium granulomatis*) — called also *donovanosis*
gran•u•lo•ma•to•sis \ˌgran-yə-ˌlō-mə-ˈtō-səs\ *n, pl* **-to•ses** \-ˌsēz\ : a chronic condition marked by the formation of numerous granulomas
granulomatosis with poly•an•gi•i•tis \-ˌpä-lē-ˌan-jē-ˈīt-əs\ *n* : a rare disease of unknown cause that is characterized by inflammation of small blood vessels and granuloma formation esp. in the kidneys and upper and lower respiratory tracts and if untreated can lead to kidney or lung failure
gran•u•lo•ma•tous \-ˈlō-mə-təs\ *adj* : of, relating to, or characterized by granuloma — see CHRONIC GRANULOMATOUS DISEASE
gran•u•lo•poi•e•sis \-(ˌ)lō-ˌpȯi-ˈē-səs\ *n, pl* **-e•ses** \-ˌsēz\ : the formation of blood granulocytes typically in the bone marrow — **gran•u•lo•poi•et•ic** \-ˌpȯi-ˈe-tik\ *adj*
gran•u•lo•sa cell \ˌgran-yə-ˈlō-sə-, -zə-\ *n* : one of the estrogen-secreting cells of the epithelial lining of a graafian follicle or its follicular precursor
granulosum — see STRATUM GRANULOSUM
grape sugar \ˈgrāp-\ *n* : DEXTROSE
-graph \ˌgraf\ *n comb form* **1** : something written ⟨mono*graph*⟩ **2** : instrument for making or transmitting records ⟨electrocardio*graph*⟩
-graph•ia \ˈgra-fē-ə\ *n comb form* : writing characteristic of a (specified) usu. psychological abnormality ⟨dys*graphia*⟩ ⟨dermo*graphia*⟩
grapho- *comb form* : writing ⟨*grapho*logy⟩
gra•phol•o•gy \gra-ˈfä-lə-jē\ *n, pl* **-gies** : the study of handwriting esp. for the purpose of character analysis — **grapho•log•i•cal** \ˌgra-fə-ˈlä-ji-kəl\ *adj* — **gra•phol•o•gist** \gra-ˈfä-lə-jist\ *n*
grapho•ma•nia \ˌgra-fō-ˈmā-nē-ə, -nyə\ *n* : a compulsive urge to write — **grapho•ma•ni•ac** \-nē-ˌak\ *n*
grapho•spasm \ˈgra-fə-ˌspa-zəm\ *n* : WRITER'S CRAMP
gras — see TULLE GRAS
GRAS *abbr* generally recognized as safe
grass \ˈgras\ *n* : MARIJUANA
grass tetany *n* : an often fatal disorder of cattle caused by low blood magnesium esp. from eating fast-growing grasses — called also *grass staggers*
grav *abbr* gravida

grave \ˈgrāv\ *adj* : very serious : dangerous to life — used of an illness or its prospects ⟨a ~ prognosis⟩

grav•el \ˈgra-vəl\ *n* **1** : a deposit of small calculous concretions in the kidneys and urinary bladder **2** : the condition that results from the presence of deposits of gravel

Graves' disease \ˈgrāvz-\ *n* : a common form of hyperthyroidism that is an autoimmune disorder characterized by goiter, rapid and irregular heartbeat, weight loss, irritability, anxiety, and often a slight protrusion of the eyeballs — called also *Basedow's disease, exophthalmic goiter*

Graves, Robert James (1796–1853), British physician.

grav•id \ˈgra-vəd\ *adj* : PREGNANT

grav•i•da \ˈgra-və-də\ *n, pl* **-das** *also* **-dae** \-ˌdē\ : a pregnant woman — often used in combination with a number or figure to indicate the number of pregnancies a woman has had ⟨a ~ four⟩; compare PARA — **gra•vid•ic** \gra-ˈvi-dik\ *adj*

gravidarum — see HYPEREMESIS GRAVIDARUM

gra•vid•i•ty \gra-ˈvi-də-tē\ *n, pl* **-ties** **1** : PREGNANCY **2** : the number of times a female has been pregnant — compare PARITY 2

gravior — see ICHTHYOSIS HYSTRIX GRAVIOR

gravis — see ICTERUS GRAVIS, ICTERUS GRAVIS NEONATORUM, MYASTHENIA GRAVIS

grav•i•ta•tion \ˌgra-və-ˈtā-shən\ *n* : a natural force of attraction that tends to draw bodies together and that occurs because of the mass of the bodies — **grav•i•ta•tion•al** \-shə-nəl\ *adj* — **grav•i•ta•tion•al•ly** *adv*

gravitational field *n* : the space around an object having mass in which the object's gravitational influence can be detected

grav•i•ty \ˈgra-və-tē\ *n, pl* **-ties** : the gravitational attraction of the mass of a celestial object (as earth) for bodies close to it; *also* : GRAVITATION

gravity drip *n* : the administration of a fluid into the body using an apparatus in which gravity provides the force moving the fluid

gray \ˈgrā\ *n* : the mks unit of absorbed dose of ionizing radiation equal to an energy of one joule per kilogram of irradiated material — abbr. *Gy*

Gray, Louis Harold (1905–1965), British radiobiologist.

gray column *n* : any of the longitudinal columns of gray matter in each lateral half of the spinal cord — called also *gray horn;* compare COLUMN A

gray commissure *n* : a transverse band of gray matter in the spinal cord appearing in sections as the transverse bar of the H-shaped mass of gray matter

gray matter *n* : neural tissue esp. of the brain and spinal cord that contains cell bodies as well as nerve fibers, has a brownish gray color, and forms most of the cortex and nuclei of the brain, the columns of the spinal cord, and the bodies of ganglia — called also *gray substance*

gray•out \ˈgrā-ˌau̇t\ *n* : a transient dimming or haziness of vision resulting from temporary impairment of cerebral circulation — compare BLACKOUT, REDOUT — **gray out** *vb*

gray ramus *n* : RAMUS COMMUNICANS b

gray substance *n* : GRAY MATTER

gray syndrome *n* : a potentially fatal toxic reaction to chloramphenicol esp. in premature infants that is characterized by abdominal distension, cyanosis, vasomotor collapse, and irregular respiration

GRE *abbr* gradient echo; gradient-recalled echo

grease heel *n* : a chronic inflammation of the skin of the fetlocks and pasterns of horses — called also *greasy heel*

great cerebral vein *n* : a broad unpaired vein formed by the junction of Galen's veins and uniting with the inferior sagittal sinus to form the straight sinus

greater cornu *n* : THYROHYAL

greater curvature *n* : the boundary of the stomach that forms a long usu. convex curve on the left from the opening for the esophagus to the opening into the duodenum — compare LESSER CURVATURE

greater multangular *n* : TRAPEZIUM — called also *greater multangular bone*

greater occipital nerve *n* : OCCIPITAL NERVE a

greater omentum *n* : a part of the peritoneum attached to the greater curvature of the stomach and to the colon and hanging down over the small intestine — called also *caul;* compare LESSER OMENTUM

greater palatine artery *n* : PALATINE ARTERY 1b

greater palatine foramen *n* : a foramen in each posterior side of the palate giving passage to the greater palatine artery and to a palatine nerve

greater petrosal nerve *n* : a mixed nerve that arises in the geniculate ganglion, joins with the deep petrosal nerve at the entrance of the pterygoid canal to form the Vidian nerve, and as part of this nerve sends sensory fibers to the soft palate with some to the eustachian tube and sends parasympathetic fibers forming the motor root of the pterygopalatine ganglion — called also *greater superficial petrosal nerve*

greater sciatic foramen *n* : SCIATIC FORAMEN a

greater sciatic notch *n* : SCIATIC NOTCH a

greater splanchnic nerve *n* : SPLANCHNIC NERVE a
greater superficial petrosal nerve *n* : GREATER PETROSAL NERVE
greater trochanter *also* **great trochanter** *n* : TROCHANTER a
greater tubercle *n* : a prominence on the upper lateral part of the end of the humerus that serves as the insertion for the supraspinatus, infraspinatus, and teres minor — compare LESSER TUBERCLE
greater vestibular gland *n* : BARTHOLIN'S GLAND
greater wing *also* **great wing** *n* : a broad curved winglike expanse on each side of the sphenoid bone — called also *alisphenoid;* compare LESSER WING
great ragweed *n* : RAGWEED b
great saphenous vein *n* : SAPHENOUS VEIN a
great toe *n* : BIG TOE
great white shark *n* : a large shark (*Carcharodon carcharias* of the family Lamnidae) that is bluish when young but becomes whitish with age and has been known to attack humans — called also *white shark*
green \ˈgrēn\ *adj* **1** *of a wound* : being recently incurred and unhealed **2** *of hemolytic streptococci* : tending to produce green pigment when cultured on blood media
green monkey *n* : a long-tailed African monkey (*Cercopithecus aethiops*) having greenish-appearing hair and often used in medical research — called also *vervet*
green monkey disease *n* : MARBURG HEMORRHAGIC FEVER
green•sick•ness \ˈgrēn-ˌsik-nəs\ *n* : CHLOROSIS — **green•sick** *adj*
green soap *n* : a soft soap made from vegetable oils and used esp. in the treatment of skin diseases
green•stick fracture \ˈgrēn-ˌstik-\ *n* : a bone fracture in a young individual in which the bone is partly broken and partly bent
grew *past of* GROW
grey•out *chiefly Brit var of* GRAYOUT
grief \ˈgrēf\ *n* : deep and poignant emotional distress caused by or as if by bereavement — **grieve** \ˈgrēv\ *vb*
[1]**gripe** \ˈgrīp\ *vb* **griped; grip•ing** : to cause or experience pinching and spasmodic pain in the bowels of
[2]**gripe** *n* : a pinching spasmodic intestinal pain — usu. used in pl.
grippe \ˈgrip\ *n* : an acute febrile contagious virus disease; *esp* : INFLUENZA 1a — **grippy** \ˈgri-pē\ *adj*
gris•eo•ful•vin \ˌgri-zē-ō-ˈfu̇l-vən, -sē-, -ˈfəl-\ *n* : a fungistatic antibiotic $C_{17}H_{17}ClO_6$ used systemically in treating superficial infections by fungi esp. of the genera *Epidermophyton, Microsporum,* and *Trichophyton*
griseum — see INDUSIUM GRISEUM
grocer's itch *n* : an itching dermatitis that results from prolonged contact with some mites (esp. family Acaridae), their products, or materials infested with them — called also *baker's itch;* compare GRAIN ITCH
groin \ˈgrȯin\ *n* : the fold or depression marking the juncture of the lower abdomen and the inner part of the thigh; *also* : the region of this line
groin pull *n* : a usu. sports-related injury characterized by intense pain in the region of the groin usu. due to abnormal straining or stretching of an adductor muscle of the thigh and esp. the adductor longus
groove \ˈgrüv\ *n* : a long narrow depression occurring naturally on the surface of an anatomical part
gross \ˈgrōs\ *adj* **1** : glaringly or flagrantly obvious **2** : visible without the aid of a microscope : MACROSCOPIC ⟨~ lesions⟩ — compare OCCULT
gross anatomy *n* : a branch of anatomy that deals with the macroscopic structure of tissues and organs — compare HISTOLOGY — **gross anatomist** *n*
ground itch *n* : an itching inflammation of the skin marking the point of entrance into the body of larval hookworms
ground substance *n* : a more or less homogeneous matrix that forms the background in which the specific differentiated elements of a system are suspended: **a** : the intercellular substance of tissues **b** : CYTOSOL
Group A *n* : the Lancefield group of beta-hemolytic streptococci comprising all strains of a species of the genus *Streptococcus* (*S. pyogenes*) — usu. used attributively ⟨*Group A* streptococcal infection⟩
Group B *n* : the Lancefield group of usu. beta-hemolytic streptococci comprising all strains of a species of the genus *Streptococcus* (*S. agalactiae*) — usu. used attributively ⟨*Group B* streptococcal sepsis of neonates⟩
group dynamics *n sing or pl* : the interacting forces within a small human group; *also* : the sociological study of these forces
group home *n* : a residence for persons (as developmentally disabled individuals) requiring care, assistance, or supervision
group practice *n* : medicine practiced by a group of associated physicians or dentists (as specialists in different fields) working as partners or as partners and employees
group psychotherapy *n* : GROUP THERAPY
group therapy *n* : therapy in the presence of a therapist in which several patients discuss and share their personal problems — **group therapist** *n*
grow \ˈgrō\ *vb* **grew** \ˈgrü\; **grown** \ˈgrōn\; **grow•ing** **1 a** : to spring up and develop to maturity **b** : to be able to grow in some place or situa-

tion **c** : to assume some relation through or as if through a process of natural growth ⟨the cut edges of the wound *grew* together⟩ **2** : to increase in size by addition of material by assimilation into the living organism or by accretion in a nonbiological process (as crystallization)

growing pains *n pl* : pains occurring in the legs of growing children having no demonstrable relation to growth

growth \ˈgrōth\ *n* **1 a** (1) : a stage in the process of growing (2) : full growth **b** : the process of growing **2 a** : something that grows or has grown **b** : an abnormal proliferation of tissue (as a tumor)

growth cone *n* : the specialized motile tip of an axon of a growing or regenerating neuron

growth factor *n* : a substance (as a vitamin B_{12} or an interleukin) that promotes growth and esp. cellular growth

growth hormone *n* : a polypeptide hormone that is secreted by the anterior lobe of the pituitary gland and regulates growth; *also* : a recombinant version of this hormone — called also *somatotropic hormone, somatotropin;* see BOVINE GROWTH HORMONE, HUMAN GROWTH HORMONE

growth hormone–releasing hormone *n* : a neuropeptide released by the hypothalamus that stimulates the release of growth hormone — abbr. *GHRH;* called also *growth hormone-releasing factor*

growth plate *n* : the region in a long bone between the epiphysis and diaphysis where growth in length occurs — called also *physis*

g's *or* **gs** *pl of* G

G6PD *abbr* glucose-6-phosphate dehydrogenase

G–spot \ˈjē-ˌspät\ *n* : a mass of tissue that is held to exist in the anterior vaginal wall and to be highly erogenous — called also *Grafenberg spot*

GSR *abbr* galvanic skin response

G suit *n* : a suit designed to counteract the physiological effects of acceleration on an aviator or astronaut

GSW *abbr* gunshot wound

GTH *abbr* gonadotropic hormone

GTP \ˌjē-(ˌ)tē-ˈpē\ *n* : an energy-rich nucleotide analogous to ATP that is composed of guanine linked to ribose and three phosphate groups and is necessary for peptide-bond formation during protein synthesis — called also *guanosine triphosphate*

G_2 phase \ˌjē-ˈtü-\ *n* : the period in the cell cycle from the completion of DNA replication to the beginning of cell division — compare G_1 PHASE, M PHASE, S PHASE

GU *abbr* genitourinary

guai·ac \ˈgwī-ˌak\ *n* : GUAIACUM

guai·a·col \ˈgwī-ə-ˌkȯl, -ˌkōl\ *n* : a liquid or solid compound $C_7H_8O_2$ with an aromatic odor used chiefly as an expectorant and as a local anesthetic

guaiac test *n* : a test for blood in urine or feces using a reagent containing guaiacum that yields a blue color when blood is present — see HEMOCCULT

guai·a·cum \ˈgwī-ə-kəm\ *n* : a resin with a faint balsamic odor obtained from either of two trees (*Guaiacum officinale* and *G. sanctum* of the family Zygophyllaceae) and used in various tests (as the guaiac test)

guai·fen·e·sin \gwī-ˈfe-nə-sən\ *n* : the glyceryl ether of guaiacol $C_{10}H_{14}O_4$ that is used esp. as an expectorant — called also *glyceryl guaiacolate*

gua·neth·i·dine \gwä-ˈne-thə-ˌdēn\ *n* : a drug used esp. in the form of its sulfate $C_{10}H_{22}N_4 \cdot H_2SO_4$ in treating severe high blood pressure

guan·fa·cine \ˈgwän-fə-ˌsēn\ *n* : a drug that is an alpha-adrenergic agonist taken orally in the form of its hydrochloride $C_9H_9Cl_2N_3O \cdot HCl$ esp. to treat hypertension and attention deficit disorder — see INTUNIV, TENEX

gua·ni·dine \ˈgwä-nə-ˌdēn\ *n* : a base CH_5N_3 that is derived from guanine and is used in the form of its hydrochloride $CH_5N_3 \cdot HCl$ to enhance acetylcholine activity

gua·nine \ˈgwä-ˌnēn\ *n* : a purine base $C_5H_5N_5O$ that codes genetic information in the polynucleotide chain of DNA or RNA — compare ADENINE, CYTOSINE, THYMINE, URACIL

gua·no·sine \ˈgwä-nə-ˌsēn\ *n* : a nucleoside $C_{10}H_{13}N_5O_5$ composed of guanine and ribose

guanosine 3′, 5′–monophosphate *n* : CYCLIC GMP

guanosine triphosphate *n* : GTP

gua·nyl·ate cy·clase \ˈgwän-ᵊl-ˌāt-ˈsī-ˌklās, -ˌklāz\ *n* : an enzyme that catalyzes the formation of cyclic GMP from GTP

guard·ing \ˈgär-diŋ\ *n* : involuntary reaction to protect an area of pain (as by spasm of muscle on palpation of the abdomen over a painful lesion)

gu·ber·nac·u·lum \ˌgü-bər-ˈna-kyü-ləm\ *n, pl* **-la** \-lə\ : a fibrous cord that connects the fetal testis with the bottom of the scrotum and by failing to elongate in proportion to the rest of the fetus causes the descent of the testis

guide \ˈgīd\ *n* : a grooved director for a surgical probe or knife

guided imagery *n* : any of various techniques (as a series of verbal suggestions) used to guide another person or oneself in imagining sensations and esp. in visualizing an image in the mind to bring about a desired physical response (as a reduction in stress, anxiety, or pain)

Guil·lain–Bar·ré syndrome \ˌgē-ˈlan-ˌbä-ˈrā-, ˌgē-ˈyaⁿ-\ *n* : a polyneuritis of unknown cause characterized esp. by muscle weakness and paralysis —

abbr. *GBS;* called also *Landry's paralysis*

Guillain \gē-ˈyaⁿ\, **Georges Charles (1876–1961),** and **Barré** \bä-ˈrā\, **Jean Alexander (1880–1967),** French neurologists.

guil•lo•tine \ˈgi-lə-ˌtēn, ˈgē-ə-\ *n* : a surgical instrument that consists of a ring and handle with a knife blade which slides down the handle and across the ring and that is used for cutting out a protruding structure (as a tonsil) capable of being placed in the ring

Guil•lo•tin \gē-yō-ˈtaⁿ\, **Joseph–Ignace (1738–1814),** French surgeon.

guillotine amputation *n* : an emergency surgical amputation (as of a leg) in which the skin is incised around the part being amputated and is allowed to retract, successive layers of muscle are then divided around the part, and finally the bone is divided

guilt \ˈgilt\ *n* : feelings of culpability esp. for imagined offenses or from a sense of inadequacy : morbid self-reproach often manifest in marked preoccupation with the moral correctness of one's behavior

Guin•ea worm \ˈgi-nē-\ *n* : a slender tropical parasitic nematode worm of the genus *Dracunculus* (*D. medinensis*) that causes dracunculiasis, has an adult female that may attain a length of several feet, and is characterized by a life cycle which includes larval development in tiny freshwater crustaceans (genus *Cyclops*), ingestion by humans in contaminated drinking water, passage from the intestine to the thorax and abdomen for maturation and mating, and migration of gravid females to subcutaneous tissues and then out through the skin — called also *Medina worm*

Guinea worm disease *n* : DRACUNCULIASIS

Gulf War syndrome *n* : a syndrome of uncertain cause including fatigue, joint pain, memory loss, skin rash, and headache that has been reported in veterans of the war fought in the Persian Gulf in 1991

gul•let \ˈgə-lət\ *n* : ESOPHAGUS; *broadly* : THROAT

gum \ˈgəm\ *n* : the tissue that surrounds the necks of teeth and covers the alveolar parts of the jaws; *broadly* : the alveolar portion of a jaw with its enveloping soft tissues

gum ar•a•bic \-ˈar-ə-bik\ *n* : a water-soluble gum obtained from several leguminous plants (genus *Acacia* and esp. *A. senegal* and *A. arabica*) and used esp. in pharmacy to suspend insoluble substances in water, to prepare emulsions, and to make pills and lozenges — called also *acacia, gum acacia*

gum•boil \ˈgəm-ˌbȯil\ *n* : an abscess in the gum

gum karaya *n* : KARAYA GUM

gum•line \ˈgəm-ˌlīn\ *n* : the line separating the gum from the exposed part of the tooth

gum•ma \ˈgə-mə\ *n, pl* **gummas** *also* **gum•ma•ta** \-mə-tə\ : a tumor of gummy or rubbery consistency that is characteristic of the tertiary stage of syphilis — **gum•ma•tous** \-mə-təs\ *adj*

gum tragacanth *n* : TRAGACANTH

gur•ney \ˈgər-nē\ *n, pl* **gurneys** : a wheeled cot or stretcher

gus•ta•tion \ˌgəs-ˈtā-shən\ *n* : the act or sensation of tasting

gus•ta•to•ry \ˈgəs-tə-ˌtōr-ē\ *adj* : relating to, affecting, associated with, or being the sense of taste

gut \ˈgət\ *n* **1 a** : DIGESTIVE TRACT; *also* : part of the digestive tract and esp. the intestine or stomach **b** : ABDOMEN 1a, BELLY — usu. used in pl.; not often in formal use **2** : CATGUT

Guth•rie test \ˈgə-thrē-\ *n* : a test for phenylketonuria in which the plasma phenylalanine of an affected individual reverses the inhibition of a strain of bacteria of the genus *Bacillus* (*B. subtilis*) needing it for growth

Guthrie, Robert (1916–1995), American microbiologist.

gut•ta–per•cha \ˌgə-tə-ˈpər-chə\ *n* : a tough plastic substance from the latex of several Malaysian trees (genera *Payena* and *Palaquium*) of the sapodilla family (Sapotaceae) that is used in dentistry esp. as a filling in root canals

gut•tate \ˈgə-ˌtāt\ *adj* : having small usu. colored spots or drops

gut•ter \ˈgə-tər\ *n* : a depressed furrow between body parts (as on the surface between a pair of adjacent ribs) — see PARACOLIC GUTTER

Gut•zeit test \ˈgüt-ˌsīt-\ *n* : a test for arsenic used esp. in toxicology

Gutzeit, Ernst Wilhelm Heinrich (1845–1888), German chemist.

GVH *abbr* graft-versus-host

GVHD *abbr* graft-versus-host disease

Gy *abbr* gray

Gym•no•din•i•um \ˌjim-nə-ˈdi-nē-əm\ *n* : a large genus of marine and freshwater dinoflagellates (family Gymnodiniidae) that includes a few forms which cause red tide

gyn *abbr* gynecologic; gynecologist; gynecology

gynaec- *or* **gynaeco-** *chiefly Brit var of* GYNEC-

gy•nae•coid, gy•nae•col•o•gy *chiefly Brit var of* GYNECOID, GYNECOLOGY

gyn•an•dro•blas•to•ma \(ˌ)gī-ˌnan-drə-bla-ˈstō-mə, (ˌ)ji-, jī-\ *n, pl* **-mas** *also* **-ma•ta** \-mə-tə\ : a rare tumor of the ovary with both masculinizing and feminizing effects — compare ARRHENOBLASTOMA

gynec- *or* **gyneco-** *comb form* : woman ⟨*gyneco*id⟩ ⟨*gyneco*logy⟩

gy•ne•cog•ra•phy \ˌgī-nə-ˈkä-grə-fē, ˌji-\ *n, pl* **-phies** : radiographic visualization of the female reproductive tract

gy•ne•coid \ˈgī-ni-ˌkȯid, ˈji-\ *adj* **1** *of the pelvis* : having the rounded form typical of the human female — compare ANDROID 1, ANTHROPOID, PLATYPELLOID **2** : relating to or characterized by the distribution of body fat chiefly in the region of the hips and thighs ⟨~ obesity⟩ — compare ANDROID 2

gy·ne·col·o·gist \ˌgī-nə-ˈkä-lə-jist, ˌji-, ˌjī-\ *n* : a specialist in gynecology

gy·ne·col·o·gy \ˌgī-nə-ˈkä-lə-jē, ˌji-, ˌjī-\ *n, pl* **-gies** : a branch of medicine that deals with the diseases and routine physical care of the reproductive system of women — **gy·ne·co·log·ic** \-ni-kə-ˈlä-jik\ *or* **gy·ne·co·log·i·cal** \-ji-kəl\ *adj*

gy·ne·co·mas·tia \ˈgī-nə-kō-ˈmas-tē-ə, ˈji-, ˈjī-\ *n* : excessive development of the breast in the male

gy·noid \ˈgī-ˌnȯid, ˈji-\ *adj* : GYNECOID 2

gyp·py tummy \ˈji-pē-\ *n* : diarrhea contracted esp. by travelers

gy·rase \ˈjī-ˌrās, -ˌrāz\ *n* : a bacterial enzyme that catalyzes the breaking and rejoining of bonds linking adjacent nucleotides in circular DNA to generate supercoiled DNA helices

gy·rate \ˈjī-ˌrāt\ *adj* : winding or coiled around : CONVOLUTED

gyrate atrophy *n* : progressive degeneration of the choroid and pigment epithelium of the retina that is inherited as an autosomal recessive trait and is characterized esp. by myopia, constriction of the visual field, night blindness, and cataracts

gy·ra·tion \jī-ˈrā-shən\ *n* : the pattern of convolutions of the brain

Gy·ro·mi·tra \ˌjī-rō-ˈmī-trə, ˌjir-ə-\ *n* : a genus of ascomycetous fungi (family Helvellaceae) that are usu. poisonous and often deadly when eaten — see FALSE MOREL

gy·rus \ˈjī-rəs\ *n, pl* **gy·ri** \-ˌrī\ : a convoluted ridge between anatomical grooves; *esp* : CONVOLUTION

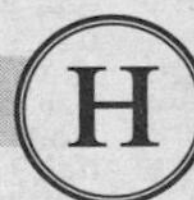

h *abbr* **1** height **2** [Latin *hora*] hour — used in writing prescriptions; see QH

H *abbr* heroin

H *symbol* hydrogen

HA *abbr* hemagglutinin

HAART \ˈhärt\ *n* : HIGHLY ACTIVE ANTIRETROVIRAL THERAPY

ha·ben·u·la \hə-ˈben-yə-lə\ *n, pl* **-lae** \-ˌlī, -ˌlē\ **1** : TRIGONUM HABENULAE **2** : either of two nuclei of which one lies on each side of the pineal gland under the corresponding trigonum habenulae, is composed of two groups of nerve cells, and forms a correlation center for olfactory stimuli — called also *habenular nucleus* — **ha·ben·u·lar** \-lər\ *adj*

habenular commissure *n* : a band of nerve fibers situated in front of the pineal gland that connects the habenular nucleus on one side with that on the other

hab·it \ˈha-bət\ *n* **1** : a behavior pattern acquired by frequent repetition or physiological exposure that shows itself in regularity or increased facility of performance **2** : an acquired mode of behavior that has become nearly or completely involuntary **3** : ADDICTION

hab·i·tat \ˈha-bə-ˌtat\ *n* : the place or environment where a plant or animal naturally occurs

habit–forming *adj* : inducing the formation of an addiction

ha·bit·u·al \hə-ˈbi-chə-wəl\ *adj* **1** : having the nature of a habit : being in accordance with habit **2** : doing, practicing, or acting in some manner by force of habit — **ha·bit·u·al·ly** *adv*

habitual abortion *n* : spontaneous abortion occurring in three or more successive pregnancies

ha·bit·u·a·tion \-ˌbi-chə-ˈwā-shən\ *n* **1** : the act or process of making habitual or accustomed **2 a** : tolerance to the effects of a drug acquired through continued use **b** : psychological dependence on a drug after a period of use — compare ADDICTION **3** : a form of nonassociative learning characterized by a decrease in responsiveness upon repeated exposure to a stimulus — compare SENSITIZATION 3 — **ha·bit·u·ate** \-ˈbi-chə-ˌwāt\ *vb*

hab·i·tus \ˈha-bə-təs\ *n, pl* **habitus** \-təs, -ˌtüs\ : HABIT; *specif* : body build and constitution esp. as related to predisposition to disease

Hab·ro·ne·ma \ˌha-brō-ˈnē-mə\ *n* : a genus of parasitic nematode worms (family Spiruridae) that are stomach parasites of horses and birds — see HABRONEMIASIS

hab·ro·ne·mi·a·sis \ˌha-brə-nē-ˈmī-ə-səs\ *n, pl* **-a·ses** \-ˌsēz\ : infestation with or disease caused by roundworms of the genus *Habronema*

hack \ˈhak\ *n* : a short dry cough — **hack** *vb*

haem- *or* **haemo-** *chiefly Brit var of* HEM-

haema- *chiefly Brit var of* HEMA-

hae·ma·cy·tom·e·ter, hae·mal, haem·an·gi·o·ma *chiefly Brit var of* HEMACYTOMETER, HEMAL, HEMANGIOMA

Hae·ma·phy·sa·lis \ˌhē-mə-ˈfī-sə-ləs, ˌhe-\ *n* : a cosmopolitan genus of small ixodid ticks including some that are disease carriers — see KYASANUR FOREST DISEASE

haemat- *or* **haemato-** *chiefly Brit var of* HEMAT-

hae•ma•tem•e•sis, hae•ma•tog•e•nous *chiefly Brit var of* HEMATEMESIS, HEMATOGENOUS

haematobium — see SCHISTOSOMIASIS HAEMATOBIUM

Hae•ma•to•pi•nus \-tə-ˈpī-nəs\ *n* : a genus of sucking lice that are parasitic on various domestic animals (as cattle and swine) — see HOG LOUSE

-hae•mia *chiefly Brit var of* -EMIA

hae•mo•bar•ton•el•la \ˌhē-mō-ˌbär-tə-ˈne-lə, ˌhe-\ *n* **1** *cap* : a genus of bacteria (family Anaplasmataceae) that are blood parasites in various mammals **2** *pl* **-lae** \-ˌlē, -ˌlī\ : a bacterium of the genus *Haemobartonella*

hae•mo•bar•ton•el•lo•sis *also* **he•mo•bar•ton•el•los•is** \-tə-nə-ˈlō-səs\ *n, pl* **-lo•ses** \-ˌsēz\ : an infection or disease caused by bacteria currently or formerly of the genus *Haemobartonella*; *esp* : FELINE INFECTIOUS ANEMIA

hae•mo•glo•bin *chiefly Brit var of* HEMOGLOBIN

Hae•mon•chus \hē-ˈmäŋ-kəs\ *n* : a genus of nematode worms (family Trichostrongylidae) including a parasite (*H. contortus*) of the stomach of ruminants (as sheep)

hae•mo•phil•ia *chiefly Brit var of* HEMOPHILIA

hae•moph•i•lus \hē-ˈmä-fə-ləs\ *n* **1** *cap* : a genus of nonmotile gram-negative rod-shaped bacteria (family Pasteurellaceae) that include several important pathogens (as *H. influenzae* associated with meningitis, pneumonia, conjunctivitis, and otitis media and *H. ducreyi* of chancroid) **2** *pl* **-li** \-ˌlī, -ˌlē\ : any bacterium of the genus *Haemophilus* — see HIB

Hae•mo•pro•te•us \ˌhē-mō-ˈprō-tē-əs, ˌhe-mə-\ *n* : a genus of protozoan parasites (family Haemoproteidae) occurring in the blood of some birds

haem•or•rhage, haem•or•rhoid *chiefly Brit var of* HEMORRHAGE, HEMORRHOID

haf•ni•um \ˈhaf-nē-əm\ *n* : a metallic element that readily absorbs neutrons — symbol *Hf;* see ELEMENT table

Hag•e•man factor \ˈha-gə-mən-, ˈhäg-mən-\ *n* : FACTOR XII

Hageman (*fl* 1963), hospital patient.

hair \ˈhar\ *n, often attrib* **1** : a slender threadlike outgrowth of the epidermis of an animal; *esp* : one of the usu. pigmented filaments that form the characteristic coat of a mammal **2** : the hairy covering of an animal or a body part; *esp* : the coating of hairs on a human head — **hairlike** *adj*

hair ball *n* : a compact mass of hair formed in the stomach esp. of a shedding animal (as a cat) that cleanses its coat by licking — called also *trichobezoar*

hair bulb *n* : the bulbous expansion at the base of a hair from which the hair shaft develops

hair cell *n* : a cell with hairlike processes; *esp* : one of the sensory cells in the auditory epithelium of the organ of Corti

haired \ˈhard\ *adj* : having hair esp. of a specified kind — usu. used in combination <red-*haired*>

hair follicle *n* : the tubular epithelial sheath that surrounds the lower part of the hair shaft and encloses at the bottom a vascular papilla supplying the growing basal part of the hair with nourishment

hair•line \ˈhar-ˈlīn\ *n* : the outline of scalp hair esp. on the forehead

hairline fracture *n* : a fracture that appears as a narrow crack along the surface of a bone

hair puller *n* : an individual affected with trichotillomania

hair•pull•ing \ˈher-ˌpu̇-liŋ\ *n* : the often pathological habit of pulling out one's hair one or a few hairs at a time — see TRICHOTILLOMANIA

hair root *n* : ROOT 2

hair shaft *n* : the part of a hair projecting beyond the surface of the skin

hair•worm \ˈhar-ˌwərm\ *n* : any nematode worm of the genus *Capillaria*

hairy cell leukemia \ˈhar-ē-\ *n* : a chronic leukemia that is usu. of B cell origin and is characterized by malignant cells with a ciliated appearance that replace bone marrow and infiltrate the spleen causing splenomegaly

hairy leukoplakia *n* : a condition that affects the mouth and esp. the edges of the tongue, is characterized by poorly demarcated white raised lesions with a corrugated appearance, is caused by infection with the Epstein-Barr virus, and is associated with HIV infection and AIDS — called also *oral hairy leukoplakia*

hal•a•zone \ˈha-lə-ˌzōn\ *n* : a white powdery acid $C_7H_5Cl_2NO_4S$ used as a disinfectant for drinking water

Hal•cion \ˈhal-sē-ˌän\ *trademark* — used for a preparation of triazolam

Hal•dol \ˈhal-ˌdȯl, -ˌdōl\ *trademark* — used for a preparation of haloperidol

half–life \ˈhaf-ˌlīf\ *n* **1** : the time required for half of the atoms of a radioactive substance to become disintegrated **2** : the time required for half the amount of a substance (as a drug or radioactive tracer) in or introduced into a living system or ecosystem to be eliminated or disintegrated by natural processes

half–moon \-ˌmün\ *n* : LUNULA a

half–value layer *n* : the thickness of an absorbing substance necessary to reduce by one half the initial intensity of the radiation passing through it

halfway house *n* : a center for individuals after institutionalization (as for mental illness or drug addiction) that is designed to facilitate their readjustment to private life

halibut–liver oil *n* : a yellowish to brownish fatty oil from the liver of the halibut used chiefly as a source of vitamin A

hal·i·to·sis \ˌha-lə-ˈtō-səs\ *n, pl* **-to·ses** \-ˌsēz\ : a condition of having fetid breath

hal·lu·ci·na·tion \hə-ˌlüs-ᵊn-ˈā-shən\ *n* **1** : a perception of something (as a visual image or a sound) with no external cause usu. arising from a disorder of the nervous system (as in delirium tremens) or in response to drugs (as LSD) **2** : the object of an hallucinatory perception — **hal·lu·ci·nate** \-ˈlüs-ᵊn-ˌāt\ *vb* — **hal·lu·ci·na·tor** \-ˈlüs-ᵊn-ˌā-tər\ *n* — **hal·lu·ci·na·to·ry** \-ˈlüs-ᵊn-ə-ˌtōr-ē\ *adj*

hal·lu·ci·no·gen \hə-ˈlüs-ᵊn-ə-jən\ *n* : a substance and esp. a drug that induces hallucinations

¹hal·lu·ci·no·gen·ic \hə-ˌlüs-ᵊn-ə-ˈje-nik\ *adj* : causing hallucinations — **hal·lu·ci·no·gen·i·cal·ly** \-ni-k(ə-)lē\ *adv*

²hallucinogenic *n* : HALLUCINOGEN

hal·lu·ci·no·sis \hə-ˌlüs-ᵊn-ˈō-səs\ *n, pl* **-no·ses** \-ˌsēz\ : a pathological mental state characterized by hallucinations

hallucis — see ABDUCTOR HALLUCIS, ADDUCTOR HALLUCIS, EXTENSOR HALLUCIS BREVIS, EXTENSOR HALLUCIS LONGUS, FLEXOR HALLUCIS BREVIS, FLEXOR HALLUCIS LONGUS

hal·lux \ˈha-ləks\ *n, pl* **hal·lu·ces** \ˈha-lə-ˌsēz, ˈhal-yə-\ : the innermost digit of the foot : BIG TOE

hallux rig·id·us \-ˈri-jə-dəs\ *n* : restricted mobility of the big toe due to stiffness of the metatarsophalangeal joint esp. when due to arthritic changes in the joint

hallux val·gus \-ˈval-gəs\ *n* : an abnormal deviation of the big toe away from the midline of the body or toward the other toes of the foot that is associated esp. with the wearing of ill-fitting shoes

ha·lo \ˈhā-(ˌ)lō\ *n, pl* **halos** *or* **haloes** **1** : a circle of light appearing to surround a luminous body; *esp* : one seen as the result of the presence of glaucoma **2** : a differentiated zone surrounding a central object **3** : an orthopedic device used to immobilize the head and neck (as to treat fracture of neck vertebrae) that consists of a metal band placed around the head and fastened to the skull usu. with metal pins and that is attached by extensions to an inflexible vest — called also *halo brace*

halo effect *n* : generalization from the perception of one outstanding personality trait to an overly favorable evaluation of the whole personality

hal·o·fan·trine \ˌha-lə-ˈfan-ˌtrēn\ *n* : an antimalarial drug used in the form of its hydrochloride $C_{26}H_{30}Cl_2F_3NO·HCl$ esp. against chloroquine-resistant falciparum malaria

halo·gen \ˈha-lə-jən\ *n* : any of the five elements fluorine, chlorine, bromine, iodine, and astatine that exist in the free state normally with two atoms per molecule

hal·o·ge·ton \ˌha-lə-ˈjē-ˌtän\ *n* : a coarse herb (*Halogeton glomeratus* of the family Chenopodiaceae) that in western U.S. ranges is dangerous to sheep and cattle because of its high oxalate content

halo·per·i·dol \ˌha-lō-ˈper-ə-ˌdȯl, -ˌdōl\ *n* : a butyrophenone antipsychotic drug $C_{21}H_{23}ClFNO_2$ used esp. to treat schizophrenia and to control the involuntary tics and vocalizations of Tourette's syndrome — see HALDOL

halo·thane \ˈha-lə-ˌthān\ *n* : a nonexplosive inhalational anesthetic $C_2HBrClF_3$

Hal·sted radical mastectomy \ˈhal-ˌsted-\ *n* : RADICAL MASTECTOMY — called also *Halsted radical*

Halsted, William Stewart (1852–1922), American surgeon.

hal·zoun \ˌhal-ˈzün, ˈhal-zün\ *n* : infestation of the larynx and pharynx esp. by tongue worms (genus *Linguatula* and esp. *L. serrata*) consumed in raw liver

ham \ˈham\ *n* **1** : the part of the leg behind the knee : the hollow of the knee : POPLITEAL SPACE **2** : a buttock with its associated thigh or with the posterior part of a thigh — usu. used in pl.

hama·dry·ad \ˌha-mə-ˈdrī-əd, -ˌad\ *n* : KING COBRA

ham·ar·to·ma \ˌha-ˌmar-ˈtō-mə\ *n, pl* **-mas** *also* **-ma·ta** \-mə-tə\ : a mass resembling a tumor that represents anomalous development of tissue natural to a part or organ rather than a true tumor

ha·mate \ˈhā-ˌmāt, ˈha-mət\ *n* : a bone on the little-finger side of the second row of the carpus — called also *hamate bone, unciform, unciform bone*

ham·mer \ˈha-mər\ *n* : MALLEUS

ham·mer·toe \ˈha-mər-ˌtō\ *n* : a deformed claw-shaped toe and esp. the second that results from permanent angular flexion between one or both phalangeal joints — called also *claw toe*

¹ham·string \ˈham-ˌstriŋ\ *n* **1 a** : either of two groups of tendons bounding the upper part of the popliteal space at the back of the knee and forming the tendons of insertion of some muscles of the back of the thigh **b** : HAMSTRING MUSCLE **2** : a large tendon above and behind the hock of a quadruped

²hamstring *vb* **-strung** \-ˌstrəŋ\; **-string·ing** \-ˌstriŋ-iŋ\ : to cripple by cutting the leg tendons

hamstring muscle *n* : any of three muscles at the back of the thigh that function to flex and rotate the leg and extend the thigh: **a** : SEMIMEMBRANOSUS **b** : SEMITENDINOSUS **c** : BICEPS b

ham•u•lus \ˈha-myə-ləs\ *n, pl* **-u•li** \-ˌlī, -ˌlē\ : a hook or hooked process

hand \ˈhand\ *n, often attrib* : the terminal part of the vertebrate forelimb when modified (as in humans) as a grasping organ

hand•ed \ˈhan-dəd\ *adj* **1** : having a hand or hands esp. of a specified kind or number — usu. used in combination ⟨a large-*handed* man⟩ **2** : using a specified hand or number of hands — used in combination ⟨right-*handed*⟩

hand•ed•ness \-nəs\ *n* : a tendency to use one hand rather than the other

hand, foot and mouth disease *n* : a usu. mild contagious viral disease esp. of young children that is characterized by fever, malaise, sore throat, and typically painful fluid-filled blisters in the mouth, on the hands and feet, and sometimes in the diaper-covered area and is caused by an enterovirus (species *Enterovirus A*, esp. serotype *coxsackievirus A16*) — compare FOOT-AND-MOUTH DISEASE

hand•i•cap \ˈhan-di-ˌkap, -dē-\ *n* **1** : a disadvantage that makes achievement unusually difficult **2** *sometimes offensive* : a physical disability

hand•i•capped \-ˌkapt\ *adj, sometimes offensive* : having a physical or mental disability; *also* : of or reserved for individuals with a physical disability

hand•piece \ˈhand-ˌpēs\ *n* : the handheld part of an electrically powered dental apparatus that holds the revolving instruments (as a bur)

Hand–Schül•ler–Chris•tian disease \ˈhand-ˈshü-lər-ˈkris-chən-\ *n* : an inflammatory histiocytosis associated with disturbances in cholesterol metabolism that occurs chiefly in young children and is marked by cystic defects of the skull and by exophthalmos and diabetes insipidus — called also *Schüller-Christian disease*

Hand, Alfred (1868–1949), American physician.

Schüller \ˈshue-ler\, **Artur (1874–1958),** Austrian neurologist.

Christian, Henry Asbury (1876–1951), American physician.

hang•nail \ˈhaŋ-ˌnāl\ *n* : a bit of skin hanging loose at the side or root of a fingernail

hang•over \-ˌō-vər\ *n* : disagreeable physical effects (as headache or nausea) following heavy consumption of alcohol or the use of drugs

hang–up \-ˌəp\ *n* : a source of mental or emotional difficulty

Han•sen's bacillus \ˈhan-sənz-\ *n* : a bacterium of the genus *Mycobacterium* (*M. leprae*) that causes leprosy

Han•sen \ˈhän-sen\, **Gerhard Henrik Armauer (1841–1912),** Norwegian physician.

Hansen's disease *n* : LEPROSY

Han•ta•an virus \ˈhan-tə-ən-\ *n* : a hantavirus (species *Hantaan virus*) that causes hemorrhagic fever with renal syndrome and esp. Korean hemorrhagic fever

han•ta•vi•rus \ˈhan-tə-ˌvī-rəs\ *n* **1** *cap* : a genus of bunyaviruses that infect rodents as their natural hosts, are transmitted to humans esp. by exposure to the virus in airborne particles of rodent feces and urine, and include viruses causing hantavirus pulmonary syndrome and hemorrhagic fever with renal syndrome **2** : any virus of the genus *Hantavirus*

hantavirus pulmonary syndrome *n* : an acute respiratory disease caused by various hantaviruses and characterized initially esp. by fatigue, fever and muscle pain which rapidly progress to pulmonary edema and hypoxia often resulting in death from shock or cardiac complications

H antigen \ˈāch-\ *n* : any of various antigens associated with the flagella of motile bacteria and used in serological identification of various bacteria — compare O ANTIGEN

HA1c \ˌāch-ˌā-ˌwən-ˈsē\ *n* : HEMOGLOBIN A1C

hap•a•lo•nych•ia \ˌha-pə-lō-ˈni-kē-ə\ *n* : abnormal softness of the fingernails or toenails

HAPE *abbr* high-altitude pulmonary edema

hap•loid \ˈha-ˌplȯid\ *adj* : having the gametic number of chromosomes or half the number characteristic of somatic cells : MONOPLOID — **haploid** *n* — **hap•loi•dy** \-ˌplȯi-dē\ *n*

hap•lo•scope \ˈha-plə-ˌskōp\ *n* : a simple stereoscope that is used in the study of depth perception

hap•lo•type \-ˌtīp\ *n* : a group of alleles of different genes (as of the major histocompatibility complex) on a single chromosome that are closely enough linked to be inherited usu. as a unit

hapt- *or* **hapto-** *comb form* : contact : touch : combination ⟨*hapt*en⟩

hap•ten \ˈhap-ˌten\ *n* : a small separable part of an antigen that reacts specif. with an antibody but is incapable of stimulating antibody production except in combination with an associated protein molecule — **hap•ten•ic** \hap-ˈte-nik\ *adj*

hap•tic \ˈhap-tik\ *adj* **1** : relating to or based on the sense of touch **2** : characterized by a predilection for the sense of touch

hap•tics \-tiks\ *n* : a science concerned with the sense of touch

hap•to•glo•bin \ˈhap-tə-ˌglō-bən\ *n* : any of several forms of an alpha globulin found in blood serum that can combine with free hemoglobin in the plasma and thereby prevent the loss of iron into the urine

hard \ˈhärd\ *adj* **1** : not easily penetrated : not easily yielding to pressure **2** : of or relating to radiation of relatively high penetrating power ⟨∼ X-rays⟩ **3** : being at once addictive and gravely detrimental to health ⟨such ∼ drugs as heroin⟩ **4** : resistant to biodegradation ⟨~ pesticides like DDT⟩ — **hard•ness** *n*

hard•en•ing \ˈhärd-ᵊn-iŋ\ *n* : SCLEROSIS 1 ⟨~ of the arteries⟩

hard–of–hearing *adj* : of or relating to a defective but functional sense of hearing

hard pad *n* : a serious and frequently fatal virus disease of dogs now considered to be a form of distemper — called also *hard pad disease*

hard palate *n* : the bony anterior part of the palate forming the roof of the mouth

Har•dy–Wein•berg law \ˈhär-dē-ˈwīn-ˌbərg-\ *n* : a fundamental principle of population genetics: population gene frequencies and population genotype frequencies remain constant from generation to generation if mating is random and if mutation, selection, immigration, and emigration do not occur — called also *Hardy-Weinberg principle*

Hardy, Godfrey Harold (1877–1947), British mathematician.

Wein•berg \ˈvīn-berk\, **Wilhelm (1862–1937),** German physician and geneticist.

hare•lip \ˈhar-ˌlip\ *n, sometimes offensive* : CLEFT LIP — **hare•lipped** \-ˌlipt\ *adj*

har•ma•line \ˈhär-mə-ˈlēn\ *n* : a hallucinogenic alkaloid $C_{13}H_{14}N_2O$ found in several plants (*Peganum harmala* of the family Zygophyllaceae and *Banisteriopsis* spp. of the family Malpighiaceae) that is a stimulant of the central nervous system

har•mine \ˈhär-ˈmēn\ *n* : a hallucinogenic alkaloid $C_{13}H_{12}N_2O$ similar to harmaline

Hart•mann's solution \ˈhärt-mənz-\ *n* : LACTATED RINGER'S SOLUTION

Hartmann, Alexis Frank (1898–1964), American pediatrician.

Hart•nup disease \ˈhärt-ˌnəp-\ *n* : an inherited metabolic disease that is caused by abnormalities of the renal tubules and is characterized esp. by aminoaciduria, a dry red scaly rash, and episodic muscular incoordination

Hartnup (*fl* 1950s), British family.

harts•horn \ˈhärts-ˌhȯrn\ *n* : a preparation of ammonia used as smelling salts — see SPIRIT OF HARTSHORN

harvest mite *n* : CHIGGER 2

Har•vo•ni \här-ˈvō-nē\ *trademark* — used for a preparation of ledipasvir and sofosbuvir

hash \ˈhash\ *n* : HASHISH

Ha•shi•mo•to's thyroiditis *also* **Hashimoto thyroiditis** \ˌhä-shē-ˈmō-(ˌ)tō(z)-\ *n* : a chronic autoimmune thyroiditis that is characterized by thyroid enlargement, thyroid fibrosis, lymphatic infiltration of thyroid tissue, and the production of antibodies which attack the thyroid — called also *Hashimoto's disease, Hashimoto's struma, struma lymphomatosa*

Hashimoto, Hakaru (1881–1934), Japanese surgeon.

hash•ish \ˈha-ˌshēsh, ha-ˈshēsh\ *n* : the concentrated resin from the flowering tops of the female hemp plant (*Cannabis sativa*) that is smoked, chewed, or drunk for its intoxicating effect — called also *charas;* compare BHANG, MARIJUANA

Has•sall's corpuscle \ˈha-səlz-\ *n* : one of the small bodies of the medulla of the thymus having granular cells at the center surrounded by concentric layers of modified epithelial cells — called also *thymic corpuscle*

Hassall, Arthur Hill (1817–1894), British physician and chemist.

has•si•um \ˈha-sē-əm\ *n* : a short-lived radioactive element produced artificially — symbol *Hs;* see ELEMENT table

hatch•et \ˈha-chət\ *n* : a dental excavator

hatha yoga \ˈhə-tə-\ *n* : a form of yoga emphasizing a system of physical postures for balancing, stretching, and strengthening the body

haus•tra•tion \hȯ-ˈstrā-shən\ *n* **1** : the property or state of having haustra **2** : HAUSTRUM

haus•trum \ˈhȯ-strəm\ *n, pl* **haus•tra** \-strə\ : one of the pouches or sacculations into which the large intestine is divided — **haus•tral** \-strəl\ *adj*

HAV *abbr* hepatitis A virus

ha•ver•sian canal \hə-ˈvər-zhən-\ *n, often cap H* : any of the small canals through which the blood vessels ramify in bone

Ha•vers \ˈhā-vərz, ˈha-\, **Clopton (1655?–1702),** British osteologist.

haversian system *n, often cap H* : a haversian canal with the laminae of bone that surround it — called also *osteon*

Hav•rix \ˈhav-riks\ *trademark* — used for a vaccine against hepatitis A

haw \ˈhȯ\ *n* : NICTITATING MEMBRANE; *esp* : an inflamed nictitating membrane of a domesticated mammal

hawk \ˈhȯk\ *vb* : to make a harsh coughing sound in or as if in clearing the throat; *also* : to raise by hawking ⟨~ up phlegm⟩ — **hawk** *n*

hay fever *n* : an acute allergic reaction to pollen that is usu. seasonal and is marked by sneezing, nasal discharge and congestion, and itching and watering of the eyes — called also *pollinosis*

haz•mat \ˈhaz-ˌmat\ *n, often attrib* : a material (as one that is flammable) that would be a danger to life or to the environment if released without necessary precautions being taken

Hb *abbr* hemoglobin

H band \ˈāch-\ *n* : a relatively pale band in the middle of the A band of striated muscle

HbA1c \ˌāch-ˌbē-ˌā-ˌwən-ˈsē\ *n* : HEMOGLOBIN A1C

HBOT *abbr* hyperbaric oxygen therapy

HBsAg *abbr* hepatitis B surface antigen

HBV *abbr* hepatitis B virus

HCG *abbr* human chorionic gonadotropin

HCM *abbr* hypertrophic cardiomyopathy

HCMV *abbr* human cytomegalovirus

HCT *abbr* hematocrit

HCTZ *abbr* hydrochlorothiazide

HCV *abbr* hepatitis C virus

HDL \ˌāch-(ˌ)dē-ˈel\ *n* : a lipoprotein of blood plasma that is composed of a high proportion of protein with little triglyceride and cholesterol and that is associated with decreased probability of developing atherosclerosis — called also *alpha-lipoprotein, good cholesterol, high-density lipoprotein;* compare LDL, VLDL

HDLC *abbr* HDL cholesterol; high density lipoprotein cholesterol

HDV *abbr* hepatitis D virus

He *symbol* helium

head \ˈhed\ *n* **1** : the division of the human body that contains the brain, the eyes, the ears, the nose, and the mouth; *also* : the corresponding anterior division of the body of all vertebrates, most arthropods, and many other animals **2** : HEADACHE **3** : a projection or extremity esp. of an anatomical part: as **a** : the rounded proximal end of a long bone (as the humerus) **b** : the end of a muscle nearest the origin **4** : the part of a boil, pimple, or abscess at which it is likely to break — **head** *adj*

head•ache \ˈhe-ˌdāk\ *n* : pain in the head — called also *cephalalgia* — **head•achy** \-ˌdā-kē\ *adj*

head cold *n* : a common cold centered in the nasal passages and adjacent mucous tissues

head louse *n* : a sucking louse of the genus *Pediculus* (*P. humanus capitis*) that lives on the human scalp

head nurse *n* : CHARGE NURSE; *esp* : one with overall responsibility for the supervision of the administrative and clinical aspects of nursing care

heal \ˈhēl\ *vb* **1** : to make or become sound or whole esp. in bodily condition **2** : to cure of disease or affliction — **heal•er** \ˈhē-lər\ *n*

[1]**heal•ing** \ˈhē-liŋ\ *n* **1** : the act or process of curing or of restoring to health **2** : the process of getting well

[2]**healing** *adj* : tending to heal or cure : CURATIVE ⟨a ~ art⟩

health \ˈhelth\ *n, often attrib* **1** : the condition of an organism or one of its parts in which it performs its vital functions normally or properly : the state of being sound in body or mind; *esp* : freedom from physical disease and pain — compare DISEASE **2** : the condition of an organism with respect to the performance of its vital functions esp. as evaluated subjectively ⟨how is your ~ today⟩

health care *n* : the maintenance and restoration of health by the treatment and prevention of disease esp. by trained and licensed professionals — **health–care** *adj*

health department *n* : a division of a local or larger government responsible for the oversight and care of matters relating to public health

health•ful \ˈhelth-fəl\ *adj* : beneficial to health of body or mind — **health•ful•ly** *adv* — **health•ful•ness** *n*

health insurance *n* : insurance against loss through illness of the insured; *esp* : insurance providing compensation for medical expenses

Health Insurance Portability and Accountability Act *n* : a federal law enacted in 1996 that protects continuity of health coverage (as when a person changes jobs), that limits health-plan exclusions for preexisting conditions, that requires patient medical information be kept private and secure, that standardizes electronic transactions involving health information, and that permits tax deduction of health insurance premiums by the self-employed — abbr. *HIPAA*

health maintenance organization *n* : HMO

health spa *n* : SPA 2; *esp* : one emphasizing health and fitness

health visitor *n, Brit* : a trained person who is usu. a qualified nurse and is employed by a local British authority to visit people in their homes and advise them on health matters

healthy \ˈhel-thē\ *adj* **health•i•er; health•i•est** **1** : enjoying health and vigor of body, mind, or spirit **2** : revealing a state of health **3** : conducive to health — **health•i•ly** \-thə-lē\ *adv* — **health•i•ness** \-thē-nəs\ *n*

hear \ˈhir\ *vb* **heard** \ˈhərd\; **hear•ing** : to perceive or have the capacity to perceive sound

hearing *n* : one of the senses that is concerned with the perception of sound, is mediated through the organ of Corti, is normally sensitive in humans to sound vibrations between 16 and 27,000 hertz but most receptive to those between 2000 and 5000 hertz, is conducted centrally by the cochlear branch of the auditory nerve, and is coordinated esp. in the medial geniculate body

hearing aid *n* : an electronic device usu. worn in or behind the ear of a hearing-impaired person for amplifying sound

hearing dog *n* : a dog trained to alert its deaf or hearing-impaired owner to sounds (as of a doorbell or telephone) — called also *hearing ear dog*

heart \ˈhärt\ *n* : a hollow muscular organ of vertebrate animals that by its rhythmic contraction acts as a pump maintaining the circulation of the blood and that in the human adult is about five inches (13 centimeters) long and three and one half inches (9 centimeters) broad, is of conical form, is enclosed in a serous pericardium, and consists as in other mammals and in birds of four chambers divided into an upper pair of rather thin-walled atria which receive blood from the veins and a lower pair of thick-walled ventricles into which the blood is forced and which in turn pump it into the arteries

heart attack *n* : an acute episode of coronary heart disease marked by the death or damage of heart muscle due to insufficient blood supply to the heart muscle itself usu. as a result of a coronary thrombosis or a coronary occlusion and that is characterized esp. by discomfort and pain in the chest — called also *acute myocardial infarction, myocardial infarction;* compare ANGINA PECTORIS, CORONARY INSUFFICIENCY, HEART FAILURE 1

heart·beat \ˈhärt-ˌbēt\ *n* : one complete pulsation of the heart

heart block *n* : incoordination of the heartbeat in which the atria and ventricles beat independently due to defective transmission through the bundle of His and which is marked by decreased cardiac output often with cerebral ischemia

heart·burn \-ˌbərn\ *n* : a burning discomfort behind the lower part of the sternum usu. related to spasm of the lower end of the esophagus or of the upper part of the stomach often in association with gastroesophageal reflux disease — called also *cardialgia, pyrosis;* compare WATER BRASH

heart disease *n* : an abnormal organic condition of the heart or of the heart and circulation

heart failure *n* **1** : a condition in which the heart is unable to pump blood at an adequate rate or in adequate volume — compare ANGINA PECTORIS, CONGESTIVE HEART FAILURE, CORONARY FAILURE, HEART ATTACK **2** : cessation of heartbeat : DEATH

heart–healthy \ˈhärt-ˌhel-thē\ *adj* : conducive to a healthy heart and circulatory system 〈a ~ diet〉

heart–lung machine *n* : a mechanical pump that maintains circulation during heart surgery by shunting blood away from the heart, oxygenating it, and returning it to the body

heart massage *n* : CARDIAC MASSAGE

heart murmur *n* : MURMUR

heart rate *n* : a measure of cardiac activity usu. expressed as number of beats per minute

heart valve *n* : any of the valves (as the atrioventricular valves) that control blood flow to and from the heart — called also *cardiac valve*

heart·wa·ter \ˈhärt-ˌwȯ-tər, -ˌwä-\ *n* : a serious febrile tick-borne disease of sheep, goats, and cattle in southern Africa that is caused by a bacterium of the genus *Ehrlichia* (*E. ruminantium*) — called also *heartwater disease*

heart·worm \-ˌwərm\ *n* : a filarial worm of the genus *Dirofilaria* (*D. immitis*) that is a parasite esp. in the right heart of dogs and is transmitted by mosquitoes; *also* : infestation with or disease caused by the heartworm

heat \ˈhēt\ *n* **1 a** : a feverish state of the body : pathological excessive bodily temperature (as from inflammation) **b** : a warm flushed condition of the body (as after exercise) **2** : sexual excitement esp. in a female mammal; *specif* : ESTRUS

heat cramps *n pl* : a condition that is marked by sudden development of cramps in skeletal muscles and that results from prolonged work or exercise in high temperatures accompanied by profuse perspiration with loss of sodium chloride from the body

heat exchanger *n* : a device (as in an apparatus for extracorporeal blood circulation) for transferring heat from one fluid to another without allowing them to mix

heat exhaustion *n* : a condition marked by faintness or fainting, palpitations, nausea, vomiting, headache, and profuse sweating that results from physical exertion in a hot environment — called also *heat prostration;* compare HEATSTROKE

heat prostration *n* : HEAT EXHAUSTION

heat rash *n* : PRICKLY HEAT

heat shock protein *n* : any of a group of proteins that are produced esp. in cells subjected to stressful conditions (as high temperature) and that serve to ensure proper protein folding

heat·stroke \ˈhēt-ˌstrōk\ *n* : a life-threatening condition marked esp. by cessation of sweating, extremely high body temperature, rapid pulse, delirium, and collapse that results from prolonged exposure to high environmental temperature which causes dysfunction of the temperature-regulating mechanism of the body — see SUNSTROKE; compare HEAT EXHAUSTION

heave \ˈhēv\ *vb* **heaved; heav·ing** : VOMIT, RETCH

heaves \ˈhēvz\ *n, sing or pl* **1** : a spell of retching or vomiting **2** : chronic emphysema of the horse affecting the alveolae of the lungs

heavy chain *n* : either of the two larger of the four polypeptide chains comprising antibodies — compare LIGHT CHAIN

he·be·phre·nia \ˌhē-bə-ˈfrē-nē-ə, -ˈfre-\ *n* : a disorganized form of schizophrenia characterized esp. by incoherence, delusions lacking an underlying theme, and affect that is flat, inappropriate, or silly — **he·be·phre·nic** \-ˈfre-nik, -ˈfrē-\ *adj or n*

Heb·er·den's node \ˈhe-bər-dənz-\ *n* : any of the bony knots at joint margins (as at the terminal joints of the fingers) commonly associated with osteoarthritis — compare BOUCHARD'S NODE

Heberden, William (1710–1801), British physician.

hec•tic \'hek-tik\ *adj* **1 :** of, relating to, or being a fluctuating but persistent fever (as in tuberculosis) **2 :** having a hectic fever

heel \'hēl\ *n* **1 :** the back of the human foot below the ankle and behind the arch **2 :** the part of the palm of the hand nearest the wrist

heel bone *n* **:** CALCANEUS

heel fly *n* **:** CATTLE GRUB; *esp* **:** one in the adult stage

Heer•fordt's syndrome \'hār-ˌfȯrts-\ *n* **:** UVEOPAROTID FEVER

Heerfordt, Christian Frederik (1871–1953), Danish ophthalmologist.

height \'hīt\ *n* **:** the distance from the bottom to the top of something standing upright; *esp* **:** the distance from the lowest to the highest point of an animal body esp. of a human being in a natural standing position or from the lowest point to an arbitrarily chosen upper point

Heim•lich maneuver \'hīm-lik-\ *n* **:** the manual application of sudden upward pressure on the upper abdomen of a choking victim to force a foreign object from the trachea

Heimlich, Henry Jay (*b* 1920), American surgeon.

Heinz body \'hīnts-, 'hīnz-\ *n* **:** a cellular inclusion in a red blood cell that consists of damaged aggregated hemoglobin and is associated with some forms of hemolytic anemia

Heinz \'hīnts\, **Robert (1865–1924),** German physician.

hela cell \'hē-lə-\ *n, often cap H & 1st L* [*He*nrietta *La*cks] **:** a cell of a continuously cultured strain isolated from a human uterine cervical carcinoma in 1951 and used in biomedical research esp. to culture viruses

Lacks \'laks\, **Henrietta (1920–1951),** American hospital patient.

heli- *or* **helio-** *comb form* **:** sun ⟨*helio*therapy⟩

helic- *or* **helico-** *comb form* **:** helix **:** spiral ⟨*helic*al⟩ ⟨*helico*trema⟩

he•li•cal \'he-li-kəl, 'hē-\ *adj* **:** of, relating to, or having the form of a helix; *broadly* **:** SPIRAL 1a — **he•li•cal•ly** *adv*

he•li•case \'he-lə-ˌkās, 'hē-\ *n* **:** any of various enzymes that catalyze the unwinding and separation of double-stranded DNA or RNA during its replication

hel•i•cine artery \'he-lə-ˌsēn-, 'hē-lə-ˌsīn-\ *n* **:** any of various convoluted and dilated arterial vessels that empty directly into the cavernous spaces of erectile tissue and function in its erection

hel•i•co•bac•ter \'he-li-kō-ˌbak-tər\ *n* **1** *cap* **:** a genus of bacteria formerly placed in the genus *Campylobacter* and including one (*H. pylori*) associated with gastritis and implicated as a causative agent of gastric and duodenal ulcers **2 :** any bacterium of the genus *Helicobacter*

hel•i•co•trema \ˌhe-lə-kō-'trē-mə\ *n* **:** the minute opening by which the scala tympani and scala vestibuli communicate at the top of the cochlea of the ear

he•lio•ther•a•py \ˌhē-lē-ō-'ther-ə-pē\ *n, pl* **-pies :** the use of sunlight or of an artificial source of ultraviolet, visible, or infrared radiation for therapeutic purposes

he•li•um \'hē-lē-əm\ *n* **:** a light nonflammable gaseous element — symbol *He;* see ELEMENT table

he•lix \'hē-liks\ *n, pl* **he•li•ces** \'he-lə-ˌsēz, 'hē-\ *also* **he•lix•es** \'hē-lik-səz\ **1 :** the inward curved rim of the external ear **2 :** a curve traced on a cylinder by the rotation of a point crossing its right sections at a constant oblique angle; *broadly* **:** SPIRAL 2 — see ALPHA-HELIX, DOUBLE HELIX

hel•le•bore \'he-lə-ˌbōr\ *n* **1 :** any of a genus (*Helleborus*) of poisonous Eurasian herbs of the buttercup family (Ranunculaceae) that have showy flowers; *also* **:** the dried rhizome of a hellebore (as *H. niger*) formerly used in medicine **2 a :** a poisonous herb of the genus *Veratrum* **b :** the dried rhizome of either of two hellebores (*Veratrum viride* of No. America and *V. album* of Eurasia) that is used as an insecticide and contains toxic alkaloids that are cardiac and respiratory depressants — called also *veratrum*

HELLP syndrome \'help-\ *n* [*h*emolysis *e*levated *l*iver enzymes, and *l*ow *p*latelet count] **:** a serious disorder of pregnancy that is of unknown etiology, that usu. occurs between the 23rd and 39th weeks, and that is characterized by a great reduction in the number of platelets per cubic millimeter, by hemolysis, and by abnormal liver function tests

hel•minth \'hel-ˌminth\ *n* **:** a parasitic worm (as a tapeworm, liver fluke, or ascarid); *esp* **:** an intestinal worm — **hel•min•thic** \hel-'min-thik\ *adj*

helminth- *or* **helmintho-** *comb form* **:** helminth ⟨*helminth*iasis⟩

hel•min•thi•a•sis \ˌhel-mən-'thī-ə-səs\ *n, pl* **-a•ses** \-ˌsēz\ **:** infestation with or disease caused by parasitic worms

hel•min•thol•o•gy \-'thä-lə-jē\ *n, pl* **-gies :** a branch of zoology concerned with helminths; *esp* **:** the study of parasitic worms — **hel•min•thol•o•gist** \-'thä-lə-jist\ *n*

Helo•der•ma \ˌhē-lō-'dər-mə, ˌhe-\ *n* **:** a genus of lizards (family Helodermatidae) including the Gila monsters

helper/inducer T cell *n* **:** T4 CELL

helper T cell *n* **:** a T cell that participates in an immune response by recognizing a foreign antigen and secreting lymphokines to activate T cell and B cell proliferation, that usu.

carries CD4 molecular markers on its cell surface, and that is reduced to 20 percent or less of normal numbers in AIDS — called also *helper cell, helper lymphocyte, helper T lymphocyte;* compare CYTOTOXIC T CELL, SUPPRESSOR T CELL

hem- *or* **hemo-** *comb form* : blood ⟨*hem*al⟩ ⟨*hem*angioma⟩ ⟨*hemo*philia⟩

hema- *comb form* : HEM- ⟨*hema*cytometer⟩

he•ma•cy•tom•e•ter \ˌhē-mə-sī-ˈtä-mə-tər\ *n* : an instrument for counting blood cells — called also *hemocytometer*

hem•ad•sorp•tion \ˌhē-(ˌ)mad-ˈsȯrp-shən, -ˈzȯrp-\ *n* : adherence of red blood cells to the surface of something (as a virus or cell) — **hem•ad•sorb•ing** \-ˈsȯr-biŋ, -ˈzȯr-\ *adj*

hem•ag•glu•ti•na•tion \ˌhē-mə-ˌglüt-ᵊn-ˈā-shən\ *n* : agglutination of red blood cells — **hem•ag•glu•ti•nate** \-ˈglüt-ᵊn-ˌāt\ *vb*

hem•ag•glu•ti•nin \ˌhē-mə-ˈglüt-ᵊn-ən\ *also* **he•mo•ag•glu•ti•nin** \ˌhē-mō-ə-\ *n* : an agglutinin (as an antibody or viral capsid protein) that causes hemagglutination — compare LEUKOAGGLUTININ — abbr. *HA*

he•mal \ˈhē-məl\ *adj* **1** : of or relating to the blood or blood vessels **2** : relating to or situated on the side of the spinal cord where the heart and chief blood vessels are placed — compare NEURAL 2

hem•an•gio•blas•to•ma \ˌhē-ˌman-jē-ō-blas-ˈtō-mə\ *n, pl* **-mas** *also* **-ma•ta** \-mə-tə\ : a hemangioma esp. of the cerebellum that tends to be associated with von Hippel-Lindau disease

he•man•gio•en•do•the•li•o•ma \ˌhē-ˌman-jē-ō-ˌen-dō-ˌthē-lē-ˈō-mə\ *n, pl* **-mas** *also* **-ma•ta** \-mə-tə\ : an often malignant tumor originating by proliferation of capillary endothelium

hem•an•gi•o•ma \ˌhē-ˌman-jē-ˈō-mə\ *n, pl* **-mas** *also* **-ma•ta** \-mə-tə\ : a usu. benign tumor made up of blood vessels that typically occurs as a purplish or reddish slightly elevated area of skin

he•man•gi•o•ma•to•sis \-jē-ˌō-mə-ˈtō-səs\ *n, pl* **-to•ses** \-ˌsēz\ : a condition in which hemangiomas are present in several parts of the body

hem•an•gio•peri•cy•to•ma \-jē-ō-ˌper-ə-ˌsī-ˈtō-mə\ *n, pl* **-mas** *also* **-ma•ta** \-mə-tə\ : a vascular tumor composed of spindle cells that are held to be derived from pericytes

he•man•gio•sar•co•ma \-jē-ō-sär-ˈkō-mə\ *n, pl* **-mas** *also* **-ma•ta** \-mə-tə\ : a malignant hemangioma

he•mar•thro•sis \ˌhē-mär-ˈthrō-səs, ˌhe-\ *n, pl* **-thro•ses** \-ˌsēz\ : hemorrhage into a joint

hemat- *or* **hemato-** *comb form* : HEM- ⟨*hemat*emesis⟩ ⟨*hemato*genous⟩

he•ma•tem•e•sis \ˌhē-mə-ˈte-mə-səs, ˌhē-mə-tə-ˈmē-səs\ *n, pl* **-e•ses** \-ˌsēz\ : the vomiting of blood

he•ma•tin \ˈhē-mə-tən\ *n* **1** : a brownish-black or bluish-black derivative $C_{34}H_{33}N_4O_5Fe$ of oxidized heme; *also* : any of several similar compounds **2** : HEME

he•ma•tin•ic \ˌhē-mə-ˈti-nik\ *n* : an agent tending to stimulate blood cell formation or to increase the hemoglobin in the blood — **hematinic** *adj*

he•ma•to•cele \ˈhē-mə-tə-ˌsēl, hi-ˈma-tə-\ *n* : a blood-filled cavity of the body; *also* : the effusion of blood into a body cavity (as the scrotum)

he•ma•to•che•zia \ˌhē-mə-tə-ˈkē-zē-ə, ˌhe-; hi-ˌma-tə-\ *n* : the passage of blood in the feces — compare MELENA

he•ma•to•col•pos \ˌhē-mə-tō-ˈkäl-pəs, ˌhe-, -ˌpäs; hi-ˌma-tə-\ *n* : an accumulation of blood within the vagina

he•mat•o•crit \hi-ˈma-tə-krət, -ˌkrit\ *n* **1** : an instrument for determining usu. by centrifugation the relative amounts of plasma and corpuscles in blood **2** : the percent of the volume of whole blood that is composed of red blood cells as determined by separation of red blood cells from the plasma usu. by centrifugation — called also *packed cell volume*

he•ma•to•gen•ic \ˌhē-mə-tə-ˈje-nik\ *adj* : HEMATOGENOUS 2

he•ma•tog•e•nous \ˌhē-mə-ˈtä-jə-nəs\ *adj* **1** : producing blood **2** : involving, spread by, or arising in the blood — **he•ma•tog•e•nous•ly** *adv*

he•ma•to•log•ic \ˌhē-mət-ᵊl-ˈä-jik\ *also* **he•ma•to•log•i•cal** \-ji-kəl\ *adj* : of or relating to blood or to hematology ⟨~ disorders⟩

he•ma•tol•o•gy \ˌhē-mə-ˈtä-lə-jē\ *n, pl* **-gies** : a medical science that deals with the blood and blood-forming organs — **he•ma•tol•o•gist** \-jist\ *n*

he•ma•to•ma \-ˈtō-mə\ *n, pl* **-mas** *also* **-ma•ta** \-mə-tə\ : a mass of usu. clotted blood that forms in a tissue, organ, or body space as a result of a broken blood vessel

he•ma•to•me•tra \ˌhē-mə-tə-ˈmē-trə, ˌhe-\ *n* : an accumulation of blood or menstrual fluid in the uterus

he•ma•to•my•e•lia \hi-ˌma-tə-ˌmī-ˈē-lē-ə, ˌhē-mə-tō-\ *n* : a hemorrhage into the spinal cord

he•ma•to•pa•thol•o•gy \hi-ˌma-tə-pə-ˈthä-lə-jē, ˌhē-mə-tō-\ *n, pl* **-gies** : the medical science concerned with diseases of the blood and related tissues — **he•ma•to•pa•thol•o•gist** \-jist\ *n*

he•ma•toph•a•gous \ˌhē-mə-ˈtä-fə-gəs\ *adj* : feeding on blood ⟨~ insects⟩

he•ma•to•poi•e•sis \hi-ˌma-tə-pȯi-ˈē-səs, ˌhē-mə-tō-\ *n, pl* **-e•ses** \-ˌsēz\ : the formation of blood or of blood cells in the living body — called also *hemopoiesis* — **he•ma•to•poi•et•ic** \-ˈe-tik\ *adj*

hematopoietic growth factor *n* : any of a group of glycoproteins that promote the proliferation and maturation of blood cells; *esp* : COLONY-STIMULATING FACTOR

he•ma•to•por•phy•rin \ˌhē-mə-tə-ˈpȯr-fə-rən, ˌhe-\ *n* : any of several isomeric porphyrins $C_{34}H_{38}O_6N_4$ that are hydrated derivatives of protoporphyrins

he•ma•to•sal•pinx \ˌhē-mə-tə-ˈsal-(ˌ)piŋks, ˌhe-, hi-ˌma-tə-\ *n, pl* **-sal•pin•ges** \-sal-ˈpin-(ˌ)jēz\ : accumulation of blood in a fallopian tube

he•ma•tox•y•lin \ˌhē-mə-ˈtäk-sə-lən\ *n* : a crystalline phenolic compound $C_{16}H_{14}O_6$ used chiefly as a biological stain

he•ma•tu•ria \ˌhē-mə-ˈtu̇r-ē-ə, -ˈtyu̇r-\ *n* : the presence of blood or blood cells in the urine

heme \ˈhēm\ *n* : the deep red iron-containing prosthetic group $C_{34}H_{32}N_4O_4Fe$ of hemoglobin and myoglobin

hem•er•a•lo•pia \ˌhe-mə-rə-ˈlō-pē-ə\ *n* **1** : a defect of vision characterized by reduced visual capacity in bright lights **2** : NIGHT BLINDNESS — not considered correct medical usage

hemi- *prefix* : half ⟨*hemi*block⟩

-hemia — see -EMIA

hemi•an•es•the•sia \ˌhe-mē-ˌa-nəs-ˈthē-zhə\ *n* : loss of sensation in either lateral half of the body

hemi•an•o•pia \-ə-ˈnō-pē-ə\ *or* **hemi•an•op•sia** \-ˈnäp-sē-ə\ *n* : blindness in one half of the visual field of one or both eyes — called also *hemiopia* — **hemi•an•op•tic** \-ə-ˈnäp-tik\ *adj*

hemi•at•ro•phy \-ˈa-trə-fē\ *n, pl* **-phies** : atrophy that affects one half of an organ or part or one side of the whole body — compare HEMIHYPERTROPHY

hemi•a•zy•gos vein *also* **hemi•a•zy•gous vein** \-(ˌ)ā-ˈzī-gəs-, -ˈa-zə-gəs-\ *n* : a vein that receives blood from the lower half of the left thoracic wall and the left abdominal wall, ascends along the left side of the spinal column, and empties into the azygos vein near the middle of the thorax

hemi•bal•lis•mus \ˌhe-mi-ba-ˈliz-məs\ *also* **hemi•bal•lism** \-ˈba-li-zəm\ *n* : violent uncontrollable movements of one lateral half of the body usu. due to a lesion in the subthalamic nucleus of the contralateral side of the body

hemi•block \ˈhe-mi-ˌbläk\ *n* : inhibition or failure of conduction of the muscular excitatory impulse in either of the two divisions of the left branch of the bundle of His

he•mic \ˈhē-mik\ *adj* : of, relating to, or produced by the blood or the circulation of the blood ⟨a ~ murmur⟩

hemi•cho•lin•ium \-kō-ˈli-nē-əm\ *n* : any of several blockers of the parasympathetic nervous system that interfere with the synthesis of acetylcholine

hemi•cho•rea \ˌhe-mi-kə-ˈrē-ə\ *n* : chorea affecting only one lateral half of the body

hemi•col•ec•to•my \-kə-ˈlek-tə-mē, -kō-\ *n, pl* **-mies** : surgical excision of part of the colon

hemi•cra•nia \-ˈkrā-nē-ə\ *n* : pain in one side of the head — **hemi•cra•ni•al** \-nē-əl\ *adj*

hemi•des•mo•some \-ˈdez-mə-ˌsōm\ *n* : a specialization of the plasma membrane of an epithelial cell that serves to connect the basal surface of the cell to the basement membrane

hemi•di•a•phragm \-ˈdī-ə-ˌfram\ *n* : one of the two lateral halves of the diaphragm separating the chest and abdominal cavities

hemi•fa•cial \-ˈfā-shəl\ *adj* : involving or affecting one lateral half of the face

hemi•field \ˈhe-mi-ˌfēld\ *n* : one of two halves of a sensory field (as of vision)

hemi•gas•trec•to•my \ˌhe-mi-ˌga-ˈstrek-tə-mē\ *n, pl* **-mies** : surgical removal of one half of the stomach

hemi•glos•sec•to•my \-ˌglä-ˈsek-tə-mē, -ˌglȯ-\ *n, pl* **-mies** : surgical excision of one lateral half of the tongue

hemi•hy•per•tro•phy \-hī-ˈpər-trə-fē\ *n, pl* **-phies** : hypertrophy of one half of an organ or part or of one side of the whole body ⟨facial ~⟩ — compare HEMIATROPHY

hemi•lam•i•nec•to•my \-ˌla-mə-ˈnek-tə-mē\ *n, pl* **-mies** : laminectomy involving the removal of vertebral laminae on only one side

hemi•me•lia \-ˈmē-lē-ə\ *n* : a congenital abnormality (as total or partial absence) affecting only the distal half of a limb

he•min \ˈhē-mən\ *n* : a crystalline salt $C_{34}H_{32}N_4O_4FeCl$ that inhibits the biosynthesis of porphyrin and is used to ameliorate the symptoms of some forms of porphyria

hemi•o•pia \ˌhe-mē-ˈō-pē-ə\ *or* **hemi•op•sia** \-ˈäp-sē-ə\ *n* : HEMIANOPIA

hemi•pa•re•sis \ˌhe-mi-pə-ˈrē-səs, -ˈpar-ə-\ *n, pl* **-re•ses** \-ˌsēz\ : muscular weakness or partial paralysis restricted to one side of the body — **hemi•pa•ret•ic** \-pə-ˈre-tik\ *adj*

hemi•pel•vec•to•my \-pel-ˈvek-tə-mē\ *n, pl* **-mies** : amputation of one leg together with removal of the half of the pelvis on the same side of the body

hemi•ple•gia \ˌhe-mi-ˈplē-jə, -jē-ə\ *n* : total or partial paralysis of one side of the body that results from disease of or injury to the motor centers of the brain

¹**hemi•ple•gic** \-ˈplē-jik\ *adj* : relating to or marked by hemiplegia

²**hemiplegic** *n* : a hemiplegic individual

hemi•ret•i•na \ˌhe-mi-ˈret-ᵊn-ə\ *n, pl* **-i•nas** *or* **-i•nae** \-ᵊn-ˌē, -ˌī\ : one half of the retina of one eye

hemi•sect \ˈhe-mi-ˌsekt\ *vb* : to divide along the mesial plane

hemi•sphere \-ˌsfir\ *n* : half of a spherical structure or organ: as **a** : CEREBRAL HEMISPHERE **b** : either of the two lobes of the cerebellum of which one projects laterally and posteriorly from each side of the vermis

hemi•spher•ec•to•my \-sfi-ˈrek-tə-mē\ *n, pl* **-mies** : surgical removal of a cerebral hemisphere

hemi•spher•ic \ˌhe-mi-ˈsfir-ik, -ˈsfer-\ *adj* : of, relating to, or affecting a hemisphere (as a cerebral hemisphere) ⟨~ lesions⟩

hemi•tho•rax \-ˈthōr-ˌaks\ *n, pl* **-tho•rax•es** *or* **-tho•ra•ces** \-ˈthōr-ə-ˌsēz\ : a lateral half of the thorax

hemi•thy•roid•ec•to•my \-ˌthī-ˌrȯi-ˈdek-tə-mē\ *n, pl* **-mies** : surgical removal of one lobe of the thyroid gland

hemi•zy•gote \-ˈzī-ˌgōt\ *n* : one that is hemizygous

hemi•zy•gous \-ˈzī-gəs\ *adj* : having or characterized by one or more genes (as in a genetic deficiency or in an X chromosome paired with a Y chromosome) that have no allelic counterparts — **hemi•zy•gos•i•ty** \-zī-ˈgä-sə-tē\ *n*

hem•lock \ˈhem-ˌläk\ *n* **1** : any of several poisonous herbs (as a poison hemlock or a water hemlock) of the carrot family (Umbelliferae) **2** : a drug or lethal drink prepared from the poison hemlock

hemo- — see HEM-

hemoagglutinin *var of* HEMAGGLUTININ

hemobartonellosis *var of* HAEMOBARTONELLOSIS

he•mo•bil•ia \ˌhē-mə-ˈbi-lē-ə\ *n* : bleeding into the bile ducts and gallbladder

he•mo•blas•to•sis \ˌhē-mə-ˌblas-ˈtō-səs\ *n, pl* **-to•ses** \-ˌsēz\ : abnormal proliferation of the blood-forming tissues

he•moc•cult \ˈhē-mə-ˌkəlt\ *adj* : relating to or being a modified guaiac test for occult blood

he•mo•cho•ri•al \ˌhē-mə-ˈkōr-ē-əl\ *adj, of a placenta* : having the fetal epithelium bathed in maternal blood

he•mo•chro•ma•to•sis \ˌhē-mə-ˌkrō-mə-ˈtō-səs\ *n, pl* **-to•ses** \-ˌsēz\ : a hereditary disorder of metabolism that involves the deposition of iron-containing pigments in the tissues, is characterized esp. by joint or abdominal pain, weakness, and fatigue, and may lead to bronzing of the skin, arthritis, diabetes, cirrhosis, or heart disease if untreated — compare HEMOSIDEROSIS — **he•mo•chro•ma•tot•ic** \-ˈtä-tik\ *adj*

he•mo•co•ag•u•la•tion \ˌhē-mō-kō-ˌa-gyə-ˈlā-shən\ *n* : coagulation of blood

he•mo•con•cen•tra•tion \ˌhē-mō-ˌkän-sən-ˈtrā-shən\ *n* : increased concentration of cells and solids in the blood usu. resulting from loss of fluid to the tissues — compare HEMODILUTION 1

he•mo•cul•ture \ˈhē-mə-ˌkəl-chər\ *n* : a culture made from blood to detect the presence of pathogenic microorganisms

he•mo•cy•to•blast \ˌhē-mə-ˈsī-tə-ˌblast\ *n* : a stem cell for blood-cellular elements; *esp* : one considered competent to produce all types of blood cell — **he•mo•cy•to•blas•tic** \-ˌsī-tə-ˈblas-tik\ *adj*

he•mo•cy•tom•e•ter \-sī-ˈtä-mə-tər\ *n* : HEMACYTOMETER

he•mo•di•al•y•sis \ˌhē-mō-dī-ˈal-ə-səs\ *n, pl* **-y•ses** \-ˌsēz\ : DIALYSIS 2a

he•mo•di•a•lyz•er \-ˈdī-ə-ˌlī-zər\ *n* : ARTIFICIAL KIDNEY

he•mo•di•lu•tion \-dī-ˈlü-shən, -də-\ *n* **1** : decreased concentration (as after hemorrhage) of cells and solids in the blood resulting from gain of fluid from the tissues — compare HEMOCONCENTRATION **2** : a medical procedure for producing hemodilution; *esp* : one performed esp. to reduce the number of red blood cells lost during surgery that involves the preoperative withdrawal of one or more units of whole blood, immediate replacement with an equal volume of intravenous fluid, and postoperative reinfusion of withdrawn blood — **he•mo•di•lute** \-ˈlüt\ *vb*

he•mo•dy•nam•ic \-dī-ˈna-mik, -də-\ *adj* **1** : of, relating to, or involving hemodynamics **2** : relating to or functioning in the mechanics of blood circulation — **he•mo•dy•nam•i•cal•ly** *adv*

he•mo•dy•nam•ics \-miks\ *n sing or pl* **1** : a branch of physiology that deals with the circulation of the blood **2 a** : the forces or mechanisms involved in circulation **b** : hemodynamic effect (as of a drug)

he•mo•fil•ter \ˈhē-mō-ˌfil-tər\ *n* : a filter used for hemofiltration

he•mo•fil•tra•tion \ˌhē-mō-fil-ˈtrā-shən\ *n* : the process of removing blood from the living body, purifying it by passing it through a system of extracorporeal filters, and returning it to the body

he•mo•glo•bin \ˈhē-mə-ˌglō-bən\ *n* : an iron-containing respiratory pigment of red blood cells that functions primarily in the transport of oxygen from the lungs to the tissues of the body, that consists of four polypeptide chains of which two are of the type designated alpha and two are of one of the types designated beta, gamma, or delta and each of which is linked to a heme molecule, that combines loosely and reversibly with oxygen in the lungs or gills to form oxyhemoglobin and with carbon dioxide in the tissues to form carbaminohemoglobin, and that in humans is present normally in blood to the extent of 14 to 16 grams in 100 milliliters — compare CARBOXYHEMOGLOBIN, METHEMOGLOBIN; see FETAL HEMOGLOBIN — **he•mo•glo•bin•ic** \ˌhē-mə-glō-ˈbi-nik\ *adj* — **he•mo•glo•bi•nous** \-ˈglō-bə-nəs\ *adj*

hemoglobin A *n* : the hemoglobin in the red blood cells of the normal human adult that consists of two alpha chains and two beta chains

hemoglobin A1c \-ˌā-ˌwən-ˈsē\ *n* : a stable glycoprotein formed when glucose binds to hemoglobin A in the blood; *also* : a test that measures the level of hemoglobin A1c in the blood as a means of determining the average blood sugar concentrations for the preceding two to three months — called also *A1c, glycated hemoglobin, glycohemoglobin, glycosylated hemoglobin, HA1c, HbA1c*

hemoglobin C *n* : an abnormal hemoglobin that differs from hemoglobin A in having a lysine residue substituted for the glutamic-acid residue at position 6 in two of the four polypeptide chains making up the hemoglobin molecule

hemoglobin C disease *n* : an inherited hemolytic anemia that occurs esp. in individuals of African descent and is characterized esp. by splenomegaly and the presence of target cells and hemoglobin C in the blood

he•mo•glo•bin•emia \-ˌglō-bə-ˈnē-mē-ə\ *n* : the presence of free hemoglobin in the blood plasma resulting from the solution of hemoglobin out of the red blood cells or from their disintegration

hemoglobin F *n* : FETAL HEMOGLOBIN

he•mo•glo•bin•om•e•ter \-ˌglō-bə-ˈnä-mə-tər\ *n* : an instrument for the colorimetric determination of hemoglobin in blood — **he•mo•glo•bin•om•e•try** \-ˈnä-mə-trē\ *n*

he•mo•glo•bin•op•a•thy \ˌhē-mə-ˌglō-bə-ˈnä-pə-thē\ *n, pl* **-thies** : a blood disorder (as sickle cell anemia or Cooley's anemia) caused by a genetically determined change in the molecular structure of hemoglobin

hemoglobin S *n* : an abnormal hemoglobin occurring in the red blood cells in sickle cell anemia and sickle cell trait and differing from hemoglobin A in having a valine residue substituted for the glutamic-acid residue in position 6 of two of the four polypeptide chains making up the hemoglobin molecule

he•mo•glo•bin•uria \ˌhē-mə-ˌglō-bə-ˈnu̇r-ē-ə, -ˈnyu̇r-\ *n* : the presence of free hemoglobin in the urine — **he•mo•glo•bin•uric** \-ˈnu̇r-ik, -ˈnyu̇r-\ *adj*

he•mo•gram \ˈhē-mə-ˌgram\ *n* : a systematic report of the findings from a blood examination

he•mol•y•sate *also* **he•mol•y•zate** \hi-ˈmä-lə-ˌzāt, -ˌsāt\ *n* : a product of hemolysis

he•mo•ly•sin \ˌhē-mə-ˈlīs-ᵊn, hi-ˈmä-lə-sən\ *n* : a substance that causes the dissolution of red blood cells — called also *hemotoxin*

he•mo•ly•sis \hi-ˈmä-lə-səs, ˌhē-mə-ˈlī-səs\ *n, pl* **-ly•ses** \-ˌsēz\ : lysis of red blood cells with liberation of hemoglobin — see BETA HEMOLYSIS — **he•mo•lyt•ic** \ˌhē-mə-ˈli-tik\ *adj*

hemolytic anemia *n* : anemia caused by excessive destruction (as in infection or sickle cell anemia) of red blood cells

hemolytic disease of the newborn *n* : ERYTHROBLASTOSIS FETALIS

hemolytic jaundice *n* : a condition characterized by excessive destruction of red blood cells accompanied by jaundice

hemolytic uremic syndrome *n* : a rare disease that is marked by the formation of thrombi in the capillaries and arterioles esp. of the kidney, that is characterized clinically by hemolytic anemia, thrombocytopenia, and progressive kidney failure, that is precipitated by a variety of etiologic factors (as infection with *Escherichia coli* or *Shigella dysenteriae*), and that primarily affects infants and young children — abbr. *HUS;* see THROMBOTIC THROMBOCYTOPENIC PURPURA

he•mo•lyze \ˈhē-mə-ˌlīz\ *vb* **-lyzed; -lyz•ing** : to cause or undergo hemolysis of

he•mo•par•a•site \ˌhē-mō-ˈpar-ə-ˌsīt\ *n* : an animal parasite (as a filarial worm) living in the blood of a vertebrate — **he•mo•par•a•sit•ic** \-ˌpar-ə-ˈsi-tik\ *adj*

he•mop•a•thy \hē-ˈmä-pə-thē\ *n, pl* **-thies** : a pathological state (as anemia or agranulocytosis) of the blood or blood-forming tissues

he•mo•per•fu•sion \ˌhē-mō-pər-ˈfyü-zhən\ *n* : blood cleansing by adsorption on an extracorporeal medium (as activated charcoal) of impurities of larger molecular size than are removed by dialysis

he•mo•peri•car•di•um \-ˌper-ə-ˈkär-dē-əm\ *n, pl* **-dia** \-dē-ə\ : blood in the pericardial cavity

he•mo•peri•to•ne•um \-ˌper-ət-ᵊn-ˈē-əm\ *n* : blood in the peritoneal cavity

he•mo•pex•in \-ˈpek-sən\ *n* : a glycoprotein that binds heme preventing its excretion in urine and that is part of the beta-globulin fraction of human serum

¹he•mo•phile \ˈhē-mə-ˌfīl\ *adj* **1** : HEMOPHILIAC **2** : HEMOPHILIC 2

²hemophile *n* **1** : HEMOPHILIAC **2** : a hemophilic organism (as a bacterium)

he•mo•phil•ia \ˌhē-mə-ˈfi-lē-ə\ *n* : a hereditary sex-linked blood disorder occurring almost exclusively in males that is marked by delayed clotting of the blood with prolonged or excessive bleeding after injury or surgery and is caused by a deficiency of clotting factors — compare VON WILLEBRAND DISEASE

hemophilia A *n* : the common form of hemophilia caused by a deficiency of factor VIII in the blood

hemophilia B *n* : a mild to severe hemophilia that is caused by a deficiency of factor IX in the blood — called also *Christmas disease*

¹he•mo•phil•i•ac \-ˈfi-lē-ˌak\ *adj* : of, resembling, or affected with hemophilia

²hemophiliac *n* : one affected with hemophilia — called also *bleeder*

[1]**he•mo•phil•ic** \-ˈfi-lik\ *adj* **1** : HEMOPHILIAC ⟨a ~ patient⟩ **2** : tending to thrive in blood ⟨~ bacteria⟩

[2]**hemophilic** *n* : HEMOPHILIAC

he•moph•i•lus \hē-ˈmä-fə-ləs\ *n* : HAEMOPHILUS 2

He•moph•i•lus \hē-ˈmä-fə-ləs\ *n, syn of* HAEMOPHILUS

he•mo•pneu•mo•tho•rax \ˌhē-mə-ˌnü-mə-ˈthōr-ˌaks, -ˌnyü-\ *n, pl* **-rax•es** *or* **-ra•ces** \-ˈthōr-ə-ˌsēz\ : the accumulation of blood and air in the pleural cavity

he•mo•poi•e•sis \ˌhē-mə-pȯi-ˈē-səs\ *n, pl* **-e•ses** \-ˌsēz\ : HEMATOPOIESIS — **he•mo•poi•et•ic** \-ˈe-tik\ *adj*

he•mo•pro•tein \-ˈprō-ˌtēn\ *n* : a conjugated protein (as hemoglobin or cytochrome) whose prosthetic group is a porphyrin combined with iron

he•mop•ty•sis \hi-ˈmäp-tə-səs\ *n, pl* **-ty•ses** \-ˌsēz\ : expectoration of blood from some part of the respiratory tract

he•mo•rhe•ol•o•gy \ˌhē-mə-rē-ˈä-lə-jē\ *n, pl* **-gies** : the science of the physical properties of blood flow in the circulatory system — **he•mo•rheo•log•i•cal** \-ˌrē-ə-ˈlä-ji-kəl\ *also* **he•mo•rheo•log•ic** \-ˈlä-jik\ *adj*

hem•or•rhage \ˈhem-rij, ˈhe-mə-\ *n* : a copious discharge of blood from the blood vessels — **hemorrhage** *vb* — **hem•or•rhag•ic** \ˌhe-mə-ˈra-jik\ *adj*

hemorrhagica — see PURPURA HEMORRHAGICA

hemorrhagic dengue *n* : DENGUE HEMORRHAGIC FEVER

hemorrhagic diathesis *n* : an abnormal tendency to spontaneous often severe bleeding

hemorrhagic fever *n* : any of a diverse group of virus diseases (as Korean hemorrhagic fever, Lassa fever, and Ebola) usu. transmitted by arthropods or rodents and characterized by a sudden onset, fever, aching, bleeding in the internal organs, petechiae, and shock

hemorrhagic fever with renal syndrome *n* : any of several clinically similar diseases that are caused by hantaviruses (as the Hantaan virus) and are characterized by fever, renal insufficiency, thrombocytopenia, and hemorrhage but not usu. by pulmonary complications

hemorrhagic septicemia *n* : any of several pasteurelloses of domestic animals that are caused by a bacterium of the genus *Pasteurella* (*P. multocida*)

hemorrhagic shock *n* : shock resulting from reduction of the volume of blood in the body due to hemorrhage

hemorrhagic stroke *n* : stroke caused by the rupture of a blood vessel in or on the surface of the brain with bleeding into the surrounding tissue that occurs most often from rupture of an aneurysm or an abnormally formed blood vessel — compare ISCHEMIC STROKE

hemorrhagicum — see CORPUS HEMORRHAGICUM

hem•or•rhoid \ˈhem-ˌrȯid, ˈhe-mə-\ *n* : an abnormal mass of dilated and engorged blood vessels in swollen tissue that occurs internally in the anal canal or externally around the anus and that may be marked by bleeding, pain, or itching — usu. used in pl.; called also *piles*

[1]**hem•or•rhoid•al** \ˌhem-ˈrȯid-ᵊl, ˌhe-mə-\ *adj* **1** : of, relating to, or involving hemorrhoids **2** : RECTAL

[2]**hemorrhoidal** *n* : a hemorrhoidal part (as an artery or vein)

hemorrhoidal artery *n* : RECTAL ARTERY

hemorrhoidal vein *n* : RECTAL VEIN

hem•or•rhoid•ec•to•my \ˌhe-mə-ˌrȯi-ˈdek-tə-mē\ *n, pl* **-mies** : surgical removal of a hemorrhoid

he•mo•sid•er•in \ˌhē-mō-ˈsi-də-rən\ *n* : a yellowish-brown granular pigment formed by breakdown of hemoglobin, found in phagocytes and in tissues esp. in disturbances of iron metabolism (as in hemochromatosis, hemosiderosis, or some anemias)

he•mo•sid•er•o•sis \-ˌsi-də-ˈrō-səs\ *n, pl* **-o•ses** \-ˌsēz\ : excessive deposition of hemosiderin in bodily tissues as a result of the breakdown of red blood cells — compare HEMOCHROMATOSIS

he•mo•sta•sis \ˌhē-mə-ˈstā-səs\ *n, pl* **-sta•ses** \-ˌsēz\ **1** : stoppage or sluggishness of blood flow **2** : the arrest of bleeding (as by a hemostatic agent)

he•mo•stat \ˈhē-mə-ˌstat\ *n* **1** : HEMOSTATIC **2** : an instrument and esp. forceps for compressing a bleeding vessel

[1]**he•mo•stat•ic** \ˌhē-mə-ˈsta-tik\ *n* : an agent that checks bleeding; *esp* : one that shortens the clotting time of blood

[2]**hemostatic** *adj* **1** : of or caused by hemostasis **2** : serving to check bleeding

he•mo•ther•a•py \-ˈther-ə-pē\ *n, pl* **-pies** : treatment involving the administration of fresh blood, a blood fraction, or a blood preparation

he•mo•tho•rax \ˌhē-mə-ˈthōr-ˌaks\ *n, pl* **-tho•rax•es** *or* **-tho•ra•ces** \-ˈthōr-ə-ˌsēz\ : blood in the pleural cavity

he•mo•tox•ic \-ˈtäk-sik\ *adj* : destructive to red blood corpuscles

he•mo•tox•in \-ˈtäk-sən\ *n* : HEMOLYSIN

he•mo•zo•in \ˌhē-mə-ˈzō-ən\ *n* : an iron-containing pigment which accumulates as cytoplasmic granules in malaria parasites and is a breakdown product of hemoglobin

hemp \ˈhemp\ *n* **1** : a tall widely grown Asian herb of the genus *Cannabis* (*C. sativa*) with a strong woody fiber used esp. for cordage **2** : the fiber of hemp **3** : a psychoactive drug (as marijuana or hashish) from hemp

hen•bane \ˈhen-ˌbān\ *n* : a poisonous fetid Old World herb of the genus *Hy-*

oscyamus (*H. niger*) that contains the alkaloids hyoscyamine and scopolamine — called also *black henbane*

Hen•le's layer \ˈhen-lēz-\ *n* : a single layer of cuboidal epithelium forming the outer boundary of the inner stratum of a hair follicle — compare HUXLEY'S LAYER

Hen•le \ˈhen-lə\, **Friedrich Gustav Jacob (1809–1885),** German anatomist and histologist.

Henle's loop *n* : LOOP OF HENLE

Henoch–Schönlein *adj* : SCHÖNLEIN-HENOCH ⟨~ purpura⟩

He•noch's purpura \ˈhe-nòks-\ *n* : Schönlein-Henoch purpura that is characterized esp. by gastrointestinal bleeding and pain — compare SCHÖNLEIN'S DISEASE

E. H. Henoch — see SCHÖNLEIN-HENOCH

HEPA \ˈhe-pə\ *adj* [*h*igh *e*fficiency *p*articulate *a*ir] : being, using, or containing a filter usu. designed to remove 99.97% of airborne particles measuring 0.3 microns or greater in diameter passing through it

hep•a•ran sulfate \ˈhe-pə-ˌran-\ *n* : a sulfated glycosaminoglycan that accumulates in bodily tissues in abnormal amounts in some mucopolysaccharidoses — called also *heparitin sulfate*

hep•a•rin \ˈhe-pə-rən\ *n* : a glycosaminoglycan sulfuric acid ester that occurs esp. in the liver and lungs, that prolongs the clotting time of blood by preventing the formation of fibrin, and that is administered parenterally in the form of its sodium salt in vascular surgery and in the treatment of postoperative thrombosis and embolism — see LIQUAEMIN; compare ANTIPROTHROMBIN, ANTITHROMBIN

he•pa•ri•nase \ˈhe-pə-rə-ˌnās, -ˌnāz\ *n* : an enzyme that breaks down heparin

hep•a•rin•ize \ˈhe-pə-rə-ˌnīz\ *vb* **-ized; -iz•ing** : to treat with heparin — **hep•a•rin•iza•tion** \-rə-nə-ˈzā-shən\ *n*

hep•a•rin•oid \-ˌnòid\ *n* : any of various sulfated polysaccharides that have anticoagulant activity resembling that of heparin — **heparinoid** *adj*

hep•a•ri•tin sulfate \ˈhe-pə-ˌrī-tin-\ *n* : HEPARAN SULFATE

hepat- *or* **hepato-** *comb form* **1** : liver ⟨*hepat*itis⟩ ⟨*hepato*toxic⟩ **2** : hepatic and ⟨*hepato*biliary⟩

hep•a•tec•to•my \ˌhe-pə-ˈtek-tə-mē\ *n, pl* **-mies** : excision of the liver or of part of the liver — **hep•a•tec•to•mized** \-tə-ˌmīzd\ *adj*

he•pat•ic \hi-ˈpa-tik\ *adj* : of, relating to, affecting, or associated with the liver ⟨~ injury⟩ ⟨~ insufficiency⟩

hepatic artery *n* : the branch of the celiac artery that supplies the liver with arterial blood

hepatic cell *n* : HEPATOCYTE

hepatic coma *n* : a coma that is induced by severe liver disease

hepatic duct *n* : a duct conveying the bile away from the liver and uniting with the cystic duct to form the common bile duct

hepatic flexure *n* : the right-angle bend in the colon on the right side of the body near the liver that marks the junction of the ascending colon and the transverse colon — called also *right colic flexure*

he•pat•i•cos•to•my \hi-ˌpa-ti-ˈkäs-tə-mē\ *n, pl* **-mies** : an operation to provide an artificial opening into the hepatic duct

he•pat•i•cot•o•my \-ˈkä-tə-mē\ *n, pl* **-mies** : surgical incision of the hepatic duct

hepatic portal system *n* : a group of veins that carry blood from the capillaries of the stomach, intestine, spleen, and pancreas to the sinusoids of the liver

hepatic portal vein *n* : a portal vein carrying blood from the digestive organs and spleen to the liver

hepaticus — see FETOR HEPATICUS

hepatic vein *n* : any of the veins that carry the blood received from the hepatic artery and from the hepatic portal vein away from the liver and that in humans are usu. three in number and open into the inferior vena cava

hepatis — see PELIOSIS HEPATIS, PORTA HEPATIS

hep•a•ti•tis \ˌhe-pə-ˈtī-təs\ *n, pl* **-tit•i•des** \-ˈti-tə-ˌdēz\ *also* **-ti•tis•es** \-ˈtī-tə-səz\ **1** : inflammation of the liver **2** : a disease or condition (as hepatitis B or hepatitis C) that is marked by inflammation of the liver, is usu. characterized by acute symptoms of fatigue, fever, nausea, vomiting, abdominal pain or tenderness, loss of appetite, darkened urine, and jaundice but may be asymptomatic, that often progresses to a chronic form leading to liver damage, failure, or cancer, and is typically transmitted by contact with infected blood (as by transfusion or illicit intravenous drug use) or other body fluids (as semen) — **hep•a•tit•ic** \-ˈti-tik\ *adj*

hepatitis A *n* : an acute usu. benign hepatitis that is caused by a picornavirus (species *Hepatitis A virus* of the genus *Hepatovirus*) transmitted esp. in food and water contaminated with infected fecal matter — called also *infectious hepatitis;* see HAVRIX

hepatitis B *n* : hepatitis that is caused by a double-stranded DNA virus (species *Hepatitis B virus* of the genus *Orthohepadnavirus*, family *Hepadnaviridae*) transmitted esp. by contact with infected blood or other infected bodily fluids and may progress from an acute mild illness to chronic infection — called also *serum hepatitis*

hepatitis B surface antigen *n* : an antigen that is usu. a surface particle from the hepatitis B virus and that is found circulating in the blood serum esp. of infected individuals — abbr. *HBsAg;* called also *Australia antigen*

hepatitis C *n* : hepatitis that is caused by a flavivirus (species *Hepatitis C virus* of the genus *Hepacivirus*), is often asymptomatic in its early stages, is usu. transmitted by contact with infected blood, and often progresses to chronic infection

hepatitis D *n* : hepatitis that is caused by the hepatitis D virus transmitted by contact with infected blood or other body fluids and when occurring simultaneously with infection of the virus causing hepatitis B is marked by a severe acute phase with decreased risk of chronic infection and when following an established hepatitis B infection is more likely to progress to a serious chronic infection — called also *delta hepatitis, hepatitis delta*

hepatitis D virus *n* : a single-stranded RNA virus (species *Hepatitis delta virus* of the genus *Deltavirus*) that is the causative agent of hepatitis D and is unable to replicate and cause infection unless the virus causing hepatitis B is also present in the body — abbr. *HDV;* called also *delta agent, delta virus, hepatitis delta virus*

hepatitis E *n* : hepatitis that is rare in the U.S. but is common in some tropical developing countries, is caused by a single-stranded RNA virus (species *Hepatitis E virus* of the genus *Hepevirus*) usu. transmitted in sewage-contaminated water, and is an acute mild illness that does not progress to a chronic infection

hep•a•ti•za•tion \ˌhe-pə-tə-ˈzā-shən\ *n* : conversion of tissue (as of the lungs in pneumonia) into a substance which resembles liver tissue — **hep•a•tized** \ˈhe-pə-ˌtīzd\ *adj*

hepato- — see HEPAT-

he•pa•to•bil•i•ary \ˌhe-pə-tō-ˈbi-lē-ˌer-ē, hi-ˌpa-tə-\ *adj* : of, relating to, situated in or near, produced in, or affecting the liver and bile, bile ducts, and gallbladder ⟨~ disease⟩

he•pa•to•blas•to•ma \-blas-ˈtō-mə\ *n, pl* **-mas** *also* **-ma•ta** \-mə-tə\ : a malignant tumor of the liver esp. of infants and young children that is composed of cells resembling embryonic hepatocytes

he•pa•to•car•cin•o•gen \-kär-ˈsi-nə-jən, -ˈkärs-ᵊn-ə-ˌjen\ *n* : a substance or agent causing cancer of the liver — **he•pa•to•car•cin•o•gen•ic** \-ˈje-nik\ *adj* — **he•pa•to•car•cin•o•ge•nic•i•ty** \-jə-ˈni-sə-tē\ *n*

he•pa•to•car•cin•o•gen•e•sis \-ˌkärs-ᵊn-ō-ˈje-nə-səs\ *n, pl* **-e•ses** \-ˌsēz\ : the production of cancer of the liver

he•pa•to•car•ci•no•ma \-ˌkärs-ᵊn-ˈō-mə\ *n, pl* **-mas** *also* **-ma•ta** \-mə-tə\ : carcinoma of the liver

he•pa•to•cel•lu•lar \ˌhep-ət-ō-ˈsel-yə-lər, hi-ˌpat-ə-ˈsel-\ *adj* : of or involving hepatocytes ⟨~ carcinomas⟩

he•pa•to•cyte \hi-ˈpa-tə-ˌsīt, ˈhe-pə-tə-\ *n* : any of the polygonal epithelial parenchymatous cells of the liver that secrete bile — called also *hepatic cell, liver cell*

he•pa•to•gen•ic \ˌhe-pə-tō-ˈje-nik, hi-ˌpa-tə-\ *or* **hep•a•tog•e•nous** \ˌhe-pə-ˈtä-jə-nəs\ *adj* : produced or originating in the liver

he•pa•to•len•tic•u•lar degeneration \hi-ˌpa-tə-len-ˌti-kyə-lər-, ˌhe-pə-tō-\ *n* : WILSON'S DISEASE

hep•a•tol•o•gy \ˌhe-pə-ˈtä-lə-jē\ *n, pl* **-gies** : a branch of medicine concerned with the structure, functions, diseases, and abnormalities of the liver — **hep•a•tol•o•gist** \-jist\ *n*

hep•a•to•ma \ˌhe-pə-ˈtō-mə\ *n, pl* **-mas** *also* **-ma•ta** \-mə-tə\ : a usu. malignant tumor of the liver — **hep•a•to•ma•tous** \-mə-təs\ *adj*

he•pa•to•meg•a•ly \ˌhe-pə-tō-ˈme-gə-lē, hi-ˌpa-tə-ˈme-\ *n, pl* **-lies** : enlargement of the liver — **he•pa•to•meg•a•lic** \-ˈme-gə-lik\ *adj*

he•pa•to•pan•cre•at•ic \hi-ˌpa-tə-ˌpaŋ-krē-ˈa-tik, ˌhe-pə-tō-, -ˌpan-\ *adj* : of or relating to the liver and the pancreas

hep•a•top•a•thy \ˌhe-pə-ˈtä-pə-thē\ *n, pl* **-thies** : an abnormal or diseased state of the liver

he•pa•to•por•tal \ˌhe-pə-tō-ˈpȯrt-ᵊl, hi-ˌpa-tə-\ *adj* : of or relating to the hepatic portal system

he•pa•to•re•nal \-ˈrē-nəl\ *adj* : of, relating to, or affecting the liver and the kidneys ⟨fatal ~ dysfunction⟩

hepatorenal syndrome *n* : functional kidney failure associated with cirrhosis of the liver and characterized typically by jaundice, ascites, hypoalbuminemia, hypoprothrombinemia, and encephalopathy

hep•a•tor•rha•phy \ˌhe-pə-ˈtȯr-ə-fē\ *n, pl* **-phies** : suture of a wound or injury to the liver

hep•a•to•sis \ˌhe-pə-ˈtō-səs\ *n, pl* **-to•ses** \-ˌsēz\ : any noninflammatory functional disorder of the liver

he•pa•to•splen•ic \ˌhe-pə-tō-ˈsple-nik, hi-ˌpa-tə-\ *adj* : of or affecting the liver and spleen ⟨~ schistosomiasis⟩

he•pa•to•spleno•meg•a•ly \-ˌsple-nō-ˈme-gə-lē\ *n, pl* **-lies** : coincident enlargement of the liver and spleen

hep•a•tot•o•my \ˌhe-pə-ˈtä-tə-mē\ *n, pl* **-mies** : surgical incision of the liver

he•pa•to•tox•ic \ˌhe-pə-tō-ˈtäk-sik, hi-ˌpa-tə-ˈtäk-\ *adj* : relating to or causing injury to the liver — **he•pa•to•tox•ic•i•ty** \-täk-ˈsi-sə-tē\ *n*

he•pa•to•tox•in \-ˈtäk-sən\ *n* : a substance toxic to the liver

Hep•se•ra \hep-ˈsir-ə\ *trademark* — used for a preparation of adefovir

hep•ta•chlor \ˈhep-tə-ˌklōr\ *n* : a persistent chlorinated hydrocarbon pesticide $C_{10}H_5Cl_7$ that causes liver disease in animals and is a suspected human carcinogen

herb \ˈərb, ˈhərb\ *n, often attrib* **1** : a seed plant that lacks woody tissue and dies to the ground at the end of a growing season **2 :** a plant or plant part valued for medicinal, savory, or aromatic qualities

[1]herb·al \ˈər-bəl, ˈhər-\ *n* **1 :** a book about plants esp. with reference to their medical properties **2 :** HERBAL REMEDY

[2]herbal *adj* **:** of, relating to, or made of herbs

herb·al·ism \ˈər-bə-ˌli-zəm, ˈhər-\ *n* **:** HERBAL MEDICINE 1

herb·al·ist \ˈər-bə-list, ˈhər-\ *n* **1 :** one who collects or grows herbs **2 :** one who practices herbal medicine

herbal medicine *n* **1 :** the art or practice of using herbs and herbal remedies to maintain health and to prevent, alleviate, or cure disease — called also *herbalism* **2 :** HERBAL REMEDY

herbal remedy *n* **:** a plant or plant part or an extract or mixture of these used in herbal medicine

herb doctor *n* **:** HERBALIST 2

Her·cep·tin \hər-ˈsep-tən\ *trademark* — used for a preparation of trastuzumab

herd immunity *n* **:** a reduction in the probability of infection that is held to apply to susceptible members of a population in which a significant proportion of the individuals are immune because the chance of coming in contact with an infected individual is less

he·red·i·tary \hə-ˈre-də-ˌter-ē\ *adj* **1 :** genetically transmitted or transmittable from parent to offspring — compare ACQUIRED 1, CONGENITAL 2, FAMILIAL **2 :** of or relating to inheritance or heredity — **he·red·i·tar·i·ly** \-ˌre-də-ˈter-ə-lē\ *adv*

hereditary hemorrhagic telangiectasia *n* **:** a hereditary abnormality that is characterized by multiple telangiectasias and by bleeding into the tissues and mucous membranes because of abnormal fragility of the capillaries — called also *Rendu-Osler-Weber disease*

hereditary spherocytosis *n* **:** a disorder of red blood cells that is inherited as a dominant trait and is characterized by anemia, small thick fragile spherocytes which are extremely susceptible to hemolysis, enlargement of the spleen, reticulocytosis, and mild jaundice

he·red·i·ty \hə-ˈre-də-tē\ *n, pl* **-ties 1 :** the sum of the qualities and potentialities genetically derived from one's ancestors **2 :** the transmission of traits from ancestor to descendant through the molecular mechanism lying primarily in the DNA or RNA of the genes — compare MEIOSIS

heredo- *comb form* **:** hereditary ⟨*heredo*familial⟩

her·e·do·fa·mil·ial \ˌher-ə-dō-fə-ˈmil-yəl\ *adj* **:** tending to occur in more than one member of a family and suspected of having a genetic basis

Her·ing–Breu·er reflex \ˈher-iŋ-ˈbrȯi-ər-\ *n* **:** any of several reflexes that control inflation and deflation of the lungs; *esp* **:** reflex inhibition of inspiration triggered by pulmonary muscle spindles upon expansion of the lungs and mediated by the vagus nerve

Hering, Karl Ewald Konstantin (1834–1918), German physiologist and psychologist.

Breuer, Josef (1842–1925), Austrian physician and physiologist.

her·i·ta·bil·i·ty \ˌher-ə-tə-ˈbi-lə-tē\ *n, pl* **-ties 1 :** the quality or state of being heritable **2 :** the proportion of observed variation in a particular trait (as intelligence) that can be attributed to inherited genetic factors in contrast to environmental ones

her·i·ta·ble \ˈher-ə-tə-bəl\ *adj* **:** HEREDITARY

her·maph·ro·dite \(ˌ)hər-ˈma-frə-ˌdīt\ *n* **:** an individual exhibiting hermaphroditism — **hermaphrodite** *adj* — **her·maph·ro·dit·ic** \-ˌma-frə-ˈdi-tik\ *adj*

her·maph·ro·dit·ism \-ˈma-frə-ˌdī-ˌti-zəm\ *n* **:** the condition of having both testicular and ovarian tissue in the same individual — compare INTERSEXUALITY, PSEUDOHERMAPHRODITISM

her·met·ic \(ˌ)hər-ˈme-tik\ *adj* **:** being airtight or impervious to air — **her·met·i·cal·ly** \-ti-k(ə-)lē\ *adv*

her·nia \ˈhər-nē-ə\ *n, pl* **-ni·as** *or* **-ni·ae** \-nē-ˌē, -nē-ˌī\ **:** a protrusion of an organ or part through connective tissue or through a wall of the cavity in which it is normally enclosed — called also *rupture;* see ABDOMINAL HERNIA, HIATAL HERNIA, STRANGULATED HERNIA — **her·ni·al** \-nē-əl\ *adj*

hernial sac *n* **:** a protruding pouch of peritoneum that contains a herniated organ or tissue

her·ni·ate \ˈhər-nē-ˌāt\ *vb* **-at·ed; -at·ing :** to protrude through an abnormal body opening **:** RUPTURE

her·ni·a·tion \ˌhər-nē-ˈā-shən\ *n* **1 :** the act or process of herniating **2 :** HERNIA

hernio- *comb form* **:** hernia ⟨*hernio*rrhaphy⟩ ⟨*hernio*tomy⟩

her·nio·plas·ty \ˈhər-nē-ə-ˌplas-tē\ *n, pl* **-ties :** HERNIORRHAPHY

her·ni·or·rha·phy \ˌhər-nē-ˈȯr-ə-fē\ *n, pl* **-phies :** an operation for hernia that involves opening the hernial sac, returning the contents to their normal place, obliterating the hernial sac, and closing the opening with strong sutures

her·ni·ot·o·my \-ˈä-tə-mē\ *n, pl* **-mies :** the operation of cutting through a band of tissue that constricts a strangulated hernia

he·ro·ic \hi-ˈrō-ik\ *adj* **1 :** of a kind that is likely to be undertaken only to save life ⟨~ surgery⟩ **2 :** having a pronounced effect — used chiefly of medicaments or dosage ⟨~ doses⟩

her•o•in \ˈher-ə-wən\ *n* : a strongly physiologically addictive narcotic $C_{21}H_{23}NO_5$ that is made by acetylation of but is more potent than morphine and that is prohibited for medical use in the U.S. but is used illicitly for its euphoric effects — called also *diacetylmorphine, diamorphine*

her•o•in•ism \-wə-ˌni-zəm\ *n* : addiction to heroin

her•pan•gi•na \ˌhər-ˌpan-ˈjī-nə, ˌhər-ˈpan-jə-nə\ *n* : a contagious disease of children characterized by fever, headache, and a vesicular eruption in the throat and caused by any of numerous Coxsackieviruses and echoviruses

her•pes \ˈhər-(ˌ)pēz\ *n* : any of several inflammatory diseases of the skin caused by herpesviruses and characterized by clusters of vesicles; *esp* : HERPES SIMPLEX

her•pes gen•i•tal•is \ˌhər-(ˌ)pēz-ˌje-nə-ˈta-ləs\ *n* : GENITAL HERPES

herpes keratitis *n* : keratitis caused by any of the herpesviruses that produce herpes simplex or shingles

herpes la•bi•al•is \-ˌlā-bē-ˈa-ləs\ *n* : herpes simplex affecting the lips and nose

herpes sim•plex \-ˈsim-ˌpleks\ *n* : either of two diseases caused by herpesviruses of the genus *Simplexvirus* that are marked esp. by watery blisters on the skin or mucous membranes of the lips, mouth, face, or genital region — see HSV-1, HSV-2

her•pes•vi•rus \-ˈvī-rəs\ *n* : any of a family (*Herpesviridae*) of double-stranded DNA viruses that include the cytomegalovirus and Epstein-Barr virus and the causative agents of chicken pox, equine coital exanthema, herpes simplex, infectious bovine rhinotracheitis, infectious laryngotracheitis, malignant catarrhal fever, Marek's disease, pseudorabies, rhinopneumonitis, roseola infantum, and shingles

herpes zos•ter \-ˈzäs-tər\ *n* : SHINGLES

herpet- *or* **herpeto-** *comb form* : herpes ⟨*herpet*iform⟩

her•pet•ic \(ˌ)hər-ˈpe-tik\ *adj* : of, relating to, or resembling herpes

her•pet•i•form \-ˈpe-tə-fȯrm\ *adj* : resembling herpes

herpetiformis — see DERMATITIS HERPETIFORMIS

hertz \ˈhərts, ˈherts\ *n* : a unit of frequency equal to one cycle per second — abbr. *Hz*

Herx•heim•er reaction \ˈhərks-ˌhī-mər-\ *n* : JARISCH-HERXHEIMER REACTION

Heschl's gyrus \ˈhe-shəlz-\ *n* : a convolution of the temporal lobe that is the cortical center for hearing and runs obliquely outward and forward from the posterior part of the lateral sulcus

Heschl, Richard Ladislaus (1824–1881), Austrian anatomist.

het•a•cil•lin \ˌhe-tə-ˈsi-lən\ *n* : a semisynthetic oral penicillin $C_{19}H_{23}N_3O_4S$ that is converted to ampicillin in the body

heter- *or* **hetero-** *comb form* : other than usual : other : different ⟨*hetero*graft⟩

Het•er•a•kis \-ˈrā-kəs\ *n* : a genus (family Heterakidae) of nematode worms including one (*H. gallinarum*) that infests esp. chickens and turkeys and serves as an intermediate host and transmitter of the protozoan causing blackhead

het•ero \ˈhe-tə-ˌrō\ *n, pl* **-er•os** : HETEROSEXUAL

het•ero•an•ti•body \ˌhe-tə-rō-ˈan-ti-ˌbä-dē\ *n, pl* **-dies** : an antibody specific for a heterologous antigen

het•ero•an•ti•gen \-ˈan-ti-jən, -ˌjen\ *n* : an antibody that is produced by an individual of one species and is capable of stimulating an immune response in an individual of another species

het•ero•chro•ma•tin \-ˈkrō-mə-tən\ *n* : densely staining chromatin that appears as nodules in or along chromosomes and contains relatively few genes — **het•ero•chro•mat•ic** \-krə-ˈma-tik\ *adj*

het•ero•chro•mia \ˌhe-tə-rō-ˈkrō-mē-ə\ *n* : a difference in coloration in two anatomical structures or two parts of the same structure which are normally alike in color ⟨∼ of the iris⟩

heterochromia ir•i•dis \-ˈir-i-dəs\ *n* : a difference in color between the irises of the two eyes or between parts of one iris

het•ero•cy•clic \ˌhe-tə-rō-ˈsī-klik, -ˈsi-\ *adj* : relating to, characterized by, or being a ring composed of atoms of more than one kind

heterocyclic amine *n* : an amine containing one or more closed rings of carbon and nitrogen; *esp* : any of various carcinogenic amines formed when creatine or creatinine reacts with free amino acids and sugar in meat cooked at high temperature

het•ero•di•mer \-ˈdī-mər\ *n* : a protein composed of two polypeptide chains differing in composition in the order, number, or kind of their amino acid residues — **het•ero•di•mer•ic** \-dī-ˈmer-ik\ *adj*

het•ero•du•plex \ˌhe-tə-rō-ˈdü-ˌpleks, -ˈdyü-\ *n* : a nucleic-acid molecule composed of two chains with each derived from a different parent molecule — **heteroduplex** *adj*

het•ero•gam•ete \ˌhe-tə-rō-ˈga-ˌmēt, -gə-ˈmēt\ *n* : either of a pair of gametes that differ in form, size, or behavior and occur typically as large nonmotile female gametes and small motile sperm

het•ero•ga•met•ic \-gə-ˈme-tik, -ˈmē-\ *adj* : forming two kinds of gametes of which one determines offspring of one sex and the other determines offspring of the opposite sex — **het•ero•gam•e•ty** \-ˈga-mə-tē\ *n*

het·er·og·a·my \ˌhe-tə-ˈrä-gə-mē\ *n, pl* **-mies** **1** : sexual reproduction involving fusion of unlike gametes **2** : the condition of reproducing by heterogamy — **het·er·og·a·mous** \-məs\ *adj*

het·ero·ge·neous \ˌhe-tə-rə-ˈjē-nē-əs\ *adj* : not uniform in structure or composition — **het·ero·ge·ne·ity** \ˌhe-tə-rō-jə-ˈnē-ə-tē\ *n*

het·ero·gen·ic \ˌhe-tər-ə-ˈje-nik\ *adj* : derived from or involving individuals of a different species ⟨∼ antigens⟩

het·er·og·e·nous \ˌhe-tə-ˈrä-jə-nəs\ *adj* **1** : originating in an outside source; *esp* : derived from another species ⟨∼ bone grafts⟩ **2** : HETEROGENEOUS

het·ero·graft \ˈhe-tə-rō-ˌgraft\ *n* : XENOGRAFT

het·er·ol·o·gous \ˌhe-tə-ˈrä-lə-gəs\ *adj* **1** : derived from a different species ⟨∼ DNA⟩ — compare AUTOLOGOUS, HOMOLOGOUS 2 **2** : characterized by cross-reactivity ⟨a ∼ vaccine⟩ — **het·er·ol·o·gous·ly** *adv*

[1]**het·ero·phile** \ˈhe-tə-rə-ˌfīl\ *also* **het·er·o·phil** \-ˌfil\ *adj* : relating to or being an antibody circulating in blood serum that is reactive with usu. weak antigen originating in a different species

[2]**heterophile** *or* **heterophil** *n* : NEUTROPHIL — used esp. in veterinary medicine

het·ero·pho·ria \ˌhe-tə-rō-ˈfōr-ē-ə\ *n* : latent strabismus in which one eye tends to deviate either medially or laterally — compare EXOPHORIA

het·ero·plas·tic \ˌhe-tə-rə-ˈplas-tik\ *adj* : HETEROLOGOUS — **het·er·o·plas·ti·cal·ly** *adv*

het·ero·plas·ty \ˈhe-tə-rə-ˌplas-tē\ *n, pl* **-ties** : XENOGRAFT

[1]**het·ero·sex·u·al** \ˌhe-tə-rō-ˈsek-shə-wəl\ *adj* **1 a** : of, relating to, or characterized by a tendency to direct sexual desire toward individuals of the opposite sex — compare HOMOSEXUAL 1 **b** : of, relating to, or involving sexual intercourse between individuals of the opposite sex — compare HOMOSEXUAL 2 **2** : of or relating to different sexes — **het·ero·sex·u·al·i·ty** \-ˌsek-shə-ˈwa-lə-tē\ *n* — **het·ero·sex·u·al·ly** *adv*

[2]**heterosexual** *n* : a heterosexual individual

het·ero·top·ic \ˌhe-tə-rə-ˈtä-pik\ *adj* **1** : occurring in an abnormal place ⟨∼ bone formation⟩ **2** : grafted or transplanted into an abnormal position ⟨∼ liver transplantation⟩ — **het·ero·to·pia** \-ˈtō-pē-ə\ *also* **het·er·ot·opy** \ˌhe-tə-ˈrä-tə-pē\ *n* — **het·ero·top·i·cal·ly** *adv*

het·ero·trans·plant \ˌhe-tə-rō-ˈtrans-ˌplant\ *n* : XENOGRAFT — **het·ero·trans·plan·ta·tion** \-ˌtrans-ˌplan-ˈtā-shən\ *n*

het·ero·tro·pia \-ˈtrō-pē-ə\ *n* : STRABISMUS

het·ero·typ·ic \ˌhe-tə-rō-ˈti-pik\ *adj* : different in kind, arrangement, or form ⟨∼ aggregations of cells⟩

het·ero·zy·go·sis \ˌhe-tə-rō-(ˌ)zī-ˈgō-səs\ *n, pl* **-go·ses** \-ˌsēz\ : HETEROZYGOSITY

het·ero·zy·gos·i·ty \-(ˌ)zī-ˈgä-sə-tē\ *n, pl* **-ties** : the state of being heterozygous

het·ero·zy·gote \-ˈzī-ˌgōt\ *n* : a heterozygous individual — **het·ero·zy·got·ic** \-(ˌ)zī-ˈgä-tik\ *adj*

het·ero·zy·gous \-ˈzī-gəs\ *adj* : having the two genes at corresponding loci on homologous chromosomes different for one or more loci — compare HOMOZYGOUS

HEV *abbr* hepatitis E virus

HEW *abbr* Department of Health, Education, and Welfare

hex A \ˌheks-ˈā\ *n* : HEXOSAMINIDASE A

hexachloride — see BENZENE HEXACHLORIDE, GAMMA BENZENE HEXACHLORIDE

hexa·chlo·ro·eth·ane \ˌhek-sə-ˌklōr-ō-ˈeth-ˌān\ *or* **hexa·chlor·eth·ane** \-ˌklōr-ˈeth-ˌān\ *n* : a toxic compound C_2Cl_6 used in the control of liver flukes in veterinary medicine

hexa·chlo·ro·phane \-ˈklōr-ə-ˌfān\ *n, Brit* : HEXACHLOROPHENE

hexa·chlo·ro·phene \-ˈklōr-ə-ˌfēn\ *n* : a powdered phenolic bacteria-inhibiting agent $C_{13}Cl_6H_6O_2$

hexa·dac·ty·ly \-ˈdak-tə-lē\ *n, pl* **-lies** : the condition of having six fingers or toes on a hand or foot

hexa·flu·o·re·ni·um \-ˌflu̇-ər-ˈē-nē-əm\ *n* : a cholinesterase inhibitor used as the bromide $C_{36}H_{12}Br_2N_2$ in surgery to extend the skeletal-muscle relaxing activity of succinylcholine

hexa·me·tho·ni·um \ˌhek-sə-mə-ˈthō-nē-əm\ *n* : either of two compounds $C_{12}H_{30}Br_2N_2$ or $C_{12}H_{30}Cl_2N_2$ used as ganglionic blocking agents in the treatment of hypertension

hexa·meth·y·lene·tet·ra·mine \-ˌme-thə-ˌlēn-ˈte-trə-ˌmēn\ *n* : METHENAMINE

hex·amine \ˈhek-sə-ˌmēn\ *n* : METHENAMINE

hexanitrate — see MANNITOL HEXANITRATE

hex B \ˌheks-ˈbē\ *n* : HEXOSAMINIDASE B

hex·es·trol \ˈhek-sə-ˌstrȯl, -ˌstrōl\ *n* : a synthetic derivative $C_{18}H_{22}O_2$ of diethylstilbestrol

hexo·bar·bi·tal \ˌhek-sə-ˈbär-bə-ˌtȯl\ *n* : a barbiturate $C_{12}H_{16}N_2O_3$ used as a sedative and hypnotic and in the form of its soluble sodium salt $C_{12}H_{15}N_2NaO_3$ as an intravenous anesthetic of short duration

hexo·bar·bi·tone \-ˈbar-bə-ˌtōn\ *n, chiefly Brit* : HEXOBARBITAL

hexo·cy·cli·um meth·yl·sul·fate \-ˈsī-klē-əm-ˌme-thəl-ˈsəl-ˌfāt\ *n* : a white crystalline anticholinergic agent $C_{21}H_{36}N_2O_5S$ that tends to suppress gastric secretion and has been used in the treatment of peptic ulcers

hex·oes·trol \ˈhek-sē-ˌstrȯl, -ˌstrōl\ *chiefly Brit var of* HEXESTROL

hexo•ki•nase \ˌhek-sə-ˈkī-ˌnās, -ˌnāz\ *n* : any of a group of enzymes that accelerate the phosphorylation of hexoses (as in the formation of glucose-6-phosphate from glucose and ATP) in carbohydrate metabolism

hex•os•a•mine \hek-ˈsä-sə-ˌmēn\ *n* : an amine (as glucosamine) derived from a hexose by replacement of hydroxyl by the amino group

hex•os•a•min•i•dase \ˌhek-ˌsä-sə-ˈmi-nə-ˌdās, -ˌdāz\ *n* : either of two hydrolytic enzymes that catalyze the splitting off of a hexose from a ganglioside and are deficient in some metabolic diseases: **a** : HEXOSAMINIDASE A **b** : HEXOSAMINIDASE B

hexosaminidase A *n* : the more thermolabile hexosaminidase that is deficient in Tay-Sachs disease and Sandhoff's disease — called also *hex A*

hexosaminidase B *n* : the more thermostable hexosaminidase that is deficient in Sandoff's disease but present in elevated quantities in Tay-Sachs disease — called also *hex B*

hex•ose \ˈhek-ˌsōs, -ˌsōz\ *n* : any monosaccharide (as glucose) containing six carbon atoms in the molecule

hex•yl•res•or•cin•ol \ˌhek-səl-rə-ˈzȯrs-ᵊn-ˌȯl, -ˌōl\ *n* : a crystalline phenol $C_{12}H_{18}O_2$ used as an anthelmintic and topical antiseptic

Hf *symbol* hafnium

HFA *abbr* hydrofluoroalkane

H5N1 \ˌāch-ˌfīv-ˌen-ˈwən\ *n* **1** : a virus that is a subtype (H5N1) of the orthomyxovirus (species *Influenza A* virus of the genus *Influenzavirus A*) which causes influenza A and that infects mainly birds but sporadically infects humans often causing severe illness and death **2** : influenza caused by the H5N1 virus; *esp* : BIRD FLU

Hg *symbol* [New Latin *hydrargyrum*] mercury — see MM HG

HGA *abbr* human granulocytic anaplasmosis

Hgb *abbr* hemoglobin

HGE *abbr* human granulocytic ehrlichiosis

HGH *or* **hGH** *abbr* human growth hormone

HHA *abbr* home health aide

HHS *abbr* Department of Health and Human Services

HHV–6 \ˌāch-ˌāch-ˌvē-ˈsiks\ *n* : a human herpesvirus (species *Human herpesvirus 6* of the genus *Roseolovirus*) that causes roseola infantum

HI *abbr* hemagglutination inhibition

5–HIAA *abbr* 5-hydroxyindoleacetic acid

hi•a•tal \hī-ˈāt-ᵊl\ *adj* : of, relating to, or involving a hiatus

hiatal hernia *n* : a hernia in which part of the stomach protrudes upward into the chest cavity through the passage in the diaphragm for the esophagus and that may be asymptomatic or accompanied by symptoms typically of gastroesophageal reflux (as heartburn) — called also *hiatus hernia*

hi•a•tus \hī-ˈā-təs\ *n* : a gap or passage through an anatomical part or organ; *esp* : an opening through which another part or organ passes

hiatus semi•lu•nar•is \-ˌse-mi-lü-ˈnar-əs\ *n* : a curved fissure in the nasal passages into which the frontal and maxillary sinuses open

Hib *n, often attrib* : a serotype of a bacterium of the genus *Haemophilus* (*H. influenzae* type B) that causes bacterial meningitis and pneumonia esp. in children ⟨a ~ vaccine⟩ ⟨~ disease⟩ — see CONJUGATE VACCINE

hi•ber•no•ma \ˌhī-bər-ˈnō-mə\ *n, pl* **-mas** *also* **-ma•ta** \-mə-tə\ : a rare benign tumor that contains fat cells

hic•cup *also* **hic•cough** \ˈhi-(ˌ)kəp\ *n* **1** : a spasmodic inhalation with closure of the glottis accompanied by a peculiar sound **2** : an attack of hiccuping — usu. used in pl. but with a sing. or pl. verb — **hiccup** *vb*

hick•ey \ˈhi-kē\ *n, pl* **hickeys** : a temporary red mark on the skin produced esp. by biting and sucking (as during sexual activity)

Hick•man \ˈhik-mən\ *trademark* — used for an indwelling venous catheter

hide•bound \ˈhīd-ˌbau̇nd\ *adj* : having or affected with scleroderma

hidr- *or* **hidro-** *comb form* : sweat glands ⟨*hidr*adenitis⟩

hi•drad•e•ni•tis \hi-ˌdrad-ᵊn-ˈī-təs, ˌhī-\ *n* : inflammation of a sweat gland

hidradenitis sup•pur•a•ti•va \-ˌsə-pyu̇r-ə-ˈtī-və\ *n* : a chronic suppurative inflammatory disease of the apocrine sweat glands

hi•drad•e•no•ma \hī-ˌdrad-ᵊn-ˈō-mə\ *n, pl* **-mas** *also* **-ma•ta** \-mə-tə\ : any benign tumor derived from epithelial cells of sweat glands

hidradenoma pa•pil•li•fer•um \-ˌpa-pi-lə-ˈfer-əm\ *n* : a benign solitary tumor of adult women that occurs in the anogenital region

hi•dro•sis \hi-ˈdrō-səs, hī-\ *n, pl* **-dro•ses** \-ˌsēz\ : excretion of sweat : PERSPIRATION

hi•drot•ic \hi-ˈdrät-ik, hī-\ *adj* : causing perspiration : DIAPHORETIC, SUDORIFIC

¹high \ˈhī\ *adj* **1** : having a complex organization : greatly differentiated or developed phylogenetically ⟨the ~*er* apes⟩ — compare LOW **2 a** : exhibiting elation or euphoric excitement **b** : being intoxicated; *also* : excited or stupefied by or as if by a drug (as marijuana or heroin)

²high *n* : an excited, euphoric, or stupefied state; *esp* : one produced by or as if by a drug (as heroin)

high blood pressure *n* : HYPERTENSION

high colonic *n* : an enema injected deeply into the colon

high–density lipoprotein *n* : HDL

high forceps *n* : a rare procedure for delivery of an infant by the use of forceps before engagement has occurred — compare LOW FORCEPS, MIDFORCEPS

high–grade \ˈhī-ˈgrād\ *adj* : being near the upper, most serious, or most life-threatening extreme of a specified range — compare LOW-GRADE

highly active antiretroviral therapy *n* : the use of a combination of antiretroviral drugs in the treatment of HIV infection — called also *HAART*

high–power *adj* : of, relating to, being, or made with a lens that magnifies an image a relatively large number of times and esp. about 40 times

high–strung \ˈhī-ˈstrəŋ\ *adj* : having an extremely nervous or sensitive temperament

hi•lar \ˈhī-lər\ *adj* : of, relating to, affecting, or located near a hilum

hill•ock \ˈhi-lək\ *n* : any small anatomical prominence or elevation

hi•lum \ˈhī-ləm\ *n, pl* **hi•la** \-lə\ : a notch in or opening from a bodily part esp. when it is where the blood vessels, nerves, or ducts leave and enter: as **a** : the indented part of a kidney **b** : the depression in the medial surface of a lung that forms the opening through which the bronchus, blood vessels, and nerves pass **c** : a shallow depression in one side of a lymph node through which blood vessels pass and efferent lymphatic vessels emerge

hi•lus \-ləs\ *n, pl* **hi•li** \-ˌlī\ : HILUM

hind•brain \ˈhīnd-ˌbrān\ *n* : the posterior division of the three primary divisions of the developing vertebrate brain or the corresponding part of the adult brain that includes the cerebellum, pons, and medulla oblongata and that controls the autonomic functions and equilibrium — called also *rhombencephalon;* see METENCEPHALON, MYELENCEPHALON

hind•foot \-ˌfu̇t\ *n* **1** *usu* **hind foot** : one of the posterior feet of a quadruped **2** : the posterior part of the human foot that contains the calcaneus, talus, navicular, and cuboid bones

hind•gut \-ˌgət\ *n* : the posterior part of the embryonic digestive tract

hind leg *n* : the posterior leg of a quadruped

hind limb *n* : a posterior limb esp. of a quadruped

hinge joint \ˈhinj-\ *n* : a joint between bones (as at the elbow or knee) that permits motion in only one plane; *esp* : GINGLYMUS

hip \ˈhip\ *n* **1** : the laterally projecting region of each side of the lower or posterior part of the mammalian trunk formed by the lateral parts of the pelvis and upper part of the femur together with the fleshy parts covering them **2** : HIP JOINT

HIPAA *abbr* Health Insurance Portability and Accountability Act

hip bone \-ˌbōn\ *n* : the large flaring bone that makes a lateral half of the pelvis in mammals and is composed of the ilium, ischium, and pubis which are consolidated into one bone in the adult — called also *innominate bone, os coxae, pelvic bone*

hip joint *n* : the ball-and-socket joint comprising the articulation between the femur and the hip bone

hipped \ˈhipt\ *adj* : having hips esp. of a specified kind — often used in combination ⟨broad-*hipped*⟩

hip•po•cam•pal \ˌhi-pə-ˈkam-pəl\ *adj* : of or relating to the hippocampus

hippocampal commissure *n* : a triangular band of nerve fibers joining the two crura of the fornix of the rhinencephalon anteriorly before they fuse to form the body of the fornix — called also *psalterium*

hippocampal convolution *n* : PARAHIPPOCAMPAL GYRUS

hippocampal gyrus *n* : PARAHIPPOCAMPAL GYRUS

hippocampal sulcus *n* : a fissure of the mesial surface of each cerebral hemisphere extending from behind the posterior end of the corpus callosum forward and downward to the parahippocampal gyrus — called also *hippocampal fissure*

hip•po•cam•pus \ˌhi-pə-ˈkam-pəs\ *n, pl* **-pi** \-ˌpī, -(ˌ)pē\ : a curved elongated ridge that is an important part of the limbic system, extends over the floor of the descending horn of each lateral ventricle of the brain, consists of gray matter covered on the ventricular surface with white matter, and is involved in forming, storing, and processing memory

Hip•po•crat•ic \ˌhi-pə-ˈkra-tik\ *adj* : of or relating to Hippocrates or to the school of medicine that took his name

Hip•poc•ra•tes \hi-ˈpä-krə-ˌtēz\ (*ca* **460** BC–*ca* **370** BC), Greek physician.

Hippocratic facies *n* : the face as it appears near death and in some debilitating conditions marked by sunken eyes and temples, pinched nose, and tense hard skin

Hippocratic oath *n* : an oath that embodies a code of medical ethics and is usu. taken by those about to begin medical practice

hip pointer *n* : a deep painful bruise to the iliac crest or to the overlying muscles attached to it that occurs from a direct blow sustained esp. in contact sports (as football)

hip•po•ther•a•py \ˌhip-ə-ˈther-ə-pē\ *n* : physical therapy in which a patient (as one affected with cerebral palsy) sits or lies on the back of a horse for the therapeutic effect of the horse's movement

hip•pu•ran \ˈhi-pyu̇-ˌran\ *n* : a white crystalline iodine-containing powder $C_9H_7INNaO_3 \cdot 2H_2O$ used as a radiopaque agent in urography of the kidney — called also *iodohippurate sodium, sodium iodohippurate*

hip•pus \'hi-pəs\ *n* : a spasmodic variation in the size of the pupil of the eye caused by a tremor of the iris

Hirsch•sprung's disease \'hirsh-ˌprůŋz-\ *n* : megacolon that is caused by congenital absence of ganglion cells in the muscular wall of the distal part of the colon with resulting loss of peristaltic function in this part and dilatation of the colon proximal to the aganglionic part — called also *congenital megacolon*

Hirschsprung, Harold (1830–1916), Danish pediatrician.

hir•sute \'hər-ˌsüt, 'hir-, ˌhər-', hir-'\ *adj* : very hairy — **hir•sute•ness** *n*

hir•sut•ism \'hər-sə-ˌti-zəm, 'hir-\ *n* : excessive growth of hair of normal or abnormal distribution : HYPERTRICHOSIS

hi•ru•din \hir-'üd-ᵊn, 'hir-yů-dən\ *n* : an anticoagulant extracted from the buccal glands of a leech

Hi•ru•do \hi-'rü-(ˌ)dō\ *n* : a genus of leeches (family Hirudinidae) that includes the common medicinal leech (*H. medicinalis*)

His bundle \'his-\ *n* : BUNDLE OF HIS

hist- *or* **histo-** *comb form* : tissue ⟨*his*tamine⟩ ⟨*histo*compatibility⟩

his•ta•mine \'his-tə-ˌmēn, -mən\ *n* : a compound $C_5H_9N_3$ esp. of mammalian tissues that causes dilatation of capillaries, contraction of smooth muscle, and stimulation of gastric acid secretion, that is released during allergic reactions, and that is formed by decarboxylation of histidine — **his•ta•min•ic** \ˌhis-tə-'mi-nik\ *adj*

histamine cephalalgia *n* : CLUSTER HEADACHE

his•ta•min•er•gic \ˌhis-tə-mə-'nər-jik\ *adj* : liberating or activated by histamine ⟨~ receptors⟩

his•ta•mi•no•lyt•ic \ˌhis-tə-ˌmi-nə-'li-tik, hi-ˌsta-mə-nə-\ *adj* : breaking down or tending to break down histamine

histi- *or* **histio-** *comb form* : tissue ⟨*his-tio*cyte⟩

his•ti•di•nae•mia *chiefly Brit var of* HISTIDINEMIA

his•ti•dine \'his-tə-ˌdēn\ *n* : a crystalline essential amino acid $C_6H_9N_3O_2$ formed by the hydrolysis of most proteins

his•ti•di•ne•mia \ˌhis-tə-də-'nē-mē-ə\ *n* : a recessive autosomal metabolic defect that results in an excess amount of histidine in the blood and urine due to an enzyme deficiency

his•ti•din•uria \-'nůr-ē-ə, -'nyůr-\ *n* : the presence of an excessive amount of histidine in the urine

his•tio•cyte \'his-tē-ə-ˌsīt\ *n* : MACROPHAGE; *esp* : a nonmotile macrophage of extravascular tissues and esp. connective tissue — **his•tio•cyt•ic** \ˌhis-tē-ə-'si-tik\ *adj*

histiocytic lymphoma *n* : a non-Hodgkin lymphoma marked by the presence of large cells that morphologically resemble histiocytes but are typically of B or T cell origin — called also *histiocytic sarcoma, reticulum cell sarcoma, reticulosarcoma*

his•tio•cy•to•ma \ˌhis-tē-ō-sī-'tō-mə\ *n, pl* **-mas** *also* **-ma•ta** \-mə-tə\ : a tumor that consists predominantly of macrophages

his•tio•cy•to•sis \-'tō-səs\ *n, pl* **-to•ses** \-ˌsēz\ : abnormal multiplication of macrophages; *broadly* : a condition characterized by such multiplication

histo- — see HIST-

his•to•chem•is•try \-'ke-mə-strē\ *n, pl* **-tries** : a science that combines the techniques of biochemistry and histology in the study of the chemical constitution of cells and tissues — **his•to•chem•i•cal** \-'ke-mə-kəl\ *adj* — **his•to•chem•i•cal•ly** *adv*

his•to•com•pat•i•bil•i•ty \ˌhis-(ˌ)tō-kəm-ˌpa-tə-'bi-lə-tē\ *n, pl* **-ties** *often attrib* : a state of mutual tolerance between tissues that allows them to be grafted effectively — see MAJOR HISTOCOMPATIBILITY COMPLEX — **his•to•com•pat•ible** \-kəm-'pa-tə-bəl\ *adj*

histocompatibility antigen *n* : any of the polymorphic glycoprotein molecules on the surface membranes of cells that aid in the ability of the immune system to determine self from nonself, that bind to and display antigenic peptide fragments for T cell recognition, and that are determined by the major histocompatibility complex

his•to•flu•o•res•cence \-ˌflōr-'es-ᵊns, -ˌflůr-\ *n* : fluorescence by a tissue upon radiation after introduction of a fluorescent substance into the body and its uptake by the tissue — **his•to•flu•o•res•cent** \-'es-ᵊnt\ *adj*

his•to•gen•e•sis \ˌhis-tə-'je-nə-səs\ *n, pl* **-e•ses** \-ˌsēz\ : the formation and differentiation of tissues — **his•to•ge•net•ic** \-jə-'ne-tik\ *adj* — **his•to•ge•net•i•cal•ly** *adv*

his•toid \'his-ˌtȯid\ *adj* **1** : resembling the normal tissues ⟨~ tumors⟩ **2** : developed from or consisting of but one tissue

his•to•in•com•pat•i•bil•i•ty \ˌhis-(ˌ)tō-ˌin-kəm-ˌpa-tə-'bi-lə-tē\ *n, pl* **-ties** : a state of mutual intolerance between tissues (as of a fetus and its mother or a graft and its host) that normally leads to reaction against or rejection of one by the other — **his•to•in•com•pat•ible** \-kəm-'pa-tə-bəl\ *adj*

his•tol•o•gy \hi-'stä-lə-jē\ *n, pl* **-gies** **1** : a branch of anatomy that deals with the minute structure of animal and plant tissues as discernible with the microscope — compare GROSS ANATOMY **2** : a treatise on histology **3** : tissue structure or organization — **his•to•log•i•cal** \ˌhis-tə-'lä-ji-kəl\ *or* **his•to•log•ic** \-'lä-jik\ *adj* — **his•to•log•i•cal•ly** *adv* — **his•tol•o•gist** \hi-'stä-lə-jist\ *n*

His•to•mo•nas \ˌhis-tə-'mō-nəs\ *n* : a genus of flagellate protozoans (family Mastigamoebidae) parasitic esp. in poultry and containing a single species (*H. meleagridis*) that causes blackhead

his•to•mo•ni•a•sis \ˌhis-tə-mə-ˈnī-ə-səs\ *n, pl* **-a•ses** \-ˌsēz\ : infection with or disease caused by protozoans of the genus *Histomonas* : BLACKHEAD 2

his•to•mor•phom•e•try \ˌhis-tō-mȯr-ˈfä-mə-trē\ *n, pl* **-tries** : the quantitative study of the microscopic organization and structure of a tissue (as bone) esp. by computer-assisted analysis of images formed by a microscope — **his•to•mor•pho•met•ric** \-ˌmȯr-fə-ˈme-trik\ *also* **his•to•mor•pho•met•ri•cal** \-tri-kəl\ *adj*

his•tone \ˈhis-ˌtōn\ *n* : any of various simple water-soluble proteins that are rich in the basic amino acids lysine and arginine and are complexed with DNA in nucleosomes

his•to•patho•gen•e•sis \ˌhis-tə-ˌpa-thə-ˈje-nə-səs\ *n, pl* **-e•ses** \-ˌsēz\ : the origin and development of diseased tissue

his•to•pa•thol•o•gist \ˌhis-tō-pə-ˈthä-lə-jist, -pa-\ *n* : a pathologist who specializes in the detection of the effects of disease on body tissues; *esp* : one who identifies tumors by their histological characteristics

his•to•pa•thol•o•gy \ˌhis-tō-pə-ˈthä-lə-jē, -pa-\ *n, pl* **-gies** **1** : a branch of pathology concerned with the tissue changes characteristic of disease **2** : the tissue changes that affect a part or accompany a disease — **his•to•path•o•log•ic** \-ˌpa-thə-ˈlä-jik\ *or* **his•to•path•o•log•i•cal** \-ji-kəl\ *adj* — **his•to•path•o•log•i•cal•ly** *adv*

his•to•plas•ma \ˌhis-tə-ˈplaz-mə\ *n* **1** *cap* : a genus of imperfect fungi that includes one (*H. capsulatum*) causing histoplasmosis and another (*H. farciminosum*) causing epizootic lymphangitis **2** : any fungus of the genus *Histoplasma*

his•to•plas•min \-ˈplaz-mən\ *n* : a sterile filtrate of a culture of a fungus of the genus *Histoplasma* (*H. capsulatum*) used in a cutaneous test for histoplasmosis

his•to•plas•mo•sis \-ˌplaz-ˈmō-səs\ *n, pl* **-mo•ses** \-ˌsēz\ : a respiratory disease with symptoms like those of influenza that is endemic in the Mississippi and Ohio river valleys of the U.S., is caused by a fungus of the genus *Histoplasma* (*H. capsulatum*), and is marked by benign involvement of lymph nodes of the trachea and bronchi usu. without symptoms or by severe progressive generalized involvement of the lymph nodes and macrophage-rich tissue with fever, anemia, leukopenia and often with local lesions (as of the skin or mouth)

his•to•ry \ˈhis-tə-rē\ *n, pl* **-ries** : an account of a patient's family and personal background and past and present health

his•to•tech•nol•o•gy \ˌhis-tə-tek-ˈnä-lə-jē\ *n, pl* **-gies** : technical histology concerned esp. with preparing and processing (as by sectioning, fixing, and staining) histological specimens — **his•to•tech•nol•o•gist** \-jəst\ *n*

his•to•tox•ic \ˌhis-tə-ˈtäk-sik\ *adj* : toxic to tissues ⟨~ agents⟩

histotoxic anoxia *n* : histotoxic hypoxia esp. when of great severity

histotoxic hypoxia *n* : a deficiency of oxygen reaching the bodily tissues due to impairment of cellular respiration esp. by a toxic agent (as cyanide or alcohol)

HIV \ˌāch-(ˌ)ī-ˈvē\ *n* : either of two retroviruses that infect and destroy helper T cells of the immune system causing the marked reduction in their numbers that is diagnostic of AIDS — called also *AIDS virus, human immunodeficiency virus;* see HIV-1, HIV-2

hive \ˈhīv\ *n* : the raised edematous red patch of skin or mucous membrane characteristic of hives : an urticarial wheal

hives \ˈhīvz\ *n sing or pl* : an allergic disorder marked by raised edematous patches of skin or mucous membrane and usu. by intense itching and caused by contact with a specific precipitating factor (as a food, drug, or inhalant) either externally or internally — called also *urticaria*

HIV–1 \ˌāch-(ˌ)ī-(ˌ)vē-ˈwən\ *n* : a retrovirus of the genus *Lentivirus* (species *Human immunodeficiency virus 1*) that is the most prevalent HIV — called also *HTLV-III, LAV*

HIV–2 \-ˈtü\ *n* : a retrovirus of the genus *Lentivirus* (species *Human immunodeficiency virus 2*) that causes AIDS esp. in western Africa, is closely related in structure to SIV of monkeys, and is less virulent and has a longer incubation period than HIV-1

HLA *also* **HL–A** \ˌāch-(ˌ)el-ˈā\ *n* [*hu*man *l*eukocyte *a*ntigen] **1** : the major histocompatibility complex in humans **2** : a genetic locus, gene, or antigen of the major histocompatibility complex in humans — often used attributively ⟨*HLA* antigens⟩ ⟨*HLA* typing⟩; often used with one or more letters to designate a locus or with letters and a number to designate an allele at the locus or the antigen corresponding to the locus and allele ⟨*HLA*-B27 antigen⟩

HMD *abbr* hyaline membrane disease

HMO \ˌāch-(ˌ)em-ˈō\ *n, pl* **HMOs** : an organization that provides comprehensive health care to voluntarily enrolled individuals and families in a particular geographic area by member physicians with limited referral to outside specialists and that is financed by fixed periodic payments determined in advance — called also *health maintenance organization*

HNPCC *abbr* hereditary nonpolyposis colon cancer; hereditary nonpolyposis colorectal cancer

Ho *symbol* holmium

hoarse \ˈhōrs\ *adj* **hoars•er; hoars•est** **1** : rough or harsh in sound ⟨a ~ voice⟩ **2** : having a hoarse voice — **hoarse•ly** *adv* — **hoarse•ness** *n*

hob•nail liver \ˈhäb-ˌnāl-\ *or* **hob•nailed liver** \ˈhäb-ˌnāld-\ *n* **1** : the liver as it appears in one form of cirrhosis in which it is shrunken and hard and covered with small projecting nodules **2** : the cirrhosis associated with hobnail liver : LAENNEC'S CIRRHOSIS

hock \ˈhäk\ *n* : the joint or region of the joint that unites the tarsal bones in the hind limb of a quadruped (as the horse) and that corresponds to the human ankle

hock disease *n* : PEROSIS

Hodg•kin's lymphoma \ˈhäj-kənz-\ *or* **Hodgkin lymphoma** *n* : a malignant lymphoma that is marked by the presence of Reed-Sternberg cells and is characterized by progressive enlargement of lymph nodes, spleen, and liver and by progressive anemia — called also *Hodgkin disease, Hodgkin's, Hodgkin's disease;* see NON-HODGKIN LYMPHOMA

Hodgkin, Thomas (1798–1866), British physician.

Hodgkin's paragranuloma *n* : PARAGRANULOMA 2

hog cholera *n* : a highly infectious often fatal disease of swine caused by a flavivirus of the genus *Pestivirus* (species *Classical swine fever virus*) and characterized by fever, loss of appetite, weakness, erythematous lesions, and severe leukopenia — called also *swine fever;* see AFRICAN SWINE FEVER

hog louse *n* : a large sucking louse of the genus *Haematopinus* (*H. suis*) that is parasitic on swine

hol- *or* **holo-** *comb form* **1** : complete : total ⟨*holo*enzyme⟩ **2** : completely : totally ⟨*holo*endemic⟩

hold•fast \ˈhōld-ˌfast\ *n* : an organ by which a parasitic animal (as a tapeworm) attaches itself to its host

ho•lism \ˈhō-ˌli-zəm\ *n* **1** : a theory that the universe and esp. living nature is correctly seen in terms of interacting wholes (as of living organisms) that are more than the mere sum of elementary particles **2** : a holistic study or method of treatment

ho•lis•tic \hō-ˈlis-tik\ *adj* **1** : of or relating to holism **2** : relating to or concerned with wholes or with complete systems rather than with the analysis of, treatment of, or dissection into parts ⟨~ medicine attempts to treat both the mind and the body⟩ — **ho•lis•ti•cal•ly** *adv*

Hol•land•er test \ˈhä-lən-dər-\ *n* : a test for function of the vagus nerve (as after vagotomy for peptic ulcer) in which insulin is administered to induce hypoglycemia and gastric acidity tends to increase if innervation by the vagus nerve remains and decrease if severance is complete

Hollander, Franklin (1899–1966), American physiologist.

hol•low \ˈhä-(ˌ)lō\ *n* : a depressed part of a surface or a concavity

hollow organ *n* : a visceral organ that is a hollow tube or pouch (as the stomach or intestine) or that includes a cavity (as of the heart or bladder) which serves a vital function

Holmes–Ad•ie syndrome \ˈhōmz-ˈā-dē-\ *n* : ADIE'S SYNDROME

W. J. Adie — see ADIE'S SYNDROME

Holmes, Gordon Morgan (1876–1965), British neurologist.

hol•mi•um \ˈhōl-mē-əm\ *n* : a metallic element that occurs with yttrium and forms highly magnetic compounds — symbol *Ho;* see ELEMENT table

ho•lo•blas•tic \ˌhō-lə-ˈblas-tik, ˌhä-\ *adj* : characterized by cleavage planes that divide the whole egg into distinct and separate though coherent blastomeres ⟨~ eggs⟩ — compare MEROBLASTIC

ho•lo•crine \ˈhō-lə-krən, ˈhä-, -ˌkrīn, -ˌkrēn\ *adj* : producing or being a secretion resulting from lysis of secretory cells ⟨~ glands⟩ — compare APOCRINE, ECCRINE, MEROCRINE

ho•lo•en•dem•ic \ˌhō-lō-en-ˈde-mik\ *adj* : affecting all or characterized by the infection of essentially all the inhabitants of a particular area

ho•lo•en•zyme \ˌhō-lō-ˈen-ˌzīm\ *n* : a catalytically active enzyme consisting of an apoenzyme combined with its cofactor

ho•lo•sys•tol•ic \ˌhō-lō-sis-ˈtä-lik\ *adj* : relating to an entire systole ⟨a ~ murmur⟩

Hol•ter monitor \ˈhōl-tər-\ *n* : a portable device that makes a continuous record of electrical activity of the heart and that can be worn by an ambulatory patient during the course of daily activities in order to detect fleeting episodes of abnormal heart rhythms — **Holter monitoring** *n*

Holter, Norman Jefferis (1914–1983), American biophysicist.

hom- — see HOMO-

Ho•mans' sign \ˈhō-mənz-\ *n* : pain in the calf of the leg upon dorsiflexion of the foot with the leg extended that is diagnostic of thrombosis in the deep veins of the area

Homans, John (1877–1954), American surgeon.

hom•at•ro•pine \hō-ˈma-trə-ˌpēn\ *n* : a poisonous drug used in the form of its hydrobromide $C_{16}H_{21}NO_3 \cdot HBr$ for dilating the pupil of the eye and in the form of its methyl bromide $C_{16}H_{21}NO_3 \cdot CH_3Br$ in combination with hydrocodone in cough suppressant preparations — see HYCODAN

home- *or* **homeo-** *also* **homoi-** *or* **homoio-** *comb form* : like : similar ⟨*homeo*stasis⟩ ⟨*homoio*thermy⟩

home care *n* : services (as nursing care) provided to individuals who are confined to the home

home health aide *n* : a trained and certified health-care worker who provides assistance to a patient in the home with personal care and light household duties and who monitors the patient's condition — abbr. *HHA*

ho•meo•box \ˈhō-mē-ō-ˌbäks\ *n* : a short usu. highly conserved DNA sequence in various genes and esp. homeotic genes that encodes a DNA-binding amino acid domain of some proteins

ho•meo•path \ˈhō-mē-ə-ˌpath\ *n* : a practitioner or adherent of homeopathy

ho•me•op•a•thy \ˌhō-mē-ˈä-pə-thē, ˌhä-\ *n, pl* **-thies** : a system of medical practice that treats a disease esp. by the administration of minute doses of a remedy that would in larger amounts produce symptoms in healthy persons similar to those of the disease — compare ALLOPATHY 2 — **ho•meo•path•ic** \ˌhō-mē-ə-ˈpa-thik\ *adj* — **ho•meo•path•i•cal•ly** *adv*

ho•meo•sta•sis \ˌhō-mē-ō-ˈstā-səs\ *n* : the maintenance of relatively stable internal physiological conditions (as body temperature or the pH of blood) under fluctuating environmental conditions — **ho•meo•stat•ic** \-ˈsta-tik\ *adj* — **ho•meo•stat•i•cal•ly** *adj*

ho•meo•ther•my \ˈhō-mē-ə-ˌthər-mē\ *also* **ho•moio•ther•my** \hō-ˈmȯi-ə-\ *n, pl* **-mies** : the condition of being warm-blooded : WARM-BLOODEDNESS — **ho•meo•therm** \-ˌthərm\ *also* **ho•moio•therm** \hō-ˈmȯi-ə-\ *n* — **ho•meo•ther•mic** \ˌhō-mē-ō-ˈthər-mik\ *also* **ho•moio•ther•mic** \hō-ˌmȯi-ə-\ *adj*

ho•me•ot•ic *also* **ho•moe•ot•ic** \ˌhō-mē-ˈä-tik\ *adj* : relating to, caused by, or being a homeotic gene

homeotic gene *n* : a gene that produces a usu. major shift in the developmental fate of an organ or body part esp. to a homologous organ or part normally found elsewhere in the organism

home remedy *n* : a simply prepared medication or tonic often of unproven effectiveness administered without prescription or professional supervision

ho•mi•cid•al \ˌhä-mə-ˈsīd-ᵊl, ˌhō-\ *adj* : of, relating to, or tending toward homicide — **ho•mi•cid•al•ly** *adv*

ho•mi•cide \ˈhä-mə-ˌsīd, ˈhō-\ *n* : a killing of one human being by another

hom•i•nid \ˈhä-mə-nəd, -ˌnid\ *n* : any of a family (Hominidae) of bipedal primate mammals comprising recent humans together with extinct ancestral and related forms — **hominid** *adj*

ho•mo \ˈhō-(ˌ)mō\ *n* **1** *cap* : a genus of primate mammals (family Hominidae) that includes modern humans (*H. sapiens*) and several extinct related species (as *H. erectus*) **2** *pl* **homos** : any primate mammal of the genus *Homo*

homo- *or* **hom-** *comb form* **1** : one and the same : similar : alike ⟨*homo*zygous⟩ **2** : derived from the same species ⟨*homo*graft⟩ **3** : homosexual ⟨*homo*phobia⟩

ho•mo•cys•te•ine \ˌhō-mō-ˈsis-tə-ˌēn, ˌhä-\ *n* : an amino acid $C_4H_9NO_2S$ that is produced in animal metabolism by removal of a methyl group from methionine and forms a complex with serine that breaks up to produce cysteine and homoserine and that appears to be associated with an increased risk of cardiovascular disease when occurring at high levels in the blood

ho•mo•cys•tine \-ˈsis-ˌtēn\ *n* : an amino acid $C_8H_{16}N_2O_4S_2$ formed by oxidation of homocysteine and excreted in the urine in homocystinuria

ho•mo•cys•tin•uria \-ˌsis-ti-ˈnu̇r-ē-ə, -ˈnyu̇r-\ *n* : a metabolic disorder inherited as a recessive autosomal trait, caused by deficiency of an enzyme important in the metabolism of homocystine with resulting accumulation of homocystine in the body and its excretion in the urine, and characterized typically by intellectual disability, dislocation of the crystalline lenses, skeletal abnormalities, and thromboembolic disease — **ho•mo•cys•tin•uric** \-ˈnu̇r-ik, -ˈnyu̇r-\ *n*

ho•mo•cy•to•tro•pic \-ˌsī-tə-ˈtrō-pik\ *adj* : of, relating to, or being any antibody that attaches to cells of the species in which it originates but not to cells of other species

ho•mo•di•mer \-ˈdī-mər\ *n* : a protein composed of two polypeptide chains that are identical in the order, number, and kind of their amino acid residues — **ho•mo•di•mer•ic** \-dī-ˈmer-ik\ *adj*

homoe- *or* **homoeo-** *chiefly Brit var of* HOME-

ho•moeo•path, ho•moe•op•a•thy, ho•moeo•sta•sis, ho•moeo•ther•my *chiefly Brit var of* HOMEOPATH, HOMEOPATHY, HOMEOSTASIS, HOMEOTHERMY

homoeotic *var of* HOMEOTIC

ho•mo•erot•ic \ˌhō-mō-i-ˈrä-tik\ *adj* : HOMOSEXUAL — **ho•mo•erot•i•cism** \-i-ˈrä-tə-ˌsi-zəm\ *also* **ho•mo•erot•ism** \-ˈer-ə-ˌti-zəm\ *n*

ho•mo•ga•met•ic \-gə-ˈme-tik, -ˈmē-\ *adj* : forming gametes which all have the same type of sex chromosome

ho•mog•e•nate \hō-ˈmä-jə-ˌnāt, hə-\ *n* : a product of homogenizing

ho•mo•ge•neous \ˌhō-mə-ˈjē-nē-əs, -nyəs\ *adj* : of uniform structure or composition throughout — **ho•mo•ge•ne•ity** \ˌhō-mə-jə-ˈnē-ə-tē, -ˌhä-, -ˈnā-\ *n* — **ho•mo•ge•neous•ly** *adv* — **ho•mo•ge•neous•ness** *n*

ho•mog•e•nize \hō-ˈmä-jə-ˌnīz, hə-\ *vb* **-nized; -niz•ing** **1** : to reduce to small particles of uniform size and distribute evenly usu. in a liquid **2** : to reduce the particles of so that they are uniformly small and evenly distributed; *specif* : to break up the fat globules of (milk) into very fine particles — **ho•mog•e•ni•za•tion** \hō-ˌmä-jə-nə-ˈzā-shən, hə-\ *n* — **ho·mog·e·niz·er** \-ˈmä-jə-ˌnī-zər\ *n*

ho·mog·e·nous \-nəs\ *adj* **1** : HOMOPLASTIC **2** : HOMOGENEOUS

ho·mo·gen·tis·ic acid \ˌhō-mō-ˌjen-ˈti-zik, ˌhä-\ *n* : a crystalline acid $C_8H_8O_4$ formed as an intermediate in the metabolism of phenylalanine and tyrosine and found esp. in the urine of those affected with alkaptonuria

ho·mo·graft \ˈhō-mə-ˌgraft, ˈhä-\ *n* : a graft of tissue from a donor of the same species as the recipient — called also *homotransplant;* compare XENOGRAFT — **homograft** *vb*

homoi- *or* **homoio-** — see HOME-

homoiothermy *var of* HOMEOTHERMY

ho·mo·lat·er·al \ˌhō-mō-ˈla-tər-əl, ˌhä-\ *adj* : IPSILATERAL

ho·mol·o·gous \hō-ˈmä-lə-gəs, hə-\ *adj* **1 a** : having the same relative position, value, or structure **b** : having the same or allelic genes with genetic loci usu. arranged in the same order ⟨~ chromosomes⟩ **2** : derived from or involving organisms of the same species ⟨~ tissue grafts⟩ — compare AUTOLOGOUS, HETEROLOGOUS 1 **3** : relating to or being immunity or a serum produced by or containing a specific antibody corresponding to a specific antigen — **ho·mol·o·gous·ly** *adv*

ho·mo·logue *or* **ho·mo·log** \ˈhō-mə-ˌlȯg, ˈhä-, -ˌläg\ *n* : something (as a chromosome) that is homologous

ho·mol·o·gy \hō-ˈmä-lə-jē, hə-\ *n, pl* **-gies** **1** : likeness in structure between parts of different organisms due to evolutionary differentiation from the same or a corresponding part of a remote ancestor — compare ANALOGY **2** : correspondence in structure between different parts of the same individual **3** : similarity of nucleotide or amino acid sequence (as in nucleic acids or proteins)

hom·on·y·mous \hō-ˈmä-nə-məs\ *adj* **1** : affecting the same part of the visual field of each eye ⟨right ~ hemianopia⟩ **2** : relating to or being diplopia in which the image that is seen by the right eye is to the right of the image that is seen by the left eye

[1]**ho·mo·phile** \ˈhō-mə-ˌfīl\ *adj* : of, relating to, or concerned with homosexuals or homosexuality ⟨~ lifestyles⟩; *also* : being homosexual

[2]**homophile** *n* : HOMOSEXUAL

ho·mo·pho·bia \ˌhō-mə-ˈfō-bē-ə\ *n* : irrational fear of, aversion to, or discrimination against homosexuality or homosexuals — **ho·mo·phobe** \ˈhō-mə-ˌfōb\ *n* — **ho·mo·pho·bic** \ˌhō-mə-ˈfō-bik\ *adj*

ho·mo·plas·tic \ˌhō-mə-ˈplas-tik, ˌhä-\ *adj* : of, relating to, or derived from another individual of the same species

ho·mo·sal·ate \ˌhō-mō-ˈsa-ˌlāt, ˌhä-\ *n* : a salicylate $C_{16}H_{22}O_3$ that is used in sunscreen lotions to absorb ultraviolet rays and promote tanning

ho·mo·ser·ine \ˌhō-mō-ˈser-ˌēn, ˌhä-, -ˈsir-\ *n* : an amino acid $C_4H_9NO_3$ that is formed in the conversion of methionine to cysteine — see HOMOCYSTEINE

[1]**ho·mo·sex·u·al** \ˌhō-mə-ˈsek-shə-wəl\ *adj* **1** : of, relating to, or characterized by a tendency to direct sexual desire toward another of the same sex — compare HETEROSEXUAL 1a **2** : of, relating to, or involving sexual intercourse between persons of the same sex — compare HETEROSEXUAL 1b — **ho·mo·sex·u·al·ly** *adv*

[2]**homosexual** *n* : a homosexual person and esp. a male

ho·mo·sex·u·al·i·ty \ˌhō-mə-ˌsek-shə-ˈwa-lə-tē\ *n, pl* **-ties** **1** : the quality or state of being homosexual **2** : erotic activity with another of the same sex

ho·mo·trans·plant \ˌhō-mō-ˈtrans-ˌplant, ˌhä-\ *n* : HOMOGRAFT — **homotransplant** *vb* — **ho·mo·trans·plan·ta·tion** \-ˌtrans-ˌplan-ˈtā-shən\ *n*

ho·mo·va·nil·lic acid \-və-ˈni-lik-\ *n* : a dopamine metabolite $C_9H_{10}O_4$ excreted in human urine

ho·mo·zy·go·sis \-zī-ˈgō-səs\ *n, pl* **-go·ses** \-ˌsēz\ : HOMOZYGOSITY

ho·mo·zy·gos·i·ty \-ˈgä-sə-tē\ *n, pl* **-ties** : the state of being homozygous

ho·mo·zy·gote \-ˈzī-ˌgōt\ *n* : a homozygous individual

ho·mo·zy·gous \-ˈzī-gəs\ *adj* : having the two genes at corresponding loci on homologous chromosomes identical for one or more loci — compare HETEROZYGOUS

H_1 antagonist \ˈāch-ˈwən-\ *n* : any of various drugs (as fexofenadine or loratadine) that bind competitively with histamine to H_1 receptors on cell membranes and are used to relieve allergic symptoms and variously as sedatives, antiemetics, and anticholinergics — called also *H_1 blocker, H_1 receptor antagonist*

H1N1 \ˈāch-ˈwən-ˈen-ˈwən\ *n* **1** : a virus that is a subtype (H1N1) of the orthomyxovirus (species *Influenza A virus*) of the genus *Influenzavirus A*) causing influenza A that infects birds, pigs, and humans and includes strains which may occur in seasonal epidemics or sometimes pandemics **2** : influenza caused by the H1N1 virus; *esp* : SWINE FLU

H_1 receptor *n* : a receptor for histamine on cell membranes that modulates the dilation of blood vessels and the contraction of smooth muscle

hon·ey·bee \ˈhə-nē-ˌbē\ *n* : a honey-producing bee (genus *Apis*); *esp* : a European bee (*A. mellifera*) introduced worldwide and kept in hives for the honey it produces

Hong Kong flu \ˈhäŋ-ˈkäŋ-\ *n* : influenza that is caused by a subtype (H3N2) of the orthomyxovirus causing influenza A and that was responsible for about 34,000 deaths in the U.S. in the influenza pandemic of

1968–1969 — called also *Hong Kong influenza;* compare ASIAN FLU, SPANISH FLU

hoof \'hu̇f, 'hüf\ *n, pl* **hooves** \'hüvz, 'hu̇vz\ *also* **hoofs** : a horny covering that protects the ends of the toes of ungulate mammals (as horses or cattle); *also* : a hoofed foot — **hoofed** \'hu̇ft, 'hüft, 'hu̇vd, 'hüvd\ *or* **hooved** \'hu̇vd, 'hüvd\ *adj*

hoof–and–mouth disease *n* : FOOT-AND-MOUTH DISEASE

hook \'hu̇k\ *n* **1** : an instrument used in surgery to take hold of tissue **2** : an anatomical part that resembles a hook

hook•worm \-ˌwərm\ *n* **1** : any of several parasitic nematode worms (family Ancylostomatidae) that have strong buccal hooks or plates for attaching to the host's intestinal lining and that include serious bloodsucking pests **2** : ANCYLOSTOMIASIS

hookworm disease *n* : ANCYLOSTOMIASIS

hoose \'hüz\ *n* : bronchitis of cattle, sheep, and goats caused by larval strongylid roundworms irritating the bronchial tubes — called also *husk*

hor•de•o•lum \hȯr-'dē-ə-ləm\ *n, pl* **-o•la** \-lə\ : STY

hore•hound \'hōr-ˌhau̇nd\ *n* **1** : an Old World bitter plant (*Marrubium vulgare*) of the mint family (Labiatae) that is used as a tonic and anthelmintic **2** : an extract or confection made from horehound and used as a remedy for coughs and colds

hor•i•zon•tal \ˌhȯr-ə-'zänt-ᵊl, ˌhär-\ *adj* **1** : relating to or being a transverse plane or section of the body **2** : relating to or being transmission (as of a disease) by physical contact or proximity — compare VERTICAL — **hor•i•zon•tal•ly** *adv*

horizontal cell *n* : any of the retinal neurons whose axons pass along a course in the plexiform layer following the contour of the retina and whose dendrites synapse with the rods and cones

horizontal fissure *n* : a fissure of the right lung that begins at the oblique fissure and runs horizontally dividing the lung into superior and middle lobes

horizontal plate *n* : a plate of the palatine bone that is situated horizontally, joins the bone of the opposite side, and forms the back part of the hard palate — compare PERPENDICULAR PLATE 2

hor•me•sis \hȯr-'mē-səs\ *n* : a theoretical phenomenon of dose-response relationships in which something (as a heavy metal or ionizing radiation) that produces harmful biological effects at moderate to high doses may produce beneficial effects at low doses — **hor•met•ic** \-'me-tik\ *adj*

hormonal therapy *n* : HORMONE THERAPY

hor•mone \'hȯr-ˌmōn\ *n* **1 a** : a product of living cells that circulates in body fluids and produces a specific often stimulatory effect on the activity of cells usu. a distance from its point of synthesis **b** : a synthetic substance that acts like a hormone **2** : SEX HORMONE — **hor•mon•al** \hȯr-'mōn-ᵊl\ *adj* — **hor•mon•al•ly** *adv* — **hor•mone•like** *adj*

hormone replacement therapy *n* : the administration of estrogen along with a synthetic progestin esp. to ameliorate the symptoms of menopause and reduce the risk of postmenopausal osteoporosis — abbr. *HRT*

hormone therapy *n* : the therapeutic use of hormones: as **a** : the administration of hormones esp. to increase diminished levels in the body; *esp* : HORMONE REPLACEMENT THERAPY **b** : therapy involving the use of drugs or surgical procedures to suppress the production of or inhibit the effects of a hormone (as estrogen or testosterone) ⟨*hormone therapy* to treat breast or prostate cancer⟩

hor•mo•no•ther•a•py \hȯr-ˌmō-nə-'ther-ə-pē\ *n* : HORMONE THERAPY

horn \'hȯrn\ *n* **1** : one of the hard projections of bone or keratin on the head of many hoofed mammals; *also* : the material of which horns are composed or a similar material **2** : CORNU — **horned** \'hȯrnd\ *adj*

horn cell *n* : a nerve cell lying in one of the gray columns of the spinal cord

horned rattlesnake *n* : SIDEWINDER

Hor•ner's syndrome \'hȯr-nərz-\ *n* : a syndrome marked by sinking in of the eyeball, contraction of the pupil, drooping of the upper eyelid, and vasodilation and anhidrosis of the face, and caused by injury to the cervical sympathetic nerve fibers on the affected side

Horner, Johann Friedrich (1831–1886), Swiss ophthalmologist.

horn fly *n* : a small black European dipteran fly (*Haematobia irritans* of the family Muscidae) that has been introduced into No. America where it is a bloodsucking pest of cattle

horny \'hȯr-nē\ *adj* **horn•i•er; -est** **1** : composed of or resembling tough fibrous material consisting chiefly of keratin : KERATINOUS ⟨~ tissue⟩ **2** : being hard or callous

horny layer *n* : STRATUM CORNEUM

hor•rip•i•la•tion \hȯ-ˌri-pə-'lā-shən, hä-\ *n* : a bristling of the hair of the head or body : GOOSE BUMPS — **hor•rip•i•late** \-'ri-pə-ˌlāt\ *vb*

horror au•to•tox•i•cus \-ˌȯ-tō-'täk-sə-kəs\ *n* : SELF-TOLERANCE

horse bot \'hȯrs-\ *n* : HORSE BOTFLY; *specif* : a larva of a horse botfly

horse botfly *n* : a cosmopolitan botfly of the genus *Gasterophilus* (*G. intestinalis*) whose larvae parasitize the stomach lining of the horse

horse•fly \ˈhȯrs-ˌflī\ *n, pl* **-flies** : any of a family (Tabanidae) of usu. large dipteran flies with bloodsucking females

horse•shoe kidney \-ˌshü\ *n* : a congenital partial fusion of the kidneys resulting in a horseshoe shape

Hor•ton's syndrome \ˈhȯr-tənz-\ *n* : CLUSTER HEADACHE

Horton, Bayard Taylor (1895–1980), American physician.

hosp *abbr* hospital

hos•pice \ˈhäs-pəs\ *n* : a facility or program designed to provide a caring environment for meeting the physical and emotional needs of the terminally ill

hos•pi•tal \ˈhäs-ˌpit-ᵊl\ *n, often attrib* **1** : a charitable institution for the needy, aged, infirm, or young **2 a** : an institution where the sick or injured are given medical or surgical care — usu. used in British English without an article after a preposition **b** : a place for the care and treatment of sick and injured animals

hospital bed *n* : a bed used for patients (as in a hospital) that can be adjusted esp. to raise the head end, foot end, or middle as required — see GATCH BED

hos•pi•tal•ism \ˈhäs-(ˌ)pit-ᵊl-ˌi-zəm\ *n* **1 a** : the factors and influences that adversely affect the health of hospitalized persons **b** : the effect of such factors on mental or physical health **2** : the deleterious physical and mental effects on infants and children resulting from their living in institutions without the benefit of a home environment and parents

hos•pi•tal•ist \ˈhäs-(ˌ)pit-ᵊl-əst\ *n* : a physician who specializes in seeing and treating other physicians' hospitalized patients in order to minimize the number of hospital visits by the patients' regular physicians

hos•pi•tal•iza•tion \ˌhäs-(ˌ)pit-ᵊl-ə-ˈzā-shən\ *n* **1** : the act or process of being hospitalized **2** : the period of stay in a hospital

hospitalization insurance *n* : insurance that provides benefits to cover or partly cover hospital expenses

hos•pi•tal•ize \ˈhäs-(ˌ)pit-ᵊl-ˌīz, häs-ˈpit-ᵊl-ˌīz\ *vb* **-ized; -iz•ing** : to place in a hospital as a patient

host \ˈhōst\ *n* **1** : a living animal or plant on or in which a parasite lives — see DEFINITIVE HOST, INTERMEDIATE HOST **2 a** : an individual into which a tissue or part is transplanted from another **b** : an individual in whom an abnormal growth (as a cancer) is proliferating

host cell *n* : a living cell invaded by or capable of being invaded by an infectious agent (as a virus)

hos•til•i•ty \hä-ˈsti-lə-tē\ *n, pl* **-ties** : conflict, opposition, or resistance in thought or principle — **hos•tile** \ˈhäs-təl, -ˌtīl\ *adj*

hot \ˈhät\ *adj* **hot•ter; hot•test** **1** : having heat in a degree exceeding normal body heat **2** : RADIOACTIVE; *esp* : exhibiting a relatively great amount of radioactivity when subjected to radionuclide scanning

hot flash *n* : a sudden brief flushing and sensation of heat caused by dilation of skin capillaries usu. associated with menopausal endocrine imbalance — called also *hot flush*

hot line *n* : a usu. toll-free telephone service available to the public for some specific purpose ⟨a poison control *hot line*⟩

hot pack *n* : absorbent material (as squares of gauze) wrung out in hot water, wrapped around the body or a portion of the body, and covered with dry material to hold in the moist heat — compare COLD PACK

hot spot *n* **1** : a patch of painful moist inflamed skin on a domestic animal and esp. a dog **2** : a site in genetic material having a high frequency of mutation or recombination

hot–water bottle *n* : a usu. rubber bag that has a stopper and is filled with hot water to provide warmth

hourglass stomach *n* : a stomach divided into two communicating cavities by a circular constriction usu. caused by the scar tissue around an ulcer

house call *n* : a visit (as by a doctor) to a home to provide medical care

house doctor *n* : a physician in residence at an establishment (as a hotel) or on the premises temporarily in the event of a medical emergency

house dust mite \ˈhau̇s-ˌdəst-\ *n* : either of two widely distributed dust mites (*Dermatophagoides farinae* and *D. pteronyssinus*) that commonly occur in house dust and often induce allergic responses (as runny nose or sneezing) and asthma

house•fly \-ˌflī\ *n, pl* **-flies** : a cosmopolitan dipteran fly of the genus *Musca* (*M. domestica*) that is often found about human habitations and may act as a mechanical vector of diseases (as typhoid fever); *also* : any of various flies of similar appearance or habitat

house•maid's knee \ˈhau̇s-ˌmādz-\ *n* : a swelling over the knee due to an enlargement of the bursa in the front of the patella

house•man \ˈhau̇s-mən\ *n, pl* **-men** \-mən\ *chiefly Brit* : INTERN

house mouse *n* : a common nearly cosmopolitan mouse of the genus *Mus* (*M. musculus*) that usu. lives and breeds about buildings, is an important laboratory animal, and is an important pest as a consumer of human food and as a vector of diseases

house officer *n* : an intern or resident employed by a hospital

house physician *n* : a physician and esp. a resident employed by a hospital

house staff *n* : interns, residents, and fellows of a hospital

house surgeon *n* : a surgeon fully qualified in a specialty and resident in a hospital

Hous·ton's valve \'hü-stənz-\ *n* : any of the usu. three but sometimes four or two permanent transverse crescent-shaped folds of the rectum

Houston, John (1802–1845), British surgeon.

How·ard test \'hau̇-ərd-\ *n* : a test of renal function that involves the catheterization of each ureter so that the urinary output of each kidney can be determined and analyzed separately

Howard, John Eager (1902–1985), American internist and endocrinologist.

How·ell–Jol·ly body \'hau̇-əl-zhȯ-'lē-, -'jä-lē-\ *n* : one of the basophilic granules that are prob. nuclear fragments, that sometimes occur in red blood cells, and that indicate by their appearance in circulating blood that red cells are leaving the marrow while incompletely mature (as in certain anemias)

Howell, William Henry (1860–1945), American physiologist.

Jolly \zhȯ-'lē\, **Justin–Marie–Jules (1870–1953),** French histologist.

How·ship's lacuna \'hau̇-ˌships-\ *n* : a groove or cavity usu. containing osteoclasts that occurs in bone which is undergoing reabsorption

Howship, John (1781–1841), British anatomist.

HPI *abbr* history of present illness

HPV \ˌāch-ˌpē-'vē\ *n* : HUMAN PAPILLOMAVIRUS

hr *abbr* [Latin *hora*] hour — used in writing prescriptions; see QH

HRT *abbr* hormone replacement therapy

hs *abbr* [Latin *hora somni*] at bedtime — used esp. in writing prescriptions

Hs *symbol* hassium

HS *abbr* house surgeon

HSA *abbr* human serum albumin

HSDD *abbr* hypoactive sexual desire disorder

HSV \ˌāch-ˌes-'vē\ *n* : either of two herpesviruses that cause herpes simplex — see HSV-1, HSV-2

HSV–1 \-ˌvē-'wən\ *n* : a herpesvirus of the genus *Simplexvirus* (species *Human herpesvirus 1*) that causes the type of herpes simplex typically involving the lips, mouth, and face

HSV–2 \-'tü\ *n* : a herpesvirus of the genus *Simplexvirus* (species *Human herpesvirus 2*) that causes the type of herpes simplex typically involving the genital region

ht *abbr* height

5–HT \'fīv-ˌāch-'tē\ *n* : SEROTONIN

HTLV \ˌāch-(ˌ)tē-(ˌ)el-'vē\ *n* : any of several retroviruses that formerly included the original strain of HIV — often used with a number or Roman numeral to indicate the type and order of discovery ⟨*HTLV*-III⟩; called also *human T-cell leukemia virus, human T-cell lymphotropic virus, human T-lymphotropic virus*

HTLV–I \-ˌvē-'wən\ *n* : an HTLV (species *Primate T-lymphotropic virus 1* of the genus *Deltaretrovirus*) that is found in association with adult T-cell leukemia and a progressive paralyzing myelopathy

HTLV–III *n* : HIV-1

H_2 antagonist \-'tü-\ *n* : a drug (as famotidine or ranitidine) that reduces or inhibits the secretion of gastric acid by binding competitively with histamine to H_2 receptors on cell membranes — called also *H_2 blocker, H_2 receptor antagonist*

H_2 receptor *n* : a receptor for histamine on cell membranes that modulates the stimulation of heart rate and the secretion of gastric acid — called also *H_2 histamine receptor*

Hub·bard tank \'hə-bərd-\ *n* : a large tank in which a patient can easily be assisted in exercises while in the water

Hubbard, Leroy Watkins (1857–1938), American orthopedic surgeon.

hue \'hyü\ *n* : the one of the three psychological dimensions of color perception that permits them to be classified as red, yellow, green, blue, or an intermediate between any contiguous pair of these colors and that is correlated with the wavelength or the combination of wavelengths comprising the stimulus — compare BRIGHTNESS, SATURATION 4

huff \'həf\ *vb* : to inhale (noxious fumes) through the mouth for the euphoric effect produced by the inhalant; *also* : to inhale the noxious fumes of (a substance) for their euphoric effect

Hughes syndrome \'hyüz-\ *n* : ANTIPHOSPHOLIPID SYNDROME

Hughes, Graham Robert Vivian (*b* 1940), British rheumatologist.

Huh·ner test \'hyü-nər-\ *n* : a test used in sterility studies that involves postcoital examination of fluid aspirated from the vagina and cervix to determine the presence or survival of spermatozoa in these areas

Huhner, Max (1873–1947), American surgeon.

Hu·ma·log \'hyü-mə-ˌlȯg\ *trademark* — used for a preparation of insulin lispro

¹hu·man \'hyü-mən, 'yü-\ *adj* **1 a** : of, relating to, or characteristic of humans **b** : primarily or usu. harbored by, affecting, or attacking humans ⟨~ parasites⟩ **2** : being or consisting of humans ⟨the ~ race⟩ **3** : consisting of hominids — **hu·man·ness** *n*

²human *n* : a bipedal primate mammal of the genus *Homo* (*H. sapiens*); *broadly* : HOMINID — **hu·man·like** \-ˌlīk\ *adj*

human being *n* : HUMAN

human botfly *n* : a large fly of the genus *Dermatobia* (*D. hominis*) that is widely distributed in tropical America and undergoes its larval development subcutaneously in some mammals including humans

human chorionic gonadotropin *n* : a glycoprotein hormone similar in structure to luteinizing hormone that is secreted by the placenta during early pregnancy to maintain corpus luteum function, is commonly tested for as an indicator of pregnancy, and is used medically to induce ovulation and to treat male hypogonadism and cryptorchidism — abbr. *HCG*

human ecology *n* : the ecology of human communities and populations esp. as concerned with preservation of environmental quality through proper application of conservation and civil engineering practices

human ehrlichiosis *n* : ehrlichiosis or anaplasmosis affecting humans — see ANAPLASMOSIS a, HUMAN MONOCYTIC EHRLICHIOSIS

human engineering *n* : ERGONOMICS 1

human factors *n* : ERGONOMICS 1

human factors engineering *n* : ERGONOMICS 1

human granulocytic anaplasmosis *n* : ANAPLASMOSIS a — abbr. *HGA*

human granulocytic ehrlichiosis *n* : ANAPLASMOSIS a — abbr. *HGE*

human growth hormone *n* : the naturally occurring growth hormone of humans or a recombinant version that is used to treat children with growth hormone deficiencies and has been used esp. by athletes to increase muscle mass — abbr. *HGH;* see SOMATROPIN

human immunodeficiency virus *n* : HIV

human leukocyte antigen *n* : any of various proteins that are encoded by genes of the major histocompatibility complex in humans and are found on the surface of many cell types (as white blood cells); *broadly* : HLA 2

human monocytic ehrlichiosis *n* : a form of ehrlichiosis that affects humans, is marked by weakness, fatigue, fever, headache, chills, muscle ache, and by an abnormally low level of white blood cells and blood platelets, and is caused by a bacterium (*Ehrlichia chaffeensis*) transmitted by the lone star tick

human papillomavirus *n* : any of numerous papillomaviruses (as of the genera *Alphapapillomavirus, Betapapillomavirus*, and *Gammapapillomavirus*) that cause human papillomas (as plantar warts and genital warts) and include some associated with the production of cervical cancer — called also *HPV*

human relations *n* **1** : the social and interpersonal relations between humans **2** : a course, study, or program designed to develop better interpersonal and intergroup adjustments

human T–cell leukemia virus *n* : HTLV

human T–cell leukemia virus type III *n* : HIV-1

human T–cell lym•pho•tro•pic virus \\-ˌlim-fə-ˈtrō-pik-\\ *n* : HTLV

human T–cell lymphotropic virus type III *n* : HIV-1

human T–lymphotropic virus *n* : HTLV

human T–lymphotropic virus type III *n* : HIV-1

hu•mec•tant \\hyü-ˈmek-tənt\\ *n* : a substance (as sorbitol) that promotes retention of moisture — **humectant** *adj*

hu•mer•al \\ˈhyü-mə-rəl\\ *adj* : of, relating to, or situated in the region of the humerus or shoulder

humeral circumflex artery — see ANTERIOR HUMERAL CIRCUMFLEX ARTERY, POSTERIOR HUMERAL CIRCUMFLEX ARTERY

hu•mer•us \\ˈhyü-mə-rəs\\ *n, pl* **hu•meri** \\-ˌrī, -ˌrē\\ : the longest bone of the upper arm or forelimb extending from the shoulder to the elbow, articulating above by a rounded head with the glenoid cavity, having below a broad articular surface divided by a ridge into a medial pulley-shaped portion and a lateral rounded eminence that articulate with the ulna and radius respectively

hu•mid•i•fi•er \\hyü-ˈmi-də-ˌfī-ər, yü-\\ *n* : a device for supplying or maintaining humidity

hu•mid•i•fy \\-ˌfī\\ *vb* **-fied; -fy•ing** : to make humid — **hu•mid•i•fi•ca•tion** \\-ˌmi-də-fə-ˈkā-shən\\ *n*

hu•mid•i•ty \\hyü-ˈmi-də-tē, yü-\\ *n, pl* **-ties** : a moderate degree of wetness esp. of the atmosphere — see ABSOLUTE HUMIDITY, RELATIVE HUMIDITY

Hu•mira \\hyü-ˈmer-ə\\ *trademark* — used for a preparation of adalimumab

hu•mor \\ˈhyü-mər, ˈyü-\\ *n* **1** : a normal functioning bodily semifluid or fluid (as the blood or lymph) **2** : a secretion (as a hormone) that is an excitant of activity

hu•mor•al \\ˈhyü-mə-rəl, ˈyü-\\ *adj* **1** : of, relating to, proceeding from, or involving a bodily humor (as a hormone) **2** : relating to or being the part of immunity or the immune response that involves antibodies secreted by B cells and circulating in bodily fluids ⟨~ immunity⟩ — compare CELL-MEDIATED

hu•mour *chiefly Brit var of* HUMOR

hump \\ˈhəmp\\ *n* : a rounded protuberance; *esp* : HUMPBACK

hump•back \\-ˌbak, *for 1 also* -ˈbak\\ *n* **1** : a humped or crooked back; *also* : KYPHOSIS **2** : HUNCHBACK 2 — **hump•backed** \\-ˌbakt\\ *adj*

Hu•mu•lin \\ˈhyü-myu̇-lən\\ *trademark* — used for a preparation of insulin produced by genetically-altered bacteria and structurally identical to insulin made by the human pancreas

hunch·back \ˈhənch-ˌbak\ *n* **1** : HUMPBACK 1 **2** : a person with a humpback — **hunch·backed** \-ˌbakt\ *adj*

hun·ger \ˈhəŋ-gər\ *n* **1** : a craving, desire, or urgent need for food **2** : an uneasy sensation occasioned normally by the lack of food and resulting directly from stimulation of the sensory nerves of the stomach by the contraction and churning movement of the empty stomach **3** : a weakened disordered condition brought about by prolonged lack of food ⟨die of ∼⟩

hunger pangs *n pl* : pains in the abdominal region which occur in the early stages of hunger or fasting and are correlated with contractions of the empty stomach or intestines

Hun·ner's ulcer \ˈhə-nərz-\ *n* : a painful ulcer affecting all layers of the bladder wall and usu. associated with inflammation of the wall

Hunner, Guy Leroy (1868–1957), American gynecologist.

Hun·ter's canal \ˈhən-tərz-\ *n* : an aponeurotic canal in the middle third of the thigh through which the femoral artery passes

Hunter, John (1728–1793), British anatomist and surgeon.

Hunter's syndrome *or* **Hunter syndrome** \ˈhən-tər-\ *n* : a mucopolysaccharidosis that is similar to Hurler syndrome but is inherited as a sex-linked recessive trait and has milder symptoms

Hunter, Charles (1873–1955), Canadian physician.

Hun·ting·ton's chorea \ˈhən-tiŋ-tənz-\ *n* : HUNTINGTON'S DISEASE

Huntington, George (1850–1916), American neurologist.

Huntington's disease *also* **Huntington disease** *n* : a hereditary brain disorder that is a progressive neurodegenerative condition marked esp. by impairments in thinking and reasoning, disturbances of emotion and behavior, and the involuntary spasmodic movements of chorea, is inherited as an autosomal dominant trait, and usu. becomes symptomatic between 30 to 50 years of age — called also *Huntington's*

Hur·ler syndrome \ˈhər-lər-, ˈhu̇r-\ *or* **Hur·ler's syndrome** \-lərz-\ *n* : a mucopolysaccharidosis that is inherited as an autosomal recessive trait and is characterized by deformities of the skeleton and features, hepatosplenomegaly, restricted joint flexibility, clouding of the cornea, intellectual disability, deafness, and death usu. in childhood or early adolescence — called also *Hurler disease, Hurler's disease*

Hur·ler \ˈhu̇r-ler\, **Gertrud (1889–1965),** German pediatrician.

HUS *abbr* hemolytic uremic syndrome

husk \ˈhəsk\ *n* : HOOSE

Hutch·in·son's teeth \ˈhə-chən-sənz-\ *n sing or pl* : peg-shaped teeth having a crescent-shaped notch in the cutting edge and occurring esp. in children with congenital syphilis

Hutchinson, Sir Jonathan (1828–1913), British surgeon and pathologist.

Hutchinson's triad *n* : a triad of symptoms that comprises Hutchinson's teeth, interstitial keratitis, and deafness and occurs in children with congenital syphilis

Hux·ley's layer \ˈhəks-lēz-\ *n* : a layer of the inner stratum of a hair follicle composed of one or two layers of horny flattened epithelial cells with nuclei and situated between Henle's layer and the cuticle next to the hair

Huxley, Thomas Henry (1825–1895), British biologist.

hy- *or* **hyo-** *comb form* : of, relating to, or connecting with the hyoid bone ⟨*hyo*glossus⟩

hyal- *or* **hyalo-** *comb form* : glass : glassy : hyaline ⟨*hyal*uronic acid⟩

[1]**hy·a·line** \ˈhī-ə-lən, -ˌlīn\ *adj* : transparent or nearly transparent and usu. homogeneous

[2]**hy·a·line** \-ə-lən\ *n* : any of several translucent nitrogenous substances that collect around cells and are capable of being stained by eosin

hyaline cartilage *n* : translucent bluish-white cartilage consisting of cells embedded in an apparently homogeneous matrix, present in joints and respiratory passages, and forming most of the fetal skeleton

hyaline cast *n* : a renal cast of mucoprotein characterized by homogeneity of structure

hyaline degeneration *n* : tissue degeneration chiefly of connective tissues in which structural elements of affected cells are replaced by homogeneous translucent material that stains intensely with acid stains

hyaline membrane disease *n* : RESPIRATORY DISTRESS SYNDROME

hy·a·lin·i·za·tion \ˌhī-ə-lə-nə-ˈzā-shən\ *n* : the process of becoming hyaline or of undergoing hyaline degeneration; *also* : the resulting state — **hy·a·lin·ized** \ˈhī-ə-lə-ˌnīzd\ *adj*

hy·a·li·no·sis \ˌhī-ə-lə-ˈnō-səs\ *n, pl* **-no·ses** \-ˌsēz\ **1** : HYALINE DEGENERATION **2** : a condition characterized by hyaline degeneration

hy·a·li·tis \ˌhī-ə-ˈlī-təs\ *n* **1** : inflammation of the vitreous body of the eye **2** : inflammation of the hyaloid membrane of the vitreous humor

hyalo- — see HYAL-

hy·a·loid \ˈhī-ə-ˌlȯid\ *adj* : being glassy or transparent ⟨a ∼ appearance⟩

hyaloid membrane *n* : a very delicate membrane enclosing the vitreous body of the eye

hy·al·o·mere \hī-ˈa-lə-ˌmir\ *n* : the pale portion of a blood platelet that is not refractile — compare CHROMOMERE

Hy·a·lom·ma \ˌhī-ə-ˈlä-mə\ *n* : a genus of Old World ticks that attack wild and domestic mammals and sometimes humans, produce severe lesions by their bites, and often serve as vectors of viral and protozoal diseases (as east coast fever)

hy·a·lo·plasm \hī-ˈa-lə-ˌpla-zəm, ˈhī-ə-lō-\ *n* : CYTOSOL — **hy·a·lo·plas·mic** \hī-ˌa-lə-ˈplaz-mik, ˌhī-ə-lō-\ *adj*

hy·al·uron·ic acid \ˌhīl-yü-ˈrä-nik-, ˌhī-əl-yü-\ *n* : a viscous glycosaminoglycan that occurs esp. in the vitreous body, the umbilical cord, and synovial fluid and as a cementing substance in the subcutaneous tissue

hy·al·uron·i·dase \-ˈrä-nə-ˌdās, -ˌdāz\ *n* : a mucolytic enzyme that facilitates the spread of fluids through tissues by lowering the viscosity of hyaluronic acid and is used esp. to aid in the dispersion of fluids (as local anesthetics) injected subcutaneously — called also *spreading factor*

H–Y antigen *n* : a male histocompatibility antigen determined by genes on the Y chromosome

hy·brid \ˈhī-brəd\ *n* **1** : an offspring of two animals or plants of different races, breeds, varieties, species, or genera **2** : something heterogeneous in origin or composition ⟨artificial ∼*s* of DNA and RNA⟩ — **hybrid** *adj* — **hy·brid·ism** \-brə-ˌdi-zəm\ *n*

hy·brid·ize \ˈhī-brə-ˌdīz\ *vb* **-ized; -iz·ing** : to cause to interbreed or combine so as to produce hybrids — **hy·brid·i·za·tion** \ˌhī-brə-də-ˈzā-shən\ *n*

hy·brid·oma \ˌhī-brə-ˈdō-mə\ *n* : a hybrid cell produced by the fusion of an antibody-producing lymphocyte with a tumor cell and used to culture continuously a specific monoclonal antibody

hy·can·thone \hī-ˈkan-ˌthōn\ *n* : a lucanthone analog $C_{20}H_{24}N_2O_2S$ used to treat schistosomiasis

Hy·co·dan \ˈhī-kə-ˌdan\ *trademark* — used for a preparation of the bitartrate of hydrocodone and the methyl bromide of homatropine

hy·dan·to·in \hī-ˈdan-tə-wən\ *n* **1** : a crystalline weakly acidic compound $C_3H_4N_2O_2$ with a sweetish taste that is found in beet juice **2** : a derivative of hydantoin (as phenytoin)

hy·da·tid \ˈhī-də-təd, -ˌtid\ *n* **1** : the larval cyst of a tapeworm of the genus *Echinococcus* that usu. occurs as a fluid-filled sac containing daughter cysts in which scolices develop but that occas. forms a proliferating spongy mass which actively metastasizes in the host's tissues — called also *hydatid cyst;* see ECHINOCOCCUS 1 **2 a** : an abnormal cyst or cystic structure; *esp* : HYDATIDIFORM MOLE **b** : HYDATID DISEASE

hydatid disease *n* : a form of echinococcosis caused by the development of hydatids of a tapeworm of the genus *Echinococcus* (*E. granulosus*) in the tissues esp. of the liver or lungs of humans and some domestic animals (as sheep and dogs)

hy·da·tid·i·form mole \ˌhī-də-ˈti-də-ˌfȯrm-\ *n* : a mass in the uterus that consists of enlarged edematous degenerated chorionic villi growing in clusters resembling grapes, that typically develops following fertilization of an enucleate egg, and that may or may not contain fetal tissue

hy·da·tid·o·sis \ˌhī-də-ˌti-ˈdō-səs\ *n, pl* **-o·ses** \-ˌsēz\ : ECHINOCOCCOSIS; *specif* : HYDATID DISEASE

Hyd·er·gine \ˈhī-dər-ˌjēn\ *trademark* — used for a preparation of ergoloid mesylates

hydr- *or* **hydro-** *comb form* **1** : water ⟨*hydro*therapy⟩ **2** : an accumulation of fluid in a (specified) bodily part ⟨*hydro*cephalus⟩ ⟨*hydro*nephrosis⟩

hy·drae·mia *chiefly Brit var of* HYDREMIA

hy·dra·gogue \ˈhī-drə-ˌgäg\ *n* : a cathartic that causes copious watery discharges from the bowels

hy·dral·azine \hī-ˈdra-lə-ˌzēn\ *n* : an antihypertensive drug that is used in the form of its hydrochloride $C_8H_8N_4{\cdot}HCl$ and produces peripheral arteriolar dilation by relaxing vascular smooth muscle

hy·dram·ni·os \hī-ˈdram-nē-ˌäs\ *n* : excessive accumulation of the amniotic fluid — called also *polyhydramnios* — **hy·dram·ni·ot·ic** \hī-ˌdram-nē-ˈä-tik\ *adj*

hy·dran·en·ceph·a·ly \ˌhī-ˌdra-nen-ˈse-fə-lē\ *n, pl* **-lies** : a congenital defect of the brain in which fluid-filled cavities take the place of the cerebral hemispheres

hy·drar·gy·rism \hī-ˈdrär-jə-ˌri-zəm\ *n* : MERCURIALISM

hy·drar·thro·sis \ˌhi-(ˌ)drär-ˈthrō-səs\ *n, pl* **-thro·ses** \-ˌsēz\ : a watery effusion into a joint cavity

[1]**hy·drate** \ˈhī-ˌdrāt\ *n* **1** : a compound or complex ion formed by the union of water with some other substance **2** : HYDROXIDE

[2]**hydrate** *vb* **hy·drat·ed; hy·drat·ing** **1** : to cause to take up or combine with water or the elements of water **2** : to become a hydrate

hy·dra·tion \hī-ˈdrā-shən\ *n* **1** : the act or process of combining or treating with water: as **a** : the introduction of additional fluid into the body **b** : a chemical reaction in which water takes part with the formation of only one product **2** : the quality or state of being hydrated; *esp* : the condition of having adequate fluid in body tissues

hy·dra·zide \ˈhī-drə-ˌzīd\ *n* : any of a class of compounds resulting from the replacement by an acid group of hydrogen in hydrazine or in one of its derivatives

hy·dra·zine \ˈhī-drə-ˌzēn\ *n* : a colorless fuming corrosive strongly reducing liquid base N_2H_4 used in the production of numerous materials (as pharmaceuticals and plastics); *also* : an organic base derived from this

hy•dra•zone \ˈhī-drə-ˌzōn\ *n* : any of a class of compounds containing the group >C=NNHR

hy•dre•mia \hī-ˈdrē-mē-ə\ *n* : an abnormally watery state of the blood — **hy•dre•mic** \-mik\ *adj*

hy•dren•ceph•a•ly \ˌhī-dren-ˈse-fə-lē\ *n, pl* **-lies** : HYDROCEPHALUS

hydro- — see HYDR-

hy•droa \hī-ˈdrō-ə\ *n* : an itching usu. vesicular eruption of the skin; *esp* : one induced by exposure to light

hy•dro•bro•mide \ˌhī-drō-ˈbrō-ˌmīd\ *n* : a salt of hydrogen bromide with an organic base

hy•dro•car•bon \-ˈkär-bən\ *n* : an organic compound (as benzene) containing only carbon and hydrogen and often occurring esp. in petroleum, natural gas, and coal

hy•dro•cele \ˈhī-drə-ˌsēl\ *n* : an accumulation of serous fluid in a sacculated cavity (as the scrotum)

hy•dro•ce•lec•to•my \ˌhī-drə-sē-ˈlek-tə-mē\ *n, pl* **-mies** : surgical removal of a hydrocele

[1]**hy•dro•ce•phal•ic** \ˌhī-drō-sə-ˈfa-lik\ *adj* : relating to, characterized by, or affected with hydrocephalus

[2]**hydrocephalic** *n* : an individual affected with hydrocephalus

hy•dro•ceph•a•lus \-ˈse-fə-ləs\ *n, pl* **-li** \-ˌlī\ : an abnormal increase in the amount of cerebrospinal fluid within the cranial cavity that is accompanied by expansion of the cerebral ventricles and often increased intracranial pressure, skull enlargement, and cognitive decline

hy•dro•ceph•a•ly \ˌhī-drō-ˈse-fə-lē\ *n, pl* **-lies** : HYDROCEPHALUS

hy•dro•chlo•ric acid \ˌhī-drə-ˈklōr-ik-\ *n* : an aqueous solution of hydrogen chloride HCl that is a strong corrosive irritating acid and is normally present in dilute form in gastric juice — called also *muriatic acid*

hy•dro•chlo•ride \-ˈklōr-ˌīd\ *n* : a salt of hydrochloric acid with an organic base used esp. as a vehicle for the administration of a drug

hy•dro•chlo•ro•thi•a•zide \-ˌklōr-ə-ˈthī-ə-ˌzīd\ *n* : a diuretic and antihypertensive drug $C_7H_8ClN_3O_4S_2$ — abbr. *HCTZ;* see ATACAND HCT, BENICAR HCT, DYAZIDE, HYZAAR, MAXZIDE, TRIBENZOR

hy•dro•cho•le•re•sis \-ˌkō-lər-ˈē-səs, -ˌkä-\ *n, pl* **-re•ses** \-ˌsēz\ : increased production of watery liver bile without necessarily increased secretion of bile solids

[1]**hy•dro•cho•le•ret•ic** \-ˈe-tik\ *adj* : of, relating to, or characterized by hydrocholeresis

[2]**hydrocholeretic** *n* : an agent that produces hydrocholeresis

hy•dro•co•done \ˌhī-drō-ˈkō-ˌdōn\ *n* : a habit-forming codeine derivative used in the form of its bitartrate $C_{18}H_{21}NO_3{\cdot}C_4H_6O_6$ usu. in combination with other drugs (as acetaminophen) as an analgesic or cough sedative — called also *dihydrocodeinone;* see HYCODAN, VICODIN

hy•dro•cor•ti•sone \-ˈkȯr-tə-ˌsōn, -ˌzōn\ *n* : CORTISOL; *esp* : cortisol used pharmaceutically

hy•dro•cy•an•ic acid \ˌhī-drō-sī-ˈa-nik-\ *n* : an aqueous solution of hydrogen cyanide HCN that is an extremely poisonous weak acid used esp. in fumigating — called also *prussic acid*

Hy•dro•di•ur•il \-ˈdī-yə-ˌril\ *n* : a preparation of hydrochlorothiazide — formerly a U.S. registered trademark

hy•dro•dy•nam•ics \ˌhī-drō-dī-ˈna-miks\ *n* : a branch of physics that deals with the motion of fluids and the forces acting on solid bodies immersed in fluids and in motion relative to them — **hy•dro•dy•nam•ic** \-mik\ *adj*

hy•dro•flu•me•thi•a•zide \-ˌflü-mə-ˈthī-ə-ˌzīd\ *n* : a diuretic and antihypertensive drug $C_8H_8F_3N_3O_4S_2$

hy•dro•fluo•ro•al•kane \-ˌflu̇r-ō-ˈal-ˌkān, -ˌflȯr-\ *n* : a gas containing carbon, fluorine, and hydrogen used esp. as an aerosol propellant in metered-dose inhalers — abbr. *HFA*

hy•dro•gel \ˈhī-drə-ˌjel\ *n* : a gel in which the liquid is water

hy•dro•gen \ˈhī-drə-jən\ *n* : a nonmetallic element that is the simplest and lightest of the elements and is normally a colorless odorless highly flammable gas having two atoms in a molecule — symbol *H;* see ELEMENT table — **hy•drog•e•nous** \hī-ˈdrä-jə-nəs\ *adj*

hy•dro•ge•nate \hī-ˈdrä-jə-ˌnāt, ˈhī-drə-jə-\ *vb* **-nat•ed; -nat•ing** : to add hydrogen to the molecule of (an unsaturated organic compound) — **hy•dro•ge•na•tion** \hī-ˌdrä-jə-ˈnā-shən, ˌhī-drə-jə-\ *n*

hydrogen bond *n* : an electrostatic attraction between a hydrogen atom in one polar molecule (as of water) and a small negatively charged atom (as of fluorine, oxygen, or nitrogen) in usu. another molecule of the same or a different polar substance

hydrogen bromide *n* : a colorless irritating gas HBr that fumes in moist air and yields a strong acid resembling hydrochloric acid when dissolved in water

hydrogen chloride *n* : a colorless pungent poisonous gas HCl that fumes in moist air and yields hydrochloric acid when dissolved in water

hydrogen cyanide *n* **1** : a poisonous usu. gaseous compound HCN that has the odor of bitter almonds **2** : HYDROCYANIC ACID

hydrogen peroxide *n* : an unstable compound H_2O_2 used esp. as an oxidizing and bleaching agent and as an antiseptic

hy•dro•lase \ˈhī-drə-ˌlās, -ˌlāz\ *n* : a hydrolytic enzyme (as an esterase)

hy·drol·o·gy \hī-ˈdrä-lə-jē\ *n, pl* **-gies** : the body of medical knowledge and practice concerned with the therapeutic use of bathing and water

hy·dro·ly·sate \hī-ˈdrä-lə-ˌsāt, ˌhī-drə-ˈlī-\ *or* **hy·dro·ly·zate** \-ˌzāt\ *n* : a product of hydrolysis

hy·dro·ly·sis \hī-ˈdrä-lə-səs, ˌhī-drə-ˈlī-\ *n* : a chemical process of decomposition involving splitting of a bond and the addition of the hydrogen cation and the hydroxide anion of water — **hy·dro·lyt·ic** \ˌhī-drə-ˈli-tik\ *adj* — **hy·dro·lyze** \ˈhī-drə-ˌlīz\ *vb* — **hy·dro·lyz·able** \ˌhī-drə-ˈlī-zə-bəl\ *adj*

hy·dro·me·tro·col·pos \ˌhī-drō-ˌmē-trō-ˈkäl-ˌpäs\ *n* : an accumulation of watery fluid in the uterus and vagina

hy·dro·mor·phone \-ˈmȯr-ˌfōn\ *n* : a morphine derivative administered in the form of its hydrochloride $C_{17}H_{19}NO_3 \cdot HCl$ as an analgesic — called also *dihydromorphinone*

hy·dro·ne·phro·sis \-ni-ˈfrō-səs\ *n, pl* **-phro·ses** \-ˌsēz\ : cystic distension of the kidney caused by the accumulation of urine in the renal pelvis as a result of obstruction to outflow and accompanied by atrophy of the kidney structure and cyst formation — **hy·dro·ne·phrot·ic** \-ni-ˈfrä-tik\ *adj*

hy·drop·a·thy \hī-ˈdrä-pə-thē\ *n, pl* **-thies** : a method of treating disease by copious and frequent use of water both externally and internally — compare HYDROTHERAPY — **hy·dro·path·ic** \ˌhī-drə-ˈpa-thik\ *adj*

hy·dro·pe·nia \ˌhī-drə-ˈpē-nē-ə\ *n* : a condition in which the body is deficient in water — **hy·dro·pe·nic** \-ˈpē-nik\ *adj*

hy·dro·peri·car·di·um \ˌhī-drō-per-ə-ˈkär-dē-əm\ *n, pl* **-dia** \-dē-ə\ : an excess of watery fluid in the pericardial cavity

hy·dro·phil·ic \-ˈfi-lik\ *adj* : of, relating to, or having a strong affinity for water ⟨~ colloids⟩ — compare LIPOPHILIC — **hy·dro·phi·lic·i·ty** \-fi-ˈli-sə-tē\ *n*

hy·dro·pho·bia \ˌhī-drə-ˈfō-bē-ə\ *n* **1** : a morbid dread of water **2 a** : extreme fearfulness of swallowing liquids that is symptomatic of rabies and results from painful spasms of the throat **b** : RABIES

hy·dro·pho·bic \-ˈfō-bik\ *adj* **1** : of, relating to, or suffering from hydrophobia **2** : resistant to or avoiding wetting ⟨a ~ lens⟩ **3** : of, relating to, or having a lack of affinity for water ⟨~ colloids⟩ — **hy·dro·pho·bic·i·ty** \-ˌfō-ˈbi-sə-tē\ *n*

hy·droph·thal·mos \ˌhī-ˌdräf-ˈthal-mäs\ *n* : general enlargement of the eyeball due to a watery effusion within it

hy·drop·ic \hī-ˈdrä-pik\ *adj* **1** : exhibiting hydrops; *esp* : EDEMATOUS **2** : characterized by swelling and taking up of fluid — used of a type of cellular degeneration

hy·dro·pneu·mo·tho·rax \ˌhī-drə-ˌnü-mə-ˈthōr-ˌaks, -ˌnyü-\ *n, pl* **-tho·rax·es** *or* **-tho·ra·ces** \-ˈthōr-ə-ˌsēz\ : the presence of gas and serous fluid in the pleural cavity

hy·drops \ˈhī-ˌdräps\ *n, pl* **hy·drop·ses** \-ˌdräp-ˌsēz\ **1** : EDEMA **2** : distension of a hollow organ with fluid **3** : HYDROPS FETALIS

hydrops fe·tal·is \-fē-ˈta-ləs\ *n* : serious and extensive edema of the fetus (as in erythroblastosis fetalis) — called also *fetal hydrops*

hy·dro·qui·none \ˌhī-drō-kwi-ˈnōn, -ˈkwi-ˌnōn\ *n* : a bleaching agent $C_6H_6O_2$ used topically to remove pigmentation from hyperpigmented areas of skin (as a lentigo or freckle)

hy·dro·sal·pinx \-ˈsal-(ˌ)piŋks\ *n, pl* **-sal·pin·ges** \-sal-ˈpin-(ˌ)jēz\ : abnormal distension of one or both fallopian tubes with fluid usu. due to inflammation

hy·dro·ther·a·py \ˌhī-drō-ˈther-ə-pē\ *n, pl* **-pies** : the therapeutic use of water (as in a whirlpool bath) — compare HYDROPATHY — **hy·dro·ther·a·peu·tic** \-ˌther-ə-ˈpyü-tik\ *adj*

hy·dro·tho·rax \-ˈthōr-ˌaks\ *n, pl* **-tho·rax·es** *or* **-tho·ra·ces** \-ˈthōr-ə-ˌsēz\ : an excess of serous fluid in the pleural cavity; *esp* : an effusion resulting from failing circulation (as in heart disease)

hy·dro·ure·ter \ˌhī-drō-ˈyu̇r-ə-tər, -yu̇-ˈrē-tər\ *n* : abnormal distension of the ureter with urine

hy·drox·ide \hī-ˈdräk-ˌsīd\ *n* **1** : the anion OH^- consisting of one atom of hydrogen and one of oxygen — called also *hydroxide ion* **2** : an ionic compound of hydroxide with an element or group

hy·droxo·co·bal·amin \hī-ˈdräk-(ˌ)sō-kō-ˈba-lə-mən\ *n* : a member $C_{62}H_{89}CoN_{13}O_{15}P$ of the vitamin B_{12} group used in treating and preventing vitamin B_{12} deficiency

hy·droxy \hī-ˈdräk-sē\ *adj* : being or containing hydroxyl; *esp* : containing hydroxyl in place of hydrogen — often used in combination ⟨*hydroxy*butyric acid⟩

hy·droxy·am·phet·amine \hī-ˌdräk-sē-am-ˈfe-tə-ˌmēn, -mən\ *n* : a sympathomimetic drug administered in the form of its hydrobromide $C_9H_{13}NO \cdot HBr$ and used esp. as a mydriatic

hydroxyanisole — see BUTYLATED HYDROXYANISOLE

hy·droxy·ap·a·tite \hī-ˌdräk-sē-ˈa-pə-ˌtīt\ *also* **hy·drox·yl·ap·a·tite** \-sə-ˈla-\ *n* : a complex phosphate of calcium $Ca_5(PO_4)_3OH$ that is the chief structural element of bone

hy·droxy·ben·zo·ic acid \-ben-ˈzō-ik-\ *n* : SALICYLIC ACID

hy·droxy·bu·ty·rate \-ˈbyü-tə-ˌrāt\ *n* : a salt or ester of hydroxybutyric acid — see GAMMA HYDROXYBUTYRATE

hy·droxy·bu·tyr·ic acid \-byu̇-ˈtir-ik-\ *or* **β–hy·droxy·bu·tyr·ic acid** \ˈbā-tə-\ *n* : a derivative $C_4H_8O_3$ of butyric acid that is excreted in urine in increased quantities in diabetes — called also *oxybutyric acid*

hy·droxy·chlor·o·quine \-ˈklōr-ə-ˌkwēn, -kwin\ *n* : a drug derived from quinoline that is administered orally in the form of its sulfate $C_{18}H_{26}ClN_3O \cdot H_2SO_4$ to treat malaria, rheumatoid arthritis, and lupus erythematosus — see PLAQUENIL

25–hy·droxy·cho·le·cal·cif·er·ol \ˈtwen-tē-ˈfīv-hī-ˌdräk-sē-ˌkō-lə-(ˌ)kal-ˈsi-fə-ˌrȯl, -ˌrōl\ *n* : a sterol $C_{27}H_{44}O_2$ that is a metabolite of cholecalciferol formed in the liver and is the circulating form of vitamin D

17–hy·droxy·cor·ti·co·ste·roid \ˌse-vən-ˈtēn-hī-ˌdräk-sē-ˌkȯrt-i-kō-ˈstir-ˌȯid, -ˈster-\ *n* : any of several adrenocorticosteroids (as cortisol) with an –OH group and an $HOCH_2CO^-$ group attached to carbon 17 of the fused ring structure of the steroid

hy·droxy·di·one sodium suc·ci·nate \hī-ˌdräk-sē-ˈdī-ˌōn . . . ˈsək-sə-ˌnāt\ *n* : a steroid $C_{25}H_{35}NaO_6$ given intravenously as a general anesthetic

6–hy·droxy·do·pa·mine \ˈsiks-hī-ˌdräk-sē-ˈdō-pə-ˌmēn\ *n* : an isomer of norepinephrine that is taken up by catecholaminergic nerve fibers and causes the degeneration of their terminals

5–hy·droxy·in·dole·ace·tic acid \ˈfīv-hī-ˌdräk-sē-ˌin-(ˌ)dō-lə-ˈsē-tik-\ *n* : a metabolite $C_{10}H_9NO_3$ of serotonin that is present in cerebrospinal fluid and in urine — abbr. *5-HIAA*

hy·drox·yl \hī-ˈdräk-səl\ *n* **1** : the chemical group or ion OH that consists of one atom of hydrogen and one of oxygen and is neutral or positively charged **2** : HYDROXIDE 1

hydroxylapatite *var of* HYDROXYAPATITE

hy·drox·y·lase \hī-ˈdräk-sə-ˌlās, -ˌlāz\ *n* : any of a group of enzymes that catalyze oxidation reactions in which one of the two atoms of molecular oxygen is incorporated into the substrate and the other is used to oxidize NADH or NADPH

hy·droxy·ly·sine \hī-ˌdräk-sē-ˈlī-ˌsēn\ *n* : an amino acid $C_6H_{14}N_2O_3$ that is found esp. in collagen

hy·droxy·pro·ges·ter·one \hī-ˌdräk-sē-prō-ˈjes-tə-ˌrōn\ *or* **17α–hydroxyprogesterone** \ˌse-vən-ˈtēn-ˈal-fə-\ *n* : a synthetic derivative of progesterone used esp. in the form of the salt of caproic acid $C_{27}H_{40}O_4$ in progestational therapy (as for amenorrhea)

hy·droxy·pro·line \-ˈprō-ˌlēn\ *n* : an amino acid $C_5H_9NO_3$ that occurs naturally as a constituent of collagen

8–hy·droxy·quin·o·line \ˈāt-hī-ˌdräk-sē-ˈkwin-ᵊl-ˌēn\ *n* : a derivative of quinoline used esp. in the form of its sulfate $(C_9H_7NO)_2 \cdot H_2SO_4$ as a disinfectant, topical antiseptic, antiperspirant, and deodorant — called also *oxyquinoline*

hy·droxy·ste·roid \-ˈstir-ˌȯid, -ˈster-\ *n* : any of several ketosteroids (as androsterone) found esp. in urine

hydroxytoluene — see BUTYLATED HYDROXYTOLUENE

5–hy·droxy·tryp·ta·mine \ˈfīv-hī-ˌdräk-sē-ˈtrip-tə-ˌmēn\ *n* : SEROTONIN

hy·droxy·urea \-yu̇-ˈrē-ə\ *n* : an antineoplastic drug $CH_4N_2O_2$ used esp. to treat myeloproliferative disorders (as chronic myelogenous leukemia, polycythemia vera, and thrombocythemia) and malignant tumors

hy·droxy·zine \hī-ˈdräk-sə-ˌzēn\ *n* : a compound that is administered usu. in the form of its dihydrochloride $C_{21}H_{27}ClN_2O_2 \cdot 2HCl$ or pamoate $C_{21}H_{27}ClN_2O_2 \cdot C_{23}H_{16}O_6$ and is used as an antihistamine and tranquilizer — see VISTARIL

hy·giene \ˈhī-ˌjēn\ *n* **1** : a science of the establishment and maintenance of health — see MENTAL HYGIENE **2** : conditions or practices (as of cleanliness) conducive to health — **hy·gien·ic** \ˌhī-jē-ˈe-nik, hī-ˈje-, hī-ˈjē-\ *adj* — **hy·gien·i·cal·ly** *adv*

hy·gien·ics \-iks\ *n* : HYGIENE 1

hy·gien·ist \hī-ˈjē-nist, -ˈje-; ˈhī-ˌjē-\ *n* : a specialist in hygiene; *esp* : one skilled in a specified branch of hygiene — see DENTAL HYGIENIST

hy·gro·ma \hī-ˈgrō-mə\ *n, pl* **-mas** *also* **-ma·ta** \-mə-tə\ : a cystic tumor of lymphatic origin

hy·gro·my·cin B \ˌhī-grə-ˈmīs-ᵊn-ˈbē\ *n* : an antibiotic $C_{20}H_{37}N_3O_{13}$ obtained from a bacterium of the genus *Streptomyces* (*S. hygroscopicus*) and used as an anthelmintic in swine and chickens

hy·gro·scop·ic \ˌhī-grə-ˈskä-pik\ *adj* : readily taking up and retaining moisture ⟨glycerol is ~⟩

Hy·gro·ton \ˈhī-grə-ˌtän\ *n* : a preparation of chlorthalidone — formerly a U.S. registered trademark

hy·men \ˈhī-mən\ *n* : a fold of mucous membrane partly or wholly closing the orifice of the vagina — **hy·men·al** \-mən-ᵊl\ *adj*

hymen- *or* **hymeno-** *comb form* : hymen : membrane ⟨*hymen*ectomy⟩

hy·men·ec·to·my \ˌhī-mə-ˈnek-tə-mē\ *n, pl* **-mies** : surgical removal of the hymen

Hy·me·nol·e·pis \ˌhī-mə-ˈnä-lə-pəs\ *n* : a genus of small taenioid tapeworms (family Hymenolepididae) that are parasites of mammals and birds and include one (*H. nana*) that is an intestinal parasite of humans

hy·me·nop·ter·an \ˌhī-mə-ˈnäp-tə-rən\ *n* : any of an order (Hymenoptera) of highly specialized and often colonial insects (as bees, wasps, and ants) that have usu. four thin transparent wings and the abdomen on a slender stalk — **hymenopteran** *adj* — **hy·me·nop·ter·ous** \-tə-rəs\ *adj*

hy·me·nop·ter·ism \-ˈnäp-tə-ˌri-zəm\ *n* : poisoning resulting from the bite or sting of a hymenopteran insect

hy·men·ot·o·my \ˌhī-mə-ˈnä-tə-mē\ *n, pl* **-mies** : surgical incision of the hymen

hyo- — see HY-

hyo·glos·sal \ˌhī-ō-ˈgläs-ᵊl, -ˈglȯs-\ *adj* : of, relating to, or connecting the tongue and hyoid bone

hyo·glos·sus \-ˈglä-səs, -ˈglȯ-\ *n, pl* **-si** \-ˌsī, -ˌsē\ : a flat muscle on each side of the tongue

hy·oid \ˈhī-ˌȯid\ *adj* : of or relating to the hyoid bone

hyoid bone *n* : a U-shaped bone or complex of bones that is situated between the base of the tongue and the larynx and that supports the tongue, the larynx, and their muscles — called also *hyoid*

hyo·man·dib·u·lar \ˌhī-ō-man-ˈdi-byu̇-lər\ *n* : a bone or cartilage that forms the columella or stapes of the ear of higher vertebrates — **hyomandibular** *adj*

hyo·scine \ˈhī-ə-ˌsēn\ *n* : SCOPOLAMINE; *esp* : the levorotatory form of scopolamine

hyo·scy·a·mine \ˌhī-ə-ˈsī-ə-ˌmēn\ *n* : a poisonous crystalline alkaloid $C_{17}H_{23}NO_3$ of which atropine is a racemic mixture; *esp* : its levorotatory form found esp. in belladonna and henbane and used similarly to atropine

hyo·scy·a·mus \-məs\ *n* **1** *cap* : a genus of poisonous Eurasian herbs of the nightshade family (Solanaceae) that includes the henbane (*H. niger*) **2** : the dried leaves of the henbane containing the alkaloids hyoscyamine and scopolamine and used as an antispasmodic and sedative

Hyo·stron·gy·lus \-ˈsträn-jə-ləs\ *n* : a genus of nematode worms (family Trichostrongylidae) that includes the stomach worm (*H. rubidus*) of swine

¹hyp·acu·sic \ˌhi-pə-ˈkü-sik, ˌhī-, -ˈkyü-\ *adj* : affected with hypoacusis

²hypacusic *n* : one affected with hypoacusis

hyp·acu·sis \-ˈkü-səs, -ˈkyü-\ *n* : HYPOACUSIS

hyp·aes·the·sia *Brit var of* HYPESTHESIA

hyp·al·ge·sia \ˌhip-ᵊl-ˈjē-zhə, ˌhī-pal-, -zē-ə, -zhē-ə\ *n* : diminished sensitivity to pain — **hyp·al·ge·sic** \-ˈjē-zik, -sik\ *adj*

Hy·paque \ˈhī-ˌpāk\ *trademark* — used for a diatrizoate preparation for use in radiographic diagnosis

hyper- *prefix* **1** : excessively ⟨*hyper*sensitive⟩ **2** : excessive ⟨*hyper*emia⟩

hy·per·acid·i·ty \ˌhī-pə-rə-ˈsi-də-tē\ *n, pl* **-ties** : the condition of containing more than the normal amount of acid — **hy·per·ac·id** \ˌhī-pə-ˈra-səd\ *adj*

¹hy·per·ac·tive \ˌhī-pə-ˈrak-tiv\ *adj* : affected with or exhibiting hyperactivity; *broadly* : more active than is usual or desirable

²hyperactive *n* : one who is hyperactive

hy·per·ac·tiv·i·ty \ˌhī-pə-ˌrak-ˈti-və-tē\ *n, pl* **-ties** : a state or condition of being excessively or pathologically active; *esp* : ATTENTION DEFICIT DISORDER

hy·per·acu·ity \ˌhī-pə-rə-ˈkyü-ə-tē\ *n, pl* **-ities** : greater than normal acuteness esp. of a sense; *specif* : visual acuity that is better than twenty-twenty

hy·per·acu·sis \ˌhī-pə-rə-ˈkü-səs, -ˈkyü-\ *n* : abnormally acute hearing

hy·per·acute \ˌhī-pə-rə-ˈkyüt\ *adj* : extremely or excessively acute ⟨~ hearing⟩

hy·per·adren·a·lin·ae·mia *chiefly Brit var of* HYPERADRENALINEMIA

hy·per·adren·a·lin·emia \ˌhī-pə-rə-ˌdren-ᵊl-ə-ˈnē-mē-ə\ *n* : the presence of an excess of adrenal hormones (as epinephrine) in the blood

hy·per·ad·re·no·cor·ti·cism \ˌhī-pə-rə-ˌdrē-nō-ˈkȯr-tə-ˌsi-zəm\ *n* : an abnormal condition marked by the presence of an excess of adrenocortical hormones and esp. cortisol in the body; *esp* : CUSHING'S SYNDROME

hy·per·ae·mia, hy·per·aes·the·sia *chiefly Brit var of* HYPEREMIA, HYPERESTHESIA

hy·per·ag·gres·sive \ˌhī-pə-rə-ˈgre-səv\ *adj* : extremely or excessively aggressive ⟨~ patients⟩

hy·per·al·do·ste·ron·ae·mia *chiefly Brit var of* HYPERALDOSTERONEMIA

hy·per·al·do·ste·ron·emia \ˌhī-pə-ral-ˌdäs-tə-ˌrō-ˈnē-mē-ə, -ˌral-dō-stə-ˌrō-\ *n* : the presence of an excess of aldosterone in the blood

hy·per·al·do·ste·ron·ism \ˌhī-pə-ˌral-ˈdäs-tə-ˌrō-ˌni-zəm, -ˌral-dō-stə-ˈrō-\ *n* : ALDOSTERONISM

hy·per·al·ge·sia \ˌhī-pə-ral-ˈjē-zhə, -zē-ə, -zhē-ə\ *n* : increased sensitivity to pain or enhanced intensity of pain sensation — **hy·per·al·ge·sic** \-ˈjē-zik, -sik\ *adj*

hy·per·al·i·men·ta·tion \ˌhī-pə-ˌra-lə-mən-ˈtā-shən\ *n* : the administration of nutrients by intravenous feeding

hy·per·ami·no·ac·id·uria \ˌhī-pə-rə-ˌmē-nō-ˌa-sə-ˈdu̇r-ē-ə, -ˈdyu̇r-\ *n* : the presence of an excess of amino acids in the urine

hy·per·am·mo·nae·mia *also* **hy·per·am·mon·i·ae·mia** *chiefly Brit var of* HYPERAMMONEMIA

hy·per·am·mo·ne·mia \ˌhī-pə-ˌra-mə-ˈnē-mē-ə\ *also* **hy·per·am·mon·i·emia** \ˌhī-pə-rə-ˌmō-ne-ˈyē-mē-ə\ *n* : the presence of an excess of ammonia in the blood — **hy·per·am·mo·ne·mic** \ˌhī-pe-ˌra-mə-ˈnē-mik\ *adj*

hy·per·am·y·las·ae·mia *chiefly Brit var of* HYPERAMYLASEMIA

hy·per·am·y·las·emia \ˌhī-pə-ˌra-mə-ˌlā-ˈsē-mē-ə\ *n* : the presence of an excess of amylase in the blood

hy·per·arous·al \ˌhī-pə-rə-ˈrau̇-zəl\ *n* : excessive arousal : an abnormal state of increased responsiveness to stimuli

hy·per·bar·ic \ˌhī-pər-ˈbar-ik\ *adj* **1** : having a specific gravity greater than that of cerebrospinal fluid — used of solutions for spinal anesthesia; compare HYPOBARIC **2** : of, relating to, or utilizing greater than normal pressure esp. of oxygen ⟨a ~ chamber⟩ ⟨~ treatment⟩ — **hy·per·bar·i·cal·ly** *adv*

hyperbaric medicine *n* : a branch of medicine dealing with the use of oxygen at a pressure greater than normal atmospheric pressure esp. in the treatment of injury and disease — see HYPERBARIC OXYGEN THERAPY

hyperbaric oxygen therapy *n* : therapy used in hyperbaric medicine that involves the administration in a sealed chamber of pure oxygen at a greater than normal atmospheric pressure — abbr. *HBOT*

hy•per•be•ta•li•po•pro•tein•emia \-ˌbā-tə-ˌlī-pō-ˌprō-ˌtē-ˈnē-mē-ə, -ˌli-, -ˌprō-tē-ə-\ *n* : the presence of excess LDLs in the blood

hy•per•bil•i•ru•bin•emia \-ˌbi-lē-ˌrü-bi-ˈnē-mē-ə\ *n* : the presence of an excess of bilirubin in the blood — called also *bilirubinemia*

hy•per•cal•cae•mia *chiefly Brit var of* HYPERCALCEMIA

hy•per•cal•ce•mia \ˌhī-pər-ˌkal-ˈsē-mē-ə\ *n* : the presence of an excess of calcium in the blood — **hy•per•cal•ce•mic** \-ˈsē-mik\ *adj*

hy•per•cal•ci•uria \-ˌkal-sē-ˈyu̇r-ē-ə\ *also* **hy•per•cal•cin•uria** \-ˌkal-sə-ˈnu̇r-ē-ə\ *n* : the presence of an excess amount of calcium in the urine

hy•per•cap•nia \-ˈkap-nē-ə\ *n* : the presence of an excess of carbon dioxide in the blood — **hy•per•cap•nic** \-nik\ *adj*

hy•per•car•bia \-ˈkär-bē-ə\ *n* : HYPERCAPNIA

hy•per•ca•tab•o•lism \-kə-ˈta-bə-ˌli-zəm\ *n* : excessive metabolic breakdown of organic molecules : excessive catabolic activity — **hy•per•cat•a•bol•ic** \-ˌka-tə-ˈbä-lik\ *adj*

hy•per•cel•lu•lar•i•ty \-ˌsel-yə-ˈlar-ə-tē\ *n, pl* **-ties** : the presence of an abnormal excess of cells (as in bone marrow) — **hy•per•cel•lu•lar** \-ˈsel-yə-lər\ *adj*

hy•per•ce•men•to•sis \-ˌsē-men-ˈtō-səs\ *n, pl* **-to•ses** \-ˌsēz\ : excessive formation of cementum at the root of a tooth

hy•per•chlor•ae•mia *chiefly Brit var of* HYPERCHLOREMIA

hy•per•chlor•emia \-ˌklōr-ˈē-mē-ə\ *n* : the presence of excess chloride ions in the blood — **hy•per•chlor•emic** \-ˈē-mik\ *adj*

hy•per•chlor•hy•dria \-ˌklōr-ˈhī-drē-ə\ *n* : the presence of a greater than typical proportion of hydrochloric acid in gastric juice — compare ACHLORHYDRIA, HYPOCHLORHYDRIA

hy•per•cho•les•ter•ol•emia \ˌhī-pər-kə-ˌles-tə-rə-ˈlē-mē-ə\ *also* **hy•per•cho•les•ter•emia** \-tə-ˈrē-mē-ə\ *n* : the presence of excess cholesterol in the blood — see FAMILIAL HYPERCHOLESTEROLEMIA — **hy•per•cho•les•ter•ol•emic** \-tə-rə-ˈlē-mik\ *also* **hy•per•cho•les•ter•emic** \-tə-ˈrē-mik\ *adj*

hy•per•chro•ma•sia \-krō-ˈmā-zhə, -zē-ə, -zhē-ə\ *n* : HYPERCHROMATISM

hy•per•chro•ma•tism \-ˈkrō-mə-ˌti-zəm\ *n* : the development of excess chromatin or of excessive nuclear staining esp. as a part of a pathological process — **hy•per•chro•mat•ic** \-krō-ˈma-tik\ *adj*

hy•per•chro•mia \-ˈkrō-mē-ə\ *n* **1** : excessive pigmentation (as of the skin) **2** : a state of the red blood cells marked by increase in the hemoglobin content — **hy•per•chro•mic** \-ˈkrō-mik\ *adj*

hyperchromic anemia *n* : an anemia with increase of hemoglobin in individual red blood cells and reduction in the number of red blood cells — see PERNICIOUS ANEMIA; compare HYPOCHROMIC ANEMIA

hy•per•chy•lo•mi•cro•ne•mia \ˌhī-pər-ˌkī-lō-ˌmī-krō-ˈnē-mē-ə\ *n* : the presence of excess chylomicrons in the blood

hy•per•co•ag•u•la•bil•i•ty \-kō-ˌa-gyə-lə-ˈbi-lə-tē\ *n, pl* **-ties** : excessive coagulability — **hy•per•co•ag•u•la•ble** \-kō-ˈa-gyə-lə-bəl\ *adj*

hy•per•cor•ti•sol•ism \-ˈkȯr-ti-ˌsȯ-ˌli-zəm, -ˌsō-\ *n* : hyperadrenocorticism produced by excess cortisol in the body

hy•per•cu•prae•mia *chiefly Brit var of* HYPERCUPREMIA

hy•per•cu•pre•mia \-kü-ˈprē-mē-ə, -kyü-\ *n* : the presence of an excess of copper in the blood

hy•per•cy•thae•mia *chiefly Brit var of* HYPERCYTHEMIA

hy•per•cy•the•mia \-sī-ˈthē-mē-ə\ *n* : the presence of an excess of red blood cells in the blood : POLYCYTHEMIA — **hy•per•cy•the•mic** \-ˈthē-mik\ *adj*

hy•per•dip•loid \-ˈdi-ˌplȯid\ *adj* : having slightly more than the diploid number of chromosomes

hy•per•dy•nam•ic \-dī-ˈna-mik\ *adj* : marked by abnormally increased muscular activity esp. when of organic origin

hy•per•eme•sis \-ˈe-mə-səs, -i-ˈmē-\ *n, pl* **-eme•ses** \-ˌsēz\ : excessive vomiting

hyperemesis grav•i•dar•um \-ˌgra-və-ˈdar-əm\ *n* : excessive vomiting during pregnancy

hy•per•emia \ˌhī-pə-ˈrē-mē-ə\ *n* : excess of blood in a body part : CONGESTION — **hy•per•emic** \-mik\ *adj*

hy•per•en•dem•ic \-en-ˈde-mik, -in-\ *adj* **1** : exhibiting a high and continued incidence — used chiefly of human diseases **2** : marked by hyperendemic disease — used of geographic areas — **hy•per•en•de•mic•i•ty** \-ˌen-ˌde-ˈmi-sə-tē\ *n*

hy•per•er•gic \ˌhī-pər-ˈər-jik\ *adj* : characterized by or exhibiting a greater than normal sensitivity to an allergen — **hy•per•er•gy** \ˈhī-pər-ˌər-jē\ *n*

hy•per•es•the•sia \ˌhī-pər-es-ˈthē-zhə, -zhē-ə\ *n* : unusual or pathological sensitivity of the skin or of a particular sense to stimulation — **hy•per•es•thet•ic** \-ˈthe-tik\ *adj*

hy•per•es•trin•ism \-ˈes-trə-ˌni-zəm\ *n* : a condition marked by the presence of excess estrins in the body

hy·per·es·tro·gen·ism \-ˈes-trə-jə-ˌni-zəm\ *n* : a condition marked by the presence of excess estrogens in the body

hy·per·ex·cit·abil·i·ty \ˌhī-pər-ik-ˌsī-tə-ˈbi-lə-tē\ *n, pl* **-ties** : the state or condition of being unusually or excessively excitable — **hy·per·ex·cit·ed** \-ik-ˈsī-təd\ *adj* — **hy·per·ex·cite·ment** *n*

hy·per·ex·cre·tion \-ik-ˈskrē-shən\ *n* : excessive secretion (as of hormones in the urine)

hy·per·ex·tend \ˌhī-pər-ik-ˈstend\ *vb* : to extend so that the angle between bones of a joint is greater than normal ⟨a ~*ed* elbow⟩; *also* : to extend (as a body part) beyond the normal range of motion — **hy·per·ex·ten·sion** \-ˈsten-chən\ *n*

hy·per·ex·ten·si·ble \-ik-ˈsten-sə-bəl\ *adj* : having the capacity to be hyperextended or stretched to a greater than normal degree — **hy·per·ex·ten·si·bil·i·ty** \-sten-sə-ˈbi-lə-tē\ *n*

hy·per·fil·tra·tion \-fil-ˈtrā-shən\ *n* : a usu. abnormal increase in the filtration rate of the renal glomeruli

hy·per·flex \ˈhī-pər-ˌfleks\ *vb* : to flex so that the angle between the bones of a joint is smaller than normal — **hy·per·flex·ion** \-ˌflek-shən\ *n*

hy·per·func·tion \-ˌfəŋk-shən\ *n* : excessive activity or function ⟨pituitary ~⟩ — **hy·per·func·tion·al** \-shə-nəl\ *adj* — **hy·per·func·tion·ing** *n*

hy·per·gam·ma·glob·u·lin·ae·mia *chiefly Brit var of* HYPERGAMMAGLOBULINEMIA

hy·per·gam·ma·glob·u·lin·emia \ˌhī-pər-ˌga-mə-ˌglä-byə-lə-ˈnē-mē-ə\ *n* : the presence of an excess of gamma globulins in the blood — **hy·per·gam·ma·glob·u·lin·emic** \-ˈnē-mik\ *adj*

hy·per·gas·trin·ae·mia *chiefly Brit var of* HYPERGASTRINEMIA

hy·per·gas·trin·emia \-ˌgas-trə-ˈnē-mē-ə\ *n* : the presence of an excess of gastrin in the blood — **hy·per·gas·trin·emic** \-ˈnē-mik\ *adj*

hy·per·glob·u·lin·ae·mia *chiefly Brit var of* HYPERGLOBULINEMIA

hy·per·glob·u·lin·emia \-ˌglä-byə-lə-ˈnē-mē-ə\ *n* : the presence of excess globulins in the blood — **hy·per·glob·u·lin·emic** \-ˈnē-mik\ *adj*

hy·per·glu·ca·gon·ae·mia *chiefly Brit var of* HYPERGLUCAGONEMIA

hy·per·glu·ca·gon·emia \-ˌglü-kə-gä-ˈnē-mē-ə\ *n* : the presence of excess glucagon in the blood

hy·per·gly·ce·mia \ˌhī-pər-glī-ˈsē-mē-ə\ *n* : an excess of sugar in the blood — **hy·per·gly·ce·mic** \-mik\ *adj*

hyperglycemic factor *n* : GLUCAGON

hy·per·gly·ci·nae·mia *chiefly Brit var of* HYPERGLYCINEMIA

hy·per·gly·ci·ne·mia \ˌhī-pər-ˌglī-sə-ˈnē-mē-ə\ *n* : a hereditary disorder characterized by the presence of excess glycine in the blood

hy·per·go·nad·ism \ˌhī-pər-ˈgō-ˌna-ˌdi-zəm\ *n* : excessive hormonal secretion by the gonads

hy·per·hi·dro·sis \-hi-ˈdrō-səs, -hī-\ *also* **hy·peri·dro·sis** \-i-ˈdrō-\ *n, pl* **-dro·ses** \-ˌsēz\ : generalized or localized excessive sweating — compare HYPOHIDROSIS

hy·per·hy·dra·tion \-hī-ˈdrā-shən\ *n* : an excess of water in the body

hy·per·i·cism \hī-ˈper-ə-ˌsi-zəm\ *n* : a severe dermatitis of domestic animals due to photosensitivity resulting from eating Saint-John's-wort

hy·per·im·mune \ˌhī-pər-i-ˈmyün\ *adj* : exhibiting an unusual degree of immunization: **a** *of a serum* : containing exceptional quantities of antibody **b** *of an antibody* : having the characteristics of a blocking antibody

hy·per·im·mu·nize \-ˈi-myə-ˌnīz\ *vb* **-nized; -niz·ing** : to induce a high level of immunity or of circulating antibodies in — **hy·per·im·mu·ni·za·tion** \-ˌi-myə-nə-ˈzā-shən\ *n*

hy·per·in·fec·tion \-in-ˈfek-shən\ *n* : repeated reinfection with larvae produced by parasitic worms already in the body — compare AUTOINFECTION

hy·per·in·fla·tion \-in-ˈflā-shən\ *n* : excessive inflation (as of the lungs)

hy·per·in·ner·va·tion \-ˌin-(ˌ)ər-ˈvā-shən, -in-ˌər-\ *n* : excessive innervation of tissue ⟨~ of muscle fibers⟩ — **hy·per·in·ner·vat·ed** \-in-ˈər-ˌvāt-əd, -ˈin-(ˌ)ər-\ *adj*

hy·per·in·su·lin·emia \-ˌin-sə-lə-ˈnē-mē-ə\ *n* : the presence of excess insulin in the blood — **hy·per·in·su·lin·emic** \-mik\ *adj*

hy·per·in·su·lin·ism \-ˈin-sə-lə-ˌni-zəm\ *n* : the presence of excess insulin in the body resulting in hypoglycemia

hy·per·in·tense \-in-ˈten(t)s\ *adj* : appearing as a bright or white spot or region in images of the brain (as those produced by MRI) ⟨~ lesions⟩ — **hy·per·in·ten·si·ty** \-in-ˈten(t)-sət-ē\ *n*

hy·per·ir·ri·ta·bil·i·ty \-ir-ə-tə-ˈbi-lə-tē\ *n, pl* **-ties** : abnormally great or uninhibited response to stimuli — **hy·per·ir·ri·ta·ble** \-ˈir-ə-tə-bəl\ *adj*

hy·per·ka·lae·mia *chiefly Brit var of* HYPERKALEMIA

hy·per·ka·le·mia \-kā-ˈlē-mē-ə\ *n* : the presence of an abnormally high concentration of potassium in the blood — called also *hyperpotassemia* — **hy·per·ka·le·mic** \-ˈlē-mik\ *adj*

hy·per·ke·ra·ti·ni·za·tion \-ˌker-ə-tə-nə-ˈzā-shən, -kə-ˌrat-ᵊn-ə-\ *n* : HYPERKERATOSIS

hy·per·ke·ra·to·sis \-ˌker-ə-ˈtō-səs\ *n, pl* **-to·ses** \-ˈtō-ˌsēz\ **1** : hypertrophy of the stratum corneum of the skin **2** : any of various conditions marked by hyperkeratosis — **hy·per·ker·a·tot·ic** \-ˈtät-ik\ *adj*

hy·per·ke·to·ne·mia \-ˌkē-tə-ˈnē-mē-ə\ *n* : KETONEMIA 1

hy·per·ki·ne·sia \-kə-ˈnē-zhə, -kī-, -zhē-ə\ *n* : HYPERKINESIS

hy·per·ki·ne·sis \-ˈnē-səs\ *n* **1** : abnormally increased and sometimes uncontrollable activity or muscular movements — compare HYPOKINESIA **2** : a condition esp. of childhood characterized by hyperactivity

hy·per·ki·net·ic \-kə-ˈne-tik, -kī-\ *adj* : of, relating to, or affected with hyperkinesis or hyperactivity

hy·per·lex·ia \-ˈlek-sē-ə\ *n* : precocious reading ability accompanied by difficulties in acquiring language and social skills — **hy·per·lex·ic** \-sik\ *adj*

hy·per·li·pe·mia \ˌhī-pər-lī-ˈpē-mē-ə\ *n* : HYPERLIPIDEMIA — **hy·per·li·pe·mic** \-mik\ *adj*

hy·per·lip·id·ae·mia *chiefly Brit var of* HYPERLIPIDEMIA

hy·per·lip·id·emia \-ˌli-pə-ˈdē-mē-ə\ *n* : the presence of excess fat or lipids in the blood — **hy·per·lip·id·emic** \-mik\ *adj*

hy·per·li·po·pro·tein·ae·mia *chiefly Brit var of* HYPERLIPOPROTEINEMIA

hy·per·li·po·pro·tein·emia \-ˌlī-pəˌprō-tē-ˈnē-mē-ə, -ˌli-\ *n* : the presence of excess lipoprotein in the blood

hy·per·lu·cent \-ˈlüs-ᵊnt\ *adj* : being excessively radiolucent ⟨a ~ lung⟩ — **hy·per·lu·cen·cy** \-ˈlüs-ᵊn-sē\ *n*

hy·per·mag·ne·sae·mia *chiefly Brit var of* HYPERMAGNESEMIA

hy·per·mag·ne·se·mia \-ˌmag-ni-ˈsē-mē-ə\ *n* : the presence of excess magnesium in the blood serum

hy·per·men·or·rhea \-ˌme-nə-ˈrē-ə\ *n* : abnormally profuse or prolonged menstrual flow — compare MENORRHAGIA

hy·per·me·tab·o·lism \-mə-ˈta-bə-ˌli-zəm\ *n* : metabolism at an increased or excessive rate — **hy·per·meta·bol·ic** \-ˌme-tə-ˈbä-lik\ *adj*

hy·per·me·tria \-ˈmē-trē-ə\ *n* : a condition of cerebellar dysfunction in which voluntary muscular movements tend to result in the movement of bodily parts (as the arm and hand) beyond the intended goal

hy·per·me·tro·pia \ˌhī-pər-mi-ˈtrō-pē-ə\ *n* : HYPEROPIA — **hy·per·me·tro·pic** \-ˈtrō-pik, -ˈträ-\ *adj*

hy·perm·ne·sia \ˌhī-(ˌ)pərm-ˈnē-zhə, -zhē-ə\ *n* : abnormally vivid or complete memory or recall of the past (as at times of extreme danger) — **hy·perm·ne·sic** \-ˈnē-zik, -sik\ *adj*

hy·per·mo·bil·i·ty \ˌhī-pər-mō-ˈbi-lə-tē\ *n, pl* **-ties** : an increase in the range of movement of which a body part and esp. a joint is capable — **hy·per·mo·bile** \-ˈmō-bəl, -ˌbīl, -ˌbēl\ *adj*

hy·per·mo·til·i·ty \ˌhī-pər-mō-ˈti-lə-tē\ *n, pl* **-ties** : abnormal or excessive movement; *specif* : excessive motility of all or part of the gastrointestinal tract — compare HYPERPERISTALSIS, HYPOMOTILITY — **hy·per·mo·tile** \-ˈmōt-ᵊl, -ˈmō-ˌtīl\ *adj*

hy·per·na·trae·mia *chiefly Brit var of* HYPERNATREMIA

hy·per·na·tre·mia \-nā-ˈtrē-mē-ə\ *n* : the presence of an abnormally high concentration of sodium in the blood — **hy·per·na·tre·mic** \-mik\ *adj*

hy·per·neph·roid \-ˈne-ˌfrȯid\ *adj* : resembling the adrenal cortex in histological structure ⟨~ tumors⟩

hy·per·ne·phro·ma \-ni-ˈfrō-mə\ *n, pl* **-mas** *also* **-ma·ta** \-mə-tə\ : a tumor of the kidney resembling the adrenal cortex in its histological structure

hy·per·oes·trin·ism, hy·per·oes·tro·gen·ism *chiefly Brit var of* HYPERESTRINISM, HYPERESTROGENISM

hy·per·ope \ˈhī-pər-ˌōp\ *n* : a person affected with hyperopia

hy·per·opia \ˌhī-pər-ˈō-pē-ə\ *n* : a condition in which visual images come to a focus behind the retina of the eye and vision is better for distant than for near objects — called also *farsightedness, hypermetropia* — **hy·per·opic** \-ˈō-pik, -ˈä-\ *adj*

hy·per·os·mia \ˌhī-pər-ˈäz-mē-ə\ *n* : extreme acuteness of the sense of smell

hy·per·os·mo·lal·i·ty \-ˌäz-mō-ˈla-lə-tē\ *n, pl* **-ties** : the condition esp. of a bodily fluid of having abnormally high osmolality

hy·per·os·mo·lar·i·ty \-ˈlar-ə-tē\ *n, pl* **-ties** : the condition esp. of a bodily fluid of having abnormally high osmolarity — **hy·per·os·mo·lar** \-ˌäz-ˈmō-lər\ *adj*

hy·per·os·mot·ic \-ˌäz-ˈmä-tik\ *adj* : HYPERTONIC 2

hy·per·os·to·sis \-ˌäs-ˈtō-səs\ *n, pl* **-to·ses** \-ˌsēz\ : excessive growth or thickening of bone tissue — **hy·per·os·tot·ic** \-ˈtä-tik\ *adj*

hy·per·ox·al·uria \-ˌäk-sə-ˈlu̇r-ē-ə\ *n* : the presence of excess oxalic acid or oxalates in the urine

hy·per·ox·ia \-ˈäk-sē-ə\ *n* : a bodily condition characterized by a greater oxygen content of the tissues and organs than normally exists at sea level

hy·per·para·thy·roid·ism \ˌhī-pər-ˌpar-ə-ˈthī-ˌrȯi-ˌdi-zəm\ *n* : the presence of excess parathyroid hormone in the body resulting in disturbance of calcium metabolism

hy·per·path·ia \-ˈpa-thē-ə\ *n* **1** : disagreeable or painful sensation in response to a normally innocuous stimulus (as touch) **2** : a condition in which the sensations of hyperpathia occur — **hy·per·path·ic** \-thik\ *adj*

hy·per·peri·stal·sis \-ˌper-ə-ˈstȯl-səs, -ˈstäl-, -ˈstal-\ *n, pl* **-stal·ses** \-ˌsēz\ : excessive or excessively vigorous peristalsis — compare HYPERMOTILITY

hy·per·pha·gia \-ˈfā-jə, -jē-ə\ *n* : abnormally increased appetite for food frequently associated with injury to the hypothalamus — compare POLYPHAGIA — **hy·per·phag·ic** \-ˈfa-jik\ *adj*

hy·per·phe·nyl·al·a·nin·ae·mia *chiefly Brit var of* HYPERPHENYLALANINEMIA

hy·per·phe·nyl·al·a·nin·emia \-ˌfen-ᵊl-ˌa-lə-nə-ˈnē-mē-ə, -ˌfēn-\ *n* : the presence of excess phenylalanine in the blood (as in phenylketonuria) — **hy-**

per•phe•nyl•al•a•nin•emic \-ˈnē-mik\ *adj*

hy•per•pho•ria \-ˈfōr-ē-ə\ *n* : latent strabismus in which one eye deviates upward in relation to the other

hy•per•phos•pha•tae•mia *chiefly Brit var of* HYPERPHOSPHATEMIA

hy•per•phos•pha•te•mia \-ˌfäs-fə-ˈtē-mē-ə\ *n* : the presence of excess phosphate in the blood

hy•per•phos•pha•tu•ria \-ˌfäs-fə-ˈtu̇r-ē-ə, -ˈtyu̇r-\ *n* : the presence of excess phosphate in the urine

hy•per•pi•e•sia \-ˌpī-ˈē-zhə, -zhē-ə\ *n* : HYPERTENSION; *esp* : ESSENTIAL HYPERTENSION

hy•per•pig•men•ta•tion \-ˌpig-mən-ˈtā-shən, -ˌmen-\ *n* : excess pigmentation in a body part or tissue (as the skin) — **hy•per•pig•ment•ed** \-ˈpig-mən-təd, -ˌmen-\ *adj*

hy•per•pi•tu•ita•rism \-pə-ˈtü-ə-tə-ˌri-zəm, -ˈtyü-, -ˌtri-zəm\ *n* : excessive production of growth hormones by the pituitary gland — **hy•per•pi•tu•itary** \-pə-ˈtü-ə-ˌter-ē, -ˈtyü-\ *adj*

hy•per•pla•sia \ˌhī-pər-ˈplā-zhə, -zhē-ə\ *n* : an abnormal or unusual increase in the elements composing a part (as cells composing a tissue) — see BENIGN PROSTATIC HYPERPLASIA — **hy•per•plas•tic** \-ˈplas-tik\ *adj*

hy•per•ploid \ˈhī-pər-ˌplȯid\ *adj* : having a chromosome number slightly greater than an exact multiple of the haploid number — **hy•per•ploi•dy** \-ˌplȯid-ē\ *n*

hy•per•pnea \ˌhī-pərp-ˈnē-ə, -ˌpər-\ *n* : abnormally rapid or deep breathing — **hy•per•pne•ic** \-ˈnē-ik\ *adj*

hy•per•pnoea *chiefly Brit var of* HYPERPNEA

hy•per•po•lar•ize \ˌhī-pər-ˈpō-lə-ˌrīz\ *vb* **-ized; -iz•ing** **1** : to produce an increase in potential difference across (a biological membrane) **2** : to undergo or produce an increase in potential difference across something — **hy•per•po•lar•i•za•tion** \-ˌpō-lə-rə-ˈzā-shən\ *n*

hy•per•po•tas•sae•mia *chiefly Brit var of* HYPERPOTASSEMIA

hy•per•po•tas•se•mia \-pə-ˌta-ˈsē-mē-ə\ *n* : HYPERKALEMIA — **hy•per•po•tas•se•mic** \-ˈsē-mik\ *adj*

hy•per•pro•duc•tion \-prə-ˈdək-shən, -prō-\ *n* : excessive production or synthesis

hy•per•pro•lac•tin•ae•mia *chiefly Brit var of* HYPERPROLACTINEMIA

hy•per•pro•lac•tin•emia \-prō-ˌlak-tə-ˈnē-mē-ə\ *n* : the presence of an abnormally high concentration of prolactin in the blood — **hy•per•pro•lac•tin•emic** \-ˈnē-mik\ *adj*

hy•per•pro•lin•ae•mia *chiefly Brit var of* HYPERPROLINEMIA

hy•per•pro•lin•emia \-ˌprō-lə-ˈnē-mē-ə\ *n* : a hereditary metabolic disorder characterized by an abnormally high concentration of proline in the blood and often associated with intellectual disability

hy•per•py•rex•ia \-pī-ˈrek-sē-ə\ *n* : exceptionally high fever

hy•per•re•ac•tive \-rē-ˈak-tiv\ *adj* : having or showing abnormally high sensitivity to stimuli — **hy•per•re•ac•tiv•i•ty** \-(ˌ)rē-ˌak-ˈti-və-tē\ *n*

hy•per•re•flex•ia \-rē-ˈflek-sē-ə\ *n* : overactivity of physiological reflexes

hy•per•re•nin•ae•mia *chiefly Brit var of* HYPERRENINEMIA

hy•per•re•nin•emia \-ˌrē-nə-ˈnē-mē-ə, -ˌre-\ *n* : the presence of an abnormally high concentration of renin in the blood

hy•per•re•spon•sive \-ri-ˈspän-siv\ *adj* : characterized by an abnormal degree of responsiveness (as to a physical stimulus) — **hy•per•re•spon•siv•i•ty** \-ri-ˌspän-ˈsi-və-tē\ *n*

hy•per•sal•i•va•tion \-ˌsa-lə-ˈvā-shən\ *n* : excessive salivation or drooling : SIALORRHEA — called also *ptyalism*

hy•per•se•cre•tion \-si-ˈkrē-shən\ *n* : excessive production of a bodily secretion — **hy•per•se•crete** \-si-ˈkrēt\ *vb* — **hy•per•se•cre•to•ry** \-ˈsē-krə-ˌtor-ē, -si-ˈkrē-tə-rē\ *adj*

hy•per•sen•si•tive \ˌhī-pər-ˈsen-sə-tiv\ *adj* **1** : excessively or abnormally sensitive **2** : abnormally susceptible physiologically to a specific agent (as a drug) — **hy•per•sen•si•tive•ness** *n* — **hy•per•sen•si•tiv•i•ty** \-ˌsen-sə-ˈti-və-tē\ *n* — **hy•per•sen•si•ti•za•tion** \-ˌsen-sə-tə-ˈzā-shən\ *n* — **hy•per•sen•si•tize** \-ˈsen-sə-ˌtīz\ *vb*

hy•per•sex•u•al \-ˈsek-shə-wəl\ *adj* : exhibiting unusual or excessive concern with or indulgence in sexual activity — **hy•per•sex•u•al•i•ty** \-ˌsek-shə-ˈwa-lə-tē\ *n*

hy•per•sid•er•ae•mia *chiefly Brit var of* HYPERSIDEREMIA

hy•per•sid•er•emia \-ˌsi-də-ˈrē-mē-ə\ *n* : the presence of an abnormally high concentration of iron in the blood — **hy•per•sid•er•e•mic** \-mik\ *adj*

hy•per•som•nia \-ˈsäm-nē-ə\ *n* **1** : sleep of excessive depth or duration **2** : the condition of sleeping for excessive periods at intervals with intervening periods of normal duration of sleeping and waking — compare NARCOLEPSY

hy•per•som•no•lence \-ˈsäm-nə-lən(t)s\ *n* : excessive sleepiness : persistent drowsiness

hy•per•sple•nism \-ˈsplē-ˌni-zəm, -ˈsple-\ *n* : a condition marked by excessive destruction of one or more kinds of blood cells in the spleen

hy•per•sthen•ic \ˌhī-pərs-ˈthe-nik\ *adj* : of, relating to, or characterized by excessive muscle tone

hy•per•stim•u•la•tion \-ˌstim-yə-ˈlā-shən\ *n* : excessive or increased stimulation — **hy•per•stim•u•late** \-ˈstim-yə-ˌlāt\ *vb*

hy•per•sus•cep•ti•ble \-sə-ˈsep-tə-bəl\ *adj* : HYPERSENSITIVE — **hy•per•sus•cep•ti•bil•i•ty** \-ˌsep-tə-ˈbi-lə-tē\ *n*

hy•per•tel•or•ism \-ˈte-lə-ˌri-zəm\ *n* : excessive width between two bodily parts or organs (as the eyes)

hy·per·tense \ˌhī-pər-ˈtens\ *adj* : excessively tense ⟨a ~ emotional state⟩

hy·per·ten·sin·ase \-ˈten-sə-ˌnās, -ˌnāz\ *n* : ANGIOTENSINASE

hy·per·ten·sin·o·gen \-ˌten-ˈsi-nə-jən, -ˌjen\ *n* : ANGIOTENSINOGEN

hy·per·ten·sion \ˌhī-pər-ˈten-chən\ *n* **1** : abnormally high arterial blood pressure that is usu. indicated by an adult systolic blood pressure of 140 mm Hg or greater or a diastolic blood pressure of 90 mm Hg or greater, is chiefly of unknown cause but may be attributable to a preexisting condition (as renal or endocrine disorder), and that is a risk factor for various pathological conditions or events (as heart attack or stroke) — see ESSENTIAL HYPERTENSION, SECONDARY HYPERTENSION, WHITE COAT HYPERTENSION **2** : a systemic condition resulting from hypertension that is either symptomless or is accompanied esp. by dizziness, palpitations, fainting, or headache

[1]**hy·per·ten·sive** \-ˈten-siv\ *adj* : marked by or due to hypertension ⟨~ renal disease⟩; *also* : affected with hypertension ⟨a ~ patient⟩

[2]**hypertensive** *n* : a person affected with hypertension

hy·per·ther·mia \-ˈthər-mē-ə\ *n* **1** : elevated temperature of the body (as that occurring in heatstroke) — see MALIGNANT HYPERTHERMIA **2** : the artificial heating of all or part of the body (as in diathermy) for therapeutic purposes (as to treat cancer) — **hy·per·ther·mic** \-mik\ *adj*

hy·per·thy·roid \-ˈthī-ˌrȯid\ *adj* : of, relating to, or affected with hyperthyroidism ⟨a ~ state⟩

hy·per·thy·roid·ism \-ˌrȯi-ˌdi-zəm\ *n* : excessive functional activity of the thyroid gland; *also* : the resulting condition marked esp. by increased metabolic rate, enlargement of the thyroid gland, rapid heart rate, and high blood pressure — called also *thyrotoxicosis;* see GRAVES' DISEASE

hy·per·to·nia \ˌhī-pər-ˈtō-nē-ə\ *n* : HYPERTONICITY

hy·per·ton·ic \-ˈtä-nik\ *adj* **1** : exhibiting excessive tone or tension ⟨a ~ bladder⟩ **2** : having a higher osmotic pressure than a surrounding medium or a fluid under comparison — compare HYPOTONIC 2, ISOTONIC 1

hy·per·to·nic·i·ty \-tə-ˈni-sə-tē\ *n, pl* **-ties** : the quality or state of being hypertonic

hy·per·to·nus \-ˈtō-nəs\ *n* : HYPERTONICITY

hy·per·tri·cho·sis \-tri-ˈkō-səs\ *n, pl* **-cho·ses** \-ˌsēz\ : excessive growth of hair

hy·per·tri·glyc·er·i·dae·mia *chiefly Brit var of* HYPERTRIGLYCERIDEMIA

hy·per·tri·glyc·er·i·de·mia \-ˌtrī-ˌgli-sə-ˌrī-ˈdē-mē-ə\ *n* : the presence of an excess of triglycerides in the blood — **hy·per·tri·glyc·er·i·de·mic** \-ˈdē-mik\ *adj*

hypertrophic arthritis *n* : OSTEOARTHRITIS

hypertrophic cardiomyopathy *n* : cardiomyopathy that is characterized by ventricular hypertrophy esp. of the left ventricle and is marked by chest pain, syncope, and palpitations — abbr. *HCM*

hypertrophic osteoarthropathy *n* : a hypertrophic condition that is marked esp. by clubbing of the fingers and toes, painful swollen joints, and periostitis and subperiosteal bone formation chiefly affecting the long bones (as the radius or fibula) and that usu. occurs secondary to another disease (as mesothelioma or cirrhosis)

hy·per·tro·phy \hī-ˈpər-trə-fē\ *n, pl* **-phies** : excessive development of an organ or part; *specif* : increase in bulk (as by thickening of muscle fibers) without multiplication of parts — **hy·per·tro·phic** \ˌhī-pər-ˈtrō-fik\ *adj* — **hypertrophy** *vb*

hy·per·tro·pia \ˌhī-pər-ˈtrō-pē-ə\ *n* : elevation of the line of vision of one eye above that of the other : upward strabismus

hy·per·uri·ce·mia \ˌhī-pər-ˌyu̇r-ə-ˈsē-mē-ə\ *n* : excess uric acid in the blood (as in gout) — called also *uricemia* — **hy·per·uri·ce·mic** \-ˈsē-mik\ *adj*

hy·per·uri·cos·uria \-ˌyu̇r-i-kō-ˈshu̇r-ē-ə, -ˈsyu̇r-\ *n* : the excretion of excessive amounts of uric acid in the urine

hy·per·vari·able \-ˈvar-ē-ə-bəl\ *adj* : relating to or being any of the relatively short extremely variable polypeptide chain segments in the variable region of an antibody light chain or heavy chain; *also* : relating to, containing, or being a highly variable nucleotide sequence

hy·per·ven·ti·late \-ˈvent-ᵊl-ˌāt\ *vb* **-lat·ed; -lat·ing** : to breathe rapidly and deeply : undergo hyperventilation

hy·per·ven·ti·la·tion \-ˌvent-ᵊl-ˈā-shən\ *n* : excessive rate and depth of respiration leading to abnormal loss of carbon dioxide from the blood — called also *overventilation*

hy·per·vig·i·lance \-ˈvi-jə-ləns\ *n* : the condition of maintaining an abnormal awareness of environmental stimuli — **hy·per·vig·i·lant** \-lənt\ *adj*

hy·per·vis·cos·i·ty \-vis-ˈkä-sə-tē\ *n, pl* **-ties** : excessive viscosity or thickness (as of the blood)

hy·per·vi·ta·min·osis \-ˌvī-tə-mə-ˈnō-səs\ *n, pl* **-oses** \-ˌsēz\ : an abnormal state resulting from excessive intake of one or more vitamins

hy·per·vol·ae·mia *chiefly Brit var of* HYPERVOLEMIA

hy·per·vol·emia \-vä-ˈlē-mē-ə\ *n* : an excessive volume of blood in the body — **hy·per·vol·emic** \-ˈlē-mik\ *adj*

hyp·es·the·sia \ˌhī-pes-ˈthē-zhə, ˌhi-, -zhē-ə\ *or* **hy·po·es·the·sia** \ˌhī-pō-es-\ *n* : impaired or decreased tactile sensibility — **hyp·es·thet·ic** *or* **hy·po·es·thet·ic** \-ˈthe-tik\ *adj*

hy·phae·ma *chiefly Brit var of* HYPHEMA

hy·phe·ma \hī-ˈfē-mə\ *n* : a hemorrhage in the anterior chamber of the eye

hypn- *or* **hypno-** *comb form* **1** : sleep ⟨*hypn*agogic⟩ **2** : hypnotism ⟨*hypno*therapy⟩

hyp·na·go·gic *also* **hyp·no·go·gic** \ˌhip-nə-ˈgä-jik, -ˈgō-\ *adj* : of, relating to, or occurring in the period of drowsiness immediately preceding sleep ⟨~ hallucinations⟩ — compare HYPNOPOMPIC

hyp·no·anal·y·sis \ˌhip-nō-ə-ˈna-lə-səs\ *n, pl* **-y·ses** \-ˌsēz\ : the treatment of mental and emotional disorders by hypnosis and psychoanalytic methods

hyp·no·pom·pic \ˌhip-nə-ˈpäm-pik\ *adj* : associated with the semiconsciousness preceding waking ⟨~ illusions⟩ — compare HYPNAGOGIC

hyp·no·sis \hip-ˈnō-səs\ *n, pl* **-no·ses** \-ˌsēz\ **1** : a trancelike state that resembles sleep but is induced by a person whose suggestions are readily accepted by the subject **2** : any of various conditions that resemble sleep **3** : HYPNOTISM 1

hyp·no·ther·a·pist \ˌhip-nō-ˈther-ə-pist\ *n* : a specialist in hypnotherapy

hyp·no·ther·a·py \-ˈther-ə-pē\ *n, pl* **-pies** **1** : treatment by hypnotism **2** : psychotherapy that facilitates suggestion, reeducation, or analysis by means of hypnosis

[1]**hyp·not·ic** \hip-ˈnä-tik\ *adj* **1** : tending to produce sleep : SOPORIFIC **2** : of or relating to hypnosis or hypnotism — **hyp·not·i·cal·ly** *adv*

[2]**hypnotic** *n* **1** : a sleep-inducing agent : SOPORIFIC **2** : one that is or can be hypnotized

hyp·no·tism \ˈhip-nə-ˌti-zəm\ *n* **1** : the study or act of inducing hypnosis — compare MESMERISM **2** : HYPNOSIS 1

hyp·no·tist \-tist\ *n* : a person who induces hypnosis

hyp·no·tize \-ˌtīz\ *vb* **-tized; -tiz·ing** : to induce hypnosis in — **hyp·no·tiz·abil·i·ty** \ˌhip-nə-ˌtī-zə-ˈbi-lə-tē\ *n* — **hyp·no·tiz·able** \ˌhip-nə-ˈtī-zə-bəl\ *adj*

[1]**hy·po** \ˈhī-(ˌ)pō\ *n, pl* **hypos** : HYPOCHONDRIA

[2]**hypo** *n, pl* **hypos** **1** : HYPODERMIC SYRINGE **2** : HYPODERMIC INJECTION

hypo- *or* **hyp-** *prefix* **1** : under : beneath : down ⟨*hypo*dermic⟩ **2** : less than normal or normally ⟨*hypo*tension⟩

hy·po·acid·i·ty \ˌhī-pō-a-ˈsi-də-tē\ *n, pl* **-ties** : abnormally low acidity

hy·po·ac·tive \-ˈak-tiv\ *adj* : less than normally active ⟨~ sexual desire⟩ — **hy·po·ac·tiv·i·ty** \-ak-ˈti-və-tē\ *n*

hypoactive sexual desire disorder *n* : persistent or recurring deficiency or absence of sexual desire and sexual thoughts or fantasies that causes marked distress or difficulties in interpersonal relationships and is not attributable to an existing medical or psychological condition, stress, or medication side effects — abbr. *HSDD*

hy·po·acu·sis \-ə-ˈkü-səs, -ˈkyü-\ *n* : partial loss of hearing — called also *hypacusis*

hy·po·adren·al·ism \-ə-ˈdren-ᵊl-ˌi-zəm\ *n* : abnormally decreased activity of the adrenal glands; *specif* : HYPOADRENOCORTICISM

hy·po·ad·re·no·cor·ti·cism \-ə-ˌdrē-nō-ˈkor-tə-ˌsi-zəm\ *n* : abnormally decreased activity of the adrenal cortex (as in Addison's disease)

hy·po·aes·the·sia \ˌhī-pō-es-ˈthē-zhə, ˌhi-, -zhē-ə\ *Brit var of* HYPESTHESIA

hy·po·al·bu·min·ae·mia *chiefly Brit var of* HYPOALBUMINEMIA

hy·po·al·bu·min·emia \-al-ˌbyü-mə-ˈnē-mē-ə\ *n* : hypoproteinemia marked by reduction in serum albumins — **hy·po·al·bu·min·emic** \-ˈnē-mik\ *adj*

hy·po·al·ge·sia \-al-ˈjē-zhə, -zhē-ə, -zē-ə\ *n* : decreased sensitivity to pain

hy·po·al·ler·gen·ic \-ˌa-lər-ˈje-nik\ *adj* : having little likelihood of causing an allergic response ⟨~ food⟩

hy·po·ami·no·ac·id·emia \-ə-ˌmē-nō-ˌa-sə-ˈdē-mē-ə\ *n* : the presence of abnormally low concentrations of amino acids in the blood

hy·po·bar·ic \-ˈbar-ik\ *adj* : having a specific gravity less than that of cerebrospinal fluid — used of solutions for spinal anesthesia; compare HYPERBARIC 1

hy·po·bar·ism \-ˈbar-ˌi-zəm\ *n* : a condition which occurs when the ambient pressure is lower than the pressure of gases within the body and which may be marked by the distension of bodily cavities and the release of gas bubbles within bodily tissues

hy·po·blast \ˈhī-pə-ˌblast\ *n* : the endoderm of an embryo — **hy·po·blas·tic** \ˌhī-pə-ˈblas-tik\ *adj*

hy·po·cal·cae·mia *chiefly Brit var of* HYPOCALCEMIA

hy·po·cal·ce·mia \ˌhī-pō-ˌkal-ˈsē-mē-ə\ *n* : a deficiency of calcium in the blood — **hy·po·cal·ce·mic** \-mik\ *adj*

hy·po·cal·ci·fi·ca·tion \-ˌkal-sə-fə-ˈkā-shən\ *n* : decreased or deficient calcification (as of tooth enamel)

hy·po·ca·lor·ic \-kə-ˈlōr-ik, -ˈlär-; -ˈka-lə-rik\ *adj* : characterized by a low number of dietary calories

hy·po·cap·nia \-ˈkap-nē-ə\ *n* : a deficiency of carbon dioxide in the blood — **hy·po·cap·nic** \-nik\ *adj*

hy·po·chlor·ae·mia *chiefly Brit var of* HYPOCHLOREMIA

hy·po·chlor·emia \ˌhī-pō-klōr-ˈē-mē-ə\ *n* : abnormal decrease of chlorides in the blood — **hy·po·chlor·emic** \-klōr-ˈē-mik\ *adj*

hy·po·chlor·hy·dria \-klōr-ˈhī-drē-ə\ *n* : deficiency of hydrochloric acid in the gastric juice — compare ACHLORHYDRIA, HYPERCHLORHYDRIA — **hy·po·chlor·hy·dric** \-ˈhī-drik\ *adj*

hy·po·chlo·rite \ˌhī-pə-ˈklōr-ˌīt\ *n* : a salt or ester of hypochlorous acid

hy·po·chlo·rous acid \-ˈklōr-əs-\ *n* : an unstable strongly oxidizing but weak acid HClO obtained in solution along with hydrochloric acid by reaction of chlorine with water and used esp. in the form of salts as an oxidizing agent, bleaching agent, disinfectant, and chlorinating agent

hy·po·cho·les·ter·ol·emia \ˌhī-pō-kə-ˌles-tə-rə-ˈlē-mē-ə\ *also* **hy·po·cho·les·ter·emia** \-tə-ˈrē-mē-ə\ *n* : an abnormal deficiency of cholesterol in the blood — **hy·po·cho·les·ter·ol·emic** \-ˈlē-mik\ *also* **hy·po·cho·les·ter·emic** \-ˈrē-mik\ *adj*

hy·po·chon·dria \ˌhī-pə-ˈkän-drē-ə\ *n* : extreme depression of mind or spirits often centered on imaginary physical ailments; *specif* : HYPOCHONDRIASIS

[1]**hy·po·chon·dri·ac** \-drē-ˌak\ *adj* **1** : HYPOCHONDRIACAL **2 a** : situated below the costal cartilages **b** : of, relating to, or being the two abdominal regions lying on either side of the epigastric region and above the lumbar regions

[2]**hypochondriac** *n* : a person affected by hypochondria or hypochondriasis

hy·po·chon·dri·a·cal \-kən-ˈdrī-ə-kəl, -ˌkän-\ *adj* : marked by unusual or excessive recurring concern about one's health : affected with or produced by hypochondria and esp. hypochondriasis

hy·po·chon·dri·a·sis \-ˈdrī-ə-səs\ *n, pl* **-a·ses** \-ˌsēz\ : morbid concern about one's health esp. when accompanied by delusions of physical disease

hy·po·chon·dri·um \-ˈkän-drē-əm\ *n, pl* **-dria** \-drē-ə\ : either hypochondriac region of the body

hy·po·chro·mia \ˌhī-pə-ˈkrō-mē-ə\ *n* **1** : deficiency of color or pigmentation **2** : deficiency of hemoglobin in the red blood cells (as in nutritional anemia) — **hy·po·chro·mic** \-ˈkrō-mik\ *adj*

hypochromic anemia *n* : an anemia marked by deficient hemoglobin and usu. microcytic red blood cells — compare HYPERCHROMIC ANEMIA

hy·po·co·ag·u·la·bil·i·ty \ˌhī-pō-kō-ˌa-gyə-lə-ˈbi-lə-tē\ *n, pl* **-ties** : decreased or deficient coagulability of blood — **hy·po·co·ag·u·la·ble** \-kō-ˈa-gyə-lə-bəl\ *adj*

hy·po·com·ple·men·tae·mia *chiefly Brit var of* HYPOCOMPLEMENTEMIA

hy·po·com·ple·men·te·mia \-ˌkäm-plə-(ˌ)men-ˈtē-mē-ə\ *n* : an abnormal deficiency of complement in the blood — **hy·po·com·ple·men·te·mic** \-ˈtē-mik\ *adj*

hy·po·cre·tin \ˌhī-pō-ˈkrē-tᵊn\ *n* : OREXIN

hy·po·cu·prae·mia *chiefly Brit var of* HYPOCUPREMIA

hy·po·cu·pre·mia \-kü-ˈprē-mē-ə, -kyü-\ *n* : an abnormal deficiency of copper in the blood

hy·po·cu·pro·sis \-kü-ˈprō-səs, -kyü-\ *n, pl* **-pro·ses** \-ˌsēz\ : HYPOCUPREMIA

hy·po·der·ma \ˌhī-pə-ˈdər-mə\ *n* **1** *cap* : a genus (family Hypodermatidae) of dipteran flies that have parasitic larvae and include the common cattle grub (*H. lineatum*) **2** : any insect or maggot of the genus *Hypoderma*

hy·po·der·ma·to·sis \-ˌdər-mə-ˈtō-səs\ *n* : infestation with maggots of flies of the genus *Hypoderma*

hy·po·der·mi·a·sis \-dər-ˈmī-ə-səs\ *n, pl* **-a·ses** \-ˌsēz\ : HYPODERMATOSIS

[1]**hy·po·der·mic** \ˌhī-pə-ˈdər-mik\ *adj* **1** : of or relating to the parts beneath the skin **2** : adapted for use in or administered by injection beneath the skin — **hy·po·der·mi·cal·ly** *adv*

[2]**hypodermic** *n* **1** : HYPODERMIC INJECTION **2** : HYPODERMIC SYRINGE

hypodermic injection *n* : an injection made into the subcutaneous tissues

hypodermic needle *n* **1** : NEEDLE 2 **2** : a hypodermic syringe complete with needle

hypodermic syringe *n* : a small syringe used with a hollow needle for injection of material into or beneath the skin

hy·po·der·mis \ˌhī-pə-ˈdər-məs\ *n* : SUPERFICIAL FASCIA

hy·po·der·moc·ly·sis \-dər-ˈmä-klə-səs\ *n, pl* **-ly·ses** \-ˌsēz\ : subcutaneous injection of fluids (as saline solution)

hy·po·dip·loid \ˌhī-pō-ˈdi-ˌplȯid\ *adj* : having slightly fewer than the diploid number of chromosomes — **hy·po·dip·loi·dy** \-ˌplȯi-dē\ *n*

hy·po·don·tia \-ˈdän-chə, -chē-ə\ *n* : an esp. congenital condition marked by a less than normal number of teeth : partial anodontia — **hy·po·don·tic** \-ˈdän-tik\ *adj*

hy·po·dy·nam·ic \-dī-ˈna-mik\ *adj* : marked by or exhibiting a decrease in strength or power ⟨the ~ heart⟩

hypoesthesia *var of* HYPESTHESIA

hy·po·es·tro·ge·ne·mia \-ˌes-trə-jə-ˈnē-mē-ə\ *n* : a deficiency of one or more estrogens (as estrone or estradiol) in the blood

hy·po·es·tro·gen·ism \-ˈes-trə-jə-ˌni-zəm\ *n* : a deficiency of estrogen in the body — **hy·po·es·tro·gen·ic** \-es-trə-ˈje-nik\ *adj*

hy·po·fer·rae·mia *chiefly Brit var of* HYPOFERREMIA

hy·po·fer·re·mia \ˌhī-pō-fə-ˈrē-mē-ə\ *n* : an abnormal deficiency of iron in the blood — **hy·po·fer·re·mic** \-ˈrē-mik\ *adj*

hy·po·fi·brin·o·gen·ae·mia *chiefly Brit var of* HYPOFIBRINOGENEMIA

hy·po·fi·brin·o·gen·emia \-fī-ˌbri-nə-jə-ˈnē-mē-ə\ *n* : an abnormal deficiency of fibrinogen in the blood

hy·po·func·tion \ˈhī-pō-ˌfəŋk-shən\ *n* : decreased or insufficient function esp. of an endocrine gland

hy·po·gam·ma·glob·u·lin·emia \-ˌga-mə-ˌglä-byə-lə-ˈnē-mē-ə\ *n* : a deficiency of gamma globulins in the blood — **hy·po·gam·ma·glob·u·lin·emic** \-ˈnē-mik\ *adj*

hy·po·gas·tric \ˌhī-pə-ˈgas-trik\ *adj* **1** : of or relating to the lower median abdominal region **2** : relating to or situated along or near the internal iliac arteries or the internal iliac veins

hypogastric artery *n* : ILIAC ARTERY 3

hypogastric nerve *n* : a nerve or several parallel nerve bundles situated dorsal and medial to the common and the internal iliac arteries

hypogastric plexus *n* : the sympathetic nerve plexus that supplies the pelvic viscera

hypogastric vein *n* : ILIAC VEIN c

hy·po·gas·tri·um \ˌhī-pə-ˈgas-trē-əm\ *n, pl* **-tria** \-trē-ə\ : the hypogastric region of the abdomen

hy·po·gen·i·tal·ism \-ˈje-nə-tə-ˌli-zəm\ *n* : subnormal development of genital organs : genital infantilism

hy·po·geu·sia \-ˈgü-sē-ə, -ˈjü-, -zē-ə\ *n* : decreased sensitivity to taste

hy·po·glos·sal \ˌhī-pə-ˈglä-səl\ *adj* : of or relating to the hypoglossal nerves

hypoglossal nerve *n* : either of the 12th and final pair of cranial nerves which are motor nerves arising from the medulla oblongata and supplying muscles of the tongue and hyoid apparatus — called also *hypoglossal, twelfth cranial nerve*

hypoglossal nucleus *n* : a nucleus in the floor of the fourth ventricle of the brain that is the origin of the hypoglossal nerve

hy·po·glos·sus \-ˈglä-səs\ *n, pl* **-glos·si** \-ˌsī, -ˌsē\ : HYPOGLOSSAL NERVE

hy·po·gly·ce·mia \ˌhī-pō-glī-ˈsē-mē-ə\ *n* : abnormal decrease of sugar in the blood

¹hy·po·gly·ce·mic \-ˈsē-mik\ *adj* **1** : of, relating to, caused by, or affected with hypoglycemia **2** : producing a decrease in the level of sugar in the blood ⟨∼ drugs⟩

²hypoglycemic *n* **1** : one affected with hypoglycemia **2** : an agent that lowers the level of sugar in the blood

hy·po·go·nad·al \-gō-ˈnad-ᵊl\ *adj* **1** : relating to or affected with hypogonadism **2** : marked by or exhibiting deficient development of secondary sex characteristics

hy·po·go·nad·ism \-ˈgō-ˌna-ˌdi-zəm\ *n* **1** : functional incompetence of the gonads esp. in the male **2** : a condition (as Klinefelter's syndrome) involving gonadal incompetence

hy·po·go·nad·o·trop·ic \-gō-ˌna-də-ˈträ-pik\ *or* **hy·po·go·nad·o·tro·phic** \-ˈtrō-fik, -ˈträ-\ *adj* : characterized by a deficiency of gonadotropins

hy·po·hi·dro·sis \-hi-ˈdrō-səs, -hī-\ *n, pl* **-dro·ses** \-ˌsēz\ : abnormally diminished sweating — compare HYPERHIDROSIS

hy·po·his·ti·di·ne·mia \-ˌhis-tə-də-ˈnē-mē-ə\ *n* : a low concentration of histidine in the blood that is characteristic of rheumatoid arthritis — **hy·po·his·ti·di·ne·mic** \-ˈnē-mik\ *adj*

hy·po·in·su·lin·emia \-ˌin-sə-lə-ˈnē-mē-ə\ *n* : an abnormally low concentration of insulin in the blood — **hy·po·in·su·lin·emic** \-ˈnē-mik\ *adj*

hy·po·ka·lae·mia *chiefly Brit var of* HYPOKALEMIA

hy·po·ka·le·mia \-kā-ˈlē-mē-ə\ *n* : a deficiency of potassium in the blood — called also *hypopotassemia* — **hy·po·ka·le·mic** \-ˈlē-mik\ *adj*

hy·po·ki·ne·sia \-kə-ˈnē-zhə, -kī-, -zhē-ə\ *n* : abnormally decreased muscular movement — compare HYPERKINESIS

hy·po·ki·ne·sis \-ˈnē-səs\ *n, pl* **-ne·ses** \-ˌsēz\ : HYPOKINESIA

hy·po·ki·net·ic \-ˈne-tik\ *adj* : characterized by, associated with, or caused by decreased motor activity

hy·po·lip·id·ae·mia *chiefly Brit var of* HYPOLIPIDEMIA

hy·po·lip·id·emia \-ˌli-pə-ˈdē-mē-ə\ *n* : a deficiency of lipids in the blood — **hy·po·lip·id·emic** \-ˈdē-mik\ *adj*

hy·po·mag·ne·sae·mia *chiefly Brit var of* HYPOMAGNESEMIA

hy·po·mag·ne·se·mia \ˌhī-pə-ˌmag-nə-ˈsē-mē-ə\ *n* : a deficiency of magnesium in the blood — **hy·po·mag·ne·se·mic** \-mik\ *adj*

hy·po·mag·ne·sia \-mag-ˈnē-shə, -zhə\ *n* : HYPOMAGNESEMIA; *also* : GRASS TETANY

hy·po·ma·nia \ˌhī-pə-ˈmā-nē-ə, -nyə\ *n* : a mild mania esp. when part of bipolar disorder

¹hy·po·man·ic \-ˈma-nik\ *adj* : of, relating to, or affected with hypomania

²hypomanic *n* : one affected with hypomania

hy·po·men·or·rhea \-ˌme-nə-ˈrē-ə\ *n* : decreased menstrual flow

hy·po·me·tab·o·lism \ˌhī-pō-mə-ˈta-bə-ˌli-zəm\ *n* : a condition (as in myxedema) marked by an abnormally low metabolic rate — **hy·po·meta·bol·ic** \-ˌme-tə-ˈbä-lik\ *adj*

hy·po·me·tria \-ˈmē-trē-ə\ *n* : a condition of cerebellar dysfunction in which voluntary muscular movements tend to result in the movement of bodily parts (as the arm and hand) short of the intended goal

hy·po·min·er·al·ized \-ˈmi-nə-rə-ˌlīzd\ *adj* : relating to or characterized by a deficiency of minerals

hy·po·mo·bil·i·ty \-mō-ˈbil-ət-ē\ *n, pl* **-ties** : a decrease in the range of movement of which a body part and esp. a joint is capable — **hy·po·mo·bile** \-ˈmō-bəl, -ˌbīl, -ˌbēl\ *adj*

hy·po·mo·til·i·ty \ˌhī-pō-mō-ˈti-lə-tē\ *n, pl* **-ties** : abnormal deficiency of movement; *specif* : decreased motility of all or part of the gastrointestinal tract — compare HYPERMOTILITY

hy·po·na·trae·mia *chiefly Brit var of* HYPONATREMIA

hy·po·na·tre·mia \-nā-ˈtrē-mē-ə\ *n* : deficiency of sodium in the blood — **hy·po·na·tre·mic** \-mik\ *adj*

hypo–oes·tro·ge·nae·mia, hypo–oes·tro·gen·ism *chiefly Brit var of* HYPOESTROGENEMIA, HYPOESTROGENISM

hypoosmolality *var of* HYPOSMOLALITY

hy·po·os·mot·ic \-ˌäz-ˈmä-tik\ *or* **hy·pos·mot·ic** \ˌhī-ˌpäz-\ *adj* : HYPOTONIC 2

hy·po·para·thy·roid·ism \-ˌpar-ə-ˈthī-ˌrȯi-ˌdi-zəm\ *n* : deficiency of parathyroid hormone in the body; *also* : the resultant abnormal state marked by low serum calcium and a tendency to chronic tetany — **hy·po·para·thy·roid** \-ˈthī-ˌrȯid\ *adj*

hy·po·per·fu·sion \ˌhī-pō-pər-ˈfyü-zhən\ *n* : decreased blood flow through an organ ⟨cerebral ~⟩

hy·po·phar·ynx \-ˈfar-iŋks\ *n, pl* **-pha·ryn·ges** \-fə-ˈrin-(ˌ)jēz\ *also* **-phar·ynx·es** : the laryngeal part of the pharynx extending from the hyoid bone to the lower margin of the cricoid cartilage — **hy·po·pha·ryn·geal** \-ˌfar-ən-ˈjē-əl; -fə-ˈrin-jəl, -jē-əl\ *adj*

hy·po·phos·pha·tae·mia *chiefly Brit var of* HYPOPHOSPHATEMIA

hy·po·phos·pha·ta·sia \ˌhī-pō-ˌfäs-fə-ˈtā-zhə, -zhē-ə\ *n* : a congenital metabolic disorder characterized by a deficiency of alkaline phosphatase and usu. resulting in demineralization of bone

hy·po·phos·pha·te·mia \-ˌfäs-fə-ˈtē-mē-ə\ *n* : deficiency of phosphates in the blood — **hy·po·phos·pha·te·mic** \-ˈtē-mik\ *adj*

hy·po·phy·se·al *also* **hy·po·phy·si·al** \(ˌ)hī-ˌpä-fə-ˈsē-əl, ˌhī-pə-fə-, -ˈzē-; ˌhī-pə-ˈfi-zē-əl\ *adj* : of or relating to the hypophysis

hypophyseal fossa *n* : the depression in the sphenoid bone that contains the hypophysis

hy·poph·y·sec·to·mize \(ˌ)hī-ˌpä-fə-ˈsek-tə-ˌmīz\ *vb* **-mized; -miz·ing** : to remove the pituitary gland from

hy·poph·y·sec·to·my \-mē\ *n, pl* **-mies** : surgical removal of the pituitary gland

hy·po·phys·io·tro·pic \ˌhī-pō-ˌfi-zē-ō-ˈtrō-pik, -ˈträ-\ *or* **hy·po·phys·io·tro·phic** \-ˈtrō-fik\ *adj* : acting on or stimulating the hypophysis

hy·poph·y·sis \hī-ˈpä-fə-səs\ *n, pl* **-y·ses** \-ˌsēz\ : PITUITARY GLAND

hypophysis ce·re·bri \-sə-ˈrē-ˌbrī, -ˈser-ə-\ *n* : PITUITARY GLAND

hy·po·pig·men·ta·tion \ˌhī-pō-ˌpig-mən-ˈtā-shən, -ˌmen-\ *n* : diminished pigmentation in a bodily part or tissue (as the skin) — **hy·po·pig·ment·ed** \-ˈpig-mən-təd, -ˌmen-\ *adj*

hy·po·pi·tu·ita·rism \ˌhī-pō-pə-ˈtü-ə-tə-ˌri-zəm, -ˈtyü-\ *n* : deficient production of growth hormones by the pituitary gland — **hy·po·pi·tu·itary** \-ˈtü-ə-ˌter-ē, -ˈtyü-\ *adj*

hy·po·pla·sia \-ˈplā-zhə, -zhē-ə\ *n* : a condition of arrested development in which an organ or part remains below the normal size or in an immature state — **hy·po·plas·tic** \-ˈplas-tik\ *adj*

hypoplastic anemia *n* : APLASTIC ANEMIA

hypoplastic left heart syndrome *n* : a congenital malformation of the heart in which the left side is underdeveloped resulting in insufficient blood flow

hy·po·pnea \ˌhī-pō-ˈnē-ə\ *n* : abnormally slow or esp. shallow respiration

hy·po·pnoea *chiefly Brit var of* HYPOPNEA

hy·po·po·tas·sae·mia *chiefly Brit var of* HYPOPOTASSEMIA

hy·po·po·tas·se·mia \-pə-ˌta-ˈsē-mē-ə\ *n* : HYPOKALEMIA — **hy·po·po·tas·se·mic** \-ˈsē-mik\ *adj*

hy·po·pro·lac·tin·ae·mia *chiefly Brit var of* HYPOPROLACTINEMIA

hy·po·pro·lac·tin·emia \-prō-ˌlak-tə-ˈnē-mē-ə\ *n* : a condition characterized by a deficiency of prolactin in the blood

hy·po·pro·tein·ae·mia *chiefly Brit var of* HYPOPROTEINEMIA

hy·po·pro·tein·emia \-ˌprō-tə-ˈnē-mē-ə, -ˌprō-ˌtē-, -ˌprō-tē-ə-\ *n* : abnormal deficiency of protein in the blood — **hy·po·pro·tein·e·mic** \-ˈnē-mik\ *adj*

hy·po·pro·throm·bin·ae·mia *chiefly Brit var of* HYPOPROTHROMBINEMIA

hy·po·pro·throm·bin·emia \-prō-ˌthräm-bə-ˈnē-mē-ə\ *n* : deficiency of prothrombin in the blood usu. due to vitamin K deficiency or liver disease and resulting in delayed clotting of blood or spontaneous bleeding (as from the nose) — **hy·po·pro·throm·bin·emic** \-ˈnē-mik\ *adj*

hy·po·py·on \hī-ˈpō-pē-ˌän\ *n* : an accumulation of white blood cells in the anterior chamber of the eye

hy·po·re·ac·tive \ˌhī-pō-rē-ˈak-tiv\ *adj* : having or showing abnormally low sensitivity to stimuli — **hy·po·re·ac·tiv·i·ty** \-(ˌ)rē-ˌak-ˈti-və-tē\ *n*

hy·po·re·flex·ia \-rē-ˈflek-sē-ə\ *n* : underactivity of bodily reflexes

hy·po·re·spon·sive \-ri-ˈspän-siv\ *adj* : characterized by a diminished degree of responsiveness (as to a physical or emotional stimulus) — **hy·po·re·spon·sive·ness** *n*

hypos *pl of* HYPO

hy·po·sal·i·va·tion \-ˌsa-lə-ˈvā-shən\ *n* : diminished salivation

hy·po·se·cre·tion \ˌhī-pō-si-ˈkrē-shən\ *n* : production of a bodily secretion at an abnormally slow rate or in abnormally small quantities

hy·po·sen·si·tive \-ˈsen-sə-tiv\ *adj* : exhibiting or marked by deficient response to stimulation — **hy·po·sen·si·tiv·i·ty** \-ˌsen-sə-ˈti-və-tē\ *n*

hy·po·sen·si·ti·za·tion \-ˌsen-sə-tə-ˈzā-shən\ *n* : the state or process of being reduced in sensitivity esp. to an allergen : DESENSITIZATION — **hy·po·sen·si·tize** \-ˈsen-sə-ˌtīz\ *vb*

hy·pos·mia \hī-ˈpäz-mē-ə, hi-\ *n* : impairment of the sense of smell

hy·pos·mo·lal·i·ty \ˌhī-ˌpäz-mō-ˈla-lə-tē\ *or* **hy·po·os·mo·lal·i·ty** \ˌhī-pō-

ˌäz-\ *n, pl* **-ties** : the condition esp. of a bodily fluid of having abnormally low osmolality

hy·pos·mo·lar·i·ty \ˌhī-ˌpäz-mō-ˈlar-ə-tē\ *n, pl* **-ties** : the condition esp. of a bodily fluid of having abnormally low osmolarity — **hy·pos·mo·lar** \ˌhī-ˌpäz-ˈmō-lər\ *adj*

hyposmotic *var of* HYPOOSMOTIC

hy·po·spa·di·as \ˌhī-pə-ˈspā-dē-əs\ *n* : an abnormality of the penis in which the urethra opens on the underside

hy·pos·ta·sis \hī-ˈpäs-tə-səs\ *n, pl* **-ta·ses** \-ˌsēz\ : the settling of blood in relatively lower parts of an organ or the body due to impaired or absent circulation — **hy·po·stat·ic** \ˌhī-pə-ˈsta-tik\ *adj*

hypostatic pneumonia *n* : pneumonia that usu. results from the collection of fluid in the dorsal region of the lungs and occurs esp. in those (as the bedridden or elderly) confined to a supine position for extended periods

hy·po·sthe·nia \ˌhī-pəs-ˈthē-nē-ə\ *n* : lack of strength : bodily weakness — **hy·po·sthen·ic** \ˌhī-pəs-ˈthe-nik\ *adj*

hy·pos·the·nu·ria \hī-ˌpäs-thə-ˈnu̇r-ē-ə, -ˈnyu̇r-\ *n* : the secretion of urine of low specific gravity due to inability of the kidney to concentrate the urine normally

hy·po·ten·sion \ˌhī-pō-ˈten-chən\ *n* **1** : abnormally low pressure of the blood — called also *low blood pressure* **2** : abnormally low pressure of the intraocular fluid

[1]**hy·po·ten·sive** \-ˈten-siv\ *adj* **1** : characterized by or due to hypotension ⟨~ shock⟩ **2** : causing low blood pressure or a lowering of blood pressure ⟨~ drugs⟩

[2]**hypotensive** *n* : one with hypotension

hy·po·tha·lam·ic \ˌhī-pō-thə-ˈla-mik\ *adj* : of or relating to the hypothalamus — **hy·po·tha·lam·i·cal·ly** *adv*

hypothalamic releasing factor *n* : any hormone that is secreted by the hypothalamus and stimulates the pituitary gland directly to secrete a hormone — called also *hypothalamic releasing hormone, releasing factor*

hypothalamo- *comb form* : hypothalamus ⟨*hypothalamo*tomy⟩

hy·po·thal·a·mol·o·my \ˌhī-pō-ˌtha-lə-ˈmä-tə-mē\ *n, pl* **-mies** : psychosurgery in which lesions are made in the hypothalamus

hy·po·thal·a·mus \-ˈtha-lə-məs\ *n, pl* **-mi** \-ˌmī\ : a basal part of the diencephalon that lies beneath the thalamus on each side, forms the floor of the third ventricle, and includes vital autonomic regulatory centers

hy·po·the·nar eminence \ˌhī-pō-ˈthē-ˌnär-, -nər-; hī-ˈpä-thə-ˌnär-, -nər-\ *n* : the prominent part of the palm of the hand above the base of the little finger

hypothenar muscle *n* : any of four muscles located in the area of the hypothenar eminence: **a** : ABDUCTOR DIGITI MINIMI **b** : FLEXOR DIGITI MINIMI BREVIS **c** : PALMARIS BREVIS **d** : OPPONENS DIGITI MINIMI

hy·po·ther·mia \-ˈthər-mē-ə\ *n* : subnormal temperature of the body — **hy·po·ther·mic** \-mik\ *adj*

hy·po·thy·reo·sis \ˌhī-pō-ˌthī-rē-ˈō-səs\ *n* : HYPOTHYROIDISM

hy·po·thy·roid·ism \ˌhī-pō-ˈthī-ˌrȯi-ˌdi-zəm\ *n* : deficient activity of the thyroid gland; *also* : a resultant bodily condition characterized by lowered metabolic rate and general loss of vigor — **hy·po·thy·roid** \-ˌrȯid\ *adj*

hy·po·thy·ro·sis \-ˌthī-ˈrō-səs\ *n* : HYPOTHYROIDISM

hy·po·thy·rox·in·ae·mia *chiefly Brit var of* HYPOTHYROXINEMIA

hy·po·thy·rox·in·emia \ˌhī-pō-thī-ˌräk-sə-ˈnē-mē-ə\ *n* : the presence of an abnormally low concentration of thyroxine in the blood — **hy·po·thy·rox·in·emic** \-ˈnē-mik\ *adj*

hy·po·to·nia \ˌhī-pə-ˈtō-nē-ə, -pō-\ *n* **1** : abnormally low pressure of the intraocular fluid **2** : the state of having hypotonic muscle tone

hy·po·ton·ic \ˌhī-pə-ˈtä-nik, -pō-\ *adj* **1** : having deficient tone or tension **2** : having a lower osmotic pressure than a surrounding medium or a fluid under comparison — compare HYPERTONIC 2

hy·po·to·nic·i·ty \-tə-ˈni-sə-tē\ *n, pl* **-ties 1** : the state or condition of having hypotonic osmotic pressure **2** : HYPOTONIA 2

hy·pot·ony \hī-ˈpä-tə-nē\ *n, pl* **-onies** : HYPOTONIA

hy·po·tri·cho·sis \-tri-ˈkō-səs\ *n, pl* **-cho·ses** \-ˌsēz\ : congenital deficiency of hair

hy·pot·ro·phy \hī-ˈpä-trə-fē\ *n, pl* **-phies** : subnormal growth

hy·po·tym·pa·num \ˌhī-pō-ˈtim-pə-nəm\ *n, pl* **-na** \-nə\ *also* **-nums** : the lower part of the middle ear — compare EPITYMPANUM

hy·po·uri·ce·mia \-ˌyu̇r-ə-ˈsē-mē-ə\ *n* : deficient uric acid in the blood — **hy·po·uri·ce·mic** \-ˈsē-mik\ *adj*

hy·po·ven·ti·la·tion \-ˌvent-ᵊl-ˈā-shən\ *n* : deficient ventilation of the lungs that results in reduction in the oxygen content or increase in the carbon dioxide content of the blood or both — **hy·po·ven·ti·lat·ed** \-ˈvent-ᵊl-ˌā-təd\ *adj*

hy·po·vi·ta·min·osis \-ˌvī-tə-mə-ˈnō-səs\ *n* : AVITAMINOSIS — **hy·po·vi·ta·min·ot·ic** \-ˈnä-tik\ *adj*

hy·po·vo·lae·mia *chiefly Brit var of* HYPOVOLEMIA

hy·po·vo·le·mia \-vä-ˈlē-mē-ə\ *n* : decrease in the volume of the circulating blood — **hy·po·vo·le·mic** \-ˈlē-mik\ *adj*

hy·pox·ae·mia *chiefly Brit var of* HYPOXEMIA

hy·po·xan·thine \ˌhī-pō-ˈzan-ˌthēn\ *n* : a purine base $C_5H_4N_4O$ of plant and animal tissues that is an intermediate in uric acid synthesis

hypoxanthine–guanine phos•pho•ri•bo•syl•trans•fer•ase \-ˌfäs-fō-ˌrī-bō-sil-ˈtrans-(ˌ)fər-ˌās, -ˌāz\ *n* : an enzyme that conserves hypoxanthine in the body by limiting its conversion to uric acid and that is lacking in Lesch-Nyhan syndrome — called also *hypoxanthine phosphoribosyltransferase*

hyp•ox•emia \ˌhi-ˌpäk-ˈsē-mē-ə, ˌhī-\ *n* : deficient oxygenation of the blood — **hyp•ox•emic** \-mik\ *adj*

hyp•ox•ia \hi-ˈpäk-sē-ə, hī-\ *n* : a deficiency of oxygen reaching the tissues of the body — **hyp•ox•ic** \-sik\ *adj*

hyps- *or* **hypsi-** *or* **hypso-** *comb form* : high ⟨*hyps*arrhythmia⟩

hyps•ar•rhyth•mia *also* **hyps•arhyth•mia** \ˌhips-ā-ˈrith-mē-ə\ *n* : an abnormal encephalogram that is characterized by slow waves of high voltage and a disorganized arrangement of spikes, occurs esp. in infants, and is indicative of a condition that leads to severe intellectual disability if left untreated

hyster- *or* **hystero-** *comb form* **1** : womb ⟨*hystero*tomy⟩ **2** : hysteria ⟨*hyster*oid⟩

hys•ter•ec•to•my \ˌhis-tə-ˈrek-tə-mē\ *n, pl* **-mies** : surgical removal of the uterus — **hys•ter•ec•to•mized** \-tə-ˌmīzd\ *adj*

hys•te•ria \hi-ˈster-ē-ə, -ˈstir-\ *n* **1** : a psychoneurosis marked by emotional excitability and disturbances of the psychic, sensory, vasomotor, and visceral functions without an organic basis **2** : behavior exhibiting overwhelming or unmanageable fear or emotional excess

hys•ter•ic \hi-ˈster-ik\ *n* : one subject to or affected with hysteria

hys•ter•i•cal \-ˈster-i-kəl\ *also* **hys•ter•ic** \-ˈster-ik\ *adj* : of, relating to, or marked by hysteria — **hys•ter•i•cal•ly** *adv*

hysterical personality *n* : a personality characterized by superficiality, egocentricity, vanity, dependence, and manipulativeness, by dramatic, reactive, and intensely expressed emotional behavior, and often by disturbed interpersonal relationships

hys•ter•ics \-iks\ *n sing or pl* : a fit of uncontrollable laughter or crying : HYSTERIA

hystericus — see GLOBUS HYSTERICUS

hys•ter•o•gram \ˈhis-tə-rō-ˌgram\ *n* : a radiograph of the uterus

hys•ter•og•ra•phy \ˌhis-tə-ˈrä-grə-fē\ *n, pl* **-phies** : examination of the uterus by radiography after the injection of an opaque medium

hys•ter•oid \ˈhis-tə-ˌroid\ *adj* : resembling or tending toward hysteria

hys•ter•o•plas•ty \ˈhis-tə-rō-ˌplas-tē\ *n, pl* **-ties** : plastic surgery of the uterus

hys•ter•or•rha•phy \ˌhis-tə-ˈror-ə-fē\ *n, pl* **-phies** : a suturing of an incised or ruptured uterus

hys•ter•o•sal•pin•go•gram \ˌhis-tə-rō-ˌsal-ˈpiŋ-gə-ˌgram\ *n* : a radiograph made by hysterosalpingography

hys•ter•o•sal•pin•gog•ra•phy \-ˌsal-ˌpin-ˈgä-gre-fē\ *n, pl* **-phies** : examination of the uterus and fallopian tubes by radiography after injection of an opaque medium — called also *uterosalpingography*

hys•ter•o•sal•pin•gos•to•my \-ˈgäs-tə-mē\ *n, pl* **-mies** : surgical establishment of an anastomosis between the uterus and an occluded fallopian tube

hys•ter•o•scope \ˈhis-tə-rō-ˌskōp\ *n* : an endoscope used for the visual examination of the cervix and the interior of the uterus — **hys•ter•o•scop•ic** \ˌhis-tə-rō-ˈskä-pik\ *adj* — **hys•ter•os•co•py** \ˌhis-tə-ˈräs-kə-pē\ *n*

hys•ter•o•sto•mat•o•my \ˌhis-tə-rō-ˌstō-ˈma-tə-mē\ *n, pl* **-mies** : surgical incision of the uterine cervix

hys•ter•ot•o•my \ˌhis-tə-ˈrä-tə-mē\ *n, pl* **-mies** : surgical incision of the uterus usu. made by transabdominal approach; *also* : a procedure (as a cesarean section) involving such an incision

hystrix — see ICHTHYOSIS HYSTRIX GRAVIOR

Hy•trin \ˈhī-trin\ *trademark* — used for a preparation of the hydrated hydrochloride of terazosin

Hy•zaar \ˈhī-ˌzär\ *trademark* — used for a preparation of hydrochlorothiazide and the potassium salt of losartan

Hz *abbr* hertz

H zone \ˈāch-ˌzōn\ *n* : a narrow and less dense zone of myosin filaments bisecting the A band in striated muscle — compare M LINE

I

i *abbr* incisor
I *symbol* iodine
-i·a·sis \ˈī-ə-səs\ *n suffix, pl* **-i·a·ses** \-ˌsēz\ : disease having characteristics of or produced by (something specified) ⟨ameb*iasis*⟩ ⟨onchocerc*iasis*⟩
-i·at·ric \ē-ˈa-trik\ *also* **-i·at·ri·cal** \-tri-kəl\ *adj comb form* : of or relating to (such) medical treatment or healing ⟨ped*iatric*⟩
-i·at·rics \ē-ˈa-triks\ *n pl comb form* : medical treatment ⟨ped*iatrics*⟩
-i·a·trist \ˈī-ə-trəst\ *n comb form* : physician : healer ⟨pod*iatrist*⟩
iatro- *comb form* : physician : medicine : healing ⟨*iatro*genic⟩
iat·ro·gen·ic \(ˌ)ī-ˌa-trə-ˈje-nik\ *adj* : induced inadvertently by a physician or surgeon or by medical treatment or diagnostic procedures ⟨an ~ rash⟩ — **iat·ro·gen·e·sis** \-ˈje-nə-səs\ *n* — **iat·ro·gen·i·cal·ly** *adv*
-i·a·try \ˈī-ə-trē\ *n comb form, pl* **-iat·ries** : medical treatment : healing ⟨pod*iatry*⟩ ⟨psych*iatry*⟩
I band \ˈī-\ *n* : a pale band across a striated muscle fiber that consists of actin and is situated between two A bands — called also *isotropic band*
iban·dro·nate \ī-ˈban-drō-ˌnāt\ *n* : a hydrated bisphosphonate sodium salt $C_9H_{22}NO_7P_2Na{\cdot}H_2O$ used in the prevention and treatment of postmenopausal osteoporosis — called also *ibandronate sodium;* see BONIVA
IBD *abbr* inflammatory bowel disease
ibo·te·nic acid \ˌī-bō-ˈtē-nik-\ *n* : a neurotoxic compound $C_5H_6N_2O_4$ found esp. in fly agaric
IBS *abbr* irritable bowel syndrome
ibu·pro·fen \ˌī-byü-ˈprō-fən\ *n* : a nonsteroidal anti-inflammatory drug $C_{13}H_{18}O_2$ used in over-the-counter preparations to relieve pain and fever and in prescription strength esp. to relieve the symptoms of rheumatoid arthritis and degenerative arthritis — see ADVIL, MOTRIN
ICD *abbr* **1** implantable cardioverter defibrillator **2** International Classification of Diseases — usu. used with a number indicating the revision ⟨*ICD*-9⟩
ice \ˈīs\ *n* : CRYSTAL METH
ice bag *n* : a waterproof bag to hold ice for local application of cold to the body
ice pack *n* : crushed ice placed in a container (as an ice bag) or folded in a towel and applied to the body
ICF *abbr* intermediate care facility
ich·tham·mol \ˈik-thə-ˌmȯl, -ˌmōl\ *n* : a brownish black viscous tarry liquid prepared from a distillate of some hydrocarbon-containing rocks and used as an antiseptic and emollient — see ICHTHYOL
ichthy- *or* **ichthyo-** *comb form* : fish ⟨*ichthyo*sarcotoxism⟩
Ich·thy·ol \ˈik-thē-ˌȯl, -ˌōl\ *trademark* — used for a preparation of ichthammol
ich·thyo·sar·co·tox·ism \ˌik-thē-ō-ˌsär-kə-ˈtäk-ˌsi-zəm\ *n* : poisoning caused by the ingestion of fish whose flesh contains a toxic substance
ich·thy·o·si·form \ˌik-thē-ˈō-sə-ˌfȯrm\ *adj* : resembling ichthyosis or that of ichthyosis ⟨~ erythroderma⟩
ich·thy·o·sis \ˌik-thē-ˈō-səs\ *n, pl* **-o·ses** \-ˌsēz\ : any of several diseases usu. of hereditary origin characterized by rough, thick, and scaly skin — **ich·thy·ot·ic** \-ˈä-tik\ *adj*
ichthyosis hys·trix gra·vi·or \-ˈhis-triks-ˈgra-vē-ˌȯr, -ˈgrä-\ *n* : a rare hereditary disorder characterized by the formation of brown, verrucose, and often linear lesions of the skin
ichthyosis vul·gar·is \-ˌvəl-ˈgar-əs\ *n* : the common hereditary form of ichthyosis that is inherited as an autosomal dominant trait
ICN *abbr* International Council of Nurses
ICP *abbr* intracranial pressure
-ics \iks\ *n sing or pl suffix* **1** : study : knowledge : skill : practice ⟨opt*ics*⟩ ⟨pediatr*ics*⟩ **2** : characteristic actions or activities ⟨hyster*ics*⟩ **3** : characteristic qualities, operations, or phenomena ⟨acoust*ics*⟩ ⟨phonet*ics*⟩
ICSH *abbr* interstitial-cell stimulating hormone
ICSI *abbr* intracytoplasmic sperm injection
ICT *abbr* insulin coma therapy
ic·tal \ˈik-təl\ *adj* : of, relating to, or caused by ictus
icter- *or* **ictero-** *comb form* : jaundice ⟨*ictero*genic⟩
ic·ter·ic \ik-ˈter-ik\ *adj* : of, relating to, or affected with jaundice
icteric index *n* : ICTERUS INDEX
ic·ter·o·gen·ic \ˌik-tə-rō-ˈje-nik, ik-ˌter-ə-\ *adj* : causing or tending to cause jaundice ⟨~ drugs⟩
ic·ter·us \ˈik-tə-rəs\ *n* : JAUNDICE
icterus gra·vis \-ˈgra-vəs, -ˈgrä-\ *n* : ICTERUS GRAVIS NEONATORUM
icterus gravis neo·na·tor·um \-ˌnē-ō-nā-ˈtȯr-əm\ *n* : severe jaundice in a newborn child due esp. to erythroblastosis fetalis
icterus index *n* : a figure representing the amount of bilirubin in the blood as determined by comparing the color of a sample of test serum with a set of color standards ⟨an *icterus index* of 15 or above indicates active jaundice⟩ — called also *icteric index*
icterus neo·na·tor·um \-ˌnē-ō-nā-ˈtȯr-əm\ *n* : jaundice in a newborn

ic•tus \ˈik-təs\ *n* **1** : a beat or pulsation esp. of the heart **2** : a sudden attack or seizure esp. of stroke
ICTV *abbr* International Committee on Taxonomy of Viruses
ICU *abbr* intensive care unit
[1]id \ˈid\ *n* : the one of the three divisions of the psyche in psychoanalytic theory that is completely unconscious and is the source of psychic energy derived from instinctual needs and drives — compare EGO, SUPEREGO
[2]id *n* : a skin rash that is an allergic reaction to an agent causing an infection ⟨a syphilitic ~⟩
ID *abbr* intradermal
[1]-id \əd, (ˌ)id\ *also* **-ide** \īd\ *n suffix* : skin rash caused by (something specified) ⟨syphil*id*⟩
[2]-id *n suffix* : structure, body, or particle of a (specified) kind ⟨chromat*id*⟩
IDA *abbr* iron-deficiency anemia
-i•da \ə-də\ *n pl suffix* : animals that are or have the form of — in names of higher taxa (as orders and classes) ⟨Arachn*ida*⟩ — **-i•dan** \ə-dən, əd-ᵊn\ *n or adj suffix*
-i•dae \ə-ˌdē\ *n pl suffix* : members of the family of — in names of zoological families ⟨Homin*idae*⟩ ⟨Ixod*idae*⟩
IDDM *abbr* insulin-dependent diabetes mellitus
idea \ī-ˈdē-ə\ *n* : something imagined or pictured in the mind
idea of reference *n* : a delusion that the remarks one overhears and people one encounters seem to be concerned with and usu. hostile to oneself — called also *delusion of reference*
ide•ation \ˌī-dē-ˈā-shən\ *n* : the capacity for or the act of forming or entertaining ideas ⟨suicidal ~⟩ — **ide•ation•al** \-shə-nəl\ *adj*
idée fixe \(ˌ)ē-ˌdā-ˈfēks\ *n, pl* **idées fixes** *same or* -ˈfēk-səz\ : a usu. delusional idea that dominates the whole mental life during a prolonged period (as in certain mental disorders) — called also *fixed idea*
iden•ti•cal \ī-ˈden-ti-kəl\ *adj* : MONOZYGOTIC ⟨~ twins⟩
iden•ti•fi•ca•tion \ī-ˌden-tə-fə-ˈkā-shən\ *n* **1** : psychological orientation of the self in regard to something (as a person or group) with a resulting feeling of close emotional association **2** : a largely unconscious process whereby an individual models thoughts, feelings, and actions after those attributed to an object that has been incorporated as a mental image — **iden•ti•fy** \ī-ˈden-tə-ˌfī\ *vb*
iden•ti•ty \ī-ˈden-tə-tē\ *n, pl* **-ties** **1** : the distinguishing character or personality of an individual **2** : the relation established by psychological identification
identity crisis *n* : personal psychosocial conflict esp. in adolescence that involves confusion about one's social role and often a sense of loss of continuity to one's personality
ideo•mo•tor \ˌī-dē-ə-ˈmō-tər, ˌi-\ *adj* **1** : not reflex but motivated by an idea ⟨~ muscular activity⟩ **2** : of, relating to, or concerned with ideomotor activity ⟨~ theory⟩
ID_{50} *symbol* — used for the dose of an infectious organism required to produce infection in 50 percent of the experimental subjects
idio- *comb form* **1** : one's own : personal : separate : distinct ⟨*idio*type⟩ ⟨*idio*syncrasy⟩ **2** : self-produced : arising within ⟨*idio*pathic⟩
id•i•o•cy \ˈi-dē-ə-sē\ *n, pl* **-cies** *dated, now offensive* : extreme intellectual disability
id•io•path•ic \ˌi-dē-ə-ˈpa-thik\ *adj* : arising spontaneously or from an obscure or unknown cause : PRIMARY ⟨~ epilepsy⟩ ⟨~ thrombocytopenic purpura⟩ — **id•io•path•i•cal•ly** *adv*
idiopathic hypertension *n* : ESSENTIAL HYPERTENSION
idiopathic intracranial hypertension *n* : an abnormal condition that is characterized by increased intracranial pressure, headaches, papilledema, and blurring or loss of vision and tends to occur in overweight women of childbearing age — called also *benign intracranial hypertension, pseudotumor cerebri*
id•io•syn•cra•sy \ˌi-dē-ə-ˈsiŋ-krə-sē\ *n, pl* **-sies** **1** : a peculiarity of physical or mental constitution or temperament **2** : individual hypersensitiveness (as to a food) — **id•io•syn•crat•ic** \ˌi-dē-ō-sin-ˈkra-tik\ *adj*
idiot sa•vant \ˈē-ˌdyō-sä-ˈvän\ *n, pl* **idiots savants** *or* **idiot savants** *same or* -ˈvänz\ : SAVANT
id•io•type \ˈi-dē-ə-ˌtīp\ *n* : the molecular structure and conformation in the variable region of an antibody that confers its antigenic specificity — compare ALLOTYPE, ISOTYPE — **id•io•typ•ic** \ˌi-dē-ə-ˈti-pik\ *adj*
id•io•ven•tric•u•lar \ˌi-dē-ə-ven-ˈtri-kyə-lər, -vən-\ *adj* : of, relating to, associated with, or arising in the ventricles of the heart independently of the atria
idox•uri•dine \ˌī-ˌdäks-ˈyu̇r-ə-ˌdēn\ *n* : a drug $C_9H_{11}IN_2O_5$ that is used to treat keratitis caused by the herpesviruses producing herpes simplex — abbr. *IDU;* called also *iododeoxyuridine, IUDR*
-i•dro•sis \i-ˈdrō-səs\ *n comb form, pl* **-i•dro•ses** \-ˌsēz\ : a specified form of sweating ⟨brom*idrosis*⟩
IDU *abbr* idoxuridine
IF *abbr* interferon
IFN *abbr* interferon
ifos•fa•mide \ˌī-ˈfäs-fə-ˌmīd\ *n* : a synthetic cyclophosphamide analog $C_7H_{15}Cl_2H_7O_2P$ that is administered by injection for the treatment esp. of testicular cancer
Ig *abbr* immunoglobulin

IgA \ˌī-(ˌ)jē-ˈā\ *n* : a class of antibodies found in external bodily secretions (as saliva, tears, and sweat); *also* : an antibody of this class — called also *immunoglobulin A*

IgD \ˌī-(ˌ)jē-ˈdē\ *n* : a minor class of antibodies that are of undetermined function except as receptors for antigen; *also* : an antibody of this class — called also *immunoglobulin D*

IgE \ˌī-(ˌ)jē-ˈē\ *n* : a class of antibodies that function esp. in allergic reactions; *also* : an antibody of this class — called also *immunoglobulin E*

IGF *abbr* insulin-like growth factor

IGF–1 *abbr* insulin-like growth factor 1

IgG \ˌī-(ˌ)jē-ˈjē\ *n* : a class of antibodies that facilitate the phagocytic destruction of microorganisms foreign to the body, that bind to and activate complement, and that are the only antibodies to cross over the placenta from mother to fetus; *also* : an antibody of this class — called also *immunoglobulin G*

IgM \ˌī-(ˌ)jē-ˈem\ *n* : a class of antibodies of high molecular weight including those appearing early in the immune response to be replaced later by IgG and that are highly efficient in binding complement; *also* : an antibody of this class — called also *immunoglobulin M*

IL *abbr* interleukin — often used with an identifying number ⟨*IL*-2⟩ ⟨*IL*-6⟩

il- — see IN-

Ile *abbr* isoleucine

ile- *also* **ileo-** *comb form* **1** : ileum ⟨*il*eitis⟩ **2** : ileal and ⟨*ileo*cecal⟩

ilea *pl of* ILEUM

il•e•al \ˈi-lē-əl\ *also* **il•e•ac** \-ˌak\ *adj* : of, relating to, or affecting the ileum

il•e•itis \ˌi-lē-ˈī-təs\ *n, pl* **-it•i•des** \-ˈi-tə-ˌdēz\ : inflammation of the ileum — see REGIONAL ILEITIS

il•eo•anal \ˌi-lē-ō-ˈā-nᵊl\ *adj* : of, relating to, or connecting the ileum and anus

il•eo•ce•cal \ˌi-lē-ō-ˈsē-kəl\ *adj* : of, relating to, or connecting the ileum and cecum

ileocecal valve *n* : the valve formed by two folds of mucous membrane at the opening of the ileum into the large intestine — called also *Bauhin's valve*

il•eo•co•lic \-ˈkō-lik, -ˈkä-\ *adj* : relating to, situated near, or involving the ileum and the colon

ileocolic artery *n* : a branch of the superior mesenteric artery that supplies the terminal part of the ileum and the beginning of the colon

il•eo•co•li•tis \ˌi-lē-ō-kō-ˈlī-təs\ *n* : inflammation of the ileum and colon

il•eo•co•los•to•my \-kə-ˈläs-tə-mē\ *n, pl* **-mies** : a surgical operation producing an artificial opening connecting the ileum and the colon

il•eo•cyto•plas•ty \-ˈsī-tə-ˌplas-tē\ *n, pl* **-ties** : plastic surgery that involves anastomosing a segment of the ileum to the bladder esp. in order to increase bladder capacity and preserve the function of the kidneys and ureters

il•eo•il•e•al \-ˈi-lē-əl\ *adj* : relating to or involving two different parts of the ileum ⟨an ∼ anastomosis⟩

il•eo•proc•tos•to•my \-ˌpräk-ˈtäs-tə-mē\ *n, pl* **-mies** : a surgical operation producing a permanent artificial opening connecting the ileum and rectum

il•e•os•to•my \ˌi-lē-ˈäs-tə-mē\ *n, pl* **-mies** **1** : surgical formation of an artificial anus by connecting the ileum to an opening in the abdominal wall **2** : the artificial opening made by ileostomy

ileostomy bag *n* : a container designed to receive feces discharged through an ileostomy

Ile•tin \ˈī-lə-tən\ *trademark* — used for a preparation of insulin

il•e•um \ˈi-lē-əm\ *n, pl* **il•ea** \-lē-ə\ : the last division of the small intestine extending between the jejunum and large intestine

il•e•us \ˈi-lē-əs\ *n* : obstruction of the bowel; *specif* : functional obstruction of the gastrointestinal tract and esp. the small intestine that is marked by the absence of peristalsis, is usu. accompanied by abdominal pain, bloating, and sometimes nausea and vomiting, and typically occurs following abdominal surgery — called also *paralytic ileus;* compare VOLVULUS

ilia *pl of* ILIUM

il•i•ac \ˈi-lē-ˌak\ *also* **il•i•al** \-əl\ *adj* **1** : of, relating to, or located near the ilium ⟨the ∼ bone⟩ **2** : of or relating to either of the lowest lateral abdominal regions

iliac artery *n* **1** : either of the large arteries supplying blood to the lower trunk and hind limbs and arising by bifurcation of the aorta to form one vessel for each side of the body — called also *common iliac artery* **2** : the outer branch of the common iliac artery on either side of the body that becomes the femoral artery — called also *external iliac artery* **3** : the inner branch of the common iliac artery on either side of the body that supplies blood chiefly to the pelvic and gluteal areas — called also *hypogastric artery, internal iliac artery*

iliac crest *n* : the thick curved upper border of the ilium

iliac fossa *n* : the inner concavity of the ilium

iliac node *n* : any of the lymph nodes grouped around the iliac arteries and the iliac veins — see EXTERNAL ILIAC NODE, INTERNAL ILIAC NODE

iliac spine *n* : any of four projections on the ilium: **a** : ANTERIOR INFERIOR ILIAC SPINE **b** : ANTERIOR SUPERIOR ILIAC SPINE **c** : POSTERIOR INFERIOR ILIAC SPINE **d** : POSTERIOR SUPERIOR ILIAC SPINE

ili•a•cus \i-ˈlī-ə-kəs\ *n, pl* **ili•a•ci** \-ə-ˌsī\ : a muscle of the iliac region of the abdomen that flexes the thigh or bends the pelvis and lumbar region forward

iliac vein *n* : any of several veins on each side of the body corresponding to and accompanying the iliac arteries: **a** : either of two veins of which one is formed on each side of the body by the union of the external and internal iliac veins and which unite to form the inferior vena cava — called also *common iliac vein* **b** : a vein that drains the leg and lower part of the anterior abdominal wall, is an upward continuation of the femoral vein, and unites with the internal iliac vein — called also *external iliac vein* **c** : a vein that drains the pelvis and gluteal and perineal regions and that unites with the external iliac vein to form the common iliac vein — called also *hypogastric vein, internal iliac vein*

ilio- *comb form* : iliac and ⟨*ilio*inguinal⟩

il•io•coc•cy•geus \ˌi-lē-ō-käk-ˈsi-jəs, -jē-əs\ *n* : a muscle of the pelvis that is a subdivision of the levator ani and helps support the pelvic viscera — compare PUBOCOCCYGEUS

il•io•cos•ta•lis \-käs-ˈtā-ləs\ *n* : the lateral division of the sacrospinalis muscle that helps to keep the trunk erect and consists of three parts: **a** : ILIOCOSTALIS CERVICIS **b** : ILIOCOSTALIS LUMBORUM **c** : ILIOCOSTALIS THORACIS

iliocostalis cer•vi•cis \-ˈsər-və-səs\ *n* : a muscle that extends from the ribs to the cervical transverse processes and acts to draw the neck to the same side and to elevate the ribs

iliocostalis dor•si \-ˈdȯr-ˌsī\ *n* : ILIOCOSTALIS THORACIS

iliocostalis lum•bor•um \-ˌləm-ˈbȯr-əm\ *n* : a muscle that extends from the ilium to the lower ribs and acts to draw the trunk to the same side or to depress the ribs

iliocostalis tho•ra•cis \-thə-ˈrā-səs\ *n* : a muscle that extends from the lower to the upper ribs and acts to draw the trunk to the same side and to approximate the ribs

il•io•fem•o•ral \ˌi-lē-ō-ˈfe-mə-rəl\ *adj* **1** : of or relating to the ilium and the femur **2** : relating to or involving an iliac vein and a femoral vein

iliofemoral ligament *n* : a ligament that extends from the anterior inferior iliac spine to the intertrochanteric line of the femur and divides below into two branches — called also *Y ligament*

il•io•hy•po•gas•tric nerve \ˌi-lē-ō-ˌhī-pə-ˈgas-trik-\ *n* : a branch of the first lumbar nerve distributed to the skin of the lateral part of the buttocks, the skin of the pubic region, and the muscles of the anterolateral abdominal wall

il•io•in•gui•nal \-ˈiŋ-gwən-ᵊl\ *adj* : of, relating to, or affecting the iliac and inguinal abdominal regions

ilioinguinal nerve *n* : a branch of the first lumbar nerve distributed to the muscles of the anterolateral wall of the abdomen, the skin of the proximal and medial part of the thigh, the base of the penis and the scrotum in the male, and the mons veneris and labia majora in the female

il•io•lum•bar artery \ˌi-lē-ō-ˈləm-bər-, -ˌbär-\ *n* : a branch of the internal iliac artery that supplies muscles in the lumbar region and the iliac fossa

iliolumbar ligament *n* : a ligament connecting the transverse process of the last lumbar vertebra with the iliac crest

il•io•pec•tin•e•al eminence \ˌi-lē-ō-pek-ˈti-nē-əl-\ *n* : a ridge on the hip bone marking the junction of the ilium and the pubis

iliopectineal line *n* : a line or ridge on the inner surface of the hip bone marking the border between the true and false pelvis

il•io•pso•as \ˌi-lē-ō-ˈsō-əs, -lē-ˈäp-sō-əs\ *n* : a muscle consisting of the iliacus and psoas major muscles

iliopsoas tendon *n* : the tendon that is common to the iliacus and psoas major

il•io•tib•i•al \ˌi-lē-ō-ˈti-bē-əl\ *adj* : of or relating to the ilium and the tibia

iliotibial band *n* : a fibrous thickening of the fascia lata that extends from the iliac crest down the lateral part of the thigh to the lateral condyle of the tibia and that provides stability to the knee and assists with flexion and extension of the knee — called also *iliotibial tract, IT band*

iliotibial band syndrome *n* : a sports injury that is marked by pain in the lateral part of the knee and results from inflammation of the iliotibial band due to overuse (as in long-distance running) as it slides across the lateral condyle of the femur as the knee is flexed and extended repeatedly — called also *iliotibial band friction syndrome*

il•i•um \ˈi-lē-əm\ *n, pl* **il•ia** \-lē-ə\ : the dorsal, upper, and largest one of the three bones composing either lateral half of the pelvis that is broad and expanded above and narrower below where it joins with the ischium and pubis to form part of the acetabulum

[1]**ill** \ˈil\ *adj* **worse** \ˈwərs\ *also* **ill•er**; **worst** \ˈwərst\ **1** : affected with some ailment : not in good health ⟨incurably ~⟩ **2** : affected with nausea often to the point of vomiting

[2]**ill** *n* : AILMENT, SICKNESS

ill•ness \ˈil-nəs\ *n* : an unhealthy condition of body or mind : SICKNESS

il•lu•sion \i-ˈlü-zhən\ *n* **1** : perception of something objectively existing in such a way as to cause misinterpretation of its actual nature; *esp* : OPTICAL ILLUSION **2** : HALLUCINATION 1 **3** : a pattern capable of reversible perspective

Il•o•sone \ˈi-lə-ˌsōn\ *n* : a preparation of erythromycin — formerly a U.S. registered trademark

Il•o•ty•cin \ˌi-lə-ˈtī-sən\ *n* : a preparation of erythromycin — formerly a U.S. registered trademark

IM *abbr* **1** infectious mononucleosis **2** internal medicine **3** intramuscular; intramuscularly

im- — see IN-

[1]**im•age** \ˈi-mij\ *n* : a mental picture or impression of something: as **a** : an idealized conception of a person and esp. a parent that is formed by an infant or child, is retained in the unconscious, and influences behavior in later life — called also *imago* **b** : the memory of a perception in psychology that is modified by subsequent experience; *also* : the representation of the source of a stimulus on a receptor mechanism

[2]**image** *vb* **im•aged; im•ag•ing** **1** : to call up a mental picture of **2** : to create a representation of; *also* : to form an image of

image intensifier *n* : a device used esp. for diagnosis in radiology that provides a more intense image for a given amount of radiation than can be obtained by the usual fluorometric methods — **image intensification** *n*

im•ag•ery \ˈi-mij-rē, -mi-jə-\ *n, pl* **-eries** : mental images; *esp* : the products of imagination <psychotic ~>

im•ag•ing *n* : the action or process of producing an image esp. of a part of the body by radiographic techniques <diagnostic ~> <cardiac ~> — see MAGNETIC RESONANCE IMAGING

ima•go \i-ˈmā-(ˌ)gō, -ˈmä-\ *n, pl* **ima•goes** *or* **ima•gi•nes** \-ˈmā-gə-ˌnēz, -ˈmä-\ : IMAGE a

imat•i•nib \i-ˈma-tə-ˌnib\ *n* : an anticancer drug that is taken orally in the form of its mesylate $C_{29}H_{31}N_7O\cdot CH_4O_3S$ to treat chronic myelogenous leukemia and metastatic or unresectable gastrointestinal stromal tumors — called also *imatinib mesylate;* see GLEEVEC

im•bal•ance \(ˌ)im-ˈba-ləns\ *n* : lack of balance : the state of being out of equilibrium or out of proportion: as **a** : loss of parallel relation between the optical axes of the eyes caused by faulty action of the extrinsic muscles and often resulting in diplopia **b** : absence of biological equilibrium <a vitamin ~> — **im•bal•anced** \-lənst\ *adj*

im•be•cile \ˈim-bə-səl, -ˌsil\ *n, dated, now offensive* : a person affected with moderate intellectual disability — **im•be•cil•i•ty** \ˌim-bə-ˈsi-lə-tē\ *n, dated, now offensive*

imbed *var of* EMBED

im•bri•ca•tion \ˌim-brə-ˈkā-shən\ *n* : an overlapping esp. of successive layers of tissue in the surgical closure of a wound — **im•bri•cate** \ˈim-brə-ˌkāt\ *vb*

im•id•az•ole \ˌi-mə-ˈda-ˌzōl\ *n* **1** : a white crystalline heterocyclic base $C_3H_4N_2$ that is an antimetabolite related to histidine **2** : any of a large class of derivatives of imidazole including histidine and histamine

im•id•az•o•line \ˌi-mə-ˈda-zə-ˌlēn\ *n* : any of three derivatives $C_3H_6N_2$ of imidazole with adrenergic blocking activity

im•i•glu•ce•rase \ˌim-ə-ˈglü-sə-ˌrās\ *n* : a modified human glucocerebrosidase produced by recombinant DNA technology and administered by injection for enzyme replacement therapy in the treatment of Gaucher disease — see CEREZYME

im•i•no•gly•cin•uria \ˌi-mə-ˌnō-ˌglī-sə-ˈnu̇r-ē-ə, -ˈnyu̇r-\ *n* : an abnormal inherited condition of the kidney associated esp. with hyperprolinemia and characterized by the presence of proline, hydroxyproline, and glycine in the urine

im•i•pen•em \ˌi-mə-ˈpe-nəm\ *n* : a semisynthetic beta-lactam $C_{12}H_{17}N_3O_4S\cdot H_2O$ that is derived from an antibiotic produced by a bacterium of the genus *Streptomyces* (*S. cattleya*) and is effective against gram-negative and gram-positive bacteria

imip•ra•mine \i-ˈmi-prə-ˌmēn\ *n* : a tricyclic antidepressant drug used esp. in the form of its hydrochloride $C_{19}H_{24}N_2\cdot HCl$ or pamoate $(C_{19}H_{24}N_2)_2\cdot C_{23}H_{16}O_6$ — see TOFRANIL

Im•i•trex \ˈi-mə-ˌtreks\ *trademark* — used for a preparation of the succinate of sumatriptan

im•ma•ture \ˌi-mə-ˈtu̇r, -ˈtyu̇r, -ˈchu̇r\ *adj* : lacking complete growth, differentiation, or development — **im•ma•ture•ly** *adv* — **im•ma•tu•ri•ty** \-ˈtu̇r-ə-tē, -ˈtyu̇r-, -ˈchu̇r-\ *n*

im•me•di•ate \i-ˈmē-dē-ət\ *adj* **1** : acting or being without the intervention of another object, cause, or agency : being direct <the ~ cause of death> **2** : present to the mind independently of other states or factors <~ awareness>

immediate auscultation *n* : auscultation performed without a stethoscope by laying the ear directly against the patient's body

immediate hypersensitivity *n, pl* **-ties** : hypersensitivity in which exposure to an antigen produces an immediate or almost immediate reaction

immersion foot *n* : a painful condition of the feet marked by inflammation and stabbing pain and followed by discoloration, swelling, ulcers, and numbness due to prolonged exposure to moist cold usu. without actual freezing

im•mo•bile \ˌi-ˈmō-bəl, -ˌbēl, -ˌbīl\ *adj* **1** : incapable of being moved **2** : not moving <keep the patient ~> — **im•mo•bil•i•ty** \ˌi-ˌmō-ˈbi-lə-tē\ *n*

im•mo•bi•lize \i-ˈmō-bə-ˌlīz\ *vb* **-ized; -iz•ing** : to make immobile; *esp* : to fix (as a body part) so as to reduce or eliminate motion usu. by means of a cast or splint, by strapping, or by strict bed rest — **im·mo·bi·li·za·tion** \ˌmō-bə-lə-ˈzā-shən\ *n*

im·mune \i-ˈmyün\ *adj* **1** : not susceptible or responsive; *esp* : having a high degree of resistance to a disease **2 a** : having or producing antibodies or lymphocytes capable of reacting with a specific antigen ⟨an ~ serum⟩ **b** : produced by, involved in, or concerned with immunity or an immune response ⟨~ agglutinins⟩

immune complex *n* : any of various molecular complexes formed in the blood by combination of an antigen and an antibody that tend to accumulate in bodily tissue and are associated with various pathological conditions (as glomerulonephritis and systemic lupus erythematosus)

immune globulin *n* : globulin from the blood of a person or animal immune to a particular disease — called also *immune serum globulin*

immune response *n* : a bodily response to an antigen that occurs when lymphocytes identify the antigenic molecule as foreign and induce the formation of antibodies and lymphocytes capable of reacting with it and rendering it harmless — called also *immune reaction*

immune serum *n* : ANTISERUM

immune system *n* : the bodily system that protects the body from foreign substances, cells, and tissues by producing the immune response and that includes esp. the thymus, spleen, lymph nodes, special deposits of lymphoid tissue (as in the gastrointestinal tract and bone marrow), lymphocytes including the B cells and T cells, and antibodies

immune therapy *n* : IMMUNOTHERAPY

im·mu·ni·ty \i-ˈmyü-nə-tē\ *n, pl* **-ties** : the quality or state of being immune; *esp* : a condition of being able to resist a particular disease esp. through preventing development of a pathogenic microorganism or by counteracting the effects of its products — see ACQUIRED IMMUNITY, ACTIVE IMMUNITY, NATURAL IMMUNITY, PASSIVE IMMUNITY

im·mu·ni·za·tion \ˌi-myə-nə-ˈzā-shən\ *n* : the creation of immunity usu. against a particular disease; *esp* : treatment (as by vaccination) of an organism for the purpose of making it immune to a particular pathogen — **im·mu·nize** \ˈi-myə-ˌnīz\ *vb*

immuno- *comb form* **1** : physiological immunity ⟨*immuno*logy⟩ **2** : immunologic ⟨*immuno*chemistry⟩ : immunologically ⟨*immuno*compromised⟩ : immunology and ⟨*immuno*genetics⟩

im·mu·no·ad·sor·bent \ˌi-myə-nō-ad-ˈsȯr-bənt, i-ˌmyü-nō-, -ˈzȯr-\ *n* : IMMUNOSORBENT — **immunoadsorbent** *adj*

im·mu·no·as·say \-ˈas-ˌā, -a-ˈsā\ *n* : a technique or test (as the enzyme-linked immunosorbent assay) used to detect the presence or quantity of a substance (as a protein) based on its capacity to act as an antigen or antibody — **immunoassay** *vb* — **im·mu·no·as·say·able** \-a-ˈsā-ə-bəl\ *adj*

im·mu·no·bi·ol·o·gy \-bī-ˈä-lə-jē\ *n, pl* **-gies** : a branch of biology concerned with the physiological reactions characteristic of the immune state — **im·mu·no·bi·o·log·i·cal** \-ˌbī-ə-ˈlä-ji-kəl\ *or* **im·mu·no·bi·o·log·ic** \-ˈlä-jik\ *adj* — **im·mu·no·bi·ol·o·gist** \-bī-ˈä-lə-jist\ *n*

im·mu·no·blast \i-ˈmyü-nō-ˌblast, ˈi-myə-nō-\ *n* : a lymphocyte that has enlarged following antigenic stimulation : LYMPHOBLAST

im·mu·no·blas·tic \ˌi-myə-nō-ˈblas-tik, im-ˌyü-nō-\ *adj* : marked by the proliferation of immunoblasts

immunoblastic lymphadenopathy *n* : ANGIOIMMUNOBLASTIC T-CELL LYMPHOMA

im·mu·no·blot \-ˌblät\ *n* : a blot (as a Western blot) in which a radioactively labeled antibody is used as the molecular probe — **im·mu·no·blot·ting** *n*

im·mu·no·chem·is·try \-ˈke-mə-strē\ *n, pl* **-tries** : a branch of chemistry that deals with the chemical aspects of immunology — **im·mu·no·chem·i·cal** \-ˈke-mə-kəl\ *adj* — **im·mu·no·chem·i·cal·ly** *adv* — **im·mu·no·chem·ist** \-ˈke-mist\ *n*

im·mu·no·che·mo·ther·a·py \-ˌkē-mō-ˈther-ə-pē\ *n, pl* **-pies** : the combined use of immunotherapy and chemotherapy in the treatment or control of disease

im·mu·no·com·pe·tence \-ˈkäm-pə-təns\ *n* : the capacity for a normal immune response — **im·mu·no·com·pe·tent** \-tənt\ *adj*

im·mu·no·com·pro·mised \-ˈkäm-prə-ˌmīzd\ *adj* : having the immune system impaired or weakened (as by drugs or illness) ⟨~ patients⟩

im·mu·no·con·ju·gate \-ˈkän-ji-gət, -ˈkän-jə-ˌgāt\ *n* : a complex of an antibody and a toxic agent (as a drug) used to kill or destroy a targeted antigen (as a cancer cell)

im·mu·no·cyte \i-ˈmyü-nō-ˌsīt, ˈi-myə-nō-\ *n* : a cell (as a lymphocyte) that has an immunologic function

im·mu·no·cy·to·chem·is·try \ˌi-myə-nō-ˌsī-tō-ˈke-mə-strē, i-ˌmyü-nō-\ *n, pl* **-tries** : the application of biochemistry to cellular immunology — **im·mu·no·cy·to·chem·i·cal** \-ˈke-mi-kəl\ *adj*

im·mu·no·de·fi·cien·cy \-di-ˈfi-shən-sē\ *n, pl* **-cies** : inability to produce a normal complement of antibodies or immunologically sensitized T cells esp. in response to specific antigens — **im·mu·no·de·fi·cient** \-shənt\ *adj*

im·mu·no·de·pres·sion \-di-ˈpre-shən\ *n* : IMMUNOSUPPRESSION — **im·mu·no·de·pres·sant** \-di-ˈpres-ᵊnt\ *n*

im·mu·no·di·ag·no·sis \-ˌdī-ig-ˈnō-səs\ *n, pl* **-no·ses** \-ˌsēz\ : diagnosis (as of cancer) by immunological methods

— **im•mu•no•di•ag•nos•tic** \-ˈnäs-tik\ *adj*

im•mu•no•dif•fu•sion \-di-ˈfyü-zhən\ *n* : any of several techniques for obtaining a precipitate between an antibody and its specific antigen by suspending one in a gel and letting the other migrate through it from a well or by letting both antibody and antigen migrate through the gel from separate wells to form an area of precipitation

im•mu•no•elec•tro•pho•re•sis \-ə-ˌlek-trə-fə-ˈrē-səs\ *n, pl* **-re•ses** \-ˌsēz\ : electrophoretic separation of proteins followed by identification by the formation of precipitates through specific immunologic reactions — **im•mu•no•elec•tro•pho•ret•ic** \-ˈre-tik\ *adj* — **im•mu•no•elec•tro•pho•ret•i•cal•ly** *adv*

im•mu•no•flu•o•res•cence \-flò-ˈres-ᵊns, -flü-\ *n* : the labeling of antibodies or antigens with fluorescent dyes esp. for the purpose of demonstrating the presence of a particular antigen or antibody in a tissue preparation or smear — **im•mu•no•flu•o•res•cent** \-ᵊnt\ *adj*

im•mu•no•gen \i-ˈmyü-nə-jən, ˈi-myə-nə-, -ˌjen\ *n* : an antigen that provokes an immune response

im•mu•no•ge•net•ics \-jə-ˈne-tiks\ *n* : a branch of immunology concerned with the interrelations of heredity, disease, and the immune system and its components (as antibodies) — **im•mu•no•ge•net•ic** \-tik\ *adj* — **im•mu•no•ge•net•i•cal•ly** *adv* — **im•mu•no•ge•net•i•cist** \-jə-ˈne-tə-sist\ *n*

im•mu•no•gen•ic \ˌi-myə-nō-ˈjen-ik, i-ˌmyü-nō-\ *adj* : relating to or producing an immune response ⟨~ substances⟩ — **im•mu•no•gen•i•cal•ly** *adv* — **im•mu•no•ge•nic•i•ty** \-jə-ˈni-sə-tē\ *n*

im•mu•no•glob•u•lin \-ˈglä-byə-lən\ *n* : ANTIBODY — abbr. *Ig*

immunoglobulin A *n* : IGA

immunoglobulin D *n* : IGD

immunoglobulin E *n* : IGE

immunoglobulin G *n* : IGG

immunoglobulin M *n* : IGM

im•mu•no•he•ma•tol•o•gy \-ˌhe-mə-ˈtä-lə-jē\ *n, pl* **-gies** : a branch of immunology that deals with the immunologic properties of blood — **im•mu•no•he•ma•to•log•ic** \-ˌhē-mə-tə-ˈlä-jik\ *or* **im•mu•no•he•ma•to•log•i•cal** \-ji-kəl\ *adj* — **im•mu•no•he•ma•tol•o•gist** \-ˌhē-mə-ˈtä-lə-jist\ *n*

im•mu•no•his•to•chem•i•cal \-ˌhis-tō-ˈke-mi-kəl\ *adj* : of or relating to the application of histochemical and immunologic methods to chemical analysis of living cells and tissues — **im•mu•no•his•to•chem•i•cal•ly** *adv* — **im-mu•no•his•to•chem•is•try** \-ˈke-mə-strē\ *n*

im•mu•no•his•to•log•i•cal \-ˌhis-tə-ˈlä-ji-kəl\ *also* **im•mu•no•his•to•log•ic** \-ˈlä-jik\ *adj* : of or relating to the application of immunologic methods to histology — **im•mu•no•his•tol•o•gy** \-hi-ˈstä-lə-jē\ *n*

immunological surveillance *n* : IMMUNOSURVEILLANCE

im•mu•nol•o•gist \ˌi-myə-ˈnä-lə-jist\ *n* : a specialist in immunology

im•mu•nol•o•gy \ˌi-myə-ˈnä-lə-jē\ *n, pl* **-gies** : a science that deals with the immune system and the cell-mediated and humoral aspects of immunity and immune responses — **im•mu•no•log•ic** \-nə-ˈlä-jik\ *or* **im•mu•no•log•i•cal** \-ji-kəl\ *adj* — **im•mu•no•log•i•cal•ly** *adv*

im•mu•no•mod•u•lat•ing \ˌi-myə-nō-ˈmä-jə-ˌlā-tiŋ, i-ˌmyü-nō-\ *adj* : of, relating to, being, or involving an immunomodulator ⟨~ agents⟩ ⟨~ therapy⟩

im•mu•no•mod•u•la•tion \-ˌmä-jə-ˈlā-shən\ *n* : modification of the immune response or the functioning of the immune system by the action of an immunomodulator

im•mu•no•mod•u•la•tor \ˌi-myə-nō-ˈmä-jə-ˌlā-tər, i-ˌmyü-nō-\ *n* : a chemical agent (as methotrexate) that modifies the immune response or the functioning of the immune system — **im•mu•no•mod•u•la•to•ry** \-ˈmä-jə-lə-ˌtōr-ē\ *adj*

im•mu•no•patho•gen•e•sis \-ˌpa-thə-ˈje-nə-səs\ *n, pl* **-e•ses** \-ˌsēz\ : the development of disease as affected by the immune system — **im•mu•no•path•o•gen•ic** \-ˈje-nik\ *adj*

im•mu•no•pa•thol•o•gist \-pə-ˈthä-lə-jist, -pa-\ *n* : a specialist in immunopathology

im•mu•no•pa•thol•o•gy \-pə-ˈthä-lə-jē, -pa-\ *n, pl* **-gies** **1** : a branch of medicine that deals with immune responses associated with disease **2** : the pathology of an organism, organ system, or disease with respect to the immune system, immunity, and immune responses — **im•mu•no•path•o•log•ic** \-ˌpa-thə-ˈlä-jik\ *or* **im•mu•no•path•o•log•i•cal** \-ji-kəl\ *adj*

im•mu•no•phe•no•type \-ˈfē-nə-ˌtīp\ *n* : the immunochemical and immunohistological characteristics of a cell or group of cells — **im•mu•no•phe•no•typ•ic** \-ˌfē-nə-ˈti-pik\ *also* **im•mu•no•phe•no•typ•i•cal** \-pi-kəl\ *adj* — **im•mu•no•phe•no•typ•i•cal•ly** \-pi-k(ə-)lē\ *adv*

im•mu•no•phe•no•typ•ing \-ˈfē-nə-ˌtī-piŋ\ *n* : the process of determining the immunophenotype of a cell or group of cells

im•mu•no•phil•in \-ˈfi-lən\ *n* : any of a group of proteins that exhibit high specificity in binding to immunosuppressive agents (as cyclosporine)

im•mu•no•pre•cip•i•ta•tion \-pri-ˌsi-pə-ˈtā-shən\ *n* : precipitation of a complex of an antibody and its specific antigen — **im•mu•no•pre•cip•i•tate** \-ˈsi-pə-tət, -ˌtāt\ *n* — **im•mu•no•pre•cip•i•tate** \-ˌtāt\ *vb*

im•mu•no•pro•lif•er•a•tive \-prə-ˈli-fə-ˌrā-tiv\ *adj* : of, relating to, or characterized by the proliferation of lymphocytes and esp. plasma cells ⟨~ disorders⟩

immunoproliferative small intestinal disease *n* : a lymphoma that arises in the small intestine, is marked esp. by abdominal pain, diarrhea, and malabsorption, is associated with the secretion by proliferating plasma cells of truncated IgA heavy chains without the accompanying light chains, and that chiefly affects individuals in Mediterranean regions — abbr. *IPSID;* called also *alpha chain disease, Mediterranean lymphoma*

im•mu•no•pro•phy•lax•is \-ˌprō-fə-ˈlak-səs, -ˌprä-\ *n, pl* **-lax•es** \-ˌsēz\ : the prevention of disease by the production of active or passive immunity

im•mu•no•ra•dio•met•ric assay \-ˌrā-dē-ō-ˈme-trik-\ *n* : immunoassay of a substance by combining it with a radioactively labeled antibody

im•mu•no•re•ac•tive \-rē-ˈak-tiv\ *adj* : reacting to particular antigens or haptens ⟨~ lymphocytes⟩ — **im•mu•no•re•ac•tion** \-ˈak-shən\ *n* — **im•mu•no•re•ac•tiv•i•ty** \-(ˌ)rē-ˌak-ˈti-və-tē\ *n*

im•mu•no•reg•u•la•to•ry \-ˈre-gyə-lə-ˌtōr-ē\ *adj* : of or relating to the regulation of the immune system ⟨~ T cells⟩ — **im•mu•no•reg•u•la•tion** \-ˌre-gyə-ˈlā-shən\ *n*

im•mu•no•sor•bent \-ˈsȯr-bənt, -ˈzȯr-\ *adj* : relating to or using a substrate consisting of a specific antibody or antigen chemically combined with an insoluble substance (as cellulose) to selectively remove the corresponding specific antigen or antibody from solution — **immunosorbent** *n*

im•mu•no•stim•u•la•tion \-ˌsti-myə-ˈlā-shən\ *n* : stimulation of an immune response — **im•mu•no•stim•u•lant** \-ˈsti-myə-lənt\ *n or adj* — **im•mu•no•stim•u•la•to•ry** \-ˈsti-myə-lə-ˌtōr-ē\ *adj*

im•mu•no•sup•pres•sion \-sə-ˈpre-shən\ *n* : suppression (as by drugs or disease) of the immune response — **im•mu•no•sup•press** \-sə-ˈpres\ *vb* — **im•mu•no•sup•pres•sant** \-ˈpres-ᵊnt\ *n or adj* — **im•mu•no•sup•pres•sive** \-ˈpre-səv\ *adj*

im•mu•no•sur•veil•lance \-sər-ˈvā-ləns\ *n* : a monitoring process of the immune system which detects and destroys neoplastic cells and which tends to break down in immunosuppressed individuals — called also *immunological surveillance*

im•mu•no•ther•a•py \-ˈther-ə-pē\ *n, pl* **-pies** : treatment or prevention of disease (as a cancer, autoimmune disorder, or allergy) that involves the stimulation, enhancement, suppression, or desensitization of the immune system — called also *immune therapy;* see ADOPTIVE IMMUNOTHERAPY — **im•mu•no•ther•a•peu•tic** \-ˌther-ə-ˈpyü-tik\ *adj*

im•mu•no•tox•ic•i•ty \-täk-ˈsi-sə-tē\ *n, pl* **-ties** : toxicity to the immune system — **im•mu•no•tox•ic** \-ˈtäk-sik\ *adj*

im•mu•no•tox•i•col•o•gy \-ˌtäk-si-ˈkä-lə-jē\ *n, pl* **-gies** : the study of the effects of toxic substances on the immune system

im•mu•no•tox•in \ˈi-myə-nō-ˌtäk-sən, i-ˈmyü-nō-\ *n* : a toxin that is linked to a monoclonal antibody and is delivered to only those cells (as cancer cells) targeted by the monoclonal antibody to which it is linked

Imo•di•um \i-ˈmō-dē-əm\ *trademark* — used for a preparation of the hydrochloride of loperamide

IMP \ˌī-(ˌ)em-ˈpē\ *n* : INOSINIC ACID

im•pact•ed \im-ˈpak-təd\ *adj* **1 a** : blocked by material (as feces) that is firmly packed or wedged in position ⟨an ~ colon⟩ **b** : wedged or lodged in a bodily passage ⟨an ~ mass of feces⟩ **2** : characterized by broken ends of bone driven together ⟨an ~ fracture⟩ **3** *of a tooth* : wedged between the jawbone and another tooth ⟨an ~ wisdom tooth⟩ — **im•pac•tion** \im-ˈpak-shən\ *n*

impaction fracture *n* : a fracture that is impacted

im•paired \im-ˈpard\ *adj* : being in an imperfect or weakened state or condition: as **a** : diminished in function or ability : lacking full functional or structural integrity ⟨~ joint movement⟩ ⟨visually ~ adults⟩ **b** : unable to function normally or safely because of intoxication by alcohol or drugs ⟨driving while ~⟩ — **im•pair•ment** \-ˈpar-mənt\ *n*

im•pal•pa•ble \(ˌ)im-ˈpal-pə-bəl\ *adj* : incapable of being felt by touch

im•ped•ance \im-ˈpēd-ᵊns\ *n* : opposition to blood flow in the circulatory system

im•ped•i•ment \im-ˈpe-də-mənt\ *n* : something that impedes; *esp* : an impairment (as a stutter) interfering with the proper articulation of speech

imperfecta — see AMELOGENESIS IMPERFECTA, OSTEOGENESIS IMPERFECTA, OSTEOGENESIS IMPERFECTA CONGENITA, OSTEOGENESIS IMPERFECTA TARDA

im•per•fect fungus \(ˌ)im-ˈpər-fikt-\ *n* : any of various fungi of which only the asexual spore-producing stage is known

im•per•fo•rate \(ˌ)im-ˈpər-fə-rət, -ˌrāt\ *adj* : having no opening or aperture; *specif* : lacking the usual or normal opening ⟨an ~ hymen⟩ ⟨an ~ anus⟩

im•pe•ri•al gallon \im-ˈpir-ē-əl-\ *n* : GALLON 2

im•per•me•able \(ˌ)im-ˈpər-mē-ə-bəl\ *adj* : not permitting passage (as of a fluid) through its substance — **im•per•me•abil•i•ty** \-mē-ə-ˈbi-lə-tē\ *n*

im•pe•tig•i•nized \ˌim-pə-ˈti-jə-ˌnīzd\ *adj* : affected with impetigo on top of an underlying dermatologic condition

im•pe•tig•i•nous \ˌim-pə-ˈti-jə-nəs\ *adj* : of, relating to, or resembling impetigo ⟨~ skin lesions⟩

im•pe•ti•go \ˌim-pə-ˈtē-(ˌ)gō, -ˈtī-\ *n* : an acute contagious staphylococcal or streptococcal skin disease characterized by vesicles, pustules, and yellowish crusts

impetigo con·ta·gi·o·sa \-kən-ˌtā-jē-ˈō-sə\ *n* : IMPETIGO

im·plant \ˈim-ˌplant\ *n* : something (as a graft, a small container of radioactive material for treatment of cancer, or a pellet containing hormones to be gradually absorbed) that is inserted or embedded esp. in tissue — **im·plant** \im-ˈplant\ *vb* — **im·plant·able** \-ˈplan-tə-bəl\ *adj*

im·plan·ta·tion \ˌim-ˌplan-ˈtā-shən\ *n* : the act or process of implanting or the state of being implanted: as **a** : the placement of a natural or artificial tooth in an artificially prepared socket in the jawbone **b** *in placental mammals* : the process of attachment of the embryo to the maternal uterine wall — called also *nidation* **c** : medical treatment by the insertion of an implant

im·plant·ee \ˌim-ˌplan-ˈtē\ *n* : the recipient of an implant

im·plan·tol·o·gist \ˌim-ˌplan-ˈtä-lə-jist\ *n* : a dentist who specializes in implantology

im·plan·tol·o·gy \-ˈtä-lə-jē\ *n, pl* **-gies** : a branch of dentistry dealing with dental implantation

im·plo·sion therapy \im-ˈplō-zhən-\ *n* : IMPLOSIVE THERAPY

im·plo·sive therapy \im-ˈplō-siv-\ *n* : exposure therapy in which visualization is utilized by the patient

imported fire ant *n* : either of two mound-building So. American fire ants of the genus *Solenopsis* (*S. invicta* and *S. richteri*) that have been introduced into the southeastern U.S. and can inflict stings requiring medical attention

im·po·tence \ˈim-pə-təns\ *n* **1** : the quality or state of not being potent ⟨the growing ~ of antibiotics⟩ **2** : an abnormal physical or psychological state of a male characterized by inability to engage in sexual intercourse because of failure to have or maintain an erection — called also *erectile dysfunction*

im·po·ten·cy \-tən-sē\ *n, pl* **-cies** : IMPOTENCE

im·po·tent \ˈim-pə-tənt\ *adj* **1** : not potent **2** : unable to engage in sexual intercourse because of inability to have and maintain an erection; *broadly* : STERILE

im·preg·nate \im-ˈpreg-ˌnāt, ˈim-ˌ\ *vb* **-nat·ed; -nat·ing 1 a** : to make pregnant **b** : to introduce sperm cells into : FERTILIZE **2** : to cause to be filled, imbued, permeated, or saturated — **im·preg·na·tion** \(ˌ)im-ˌpreg-ˈnā-shən\ *n*

im·pres·sion \im-ˈpre-shən\ *n* : an imprint in plastic material of the surfaces of the teeth and adjacent portions of the jaw from which a likeness may be produced in dentistry

im·print·ing \ˈim-ˌprint-iŋ, im-ˈ\ *n* **1** : a rapid learning process that takes place early in the life of a social animal and establishes a behavior pattern (as recognition of and attraction to its own kind or a substitute) **2** : GENOMIC IMPRINTING — **imprint** *vb*

im·pulse \ˈim-ˌpəls\ *n* **1** : a wave of excitation transmitted through tissues and esp. nerve fibers and muscles that results in physiological activity or inhibition — see CARDIAC IMPULSE, NERVE IMPULSE **2** : a sudden spontaneous inclination or incitement to some usu. unpremeditated action

im·pul·sive \im-ˈpəl-siv\ *adj* **1** : actuated by or prone to act on impulse ⟨~ behavior⟩ **2** : acting momentarily ⟨brief ~ auditory stimuli⟩ — **im·pul·sive·ly** *adv* — **im·pul·sive·ness** *n* — **im·pul·siv·i·ty** \-ˌpəl-ˈsi-və-tē\ *n*

Im·u·ran \ˈi-myə-ˌran\ *trademark* — used for a preparation of azathioprine

in *abbr* inch

In *symbol* indium

[1]**in-** *or* **il-** *or* **im-** *or* **ir-** *prefix* : not — usu. *il-* before *l* ⟨*il*legitimate⟩ and *im-* before *b, m,* or *p* ⟨*im*balance⟩ ⟨*im*mobile⟩ ⟨*im*palpable⟩ and *ir-* before *r* ⟨*ir*reducible⟩ and *in-* before other sounds ⟨*in*operable⟩

[2]**in-** *or* **il-** *or* **im-** *or* **ir-** *prefix* : in : within : into : toward : on ⟨*ir*radiation⟩ — usu. *il-* before *l, im-* before *b, m,* or *p, ir-* before *r,* and *in-* before other sounds

-in \ən,ᵊn, ˌin\ *n suffix* **1 a** : neutral chemical compound ⟨insul*in*⟩ **b** : enzyme ⟨pancreat*in*⟩ **c** : antibiotic ⟨penicill*in*⟩ **2** : pharmaceutical product ⟨niac*in*⟩

in·ac·ti·vate \(ˌ)i-ˈnak-tə-ˌvāt\ *vb* **-vat·ed; -vat·ing** : to make inactive: as **a** : to destroy certain biological activities of ⟨~ the complement of normal serum by heat⟩ **b** : to cause (as an infective agent) to lose disease-producing capacity ⟨~ bacteria⟩ — **in·ac·ti·va·tion** \i-ˌnak-tə-ˈvā-shən\ *n*

in·ac·tive \i-ˈnak-tiv\ *adj* : not active: as **a** : marked by deliberate or enforced absence of activity or effort ⟨forced by illness to lead an ~ life⟩ **b** *of a disease* : not progressing or fulminant : QUIESCENT **c** : chemically inert ⟨~ charcoal⟩ **d** : biologically inert esp. because of the loss of some quality (as infectivity or antigenicity) — **in·ac·tiv·ity** \i-ˌnak-ˈti-və-tē\ *n*

in·ad·e·quate \i-ˈna-də-kwət\ *adj* : not adequate; *specif* : lacking the capacity for psychological maturity or adequate social adjustment

in·a·ni·tion \ˌi-nə-ˈni-shən\ *n* : the exhausted condition that results from lack of food and water

in·ap·pe·tence \i-ˈna-pə-təns\ *n* : loss or lack of appetite

in·ap·pro·pri·ate \ˌi-nə-ˈprō-prē-ət\ *adj* : ABNORMAL 1

in·born \ˈin-ˈbȯrn\ *adj* : HEREDITARY, INHERITED ⟨~ errors of metabolism⟩

in·breed·ing \ˈin-ˌbrē-diŋ\ *n* : the interbreeding of closely related individuals — **in·bred** \-ˌbred\ *adj* — **in·breed** \-ˌbrēd\ *vb*

in·ca·pac·i·tant \ˌin-kə-ˈpa-sə-tənt\ *n* : a chemical or biological agent (as tear gas) used to temporarily incapacitate people or animals (as in a riot)

in·car·cer·at·ed \in-ˈkär-sə-ˌrā-təd\ *adj, of a hernia* : constricted but not strangulated

in·car·cer·a·tion \in-ˌkär-sə-ˈrā-shən\ *n* **1** : a confining or state of being confined **2** : abnormal retention or confinement of a body part; *specif* : a constriction of the neck of a hernial sac so that the hernial contents become irreducible

in·cest \ˈin-ˌsest\ *n* : sexual intercourse between persons so closely related that they are forbidden by law to marry; *also* : the statutory crime of engaging in such sexual intercourse — **in·ces·tu·ous** \in-ˈses-chə-wəs\ *adj*

inch \ˈinch\ *n* : a unit of length equal to 1/36 yard or 2.54 centimeters

in·ci·dence \ˈin-sə-dəns, -ˌdens\ *n* : rate of occurrence or influence; *esp* : the rate of occurrence of new cases of a particular disease in a population being studied — compare PREVALENCE

in·cip·i·ent \in-ˈsi-pē-ənt\ *adj* : beginning to come into being or to become apparent ⟨the ~ stage of a fever⟩

in·ci·sal \in-ˈsī-zəl\ *adj* : relating to, being, or involving the cutting edge or surface of a tooth (as an incisor)

in·cise \in-ˈsīz, -ˈsīs\ *vb* **in·cised; in·cis·ing** : to cut into : make an incision in ⟨*incised* the swollen tissue⟩

incised *adj, of a cut or wound* : made with or as if with a sharp knife or scalpel : clean and well-defined

in·ci·sion \in-ˈsi-zhən\ *n* **1** : a cut or wound of body tissue made esp. in surgery **2** : an act of incising something — **in·ci·sion·al** \-zhə-nəl\ *adj*

in·ci·sive \in-ˈsī-siv\ *adj* : INCISAL; *also* : of, relating to, or situated near the incisors

incisive canal *n* : a narrow branched passage that extends from the floor of the nasal cavity to the incisive fossa and transmits the nasopalatine nerve and a branch of the greater palatine artery

incisive fossa *n* : a depression on the front of the maxillary bone above the incisor teeth

in·ci·sor \in-ˈsī-zər\ *n* : a front tooth adapted for cutting; *esp* : any of the eight cutting human teeth that are located between the canines with four in the lower and four in the upper jaw

in·ci·su·ra \ˌin-ˌsī-ˈzhu̇r-ə, -sə-\ *n, pl* **in·ci·su·rae** \-ˌē, -ˌī\ **1** : a notch, cleft, or fissure of a body part or organ **2** : a downward notch in the curve recording aortic blood pressure that occurs between systole and diastole and is caused by backward flow of blood for a short time before the aortic valve closes

incisura an·gu·lar·is \-ˌaŋ-gyə-ˈlar-əs\ *n* : a notch or bend in the lesser curvature of the stomach near its pyloric end

in·cli·na·tion \ˌin-klə-ˈnā-shən\ *n* : a deviation from the true vertical or horizontal; *esp* : the deviation of the long axis of a tooth or of the slope of a cusp from the vertical

in·clu·sion \in-ˈklü-zhən\ *n* : something that is included; *esp* : a passive usu. temporary product of cell activity (as a starch grain) within the cytoplasm or nucleus

inclusion blennorrhea *n* : INCLUSION CONJUNCTIVITIS

inclusion body *n* : an inclusion, abnormal structure, or foreign cell within a cell; *specif* : an intracellular body that is characteristic of some virus diseases and that is the site of virus multiplication

inclusion body myositis *n* : an inflammatory muscle disease of unknown cause that is marked physically by slowly progressive muscle weakness and atrophy esp. of the limbs and histologically by abnormal inclusions (as vacuoles, amyloid deposits, or T cell infiltrates) in muscle fibers

inclusion conjunctivitis *n* : an infectious disease esp. of newborn infants characterized by acute conjunctivitis and the presence of large inclusion bodies and caused by a chlamydia (*C. trachomatis*)

inclusion disease *n* : CYTOMEGALIC INCLUSION DISEASE

in·co·her·ent \ˌin-kō-ˈhir-ənt, -ˈher-\ *adj* : lacking clarity or intelligibility usu. by reason of some emotional stress ⟨~ speech⟩ — **in·co·her·ence** \-əns\ *n* — **in·co·her·ent·ly** *adv*

in·com·pat·i·ble \ˌin-kəm-ˈpa-tə-bəl\ *adj* **1** : unsuitable for use together because of chemical interaction or antagonistic physiological effects ⟨~ drugs⟩ **2** *of blood or serum* : unsuitable for use in a particular transfusion because of the presence of agglutinins that act against the recipient's red blood cells — **in·com·pat·i·bil·i·ty** \-ˌpa-tə-ˈbi-lə-tē\ *n*

in·com·pe·tence \in-ˈkäm-pə-təns\ *n* **1** : lack of legal qualification **2** : inability of an organ or part to perform its function adequately ⟨venous ~⟩ — **in·com·pe·tent** \-tənt\ *adj*

in·com·pe·ten·cy \-tən-sē\ *n, pl* **-cies** : INCOMPETENCE

in·com·plete \ˌin-kəm-ˈplēt\ *adj* **1** *of a bone fracture* : not broken entirely across — compare COMPLETE 1 **2** *of a protein* : deficient in one or more essential amino acids — compare COMPLETE 2

incomplete dominance *n* : the property of being expressed or inherited as a semidominant gene or trait

in·con·stant \in-ˈkän-stənt\ *adj* : not always present ⟨an ~ muscle⟩

in·con·ti·nence \in-ˈkänt-ᵊn-əns\ *n* **1** : inability or failure to restrain sexual appetite **2** : inability of the body to control the evacuative functions — see STRESS INCONTINENCE, URGE INCONTINENCE — **in·con·ti·nent** \-ənt\ *adj*

in·co·or·di·na·tion \ˌin-kō-ˌȯrd-ᵊn-ˈā-shən\ *n* : lack of coordination esp. of muscular movements resulting from loss of voluntary control

in·cre·men·tal lines \ˌiŋ-krə-ˈment-ᵊl-, ˌin-\ *n pl* : lines seen in a tooth in section showing the periodic depositions of dentin, enamel, and cementum occurring during growth

incremental lines of Ret·zi·us \-ˈret-sē-əs\ *n pl* : incremental lines in the enamel of a tooth

Retzius, Magnus Gustaf (1842–1919), Swedish anatomist and anthropologist.

in·cre·tin \in-ˈkre-tᵊn\ *n* : any of various gastrointestinal hormones that stimulate the secretion of insulin by the pancreas

in·crus·ta·tion \ˌin-ˌkrəs-ˈtā-shən\ *or* **en·crus·ta·tion** \ˌen-\ *n* **1** : the act of encrusting : the state of being encrusted **2** : a crust or hard coating

in·cu·bate \ˈiŋ-kyə-ˌbāt, ˈin-\ *vb* **-bat·ed; -bat·ing** **1** : to maintain (as embryos or bacteria) under conditions favorable for hatching or development **2** : to undergo incubation

in·cu·ba·tion \ˌiŋ-kyə-ˈbā-shən, ˌin-\ *n* **1** : the act or process of incubating **2** : INCUBATION PERIOD

incubation period *n* : the period between the infection of an individual by a pathogen and the manifestation of the disease it causes

in·cu·ba·tor \ˈiŋ-kyə-ˌbā-tər, ˈin-\ *n* : one that incubates; *esp* : an apparatus with a chamber used to provide controlled environmental conditions esp. for the cultivation of microorganisms or the care and protection of premature or sick babies

in·cur·able \in-ˈkyu̇r-ə-bəl\ *adj* : impossible to cure ⟨~ diseases⟩ — **in·cur·ably** \-blē\ *adv*

in·cus \ˈiŋ-kəs\ *n, pl* **in·cu·des** \iŋ-ˈkyü-(ˌ)dēz, ˈiŋ-kyə-ˌdēz\ : the middle bone of a chain of three small bones in the middle ear — called also *anvil*

IND \ˌī-(ˌ)en-ˈdē\ *abbr* investigational new drug

in·dane·di·one \ˌin-dān-ˈdī-ˌōn\ *or* **in·dan·di·one** \ˌin-dan-\ *n* : any of a group of synthetic anticoagulants

indecent assault *n* : an offensive sexual act or series of acts exclusive of rape committed against another person without consent

indecent exposure *n* : intentional exposure of part of one's body (as the genitalia) in a place where such exposure is likely to be an offense against the generally accepted standards of decency in a community

independent assortment *n* : formation of random combinations of chromosomes in meiosis and of genes on different pairs of homologous chromosomes by the passage at random of one of each diploid pair of homologous chromosomes into each gamete independently of each other pair

independent practice association *n* : an organization providing health care by doctors who maintain their own offices and continue to see their own patients but agree to treat enrolled members of the organization for a negotiated lump sum payment or a fixed payment per member or per service provided — abbr. *IPA*

In·der·al \ˈin-də-ˌral\ *trademark* — used for a preparation of the hydrochloride of propranolol

in·de·ter·mi·nate \ˌin-di-ˈtər-mə-nət\ *adj* : relating to, being, or undergoing indeterminate cleavage ⟨an ~ egg⟩

indeterminate cleavage *n* : cleavage in which all the early divisions produce blastomeres with the potencies of the entire zygote — compare DETERMINATE CLEAVAGE

in·dex \ˈin-ˌdeks\ *n, pl* **in·dex·es** *or* **in·di·ces** \-də-ˌsēz\ **1** : a number (as a ratio) derived from a series of observations and used as an indicator or measure (as of a condition, property, or phenomenon) **2** : the ratio of one dimension of a thing (as an anatomical structure) to another dimension — see CEPHALIC INDEX, CRANIAL INDEX

index case *n* **1** : an instance of a disease or a genetically determined condition that is discovered first and leads to the discovery of others in a family or group **2** : INDEX PATIENT

index finger *n* : the finger next to the thumb — called also *forefinger*

index of refraction *n* : the ratio of the speed of radiation (as light) in one medium to that in another medium — called also *refractive index*

index patient *n* : a patient whose disease or condition provides an index case — called also *index case-patient*

Indian hemp *n* : HEMP 1

indica — see CANNABIS INDICA

in·di·can \ˈin-də-ˌkan\ *n* : an indigo-forming substance $C_8H_7NO_4S$ found as a salt in urine and other animal fluids; *also* : its potassium salt $C_8H_6KNO_4S$

in·di·cate \ˈin-də-ˌkāt\ *vb* **-cat·ed; -cat·ing** **1** : to be a fairly certain symptom of : show the presence or existence of **2** : to call for esp. as treatment for a particular condition ⟨radical surgery is *indicated*⟩

in·di·ca·tion \ˌin-də-ˈkā-shən\ *n* **1** : a symptom or particular circumstance that indicates the advisability or necessity of a specific medical treatment or procedure **2** : something that is indicated as advisable or necessary

in·di·ca·tor \ˈin-də-ˌkā-tər\ *n* : a substance (as a dye) used to show visually (as by change of color) the condition of a solution with respect to the presence of a particular material (as a free acid or alkali)

indices *pl of* INDEX

indicis — see EXTENSOR INDICIS, EXTENSOR INDICIS PROPRIUS

in•dig•e•nous \in-ˈdi-jə-nəs\ *adj* : having originated in and being produced, growing, or living naturally in a particular region or environment ⟨a disease ~ to the tropics⟩

in•di•gest•ible \ˌin-(ˌ)dī-ˈjes-tə-bəl, -də-\ *adj* : not digestible : not easily digested ⟨~ fiber⟩ — **in•di•gest•ibil•i•ty** \-ˌjes-tə-ˈbi-lə-tē\ *n*

in•di•ges•tion \-ˈjes-chən\ *n* **1** : inability to digest or difficulty in digesting food : incomplete or imperfect digestion of food **2** : a case or attack of indigestion marked esp. by pain, discomfort, or a burning sensation in the upper abdomen often accompanied by abdominal bloating, nausea, belching, flatulence, or uncomfortable fullness

in•di•go car•mine \ˈin-di-ˌgō-ˈkär-mən, -ˌmīn\ *n* : a soluble blue dye $C_{16}H_8N_2Na_2O_8S_2$ that is used chiefly as a biological stain and food color and since it is rapidly excreted by the kidneys is used as a dye to mark ureteral structures (as in cystoscopy and catheterization)

in•din•a•vir \in-ˈdi-nə-ˌvir\ *n* : a protease inhibitor used in the form of its sulfate $C_{36}H_{47}N_5O_4·H_2SO_4$ in combination therapy with antiretroviral drugs (as lamivudine) to treat HIV infection — see CRIXIVAN

in•dis•posed \ˌin-di-ˈspōzd\ *adj* : being usu. temporarily in poor physical health : slightly ill — **in•dis•po•si•tion** \(ˌ)in-ˌdis-pə-ˈzi-shən\ *n*

in•di•um \ˈin-dē-əm\ *n* : a malleable fusible silvery metallic element — symbol *In;* see ELEMENT table

individual psychology *n* : a modification of psychoanalysis developed by the Austrian psychologist Alfred Adler emphasizing feelings of inferiority and a desire for power as the primary motivating forces in human behavior

in•di•vid•u•a•tion \ˌin-də-ˌvi-jə-ˈwā-shən\ *n* : the process in the analytic psychology of C. G. Jung by which the self is formed by integrating elements of the conscious and unconscious mind — **in•di•vid•u•ate** \-ˈvi-jə-ˌwāt\ *vb*

In•do•cin \ˈin-də-sən\ *trademark* — used for a preparation of indomethacin

in•do•cy•a•nine green \ˌin-dō-ˈsī-ə-ˌnēn-, -nən-\ *n* : a green dye $C_{43}H_{47}N_2NaO_6S_2$ used esp. in testing liver blood flow and cardiac output

in•dole \ˈin-ˌdōl\ *n* : a crystalline compound C_8H_7N that is found in the intestines and feces as a decomposition product of proteins containing tryptophan; *also* : a derivative of indole

in•dole•ace•tic acid \ˌin-ˌdō-lə-ˈsē-tik-\ *n* : a compound $C_{10}H_9NO_2$ formed from tryptophan in plants and animals that is present in small amounts in normal urine and acts as a growth hormone in plants

in•do•lent \ˈin-də-lənt\ *adj* **1** : causing little or no pain ⟨an ~ tumor⟩ **2 a** : growing or progressing slowly ⟨an ~ disease⟩ **b** : slow to heal ⟨an ~ ulcer⟩ — **in•do•lence** \-ləns\ *n*

in•do•meth•a•cin \ˌin-dō-ˈme-thə-sən\ *n* : an NSAID $C_{19}H_{16}ClNO_4$ with analgesic and antipyretic properties used esp. to treat painful inflammatory conditions (as rheumatoid arthritis and osteoarthritis) — see INDOCIN

in•duce \in-ˈdüs, -ˈdyüs\ *vb* **in•duced; in•duc•ing** **1** : to cause or bring about: as **a** : to cause to form through embryonic induction **b** : to cause or initiate by artificial means ⟨*induced* labor⟩ **2** : to produce anesthesia in

in•duc•er \-ˈdü-sər, -ˈdyü-\ *n* : one that induces; *specif* : a substance capable of activating the transcription of a gene by combining with and inactivating a genetic repressor

in•duc•ible \in-ˈdü-sə-bəl, -ˈdyü-\ *adj* : capable of being formed, activated, or expressed in response to a stimulus esp. of a molecular kind ⟨~ enzymes⟩ — **in•duc•ibil•i•ty** \in-ˌdü-sə-ˈbi-lə-tē, -ˌdyü-\ *n*

in•duc•tion \in-ˈdək-shən\ *n* **1** : the act of causing or bringing on or about ⟨~ of labor⟩; *specif* : the establishment of the initial state of anesthesia often with an agent other than that used subsequently to maintain the anesthetic state **2 a** : arousal of a part or area (as of the retina) by stimulation of an adjacent part or area **b** : the sum of the processes by which the fate of embryonic cells is determined and differentiation brought about — **in•duct** \in-ˈdəkt\ *vb* — **in•duc•tive** \in-ˈdək-tiv\ *adj* — **in•duc•tive•ly** *adv*

induction chemotherapy *n* : chemotherapy usu. with high doses of anticancer drugs in the initial treatment esp. of advanced cancers in order to make subsequent treatment (as surgery or radiotherapy) more effective

induction therapy *n* : the initial therapy used when treating a disease; *specif* : INDUCTION CHEMOTHERAPY

in•duc•tor \in-ˈdək-tər\ *n* : one that inducts; *esp* : ORGANIZER

in•du•rat•ed \ˈin-dü-ˌrā-təd, -dyü-\ *adj* : having become firm or hard esp. by increase of fibrous elements ⟨~ tissue⟩ ⟨an ulcer with an ~ border⟩

in•du•ra•tion \ˌin-dü-ˈrā-shən, -dyü-\ *n* **1** : an increase in the fibrous elements in tissue commonly associated with inflammation and marked by loss of elasticity and pliability : SCLEROSIS **2** : a hardened mass or formation — **in•du•ra•tive** \ˈin-dü-ˌrā-tiv, -dyü-; in-ˈdür-ə-tiv, -ˈdyür-\ *adj*

in·du·si·um gris·e·um \in-ˈdü-zē-əm-ˈgri-zē-əm, -ˈdyü-, -zhē-\ *n* : a thin layer of gray matter over the dorsal surface of the corpus callosum

industrial disease *n* : OCCUPATIONAL DISEASE

industrial hygiene *n* : a science concerned with the protection and improvement of the health and well-being of workers in their vocational environment — **industrial hygienist** *n*

industrial psychologist *n* : a psychologist who specializes in workplace problems and issues (as employee satisfaction and motivation)

in·dwell·ing \ˈin-ˌdwe-liŋ\ *adj* : left within a bodily organ or passage to maintain drainage, prevent obstruction, or provide a route for administration of food or drugs — used of an implanted tube (as a catheter)

in·elas·tic \ˌi-nə-ˈlas-tik\ *adj* : not elastic

in·ert \i-ˈnərt\ *adj* **1** : lacking the power to move **2** : deficient in active properties; *esp* : lacking a usual or anticipated chemical or biological action ⟨an ~ drug⟩ — **in·ert·ness** *n*

inert gas *n* : NOBLE GAS

in·er·tia \i-ˈnər-shə\ *n* : lack of activity or movement — used esp. of the uterus in labor when its contractions are weak or irregular

in ex·tre·mis \ˌin-ik-ˈstrē-məs, -ˈstrā-\ *adv* : at the point of death

in·fan·cy \ˈin-fən-sē\ *n, pl* **-cies** **1** : early childhood **2** : the legal status of an infant

in·fant \ˈin-fənt\ *n* **1 a** : a child in the first year of life : BABY **b** : a child several years of age **2** : a person who is not of full age : MINOR — **infant** *adj*

in·fan·ti·cide \in-ˈfan-tə-ˌsīd\ *n* : the killing of an infant — **in·fan·ti·ci·dal** \-ˌfan-tə-ˈsīd-ᵊl\ *adj*

in·fan·tile \ˈin-fən-ˌtīl, -ˌtēl, -(ˌ)til\ *adj* **1** : of, relating to, or occurring in infants or infancy ⟨~ eczema⟩ **2** : suitable to or characteristic of an infant; *esp* : very immature

infantile amaurotic idiocy *n, dated, now usu. offensive* **1** : TAY-SACHS DISEASE **2** : SANDHOFF'S DISEASE

infantile autism *n* : AUTISM

infantile paralysis *n* : POLIO

infantile scurvy *n* : acute scurvy during infancy caused by malnutrition — called also *Barlow's disease*

in·fan·til·ism \ˈin-fən-ˌtī-ˌli-zəm, -tə-; in-ˈfant-ᵊl-ˌi-\ *n* : retention of childish physical, mental, or emotional qualities in adult life; *esp* : failure to attain sexual maturity

infantum — see ROSEOLA INFANTUM

in·farct \ˈin-ˌfärkt, in-ˈ\ *n* : an area of necrosis in a tissue or organ resulting from obstruction of the local circulation by a thrombus or embolus — **in·farct·ed** \in-ˈfärk-təd\ *adj*

in·farc·tion \in-ˈfärk-shən\ *n* **1** : the process of forming an infarct **2** : INFARCT

in·fect \in-ˈfekt\ *vb* **1** : to contaminate with a disease-producing substance or agent (as bacteria) **2 a** : to communicate a pathogen or a disease to **b** *of a pathogenic organism* : to invade (an individual or organ) usu. by penetration — compare INFEST

in·fec·tant \in-ˈfek-tənt\ *n* : an agent of infection (as a bacterium or virus)

in·fec·tion \in-ˈfek-shən\ *n* **1** : an infective agent or material contaminated with an infective agent **2 a** : the state produced by the establishment of an infective agent in or on a suitable host **b** : a disease resulting from infection : INFECTIOUS DISEASE **3** : an act or process of infecting; *also* : the establishment of a pathogen in its host after invasion

infection stone *n* : a kidney stone composed of struvite

infectiosum — see ERYTHEMA INFECTIOSUM

in·fec·tious \in-ˈfek-shəs\ *adj* **1** : capable of causing infection **2** : communicable by invasion of the body of a susceptible organism — compare CONTAGIOUS 1 — **in·fec·tious·ly** *adv* — **in·fec·tious·ness** *n*

infectious anemia *n* **1** : EQUINE INFECTIOUS ANEMIA **2** : FELINE INFECTIOUS ANEMIA

infectious bovine rhinotracheitis *n* : a highly contagious disease of cattle caused by a herpesvirus of the genus *Varicellovirus* (species *Bovine herpesvirus 1*) and characterized esp. by fever and by inflammation and ulceration of the nasal cavities and trachea

infectious coryza *n* : an acute infectious respiratory disease of chickens that is caused by a bacterium of the genus *Haemophilus* (*H. paragallinarum* syn. *H. gallinarum*)

infectious disease *n* : a disease caused by the entrance into the body of organisms (as bacteria) which grow and multiply there — see COMMUNICABLE DISEASE, CONTAGIOUS DISEASE

infectious enterohepatitis *n* : BLACKHEAD 2

infectious hepatitis *n* : HEPATITIS A

infectious jaundice *n* **1** : HEPATITIS A **2** : WEIL'S DISEASE

infectious laryngotracheitis *n* : a severe highly contagious and often fatal respiratory disease of chickens and pheasants that is caused by a herpesvirus (species *Gallid herpesvirus 1* of the genus *Iltovirus*)

infectious mononucleosis *n* : an acute infectious disease associated with Epstein-Barr virus that is characterized esp. by fever, sore throat, swollen lymph nodes, fatigue, and lymphocytosis and occurs primarily in adolescents and young adults — abbr. *IM;* called also *glandular fever, kissing disease, mono*

in·fec·tive \in-ˈfek-tiv\ *adj* : producing or capable of producing infection : INFECTIOUS

in·fec·tiv·i·ty \ˌin-ˌfek-ˈti-və-tē\ *n, pl* **-ties** : the quality of being infective : the ability to produce infection; *specif* : a tendency to spread rapidly from host to host — compare VIRULENCE b

in·fec·tor \in-ˈfek-tər\ *n* : one that infects

in·fe·ri·or \in-ˈfir-ē-ər\ *adj* **1** : situated below and closer to the feet than another and esp. another similar part of an upright body esp. of a human being — compare SUPERIOR 1 **2** : situated in a more posterior or ventral position in the body of a quadruped — compare SUPERIOR 2

inferior alveolar artery *n* : a branch of the maxillary artery that is distributed to the mucous membrane of the mouth and to the teeth of the lower jaw — called also *mandibular artery, inferior dental artery*

inferior alveolar nerve *n* : a branch of the mandibular nerve that is distributed to the teeth of the lower jaw and to the skin of the chin and the skin and mucous membrane of the lower lip — called also *inferior alveolar, inferior dental nerve*

inferior alveolar vein *n* : a vein that accompanies the inferior alveolar artery and drains the lower jaw and lower teeth

inferior articular process *n* : ARTICULAR PROCESS b

inferior cerebellar peduncle *n* : CEREBELLAR PEDUNCLE c

inferior colliculus *n* : either member of the posterior and lower pair of corpora quadrigemina that are situated next to the pons and together constitute one of the lower centers for hearing — compare SUPERIOR COLLICULUS

inferior concha *n* : NASAL CONCHA a

inferior constrictor *n* : a muscle of the pharynx that acts to constrict part of the pharynx in swallowing — called also *constrictor pharyngis inferior, inferior pharyngeal constrictor muscle;* compare MIDDLE CONSTRICTOR, SUPERIOR CONSTRICTOR

inferior dental artery *n* : INFERIOR ALVEOLAR ARTERY

inferior dental nerve *n* : INFERIOR ALVEOLAR NERVE

inferior extensor retinaculum *n* : EXTENSOR RETINACULUM 1a

inferior ganglion *n* **1** : the lower and larger of the two sensory ganglia of the glossopharyngeal nerve — called also *petrosal ganglion;* compare SUPERIOR GANGLION 1 **2** : the lower of the two ganglia of the vagus nerve that forms a swelling just beyond the exit of the nerve from the jugular foramen — called also *inferior vagal ganglion, nodose ganglion;* compare SUPERIOR GANGLION 2

inferior gluteal artery *n* : GLUTEAL ARTERY b

inferior gluteal nerve *n* : GLUTEAL NERVE b

inferior hemorrhoidal artery *n* : RECTAL ARTERY a

inferior hemorrhoidal vein *n* : RECTAL VEIN a

inferior horn *n* : the cornu in the lateral ventricle of each cerebral hemisphere that curves downward into the temporal lobe — compare ANTERIOR HORN 2, POSTERIOR HORN 2

in·fe·ri·or·i·ty \(ˌ)in-ˌfir-ē-ˈȯr-ə-tē, -ˈär-\ *n, pl* **-ties** : a condition or state of being or having a sense of being inferior or inadequate esp. with respect to one's apparent equals or to the world at large

inferiority complex *n* : an acute sense of personal inferiority resulting either in timidity or through overcompensation in exaggerated aggressiveness

inferior laryngeal artery *n* : LARYNGEAL ARTERY a

inferior laryngeal nerve *n* **1** : LARYNGEAL NERVE b — called also *inferior laryngeal* **2** : any of the terminal branches of the inferior laryngeal nerve

inferior longitudinal fasciculus *n* : a band of association fibers in each cerebral hemisphere that connects the occipital and temporal lobes

in·fe·ri·or·ly *adv* : in a lower position

inferior maxillary bone *n* : JAW 1b

inferior maxillary nerve *n* : MANDIBULAR NERVE

inferior meatus *n* : a space extending along the lateral wall of the nasal cavity between the inferior nasal concha and the floor of the nasal cavity — compare MIDDLE MEATUS, SUPERIOR MEATUS

inferior mesenteric artery *n* : MESENTERIC ARTERY a

inferior mesenteric ganglion *n* : MESENTERIC GANGLION a

inferior mesenteric plexus *n* : MESENTERIC PLEXUS a

inferior mesenteric vein *n* : MESENTERIC VEIN a

inferior nasal concha *n* : NASAL CONCHA a

inferior nuchal line *n* : NUCHAL LINE c

inferior oblique *n* : OBLIQUE b(2) — called also *inferior oblique muscle*

inferior olive *n* : a large gray nucleus that forms the interior of the olive on each side of the medulla oblongata — called also *inferior olivary nucleus;* see ACCESSORY OLIVARY NUCLEUS; compare SUPERIOR OLIVE

inferior ophthalmic vein *n* : OPHTHALMIC VEIN b

inferior orbital fissure *n* : ORBITAL FISSURE b

inferior pancreaticoduodenal artery *n* : PANCREATICODUODENAL ARTERY a

inferior pectoral nerve *n* : PECTORAL NERVE b

inferior peroneal retinaculum *n* : PERONEAL RETINACULUM b
inferior petrosal sinus *n* : PETROSAL SINUS b
inferior pharyngeal constrictor muscle *n* : INFERIOR CONSTRICTOR
inferior phrenic artery *n* : PHRENIC ARTERY b
inferior phrenic vein *n* : PHRENIC VEIN b
inferior radioulnar joint *n* : DISTAL RADIOULNAR JOINT
inferior ramus *n* : RAMUS b(2), c
inferior rectal artery *n* : RECTAL ARTERY a
inferior rectal vein *n* : RECTAL VEIN a
inferior rectus *n* : RECTUS 2d
inferior sagittal sinus *n* : SAGITTAL SINUS b
inferior temporal gyrus *n* : TEMPORAL GYRUS c
inferior thyroarytenoid ligament *n* : VOCAL LIGAMENT
inferior thyroid artery *n* : THYROID ARTERY b
inferior turbinate *n* : NASAL CONCHA a
inferior turbinate bone *also* **inferior tur•bi•nat•ed bone** \-ˈtər-bə-ˌnā-təd-\ *n* : NASAL CONCHA a
inferior ulnar collateral artery *n* : a small artery that arises from the brachial artery just above the elbow and branches to anastomose with other arteries in the region of the elbow — compare SUPERIOR ULNAR COLLATERAL ARTERY
inferior vagal ganglion *n* : INFERIOR GANGLION 2
inferior vena cava *n* : a vein that is the largest vein in the human body, is formed by the union of the two common iliac veins at the level of the fifth lumbar vertebra, and returns blood to the right atrium of the heart from bodily parts below the diaphragm
inferior vermis *n* : VERMIS 1b
inferior vesical *n* : VESICAL ARTERY b
inferior vesical artery *n* : VESICAL ARTERY b
inferior vestibular nucleus *n* : the one of the four vestibular nuclei on each side of the medulla oblongata that sends fibers down both sides of the spinal cord to synapse with motor neurons of the ventral roots
inferior vocal cords *n pl* : TRUE VOCAL CORDS
infero- *comb form* : below and ⟨*inferomedial*⟩
in•fe•ro•me•di•al \ˌin-fə-rō-ˈmē-dē-əl\ *adj* : situated below and in the middle
in•fe•ro•tem•po•ral \-ˈtem-p(ə-)rəl\ *adj* **1** : being the inferior part of the temporal lobe of the cerebral cortex; *also* : situated or occurring in, on, or under this part **2** : of, relating to, or being the lower lateral quadrant of the eye or visual field
in•fer•tile \in-ˈfərt-ᵊl\ *adj* : not fertile : incapable of or unsuccessful in achieving pregnancy over a considerable period of time (as a year) in spite of determined attempts by heterosexual intercourse without contraception — **in•fer•til•i•ty** \ˌin-(ˌ)fər-ˈti-lə-tē\ *n*
in•fest \in-ˈfest\ *vb* : to live in or on as a parasite — compare INFECT — **in•fes•tant** \in-ˈfes-tənt\ *n* — **in•fes•ta•tion** \ˌin-ˌfes-ˈtā-shən\ *n*
in•fib•u•la•tion \(ˌ)in-ˌfi-byə-ˈlā-shən\ *n* : an act or practice of fastening by ring, clasp, or stitches the labia majora in girls and the foreskin in boys in order to prevent sexual intercourse
in•fil•trate \in-ˈfil-ˌtrāt, ˈin-(ˌ)fil-\ *n* : something that passes or is caused to pass into or through something by permeating or filtering; *esp* : a substance that passes into the bodily tissues and forms an abnormal accumulation ⟨a lung ~⟩ — **infiltrate** *vb* — **in•fil•tra•tion** \ˌin-(ˌ)fil-ˈtrā-shən\ *n* — **in•fil•tra•tive** \ˈin-fil-ˌtrā-tiv, in-ˈfil-trə-\ *adj*
infiltration anesthesia *n* : anesthesia of an operative site accomplished by local injection of anesthetics
in•firm \in-ˈfərm\ *adj* : of poor or deteriorated vitality; *esp* : feeble from age
in•fir•ma•ry \in-ˈfər-mə-rē\ *n, pl* **-ries** : a place esp. in a school or college for the care and treatment of the sick
in•fir•mi•ty \in-ˈfər-mə-tē\ *n, pl* **-ties** : the quality or state of being infirm; *esp* : an unsound, unhealthy, or debilitated state
in•flame \in-ˈflām\ *vb* **in•flamed; in•flam•ing** **1** : to cause inflammation in (bodily tissue) **2** : to become affected with inflammation
in•flam•ma•tion \ˌin-flə-ˈmā-shən\ *n* : a local response to cellular injury that is marked by capillary dilatation, leukocytic infiltration, redness, heat, pain, swelling, and often loss of function and that serves as a mechanism initiating the elimination of noxious agents and of damaged tissue — **in•flam•ma•to•ry** \in-ˈfla-mə-ˌtōr-ē\ *adj*
inflammatory bowel disease *n* : either of two inflammatory diseases of the bowel: **a** : CROHN'S DISEASE **b** : ULCERATIVE COLITIS
in•flix•i•mab \in-ˈflik-si-ˌmab\ *n* : an immunosuppressive drug that blocks the activity of tumor necrosis factor and is administered by intravenous injection esp. to treat the symptoms of Crohn's disease, ulcerative colitis, and rheumatoid arthritis — see REMICADE
in•flu•en•za \ˌin-(ˌ)flü-ˈen-zə\ *n* **1 a** : an acute highly contagious respiratory disease caused by an orthomyxovirus: (1) : INFLUENZA A (2) : INFLUENZA B (3) : INFLUENZA C **b** : any human respiratory infection of undetermined cause — not used technically **2** : any of various virus diseases of domestic animals marked esp. by fever and respiratory symptoms — **in•flu•en•zal** \-zəl\ *adj*
influenza A *n* : moderate to severe influenza that in humans is marked esp.

by sudden onset, fever, sore throat, fatigue, muscle aches, inflammation of the respiratory mucous membranes, and cough, that is caused by any of several subtypes (as H1N1, H2N2, or H3N2) of an orthomyxovirus (species *Influenza A virus* of the genus *Influenzavirus A*) infecting humans and various animals (as birds), and that may occur in seasonal epidemics or sometimes pandemics following mutation of the causative virus — see ASIAN FLU, BIRD FLU, HONG KONG FLU, SPANISH FLU, SWINE INFLUENZA

influenza B *n* : influenza that causes less severe symptoms than influenza A, that may occur in seasonal epidemics but not pandemics, and that is caused by an orthomyxovirus (species *Influenza B virus* of the genus *Influenzavirus B*) infecting only humans and esp. children

influenza C *n* : mild influenza that is often asymptomatic, that does not occur in epidemics or pandemics, and that is caused by an orthomyxovirus (species *Influenza C virus* of the genus *Influenzavirus C*) infecting only humans

influenza vaccine *n* : a vaccine against influenza that typically contains a mixture of strains of influenza virus cultured in chick embryos: **a** : one that is injectable and contains formaldehyde-inactivated influenza viruses **b** : one that is delivered as a nasal spray and contains live attenuated influenza viruses

influenza virus *n* : any of the orthomyxoviruses that belong to three genera (*Influenzavirus A, Influenzavirus B*, and *Influenzavirus C*) and that cause influenza A, influenza B, and influenza C

informed consent *n* : consent to surgery by a patient or to participation in a medical experiment by a subject after achieving an understanding of what is involved

infra- *prefix* **1** : below ⟨*infra*hyoid⟩ **2** : below in a scale or series ⟨*infra*red⟩

in•fra•car•di•ac \ˌin-frə-ˈkär-dē-ˌak\ *adj* : situated below the heart

in•fra•cla•vic•u•lar \ˌin-frə-kla-ˈvi-kyə-lər\ *adj* : situated or occurring below the clavicle

in•fra•dia•phrag•mat•ic \ˌin-frə-ˌdī-ə-frə-ˈma-tik, -ˌfrag-\ *adj* : situated, occurring, or performed below the diaphragm ⟨an ~ abscess⟩

in•fra•gle•noid tubercle \ˌin-frə-ˈglē-ˌnȯid-, -ˈgle-\ *n* : a tubercle on the scapula for the attachment of the long head of the triceps muscle

in•fra•hy•oid \ˌin-frə-ˈhī-ˌȯid\ *adj* : situated below the hyoid bone

infrahyoid muscle *n* : any of four muscles on each side that are situated next to the larynx and comprise the sternohyoid, sternothyroid, thyrohyoid, and omohyoid muscles

in•fra•mam•ma•ry \ˌin-frə-ˈma-mə-rē\ *adj* : situated or occurring below the mammary gland ⟨~ pain⟩

in•fra•or•bit•al \ˌin-frə-ˈȯr-bət-ᵊl\ *adj* : situated beneath the orbit

infraorbital artery *n* : a branch or continuation of the maxillary artery that runs along the infraorbital groove with the infraorbital nerve and passes through the infraorbital foramen to give off branches which supply the face just below the eye

infraorbital fissure *n* : ORBITAL FISSURE b

infraorbital foramen *n* : an opening in the maxillary bone just below the lower rim of the orbit that gives passage to the infraorbital artery, nerve, and vein

infraorbital groove *n* : a groove in the middle of the posterior part of the bony floor of the orbit that gives passage to the infraorbital artery, vein, and nerve

infraorbital nerve *n* : a branch of the maxillary nerve that divides into branches distributed to the skin of the upper part of the cheek, the upper lip, and the lower eyelid

infraorbital vein *n* : a vein that drains the inferior structures of the orbit and the adjacent area of the face and that empties into the pterygoid plexus

in•fra•pa•tel•lar \ˌin-frə-pə-ˈte-lər\ *adj* : situated below the patella or its ligament

in•fra•red \ˌin-frə-ˈred\ *adj* **1** : lying outside the visible spectrum at its red end — used of radiation having a wavelength between about 700 nanometers and 1 millimeter **2** : relating to, producing, or employing infrared radiation ⟨~ therapy⟩ — **infrared** *n*

in•fra•re•nal \ˌin-frə-ˈrēn-ᵊl\ *adj* : situated or occurring below the kidneys

in•fra•spi•na•tus \ˌin-frə-spī-ˈnā-təs\ *n, pl* **-na•ti** \-ˈnā-ˌtī\ : a muscle that occupies the chief part of the infraspinous fossa of the scapula and rotates the arm laterally

in•fra•spi•nous \ˌin-frə-ˈspī-nəs\ *adj* : lying below a spine; *esp* : lying below the spine of the scapula

infraspinous fossa *n* : the part of the dorsal surface of the scapula below the spine of the scapula

in•fra•tem•po•ral \ˌin-frə-ˈtem-pə-rəl\ *adj* : situated below the temporal fossa

infratemporal crest *n* : a transverse ridge on the outer surface of the greater wing of the sphenoid bone that divides it into a superior portion that contributes to the formation of the temporal fossa and an inferior portion that contributes to the formation of the infratemporal fossa

infratemporal fossa *n* : a fossa that is bounded above by the plane of the zygomatic arch, laterally by the ramus of the mandible, and medially by the pterygoid plate, and that contains the masseter and pterygoid muscles and the mandibular nerve

in•fra•ten•to•ri•al \ˌin-frə-ten-ˈtōr-ē-əl\ *adj* : occurring or made below the tentorium cerebelli ⟨~ burr holes⟩

in•fun•dib•u•lar \ˌin-(ˌ)fən-ˈdi-byə-lər\ *adj* : of, relating to, affecting, situated near, or having an infundibulum

infundibular process *n* : NEURAL LOBE

infundibular recess *n* : a funnel-shaped downward prolongation of the floor of the third ventricle of the brain

in•fun•dib•u•lo•pel•vic ligament \ˌin-fən-ˌdi-byə-lō-ˈpel-vik-\ *n* : SUSPENSORY LIGAMENT OF THE OVARY

in•fun•dib•u•lum \ˌin-(ˌ)fən-ˈdi-byə-ləm\ *n, pl* **-la** \-lə\ : any of various conical or dilated organs or parts: as **a** : the hollow conical process of gray matter that constitutes the stalk of the neurohypophysis by which the pituitary gland is continuous with the brain **b** : any of the small spaces having walls with alveoli in which the bronchial tubes terminate in the lungs **c** : CONUS ARTERIOSUS **d** : the abdominal opening of a fallopian tube

in•fusion \in-ˈfyü-zhən\ *n* **1** : the introducing of a solution (as of glucose) esp. into a vein; *also* : the solution so used **2 a** : the steeping or soaking usu. in water of a substance (as a plant drug) in order to extract its soluble constituents or principles — compare DECOCTION 1 **b** : the liquid extract obtained by this process — **in•fuse** \in-ˈfyüz\ *vb*

infusion pump *n* : a device that releases a measured amount of a substance in a specific period of time

in•ges•ta \in-ˈjes-tə\ *n pl* : material taken into the body by way of the digestive tract

in•gest•ible \in-ˈjes-tə-bəl\ *adj* : capable of being ingested ⟨~ capsules⟩

in•ges•tion \in-ˈjes-chən\ *n* : the taking of material (as food) into the digestive system — **in•gest** \-ˈjest\ *vb* — **in•gest•ive** \in-ˈjes-tiv\ *adj*

in•grow•ing \ˈin-ˌgrō-iŋ\ *adj* : INGROWN

in•grown \ˈin ˌgrōn\ *adj* : grown in; *specif* : having the normally free tip or edge embedded in the flesh ⟨an ~ toenail⟩

in•growth \ˈin-ˌgrōth\ *n* **1** : a growing inward (as to fill a void) ⟨~ of cells⟩ **2** : something that grows in or into a space ⟨lymphoid ~*s*⟩

in•gui•nal \ˈiŋ-gwən-ᵊl\ *adj* **1** : of, relating to, or situated in the region of the groin ⟨an ~ rash⟩ **2** : ILIAC 2

inguinal canal *n* **1** : a passage in the male through which the testis descends into the scrotum and in which the spermatic cord lies **2** : a passage in the female accommodating the round ligament

inguinale — see GRANULOMA INGUINALE, LYMPHOGRANULOMA INGUINALE

inguinal hernia *n* : a hernia in which part of the intestine protrudes into the inguinal canal

inguinal ligament *n* : the thickened lower border of the aponeurosis of the external oblique muscle of the abdomen — called also *Poupart's ligament*

inguinal node *n* : any of the superficial lymph nodes of the groin

inguinal ring *n* : either of two openings in the fasciae of the abdominal muscles on each side of the body that are the inlet and outlet of the inguinal canal, give passage to the spermatic cord in the male and the round ligament in the female, and are a frequent site of hernia formation: **a** : DEEP INGUINAL RING **b** : SUPERFICIAL INGUINAL RING

INH *abbr* isoniazid

[1]**in•hal•ant** *also* **in•hal•ent** \in-ˈhā-lənt\ *n* **1** : something (as an allergen) that is inhaled **2** : any of various often toxic volatile substances (as spray paint or glue) whose fumes are sometimes inhaled for their euphoric effect

[2]**inhalant** *also* **inhalent** *adj* : used for inhaling or constituting an inhalant ⟨~ anesthetics⟩

in•ha•la•tion \ˌin-hə-ˈlā-shən, ˌin-ᵊl-ˈā-\ *n* **1** : the act or an instance of inhaling; *specif* : the action of drawing air into the lungs by means of a complex of essentially reflex actions **2** : material (as medication) to be taken in by inhaling — **in•ha•la•tion•al** \-shə-nəl\ *adj*

inhalation therapist *n* : a specialist in inhalation therapy

inhalation therapy *n* : the therapeutic use of inhaled gases and esp. oxygen (as in the treatment of respiratory disease)

in•ha•la•tor \ˈin-hə-ˌlā-tər, ˈin-ᵊl-ˌā-\ *n* : a device providing a mixture of oxygen and carbon dioxide for breathing that is used esp. in conjunction with artificial respiration

in•hale \in-ˈhāl\ *vb* **in•haled; in•hal•ing** : to breathe in

in•hal•er \in-ˈhā-lər\ *n* : a device by means of which usu. medicinal material is inhaled

in•her•it \in-ˈher-ət\ *vb* : to receive from a parent or ancestor by genetic transmission — **in•her•it•able** \in-ˈher-ə-tə-bəl\ *adj* — **in•her•it•abil•i•ty** \-ˌher-ə-tə-ˈbi-lə-tē\ *n*

in•her•i•tance \in-ˈher-ə-təns\ *n* **1** : the reception of genetic qualities by transmission from parent to offspring **2** : all the genetic characters or qualities transmitted from parent to offspring

in•hib•in \in-ˈhi-bən\ *n* : a hormone that is secreted by the pituitary gland and in the male by the Sertoli cells and in the female by the granulosa cells and that inhibits the secretion of follicle-stimulating hormone

in•hib•it \in-ˈhi-bət\ *vb* **1 a** : to restrain from free or spontaneous activity esp.

through the operation of inner psychological or external social constraints **b** : to check or restrain the force or vitality of ⟨~ aggressive tendencies⟩ **2 a** : to reduce or suppress the activity of ⟨~ a nerve⟩ **b** : to retard or prevent the formation of **c** : to retard, interfere with, or prevent (a process or reaction) ⟨~ ovulation⟩ — **in·hib·i·tor** \in-ˈhi-bə-tər\ *n* — **in·hib·i·to·ry** \in-ˈhi-bə-ˌtōr-ē\ *adj*

in·hib·it·able \-bə-tə-bəl\ *adj* : capable of being inhibited

in·hi·bi·tion \ˌin-hə-ˈbi-shən, ˌi-nə-\ *n* : the act or an instance of inhibiting or the state of being inhibited: as **a** (1) : a restraining of the function of a bodily organ or an agent (as an enzyme) ⟨~ of the heartbeat⟩ (2) : interference with or retardation or prevention of a process or activity ⟨~ of bacterial growth⟩ **b** (1) : a desirable restraint or check upon the free or spontaneous instincts or impulses of an individual guided or directed by social and cultural forces (2) : a neurotic restraint upon a normal or beneficial impulse or activity caused by psychological inner conflicts or by sociocultural forces

inhibitory postsynaptic potential *n* : increased negativity of the membrane potential of a neuron on the postsynaptic side of a nerve synapse that is caused by a neurotransmitter and that tends to inhibit the neuron — abbr. *IPSP*

in·i·en·ceph·a·lus \ˌi-nē-in-ˈse-fə-ləs\ *n* : a teratological fetus with a fissure in the occiput through which the brain protrudes — **in·i·en·ceph·a·ly** \-lē\ *n*

in·i·on \ˈi-nē-ˌän, -ən\ *n* : OCCIPITAL PROTUBERANCE a

initiation codon *n* : START CODON — called also *initiator codon*

ini·ti·a·tor \i-ˈni-shē-ˌā-tər\ *n* **1** : a substance that initiates a chemical reaction **2** : a substance that produces an irreversible change in bodily tissue causing it to respond to other substances which promote the growth of tumors

in·ject \in-ˈjekt\ *vb* : to introduce a fluid into (a living body); *also* : to treat (an individual) with injections

[1]**in·ject·able** \-ˈjek-tə-bəl\ *adj* : capable of being injected ⟨~ medications⟩

[2]**injectable** *n* : an injectable substance

in·jec·tion \in-ˈjek-shən\ *n* **1 a** : the act or an instance of injecting a drug or other substance into the body **b** : a solution (as of a drug) intended for injection (as by catheter or hypodermic syringe) either under or through the skin or into the tissues, a vein, or a body cavity **2** : CONGESTION — see CIRCUMCORNEAL INJECTION

in·jure \ˈin-jər\ *vb* **in·jured; in·jur·ing 1** : to inflict bodily hurt on **2** : to impair the soundness of — **in·ju·ri·ous** \in-ˈjůr-ē-əs\ *adj* — **in·ju·ri·ous·ly** *adv*

in·ju·ry \ˈin-jə-rē\ *n, pl* **-ries** : hurt, damage, or loss sustained

injury potential *n* : the difference in electrical potential between the injured and uninjured parts of a nerve or muscle

inkblot test *n* : any of several psychological tests (as a Rorschach test) based on the interpretation of irregular figures (as blots of ink)

in·lay \ˈin-ˌlā\ *n* **1** : a tooth filling shaped to fit a cavity and then cemented into place **2** : a piece of tissue (as bone) laid into the site of missing tissue to cover a defect

in·let \ˈin-ˌlet, -lət\ *n* : the upper opening of a bodily cavity; *esp* : that of the cavity of the true pelvis bounded by the pelvic brim

in·mate \ˈin-ˌmāt\ *n* : a person confined (as in a psychiatric hospital) esp. for a long time

in·nards \ˈi-nərdz\ *n pl* : the internal organs of a human being or animal; *esp* : VISCERA

in·nate \i-ˈnāt, ˈi-ˌ\ *adj* : existing in, belonging to, or determined by factors present in an individual from birth : INBORN ⟨~ behavior⟩ — **in·nate·ly** *adv* — **in·nate·ness** *n*

innate immunity *n* : immunity that is present in an individual at birth prior to exposure to a pathogen or antigen and that includes components (as intact skin, salivary enzymes, neutrophils, and natural killer cells) which provide an initial response against infection — called also *natural immunity;* compare ACQUIRED IMMUNITY, ACTIVE IMMUNITY, PASSIVE IMMUNITY

inner cell mass *n* : the portion of the blastocyst of an embryo that is destined to become the embryo proper

inner–directed *adj* : directed in thought and action by one's own scale of values as opposed to external norms — compare OTHER-DIRECTED — **inner–direction** *n*

inner ear *n* : the essential part of the organ of hearing and equilibrium that is typically located in the temporal bone, is innervated by the auditory nerve, and includes the vestibule, the semicircular canals, and the cochlea — called also *internal ear*

in·ner·vate \i-ˈnər-ˌvāt, ˈi-(ˌ)nər-\ *vb* **-vat·ed; -vat·ing 1** : to supply with nerves **2** : to arouse or stimulate (a nerve or an organ) to activity — **in·ner·va·tion** \ˌi-(ˌ)nər-ˈvā-shən, iˌnər-\ *n*

in·no·cent \ˈi-nə-sənt\ *adj* : lacking capacity to injure : BENIGN ⟨an ~ tumor⟩ ⟨~ heart murmurs⟩

innominata — see SUBSTANTIA INNOMINATA

in·nom·i·nate artery \i-ˈnä-mə-nət-\ *n* : BRACHIOCEPHALIC ARTERY

innominate bone *n* : HIP BONE

innominate vein *n* : BRACHIOCEPHALIC VEIN

In•no•pran \ˈi-nō-ˌpran\ *trademark* — used for a preparation of the hydrochloride of propranolol

ino- *comb form* : fiber : fibrous ⟨*ino*tropic⟩

in•oc•u•lant \i-ˈnä-kyə-lənt\ *n* : INOCULUM

in•oc•u•late \-ˌlāt\ *vb* **-lat•ed; -lat•ing** **1** : to introduce a microorganism or virus into ⟨∼ mice with anthrax⟩ **2** : to introduce (as a microorganism) into a suitable situation for growth **3** : to introduce immunologically active material (as an antibody or antigen) into esp. in order to treat or prevent a disease ⟨∼ children against diphtheria⟩

in•oc•u•la•tion \i-ˌnä-kyə-ˈlā-shən\ *n* **1** : the act or process or an instance of inoculating: as **a** : the introduction of a pathogen or antigen into a living organism to stimulate the production of antibodies **b** : the introduction of a vaccine or serum into a living organism to confer immunity **2** : INOCULUM

in•oc•u•lum \i-ˈnä-kyə-ləm\ *n, pl* **-la** \-lə\ : material used for inoculation

in•op•er•a•ble \i-ˈnä-pə-rə-bəl\ *adj* : not treatable or remediable by surgery ⟨∼ cancer⟩ — **in•op•er•a•bil•i•ty** \i-ˌnä-pə-rə-ˈbi-lə-tē\ *n*

in•or•gan•ic \ˌin-ˌȯr-ˈga-nik\ *adj* **1** : being or composed of matter other than plant or animal ⟨an ∼ heart⟩ **2** : of, relating to, or dealt with by a branch of chemistry concerned with substances not usu. classed as organic — **in•or•gan•i•cal•ly** *adv*

in•or•gas•mic \ˌin-ˌȯr-ˈgaz-mik\ *adj* : not experiencing or having experienced orgasm

ino•sin•ate \i-ˈnō-si-ˌnāt\ *n* : a salt or ester of inosinic acid

ino•sine \ˈi-nə-ˌsēn, ˈī-, -sən\ *n* : a crystalline nucleoside $C_{10}H_{12}N_4O_5$

ino•sin•ic acid \ˌi-nə-ˈsi-nik-, ˌī-\ *n* : a nucleotide $C_{10}H_{13}N_4O_8P$ that is found in muscle and is formed by deamination of AMP — called also *IMP*

ino•si•tol \i-ˈnō-sə-ˌtȯl, ī-, -ˌtōl\ *n* : any of several stereoisomeric cyclic alcohols $C_6H_{12}O_6$; *esp* : MYOINOSITOL

ino•trope \ˈī-nə-ˌtrōp\ *n* : an agent (as epinephrine or a beta-blocker) that either increases or decreases the force of muscular contraction

ino•tro•pic \ˌē-nə-ˈtrō-pik, ˌī-, -ˈträ-\ *adj* : relating to or influencing the force of muscular contractions

in•pa•tient \ˈin-ˌpā-shənt\ *n* : a hospital patient who receives lodging and food as well as treatment — compare OUTPATIENT

in•quest \ˈin-ˌkwest\ *n* : a judicial or official inquiry esp. before a jury to determine the cause of a violent or unexpected death ⟨a coroner's ∼⟩

in•sane \(ˌ)in-ˈsān\ *adj, dated* : exhibiting a severely disordered state of mind — **in•sane•ly** *adv*

in•san•i•tary \(ˌ)in-ˈsa-nə-ˌter-ē\ *adj* : unclean enough to endanger health

in•san•i•ty \in-ˈsa-nə-tē\ *n, pl* **-ties** **1** *dated* : a severely disordered state of the mind usu. occurring as a specific disorder **2** *law* : unsoundness of mind or lack of the ability to understand that prevents one from having the mental capacity required by law to enter into a particular relationship, status, or transaction or that removes one from criminal or civil responsibility

in•scrip•tion \in-ˈskrip-shən\ *n* : the part of a medical prescription that contains the names and quantities of the drugs to be compounded

in•sect \ˈin-ˌsekt\ *n* : any of a class (Insecta) of arthropods with well-defined head, thorax, and abdomen, three pairs of legs, and typically one or two pairs of wings — **insect** *adj*

in•sec•ti•cide \in-ˈsek-tə-ˌsīd\ *n* : an agent that destroys insects — **in•sec•ti•cid•al** \(ˌ)in-ˌsek-tə-ˈsīd-ᵊl\ *adj*

in•se•cu•ri•ty \ˌin-si-ˈkyu̇r-ə-tē\ *n, pl* **-ties** : a feeling of apprehensiveness and uncertainty : lack of assurance or stability — **in•se•cure** \-ˈkyu̇r\ *adj*

in•sem•i•nate \in-ˈse-mə-ˌnāt\ *vb* **-nat•ed; -nat•ing** : to introduce semen into the genital tract of (a female) — **in•sem•i•na•tion** \-ˌse-mə-ˈnā-shən\ *n*

in•sem•i•na•tor \-ˌnā-tər\ *n* : one that inseminates cattle artificially

in•sen•si•ble \(ˌ)in-ˈsen-sə-bəl\ *adj* **1** : incapable or bereft of feeling or sensation: as **a** : UNCONSCIOUS **b** : lacking sensory perception or ability to react **c** : lacking emotional response : APATHETIC **2** : not perceived by the senses ⟨∼ perspiration⟩ — **in•sen•si•bil•i•ty** \(ˌ)in-ˌsen-sə-ˈbi-lə-tē\ *n*

in•sert \in-ˈsərt\ *vb, of a muscle* : to be in attachment to the part to be moved

inserted *adj* : attached by natural growth (as a muscle or tendon)

in•ser•tion \in-ˈsər-shən\ *n* **1** : the part of a muscle by which it is attached to the part to be moved — compare ORIGIN 2 **2** : the mode or place of attachment of an organ or part **3 a** : a section of genetic material inserted into an existing gene sequence **b** : the mutational process producing a genetic insertion — **in•ser•tion•al** \-shə-nəl\ *adj*

in•sid•i•ous \in-ˈsi-dē-əs\ *adj* : developing so gradually as to be well established before becoming apparent ⟨an ∼ disease⟩ — **in•sid•i•ous•ly** *adv*

in•sight \ˈin-ˌsīt\ *n* **1** : understanding or awareness of one's mental or emotional state or condition **2** : immediate and clear understanding (as seeing the solution to a problem) that takes place without recourse to overt trial-and-error behavior — **in•sight•ful** \ˈin-ˌsīt-fəl, in-ˈ\ *adj* — **in•sight•ful•ly** *adv*

insipidus — see CENTRAL DIABETES INSIPIDUS, DIABETES INSIPIDUS, NEPHROGENIC DIABETES INSIPIDUS

in si·tu \ˌin-ˈsī-(ˌ)tü, -ˈsi-, -ˈsē-, -(ˌ)tyü, -(ˌ)chü\ *adv or adj* : in the natural or original position or place — see CARCINOMA IN SITU

in·sol·u·ble \in-ˈsäl-yə-bəl\ *adj* : incapable of being dissolved in a liquid; *also* : soluble only with difficulty or to a slight degree

in·som·nia \in-ˈsäm-nē-ə\ *n* : prolonged and usu. abnormal inability to obtain adequate sleep

[1]**in·som·ni·ac** \-nē-ˌak\ *n* : one affected with insomnia

[2]**insomniac** *adj* : affected with insomnia ⟨an ~ patient⟩

in·spec·tion \in-ˈspek-shən\ *n* : visual observation of the body during a medical examination — compare PALPATION 2 — **in·spect** \in-ˈspekt\ *vb*

in·spi·ra·tion \ˌin-spə-ˈrā-shən\ *n* : the drawing of air into the lungs — **in·spi·ra·to·ry** \in-ˈspī-rə-ˌtōr-ē, ˈin-spə-rə-\ *adj*

inspiratory capacity *n* : the total amount of air that can be drawn into the lungs after normal expiration

inspiratory reserve volume *n* : the maximal amount of additional air that can be drawn into the lungs by determined effort after normal inspiration — compare EXPIRATORY RESERVE VOLUME

in·spire \in-ˈspīr\ *vb* **in·spired; in·spir·ing** : to draw in by breathing : breathe in : INHALE

in·spis·sat·ed \in-ˈspi-ˌsā-təd, ˈin-spə-ˌsā-\ *adj* : thick or thickened in consistency

in·sta·bil·i·ty \ˌin-stə-ˈbi-lə-tē\ *n, pl* **-ties** : lack of emotional or mental stability

in·step \ˈin-ˌstep\ *n* : the arched middle portion of the human foot in front of the ankle joint; *esp* : its upper surface

in·still \in-ˈstil\ *vb* **in·stilled; in·still·ing** : to cause to enter esp. drop by drop ⟨~ medication into the eye⟩ — **in·stil·la·tion** \ˌin-stə-ˈlā-shən\ *n*

in·stinct \ˈin-ˌstiŋkt\ *n* **1** : a largely inheritable and unalterable tendency of an organism to make a complex and specific response to environmental stimuli without involving reason **2** : behavior that is mediated by reactions below the conscious level — **in·stinc·tive** \in-ˈstiŋk-tiv\ *adj* — **in·stinc·tive·ly** *adv* — **in·stinc·tu·al** \in-ˈstiŋk-chə-wəl\ *adj*

in·sti·tu·tion \ˌin-stə-ˈtü-shən, -ˈtyü-\ *n* : a facility or establishment in which people (as the sick or needy) live and receive care typically in a confined setting and often without individual consent

in·sti·tu·tion·al·ize \-ˈtü-shə-nə-ˌlīz, -ˈtyü-\ *vb* : to place in or commit to the care of a specialized institution — **in·sti·tu·tion·al·iza·tion** \-ˌtü-shə-nə-lə-ˈzā-shən, -ˌtyü-\ *n*

in·sti·tu·tion·al·ized \-ˈtü-shə-nə-ˌlīzd, -ˈtyü-\ *adj* : accustomed so firmly to the care and routine of an institution as to find independent life in the outside world difficult or unmanageable

in·stru·men·tal \ˌin-strə-ˈmen-təl\ *adj* : OPERANT ⟨~ conditioning⟩

in·stru·men·ta·tion \ˌin-strə-mən-ˈtā-shən, -ˌmen-\ *n* : a use of or operation with instruments

in·suf·fi·cien·cy \ˌin-sə-ˈfi-shən-sē\ *n, pl* **-cies** : the quality or state of not being sufficient: as **a** : lack of adequate supply of something **b** : lack of physical power or capacity; *esp* : inability of an organ or bodily part to function normally ⟨renal ~⟩ — **in·suf·fi·cient** \-shənt\ *adj*

in·suf·fla·tion \ˌin-sə-ˈflā-shən\ *n* : the act of blowing something (as a drug in powdered form) into a body cavity; *specif* : the introduction of a flow of gas into a body cavity ⟨oxygen for tracheal gas ~⟩ ⟨abdominal ~ with carbon dioxide⟩ — **in·suf·flate** \ˈin-sə-ˌflāt, in-ˈsə-ˌflāt\ *vb* — **in·suf·fla·tor** \ˈin-sə-ˌflā-tər, in-ˈsə-ˌflā-tər\ *n*

in·su·la \ˈin-sü-lə, -syü-, -shü-\ *n, pl* **in·su·lae** \-ˌlē, -ˌlī\ : the lobe in the center of the cerebral hemisphere that is situated deeply between the lips of the sylvian fissure — called also *central lobe, island of Reil*

in·su·lar \-lər\ *adj* : of or relating to an island of cells or tissue (as the islets of Langerhans or the insula)

in·su·lin \ˈin-sə-lən\ *n* : a protein hormone that is synthesized in the pancreas from proinsulin and secreted by the beta cells of the islets of Langerhans, that is essential for the metabolism of carbohydrates, lipids, and proteins, that regulates blood sugar levels by facilitating the uptake of glucose into tissues, by promoting its conversion into glycogen, fatty acids, and triglycerides, and by reducing the release of glucose from the liver, and that when produced in insufficient quantities results in diabetes mellitus — see ILETIN

in·su·lin·ae·mia *chiefly Brit var of* INSULINEMIA

in·su·lin·ase \-lə-ˌnās, -ˌnāz\ *n* : an enzyme found esp. in the liver that inactivates insulin

insulin as·part \-ˈas-ˌpärt\ *n* : a short-acting recombinant form of insulin administered by subcutaneous injection in the treatment of type 1 and type 2 diabetes — see NOVOLOG

insulin coma therapy *n* : INSULIN SHOCK THERAPY

insulin–dependent diabetes *n* : TYPE 1 DIABETES

insulin–dependent diabetes mellitus *n* : TYPE 1 DIABETES — abbr. *IDDM*

insulin det·e·mir \-ˈdet-ə-ˌmir\ *n* : a long-acting recombinant form of insulin administered by subcutaneous injection in the treatment of type 1 and type 2 diabetes — see LEVEMIR

in·su·lin·emia \ˌin-sə-lə-ˈnē-mē-ə\ *n* : the presence of an abnormally high concentration of insulin in the blood

insulin glar·gine \-ˈglär-ˌjēn\ *n* : a long-acting recombinant form of insulin administered by subcutaneous injection for the management of type 1 and type 2 diabetes — see LANTUS

insulin isophane *n* : ISOPHANE INSULIN

insulin–like growth factor *n* : either of two polypeptides structurally similar to insulin that are secreted either during fetal development or during childhood and that mediate growth hormone activity; *esp* : INSULIN-LIKE GROWTH FACTOR 1

insulin–like growth factor 1 *n* : the juvenile form of insulin-like growth factor that is produced chiefly by the liver with production declining after puberty — abbr. *IGF-1*

insulin lis·pro \-ˈlis-ˌprō\ *n* : a short-acting recombinant form of insulin administered by injection in the treatment of type 1 and type 2 diabetes — see HUMALOG

in·su·lin·o·ma \ˌin-sə-lə-ˈnō-mə\ *n, pl* **-mas** *also* **-ma·ta** \-mə-tə\ : a usu. benign insulin-secreting tumor of the islets of Langerhans

in·su·li·no·tro·pic \ˌin-sə-ˌli-nə-ˈtrō-pik, -ˈträ-\ *adj* : stimulating or affecting the production and activity of insulin ⟨an ∼ hormone⟩

insulin resistance *n* : reduced sensitivity to insulin by the body's insulin-dependent processes (as glucose uptake, lipolysis, and inhibition of glucose production by the liver) that is typical of type 2 diabetes but often occurs in the absence of diabetes

insulin resistance syndrome *n* : METABOLIC SYNDROME

insulin shock *n* : severe hypoglycemia that is associated with the presence of excessive insulin in the system and that if left untreated may result in convulsions and progressive development of coma

insulin shock therapy *n* : the treatment of mental illness (as schizophrenia) by insulin in doses sufficient to produce deep coma — called also *insulin coma therapy*

insulin zinc suspension *n* : a suspension of insulin in a solution containing zinc in the form of a salt that is used for injection and has a slow onset and intermediate to long duration of action — see LENTE INSULIN, ULTRALENTE INSULIN

in·su·li·tis \ˌin-sə-ˈlī-təs\ *n* : invasion of the pancreatic islets of Langerhans by lymphocytes that results in destruction of the beta cells of the pancreas

in·su·lo·ma \ˌin-sə-ˈlō-mə\ *n, pl* **-mas** *also* **-ma·ta** \-mə-tə\ : INSULINOMA

in·sult \ˈin-ˌsəlt\ *n* **1** : injury to the body or one of its parts **2** : something that causes or has a potential for causing insult to the body — **insult** *vb*

in·tact \in-ˈtakt\ *adj* **1** : physically and functionally complete **2** : mentally unimpaired — **in·tact·ness** *n*

In·tal \ˈin-ˌtal\ *trademark* — used for a preparation of cromolyn

in·te·gra·tion \ˌin-tə-ˈgrā-shən\ *n* **1** : coordination of mental processes into a normal effective personality or with the individual's environment **2** : the process by which the different parts of an organism are made a functional and structural whole esp. through the activity of the nervous system and of hormones — **in·te·grate** \ˈin-tə-ˌgrāt\ *vb* — **in·te·gra·tive** \ˈin-tə-ˌgrā-tiv\ *adj*

integrative medicine *n* : medicine that integrates the therapies of alternative medicine with those practiced by mainstream medical practitioners

in·te·grin \ˈin-tə-grən\ *n* : any of various glycoproteins found on cell surfaces that are involved in the adhesion of cells (as T cells) to other cells (as endothelial cells) or to extracellular material (as fibronectin) and mediate various biological processes (as phagocytosis and wound healing)

in·teg·ri·ty \in-ˈte-grə-tē\ *n, pl* **-ties** : an unimpaired condition ⟨vascular ∼⟩

in·teg·u·ment \in-ˈte-gyə-mənt\ *n* : an enveloping layer (as a skin or membrane) of an organism or one of its parts — **in·teg·u·men·ta·ry** \-ˈmen-tə-rē\ *adj*

intellectual disability *n* : mild to severe intellectual impairment equivalent to an IQ of 70 to 75 or below that is accompanied by significant limitations in social, practical, and conceptual skills (as in communication, reasoning, and self-care) necessary for independent daily functioning

in·tel·lec·tu·al·ize \ˌint-ᵊl-ˈek-chə-wə-ˌlīz\ *vb* **-ized; -iz·ing** : to avoid conscious recognition of the emotional basis of (an act or feeling) by substituting a superficially plausible explanation — **in·tel·lec·tu·al·iza·tion** \-ˌek-chə-wə-lə-ˈzā-shən\ *n*

in·tel·li·gence \in-ˈte-lə-jəns\ *n* **1 a** : the ability to learn or understand or to deal with new or trying situations **b** : the ability to apply knowledge to manipulate one's environment or to think abstractly as measured by objective criteria (as tests) **2** : mental acuteness — **in·tel·li·gent** \-jənt\ *adj* — **in·tel·li·gent·ly** *adv*

intelligence quotient *n* : IQ

intelligence test *n* : a test designed to determine the relative mental capacity of a person

intensifying screen *n* : a fluorescent screen placed next to an X-ray photographic film in order to intensify the image initially produced on the film by the action of X-rays

in·ten·si·ty \in-ˈten-sə-tē\ *n, pl* **-ties** : SATURATION 4

in•ten•sive \in-ˈten-siv\ *adj* : of, relating to, or marked by an extreme degree esp. of dosage, duration, or frequency ⟨high-dose ~ chemotherapy⟩ ⟨~ counseling for eating disorders⟩ — **in•ten•sive•ly** *adv*

intensive care *adj* : having special medical facilities, services, and monitoring devices to meet the needs of gravely ill patients ⟨an *intensive care* unit⟩ — **intensive care** *n*

in•ten•siv•ist \in-ˈten-sə-vəst\ *n* : a physician specializing in the care and treatment of patients in intensive care

in•ten•tion \in-ˈten-chən\ *n* : a process or manner of healing of incised wounds — see FIRST INTENTION, SECOND INTENTION

intention tremor *n* : a slow tremor of the extremities that increases on attempted voluntary movement and is observed in certain diseases (as multiple sclerosis) of the nervous system

inter- *comb form* : between : among ⟨*inter*cellular⟩ ⟨*inter*costal⟩

in•ter•al•ve•o•lar \ˌin-tə-ral-ˈvē-ə-lər\ *adj* : situated between alveoli esp. of the lungs

in•ter•atri•al \ˌin-tər-ˈā-trē-əl\ *adj* : situated between the atria of the heart

interatrial septum *n* : the wall separating the right and left atria of the heart — called also *atrial septum*

in•ter•au•ral \-ˈȯr-əl\ *adj* **1** : situated between or connecting the ears **2** : of or relating to sound reception and perception by each ear considered separately

in•ter•body \ˈin-tər-ˌbä-dē\ *adj* : performed between the bodies of two contiguous vertebrae ⟨an ~ fusion⟩

in•ter•breed \ˌin-tər-ˈbrēd\ *vb* **-bred** \-ˈbred\; **-breed•ing** : to breed together: as **a** : CROSSBREED **b** : to breed within a closed population

in•ter•ca•lat•ed disk \in-ˈtər-kə-ˌlā-təd-\ *n* : any of the regions of the sarcolemma and underlying cytoplasm of cardiac muscle cells that comprise the junctions between adjacent cells and that function to connect them mechanically and electrically across cardiac muscle

intercalated duct *n* : a duct from a tubule or acinus of the pancreas that drains into an intralobular duct

in•ter•cap•il•lary \ˌin-tər-ˈka-pə-ˌler-ē\ *adj* : situated between capillaries

in•ter•car•pal \-ˈkär-pəl\ *adj* : situated between, occurring between, or connecting carpal bones ⟨an ~ joint⟩

in•ter•cav•ern•ous \-ˈka-vər-nəs\ *adj* : situated between and connecting the cavernous sinuses behind and in front of the pituitary gland ⟨an ~ sinus⟩

in•ter•cel•lu•lar \-ˈsel-yə-lər\ *adj* : occurring between cells ⟨~ spaces⟩ — **in•ter•cel•lu•lar•ly** *adv*

in•ter•con•dy•lar \-ˈkän-də-lər\ *adj* : situated between two condyles

in•ter•con•dy•loid \-ˈkän-də-ˌlȯid\ *adj* : INTERCONDYLAR

¹in•ter•cos•tal \ˌin-tər-ˈkäs-tᵊl\ *adj* : situated or extending between the ribs

²intercostal *n* : an intercostal part or structure (as a muscle or nerve)

intercostal artery *n* : any of the arteries supplying or lying in the intercostal spaces: **a** : any of the arteries branching in front directly from the internal mammary artery — called also *anterior intercostal artery* **b** : any of the arteries that branch from the costocervical trunk of the subclavian artery — called also *posterior intercostal artery*

intercostal muscle *n* : any of the short muscles that extend between the ribs and serve to move the ribs in respiration: **a** : any of 11 muscles on each side between the vertebrae and the junction of the ribs and their cartilages — called also *external intercostal muscle* **b** : any of 11 muscles on each side between the sternum and the line on a rib marking an insertion of the iliocostalis — called also *internal intercostal muscle*

intercostal nerve *n* : any of 11 nerves on each side of which each is an anterior division of a thoracic nerve lying between a pair of adjacent ribs

intercostal vein *n* : any of the veins of the intercostal spaces — see SUPERIOR INTERCOSTAL VEIN

in•ter•cos•to•bra•chi•al nerve \ˌin-tər-ˌkäs-tō-ˈbrā-kē-əl-\ *n* : a branch of the second intercostal nerve that supplies the skin of the inner and back part of the upper half of the arm

in•ter•course \ˈin-tər-ˌkōrs\ *n* : physical sexual contact between individuals that involves the genitalia of at least one person ⟨anal ~⟩; *esp* : SEXUAL INTERCOURSE 1 ⟨heterosexual ~⟩

in•ter•cris•tal \ˌin-tər-ˈkris-tᵊl\ *adj* : measured between two crests (as of bone)

in•ter•crit•i•cal \-ˈkri-ti-kəl\ *adj* : being in the period between attacks ⟨~ gout⟩

in•ter•cur•rent \-ˈkər-ənt\ *adj* : occurring during and modifying the course of another disease ⟨an ~ infection⟩

in•ter•den•tal \-ˈdent-ᵊl\ *adj* : situated or intended for use between the teeth — **in•ter•den•tal•ly** \-ᵊl-ē\ *adv*

interdental papilla *n* : the triangular wedge of gingiva between two adjacent teeth — called also *gingival papilla*

in•ter•dig•i•tal \-ˈdi-jə-təl\ *adj* : occurring between digits ⟨an ~ neuroma⟩

in•ter•dig•i•tate \-ˈdi-jə-ˌtāt\ *vb* **-tat•ed; -tat•ing** : to become interlocked like the fingers of folded hands — **in•ter•dig•i•ta•tion** \-ˌdij-ə-ˈtā-shən\ *n*

in•ter•fere \ˌin-tər-ˈfir\ *vb* **-fered; -fer•ing** : to be inconsistent with and disturb the performance of previously learned behavior

in•ter•fer•ence \-ˈfir-əns\ *n* **1** : partial or complete inhibition or sometimes facilitation of other genetic crossovers in the vicinity of a chromosomal locus where a preceding crossover has occurred **2** : the disturbing effect of new learning on the performance of previously learned behavior with which it is inconsistent — compare NEGATIVE TRANSFER **3** : prevention of typical growth and development of a virus in a suitable host by the presence of another virus in the same host individual

in•ter•fer•on \ˌin-tər-ˈfir-ˌän\ *n* : any of a group of heat-stable soluble basic antiviral glycoproteins of low molecular weight that are produced usu. by cells exposed to the action of a virus, sometimes to the action of another intracellular parasite (as a bacterium), or experimentally to the action of some chemicals, and that include some used medically as antiviral or antineoplastic agents — see ALPHA INTERFERON, BETA INTERFERON, GAMMA INTERFERON

interferon al•fa \-ˈal-fə\ *n* : alpha interferon produced by recombinant DNA technology

interferon alpha *n* : ALPHA INTERFERON

interferon beta *n* : BETA INTERFERON

interferon gamma *n* : GAMMA INTERFERON

in•ter•fi•bril•lar \ˌin-tər-ˈfi-brə-lər, -ˈfī-\ *or* **in•ter•fi•bril•lary** \-ˈfi-brə-ˌler-ē, -ˈfī\ *adj* : situated between fibrils

in•ter•ge•nic \-ˈjē-nik\ *adj* : occurring between genes : involving more than one gene

in•ter•glob•u•lar \-ˈglä-byə-lər\ *adj* : resulting from or situated in an area of faulty dentin formation ⟨~ dentin⟩

in•ter•hemi•spher•ic \-ˌhe-mə-ˈsfir-ik, -ˈsfer-\ *also* **in•ter•hemi•spher•al** \-əl\ *adj* : extending or occurring between hemispheres (as of the cerebrum)

in•ter•ic•tal \-ˈik-təl\ *adj* : occurring between seizures (as of epilepsy)

in•ter•ki•ne•sis \-kə-ˈnē-səs, -kī-\ *n, pl* **-ne•ses** \-ˌsēz\ : the period between the first and second meiotic divisions

in•ter•lam•i•nar \ˌin-tər-ˈlam-ə-nər\ *adj* : administered or occurring between two laminae (as of vertebra) : involving two or more laminae

in•ter•leu•kin \ˌin-tər-ˈlü-kən\ *n* : any of several compounds of low molecular weight that are produced by lymphocytes, macrophages, and monocytes and that function esp. in regulation of the immune system and esp. cell-mediated immunity — often used with an identifying number ⟨*interleukin*-6 induces maturation of B cells and proliferation of T cells⟩

in•ter•lo•bar \ˌin-tər-ˈlō-bər, -ˌbär\ *adj* : situated between the lobes of an organ or structure

interlobar artery *n* : any of various secondary branches of the renal arteries that branch to form the arcuate arteries

interlobar vein *n* : any of the veins of the kidney that are formed by convergence of arcuate veins and empty into the renal veins or their branches

in•ter•lob•u•lar \-ˈlä-byə-lər\ *adj* : lying between, connecting, or transporting the secretions of lobules

interlobular artery *n* **1** : any of the branches of an arcuate artery that pass through the cortex of the kidney toward the surface and supply the glomeruli **2** : any of the branches of the hepatic artery that form a network around each lobule of the liver

interlobular vein *n* **1** : any of the veins in the cortex of the kidney that empty into the arcuate veins **2** : any of the branches of the hepatic portal vein that empty into minute spaces in the liver

in•ter•max•il•lary \-ˈmak-sə-ˌler-ē\ *adj* **1** : lying between maxillae; *esp* : joining the two maxillary bones ⟨~ sutures⟩ **2** : of or relating to the premaxillae

intermedia — see MASSA INTERMEDIA, PARS INTERMEDIA

intermediary metabolism *n* : the intracellular process by which nutritive material is converted into cellular components

intermediate cuneiform bone *n* : CUNEIFORM BONE 1b — called also *intermediate cuneiform*

intermediate filament *n* : any of a class of usu. insoluble cellular protein fibers (as a neurofilament or cytokeratin) that serve esp. to provide structural stability and strength to the cytoskeleton and are intermediate in diameter between microfilaments and microtubules

intermediate host *n* **1** : a host which is normally used by a parasite in the course of its life cycle and in which it may multiply asexually but not sexually — compare DEFINITIVE HOST **2 a** : RESERVOIR 2 **b** : VECTOR 1

intermediate metabolism *n* : INTERMEDIARY METABOLISM

intermediate temporal artery *n* : TEMPORAL ARTERY 3b

in•ter•me•din \ˌin-tər-ˈmēd-ᵊn\ *n* : MELANOCYTE-STIMULATING HORMONE

in•ter•me•dio•lat•er•al \ˌin-tər-ˌmē-dē-ō-ˈla-tə-rəl\ *adj* : of, relating to, or being the lateral column of gray matter in the spinal cord

intermedium — see STRATUM INTERMEDIUM

intermedius — see NERVUS INTERMEDIUS, VASTUS INTERMEDIUS

in•ter•men•stru•al \-ˈmen-strə-wəl\ *adj* : occurring between menstrual periods ⟨~ pain⟩

in•ter•mis•sion \ˌin-tər-ˈmi-shən\ *n* : the space of time between two paroxysms of a disease

in•ter•mit•tent \-ˈmit-ᵊnt\ *adj* : coming and going at intervals : not continuous ⟨~ fever⟩ — **in•ter•mit•tence** \-ᵊns\ *n*

intermittent claudication *n* : cramping pain and weakness in the legs and esp. the calves on walking that disappears after rest and is usu. associated with inadequate blood supply to the muscles

intermittent explosive disorder *n* : a personality disorder characterized by repeated episodes of violent aggressive behavior that is out of proportion to the events provoking it

intermittent positive pressure breathing *n* : enforced periodic inflation of the lungs by the intermittent application of an increase of pressure to a reservoir of air (as in a bag) supplying the lungs — abbr. *IPPB*

in·ter·mus·cu·lar \-ˈməs-kyə-lər\ *adj* : lying between and separating muscles ⟨∼ fat⟩

in·tern *also* **in·terne** \ˈin-ˌtərn\ *n* : a physician gaining supervised practical experience in a hospital after graduating from medical school — **intern** *vb*

interna — see THECA INTERNA

in·ter·nal \in-ˈtərn-ᵊl\ *adj* **1 a** : situated near the inside of the body **b** : situated on the side toward the midsagittal plane of the body ⟨the ∼ surface of the lung⟩ **2** : present or arising within an organism or one of its parts ⟨∼ stimulus⟩ **3** : applied or intended for application through the stomach by being swallowed ⟨an ∼ remedy⟩ — **in·ter·nal·ly** *adv*

internal acoustic meatus *n* : INTERNAL AUDITORY CANAL

internal anal sphincter *n* : ANAL SPHINCTER b

internal auditory artery *n* : a long slender artery that arises from the basilar artery or one of its branches and is distributed to the inner ear — called also *labyrinthine artery*

internal auditory canal *n* : a short auditory canal in the petrous portion of the temporal bone through which pass the facial and auditory nerves and the internal auditory artery — called also *internal acoustic meatus, internal auditory meatus*

internal capsule *n* : CAPSULE 1b(1)

internal carotid artery *n* : the inner branch of the carotid artery that supplies the brain, eyes, and other internal structures of the head — called also *internal carotid*

internal ear *n* : INNER EAR

internal iliac artery *n* : ILIAC ARTERY 3

internal iliac node *n* : any of the lymph nodes grouped around the internal iliac artery and the internal iliac vein — compare EXTERNAL ILIAC NODE

internal iliac vein *n* : ILIAC VEIN c

internal inguinal ring *n* : DEEP INGUINAL RING

internal intercostal muscle *n* : INTERCOSTAL MUSCLE b — called also *internal intercostal*

in·ter·nal·ize \in-ˈtərn-ᵊl-ˌīz\ *vb* **-ized; -iz·ing** : to incorporate (as values) within the self as conscious or subconscious guiding principles through learning or socialization — **in·ter·nal·iza·tion** \-ˌtərn-ᵊl-ə-ˈzā-shən\ *n*

internal jugular vein *n* : JUGULAR VEIN a — called also *internal jugular*

internal malleolus *n* : MALLEOLUS b

internal mammary artery *n* : a branch of the subclavian artery of each side that runs down along the anterior wall of the thorax — called also *internal thoracic artery*

internal mammary vein *n* : a vein of the thorax on each side that accompanies the corresponding internal mammary artery and empties into the brachiocephalic vein — called also *internal thoracic vein*

internal maxillary artery *n* : MAXILLARY ARTERY

internal medicine *n* : a branch of medicine that deals with the diagnosis and treatment of nonsurgical diseases — abbr. *IM*

internal oblique *n* : OBLIQUE a(2) — called also *internal oblique muscle*

internal occipital crest *n* : OCCIPITAL CREST b

internal occipital protuberance *n* : OCCIPITAL PROTUBERANCE b

internal os *n* : the opening of the cervix into the body of the uterus

internal pterygoid muscle *n* : PTERYGOID MUSCLE b

internal pudendal artery *n* : a branch of the internal iliac artery that is distributed esp. to the external genitalia and the perineum — compare EXTERNAL PUDENDAL ARTERY

internal pudendal vein *n* : any of several veins that receive blood from the external genitalia and the perineum and unite to form a single vein that empties into the internal iliac vein

internal respiration *n* : the exchange of gases (as oxygen and carbon dioxide) between the cells of the body and the blood — compare EXTERNAL RESPIRATION

internal spermatic artery *n* : TESTICULAR ARTERY

internal thoracic artery *n* : INTERNAL MAMMARY ARTERY

internal thoracic vein *n* : INTERNAL MAMMARY VEIN

In·ter·na·tion·al System of Units \ˌin-tər-ˈnash-nəl-, -ən-ᵊl-\ *n* : a system of units based on the metric system and developed and refined by international convention esp. for scientific work

international unit *n* : a quantity of a biologic (as a vitamin) that produces a particular biological effect agreed upon as an international standard

interne, interneship *var of* INTERN, INTERNSHIP

in·ter·neu·ron \ˌin-tər-ˈnü-ˌrän, -ˈnyü-\ *n* : a neuron that conveys impulses from one neuron to another — called also *associative neuron, internuncial, internuncial neuron;* compare MOTOR

NEURON, SENSORY NEURON — **in·ter·neu·ro·nal** \-ˈnu̇r-ən-ᵊl, -ˈnyu̇r-ən-, -nyu̇-ˈrōn-\ *adj*

in·ter·nist \ˈin-ˌtər-nist\ *n* : a specialist in internal medicine esp. as distinguished from a surgeon

in·tern·ship *also* **in·terne·ship** *n* **1** : the state or position of being an intern **2 a** : a period of service as an intern **b** : the phase of medical training covered during such service

[1]**in·ter·nun·ci·al** \ˌin-tər-ˈnən-sē-əl, -ˈnu̇n-\ *adj* : of, relating to, or being interneurons ⟨~ fibers⟩

[2]**internuncial** *n* : INTERNEURON

internuncial neuron *n* : INTERNEURON

internus — see OBLIQUUS INTERNUS ABDOMINIS, OBTURATOR INTERNUS, SPHINCTER ANI INTERNUS, VASTUS INTERNUS

in·ter·oc·clu·sal \-ə-ˈklü-səl, -zəl\ *adj* : situated or occurring between the occlusal surfaces of opposing teeth

in·tero·cep·tive \ˌin-tə-rō-ˈsep-tiv\ *adj* : of, relating to, or being stimuli arising within the body and esp. in the viscera

in·tero·cep·tor \-tər\ *n* : a sensory receptor excited by interoceptive stimuli — compare EXTEROCEPTOR

in·ter·os·se·ous \ˌin-tər-ˈä-sē-əs\ *adj* : situated between bones

interosseous artery — see COMMON INTEROSSEOUS ARTERY

interosseous membrane *n* : either of two thin strong sheets of fibrous tissue: **a** : one extending between and connecting the shafts of the radius and ulna **b** : one extending between and connecting the shafts of the tibia and fibula

interosseous muscle *n* : INTEROSSEUS

in·ter·os·se·us \ˌin-tər-ˈä-sē-əs\ *n, pl* **-sei** \-sē-ˌī\ : any of various small muscles arising from the metacarpals and metatarsals and inserted into the bases of the first phalanges: **a** : DORSAL INTEROSSEUS **b** : PALMAR INTEROSSEUS **c** : PLANTAR INTEROSSEUS

interosseus dorsalis *n, pl* **interossei dorsales** : DORSAL INTEROSSEUS

interosseus palmaris *n, pl* **interossei palmares** : PALMAR INTEROSSEUS

interosseus plantaris *n, pl* **interossei plantares** : PLANTAR INTEROSSEUS

in·ter·par·ox·ys·mal \-ˌpar-ək-ˈsiz-məl, -pə-ˌräk-\ *adj* : occurring between paroxysms

in·ter·pe·dun·cu·lar nucleus \ˌin-tər-pi-ˈdəŋ-kyə-lər-\ *n* : a mass of nerve cells lying between the cerebral peduncles in the midsagittal plane just dorsal to the pons — called also *interpeduncular ganglion*

in·ter·per·son·al \-ˈpərs-ᵊn-əl\ *adj* : being, relating to, or involving relations between persons — **in·ter·per·son·al·ly** *adv*

interpersonal therapy *n* : psychotherapy that focuses on a patient's interpersonal relationships and is used esp. to treat depression — abbr. *IPT;* called also *interpersonal psychotherapy*

in·ter·pha·lan·ge·al \ˌin-tər-ˌfā-lən-ˈjē-əl, -ˌfa-; -fə-ˈlan-jē-əl, -fā-\ *adj* : situated or occurring between phalanges; *also* : of or relating to an interphalangeal joint

in·ter·phase \ˈin-tər-ˌfāz\ *n* : the interval between the end of one mitotic or meiotic division and the beginning of another — called also *resting stage*

in·ter·po·lat·ed \in-ˈtər-pə-ˌlā-təd\ *adj* : occurring between normal heartbeats without disturbing the succeeding beat or the basic rhythm of the heart ⟨an ~ ventricular extrasystole⟩

in·ter·pris·mat·ic \ˌin-tər-priz-ˈma-tik\ *adj* : situated or occurring between prisms esp. of enamel

in·ter·prox·i·mal \-ˈpräk-sə-məl\ *adj* : situated, occurring, or used in the areas between adjoining teeth

in·ter·pu·pil·lary \-ˈpyü-pə-ˌler-ē\ *adj* : extending between the pupils of the eyes; *also* : extending between the centers of a pair of spectacle lenses ⟨~ distance⟩

in·ter·ra·dic·u·lar \-rə-ˈdi-kyə-lər\ *adj* : situated between the roots of a tooth

interruptus — see COITUS INTERRUPTUS

in·ter·scap·u·lar \ˌin-tər-ˈska-pyə-lər\ *adj* : of, relating to, situated in, or occurring in the region between the scapulae ⟨~ pain⟩

in·ter·sen·so·ry \-ˈsens-ə-rē\ *adj* : involving two or more sensory systems

in·ter·sep·tal \-ˈsept-ᵊl\ *adj* : situated between septa

[1]**in·ter·sex** \ˈin-tər-ˌseks\ *n* **1** : an intersexual individual **2** : INTERSEXUALITY

[2]**intersex** *adj* : of or relating to intersexuality; *also* : exhibiting intersexuality ⟨an ~ individual⟩

[1]**in·ter·sex·u·al** \ˌin-tər-ˈsek-shə-wəl\ *adj* **1** : existing between sexes ⟨~ hostility⟩ **2** : INTERSEX

[2]**intersexual** *n* : an individual exhibiting intersexuality

in·ter·sex·u·al·i·ty \-ˌsek-shə-ˈwa-lə-tē\ *n* : the condition (as that occurring in congenital adrenal hyperplasia) of either having both male and female gonadal tissue in one individual or of having the gonads of one sex and external genitalia that is of the other sex or is ambiguous

in·ter·space \ˈin-tər-ˌspās\ *n* : the space between two related body parts whether void or filled by another kind of structure

in·ter·spi·na·lis \ˌin-tər-ˌspī-ˈna-ləs, -ˈnā-\ *n, pl* **-na·les** \-ˌlēz\ : any of various short muscles that have their origin on the superior surface of the spinous process of one vertebra and their insertion on the inferior surface of the contiguous vertebra above

in·ter·spi·nal ligament \ˌin-tər-ˈspīn-ᵊl-\ *n* : any of the thin membranous ligaments that connect the spinous processes of contiguous vertebrae — called also *interspinous ligament*

in·ter·stim·u·lus \-ˈstim-yə-ləs\ *adj* : of, relating to, or being the interval between the presentation of two discrete stimuli

in·ter·sti·tial \-ˈsti-shəl\ *adj* **1** : situated within but not restricted to or characteristic of a particular organ or tissue — used esp. of fibrous tissue **2** : affecting the interstitial tissues of an organ or part ⟨~ hepatitis⟩ **3** : occurring in the part of a fallopian tube in the wall of the uterus ⟨~ pregnancy⟩ — **in·ter·sti·tial·ly** *adv*

interstitial cell *n* : a cell situated between the germ cells of the gonads; *esp* : LEYDIG CELL

interstitial cell of Leydig *n* : LEYDIG CELL

interstitial–cell stimulating hormone *n* : LUTEINIZING HORMONE

interstitial cystitis *n* : a chronic idiopathic cystitis characterized by painful inflammation of the subepithelial connective tissue and often accompanied by Hunner's ulcer

interstitial keratitis *n* : a chronic progressive keratitis of the corneal stroma often resulting in blindness and frequently associated with congenital syphilis

interstitial pneumonia *n* : any of several chronic lung diseases of unknown etiology that affect interstitial tissues of the lung

in·ter·sti·tium \ˌin-tər-ˈsti-shē-əm\ *n, pl* **-tia** \-ē-ə\ : interstitial tissue

in·ter·sub·ject \ˈin-tər-ˌsəb-jekt\ *adj* : occurring between subjects in an experiment ⟨~ variability⟩

in·ter·tar·sal \ˌin-tər-ˈtär-səl\ *adj* : situated, occurring, or performed between tarsal bones ⟨~ joint⟩

in·ter·trans·ver·sar·ii \-ˌtrans-vər-ˈser-ē-ˌī\ *n pl* : a series of small muscles connecting the transverse processes of contiguous vertebrae

in·ter·tri·go \-ˈtrī-ˌgō\ *n* : inflammation produced by chafing of adjacent areas of skin — **in·ter·trig·i·nous** \-ˈtri-jə-nəs\ *adj*

in·ter·tro·chan·ter·ic \-ˌtrō-kən-ˈter-ik, -ˌkan-\ *adj* : situated, performed, or occurring between trochanters ⟨~ fractures⟩

intertrochanteric line *n* : a line on the anterior surface of the femur that runs obliquely from the greater trochanter to the lesser trochanter

in·ter·tu·ber·cu·lar groove \ˌin-tər-tü-ˈbər-kyə-lər-, -tyü-\ *n* : BICIPITAL GROOVE

intertubercular line *n* : an imaginary line passing through the iliac crests of the hip bones that separates the umbilical and lumbar regions of the abdomen from the hypogastric and iliac regions

in·ter·ven·tion \ˌin-tər-ˈven-chən\ *n* : the act or fact or a means of interfering with the outcome or course esp. of a condition or process (as to prevent harm or improve functioning) — **in·ter·ven·tion·al** \-ˈven-chə-nəl\ *adj*

in·ter·ven·tric·u·lar \-ven-ˈtri-kyə-lər\ *adj* : situated between ventricles

interventricular foramen *n* : the opening from each lateral ventricle into the third ventricle of the brain — called also *foramen of Monro*

interventricular groove *n* : INTERVENTRICULAR SULCUS

interventricular septum *n* : the curved slanting wall that separates the right and left ventricles of the heart

interventricular sulcus *n* : either of the anterior and posterior grooves on the surface of the heart that lie over the interventricular septum and join at the apex

in·ter·ver·te·bral \ˌin-tər-ˈvər-tə-brəl, -(ˌ)vər-ˈtē-\ *adj* : situated between vertebrae — **in·ter·ver·te·bral·ly** *adv*

intervertebral disk *n* : any of the tough elastic disks that are interposed between the centra of adjoining vertebrae

intervertebral foramen *n* : any of the openings that give passage to the spinal nerves from the vertebral canal

in·tes·ti·nal \in-ˈtes-tən-ᵊl\ *adj* **1 a** : affecting or occurring in the intestine **b** : living in the intestine ⟨the ~ flora⟩ **2** : of, relating to, or being the intestine ⟨the ~ canal⟩ — **in·tes·ti·nal·ly** *adv*

intestinal artery *n* : any of 12 to 15 arteries that arise from the superior mesenteric artery and supply the jejunum and ileum

intestinal flu *n* : an acute usu. transitory attack of gastroenteritis that is marked by nausea, vomiting, diarrhea, and abdominal cramping and is typically caused by a virus (as the Norwalk virus) or a bacterium (as E. coli) — not usu. used technically

intestinal gland *n* : CRYPT OF LIEBERKÜHN

intestinal juice *n* : a fluid that is secreted in small quantities by the small intestine and contains various enzymes (as lipase and amylase) — called also *succus entericus*

intestinal lipodystrophy *n* : WHIPPLE'S DISEASE

in·tes·tine \in-ˈtes-tən\ *n* : the tubular portion of the digestive tract that lies posterior to the stomach from which it is separated by the pyloric sphincter and consists of a slender but long anterior part made up of the duodenum, jejunum, and ileum and a broader shorter posterior part made up of the cecum, colon, and rectum — often used in pl.; see LARGE INTESTINE, SMALL INTESTINE

in·ti·ma \ˈin-tə-mə\ *n, pl* **-mae** \-ˌmē, -ˌmī\ *or* **-mas** : the innermost coat of an organ (as a blood vessel) consisting usu. of an endothelial layer backed by connective tissue and elastic tissue — called also *tunica intima* — **in·ti·mal** \-məl\ *adj*

in·tol·er·ance \(ˌ)in-ˈtä-lə-rəns\ *n* **1** : lack of an ability to endure ⟨an ~ to light⟩ **2** : exceptional sensitivity (as to a drug); *specif* : inability to properly metabolize or absorb a substance ⟨glucose ~⟩ — **in·tol·er·ant** \-rənt\ *adj*

in·tox·i·cant \in-ˈtäk-si-kənt\ *n* : something that intoxicates; *esp* : an alcoholic drink — **intoxicant** *adj*

in·tox·i·cate \-sə-ˌkāt\ *vb* **-cat·ed; -cat·ing** **1** : POISON **2** : to excite or stupefy by alcohol or a drug esp. to the point where physical and mental control is markedly diminished

in·tox·i·cat·ed \-ˌkā-təd\ *adj* : affected by an intoxicant and esp. by alcohol

in·tox·i·ca·tion \in-ˌtäk-sə-ˈkā-shən\ *n* **1** : an abnormal state that is essentially a poisoning ⟨intestinal ~⟩ **2** : the condition of being drunk

in·tra- \ˌin-trə, -(ˌ)trä\ *prefix* **1 a** : within ⟨*intra*cerebellar⟩ **b** : during ⟨*intra*operative⟩ **c** : between layers of ⟨*intra*dermal⟩ **2** : INTRO- ⟨an *intra*muscular injection⟩

in·tra–ab·dom·i·nal \ˌin-trə-ab-ˈdä-mən-ᵊl\ *adj* : situated within, occurring within, or administered by entering the abdomen ⟨~ pressure⟩

in·tra–al·ve·o·lar \ˌin-trə-al-ˈvē-ə-lər\ *adj* : situated or occurring within an alveolus ⟨~ hemorrhage⟩

in·tra–am·ni·ot·ic \-ˌam-nē-ˈä-tik\ *adj* : situated within, occurring within, or administered by entering the amnion — **in·tra–am·ni·ot·i·cal·ly** *adv*

in·tra–aor·tic \-ā-ˈȯr-tik\ *adj* **1** : situated or occurring within the aorta **2** : of, relating to, or used in intra-aortic balloon counterpulsation

intra–aortic balloon counterpulsation *n* : counterpulsation in which cardiocirculatory assistance is provided by a balloon inserted in the thoracic aorta which is inflated during diastole and deflated just before systole

in·tra–ar·te·ri·al \-är-ˈtir-ē-əl\ *adj* : situated or occurring within, administered into, or involving entry by way of an artery ⟨an ~ catheter⟩ — **in·tra–ar·te·ri·al·ly** *adv*

in·tra–ar·tic·u·lar \-är-ˈti-kyə-lər\ *adj* : situated within, occurring within, or administered by entering a joint — **in·tra–ar·tic·u·lar·ly** *adv*

in·tra–atri·al \-ˈā-trē-əl\ *adj* : situated or occurring within an atrium esp. of the heart ⟨an ~ block⟩

in·tra·bron·chi·al \-ˈbräŋ-kē-əl\ *adj* : situated or occurring within the bronchial tubes ⟨~ foreign bodies⟩

in·tra·can·a·lic·u·lar \-ˌkan-ᵊl-ˈi-kyə-lər\ *adj* : situated or occurring within a canaliculus ⟨~ biliary stasis⟩

in·tra·cap·su·lar \-ˈkap-sə-lər\ *adj* **1** : situated or occurring within a capsule **2** *of a cataract operation* : involving removal of the entire lens and its capsule — compare EXTRACAPSULAR 2

in·tra·car·di·ac \-ˈkär-dē-ˌak\ *also* **in·tra·car·di·al** \-dē-əl\ *adj* : situated within, occurring within, introduced into, or involving entry into the heart

in·tra·ca·rot·id \-kə-ˈrä-təd\ *adj* : situated within, occurring within, or administered by entering a carotid artery

in·tra·cav·i·tary \-ˈka-və-ˌter-ē\ *adj* : situated or occurring within a body cavity; *esp* : of, relating to, or being treatment (as of cancer) characterized by the insertion of esp. radioactive substances in a cavity

in·tra·cel·lu·lar \-ˈsel-yə-lər\ *adj* : existing, occurring, or functioning within a cell — **in·tra·cel·lu·lar·ly** *adv*

in·tra·cer·e·bel·lar \-ˌser-ə-ˈbe-lər\ *adj* : situated or occurring within the cerebellum ⟨~ hematoma⟩

in·tra·ce·re·bral \-sə-ˈrē-brəl, -ˈser-ə-\ *adj* : situated within, occurring within, or administered by entering the cerebrum ⟨~ injections⟩ ⟨~ bleeding⟩ — **in·tra·ce·re·bral·ly** *adv*

intracerebral hemorrhage *n* : CEREBRAL HEMORRHAGE

in·tra·cis·ter·nal \-sis-ˈtər-nəl\ *adj* : situated within, occurring within, or administered by entering a cisterna — **in·tra·cis·ter·nal·ly** *adv*

in·tra·cor·ne·al \-ˈkȯr-nē-əl\ *adj* : occurring within, situated within, or implanted in the cornea ⟨an ~ lens⟩

in·tra·co·ro·nal \-ˈkȯr-ən-ᵊl, -ˈkär-; -kə-ˈrōn-\ *adj* : situated or made within the crown of a tooth

in·tra·cor·o·nary \-ˈkȯr-ə-ˌner-ē, -ˈkär-\ *adj* : situated within, occurring within, or administered by entering the heart ⟨~ pressure⟩

in·tra·cor·ti·cal \-ˈkȯr-ti-kəl\ *adj* : situated or occurring within a cortex and esp. the cerebral cortex ⟨~ injection⟩

in·tra·cra·ni·al \-ˈkrā-nē-əl\ *adj* : situated or occurring within the cranium ⟨~ pressure⟩; *also* : affecting or involving intracranial structures — **in·tra·cra·ni·al·ly** *adv*

intracranial hemorrhage *n* : bleeding from a ruptured blood vessel within the brain or in the space between the brain and the skull

in·trac·ta·ble \(ˌ)in-ˈtrak-tə-bəl\ *adj* **1** : not easily managed or controlled (as by antibiotics or psychotherapy) **2** : not easily relieved or cured ⟨~ pain⟩ — **in·trac·ta·bil·i·ty** \(ˌ)in-ˌtrak-tə-ˈbi-lə-tē\ *n*

in·tra·cu·ta·ne·ous \ˌin-trə-kyu̇-ˈtā-nē-əs, -(ˌ)trä-\ *adj* : INTRADERMAL ⟨~ lesions⟩ — **in·tra·cu·ta·ne·ous·ly** *adv*

intracutaneous test *n* : INTRADERMAL TEST

in·tra·cy·to·plas·mic \-ˌsī-tə-ˈplaz-mik\ *adj* : lying or occurring in the cytoplasm ⟨~ inclusions⟩
intracytoplasmic sperm injection *n* : injection of a single sperm into an egg that has been obtained from an ovary followed by transfer of the egg to an incubator where fertilization takes place and then by introduction of the fertilized egg into a female's uterus — abbr. *ICSI*
in·tra·der·mal \-ˈdər-məl\ *adj* : situated, occurring, or done within or between the layers of the skin; *also* : administered by entering the skin ⟨~ injections⟩ — **in·tra·der·mal·ly** *adv*
intradermal test *n* : a test for immunity or hypersensitivity made by injecting a minute amount of diluted antigen into the skin — called also *intracutaneous test;* compare PATCH TEST, PRICK TEST, SCRATCH TEST
in·tra·di·a·lyt·ic \-ˌdī-ə-ˈli-tik\ *adj* : occurring or carried out during hemodialysis ⟨~ hypotension⟩
in·tra·duc·tal \ˌin-trə-ˈdəkt-ᵊl\ *adj* : situated within, occurring within, or introduced into a duct ⟨~ carcinoma⟩
in·tra·du·o·de·nal \-ˌdü-ə-ˈdēn-ᵊl, -ˌdyü-, -ˈäd-ᵊn-əl\ *adj* : situated in or introduced into the duodenum
in·tra·du·ral \-ˈdu̇r-əl, -ˈdyu̇r-\ *adj* : situated, occurring, or performed within or between the membranes of the dura mater ⟨an ~ tumor⟩
in·tra·epi·der·mal \-ˌe-pə-ˈdər-məl\ *adj* : located or occurring within the epidermis ⟨~ nerve fibers⟩
in·tra·ep·i·the·li·al \-ˌe-pə-ˈthē-lē-əl\ *adj* : occurring in or situated among the cells of the epithelium — see PROSTATIC INTRAEPITHELIAL NEOPLASIA
in·tra·eryth·ro·cyt·ic \-i-ˌri-thrə-ˈsi-tik\ *adj* : situated or occurring within the red blood cells
in·tra·esoph·a·ge·al \-i-ˌsä-fə-ˈjē-əl\ *adj* : occurring within the esophagus
intrafallopian — see GAMETE INTRAFALLOPIAN TRANSFER, ZYGOTE INTRAFALLOPIAN TRANSFER
in·tra·fa·mil·ial \-fə-ˈmil-yəl\ *adj* : occurring within a family ⟨~ conflict⟩
in·tra·fol·lic·u·lar \-fə-ˈli-kyə-lər, -fä-\ *adj* : situated within a follicle
in·tra·fu·sal \-ˈfyü-zəl\ *adj* : situated within a muscle spindle ⟨~ muscle fibers⟩ — compare EXTRAFUSAL
in·tra·gas·tric \-ˈgas-trik\ *adj* : situated or occurring within the stomach
in·tra·gen·ic \-ˈje-nik\ *adj* : being or occurring within a gene
in·tra·he·pat·ic \-hi-ˈpa-tik\ *adj* : situated or occurring within or originating in the liver ⟨~ cholestasis⟩
in·tra·le·sion·al \-ˈlē-zhən-ᵊl\ *adj* : introduced into or performed within a lesion — **in·tra·le·sion·al·ly** *adv*
in·tra·lo·bar \-ˈlō-bər, -ˌbär\ *adj* : situated within a lobe
in·tra·lob·u·lar \-ˈlä-byə-lər\ *adj* : situated or occurring within a lobule (as of the liver, pancreas, or lung)
intralobular vein *n* : CENTRAL VEIN
in·tra·lu·mi·nal \-ˈlü-mən-ᵊl\ *adj* : situated within, occurring within, or introduced into the lumen
in·tra·mam·ma·ry \-ˈma-mə-rē\ *adj* : situated or introduced within the mammary tissue ⟨an ~ infusion⟩
in·tra·med·ul·lary \-ˈmed-ᵊl-ˌer-ē, -ˈmej-ᵊl-; -mə-ˈdə-lə-rē\ *adj* : situated or occurring within a medulla; *esp* : involving use of the marrow space of a bone for support ⟨~ pinning of a fracture⟩
in·tra·mem·brane \-ˈmem-ˌbrān\ *adj* : INTRAMEMBRANOUS 2
in·tra·mem·bra·nous \-ˈmem-brə-nəs\ *adj* **1** : relating to, formed by, or being ossification of a membrane ⟨~ bone development⟩ **2** : situated within a membrane
in·tra·mi·to·chon·dri·al \-ˌmī-tə-ˈkän-drē-əl\ *adj* : situated or occurring within mitochondria ⟨~ inclusions⟩
in·tra·mu·co·sal \-myü-ˈkō-zəl\ *adj* : situated within, occurring within, or administered by entering a mucous membrane ⟨~ gastric carcinoma⟩
in·tra·mu·ral \-ˈmyu̇r-əl\ *adj* : situated or occurring within the substance of the walls of an organ ⟨~ infarction⟩
in·tra·mus·cu·lar \-ˈməs-kyə-lər\ *adj* : situated within, occurring within, or administered by entering a muscle — **in·tra·mus·cu·lar·ly** *adv*
in·tra·myo·car·di·al \-ˌmī-ə-ˈkär-dē-əl\ *adj* : situated within, occurring within, or administered by entering the myocardium ⟨an ~ injection⟩
in·tra·na·sal \-ˈnā-zəl\ *adj* : lying within or administered by way of the nasal structures ⟨~ corticosteroids⟩ — **in·tra·na·sal·ly** *adv*
in·tra·neu·ral \-ˈnu̇r-əl, -ˈnyu̇r-\ *adj* : situated within, occurring within, or administered by entering a nerve or nervous tissue — **in·tra·neu·ral·ly** *adv*
in·tra·neu·ro·nal \-ˈnu̇r-ən-ᵊl, -ˈnyu̇r-; -nu̇-ˈrōn-ᵊl, -nyu̇-\ *adj* : situated or occurring within a neuron
in·tra·nu·cle·ar \-ˈnü-klē-ər, -ˈnyü-\ *adj* : situated or occurring within a nucleus ⟨cells with ~ inclusions⟩
in·tra·oc·u·lar \ˌin-trə-ˈä-kyə-lər\ *adj* : implanted in, occurring within, or administered by entering the eyeball — **in·tra·oc·u·lar·ly** *adv*
intraocular pressure *n* : the pressure within the eyeball that gives it a round firm shape and is caused by the aqueous humor and vitreous body — called also *intraocular tension*
in·tra·op·er·a·tive \ˌin-trə-ˈä-pə-rə-tiv\ *adj* : occurring, carried out, or encountered in the course of surgery ⟨~ irradiation⟩ ⟨~ infarction⟩ — **in·tra·op·er·a·tive·ly** *adv*
in·tra·oral \-ˈōr-əl, -ˈär-\ *adj* : situated, occurring, or performed within the mouth ⟨~ ulcerations⟩

in·tra·os·se·ous \-ˈä-sē-əs\ *adj* : situated within, occurring within, or administered by entering a bone

in·tra·ovar·i·an \-ō-ˈvar-ē-ən\ *adj* : situated or occurring within the ovary

in·tra·ovu·lar \-ˈä-vyə-lər, -ˈō-\ *adj* : situated or occurring within the ovum

in·tra·pan·cre·at·ic \-ˌpaŋ-krē-ˈa-tik, -ˌpan-\ *adj* : situated or occurring within the pancreas

in·tra·pa·ren·chy·mal \-pə-ˈreŋ-kə-məl, -ˌpar-ən-ˈkī-\ *adj* : situated or occurring within the parenchyma of an organ

in·tra·par·tum \-ˈpär-təm\ *adj* : occurring or provided during the act of birth ⟨~ fetal monitoring⟩ ⟨~ care⟩

in·tra·pel·vic \-ˈpel-vik\ *adj* : situated or performed within the pelvis

in·tra·peri·car·di·al \-ˌper-ə-ˈkär-dē-əl\ *adj* : situated within or administered by entering the pericardium

in·tra·per·i·to·ne·al \ˌin-trə-ˌper-ət-ᵊn-ˈē-əl\ *adj* : situated within or administered by entering the peritoneum — **in·tra·per·i·to·ne·al·ly** *adv*

in·tra·pleu·ral \-ˈplu̇r-əl\ *adj* : situated within, occurring within, or administered by entering the pleura or pleural cavity — **in·tra·pleu·ral·ly** *adv*

intrapleural pneumonolysis *n* : PNEUMONOLYSIS b

in·tra·psy·chic \ˌin-trə-ˈsī-kik\ *adj* : being or occurring within the psyche, mind, or personality

in·tra·pul·mo·nary \-ˈpu̇l-mə-ˌner-ē, -ˈpəl-\ *also* **in·tra·pul·mon·ic** \-pu̇l-ˈmä-nik, -pəl-\ *adj* : situated within, occurring within, or administered by entering the lungs — **in·tra·pul·mo·nar·i·ly** \-ˌpu̇l-mə-ˈner-ə-ˌlē\ *adv*

in·tra·rec·tal \-ˈrekt-ᵊl\ *adj* : situated within, occurring within, or administered by entering the rectum

in·tra·re·nal \-ˈrēn-ᵊl\ *adj* : situated within, occurring within, or administered by entering the kidney — **in·tra·re·nal·ly** *adv*

in·tra·ret·i·nal \-ˈret-ᵊn-əl\ *adj* : situated or occurring within the retina

in·tra·scro·tal \-ˈskrōt-ᵊl\ *adj* : situated or occurring within the scrotum

in·tra·spi·nal \-ˈspī-nᵊl\ *adj* : situated within, occurring within, or introduced into the spinal column and esp. the vertebral canal ⟨~ nerve terminals⟩

in·tra·splen·ic \-ˈsple-nik\ *adj* : situated within or introduced into the spleen — **in·tra·splen·i·cal·ly** *adv*

in·tra·tes·tic·u·lar \-tes-ˈti-kyə-lər\ *adj* : situated within, performed within, or administered into a testis — **in·tra·tes·tic·u·lar·ly** *adv*

in·tra·the·cal \-ˈthē-kəl\ *adj* : introduced into or occurring in the space under the arachnoid membrane of the brain or spinal cord — **in·tra·the·cal·ly** *adv*

in·tra·tho·rac·ic \-thə-ˈra-sik\ *adj* : situated, occurring, or performed within the thorax ⟨~ pressure⟩

in·tra·thy·roi·dal \-thī-ˈroid-ᵊl\ *adj* : situated or occurring within the thyroid

in·tra·tra·che·al \-ˈtrā-kē-əl\ *adj* : occurring within or introduced into the trachea — **in·tra·tra·che·al·ly** *adv*

in·tra·ure·thral \-yu̇-ˈrē-thrəl\ *adj* : situated within, introduced into, or done in the urethra

in·tra·uter·ine \-ˈyü-tə-rən, -ˌrīn\ *adj* : of, situated in, used in, or occurring within the uterus; *also* : involving or occurring during the part of development that takes place in the uterus

intrauterine contraceptive device *n* : INTRAUTERINE DEVICE

intrauterine device *n* : a usu. T-shaped plastic device inserted into and left in the uterus for an extended time to prevent effective conception — called also *IUCD, IUD*

in·tra·vag·i·nal \-ˈva-jən-ᵊl\ *adj* : situated within, occurring within, or introduced into the vagina — **in·tra·vag·i·nal·ly** *adv*

in·trav·a·sa·tion \in-ˌtra-və-ˈsā-shən\ *n* : the entrance of foreign matter into a vessel of the body and esp. a blood vessel

in·tra·vas·cu·lar \ˌin-trə-ˈvas-kyə-lər\ *adj* : situated in, occurring in, or administered by entry into a blood vessel — **in·tra·vas·cu·lar·ly** *adv*

in·tra·ve·nous \ˌin-trə-ˈvē-nəs\ *adj* **1** : situated within, performed within, occurring within, or administered by entering a vein ⟨an ~ feeding⟩ **2** : used in intravenous procedures ⟨an ~ needle⟩ — **in·tra·ve·nous·ly** *adv*

intravenous pyelogram *n* : a pyelogram in which radiographic visualization is obtained after intravenous administration of a radiopaque medium which collects in the kidneys

in·tra·ven·tric·u·lar \ˌin-trə-ven-ˈtri-kyə-lər\ *adj* : situated within, occurring within, or administered into a ventricle — **in·tra·ven·tric·u·lar·ly** *adv*

in·tra·ver·te·bral \-(ˌ)vər-ˈtē-brəl, -ˈvər-tə-\ *adj* : situated or occurring within a vertebra

in·tra·ves·i·cal \-ˈve-si-kəl\ *adj* : situated or occurring within the bladder

in·tra·vi·tal \-ˈvīt-ᵊl\ *adj* **1** : performed upon or found in a living subject **2** : having or utilizing the property of staining cells without killing them — compare SUPRAVITAL — **in·tra·vi·tal·ly** *adv*

in·tra·vi·tam \-ˈvī-ˌtam, -ˈwē-ˌtäm\ *adj* : INTRAVITAL

in·tra·vit·re·al \-ˈvi-trē-əl\ *adj* : INTRAVITREOUS ⟨~ injection⟩

in·tra·vit·re·ous \-trē-əs\ *adj* : situated within, occurring within, or introduced into the vitreous body ⟨~ hemorrhage⟩

in·trin·sic \in-ˈtrin-zik, -sik\ *adj* **1** : originating or due to causes or factors within a body, organ, or part ⟨~ asthma⟩ **2** : originating and included wholly within an organ or part ⟨~ muscles⟩ — compare EXTRINSIC 2

intrinsic factor *n* : a substance produced by the normal gastrointestinal mucosa that facilitates absorption of vitamin B_{12}

intro- *prefix* **1** : in : into ⟨*intro*jection⟩ **2** : inward : within ⟨*intro*vert⟩ — compare EXTRO-

in•troi•tus \in-ˈtrō-ə-təs\ *n, pl* **introitus** : the vaginal opening — **in•troi•tal** \in-ˈtrō-ət-ᵊl\ *adj*

in•tro•ject \ˌin-trə-ˈjekt\ *vb* **1** : to incorporate (attitudes or ideas) into one's personality unconsciously **2** : to turn toward oneself (the love felt for another) or against oneself (the hostility felt toward another) — **in•tro•jec•tion** \-ˈjek-shən\ *n*

in•tro•mis•sion \ˌin-trə-ˈmi-shən\ *n* : the insertion or period of insertion of the penis in the vagina in copulation

in•tron \ˈin-ˌträn\ *n* : a polynucleotide sequence in a nucleic acid that does not code information for protein synthesis and is removed before translation of messenger RNA — compare EXON — **in•tron•ic** \-ˈträ-nik\ *adj*

In•tro•pin \ˈin-trə-ˌpin\ *trademark* — used for a preparation of the hydrochloride of dopamine

in•tro•spec•tion \ˌin-trə-ˈspek-shən\ *n* : an examination of one's own thoughts and feelings — **in•tro•spec•tive** \-tiv\ *adj*

in•tro•ver•sion \ˌin-trə-ˈvər-zhən, -shən\ *n* **1** : the act of directing one's attention toward or getting gratification from one's own interests, thoughts, and feelings **2** : the state or tendency toward being wholly or predominantly concerned with and interested in one's own mental life — compare EXTROVERSION

in•tro•vert \ˈin-trə-ˌvərt\ *n* : one whose attention and interests are directed toward one's own thoughts and feelings : one characterized by introversion; *broadly* : a reserved or shy person — compare EXTROVERT — **in•tro•vert•ed** \ˈin-trə-ˌvər-təd\ *also* **in•tro•vert** \ˈin-trə-ˌvərt\ *adj*

in•tu•ba•tion \ˌin-tü-ˈbā-shən, -tyü-\ *n* : the introduction of a tube into a hollow organ (as the trachea or intestine) to keep it open or restore its patency if obstructed — compare EXTUBATION — **in•tu•bate** \ˈin-tü-ˌbāt, -tyü-\ *vb*

in•tu•mes•cence \ˌin-tu̇-ˈmes-ᵊns, -tyu̇-\ *n* **1 a** : the action or process of becoming enlarged or swollen **b** : the state of being swollen **2** : something (as a tumor) that is swollen or enlarged

In•tu•niv \in-ˈtü-niv\ *trademark* — used for a preparation of guanfacine

in•tus•sus•cep•tion \ˌin-tə-sə-ˈsep-shən\ *n* : INVAGINATION; *esp* : the slipping of a length of intestine into an adjacent portion usu. producing obstruction — **in•tus•sus•cept** \ˌin-tə-sə-ˈsept\ *vb*

in•u•lin \ˈin-yə-lən\ *n* : a white mildly sweet plant polysaccharide that is used as a source of levulose, as a diagnostic agent in a test for kidney function, and as an additive in low-fat and low-sugar processed foods

in•unc•tion \i-ˈnəŋk-shən\ *n* **1** : the rubbing of an ointment into the skin for therapeutic purposes **2** : OINTMENT, UNGUENT

in utero \in-ˈyü-tə-ˌrō\ *adv or adj* : in the uterus : before birth

in•vade \in-ˈvād\ *vb* **in•vad•ed; in•vad•ing** **1** : to enter and spread within either normally (as in development) or abnormally (as in infection) often with harmful effects **2** : to affect injuriously and progressively

in•vag•i•na•tion \in-ˌva-jə-ˈnā-shən\ *n* **1** : an act or process of folding in so that an outer surface becomes an inner surface: as **a** : the formation of a gastrula by an infolding of part of the wall of the blastula **b** : intestinal intussusception **2** : an invaginated part — **in•vag•i•nate** \in-ˈva-jə-ˌnāt\ *vb*

[1]**in•va•lid** \ˈin-və-ləd\ *adj* **1** : suffering from disease or disability : SICKLY **2** : of, relating to, or suited to one that is sick ⟨an ~ chair⟩

[2]**invalid** *n* : one that is sickly or disabled

[3]**in•va•lid** \ˈin-və-ləd, -ˌlid\ *vb* **1** : to remove from active duty by reason of sickness or disability **2** : to make sickly or disabled

in•va•lid•ism \ˈin-və-lə-ˌdi-zəm\ *n* : a chronic condition of being an invalid

in•va•sion \in-ˈvā-zhən\ *n* : the act of invading: as **a** : the penetration of the body of a host by a microorganism **b** : the spread and multiplication of a pathogenic microorganism or of malignant cells in the body of a host

in•va•sive \-siv, -ziv\ *adj* **1** : tending to spread; *esp* : tending to invade healthy tissue ⟨~ cancer cells⟩ **2** : involving entry into the living body (as by incision or by insertion of an instrument) ⟨~ diagnostic techniques⟩ — **in•va•sive•ness** *n*

in•ven•to•ry \ˈin-vən-ˌtōr-ē\ *n, pl* **-ries** **1** : a questionnaire designed to provide an index of individual interests or personality traits **2** : a list of traits, preferences, attitudes, interests, or abilities that is used in evaluating personal characteristics or skills

in•ver•sion \in-ˈvər-zhən, -shən\ *n* **1** : a reversal of position, order, form, or relationship: as **a** : a dislocation of a bodily structure in which it is turned partially or wholly inside out ⟨~ of the uterus⟩ **b** : the condition (as of the foot) of being turned or rotated inward — compare EVERSION 2 **c** : a breaking off of a chromosome section and its subsequent reattachment in inverted position; *also* : a chromosomal section that has undergone this process **2** : HOMOSEXUALITY — **in•vert** \in-ˈvərt\ *vb*

inversus — see SITUS INVERSUS

in•vert•ase \in-ˈvər-ˌtās, ˈin-vər-, -ˌtāz\ *n* : an enzyme found in many microorganisms and plants and in animal intestines that catalyzes the hydrolysis of sucrose — called also *saccharase, sucrase*

[1]**in•ver•te•brate** \(ˌ)in-ˈvər-tə-brət, -ˌbrāt\ *n* : an animal having no backbone or internal skeleton

[2]**invertebrate** *adj* : lacking a spinal column; *also* : of or relating to invertebrate animals

in•vest \in-ˈvest\ *vb* : to envelop or cover completely ⟨the pleura ~*s* the lung⟩

in•ves•ti•ga•tion•al new drug \in-ˌves-ti-ˈgā-shə-nəl-\ *n* : a drug that has not been approved for general use by the Food and Drug Administration but is under investigation in clinical trials regarding its safety and effectiveness first by clinical investigators and then by practicing physicians using patients who have given informed consent to participate — abbr. *IND;* called also *investigational drug*

in•vest•ment \-mənt\ *n* : an external covering of a cell, part, or organism

in•vi•a•ble \(ˌ)in-ˈvī-ə-bəl\ *adj* : incapable of surviving esp. because of a deleterious genetic constitution — **in•vi•a•bil•i•ty** \-ˌvī-ə-ˈbi-lə-tē\ *n*

in vi•tro \in-ˈvē-(ˌ)trō, -ˈvi-\ *adv or adj* : outside the living body and in an artificial environment

in vitro fertilization *n* : mixture usu. in a laboratory dish of sperm with eggs which have been obtained from an ovary that is followed by transfer of one or more of the resulting fertilized eggs into the uterus — abbr. *IVF*

in vi•vo \in-ˈvē-(ˌ)vō\ *adv or adj* **1** : in the living body of a plant or animal **2** : in a real-life situation

In•vo•ka•met \in-ˈvō-kə-ˌmet\ *trademark* — used for a preparation containing canagliflozin and metformin

In•vo•ka•na \ˌin-vō-ˈkä-nə\ *trademark* — used for a preparation of canagliflozin

in•vo•lu•crum \ˌin-və-ˈlü-krəm\ *n, pl* **-cra** \-krə\ : a formation of new bone about a sequestrum (as in osteomyelitis)

in•vol•un•tary \(ˌ)in-ˈvä-lən-ˌter-ē\ *adj* : not subject to control of the will : REFLEX ⟨~ contractions⟩

involuntary muscle *n* : muscle governing reflex functions and not under direct voluntary control; *esp* : SMOOTH MUSCLE

in•vo•lute \ˌin-və-ˈlüt\ *vb* **-lut•ed; -lut•ing 1** : to return to a former condition **2** : to become cleared up

in•vo•lu•tion \ˌin-və-ˈlü-shən\ *n* **1 a** : an inward curvature or penetration **b** : the formation of a gastrula by ingrowth of cells formed at the dorsal lip **2** : a shrinking or return to a former size ⟨~ of the uterus after pregnancy⟩ **3** : the regressive alterations of a body or its parts characteristic of the aging process; *specif* : decline marked by a decrease of bodily vigor and in women by menopause

in•vo•lu•tion•al \ˌin-və-ˈlü-shə-nəl\ *adj* **1** : of or relating to involutional melancholia **2** : of or relating to the climacterium and its associated bodily and mental changes

involutional melancholia *n* : agitated depression occurring at about the time of menopause or andropause — called also *involutional psychosis*

in•volve \in-ˈvälv, -ˈvȯlv\ *vb* **in•volved; in•volv•ing** : to affect with a disease or condition : include in an area of damage, trauma, or insult ⟨herpes *involved* the trigeminal nerve⟩ — **in•volve•ment** \-mənt\ *n*

Iod•amoe•ba \(ˌ)ī-ˌō-də-ˈmē-bə\ *n* : a genus of amoebas including one (*I. butschlii*) commensal in the intestine of mammals including humans

io•dide \ˈī-ə-ˌdīd\ *n* : a compound of iodine usu. with a more electrically positive element or radical

io•dine \ˈī-ə-ˌdīn, -dən, -ˌdēn\ *n* **1** : a nonmetallic halogen element used in medicine (as in antisepsis and in the treatment of goiter) — symbol *I;* see ELEMENT table **2** : a tincture of iodine used esp. as a topical antiseptic

iodine–131 *n* : a heavy radioactive isotope of iodine that has the mass number 131 and a half-life of eight days, gives off beta and gamma rays, and is used esp. in the form of its sodium salt in the diagnosis of thyroid disease and the treatment of goiter

iodine–125 *n* : a light radioactive isotope of iodine that has a mass number of 125 and a half-life of 60 days, gives off soft gamma rays, and is used as a tracer in thyroid studies and as therapy in hyperthyroidism

io•dip•amide \ˌī-ə-ˈdi-pə-ˌmīd\ *n* : a radiopaque substance $C_{20}H_{14}I_6N_2O_6$ used as the sodium or meglumine salts esp. in cholecystography

io•dism \ˈī-ə-ˌdi-zəm\ *n* : an abnormal local and systemic condition resulting from overdosage with, prolonged use of, or sensitivity to iodine or iodine compounds and marked by hypersalivation, coryza, frontal headache, emaciation, and skin eruptions

io•dize \ˈī-ə-ˌdīz\ *vb* **io•dized; io•diz•ing** : to treat with iodine or an iodide ⟨*iodized* salt⟩

io•do•chlor•hy•droxy•quin \ī-ˌō-də-ˌklōr-hi-ˈdräk-sē-ˌkwin, ī-ˌä-də-\ *n* : an antimicrobial and mildly irritant drug C_9H_5ClINO formerly used esp. as an antidiarrheal but now used mainly as an antiseptic

io•do•de•oxy•uri•dine \ī-ˌō-də-ˌdē-ˌäk-sē-ˈyu̇r-ə-ˌdēn\ *or* **5–io•do•de•oxy•uri•dine** \ˌfīv-\ *n* : IDOXURIDINE

io•do•form \ī-ˈō-də-ˌfȯrm, -ˈä-\ *n* : a yellow crystalline volatile compound CHI_3 used as an antiseptic dressing

io•do•hip•pur•ate sodium \ī-ˌō-də-ˈhi-pyə-ˌrāt-, ī-ˌä-, -hi-ˈpyu̇r-ˌāt-\ *n* : HIPPURAN

io·do·phor \ī-ˈō-də-ˌfȯr, ī-ˈä-\ *n* : a complex of iodine and a surface-active agent that releases iodine gradually and serves as a disinfectant

io·dop·sin \ˌī-ə-ˈdäp-sən\ *n* : a photosensitive violet pigment in the retinal cones that is similar to rhodopsin but more labile, is formed from vitamin A, and is important in photopic vision

io·do·pyr·a·cet \ī-ˌō-də-ˈpir-ə-ˌset, ī-ˌä-\ *n* : a salt $C_8H_{19}I_2N_2O_3$ used as a radiopaque medium esp. in urography

io·do·quin·ol \ī-ˌō-də-ˈkwi-ˌnȯl, -ˌä-, -ˌnōl\ *n* : a drug $C_9H_5I_2NO$ used esp. in the treatment of amebic dysentery — called also *diiodohydroxyquin, diiodohydroxyquinoline*

IOM *abbr* Institute of Medicine

ion \ˈī-ˌän, ˈī-ən\ *n* : an electrically charged particle, atom, or group of atoms — **ion·ic** \ī-ˈä-nik\ *adj* — **ion·i·cal·ly** *adv*

ion channel *n* : a cell membrane channel that is selectively permeable to certain ions (as of calcium or sodium)

ion·ize \ˈī-ə-ˌnīz\ *vb* **ion·ized; ion·iz·ing 1** : to convert wholly or partly into ions **2** : to become ionized — **ion·iz·able** \ˌī-ə-ˈnī-zə-bəl\ *adj* — **ion·iza·tion** \ˌī-ə-nə-ˈzā-shən\ *n*

ion·o·phore \ī-ˈä-nə-ˌfōr\ *n* : a compound that facilitates transmission of an ion (as of calcium) across a lipid barrier (as in a cell membrane) by combining with the ion or by increasing the permeability of the barrier to it — **io·noph·or·ous** \ī-ə-ˈnä-fə-rəs\ *adj*

ion·to·pho·re·sis \(ˌ)ī-ˌän-tə-fə-ˈrē-səs\ *n, pl* **-re·ses** \-ˌsēz\ : the introduction of an ionized substance (as a drug) through intact skin by the application of a direct electric current — **ion·to·pho·ret·ic** \-ˈre-tik\ *adj* — **ion·to·pho·ret·i·cal·ly** *adv*

io·pa·no·ic acid \ˌī-ə-pə-ˈnō-ik-\ *n* : a crystalline powder $C_{11}H_{12}I_3NO_2$ used as a radiopaque medium in cholecystography

io·phen·dyl·ate \ˌī-ə-ˈfen-də-ˌlāt\ *n* : a radiopaque liquid $C_{19}H_{29}IO_2$ used esp. in myelography

io·thal·a·mate \ˌī-ə-ˈtha-lə-ˌmāt\ *n* : any of several salts of iothalamic acid that are administered by injection as radiopaque media

io·tha·lam·ic acid \ˌī-ə-thə-ˈla-mik-\ *n* : a white odorless powder $C_{11}H_9I_3N_2O_4$ used as a radiopaque medium

IP *abbr* intraperitoneal; intraperitoneally

IPA *abbr* independent practice association; individual practice association

ip·e·cac \ˈi-pi-ˌkak\ *also* **ipe·ca·cu·a·nha** \ˌi-pi-ˌka-kü-ˈa-nə\ *n* **1** : the dried rhizome and roots of either of two tropical American plants (*Cephaelis acuminata* and *C. ipecacuanha*) of the madder family (Rubiaceae) used esp. as a source of emetine **2** : an emetic and expectorant preparation of ipecac; *esp* : IPECAC SYRUP

ipecac syrup *n* : an emetic and expectorant liquid preparation that is used to induce vomiting in accidental poisoning and is prepared by extracting the ether-soluble alkaloids from powdered ipecac and mixing them with glycerol and a syrup — called also *syrup of ipecac*

ipo·date \ˈī-pə-ˌdāt\ *n* : a compound $C_{12}H_{13}I_3N_2O_2$ that is administered as the sodium or calcium salt for use as a radiopaque medium in cholecystography and cholangiography

IPPB *abbr* intermittent positive pressure breathing

ip·ra·tro·pi·um bromide \ˌi-prə-ˌtrō-pē-əm-\ *n* : an anticholinergic drug $C_{20}H_{30}BrNO_3{\cdot}H_2O$ used as an inhalational aerosol for bronchodilation esp. in the treatment of chronic obstructive pulmonary disease and as a nasal spray in the treatment of runny nose associated with rhinitis — see ATROVENT, COMBIVENT

ipri·fla·vone \ˌī-pri-ˈflā-ˌvōn\ *n* : a semisynthetic isoflavone $C_{18}H_{16}O_3$ used to prevent postmenopausal bone loss

ipro·ni·a·zid \ˌī-prə-ˈnī-ə-zəd\ *n* : a derivative $C_9H_{13}N_3O$ of isoniazid that is a monoamine oxidase inhibitor used as an antidepressant and formerly used in treating tuberculosis

IPSID *abbr* immunoproliferative small intestinal disease

ip·si·lat·er·al \ˌip-si-ˈla-tə-rəl\ *adj* : situated or appearing on or affecting the same side of the body — compare CONTRALATERAL — **ip·si·lat·er·al·ly** *adv*

IPSP *abbr* inhibitory postsynaptic potential

IPT *abbr* interpersonal psychotherapy; interpersonal therapy

IQ \ˌī-ˈkyü\ *n* [*i*ntelligence *q*uotient] : a number used to express the apparent relative intelligence of a person: as **a** : the ratio of the mental age (as reported on a standardized test) to the chronological age multiplied by 100 **b** : a score determined by one's performance on a standardized intelligence test relative to the average performance of others of the same age

Ir *symbol* iridium

IR *abbr* infrared

ir- — see IN-

ir·be·sar·tan \ˌər-bə-ˈsär-tᵊn\ *n* : an antihypertensive drug $C_{25}H_{28}N_6O$ that is taken orally and blocks the action of angiotensin II — see AVAPRO

irid- *or* **irido-** *comb form* **1** : iris of the eye ⟨*irid*ectomy⟩ **2** : iris and ⟨*irido*cyclitis⟩

iri·dec·to·my \ˌir-ə-ˈdek-tə-mē, ˌīr-\ *n, pl* **-mies** : the surgical removal of part of the iris of the eye

iri·den·clei·sis \ˌir-ə-den-ˈklī-səs, ˌīr-\ *n, pl* **-clei·ses** \-ˌsēz\ : a surgical procedure esp. for relief of glaucoma in which a small portion of the iris is implanted in a corneal incision to facilitate drainage of aqueous humor

irides *pl of* IRIS

irid•ic \ī-ˈri-dik, i-\ *adj* : of or relating to the iris of the eye

iridis — see HETEROCHROMIA IRIDIS, RUBEOSIS IRIDIS

irid•i•um \ir-ˈi-dē-əm\ *n* : a silver-white brittle metallic element of the platinum group — symbol *Ir;* see ELEMENT table

iri•do•cy•cli•tis \ˌir-ə-dō-sī-ˈklī-təs, ˌīr-, -si-\ *n* : inflammation of the iris and the ciliary body

iri•do•di•al•y•sis \ˌir-ə-dō-dī-ˈa-lə-səs, ˌīr-\ *n, pl* **-y•ses** \-ˌsēz\ : separation of the iris from its attachments to the ciliary body

ir•i•dol•o•gy \ˌī-rə-ˈdä-lə-jē\ *n, pl* **-gies** : the study of the iris of the eye for indications of bodily health and disease — **ir•i•dol•o•gist** \-jist\ *n*

iri•do•ple•gia \ˌir-ə-dō-ˈplē-jə, ˌīr-, -jē-ə\ *n* : paralysis of the sphincter of the iris

iri•dot•o•my \ˌir-ə-ˈdä-tə-mē, ˌīr-\ *n, pl* **-mies** : incision of the iris

iris \ˈī-rəs\ *n, pl* **iris•es** *or* **iri•des** \ˈī-rə-ˌdēz, ˈir-ə-\ : the opaque muscular contractile diaphragm that is suspended in the aqueous humor in front of the lens of the eye, is perforated by the pupil and is continuous peripherally with the ciliary body, has a deeply pigmented posterior surface which excludes the entrance of light except through the pupil and a colored anterior surface which determines the color of the eyes

iris bom•bé \-ˌbäm-ˈbā\ *n* : a condition in which the iris is bowed forward by an accumulation of fluid between the iris and the lens

Irish moss *n* **1** : the dried and bleached plants of a red alga (esp. *Chondrus crispus*) used as an agent for thickening or emulsifying or as a demulcent **2** : a red alga (esp. *Chondrus crispus*) that is a source of Irish moss

iri•tis \ī-ˈrī-təs\ *n* : inflammation of the iris of the eye

iron \ˈīrn, ˈī-ərn\ *n* **1** : a heavy malleable ductile magnetic silver-white metallic element vital to biological processes (as in transport of oxygen in the body) — symbol *Fe;* see ELEMENT table **2** : iron chemically combined ⟨~ in the blood⟩ — **iron** *adj*

iron–deficiency anemia *n* : anemia that is caused by a deficiency of iron and characterized by hypochromic microcytic red blood cells

iron lung *n* : a device for artificial respiration in which rhythmic alternations in the air pressure in a chamber surrounding a patient's chest force air into and out of the lungs esp. when the nerves governing the chest muscles fail to function because of polio — called also *Drinker respirator*

ir•ra•di•ate \i-ˈrā-dē-ˌāt\ *vb* **-at•ed; -at•ing** : to affect or treat by radiant energy (as heat); *specif* : to treat by exposure to radiation (as ultraviolet light or gamma rays) — **ir•ra•di•a•tor** \-ā-tər\ *n*

ir•ra•di•a•tion \ir-ˌā-dē-ˈā-shən\ *n* **1** : the radiation of a physiologically active agent from a point of origin within the body; *esp* : the spread of a nerve impulse beyond the usual conduction path **2 a** : exposure to radiation (as X-rays or alpha particles) **b** : application of radiation (as X-rays or gamma rays) for therapeutic purposes or for sterilization (as of food)

ir•re•duc•ible \ˌir-i-ˈdü-sə-bəl, -ˈdyü-\ *adj* : impossible to bring into a desired or normal position or state ⟨an ~ hernia⟩

ir•reg•u•lar \i-ˈre-gyə-lər\ *adj* **1** : lacking perfect symmetry of form : not straight, smooth, even, or regular ⟨~ teeth⟩ **2 a** : lacking continuity or regularity of occurrence, activity, or function ⟨~ breathing⟩ **b** *of a physiological function* : failing to occur at regular or normal intervals **c** *of an individual* : failing to defecate at regular or normal intervals — **ir•reg•u•lar•ly** *adv*

ir•reg•u•lar•i•ty \i-ˌre-gyə-ˈlar-ə-tē\ *n, pl* **-ties** **1** : the quality or state of being irregular ⟨~ of breathing⟩ **2** : occasional constipation

ir•re•me•di•a•ble \ˌir-i-ˈmē-dē-ə-bəl\ *adj* : impossible to remedy or cure

ir•re•vers•ible \ˌir-i-ˈvər-sə-bəl\ *adj, of a pathological process* : of such severity that recovery is impossible ⟨~ brain damage⟩ — **ir•re•vers•ibil•i•ty** \-ˌvər-sə-ˈbi-lə-tē\ *n* — **ir•re•vers•ibly** \-ˈvər-sə-blē\ *adv*

ir•ri•gate \ˈir-ə-ˌgāt\ *vb* **-gat•ed; -gat•ing** : to flush (a body part) with a stream of liquid (as in removing a foreign body or medicating) — **ir•ri•ga•tion** \ˌir-ə-ˈgā-shən\ *n* — **ir•ri•ga•tor** \ˈir-ə-ˌgā-tər\ *n*

ir•ri•ta•bil•i•ty \ˌir-ə-tə-ˈbi-lə-tē\ *n, pl* **-ties** **1** : the property of protoplasm and of living organisms that permits them to react to stimuli **2 a** : quick excitability to annoyance, impatience, or anger **b** : abnormal or excessive excitability of an organ or part of the body (as the stomach or bladder) — **ir•ri•ta•ble** \ˈir-ə-tə-bəl\ *adj*

irritable bowel syndrome *n* : a chronic functional disorder of the colon that is of unknown etiology but is often associated with abnormal intestinal motility and increased sensitivity to visceral pain and that is characterized by diarrhea or constipation or diarrhea alternating with constipation, abdominal pain or discomfort, abdominal bloating, and passage of mucus in the stool — abbr. *IBS;* called also *irritable colon, irritable colon syndrome, mucous colitis, spastic colon*

ir·ri·tant \ˈir-ə-tənt\ *adj* : causing irritation; *specif* : tending to produce inflammation — **irritant** *n*

irritant contact dermatitis *n* : inflammation of the skin that follows direct contact of an irritant (as soap or acid) with the skin and is typically marked by a burning red rash often with dry scales, crusting, and pustules — compare ALLERGIC CONTACT DERMATITIS

ir·ri·tate \ˈir-ə-ˌtāt\ *vb* **-tat·ed; -tat·ing 1** : to provoke impatience, anger, or displeasure in **2** : to cause (an organ or tissue) to be irritable : produce irritation in **3** : to produce excitation in (as a nerve) : cause (as a muscle) to contract — **ir·ri·ta·tion** \ˌir-ə-ˈtā-shən\ *n*

ir·ri·ta·tive \ˈir-ə-ˌtā-tiv\ *adj* **1** : serving to excite : IRRITATING ⟨an ~ agent⟩ **2** : accompanied with or produced by irritation ⟨~ coughing⟩

is- *or* **iso-** *comb form* **1** : equal : homogeneous : uniform ⟨*is*osmotic⟩ **2** : for or from different individuals of the same species ⟨*iso*agglutinin⟩

isch·ae·mia *chiefly Brit var of* ISCHEMIA

isch·emia \is-ˈkē-mē-ə\ *n* : deficient supply of blood to a body part (as the heart or brain) that is due to obstruction of the inflow of arterial blood (as by the narrowing of arteries by spasm or disease) — **isch·emic** \-mik\ *adj* — **isch·emi·cal·ly** *adv*

ischemic stroke *n* : stroke caused by the narrowing or blockage of a blood vessel supplying the brain as a result of thrombosis or embolism — compare HEMORRHAGIC STROKE

ischi- *or* **ischio-** *comb form* **1** : ischium ⟨*ischi*ectomy⟩ **2** : ischial and ⟨*ischio*rectal⟩

ischia *pl of* ISCHIUM

is·chi·al \ˈis-kē-əl\ *adj* : of, relating to, or situated near the ischium

ischial spine *n* : a thin pointed triangular eminence that projects from the dorsal border of the ischium and gives attachment to the gemellus superior on its external surface and to the coccygeus, levator ani, and pelvic fascia on its internal surface

ischial tuberosity *n* : a bony swelling on the posterior part of the superior ramus of the ischium that gives attachment to various muscles and bears the weight of the body in sitting

is·chi·ec·to·my \ˌis-kē-ˈek-tə-mē\ *n, pl* **-mies** : surgical removal of a segment of the hip bone including the ischium

is·chio·cav·er·no·sus \ˌis-kē-ō-ˌka-vər-ˈnō-səs\ *n, pl* **-no·si** \-ˌsī\ : a muscle on each side that arises from the ischium near the crus of the penis or clitoris and is inserted on the crus near the pubic symphysis

is·chio·coc·cy·geus \-käk-ˈsi-jē-əs\ *n, pl* **-cy·gei** \-jē-ˌī, -ˌē\ : COCCYGEUS

is·chio·fem·o·ral \-ˈfe-mə-rəl\ *adj* : of, relating to, or being an accessory ligament of the hip joint passing from the ischium below the acetabulum to blend with the joint capsule

is·chio·pu·bic ramus \ˌis-kē-ō-ˈpyü-bik-\ *n* : the flattened inferior projection of the hip bone below the obturator foramen consisting of the united inferior rami of the pubis and ischium

is·chio·rec·tal \ˌis-kē-ō-ˈrekt-ᵊl\ *adj* : of, relating to, or adjacent to both ischium and rectum ⟨an ~ abscess⟩

is·chi·um \ˈis-kē-əm\ *n, pl* **is·chia** \-ə\ : the dorsal and posterior of the three principal bones composing either half of the pelvis consisting in humans of a thick portion, a large rough eminence on which the body rests when sitting, and a forwardly directed ramus which joins that of the pubis

Isen·tress \ī-ˈsen-ˌtres\ *trademark* — used for a preparation of raltegravir

Ishi·ha·ra \ˌi-shē-ˈhär-ə\ *adj* : of, relating to, or used in an Ishihara test

Ishihara, Shinobu (1879–1963), Japanese ophthalmologist.

Ishihara test *n* : a widely used test for color blindness that consists of a set of plates covered with colored dots which the test subject views in order to find a number composed of dots of one color which a person with various defects of color vision will confuse with surrounding dots of color

is·land \ˈī-lənd\ *n* : an isolated anatomical structure, tissue, or group of cells

island of Lang·er·hans \-ˈläŋ-ər-ˌhänz, -ˌhäns\ *n* : ISLET OF LANGERHANS

island of Reil \-ˈrīl\ *n* : INSULA

Reil, Johann Christian (1759–1813), German anatomist.

is·let \ˈī-lət\ *n* : ISLET OF LANGERHANS

islet amyloid polypeptide *n* : AMYLIN

islet cell *n* : one of the endocrine cells making up an islet of Langerhans

islet of Lang·er·hans \-ˈläŋ-ər-ˌhänz, -ˌhäns\ *n* : any of the groups of small slightly granular endocrine cells that form anastomosing trabeculae among the tubules and alveoli of the pancreas and secrete insulin and glucagon — called also *islet*

Langerhans, Paul (1847–1888), German pathologist.

-ism \ˌi-zəm\ *n suffix* **1** : act, practice, or process ⟨hypnot*ism*⟩ **2 a** : state, condition, or property ⟨polymorph*ism*⟩ **b** : abnormal state or condition resulting from excess of a (specified) thing or marked by resemblance to a (specified) person or thing ⟨alcohol*ism*⟩ ⟨morphin*ism*⟩

iso- — see IS-

iso·ag·glu·ti·na·tion \ˌī-(ˌ)sō-ə-ˌglüt-ᵊn-ˈā-shən\ *n* : agglutination of an agglutinogen of one individual by the serum of another of the same species

iso·ag·glu·ti·nin \-ə-ˈglüt-ᵊn-ən\ *n* : an antibody produced by one individual that causes agglutination of cells (as red blood cells) of other individuals of the same species

iso·ag·glu·tin·o·gen \-ˌa-glü-ˈti-nə-jən\ *n* : an antigenic substance capable of provoking formation of or reacting with an isoagglutinin

iso·al·lox·a·zine \-ə-ˈläk-sə-ˌzēn\ *n* : a yellow solid $C_{10}H_6N_4O_2$ that is the precursor of various flavins (as riboflavin)

iso·am·yl nitrite \ˌī-sō-ˈa-məl-\ *n* : AMYL NITRITE

iso·an·ti·body \ˌī-(ˌ)sō-ˈan-ti-ˌbä-dē\ *n, pl* **-bod·ies** : ALLOANTIBODY

iso·an·ti·gen \-ˈan-ti-jən\ *n* : ALLOANTIGEN

iso·bor·nyl thio·cyano·ace·tate \ˌī-sō-ˈbȯr-nil-ˌthī-ō-ˌsī-ə-nō-ˈa-sə-ˌtāt, -sī-ˌa-nō-\ *n* : a yellow oily liquid $C_{13}H_{19}N_2OS$ used as a pediculicide

iso·bu·tyl nitrite \ˌī-sō-ˈbyüt-ᵊl-\ *n* : BUTYL NITRITE

iso·car·box·az·id \-ˌkär-ˈbäk-sə-zəd\ *n* : a hydrazide monoamine oxidase inhibitor $C_{12}H_{13}N_3O_2$ used as an antidepressant — see MARPLAN

iso·chro·mo·some \-ˈkrō-mə-ˌsōm, -ˌzōm\ *n* : a chromosome produced by transverse splitting of the centromere so that both arms are from the same side of the centromere, are of equal length, and possess identical genes

iso·cit·rate \ˌī-sō-ˈsi-ˌtrāt\ *n* : any salt or ester of isocitric acid; *also* : ISOCITRIC ACID

isocitrate de·hy·dro·ge·nase \-ˌdē-(ˌ)hī-ˈdrä-je-ˌnās, -ˈhī-drə-jə-, -ˌnāz\ *n* : either of two enzymes which catalyze the oxidation of isocitric acid (as in the Krebs cycle) — called also *isocitric dehydrogenase*

iso·cit·ric acid \ˌī-sə-ˈsi-trik-\ *n* : a crystalline isomer of citric acid that occurs esp. as an intermediate stage in the Krebs cycle

isocitric dehydrogenase *n* : ISOCITRATE DEHYDROGENASE

iso·dose \ˈī-sə-ˌdōs\ *adj* : of or relating to points or zones in a medium that receive equal doses of radiation

iso·elec·tric \ˌī-sō-i-ˈlek-trik\ *adj* **1** : relating to or being a flat line on an electroencephalogram **2** : being the pH at which the electrolyte will not migrate in an electrical field ⟨the ~ point of a protein⟩

isoelectric focusing *n* : an electrophoretic technique for separating proteins by causing them to migrate under the influence of an electric field through a medium (as a gel) having a pH gradient to locations with pH values corresponding to their isoelectric points

iso·en·zyme \ˌī-sō-ˈen-ˌzīm\ *n* : any of two or more chemically distinct but functionally similar enzymes — called also *isozyme* — **iso·en·zy·mat·ic** \ˌī-sō-ˌen-zə-ˈma-tik, -zī-\ *adj* — **iso·en·zy·mic** \-en-ˈzī-mik\ *adj*

iso·eth·a·rine \-ˈe-thə-ˌrēn\ *n* : a beta-adrenergic bronchodilator administered by oral inhalation esp. in the form of its hydrochloride $C_{13}H_{21}NO_3 \cdot HCl$ to treat asthma and bronchospasm

iso·fla·vone \-ˈflā-ˌvōn\ *n* : a bioactive ketone $C_{15}H_{10}O_2$ having numerous derivatives that are found in plants (as the soybean) and have antioxidant and estrogenic activity; *also* : any of these derivatives (as genistein)

iso·fluro·phate \-ˈflu̇r-ə-ˌfāt\ *n* : a volatile irritating liquid ester $C_6H_{14}FO_3P$ that acts as a nerve gas by inhibiting cholinesterases and as a miotic and that is used chiefly in treating glaucoma — called also *DFP, diisopropyl fluorophosphate*

iso·form \ˈī-sə-ˌfȯrm\ *n* : any of two or more functionally similar proteins that have a similar but not identical amino acid sequence

iso·ge·ne·ic \ˌī-sō-jə-ˈnē-ik, -ˈnā-\ *adj* : SYNGENEIC ⟨an ~ graft⟩

iso·gen·ic \-ˈje-nik\ *adj* : characterized by essentially identical genes

iso·graft \ˈī-sə-ˌgraft\ *n* : a homograft between genetically identical or nearly identical individuals — **isograft** *vb*

iso·hem·ag·glu·ti·nin \-ˌhē-mə-ˈglüt-ᵊn-ən\ *n* : a hemagglutinin causing isoagglutination

iso·hy·dric shift \ˌī-sō-ˈhī-drik-\ *n* : the set of chemical reactions in a red blood cell by which oxygen is released to the tissues and carbon dioxide is taken up while the blood remains at constant pH

iso·im·mu·ni·za·tion \ˌī-sō-ˌi-myə-nə-ˈzā-shən\ *n* : production by an individual of antibodies against constituents of the tissues of another individual of the same species (as when transfused with blood from one belonging to a different blood group) — called also *alloimmunization*

[1]**iso·late** \ˈī-sə-ˌlāt\ *vb* **-lat·ed; -lat·ing** : to set apart from others: as **a** : to separate (one with a contagious disease) from others not similarly infected **b** : to separate (as a chemical compound) from all other substances : obtain pure or in a free state

[2]**iso·late** \ˈī-sə-lət, -ˌlāt\ *n* **1** : an individual (as a single organism), a viable part of an organism (as a cell), or a strain that has been isolated (as from diseased tissue); *also* : a pure culture produced from such an isolate **2** : a socially withdrawn individual

iso·la·tion \ˌī-sə-ˈlā-shən\ *n* **1** : the action of isolating or condition of being isolated **2** : a psychological defense mechanism consisting of the separating of ideas or memories from the emotions connected with them

Iso·lette \ˌī-sə-ˈlet\ *trademark* — used for an incubator for premature infants that provides controlled temperature and humidity and an oxygen supply

iso·leu·cine \ˌī-sō-ˈlü-ˌsēn\ *n* : a crystalline essential amino acid $C_6H_{13}NO_2$ isomeric with leucine — abbr. *Ile*

isol·o·gous \ī-ˈsä-lə-gəs\ *adj* : SYNGENEIC

iso·mer \ˈī-sə-mər\ *n* : any of two or more compounds, radicals, or ions that contain the same number of atoms of the same elements but differ in structural arrangement and properties — **iso·mer·ic** \ˌī-sə-ˈmer-ik\ *adj* — **isom·er·ism** \ī-ˈsä-mə-ˌri-zəm\ *n*

iso·me·thep·tene \ˌī-sō-me-ˈthep-ˌtēn\ *n* : a vasoconstrictive and antispasmodic drug administered esp. in the form of its mucate $C_{24}H_{48}N_2O_8$

iso·met·ric \ˌī-sə-ˈme-trik\ *adj* : of, relating to, involving, or being muscular contraction (as in isometrics) against resistance, without significant change of length of muscle fibers, and with marked increase in muscle tone — compare ISOTONIC 2 — **iso·met·ri·cal·ly** *adv*

iso·met·rics \ˌī-sə-ˈme-triks\ *n sing or pl* : isometric exercise or an isometric system of exercises

iso·ni·a·zid \ˌī-sə-ˈnī-ə-zəd\ *n* : a crystalline compound $C_6H_7N_3O$ used in treating tuberculosis

isonicotinic acid hydrazide *n* : ISONIAZID

iso·nip·e·caine \ˌī-sō-ˈni-pə-ˌkān\ *n* : MEPERIDINE

iso·os·mot·ic \ˌī-sō-äz-ˈmä-tik\ *adj* : ISOTONIC 1

Iso·paque \ˌī-sō-ˈpāk\ *trademark* — used for a preparation of metrizoate sodium

iso·peri·stal·tic \ˌī-sō-ˌper-ə-ˈstȯl-tik, -ˈstäl-, -ˈstal-\ *adj* : performed or arranged so that the grafted or anastomosed parts exhibit peristalsis in the same direction ⟨~ gastroenterostomy⟩ — **iso·peri·stal·ti·cal·ly** *adv*

iso·phane insulin \ˈī-sō-ˌfān-\ *n* : a crystalline suspension of insulin, protamine, and zinc in a buffered aqueous solution that is used for injection and has a slow onset and long duration of action — called also *insulin isophane, isophane, NPH insulin*

iso·preg·nen·one \-ˈpreg-ne-ˌnōn\ *n* : DYDROGESTERONE

iso·pren·a·line \ˌī-sə-ˈpren-ᵊl-ən\ *n* : ISOPROTERENOL

iso·pro·pa·mide iodide \ˌī-sō-ˈprō-pə-mēd-\ *n* : an anticholinergic $C_{23}H_{33}IN_2O$ used esp. for its antispasmodic and antisecretory effect on the gastrointestinal tract — called also *isopropamide*

iso·pro·pa·nol \-ˈprō-pə-ˌnȯl, -ˌnōl\ *n* : ISOPROPYL ALCOHOL

iso·pro·pyl alcohol \ˌī-sə-ˈprō-pəl-\ *n* : a volatile flammable alcohol C_3H_8O used as a rubbing alcohol

iso·pro·pyl·ar·te·re·nol \ˌī-sə-ˌprō-pə-ˌlär-tə-ˈrē-ˌnȯl, -ˌnōl\ *n* : ISOPROTERENOL

isopropyl my·ris·tate \-mə-ˈris-ˌtāt\ *n* : an ester $C_{17}H_{34}O_2$ of isopropyl alcohol that is used as an emollient to promote absorption through the skin

iso·pro·ter·e·nol \ˌī-sə-prō-ˈter-ə-ˌnȯl, -nəl\ *n* : a sympathomimetic agent that is used in the form of its hydrochloride $C_{11}H_{17}NO_3{\cdot}HCl$ or sulfate $(C_{11}H_{17}NO_3)_2{\cdot}H_2SO_4$ esp. as a bronchodilator in the treatment of asthma, bronchitis, and emphysema — called also *isoprenaline, isopropylarterenol;* see ISUPREL

isop·ter \ī-ˈsäp-tər\ *n* : a contour line in a representation of the visual field around the points representing the macula that passes through the points of equal visual acuity

Isor·dil \ˈī-sȯr-ˌdil\ *trademark* — used for a preparation of isosorbide dinitrate

is·os·mot·ic \ˌī-ˌsäz-ˈmä-tik, -ˌsäs-\ *adj* : ISOTONIC 1 — **is·os·mot·i·cal·ly** *adv*

iso·sor·bide \ˌī-sō-ˈsȯr-ˌbīd\ *n* **1** : a diuretic $C_6H_{10}O_4$ **2** : ISOSORBIDE DINITRATE

isosorbide di·ni·trate \-dī-ˈnī-ˌtrāt\ *n* : a coronary vasodilator $C_6H_8N_2O_8$ used esp. in the treatment of angina pectoris — see ISORDIL

Isos·po·ra \ī-ˈsäs-pə-rə\ *n* : a genus of coccidian protozoans closely related to the genus *Eimeria* and including the only coccidian (*I. hominis*) known to be parasitic in humans

isothiocyanate — see ALLYL ISOTHIOCYANATE

iso·thi·pen·dyl \ˌī-sō-ˌthī-ˈpen-ˌdil\ *n* : an antihistamine drug $C_{16}H_{19}N_3S$

iso·ton·ic \ˌī-sə-ˈtä-nik\ *adj* **1** : of, relating to, or exhibiting equal osmotic pressure ⟨~ solutions⟩ — compare HYPERTONIC 2, HYPOTONIC 2 **2** : of, relating to, or being muscular contraction in the absence of significant resistance, with marked shortening of muscle fibers, and without great increase in muscle tone — compare ISOMETRIC — **iso·ton·i·cal·ly** *adv* — **iso·to·nic·i·ty** \-tō-ˈni-sə-tē\ *n*

iso·tope \ˈī-sə-ˌtōp\ *n* **1** : any of two or more species of atoms of a chemical element with the same atomic number that differ in the number of neutrons in an atom and have different physical properties **2** : NUCLIDE — **iso·to·pic** \ˌī-sə-ˈtä-pik, -ˈtō-\ *adj* — **iso·to·pi·cal·ly** *adv*

iso·trans·plant \ˌī-sō-ˈtrans-ˌplant\ *n* : a graft between syngeneic individuals

iso·tret·i·no·in \ˌī-sō-ˈtre-tə-ˌnȯin\ *n* : an isomer of retinoic acid that is a synthetic derivative of vitamin A, that inhibits sebaceous gland function and keratinization, and that is used in the treatment of severe inflammatory acne but is contraindicated in pregnancy because of its implication as a cause of birth defects — called also *13-cis-retinoic acid, retinoic acid;* see ACCUTANE

isotropic band *n* : I BAND

iso·type \ˈī-sə-ˌtīp\ *n* : any of the categories of antibodies determined by their physicochemical properties (as molecular weight) and antigenic characteristics that occur in all individuals of a species — compare ALLOTYPE, IDIOTYPE — **iso·typ·ic** \ˌī-sə-ˈti-pik\ *adj*

iso·va·ler·ic acid \ˌī-sō-və-ˈlir-ik-, -ˈler-\ *n* : a liquid acid $C_5H_{10}O_2$ that has a disagreeable odor

isovaleric ac·i·de·mia \-ˌa-sə-ˈdē-mē-ə\ *n* : a metabolic disorder characterized by the presence of an abnormally high concentration of isovaleric acid in the blood causing acidosis, coma, and an unpleasant body odor

iso·vol·ume \ˈī-sə-ˌväl-yəm, -(ˌ)yüm\ *adj* : ISOVOLUMETRIC

iso·vol·u·met·ric \ˌī-sə-ˌväl-yu̇-ˈme-trik\ *adj* : of, relating to, or characterized by unchanging volume; *esp* : relating to or being an early phase of ventricular systole in which the cardiac muscle exerts increasing pressure on the contents of the ventricle without significant change in the muscle fiber length and the ventricular volume remains constant

iso·vo·lu·mic \-və-ˈlü-mik\ *adj* : ISOVOLUMETRIC

is·ox·az·o·lyl \(ˌ)ī-ˌsäk-ˈsa-zə-ˌlil\ *adj* : relating to or being any of a group of semisynthetic penicillins (as oxacillin and cloxacillin) that are resistant to beta-lactamase, stable in acids, and active against gram-positive bacteria

is·ox·su·prine \ī-ˈsäk-sə-ˌprēn\ *n* : a sympathomimetic drug $C_{18}H_{23}NO_3$ used chiefly as a vasodilator

iso·zyme \ˈī-sə-ˌzīm\ *n* : ISOENZYME — **iso·zy·mic** \ˌī-sə-ˈzī-mik\ *adj*

is·sue \ˈi-(ˌ)shü\ *n* : a discharge (as of blood) from the body that is caused by disease or other physical disorder or that is produced artificially; *also* : an incision made to produce such a discharge

isth·mus \ˈis-məs\ *n* : a contracted anatomical part or passage connecting two larger structures or cavities: as **a** : an embryonic constriction separating the midbrain from the hindbrain **b** : the lower portion of the uterine corpus — **isth·mic** \ˈis-mik\ *adj*

isthmus of the fauces *n* : FAUCES

Isu·prel \ˈī-su̇-ˌprel\ *trademark* — used for a preparation of the hydrochloride of isoproterenol

itai–itai \i-ˈtī-i-ˌtī\ *n* : an extremely painful condition caused by poisoning following the ingestion of cadmium and characterized by bone decalcification — called also *itai-itai disease*

IT band \ˌī-ˈtē-\ *n* : ILIOTIBIAL BAND

itch \ˈich\ *n* **1** : an uneasy irritating sensation in the upper surface of the skin usu. held to result from mild stimulation of pain receptors **2** : a skin disorder accompanied by an itch; *esp* : a contagious eruption caused by an itch mite of the genus *Sarcoptes* (*S. scabiei*) that burrows in the skin and causes intense itching — **itch** *vb* — **itch·i·ness** \ˈi-chē-nəs\ *n* — **itchy** \ˈi-chē\ *adj*

¹itch·ing *adj* : having, producing, or marked by an uneasy sensation in the skin ⟨an ~ skin eruption⟩

²itching *n* : ITCH 1

itch mite *n* : any of several minute parasitic mites that burrow into the skin and cause itch; *esp* : a mite of any of several varieties of a species of the genus *Sarcoptes* (*S. scabiei*) that causes the itch

-ite \ˌīt\ *n suffix* **1** : substance produced through some (specified) process ⟨catabol*ite*⟩ **2** : segment or constituent part of a body or of a bodily part ⟨so*mite*⟩ ⟨dendr*ite*⟩

-it·ic \ˈi-tik\ *adj suffix* : of, resembling, or marked by — in adjectives formed from nouns usu. ending in *-ite* ⟨dendr*itic*⟩ and *-itis* ⟨bronch*itic*⟩

-i·tis \ˈī-təs\ *n suffix, pl* **-i·tis·es** *also* **-it·i·des** \ˈi-tə-ˌdēz\ *or* **-i·tes** \ˈī-(ˌ)tēz\ : disease usu. inflammatory of a (specified) part or organ : inflammation of ⟨laryng*itis*⟩ ⟨appendic*itis*⟩

ITP *abbr* idiopathic thrombocytopenic purpura

it·ra·con·a·zole \ˌi-trə-ˈkä-nə-ˌzōl\ *n* : a triazole antifungal agent $C_{35}H_{38}Cl_2N_8O_4$ used orally esp. to treat blastomycosis and histoplasmosis — see SPORANOX

IU *abbr* international unit

IUCD \ˌī-(ˌ)yü-(ˌ)sē-ˈdē\ *n* : INTRAUTERINE DEVICE

IUD \ˌī-(ˌ)ü-ˈdē\ *n* : INTRAUTERINE DEVICE

IUDR \ˌī-(ˌ)yü-(ˌ)dē-ˈär\ *n* : IDOXURIDINE

IV \ˈī-ˈvē\ *n, pl* **IVs** : an apparatus used to administer a fluid (as of medication, blood, or nutrients) intravenously; *also* : a fluid administered by IV

IV *abbr* **1** intravenous; intravenously **2** intraventricular

iver·mec·tin \ˌī-vər-ˈmek-tən\ *n* : a drug mixture of two structurally similar semisynthetic lactones that is used in veterinary medicine as an anthelmintic, acaricide, and insecticide and in human medicine to treat onchocerciasis

IVF *abbr* in vitro fertilization

IVP *abbr* intravenous pyelogram

Ix·o·des \ˌik-ˈsō-(ˌ)dēz\ *n* : a widespread genus of ixodid ticks including bloodsucking parasites of humans and animals which may transmit disease-causing microorganisms — see DEER TICK, WESTERN BLACK-LEGGED TICK

ix·od·i·cide \ik-ˈsä-di-ˌsīd, -ˈsō-\ *n* : an agent that destroys ticks

ixo·did \ik-ˈsä-did, -ˈsō-\ *adj* : of or relating to a family (Ixodidae) of ticks (as the deer tick and American dog tick) having a hard outer shell and feeding on two or three hosts during the life cycle — **ixodid** *n*

J

jaag·siek·te *also* **jag·siek·te** *or* **jaag·ziek·te** *or* **jag·ziek·te** \ˈyäg-ˌsēk-tə, -ˌzēk-\ *n* : a chronic contagious pneumonitis of sheep and sometimes goats that is caused by a retrovirus (species *Ovine pulmonary adenocarcinoma virus* of the genus *Betaretrovirus*) — called also *pulmonary adenomatosis*
jack·et \ˈja-kət\ *n* **1** : a rigid covering that envelops the upper body and provides support, correction, or restraint **2** : JACKET CROWN
jacket crown *n* : an artificial crown that is placed over the remains of a natural tooth
jack·so·ni·an \jak-ˈsō-nē-ən\ *adj, often cap* : of, relating to, associated with, or resembling Jacksonian epilepsy
Jack·son \ˈjak-sən\, **John Hughlings (1835–1911)**, British neurologist.
Jacksonian epilepsy *n* : epilepsy that is characterized by progressive spreading of the abnormal movements or sensations from a focus affecting a muscle group on one side of the body to adjacent muscles or by becoming generalized and that corresponds to the spread of epileptic activity in the motor cortex
Ja·cob·son's nerve \ˈjā-kəb-sənz-\ *n* : TYMPANIC NERVE
Jacobson \ˈyä-kȯp-sən\, **Ludwig Levin (1783–1843)**, Danish anatomist.
Jacobson's organ *n* : VOMERONASAL ORGAN
jac·ti·ta·tion \ˌjak-tə-ˈtā-shən\ *n* : a tossing to and fro or jerking and twitching of the body or its parts : excessive restlessness esp. in certain psychiatric disorders — **jac·ti·tate** \ˈjak-tə-ˌtāt\ *vb*
Jaf·fé reaction \yä-ˈfā-, zhä-\ *also* **Jaf·fé's reaction** \-ˈfāz-\ *n* : a reaction between creatinine and picric acid in alkaline solution that results in the formation of a red compound and is used to measure the amount of creatinine (as in creatinuria)
Jaffé \yä-ˈfā\, **Max (1841–1911)**, German biochemist.
jail fever \ˈjāl-\ *n* : TYPHUS a
jake leg \ˈjāk-\ *n* : a paralysis caused by drinking improperly distilled or contaminated liquor
Ja·kob–Creutz·feldt disease \ˈyä-(ˌ)kōb-ˈkrȯits-ˌfelt-\ *n* : CREUTZFELDT-JAKOB DISEASE
jal·ap \ˈja-ləp, ˈjä-\ *n* **1** : the dried tuberous root of a Mexican plant (*Ipomoea purga*) of the morning-glory family (Convolvulaceae); *also* : a powdered purgative drug prepared from it that contains resinous glycosides **2** : a plant yielding jalap
JAMA *abbr Journal of the American Medical Association*
ja·mais vu \ˌzhȧ-ˌme-ˈvūē, ˌjä-ˌmā-ˈvü\ *n* : a disorder of memory characterized by the illusion that the familiar is being encountered for the first time — compare PARAMNESIA b
James·town weed \ˈjāmz-tau̇n-\ *n* : JIMSONWEED
jani·ceps \ˈja-nə-ˌseps, ˈjā-\ *n* : conjoined twins united at the thorax and skull and having two equal faces looking in opposite directions
Jan·u·met \ˈjan-yu̇-ˌmet\ *trademark* — used for a preparation of sitagliptin and metformin
Ja·nu·via \jə-ˈnü-vē-ə\ *trademark* — used for a preparation of sitagliptin
Japanese B encephalitis *n* : an encephalitis that occurs epidemically in Japan and other Asian countries in the summer, is caused by a virus of the genus *Flavivirus* (species *Japanese encephalitis virus*) transmitted by mosquitoes (esp. *Culex tritaeniorhynchus*), and usu. produces a subclinical infection but may cause acute meningoencephalomyelitis — called also *Japanese encephalitis*
japonica — see SCHISTOSOMIASIS JAPONICA
jar·gon \ˈjär-gən\ *n* : unintelligible, meaningless, or incoherent speech (as that associated with Wernicke's aphasia or some forms of schizophrenia)
Ja·risch–Herx·hei·mer reaction \ˈyä-rish-ˈherks-ˌhī-mər-\ *n* : an increase in the symptoms of a spirochetal disease (as syphilis or Lyme disease) occurring in some persons when treatment with spirocheticidal drugs is started — called also *Herxheimer reaction*
Jarisch, Adolf (1850–1902), Austrian dermatologist.
Herxheimer, Karl (1861–1944), German dermatologist.
Jar·vik–7 \jär-vik-ˈse-vən\ *n* : an air-driven artificial heart that remains tethered to an external console after implantation and that was formerly implanted in human patients in a clinical study — called also *Jarvik heart*
Jarvik, Robert Koffler (*b* 1946), American physician and inventor.
jaun·dice \ˈjȯn-dəs, ˈjän-\ *n* **1** : a yellowish pigmentation of the skin, tissues, and certain body fluids caused by the deposition of bilirubin that follows interference with normal production and discharge of bile (as in certain liver diseases) or excessive breakdown of red blood cells (as after internal hemorrhage or in various hemolytic states) **2** : any disease or abnormal condition (as hepatitis A or leptospirosis) that is characterized by jaundice — **jaun·diced** \-dəst\ *adj*
jaw \ˈjȯ\ *n* **1** : either of two complex cartilaginous or bony structures in most vertebrates that border the mouth, support the soft parts enclosing it, and usu. bear teeth on their oral margin: **a** : an upper structure

more or less firmly fused with the skull — called also *upper jaw, maxilla* **b** : a lower structure that consists of a single bone or of completely fused bones and that is hinged, movable, and articulated by a pair of condyles with the temporal bone of either side — called also *inferior maxillary bone, lower jaw, mandible* **2** : the parts constituting the walls of the mouth and serving to open and close it — usu. used in pl.

jaw·bone \ˈjȯ-ˌbōn\ *n* : JAW 1; *esp* : MANDIBLE

jawed \ˈjȯd\ *adj* : having jaws — usu. used in combination ⟨square-*jawed*⟩

Jaws of Life *trademark* — used for a hydraulic tool that is used esp. to free victims trapped inside wrecked motor vehicles

JCAH *abbr* Joint Commission on Accreditation of Hospitals

JCAHO *abbr* Joint Commission on Accreditation of Healthcare Organizations

J chain \ˈjā-\ *n* : a relatively short polypeptide chain with a high number of cysteine residues that is found in antibodies of the IgM and IgA classes

jejun- *or* **jejuno-** *comb form* **1** : jejunum ⟨*jejun*itis⟩ **2** : jejunum and ⟨*jejuno*ileitis⟩

je·ju·nal \ji-ˈjün-ᵊl\ *adj* : of or relating to the jejunum

je·ju·ni·tis \ˌje-jü-ˈnī-təs\ *n* : inflammation of the jejunum

je·ju·no·il·e·al bypass \ji-ˌjü-nō-ˈi-lē-əl-\ *n* : a surgical bypass operation performed esp. to reduce absorption in the small intestine that involves joining the first part of the jejunum with the more distal segment of the ileum

je·ju·no·il·e·it·is \ji-ˌjü-nō-ˌi-lē-ˈī-təs, ˌje-jü-nō-\ *n* : inflammation of the jejunum and the ileum

je·ju·no·il·e·os·to·my \ji-ˌjü-nō-ˌi-lē-ˈäs-tə-mē, ˌje-jü-nō-\ *n, pl* **-mies** : the formation of an anastomosis between the jejunum and the ileum

je·ju·nos·to·my \ji-ˌjü-ˈnäs-tə-mē, ˌje-jü-\ *n, pl* **-mies** **1** : the surgical formation of an opening through the abdominal wall into the jejunum **2** : the opening made by jejunostomy

je·ju·num \ji-ˈjü-nəm\ *n, pl* **je·ju·na** \-nə\ : the section of the small intestine that comprises the first two fifths beyond the duodenum and that is larger, thicker-walled, and more vascular and has more circular folds and fewer Peyer's patches than the ileum

jel·ly \ˈje-lē\ *n, pl* **jellies** : a semisolid gelatinous substance: as **a** : a medicated preparation usu. intended for local application ⟨ephedrine ~⟩ **b** : a jellylike preparation used in electrocardiography to obtain better conduction of electricity ⟨electrode ~⟩

jel·ly·fish \-ˌfish\ *n* : a free-swimming marine sexually reproducing coelenterate of either of two classes (Hydrozoa and Scyphozoa) that has a nearly transparent saucer-shaped body and tentacles studded with stinging cells

Jen·ta·du·eto \ˌjen-tə-dü-ˈet-ō\ *trademark* — used for a preparation of linagliptin and metformin

je·quir·i·ty bean \jə-ˈkwir-ə-tē-\ *n* **1** : the poisonous scarlet and black seed of the rosary pea **2** : ROSARY PEA 1

jerk \ˈjərk\ *n* : an involuntary spasmodic muscular movement due to reflex action; *esp* : one induced by an external stimulus — see KNEE JERK

jet fa·tigue \ˈjet-fə-ˌtēg\ *n* : JET LAG

jet in·jec·tor \-in-ˈjek-tər\ *n* : a device used to inject subcutaneously a fine stream of fluid under high pressure without puncturing the skin — **jet injec·tion** \-ˈjek-shən\ *n*

jet lag \ˈjet-ˌlag\ *n* : a condition that is characterized by various psychological and physiological effects (as fatigue and irritability), occurs following long flight through several time zones, and prob. results from disruption of circadian rhythms in the human body — called also *jet fatigue* — **jet–lagged** *adj*

jig·ger \ˈji-gər\ *n* : CHIGGER

jim·son·weed \ˈjim-sən-ˌwēd\ *n* : a poisonous tall annual weed of the genus *Datura* (*D. stramonium*) with rank-smelling foliage and globe-shaped prickly fruits — called also *Jamestown weed;* see STRAMONIUM 1

jit·ters \ˈji-tərz\ *n pl* : a state of extreme nervousness or nervous shaking — **jit·ter** \-tər\ *vb* — **jit·teri·ness** \-tə-rē-nəs\ *n* — **jit·tery** *adj*

JND *abbr* just noticeable difference

job \ˈjäb\ *n* : plastic surgery for cosmetic purposes ⟨an eye ~⟩

jock itch \ˈjäk-\ *n* : ringworm of the crotch : TINEA CRURIS — called also *jockey itch*

jock·strap \ˈjäk-ˌstrap\ *n* : ATHLETIC SUPPORTER

jogger's nipple *n* : pain and often dermatitis due to chafing of the nipples by clothing worn while jogging — called also *jogger's nipples*

Joh·ne's bacillus \ˈyō-ˌnēz-\ *n* : a bacillus of the genus *Mycobacterium* (*M. paratuberculosis*) that causes Johne's disease

Johne \ˈyō-nə\, **Heinrich Albert (1839–1910),** German bacteriologist.

Joh·ne's disease \ˈyō-nəz-\ *n* : a chronic often fatal enteritis esp. of cattle that is caused by Johne's bacillus — called also *paratuberculosis*

john·ny *also* **john·nie** \ˈjä-nē\ *n, pl* **johnnies** : a short-sleeved collarless gown that is open in the back and is worn by persons (as hospital patients) undergoing medical examination or treatment

joint \ˈjȯint\ *n* : : the point of contact between skeletal elements whether movable or rigidly fixed together with the surrounding and supporting parts (as membranes, tendons, and ligaments) — **out of joint** *of a bone* : having the head slipped from its socket

joint capsule *n* : a ligamentous sac that surrounds the articular cavity of a freely movable joint, is attached to the bones, completely encloses the joint, and is composed of an outer fibrous membrane and an inner synovial membrane — called also *articular capsule*

joint·ed \ˈjȯin-təd\ *adj* : having joints

joint fluid *n* : SYNOVIAL FLUID

joint ill *n* : NAVEL ILL

joint mouse \-ˈmau̇s\ *n* : a loose fragment (as of cartilage) within a synovial space

joule \ˈjül\ *n* : a unit of work or energy equal to the work done by a force of one newton acting through a distance of one meter

Joule, James Prescott (1818–1889), British physicist.

Ju·blia \ˈjü-blē-ə\ *trademark* — used for a preparation of efinaconazole

¹ju·gal \ˈjü-gəl\ *adj* : MALAR

²jugal *n* : ZYGOMATIC BONE — called also *jugal bone*

¹jug·u·lar \ˈjə-gyə-lər, ˈjü-\ *adj* **1** : of or relating to the throat or neck **2** : of or relating to the jugular vein

²jugular *n* : JUGULAR VEIN

jugulare — see GLOMUS JUGULARE

jugular foramen *n* : a large irregular opening from the posterior cranial fossa that is bounded anteriorly by the petrous part of the temporal bone and posteriorly by the jugular notch of the occipital bone and that transmits the inferior petrosal sinus, the glossopharyngeal, vagus, and accessory nerves, and the internal jugular vein

jugular fossa *n* : a depression on the basilar surface of the petrous portion of the temporal bone that contains a dilation of the internal jugular vein

jugular ganglion *n* : SUPERIOR GANGLION

jugular notch \-ˈnäch\ *n* **1** : SUPRASTERNAL NOTCH **2 a** : a notch in the inferior border of the occipital bone behind the jugular process that forms the posterior part of the jugular foramen **b** : a notch in the petrous portion of the temporal bone that corresponds to the jugular notch of the occipital bone and with it makes up the jugular foramen

jugular process *n* : a quadrilateral or triangular process of the occipital bone on each side that articulates with the temporal bone and is situated lateral to the condyle of the occipital bone on each side articulating with the atlas

jugular trunk *n* : either of two major lymph vessels of which one lies on each side of the body and drains the head and neck

jugular vein *n* : any of several veins of each side of the neck: as **a** : a vein that collects the blood from the interior of the cranium, the superficial part of the face, and the neck, runs down the neck on the outside of the internal and common carotid arteries, and unites with the subclavian vein to form the brachiocephalic vein — called also *internal jugular vein* **b** : a smaller and more superficial vein that collects most of the blood from the exterior of the cranium and deep parts of the face and opens into the subclavian vein — called also *external jugular vein* **c** : a vein that commences near the hyoid bone and joins the terminal part of the external jugular vein or the subclavian vein — called also *anterior jugular vein*

juice \ˈjüs\ *n* : a natural bodily fluid — see GASTRIC JUICE, INTESTINAL JUICE, PANCREATIC JUICE

jumper's knee *n* : PATELLAR TENDINITIS

jumping gene *n* : TRANSPOSABLE ELEMENT; *also* : TRANSPOSON

junc·tion \ˈjəŋk-shən\ *n* : a place or point of meeting — see NEUROMUSCULAR JUNCTION — **junc·tion·al** \-shə-nəl\ *adj*

junctional epidermolysis bullosa *n* : any of several forms of epidermolysis bullosa that are marked esp. by usu. severe blister formation between the epidermis and basement membrane often accompanied by involvement of the mucous membranes (as of the mouth) and that are inherited as an autosomal recessive trait

junctional nevus *n* : a nevus that develops at the junction of the dermis and epidermis and is potentially cancerous — called also *junction nevus*

junctional rhythm *n* : a cardiac rhythm resulting from impulses coming from a locus of tissue in the area of the atrioventricular node

junctional tachycardia *n* : tachycardia associated with the generation of impulses in a locus in the region of the atrioventricular node

Jung·ian \ˈyu̇ŋ-ē-ən\ *adj* : of, relating to, or characteristic of C. G. Jung or his psychological doctrines — **Jungian** *n*

Jung \ˈyu̇ŋ\, **Carl Gustav (1875–1961),** Swiss psychologist and psychiatrist.

jungle fever *n* : a severe form of malaria or yellow fever — compare JUNGLE YELLOW FEVER

jungle rot *n* : any of various esp. pyogenic skin infections contracted in tropical environments

jungle yellow fever *n* : yellow fever endemic in or near forest or jungle areas in Africa and So. America and transmitted by mosquitoes (esp. genus *Haemagogus*) other than members of the genus *Aedes*

Ju·nin virus \hü-ˈnēn-\ *n* : a virus of the genus *Arenavirus* (species *Junin virus*) that is the causative agent of a hemorrhagic fever endemic in Argentina and that is transmitted to humans chiefly by rodents

ju•ni•per \ˈjü-nə-pər\ *n* : an evergreen shrub or tree (genus *Juniperus*) of the cypress family (Cupressaceae)

juniper tar *n* : a dark tarry liquid used topically in treating skin diseases and obtained by distillation from the wood of a Eurasian juniper (*Juniperus oxycedrus*) — called also *cade oil, juniper tar oil*

junk DNA *n* : a region of DNA that usu. consists of a repeating DNA sequence, does not code for a protein, and has no known function

just noticeable difference *n* : the minimum amount of change in a physical stimulus required for a subject to detect reliably a difference in the level of stimulation

jus•to ma•jor \ˈjəs-tō-ˈmā-jər\ *adj, of pelvic dimensions* : greater than normal

justo mi•nor \-ˈmī-nər\ *adj, of pelvic dimensions* : smaller than normal

ju•ve•nile \ˈjü-və-ˌnīl, -nəl\ *adj* **1** : physiologically immature or undeveloped **2** : of, relating to, characteristic of, or affecting children or young people ⟨~ arthritis⟩ **3** : reflecting psychological or intellectual immaturity — **juvenile** *n*

juvenile absence epilepsy *n* : epilepsy that typically begins between the ages of 10 and 16 and is marked by the daily occurrence of absence seizures and usu. by tonic-clonic seizures

juvenile amaurotic idiocy *n, dated, now usu. offensive* : BATTEN DISEASE

juvenile delinquency *n* **1** : conduct by a juvenile characterized by antisocial behavior that is subject to legal action **2** : a violation of the law committed by a juvenile that would have been a crime if committed by an adult — **juvenile delinquent** *n*

juvenile diabetes *n* : TYPE 1 DIABETES

juvenile myoclonic epilepsy *n* : epilepsy that typically begins during adolescence or late childhood and is marked by myoclonic seizures which occur shortly after awakening and are often followed by tonic-clonic seizures or sometimes by absence seizures

juvenile–onset diabetes *n* : TYPE 1 DIABETES

juxta- *comb form* : situated near ⟨*juxta*glomerular⟩

jux•ta–ar•tic•u•lar \ˌjək-stə-är-ˈti-kyə-lər\ *adj* : situated near a joint

jux•ta•glo•mer•u•lar \-glə-ˈmer-yə-lər, -glō-, -ə-lər\ *adj* : situated near a kidney glomerulus

juxtaglomerular apparatus *n* : a functional unit near a kidney glomerulus that controls renin release and is composed of juxtaglomerular cells and a macula densa

juxtaglomerular cell *n* : any of a group of cells that are situated in the wall of each afferent arteriole of a kidney glomerulus near its point of entry adjacent to a macula densa and that produce and secrete renin

jux•ta•med•ul•lary \ˌjək-stə-ˈmed-ᵊl-ˌer-ē, -ˈmej-ᵊl-; -mə-ˈdə-lə-rē\ *adj* : situated or occurring near the edge of the medulla of the kidney

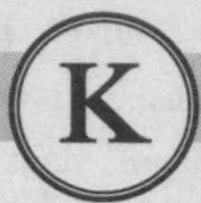

K *symbol* [New Latin *kalium*] potassium

Kahn test \ˈkän-\ *n* : a serum-precipitation reaction for the diagnosis of syphilis — called also *Kahn, Kahn reaction*

Kahn, Reuben Leon (1887–1979), American immunologist.

kai•nate \ˈkī-ˌnāt, ˈkā-\ *n* : KAINIC ACID

kai•nic acid \ˈkī-nik-, ˈkā-\ *n* : an excitatory neurotoxin $C_{10}H_{15}NO_4$ that is a glutamate analog orig. isolated from a dried red alga (*Digenia simplex*) and is used as an anthelmintic and experimentally to induce seizures and neurodegeneration in laboratory animals

kala–azar \ˈkä-lə-ə-ˈzär, ˈka-\ *n* : a severe parasitic disease chiefly of Asia marked by fever, progressive anemia, leukopenia, and enlargement of the spleen and liver and caused by a flagellate of the genus *Leishmania* (*L. donovani*) that is transmitted by the bite of sand flies — called also *dumdum fever, visceral leishmaniasis;* see LEISHMAN-DONOVAN BODY

ka•li•ure•sis \ˌkā-lē-yu̇-ˈrē-səs, ˌka-\ *also* **kal•ure•sis** \ˌkāl-(y)ü-ˈre-, ˌkal-\ *n, pl* **-ure•ses** \-ˌsēz\ : excretion of potassium in the urine esp. in excessive amounts — **ka•li•uret•ic** \-ˈre-tik\ *adj*

kal•li•din \ˈka-lə-din\ *n* : either of two vasodilator kinins formed from blood plasma globulin by the action of kallikrein

kal•li•kre•in \ˌka-lə-ˈkrē-ən, kə-ˈli-krē-ən\ *n* : a hypotensive protease that liberates kinins from blood plasma proteins and is used therapeutically for vasodilation

Kall•mann syndrome \ˈkȯl-mən-\ *or* **Kall•mann's syndrome** \-mənz-\ *n* : a hereditary condition marked by hypogonadism caused by a deficiency of gonadotropins and anosmia caused by failure of the olfactory lobes to develop

Kallmann, Franz Josef (1897–1965), American geneticist and psychiatrist.

kana•my•cin \ˌka-nə-ˈmīs-ᵊn\ *n* : a broad-spectrum antibiotic from a Japanese soil bacterium of the genus *Streptomyces* (*S. kanamyceticus*)

Kan•ner's syndrome \ˈka-nərz-\ *n* : AUTISM

Kanner, Leo (1894–1981), American psychiatrist.

Kan•trex \ˈkan-ˌtreks\ *trademark* — used for a preparation of kanamycin

ka•olin \ˈkā-ə-lin\ *n* : a fine usu. white clay that is used in medicine esp. as an adsorbent in the treatment of diarrhea (as from food poisoning)

Kao•pec•tate \ˌkā-ō-ˈpek-ˌtāt\ *trademark* — used for a preparation of kaolin used as an antidiarrheal

Ka•po•si's sarcoma \ˈka-pə-zēz-, kə-ˈpō-, -sēz-\ *n* : a neoplastic disease that occurs esp. in individuals coinfected with HIV and a specific herpesvirus (species *Human herpesvirus 8* of the genus *Rhadinovirus*), that affects esp. the skin and mucous membranes, and is marked usu. by pink to red-dish-brown or bluish plaques, macules, papules, or nodules esp. on the lower extremities — abbr. *KS*

Kaposi \ˈkȯ-pō-sē\, **Moritz (1837–1902),** Hungarian dermatologist.

kap•pa chain *or* **κ chain** \ˈka-pə-\ *n* : a polypeptide chain of one of the two types of light chain that are found in antibodies and can be distinguished antigenically and by the sequence of amino acids in the chain — compare LAMBDA CHAIN

ka•ra•ya gum \kə-ˈrī-ə-\ *n* : any of several laxative vegetable gums obtained from tropical Asian trees (genera *Sterculia* of the family Sterculiaceae and *Cochlospermum* of the family Bixaceae) — called also *gum karaya, karaya, sterculia gum*

ka•rez•za \kä-ˈret-sə\ *n* : COITUS RESERVATUS

Kar•ta•ge•ner's syndrome \kär-ˈtä-gə-nərz-, ˌkär-tə-ˈgā-nərz-\ *n* : an abnormal condition inherited as an autosomal recessive trait and characterized by situs inversus, abnormalities in the protein structure of cilia, and chronic bronchiectasis and sinusitis

Kartagener, Manes (1897–1975), Swiss physician.

kary- *or* **karyo-** *also* **cary-** *or* **caryo-** *comb form* : nucleus of a cell ⟨*karyo*kinesis⟩ ⟨*karyo*type⟩

kary•og•a•my \ˌkar-ē-ˈä-gə-mē\ *n, pl* **-mies** : the fusion of cell nuclei (as in fertilization)

karyo•gram \ˈkar-ē-ō-ˌgram\ *n* : KARYOTYPE; *esp* : a diagrammatic representation of the chromosome complement of an organism

karyo•ki•ne•sis \ˌkar-ē-ō-kə-ˈnē-səs, -kī-\ *n, pl* **-ne•ses** \-ˌsēz\ **1** : the nuclear phenomena characteristic of mitosis **2** : the whole process of mitosis — compare CYTOKINESIS — **karyo•ki•net•ic** \-ˈne-tik\ *adj*

kary•ol•o•gy \ˌkar-ē-ˈä-lə-jē\ *n, pl* **-gies** **1** : the minute cytological characteristics of the cell nucleus esp. with regard to the chromosomes of a single cell or of the cells of an organism or group of organisms **2** : a branch of cytology concerned with the karyology of cell nuclei — **kary•o•log•i•cal** \-ē-ə-ˈlä-ji-kəl\ *also* **kary•o•log•ic** \-jik\ *adj* — **kary•o•log•i•cal•ly** *adv*

karyo•lymph \ˈkar-ē-ō-ˌlimf\ *n* : NUCLEOPLASM

kary•ol•y•sis \ˌkar-ē-ˈä-lə-səs\ *n, pl* **-y•ses** \-ˌsēz\ : dissolution of the cell nucleus with loss of its affinity for basic stains sometimes occurring normally but usu. in necrosis — compare KARYORRHEXIS

karyo•plasm \ˈkar-ē-ō-ˌpla-zəm\ *n* : NUCLEOPLASM

karyo•pyk•no•sis \ˌkar-ē-(ˌ)ō-pik-ˈnō-səs\ *n* : shrinkage of the cell nuclei of epithelial cells (as of the vagina) with breakup of the chromatin into unstructured granules — **karyo•pyk•not•ic** \-ˈnä-tik\ *adj*

karyopyknotic index *n* : an index that is calculated as the percentage of epithelial cells with karyopyknotic nuclei exfoliated from the vagina and is used in the hormonal evaluation of a patient

kary•or•rhex•is \ˌkar-ē-ȯ-ˈrek-səs\ *n, pl* **-rhex•es** \-ˌsēz\ : a degenerative cellular process involving fragmentation of the nucleus and the breakup of the chromatin into unstructured granules — compare KARYOLYSIS

karyo•some \ˈkar-ē-ə-ˌsōm\ *n* : a mass of chromatin in a cell nucleus that resembles a nucleolus

1**karyo•type** \ˈkar-ē-ə-ˌtīp\ *n* : the chromosomal characteristics of a cell; *also* : the chromosomes themselves or a representation of them — **karyo•typ•ic** \ˌkar-ē-ə-ˈti-pik\ *adj* — **karyo•typ•i•cal•ly** *adv*

2**karyotype** *vb* **-typed; -typ•ing** : to determine the karyotype of

karyo•typ•ing \-ˌtīp-iŋ\ *n* : the action or process of studying karyotypes or of making representations of them

Ka•ta•ya•ma syndrome \ˌkä-tə-ˈyä-mə-\ *n* : SCHISTOSOMIASIS JAPONICA; *specif* : an acute form usu. occurring several weeks after initial infection with the causative schistosome (*Schistosoma japonicum*) — called also *Katayama disease, Katayama fever*

ka•va \ˈkä-və\ *n* **1** : an Australasian pepper (*Piper methysticum*) from whose crushed root an intoxicating beverage is made; *also* : the beverage **2** : a preparation consisting of the ground dried rhizome and roots of the kava plant that is used esp. as a dietary supplement chiefly to relieve stress, anxiety, and sleeplessness and that has been linked to cases of severe liver injury

kava kava \ˈkä-və-ˈkä-və\ *n* : KAVA

Ka•wa•sa•ki disease \ˌkä-wə-ˈsä-kē-\ *also* **Ka•wa•sa•ki's disease** \-kēz-\ *n* : an acute febrile disease of unknown cause affecting esp. infants and children that is characterized by a reddish macular rash esp. on the trunk, conjunctivitis, inflammation of mucous membranes (as of the tongue), erythema of the palms and soles followed by desquamation, edema of the hands and feet, and swollen lymph nodes in the neck — called also *Kawasaki's syndrome, Kawasaki syndrome, mucocutaneous lymph node disease, mucocutaneous lymph node syndrome*

Kawasaki, Tomisaku (*fl* **1961**), Japanese pediatrician.

Kay•ser–Flei•scher ring \ˈkī-zər-ˈflī-shər-\ *n* : a brown or greenish-brown ring of copper deposits around the cornea that is characteristic of Wilson's disease

Kayser, Bernhard (1869–1954) and **Fleischer, Bruno Otto (1874–1965),** German ophthalmologists.

kb *abbr* kilobase

K–Dur \ˈkā-ˌdu̇r\ *trademark* — used for a sustained-release preparation of potassium chloride for oral administration

ked \ˈked\ *n* : SHEEP KED

Kef•lex \ˈkef-ˌleks\ *trademark* — used for a preparation of the monohydrate of cephalexin

Ke•gel exercises \ˈkā-gəl-, ˈkē-\ *n pl* : repetitive contractions of the muscles that control flow in urination in order to increase the tone of the pubococcygeus muscle esp. to prevent or control incontinence or to enhance sexual responsiveness during intercourse

Kegel, Arnold Henry (1894–1976), American physician.

Kell \ˈkel\ *adj* : of, relating to, or being a group of allelic red-blood-cell antigens of which some are important causes of transfusion reactions and some forms of erythroblastosis fetalis

Kell, medical patient.

Kel•ler \ˈke-lər\ *adj* : relating to or being an operation to correct hallux valgus by excision of the proximal part of the proximal phalanx of the big toe with resulting shortening of the toe

Keller, William Lorden (1874–1959), American surgeon.

ke•loid \ˈkē-ˌlȯid\ *n* : a thick scar resulting from excessive growth of fibrous tissue and occurring esp. after burns or radiation injury — **keloid** *adj* — **ke•loi•dal** \kē-ˈlȯid-ᵊl\ *adj*

kelp \ˈkelp\ *n* : any of various large brown seaweeds (order Laminariales) and esp. laminarias

kel•vin \ˈkel-vin\ *n* : the base unit of temperature in the International System of Units that is equal to $^{1}/_{273.16}$ of the Kelvin scale temperature of the triple point of water

Thom•son \ˈtäm-sən\, **Sir William (1st Baron Kelvin of Largs) (1824–1907),** British physicist.

Kelvin *adj* : relating to, conforming to, or being a temperature scale according to which absolute zero is 0 K, the equivalent of −273.15°C

Ken•a•cort \ˈke-nə-ˌkȯrt\ *n* : a preparation of triamcinolone — formerly a U.S. registered trademark

Ken•ne•dy's disease \ˈke-nə-dēz-\ *also* **Ken•ne•dy disease** \-dē-\ *n* : a progressive muscular and neurological disorder that is characterized esp. by muscular weakness and atrophy and by neural degeneration, that is inherited as an X-linked recessive trait, and that chiefly affects adult males — called also *spinal and bulbar muscular atrophy*

Kennedy, William Robert (*b* 1927), American neurologist.

kennel cough *n* : tracheobronchitis of dogs or cats

Ken•ny method \ˈke-nē-\ *n* : a method of treating polio consisting basically of application of hot fomentations and rehabilitation of muscular activity by passive movement and then guided active coordination — called also *Kenny treatment*

Kenny, Elizabeth (1880–1952), Australian nurse.

ker•a•sin \ˈker-ə-sən\ *n* : a cerebroside $C_{48}H_{93}NO_8$ that occurs esp. in Gaucher disease

ker•a•tan sulfate \ˈker-ə-ˌtan-\ *n* : any of several sulfated glycosaminoglycans that have been found esp. in the cornea, cartilage, and bone

ker•a•tec•to•my \ˌker-ə-ˈtek-tə-mē\ *n, pl* **-mies** : surgical excision of part of the cornea

ke•rat•ic precipitates \kə-ˈra-tik-\ *n pl* : accumulations on the posterior surface of the cornea esp. of macrophages and epithelial cells that occur in chronic inflammatory conditions — called also *keratitis punctata*

ker•a•tin \ˈker-ət-ᵊn\ *n* : any of various sulfur-containing fibrous proteins that form the chemical basis of horny epidermal tissues (as hair and nails)

ke•ra•ti•ni•za•tion \ˌker-ə-tə-nə-ˈzā-shən, kə-ˌrat-ᵊn-ə-\ *n* : conversion into keratin or keratinous tissue — **ke•ra•ti•nize** \ˈker-ə-tə-ˌnīz, kə-ˈrat-ᵊn-ˌīz\ *vb*

ke•ra•ti•no•cyte \kə-ˈrat-ᵊn-ə-ˌsīt, ˌker-ə-ˈti-nə-\ *n* : an epidermal cell that produces keratin

ke•ra•ti•nous \kə-ˈrat-ᵊn-əs, ˌker-ə-ˈtī-nəs\ *adj* : composed of or containing keratin : HORNY ⟨∼ tissue⟩

ker•a•ti•tis \ˌker-ə-ˈtī-təs\ *n, pl* **-tit•i•des** \-ˈti-tə-ˌdēz\ : inflammation of the cornea of the eye characterized by burning or smarting, blurring of vision, and sensitiveness to light and caused by infectious or noninfectious agents

keratitis punc•ta•ta \-pəŋk-ˈtä-tə, -ˈtā-\ *n* : KERATIC PRECIPITATES

ker•a•to•ac•an•tho•ma \ˌker-ə-tō-ˌa-ˌkan-ˈthō-mə\ *n, pl* **-mas** *also* **-ma•ta** \-mə-tə\ : a rapidly growing skin tumor that occurs esp. in elderly individuals, resembles a carcinoma of squamous epithelial cells but does not spread, and tends to heal spontaneously with some scarring if left untreated

ker•a•to•con•junc•ti•vi•tis \ˈker-ə-(ˌ)tō-kən-ˌjəŋk-tə-ˈvī-təs\ *n* : combined inflammation of the cornea and conjunctiva; *esp* : EPIDEMIC KERATOCONJUNCTIVITIS

keratoconjunctivitis sic•ca \-ˈsi-kə\ *n* : DRY EYE

ker•a•to•co•nus \ˌker-ə-tō-ˈkō-nəs\ *n* : cone-shaped protrusion of the cornea

ker•a•to•der•ma \-ˈdər-mə\ *n* : a horny condition of the skin

keratoderma blen•nor•rhag•i•cum \-ˌble-nò-ˈra-ji-kəm\ *n* : KERATOSIS BLENNORRHAGICA

ker•a•to•der•mia \ˌker-ə-tō-ˈdər-mē-ə\ *n* : KERATODERMA

ker•a•to•hy•a•lin \-ˈhī-ə-lən\ *also* **ker•a•to•hy•a•line** \-lən, -ˌlēn\ *n* : a colorless translucent protein that occurs esp. in granules of the stratum granulosum of the epidermis

ker•a•tol•y•sis \ˌker-ə-ˈtä-lə-səs\ *n, pl* **-y•ses** \-ˌsēz\ **1** : the process of breaking down or dissolving keratin **2** : a skin disease marked by peeling of the horny layer of the epidermis

[1]**ker•a•to•lyt•ic** \ˌker-ə-tō-ˈli-tik\ *adj* : relating to or causing keratolysis

[2]**keratolytic** *n* : a keratolytic agent

ker•a•to•ma•la•cia \ˌker-ə-tō-mə-ˈlā-shə, -sē-ə\ *n* : a softening and ulceration of the cornea of the eye resulting from severe systemic deficiency of vitamin A — compare XEROPHTHALMIA

ker•a•tome \ˈker-ə-ˌtōm\ *n* : a surgical instrument used for making an incision in the cornea in cataract operations

ker•a•tom•e•ter \ˌker-ə-ˈtä-mə-tər\ *n* : an instrument for measuring the curvature of the cornea

ker•a•tom•e•try \ˌker-ə-ˈtä-mə-trē\ *n, pl* **-tries** : measurement of the form and curvature of the cornea — **ker•a•to•met•ric** \-tō-ˈme-trik\ *adj*

ker•at•o•mil•eu•sis \ˌker-ət-ō-mi-ˈlü-səs, -ˈlyü-\ *n* : a surgical procedure for correcting the refractive power of the eye to improve vision that formerly involved removing, freezing, reshaping, and reinserting a section of the cornea but now typically involves reshaping the cornea in place with the use of an excimer laser — see LASIK

ker•a•top•a•thy \ˌker-ə-ˈtä-pə-thē\ *n, pl* **-thies** : any noninflammatory disease of the eye — see BAND KERATOPATHY

ker•a•to•pha•kia \ˌker-ə-tō-ˈfā-kē-ə\ *n* : keratoplasty in which corneal tissue from a donor is frozen, shaped, and inserted into the cornea of a recipient

ker•a•to•plas•ty \ˈker-ə-tō-ˌplas-tē\ *n, pl* **-ties** : plastic surgery on the cornea; *esp* : corneal grafting

ker•a•to•pros•the•sis \ˌker-ə-tō-präs-ˈthē-səs, -ˈpräs-thə-\ *n, pl* **-the•ses** \-ˌsēz\ : a plastic replacement for an opacified inner part of a cornea

ker•a•to•scope \ˈker-ə-tō-ˌskōp\ *n* : an instrument for examining the cornea esp. to detect irregularities of its anterior surface

ker•a•to•sis \ˌker-ə-ˈtō-səs\ *n, pl* **-to•ses** \-ˌsēz\ **1** : a disease of the skin marked by overgrowth of horny tissue **2** : an area of the skin affected with keratosis — **ker•a•tot•ic** \-ˈtä-tik\ *adj*

keratosis blen•nor•rhag•i•ca \-ˌble-nò-ˈra-ji-kə\ *n* : a disease that is characterized by a scaly rash esp. on the palms and soles and is associated esp. with reactive arthritis — called also *keratoderma blennorrhagicum*

keratosis fol·li·cu·lar·is \-ˌfä-lə-kyə-ˈler-əs\ *n* : DARIER'S DISEASE

keratosis pi·la·ris \-pi-ˈler-əs\ *n* : a condition marked by the formation of hard conical elevations in the openings of the sebaceous glands esp. of the thighs and arms that resemble permanent goose bumps

ker·a·tot·o·mist \ˌker-ə-ˈtä-tə-mist\ *n* : a surgeon who performs keratotomies

ker·a·tot·o·my \-mē\ *n, pl* **-mies** : incision of the cornea

ke·ri·on \ˈkir-ē-ˌän\ *n* : inflammatory ringworm of the hair follicles of the beard and scalp usu. accompanied by secondary bacterial infection

ker·nic·ter·us \kər-ˈnik-tə-rəs\ *n* : a condition marked by the deposit of bile pigments in the nuclei of the brain and spinal cord and by degeneration of nerve cells that occurs usu. in infants as a part of the syndrome of erythroblastosis fetalis — **ker·nic·ter·ic** \-rik\ *adj*

Ker·nig sign \ˈker-nig-\ *or* **Kernig's sign** \ˈker-nigz-\ *n* : an indication usu. present in meningitis that consists of pain and resistance on attempting to extend the leg at the knee with the thigh flexed at the hip

Kernig, Vladimir Mikhailovich (1840–1917), Russian physician.

ke·ta·mine \ˈkē-tə-ˌmēn\ *n* : a general anesthetic that is administered intravenously or intramuscularly in the form of its hydrochloride $C_{13}H_{16}ClNO \cdot HCl$ and is used illicitly usu. by being inhaled in powdered form esp. for the dreamlike or hallucinogenic state it produces— see SPECIAL K

ke·thox·al \kē-ˈthäk-səl\ *n* : an antiviral agent $C_6H_{12}O_4$

ke·to \ˈkē-(ˌ)tō\ *adj* : of or relating to a ketone; *also* : containing a ketone group

keto acid *n* : a compound that is both a ketone and an acid

ke·to·ac·i·do·sis \ˌkē-tō-ˌa-sə-ˈdō-səs\ *n, pl* **-do·ses** \-ˌsēz\ : acidosis resulting from increased levels of ketone bodies in the blood ⟨diabetic ~⟩ — **ke·to·ac·i·dot·ic** \-ˈdä-tik\ *adj*

ke·to·co·na·zole \ˌkē-tō-ˈkō-nə-ˌzōl\ *n* : a synthetic broad-spectrum antifungal agent $C_{26}H_{28}Cl_2N_4O_4$ used to treat chronic internal and cutaneous disorders — see NIZORAL

ke·to·gen·e·sis \ˌkē-tō-ˈje-nə-səs\ *n, pl* **-e·ses** \-ˌsēz\ : the production of ketone bodies (as in diabetes mellitus) — **ke·to·gen·ic** \-ˈje-nik\ *adj*

ketogenic diet *n* : a diet supplying a large amount of fat and minimal amounts of carbohydrate and protein

ke·to·glu·tar·ic acid \ˌkē-tō-glü-ˈtar-ik-\ *n* : either of two crystalline keto derivatives $C_5H_6O_5$ of glutaric acid; *esp* : ALPHA-KETOGLUTARIC ACID

α–ketoglutaric acid *var of* ALPHA-KETOGLUTARIC ACID

ke·to·nae·mia *chiefly Brit var of* KETONEMIA

ke·tone \ˈkē-ˌtōn\ *n* : an organic compound (as acetone) with a CO group attached to two carbon atoms

ketone body *n* : any of the three compounds acetoacetic acid, acetone, and the beta derivative of hydroxybutyric acid which are normal intermediates in lipid metabolism and accumulate in the blood and urine in abnormal amounts in conditions of impaired metabolism (as diabetes mellitus) — called also *acetone body*

ke·to·ne·mia \ˌkē-tə-ˈnē-mē-ə\ *n* **1** : a condition marked by an abnormal increase of ketone bodies in the circulating blood — called also *hyperketonemia* **2** : KETOSIS 2 — **ke·to·ne·mic** \-ˈnē-mik\ *adj*

ke·ton·uria \ˌkē-tə-ˈnu̇r-ē-ə, -ˈnyu̇r-\ *n* : the presence of excess ketone bodies in the urine in conditions (as diabetes mellitus and starvation acidosis) involving reduced or disturbed carbohydrate metabolism — called also *acetonuria*

ke·to·pro·fen \ˌkē-tə-ˈprō-fən\ *n* : an analgesic nonsteroidal anti-inflammatory drug $C_{16}H_{14}O_3$ used to treat dysmenorrhea and the symptoms of rheumatoid arthritis and osteoarthritis

ke·tose \ˈkē-ˌtōs, -ˌtōz\ *n* : a sugar (as fructose) containing one ketone group per molecule

ke·to·sis \kē-ˈtō-səs\ *n, pl* **-to·ses** \-ˌsēz\ **1** : an abnormal increase of ketone bodies in the body in conditions of reduced or disturbed carbohydrate metabolism (as in diabetes mellitus) — compare ACIDOSIS, ALKALOSIS **2** : a nutritional disease esp. of cattle that is marked by reduction of blood sugar and the presence of ketone bodies — **ke·tot·ic** \-ˈtä-tik\ *adj*

ke·to·ste·roid \ˌkē-tō-ˈstir-ˌȯid, -ˈster-\ *n* : a steroid (as cortisone or estrone) containing a ketone group; *esp* : 17-KETOSTEROID

17–ketosteroid *n* : any of the ketosteroids (as androsterone, dehydroepiandrosterone, and estrone) that have the keto group attached to carbon atom 17 of the steroid ring structure, are present in normal human urine, and may be an indication of a tumor of the adrenal cortex or ovary when present in excess

Ke·ty method \ˈkē-tē-\ *n* : a method of determining coronary blood flow by measurement of nitrous oxide levels in the blood of a patient breathing nitrous oxide

Kety, Seymour Solomon (1915–2000), American physiologist.

key·hole \ˈkē-ˌhōl\ *adj* **1** : relating to, used in, or being a minimally invasive operation or surgical procedure (as laparoscopy or arthroscopy) in which one or more small incisions are made to permit passage of instruments (as an endoscope and forceps) into the body ⟨~ surgery for gall bladder removal⟩ **2** : being a small incision made in keyhole surgery

kg *abbr* kilogram

khel·lin \ˈke-lən\ *n* : a crystalline compound $C_{14}H_{12}O_5$ obtained from the fruit of a Middle Eastern plant (*Ammi visnaga*) of the carrot family (Umbelliferae) and used esp. as a coronary vasodilator

kid·ney \ˈkid-nē\ *n, pl* **kidneys** : one of a pair of vertebrate organs situated in the body cavity near the spinal column that excrete waste products of metabolism, in humans are bean-shaped organs about 4½ inches (11½ centimeters) long lying behind the peritoneum in a mass of fatty tissue, and consist chiefly of nephrons by which urine is secreted, collected, and discharged into the renal pelvis where it is conveyed by the ureter to the bladder — compare MESONEPHROS, METANEPHROS, PRONEPHROS

kidney stone *n* : a calculus in the kidney — called also *renal calculus*

kidney worm *n* : any of several nematode worms parasitic in the kidneys: as **a** : GIANT KIDNEY WORM **b** : a common worm of the genus *Stephanurus* (*S. dentatus*) that is related to the gapeworm and is parasitic in the kidneys, lungs, and other viscera of the hog in warm regions

Kien·böck's disease \ˈkēn-ˌbeks-\ *n* : osteochondrosis affecting the lunate bone

Kien·böck \ˈkēn-ˌbœk\, **Robert (1871–1953)**, Austrian radiologist.

killed \ˈkild\ *adj* : being or containing a virus that has been inactivated (as by chemicals) so that it is no longer effective ⟨~ vaccines⟩

killer bee *n* : AFRICANIZED BEE

killer cell *n* : a lymphocyte (as a cytotoxic T cell or a natural killer cell) with cytotoxic activity

killer T cell *n* : CYTOTOXIC T CELL

killer T lymphocyte *n* : CYTOTOXIC T CELL

ki·lo·base \ˈki-lə-ˌbās\ *n* : a unit of measure of the length of a nucleic-acid chain (as of DNA or RNA) that equals one thousand base pairs

ki·lo·cal·o·rie \-ˌka-lə-rē\ *n* : CALORIE 1b

ki·lo·gram \ˈki-lə-ˌgram, ˈkē-\ *n* **1** : the base unit of mass in the International System of Units that is nearly equal to the mass of 1000 cubic centimeters of water at the temperature of its maximum density **2** : a unit of force or weight equal to the weight of a kilogram mass under a gravitational attraction equal to that of the earth

kilogram calorie *n* : CALORIE 1b

ki·lo·joule \ˈki-lə-ˌjül\ *n* : 1000 joules

ki·lo·me·ter \ˈki-lə-ˌmē-tər, kə-ˈlä-mə-tər\ *n* : 1000 meters

ki·lo·rad \ˈki-lə-ˌrad\ *n* : 1000 rads

ki·lo·volt \-ˌvōlt\ *n* : a unit of potential difference equal to 1000 volts

kin- *or* **kine-** *or* **kino-** *or* **cin-** *or* **cino-** *comb form* : motion : action ⟨*kin*esthesia⟩

kin·aes·the·sia *chiefly Brit var of* KINESTHESIA

ki·nase \ˈkī-ˌnās, -ˌnāz\ *n* : an enzyme that catalyzes the transfer of phosphate groups from a high-energy phosphate-containing molecule (as ATP or ADP) to a substrate — called also *phosphokinase*

kind·ling \ˈkin-dliŋ\ *n* : the electrophysiological changes that occur in the brain as a result of repeated intermittent exposure to a subthreshold electrical or chemical stimulus (as one causing seizures) so that there develops a usu. permanent decrease in the threshold of excitability

ki·ne·mat·ics \ˌki-nə-ˈma-tiks, ˌkī-\ *n* **1** : a science that deals with aspects of motion apart from considerations of mass and force **2** : the properties and phenomena of an object or system in motion of interest to kinematics ⟨the ~ of a joint⟩ — **ki·ne·mat·ic** \-tik\ *or* **ki·ne·mat·i·cal** \-ti-kəl\ *adj*

kineplasty *var of* CINEPLASTY

Kin·e·ret \ˈki-nə-ˌret\ *trademark* — used for a preparation of anakinra

kinesi- *or* **kinesio-** *comb form* : movement ⟨*kinesio*logy⟩

-ki·ne·sia \kə-ˈnē-zhə, kī-, -zhē-ə\ *n comb form* : movement : motion ⟨hyper*kinesia*⟩

ki·ne·sin \ki-ˈnē-sən\ *n* : an ATPase similar to dynein that functions as a motor protein in the intracellular transport esp. of cell organelles and molecules along microtubules

ki·ne·si·ol·o·gy \kə-ˌnē-sē-ˈä-lə-jē, kī-, -zē-\ *n, pl* **-gies** : the study of the principles of mechanics and anatomy in relation to human movement — **ki·ne·si·o·log·ic** \-ō-ˈlä-jik\ *or* **ki·ne·si·o·log·i·cal** \-ji-kəl\ *adj* — **ki·ne·si·ol·o·gist** \kə-ˌnē-sē-ˈä-lə-jist, kī-, -zē-\ *n*

ki·ne·sis \kə-ˈnē-səs, kī-\ *n, pl* **ki·ne·ses** \-ˌsēz\ : a movement that lacks directional orientation and depends upon the intensity of stimulation

-ki·ne·sis \kə-ˈnē-sis, kī-\ *n, pl* **-ki·ne·ses** \-ˌsēz\ **1** : division ⟨karyo*kinesis*⟩ **2** : production of motion ⟨psycho*kinesis*⟩ ⟨tele*kinesis*⟩

kin·es·the·sia \ˌki-nəs-ˈthē-zhə, ˌkī-, -zhē-ə\ *or* **kin·es·the·sis** \-ˈthē-səs\ *n, pl* **-the·sias** *or* **-the·ses** \-ˌsēz\ : a sense mediated by end organs located in muscles, tendons, and joints and stimulated by bodily movements and tensions; *also* : sensory experience derived from this sense — see MUSCLE SENSE — **kin·es·thet·ic** \-ˈthe-tik\ *adj* — **kin·es·thet·i·cal·ly** *adv*

kinet- *or* **kineto-** *comb form* : movement : motion ⟨*kineto*chore⟩

ki·net·ic \kə-ˈne-tik, kī-\ *adj* : of or relating to the motion of material bodies and the forces and energy associated therewith — **ki•net•i•cal•ly** *adv*

ki•net•ics \kə-ˈne-tiks, kī-\ *n sing or pl* **1 a** : a science that deals with the effects of forces upon the motions of material bodies or with changes in a physical or chemical system **b** : the rate of change in such a system **2** : the mechanism by which a physical or chemical change is effected

ki•net•o•chore \kə-ˈne-tə-ˌkōr, kī-\ *n* **1** : CENTROMERE **2** : a specialized structure on the centromere to which the microtubular spindle fibers attach during mitosis and meiosis

king co•bra \-ˈkō-brə\ *n* : a large cobra (*Ophiophagus hannah* syn. *Naja hannah*) of southeastern Asia and the Philippines — called also *hamadryad*

king•dom \ˈkiŋ-dəm\ *n* : any of the three primary divisions of lifeless material, plants, and animals into which natural objects are grouped; *also* : a biological category (as Animalia) that ranks above the phylum and below the domain

king's evil *n, often cap K&E* : SCROFULA

ki•nin \ˈkī-nən\ *n* : any of various polypeptide hormones that are formed locally in the tissues and cause dilation of blood vessels and contraction of smooth muscle

ki•ni•nase \ˈkī-nə-ˌnās, -ˌnāz\ *n* : an enzyme in blood that destroys a kinin

ki•nin•o•gen \kī-ˈni-nə-jən\ *n* : an inactive precursor of a kinin — **ki•nin•o•gen•ic** \(ˌ)kī-ˌni-nə-ˈje-nik\ *adj*

kino- — see KIN-

ki•no•cil•i•um \ˌkī-nō-ˈsi-lē-əm\ *n, pl* **-cil•ia** \-lē-ə\ : a motile cilium that occurs alone at the end of a sensory hair cell of the inner ear among numerous nonmotile stereocilia

Kirsch•ner wire \ˈkərsh-nər-\ *n* : metal wire inserted through bone and used to achieve internal traction or immobilization of bone fractures

Kirschner, Martin (1879–1942), German surgeon.

kissing bug *n* : CONENOSE

kissing disease *n* : INFECTIOUS MONONUCLEOSIS

kiss of life *n, chiefly Brit* : artificial respiration by the mouth-to-mouth method

kleb•si•el•la \ˌkleb-zē-ˈe-lə\ *n* **1** *cap* : a genus of nonmotile gram-negative rod-shaped bacteria (family Enterobacteriaceae) that include causative agents of respiratory and urinary infections — see DONOVAN BODY, PNEUMOBACILLUS **2** : any bacterium of the genus *Klebsiella*

Klebs \ˈkleps\, **(Theodor Albrecht) Edwin (1834–1913),** German bacteriologist.

Klebs–Löff•ler bacillus \ˈkleps-ˈlef-lər-, ˈklebz-\ *n* : a bacterium of the genus *Corynebacterium* (*C. diphtheriae*) that causes human diphtheria

Löff•ler \ˈlœf-lər\, **Friedrich August Johannes (1852–1915),** German bacteriologist.

klee•blatt•schädel \ˈklā-ˌblät-ˌshād-ᵊl\ *n* : CLOVERLEAF SKULL

Klein•ian \ˈklī-nē-ən\ *adj* : of, relating to, or according with the psychoanalytic theories or practices of Melanie Klein — **Kleinian** *n*

Klein \ˈklīn\, **Melanie (1882–1960),** Austrian psychoanalyst.

klept- *or* **klepto-** *comb form* : stealing : theft ⟨*klepto*mania⟩

klep•to•lag•nia \ˌklep-tə-ˈlag-nē-ə\ *n* : sexual arousal and gratification produced by committing an act of theft

klep•to•ma•nia \ˌklep-tə-ˈmā-nē-ə, -nyə\ *n* : a persistent neurotic impulse to steal esp. without economic motive

klep•to•ma•ni•ac \-nē-ˌak\ *n* : an individual exhibiting kleptomania

Kline•fel•ter's syndrome \ˈklīn-ˌfel-tərz-\ *also* **Kline•fel•ter syndrome** \-tər-\ *n* : an abnormal condition in a male characterized by two X chromosomes and one Y chromosome, infertility, smallness of the testes, sparse facial and body hair, and gynecomastia

Klinefelter, Harry Fitch (1912–1990), American physician.

Kline reaction \ˈklīn-\ *n* : KLINE TEST

Kline test *n* : a rapid precipitation test for the diagnosis of syphilis

Kline, Benjamin Schoenbrun (*b* 1886), American pathologist.

Klip•pel–Feil syndrome \kli-ˈpel-ˈfīl-\ *n* : congenital fusion of the cervical vertebrae resulting in a short and relatively immobile neck

Klip•pel \klē-ˈpel\, **Maurice (1858–1942)** and **Feil** \ˈfāl\, **André (*b* 1884),** French neurologists.

Klor–Con \ˈklȯr-ˌkän\ *trademark* — used for a preparation of potassium chloride or potassium bicarbonate

Klump•ke's paralysis \ˈklümp-kēz-\ *n* : atrophic paralysis of the forearm and the hand due to injury to the eighth cervical and first thoracic nerves

Dé•jé•rine–Klump•ke \dā-zhā-ˌrēn-klüm-ˈkē\, **Augusta (1859–1927),** French neurologist.

Klüver–Bu•cy syndrome \ˈklü-vər-ˈb(y)ü-sē-\ *n* : a group of symptoms (as excessive reactivity to visual stimuli, hypersexuality, and diminished emotional responses) that are caused by bilateral removal of the temporal lobes induced experimentally in monkeys and that sometimes occur in humans with severe injuries to the temporal lobes

Klüver, Heinrich (1897–1979), American neurologist and psychologist.

Bucy, Paul Clancy (1904–1992), American neurologist.

km *abbr* kilometer

knee \ˈnē\ *n* **1** : a joint in the middle part of the leg that is the articulation between the femur, tibia, and patella — called also *knee joint* **2** : the part of the leg that includes this joint — **kneed** \ˈnēd\ *adj*

knee•cap \ˈnē-ˌkap\ *n* : PATELLA

knee jerk *n* : an involuntary forward jerk or kick produced by a light blow or sudden strain upon the patellar tendon of the knee that causes a reflex contraction of the quadriceps muscle — called also *patellar reflex*

knee joint *n* : KNEE 1

Kne·mi·do·kop·tes \ˌnē-mə-dō-ˈkäp-(ˌ)tēz\ *n* : a genus of itch mites (family Sarcoptidae) that attack birds

knife \ˈnīf\ *n, pl* **knives** \ˈnīvz\ **1** : any of various instruments used in surgery primarily to sever tissues: as **a** : a cutting instrument consisting of a sharp blade attached to a handle **b** : an instrument that cuts by means of an electrical current **2** : SURGERY 3 — usu. used in the phrase *under the knife* ⟨went under the ~ this morning⟩

knit \ˈnit\ *vb* **knit** *or* **knit·ted; knit·ting** : to grow or cause to grow together ⟨a fracture that *knitted* slowly⟩

knock–knee \ˈnäk-ˌnē\ *n* : a condition in which the legs curve inward at the knees — called also *genu valgum* — **knock–kneed** \-ˌnēd\ *adj*

knock·out \ˈnäk-ˌau̇t\ *adj* : having all or part of a gene eliminated or inactivated by genetic engineering ⟨~ mice⟩

knot \ˈnät\ *n* **1** : an interlacing of the parts of one or more flexible bodies (as threads or sutures) in a lump to prevent their spontaneous separation **2** : a usu. firm or hard lump, swelling, or protuberance (as in a muscle or on the surface of a bone) — **knot** *vb*

knuck·le \ˈnə-kəl\ *n* **1 a** : the rounded prominence formed by the ends of the two adjacent bones at a joint — used esp. of those at the joints of the fingers **b** : the joint of a knuckle **2** : a sharply flexed loop of intestines incarcerated in a hernia

Koch·er's forceps \ˈkō-kərz-\ *n* : a strong forceps for controlling bleeding in surgery having serrated blades with interlocking teeth at the tips

Kocher \ˈkȯ-k̲ər\, **Emil Theodor (1841–1917)**, Swiss surgeon.

Koch's bacillus \ˈkōks-, ˈkä-chəz-\ *or* **Koch bacillus** \ˈkōk-, ˈkäch-\ *n* : a bacillus of the genus *Mycobacterium* (*M. tuberculosis*) that causes human tuberculosis

Koch \ˈkȯk̲\, **(Heinrich Hermann) Robert (1843–1910)**, German bacteriologist.

Koch's postulates *n pl* : a statement of the steps required to establish a microorganism as the cause of a disease: (1) it must be found in all cases of the disease; (2) it must be isolated from the host and grown in pure culture; (3) it must reproduce the original disease when introduced into a susceptible host; (4) it must be found present in the experimental host so infected — called also *Koch's laws*

Koch–Weeks bacillus \-ˈwēks-\ *n* : a bacterium of the genus *Haemophilus* (*H. aegyptius*) associated with an infectious form of human conjunctivitis

Weeks, John Elmer (1853–1949), American ophthalmologist.

Koch–Weeks conjunctivitis *n* : conjunctivitis caused by the Koch-Weeks bacillus

koi·lo·cyte \ˈkȯi-lə-ˌsīt\ *n* : a vacuolated pyknotic epithelial cell associated with certain human papillomavirus infections (as of the genitals)

koi·lo·cy·to·sis \ˌkȯi-lə-sī-ˈtō-səs\ *n* : the presence of koilocytes usu. in the anogenital region or the uterine cervix

koil·onych·ia \ˌkȯi-lō-ˈni-kē-ə\ *n* : abnormal thinness and concavity of fingernails occurring esp. in hypochromic anemias — called also *spoon nails*

Kom·bi·glyze \ˈkäm-bə-ˌglīz\ *trademark* — used for a preparation of saxagliptin and the hydrochloride of metformin

Kop·lik's spots \ˈkä-pliks-\ *or* **Kop·lik spots** \-plik-\ *n pl* : small bluish-white dots surrounded by a reddish zone that appear on the mucous membrane of the cheeks and lips before the appearance of the skin eruption in a case of measles

Koplik, Henry (1858–1927), American pediatrician.

Korean hemorrhagic fever *n* : a hemorrhagic fever that is endemic in Korea, Manchuria, and Siberia, is caused by the Hantaan virus, and is characterized by acute renal failure in addition to the usual symptoms of the hemorrhagic fevers — called also *epidemic hemorrhagic fever*

Ko·rot·koff sounds *also* **Ko·rot·kow sounds** *or* **Ko·rot·kov sounds** \kȯ-ˈrȯt-kȯf-\ *n pl* : arterial sounds heard through a stethoscope applied to the brachial artery distal to the cuff of a sphygmomanometer that change with varying cuff pressure and that are used to determine systolic and diastolic blood pressure

Korotkoff, Nikolai Sergeievich (1874–1920), Russian physician.

Kor·sa·koff psychosis \ˈkȯr-sə-ˌkȯf-\ *also* **Kor·sa·koff's psychosis** \-ˌkȯfs-\ *n* : KORSAKOFF SYNDROME

Korsakoff *or* **Korsakov, Sergei Sergeievich (1853–1900)**, Russian psychiatrist.

Korsakoff syndrome *also* **Korsakoff's syndrome** *n* : a chronic memory disorder that is caused by brain damage related to a severe deficiency of thiamine (as that associated with alcoholism or malnutrition) and is characterized by impaired ability to form new memories and by memory loss for which the patient often attempts to compensate through confabulation and that is often preceded by Wernicke's encephalopathy

Kr *symbol* krypton

Krab•be's disease \ˈkra-bēz-\ *n* : a rapidly progressive demyelinating familial leukoencephalopathy with onset in infancy characterized by irritability followed by tonic convulsions, quadriplegia, blindness, deafness, dementia, and death

Krabbe \ˈkrä-bə\, **Knud H. (1885–1961),** Danish neurologist.

krad \ˈkā-ˌrad\ *n, pl* **krad** *also* **krads** : KILORAD

krait \ˈkrīt\ *n* : any of a genus (*Bungarus*) of brightly banded extremely venomous nocturnal elapid snakes of southern Asia and adjacent islands

krau•ro•sis \krȯ-ˈrō-səs\ *n, pl* **-ro•ses** \-ˌsēz\ : atrophy and shriveling of the skin or mucous membrane esp. of the vulva where it is often a precancerous lesion — **krau•rot•ic** \-ˈrä-tik\ *adj*

kraurosis vul•vae \-ˈvəl-vē\ *n* : kraurosis of the vulva

Krau•se's corpuscle \ˈkrau̇-zəz-\ *n* : any of various rounded sensory end organs occurring in mucous membranes (as of the conjunctiva or genitals) — called also *corpuscle of Krause*

Krause, Wilhelm Johann Friedrich (1833–1910), German anatomist.

Krause's end–bulb *n* : KRAUSE'S CORPUSCLE

kre•bi•o•zen \krə-ˈbī-ə-zən\ *n* : a drug formerly used in the treatment of cancer that was of unproved effectiveness and was of undisclosed formulation but was reported to contain creatine

Krebs cycle \ˈkrebz-\ *n* : a sequence of reactions in the living organism in which oxidation of acetic acid or acetyl equivalent provides energy for storage in phosphate bonds (as in ATP) — called also *citric acid cycle, tricarboxylic acid cycle*

Krebs, Sir Hans Adolf (1900–1981), German-British biochemist.

Kru•ken•berg tumor \ˈkrü-kən-ˌbərg-\ *n* : a metastatic ovarian tumor of mucin-producing epithelial cells usu. derived from a primary gastrointestinal tumor

Kru•ken•berg \-ˌberk\, **Friedrich Ernst (1871–1946),** German pathologist.

kryp•ton \ˈkrip-ˌtän\ *n* : a colorless relatively inert gaseous element — symbol *Kr;* see ELEMENT table

KS *abbr* Kaposi's sarcoma

KUB *abbr* kidney, ureter, and bladder

Ku•gel•berg–Wel•an•der disease \ˈkü-gəl-ˌbərg-ˈve-lən-dər-\ *n* : muscular weakness and atrophy that is caused by degeneration of motor neurons in the ventral horn of the spinal cord, is usu. inherited as an autosomal recessive trait, and that becomes symptomatic during childhood or adolescence typically progressing slowly during adulthood — compare WERDNIG-HOFFMANN DISEASE

Kugelberg, Eric Klas Henrik (1913–1983), and **Welander, Lisa (1909–2001),** Swedish neurologists.

Kupf•fer cell \ˈku̇p-fər-\ *also* **Kupffer's cell** \-fərz-\ *n* : a fixed macrophage of the walls of the liver sinusoids that is stellate with a large oval nucleus and the cytoplasm commonly packed with fragments resulting from phagocytic action

Kupffer, Karl Wilhelm von (1829–1902), German anatomist.

ku•ru \ˈkü-ˌrü, ˈku̇r-ü\ *n* : a rare progressive fatal prion disease that resembles Creutzfeldt-Jakob disease and has occurred among tribespeople in eastern New Guinea who engaged in a form of ritual cannibalism — called also *laughing death, laughing sickness*

Kuss•maul breathing \ˈku̇s-ˌmau̇l-\ *or* **Kuss•maul's breathing** \-ˌmau̇lz-\ *n* : deep rapid labored breathing that occurs as an involuntary response to severe acidosis (as that associated with diabetes or kidney failure) — called also *Kussmaul respiration*

Kussmaul, Adolf (1822–1902), German physician.

Kveim test \ˈkvām-\ *n* : a test for sarcoidosis used esp. formerly in which a suspension of sarcoid-containing tissue (as of the lymph nodes or spleen) is injected intradermally and which is positive when the formation of sarcoid granulomas are detected at the site of injection

Kveim, Morten Ansgar (1892–1966), Norwegian physician.

kwa•shi•or•kor \ˌkwä-shē-ˈȯr-kȯr, -ȯr-ˈkȯr\ *n* : severe malnutrition chiefly affecting young children esp. of impoverished regions that is characterized by failure to grow and develop, changes in the pigmentation of the skin and hair, edema, fatty degeneration of the liver, anemia, and apathy and is caused by a diet excessively high in carbohydrate and extremely low in protein — compare PELLAGRA

Kwell \ˈkwel\ *trademark* — used for a preparation of lindane

Kya•sa•nur For•est disease \ˌkya-sə-ˈnu̇r-ˈfȯr-əst-\ *n* : a disease caused by a virus of the genus *Flavivirus* (*Kyasanur Forest disease virus*) that is characterized by fever, headache, diarrhea, and intestinal bleeding and is transmitted by immature ticks of the genus *Haemaphysalis*

ky•mo•gram \ˈkī-mə-ˌgram\ *n* : a record made by a kymograph

ky•mo•graph \-ˌgraf\ *n* : a device which graphically records motion or pressure (as of blood) — **ky•mo•graph•ic** \ˌkī-mə-ˈgra-fik\ *adj* — **ky•mog•ra•phy** \kī-ˈmä-grə-fē\ *n*

kyn•uren•ic acid \ˌkīn-yu̇-ˌren-ik-, ˌkin-\ *n* : a crystalline acid $C_{10}H_7NO_3$ that is one of the normal products of tryptophan metabolism and is excreted in the urine

ky•pho•plas•ty \ˈkī-fō-ˌplas-tē\ *n, pl* **-ties** : a medical procedure that is similar to vertebroplasty in the use of acrylic cement to stabilize and reduce pain associated with a vertebral compression fracture but that additionally seeks to restore vertebral height and lessen spinal deformity by injecting the cement into a cavity created (as by a mechanical device) in the fractured bone

ky•pho•sco•li•o•sis \ˌkī-fō-ˌskō-lē-ˈō-səs\ *n, pl* **-o•ses** \-ˌsēz\ : backward and lateral curvature of the spine

ky•pho•sis \kī-ˈfō-səs\ *n, pl* **-pho•ses** \-ˌsēz\ : exaggerated backward curvature of the thoracic region of the spinal column — compare LORDOSIS 2, SCOLIOSIS — **ky•phot•ic** \-ˈfä-tik\ *adj*

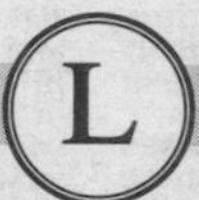

L *abbr* lumbar — used esp. with a number from 1 to 5 to indicate a vertebra or segment of the spinal cord in the lumbar region

L *symbol* lithium

l- *prefix* **1** \ˌlē-(ˌ)vō, ˌel, ˈel\ : levorotatory — usu. printed in italic ⟨*l*-tartaric acid⟩ **2** \ˌel, ˈel\ : having a similar configuration at a selected carbon atom to the configuration of levorotatory glyceraldehyde — usu. printed as a small capital ⟨L-fructose⟩

La *symbol* lanthanum

LA *abbr* long-acting

lab \ˈlab\ *n* : LABORATORY

[1]**la•bel** \ˈlā-bəl\ *n* : a usu. radioactive isotope used in labeling

[2]**label** *vb* **la•beled** *or* **la•belled; la•bel•ing** *or* **la•bel•ling** **1** : to distinguish (an element or atom) by using an isotope distinctive in some manner (as in mass or radioactivity) **2** : to distinguish (as a compound or cell) by introducing a traceable constituent (as a dye or labeled atom)

la•bet•a•lol \lə-ˈbe-tə-ˌlȯl, -ˌlōl\ *n* : a beta-adrenergic blocking agent used in the form of its hydrochloride $C_{19}H_{24}O_3 \cdot HCl$ to treat hypertension

labia *pl of* LABIUM

la•bi•al \ˈlā-bē-əl\ *adj* : of, relating to, or situated near the lips or labia — **la•bi•al•ly** *adv*

labial artery *n* : either of two branches of the facial artery of which one is distributed to the upper and one to the lower lip

labial gland *n* : one of the small tubular mucous and serous glands lying beneath the mucous membrane of the lips

labialis — see HERPES LABIALIS

la•bia ma•jo•ra \ˈlā-bē-ə-mə-ˈjōr-ə\ *n pl* : the outer fatty folds of the vulva bounding the vestibule

labia mi•no•ra \-mə-ˈnōr-ə\ *n pl* : the inner highly vascular largely connective-tissue folds of the vulva bounding the vestibule — called also *nymphae*

labii — see LEVATOR LABII SUPERIORIS, LEVATOR LABII SUPERIORIS ALAEQUE NASI, QUADRATUS LABII SUPERIORIS

la•bile \ˈlā-ˌbīl, -bəl\ *adj* : readily or frequently changing: as **a** : readily or continually undergoing chemical, physical, or biological change or breakdown ⟨a ∼ antigen⟩ **b** : characterized by wide fluctuations (as in blood pressure or glucose tolerance) ⟨∼ hypertension⟩ **c** : emotionally unstable — **la•bil•i•ty** \lā-ˈbi-lə-tē\ *n*

labile factor *n* : FACTOR V

labio- *comb form* : labial and ⟨*labio*lingual⟩

la•bio–buc•cal \ˌlā-bē-ō-ˈbə-kəl\ *adj* : of, relating to, or lying against the inner surface of the lips and cheeks; *also* : administered to labio-buccal tissue ⟨a ∼ injection⟩

la•bio•glos•so•pha•ryn•geal \ˌlā-bē-ō-ˌglä-sō-ˌfar-ən-ˈjē-əl, -ˌglȯ-, -fə-ˈrin-jəl, -jē-əl\ *adj* : of, relating to, or affecting the lips, tongue, and pharynx

la•bio•lin•gual \-ˈliŋ-gwəl, -gyə-wəl\ *adj* **1** : of or relating to the lips and the tongue **2** : of or relating to the labial and lingual aspects of a tooth — **la•bio•lin•gual•ly** *adv*

la•bio•scro•tal \-ˈskrōt-ᵊl\ *adj* : relating to or being a swelling or ridge on each side of the embryonic rudiment of the penis or clitoris which develops into one of the scrotal sacs in the male and one of the labia majora in the female

la•bi•um \ˈlā-bē-əm\ *n, pl* **la•bia** \-ə\ : any of the folds at the margin of the vulva — compare LABIA MAJORA, LABIA MINORA

la•bor \ˈlā-bər\ *n* : the physical activities involved in childbirth consisting essentially of a prolonged series of involuntary contractions of the uterine musculature together with both reflex and voluntary contractions of the abdominal wall; *also* : the period of time during which such labor takes place — **labor** *vb*

lab•o•ra•to•ry \ˈla-brə-ˌtōr-ē\ *n, pl* **-ries** *often attrib* : a place equipped for experimental study in a science or for testing and analysis

la•bored \ˈlā-bərd\ *adj* : produced or performed with difficulty or strain ⟨∼ breathing⟩

labor room *n* : a hospital room where a woman in labor stays before being taken to the delivery room

la•brum \ˈlā-brəm\ *n* : a fibrous ring of cartilage attached to the rim of a joint; *esp* : GLENOID LABRUM

lab•y•rinth \ˈla-bə-ˌrinth\ *n* : an anatomical structure with a series of interconnecting canals or cavities; *esp* : the internal ear or its bony or membranous part — see BONY LABYRINTH, MEMBRANOUS LABYRINTH

lab•y•rin•thec•to•my \ˌlab-ə-ˌrin-ˈthek-tə-mē\ *n, pl* **-mies** : surgical removal of the labyrinth of the ear

lab•y•rin•thine \-ˈrin-thən, -ˌthīn, -ˌthēn\ *adj* : of, relating to, affecting, or originating in the internal ear

labyrinthine artery *n* : INTERNAL AUDITORY ARTERY

labyrinthine sense *n* : VESTIBULAR SENSE

lab•y•rin•thi•tis \ˌla-bə-rin-ˈthī-təs\ *n* : inflammation of the labyrinth of the internal ear

lab•y•rin•thot•o•my \ˌla-bə-rin-ˈthä-tə-mē\ *n, pl* **-mies** : surgical incision into the labyrinth of the internal ear

lac•er•a•tion \ˌla-sə-ˈrā-shən\ *n* **1** : the act of making a rough or jagged wound or tear **2** : a torn and ragged wound — **lac•er•ate** \ˈla-sə-ˌrāt\ *vb*

lacerum — see FORAMEN LACERUM

lachrymal, lachrymation, lachrymator, lachrymatory *var of* LACRIMAL, LACRIMATION, LACRIMATOR, LACRIMATORY

lac operon \ˈlak-\ *n* : the operon which controls lactose metabolism and has been isolated from E. coli

[1]**lac•ri•mal** *also* **lach•ry•mal** \ˈla-krə-məl\ *adj* **1** : of, relating to, associated with, located near, or constituting the glands that produce tears **2** : of or relating to tears ⟨∼ effusions⟩

[2]**lacrimal** *also* **lachrymal** *n* : a lacrimal anatomical part (as a lacrimal bone)

lacrimal apparatus *n* : the bodily parts which function in the production of tears including the lacrimal glands, lacrimal ducts, lacrimal sacs, nasolacrimal ducts, and lacrimal puncta

lacrimal artery *n* : a large branch of the ophthalmic artery that arises near the optic foramen and supplies the lacrimal gland

lacrimal bone *n* : a small thin bone making up part of the front inner wall of each orbit and providing a groove for the passage of the lacrimal ducts

lacrimal canal *n* : LACRIMAL DUCT 1

lacrimal canaliculus *n* : LACRIMAL DUCT 1

lacrimal caruncle *n* : a small reddish follicular elevation at the medial angle of the eye

lacrimal duct *n* **1** : a short canal leading from a minute orifice on a small elevation at the medial angle of each eyelid to the lacrimal sac — called also *lacrimal canal, lacrimal canaliculus* **2** : any of several small ducts that carry tears from the lacrimal gland to the fornix of the conjunctiva

lacrimal gland *n* : an acinous gland that is about the size and shape of an almond, secretes tears, and is situated laterally and superiorly to the bulb of the eye in a shallow depression on the inner surface of the frontal bone — called also *tear gland*

lacrimal nerve *n* : a small branch of the ophthalmic nerve that enters the lacrimal gland with the lacrimal artery and supplies the lacrimal gland and the adjacent conjunctiva and the skin of the upper eyelid

lacrimal punc•tum \-ˈpəŋk-təm\ *n* : the opening of either the upper or the lower lacrimal duct at the inner canthus of the eye

lacrimal sac *n* : the dilated oval upper end of the nasolacrimal duct that is situated in a groove formed by the lacrimal bone and the frontal process of the maxilla, is closed at its upper end, and receives the lacrimal ducts

lac•ri•ma•tion *also* **lach•ry•ma•tion** \ˌla-krə-ˈmā-shən\ *n* : the secretion of tears; *specif* : abnormal or excessive secretion of tears due to local or systemic disease

lac•ri•ma•tor *also* **lach•ry•ma•tor** \ˈla-krə-ˌmā-tər\ *n* : a tear-producing substance (as tear gas)

lac•ri•ma•to•ry *also* **lach•ry•ma•to•ry** \ˈla-kri-mə-ˌtōr-ē\ *adj* : of, relating to, or prompting tears

La Crosse encephalitis \lə-ˈkrȯs-\ *n* : an encephalitis typically affecting children that is caused by the La Crosse virus transmitted esp. by a mosquito of the genus *Aedes* (*A. triseriatus*)

La Crosse virus *n* : a virus that causes La Crosse encephalitis and that belongs to a strain of a virus of the genus *Orthobunyavirus* (species *California encephalitis virus*)

lact- *or* **lacti-** *or* **lacto-** *comb form* **1** : milk ⟨*lacto*genesis⟩ **2 a** : lactic acid ⟨*lact*ate⟩ **b** : lactose ⟨*lact*ase⟩

lact•aci•de•mia \ˌlak-ˌta-sə-ˈdē-mē-ə\ *n* : the presence of excess lactic acid in the blood

lact•al•bu•min \ˌlak-ˌtal-ˈbyü-mən\ *n* : an albumin that is found in milk and is similar to serum albumin; *esp* : a protein fraction from whey

lac•tam \ˈlak-ˌtam\ *n* : any of a class of amides of amino carboxylic acids that are characterized by the group –CONH– in a ring and that include many antibiotics

β–lactam *var of* BETA-LACTAM

β–lactamase *var of* BETA-LACTAMASE

lac•tase \ˈlak-ˌtās, -ˌtāz\ *n* : an enzyme that hydrolyzes lactose to glucose and galactose and occurs esp. in the intestines of young mammals and in yeasts

[1]**lac•tate** \ˈlak-ˌtāt\ *n* : a salt or ester of lactic acid

[2]**lactate** *vb* **lac•tat•ed; lac•tat•ing** : to secrete milk

lactate dehydrogenase *n* : any of a group of isoenzymes that catalyze reversibly the conversion of pyruvic acid to lactic acid, are found esp. in the liver, kidneys, striated muscle, and the myocardium, and tend to accumulate in the body when these organs or tissues are diseased or injured — called also *lactic dehydrogenase*

lactated Ringer's solution *n* : a sterile aqueous solution that is similar to Ringer's solution but contains sodium lactate in addition to calcium chloride, sodium chloride, and potassium chloride — called also *Hartmann's solution, lactated Ringer's, Ringer's lactate, Ringer's lactate solution*

S. Ringer — see RINGER'S FLUID

lac•ta•tion \lak-ˈtā-shən\ *n* **1** : the secretion and yielding of milk by the mammary gland **2** : one complete period of lactation extending from about the time of parturition to weaning

lactation tetany *n* : MILK FEVER 1

[1]**lac•te•al** \ˈlak-tē-əl\ *adj* **1** : relating to, consisting of, producing, or resembling milk ⟨~ fluid⟩ **2 a** : conveying or containing a milky fluid (as chyle) ⟨a ~ channel⟩ **b** : of or relating to the lacteals ⟨impaired ~ function⟩

[2]**lacteal** *n* : any of the lymphatic vessels arising from the villi of the small intestine and conveying chyle to the thoracic duct

lacti- — see LACT-

lac•tic acid \ˈlak-tik-\ *n* : an organic acid $C_3H_6O_3$ that is known in three optically isomeric forms: **a** *or* **D–lactic acid** \ˈdē-\ : the dextrorotatory form present normally in blood and muscle tissue as a product of the metabolism of glucose and glycogen **b** *or* **L–lactic acid** \ˈel-\ : the levorotatory form obtained by biological fermentation of sucrose **c** *or* **DL–lactic acid** \ˈdē-ˈel-\ : the racemic form present in food products and made usu. by bacterial fermentation

lactic acidosis *n* : a condition characterized by the accumulation of lactic acid in bodily tissues

lactic dehydrogenase *n* : LACTATE DEHYDROGENASE

lac•tif•er•ous duct \lak-ˈti-fə-rəs-\ *n* : any of the milk-carrying ducts of the mammary gland that open on the nipple

lactiferous sinus *n* : an expansion in a lactiferous duct at the base of the nipple in which milk accumulates

lacto- — see LACT-

lac•to•ba•cil•lus \ˌlak-tō-bə-ˈsi-ləs\ *n* **1** *cap* : a genus of gram-positive nonmotile lactic-acid-forming bacteria (family Lactobacillaceae) **2** *pl* **-li** \-ˌī *also* -ˌē\ : any bacterium of the genus Lactobacillus

lac•to•fer•rin \ˌlak-tō-ˈfer-ən\ *n* : a red iron-binding protein synthesized by neutrophils and glandular epithelial cells, found in many human secretions (as tears and milk), and retarding bacterial and fungal growth

lac•to•fla•vin \ˌlak-tō-ˈflā-vən\ *n* : RIBOFLAVIN

lac•to•gen \ˈlak-tə-jən, -ˌjen\ *n* : any hormone (as prolactin) that stimulates the production of milk — see PLACENTAL LACTOGEN

lac•to•gen•e•sis \ˌlak-tō-ˈje-nə-səs\ *n, pl* **-e•ses** \-ˌsēz\ : initiation of lactation

lac•to•gen•ic \ˌlak-tō-ˈje-nik\ *adj* : stimulating lactation

lactogenic hormone *n* : LACTOGEN; *esp* : PROLACTIN

lac•tone \ˈlak-ˌtōn\ *n* : any of various cyclic esters formed from acids containing one or more OH groups

lac•to–ovo–veg•e•tar•i•an \ˌlak-tō-ˌō-vō-ˌve-jə-ˈter-ē-ən\ *n* : a vegetarian whose diet includes milk, eggs, vegetables, fruits, grains, and nuts — compare LACTO-VEGETARIAN — **lacto–ovo–vegetarian** *adj*

lac•to•per•ox•i•dase \ˌlak-tō-pə-ˈräk-sə-ˌdās, -ˌdāz\ *n* : a peroxidase found in milk and saliva that catalyzes the oxidation of the anions thiocyanate or iodide by hydrogen peroxide resulting in the production of antimicrobial compounds

lac•tose \ˈlak-ˌtōs, -ˌtōz\ *n* : a disaccharide sugar $C_{12}H_{22}O_{11}$ that is present in milk, yields glucose and galactose upon hydrolysis, yields esp. lactic acid upon fermentation, and is used chiefly in foods, medicines, and culture media (as for the production of penicillin) — called also *milk sugar*

lac•tos•uria \ˌlak-tō-ˈshu̇r-ē-ə, -ˈsyu̇r-\ *n* : the presence of lactose in the urine

lac•to–veg•e•tar•i•an \ˌlak-tō-ˌve-jə-ˈter-ē-ən\ *n* : a vegetarian whose diet includes milk, vegetables, fruits, grains, and nuts — compare LACTO-OVO-VEGETARIAN — **lacto–vegetarian** *adj*

lac•tu•lose \ˈlak-tyu̇-ˌlōs, -tu̇-, -ˌlōz\ *n* : a synthetic disaccharide $C_{12}H_{22}O_{11}$ used as a laxative for chronic constipation and as an acidifier to reduce blood ammonia levels causing neurological symptoms in advanced liver disease

la•cu•na \lə-ˈkü-nə, -ˈkyü-\ *n, pl* **la•cu•nae** \-ˌnē, -ˌnī\ : a small cavity, pit, or discontinuity in an anatomical structure: as **a** : one of the follicles in the mucous membrane of the urethra **b** : one of the minute cavities in bone or cartilage occupied by the osteocytes — **la•cu•nar** \-nər\ *adj*

Laen•nec's cirrhosis *or* **Laën•nec's cirrhosis** \ˈlā-neks-\ *n* : hepatic cirrhosis in which increased connective tissue spreads out from the portal spaces compressing and distorting the lobules, causing impairment of liver function, and ultimately producing the typical hobnail liver — called also *portal cirrhosis*

Laennec, René–Théophile–Hyacinthe (1781–1826), French physician.

la•e•trile \ˈlā-ə-(ˌ)tril\ *n, often cap* : a drug that is derived esp. from pits of the apricot (*Prunus armeniaca* of the rose family, Rosaceae), that contains amygdalin, and that has been used in the treatment of cancer although of unproved effectiveness

laev- *or* **laevo-** *Brit var of* LEV-

lae•vo•car•dia, lae•vo•do•pa *Brit var of* LEVOCARDIA, LEVODOPA

La•fora body \lä-ˈfȯr-ə-\ *n* : any of the cytoplasmic inclusion bodies found in neurons of parts of the central nervous system in Lafora disease and consisting of a complex of glycoprotein and glycosaminoglycan

Lafora, Gonzalo Rodriguez (1886–1971), Spanish neurologist.

Lafora disease *or* **Lafora's disease** *n* : an inherited form of myoclonic epilepsy that typically begins during adolescence or late childhood and is characterized by progressive neurological deterioration and the presence of Lafora bodies in parts of the central nervous system

-lag•nia \ˈlag-nē-ə\ *comb form* : sexual excitement ⟨uro*lagnia*⟩

lag•oph•thal•mos *or* **lag•oph•thal•mus** \ˌla-ˌgäf-ˈthal-məs\ *n* : pathological incomplete closure of the eyelids : inability to close the eyelids fully

la grippe \lä-ˈgrip\ *n* : INFLUENZA

LAK \ˈlak; ˌel-(ˌ)ā-ˈkā\ *n* : LYMPHOKINE-ACTIVATED KILLER CELL

LAK cell *n* : LYMPHOKINE-ACTIVATED KILLER CELL

lake \ˈlāk\ *vb* **laked; lak•ing** : to undergo or cause (blood) to undergo a physiological change in which the hemoglobin becomes dissolved in the plasma

-la•lia \ˈlā-lē-ə\ *n comb form* : speech disorder (of a specified type) ⟨echo*lalia*⟩

lal•la•tion \la-ˈlā-shən\ *n* **1** : infantile speech whether in infants or in older speakers **2** : a defective articulation of the letter *l*, the substitution of \l\ for another sound, or the substitution of another sound for \l\

La•maze \lə-ˈmäz\ *adj* : relating to or being a method of childbirth that involves psychological and physical preparation by the mother in order to suppress pain and facilitate delivery without drugs

Lamaze, Fernand (1890–1957), French obstetrician.

lamb•da \ˈlam-də\ *n* **1** : the point of junction of the sagittal and lambdoid sutures of the skull **2** : BACTERIOPHAGE LAMBDA

lambda chain *or* **λ chain** *n* : a polypeptide chain of one of the two types of light chain that are found in antibodies and can be distinguished antigenically and by the sequence of amino acids in the chain — compare KAPPA CHAIN

lamb•da•cism \ˈlam-də-ˌsi-zəm\ *n* : a defective articulation of \l\, the substitution of other sounds for it, or the substitution of \l\ for another sound

lambda phage *n* : BACTERIOPHAGE LAMBDA

lamb•doid \ˈlam-ˌdȯid\ *or* **lamb•doi•dal** \ˌlam-ˈdȯid-ᵊl\ *adj* : of, relating to, or being the suture shaped like the Greek letter lambda (λ) that connects the occipital and parietal bones

Lam•bert–Ea•ton syndrome \ˈlam-bərt-ˈē-tᵊn-\ *n* : an autoimmune disorder that is caused by impaired presynaptic release of acetylcholine at nerve synapses, that is characterized by progressive weakness esp. of the limbs, and that is often associated with a malignant condition (as small-cell lung cancer) — called also *Eaton-Lambert syndrome, Lambert-Eaton myasthenic syndrome*

Lambert, Edward Howard (1915–2003), and **Eaton, Lealdes McKendree (1905–1958),** American physicians.

lam•bli•a•sis \lam-ˈblī-ə-səs\ *n, pl* **-a•ses** \-ˌsēz\ : GIARDIASIS

Lambl \ˈlämb-ᵊl\, **Wilhelm Dusan (1824–1895),** Austrian physician.

lame \ˈlām\ *adj* **lam•er; lam•est** : having a body part and esp. a limb so disabled as to impair freedom of movement : physically disabled — **lame•ly** *adv* — **lame•ness** *n*

la•mel•la \lə-ˈme-lə\ *n, pl* **la•mel•lae** \-ˌlē, -ˌlī\ *also* **lamellas 1** : an organ, process, or part resembling a plate: as **a** : one of the bony concentric layers surrounding the haversian canals in bone **b** (1) : one of the incremental layers of cementum laid down in a tooth (2) : a thin sheetlike organic structure in the enamel of a tooth extending inward from a surface crack **2** : a small medicated disk prepared from gelatin and glycerin for use esp. in the eyes — **la•mel•lar** \lə-ˈme-lər\ *adj* — **lam•el•lat•ed** \ˈla-mə-ˌlā-təd\ *adj*

lamellar ichthyosis *n* : a rare inherited form of ichthyosis characterized by large coarse scales

lamin- *or* **lamini-** *or* **lamino-** *comb form* : lamina ⟨*lamin*itis⟩

lam•i•na \ˈla-mə-nə\ *n, pl* **-nae** \-ˌnē, -ˌnī\ *or* **-nas** : a thin plate or layer esp. of an anatomical part

lamina cri•bro•sa \-kri-ˈbrō-sə\ *n, pl* **laminae cri•bro•sae** \-ˌsē, -ˌsī\ : any of several anatomical structures having the form of a perforated plate: as **a** : CRIBRIFORM PLATE 1 **b** : the part of the sclera of the eye penetrated by the fibers of the optic nerve **c** : a perforated plate that closes the internal auditory canal

lamina du•ra \-ˈdu̇r-ə, -ˈdyu̇r-\ *n* : the thin hard layer of bone that lines the socket of a tooth and that appears as a dense white line in radiography

laminagram, laminagraph *var of* LAMINOGRAM, LAMINOGRAPH

lamina pro•pria \-ˈprō-prē-ə\ *n, pl* **laminae pro•pri•ae** \-prē-ˌē, -ˌī\ : a highly vascular layer of connective tissue under the basement membrane lining a layer of epithelium

lam•i•nar \ˈla-mə-nər\ *adj* : arranged in, consisting of, or resembling laminae

lam•i•nar•ia \ˌla-mə-ˈnar-ē-ə\ *n* : any of a genus (*Laminaria*) of kelps of which some have been used to dilate the cervix in performing an abortion

lamina spi•ral•is \-spə-ˈra-ləs, -ˈrā-\ *n* : SPIRAL LAMINA

lam•i•nat•ed \ˈla-mə-ˌnā-təd\ *adj* : composed or arranged in layers or laminae ⟨~ membranes⟩

lamina ter•mi•nal•is \-ˌtər-mi-ˈna-ləs, -ˈnā-\ *n* : a thin layer of gray matter in the telencephalon that extends backward from the corpus callosum above the optic chiasma and forms the median portion of the rostral wall of the third ventricle of the cerebrum

lam•i•na•tion \ˌla-mə-ˈnā-shən\ *n* : a laminated structure or arrangement

lam•i•nec•to•my \ˌla-mə-ˈnek-tə-mē\ *n, pl* **-mies** : surgical removal of the posterior arch of a vertebra (as to relieve compression of a spinal nerve root) ⟨lumbar ~⟩

lamini- *or* **lamino-** — see LAMIN-

lam•i•nin \ˈla-mə-nən\ *n* : a glycoprotein that is a component of connective tissue basement membrane and that promotes cell adhesion

lam•i•ni•tis \ˌla-mə-ˈnī-təs\ *n* : painful inflammation of a lamina esp. in the hoof of a horse, cow, or goat — called also *founder*

lam•i•no•gram *or* **lam•i•na•gram** \ˈla-mə-nə-ˌgram\ *n* : a radiograph of a layer of the body made by means of a laminograph; *broadly* : TOMOGRAM

lam•i•no•graph *or* **lam•i•na•graph** \-ˌgraf\ *n* : an X-ray machine that makes radiography of body tissue possible at any desired depth; *broadly* : TOMOGRAPH — **lam•i•no•graph•ic** \ˌla-mə-nə-ˈgra-fik\ *adj* — **lam•i•nog•ra•phy** \ˌla-mə-ˈnä-grə-fē\ *n*

lam•i•not•o•my \ˌla-mə-ˈnä-tə-mē\ *n, pl* **-mies** : surgical division of a vertebral lamina

Lam•i•sil \ˈla-mə-ˌsil\ *trademark* — used for a preparation of the hydrochloride of terbinafine

la•miv•u•dine \lə-ˈmi-vyü-ˌdēn\ *n* : an antiviral drug $C_8H_{11}N_3O_3S$ that inhibits its reverse transcriptase and is taken orally in the treatment of hepatitis B and HIV— see EPIVIR, 3TC

lamp \ˈlamp\ *n* : any of various devices for producing light or heat — see SLIT LAMP

la•nat•o•side \lə-ˈna-tə-ˌsīd\ *n* : any of three poisonous crystalline cardiac steroid glycosides occurring in the leaves of a foxglove (*Digitalis lanata*): **a** : the glycoside $C_{49}H_{76}O_{19}$ yielding digitoxin, glucose, and acetic acid on hydrolysis — called also *digilanid A, lanatoside A* **b** : the glycoside $C_{49}H_{76}O_{20}$ yielding gitoxin, glucose, and acetic acid on hydrolysis — called also *digilanid B, lanatoside B* **c** : the bitter glycoside $C_{49}H_{76}O_{20}$ yielding digoxin, glucose, and acetic acid on hydrolysis and used similarly to digitalis — called also *digilanid C, lanatoside C*

[1]**lance** \ˈlans\ *n* : LANCET

[2]**lance** *vb* **lanced; lanc•ing** : to open with a lancet : make an incision in or into ⟨~ a boil⟩ ⟨~ a vein⟩

Lance•field group \ˈlans-ˌfēld-\ *also* **Lance•field's group** \-ˌfēldz-\ *n* : any of the serologically distinguishable groups into which streptococci can be divided — see GROUP A, GROUP B

Lancefield, Rebecca Craighill (1895–1981), American bacteriologist.

lan•cet \ˈlan-sət\ *n* : a sharp-pointed and commonly two-edged surgical instrument used to make small incisions

lancet fluke *n* : a liver fluke of the genus *Dicrocoelium* (*D. dendriticum*) common in sheep and cattle and rarely infecting humans

lan•ci•nat•ing \ˈlan-sə-ˌnā-tiŋ\ *adj* : characterized by piercing or stabbing sensations ⟨~ pain⟩

land•mark \ˈland-ˌmärk\ *n* : an anatomical structure used as a point of orientation in locating other structures (as in surgical procedures)

Lan•dolt ring \ˈlän-dōlt-\ *n* : one of a series of incomplete rings or circles used in some eye charts to determine visual discrimination or acuity

Landolt, Edmond (1846–1926), French ophthalmologist.

Lan•dry's paralysis \ˈlan-drēz-\ *n* : GUILLAIN-BARRÉ SYNDROME

Landry, Jean–Baptiste–Octave (1826–1865), French physician.

Lang•er•hans cell \ˈläŋ-ər-ˌhäns-\ *n* : a dendritic cell of the interstitial spaces of the epidermis that functions as an antigen-presenting cell

P. Langerhans — see ISLET OF LANGERHANS

Lang•hans cell \ˈläŋ-häns-\ *n* : any of the cells of cuboidal epithelium that make up the cytotrophoblast

Langhans, Theodor (1839–1915), German pathologist and anatomist.

Langhans giant cell *n* : any of the large cells found in the lesions of some granulomatous conditions (as leprosy) and containing a number of peripheral nuclei arranged in a circle or in the shape of a horseshoe

lan•o•lin \ˈlan-ᵊl-ən\ *n* : wool grease esp. when refined for use in ointments and cosmetics

Lan•ox•in \la-ˈnäk-sən\ *trademark* — used for a preparation of digoxin

lan•so•praz•ole \lan-ˈsō-prə-ˌzōl\ *n* : a benzimidazole derivative $C_{16}H_{14}F_3N_3O_2S$ that inhibits gastric acid secretion and is used similarly to omeprazole — see PREVACID

lan•tha•num \ˈlan-thə-nəm\ *n* : a white soft malleable metallic element — symbol *La;* see ELEMENT table

Lan•tus \ˈlan-təs\ *trademark* — used for a preparation of insulin glargine

la•nu•go \lə-ˈnü-(ˌ)gō, -ˈnyü-\ *n* : a dense cottony or downy growth; *specif* : the soft downy hair that covers the fetus

lap *abbr* laparotomy

lap•a•ro•scope \ˈla-pə-rə-ˌskōp\ *n* : a usu. rigid endoscope that is inserted through an incision in the abdominal wall and is used to examine visually the interior of the peritoneal cavity — called also *peritoneoscope*

lap•a•ros•co•pist \ˌla-pə-ˈräs-kə-pist\ *n* : a physician or surgeon who performs laparoscopies

lap•a•ros•co•py \-pē\ *n, pl* **-pies 1** : visual examination of the abdomen by means of a laparoscope **2** : an operation (as tubal ligation or gallbladder removal) involving laparoscopy — **lap•a•ro•scop•ic** \-rə-ˈskä-pik\ *adj* — **lap•a•ro•scop•i•cal•ly** *adv*

lap•a•rot•o•my \ˌla-pə-ˈrä-tə-mē\ *n, pl* **-mies** : surgical section of the abdominal wall

La•place's law \lä-ˈplä-səz-\ *n* : LAW OF LAPLACE

Lar•gac•til \lär-ˈgak-til\ *n* : a preparation of the hydrochloride of chlorpromazine — formerly a U.S. registered trademark

large bowel *n* : LARGE INTESTINE

large calorie *n* : CALORIE 1b

large–cell carcinoma *n* : a non-small cell lung cancer usu. arising in the bronchi and composed of large undifferentiated cells — called also *large-cell lung carcinoma*

large intestine *n* : the more terminal division of the intestine that is wider and shorter than the small intestine, typically divided into cecum, colon, and rectum, and concerned esp. with the resorption of water and the formation of feces

lark•spur \ˈlärk-ˌspər\ *n* : DELPHINIUM 2

Lar•sen's syndrome \ˈlär-sənz-\ *n* : a syndrome characterized by cleft palate, flattened facies, multiple congenital joint dislocations, and deformities of the foot

Larsen, Loren Joseph (1914–2001), American orthopedic surgeon.

lar•va \ˈlär-və\ *n, pl* **lar•vae** \-(ˌ)vē, -ˌvī\ *also* **larvas** : the immature, wingless, and often wormlike feeding form that hatches from the egg of many insects — **lar•val** \-vəl\ *adj*

larval mi•grans \-ˈmī-ˌgranz\ *n* : CREEPING ERUPTION

larva migrans *n, pl* **larvae mi•gran•tes** \-ˌmī-ˈgran-ˌtēz\ : CREEPING ERUPTION

lar•vi•cide *also* **lar•va•cide** \ˈlär-və-ˌsīd\ *n* : an agent for killing larvae — **lar•vi•cid•al** \ˌlär-və-ˈsīd-ᵊl\ *adj* — **lar•vi•cid•al•ly** *adv*

laryng- *or* **laryngo-** *comb form* **1** : larynx ⟨*laryng*itis⟩ **2 a** : laryngeal ⟨*laryngo*spasm⟩ **b** : laryngeal and ⟨*laryngo*pharyngeal⟩

[1]**la•ryn•geal** \lə-ˈrin-jəl, -jē-əl; ˌlar-ən-ˈjē-əl\ *adj* : of, relating to, affecting, or used on the larynx — **la•ryn•geal•ly** *adv*

[2]**laryngeal** *n* : an anatomical part (as a nerve or artery) that supplies or is associated with the larynx

laryngeal artery *n* : either of two arteries supplying blood to the larynx: **a** : a branch of the inferior thyroid artery that supplies the muscles and mucous membranes of the dorsal part of the larynx — called also *inferior laryngeal artery* **b** : a branch of the superior thyroid artery or sometimes of the external carotid artery that supplies the muscles, mucous membranes, and glands of the larynx — called also *superior laryngeal artery*

laryngeal nerve *n* : either of two branches of the vagus nerve supplying the larynx: **a** : one that arises from the ganglion of the vagus situated below the jugular foramen and supplies the cricothyroid muscle — called also *superior laryngeal nerve* **b** : one that arises below the larynx and supplies all the muscles of the thyroid except the cricothyroid — called also *inferior laryngeal nerve, recurrent laryngeal nerve;* see INFERIOR LARYNGEAL NERVE 2

lar•yn•gec•to•mee \ˌlar-ən-ˌjek-tə-ˈmē\ *n* : a person who has undergone laryngectomy

lar•yn•gec•to•my \-ˈjek-tə-mē\ *n, pl* **-mies** : surgical removal of all or part of the larynx — **lar•yn•gec•to•mized** \-tə-ˌmīzd\ *adj*

larynges *pl of* LARYNX

lar•yn•gis•mus stri•du•lus \ˌlar-ən-ˈjiz-məs-ˈstri-jə-ləs\ *n, pl* **lar•yn•gis•mi strid•u•li** \-ˌmī-ˈstri-jə-ˌlī\ : a sudden spasm of the larynx that occurs in children esp. in rickets and is marked by difficult breathing with prolonged noisy inspiration — compare LARYNGOSPASM

lar•yn•gi•tis \ˌlar-ən-ˈjī-təs\ *n, pl* **-git•i•des** \-ˈji-tə-ˌdēz\ : inflammation of the larynx

laryngo- — see LARYNG-

la•ryn•go•cele \lə-ˈriŋ-gə-ˌsēl\ *n* : an air-containing evagination of laryngeal mucous membrane having its opening communicating with the ventricle of the larynx

la•ryn•go•fis•sure \lə-ˌriŋ-gō-ˈfi-shər\ *n* : surgical opening of the larynx by an incision through the thyroid cartilage esp. for the removal of a tumor

lar•yn•gog•ra•phy \ˌlar-ən-ˈgä-grə-fē\ *n, pl* **-phies** : X-ray depiction of the larynx after use of a radiopaque material

laryngol *abbr* laryngological

la•ryn•go•log•i•cal \lə-ˌriŋ-gə-ˈlä-ji-kəl\ *also* **la•ryn•go•log•ic** \-ˈlä-jik\ *adj* : of or relating to laryngology or the larynx

lar•yn•gol•o•gist \ˌlar-ən-ˈgä-lə-jist\ *n* : a physician specializing in laryngology

lar•yn•gol•o•gy \ˌlar-ən-ˈgä-lə-jē\ *n, pl* **-gies** : a branch of medicine dealing with diseases of the larynx and nasopharynx

la•ryn•go•pha•ryn•ge•al \lə-ˌriŋ-gō-ˌfar-ən-ˈjē-əl, -fə-ˈrin-jəl, -jē-əl\ *adj* : of or common to both the larynx and the pharynx ⟨~ cancer⟩

la•ryn•go•phar•yn•gi•tis \-ˌfar-ən-ˈjī-təs\ *n, pl* **-git•i•des** \-ˈji-tə-ˌdēz\ : inflammation of both the larynx and the pharynx

la•ryn•go•phar•ynx \-ˈfar-iŋks\ *n* : the lower part of the pharynx lying behind or adjacent to the larynx — compare NASOPHARYNX

la•ryn•go•plas•ty \lə-ˈriŋ-gə-ˌplas-tē\ *n, pl* **-ties** : plastic surgery to repair laryngeal defects

la•ryn•go•scope \lə-ˈriŋ-gə-ˌskōp, -ˈrin-jə-\ *n* : an endoscope for visually examining the interior of the larynx — **la•ryn•go•scop•ic** \-ˌriŋ-gə-ˈskä-pik, -ˌrin-jə-\ *or* **la•ryn•go•scop•i•cal** \-pi-kəl\ *adj*

lar•yn•gos•co•py \ˌlar-ən-ˈgäs-kə-pē\ *n, pl* **-pies** : examination of the interior of the larynx (as with a laryngoscope)

la•ryn•go•spasm \lə-ˈriŋ-gə-ˌspa-zəm\ *n* : spasmodic closure of the larynx — compare LARYNGISMUS STRIDULUS

lar•yn•got•o•my \ˌlar-ən-ˈgä-tə-mē\ *n, pl* **-mies** : surgical incision of the larynx

la•ryn•go•tra•che•al \lə-ˌriŋ-gō-ˈtrā-kē-əl\ *adj* : of or common to the larynx and trachea ⟨~ stenosis⟩

la•ryn•go•tra•che•itis \-ˌtrā-kē-ˈī-təs\ *n* : inflammation of both larynx and trachea — see INFECTIOUS LARYNGOTRACHEITIS

la•ryn•go•tra•cheo•bron•chi•tis \-ˌtrā-kē-ō-brän-ˈkī-təs, -bräŋ-\ *n, pl* **-chit•i•des** \-ˈki-tə-ˌdēz\ : inflammation of the larynx, trachea, and bronchi

lar•ynx \ˈlar-iŋks\ *n, pl* **la•ryn•ges** \lə-ˈrin-(ˌ)jēz\ *or* **lar•ynx•es** : the modified upper part of the respiratory passage that is bounded above by the glottis, is continuous below with the trachea, has a complex cartilaginous or bony skeleton capable of limited motion through the action of associated muscles, and has a set of elastic vocal cords that play a major role in sound production and speech — called also *voice box*

[1]la•ser \ˈlā-zər\ *n* : a device that utilizes the natural oscillations of atoms or molecules between energy levels for generating coherent electromagnetic radiation usu. in the ultraviolet, visible, or infrared regions of the spectrum

[2]laser *vb* : to subject to the action of a laser : treat with a laser

laser–assisted in–situ keratomileusis *n* : LASIK

lash \ˈlash\ *n* : EYELASH

LA•SIK \ˈlā-sik\ *n* : a surgical operation to reshape the cornea for correction of nearsightedness, farsightedness, or astigmatism that involves use of an excimer laser to remove varying degrees of tissue from the inner part of the cornea — called also *laser-assisted in-situ keratomileusis*

La•six \ˈlā-ziks, -siks\ *trademark* — used for a preparation of furosemide

L–as•par•a•gi•nase \ˈel-as-ˈpar-ə-jə-ˌnās, -ˌnāz\ *n* : an enzyme that breaks down the physiologically commoner form of asparagine, is obtained esp. from bacteria, and is used esp. to treat leukemia

Las•sa fever \ˈla-sə-\ *n* : a disease esp. of Africa that is caused by the Lassa virus and is characterized by a high fever, headaches, mouth ulcers, muscle aches, small hemorrhages under the skin, heart and kidney failure, and a high mortality rate

Lassa virus *n* : a virus of the genus *Arenavirus* (species *Lassa virus*) that causes Lassa fever

las•si•tude \ˈla-sə-ˌtüd, -ˌtyüd\ *n* : a condition of weariness, debility, or fatigue

lat \ˈlat\ *n* : LATISSIMUS DORSI — usu. used in pl.

lata — see FASCIA LATA

latae — see FASCIA LATA, TENSOR FASCIAE LATAE

la•tah \ˈlä-tə\ *n* : a neurotic condition marked by automatic obedience, echolalia, and echopraxia observed esp. among the Malayan people

la•tan•o•prost \lə-ˈta-nə-ˌpräst\ *n* : a prostaglandin analog $C_{26}H_{40}O_5$ used topically to reduce elevated intraocular pressure — see XALATAN

la•ten•cy \ˈlāt-ᵊn-sē\ *n, pl* **-cies** **1 a** : the quality or state of being latent; *esp* : the state or period of living or developing in a host without producing symptoms ⟨viral ~⟩ **b** : the time or period between exposure to a disease-causing agent or process and the onset of symptoms or disease ⟨a 10 to 20-year ~⟩ **2** : LATENCY PERIOD 1 **3** : the time interval between application of a stimulus and the beginning of an identifiable response (as muscle contraction) : REACTION TIME — called also *latent period*

latency period *n* **1** : a stage of psychosexual development that follows the phallic stage and precedes the genital stage, extends from about the age of five or six to the beginning of puberty, and during which sexual urges often appear to lie dormant — called also *latency, latency stage* **2** : LATENCY 1

la•tent \ˈlāt-ᵊnt\ *adj* : existing in hidden or dormant form: as **a** : present or capable of living or developing in a host without producing visible symptoms of disease ⟨a ~ virus⟩ **b** : not consciously expressed **c** : relating to or being the latent content of a dream or thought — **la•tent•ly** *adv*

latent content *n* : the underlying meaning of a dream or thought that is exposed in psychoanalysis by interpretation of its symbols or by free association — compare MANIFEST CONTENT

latent learning *n* : learning that is not demonstrated by behavior at the time it is held to take place but that is inferred to exist based on a greater than expected number of favorable or desired responses at a later time when reinforcement is given

latent period *n* : LATENCY 1, 3

late–onset diabetes *n* : TYPE 2 DIABETES

lat•er•al \ˈla-tə-rəl, -trəl\ *adj* : of or relating to the side; *esp, of a body part* : lying at or extending toward the right or left side : lying away from the median axis of the body

lateral arcuate ligament *n* : a fascial band that extends from the tip of the transverse process of the first lumbar vertebra to the twelfth rib and provides attachment for part of the diaphragm — compare MEDIAL ARCUATE LIGAMENT, MEDIAN ARCUATE LIGAMENT

lateral brachial cutaneous nerve *n* : a continuation of the posterior branch of the axillary nerve that supplies the skin of the lateral aspect of the upper arm over the distal part of the deltoid muscle and the adjacent head of the triceps brachii

lateral collateral ligament *n* **1** : a ligament of the outer knee that connects the lateral epicondyle of the femur with the lateral side of the head of the fibula and helps to stabilize the knee by preventing lateral dislocation — called also *fibular collateral ligament, LCL;* compare MEDIAL COLLATERAL LIGAMENT 1 **2** : RADIAL COLLATERAL LIGAMENT 1 — called also *LCL*

lateral column *n* **1** : a lateral extension of the gray matter in each lateral half of the spinal cord present in the thoracic and upper lumbar regions — called also *lateral horn;* compare DORSAL HORN, VENTRAL HORN **2** : LATERAL FUNICULUS

lateral condyle *n* : a condyle on the outer side of the lower extremity of the femur; *also* : a corresponding eminence on the upper part of the tibia that articulates with the lateral condyle of the femur — compare MEDIAL CONDYLE

lateral cord *n* : a cord of nerve tissue that is formed by union of the superior and middle trunks of the brachial plexus and that forms one of the two roots of the median nerve — compare MEDIAL CORD, POSTERIOR CORD

lateral corticospinal tract *n* : a band of nerve fibers that descends in the lateral funiculus of the spinal cord and consists mostly of fibers arising in the motor cortex of the contralateral side of the brain

lateral cricoarytenoid *n* : CRICOARYTENOID 1

lateral cuneiform bone *n* : CUNEIFORM BONE 1c — called also *lateral cuneiform*

lateral decubitus *n* : a position in which a patient lies on his or her side and which is used esp. in radiography and in making a lumbar puncture

lateral epicondyle *n* : EPICONDYLE a

lateral epicondylitis *n* : TENNIS ELBOW

lateral femoral circumflex artery *n* : an artery that branches from the deep femoral artery or from the femoral artery itself and that supplies the muscles of the lateral part of the thigh and hip joint — compare MEDIAL FEMORAL CIRCUMFLEX ARTERY

lateral femoral circumflex vein *n* : a vein accompanying the lateral femoral circumflex artery and emptying into the femoral vein — compare MEDIAL FEMORAL CIRCUMFLEX VEIN

lateral femoral cutaneous nerve *n* : a nerve that arises from the lumbar plexus and that supplies the anterior and lateral aspects of the thigh down to the knee — compare POSTERIOR FEMORAL CUTANEOUS NERVE

lateral fissure *n* : SYLVIAN FISSURE

lateral funiculus *n* : a longitudinal division on each side of the spinal cord comprising white matter between the dorsal and ventral roots — compare POSTERIOR FUNICULUS, VENTRAL FUNICULUS

lateral gastrocnemius bursa *n* : a bursa of the knee joint that is situated between the lateral head of the gastrocnemius muscle and the joint capsule

lateral geniculate body *n* : a part of the metathalamus that consists of an oval elevation produced by the underlying lateral geniculate nucleus— compare MEDIAL GENICULATE BODY

lateral geniculate nucleus *n* : a nucleus of the lateral geniculate body that is the terminus of most nerve fibers of the optic tract and receives nerve impulses from the retinas which are relayed to the visual cortex by way of the geniculocalcarine tracts

lateral horn *n* : LATERAL COLUMN 1

lateral humeral epicondylitis *n* : TENNIS ELBOW

lateral inhibition *n* : a visual process in which the firing of a retinal cell inhibits the firing of surrounding retinal cells and which is held to enhance the perception of areas of contrast

lateralis — see RECTUS LATERALIS, VASTUS LATERALIS

lat•er•al•i•ty \ˌla-tə-ˈra-lə-tē\ *n, pl* **-ties** : preference in use of homologous parts on one lateral half of the body over those on the other : dominance in function of one of a pair of lateral homologous parts

lat•er•al•i•za•tion \ˌla-tə-rə-lə-ˈzā-shən, ˌla-trə-lə-\ *n* : localization of function or activity (as of verbal processes in the brain) on one side of the body in preference to the other — **lat•er•al•ize** \ˈla-tə-rə-ˌlīz, -trə-\ *vb*

lateral lemniscus *n* : a band of nerve fibers that arises in the cochlear nuclei and terminates in the inferior colliculus and the lateral geniculate body of the opposite side of the brain

lateral ligament *n* : any of various ligaments (as the lateral collateral ligament of the knee) that are in a lateral position or that prevent lateral dislocation of a joint

lateral malleolus *n* : MALLEOLUS a

lateral meniscus *n* : MENISCUS a(1)

lateral nucleus *n* : any of a group of nuclei of the thalamus situated in the dorsolateral region extending from its anterior to posterior ends

lateral pectoral nerve *n* : PECTORAL NERVE a

lateral plantar artery *n* : PLANTAR ARTERY a

lateral plantar nerve *n* : PLANTAR NERVE a

lateral plantar vein *n* : PLANTAR VEIN a

lateral popliteal nerve *n* : COMMON PERONEAL NERVE

lateral pterygoid muscle *n* : PTERYGOID MUSCLE a

lateral pterygoid nerve *n* : PTERYGOID NERVE a

lateral pterygoid plate *n* : PTERYGOID PLATE a

lateral rectus *n* : RECTUS 2b

lateral reticular nucleus *n* : a nucleus of the reticular formation that receives fibers esp. from the dorsal horn of the spinal cord and sends axons to the cerebellum on the same side of the body

lateral sacral artery *n* : either of two arteries on each side which arise from the posterior division of the internal iliac artery and supply muscles and skin in the area

lateral sacral crest *n* : SACRAL CREST b

lateral sacral vein *n* : any of several veins that accompany the corresponding lateral sacral arteries and empty into the internal iliac veins

lateral semilunar cartilage *n* : MENISCUS a(1)

lateral spinothalamic tract *n* : SPINOTHALAMIC TRACT b

lateral sulcus *n* : SYLVIAN FISSURE

lateral thoracic artery *n* : THORACIC ARTERY 1b

lateral umbilical ligament *n* : MEDIAL UMBILICAL LIGAMENT

lateral ventricle *n* : an internal cavity in each cerebral hemisphere that consists of a central body and three cornua — see ANTERIOR HORN 2, INFERIOR HORN, POSTERIOR HORN 2

lateral vestibular nucleus *n* : the one of the four vestibular nuclei on each side of the medulla oblongata that sends fibers down the same side of the spinal cord through the vestibulospinal tract — called also *Deiters' nucleus*

latex agglutination test *n* : a test for a specific antibody and esp. rheumatoid factor in which the corresponding antigen is adsorbed on spherical polystyrene latex particles which undergo agglutination upon addition of the specific antibody — called also *latex fixation test, latex test*

lath•y•rism \ˈla-thə-ˌri-zəm\ *n* : a neurotoxic disorder chiefly affecting people and domestic animals (as cows and horses) that is characterized esp. by irreversible spastic paralysis of the hind or lower limbs and that results from poisoning by an amino acid found in some legumes (genus *Lathyrus* and esp. *L. sativus*) — **lath•y•rit•ic** \ˌla-thə-ˈri-tik\ *adj*

lath•y•ro•gen \ˈla-thə-rə-jən, -ˌjen\ *n* : any of a group of compounds that tend to cause lathyrism and inhibit the formation of links between chains of collagen

La•tisse \lə-ˈtēs\ *trademark* — used for a preparation of bimatoprost

la•tis•si•mus dor•si \lə-ˈti-sə-məs-ˈdȯr-ˌsī\ *n, pl* **la•tis•si•mi dorsi** \-ˌmī-\ : a broad flat superficial muscle of the lower part of the back that extends, adducts, and rotates the arm medially and draws the shoulder downward and backward

Lat•ro•dec•tus \ˌla-trō-ˈdek-təs\ *n* : a genus of venomous spiders (family Theridiidae) including the black widow (*L. mactans*)

lats \ˈlats\ *pl of* LAT

LATS *abbr* long-acting thyroid stimulator

La•tu•da \lə-ˈtü-də\ *trademark* — used for a preparation of lurasidone

latum — see CONDYLOMA LATUM

laud•able pus \ˈlȯ-də-bəl-\ *n* : pus discharged freely (as from a wound) and formerly supposed to facilitate the elimination of unhealthy humors from the injured body

lau•da•num \ˈlȯd-nəm, -ᵊn-əm\ *n* **1** : any of various formerly used preparations of opium **2** : a tincture of opium

laughing death *n* : KURU

laughing gas *n* : NITROUS OXIDE

laughing sickness *n* : KURU

Lau•rence–Moon syndrome \ˈlȯr-əns-ˈmün-\ *n* : a genetic disorder that is a ciliopathy characterized esp. by obesity, ataxia, learning disabilities, kidney abnormalities, short stature, subnormal development of the genital organs, and retinitis pigmentosa, is inherited as an autosomal recessive trait, and is sometimes considered a variant of Bardet-Biedl syndrome

Laurence, John Zachariah (1830–1874), British physician.

Moon, Robert Charles (1844–1914), American ophthalmologist.

lau•ryl \ˈlȯr-əl, ˈlär-\ *n* : the monovalent chemical group $C_{12}H_{25}$– — see SODIUM LAURYL SULFATE

LAV \ˌel-(ˌ)ā-ˈvē\ *n* : HIV-1

la•vage \lə-ˈväzh, ˈla-vij\ *n* : the act or action of washing; *esp* : the therapeutic washing out of an organ or part ⟨gastric ~⟩ — **lavage** *vb*

law of dominance *n* : MENDEL'S LAW 3

law of independent assortment *n* : MENDEL'S LAW 2

law of La•place \-lä-ˈpläs\ *n* : a law in physics that in medicine is applied in the physiology of blood flow: under equilibrium conditions the pressure tangent to the circumference of a vessel storing or transmitting fluid equals the product of the pressure across the wall and the radius of the vessel for a sphere and half this for a tube — called also *Laplace's law*

Laplace, Pierre–Simon (1749–1827), French astronomer and mathematician.

law of segregation *n* : MENDEL'S LAW 1

law·ren·ci·um \lȯ-ˈren-sē-əm\ *n* : a short-lived radioactive element that is produced artificially from californium — symbol *Lr;* see ELEMENT table

Law·rence \ˈlȯr-əns, ˈlär-\, **Ernest Orlando (1901–1958),** American physicist.

lax \ˈlaks\ *adj* **1** *of the bowels* : LOOSE 3 **2** : having loose bowels

lax·a·tion \lak-ˈsā-shən\ *n* : a bowel movement

[1]**lax·a·tive** \ˈlak-sə-tiv\ *adj* **1** : having a tendency to loosen or relax; *specif* : relieving constipation **2** : LAX 2 — **lax·a·tive·ly** *adv*

[2]**laxative** *n* : a usu. mild laxative drug

lax·i·ty \ˈlak-sə-tē\ *n, pl* **-ties** : the quality or state of being loose ⟨a certain ~ of the bowels⟩ ⟨ligamentous ~⟩

la·zar \ˈla-zər, ˈlā-\ *n* : LEPER

lazy eye *n* : AMBLYOPIA; *also* : an eye affected with amblyopia

lazy–eye blindness *n* : AMBLYOPIA

lb *abbr* pound

L chain *n* : LIGHT CHAIN

LCL \ˌel-ˌsē-ˈel\ *n* : LATERAL COLLATERAL LIGAMENT

LCMV *abbr* lymphocytic choriomeningitis virus

LD *abbr* **1** learning difference; learning disability; learning disabled **2** lethal dose

LD50 *or* **LD_{50}** \ˌel-ˌdē-ˈfif-tē\ *n* : the amount of a toxic agent (as a poison, virus, or radiation) that is sufficient to kill 50 percent of a population of animals usu. within a certain time — called also *median lethal dose*

LDH *abbr* lactate dehydrogenase; lactic dehydrogenase

LDL \ˌel-(ˌ)dē-ˈel\ *n* : a lipoprotein of blood plasma that is composed of a moderate proportion of protein with little triglyceride and a high proportion of cholesterol and that is associated with increased probability of developing atherosclerosis — called also *bad cholesterol, beta-lipoprotein, low-density lipoprotein;* compare HDL, VLDL

L–do·pa \ˈel-ˈdō-pə\ *n* : the levorotatory form of dopa that is obtained esp. from broad beans or prepared synthetically, is converted to dopamine in the brain, and is used esp. in combination with carbidopa in the treatment of Parkinson's disease — called also *levodopa;* see DUOPA, PARCOPA, RYTARY, SINEMET, STALEVO

LE *abbr* lupus erythematosus

[1]**lead** \ˈlēd\ *n* : a flexible or solid insulated conductor connected to or leading out from an electrical device (as an electroencephalograph)

[2]**lead** \ˈled\ *n, often attrib* : a heavy soft malleable bluish-white metallic element found mostly in combination and used esp. in pipes, cable sheaths, batteries, solder, type metal, and shields against radioactivity — symbol *Pb;* see ELEMENT table

lead acetate \ˈled-\ *n* : a poisonous soluble lead salt $PbC_4H_6O_4·3H_2O$ used in medicine esp. formerly as an astringent

lead arsenate *n* : an arsenate of lead; *esp* : either of the two salts $PbHAsO_4$ and $Pb_3(AsO_4)_2$ formerly used as insecticides

lead carbonate *n* : a carbonate of lead; *esp* : a poisonous basic salt $Pb_3(OH)_2(CO_3)_2$ that was formerly used as a white pigment in paints

lead palsy *n* : localized paralysis caused by lead poisoning esp. of the extensor muscles of the forearm

lead poisoning *n* : a serious acute or chronic condition that is caused by exposure to and absorption of lead (as lead carbonate) and is characterized by variable symptoms including fatigue, abdominal pain, vomiting, constipation, impaired cognitive development or function, joint and muscle pain, loss of appetite, anemia, a dark line along the gums, encephalopathy, seizures, paralysis, and kidney damage — called also *plumbism, saturnism*

leaf·let \ˈlē-flət\ *n* : a leaflike organ, structure, or part; *esp* : any of the flaps of the biscuspid valve or the tricuspid valve

learn·ing \ˈlər-niŋ\ *n* : the process of acquiring a modification in a behavioral tendency by experience (as exposure to conditioning); *also* : the modified behavioral tendency itself — **learn** \ˈlərn\ *vb*

learning difference *n* : LEARNING DISABILITY — abbr. *LD*

learning disability *n* : any of various disorders (as dyslexia or dysgraphia) that interfere with an individual's ability to learn resulting in impaired functioning in verbal language, reasoning, or academic skills (as reading and mathematics) and are thought to be caused by difficulties in processing and integrating information — abbr. *LD* — **learning disabled** *adj*

least splanchnic nerve \ˈlēst-\ *n* : SPLANCHNIC NERVE C

Le·boy·er \lə-bȯi-ˈā\ *adj* : of or relating to a method of childbirth designed to reduce trauma for the newborn esp. by avoiding use of forceps and bright lights in the delivery room and by giving the newborn a warm bath

Leboyer, Frédérick (*b* 1918), French obstetrician.

LE cell \ˌel-ˈē-ˌsel\ *n* : a neutrophil that is found esp. in patients with lupus erythematosus — called also *lupus erythematosus cell*

lecith- *or* **lecitho-** *comb form* : yolk of an egg ⟨*lecith*al⟩ ⟨ovo*lecith*in⟩

lec•i•thal \ˈle-sə-thəl\ *adj* : having a yolk — often used in combination

lec•i•thin \ˈle-sə-thən\ *n* : any of several waxy hygroscopic phospholipids that are widely distributed in animals and plants, form colloidal solutions in water, and have emulsifying, wetting, and antioxidant properties; *also* : a mixture of or a substance rich in lecithins — called also *phosphatidylcholine*

lec•i•thin•ase \-thə-ˌnās, -ˌnāz\ *n* : PHOSPHOLIPASE

lec•tin \ˈlek-tin\ *n* : any of a group of proteins esp. of plants that are not antibodies and do not originate in an immune system but bind specif. to carbohydrate-containing receptors on cell surfaces (as of red blood cells)

le•dip•as•vir \lə-ˈdi-pəs-ˌvir\ *n* : an antiviral drug $C_{49}H_{54}F_2N_8O_6$ taken orally in combination with sofosbuvir in the treatment of hepatitis C infection — see HARVONI

leech \ˈlēch\ *n* : any of numerous carnivorous or bloodsucking usu. freshwater annelid worms (class Hirudinea) that typically have a flattened segmented lance-shaped body with a sucker at each end — see MEDICINAL LEECH

LE factor \ˌel-ˈē-\ *n* : an antibody found in the serum esp. of patients with systemic lupus erythematosus

Le•Fort \lə-ˈfȯrt\ *n* **1** : a fracture of the maxilla and associated bones of the middle face region: **a** *or* **LeFort I** : a horizontal fracture of the maxilla above the apices of the teeth **b** *or* **LeFort II** : a pyramid-shaped fracture of the maxilla in which the lines of fracture meet at an apex near the bridge of the nose **c** *or* **LeFort III** : a fracture of the maxilla and one or more facial bones so that complete separation from the skull occurs **2** : an operation that involves reconstructing the middle face region by moving the maxilla and associated bones forward: **a** *or* **LeFort I** : one in which the teeth-bearing part of the maxilla is repositioned **b** *or* **LeFort II** : one in which the maxilla and adjacent nasal bones are repositioned **c** *or* **LeFort III** : one in which the maxilla, nasal bones, and both zygomatic bones are repositioned

Le Fort, René (1869–1951), French surgeon.

left atrioventricular valve *n* : MITRAL VALVE

left colic flexure *n* : SPLENIC FLEXURE

left gastric artery *n* : GASTRIC ARTERY 1

left gastroepiploic artery *n* : GASTROEPIPLOIC ARTERY b

left–hand•ed \ˈleft-ˈhan-dəd\ *adj* **1** : using the left hand habitually or more easily than the right **2** : relating to, designed for, or done with the left hand **3** : having a direction contrary to that of movement of the hands of a watch viewed from in front **4** : LEVOROTATORY — **left–handed** *adv* — **left–hand•ed•ness** *n*

left heart *n* : the left atrium and ventricle : the half of the heart that receives oxygenated blood from the pulmonary circulation and passes it to the aorta

left lymphatic duct *n* : THORACIC DUCT

left pulmonary artery *n* : PULMONARY ARTERY c

left subcostal vein *n* : SUBCOSTAL VEIN b

leg \ˈleg\ *n* : a limb of an animal used esp. for supporting the body and for walking: as **a** : either of the two lower human limbs that extend from the top of the thigh to the foot and esp. the part between the knee and the ankle **b** : any of the rather generalized appendages of an arthropod used in walking and crawling — **leg•ged** \ˈle-gəd, ˈlegd\ *adj*

legal age *n* : the age at which a person enters into full adult legal rights and responsibilities

legal blindness *n* : blindness as recognized by law which in most states of the U.S. means that the better eye using the best possible methods of correction has visual acuity of 20/200 or worse or that the visual field is restricted to 20 degrees or less — **le•gal•ly blind** *adj*

Legg–Cal•vé–Per•thes disease \ˈleg-ˌkal-ˈvā-ˈpər-ˌtēz-\ *n* : osteochondritis affecting the bony knob at the upper end of the femur — called also *Legg-Perthes disease, Perthes disease*

Legg, Arthur Thornton (1874–1939), American orthopedic surgeon.

Calvé, Jacques (1875–1954), French surgeon.

Perthes, Georg Clemens (1869–1927), German surgeon.

Legg–Perthes disease *n* : LEGG-CALVÉ-PERTHES DISEASE

le•gion•el•la \ˌlē-jə-ˈne-lə\ *n* **1** *cap* : a genus of gram-negative rod-shaped bacteria (family Legionellaceae) that includes the causative agent (*L. pneumophila*) of Legionnaires' disease **2** *pl* **-lae** *also* **-las** : a bacterium of the genus *Legionella*

le•gion•el•lo•sis \ˌlē-jə-ˌne-ˈlō-səs\ *n* : LEGIONNAIRES' DISEASE

Le•gion•naires' bacillus \ˌlē-jə-ˈnarz-\ *n* : a bacterium of the genus *Legionella* (*L. pneumophila*) that causes Legionnaires' disease

Legionnaires' disease *also* **Legionnaire's disease** *n* : pneumonia that is caused by a bacterium of the genus *Legionella* (*L. pneumophila*), that is characterized initially by symptoms resembling influenza (as malaise and muscular aches) followed by high fever, cough, diarrhea, lobar pneumonia, and mental confusion, and that may be fatal esp. in elderly and immunocompromised individuals — see PONTIAC FEVER

le•gume \ˈle-ˌgyüm, li-ˈgyüm\ *n* : any of a large family (Leguminosae) of plants having fruits that are dry pods and split when ripe and including important food and forage plants (as beans and clover); *also* : the fruit or seed of a legume used as food — **le•gu•mi•nous** \li-ˈgyü-mə-nəs, le-\ *adj*

leio- *or* **lio-** *comb form* : smooth ⟨*leiomyoma*⟩

leio•myo•blas•to•ma \ˌlī-ō-ˌmī-ō-blas-ˈtō-mə\ *n, pl* **-mas** *also* **-ma•ta** \-mə-tə\ : LEIOMYOMA; *esp* : one resembling epithelium

leio•my•o•ma \ˌlī-ō-mī-ˈō-mə\ *n, pl* **-mas** *also* **-ma•ta** \-mə-tə\ : a benign tumor (as a fibroid) consisting of smooth muscle fibers — **leio•my•o•ma•tous** \-mə-təs\ *adj*

leio•myo•sar•co•ma \ˌlī-ō-ˌmī-ō-sär-ˈkō-mə\ *n, pl* **-mas** *also* **-ma•ta** \-mə-tə\ : a sarcoma composed in part of smooth muscle cells

Leish•man–Don•o•van body \ˈlēsh-mən-ˈdä-nə-vən-\ *n* : a protozoan of the genus *Leishmania* (esp. *L. donovani*) in its nonmotile stage that is found esp. in cells of the skin, spleen, and liver of individuals affected with leishmaniasis and esp. kala-azar — compare DONOVAN BODY

Leishman, Sir William Boog (1865–1926), British bacteriologist.

Donovan, Charles (1863–1951), British surgeon.

leish•man•ia \lēsh-ˈma-nē-ə, -ˈmā-\ *n* **1** *cap* : a genus of flagellate protozoans (family Trypanosomatidae) that are parasitic in the tissues of vertebrates, are transmitted by sand flies (genera *Phlebotomus* and *Lutzomyia*), and include one (*L. donovani*) causing kala-azar and another (*L. tropica*) causing oriental sore **2** : any protozoan of the genus *Leishmania; broadly* : a protozoan resembling the leishmanias that is included in the family (Trypanosomatidae) to which they belong — **leish•man•ial** \-nē-əl\ *adj*

leish•man•i•a•sis \ˌlēsh-mə-ˈnī-ə-səs\ *n, pl* **-a•ses** \-ˌsēz\ : infection with or disease (as kala-azar or oriental sore) caused by leishmanias

lem•nis•cus \lem-ˈnis-kəs\ *n, pl* **-nis•ci** \-ˈnis-ˌkī, -ˌkē; -ˈni-ˌsī\ : a band of fibers and esp. nerve fibers — called also *fillet;* see LATERAL LEMNISCUS, MEDIAL LEMNISCUS — **lem•nis•cal** \-ˈnis-kəl\ *adj*

len•i•tive \ˈle-nə-tiv\ *adj* : alleviating pain or harshness — **lenitive** *n*

Len•nox–Gas•taut syndrome \ˈle-nəks-gas-ˈtō-\ *n* : an epileptic syndrome esp. of young children that is marked by tonic, atonic, and myoclonic seizures and by atypical absence seizures and that is associated with impaired intellectual functioning and developmental delays

Lennox, William Gordon (1884–1960), American neurologist.

Gas•taut \gȧs-tō\, **Henri Jean–Pascal (1915–1995),** French neurologist.

lens *also* **lense** \ˈlenz\ *n* **1** : a curved piece of glass or plastic used singly or combined in eyeglasses or an optical instrument (as a microscope) for forming an image; *also* : a device for focusing radiation other than light **2** : a highly transparent biconvex lens-shaped or nearly spherical body in the eye that focuses light rays entering the eye typically onto the retina and that lies immediately behind the pupil — **lensed** *adj* — **lens•less** *adj*

lens•om•e•ter \len-ˈzä-mə-tər\ *n* : an instrument used to determine the optical properties (as the focal length and axis) of ophthalmic lenses

len•te insulin \ˈlen-tā-\ *n, often cap* : a preparation of insulin zinc suspension that contains insulin in both crystalline and amorphous form and has a duration of action that is relatively shorter than ultralente insulin — formerly a U.S. registered trademark; called also *lente*

len•ti•co•nus \ˌlen-tə-ˈkō-nəs\ *n* : a rare abnormal and usu. congenital condition of the lens of the eye in which the surface is conical esp. on the posterior side

len•tic•u•lar \len-ˈti-kyə-lər\ *adj* **1** : having the shape of a double-convex lens **2** : of or relating to a lens esp. of the eye **3** : relating to or being the lentiform nucleus of the brain

lenticular nucleus *n* : LENTIFORM NUCLEUS

lenticular process *n* : the tip of the long process of the incus which articulates with the stapes

lentiform nucleus *n* : the one of the four basal ganglia in each cerebral hemisphere that comprises the larger and external nucleus of the corpus striatum — called also *lenticular nucleus*

len•ti•go \len-ˈtī-(ˌ)gō, -ˈtē-\ *n, pl* **len•tig•i•nes** \len-ˈti-jə-ˌnēz\ **1** : a small melanotic spot in the skin in which the formation of pigment is unrelated to exposure to sunlight and which is potentially malignant; *esp* : NEVUS — compare FRECKLE **2** : FRECKLE

lentigo ma•lig•na \-mə-ˈlig-nə\ *n* : a precancerous lesion on the skin esp. in areas exposed to the sun (as the face) that is flat, mottled, and brownish with an irregular outline and grows slowly over a period of years

lentigo se•nil•is \-sə-ˈni-ləs\ *n* : AGE SPOTS

len•ti•vi•rus \ˈlen-tə-ˌvī-rəs\ *n* **1** *cap* : a genus of retroviruses that cause progressive often fatal disease and include SIV and HIV **2** : any virus of the genus *Lentivirus* — **len•ti•vi•ral** \-rəl\ *adj*

le•on•ti•a•sis os•sea \ˌlē-ən-ˈtī-ə-səs-ˈä-sē-ə\ *n* : an overgrowth of the bones of the head producing enlargement and distortion of the face

lep•er \ˈle-pər\ *n* : an individual affected with leprosy

LE phenomenon \ˌel-ˈē-\ *n* : the process which a white blood cell undergoes in becoming a lupus erythematosus cell

lep•ra \ˈle-prə\ *n* : LEPROSY

lep•re•chaun•ism \ˈle-prə-ˌkä-ˌni-zəm, -ˌkȯ-\ *n* : a rare inherited disorder of insulin resistance characterized by growth retardation, by endocrine disorders, by hirsutism, and by a facies marked by large wide-set eyes and large low-set ears

lep•rol•o•gist \le-ˈprä-lə-jist\ *n* : a specialist in the study of leprosy and its treatment — **lep•rol•o•gy** \-jē\ *n*

lep•ro•ma \le-ˈprō-mə\ *n, pl* **-mas** *also* **-ma•ta** \-mə-tə\ : a nodular lesion of leprosy

le•pro•ma•tous \lə-ˈprä-mə-təs, -ˈprō-\ *adj* : of, relating to, characterized by, or affected with lepromas or lepromatous leprosy ⟨~ patients⟩

lepromatous leprosy *n* : the one of the two major forms of leprosy that is characterized by the formation of lepromas, the presence of numerous Hansen's bacilli in the lesions, and a negative skin reaction to lepromin and that remains infectious to others until treated — compare TUBERCULOID LEPROSY

lep•ro•min \le-ˈprō-mən\ *n* : an extract of human leprous tissue used in a skin test for leprosy infection

lep•ro•sar•i•um \ˌle-prə-ˈser-ē-əm\ *n, pl* **-i•ums** *or* **-ia** \-ē-ə\ : a hospital for leprosy patients

lep•ro•stat•ic \ˌle-prə-ˈsta-tik\ *n* : an agent that inhibits the growth of Hansen's bacillus

lep•ro•sy \ˈle-prə-sē\ *n, pl* **-sies** : a chronic infectious disease that is caused by a mycobacterium (*Mycobacterium leprae*), affects esp. the skin and peripheral nerves, and is characterized by the formation of nodules or macules that enlarge and spread and are accompanied by loss of sensation with eventual paralysis, wasting of muscle, and production of deformities — called also *Hansen's disease, lepra;* see LEPROMATOUS LEPROSY, TUBERCULOID LEPROSY

lep•rot•ic \le-ˈprä-tik\ *adj* : of, caused by, or infected with leprosy

lep•rous \ˈle-prəs\ *adj* **1** : infected with leprosy **2** : of, relating to, or associated with leprosy or a leper

-lep•sy \ˌlep-sē\ *n comb form, pl* **-lep•sies** : taking : seizure ⟨narco*lepsy*⟩

lept- *or* **lepto-** *comb form* : small : weak : thin : fine ⟨*lepto*meninges⟩

lep•ta•zol \ˈlep-tə-ˌzȯl, -ˌzōl\ *n, chiefly Brit* : PENTYLENETETRAZOL

lep•tin \ˈlep-tən\ *n* : a peptide hormone that is produced by fat cells and plays a role in body weight regulation by acting on the hypothalamus to suppress appetite and burn fat stored in adipose tissue

lep•to \ˈlep-ˌtō\ *n* : LEPTOSPIROSIS

lep•to•me•nin•ges \ˌlep-tō-mə-ˈnin-(ˌ)jēz\ *n pl* : the pia mater and the arachnoid considered together as investing the brain and spinal cord — called also *pia-arachnoid* — **lep•to•men•in•ge•al** \-ˌme-nən-ˈjē-əl\ *adj*

lep•to•men•in•gi•tis \-ˌme-nən-ˈjī-təs\ *n, pl* **-git•i•des** \-ˈji-tə-ˌdēz\ : inflammation of the pia mater and the arachnoid membrane

lep•to•ne•ma \ˌlep-tə-ˈnē-mə\ *n* : a chromatin thread or chromosome at the leptotene stage of meiotic prophase

lep•to•phos \ˈlep-tō-ˌfäs\ *n* : a neurotoxic pesticide $C_{13}H_{10}BrCl_2O_2PS$

lep•to•spi•ra \ˌlep-tō-ˈspī-rə\ *n* **1** *cap* : a genus of extremely slender aerobic spirochetes (family Leptospiraceae) that are free-living or parasitic in mammals and include a number of important pathogens (as *L. icterohaemorrhagiae* of Weil's disease or *L. canicola* of canicola fever) **2** *pl* **-ra** *or* **-ras** *or* **-rae** \-ˌrē\ : LEPTOSPIRE

lep•to•spire \ˈlep-tə-ˌspīr\ *n* : any spirochete of the genus *Leptospira* — called also *leptospira* — **lep•to•spi•ral** \ˌlep-tə-ˈspī-rəl\ *adj*

lep•to•spi•ro•sis \ˌlep-tə-spī-ˈrō-səs\ *n, pl* **-ro•ses** \-ˌsēz\ : any of several diseases of humans and domestic animals that are caused by infection with spirochetes of the genus *Leptospira* — called also *lepto;* see WEIL'S DISEASE

lep•to•tene \ˈlep-tə-ˌtēn\ *n* : a stage of meiotic prophase immediately preceding synapsis in which the chromosomes appear as fine discrete threads — **leptotene** *adj*

Le•riche's syndrome \lə-ˈrē-shəz-\ *n* : occlusion of the descending continuation of the aorta in the abdomen typically resulting in impotence, the absence of a pulse in the femoral arteries, and weakness and numbness in the lower back, buttocks, hips, thighs, and calves

Leriche, René (1879–1955), French surgeon.

[1]**les•bi•an** \ˈlez-bē-ən\ *adj* : of or relating to homosexuality between females

[2]**lesbian** *n* : a female homosexual

les•bi•an•ism \ˈlez-bē-ə-ˌni-zəm\ *n* : female homosexuality

Lesch–Ny•han syndrome \ˈlesh-ˈnī-ən-\ *n* : a rare and usu. fatal genetic disorder of male children that is inherited as an X-linked recessive trait and is characterized by hyperuricemia, intellectual disability, spasticity, compulsive biting of the lips and fingers, and a deficiency of hypoxanthine-guanine phosphoribosyltransferase — called also *Lesch-Nyhan disease*

Lesch, Michael (1939–2008), and **Nyhan, William Leo (*b* 1926),** American pediatricians.

Les•col \ˈles-ˌkȯl\ *trademark* — used for a preparation of the sodium salt of fluvastatin

[1]**le•sion** \ˈlē-zhən\ *n* : an abnormal change in structure of an organ or part due to injury or disease; *esp* : one

that is circumscribed and well defined — **le•sioned** \-zhənd\ *adj*

[2]**lesion** *vb* : to produce lesions in

lesser cornu *n* : CERATOHYAL

lesser curvature *n* : the boundary of the stomach that in humans forms a relatively short concave curve on the right from the opening for the esophagus to the opening into the duodenum — compare GREATER CURVATURE

lesser multangular *n* : TRAPEZOID — called also *lesser multangular bone*

lesser occipital nerve *n* : OCCIPITAL NERVE b

lesser omentum *n* : a part of the peritoneum attached to the liver and to the lesser curvature of the stomach and supporting the hepatic vessels — compare GREATER OMENTUM

lesser petrosal nerve *n* : the continuation of the tympanic nerve beyond the inferior ganglion of the glossopharyngeal nerve that terminates in the otic ganglion which it supplies with preganglionic parasympathetic fibers

lesser sciatic foramen *n* : SCIATIC FORAMEN b

lesser sciatic notch *n* : SCIATIC NOTCH b

lesser splanchnic nerve *n* : SPLANCHNIC NERVE b

lesser trochanter *n* : TROCHANTER b

lesser tubercle *n* : a prominence on the upper anterior part of the end of the humerus that serves as the insertion for the subscapularis — compare GREATER TUBERCLE

lesser wing *n* : an anterior triangular process on each side of the sphenoid bone in front of and much smaller than the corresponding greater wing

let•down \ˈlet-ˌdau̇n\ *n* : a physiological response of a lactating mammal to suckling and allied stimuli whereby increased intramammary pressure forces previously secreted milk from the acini and finer tubules into larger ducts from where it can be drawn through the nipple

let down *vb* : to release (formed milk) within the mammary gland or udder

[1]**le•thal** \ˈlē-thəl\ *adj* : of, relating to, or causing death ⟨a ~ injury⟩; *also* : capable of causing death ⟨~ chemicals⟩ ⟨a ~ dose⟩ — **le•thal•i•ty** \lē-ˈtha-lə-tē\ *n* — **le•thal•ly** *adv*

[2]**lethal** *n* **1** : an abnormality of genetic origin causing the death of the organism possessing it usu. before maturity **2** : LETHAL GENE

lethal gene *n* : a gene that in some (as homozygous) conditions may prevent development or cause the death of an organism or its germ cells — called also *lethal factor, lethal mutant, lethal mutation*

lethargica — see ENCEPHALITIS LETHARGICA

leth•ar•gy \ˈle-thər-jē\ *n, pl* **-gies** **1** : abnormal drowsiness **2** : the quality or state of being lazy, sluggish, or indifferent — **lethargic** *adj*

let•ro•zole \ˈle-trə-ˌzōl\ *n* : a nonsteroidal aromatase inhibitor $C_{17}H_{11}N_5$ that is administered orally to treat breast cancer in postmenopausal women — see FEMARA

Let•ter•er–Si•we disease \ˈle-tər-ər-ˈsē-və-\ *n* : an acute often fatal disease of young children that is marked by proliferation of Langerhans cells and is characterized esp. by fever, anemia, hepatosplenomegaly, and a eczematous skin rash

Letterer, Erich (1895–1982), German physician.

Siwe, Sture August (1897–1966), Swedish pediatrician.

Leu *abbr* leucine

leuc- *or* **leuco-** *chiefly Brit var of* LEUK-

leu•cine \ˈlü-ˌsēn\ *n* : a white crystalline essential amino acid $C_6H_{13}NO_2$ obtained by the hydrolysis of most dietary proteins — abbr. *Leu*

leucine aminopeptidase *n* : an aminopeptidase that is found in all bodily tissues and is increased in the serum in some conditions or diseases (as pancreatic carcinoma)

leucine–en•keph•a•lin \-en-ˈke-fə-lən\ *n* : a pentapeptide having a terminal leucine residue that is one of the two enkephalins occurring naturally in the brain — called also *Leu-enkephalin*

leu•ci•no•sis \ˌlü-sə-ˈnō-səs\ *n, pl* **-no•ses** \-ˌsēz\ *or* **-no•sis•es** : a condition characterized by an abnormally high concentration of leucine in bodily tissues and the presence of leucine in the urine

leucocyt- *or* **leucocyto-** *chiefly Brit var of* LEUKOCYT-

leu•co•cy•to•zo•on \ˌlü-kō-ˌsī-tə-ˈzō-ˌän, -ən\ *n* **1** *cap* : a genus of sporozoans parasitic in birds **2** *pl* **-zoa** \-ˈzō-ə\ : any sporozoan of the genus *Leucocytozoon*

leu•cov•o•rin \lü-ˈkä-və-rin\ *n* : a metabolically active form of folic acid that has been used in cancer therapy to protect normal cells against methotrexate — called also *citrovorum factor, folinic acid*

Leu–en•keph•a•lin \ˌlü-en-ˈke-fə-lin\ *n* : LEUCINE-ENKEPHALIN

leuk- *or* **leuko-** *comb form* **1** : white : colorless : weakly colored ⟨*leuko*cyte⟩ ⟨*leuko*rrhea⟩ **2** : leukocyte ⟨*leu*kemia⟩ **3** : white matter of the brain ⟨*leuko*encephalopathy⟩

leu•kae•mia, leu•kae•mic *chiefly Brit var of* LEUKEMIA, LEUKEMIC

leu•ka•phe•re•sis \ˌlü-kə-fə-ˈrē-səs\ *n, pl* **-phe•re•ses** \-ˌsēz\ : apheresis used to remove white blood cells (as in the treatment of chronic lymphocytic leukemia) — called also *leukopheresis*

leu•ke•mia \lü-ˈkē-mē-ə\ *n* : an acute or chronic disease characterized by an abnormal increase in the number of white blood cells in bodily tissues with or without a corresponding increase of those in the circulating blood — see ACUTE LYMPHOBLASTIC LEUKEMIA, ACUTE MYELOGENOUS LEUKEMIA, CHRONIC LYMPHOCYTIC LEUKEMIA, CHRONIC MYELOGENOUS LEUKEMIA, FELINE LEUKEMIA, LYMPHOBLASTIC LEUKEMIA, LYMPHOCYTIC LEUKEMIA, MONOCYTIC LEUKEMIA, MYELOGENOUS LEUKEMIA, PROMYELOCYTIC LEUKEMIA

[1]**leu•ke•mic** \lü-ˈkē-mik\ *adj* **1** : of, relating to, or affected by leukemia **2** : characterized by an increase in white blood cells ⟨∼ blood⟩

[2]**leukemic** *n* : a person affected with leukemia

leu•ke•mo•gen•e•sis \lü-ˌkē-mə-ˈje-nə-səs\ *n, pl* **-e•ses** \-ˌsēz\ : induction or production of leukemia — **leu•ke•mo•gen•ic** \-ˈjen-ik\ *adj*

leu•ke•moid \lü-ˈkē-mȯid\ *adj* : resembling leukemia

leuko- — see LEUK-

leu•ko•ag•glu•ti•nin \ˌlü-kō-ə-ˈglüt-ᵊn-ən\ *n* : an antibody that agglutinates white blood cells — compare HEMAGGLUTININ

leukocyt- *or* **leukocyto-** *comb form* : leukocyte ⟨*leukocyt*osis⟩

leu•ko•cyte \ˈlü-kə-ˌsīt\ *n* : any of the colorless blood cells of the immune system including the neutrophils, lymphocytes, monocytes, eosinophils, basophils, and their derivatives : WHITE BLOOD CELL

leu•ko•cyt•ic \ˌlü-kə-ˈsi-tik\ *adj* **1** : of, relating to, or involving leukocytes or white blood cells **2** : characterized by an excess of leukocytes or white blood cells

leu•ko•cy•to•sis \ˌlü-kə-sī-ˈtō-səs, -kə-sə-\ *n, pl* **-to•ses** \-ˌsēz\ : an increase in the number of white blood cells in the circulating blood that occurs normally (as after meals) or abnormally (as in some infections) — **leu•ko•cy•tot•ic** \-ˈtä-tik\ *adj*

leu•ko•der•ma \ˌlü-kə-ˈdər-mə\ *n* : partial or total loss or absence of pigmentation that is marked esp. by white patches of skin — see VITILIGO

leu•ko•dys•tro•phy \ˌlü-kō-ˈdis-trə-fē\ *n, pl* **-phies** : any of several inherited diseases characterized by progressive degeneration of myelin in the brain, spinal cord, and peripheral nerves

leu•ko•en•ceph•a•lop•a•thy \-in-ˌse-fə-ˈlä-pə-thē\ *n, pl* **-thies** : any of various diseases affecting the brain's white matter; *esp* : PROGRESSIVE MULTIFOCAL LEUKOENCEPHALOPATHY

leuk•onych•ia \ˌlü-kō-ˈni-kē-ə\ *n* : a white spotting, streaking, or discoloration of the fingernails caused by injury or ill health

leu•ko•pe•nia \ˌlü-kō-ˈpē-nē-ə\ *n* : a condition in which the number of white blood cells circulating in the blood is abnormally low and which is most commonly due to a decreased production of new cells in conjunction with various infectious diseases, as a reaction to various drugs or other chemicals, or in response to irradiation — **leu•ko•pe•nic** \-ˈpē-nik\ *adj*

leu•ko•phe•re•sis \-fə-ˈrē-səs\ *n, pl* **-re•ses** \-ˌsēz\ : LEUKAPHERESIS

leu•ko•pla•kia \ˌlü-kō-ˈplā-kē-ə\ *n* : a condition commonly considered precancerous in which thickened white patches of epithelium occur on the mucous membranes esp. of the mouth, vulva, and renal pelvis; *also* : a lesion or lesioned area of leukoplakia — **leu•ko•pla•kic** \-ˈplā-kik\ *adj*

leu•ko•poi•e•sis \-pȯi-ˈē-səs\ *n, pl* **-e•ses** \-ˌsēz\ : the formation of white blood cells — **leu•ko•poi•et•ic** \-ˈe-tik\ *adj*

leu•kor•rhea \ˌlü-kə-ˈrē-ə\ *n* : a white, yellowish, or greenish-white viscid discharge from the vagina resulting from inflammation or congestion of the uterine or vaginal mucous membrane — **leu•kor•rhe•al** \-ˈrē-əl\ *adj*

leu•ko•sar•co•ma \ˌlü-kō-sär-ˈkō-mə\ *n, pl* **-mas** *also* **-ma•ta** \-mə-tə\ : lymphosarcoma accompanied by leukemia — **leu•ko•sar•co•ma•to•sis** \-sär-ˌkō-mə-ˈtō-səs\ *n*

leu•ko•sis \lü-ˈkō-səs\ *n, pl* **-ko•ses** \-ˌsēz\ : LEUKEMIA; *esp* : any of various leukemic diseases of poultry — **leu•kot•ic** \-ˈkä-tik\ *adj*

leu•ko•tac•tic \ˌlü-kō-ˈtak-tik\ *adj* : tending to attract white blood cells

leu•ko•tome \ˈlü-kə-ˌtōm\ *n* : a cannula through which a wire is inserted and used to cut the white matter in the brain in lobotomy

leu•kot•o•my \lü-ˈkä-tə-mē\ *n, pl* **-mies** : LOBOTOMY

leu•ko•tox•in \ˌlü-kō-ˈtäk-sən\ *n* : a substance specif. destructive to white blood cells

leu•ko•tri•ene \ˌlü-kə-ˈtrī-ˌēn\ *n* : any of a group of eicosanoids that are generated in basophils, mast cells, macrophages, and human lung tissue by lipoxygenase-catalyzed oxygenation esp. of arachidonic acid and that participate in allergic responses (as bronchoconstriction in asthma) — see SLOW-REACTING SUBSTANCE OF ANAPHYLAXIS

leu•pro•lide \lü-ˈprō-ˌlīd\ *n* : a synthetic analog of gonadotropin-releasing hormone administered by injection in the form of its acetate $C_{59}H_{84}N_{16}O_{12}{\cdot}C_2H_4O_2$ to treat cancer of the prostate gland, endometriosis, uterine fibroids, and precocious puberty — see ELIGARD, LUPRON

leu•ro•cris•tine \ˌlu̇r-ō-ˈkris-ˌtēn\ *n* : VINCRISTINE

lev- *or* **levo-** *comb form* : left : on the left side : to the left ⟨*levo*cardia⟩

lev•al•bu•te•rol \ˌlev-al-ˈbyü-tə-ˌrȯl, -ˌrōl\ *n* : a beta-agonist bronchodilator administered by oral inhalation in the form of its hydrochloride $C_{13}H_{21}NO_3{\cdot}HCl$ or tartrate $(C_{13}H_{21}NO_3)_2{\cdot}C_4H_6O_6$ to treat bronchospasm associated esp. with asthma — called also *levosalbutamol;* see XOPENEX

lev·al·lor·phan \ˌle-və-ˈlȯr-ˌfan, -fən\ *n* : a drug $C_{19}H_{25}NO$ related to morphine that is used to counteract morphine poisoning

le·vam·i·sole \lə-ˈva-mə-ˌsōl\ *n* : an anthelmintic drug administered in the form of its hydrochloride $C_{11}H_{12}N_2S{\cdot}HCl$ that also possesses immunostimulant properties and is used esp. in the treatment of colon cancer

Le·vant storax \lə-ˈvant-\ *n* : STORAX 1

Le·va·quin \ˈle-və-kwən\ *trademark* — used for a preparation of levofloxacin

lev·ar·ter·e·nol \ˌle-vär-ˈtir-ə-ˌnȯl, -ˈter-, -ˌnōl\ *n* : levorotatory norepinephrine

le·va·tor \li-ˈvā-tər\ *n, pl* **lev·a·to·res** \ˌle-və-ˈtōr-(ˌ)ēz\ *or* **le·va·tors** \li-ˈvā-tərz\ : a muscle that serves to raise a body part — compare DEPRESSOR a

levator an·gu·li oris \-ˈaŋ-gyə-ˌlī-ˈȯr-əs\ *n* : a facial muscle that arises from the maxilla, inclines downward to be inserted into the corner of the mouth, and draws the lips up and back — called also *caninus*

levator ani \-ˈā-ˌnī\ *n* : a broad thin muscle that is attached in a sheet to each side of the inner surface of the pelvis and descends to form the floor of the pelvic cavity where it supports the viscera and surrounds structures which pass through it and inserts into the sides of the apex of the coccyx, the margins of the anus, the side of the rectum, and the central tendinous point of the perineum — see ILIOCOCCYGEUS, PUBOCOCCYGEUS

levatores cos·tar·um \-ˌkäs-ˈtār-əm, -ˈtär-\ *n pl* : a series of 12 muscles on each side that arise from the transverse processes of the seventh cervical and upper 11 thoracic vertebrae, that insert into the ribs, and that raise the ribs increasing the volume of the thoracic cavity and extend, bend, and rotate the spinal column

levator la·bii su·pe·ri·or·is \-ˈlā-bē-ˌī-sü-ˌpir-ē-ˈȯr-əs\ *n* : a facial muscle arising from the lower margin of the orbit and inserting into the muscular substance of the upper lip which it elevates — called also *quadratus labii superioris*

levator labii superioris alae·que na·si \-ā-ˈlē-kwē-ˈnā-ˌzī\ *n* : a muscle that arises from the nasal process of the maxilla, that passes downward and laterally, that divides into a part inserting into the alar cartilage and one inserting into the upper lip, and that dilates the nostril and raises the upper lip

levator pal·pe·brae su·pe·ri·or·is \-ˌpal-ˈpē-ˌbrē-sü-ˌpir-ē-ˈȯr-əs\ *n* : a thin flat extrinsic muscle of the eye arising from the lesser wing of the sphenoid bone and inserting into the tarsal plate of the skin of the upper eyelid which it raises

levator pros·ta·tae \-ˈpräs-tə-ˌtē\ *n* : a part of the pubococcygeus comprising the more medial and ventral fasciculi that insert into the tissue in front of the anus and serve to support and elevate the prostate gland

levator scap·u·lae \-ˈska-pyə-ˌlē\ *n* : a back muscle that arises in the transverse processes of the first four cervical vertebrae and descends to insert into the vertebral border of the scapula which it elevates

levator ve·li pal·a·ti·ni \-ˈvē-ˌlī-ˌpa-lə-ˈtī-ˌnī\ *n* : a muscle arising from the temporal bone and the cartilage of the eustachian tube and descending to insert into the midline of the soft palate which it elevates esp. to close the nasopharynx while swallowing is taking place

Le·Veen shunt \lə-ˈvēn-ˈshənt\ *n* : a plastic tube that passes from the jugular vein to the peritoneal cavity where a valve permits absorption of ascitic fluid which is carried back to venous circulation by way of the superior vena cava

LeVeen, Harry Henry (1914–1996), American surgeon.

Lev·e·mir \ˈlev-ə-ˌmir\ *trademark* — used for a preparation of insulin detemir

Le·vin tube \lə-ˈvēn-, lə-ˈvin-\ *n* : a tube designed to be passed into the stomach or duodenum through the nose

Levin, Abraham Louis (1880–1940), American physician.

Le·vi·tra \lə-ˈvē-trə\ *trademark* — used for a preparation of the hydrated hydrochloride of vardenafil

le·vo \ˈlē-(ˌ)vō\ *adj* : LEVOROTATORY

levo- — see LEV-

le·vo·car·dia \ˌlē-və-ˈkär-dē-ə\ *n* : normal position of the heart when associated with situs inversus of other abdominal viscera and usu. with structural defects of the heart itself

le·vo–di·hy·droxy·phe·nyl·al·a·nine \ˌlē-vō-ˌdī-hī-ˌdräk-sē-ˌfen-ᵊl-ˈa-lə-ˌnēn, -ˌfēn \ *n* : L-DOPA

levo·do·pa \ˈle-və-ˌdō-pə, ˌlē-və-ˈdō-pə\ *n* : L-DOPA

Le·vo–Dro·mo·ran \ˌlē-vō-ˈdrō-mə-ˌran\ *trademark* — used for a preparation of levorphanol

le·vo·flox·a·cin \ˌlē-və-ˈfläk-sə-sən\ *n* : a broad-spectrum antibacterial agent that is the levorotatory isomer of ofloxacin — see LEVAQUIN

le·vo·nor·ges·trel \ˌlē-və-nȯr-ˈjes-trəl\ *n* : a synthetic progestin $C_{21}H_{28}O_2$ that is used esp. in birth control pills and contraceptive implants and that is the levorotatory form of norgestrel — see MIRENA, PLAN B, SEASONALE, SEASONIQUE

Levo·phed \ˈle-və-ˌfed\ *trademark* — used for a preparation of norepinephrine

Le·vo·prome \ˈlē-və-ˌprōm\ *trademark* — used for a preparation of methotrimeprazine

le·vo·pro·poxy·phene \ˌlē-və-ˌprō-ˈpäk-si-ˌfēn\ *n* : a drug used esp. in the form of the napsylate $C_{22}H_{29}NO_2 \cdot C_{10}H_8SO_3$ as an antitussive

le·vo·ro·ta·to·ry \-ˈrō-tə-ˌtōr-ē\ *or* **le·vo·ro·ta·ry** \-ˈrō-tə-rē\ *adj* : turning toward the left or counterclockwise; *esp* : rotating the plane of polarization of light to the left — compare DEXTROROTATORY

lev·or·pha·nol \ˌle-ˈvȯr-fə-ˌnȯl\ *n* : an addictive drug used esp. in the form of its hydrated tartrate $C_{17}H_{23}NO \cdot C_4H_6O_6 \cdot 2H_2O$ as a potent analgesic with properties similar to morphine — see LEVO-DROMORAN

le·vo·sal·bu·ta·mol \ˌlē-vō-sal-ˈbyüt-ə-ˌmȯl, -ˌmōl\ *n* : LEVALBUTEROL

Le·vo·throid \ˈlē-və-ˌthrȯid\ *trademark* — used for a preparation of the sodium salt of levothyroxine

le·vo·thy·rox·ine \ˌlē-vō-thī-ˈräk-ˌsēn, -sən\ *n* : the levorotatory isomer of thyroxine that is administered in the form of its sodium salt $C_{15}H_{10}I_4NNaO_4$ in the treatment of hypothyroidism — see LEVOTHROID, LEVOXYL, SYNTHROID

Le·vox·yl \lə-ˈväk-səl\ *trademark* — used for a preparation of the sodium salt of levothyroxine

Lev·u·lan \ˈle-vyə-ˌlan\ *trademark* — used for a preparation of aminolevulinic acid

lev·u·lose \ˈle-vyə-ˌlōs, -ˌlōz\ *n* : FRUCTOSE 2

lev·u·los·uria \ˌle-vyə-lō-ˈsyu̇r-ē-ə, -ˈshu̇r-\ *n* : the presence of fructose in the urine

Lew·is blood group \ˈlü-əs-\ *n* : any of a system of blood groups controlled by a pair of dominant-recessive alleles and characterized by antigens which are adsorbed onto the surface of red blood cells and tend to interreact with the antigens produced by secretors although they are genetically independent of them

Lewis, H. D. G., British hospital patient.

lew·is·ite \ˈlü-ə-ˌsīt\ *n* : a colorless or brown vesicant liquid $C_2H_2AsCl_3$ developed as a poison gas for war use

Lewis, Winford Lee (1878–1943), American chemist.

Lewy body \ˈlü-ē-, ˈlā-vē-\ *n* : an eosinophilic inclusion body found in the cytoplasm of neurons of the cortex and brain stem in Parkinson's disease, Lewy body disease, and other neurodegenerative disorders

Lew·ey \ˈlü-ē\, **Frederic Henry** (*orig.* **Friedrich Heinrich Lewy) (1885–1950),** American neurologist.

Lewy body disease *n* : a dementia with onset typically after the age of 60 that is marked by the presence of Lewy bodies and is characterized chiefly by a progressive decline in cognitive functioning, fluctuations in attention and alertness, recurrent visual hallucinations, and parkinsonian symptoms (as tremor and muscle rigidity) — called also *Lewy body dementia*

Lex·a·pro \ˈlek-sə-ˌprō\ *trademark* — used for a preparation of the oxalate of escitalopram

-lex·ia \ˈlek-sē-ə\ *n comb form* : reading of (such) a kind or with (such) an impairment ⟨dys*lexia*⟩

Ley·dig cell \ˈlī-dig-\ *also* **Ley·dig's cell** \-digz-\ *n* : a cell of interstitial tissue of the testis that is usu. considered the chief source of testicular androgens and esp. testosterone — called also *cell of Leydig, interstitial cell of Leydig*

Leydig, Franz von (1821–1908), German anatomist.

L–form \ˈel-ˌfȯrm\ *n* : a variant form of some bacteria (as those causing anthrax and tuberculosis) that usu. lacks a cell wall and typically displays resistance to antibiotics — called also *L-phase*

LGL syndrome \ˌel-ˌjē-ˈel-\ *n* : LOWN-GANONG-LEVINE SYNDROME

LH *abbr* luteinizing hormone

LHRH *abbr* luteinizing hormone-releasing hormone

Li *symbol* lithium

lib — see AD LIB

li·bi·do \lə-ˈbē-(ˌ)dō, -ˈbī-, ˈli-bə-ˌdō\ *n, pl* **-dos** **1** : instinctual psychic energy that in psychoanalytic theory is derived from primitive biological urges (as for sexual pleasure or self-preservation) and is expressed in conscious activity **2** : sexual drive — **li·bid·i·nal** \lə-ˈbid-ᵊn-əl\ *adj*

libitum — see AD LIBITUM

Lib·man–Sacks endocarditis \ˈlib-mən-ˈsaks-\ *n* : a noninfectious form of verrucous endocarditis associated with systemic lupus erythematosus — called also *Libman-Sacks disease, Libman-Sacks syndrome*

Libman, Emanuel (1872–1946), and **Sacks, Benjamin (1896–1939),** American physicians.

li·brary \ˈlī-ˌbrer-ē\ *n, pl* **-brar·ies** : a collection of cloned DNA fragments that are maintained in a suitable cellular environment and that represent the genetic material of a particular organism or tissue

Lib·ri·um \ˈli-brē-əm\ *trademark* — used for a preparation of the hydrochloride of chlordiazepoxide

lice *pl of* LOUSE

licensed practical nurse *n* : a person who has undergone training and obtained a license (as from a state) to provide routine care for the sick — called also *LPN*

licensed vocational nurse *n* : a licensed practical nurse authorized by license to practice in the states of California or Texas — called also *LVN*

li·cen·sure \ˈlī-sᵊn-shər\ *n* : the state or condition of having a license granted by official or legal authority to perform medical acts and procedures not permitted by persons without such a license ⟨RN ~⟩; *also* : the granting of such licenses

li·chen \'lī-kən\ *n* **1** : any of several skin diseases characterized by the eruption of flat papules; *esp* : LICHEN PLANUS **2** : any of numerous complex plantlike organisms made up of an alga and a fungus growing in symbiotic association

li·chen·i·fi·ca·tion \lī-ˌke-nə-fə-'kā-shən, ˌlī-kə-\ *n* : the process by which skin becomes hardened and leathery or lichenoid usu. as a result of chronic irritation; *also* : a patch of skin so modified — **li·chen·i·fied** \lī-'ke-nə-ˌfīd, 'lī-kə-\ *adj*

li·chen·oid \'lī-kə-ˌnȯid\ *adj* : resembling lichen ⟨a ~ eruption⟩

lichenoides — see PITYRIASIS LICHENOIDES ET VARIOLIFORMIS ACUTA

lichen pla·nus \-'plā-nəs\ *n* : a skin disease characterized by an eruption of wide flat papules covered by a horny glazed film, marked by intense itching, and often accompanied by lesions on the oral mucosa

lichen scle·ro·sus et atro·phi·cus \-sklə-'rō-səs-et-ˌā-'trō-fi-kəs\ *n* : a chronic skin disease that is characterized by the eruption of flat white hardened papules with central hair follicles often having black keratotic plugs

lichen sim·plex chron·i·cus \-'sim-ˌpleks-'krä-ni-kəs\ *n* : NEURODERMATITIS; *specif* : neurodermatitis marked by raised scaly patches of thickened leathery skin

lic·o·rice \'li-kə-rish, -ris\ *n* : the dried root of a European herb (*Glycyrrhiza glabra* of the legume family, Leguminosae) that is the source of extracts used to mask unpleasant flavors (as in drugs) or to give a pleasant taste (as to confections) — called also *licorice root*

lid \'lid\ *n* : EYELID

li·do·caine \'lī-də-ˌkān\ *n* : a crystalline compound $C_{14}H_{22}N_2O$ used as a local anesthetic often in the form of its hydrochloride $C_{14}H_{22}N_2O·HCl$ — called also *lignocaine;* see XYLOCAINE

Lie·ber·mann–Bur·chard test \'lē-bər-mən-'bu̇r-ˌkärt-\ *n* : a test for unsaturated steroids (as cholesterol) and for terpenes having the formula $C_{30}H_{48}$ — called also *Liebermann-Burchard reaction*

Liebermann, Carl Theodore (1842–1914), German chemist. H. Burchard may have been one of his many student-research assistants.

lie detector \'lī-di-ˌtek-tər\ *n* : a polygraph for detecting physiological evidence (as changes in heart rate) of the tension that accompanies lying

li·en \'lī-ən, 'lī-ˌen\ *n* : SPLEEN — **li·en·al** \-ᵊl\ *adj*

lienal vein *n* : SPLENIC VEIN

life \'līf\ *n, pl* **lives** \'līvz\ **1 a** : the quality that distinguishes a vital and functional plant or animal from a dead body **b** : a state of living characterized by capacity for metabolism, growth, reaction to stimuli, and reproduction **2 a** : the sequence of physical and mental experiences that make up the existence of an individual **b** : a specific part or aspect of the process of living ⟨sex ~⟩ ⟨adult ~⟩ — **life·less** \'līf-ləs\ *adj*

life cycle *n* : the series of stages in form and functional activity through which an organism passes between successive recurrences of a specified primary stage

life expectancy *n* : an expected number of years of life based on statistical probability

[1]**life·sav·ing** \'līf-ˌsā-viŋ\ *adj* : designed for or used in saving lives ⟨~ drugs⟩

[2]**lifesaving** *n* : the skill or practice of saving or protecting the lives esp. of drowning persons

life science *n* : a branch of science (as biology or medicine) that deals with living organisms and life processes — usu. used in pl. — **life scientist** *n*

life space *n* : the physical and psychological environment of an individual or group

life span \'līf-ˌspan\ *n* **1** : the duration of existence of an individual **2** : the average length of life of a kind of organism or of a material object

life–sup·port \'līf-sə-ˌpȯrt\ *adj* : providing support necessary to sustain life; *esp* : of, relating to, or being a life-support system ⟨~ equipment⟩

life support *n* : equipment, material, and treatment needed to keep a seriously ill or injured patient alive ⟨the patient was placed on *life support*⟩

life–support system *n* : a system that provides all or some of the items (as oxygen, food, water, and disposition of carbon dioxide and body wastes) necessary for maintaining life or health

life–threat·en·ing \'līf-ˌthret-ən-iŋ\ *adj* : capable of causing death : potentially fatal ⟨~ injuries⟩ ⟨a ~ allergic reaction⟩ ⟨~ arrhythmia⟩

Li–Frau·me·ni syndrome \'lē frau̇ 'mē-nē-\ *n* : a rare familial syndrome that is characterized esp. by a high risk of developing early breast cancer and sarcomas of soft tissue

Li, Frederick P. (*b* 1940), and Fraumeni, Joseph F., Jr. (*b* 1933), American epidemiologists.

lift \'lift\ *n* : plastic surgery on a part of the body typically to improve a drooping or sagging appearance esp. by reducing excess skin and fat — compare BRACHIOPLASTY, FACELIFT, BREAST LIFT — **lift** *vb*

lig·a·ment \'li-gə-mənt\ *n* **1** : a tough band of tissue that serves to connect the articular extremities of bones or to support or retain an organ in place and is usu. composed of coarse bundles of dense white fibrous tissue parallel or closely interlaced, pliant, and flexible, but not extensible **2** : any of various folds or bands of pleura, peritoneum, or mesentery connecting parts or organs

ligament of the ovary *n* : a rounded cord of fibrous and muscular tissue extending from each superior angle of the uterus to the inner extremity of the ovary of the same side — called also *ovarian ligament;* see SUSPENSORY LIGAMENT OF THE OVARY

ligament of Treitz \-ˈtrīts\ *n* : a band of smooth muscle extending from the junction of the duodenum and jejunum to the left crus of the diaphragm and functioning as a suspensory ligament

Treitz, Wenzel (1819–1872), Austrian physician.

ligament of Zinn \-ˈzin, -ˈtsin\ *n* : the common tendon of the inferior rectus and the internal rectus muscles of the eye — called also *tendon of Zinn*

Zinn \ˈtsin\, **Johann Gottfried (1727–1759),** German anatomist and botanist.

lig•a•men•tous \ˌli-gə-ˈmen-təs\ *adj* **1** : of or relating to a ligament **2** : forming or formed of a ligament

lig•a•men•tum \ˌli-gə-ˈmen-təm\ *n, pl* **-ta** \-tə\ : LIGAMENT

ligamentum ar•te•rio•sum \-är-ˌtir-ē-ˈō-səm\ *n* : a cord of tissue that connects the pulmonary trunk and the aorta and that is the vestige of the ductus arteriosus

ligamentum fla•vum \-ˈflā-vəm\ *n, pl* **ligamenta fla•va** \-və\ : any of a series of ligaments of yellow elastic tissue connecting the laminae of adjacent vertebrae from the axis to the sacrum

ligamentum nu•chae \-ˈnü-ˌkē, -ˈnyü-, -ˌkī\ *n, pl* **ligamenta nuchae** : a medium ligament of the back of the neck that is rudimentary in humans but highly developed and composed of yellow elastic tissue in many quadrupeds where it assists in supporting the head

ligamentum te•res \-ˈtē-ˌrēz\ *n* : ROUND LIGAMENT; *esp* : ROUND LIGAMENT 1

ligamentum ve•no•sum \-vē-ˈnō-səm\ *n* : a cord of tissue connected to the liver that is the vestige of the ductus venosus

li•gase \ˈlī-ˌgās, -ˌgāz\ *n* : SYNTHETASE

li•ga•tion \lī-ˈgā-shən\ *n* **1 a** : the surgical process of tying up an anatomical channel (as a blood vessel) **b** : the process of joining together chemical chains (as of DNA or protein) **2** : something that binds : LIGATURE — **li•gate** \ˈlī-ˌgāt, lī-ˈ\ *vb*

lig•a•ture \ˈli-gə-ˌchu̇r, -chər, -ˌtyu̇r\ *n* **1** : something that is used to bind; *specif* : a filament (as a thread) used in surgery (as for tying blood vessels) **2** : the action or result of binding or tying — **ligature** *vb*

[1]light \ˈlīt\ *n* **1 a** : the sensation aroused by stimulation of the visual receptors **b** : an electromagnetic radiation in the wavelength range including infrared, visible, ultraviolet, and X-rays and traveling in a vacuum with a speed of about 186,281 miles (300,000 kilometers) per second; *specif* : the part of this range that is visible to the human eye **2** : a source of light

[2]light *or* **lite** *adj* : made with a lower calorie content or with less of some ingredient (as salt, fat, or alcohol) than usual ⟨~ salad dressing⟩

light adaptation *n* : the adjustments including narrowing of the pupillary opening and decrease in rhodopsin by which the retina of the eye is made efficient as a visual receptor under conditions of strong illumination — compare DARK ADAPTATION — **light–adapt•ed** \ˈlīt-ə-ˌdap-təd\ *adj*

light chain *n* : either of the two smaller of the four polypeptide chains that are subunits of antibodies — called also *L chain;* compare HEAVY CHAIN

light•en•ing \ˈlīt-ᵊn-iŋ\ *n* : a sense of decreased weight and abdominal tension felt by a pregnant woman on descent of the fetus into the pelvic cavity prior to labor

light–head•ed•ness \ˈlīt-ˈhe-dəd-nəs\ *n* : the condition of being dizzy or on the verge of fainting — **light–head•ed** *adj*

light microscope *n* : an ordinary microscope that uses light as distinguished from an electron microscope — **light microscopy** *n*

light•ning pains \ˈlīt-niŋ-\ *n pl* : intense shooting or lancinating pains occurring in tabes dorsalis

light therapy *n* : PHOTOTHERAPY; *esp* : the use of strong light for the treatment of depression (as in seasonal affective disorder) — called also *light treatment*

lig•nan \ˈlig-ˌnan\ *n* : any of a class of compounds including many found in plants and noted for having antioxidant and estrogenic activity

lig•no•caine \ˈlig-nə-ˌkān\ *n, Brit* : LIDOCAINE

limb \ˈlim\ *n* **1** : one of the projecting paired appendages of an animal body concerned esp. with movement and grasping; *esp* : a human leg or arm **2** : a branch or arm of something (as an anatomical part)

lim•bal \ˈlim-bəl\ *adj* : of or relating to the limbus ⟨a ~ incision⟩

limb bud *n* : a proliferation of embryonic tissue shaped like a mound from which a limb develops

lim•ber•neck \ˈlim-bər-ˌnek\ *n* : a botulism of birds (esp. poultry) characterized by paralysis of the neck muscles and pharynx

lim•bic \ˈlim-bik\ *adj* : of, relating to, or being the limbic system of the brain

limbic lobe *n* : the marginal medial portion of the cortex of a cerebral hemisphere

limbic system *n* : a group of subcortical structures (as the hypothalamus, the hippocampus, and the amygdala) of the brain that are concerned esp. with emotion and motivation

lim•bus \ˈlim-bəs\ *n* : a border distinguished by color or structure; *esp* : the marginal region of the cornea of the eye by which it is continuous with the sclera

lime \ˈlīm\ *n* : a caustic powdery white solid that consists of the oxide of calcium often together with magnesia

li•men \ˈlī-mən\ *n* : THRESHOLD

lim•i•nal \ˈli-mə-nəl\ *adj* : of, relating to, or situated at a sensory threshold : barely perceptible or capable of eliciting a response ⟨~ visual stimuli⟩

limp \ˈlimp\ *vb* **1** : to walk lamely; *esp* : to walk favoring one leg **2** : to go unsteadily — **limp** *n*

lin•a•clo•tide \ˌlin-ə-ˈklō-ˌtīd\ *n* : a drug $C_{59}H_{79}N_{15}O_{21}S_6$ that is taken orally to relieve symptoms of constipation of unknown cause and constipation associated with irritable bowel syndrome and that acts by binding to guanylate cyclase receptors to increase intestinal secretions, decrease abdominal pain, and accelerate the movement of waste through the intestines — see LINZESS

lin•a•glip•tin \ˌlin-ə-ˈglip-tən\ *n* : a hypoglycemic drug $C_{25}H_{28}N_8O_2$ that inhibits the breakdown of incretin and is taken orally in the treatment of type 2 diabetes — see JENTADUETO, TRADJENTA

Lin•co•cin \liŋ-ˈkō-sən\ *trademark* — used for a preparation of the hydrated hydrochloride of lincomycin

lin•co•my•cin \ˌliŋ-kə-ˈmīs-ᵊn\ *n* : an antibiotic effective esp. against gram-positive bacteria that is obtained from an actinomycete of the genus *Streptomyces* (*S. lincolnensis*) and is used in the form of its hydrated hydrochloride $C_{18}H_{34}N_2O_6S{\cdot}HCl{\cdot}H_2O$

linc•tus \ˈliŋk-təs\ *n, pl* **linc•tus•es** : a syrupy or sticky medicated preparation exerting a local action on the mucous membrane of the throat

lin•dane \ˈlin-ˌdān\ *n* : a compound consisting of not less than 99 percent gamma benzene hexachloride that is sometimes used topically in medicine to treat scabies and was formerly used as an agricultural insecticide

Lin•dau's disease \ˈlin-ˌdau̇z-\ *n* : VON HIPPEL-LINDAU DISEASE

line \ˈlīn\ *n* **1** : a strain produced and maintained esp. by selective breeding or biological culture **2** : a narrow short synthetic tube (as of plastic) that is inserted approximately one inch into a vein (as of the arm) to provide temporary intravenous access for the administration of fluid, medication, or nutrients

lin•ea al•ba \ˈli-nē-ə-ˈal-bə\ *n, pl* **lin•e•ae al•bae** \ˈli-nē-ˌē-ˈal-ˌbē\ : a median vertical tendinous line on the abdomen formed of fibers from the aponeuroses of the two rectus abdominis muscles and extending from the xiphoid process to the pubic symphysis

linea as•pe•ra \-ˈas-pə-rə\ *n, pl* **lineae as•pe•rae** \-ˌrē\ : a longitudinal ridge on the posterior surface of the middle third of the femur

lineae al•bi•can•tes \-ˌal-bə-ˈkan-ˌtēz\ *n pl* : whitish marks in the skin esp. of the abdomen and breasts that often follow pregnancy

linea semi•lu•nar•is \-ˌse-mi-lü-ˈnar-əs\ *n, pl* **lineae semi•lu•nar•es** \-ˈnar-ˌēz\ : a curved line on the ventral abdominal wall parallel to the midline and halfway between it and the side of the body that marks the lateral border of the rectus abdominis muscle — called also *semilunar line*

line of sight *n* : a line from an observer's eye to a distant point

line of vision *n* : a straight line joining the fovea of the eye with the fixation point

linguae — see LONGITUDINALIS LINGUAE

lin•gual \ˈliŋ-gwəl, -gyə-wəl\ *adj* **1** : of, relating to, or resembling the tongue **2** : lying near or next to the tongue; *esp* : relating to or being the surface of a tooth next to the tongue

lingual artery *n* : an artery arising from the external carotid artery between the superior thyroid and facial arteries and supplying the tongue

lingual gland *n* : any of the mucous, serous, or mixed glands that empty their secretions onto the surface of the tongue

lin•gual•ly \ˈliŋ-gwə-lē\ *adv* : toward the tongue ⟨a tooth displaced ~⟩

lingual nerve *n* : a branch of the mandibular division of the trigeminal nerve supplying the anterior two thirds of the tongue and responding to stimuli of pressure, touch, and temperature

lingual tonsil *n* : a variable mass or group of small nodules of lymphoid tissue lying at the base of the tongue just anterior to the epiglottis

lin•gu•la \ˈliŋ-gyə-lə\ *n, pl* **lin•gu•lae** \-ˌlē\ : a tongue-shaped process or part: as **a** : a ridge of bone in the angle between the body and the greater wing of the sphenoid **b** : an elongated prominence of the superior vermis of the cerebellum **c** : a dependent projection of the upper lobe of the left lung — **lin•gu•lar** \-lər\ *adj*

lin•i•ment \ˈli-nə-mənt\ *n* : a liquid or semifluid preparation that is applied to the skin as an anodyne or a counterirritant — called also *embrocation*

li•ni•tis plas•ti•ca \lə-ˈnī-təs-ˈplas-ti-kə\ *n* : carcinoma of the stomach marked by thickening and diffuse infiltration of the wall rather than localization of the tumor in a discrete lump

link•age \ˈliŋ-kij\ *n* : the relationship between genes on the same chromo-

some that causes them to be inherited together — compare MENDEL'S LAW 2
linkage group *n* : a set of linked genes at different loci on the same chromosome
linked \ˈliŋkt\ *adj* : marked by linkage ⟨~ genes⟩
Li•nog•na•thus \li-ˈnäg-nə-thəs\ *n* : a genus of sucking lice including parasites of several domestic mammals
Lin•zess \ˌlin-ˈzes\ *trademark* — used for a preparation of linaclotide
lio- — see LEIO-
li•o•thy•ro•nine \ˌlī-ō-ˈthī-rə-ˌnēn\ *n* : TRIIODOTHYRONINE
lip \ˈlip\ *n* **1** : either of the two fleshy folds which surround the mouth and in humans are organs of speech essential to certain articulations; *also* : the pink or reddish margin of the human lip composed of nonglandular mucous membrane **2** : an edge of a wound **3** : either of a pair of fleshy folds surrounding an orifice **4** : an anatomical part or structure (as a labium) resembling a lip — **lip•like** \ˈlip-ˌlīk\ *adj*
lip- *or* **lipo-** *comb form* : fat : fatty tissue : fatty ⟨*lipoid*⟩ ⟨*lipoprotein*⟩
li•pae•mia *chiefly Brit var of* LIPEMIA
li•pase \ˈli-ˌpās, ˈlī-, -ˌpāz\ *n* : an enzyme (as one secreted by the pancreas) that catalyzes the breakdown of fats and lipoproteins usu. into fatty acids and glycerol
li•pec•to•my \lī-ˈpek-tə-mē, li-\ *n, pl* **-mies** : the excision of subcutaneous fatty tissue esp. as a cosmetic surgical procedure
li•pe•mia \li-ˈpē-mē-ə\ *n* : the presence of an excess of fats or lipids in the blood; *specif* : HYPERCHOLESTEROLEMIA — **li•pe•mic** \-mik\ *adj*
lip•id \ˈli-pəd\ *also* **lip•ide** \-ˌpīd\ *n* : any of various substances that are soluble in nonpolar organic solvents, that with proteins and carbohydrates constitute the principal structural components of living cells, and that include fats, waxes, phospholipids, cerebrosides, and related and derived compounds — **li•pid•ic** \li-ˈpi-dik\ *adj*
lip•i•do•sis \ˌli-pə-ˈdō-səs\ *n, pl* **-do•ses** \-ˌsēz\ : a disorder of fat metabolism esp. involving the deposition of fat in an organ (as the liver or spleen) — called also *lipoidosis*
Lip•i•tor \ˈli-pə-ˌtȯr\ *trademark* — used for a preparation of the calcium salt of atorvastatin
li•po•at•ro•phy \ˌli-pō-ˈa-trə-fē\ *n, pl* **-phies** : loss of subcutaneous fat (as that occurring from subcutaneous injections esp. of insulin or corticosteroids or from long-term use of protease inhibitors in the treatment of HIV) — **li•po•atro•phic** \-(ˌ)ā-ˈtrō-fik\ *adj*
li•po•chon•dro•dys•tro•phy \-ˌkän-drə-ˈdis-trə-fē\ *n, pl* **-phies** : MUCOPOLYSACCHARIDOSIS; *esp* : HURLER SYNDROME
li•po•chrome \ˈli-pə-ˌkrōm, ˈlī-\ *n* : any of the naturally occurring pigments soluble in fats or in solvents for fats; *esp* : CAROTENOID
li•po•dys•tro•phy \ˌli-pō-ˈdis-trə-fē, ˌlī-\ *n, pl* **-phies** : a disorder of fat metabolism esp. involving loss of fat from or deposition of fat in tissue
lipodystrophy syndrome *n* : a group of side effects of antiretroviral therapy for HIV infection that include high triglyceride levels in the blood, diabetes, and redistribution of fat in the body
Li•po•fen \ˈlī-pə-ˌfen\ *trademark* — used for a preparation of fenofibrate
li•po•fi•bro•ma \ˌli-pō-fī-ˈbrō-mə, ˌlī-\ *n, pl* **-mas** *also* **-ma•ta** \-mə-tə\ : a lipoma containing fibrous tissue
li•po•fus•cin \ˌli-pə-ˈfəs-ᵊn, ˌlī-, -ˈfyü-sᵊn\ *n* : a usu. yellowish-brown insoluble granule that contains protein and lipid and accumulates in cells (as of the heart or brain) as part of the normal aging process or sometimes in association with diseased states
li•po•fus•cin•o•sis \-ˌfə-sə-ˈnō-səs, -ˌfyü-\ *n, pl* **-o•ses** \-ˌsēz\ : a storage disease (as Batten disease) marked by abnormal accumulation of lipofuscin in tissues esp. of the brain
li•po•gen•e•sis \-ˈje-nə-səs\ *n, pl* **-e•ses** \-ˌsēz\ : the formation of fat; *specif* : the formation of fatty acids from acetyl coenzyme A esp. in adipose tissue and the liver
li•po•ic acid \li-ˈpō-ik-, lī-\ *n* : any of several microbial growth factors; *esp* : a crystalline compound $C_8H_{14}O_2S_2$ that is essential for the oxidation of alpha-keto acids (as pyruvic acid) in metabolism
[1]**li•poid** \ˈli-ˌpȯid, ˈlī-\ *or* **li•poi•dal** \li-ˈpȯid-ᵊl\ *adj* : resembling fat
[2]**lipoid** *n* : LIPID
lipoidica — see NECROBIOSIS LIPOIDICA, NECROBIOSIS LIPOIDICA DIABETICORUM
li•poid•o•sis \ˌli-ˌpȯi-ˈdō-səs, ˌlī-\ *n, pl* **-o•ses** \-ˌsēz\ : LIPIDOSIS
li•pol•y•sis \li-ˈpä-lə-səs, lī-\ *n, pl* **-y•ses** \-ˌsēz\ : the hydrolysis of fat — **li•po•lyt•ic** \ˌli-pə-ˈli-tik, ˌlī-\ *adj*
li•po•ma \li-ˈpō-mə, lī-\ *n, pl* **-mas** *also* **-ma•ta** \-mə-tə\ : a tumor of fatty tissue — **li•po•ma•tous** \-mə-təs\ *adj*
li•po•ma•to•sis \li-ˌpō-mə-ˈtō-səs, lī-\ *n, pl* **-to•ses** \-ˌsēz\ : any of several abnormal conditions marked by local or generalized deposits of fat or replacement of other tissue by fat; *specif* : the presence of multiple lipomas
li•po•phil•ic \ˌli-pə-ˈfi-lik, ˌlī-\ *adj* : having an affinity for lipids (as fats) ⟨a ~ metabolite⟩ — compare HYDROPHILIC — **li•po•phi•lic•i•ty** \-fi-ˈli-sə-tē\ *n*
li•po•poly•sac•cha•ride \ˌli-pō-ˌpä-li-ˈsa-kə-ˌrīd, ˌlī-\ *n* : a large molecule consisting of lipids and sugars joined by chemical bonds
li•po•pro•tein \-ˈprō-ˌtēn\ *n* : any of a large class of conjugated proteins

composed of a complex of protein and lipid — see HDL, LDL, VLDL

li·po·sar·co·ma \-sär-ˈkō-mə\ *n, pl* **-mas** *also* **-ma·ta** \-mə-tə\ : a sarcoma arising from immature fat cells of the bone marrow

li·po·some \ˈli-pə-ˌsōm, ˈlī-\ *n* **1** : one of the fatty droplets in the cytoplasm of a cell **2** : an artificial vesicle that is composed of one or more concentric phospholipid bilayers and is used esp. to deliver microscopic substances (as DNA or drugs) to body cells — **li·po·so·mal** \ˌli-pə-ˈsō-məl, ˌlī-\ *adj*

li·po·suc·tion \-ˌsək-shən\ *n* : surgical removal of local fat deposits (as in the thighs) esp. for cosmetic purposes by applying suction through a small tube inserted into the body — **liposuction** *vb*

li·po·tro·pin \ˌli-pə-ˈtrō-pən, ˌlī-\ *n* : either of two protein hormones of the anterior part of the pituitary gland that function in the mobilization of fat reserves; *esp* : BETA-LIPOTROPIN

li·pox·y·gen·ase \li-ˈpäk-sə-jə-ˌnās, lī-, -ˌnāz\ *n* : a crystallizable enzyme that catalyzes the oxidation primarily of unsaturated fatty acids or unsaturated fats by oxygen

Lippes loop \ˈli-pēz-\ *n* : an S-shaped plastic intrauterine device

Lippes, Jack (*b* 1924), American obstetrician and gynecologist.

lip–read \ˈlip-ˌrēd\ *vb* **-read** \-ˌred\; **-read·ing** \-ˌrē-diŋ\ : to understand by lipreading; *also* : to use lipreading — **lip–read·er** \-ˌrē-dər\ *n*

lip·read·ing \-ˌrē-diŋ\ *n* : the interpreting of spoken words by watching the speaker's lip and facial movements without hearing the voice

Li·quae·min \ˈli-kwə-ˌmin\ *n* : a preparation of heparin — formerly a U.S. registered trademark

liq·ue·fac·tion \ˌli-kwə-ˈfak-shən\ *n* **1** : the process of making or becoming liquid **2** : the state of being liquid

[1]liq·uid \ˈlik-wəd\ *adj* **1** : flowing freely like water **2** : having the properties of a liquid

[2]liquid *n* : a fluid (as water) that has no independent shape but has a definite volume, does not expand indefinitely, and is only slightly compressible

liq·uid·am·bar \ˌli-kwə-ˈdam-bər\ *n* **1** *cap* : a genus of trees of the witch hazel family (Hamamelidaceae) **2** : STORAX 2

liquid protein diet *n* : a reducing diet consisting of high-protein liquids

Li·qui·prin \ˈli-kwə-ˌprin\ *n* : a preparation of acetaminophen — formerly a U.S. registered trademark

li·quor \ˈli-kər\ *n* : a liquid substance (as a medicinal solution usu. in water) — compare TINCTURE

li·quor am·nii \ˈlī-ˌkwȯr-ˈam-nē-ˌī, ˈli-\ *n* : AMNIOTIC FLUID

liquor fol·li·cu·li \-fä-ˈli-kyə-ˌlī\ *n* : the fluid surrounding the ovum in the ovarian follicle

li·quo·rice *chiefly Brit var of* LICORICE

li·rag·lu·tide \ˌli-ˈrag-lü-ˌtīd\ *n* : an antidiabetic drug $C_{172}H_{265}N_{43}O_{51}$ that is administered by injection to treat type 2 diabetes and obesity — see VICTOZA

lis·dex·am·fet·a·mine di·mes·y·late \ˌlis-ˌdeks-ˌam-ˈfet-ə-ˌmēn-dī-ˈmes-i-ˌlāt\ *n* : a prodrug $C_{15}H_{25}N_3O{\cdot}(CH_4O_3S)_2$ of dextroamphetamine taken orally in the treatment of attention deficit disorder and binge eating disorder — called also *lisdexamfetamine;* see VYVANSE

li·sin·o·pril \li-ˈsi-nə-ˌpril, lī-\ *n* : an antihypertensive drug $C_{21}H_{31}N_3O_5{\cdot}2H_2O$ that is an ACE inhibitor — see PRINIVIL, ZESTRIL

lisp \ˈlisp\ *vb* **1** : to pronounce the sibilants \s\ and \z\ imperfectly esp. by giving them the sounds \th\ and \t͟h\ **2** : to speak with a lisp — **lisp** *n* — **lisp·er** \ˈlis-pər\ *n*

liss- *or* **lisso-** *comb form* : smooth ⟨*lis*sencephaly⟩

lis·sen·ceph·a·ly \ˌli-sen-ˈse-fə-lē\ *n, pl* **-lies** : an abnormality of brain development marked by the presence of a smooth cerebral cortex with few or no convolutions — see AGYRIA, PACHYGYRIA — **lis·sen·ce·phal·ic** \-sə-ˈfa-lik\ *adj*

lis·te·ria \li-ˈstir-ē-ə\ *n* **1** *cap* : a genus of small gram-positive flagellated rod-shaped bacteria including one (*L. monocytogenes*) causing listeriosis **2** : any bacterium of the genus *Listeria* — **lis·te·ri·al** \li-ˈstir-ē-əl\ *adj* — **lis·te·ric** \-ik\ *adj*

Lis·ter \ˈlis-tər\, **Joseph (1827–1912)**, British surgeon and medical scientist.

lis·te·ri·o·sis \(ˌ)li-ˌstir-ē-ˈō-səs\ *n, pl* **-ri·o·ses** \-ˌsēz\ : a serious disease that is caused by a bacterium of the genus *Listeria* (*L. monocytogenes*), that in animals causes severe encephalitis and is often fatal, that is contracted by humans esp. from contaminated food (as processed meats or unpasteurized milk), that in otherwise healthy people typically takes the form of a mild flu-like illness or has no noticeable symptoms, that in neonates, the elderly, and the immunocompromised often causes serious sometimes fatal illness with symptoms including meningitis and sepsis, and that in pregnant women usu. causes only mild illness in the mother but often results in miscarriage, stillbirth, or premature birth

li·ter \ˈlē-tər\ *n* : a metric unit of capacity equal to the volume of one kilogram of water at 4°C (39°F) and at standard atmospheric pressure of 760 millimeters of mercury

lith- *or* **litho-** *comb form* : calculus ⟨*lith*iasis⟩ ⟨*litho*tripsy⟩

-lith \ˌlith\ *n comb form* : calculus ⟨uro*lith*⟩

li·thi·a·sis \li-ˈthī-ə-səs\ *n, pl* **-a·ses** \-ˌsēz\ : the formation of stony concretions in the body (as in the urinary tract or gallbladder) — often used in combination ⟨chole*lithiasis*⟩

lith•i•um \ˈli-thē-əm\ *n* **1** : a soft silver-white element that is the lightest metal known — symbol *Li;* see ELEMENT table **2** : a lithium salt and esp. lithium carbonate used in psychiatric medicine

lithium carbonate *n* : a crystalline salt Li_2CO_3 used in medicine in the treatment of mania and hypomania in bipolar disorder

lith•o•gen•ic \ˌli-thə-ˈje-nik\ *adj* : of, promoting, or undergoing the formation of calculi ⟨a ~ diet⟩ — **lith•o•gen•e•sis** \-ˈje-nə-səs\ *n*

lith•ol•a•paxy \li-ˈthä-lə-ˌpak-sē, ˈli-thə-lə-\ *n, pl* **-pax•ies** : LITHOTRIPSY

lith•o•pe•di•on \ˌli-thə-ˈpē-dē-ˌän\ *n* : a fetus calcified in the body of the mother

li•thot•o•my \li-ˈthä-tə-mē\ *n, pl* **-mies** : surgical incision of the urinary bladder for removal of a calculus

lithotomy position *n* : a position of the body for medical examination, pelvic or abdominal surgery, or childbirth in which the individual lies on the back with the hips and knees flexed and the legs spread and raised above the hips

lith•o•trip•sy \ˈli-thə-ˌtrip-sē\ *n, pl* **-sies** : the breaking of a calculus (as by shock waves or crushing with a surgical instrument) in the urinary system into pieces small enough to be voided or washed out — called also *litholapaxy*

lith•o•trip•ter *also* **lith•o•trip•tor** \ˈli-thə-ˌtrip-tər\ *n* : a device for performing lithotripsy; *esp* : a noninvasive device that pulverizes calculi by focusing shock waves on a patient immersed in a water bath

lit•mus \ˈlit-məs\ *n* : a coloring matter from lichens that turns red in acid solutions and blue in alkaline solutions and is used as an acid-base indicator

litmus paper *n* : paper colored with litmus and used as an acid-base indicator

li•tre \ˈlē-tər\ *chiefly Brit var of* LITER

[1]lit•ter \ˈli-tər\ *n* **1** : a device (as a stretcher) for carrying a sick or injured person **2** : the offspring at one birth of a multiparous animal

[2]litter *vb* : to give birth to young

little finger *n* : the fourth and smallest finger of the hand counting the index finger as the first

Little League elbow *n* : inflammation of the medial epicondyle and adjacent tissues of the elbow esp. in preteen and teenage baseball players who make too strenuous use of the muscles of the forearm — called also *Little Leaguer's elbow*

Lit•tle's disease \ˈli-tᵊlz-\ *n* : a form of spastic cerebral palsy marked by spastic diplegia in which the legs are typically more severely affected than the arms; *broadly* : CEREBRAL PALSY

Little, William John (1810–1894), British physician.

little stroke *n* : TRANSIENT ISCHEMIC ATTACK

little toe *n* : the outermost and smallest digit of the foot

Li•valo \li-ˈva-lō\ *trademark* — used for a preparation of pitavastatin

live birth \ˈlīv-\ *n* : birth in such a state that processes of life are manifested after the emergence of the whole body : birth of a live fetus — compare STILLBIRTH

live–born \ˈlīv-ˈbȯrn\ *adj* : born alive — compare STILLBORN

li•ve•do re•tic•u•lar•is \li-ˈvē-dō-ri-ˌti-kyə-ˈlar-əs\ *n* : a condition of the peripheral blood vessels characterized by reddish-blue mottling of the skin esp. of the extremities usu. upon exposure to cold

liv•er \ˈli-vər\ *n* : a large very vascular glandular organ of vertebrates that secretes bile and causes important changes in many of the substances contained in the blood which passes through it (as by converting sugars into glycogen which it stores up until required and by forming urea) that in humans is the largest gland in the body, weighs from 40 to 60 ounces (1100 to 1700 grams), is a dark red color, and occupies the upper right portion of the abdominal cavity immediately below the diaphragm

liver cell *n* : HEPATOCYTE

liver fluke *n* : any of various trematode worms that invade the mammalian liver; *esp* : one of the genus *Fasciola* (*F. hepatica*) that is a major parasite of the liver, bile ducts, and gallbladder of cattle and sheep, causes fascioliasis in humans, and uses snails of the genus *Lymnaea* as an intermediate host — see CHINESE LIVER FLUKE

liv•er•mo•ri•um \ˌli-vər-ˈmȯr-ē-əm\ *n* : a short-lived radioactive element that is artificially produced — symbol *Lv;* see ELEMENT table

liver rot *n* : a disease caused by liver flukes esp. in sheep and cattle and marked by great local damage to the liver — see DISTOMATOSIS

liver spots *n pl* : AGE SPOTS

lives *pl of* LIFE

liv•id \ˈli-vəd\ *adj* : discolored by bruising : BLACK-AND-BLUE — **li•vid•i•ty** \li-ˈvi-də-tē\ *n*

living will *n* : a document in which the signer requests to be allowed to die rather than be kept alive by artificial means in the event of becoming disabled beyond a reasonable expectation of recovery

livor mor•tis \ˈlī-ˌvȯr-ˈmȯr-təs\ *n* : hypostasis of the blood following death that causes a purplish-red discoloration of the skin — called also *dependent lividity, postmortem lividity*

LLQ *abbr* left lower quadrant (abdomen)

LMP *abbr* last menstrual period

Loa \ˈlō-ə\ *n* : a genus of African filarial worms (family Dipetalonematidae) that infect the subcutaneous tissues and blood, include the eye worm (*L. loa*) causing Calabar swellings, and are transmitted by the bite of flies of the genus *Chrysops*

load \ˈlōd\ *n* **1** : the amount of a deleterious microorganism, parasite, growth, or substance present in a human or animal body ⟨measure viral ~ in the blood⟩ — called also *burden* **2** : GENETIC LOAD

load·ing \ˈlō-diŋ\ *n* **1** : administration of a factor or substance to the body or a bodily system in sufficient quantity to test capacity to deal with it **2** : the relative contribution of each component factor in a psychological test or in an experimental, clinical, or social situation

lo·a·i·a·sis \ˌlō-ə-ˈī-ə-səs\ *or* **lo·i·a·sis** \ˌlō-ˈī-\ *n, pl* **-a·ses** \-ˌsēz\ : infestation with or disease caused by an eye worm of the genus *Loa* (*L. loa*) that migrates through the subcutaneous tissue and across the cornea of the eye — compare CALABAR SWELLING

loa loa \ˈlō-ə-ˈlō-ə\ *n* : LOAIASIS

lob- *or* **lobi-** *or* **lobo-** *comb form* : lobe ⟨*lob*ectomy⟩ ⟨*lobo*tomy⟩

lo·bar \ˈlō-bər, -ˌbär\ *adj* : of or relating to a lobe

lobar pneumonia *n* : acute pneumonia involving one or more lobes of the lung characterized by sudden onset, chill, fever, difficulty in breathing, cough, and blood-stained sputum, marked by consolidation, and normally followed by resolution and return to normal of the lung tissue

lobe \ˈlōb\ *n* : a curved or rounded projection or division: as **a** : a more or less rounded projection of a body organ or part ⟨~ of the ear⟩ **b** : a division of a body organ (as the brain or lungs) marked off by a fissure on the surface — **lobed** \ˈlōbd\ *adj*

lo·bec·to·my \lō-ˈbek-tə-mē\ *n, pl* **-mies** : surgical removal of a lobe of an organ (as a lung) or gland (as the thyroid); *specif* : excision of a lobe of the lung

lo·be·line \ˈlō-bə-ˌlēn\ *n* : an alkaloid $C_{22}H_{27}NO_2$ that is obtained from an American herb (*Lobelia inflata* of the family Lobeliaceae) and is used esp. as a smoking deterrent

lobi-, lobo- — see LOB-

lo·bot·o·my \lō-ˈbä-tə-mē\ *n, pl* **-mies** : surgical severance of nerve fibers connecting the frontal lobes to the thalamus that has been performed esp. formerly chiefly to treat mental illness — called also *leukotomy* — **lo·bot·o·mize** \-ˌmīz\ *vb*

lobster claw \ˈläb-stər-ˌklȯ\ *n* : ectrodactyly that is marked by one or more missing or underdeveloped middle digits with cleaving of the hand or foot into two segments and syndactyly of the remaining digits and is inherited esp. as an autosomal dominant trait

lob·u·lar \ˈlä-byə-lər\ *adj* : of, relating to, affecting, or resembling a lobule

lob·u·lat·ed \ˈlä-byə-ˌlā-təd\ *adj* : made up of, provided with, or divided into lobules ⟨a ~ tumor⟩ — **lob·u·la·tion** \ˌlä-byə-ˈlā-shən\ *n*

lob·ule \ˈlä-ˌbyül\ *n* **1** : a small lobe ⟨the ~ of the ear⟩ **2** : a subdivision of a lobe; *specif* : one of the small masses of tissue of which various organs (as the liver) are made up

lob·u·lus \ˈlä-byə-ləs\ *n, pl* **lob·u·li** \-ˌlī\ **1** : LOBE **2** : LOBULE

[1]**lo·cal** \ˈlō-kəl\ *adj* : involving or affecting only a restricted part of the organism ⟨~ inflammation⟩ — compare SYSTEMIC a — **lo·cal·ly** *adv*

[2]**local** *n* : LOCAL ANESTHETIC; *also* : LOCAL ANESTHESIA

local anesthesia *n* : loss of sensation in a limited and usu. superficial area esp. from the effect of a local anesthetic

local anesthetic *n* : an anesthetic for use on a limited and usu. superficial area of the body

lo·cal·ize \ˈlō-kə-ˌlīz\ *vb* **-ized; -iz·ing 1** : to make local; *esp* : to fix in or confine to a definite place or part **2** : to accumulate in or be restricted to a specific or limited area — **lo·cal·i·za·tion** \ˌlō-kə-lə-ˈzā-shən\ *n*

lo·chia \ˈlō-kē-ə, ˈlä-\ *n, pl* **lochia** : a discharge from the uterus and vagina following delivery — **lo·chi·al** \-əl\ *adj*

loci *pl of* LOCUS

loci cerulei, loci coerulei *pl of* LOCUS CERULEUS, LOCUS COERULEUS

locked \ˈläkt\ *adj, of the knee joint* : having a restricted mobility and incapable of complete extension

locked–in syndrome *n* : the condition of an awake and conscious patient who because of motor paralysis throughout the body is unable to communicate except possibly by coded eye movements

lock·jaw \ˈläk-ˌjȯ\ *n* : an early symptom of tetanus marked by spasm of the jaw muscles and inability to open the jaws; *also* : TETANUS 1a

lo·co·mo·tion \ˌlō-kə-ˈmō-shən\ *n* : an act or the power of moving from place to place — **lo·co·mo·tor** \ˌlō-kə-ˈmō-tər\ *adj* — **lo·co·mo·to·ry** \ˌlō-kə-ˈmō-tə-rē\ *adj*

locomotor ataxia *n* : TABES DORSALIS

lo·co·re·gion·al \-ˈrēj-ən-ᵊl\ *adj* : restricted to a localized region of the body ⟨~ anesthesia⟩

lo·co·weed \ˈlō-(ˌ)kō-ˌwēd\ *n* : any of several neurotoxic leguminous plants (genera *Astragalus* and *Oxytropis*) of western No. America that cause poisoning in grazing animals

loc·u·lus \ˈlä-kyə-ləs\ *n, pl* **-li** \-ˌlī, -ˌlē\ : a small chamber or cavity esp. in a plant or animal body — **loc·u·lat·ed** \ˈlä-kyə-ˌlā-təd\ *adj* — **loc·u·la·tion** \ˌlä-kyə-ˈlā-shən\ *n*

lo·cum te·nens \ˌlō-kəm-ˈtē-ˌnenz, -nənz\ *n, pl* **locum te·nen·tes** \-ti-ˈnen-ˌtēz\ : a medical practitioner who temporarily takes the place of another

lo•cus \ˈlō-kəs\ *n, pl* **lo•ci** \ˈlō-ˌsī, -ˌkī, -ˌkē\ **1** : a place or site of an event, activity, or thing **2** : the position in a chromosome of a particular gene or allele

lo•cus coe•ru•le•us *also* **lo•cus ce•ru•le•us** \ˌlō-kəs-si-ˈrü-lē-əs\ *n, pl* **loci coe•ru•lei** *also* **loci ce•ru•lei** \-lē-ˌī\ : a blue area of the brain stem with many norepinephrine-containing neurons

Lo•do•syn \ˈlō-dō-ˌsin\ *trademark* — used for a preparation containing carbidopa

Loef•fler's syndrome \ˈle-flərz-\ *n* : a mild pneumonitis marked by eosinophilia and transitory pulmonary infiltrates and usu. occurring as an allergic reaction to drugs or parasitic infection — called also *Loeffler's pneumonia*

Löf•fler \ˈlœ-fler\, **Wilhelm (1887–1972)**, Swiss physician.

Lo•es•trin \lō-ˈes-trən\ *trademark* — used for a preparation of ethinyl estradiol and the acetate of norethindrone

Lo•fi•bra \lō-ˈfī-brə\ *trademark* — used for a preparation of fenofibrate

log- *or* **logo-** *comb form* : word : thought : speech ⟨*logo*rrhea⟩

log•o•pe•dics \ˌlȯ-gə-ˈpē-diks, ˌlä-\ *n sing or pl* : the scientific study and treatment of speech defects

log•or•rhea \ˌlȯ-gə-ˈrē-ə, ˌlä-\ *n* : pathologically excessive and often incoherent talkativeness or wordiness

log•or•rhoea *chiefly Brit var of* LOGORRHEA

log•o•ther•a•py \ˌlȯ-gə-ˈther-ə-pē, ˌlä-\ *n, pl* **-pies** : a highly directive existential psychotherapy that emphasizes the importance of meaning in the patient's life esp. as gained through spiritual values

-l•o•gy \l-ə-jē\ *n comb form, pl* **-logies** : doctrine : theory : science ⟨physio*logy*⟩

loiasis *var of* LOAIASIS

loin \ˈlȯin\ *n* **1** : the part of the body on each side of the spinal column between the hip bone and the false ribs **2** *pl* **a** : the upper and lower abdominal regions and the region about the hips **b** (1) : the pubic region (2) : the generative organs — not usu. used technically in senses 2a, b

Lo•mo•til \ˈlō-mə-ˌtil, lō-ˈmōt-ᵊl\ *trademark* — used for a preparation of the hydrochloride of diphenoxylate and the sulfate of atropine

lo•mus•tine \lō-ˈməs-ˌtēn\ *n* : an antineoplastic drug $C_9H_{16}ClN_3O_2$ used esp. in the treatment of brain tumors and Hodgkin's lymphoma

lone star tick *n* : an ixodid tick of the genus *Amblyomma* (*A. americanum*) of the southern, central, and eastern U.S. that is a vector of several diseases (as Rocky Mountain spotted fever, ehrlichiosis, and anaplasmosis) and in which the adult female has a single white spot on the back

long–acting thyroid stimulator *n* : an IgG antibody that often occurs in the plasma of patients with Graves' disease — abbr. *LATS*

long bone *n* : any of the elongated bones supporting a limb and consisting of an essentially cylindrical shaft that contains marrow and ends in enlarged heads for articulation with other bones

long ciliary nerve *n* : any of two or three nerves that are given off by the nasociliary nerve and are distributed to the iris and cornea — compare SHORT CILIARY NERVE

long head *n* : the longest of the three heads of the triceps muscle that arises from the infraglenoid tubercle of the scapula

longi *pl of* LONGUS

lon•gis•si•mus \län-ˈji-si-məs\ *n, pl* **lon•gis•si•mi** \-ˌmī\ : the intermediate division of the sacrospinalis muscle that consists of the longissimus capitis, longissimus cervicis, and longissimus thoracis; *also* : any of these three muscles

longissimus cap•i•tis \-ˈka-pi-təs\ *n* : a muscle that arises by tendons from the upper thoracic and lower cervical vertebrae, is inserted into the posterior margin of the mastoid process, and extends the head and bends and rotates it to one side — called also *trachelomastoid muscle*

longissimus cer•vi•cis \-ˈsər-vi-səs\ *n* : a muscle medial to the longissimus thoracis that arises by long thin tendons from the transverse processes of the upper four or five thoracic vertebrae, is inserted by similar tendons into the transverse processes of the second to sixth cervical vertebrae, and extends the spinal column and bends it to one side

longissimus dor•si \-ˈdȯr-sī\ *n* : LONGISSIMUS THORACIS

longissimus thor•a•cis \-ˈthȯr-ə-səs, -thȯ-ˈrā-səs\ *n* : a muscle that arises as the middle and largest division of the sacrospinalis muscle, that is attached by some of its fibers to the lumbar vertebrae, that is inserted into all the thoracic vertebrae and the lower 9 or 10 ribs, and that depresses the ribs and with the longissimus cervicis extends the spinal column and bends it to one side

lon•gi•tu•di•nal \ˌlän-jə-ˈtüd-ᵊn-əl, -ˈtyüd-\ *adj* **1** : of, relating to, or occurring in the lengthwise dimension ⟨a ~ fracture⟩ **2** : extending along or relating to the anteroposterior axis of a body or part **3** : involving the repeated observation or examination of a set of subjects over time with respect to one or more study variables — **lon•gi•tu•di•nal•ly** *adv*

longitudinal fissure *n* : the deep groove that divides the cerebrum into right and left hemispheres

lon•gi•tu•di•na•lis linguae \ˌlän-jə-ˌtü-də-ˈnā-ləs-, -ˌtyü-\ *n* : either of two bands of muscle comprising the intrinsic musculature of the tongue — called also *longitudinalis*

long posterior ciliary artery *n* : either of usu. two arteries of which one arises from the ophthalmic artery on each side of the optic nerve, passes forward along the optic nerve, enters the sclera, and at the junction of the ciliary process and the iris divides into upper and lower branches which form a ring of arteries around the iris — compare SHORT POSTERIOR CILIARY ARTERY

long QT syndrome *n* : any of several inherited cardiac arrhythmias that are characterized by abnormal duration and shape of the QT interval and that place the subject at risk for torsades de pointes — abbr. *LQTS*

long saphenous vein *n* : SAPHENOUS VEIN a

long•sight•ed \ˈlȯŋ-ˈsī-təd\ *adj* : FARSIGHTED — **long•sight•ed•ness** *n*

long terminal repeat *n* : an identical sequence of several hundred base pairs at each end of the DNA synthesized by the reverse transcriptase of a retrovirus that controls integration of the viral DNA into the host DNA and expression of the genes of the virus — called also *LTR*

long–term memory *n* : memory that involves the storage and recall of information over a long period of time (as days, weeks, or years) — abbr. *LTM*

long–term nonprogressor *n* : an HIV-infected individual who remains symptom-free over the long term and does not progress to develop AIDS — called also *nonprogressor*

long–term potentiation *n* : a long-lasting strengthening of the response of a postsynaptic neuron to stimulation across the synapse that occurs with repeated stimulation and is thought to be related to learning and long-term memory — abbr. *LTP*

lon•gus \ˈlȯŋ-gəs\ *n, pl* **lon•gi** \-ˌgī\ : a long structure (as a muscle) in the body — see ABDUCTOR POLLICIS LONGUS, ADDUCTOR LONGUS, EXTENSOR CARPI RADIALIS LONGUS, EXTENSOR DIGITORUM LONGUS, EXTENSOR HALLUCIS LONGUS, EXTENSOR POLLICIS LONGUS, FLEXOR DIGITORUM LONGUS, FLEXOR HALLUCIS LONGUS, FLEXOR POLLICIS LONGUS, PALMARIS LONGUS, PERONEUS LONGUS

longus cap•i•tis \-ˈka-pi-təs\ *n* : a muscle of either side of the front and upper portion of the neck that arises from the third to sixth cervical vertebrae, is inserted into the basilar portion of the occipital bone, and bends the neck forward

Lon•i•ten \ˈlä-ni-tən\ *trademark* — used for a preparation of minoxidil

loop — see LIPPES LOOP

loop diuretic *n* : a diuretic that inhibits reabsorption in the ascending limb of the loop of Henle causing greatly increased excretion of sodium chloride in the urine

loop of Hen•le \-ˈhen-lē\ *n* : the U-shaped part of a nephron that lies between and is continuous with the proximal and distal convoluted tubules, that leaves the cortex of the kidney descending into the medullary tissue and then bending back and reentering the cortex, and that functions in water resorption — called also *Henle's loop*

F. G. J. Henle — see HENLE'S LAYER

loose \ˈlüs\ *adj* **loos•er; loos•est** **1 a** (1) : having worked partly free from attachments ⟨a ∼ tooth⟩ (2) : having relative freedom of movement **b** : produced freely and accompanied by raising of mucus ⟨a ∼ cough⟩ **2 a** : not dense, close, or compact in structure or arrangement ⟨∼ connective tissue⟩ **b** : not solid : WATERY ⟨∼ stools⟩ **3** : OVERACTIVE; *specif* : marked by frequent voiding esp. of watery stools ⟨∼ bowels⟩ **4** : not tightly drawn or stretched ⟨∼ skin⟩ — **loose•ly** *adv* — **loose•ness** *n*

loose–joint•ed \ˈlüs-ˈjȯin-təd\ *adj* **1** : having or marked by one or more joints with an increased range of motion **2** : moving or able to move and bend in a free and relaxed way : very flexible — **loose–joint•ed•ness** *n*

lo•per•a•mide \lō-ˈper-ə-ˌmīd\ *n* : a synthetic antidiarrheal agent that slows intestinal peristalsis and is taken orally in the form of its hydrochloride $C_{29}H_{33}ClN_2O_2 \cdot HCl$ — called also *loperamide hydrochloride;* see IMODIUM

Lo•pid \ˈlō-pid\ *trademark* — used for a preparation of gemfibrozil

Lo•pres•sor \lō-ˈpre-sər, -ˌsȯr\ *trademark* — used for a preparation of the tartrate of metoprolol

Lo•prox \ˈlō-ˌpräks\ *trademark* — used for a preparation of ciclopirox or ciclopirox olamine

lo•rat•a•dine \lə-ˈra-tə-ˌdēn\ *n* : a long-acting nonsedating antihistamine drug $C_{22}H_{23}ClN_2O_2$ that is an H_1 antagonist taken orally esp. to relieve the symptoms of seasonal allergic rhinitis and chronic hives— see CLARITIN

lor•az•e•pam \lȯr-ˈa-zə-ˌpam\ *n* : a benzodiazepine tranquilizer $C_{15}H_{10}Cl_2N_2O_2$ used esp. to relieve anxiety and insomnia, to control status epilepticus, and as a premedication before surgery— see ATIVAN

lor•cas•e•rin \lȯr-ˈka-sə-rən\ *n* : a serotonin agonist $C_{11}H_{15}Cl_2NO \cdot 5H_2O$ that is taken orally to promote satiety and reduce food consumption in the treatment of overweight and obese individuals — called also *lorcaserin hydrochloride;* see BELVIQ

lor•do•sis \lȯr-ˈdō-səs\ *n* **1** : the normal convex curvature of the cervical and lumbar regions of the spine **2** : abnormally exaggerated forward curvature of the lumbar and cervical regions of the spine resulting in a concave back when viewed from the side — called also *swayback;* compare KYPHOSIS, SCOLIOSIS — **lor•dot•ic** \-ˈdä-tik\ *adj*

lo•sar•tan \lō-ˈsär-ˌtan\ *n* : an antihypertensive drug that is taken orally in the form of its potassium salt $C_{22}H_{22}ClKN_6O$ and blocks the action of angiotensin II — see COZAAR, HYZAAR

Lo•te•max \ˈlōt-ə-ˌmaks\ *trademark* — used for a preparation of loteprednol

Lo•ten•sin \lō-ˈten-sən\ *trademark* — used for a preparation of the hydrochloride of benazepril

lo•te•pred•nol \ˌlōt-ə-ˈpred-ˌnȯl\ *n* : a synthetic corticosteroid $C_{24}H_{31}ClO_7$ applied topically to the eye to treat inflammatory conditions (as allergic conjunctivitis and keratitis) — see ALREX, LOTEMAX, ZYLET

lo•tion \ˈlō-shən\ *n* **1** : a liquid usu. aqueous medicinal preparation containing one or more insoluble substances and applied externally for skin disorders **2** : a liquid cosmetic preparation usu. containing a cleansing, softening, or astringent agent and applied to the skin

Lo•trel \ˈlō-ˌtrel\ *trademark* — used for a preparation of amlodipine and benazepril

Lo•tri•min \ˈlō-trə-min\ *trademark* — used for a preparation of clotrimazole

Lou Geh•rig's disease \ˈlü-ˈger-igz-\ *n* : AMYOTROPHIC LATERAL SCLEROSIS

Gehrig, Lou (1903–1941), American baseball player.

loupe \ˈlüp\ *n* : a magnifying lens worn esp. by surgeons performing microsurgery; *also* : two such lenses mounted on a single frame

loup•ing ill \ˈlau̇-piŋ-, ˈlō-\ *n* : a tick-borne virus disease that occurs esp. in domestic animals (as sheep) and sporadically in humans, primarily affects the central nervous system, and is caused by a flavivirus (species *Louping ill virus* of the genus *Flavivirus*)

louse \ˈlau̇s\ *n, pl* **lice** \ˈlīs\ : any of the small wingless usu. flattened insects that are parasitic on warm-blooded animals and constitute two orders (Anoplura and Mallophaga)

louse–borne typhus *n* : TYPHUS a

lousy \ˈlau̇-zē\ *adj* **lous•i•er; -est** : infested with lice — **lous•i•ness** \ˈlau̇-zē-nəs\ *n*

lov•a•stat•in \ˈlō-və-ˌsta-tən, ˈlə-\ *n* : a statin $C_{24}H_{36}O_8$ that decreases the level of cholesterol in the bloodstream by inhibiting the liver enzyme that controls cholesterol synthesis and is used in the treatment of hypercholesterolemia — see MEVACOR

Lo•va•za \lō-ˈvā-zə\ *trademark* — used for a preparation of ethyl esters of omega-3 fatty acids

love handles *n pl* : fatty bulges along the sides at the waist

Lo•ve•nox \ˈlō-və-ˌnäks\ *trademark* — used for a preparation of enoxaparin

love object *n* : a person on whom affection is centered or on whom one is dependent for affection or needed help

low \ˈlō\ *adj* **low•er** \ˈlō-ər\; **low•est** \ˈlō-əst\ : having a relatively less complex organization : not greatly differentiated or developed phylogenetically ⟨the ~*er* vertebrates⟩ — compare HIGH 1

low–back \ˈlō-ˈbak\ *adj* : of, relating to, suffering, or being pain in the lowest portion of the back ⟨~ pain⟩

low blood pressure *n* : HYPOTENSION 1

low–density lipoprotein *n* : LDL

low•er \ˈlō-ər\ *n* : the lower member of a pair; *esp* : a lower denture

lower jaw *n* : JAW 1b

lower respiratory *adj* : of, relating to, or affecting the lower respiratory tract ⟨*lower respiratory* infections⟩

lower respiratory tract *n* : the part of the respiratory system including the larynx, trachea, bronchi, and lungs — compare UPPER RESPIRATORY TRACT

lowest splanchnic nerve *n* : SPLANCHNIC NERVE c

Lowe syndrome *also* **Lowe's syndrome** \ˈlō(z)-\ *n* : OCULOCEREBRORENAL SYNDROME

Lowe, Charles Upton (1921–2012), American pediatrician.

low forceps *n* : a procedure for delivery of an infant by the use of forceps when the head is visible at the outlet of the birth canal — called also *outlet forceps;* compare HIGH FORCEPS, MIDFORCEPS

low–grade \ˈlō-ˈgrād\ *adj* : being near that extreme of a specified range which is lowest, least intense, or least competent ⟨a ~ fever⟩ ⟨a ~ infection⟩ — compare HIGH-GRADE

Lown–Gan•ong–Le•vine syndrome \ˈlau̇n-ˈgan-ˌȯŋ-lə-ˈvīn-, -ˈvēn-\ *n* : a preexcitation syndrome characterized by atrial tachycardia together with a short P-R interval and a QRS complex of normal duration — called also *LGL syndrome*

Lown \ˈlau̇n\, **Bernard (*b* 1921),** American cardiologist.

Gan•ong \ˈgan-ˌȯŋ\, **William Francis (1924–2007),** American physiologist.

Le•vine \lə-ˈvīn, -ˈvēn\, **Samuel Albert (1891–1966),** American cardiologist.

low–power *adj* : of, relating to, or being a lens that magnifies an image a relatively small number of times and esp. 10 times — compare HIGH-POWER

low–salt diet *n* : LOW-SODIUM DIET

low–sodium diet *n* : a diet restricted to foods naturally low in sodium content and prepared without added salt that is used esp. in the management of hypertension, heart failure, and kidney or liver dysfunction

low vision *n* : impaired vision in which there is a significant reduction in visual function that cannot be corrected by conventional glasses but which may be improved with special aids or devices

Lox•os•ce•les \ˌläk-ˈsä-sə-ˌlēz\ *n* : a genus of spiders (family Loxoscelidae) that includes the brown recluse spider (*L. reclusa*)

lox•os•ce•lism \läk-ˈsä-sə-ˌli-zəm\ *n* : a painful condition resulting from the bite of a spider of the genus *Loxosceles* and esp. the brown recluse spider (*L. reclusa*) that is characterized esp. by local necrosis of tissue

loz•enge \ˈläz-ᵊnj\ *n* : a small usu. sweetened solid piece of medicated material that is designed to be held in the mouth for slow dissolution and often contains a demulcent — called also *pastille, troche*

L–PAM \ˈel-ˌpam\ *n* : MELPHALAN

L–phase \ˈel-ˌfāz\ *n* : L-FORM

LPN \ˌel-(ˌ)pē-ˈen\ *n* : LICENSED PRACTICAL NURSE

LQTS *abbr* long QT syndrome

Lr *symbol* lawrencium

LSD \ˌel-(ˌ)es-ˈdē\ *n* : a semisynthetic illicit organic compound $C_{20}H_{25}N_3O$ derived from ergot that induces extreme sensory distortions, altered perceptions of reality, and intense emotional states, that may also produce delusions or paranoia, and that may sometimes cause panic reactions in response to the effects experienced — called also *acid, lysergic acid diethylamide, lysergide*

LSD–25 *n* : LSD

LTH *abbr* luteotropic hormone

LTM *abbr* long-term memory

LTP *abbr* long-term potentiation

LTR \ˌel-ˌtē-ˈär\ *n* : LONG TERMINAL REPEAT

L–tryp•to•phan \ˈel-ˈtrip-tə-ˌfan\ *n* : the levorotatory form of tryptophan that is a precursor of serotonin and was formerly used in some health food preparations in the belief that it promoted sleep and relieved depression — see EOSINOPHILA-MYALGIA SYNDROME

Lu *symbol* lutetium

lubb–dupp *also* **lub–dup** *or* **lub–dub** \ˌləb-ˈdəp, -ˈdəb\ *n* : the characteristic sounds of a normal heartbeat as heard in auscultation

lu•bi•pros•tone \ˌlü-bə-ˈpräs-ˌtōn\ *n* : a laxative drug $C_{20}H_{32}F_2O_5$ taken orally in the treatment of chronic constipation and irritable bowel syndrome — see AMITIZA

lu•can•thone \lü-ˈkan-ˌthōn\ *n* : an antischistosomal drug administered in the form of its hydrochloride $C_{20}H_{24}N_2OS{\cdot}HCl$ — called also *miracil D*

Lu•cen•tis \lü-ˈsen-təs\ *trademark* — used for a preparation of ranibizumab

lu•cid \ˈlü-səd\ *adj* : having, showing, or characterized by an ability to think clearly and rationally — **lu•cid•i•ty** \lü-ˈsi-də-tē\ *n*

lucid interval *n* : a temporary period of rationality or neurological normality (as between periods of dementia or immediately following a fatal head injury)

lucidum — see STRATUM LUCIDUM

Lu•cil•ia \lü-ˈsi-lē-ə\ *n* : a genus of blowflies whose larvae are sometimes the cause of intestinal myiasis and infest open wounds

lüc•ken•schä•del \ˈlæ-kən-ˌshād-ᵊl\ *n* : a condition characterized by incomplete ossification of the bones of the skull

Lud•wig's angina \ˈlüd-(ˌ)vigz-\ *n* : an acute streptococcal or sometimes staphylococcal infection of the deep tissues of the floor of the mouth and adjoining parts of the neck and lower jaw that is marked by severe rapid swelling which may close the respiratory passage and that is accompanied by chills and fever

Ludwig, Wilhelm Friedrich von (1790–1865), German surgeon.

Lu•er syringe \ˈlü-ər-\ *n* : a glass syringe with a glass piston that has the apposing surfaces ground and that is used esp. for hypodermic injection

Luer (*d* 1883), German instrument maker.

lu•es \ˈlü-(ˌ)ēz\ *n, pl* **lues** : SYPHILIS

lu•et•ic \lü-ˈe-tik\ *adj* : SYPHILITIC

Lu•gol's solution \lü-ˈgólz-\ *n* : any of several deep brown solutions of iodine and potassium iodide in water or alcohol — called also *Lugol's iodine, Lugol's iodine solution*

Lugol, Jean Guillaume Auguste (1786–1851), French physician.

lumb- *or* **lumbo-** *comb form* : lumbar and ⟨*lumbo*sacral⟩

lum•ba•go \ˌləm-ˈbā-(ˌ)gō\ *n* : acute or chronic pain (as that caused by muscle strain) in the lower back

lum•bar \ˈləm-bər, -ˌbär\ *adj* **1** : of, relating to, or constituting the loins or the vertebrae between the thoracic vertebrae and sacrum **2** : of, relating to, or being the abdominal region lying on either side of the umbilical region and above the corresponding iliac region

lumbar artery *n* : any artery of the usu. four pairs that arise from the back of the aorta opposite the lumbar vertebrae and supply the muscles of the loins, the skin of the sides of the abdomen, and the spinal cord

lum•bar•i•za•tion \ˌləm-bə-rə-ˈzā-shən\ *n* : a condition in which the first segment of the sacrum fails to fuse with the second segment so it appears to be part of the lumbar vertebrae

lumbar nerve *n* : any nerve of the five pairs of spinal nerves of the lumbar region of which one on each side passes out below each lumbar vertebra and the upper four unite by connecting branches into a lumbar plexus

lumbar plexus *n* : a plexus embedded in the psoas major and formed by the anterior or ventral divisions of the four upper lumbar nerves of which the first is usu. supplemented by a communication from the twelfth thoracic nerve

lumbar puncture *n* : puncture of the subarachnoid space in the lumbar region of the spinal cord to withdraw cerebrospinal fluid or inject anesthetic drugs — called also *spinal tap*

lumbar vein *n* : any vein of the four pairs collecting blood from the muscles and integument of the loins, the walls of the abdomen, and adjacent parts and emptying into the dorsal part of the inferior vena cava — see ASCENDING LUMBAR VEIN

lumbar vertebra *n* : any of the five vertebrae situated between the thoracic vertebrae above and the sacrum below

lumbo- — see LUMB-

lum•bo•dor•sal fascia \ˌləm-bō-ˈdȯr-səl-\ *n* : a large fascial band on each side of the back extending from the iliac crest and the sacrum to the ribs and the intermuscular septa of the muscles of the neck

lumborum — see ILIOCOSTALIS LUMBORUM, QUADRATUS LUMBORUM

lum•bo•sa•cral \ˌləm-bō-ˈsa-krəl, -ˈsā-\ *adj* : of, relating to, or being the lumbar and sacral regions or parts ⟨the ~ spinal cord⟩

lumbosacral joint *n* : the joint between the fifth lumbar vertebra and the sacrum

lumbosacral plexus *n* : a network of nerves comprising the lumbar plexus and the sacral plexus

lumbosacral trunk *n* : a nerve trunk formed by the fifth lumbar nerve and a smaller branch of the fourth lumbar nerve and connecting the lumbar plexus to the sacral plexus

lum•bri•ca•lis \ˌləm-brə-ˈkā-ləs\ *n, pl* **-les** \-ˌlēz\ **1** : any of the four small muscles of the palm of the hand that arise from tendons of the flexor digitorum profundus, are inserted at the base of the digit to which the tendon passes, and flex the proximal phalanx and extend the two distal phalanges of each finger **2** : any of four small muscles of the foot homologous to the lumbricales of the hand that arise from tendons of the flexor digitorum longus and are inserted into the first phalanges of the four small toes of which they flex the proximal phalanges and extend the two distal phalanges — **lum•bri•cal** \ˈləm-bri-kəl\ *adj*

lu•me•fan•trine \ˌlü-mə-ˈfan-ˌtrēn\ *n* : an antimalarial drug $C_{30}H_{32}Cl_3NO$ taken orally in combination with artemether — see COARTEM

lu•men \ˈlü-mən\ *n, pl* **lu•mi•na** \-mə-nə\ *or* **lumens** **1** : the cavity of a tubular organ or part ⟨the ~ of a blood vessel⟩ **2** : the bore of a tube (as of a hollow needle or catheter) — **lu•mi•nal** *also* **lu•me•nal** \ˈlü-mən-ᵊl\ *adj*

Lu•mi•gan \ˈlü-mə-ˌgan\ *trademark* — used for a preparation of bimatoprost

Lu•mi•nal \ˈlü-mə-ˌnal, -ˌnȯl\ *trademark* — used for a preparation of the sodium salt of phenobarbital

lump \ˈləmp\ *n* **1** : a piece or mass of indefinite size and shape **2** : an abnormal mass or swelling

lump•ec•to•my \ˌləm-ˈpek-tə-mē\ *n, pl* **-mies** : excision of a breast tumor with a limited amount of associated tissue — called also *tylectomy*

lumpy jaw \ˈləm-pē-\ *also* **lump jaw** *n* : ACTINOMYCOSIS; *esp* : actinomycosis of the head in cattle

lu•na•cy \ˈlü-nə-sē\ *n, pl* **-cies** *dated* : a severely disordered state of mind esp. once believed to be related to phases of the moon

lu•nar caustic \ˈlü-nər-, -ˌnär-\ *n* : silver nitrate esp. when fused and molded into sticks or small cones for use as a caustic

lu•nate bone \ˈlü-ˌnāt-\ *n* : a crescent-shaped bone that is the middle bone in the proximal row of the carpus between the scaphoid bone and the triquetral bone and that has a deep concavity on the distal surface articulating with the capitate — called also *lunate, semilunar bone*

lunate sulcus *n* : a sulcus of the cerebrum on the lateral part of the occipital lobe that marks the front boundary of the visual cortex

Lu•nes•ta \lü-ˈnes-tə\ *trademark* — used for a preparation of eszopiclone

lung \ˈləŋ\ *n* **1** : one of the usu. two compound saccular organs that constitute the basic respiratory organ of air-breathing vertebrates, that normally occupy the entire lateral parts of the thorax and consist essentially of an inverted tree of intricately branched bronchioles communicating with thin-walled terminal alveoli swathed in a network of delicate capillaries where the actual gaseous exchange of respiration takes place, and that in humans are somewhat flattened with a broad base resting against the diaphragm and have the right lung divided into three lobes and the left into two lobes **2** : a mechanical device for regularly introducing fresh air into and withdrawing stale air from the lungs : RESPIRATOR — see IRON LUNG — **lunged** *adj*

lung•er \ˈləŋ-ər\ *n* : one affected with a chronic disease of the lungs; *esp* : one who is tubercular

lung fluke *n* : a fluke invading the lungs; *esp* : either of two forms of the genus *Paragonimus* (*P. westermani* and *P. kellicotti*) that produce lesions in humans which are comparable to those of tuberculosis and that are acquired by eating inadequately cooked freshwater crustaceans which act as intermediate hosts

lung•worm \ˈləŋ-ˌwərm\ *n* : any of various nematodes (esp. genera *Dictyocaulus* and *Metastrongylus* of the family Metastrongylidae) that infest the lungs and air passages of mammals

lu•nu•la \ˈlü-nyə-lə\ *n, pl* **-lae** \-(ˌ)lē *also* -ˌlī\ : a crescent-shaped body part: as **a** : the whitish mark at the base of a fingernail — called also *half-moon* **b** : the crescentic unattached border of a semilunar valve

lu•nule \ˈlü-(ˌ)nyül\ *n* : LUNULA

lu•pine *also* **lu•pin** \ˈlü-pən\ *n* : any of a genus (*Lupinus*) of leguminous herbs some of which cause lupinosis

lu•pi•no•sis \ˌlü-pə-ˈnō-səs\ *n, pl* **-no•ses** \-ˌsēz\ : acute liver atrophy of domestic animals (as sheep) due to poisoning by ingestion of various lupines

lu•poid hepatitis \ˈlü-ˌpȯid-\ *n* : chronic active hepatitis associated with lupus erythematosus

Lu•pron \ˈlü-ˌprän\ *trademark* — used for a preparation of the acetate of leuprolide

lu•pus \ˈlü-pəs\ *n* : any of several diseases (as lupus vulgaris or systemic lupus erythematosus) characterized by skin lesions

lupus band test *n* : a test to determine the presence of antibodies and complement deposits at the junction of the dermal and epidermal skin layers of patients with systemic lupus erythematosus

lupus er•y•the•ma•to•sus \-ˌer-ə-ˌthē-mə-ˈtō-səs\ *n* : a disorder characterized by skin inflammation; *esp* : SYSTEMIC LUPUS ERYTHEMATOSUS

lupus erythematosus cell *n* : LE CELL

lupus ne•phri•tis \-ni-ˈfrī-təs\ *n* : glomerulonephritis associated with systemic lupus erythematosus that is typically characterized by proteinuria and hematuria and that often leads to renal failure

lupus vul•gar•is \-ˌvəl-ˈgar-əs\ *n* : a tuberculous disease of the skin marked by formation of soft brownish nodules with ulceration and scarring

LUQ *abbr* left upper quadrant (abdomen)

lu•ras•i•done \lu̇-ˈras-ə-ˌdōn\ *n* : an atypical antipsychotic taken orally in the form of its hydrochloride $C_{28}H_{36}N_4O_2S·HCl$ to treat depression associated with bipolar disorder and to treat schizophrenia — see LATUDA

Lur•ide \ˈlu̇r-ˌīd\ *trademark* — used for a preparation of sodium fluoride

lute- *or* **luteo-** *comb form* : corpus luteum ⟨*lute*al⟩ ⟨*luteo*lysis⟩

lutea — see MACULA LUTEA

lu•te•al \ˈlü-tē-əl\ *adj* : of, relating to, characterized by, or involving the corpus luteum ⟨∼ activity⟩

lutecium *var of* LUTETIUM

lu•tein \ˈlü-tē-ən, ˈlü-ˌtēn\ *n* : an orange xanthophyll $C_{40}H_{56}O_2$ occurring in plants usu. with carotenes and chlorophylls and in animal fat, egg yolk, and the corpus luteum

lu•tein•i•za•tion \ˌlü-tē-ə-nə-ˈzā-shən, ˌlü-ˌtē-\ *n* : the process of forming corpora lutea — **lu•tein•ize** \ˈlü-tē-ə-ˌnīz, ˈlü-ˌtē-ˌnīz\ *vb*

luteinizing hormone *n* : a hormone that is secreted by the adenohypophysis of the pituitary gland and that in the female stimulates ovulation and the development of the corpora lutea and together with follicle-stimulating hormone the secretion of estrogen from developing ovarian follicles and in the male the development of interstitial tissue in the testis and the secretion of testosterone — abbr. *LH;* called also *interstitial-cell stimulating hormone, lutropin*

luteinizing hormone–releasing factor *n* : GONADOTROPIN-RELEASING HORMONE

luteinizing hormone–releasing hormone *n* : GONADOTROPIN-RELEASING HORMONE

lu•te•ol•y•sis \ˌlü-tē-ˈä-lə-səs\ *n, pl* **-y•ses** \-ˌsēz\ : regression of the corpus luteum — **lu•teo•lyt•ic** \ˌlü-tē-ə-ˈli-tik\ *adj*

lu•te•o•ma \ˌlü-tē-ˈō-mə\ *n, pl* **-mas** *also* **-ma•ta** \-mə-tə\ : an ovarian tumor derived from a corpus luteum — **lu•te•o•ma•tous** \-mə-təs\ *adj*

lu•teo•tro•pic \ˌlü-tē-ə-ˈtrō-pik, -ˈträ-\ *or* **lu•teo•tro•phic** \-ˈtrō-fik, -ˈträ-\ *adj* : acting on the corpora lutea

luteotropic hormone *n* : PROLACTIN

lu•teo•tro•pin \ˌlü-tē-ə-ˈtrō-pən\ *or* **lu•teo•tro•phin** \-fən\ *n* : PROLACTIN

lu•te•tium *also* **lu•te•cium** \lü-ˈtē-shē-əm, -shəm\ *n* : a metallic element — symbol *Lu;* see ELEMENT table

luteum — see CORPUS LUTEUM

lu•tro•pin \lü-ˈtrō-pən\ *n* : LUTEINIZING HORMONE

Lu•vox \ˈlü-ˌväks\ *trademark* — used for a preparation of the maleate of fluvoxamine

lux•a•tion \ˌlək-ˈsā-shən\ *n* : dislocation of an anatomical part — **lux•ate** \ˈlək-ˌsāt\ *vb*

Lv *symbol* livermorium

LV *abbr* left ventricle

LVN \ˌel-(ˌ)vē-ˈen\ *n* : LICENSED VOCATIONAL NURSE

ly•can•thro•py \lī-ˈkan-thrə-pē\ *n, pl* **-pies** : a delusion that one has become or has assumed the characteristics of a wolf

ly•co•pene \ˈlī-kə-ˌpēn\ *n* : a red pigment $C_{40}H_{56}$ isomeric with carotene

Ly•ell's syndrome \ˈlī-əlz-\ *n* : TOXIC EPIDERMAL NECROLYSIS

Lyell, Alan (1917–2007), British dermatologist.

ly•ing–in \ˌlī-iŋ-ˈin\ *n, pl* **lyings–in** *or* **lying–ins** : the state attending and consequent to childbirth : CONFINEMENT

Lyme arthritis \ˈlīm-\ *n* : arthritis as a symptom of or caused by Lyme disease; *also* : LYME DISEASE

Lyme disease *n* : an acute inflammatory disease that is usu. characterized initially by the skin lesion erythema migrans and by fatigue, fever, and chills and if left untreated may later manifest itself in cardiac and neurological disorders, joint pain, and arthritis and that is caused by a spirochete of the genus *Borrelia* (*B. burgdorferi*) transmitted by the bite of a tick esp. of the genus *Ixodes* (*I. scapularis* syn. *I. dammini* in the eastern and midwestern U.S., *I. pacificus* esp. in some parts of the Pacific coastal states of the U.S., and *I. ricinus* in Europe) — called also *Lyme, Lyme borreliosis*

Lym•naea \lim-ˈnē-ə, ˈlim-nē-ə\ *n* : a genus of snails (family Lymnaeidae) including some medically important intermediate hosts of flukes

lymph \ˈlimf\ *n* : a usu. clear coagulable fluid that passes from intercellular spaces of body tissue into lymphatic vessels, is discharged into the blood by way of the thoracic duct, and resembles blood plasma in containing white blood cells and esp. lymphocytes but normally few red blood cells and no plateletes — see CHYLE

lymph- *or* **lympho-** *comb form* : lymph : lymphatic tissue ⟨*lymph*edema⟩

lymph•ad•e•nec•to•my \ˌlim-ˌfad-ᵊn-ˈek-tə-mē\ *n, pl* **-mies** : surgical removal of a lymph node

lymph•ad•e•ni•tis \ˌlim-ˌfad-ᵊn-ˈī-təs\ *n* : inflammation of lymph nodes — **lymph•ad•e•nit•ic** \-ˈi-tik\ *adj*

lymph•ad•e•nop•a•thy \ˌlim-ˌfad-ᵊn-ˈä-pə-thē\ *n, pl* **-thies** : abnormal enlargement of the lymph nodes — **lymph•ad•e•no•path•ic** \ˌlim-ˌfad-ᵊn-ō-ˈpa-thik\ *adj*

lymphadenopathy–associated virus *n* : HIV-1

lymph•ad•e•no•sis \ˌlim-ˌfad-ᵊn-ˈō-səs\ *n, pl* **-no•ses** \-ˌsēz\ : any of certain abnormalities or diseases affecting the lymphatic system: as **a** : leukosis involving lymphatic tissues **b** : LYMPHOCYTIC LEUKEMIA

lymphangi- *or* **lymphangio-** *comb form* : lymphatic vessels ⟨*lymphangi*oma⟩

lymph•an•gi•ec•ta•sia \ˌlim-ˌfan-jē-ek-ˈtā-zhə, -zhē-ə\ *or* **lymph•an•gi•ec•ta•sis** \-ˈek-tə-səs\ *n, pl* **-ta•sias** *or* **-ta•ses** \-ˌsēz\ : dilatation of the lymphatic vessels

lymph•an•gio•gram \(ˌ)lim-ˈfan-jē-ə-ˌgram\ *n* : an X-ray picture made by lymphangiography

lymph•an•gi•og•ra•phy \ˌlim-ˌfan-jē-ˈä-grə-fē\ *n, pl* **-phies** : X-ray depiction of lymphatic vessels and lymph nodes after use of a radiopaque material — called also *lymphography* — **lymph•an•gio•graph•ic** \ˌlim-ˌfan-jē-ə-ˈgra-fik\ *adj*

lymph•an•gi•o•ma \ˌlim-ˌfan-jē-ˈō-mə\ *n, pl* **-mas** *also* **-ma•ta** \-mə-tə\ : a tumor formed of dilated lymphatic vessels

lymph•an•gio•sar•co•ma \ˌlim-ˌfan-jē-ō-(ˌ)sär-ˈkō-mə\ *n, pl* **-mas** *also* **-ma•ta** \-mə-tə\ : a sarcoma arising from the endothelial cells of lymphatic vessels

lymph•an•gi•ot•o•my \ˌlim-ˌfan-jē-ˈä-tə-mē\ *n, pl* **-mies** : incision of a lymphatic vessel

lym•phan•gi•tis \ˌlim-ˌfan-ˈjī-təs\ *n, pl* **-git•i•des** \-ˈji-tə-ˌdēz\ : inflammation of the lymphatic vessels

¹lym•phat•ic \lim-ˈfa-tik\ *adj* **1** : of, relating to, or produced by lymph, lymphoid tissue, or lymphocytes **2** : conveying lymph — **lym•phat•i•cal•ly** *adv*

²lymphatic *n* : a vessel that contains or conveys lymph, that originates as an interfibrillar or intercellular cleft or space in a tissue or organ, and that if small has no distinct walls or walls composed only of endothelial cells and if large resembles a vein in structure — called also *lymphatic vessel, lymph vessel;* see THORACIC DUCT

lymphatic capillary *n* : any of the smallest lymphatic vessels that are blind at one end and collect lymph in organs and tissues — called also *lymph capillary*

lymphatic duct *n* : any of the lymphatic vessels that are part of the system collecting lymph from the lymphatic capillaries and draining it into the subclavian veins by way of the right lymphatic duct and the thoracic duct — called also *lymph duct*

lymphatic leukemia *n* : LYMPHOCYTIC LEUKEMIA

lym•phat•i•co•ve•nous \lim-ˌfa-ti-kō-ˈvē-nəs\ *adj* : of, relating to, or connecting the veins and lymphatic vessels ⟨∼ anastomoses⟩

lymphatic system *n* : the part of the circulatory system that is concerned esp. with collecting fluids and proteins that have escaped from cells and tissues and returning them to the blood, with the phagocytic removal of cellular debris and foreign material, and with immune responses, and that consists mainly of the thymus, spleen, tonsils, lymph, lymph nodes, lymphatic vessels, lymphocytes, and bone marrow — called also *lymphoid system, lymph system*

lymphatic vessel *n* : LYMPHATIC

lymph capillary *n* : LYMPHATIC CAPILLARY

lymph duct *n* : LYMPHATIC DUCT

lymph•ede•ma \ˌlim-fi-ˈdē-mə\ *n* : edema due to faulty lymphatic drainage — **lymph•edem•a•tous** \ˌlim-fi-ˈde-mə-təs\ *adj*

lymph follicle *n* : LYMPH NODE; *esp* : LYMPH NODULE

lymph gland *n* : LYMPH NODE

lymph node *n* : any of the rounded masses of lymphoid tissue that are surrounded by a capsule of connective tissue, are distributed along the lymphatic vessels, and contain numerous lymphocytes which filter the flow of lymph passing through the node — called also *lymph gland*

lymph nodule *n* : a small simple lymph node

lympho- — see LYMPH-

lym•pho•blast \ˈlim-fə-ˌblast\ *n* : a lymphocyte that has enlarged following stimulation by an antigen, has the capacity to recognize the stimulating antigen, and is undergoing proliferation and differentiation either to an effector state in which it functions to eliminate the antigen or to a memory state in which it functions to recognize the future reappearance of the antigen — called also *immunoblast* — **lym•pho•blas•tic** \ˌlim-fə-ˈblas-tik\ *adj*

lymphoblastic leukemia *n* : lymphocytic leukemia characterized by an abnormal increase in the number of lymphoblasts; *specif* : ACUTE LYMPHOBLASTIC LEUKEMIA

lym•pho•blas•toid \ˌlim-fə-ˈblas-ˌtȯid\ *adj* : resembling a lymphoblast

lym•pho•blas•to•ma \ˌlim-fə-ˌblas-ˈtō-mə\ *n, pl* **-mas** *also* **-ma•ta** \-mə-tə\ : any of several diseases of lymph nodes marked by the formation of tumorous masses composed of mature or immature lymphocytes

lym•pho•blas•to•sis \-ˌblas-ˈtō-səs\ *n, pl* **-to•ses** \-ˌsēz\ : the presence of lymphoblasts in the peripheral blood

lym•pho•cele \ˈlim-fə-ˌsēl\ *n* : a cyst containing lymph

lym•pho•cyte \ˈlim-fə-ˌsīt\ *n* : any of the colorless weakly motile cells originating from stem cells and differentiating in lymphoid tissue (as of the thymus or bone marrow) that are the typical cellular elements of lymph, include the cellular mediators of immunity, and constitute 20 to 30 percent of the white blood cells of normal human blood — see B CELL, T CELL — **lym•pho•cyt•ic** \ˌlim-fə-ˈsi-tik\ *adj*

lymphocyte transformation *n* : a transformation caused in lymphocytes by a mitosis-inducing agent (as phytohemagglutinin) or by a second exposure to an antigen and characterized by an increase in size and in the amount of cytoplasm, by visibility of nucleoli in the nucleus, and after about 72 hours by a marked resemblance to blast cells

lymphocytic cho•rio•men•in•gi•tis \-ˌkȯr-ē-ō-ˌme-nən-ˈjī-təs\ *n* : an acute disease that is caused by an arenavirus (species *Lymphocytic choriomeningitis virus* of the genus *Arenavirus*), is characterized by fever, nausea, vomiting, headache, stiff neck, and slow pulse, and is transmitted esp. by rodents

lymphocytic leukemia *n* : leukemia of either of two types marked by an abnormal increase in the number of white blood cells (as lymphocytes) which accumulate in bone marrow, lymphoid tissue (as of the lymph nodes and spleen), and circulating blood — called also *lymphatic leukemia, lymphoid leukemia;* see ACUTE LYMPHOBLASTIC LEUKEMIA, CHRONIC LYMPHOCYTIC LEUKEMIA

lym•pho•cy•to•pe•nia \ˌlim-fō-ˌsī-tə-ˈpē-nē-ə\ *n* : a decrease in the normal number of lymphocytes in the circulating blood

lym•pho•cy•to•poi•e•sis \-pȯi-ˈē-səs\ *n, pl* **-e•ses** \-ˌsēz\ : formation of lymphocytes usu. in the lymph nodes

lym•pho•cy•to•sis \ˌlim-fə-ˌsī-ˈtō-səs, -fə-sə-\ *n, pl* **-to•ses** \-ˌsēz\ : an increase in the number of lymphocytes in the blood usu. associated with chronic infections or inflammations — compare GRANULOCYTOSIS, MONOCYTOSIS

lym•pho•cy•to•tox•ic \ˌlim-fə-ˌsī-tə-ˈtäk-sik\ *adj* **1** : being or relating to toxic effects on lymphocytes **2** : being toxic to lymphocytes — **lym•pho•cy•to•tox•ic•i•ty** \-täk-ˈsi-sə-tē\ *n*

lym•phog•e•nous \lim-ˈfä-jə-nəs\ *also* **lym•pho•gen•ic** \ˌlim-fə-ˈje-nik\ *adj* **1** : producing lymph or lymphocytes **2** : arising, resulting from, or spread by way of lymphocytes or lymphatic vessels 〈~ metastases〉

lym•pho•gran•u•lo•ma \ˌlim-fō-ˌgran-yə-ˈlō-mə\ *n, pl* **-mas** *also* **-ma•ta** \-mə-tə\ **1** : a nodular swelling of a lymph node **2** : LYMPHOGRANULOMA VENEREUM — **lym•pho•gran•u•lo•mat•ous** \-ˈlō-mə-təs\ *adj*

lymphogranuloma in•gui•na•le \-ˌiŋ-gwə-ˈnä-lē, -ˈna-, -ˈnā-\ *n* : LYMPHOGRANULOMA VENEREUM

lym•pho•gran•u•lo•ma•to•sis \-ˌlō-mə-ˈtō-səs\ *n, pl* **-to•ses** \-ˌsēz\ : the development of benign or malignant lymphogranulomas in various parts of the body; *also* : a condition characterized by lymphogranulomas

lymphogranuloma ve•ne•re•um \-və-ˈnir-ē-əm\ *n* : a contagious venereal disease that is caused by various strains of a bacterium of the genus *Chlamydia* (*C. trachomatis*) and is marked by painful swelling and inflammation of the lymph nodes esp. in the region of the groin — called also *lymphogranuloma inguinale, lymphopathia venereum*

lym•phog•ra•phy \lim-ˈfä-grə-fē\ *n, pl* **-phies** : LYMPHANGIOGRAPHY — **lym•pho•graph•ic** \ˌlim-fə-ˈgra-fik\ *adj*

lym•phoid \ˈlim-ˌfȯid\ *adj* **1** : of, relating to, or being tissue (as the lymph nodes or thymus) containing lymphocytes **2** : of, relating to, or resembling lymph

lymphoid cell *n* : any of the cells responsible for the production of immunity mediated by cells or antibodies and including lymphocytes, lymphoblasts, and plasma cells

lymphoid leukemia *n* : LYMPHOCYTIC LEUKEMIA

lymphoid system *n* : LYMPHATIC SYSTEM

lym•pho•kine \ˈlim-fə-ˌkīn\ *n* : any of various substances (an interleukin) of low molecular weight that are not antibodies, are secreted by T cells in response to stimulation by antigens, and have a role (as the activation of macrophages or the enhancement or inhibition of antibody production) in cell-mediated immunity

lym•pho•kine–activated killer cell *n* : a lymphocyte that has been turned into a tumor-killing cell by being cultured with interleukin-2 — called also *LAK*

lym•pho•ma \lim-ˈfō-mə\ *n, pl* **-mas** *also* **-ma•ta** \-mə-tə\ : a usu. malignant tumor of lymphoid tissue — see HODGKIN'S LYMPHOMA, NON-HODGKIN LYMPHOMA — **lym•pho•ma•tous** \-mə-təs\ *adj*

lym•pho•ma•toid \lim-ˈfō-mə-ˌtȯid\ *adj* : characterized by or resembling lymphomas ⟨a ~ tumor⟩

lymphomatosa — see STRUMA LYMPHOMATOSA

lym•pho•ma•to•sis \(ˌ)lim-ˌfō-mə-ˈtō-səs\ *n, pl* **-to•ses** \-ˌsēz\ : the presence of multiple lymphomas in the body

lym•pho•path•ia ve•ne•re•um \ˌlim-fə-ˌpa-thē-ə-və-ˈnir-ē-əm\ *n* : LYMPHOGRANULOMA VENEREUM

lym•pho•pe•nia \ˌlim-fə-ˈpē-nē-ə\ *n* : reduction in the number of lymphocytes circulating in the blood — **lym•pho•pe•nic** \-ˈpē-nik\ *adj*

lym•pho•plas•ma•cyt•ic *also* **lym•pho•plas•mo•cyt•ic** \-ˌplaz-mə-ˈsi-tik\ *adj* : of, relating to, or consisting of lymphocytes and plasma cells

lymphoplasmacytic lymphoma *n* : a slowly progressive non-Hodgkin lymphoma marked by proliferation of small lymphocytes, plasmacytoid lymphocytes, and plasma cells — see WALDENSTRÖM'S MACROGLOBULINEMIA

lym•pho•poi•e•sis \ˌlim-fə-pȯi-ˈē-səs\ *n, pl* **-e•ses** \-ˌsēz\ : the formation of lymphocytes or lymphatic tissue — **lym•pho•poi•et•ic** \-pȯi-ˈe-tik\ *adj*

lym•pho•pro•lif•er•a•tive \ˌlim-fō-prə-ˈli-fə-ˌrā-tiv, -rə-tiv\ *adj* : of or relating to the proliferation of lymphoid tissue ⟨a ~ disorder⟩ — **lym•pho•pro•lif•er•a•tion** \prə-ˌli-fə-ˈrā-shən\ *n*

lym•pho•re•tic•u•lar \ˌlim-fō-ri-ˈti-kyə-lər\ *adj* : RETICULOENDOTHELIAL

lymphoreticular system *n* : RETICULOENDOTHELIAL SYSTEM

lym•pho•sar•co•ma \ˌlim-fō-sär-ˈkō-mə\ *n, pl* **-mas** *also* **-ma•ta** \-mə-tə\ : a malignant lymphoma that tends to metastasize freely

lym•pho•tox•in \ˌlim-fō-ˈtäk-sən\ *n* : a lymphokine that lyses various cells and esp. tumor cells — **lym•pho•tox•ic** \-ˈtäk-sik\ *adj*

lym•pho•tro•pic \-ˈtrō-pik, -ˈträ-pik\ *adj* : having an affinity for lymphocytes — see HUMAN T-CELL LYMPHOTROPIC VIRUS, HUMAN T-LYMPHOTROPIC VIRUS

lymph system *n* : LYMPHATIC SYSTEM

lymph vessel *n* : LYMPHATIC

lyn•es•tre•nol \lin-ˈes-trə-ˌnȯl\ *n* : a progestational steroid $C_{20}H_{28}O$ used esp. in birth control pills

ly•oph•i•lize \lī-ˈä-fə-ˌlīz\ *vb* **-lized; -liz•ing** : FREEZE-DRY — **ly•oph•i•li•za•tion** *n*

ly•pres•sin \ˌlī-ˈpres-ᵊn\ *n* : a lysine-containing vasopressin $C_{46}H_{65}N_{13}O_{12}S_2$ used esp. as a nasal spray in the control of diabetes insipidus

Lyr•i•ca \ˈlir-i-kə\ *trademark* — used for a preparation of pregabalin

Lys *abbr* lysine

lys- *or* **lysi-** *or* **lyso-** *comb form* : lysis ⟨*lys*in⟩ ⟨*lyso*lecithin⟩

lyse \ˈlīs, ˈlīz\ *vb* **lysed; lys•ing** : to cause to undergo lysis : produce lysis in ⟨cells were *lysed*⟩

ly•ser•gic acid \lə-ˈsər-jik-, (ˌ)lī-\ *n* : a crystalline acid $C_{16}H_{16}N_2O_2$ that is an ergot alkaloid; *also* : LSD

lysergic acid di•eth•yl•am•ide \-ˌdī-ˌe-thə-ˈla-ˌmīd\ *n* : LSD

ly•ser•gide \lə-ˈsər-ˌjīd, lī-\ *n* : LSD

lysi- — see LYS-

ly•sin \ˈlīs-ᵊn\ *n* : a substance (as an antibody) capable of causing lysis

ly•sine \ˈlī-ˌsēn\ *n* : a crystalline essential amino acid $C_6H_{14}N_2O_2$ obtained from the hydrolysis of various proteins — abbr. *Lys*

lysine vasopressin *n* : LYPRESSIN

ly•sis \ˈlī-səs\ *n, pl* **ly•ses** \-ˌsēz\ **1** : the gradual decline of a disease process (as fever) — compare CRISIS 1 **2** : a process of disintegration or dissolution (as of cells)

-ly•sis \l-ə-səs, ˈlī-səs\ *n comb form, pl* **-ly•ses** \l-ə-ˌsēz\ **1** : decomposition ⟨hydro*lysis*⟩ **2** : disintegration : breaking down ⟨auto*lysis*⟩ **3 a** : relief or reduction ⟨neuro*lysis*⟩ **b** : detachment ⟨epidermo*lysis*⟩

lyso- — see LYS-

ly•so•gen \ˈlī-sə-jən\ *n* : a lysogenic bacterium or bacterial strain

ly•so•gen•ic \ˌlī-sə-ˈje-nik\ *adj* **1** : harboring a prophage as hereditary material ⟨~ bacteria⟩ **2** : TEMPERATE — **ly•sog•e•ny** \lī-ˈsä-jə-nē\ *n*

Ly•sol \ˈlī-ˌsȯl, -ˌsōl\ *trademark* — used for a disinfectant consisting of a brown solution containing cresols

ly•so•lec•i•thin \ˌlī-sə-ˈle-sə-thən\ *n* : LYSOPHOSPHATIDYLCHOLINE

ly•so•phos•pha•ti•dyl•cho•line \ˌlī-sō-ˌfäs-fə-ˌtīd-ᵊl-ˈkō-ˌlēn, -(ˌ)fäs-ˌfa-təd-ᵊl-\ *n* : a hemolytic substance produced by the removal of a fatty acid group from a lecithin

ly•so•some \ˈlī-sə-ˌsōm\ *n* : a saclike cellular organelle that contains various hydrolytic enzymes — **ly•so•som•al** \ˌlī-sə-ˈsō-məl\ *adj* — **ly•so•so•mal•ly** *adv*

ly•so•zyme \ˈlī-sə-ˌzīm\ *n* : a basic bacteriolytic protein that hydrolyzes peptidoglycan and is present in egg white and in saliva and tears — called also *muramidase*

-lyte \ˌlīt\ *n comb form* : substance capable of undergoing (such) decomposition ⟨electro*lyte*⟩

lyt•ic \ˈli-tik\ *adj* : of or relating to lysis or a lysin; *also* : productive of or effecting lysis (as of cells) ⟨~ viruses⟩ — **ly•ti•cal•ly** *adv*

-lyt•ic \ˈli-tik\ *adj suffix* : of, relating to, or effecting (such) decomposition ⟨hydro*lytic*⟩

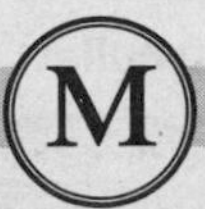

m *abbr* **1** meter **2** molar **3** molarity **4** mole **5** muscle
M *abbr* [Latin *misce*] mix — used in writing prescriptions
MA *abbr* mental age
McArdle's disease, McBurney's point — see entries alphabetized as MC-
Mace \ˈmās\ *trademark* — used for a temporarily disabling liquid that is usu. used as a spray and causes tears, dizziness, and burning sensation
mac•er•ate \ˈma-sə-ˌrāt\ *vb* **-at•ed; -at•ing :** to soften (as tissue) by steeping or soaking so as to separate into constituent elements — **mac•er•at•ed** \-ˌrā-təd\ *adj* — **mac•er•a•tion** \ˌma-sə-ˈrā-shən\ *n*
Ma•cha•do–Jo•seph disease \mə-ˌshä-dō-ˈjō-səf-\ *n* **:** ataxia of any of several phenotypically variant forms that are inherited as autosomal dominant traits, have an onset usu. early in adult life, tend to occur in families of Portuguese and esp. Azorean ancestry, and are characterized by progressive degeneration of the central nervous system
Machado and **Joseph** (*fl* **1970s),** Azorean-Portuguese families.
Ma•chu•po virus \mä-ˈchü-pō-\ *n* **:** a virus of the genus *Arenavirus* (species *Machupo virus*) that causes a hemorrhagic fever endemic in Bolivia and is transmitted by infected mice
mackerel shark *n* **:** any of a family (Lamnidae) of large aggressive sharks including the great white shark
Mac•leod's syndrome \mə-ˈklaủdz-\ *n* **:** abnormally increased translucence of one lung usu. accompanied by reduction in ventilation and in perfusion with blood
Macleod, William Mathieson (1911–1977), British physician.
macr- *or* **macro-** *comb form* **:** large ⟨*macro*molecule⟩ ⟨*macro*cyte⟩
Mac•ra•can•tho•rhyn•chus \ˌma-krə-ˌkan-thə-ˈriŋ-kəs\ *n* **:** a genus of acanthocephalan worms including one (*M. hirudinaceus*) parasitic in swine
mac•ro•ad•e•no•ma \ˌma-krō-ˌa-dᵊn-ˈō-mə\ *n, pl* **-mas** *also* **-ma•ta** \-mə-tə\ **:** an adenoma of the pituitary gland that is greater than ten millimeters in diameter
mac•ro•al•bu•min•uria \ˌma-krō-al-ˌbyü-mə-ˈnůr-ē-ə, -ˈnyůr-\ *n* **:** albuminuria characterized by a relatively high rate of urinary excretion of albumin typically greater than 300 milligrams per 24-hour period — compare MICROALBUMINURIA
mac•ro•an•gi•op•a•thy \ˌma-krō-ˌan-jē-ˈä-pə-thē\ *n, pl* **-thies :** an angiopathy affecting blood vessels of large and medium size
Mac•rob•del•la \ˌma-ˌkräb-ˈde-lə\ *n* **:** a genus of leeches including one (*M. decora*) formerly used in medicine
mac•ro•bi•ot•ic \ˌma-krō-bī-ˈä-tik, -bē-\ *adj* **:** of, relating to, or being a diet that consists of whole cereals and grains supplemented esp. with beans and vegetables
mac•ro•bi•ot•ics \-tiks\ *n* **:** a macrobiotic dietary system
mac•ro•ceph•a•lous \ˌma-krō-ˈse-fə-ləs\ *or* **mac•ro•ce•phal•ic** \-sə-ˈfa-lik\ *adj* **:** having or being an exceptionally large head or cranium — **mac•ro•ceph•a•ly** \-ˈse-fə-lē\ *n*
mac•ro•cy•clic \ˌma-krō-ˈsi-klik, -ˈsī-\ *adj* **:** containing or being a chemical ring that consists usu. of 15 or more atoms ⟨~ esters⟩ — **macrocyclic** *n*
mac•ro•cyte \ˈma-krə-ˌsīt\ *n* **:** an exceptionally large red blood cell occurring chiefly in anemias (as pernicious anemia) — called also *megalocyte*
mac•ro•cyt•ic \ˌma-krə-ˈsi-tik\ *adj* **:** of or relating to macrocytes; *specif, of an anemia* **:** characterized by macrocytes in the blood
mac•ro•cy•to•sis \ˌma-krə-sī-ˈtō-səs\ *n, pl* **-to•ses** \-ˌsēz\ **:** the occurrence of macrocytes in the blood
mac•ro•ga•mete \ˌma-krō-gə-ˈmēt, -ˈga-ˌmēt\ *n* **:** the larger and usu. female gamete of a heterogamous organism — compare MICROGAMETE
mac•ro•gen•i•to•so•mia \ˌma-krō-ˌje-ni-tə-ˈsō-mē-ə\ *n* **:** premature excessive development of the external genitalia
mac•ro•glia \ma-ˈkrä-glē-ə, ˌma-krō-ˈglī-ə\ *n* **:** glia of ectodermal origin made up of astrocytes and oligodendrocytes — **mac•ro•gli•al** \-əl\ *adj*
mac•ro•glob•u•lin \ˌma-krō-ˈglä-byə-lən\ *n* **:** a highly polymerized globulin (as IgM) of high molecular weight
mac•ro•glob•u•lin•ae•mia *chiefly Brit var of* MACROGLOBULINEMIA
mac•ro•glob•u•lin•emia \-ˌglä-byə-lə-ˈnē-mē-ə\ *n* **:** a disorder characterized by increased blood serum viscosity and the presence of macroglobulins in the serum — **mac•ro•glob•u•lin•emic** \-mik\ *adj*
mac•ro•glos•sia \ˌma-krō-ˈglä-sē-ə, -ˈglȯ-\ *n* **:** pathological and commonly congenital enlargement of the tongue
mac•ro•lide \ˈma-krə-ˌlīd\ *n* **:** any of several antibiotics (as erythromycin and clarithromycin) that are effective esp. against gram-positive bacteria (as staphylococci)
mac•ro•mol•e•cule \ˌma-krō-ˈmä-li-ˌkyül\ *n* **:** a very large molecule (as of a protein) built up from smaller chemical structures — compare MICROMOLECULE — **mac•ro•mo•lec•u•lar** \-mə-ˈle-kyə-lər\ *adj*
mac•ro•nu•tri•ent \-ˈnü-trē-ənt, -ˈnyü-\ *n* **:** a substance (as protein, carbohydrate, or fat) required in relatively large quantities in nutrition — compare MICRONUTRIENT

mac•ro•or•chid•ism \-ˈȯr-kə-ˌdi-zəm\ *n* : the condition (as in fragile X syndrome) of having large testicles

mac•ro•phage \ˈma-krə-ˌfāj, -ˌfäzh\ *n* : a phagocytic tissue cell of the immune system that may be fixed or freely motile, is derived from a monocyte, functions in the destruction of foreign antigens (as bacteria and viruses), and serves as an antigen-presenting cell — see HISTIOCYTE, MONONUCLEAR PHAGOCYTE SYSTEM — **mac•ro•phag•ic** \ˌma-krə-ˈfa-jik\ *adj*

macrophage colony–stimulating factor *n* : a colony-stimulating factor produced by macrophages, endothelial cells, and fibroblasts that stimulates production and maturation of macrophages — abbr. *M-CSF*

mac•ro•scop•ic \ˌma-krə-ˈskä-pik\ *adj* : large enough to be observed by the naked eye — compare MICROSCOPIC 2 — **mac•ro•scop•i•cal•ly** *adv*

mac•ro•so•mia \ˌma-krə-ˈsō-mē-ə\ *n* : GIGANTISM — **mac•ro•so•mic** \-ˈsō-mik\ *adj*

mac•ro•struc•ture \ˈma-krō-ˌstrək-chər\ *n* : the structure (as of a body part) revealed by visual examination with little or no magnification — **mac•ro•struc•tur•al** \ˌma-krō-ˈstrək-chə-rəl, -shə-rəl\ *adj*

macul- *or* **maculo-** *comb form* : macule : macular and ⟨*maculo*papular⟩

mac•u•la \ˈma-kyə-lə\ *n, pl* **-lae** \-ˌlē, -ˌlī\ *also* **-las** **1** : a spot or blotch; *esp* : MACULE 2 **2** : an anatomical structure having the form of a spot differentiated from surrounding tissues: as **a** : MACULA ACUSTICA **b** : a small yellowish area lying slightly lateral to the center of the retina that is made up mostly of cones, plays a key role in visual acuity, and has the fovea at is center — called also *macula lutea*

macula acu•sti•ca \-ə-ˈküs-ti-kə\ *n, pl* **maculae acu•sti•cae** \-ti-ˌsē\ : either of two small areas of sensory hair cells in the ear that are covered with gelatinous material on which are located crystals or concretions of calcium carbonate and that are associated with the perception of equilibrium: **a** : one located in the saccule — called also *macula sacculi* **b** : one located in the utricle — called also *macula utriculi*

macula den•sa \-ˈden-sə\ *n* : a group of modified epithelial cells in the distal convoluted tubule of the kidney that control renin release by relaying information about the sodium concentration in the fluid passing through the convoluted tubule to the renin-producing juxtaglomerular cells of the afferent arteriole

macula lu•tea \-ˈlü-tē-ə\ *n, pl* **maculae lu•te•ae** \-tē-ˌē, -tē-ˌī\ : MACULA 2b

mac•u•lar \ˈma-kyə-lər\ *adj* **1** : of, relating to, or characterized by a spot or spots ⟨a ~ skin rash⟩ **2** : of, relating to, affecting, or mediated by the macula of the eye ⟨~ vision⟩

macular degeneration *n* : progressive deterioration of the macula of the eye resulting in the gradual loss of the central part of the visual field; *esp* : AGE-RELATED MACULAR DEGENERATION

macula sac•cu•li \-ˈsa-kyə-ˌlī\ *n* : MACULA ACUSTICA a

macula utriculi \-yu̇-ˈtri-kyə-ˌlī\ *n* : MACULA ACUSTICA b

mac•ule \ˈma-(ˌ)kyül\ *n* **1** : MACULA 2 **2** : a patch of skin that is altered in color but usu. not elevated

maculo- — see MACUL-

mac•u•lo•pap•u•lar \ˌma-kyə-(ˌ)lō-ˈpa-pyə-lər\ *adj* : combining the characteristics of macules and papules ⟨a ~ rash⟩ ⟨a ~ lesion⟩

mac•u•lo•pap•ule \-ˈpa-(ˌ)pyül\ *n* : a maculopapular elevation of the skin

mac•u•lop•a•thy \ˌma-kyə-ˈlä-pə-thē\ *n, pl* **-thies** : any pathological condition of the macula of the eye

mad \ˈmad\ *adj* **mad•der; mad•dest** **1** : arising from, indicative of, or marked by mental disorder — not used technically **2** : affected with rabies : RABID

Mad•a•gas•car periwinkle \ˌma-də-ˈgas-kər-\ *n* : ROSY PERIWINKLE

mad cow disease *n* : BOVINE SPONGIFORM ENCEPHALOPATHY

mad itch *n* : PSEUDORABIES

mad•ness \ˈmad-nəs\ *n* **1** : a severely disordered state of mind — not used technically **2** : any of several ailments of animals marked by frenzied behavior; *specif* : RABIES

Ma•du•ra foot \ˈma-dyu̇r-ə-, -du̇r-; mə-ˈ\ *n* : maduromycosis of the foot

mad•u•ro•my•co•sis \ˈma-dyu̇-rō-mī-ˈkō-səs, -du̇-\ *n, pl* **-co•ses** \-ˌsēz\ : a destructive chronic disease usu. restricted to the feet, marked by swelling and deformity resulting from the formation of granulomatous nodules and caused by various actinomycetes (as of the genus *Nocardia*) and fungi (as of the genus *Madurella*) — called also *mycetoma* — **mad•u•ro•my•cot•ic** \-ˈkä-tik\ *adj*

mae•di \ˈmī-t͟hē\ *n* : ovine progressive pneumonia esp. as manifested by respiratory symptoms

maf•e•nide \ˈma-fə-ˌnīd\ *n* : an antibacterial sulfonamide applied topically in the form of its acetate $C_7H_{10}N_2O_2S{\cdot}C_2H_4O_2$ esp. in the treatment of burns — see SULFAMYLON

ma•ga•i•nin \mə-ˈgā-(ə-)nən\ *n* : any of a group of peptide antibiotics isolated from the skin of frogs (esp. *Xenopus laevis*)

mag•got \ˈma-gət\ *n* : a soft-bodied legless grub that is the larva of a dipteran fly (as the housefly) and develops usu. in decaying matter or as a parasite in plants or animals

magic bullet *n* : a substance or therapy capable of destroying pathogens (as cancer cells) or providing an effective remedy for a disease or condition without deleterious side effects

magic mushroom *n* : any fungus containing hallucinogenic alkaloids (as psilocybin)

mag•ma \ˈmag-mə\ *n* : a suspension of a large amount of precipitated material (as in milk of magnesia) in a small volume of a watery vehicle

magna — see CISTERNA MAGNA

mag•ne•sia \mag-ˈnē-shə, -ˈnē-zhə\ *n* : MAGNESIUM OXIDE

magnesia magma *n* : MILK OF MAGNESIA

mag•ne•sium \mag-ˈnē-zē-əm, -zhəm\ *n* : a silver-white light malleable ductile metallic element that occurs abundantly in nature (as in bones) — symbol *Mg;* see ELEMENT table

magnesium carbonate *n* : a carbonate of magnesium; *esp* : the very white crystalline salt $MgCO_3$ used as an antacid and laxative

magnesium chloride *n* : a bitter crystalline salt $MgCl_2$ used esp. to replenish body electrolytes

magnesium citrate *n* : a crystalline salt $C_{12}H_{10}Mg_3O_{14}$ used in the form of a lemony effervescent solution as a saline laxative

magnesium hydroxide *n* : a slightly alkaline crystalline compound $Mg(OH)_2$ used as an antacid and laxative — see MILK OF MAGNESIA

magnesium oxide *n* : a white compound MgO used as an antacid and mild laxative

magnesium si•li•cate \-ˈsi-lə-ˌkāt, -kət\ *n* : a silicate that is approximately $Mg_2Si_3O_8 \cdot nH_2O$ and that is used chiefly in medicine as a gastric antacid adsorbent and coating (as in the treatment of ulcers)

magnesium sulfate *n* : a white anhydrous salt $MgSO_4$ that occurs naturally in hydrated form as Epsom salts and that in the hydrated form $MgSO_4 \cdot 7H_2O$ is used esp. to relieve constipation, to treat magnesium deficiency, and to control convulsions (as those associated with eclampsia)

mag•net•ic field \mag-ˈne-tik-\ *n* : the portion of space near a magnetic body or a current-carrying body in which the magnetic forces due to the body or current can be detected

magnetic resonance *n* : the excitation of particles (as atomic nuclei or electrons) in a magnetic field by exposure to electromagnetic radiation of a specific frequency — abbr. *MR;* see NUCLEAR MAGNETIC RESONANCE

magnetic resonance angiogram *n* : MAGNETIC RESONANCE ANGIOGRAPHY

magnetic resonance angiography *n* : magnetic resonance imaging used to visualize noninvasively the heart, blood vessels, or blood flow in the circulatory system — abbr. *MRA*; called also *magnetic resonance angiogram, MR angiography*

magnetic resonance imaging *n* : a noninvasive diagnostic technique that produces computerized images of internal body tissues and is based on nuclear magnetic resonance of atoms within the body induced by the application of radio waves — abbr. *MRI*

magnetic resonance spectroscopy *n* : a noninvasive technique that is similar to magnetic resonance imaging but uses a stronger field and is used to monitor body chemistry (as in metabolism or blood flow) — abbr. *MRS*

magnetic therapy *n* : the therapeutic use of magnets or magnetic fields in the practice of alternative medicine to treat illness, relieve pain, and promote health — called also *biomagnetic therapy, biomagnetism, magnet therapy*

mag•ne•to•en•ceph•a•log•ra•phy \mag-ˌnē-tō-in-ˌse-fə-ˈlä-grə-fē\ *n, pl* **-phies** : a noninvasive technique that detects and records the magnetic field associated with electrical activity in the brain — abbr. *MEG*

mag•ni•fi•ca•tion \ˌmag-nə-fə-ˈkā-shən\ *n* : the apparent enlargement of an object by an optical instrument that is the ratio of the dimensions of an image formed by the instrument to the corresponding dimensions of the object — called also *power* — **mag•ni•fy** \ˈmag-nə-ˌfī\ *vb*

mag•no•cel•lu•lar \ˌmag-nō-ˈsel-yə-lər\ *adj* : being or containing neurons with large cell bodies — compare PARVOCELLULAR

magnum — see FORAMEN MAGNUM

magnus — see ADDUCTOR MAGNUS

ma huang \ˈmä-ˈhwäŋ\ *n* : EPHEDRA 2

maid•en•head \ˈmād-ᵊn-ˌhed\ *n* : HYMEN

maim \ˈmām\ *vb* **1** : to commit the felony of mayhem upon **2** : to wound seriously : MUTILATE, DISABLE

main•line \ˈmān-ˌlīn\ *vb* **-lined; -lin•ing** *slang* : to inject a narcotic drug (as heroin) into a vein

main•stream \-ˌstrēm\ *adj* : relating to or being tobacco smoke that is drawn (as from a cigarette) directly into the mouth of the smoker and is usu. inhaled into the lungs — compare SIDESTREAM

main•te•nance \ˈmānt-ᵊn-əns\ *adj* : designed or adequate to maintain a patient in a stable condition : serving to maintain a gradual process of healing or to prevent a relapse ⟨a ~ dose⟩

ma•jor \ˈmā-jər\ *adj* : involving grave risk : SERIOUS ⟨a ~ illness⟩ — compare MINOR

majora — see LABIA MAJORA

major basic protein *n* : a toxic cationic protein that is the principal protein found in the granules of eosinophils and that is capable of damaging tissue (as of the eye) if released into extracellular spaces

major depression *n* **1** : MAJOR DEPRESSIVE DISORDER **2** : an episode of depression characteristic of major depressive disorder

[1]**major depressive** *adj* : of, relating to, or affected with major depressive disorder

[2]**major depressive** *n* : an individual affected with or subject to episodes of major depressive disorder

major depressive disorder *n* : a mood disorder having a clinical course involving one or more episodes of serious psychological depression that last two or more weeks each and do not have intervening episodes of mania or hypomania

major histocompatibility complex *n* : a group of genes that function esp. in determining the histocompatibility antigens found on cell surfaces and that in humans comprise the alleles occurring at four loci on the short arm of chromosome 6 — abbr. *MHC*

major labia *n pl* : LABIA MAJORA

major–medical *adj* : of, relating to, or being a form of insurance designed to pay all or part of the medical bills of major illnesses usu. after deduction of a fixed initial sum

major surgery *n* : surgery involving a risk to the life of the patient; *specif* : an operation upon an organ within the cranium, chest, abdomen, or pelvic cavity — compare MINOR SURGERY

mal \ˈmäl, ˈmal\ *n* : DISEASE, SICKNESS

mal- *comb form* **1** : bad ⟨*mal*practice⟩ **2 a** : abnormal ⟨*mal*formation⟩ **b** : abnormally ⟨*mal*formed⟩ **3 a** : inadequate ⟨*mal*adjustment⟩ **b** : inadequately ⟨*mal*nourished⟩

mal•ab•sorp•tion \ˌma-ləb-ˈsȯrp-shən, -ˈzȯrp-\ *n* : faulty absorption of nutrient materials from the digestive tract — **mal•ab•sorp•tive** \-tiv\ *adj*

malabsorption syndrome *n* : a syndrome resulting from malabsorption that is typically characterized by weakness, diarrhea, muscle cramps, edema, and loss of weight

malac- *or* **malaco-** *comb form* : soft ⟨*malaco*plakia⟩

ma•la•cia \mə-ˈlā-shə, -shē-ə\ *n* : abnormal softening of a tissue — often used in combination ⟨osteo*malacia*⟩ — **ma•lac•ic** \-sik\ *adj*

mal•a•co•pla•kia *also* **mal•a•ko•pla•kia** \ˌma-lə-kō-ˈplā-kē-ə\ *n* : inflammation of the mucous membrane of a hollow organ (as the urinary bladder) characterized by the formation of soft granulomatous lesions

mal•ad•ap•ta•tion \ˌmal-ˌa-ˌdap-ˈtā-shən\ *n* : poor or inadequate adaptation ⟨psychological ~⟩ — **mal•adap•tive** \ˌma-lə-ˈdap-tiv\ *adj* — **mal•adap•tive•ly** *adv*

mal•a•die de Ro•ger \ˌma-lə-ˈdē-də-rō-ˈzhā\ *n* : a small usu. asymptomatic ventricular septal defect

Roger, Henri–Louis (1809–1891), French physician.

mal•ad•just•ment \ˌma-lə-ˈjəst-mənt\ *n* : poor, faulty, or inadequate adjustment — **mal•ad•just•ed** \-ˈjəs-təd\ *adj*

mal•ad•min•is•tra•tion \ˌma-ləd-ˌmi-nə-ˈstrā-shən\ *n* : incorrect administration (as of a drug) ⟨~ of insulin⟩

mal•a•dy \ˈma-lə-dē\ *n, pl* **-dies** : DISEASE, SICKNESS ⟨a fatal ~⟩

mal•aise \mə-ˈlāz, ma-, -ˈlez\ *n* : an indefinite feeling of debility or lack of health often indicative of or accompanying the onset of an illness

mal•align•ment \ˌma-lə-ˈlīn-mənt\ *n* : incorrect or imperfect alignment (as of teeth) — **mal•aligned** \-ˈlīnd\ *adj*

ma•lar \ˈmā-lər, -ˌlär\ *adj* : of or relating to the cheek, the side of the head, or the zygomatic bone

malar bone *n* : ZYGOMATIC BONE — called also *malar*

malari- *or* **malario-** *comb form* : malaria ⟨*malario*logy⟩

ma•lar•ia \mə-ˈler-ē-ə\ *n* **1** : an acute or chronic disease caused by the presence of sporozoan parasites of the genus *Plasmodium* in the red blood cells, transmitted from an infected to an uninfected individual by the bite of anopheline mosquitoes, and characterized by periodic attacks of chills and fever that coincide with mass destruction of blood cells and the release of toxic substances by the parasite at the end of each reproductive cycle — see FALCIPARUM MALARIA, VIVAX MALARIA **2** : any of various diseases of birds and mammals that are more or less similar to malaria of humans and are caused by blood protozoans — **ma•lar•ial** \-əl\ *adj*

ma•lar•i•ae malaria \mə-ˈler-ē-ˌē-\ *n* : malaria caused by a malaria parasite (*Plasmodium malariae*) and marked by recurrence of paroxysms at 72-hour intervals — called also *quartan malaria*

malarial mosquito *or* **malaria mosquito** *n* : a mosquito of the genus *Anopheles* (esp. *A. quadrimaculatus*) that transmits the malaria parasite

malaria parasite *n* : a protozoan of the sporozoan genus *Plasmodium* that is transmitted to humans or to certain other mammals or birds by the bite of a mosquito in which its sexual reproduction takes place, that multiplies asexually in the vertebrate host by schizogony in the red blood cells or in certain tissue cells, and that causes destruction of red blood cells and the febrile disease malaria — see MEROZOITE, PHANEROZOITE, SCHIZONT, SPOROZOITE

ma•lar•i•ol•o•gy \mə-ˌler-ē-ˈä-lə-jē\ *n, pl* **-gies** : the scientific study of malaria — **ma•lar•i•ol•o•gist** \-jist\ *n*

ma•lar•i•ous \mə-ˈler-ē-əs\ *adj* : characterized by the presence of or infected with malaria ⟨~ regions⟩

Mal•a•rone \ˈma-lə-ˌrōn\ *trademark* — used for a preparation of atovaquone and the hydrochloride of proguanil

Mal•as•se•zia \ˌma-lə-ˈsā-zē-ə\ *n* : a genus of lipophilic yeastlike fungi including one (*M. furfur* syn. *Pityrosporum oribiculare*) causing tinea versicolor and another (*M. ovalis* syn. *Pityrosporum ovale*) associated with seborrheic dermatitis

ma•late \ˈma-ˌlāt, ˈmā-\ *n* : a salt or ester of malic acid

mal•a•thi•on \ˌma-lə-ˈthī-ən, -ˌän\ *n* : an insecticide $C_{10}H_{19}O_6PS_2$ that is less toxic to mammals than parathion

mal del pin•to \ˌmal-del-ˈpin-tō\ *n* : PINTA

mal de mer \ˌmal-də-ˈmer\ *n* : SEASICKNESS

mal•des•cent \ˌmal-di-ˈsent\ *n* : an improper or incomplete descent of a testis into the scrotum — **mal•des•cend•ed** \-ˈsen-dəd\ *adj*

mal•de•vel•op•ment \ˌmal-di-ˈve-ləp-mənt\ *n* : abnormal growth or development : DYSPLASIA

[1]**male** \ˈmāl\ *n* : an individual that produces small usu. motile gametes (as sperm or spermatozoa) which fertilize the eggs of a female

[2]**male** *adj* : of, relating to, or being the sex that produces gametes which fertilize the eggs of a female

ma•le•ate \ˈmā-lē-ˌāt, -lē-ət\ *n* : a salt or ester of maleic acid

male bonding *n* : bonding between males through shared activities excluding females

male climacteric *n* : ANDROPAUSE

ma•le•ic acid \mə-ˈlē-ik-, -ˈlā-\ *n* : an isomer of fumaric acid

male menopause *n* : ANDROPAUSE

male–pattern baldness *n* : typical hereditary baldness in the male characterized by loss of hair on the crown and temples : androgenetic alopecia in men

mal•for•ma•tion \ˌmal-fȯr-ˈmā-shən\ *n* : irregular, anomalous, abnormal, or faulty formation or structure — **mal•formed** \(ˌ)mal-ˈfȯrmd\ *adj*

mal•func•tion \(ˌ)mal-ˈfəŋk-shən\ *vb* : to function imperfectly or badly : fail to operate in the normal or usual manner — **malfunction** *n*

ma•lic acid \ˈma-lik, ˈmā-\ *n* : any of three optical isomers of an acid $C_4H_6O_5$; *esp* : the one formed as an intermediate in the Krebs cycle

maligna — see LENTIGO MALIGNA

ma•lig•nan•cy \mə-ˈlig-nən-sē\ *n, pl* **-cies** **1** : the quality or state of being malignant **2 a** : exhibition (as by a tumor) of malignant qualities : VIRULENCE **b** : a malignant tumor

ma•lig•nant \-nənt\ *adj* **1** : tending to produce death or deterioration; *esp* : tending to infiltrate, metastasize, and terminate fatally ⟨~ tumors⟩ — compare BENIGN 1 **2** : of unfavorable prognosis : not responding favorably to treatment ⟨a ~ trend⟩

malignant catarrhal fever *n* : an acute infectious often fatal disease esp. of cattle and deer that is caused by several herpesviruses (genus *Rhadinovirus*) and is characterized esp. by fever, depression, enlarged lymph nodes, and discharge from the eyes and nose — called also *catarrhal fever, malignant catarrh*

malignant edema *n* : an acute often fatal toxemia of wild and domestic animals that follows wound infection by an anaerobic toxin-producing bacterium of the genus *Clostridium* (*C. septicum*)

malignant hypertension *n* : essential hypertension characterized by acute onset, severe symptoms, rapidly progressive course, and poor prognosis

malignant hyperthermia *n* : a rare inherited condition characterized by a rapid, extreme, and often fatal rise in body temperature following the administration of general anesthesia

malignant malaria *n* : FALCIPARUM MALARIA

malignant malnutrition *n* : KWASHIORKOR

malignant melanoma *n* : MELANOMA 2

malignant pustule *n* : localized anthrax of the skin taking the form of a pimple surrounded by a zone of edema and hyperemia and tending to become necrotic and ulcerated

malignant tertian malaria *n* : FALCIPARUM MALARIA

malignant transformation *n* : the transformation that a cell undergoes to become a rapidly dividing tumor-producing cell; *also* : the transformation of a mass of cells or a tissue into a rapidly growing tumor

ma•lig•ni•za•tion \mə-ˌlig-nə-ˈzā-shən\ *n* : a process or instance of becoming malignant ⟨~ of a tumor⟩

ma•lin•ger \mə-ˈliŋ-gər\ *vb* **-gered; -gering** : to pretend or exaggerate incapacity or illness (as to avoid duty or work) — **ma•lin•ger•er** \-ər\ *n*

mal•le•o•lar \mə-ˈlē-ə-lər\ *adj* : of or relating to a malleolus ⟨~ fracture⟩

mal•le•o•lus \mə-ˈlē-ə-ləs\ *n, pl* **-li** \-ˌlī\ : an expanded projection or process at the distal end of the fibula or tibia at the level of the ankle: **a** : the expanded lower end of the fibula situated on the lateral side of the leg at the ankle — called also *external malleolus, lateral malleolus* **b** : a strong pyramid-shaped process of the tibia that projects distally on the medial side of its lower end at the ankle — called also *internal malleolus, medial malleolus* **c** : a small projection of the tibia on the posterior side of its lower end at the ankle — called also *posterior malleolus*

mal•let finger \ˈma-lət-\ *n* : involuntary flexion of the distal phalanx of a finger caused by avulsion of the extensor tendon

mal•le•us \ˈma-lē-əs\ *n, pl* **mal•lei** \-lē-ˌī, -lē-ˌē\ : the outermost of the chain of three ossicles in the middle ear consisting of a head, neck, short process, long process, and handle with the short process and handle being fastened to the tympanic membrane and the head articulating with the head of the incus — called also *hammer*

mal•nour•ished \(ˌ)mal-ˈnər-isht\ *adj* : UNDERNOURISHED

mal·nour·ish·ment \-ˈnər-ish-mənt\ *n* : MALNUTRITION

mal·nu·tri·tion \ˌmal-nu̇-ˈtri-shən, -nyu̇-\ *n* : faulty nutrition due to inadequate or unbalanced intake of nutrients or their impaired assimilation or utilization — **mal·nu·tri·tion·al** \-ᵊl\ *adj*

mal·oc·clu·sion \ˌma-lə-ˈklü-zhən\ *n* : improper occlusion; *esp* : abnormality in the coming together of teeth — **mal·oc·clu·ded** \-ˈklü-dəd\ *adj*

Mal·pi·ghi·an body \mal-ˈpi-gē-ən-, -ˈpē-\ *n* : RENAL CORPUSCLE; *also* : MALPIGHIAN CORPUSCLE 2

Malpighi \mäl-ˈpē-gē\, **Marcello (1628–1694),** Italian anatomist.

Malpighian corpuscle *n* **1** : RENAL CORPUSCLE **2** : any of the small masses of adenoid tissue formed around the branches of the splenic artery in the spleen

Malpighian layer *n* : the deepest part of the epidermis that consists of the stratum basale and stratum spinosum and is the site of mitotic activity

Malpighian pyramid *n* : RENAL PYRAMID

mal·posed \ˌmal-ˈpōzd\ *adj* : characterized by malposition ⟨~ teeth⟩

mal·po·si·tion \ˌmal-pə-ˈzi-shən\ *n* : wrong or faulty position — **mal·po·si·tion·ing** \-shə-niŋ\ *n*

mal·prac·tice \(ˌ)mal-ˈprak-təs\ *n* : a dereliction of professional duty or a failure to exercise an accepted degree of professional skill or learning by a physician rendering professional services which results in injury, loss, or damage — **malpractice** *vb*

mal·pre·sen·ta·tion \ˌmal-ˌprē-zen-ˈtā-shən, -ˌpre-\ *n* : abnormal presentation of the fetus at birth

mal·ro·ta·tion \ˌmal-rō-ˈtā-shən\ *n* : improper rotation of a bodily part and esp. of the intestines — **mal·ro·ta·ted** \-ˈrō-ˌtāt-əd\ *adj*

MALT *abbr* mucosa-associated lymphoid tissue

Mal·ta fever \ˈmȯl-tə-\ *n* : BRUCELLOSIS 2

malt·ase \ˈmȯl-ˌtās, -ˌtāz\ *n* : an enzyme that catalyzes the hydrolysis of maltose to glucose

mal·ti·tol \ˈmȯl-tə-ˌtȯl\ *n* : a crystalline sweet alcohol $C_{12}H_{24}O_{11}$ that is used as a sugar substitute in reduced-calorie or sugar-free food products

malt·ose \ˈmȯl-ˌtōs, -ˌtōz\ *n* : a crystalline dextrorotatory sugar $C_{12}H_{22}O_{11}$ formed esp. from starch by amylase (as in saliva)

mal·union \ˌmal-ˈyün-yən\ *n* : incomplete or faulty union (as of the fragments of a fractured bone)

mam·ba \ˈmäm-bə, ˈmam-\ *n* : any of several venomous elapid snakes (genus *Dendroaspis*) of Africa

mamillary, mamillated, mamillothalamic tract *var of* MAMMILLARY, MAMMILLATED, MAMMILLOTHALAMIC TRACT

mamm- *or* **mamma-** *or* **mammi-** *or* **mammo-** *comb form* : breast ⟨*mammo*gram⟩

mam·ma \ˈma-mə\ *n, pl* **mam·mae** \ˈma-ˌmē, -ˌmī\ : a mammary gland and its accessory parts

mam·mal \ˈma-məl\ *n* : any of a class (Mammalia) of warm-blooded higher vertebrates (as dogs, cats, and humans) that nourish their young with milk secreted by mammary glands and have the skin more or less covered by hair — **mam·ma·li·an** \mə-ˈmā-lē-ən, ma-\ *adj or n*

mam·ma·plas·ty *or* **mam·mo·plas·ty** \ˈma-mə-ˌplas-tē\ *n, pl* **-ties** : plastic surgery of the breast

[1]**mam·ma·ry** \ˈma-mə-rē\ *adj* : of, relating to, lying near, or affecting the mammae

[2]**mammary** *n, pl* **-aries** : MAMMARY GLAND

mammary artery — see INTERNAL MAMMARY ARTERY

mammary gland *n* : any of the large compound sebaceous glands that in female mammals are modified to secrete milk, are situated ventrally in pairs, and usu. terminate in a nipple

mam·mil·la·ry *or* **mam·il·la·ry** \ˈma-mə-ˌler-ē, ma-ˈmi-lə-rē\ *adj* **1** : of, relating to, or resembling the breasts **2** : studded with breast-shaped protuberances

mammillary body *n* : either of two small rounded eminences on the underside of the brain behind the tuber cinereum

mam·mil·lat·ed *or* **mam·il·lat·ed** \ˈma-mə-ˌlā-təd\ *adj* **1** : having nipples or small protuberances **2** : having the form of a bluntly rounded protuberance

mam·mil·lo·tha·lam·ic tract *or* **ma·mil·lo·tha·lam·ic tract** \mə-ˌmi-lō-thə-ˈla-mik-\ *n* : a bundle of nerve fibers that runs from the mammillary body to the anterior nucleus of the thalamus — called also *mammillothalamic fasciculus*

mammo- — see MAMM-

mam·mo·gram \ˈma-mə-ˌgram\ *n* **1** : a photograph of the breasts made by X-rays **2** : the procedure for producing a mammogram

mam·mo·graph \-ˌgraf\ *n* : MAMMOGRAM 1

mam·mog·raph·er \ma-ˈmä-grə-fər\ *n* : a physician or radiological technologist who prepares and interprets mammograms

mam·mog·ra·phy \ma-ˈmä-grə-fē\ *n, pl* **-phies** : X-ray examination of the breasts (as for early detection of cancer) — **mam·mo·graph·ic** \ˌma-mə-ˈgra-fik\ *adj*

mammoplasty *var of* MAMMAPLASTY

mam·mo·tro·pin \ˌma-mə-ˈtrōp-ᵊn\ *n* : PROLACTIN

managed care *n* : a system of providing health care (as by an HMO or a PPO) that is designed to control costs through managed programs in which the physician accepts constraints on the amount charged for medical care and the patient is limited in the choice of a physician

managed care organization *n* : a company (as an HMO or PPO) offering health-care plans with cost controls using managed care — called also *MCO*

man·age·ment \ˈma-nij-mənt\ *n* : the whole system of care and treatment of a disease or a sick individual — **man·age** \ˈma-nij\ *vb*

Man·del·amine \man-ˈde-lə-mēn\ *trademark* — used for a preparation of the mandelate of methenamine

man·del·ate \ˈman-də-ˌlāt\ *n* : a salt or ester of mandelic acid

man·del·ic acid \man-ˈde-lik-\ *n* : an acid $C_8H_8O_3$ that is used chiefly in the form of its salts as a urinary antiseptic

man·di·ble \ˈman-də-bəl\ *n* **1** : JAW 1; *esp* : JAW 1b **2** : the lower jaw with its investing soft parts — **man·dib·u·lar** \man-ˈdi-byə-lər\ *adj*

mandibul- *or* **mandibuli-** *or* **mandibulo-** *comb form* : mandibular and ⟨*mandibulo*facial dysostosis⟩

mandibular arch *n* : the first branchial arch of the vertebrate embryo from which in humans are developed the lower lip, the mandible, the masticatory muscles, and the anterior part of the tongue

mandibular artery *n* : INFERIOR ALVEOLAR ARTERY

mandibular canal *n* : a bony canal within the mandible that gives passage to blood vessels and nerves supplying the lower teeth

mandibular foramen *n* : the opening on the medial surface of the ramus of the mandible that leads into the mandibular canal and transmits blood vessels and nerves supplying the lower teeth

mandibular fossa *n* : GLENOID FOSSA

mandibular nerve *n* : the one of the three major branches or divisions of the trigeminal nerve that supplies sensory fibers to the lower jaw, the floor of the mouth, the anterior two-thirds of the tongue, and the lower teeth and motor fibers to the muscles of mastication — called also *inferior maxillary nerve;* compare MAXILLARY NERVE, OPHTHALMIC NERVE

mandibular notch *n* : a curved depression on the upper border of the lower jaw between the coronoid process and the condyloid process — called also *sigmoid notch*

mandibuli-, mandibulo- — see MANDIBUL-

man·di·bu·lo·fa·cial dysostosis \man-ˌdi-byə-lō-ˈfā-shəl-\ *n* : a dysostosis of the face and lower jaw inherited as an autosomal dominant trait and characterized by bilateral malformations, deformities of the outer and middle ear, and a usu. smaller lower jaw — called also *Treacher Collins syndrome*

ma·neu·ver \mə-ˈnü-vər, -ˈnyü-\ *n* **1** : a movement, procedure, or method performed to achieve a desired result and esp. to restore a normal physiological state or to promote normal function — see HEIMLICH MANEUVER, VALSALVA MANEUVER **2** : a manipulation to accomplish a change of position; *specif* : rotational or other movement applied to a fetus within the uterus to alter its position and facilitate delivery — see SCANZONI MANEUVER

man·ga·nese \ˈmaŋ-gə-ˌnēz, -ˌnēs\ *n* : a grayish-white usu. hard and brittle metallic element — symbol *Mn;* see ELEMENT table

mange \ˈmānj\ *n* : any of various persistent contagious skin diseases that are marked esp. by eczematous inflammation and loss of hair, that affect domestic animals or sometimes humans, and that are caused by a minute parasitic mite of *Sarcoptes, Psoroptes, Chorioptes,* or related genera which burrows in or lives on the skin or by one of the genus *Demodex* which lives in the hair follicles or sebaceous glands — see CHORIOPTIC MANGE, DEMODECTIC MANGE, SARCOPTIC MANGE, SCABIES

mange mite *n* : any of the small parasitic mites that infest the skin of animals and cause mange

man·go fly \ˈmaŋ-gō-\ *n* : any of various horseflies of the genus *Chrysops* that are vectors of filarial worms

man·gy \ˈmān-jē\ *adj* **man·gi·er; -est** **1** : infected with mange ⟨a ~ dog⟩ **2** : relating to, characteristic of, or resulting from mange ⟨a ~ itch⟩

ma·nia \ˈmā-nē-ə, -nyə\ *n* : excitement of psychotic proportions manifested by mental and physical hyperactivity, disorganization of behavior, and elevation of mood; *specif* : the manic phase of bipolar disorder

ma·ni·a·cal \mə-ˈnī-ə-kəl\ *adj* : MANIC

[1]**man·ic** \ˈma-nik\ *adj* : affected with, relating to, or resembling mania — **man·i·cal·ly** *adv*

[2]**manic** *n* : an individual affected with mania

manic depression *n* : BIPOLAR DISORDER

[1]**manic–depressive** *adj* : characterized by or affected with either mania or depression or alternating mania and depression (as in bipolar disorder)

[2]**manic–depressive** *n* : a manic-depressive person

manic–depressive illness *n* : BIPOLAR DISORDER

manic–depressive psychosis *n* : BIPOLAR DISORDER

man·i·fes·ta·tion \ˌma-nə-fə-ˈstā-shən, -ˌfe-\ *n* : a perceptible, outward, or visible expression (as of a disease or abnormal condition)

manifest content *n* : the content of a dream as it is recalled by the dreamer in psychoanalysis — compare LATENT CONTENT

ma•nip•u•late \mə-ˈni-pyə-ˌlāt\ *vb* **-lat•ed; -lat•ing 1** : to treat or operate with the hands or by mechanical means esp. in a skillful manner **2** : to control or play upon by artful, unfair, or insidious means esp. to one's own advantage — **ma•nip•u•la•tive** \mə-ˈni-pyə-ˌlā-tiv, -lə-\ *adj* — **ma•nip•u•la•tive•ness** *n*

ma•nip•u•la•tion \mə-ˌni-pyə-ˈlā-shən\ *n* **1** : the act, process, or an instance of manipulating esp. a body part by manual examination and treatment; *esp* : adjustment of faulty structural relationships by manual means (as in the reduction of fractures or dislocations) **2** : the condition of being manipulated

man•ner•ism \ˈma-nə-ˌri-zəm\ *n* : a characteristic and often unconscious mode or peculiarity of action, bearing, or treatment; *esp* : any pointless and compulsive activity performed repeatedly

man•ni•tol \ˈma-nə-ˌtȯl, -ˌtōl\ *n* : a slightly sweet crystalline alcohol $C_6H_{14}O_6$ found in many plants and used esp. as a diuretic and in testing kidney function

mannitol hexa•ni•trate \-ˌhek-sə-ˈnī-ˌtrāt\ *n* : an explosive crystalline ester $C_6H_8(NO_3)_6$ made from mannitol and used mixed with a carbohydrate (as lactose) in the treatment of angina pectoris and vascular hypertension

man•nose \ˈma-ˌnōs, -ˌnōz\ *n* : an aldose $C_6H_{12}O_6$ found esp. in plants

man•nos•i•do•sis \mə-ˌnō-sə-ˈdō-səs\ *n, pl* **-do•ses** \-ˌsēz\ : a rare inherited metabolic disease characterized by deficiency of an enzyme catalyzing the metabolism of mannose with resulting accumulation of mannose in the body and marked esp. by facial and skeletal deformities and by intellectual disability

ma•noeu•vre *chiefly Brit var of* MANEUVER

ma•nom•e•ter \mə-ˈnä-mə-tər\ *n* **1** : an instrument for measuring the pressure of gases and vapors **2** : SPHYGMOMANOMETER — **mano•met•ric** \ˌma-nə-ˈme-trik\ *adj* — **mano•met•ri•cal•ly** *adv* — **ma•nom•e•try** \mə-ˈnä-mə-trē\ *n*

Man•son•el•la \ˌman-sə-ˈne-lə\ *n* : a genus of filarial worms (as *M. ozzardi*, *M. perstans*, and *M. streptocerca*) of Africa, So. America, and Central America that are parasitic in humans, are transmitted by biting midges and blackflies, and produce microfilariae which are found in the bloodstream and subcutaneous tissue

Man•son \ˈman-sən\, **Sir Patrick (1844–1922),** British parasitologist.

mansoni — see SCHISTOSOMIASIS MANSONI

Man•son's disease \ˈman-sənz-\ *n* : SCHISTOSOMIASIS MANSONI

man•tle \ˈmant-ᵊl\ *n* **1** : something that covers, enfolds, or envelops **2** : CEREBRAL CORTEX

Man•toux test \ˌman-ˈtü-, ˌmäⁿ-\ *n* : an intradermal test for hypersensitivity to tuberculin that indicates past or present infection with tubercle bacilli — see TUBERCULIN TEST

Mantoux, Charles (1877–1947), French physician.

ma•nu•bri•um \mə-ˈnü-brē-əm, -ˈnyü-\ *n, pl* **-bria** \-brē-ə\ *also* **-bri•ums** : an anatomical process or part shaped like a handle: as **a** : the uppermost segment of the sternum that is a somewhat triangular flattened bone with anterolateral borders which articulate with the clavicles **b** : the process of the malleus of the ear

ma•nus \ˈmā-nəs, ˈmä-\ *n, pl* **ma•nus** \-nəs, -ˌnüs\ : the segment of the vertebrate forelimb from the carpus to the distal end

MAO *abbr* monoamine oxidase

MAOI *abbr* monoamine oxidase inhibitor

MAO inhibitor \ˈem-ˈā-ˈō-\ *n* : MONOAMINE OXIDASE INHIBITOR

[1]**map** \ˈmap\ *n* : the arrangement of genes on a chromosome — called also *genetic map*

[2]**map** *vb* **mapped; map•ping 1** : to locate (a gene) on a chromosome **2** *of a gene* : to be located ⟨the mutated locus ~*s* to chromosome 7⟩

maple syrup urine disease *n* : a disorder of amino acid metabolism that is inherited as an autosomal recessive trait, is caused by a deficiency of decarboxylase resulting in high concentrations of certain amino acids (as valine and leucine) in the body, is characterized initially by a maple syrup odor in the urine and earwax and by vomiting, fatigue, irritability, and hypertonicity, and that unless treated with dietary measures leads to seizures, brain damage, coma, and death

ma•pro•ti•line \mə-ˈprō-tə-ˌlēn\ *n* : an antidepressant drug used in the form of its hydrochloride $C_{20}H_{23}N·HCl$ to relieve major depression (as in bipolar disorder) and anxiety associated with depression

ma•ras•mus \mə-ˈraz-məs\ *n* : severe malnutrition affecting infants and children esp. of impoverished regions that is characterized by poor growth, loss of subcutaneous fat, muscle atrophy, apathy, and pronounced weight loss and is usu. caused by a diet deficient in calories and proteins but sometimes by disease (as dysentery or giardiasis) — **ma•ras•mic** \-mik\ *adj*

marble bone disease *n* : OSTEOPETROSIS

Mar•burg hemorrhagic fever \ˈmär-bərg-\ *n* : an often fatal hemorrhagic fever that is caused by the Marburg virus, is an acute febrile illness often progressing to severe hemorrhaging, is spread esp. by contact with the body fluids (as blood or saliva) of infected individuals, and was orig. reported in humans infected by green monkeys — called also *green monkey disease, Marburg disease, Marburg fever, Marburg virus disease*

Marburg virus *n* : a filovirus (species *Lake Victoria marburgvirus* of the genus *Marburgvirus*) that causes Marburg hemorrhagic fever

march \ˈmärch\ *n* : the progression of epileptic activity through the motor centers of the cerebral cortex that is manifested in localized convulsions in first one and then an adjacent part of the body

Mar•ek's disease \ˈmar-iks-\ *n* : a highly contagious virus disease of poultry that is caused by either of two herpesviruses (species *Gallid herpesvirus 2* and *Gallid herpesvirus 3* of the genus *Mardivirus*)

Marek, Jozsef (1867–1952), Hungarian veterinarian.

Ma•rey's law \mə-ˈrāz-\ *n* : a statement in physiology: heart rate is related inversely to arterial blood pressure

Marey, Étienne–Jules (1830–1904), French physiologist.

Mar•e•zine \ˈmar-ə-ˌzēn\ *n* : a preparation of the hydrochloride of cyclizine — formerly a U.S. registered trademark

mar•fa•noid \ˈmär-fə-ˌnȯid\ *adj* : exhibiting the typical characteristics of Marfan syndrome ⟨~ habitus⟩

Mar•fan syndrome \ˈmär-ˌfan-\ *or* **Mar•fan's syndrome** \-ˌfanz-\ *n* : a disorder of connective tissue that is inherited as a simple dominant trait, is caused by a defect in the gene controlling the production of fibrillin, and is characterized by abnormal elongation of the long bones and often by ocular and circulatory defects

Marfan \mär-ˈfäⁿ\, **Antonin Bernard Jean (1858–1942),** French pediatrician.

mar•gin \ˈmär-jən\ *n* **1** : the outside limit or edge of something (as a bodily part or a wound) **2** : the part of consciousness at a particular moment that is felt only vaguely and dimly — **mar•gin•al** \ˈmär-jə-nəl\ *adj*

mar•gin•ation \ˌmär-jə-ˈnā-shən\ *n* **1** : the act or process of forming a margin; *specif* : the adhesion of white blood cells to the walls of damaged blood vessels **2** : the action of finishing a dental restoration or a filling for a cavity

Ma•rie–Strüm•pell disease *also* **Ma•rie–Strüm•pell's disease** \mä-ˈrē-ˈstrüm-pəl(z)-\ *n* : ANKYLOSING SPONDYLITIS

Marie, Pierre (1853–1940), French neurologist.

Strümpell \ˈshtruem-pəl\, **Ernst Adolf Gustav Gottfried von (1853–1925),** German neurologist.

mar•i•jua•na *also* **mar•i•hua•na** \ˌmar-ə-ˈwä-nə, -ˈhwä-\ *n* **1** : HEMP 1 **2** : the dried leaves and flowering tops of the hemp plant that yield THC and are typically smoked for their intoxicating effect — compare BHANG, CANNABIS, HASHISH

Mar•i•nol \ˈmar-ə-ˌnȯl\ *trademark* — used for a preparation of dronabinol

mark \ˈmärk\ *n* : an impression or trace made or occurring on something — see BIRTHMARK, STRAWBERRY MARK

mark•er \ˈmär-kər\ *n* : something that serves to identify, predict, or characterize: as **a** : BIOMARKER **b** : GENETIC MARKER — called also *marker gene*

Mar•o•teaux–La•my syndrome \mär-ō-ˈtō-lä-ˈmē-\ *n* : a mucopolysaccharidosis that is inherited as an autosomal recessive trait and that is similar to Hurler syndrome except that intellectual development is not retarded

Maroteaux, Pierre (*b* 1926), French physician.

Lamy, Maurice Emile Joseph (1895–1975), French physician.

Mar•plan \ˈmär-ˌplan\ *trademark* — used for a preparation of isocarboxazid

mar•riage counseling \ˈmer-ij-, ˈma-rij-\ *n* : counseling for married and unmarried couples designed to address problems in their relationship : COUPLES THERAPY — **marriage counselor** *n*

mar•row \ˈmar-(ˌ)ō\ *n* **1** : BONE MARROW **2** : the substance of the spinal cord

Mar•seilles fever \mär-ˈsā-\ *n* : BOUTONNEUSE FEVER

mar•su•pi•al•ize \mär-ˈsü-pē-ə-ˌlīz\ *vb* **-ized; -iz•ing** : to open (as the bladder or a cyst) and sew by the edges to the abdominal wound to permit further treatment (as of an enclosed tumor) or to discharge pathological matter (as from a hydatid cyst) — **mar•su•pi•al•i•za•tion** \-ˌsü-pē-ə-li-ˈzā-shən\ *n*

mas•cu•line \ˈmas-kyə-lən\ *adj* **1** : MALE **2** : having the qualities distinctive of or appropriate to a male — **mas•cu•lin•i•ty** \ˌmas-kyə-ˈli-nə tē\ *n*

mas•cu•lin•ize \ˈmas-kyə-lə-ˌnīz\ *vb* **-ized; -iz•ing** : to give a preponderantly masculine character to; *esp* : to cause (a female) to take on male characteristics — **mas•cu•lin•i•za•tion** \ˌmas-kyə-lə-nə-ˈzā-shən\ *n*

MASH *abbr* mobile army surgical hospital

¹mask \ˈmask\ *n* **1** : a protective covering for the face **2 a** : any of various devices that cover the mouth and nose and are used to prevent inhalation of dangerous substances, to facilitate delivery of a gas, or to prevent the dispersal of exhaled infective material — see GAS MASK, OXYGEN MASK **b** : a cosmetic preparation for the skin of the face that produces a tightening effect as it dries

²mask *vb* **1** : to modify or reduce the effect or activity of (as a process or a reaction) **2** : to raise the audibility

threshold of (a sound) by the simultaneous presentation of another sound
masked *adj* : failing to present or produce the usual symptoms : not obvious : LATENT ⟨a ~ fever⟩
mas•och•ism \ˈma-sə-ˌki-zəm, ˈma-zə-, ˈmā-sə-\ *n* : a sexual perversion characterized by pleasure in being subjected to pain or humiliation esp. by a love object — compare ALGOLAGNIA, SADISM — **mas•och•is•tic** \ˌma-sə-ˈkis-tik, ˌma-zə-, ˌmā-sə-\ *adj* — **mas•och•is•ti•cal•ly** *adv*

Sa•cher–Ma•soch \ˈzä-k̲ər-ˈmä-zȯk̲\, **Leopold von (1836–1895),** Austrian novelist.

mas•och•ist \-kist\ *n* : an individual who is given to masochism
mass \ˈmas\ *n* **1** : the property of a body that is a measure of its inertia, that is commonly taken as a measure of the amount of material it contains and causes it to have weight in a gravitational field **2** : a homogeneous pasty mixture compounded for making pills, lozenges, and plasters
mas•sage \mə-ˈsäzh, -ˈsäj\ *n* : manipulation of tissues (as by rubbing, stroking, kneading, or tapping) with the hand or an instrument for therapeutic purposes — **massage** *vb*
mas•sa in•ter•me•dia \ˈma-sə-ˌin-tər-ˈmē-dē-ə\ *n* : an apparently functionless mass of gray matter in the midline of the third ventricle that is found in many but not all human brains and is formed when the surfaces of the thalami protruding inward from opposite sides of the third ventricle make contact and fuse
mas•sa•sau•ga \ˌma-sə-ˈsȯ-gə\ *n* : a No. American rattlesnake of the genus *Sistrurus* (*S. catenatus*)
mas•se•ter \mə-ˈsē-tər, ma-\ *n* : a large muscle that raises the lower jaw and assists in mastication, arises from the zygomatic arch and the zygomatic process of the temporal bone, and is inserted into the mandibular ramus and gonial angle — **mas•se•ter•ic** \ˌma-sə-ˈter-ik\ *adj*
mas•seur \ma-ˈsər, mə-\ *n* : a man who practices massage
mas•seuse \-ˈsərz, -ˈsüz\ *n* : a person who practices massage — usu. used of a woman
mas•sive \ˈma-siv\ *adj* **1** : large in comparison to what is typical — used esp. of medical dosage or of an infective agent ⟨a ~ dose of penicillin⟩ **2** : being extensive and severe — used of a pathologic condition ⟨a ~ hemorrhage⟩
mass number *n* : an integer that approximates the mass of an isotope and designates the total number of protons and neutrons in the nucleus ⟨the symbol for carbon of *mass number* 14 is ^{14}C or C^{14}⟩
mas•so•ther•a•py \ˌma-sō-ˈther-ə-pē\ *n, pl* **-pies** : the practice of therapeutic massage
mass spectrometry *n* : an instrumental method for identifying the chemical constitution of a substance by means of the separation of gaseous ions according to their differing mass and charge — **mass spectrometer** *n* — **mass spectrometric** *adj*
mass spectroscopy *n* : MASS SPECTROMETRY — **mass spectroscope** *n* — **mass spectroscopic** *adj*
mast- *or* **masto-** *comb form* : breast : nipple : mammary gland ⟨*mast*itis⟩
Mas•tad•e•no•vi•rus \ma-ˈsta-də-nō-ˌvī-rəs\ *n* : a genus of adenoviruses that include the causative agents of epidemic keratoconjunctivitis and pharyngoconjunctival fever
mas•tal•gia \mas-ˈtal-jə\ *n* : MASTODYNIA
mast cell \ˈmast-\ *n* : a large cell that occurs esp. in connective tissue and has basophilic granules containing substances (as histamine and heparin) which mediate allergic reactions
mas•tec•to•mee \ma-ˌstek-tə-ˈmē\ *n* : a person who has had a mastectomy
mas•tec•to•my \ma-ˈstek-tə-mē\ *n, pl* **-mies** : surgical removal of all or part of the breast and sometimes associated lymph nodes and muscles
master gland *n* : PITUITARY GLAND
-mas•tia \ˈmas-tē-ə\ *n comb form* : condition of having (such or so many) breasts or mammary glands ⟨gyneco*mastia*⟩
mas•ti•cate \ˈmas-tə-ˌkāt\ *vb* **-cat•ed; -cat•ing** **1** : to grind, crush, and chew (food) with or as if with the teeth in preparation for swallowing **2** : to soften or reduce to pulp by crushing or kneading — **mas•ti•ca•tion** \ˌmas-tə-ˈkā-shən\ *n* — **mas•ti•ca•to•ry** \ˈmas-ti-kə-ˌtōr-ē\ *adj*
mas•ti•tis \ma-ˈstī-təs\ *n, pl* **-tit•i•des** \-ˈti-tə-ˌdēz\ : inflammation of the mammary gland or udder usu. caused by infection — **mas•tit•ic** \ma-ˈsti-tik\ *adj*
masto- — see MAST-
mas•to•cy•to•ma \ˌmas-tə-ˌsī-ˈtō-mə\ *n, pl* **-mas** *also* **-ma•ta** \-mə-tə\ : a tumorous mass produced by proliferation of mast cells
mas•to•cy•to•sis \-ˈtō-səs\ *n, pl* **-to•ses** \-ˌsēz\ : excessive proliferation of mast cells in the tissues; *specif* : a rare variable disorder marked by the abnormal proliferation and accumulation of mast cells in the skin, bone marrow, or internal organs
mas•to•dyn•ia \ˌmas-tə-ˈdī-nē-ə\ *n* : pain in the breast — called also *mastalgia*
[1]mas•toid \ˈmas-ˌtȯid\ *adj* : of, relating to, or being the mastoid process; *also* : occurring in the region of the mastoid process
[2]mastoid *n* : a mastoid bone or process
mastoid air cell *n* : MASTOID CELL
mastoid antrum *n* : TYMPANIC ANTRUM
mastoid cell *n* : one of the small cavities in the mastoid process that develop after birth and are filled with air — called also *mastoid air cell*

mas•toid•ec•to•my \ˌmas-ˌtȯi-ˈdek-tə-mē\ *n, pl* **-mies** : surgical removal of the mastoid cells or of the mastoid process of the temporal bone

mas•toid•itis \ˌmas-ˌtȯi-ˈdī-təs\ *n, pl* **-it•i•des** \-ˈdi-tə-ˌdēz\ : inflammation of the mastoid and esp. of the mastoid cells

mas•toid•ot•o•my \ˌmas-ˌtȯi-ˈdä-tə-mē\ *n, pl* **-mies** : incision of the mastoid

mastoid process *n* : the process of the temporal bone behind the ear that is well developed and of somewhat conical form in adults but inconspicuous in children

mas•top•a•thy \ma-ˈstä-pə-thē\ *n, pl* **-thies** : a disorder of the breast; *esp* : a painful disorder of the breast

mas•to•pexy \ˈmas-tō-ˌpek-sē\ *n, pl* **-pex•ies** : BREAST LIFT

mas•tot•o•my \ma-ˈstä-tə-mē\ *n, pl* **-mies** : incision of the breast

mas•tur•ba•tion \ˌmas-tər-ˈbā-shən\ *n* : erotic stimulation esp. of one's own genital organs commonly resulting in orgasm and achieved by manual or other bodily contact exclusive of sexual intercourse, by instrumental manipulation, occas. by sexual fantasies, or by various combinations of these agencies — **mas•tur•bate** \ˈmas-tər-ˌbāt\ *vb* — **mas•tur•ba•tor** \-ˌbā-tər\ *n*

mas•tur•ba•tory \ˈmas-tər-bə-ˌtōr-ē\ *adj* : of, relating to, or associated with masturbation ⟨~ fantasies⟩

mate \ˈmāt\ *vb* **mat•ed; mat•ing** **1** : to pair or join for breeding **2** : COPULATE

ma•te•ria al•ba \mə-ˈtir-ē-ə-ˈal-bə\ *n pl* : a soft whitish deposit of epithelial cells, white blood cells, and microorganisms esp. at the gumline

materia med•i•ca \-ˈme-di-kə\ *n* **1** : substances used in the composition of medical remedies : DRUGS, MEDICINE **2 a** : a branch of medical science that deals with the sources, nature, properties, and preparation of drugs **b** : a treatise on materia medica

ma•ter•nal \mə-ˈtərn-ᵊl\ *adj* **1** : of, relating to, belonging to, or characteristic of a mother ⟨~ instinct⟩ **2 a** : related through a mother **b** : inherited or derived from the female parent ⟨~ genes⟩ — **ma•ter•nal•ly** *adv*

maternal inheritance *n* : inheritance of characters transmitted through extranuclear elements (as mitochondrial DNA) in the cytoplasm of the egg

maternal rubella *n* : German measles in a pregnant woman that may cause developmental anomalies in the fetus when occurring during the first trimester

¹ma•ter•ni•ty \mə-ˈtər-nə-tē\ *n, pl* **-ties** : a hospital facility designed for the care of women before and during childbirth and for the care of newborn babies

²maternity *adj* **1** : being or providing care during and immediately before and after childbirth ⟨a ~ unit⟩ **2** : designed for wear during pregnancy **3** : effective for the period close to and including childbirth ⟨~ leave⟩

ma•ter•no•fe•tal \me-ˌtər-nō-ˈfēt-ᵊl\ *adj* : involving a fetus and its mother ⟨the human ~ interface⟩; *also* : passing or transferred from the mother to the fetus ⟨~ transmission of HIV⟩

ma•trix \ˈmā-triks\ *n, pl* **ma•tri•ces** \ˈmā-trə-ˌsēz, ˈma-\ *or* **matrixes** **1 a** : the extracellular substance in which tissue cells (as of connective tissue) are embedded **b** : the thickened epithelium at the base of a fingernail or toenail from which new nail substance develops — called also *nail bed, nail matrix* **2** : a mass by which something is enclosed or in which something is embedded **3 a** : a strip or band placed so as to serve as a retaining outer wall of a tooth in filling a cavity **b** : a metal or porcelain pattern in which an inlay is cast or fused

mat•ter \ˈma-tər\ *n* **1** : material (as feces or urine) discharged or for discharge from the living body **2** : material discharged by suppuration : PUS

mattress suture *n* : a surgical stitch in which the suture is passed back and forth through both edges of a wound so that the needle is reinserted each time on the side of exit and passes through to the side of insertion

mat•u•rate \ˈma-chə-ˌrāt\ *vb* **-rat•ed; -rat•ing** : MATURE

mat•u•ra•tion \ˌma-chə-ˈrā-shən\ *n* **1 a** : the process of becoming mature **b** : the emergence of personal and behavioral characteristics through growth processes **c** : the final stages of differentiation of cells, tissues, or organs **d** : the achievement of intellectual or emotional maturity **2 a** : the entire process by which diploid gamete-producing cells are transformed into haploid gametes that includes both meiosis and physiological and structural changes fitting the gamete for its future role **b** : SPERMIOGENESIS 2 — **mat•u•ra•tion•al** \ˌma-chə-ˈrā-shə-nəl\ *adj*

maturation promoting factor *n* : a protein complex that in its active form causes eukaryotic cells to undergo mitosis

ma•ture \mə-ˈtu̇r, -ˈtyu̇r, -ˈchu̇r\ *adj* **ma•tur•er; -est** **1** : having completed natural growth and development ⟨a ~ ovary⟩ **2** : having undergone maturation ⟨~ germ cells⟩ — **mature** *vb*

ma•tu•ri•ty \mə-ˈtu̇r-ə-tē, -ˈtyu̇r-, -ˈchu̇r-\ *n, pl* **-ties** : the quality or state of being mature; *esp* : full development

maturity–onset diabetes *n* : TYPE 2 DIABETES

maturity–onset diabetes of the young *n* : type 2 diabetes of a relatively mild form that is inherited as an autosomal dominant trait and occurs in late adolescence or early adulthood — abbr. *MODY*

Ma•vik \ˈmä-vik\ *trademark* — used for a preparation of trandolapril

max *abbr* maximum

maxill- *or* **maxilli-** *or* **maxillo-** *comb form* **1** : maxilla ⟨*maxill*ectomy⟩ **2** : maxillary and ⟨*maxillo*facial⟩

max•il•la \mak-ˈsi-lə\ *n, pl* **max•il•lae** \-ˈsi-(ˌ)lē, -ˌlī\ *or* **maxillas** **1** : JAW 1a **2 a** : an upper jaw esp. of humans or other mammals in which the bony elements are closely fused **b** : either of two membrane bone elements of the upper jaw that lie lateral to the premaxillae and bear most of the teeth

[1]**max•il•lary** \ˈmak-sə-ˌler-ē\ *adj* : of, relating to, being, or associated with a maxilla ⟨∼ blood vessels⟩

[2]**maxillary** *n, pl* **-lar•ies** **1** : MAXILLA 2b **2** : a maxillary part (as a nerve or blood vessel)

maxillary air sinus *n* : MAXILLARY SINUS

maxillary artery *n* : an artery supplying the deep structures of the face (as the nasal cavities, palate, tonsils, and pharynx) and sending a branch to the meninges of the brain — called also *internal maxillary artery;* compare FACIAL ARTERY

maxillary bone *n* : MAXILLA 2b

maxillary nerve *n* : the one of the three major branches or divisions of the trigeminal nerve that supplies sensory fibers to the skin areas of the middle part of the face, the upper jaw and its teeth, and the mucous membranes of the palate, nasal cavities, and nasopharynx — called also *maxillary division;* compare MANDIBULAR NERVE, OPHTHALMIC NERVE

maxillary process *n* : a triangular embryonic process that grows out from the dorsal end of the mandibular arch on each side and forms the lateral part of the upper lip, the cheek, and the upper jaw except the premaxilla

maxillary sinus *n* : an air cavity in the body of the maxilla that communicates with the middle meatus of the nose — called also *antrum of Highmore*

maxillary vein *n* : a short venous trunk of the face that is formed by the union of veins from the pterygoid plexus and that joins with the superficial temporal vein to form a vein which contributes to the formation of the external jugular vein

max•il•lec•to•my \ˌmak-sə-ˈlek-tə-mē\ *n, pl* **-mies** : surgical removal of the maxilla

maxilli-, maxillo- — see MAXILL-

max•il•lo•fa•cial \mak-ˌsi-(ˌ)lō-ˈfā-shəl, ˌmak-sə-(ˌ)lō-\ *adj* : of, relating to, treating, or affecting the maxilla and the face ⟨∼ lesions⟩

max•i•mal \ˈmak-sə-məl\ *adj* **1** : most complete or effective ⟨∼ vasodilation⟩ **2** : being an upper limit — **max•i•mal•ly** *adv*

maximal oxygen consumption *or* **maximum oxygen consumption** *n* : VO_2 MAX

maximal oxygen uptake *or* **maximum oxygen uptake** *n* : VO_2 MAX

max•i•mum \ˈmak-sə-məm\ *n, pl* **max•i•ma** \-sə-mə\ *or* **maximums** **1 a** : the greatest quantity or value attainable or attained **b** : the period of highest, greatest, or utmost development **2** : an upper limit allowed (as by a legal authority) or allowable (as by the circumstances of a particular case) — **maximum** *adj*

maximum heart rate *n* : the age-related number of beats per minute of the heart when working at its maximum that is usu. estimated as 220 minus one's age

maximum permissible concentration *n* : the maximum concentration of radioactive material in body tissue that is regarded as acceptable and not producing significant deleterious effects on the human organism — abbr. *MPC*

maximum permissible dose *n* : the amount of ionizing radiation a person may be exposed to supposedly without being harmed

max VO_2 *n* : VO_2 MAX

Max•zide \ˈmaks-ˌzīd\ *trademark* — used for a preparation of triamterene and hydrochlorothiazide

may•ap•ple \ˈmā-ˌap-ᵊl\ *n, often cap* : a No. American herb of the genus *Podophyllum* (*P. peltatum*) having a poisonous rootstock and rootlets that are a source of the drug podophyllum

Ma•ya•ro virus \mä-ˈyä-rō-\ *n* : a virus of the genus *Alphavirus* (species *Mayaro virus*) that is found in tropical So. America, is transmitted by mosquitoes, and is the causative agent of an acute illness marked chiefly by fever, joint pain, and rash

May•er–Ro•ki•tan•sky–Kü•ster–Hau•ser syndrome \ˈmī-ər-ˌrō-kə-ˈtän-skē-ˈkes-tər-ˈhau̇-zər-\ *n* : a congenital disorder that is marked esp. by absence of the vagina, primary amenorrhea, absent or rudimentary uterus, and morphologically normal ovaries and external genitalia and that results from arrested development of the Müllerian ducts during early embryogenesis — called also *Mayer-Rokitansky syndrome, MRKH syndrome, Müllerian agenesis*

Mayer, August Franz Josef Karl (1787–1865), German anatomist and physiologist.

Rokitansky, Karl Freiherr von (1804–1878), Austrian pathologist.

Küster, Hermann (*fl* 1910), German gynecologist.

Hauser, Georges A. (*fl* 1961), Swiss gynecologist.

may•hem \ˈmā-ˌhem, ˈmā-əm\ *n* : willful and permanent crippling, mutilation, or disfiguring of any part of another's body; *also* : the crime of engaging in mayhem

may•tan•sine \ˈmā-ˌtan-ˌsēn\ *n* : an antineoplastic agent $C_{34}H_{46}ClN_3O_{10}$ isolated from any of several tropical shrubs and trees (genus *Maytenus* of the family Celastraceae)

maz- *or* **mazo-** *comb form* : breast ⟨*mazo*plasia⟩

ma•zin•dol \ˈmā-zin-ˌdōl\ *n* : an adrenergic drug $C_{16}H_{13}ClN_2O$ used as an appetite suppressant

ma•zo•pla•sia \ˌmā-zə-ˈplā-zhə, -zhē-ə\ *n* : a degenerative condition of breast tissue

Maz•zi•ni test \mə-ˈzē-nē-\ *n* : a flocculation test for the diagnosis of syphilis
Mazzini, Louis Yolando (1894–1973), American serologist.

MB *abbr* [New Latin *medicinae baccalaureus*] bachelor of medicine

M band \ˈem-ˌband\ *n* : M LINE

MBD *abbr* minimal brain dysfunction

mc *abbr* millicurie

MC *abbr* **1** medical corps **2** [New Latin *magister chirurgiae*] master of surgery

Mc•Ar•dle's disease \mə-ˈkärd-ᵊlz-\ *n* : a glycogen storage disease that is inherited as an autosomal recessive trait, is marked esp. by muscle weakness and myoglobinuria, and is caused by a deficiency of muscle phosphorylase — called also *McArdle's syndrome*
McArdle, Brian (1911–2002), British physician.

MCAT *abbr* Medical College Admissions Test

Mc•Bur•ney's point \mək-ˈbər-nēz-\ *n* : a point on the abdominal wall that lies between the navel and the right anterior superior iliac spine and that is the point where most pain is elicited by pressure in acute appendicitis
McBurney, Charles (1845–1913), American surgeon.

mcg *abbr* microgram

MCh *abbr* [New Latin *magister chirurgiae*] master of surgery

MCH *abbr* **1** maternal and child health **2** mean corpuscular hemoglobin (concentration)

MCHC *abbr* mean corpuscular hemoglobin concentration

mCi *abbr* millicurie

MCI *abbr* mild cognitive impairment

MCL \ˌem-ˌsē-ˈel\ *n* : MEDIAL COLLATERAL LIGAMENT

MCO \ˌem-ˌsē-ˈō\ *n* : MANAGED CARE ORGANIZATION

M–CSF *abbr* macrophage colony-stimulating factor

MCV *abbr* mean corpuscular volume

Md *symbol* mendelevium

MD \ˌem-ˈdē\ *n* **1** [Latin *medicinae doctor*] : an earned academic degree conferring the rank and title of doctor of medicine **2** : a person who has a doctor of medicine

MD *abbr* muscular dystrophy

MDA \ˌem-ˌdē-ˈā\ *n* : a synthetic amphetamine derivative $C_{10}H_{13}NO_2$ used illicitly for its mood-enhancing and hallucinogenic properties — called also *methylenedioxyamphetamine*

MDI *abbr* metered-dose inhaler

MDMA \ˌem-(ˌ)dē-(ˌ)em-ˈā\ *n* : ECSTASY 2

MDPV \ˌem-ˌdē-ˌpē-ˈvē\ *n* : a synthetic compound $C_{16}H_{21}NO_3$ that is an analog of cathinone and is used illicitly as a stimulant with effects similar to those of cocaine — called also *methylenedioxypyrovalerone*

MDR *abbr* **1** minimum daily requirement **2** multidrug resistance; multidrug-resistant

MDS *abbr* master of dental surgery

ME *abbr* medical examiner

meadow mushroom *n* : a common edible brown-spored mushroom (*Agaricus campestris*) that occurs naturally in moist open organically rich soil

mean corpuscular hemoglobin concentration *n* : the number of grams of hemoglobin per unit volume and usu. 100 milliliters of packed red blood cells that is found by multiplying the number of grams of hemoglobin per unit volume of the original blood sample of whole blood by 100 and dividing by the hematocrit — abbr. *MCHC*

mean corpuscular volume *n* : the volume of the average red blood cell in a given blood sample that is found by multiplying the hematocrit by 10 and dividing by the estimated number of red blood cells — abbr. *MCV*

mea•sle \ˈmē-zəl\ *n* : CYSTICERCUS; *specif* : one found in the muscles of a domesticated mammal

mea•sles \ˈmē-zəlz\ *n sing or pl* **1 a** : an acute contagious disease that is caused by a paramyxovirus of the genus *Morbillivirus* (species *Measles virus*), that commences with catarrhal symptoms, conjunctivitis, cough, and Koplik's spots on the oral mucous membrane, and that is marked by the appearance on the third or fourth day of an eruption of distinct red circular spots which coalesce in a crescentic form, are slightly raised, and after the fourth day of the eruption gradually decline — called also *rubeola* **b** : any of various eruptive diseases (as German measles) **2** : infestation with or disease caused by larval tapeworms in the muscles and tissues; *specif* : infestation of cattle and swine with cysticerci of tapeworms that as adults parasitize humans

mea•sly \ˈmē-zə-lē, ˈmēz-lē\ *adj* **mea•sli•er; -est 1** : infected with measles **2 a** : containing larval tapeworms **b** : infected with trichinae

meat- *or* **meato-** *comb form* : meatus ⟨*meato*plasty⟩

me•a•tal \mē-ˈāt-ᵊl\ *adj* : of, relating to, or forming a meatus

me•ato•plas•ty \mē-ˈa-tə-ˌplast-ē\ *n, pl* **-ties** : plastic surgery of a meatus

me•a•tot•o•my \ˌmē-ə-ˈtä-tə-mē\ *n, pl* **-mies** : incision of the urethral meatus esp. to enlarge it

me•atus \mē-ˈā-təs\ *n, pl* **me•atus•es** \-tə-səz\ *or* **me•atus** \-ˈā-təs, -ˌtüs\ : a natural body passage : CANAL, DUCT

me•ban•a•zine \me-ˈba-nə-ˌzēn\ *n* : a monoamine oxidase inhibitor $C_8H_{12}N_2$ used as an antidepressant

Meb•a•ral \ˈme-bə-ˌral\ *trademark* — used for a preparation of mephobarbital

me•ben•da•zole \me-ˈben-də-ˌzōl\ *n* : a broad-spectrum anthelmintic agent $C_{16}H_{13}N_3O_3$

me•bu•ta•mate \me-ˈbyü-tə-ˌmāt\ *n* : a central nervous system depressant $C_{10}H_{20}N_2O_4$ used to treat mild hypertension

mec•a•myl•a•mine \ˌme-kə-ˈmi-lə-ˌmēn\ *n* : a drug administered orally in the form of its hydrochloride $C_{11}H_{21}N{\cdot}HCl$ as a ganglionic blocking agent to effect a rapid lowering of severely elevated blood pressure

me•chan•i•cal \mi-ˈka-ni-kəl\ *adj* : caused by, resulting from, or relating to physical as opposed to biological or chemical processes or change ⟨~ injury⟩ ⟨~ asphyxiation⟩ — **me•chan•i•cal•ly** *adv*

mechanical heart *n* : a mechanism designed to maintain the flow of blood to the tissues of the body esp. during a surgical operation on the heart; *also* : an artificial heart

mechanical ventilation *n* : artificial ventilation of the lungs (as by positive end-expiratory pressure) using means external to the body

mech•a•nism \ˈme-kə-ˌni-zəm\ *n* **1** : a piece of machinery **2 a** : a bodily process or function ⟨the ~ of healing⟩ **b** : the combination of mental processes by which a result is obtained ⟨psychological ~*s*⟩ **3** : the fundamental physical or chemical processes involved in or responsible for an action, reaction, or other natural phenomenon — **mech•a•nis•tic** \ˌme-kə-ˈnis-tik\ *adj*

mech•a•no•chem•is•try \ˌme-kə-nō-ˈke-mə-strē\ *n, pl* **-tries** : chemistry dealing with the conversion of chemical energy into mechanical work (as in muscle contraction) — **mech•a•no•chem•i•cal** \-ˈke-mi-kəl\ *adj*

mech•a•no•re•cep•tor \-ri-ˈsep-tər\ *n* : a neural end organ (as a Pacinian corpuscle) that responds to a mechanical stimulus (as a change in pressure) — **mech•a•no•re•cep•tion** \-ˈsep-shən\ *n* — **mech•a•no•re•cep•tive** \-ˈsep-tiv\ *adj*

mech•a•no•sen•so•ry \-ˈsen-sə-rē\ *adj* : of, relating to, or functioning in the sensing of mechanical stimuli (as pressure or vibration) ⟨~ neurons⟩

mech•lor•eth•amine \ˌme-ˌklōr-ˈe-thə-ˌmēn\ *n* : a nitrogen mustard administered by injection in the form of its hydrochloride $C_5H_{11}Cl_2N{\cdot}HCl$ in the palliative treatment of neoplastic diseases (as Hodgkin's lymphoma) — see BENDAMUSTINE, MOPP

mech•o•lyl \ˈme-kə-ˌlil\ *n* : a preparation of the chloride of methacholine

Me•cis•to•cir•rus \mə-ˌsis-tō-ˈsir-əs\ *n* : a genus of nematode worms (family Trichostrongylidae) including a common parasite (*M. digitatus*) of the stomach of domesticated ruminants and swine

Meck•el–Gru•ber syndrome \ˈme-kəl-ˈgrü-bər-\ *n* : a syndrome inherited as an autosomal recessive trait and typically characterized by occipital encephalocele, microcephaly, cleft palate, polydactyly, and polycystic kidneys — called also *Meckel's syndrome*

Meckel, Johann Friedrich, the Younger (1781–1833), German anatomist.

Gruber, Georg Benno Otto (1884–1977), German pathologist.

Meck•el's cartilage \ˈme-kəlz-\ *n* : the cartilaginous bar of the embryonic mandibular arch of which the distal end ossifies to form the malleus

J. F. Meckel the Younger — see MECKEL-GRUBER SYNDROME

Meckel's diverticulum *n* : the proximal part of the omphalomesenteric duct when persistent as a blind fibrous tube connected with the lower ileum

J. F. Meckel the Younger — see MECKEL-GRUBER SYNDROME

Meckel's ganglion *n* : PTERYGOPALATINE GANGLION

Meckel, Johann Friedrich, the Elder (1724–1774), German anatomist.

mec•li•zine \ˈme-klə-ˌzēn\ *n* : a drug used usu. in the form of its hydrated hydrochloride $C_{25}H_{27}ClN_2{\cdot}2HCl{\cdot}H_2O$ to treat nausea and vertigo — see ANTIVERT, BONINE

mec•lo•fen•a•mate sodium \ˌme-klō-ˈfe-nə-ˌmāt-\ *n* : a mild analgesic and anti-inflammatory drug $C_{14}H_{10}Cl_2NNaO_2{\cdot}H_2O$ used orally to treat rheumatoid arthritis and osteoarthritis — called also *meclofenamate*

mec•lo•zine \ˈme-klō-ˌzēn\ *Brit var of* MECLIZINE

me•co•ni•um \mi-ˈkō-nē-əm\ *n* : a dark greenish mass of desquamated cells, mucus, and bile that accumulates in the bowel of a fetus and is typically discharged shortly after birth

meconium ileus *n* : congenital intestinal obstruction by viscous meconium that is often associated with cystic fibrosis of newborn infants

[1]med \ˈmed\ *adj* : MEDICAL ⟨~ school⟩

[2]med *n* : MEDICATION 2 — usu. used in pl. ⟨took pain ~*s*⟩

me•daz•e•pam \me-ˈda-zə-ˌpam\ *n* : a drug used in the form of its hydrochloride $C_{16}H_{15}ClN_2{\cdot}HCl$ esp. formerly as a tranquilizer

med•e•vac *also* **med•i•vac** \ˈme-də-ˌvak\ *n* **1** : emergency evacuation of the sick or wounded (as from a combat area) **2** : a helicopter used for medevac — **medevac** *vb*

medi- *or* **medio-** *comb form* : middle ⟨*medio*lateral⟩

[1]media *pl of* MEDIUM

[2]me•dia \ˈmē-dē-ə\ *n, pl* **me•di•ae** \-dē-ˌē\ : the middle coat of the wall of a blood or lymph vessel consisting chiefly of circular muscle fibers — called also *tunica media*

media — see AERO-OTITIS MEDIA, OTITIS MEDIA, SCALA MEDIA, SEROUS OTITIS MEDIA

me·di·ad \ˈmē-dē-ˌad\ *adv* : toward the median line or plane of a body or part

me·di·al \ˈmē-dē-əl\ *adj* **1** : lying or extending in the middle; *esp, of a body part* : lying or extending toward the median axis of the body ⟨the ~ surface of the tibia⟩ **2** : of or relating to the media of a blood vessel — **me·di·al·ly** *adv*

medial arcuate ligament *n* : an arched band of fascia that covers the upper part of the psoas major muscle, extends from the body of the first or second lumbar vertebra to the transverse process of the first and sometimes also the second lumbar vertebra, and provides attachment for part of the lumbar portion of the diaphragm — compare LATERAL ARCUATE LIGAMENT

medial collateral ligament *n* **1** : a ligament that connects the medial epicondyle of the femur with the medial condyle and medial surface of the tibia and that helps to stabilize the knee by preventing lateral dislocation — called also *MCL, tibial collateral ligament;* compare LATERAL COLLATERAL LIGAMENT 1 **2** : ULNAR COLLATERAL LIGAMENT 1 — called also *MCL*

medial condyle *n* : a condyle on the inner side of the lower extremity of the femur; *also* : a corresponding eminence on the upper part of the tibia that articulates with the medial condyle of the femur — compare LATERAL CONDYLE

medial cord *n* : a cord of nerve tissue that is continuous with the anterior division of the inferior trunk of the brachial plexus and that is one of the two roots forming the median nerve — compare LATERAL CORD, POSTERIOR CORD

medial cuneiform bone *n* : CUNEIFORM BONE 1a — called also *medial cuneiform*

medial epicondyle *n* : EPICONDYLE b

medial femoral circumflex artery *n* : an artery that branches from the deep femoral artery or from the femoral artery itself and that supplies the muscles of the medial part of the thigh and hip joint — compare LATERAL FEMORAL CIRCUMFLEX ARTERY

medial femoral circumflex vein *n* : a vein accompanying the medial femoral circumflex artery and emptying into the femoral vein or sometimes into one of its tributaries corresponding to the deep femoral artery — compare LATERAL FEMORAL CIRCUMFLEX VEIN

medial forebrain bundle *n* : a prominent tract of nerve fibers that connects the subcallosal area of the cerebral cortex with the lateral areas of the hypothalamus and that has fibers passing to the tuber cinereum, the brain stem, and the mammillary bodies

medial geniculate body *n* : a part of the metathalamus consisting of a small oval tubercle situated between the pulvinar, colliculi, and cerebral peduncle that receives nerve impulses from the inferior colliculus and relays them to the auditory cortex — compare LATERAL GENICULATE BODY

medialis — see RECTUS MEDIALIS, VASTUS MEDIALIS

medial lemniscus *n* : a band of nerve fibers that transmits proprioceptive impulses from the spinal cord to the thalamus

medial longitudinal fasciculus *n* : any of four longitudinal bundles of white matter of which there are two on each side that extend from the midbrain to the upper parts of the spinal cord where they are located close to the midline ventral to the gray commissure and that are composed of fibers esp. from the vestibular nuclei

medial malleolus *n* : MALLEOLUS b

medial meniscus *n* : MENISCUS a(2)

medial pectoral nerve *n* : PECTORAL NERVE b

medial plantar artery *n* : PLANTAR ARTERY b

medial plantar nerve *n* : PLANTAR NERVE b

medial plantar vein *n* : PLANTAR VEIN b

medial popliteal nerve *n* : TIBIAL NERVE

medial pterygoid muscle *n* : PTERYGOID MUSCLE b

medial pterygoid nerve *n* : PTERYGOID NERVE b

medial pterygoid plate *n* : PTERYGOID PLATE b

medial rectus *n* : RECTUS 2c

medial semilunar cartilage *n* : MENISCUS a(2)

medial umbilical ligament *n* : a fibrous cord sheathed in peritoneum and extending from the pelvis to the navel that is a remnant of part of the umbilical artery in the fetus — called also *lateral umbilical ligament*

medial vestibular nucleus *n* : the one of the four vestibular nuclei on each side of the medulla oblongata that sends ascending fibers to the oculomotor and trochlear nuclei in the cerebrum on the opposite side of the brain and sends descending fibers down both sides of the spinal cord to synapse with motor neurons of the ventral roots

[1]me·di·an \ˈmē-dē-ən\ *n* : a medial part (as a vein or nerve)

[2]median *adj* : situated in the middle; *specif* : lying in a plane dividing a bilateral animal into right and left halves

median an·te·bra·chi·al vein \-ˌan-ti-ˈbrā-kē-əl-\ *n* : a vein usu. present in the forearm that drains the plexus of veins in the palm of the hand and that runs up the little finger side of the forearm

median arcuate ligament *n* : a tendinous arch that lies in front of the aorta and that connects the attachments of the lumbar portion of the diaphragm to the lumbar vertebrae on each side — compare LATERAL ARCUATE LIGAMENT

median cubital vein *n* : a continuation of the cephalic vein of the forearm that passes obliquely toward the inner side of the arm in the bend of the elbow to join with the ulnar veins in forming the basilic vein and is often selected for venipuncture

median eminence *n* : a raised area in the floor of the third ventricle of the brain produced by the infundibulum of the hypothalamus

median lethal dose *n* : LD50

median nerve *n* : a nerve that arises by two roots from the brachial plexus and passes down the middle of the front of the arm

median nuchal line *n* : OCCIPITAL CREST a

median plane *n* : MIDSAGITTAL PLANE

median sacral crest *n* : SACRAL CREST a

median sacral vein *n* : an unpaired vein that accompanies the middle sacral artery and usu. empties into the left common iliac vein

median umbilical ligament *n* : a fibrous cord extending from the urinary bladder to the umbilicus that is the remnant of the fetal urachus

me·di·as·ti·nal \ˌmē-dē-ə-ˈstī-nəl\ *adj* : of, relating to, or affecting the mediastinum 〈~ fibrosis〉

me·di·as·ti·ni·tis \ˌmē-dē-ˌas-tə-ˈnī-təs\ *n, pl* **-nit·i·des** \-ˈni-tə-ˌdēz\ : inflammation of the tissues of the mediastinum

me·di·as·tin·o·scope \ˌmē-dē-a-ˈsti-nə-ˌskōp\ *n* : an endoscope used in mediastinoscopy

me·di·as·ti·nos·co·py \ˌmē-dē-ˌas-tə-ˈnäs-kə-pē\ *n, pl* **-pies** : examination of the mediastinum through an incision above the sternum

me·di·as·ti·not·o·my \-ˈnä-tə-mē\ *n, pl* **-mies** : surgical incision into the mediastinum

me·di·as·ti·num \ˌmē-dē-ə-ˈstī-nəm\ *n, pl* **-na** \-nə\ **1** : the space in the chest between the pleural sacs of the lungs that contains all the viscera of the chest except the lungs and pleurae; *also* : this space with its contents **2** : MEDIASTINUM TESTIS

mediastinum testis *n* : a mass of connective tissue at the back of the testis that is continuous externally with the tunica albuginea and internally with the interlobular septa and encloses the rete testis

[1]**me·di·ate** \ˈmē-dē-ət\ *adj* **1** : occupying a middle position **2** : acting through an intervening agency : exhibiting indirect causation, connection, or relation

[2]**me·di·ate** \ˈmē-dē-ˌāt\ *vb* **-at·ed; -at·ing** : to transmit or carry (as a physical process or effect) as an intermediate mechanism or agency — **me·di·a·tion** \ˌmē-dē-ˈā-shən\ *n*

me·di·a·tor \ˈmē-dē-ˌā-tər\ *n* : one that mediates; *esp* : a mediating agent (as an enzyme or hormone) in a chemical or biological process

med·ic \ˈme-dik\ *n* : one engaged in medical work; *esp* : CORPSMAN

medica — see MATERIA MEDICA

med·i·ca·ble \ˈme-di-kə-bəl\ *adj* : CURABLE, REMEDIABLE

Med·ic·aid \ˈme-di-ˌkād\ *n* : a program of medical aid designed for those unable to afford regular medical service and financed jointly by the state and federal governments

[1]**med·i·cal** \ˈme-di-kəl\ *adj* **1** : of, relating to, or concerned with physicians or the practice of medicine often as distinguished from surgery **2** : requiring or devoted to medical treatment — **med·i·cal·ly** *adv*

[2]**medical** *n* : a medical examination

med·i·cal·ese \ˌme-di-kə-ˈlēz\ *n* : the specialized terminology of the medical profession

medical examiner *n* **1** : a usu. appointed public officer with duties similar to those of a coroner but who is required to have specific medical training (as in pathology) and is qualified to conduct medical examinations and autopsies **2** : a physician employed to make medical examinations (as of applicants for military service or of claimants of workers' compensation) **3** : a physician appointed to examine and license candidates for the practice of medicine in a political jurisdiction (as a state)

med·i·cal·ise *Brit var of* MEDICALIZE

med·i·cal·ize \ˈme-də-kə-ˌlīz\ *vb* **-ized; -iz·ing** : to view or treat as a medical concern, problem, or disorder — **med·i·cal·i·za·tion** \ˌme-də-kə-lə-ˈzā-shən\ *n*

medical mall *n* : a facility offering comprehensive ambulatory medical services (as primary care, diagnostic procedures, and outpatient surgery)

medical psychology *n* : theories of personality and behavior not necessarily derived from academic psychology that provide a basis for psychotherapy in psychiatry and in general medicine

medical record *n* : a record of a patient's medical information (as past diagnoses and treatments received)

medical tran·scrip·tion·ist \-tran-ˈskrip-shə-nist\ *n* : a typist who transcribes dictated medical reports

me·di·ca·ment \mi-ˈdi-kə-mənt, ˈme-di-kə-\ *n* : a substance used in therapy — **med·i·ca·men·tous** \mi-ˌdi-kə-ˈmen-təs, ˌme-di-kə-\ *adj*

med·i·cant \ˈme-di-kənt\ *n* : a medicinal substance

Medi•care \ˈme-di-ˌkar\ *n* : a government program of medical care esp. for the elderly

med•i•cate \ˈme-də-ˌkāt\ *vb* **-cat•ed; -cat•ing** **1** : to treat medicinally **2** : to impregnate with a medicinal substance ⟨*medicated* soap⟩

med•i•ca•tion \ˌme-də-ˈkā-shən\ *n* **1** : the act or process of medicating **2** : a medicinal substance : MEDICAMENT

[1]**me•dic•i•nal** \mə-ˈdis-ᵊn-əl\ *adj* : of, relating to, or being medicine : tending or used to cure disease or relieve pain — **me•dic•i•nal•ly** *adv*

[2]**medicinal** *n* : a medicinal substance : MEDICINE

medicinal leech *n* : a large European freshwater leech of the genus *Hirudo* (*H. medicinalis*) that is a source of hirudin, is now sometimes used to drain blood (as from a hematoma), and was formerly used to bleed patients thought to have excess blood

med•i•cine \ˈme-də-sən\ *n* **1** : a substance or preparation used in treating disease **2 a** : the science and art dealing with the maintenance of health and the prevention, alleviation, or cure of disease **b** : the branch of medicine concerned with the nonsurgical treatment of disease

medicine chest *n* : a cupboard used esp. for storing medicines or first-aid supplies — called also *medicine cabinet*

medicine dropper *n* : DROPPER

med•i•co \ˈme-di-ˌkō\ *n, pl* **-cos** : a medical practitioner : PHYSICIAN; *also* : a medical student

medico- *comb form* : medical : medical and ⟨*medico*legal⟩

med•i•co•le•gal \ˌme-di-kō-ˈlē-gəl\ *adj* : of or relating to both medicine and law

med•i•gap \ˈme-də-ˌgap\ *n, often attrib* : supplemental health insurance that covers costs (as of a hospital stay) not covered by Medicare ⟨∼ plans⟩

Me•di•na worm \mə-ˈdē-nə-\ *n* : GUINEA WORM

medio- — see MEDI-

me•dio•car•pal \ˌmē-dē-ō-ˈkär-pəl\ *adj* : located between the two rows of the bones of the carpus ⟨the ∼ joint⟩

me•dio•lat•er•al \-ˈla-tə-rəl\ *adj* : relating to, extending along, or being a direction or axis from side to side or from median to lateral — **me•dio•lat•er•al•ly** *adv*

Med•i•ter•ra•nean anemia \ˌme-də-tə-ˈrā-nē-ən-\ *n* : THALASSEMIA

Mediterranean diet *n* : a diet typical of many Mediterranean countries (as Italy and Spain) that consists mainly of cereals, grains, vegetables, beans, fruits, and nuts along with moderate amounts of fish, cheese, olive oil, and wine and little red meat

Mediterranean fever *n* : any of several febrile conditions often endemic in parts of the Mediterranean region; *specif* : BRUCELLOSIS 2

Mediterranean lymphoma *n* : IMMUNOPROLIFERATIVE SMALL INTESTINAL DISEASE

Mediterranean spotted fever *n* : BOUTONNEUSE FEVER

me•di•um \ˈmē-dē-əm\ *n, pl* **mediums** *or* **me•dia** \-dē-ə\ **1** : a means of effecting or conveying something **2** *pl media* : a nutrient system for the artificial cultivation of cells or organisms and esp. bacteria

medius — see CONSTRICTOR PHARYNGIS MEDIUS, GLUTEUS MEDIUS, PEDUNCULUS CEREBELLARIS MEDIUS, SCALENUS MEDIUS

medivac *var of* MEDEVAC

MED•LINE \ˈmed-ˌlīn\ *service mark* — used for an online computer database of abstracts and references from biomedical journals

med•ro•ges•tone \ˌme-drō-ˈjes-ˌtōn\ *n* : a synthetic progestin $C_{23}H_{32}O_2$ that has been used in the treatment of fibroid uterine tumors

Med•rol \ˈme-ˌdrȯl\ *trademark* — used for a preparation of methylprednisolone

me•droxy•pro•ges•ter•one acetate \me-ˌdräk-sē-prō-ˈjes-tə-ˌrōn-\ *n* : a synthetic progesterone $C_{24}H_{34}O_4$ that is administered orally esp. to treat amenorrhea and abnormal uterine bleeding and in conjunction with conjugated estrogens to relieve the symptoms of menopause and to prevent osteoporosis and that is administered by injection as a long-acting contraceptive — called also *medroxyprogesterone;* see DEPO-PROVERA, PREMPHASE, PREMPRO, PROVERA

me•dul•la \mə-ˈdə-lə, -ˈdu̇-\ *n, pl* **-las** *or* **-lae** \-(ˌ)lē, -ˌlī\ **1** *pl medullae* **a** : BONE MARROW **b** : MEDULLA OBLONGATA **2 a** : the inner or deep part of an organ or structure **b** : MYELIN SHEATH

medulla ob•lon•ga•ta \-ˌä-ˌblȯŋ-ˈgä-tə\ *n, pl* **medulla oblongatas** *or* **medullae ob•lon•ga•tae** \-ˈgä-tē, -ˌtī\ : the somewhat pyramidal last part of the vertebrate brain developed from the posterior portion of the hindbrain and continuous posteriorly with the spinal cord, enclosing the fourth ventricle, and containing nuclei associated with most of the cranial nerves, major fiber tracts and decussations that link spinal with higher centers, and various centers mediating the control of involuntary vital functions (as respiration)

medullaris — see CONUS MEDULLARIS

med•ul•lary \ˈmed-ᵊl-ˌer-ē, ˈme-jə-ˌler-ē; mə-ˈdə-lə-rē\ *adj* **1 a** : of or relating to the medulla of any body part or organ **b** : containing, consisting of, or resembling bone marrow **c** : of or relating to the medulla oblongata or the spinal cord **d** : of, relating to, or formed of the dorsally located embryonic ectoderm destined to sink below the surface and become neural tissue **2** : resembling bone marrow in consistency — used of cancers

medullary canal *n* : the marrow cavity of a bone

medullary cavity *n* : MEDULLARY CANAL

medullary cystic disease *n* : a progressive familial kidney disease that is characterized by renal medullary cysts and that manifests itself in anemia and uremia

medullary fold *n* : NEURAL FOLD

medullary groove *n* : NEURAL GROOVE

medullary plate *n* : the longitudinal dorsal zone of epiblast in the early vertebrate embryo that constitutes the primordium of the neural tissue

medulla spi•na•lis \-ˌspī-ˈnā-ləs\ *n* : SPINAL CORD

med•ul•lat•ed \ˈmed-ᵊl-ˌā-təd, ˈme-jə-ˌlā-\ *adj* **1** : MYELINATED **2** : having a medulla — used of fibers other than nerve fibers

med•ul•lec•to•my \ˌmed-ᵊl-ˈek-tə-mē, ˌme-jə-ˈlek-\ *n, pl* **-mies** : surgical excision of a medulla (as of the adrenal glands)

me•dul•lin \me-ˈdə-lən, ˈmed-ᵊl-in, ˈme-jə-lin\ *n* : a renal prostaglandin effective in reducing blood pressure

me•dul•lo•blas•to•ma \mə-ˌdə-lō-ˌblas-ˈtō-mə\ *n, pl* **-to•mas** *also* **-to•ma•ta** \-ˈtō-mə-tə\ : a malignant tumor of the central nervous system arising in the cerebellum esp. in children

mef•e•nam•ic acid \ˌme-fə-ˈna-mik-\ *n* : a drug $C_{15}H_{15}NO_2$ used as an anti-inflammatory

mef•lo•quine \ˈme-flə-ˌkwīn\ *n* : an antimalarial drug related to quinine that is administered in the form of its hydrochloride $C_{17}H_{16}F_6N_2O·HCl$

MEG *abbr* magnetoencephalography

mega- *or* **meg-** *comb form* **1** : great : large ⟨*mega*colon⟩ ⟨*mega*dose⟩ **2** : million : multiplied by one million ⟨*mega*curie⟩

mega•co•lon \ˈme-gə-ˌkō-lən\ *n* : extreme dilation of the colon that may be congenital or acquired — see HIRSCHSPRUNG'S DISEASE

mega•cu•rie \ˈme-gə-ˌkyu̇r-ē, -kyu̇-ˌrē\ *n* : one million curies

mega•dose \-ˌdōs\ *n* : a large dose (as of a vitamin) — **mega•dos•ing** \-ˌdō-siŋ\ *n*

mega•esoph•a•gus \ˌme-gə-i-ˈsä-fə-gəs\ *n, pl* **-gi** \-ˌgī, -ˌjī\ : enlargement and hypertrophy of the lower portion of the esophagus

mega•kary•o•blast \ˌme-gə-ˈkar-ē-ō-ˌblast\ *n* : a large cell with large reticulate nucleus that gives rise to megakaryocytes

mega•kary•o•cyte \ˌme-gə-ˈkar-ē-ō-ˌsīt\ *n* : a large cell that has a lobulated nucleus, is found esp. in the bone marrow, and is the source of blood platelets — **mega•kary•o•cyt•ic** \-ˌkar-ē-ō-ˈsi-tik\ *adj*

megal- *or* **megalo-** *comb form* **1** : large ⟨*megalo*cyte⟩ : abnormally large ⟨*megalo*cephaly⟩ **2** : grandiose ⟨*megalo*mania⟩

meg•a•lo•blast \ˈme-gə-lō-ˌblast\ *n* : a large erythroblast that appears in the blood esp. in pernicious anemia — **meg•a•lo•blas•tic** \ˌme-gə-lō-ˈblas-tik\ *adj*

megaloblastic anemia *n* : an anemia (as pernicious anemia) characterized by the presence of megaloblasts in the circulating blood

meg•a•lo•ceph•a•ly \ˌme-gə-lō-ˈse-fə-lē\ *n, pl* **-lies** : largeness and esp. abnormal largeness of the head

meg•a•lo•cyte \ˈme-gə-lə-ˌsīt\ *n* : MACROCYTE — **meg•a•lo•cyt•ic** \ˌme-gə-lə-ˈsi-tik\ *adj*

meg•a•lo•ma•nia \ˌme-gə-lō-ˈmā-nē-ə, -nyə\ *n* : a delusional mental illness that is marked by infantile feelings of personal omnipotence and grandeur — **meg•a•lo•ma•ni•a•cal** \-mə-ˈnī-ə-kəl\ *or* **megalomaniac** *also* **meg•a•lo•man•ic** \-ˈma-nik\ *adj* — **meg•a•lo•ma•ni•a•cal•ly** *adv*

meg•a•lo•ma•ni•ac \-ˈmā-nē-ˌak\ *n* : an individual affected with or exhibiting megalomania

-meg•a•ly \ˈme-gə-lē\ *n comb form, pl* **-meg•a•lies** : abnormal enlargement (of a specified part) ⟨hepato*megaly*⟩

mega•rad \ˈme-gə-ˌrad\ *n* : one million rads — abbr. *Mrad*

mega•vi•ta•min \ˌme-gə-ˈvī-tə-mən\ *adj* : relating to or consisting of very large doses of vitamins and esp. doses many times greater than the recommended daily allowances

mega•vi•ta•mins \-mənz\ *n pl* : a large quantity of vitamins

me•ges•trol acetate \me-ˈjes-ˌtrȯl-\ *n* : a synthetic progestational hormone $C_{24}H_{32}O_4$ used in palliative treatment of advanced carcinoma of the breast and in endometriosis

meg•lu•mine \ˈme-glu̇-ˌmēn, me-ˈglü-\ *n* : a crystalline base $C_7H_{17}NO_5$ used to prepare salts used in radiopaque and therapeutic substances — see IODIPAMIDE

me•grim \ˈmē-grəm\ *n* **1** : MIGRAINE **2** : VERTIGO

mei•bo•mian gland \mī-ˈbō-mē-ən-\ *n, often cap M* : one of the long sebaceous glands of the eyelids that discharge a fatty secretion which lubricates the eyelids — called also *tarsal gland;* see CHALAZION

Mei•bom \ˈmī-ˌbōm\, **Heinrich (1638–1700)**, German physician.

mei•o•sis \mī-ˈō-səs\ *n, pl* **mei•o•ses** \-ˌsēz\ : the cellular process that results in the number of chromosomes in gamete-producing cells being reduced to one half and that involves a reduction division in which one of each pair of homologous chromosomes passes to each daughter cell and a mitotic division — compare MITOSIS 1 — **mei•ot•ic** \mī-ˈä-tik\ *adj* — **mei•ot•i•cal•ly** *adv*

Meiss•ner's corpuscle \ˈmīs-nərz-\ *n* : any of the small elliptical tactile end organs in hairless skin containing numerous transversely placed tactile cells and fine flattened nerve endings

Meissner, Georg (1829–1905), German anatomist and physiologist.

Meissner's plexus *n* : a plexus of ganglionated nerve fibers lying between the muscular and mucous coats of the intestine — compare MYENTERIC PLEXUS

meit•ner•i•um \mīt-ˈnir-ē-əm\ *n* : a short-lived radioactive element produced artificially — symbol *Mt;* see ELEMENT table

Meitner, Lise (1878–1968), German physicist.

mel \ˈmel\ *n* : a subjective unit of tone pitch equal to $^{1}/_{1000}$ of the pitch of a tone having a frequency of 1000 hertz — used esp. in audiology

me•lae•na *chiefly Brit var of* MELENA

melan- *or* **melano-** *comb form* **1** : black : dark ⟨*melan*in⟩ ⟨*melan*oma⟩ **2** : melanin ⟨*melano*genesis⟩

mel•an•cho•lia \ˌme-lən-ˈkō-lē-ə\ *n* : a mental condition and esp. a manic-depressive condition characterized by extreme depression, psychomotor agitation, and often hallucinations and delusions

mel•an•cho•li•ac \-lē-ˌak\ *n* : an individual affected with melancholia

[1]**mel•an•chol•ic** \ˌme-lən-ˈkä-lik\ *adj* **1** : of, relating to, or subject to melancholy : DEPRESSED **2** : of or relating to melancholia

[2]**melancholic** *n* **1** : a melancholy person **2** : MELANCHOLIAC

mel•an•choly \ˈme-lən-ˌkä-lē\ *n, pl* **-chol•ies** **1** : MELANCHOLIA **2** : depression or dejection of spirits — **melancholy** *adj*

mel•a•nin \ˈme-lə-nən\ *n* : any of various black, dark brown, reddish-brown, or yellow pigments of animal or plant structures (as skin or hair); *esp* : any of numerous animal pigments that are essentially polymeric derivatives of indole formed by enzymatic modification of tyrosine

mel•a•nism \ˈme-lə-ˌni-zəm\ *n* **1** : an increased amount of black or nearly black pigmentation (as of skin, feathers, or hair) of an individual or kind of organism **2** : intense human pigmentation in skin, eyes, and hair — **mel•a•nis•tic** \ˌme-lə-ˈnis-tik\ *adj*

mel•a•nize \ˈme-lə-ˌnīz\ *vb* **-nized; -niz•ing** : to convert into or infiltrate with melanin ⟨*melanized* cell granules⟩ — **mel•a•ni•za•tion** \ˌme-lə-nə-ˈzā-shən\ *n*

melano- — see MELAN-

me•la•no•blast \mə-ˈla-nə-ˌblast, ˈme-lə-nō-\ *n* : a cell that is a precursor of a melanocyte

me•la•no•blas•to•ma \mə-ˌla-nə-blas-ˈtō-mə, ˌme-lə-nō-\ *n, pl* **-mas** *also* **-ma•ta** \-mə-tə\ : a malignant tumor derived from melanoblasts

mel•a•no•car•ci•no•ma \-ˌkärs-ᵊn-ˈō-mə\ *n, pl* **-mas** *also* **-ma•ta** \-mə-tə\ : MELANOMA 2

me•la•no•cyte \mə-ˈla-nə-ˌsīt, ˈme-lə-nō-\ *n* : an epidermal cell that produces melanin

melanocyte–stimulating hormone *n* : either of two vertebrate hormones of the pituitary gland that darken the skin by stimulating melanin dispersion in pigment-containing cells — abbr. *MSH;* called also *intermedin, melanophore-stimulating hormone, melanotropin*

me•la•no•cyt•ic \mə-ˌla-nə-ˈsi-tik, ˌme-lə-nō-\ *adj* : similar to or characterized by the presence of melanocytes

me•la•no•cy•to•ma \-sī-ˈtō-mə\ *n, pl* **-mas** *also* **-ma•ta** \-mə-tə\ : a benign tumor composed of melanocytes

mel•a•no•der•ma \ˌme-lə-nō-ˈdər-mə, mə-ˌla-\ *n* : abnormally intense pigmentation of the skin

me•la•no•gen•e•sis \mə-ˌla-nə-ˈje-nə-səs, ˌme-lə-nō-\ *n, pl* **-e•ses** \-ˌsēz\ : the formation of melanin

me•la•no•gen•ic \-ˈje-nik\ *adj* **1** : of, relating to, or characteristic of melanogenesis **2** : producing melanin

mel•a•no•ma \ˌme-lə-ˈnō-mə\ *n, pl* **-mas** *also* **-ma•ta** \-mə-tə\ **1** : a benign or malignant skin tumor containing dark pigment **2** : a tumor of high malignancy that starts in melanocytes of normal skin or moles and metastasizes rapidly and widely — called also *malignant melanoma, melanocarcinoma, melanosarcoma*

me•la•no•phage \mə-ˈla-nə-ˌfāj, ˈme-lə-nə-\ *n* : a melanin-containing macrophage found in pigmented skin lesions

me•la•no•phore–stimulating hormone \mə-ˈla-nō-ˌfōr-, ˈme-lə-nə-\ *n* : MELANOCYTE-STIMULATING HORMONE

me•la•no•sar•co•ma \-sär-ˈkō-mə\ *n, pl* **-mas** *also* **-ma•ta** \-mə-tə\ : MELANOMA 2

mel•a•no•sis \ˌme-lə-ˈnō-səs\ *n, pl* **-no•ses** \-ˈnō-ˌsēz\ : a condition characterized by abnormal deposition of melanins or sometimes other pigments in the tissues of the body

melanosis co•li \-ˈkō-ˌlī\ *n* : dark brownish-black pigmentation of the mucous membrane of the colon due to the deposition of pigment in macrophages

me•la•no•some \mə-ˈla-nə-ˌsōm, ˈme-lə-nō-\ *n* : a melanin-producing granule in a melanocyte — **me•la•no•som•al** \mə-ˌla-nə-ˈsō-məl, ˌme-lə-nō-\ *adj*

mel•a•not•ic \ˌme-lə-ˈnä-tik\ *adj* : having or characterized by black pigmentation ⟨a ~ sarcoma⟩

me•la•no•tro•pin \mə-ˌla-nə-ˈtrō-pən, ˌme-lə-nō-\ *n* : MELANOCYTE-STIMULATING HORMONE

me•lar•so•prol \me-ˈlar-sə-ˌpröl\ *n* : a drug $C_{12}H_{15}AsN_6OS_2$ used in the treatment of trypanosomiasis esp. in advanced stages

me•las•ma \mə-ˈlaz-mə\ *n* : a dark pigmentation of the skin (as in Addison's disease) — **me•las•mic** \-mik\ *adj*

mel•a•to•nin \ˌme-lə-ˈtō-nən\ *n* : a vertebrate hormone $C_{13}H_{16}N_2O_2$ that is derived from serotonin, is secreted by the pineal gland esp. in response to darkness, and has been linked to the regulation of circadian rhythms

me•le•na \mə-ˈlē-nə\ *n* : the passage of dark tarry stools containing decomposing blood that is usu. an indication of bleeding in the upper part of the digestive tract and esp. the esophagus, stomach, and duodenum — compare HEMATOCHEZIA — **me•le•nic** \-nik\ *adj*

mel•en•ges•trol acetate \ˌme-lən-ˈjes-ˌtrȯl-, -ˌtrōl-\ *n* : a progestational and antineoplastic agent $C_{25}H_{32}O_4$ that has been used as a growth-stimulating feed additive for beef cattle

-me•lia \ˈmē-lē-ə\ *n comb form* : condition of the limbs ⟨micro*melia*⟩

mel•i•oi•do•sis \ˌme-lē-ˌȯi-ˈdō-səs\ *n, pl* **-do•ses** \-ˌsēz\ : an infectious disease chiefly of southeastern Asia that is closely related to glanders, that is caused by a bacterium of the genus *Burkholderia* (*B. pseudomallei* syn. *Pseudomonas pseudomallei*) which is found esp. in water and moist soil and transmitted to mammals including humans chiefly by direct contact, ingestion, or inhalation, and that may occur as an acute pulmonary infection, as a localized infection (as of the skin), or as a sometimes fatal septicemia

me•lit•tin \mə-ˈlit-ᵊn\ *n* : a toxic protein in bee venom that causes localized pain and inflammation

Mel•la•ril \ˈme-lə-ˌril\ *trademark* — used for a preparation of thioridazine

mellitus — see DIABETES MELLITUS, INSULIN-DEPENDENT DIABETES MELLITUS, NON-INSULIN-DEPENDENT DIABETES MELLITUS

Me•loph•a•gus \mə-ˈlä-fə-gəs\ *n* : a genus of wingless flies (family Hippoboscidae) that includes the sheep ked (*M. ovinus*)

melo•rhe•os•to•sis \ˌme-lə-ˌrē-ä-ˈstō-səs\ *n, pl* **-to•ses** \-ˌsēz\ *or* **-tosises** : an extremely rare form of osteosclerosis characterized by asymmetrical or local enlargement and sclerotic changes in the long bones of one extremity

me•lox•i•cam \mə-ˈläk-si-ˌkam\ *n* : an NSAID $C_{14}H_{13}N_3O_4S_2$ that is a COX-2 inhibitor taken orally esp. to treat osteoarthritis and rheumatoid arthritis — see MOBIC

mel•pha•lan \ˈmel-fə-ˌlan\ *n* : an antineoplastic drug $C_{13}H_{18}Cl_2N_2O_2$ that is a derivative of nitrogen mustard and is used esp. in the treatment of multiple myeloma — called also *L-PAM, phenylalanine mustard, sarcolysin*

melting point *n* : the temperature at which a solid melts

-m•e•lus \mə-ləs\ *n comb form, pl* **-m•e•li** \-ˌlī\ : one having a (specified) abnormality of the limbs ⟨phoco*melus*⟩

mem•an•tine \ˈmem-an-ˌtēn\ *n* : a drug $C_{12}H_{21}N{\cdot}HCl$ that blocks the action of glutamate and is taken orally in the treatment of moderate to severe Alzheimer's disease — see NAMENDA, NAMZARIC

mem•ber \ˈmem-bər\ *n* : a body part or organ: as **a** : LIMB **b** : PENIS

membran- *or* **membrani-** *or* **membrano-** *comb form* : membrane ⟨*membrano*proliferative glomerulonephritis⟩

mem•bra•na \mem-ˈbrā-nə, -ˈbrä-\ *n, pl* **mem•bra•nae** \-ˌnē, -ˌnī\ : MEMBRANE

membrana nic•ti•tans \-ˈnik-tə-ˌtanz\ *n* : NICTITATING MEMBRANE

mem•brane \ˈmem-ˌbrān\ *n* **1** : a thin soft pliable sheet or layer esp. of animal or plant origin **2** : a limiting protoplasmic surface or interface — see NUCLEAR MEMBRANE, PLASMA MEMBRANE — **mem•braned** \ˈmem-ˌbrānd\ *adj*

membrane bone *n* : a bone that ossifies directly in connective tissue without previous existence as cartilage

membrane of Descemet *n* : DESCEMET'S MEMBRANE

membrane oxygenator *n* : a device that adds oxygen and removes carbon dioxide from the blood of a patient esp. during cardiac surgery and extracorporeal membrane oxygenation and that consists of a semipermeable membrane which allows for the exchange of respiratory gases

membrane potential *n* : the difference in electrical potential between the interior of a cell and the interstitial fluid beyond the membrane

mem•bra•no•pro•lif•er•a•tive glomerulonephritis \mem-ˌbrā-nō-prə-ˈli-fə-rə-tiv-\ *n* : a slowly progressive chronic glomerulonephritis characterized by proliferation of mesangial cells and irregular thickening of glomerular capillary walls and narrowing of the capillary lumina

mem•bra•nous \ˈmem-brə-nəs\ *adj* **1** : of, relating to, or resembling membranes **2** : characterized or accompanied by the formation of a usu. abnormal membrane or membranous layer — **mem•bra•nous•ly** *adv*

membranous glomerulonephritis *n* : a form of glomerulonephritis characterized by thickening of glomerular capillary basement membranes and nephrotic syndrome

membranous labyrinth *n* : the system of membrane-lined interconnected sacs and passages that is suspended within the bony labyrinth of the inner ear, is filled with endolymph and surrounded by perilymph, and includes the cochlear duct, utricle, saccule, and semicircular ducts

membranous urethra *n* : the part of the male urethra that is situated between the layers of the urogenital diaphragm and that connects the parts of the urethra passing through the prostate gland and the penis

mem•o•ry \ˈmem-rē, ˈme-mə-\ *n, pl* **-ries** **1** : the power or process of reproducing or recalling what has been learned and retained esp. through associative mechanisms **2** : the store of things learned and retained from an organism's activity or experience as indicated by modification of structure or behavior or by recall and recognition

memory cell *n* : a long-lived lymphocyte that carries the antibody or receptor for a specific antigen after a first exposure to the antigen and that remains in a less than mature state until stimulated by a second exposure to the antigen at which time it mounts a more effective immune response than a cell which has not been exposed previously

memory trace *n* : a transient or long-term change in the brain that represents something (as an experience) stored as a memory : ENGRAM

men- *or* **meno-** *comb form* : menstruation ⟨*meno*pause⟩ ⟨*meno*rrhagia⟩

men•a•di•one \ˌme-nə-ˈdī-ˌōn, -dī-ˈ\ *n* : a yellow compound $C_{11}H_8O_2$ with the biological activity of natural vitamin K — called also *vitamin K_3*

me•naph•thone \mə-ˈnaf-ˌthōn\ *n, Brit* : MENADIONE

men•a•quin•one \ˌme-nə-ˈkwi-ˌnōn\ *n* : VITAMIN K 1b; *also* : a synthetic derivative of vitamin K_2

men•ar•che \ˈme-ˌnär-kē\ *n* : the beginning of the menstrual function; *esp* : the first menstrual period of an individual — **men•ar•che•al** \ˌme-ˈnär-kē-əl\ *or* **men•ar•chal** \-kəl\ *adj*

[1]**mend** \ˈmend\ *vb* **1** : to restore to health : CURE **2** : to improve in health; *also* : HEAL

[2]**mend** *n* : an act of mending or repair — **on the mend** : getting better or improving esp. in health

men•de•le•vi•um \ˌmen-də-ˈlē-vē-əm, -ˈlā-\ *n* : a radioactive element that is artificially produced — symbol *Md;* see ELEMENT table

Men•de•lian \men-ˈdē-lē-ən, -ˈdēl-yən\ *adj* : of, relating to, or according with Mendel's laws or Mendelism — **Mendelian** *n*

Men•del \ˈmend-ᵊl\, **Gregor Johann (1822–1884),** Austrian botanist and geneticist.

Mendelian factor *n* : GENE

Mendelian inheritance *n* : inheritance of characters specif. transmitted by genes in accord with Mendel's law — called also *particulate inheritance*

Men•del•ism \ˈmend-ᵊl-ˌi-zəm\ *n* : the principles or the operations of Mendel's laws; *also* : MENDELIAN INHERITANCE

Men•del's law \ˈmen-dᵊlz-\ *n* **1** : a principle in genetics: hereditary units occur in pairs that separate during gamete formation so that every gamete receives but one member of a pair — called also *law of segregation* **2** : a principle in genetics limited and modified by the subsequent discovery of the phenomenon of linkage: the different pairs of hereditary units are distributed to the gametes independently of each other, the gametes combine at random, and the various combinations of hereditary pairs occur in the zygotes according to the laws of chance — called also *law of independent assortment* **3** : a principle in genetics proved subsequently to be subject to many limitations: because one of each pair of hereditary units dominates the other in expression, characters are inherited as alternatives on an all or nothing basis — called also *law of dominance*

men•go•vi•rus \ˈmeŋ-gō-ˌvī-rəs\ *n* : a picornavirus (species *Encephalomyocarditis virus* of the genus *Cardiovirus*) that causes encephalomyocarditis

Mé•nière's disease \mən-ˈyerz-, ˈmen-yərz-\ *n* : a disorder of the membranous labyrinth of the inner ear that is marked by recurrent attacks of dizziness, tinnitus, and deafness — called also *Ménière's syndrome*

Ménière, Prosper (1799–1862), French physician.

mening- *or* **meningo-** *also* **meningi-** *comb form* **1** : meninges ⟨*meningo*coccus⟩ ⟨*mening*itis⟩ **2** : meninges and ⟨*meningo*encephalitis⟩

men•in•ge•al \ˌme-nən-ˈjē-əl\ *adj* : of, relating to, or affecting the meninges

meningeal artery *n* : any of several arteries supplying the meninges of the brain and neighboring structures; *esp* : MIDDLE MENINGEAL ARTERY

meningeal vein *n* : any of several veins draining the meninges of the brain and neighboring structures

meninges *pl of* MENINX

me•nin•gi•o•ma \mə-ˌnin-jē-ˈō-mə\ *n, pl* **-mas** *also* **-ma•ta** \-tə\ : a slow-growing encapsulated tumor arising from the meninges and often causing damage by pressing upon the brain and adjacent parts

men•in•gism \ˈme-nən-ˌji-zəm, mə-ˈnin-\ *n* : MENINGISMUS

men•in•gis•mus \ˌme-nən-ˈjiz-məs\ *n, pl* **-gis•mi** \-ˌmī\ : a state of meningeal irritation with symptoms suggesting meningitis that often occurs at the onset of acute febrile diseases esp. in children

men•in•gi•tis \ˌme-nən-ˈjī-təs\ *n, pl* **-git•i•des** \-ˈji-tə-ˌdēz\ : inflammation of the meninges and esp. of the pia mater and the arachnoid; *specif* : a disease marked by inflammation of the meninges that is either a relatively mild illness caused by a virus (as various Coxsackieviruses) or a more severe usu. life-threatening illness caused by a bacterium (esp. the meningococcus or the serotype designated B of *Haemophilus influenzae*) and that is often marked by fever, headache, vomiting, malaise, and stiff neck and if left untreated in bacterial forms may progress to confusion, stupor, convulsions, coma, and death — **men·in·git·ic** \-ˈji-tik\ *adj*

me·nin·go·cele *also* **me·nin·go·coele** \me-ˈniŋ-gə-ˌsēl, mə-ˈnin-jə-\ *n* : a protrusion of meninges through a defect in the skull or spinal column forming a cyst filled with cerebrospinal fluid

me·nin·go·coc·cae·mia *chiefly Brit var of* MENINGOCOCCEMIA

me·nin·go·coc·ce·mia \mə-ˌniŋ-gō-käk-ˈsē-mē-ə, -ˌnin-jə-\ *n* : an abnormal condition characterized by the presence of meningococci in the blood

me·nin·go·coc·cus \mə-ˌniŋ-gə-ˈkä-kəs, -ˌnin-jə-\ *n, pl* **-coc·ci** \-ˈkä-ˌkī, -ˌkē; -ˈkäk-ˌsī, -ˌsē\ : a bacterium of the genus *Neisseria* (*N. meningitidis*) that causes cerebrospinal meningitis — **me·nin·go·coc·cal** \-ˈkä-kəl\ *also* **me·nin·go·coc·cic** \-ˈkä-kik, -ˈkäk-sik\ *adj*

me·nin·go·en·ceph·a·li·tis \-in-ˌse-fə-ˈlī-təs\ *n, pl* **-lit·i·des** \-ˈli-tə-ˌdēz\ : inflammation of the brain and meninges — **me·nin·go·en·ceph·a·lit·ic** \mə-ˌniŋ-(ˌ)gō-ən-ˌse-fə-ˈli-tik, -ˌnin-(ˌ)jō-\ *adj*

me·nin·go·en·ceph·a·lo·cele \-in-ˈse-fə-lō-ˌsēl\ *n* : a protrusion of meninges and brain through a defect in the skull

me·nin·go·en·ceph·a·lo·my·eli·tis \-in-ˌse-fə-lō-ˌmī-ə-ˈlī-təs\ *n, pl* **-elit·i·des** \-ə-ˈli-tə-ˌdēz\ : inflammation of the meninges, brain, and spinal cord

me·nin·go·my·elo·cele \-ˈmī-ə-lō-ˌsēl\ *n* : a protrusion of meninges and spinal cord through a defect in the spinal column

me·nin·go·vas·cu·lar \-ˈvas-kyə-lər\ *adj* : of, relating to, or affecting the meninges and cerebral blood vessels

me·ninx \ˈmē-niŋks, ˈme-\ *n, pl* **me·nin·ges** \mə-ˈnin-(ˌ)jēz\ : any of the three membranes that envelop the brain and spinal cord and include the arachnoid, dura mater, and pia mater

me·nis·cal \mə-ˈnis-kəl\ *adj* : of or relating to a meniscus ⟨a ~ tear⟩

men·is·cec·to·my \ˌme-ni-ˈsek-tə-mē\ *n, pl* **-mies** : surgical excision of a meniscus of the knee or temporomandibular joint

me·nis·cus \mə-ˈnis-kəs\ *n, pl* **me·nis·ci** \-ˈnis-ˌkī, -ˌkē; -ˈni-ˌsī\ *also* **me·nis·cus·es** : a fibrous cartilage within a joint: **a** : either of two crescent-shaped lamellae of fibrocartilage that border and partly cover the articulating surfaces of the tibia and femur at the knee : SEMILUNAR CARTILAGE: (1) : one mostly between the lateral condyles of the tibia and femur — called also *lateral meniscus, lateral semilunar cartilage* (2) : one mostly between the medial condyles of the tibia and femur — called also *medial meniscus, medial semilunar cartilage* **b** : a thin oval ligament of the temporomandibular joint that is situated between the condyle of the mandible and the mandibular fossa and separates the joint into two cavities

Men·kes' disease \ˈmeŋ-kəz-\ *n* : a disorder of copper metabolism that is inherited as a recessive X-linked trait and is characterized by a deficiency of copper in the liver and of copper-containing proteins (as ceruloplasmin) which results in intellectual disability, brittle kinky hair, and a typically fatal outcome early in life — called also *Menkes' syndrome*

Menkes, John Hans (1928–2008), American (Austrian-born) pediatric neurologist.

meno·met·ror·rha·gia \ˌme-nō-ˌmē-trə-ˈrā-jə, -ˈrä-, -jē-ə, -zhə\ *n* : a combination of menorrhagia and metrorrhagia

meno·pause \ˈme-nə-ˌpȯz, ˈmē-\ *n* **1 a** (1) : the natural cessation of menstruation occurring usu. between the ages of 45 and 55 (2) : the physiological period in the life of a woman in which such cessation occurs — called also *climacteric, climax;* compare PERIMENOPAUSE **b** : cessation of menstruation from other than natural causes (as from surgical removal of the ovaries) **2** : ANDROPAUSE — **meno·paus·al** \ˌme-nə-ˈpȯ-zəl, ˌmē-\ *adj*

Men·o·pon \ˈme-nə-ˌpän\ *n* : a genus of biting lice — see SHAFT LOUSE

men·or·rha·gia \ˌme-nə-ˈrā-jə, -ˈrä-, -jē-ə, -zhə\ *n* : abnormally profuse menstrual flow — compare HYPERMENORRHEA, METRORRHAGIA — **men·or·rhag·ic** \-ˈra-jik\ *adj*

men·or·rhea \ˌme-nə-ˈrē-ə\ *n* : normal menstrual flow

men·or·rhoea *chiefly Brit var of* MENORRHEA

men·ses \ˈmen-ˌsēz\ *n sing or pl* : the menstrual flow

men·stru·al \ˈmen-strə-wəl\ *adj* : of or relating to menstruation — **men·stru·al·ly** *adv*

menstrual cycle *n* : the whole cycle of physiologic changes from the beginning of one menstrual period to the beginning of the next

menstrual extraction *n* : a procedure for early termination of pregnancy by withdrawing the uterine lining and a fertilized egg if present by means of suction

men·stru·a·tion \ˌmen-strə-ˈwā-shən\ *n* : a discharging of blood, secretions, and tissue debris from the uterus that recurs in nonpregnant human and other primate females of breeding age at approximately monthly intervals and that is considered to represent a readjustment of the uterus to the nonpregnant state following proliferative changes accompanying the preceding ovulation; *also* : PERIOD 1b — **men·stru·ate** \ˈmen-strə-ˌwāt\ *vb* — **men·stru·ous** \ˈmen-strə-wəs\ *adj*

men·stru·um \ˈmen-strə-wəm\ *n, pl* **-stru·ums** *or* **-strua** \-strə-wə\ : a substance that dissolves a solid or holds it in suspension : SOLVENT

menta *pl of* MENTUM

[1]**men•tal** \ˈment-ᵊl\ *adj* **1 a :** of or relating to the mind; *specif* : of or relating to the total emotional and intellectual response of an individual to external reality **b :** of or relating to intellectual as contrasted with emotional activity **2 a :** of, relating to, or affected by a psychiatric disorder ⟨~ diagnoses⟩ **b :** intended for the care or treatment of persons affected by psychiatric disorders ⟨~ hospitals⟩ — **men•tal•ly** *adv*

[2]**mental** *adj* : of or relating to the chin : GENIAL

mental age *n* : a measure used in psychological testing that expresses an individual's mental attainment in terms of the number of years it takes an average child to reach the same level

mental artery *n* : a branch of the inferior alveolar artery on each side that emerges from the mental foramen and supplies blood to the chin — called also *mental branch*

mental capacity *n* **1 :** sufficient understanding and memory to comprehend in a general way the situation in which one finds oneself and the nature, purpose, and consequence of any act or transaction into which one proposes to enter **2 :** the degree of understanding and memory the law requires to uphold the validity of or to charge one with responsibility for a particular act or transaction

mental competence *n* : MENTAL CAPACITY

mental deficiency *n* : INTELLECTUAL DISABILITY

mental disorder *n* : MENTAL ILLNESS — called also *mental disease*

mentales *pl of* MENTALIS

mental foramen *n* : a foramen for the passage of blood vessels and a nerve on the outside of the lower jaw on each side near the chin

mental health *n* **1 :** the condition of being sound mentally and emotionally that is characterized by the absence of mental illness and by adequate adjustment esp. as reflected in feeling comfortable about oneself, having positive feelings about others, and being able to meet the demands of daily life; *also* : the general condition of one's mental and emotional state **2 :** health care dealing with the promotion and improvement of mental health and the treatment of mental illness : MENTAL HYGIENE

mental hygiene *n* : the science of maintaining mental health and preventing the development of mental illness

mental illness *n* : any of a broad range of medical conditions (as major depression, schizophrenia, or obsessive-compulsive disorder) that are marked primarily by sufficient disorganization of personality, mind, or emotions to impair normal psychological functioning and cause marked distress or disability and that are typically associated with a disruption in normal thinking, feeling, mood, behavior, interpersonal interactions, or daily functioning — called also *mental disease, mental disorder* — **mentally ill** *adj*

mental incapacity *n* **1 :** an absence of mental capacity **2 :** an inability through mental illness or significant cognitive impairment to carry on the everyday affairs of life or to care for one's person or property with reasonable discretion ⟨treatment consent was not possible due to the patient's *mental incapacity*⟩ — called also *mental incompetence*

men•ta•lis \men-ˈtā-lis\ *n, pl* **men•ta•les** \-ˌlēz\ : a muscle that originates in the incisive fossa of the mandible, inserts in the skin of the chin, and raises the chin and pushes up the lower lip

men•tal•i•ty \men-ˈta-lə-tē\ *n, pl* **-ties 1 :** mental power or capacity **2 :** mode or way of thought

mental nerve *n* : a branch of the inferior alveolar nerve that emerges from the bone of the mandible near the mental protuberance and divides into branches which are distributed to the skin of the chin and to the skin and mucous membranes of the lower lip

mental protuberance *n* : the bony protuberance at the front of the lower jaw forming the chin

mental retardation *n, now sometimes offensive* : INTELLECTUAL DISABILITY — **mentally retarded** *adj*

mental spine *n* : either of two small elevations on the inner surface of each side of the symphysis of the lower jaw of which the superior one on each side provides attachment for the genioglossus and the inferior for the geniohyoid muscle

mental test *n* : any of various standardized procedures applied to an individual in order to ascertain ability or evaluate behavior in comparison with other individuals or with the average of any class of individuals

mental tubercle *n* : a prominence on each side of the mental protuberance of the mandible — called also *genial tubercle*

men•ta•tion \men-ˈtā-shən\ *n* : mental activity ⟨unconscious ~⟩

men•thol \ˈmen-ˌthȯl, -ˌthōl\ *n* : a crystalline alcohol $C_{10}H_{20}O$ that occurs esp. in mint oils, has the odor and cooling properties of peppermint, and is used in flavoring and in medicine (as locally to relieve pain, itching, and nasal congestion)

men•tho•lat•ed \ˈmen-thə-ˌlā-təd\ *adj* : containing or impregnated with menthol ⟨a ~ salve⟩ ⟨~ cough drops⟩

mentis — see COMPOS MENTIS, NON COMPOS MENTIS

men•tum \ˈmen-təm\ *n, pl* **men•ta** \-tə\ : CHIN

mep•a•crine \ˈme-pə-ˌkrēn, -krən\ *n, chiefly Brit* : QUINACRINE

mep•a•zine \ˈme-pə-ˌzēn\ *n* : a phenothiazine $C_{19}H_{22}N_2S$ formerly used as a tranquilizer

me•pen•zo•late bromide \mə-ˈpen-zə-ˌlāt-\ *n* : an anticholinergic drug $C_{21}H_{26}BrNO_3$ used to treat peptic ulcer

me•per•i•dine \mə-ˈper-ə-ˌdēn\ *n* : a synthetic narcotic drug used in the form of its hydrochloride $C_{15}H_{21}NO_2 \cdot HCl$ as an analgesic, sedative, and antispasmodic — called also *isonipecaine, pethidine*

me•phen•e•sin \mə-ˈfe-nə-sin\ *n* : a muscle relaxant $C_{10}H_{14}O_3$ used esp. to treat spasticity and painful muscle spasm — called also *myanesin*

meph•en•ox•a•lone \ˌme-fə-ˈnäk-sə-ˌlōn\ *n* : a tranquilizing drug $C_{11}H_{13}NO_4$

me•phen•ter•mine \mə-ˈfen-tər-ˌmēn\ *n* : an adrenergic drug administered often in the form of the sulfate $C_{11}H_{17}N \cdot H_2SO_4$ as a vasopressor and nasal decongestant

me•phen•y•to•in \mə-ˈfe-ni-ˌtō-in\ *n* : an anticonvulsant drug $C_{12}H_{14}N_2O_2$ — see MESANTOIN

mepho•bar•bi•tal \ˌme-fō-ˈbär-bə-ˌtäl\ *n* : a crystalline barbiturate $C_{13}H_{14}N_2O_3$ used as a sedative and in the treatment of epilepsy

Meph•y•ton \ˈme-fə-ˌtän\ *trademark* — used for a preparation of vitamin K_1

me•piv•a•caine \me-ˈpi-və-ˌkān\ *n* : a drug used esp. in the form of the hydrochloride $C_{15}H_{22}N_2O \cdot HCl$ as a local anesthetic

mep•ro•bam•ate \ˌme-prō-ˈba-ˌmāt, mə-ˈprō-bə-ˌmāt\ *n* : a bitter carbamate $C_9H_{18}N_2O_4$ used as a tranquilizer — see EQUANIL, MILTOWN

¹**mer-** *or* **mero-** *comb form* : thigh ⟨*me*ralgia⟩

²**mer-** *or* **mero-** *comb form* : part : partial ⟨*mero*blastic⟩

me•ral•gia \mə-ˈral-jə, -jē-ə\ *n* : pain esp. of a neuralgic kind in the thigh

meralgia par•aes•thet•i•ca *Brit var of* MERALGIA PARESTHETICA

meralgia par•es•thet•i•ca \-ˌpar-əs-ˈthe-ti-kə\ *n* : an abnormal condition characterized by pain and paresthesia in the outer surface of the thigh

mer•al•lu•ride \mə-ˈral-yə-ˌrīd, -ˌrid\ *n* : a mercurial compound $C_9H_{16}HgN_2O_6$ combined with theophylline and formerly used as a diuretic

mer•bro•min \ˌmər-ˈbrō-mən\ *n* : a green crystalline mercurial compound $C_{20}H_8Br_2HgNa_2O_6$ used as a topical antiseptic and germicide in the form of its red solution — see MERCUROCHROME

mer•cap•tom•er•in \(ˌ)mər-ˌkap-ˈtä-mə-rən\ *n* : a mercurial compound $C_{16}H_{25}HgNNa_2O_6S$ formerly used as a diuretic

mer•cap•to•pu•rine \(ˌ)mər-ˌkap-tə-ˈpyu̇r-ˌēn\ *n* : an antimetabolite $C_5H_4N_4S$ that interferes esp. with the metabolism of purine bases and the biosynthesis of nucleic acids and that is sometimes useful in the treatment of acute leukemia

mer•cu•mat•i•lin \ˌmər-kyu̇-ˈmat-ᵊl-ən, mər-ˌkyü-mə-ˈti-lən\ *n* : a chemical combination of a mercury-containing acid $C_{14}H_{14}HgO_6$ and theophylline formerly used as a diuretic

¹**mer•cu•ri•al** \(ˌ)mər-ˈkyu̇r-ē-əl\ *adj* : of, relating to, containing, or caused by mercury ⟨~ salves⟩

²**mercurial** *n* : a pharmaceutical or chemical containing mercury

mer•cu•ri•al•ism \(ˌ)mər-ˈkyu̇r-ē-ə-ˌli-zəm\ *n* : chronic poisoning with mercury — called also *hydrargyrism*

mer•cu•ric chloride \(ˌ)mər-ˈkyu̇r-ik-\ *n* : a poisonous compound $HgCl_2$ used as a disinfectant and fungicide — called also *bichloride of mercury, corrosive sublimate, mercury bichloride*

mercuric cyanide *n* : the mercury cyanide $Hg(CN)_2$ which has been used as an antiseptic

mercuric iodide *n* : a red crystalline poisonous salt HgI_2 which has been used as a topical antiseptic

mercuric oxide *n* : either of two forms of a slightly water-soluble poisonous compound HgO which have been used in antiseptic ointments

Mer•cu•ro•chrome \(ˌ)mər-ˈkyu̇r-ə-ˌkrōm\ *trademark* — used for a preparation of merbromin

mer•cu•ro•phyl•line \ˌmər-kyə-rō-ˈfi-ˌlēn, -lən\ *n* : a chemical combination of a mercurial compound $C_{14}H_{24}HgNNaO_5$ and theophylline formerly used as a diuretic

mer•cu•rous chloride \mər-ˈkyu̇r-əs-, ˈmər-kyə-rəs-\ *n* : CALOMEL

mer•cu•ry \ˈmər-kyə-rē\ *n, pl* **-ries** **1** : a heavy silver-white poisonous metallic element that is liquid at ordinary temperatures — symbol *Hg;* called also *quicksilver;* see ELEMENT table **2** : a pharmaceutical preparation containing mercury or a compound of it

mercury bi•chlo•ride \-ˌbī-ˈklōr-ˌīd\ *n* : MERCURIC CHLORIDE

mercury chloride *n* : a chloride of mercury: as **a** : CALOMEL **b** : MERCURIC CHLORIDE

mercury–vapor lamp *n* : an electric lamp in which the discharge takes place through mercury vapor and which has been used therapeutically as a source of ultraviolet radiation

mercy killing *n* : EUTHANASIA

-mere \ˌmir\ *n comb form* : part : segment ⟨blasto*mere*⟩ ⟨centro*mere*⟩

Me•rid•ia \mə-ˈrid-ē-ə\ *trademark* — used for a preparation of the hydrated hydrochloride of sibutramine

me•rid•i•an \mə-ˈri-dē-ən\ *n* **1** : an imaginary circle or closed curve on the surface of a sphere or globe=

shaped body (as the eyeball) that lies in a plane passing through the poles **2** : any of the pathways along which the body's vital energy flows according to the theory of acupuncture — **merid·ian** *adj* — **me·rid·i·o·nal** \mə-ˈri-dē-ən-ᵊl\ *adj*

Mer·kel cell *also* **Merkel's cell** \ˈmər-kəl(z)-\ *n* : a cell that occurs in the basal part of the epidermis, is characterized by dense granules in its cytoplasm, is closely associated with the unmyelinated tip of a nerve fiber, and prob. functions in tactile sensory perception

Merkel, Friedrich Siegmund (1845–1919), German anatomist.

Merkel's disk *n* : the disklike expansion of the end of a nerve fiber together with a closely associated Merkel cell that has a presumed tactile function — called also *Merkel's corpuscle*

mero- — see MER-

mero·blas·tic \ˌmer-ə-ˈblas-tik\ *adj* : characterized by or being incomplete cleavage as a result of the presence of an impeding mass of yolk material (as in the eggs of birds) — compare HOLOBLASTIC — **mero·blas·ti·cal·ly** *adv*

mero·crine \ˈmer-ə-krən, -ˌkrīn, -ˌkrēn\ *adj* : producing a secretion that is discharged without major damage to the secreting cells ⟨~ glands⟩; *also* : of or produced by a merocrine gland ⟨a ~ secretion⟩ — compare APOCRINE, ECCRINE, HOLOCRINE

mero·my·o·sin \ˌmer-ə-ˈmī-ə-sən\ *n* : either of two structural subunits of myosin that are obtained esp. by tryptic digestion

mero·zo·ite \ˌmer-ə-ˈzō-ˌīt\ *n* : a small amoeboid sporozoan trophozoite (as of a malaria parasite) produced by schizogony that is capable of initiating a new sexual or asexual cycle of development

MERS \ˈmərz\ *n* : a serious viral respiratory illness that is caused by a coronavirus (species *Middle East respiratory syndrome coronavirus* of the genus *Betacoronavirus*), that is marked by fever, cough, and shortness of breath, and may often progress to severe pneumonia with acute respiratory distress syndrome and organ failure, and that typically occurs in or near the Arabian peninsula — called also *Middle East respiratory syndrome*

mer·sal·yl \(ˌ)mər-ˈsa-lil\ *n* : an organic mercurial $C_{13}H_{16}HgNNaO_6$ administered by injection in combination with theophylline as a diuretic

Mer·thi·o·late \(ˌ)mər-ˈthī-ə-ˌlāt, -lət\ *n* : a preparation of thimerosal — formerly a U.S. registered trademark

mes- *or* **meso-** *comb form* **1 a** : mid : in the middle ⟨*meso*derm⟩ **b** : mesentery or membrane supporting a (specified) part ⟨*meso*appendix⟩ ⟨*meso*colon⟩ **2** : intermediate (as in size or type) ⟨*meso*morph⟩

mes·an·gi·um \ˌme-ˈsan-jē-əm, ˌmē-\ *n, pl* **-gia** \-jē-ə\ : a thin membrane that gives support to the capillaries surrounding the tubule of a nephron — **mes·an·gi·al** \-jē-əl\ *adj*

Mes·an·to·in \me-ˈsan-tō-in\ *trademark* — used for a preparation of mephenytoin

mes·aor·ti·tis \ˌme-ˌsā-ȯr-ˈtī-təs, ˌmē-\ *n, pl* **-tit·i·des** \-ˈti-tə-ˌdēz\ : inflammation of the middle layer of the aorta

mes·ar·ter·i·tis \-ˌsär-tə-ˈrī-təs\ *n, pl* **-it·i·des** \-ˈri-tə-ˌdēz\ : inflammation of the middle layer of an artery

mes·cal \me-ˈskal, mə-\ *n* **1** : PEYOTE 2 **2** : a usu. colorless Mexican liquor distilled esp. from the central leaves of any of various fleshy-leaved agaves (genus *Agave* of the family Agavaceae); *also* : a plant from which mescal is produced

mescal button *n* : PEYOTE BUTTON

mes·ca·line \ˈmes-kə-lən, -ˌlēn\ *n* : a hallucinatory crystalline alkaloid $C_{11}H_{17}NO_3$ that is the chief active principle in peyote buttons

mes·en·ceph·a·lon \ˌme-zən-ˈse-fə-ˌlän, ˌmē-, -sən-, -lən\ *n* : MIDBRAIN — **mes·en·ce·phal·ic** \-zen-sə-ˈfa-lik, -sen-\ *adj*

mes·en·chyme \ˈme-zən-ˌkīm, ˈmē-, -sən-\ *n* : loosely organized undifferentiated mesodermal cells that give rise to such structures as connective tissues, blood, lymphatics, bone, and cartilage — **mes·en·chy·mal** \ˌme-zən-ˈkī-məl, ˌmē-, -sən-\ *adj* — **mes·en·chy·ma·tous** \-mə-təs\ *adj*

mes·en·chy·mo·ma \ˌme-zən-ˌkī-ˈmō-mə, ˌmē-, -sən-\ *n, pl* **-mas** *also* **-ma·ta** \-mə-tə\ : a benign or malignant tumor consisting of a mixture of at least two types of embryonic connective tissue

[1]**mes·en·ter·ic** \ˌme-zən-ˈter-ik, -sən-\ *adj* : of, relating to, or located in or near a mesentery

[2]**mesenteric** *n* : a mesenteric part; *esp* : MESENTERIC ARTERY

mesenteric artery *n* : either of two arteries arising from the aorta and passing between the two layers of the mesentery to the intestine: **a** : one that arises just above the bifurcation of the abdominal aorta into the common iliac arteries and supplies the left half of the transverse colon, the descending colon, the sigmoid colon, and most of the rectum — called also *inferior mesenteric artery* **b** : one that arises from the aorta just below the celiac artery at the level of the first lumbar vertebra and supplies the greater part of the small intestine, the cecum, the ascending colon, and the right half of the transverse colon — called also *superior mesenteric artery*

mesenteric ganglion *n* : either of two ganglionic masses of the sympathetic nervous system associated with the corresponding mesenteric plexus: **a** : a variable amount of massed ganglionic tissue of the inferior mesenteric plexus near the origin of the inferior mesenteric artery — called also *inferior mesenteric ganglion* **b :** a usu. discrete ganglionic mass of the superior mesenteric plexus near the origin of the superior mesenteric artery — called also *superior mesenteric ganglion*

mesenteric node *n* **:** any of the lymphatic glands of the mesentery — called also *mesenteric gland, mesenteric lymph node*

mesenteric plexus *n* **:** either of two plexuses of the sympathetic nervous system lying mostly in the mesentery in close proximity to and distributed to the same structures as the corresponding mesenteric arteries: **a :** one associated with the inferior mesenteric artery — called also *inferior mesenteric plexus* **b :** a subdivision of the celiac plexus associated with the superior mesenteric artery — called also *superior mesenteric plexus*

mesenteric vein *n* **:** either of two veins draining the intestine, passing between the two layers of the mesentery, and associated with the corresponding mesenteric arteries: **a :** one that is a continuation of the superior rectal vein, that returns blood from the rectum, the sigmoid colon, and the descending colon, that accompanies the inferior mesenteric artery, and that usu. empties into the splenic vein — called also *inferior mesenteric vein* **b :** one that drains blood from the small intestine, the cecum, the ascending colon, and the transverse colon, that accompanies the superior mesenteric artery, and that joins with the splenic vein to form the portal vein — called also *superior mesenteric vein*

mes•en•tery \ˈme-zən-ˌter-ē, -sən-\ *n, pl* **-ter•ies** **1 :** one or more vertebrate membranes that consist of a double fold of the peritoneum and invest the intestines and their appendages and connect them with the dorsal wall of the abdominal cavity; *specif* **:** such membranes connected with the jejunum and ileum in humans **2 :** a fold of membrane comparable to a mesentery and supporting a viscus (as the heart) that is not a part of the digestive tract

mesh \ˈmesh\ *n* **:** a flexible netting of fine wire used in surgery (as in the repair of large hernias)

me•si•al \ˈmē-zē-əl, -sē-\ *adj* **1 :** being or located in the middle or a median part ⟨the ~ aspect of the metacarpal head⟩ **2 :** situated in or near or directed toward the median plane of the body ⟨the heart is ~ to the lungs⟩ — compare DISTAL 1b **3 :** of, relating to, or being the surface of a tooth that is next to the tooth in front of it or that is closest to the middle of the front of the jaw — compare DISTAL 1c, PROXIMAL 1b — **me•si•al•ly** *adv*

mesio- *comb form* **:** mesial and ⟨*mesio*distal⟩ ⟨*mesio*buccal⟩

me•sio•buc•cal \ˌmē-zē-ō-ˈbək-əl, -sē-\ *adj* **:** of or relating to the mesial and buccal surfaces of a tooth — **me•sio•buc•cal•ly** *adv*

me•sio•clu•sion *also* **me•si•oc•clu•sion** \ˌmē-zē-ə-ˈklü-zhən, -sē-\ *n* **:** malocclusion characterized by mesial displacement of one or more of the lower teeth

me•sio•dis•tal \ˌmē-zē-ō-ˈdist-əl\ *adj* **:** of or relating to the mesial and distal surfaces of a tooth; *esp* **:** relating to, lying along, containing, or being a diameter joining the mesial and distal surfaces — **me•sio•dis•tal•ly** *adv*

me•sio•lin•gual \-ˈliŋ-gwəl\ *adj* **:** of or relating to the mesial and lingual surfaces of a tooth — **me•sio•lin•gual•ly** *adv*

mes•mer•ism \ˈmez-mə-ˌri-zəm, ˈmes-\ *n* **:** hypnotic induction by the practices of F. A. Mesmer; *broadly* **:** HYPNOTISM — **mes•mer•ist** \-rist\ *n* — **mes•mer•ize** \-ˌrīz\ *vb*

Mes•mer \ˈmes-mər\, **Franz** *or* **Friedrich Anton (1734–1815),** German physician.

meso- — see MES-

me•so•ap•pen•dix \ˌme-zō-ə-ˈpen-diks, ˌmē-, -sō-\ *n, pl* **-dix•es** *or* **-di•ces** \-də-ˌsēz\ **:** the mesentery of the vermiform appendix — **me•so•ap•pen•di•ce•al** \-ˌpen-də-ˈsē-əl\ *adj*

me•so•blast \ˈme-zə-ˌblast, ˈmē-, -sə-\ *n* **:** the embryonic cells that give rise to mesoderm; *broadly* **:** MESODERM — **me•so•blas•tic** \ˌme-zō-ˈblas-tik, ˌmē-, -sō-\ *adj*

me•so•car•di•um \ˌme-zō-ˈkär-dē-əm, ˌmē-, -sō-\ *n* **1 :** the transitory mesentery of the embryonic heart **2 :** either of two tubular prolongations of the epicardium that enclose the aorta and pulmonary trunk and the venae cavae and pulmonary veins

Me•so•ces•toi•des \-ˌses-ˈtȯi-(ˌ)dēz\ *n* **:** a genus (family Mesocestoididae) of tapeworms parasitic in mammals and birds

me•so•co•lon \ˌme-zə-ˈkō-lən, ˌmē-, -sə-\ *n* **:** a mesentery joining the colon to the dorsal abdominal wall

me•so•derm \ˈme-zə-ˌdərm, ˈmē-, -sə-\ *n* **:** the middle of the three primary germ layers of an embryo that is the source esp. of bone, muscle, connective tissue, and dermis; *broadly* **:** tissue derived from this germ layer — **me•so•der•mal** \ˌme-zə-ˈdər-məl, ˌmē-, -sə-\ *adj* — **me•so•der•mal•ly** *adv*

me•so•duo•de•num \ˌme-zə-ˌdü-ə-ˈdē-nəm, ˌmē-, -sə-, -ˌdyü-; -dü-ˈäd-ən-əm, -dyü-\ *n, pl* **-de•na** \-ə-ˈdē-nə, -ˈäd-ən-ə\ *or* **-de•nums** **:** the mesentery of the duodenum usu. not persisting in adult life in humans and other mammals in which the developing intestine undergoes a counterclockwise rotation

me•so•gas•tri•um \-ˈgas-trē-əm\ *n, pl* **-tria** \-trē-ə\ **1 :** a ventral mesentery of the embryonic stomach that persists as the falciform ligament and the lesser omentum — called also *ventral mesogastrium* **2** : a dorsal mesentery of the embryonic stomach that gives rise to ligaments between the stomach and spleen and the spleen and kidney — called also *dorsal mesogastrium*

me•so•ino•si•tol \ˌme-zō-i-ˈnō-sə-ˌtȯl, ˌmē-, -ī-ˈnō-, -ˌtōl\ *n* : MYOINOSITOL

me•so•lim•bic \-ˈlim-bik\ *adj* : of, relating to, or being the more central portion of the limbic system of the brain that arises mainly in the ventral tegmental area, consists esp. of dopaminergic neurons, and innervates the amygdala, nucleus accumbens, and olfactory tubercle

me•so•morph \ˈme-zə-ˌmȯrf, ˈmē-, -sə-\ *n* : a mesomorphic body or person

me•so•mor•phic \ˌme-zə-ˈmȯr-fik, ˌmē-, -sə-\ *adj* : having a husky muscular body build — compare ECTOMORPHIC, ENDOMORPHIC — **me•so•mor•phy** \ˈme-zə-ˌmȯr-fē, ˈmē-, -sə-\ *n*

me•so•neph•ric \ˌme-zə-ˈne-frik, ˌmē-, -sə-\ *adj* : of or relating to the mesonephros

mesonephric duct *n* : WOLFFIAN DUCT

me•so•ne•phro•ma \-ni-ˈfrō-mə\ *n, pl* **-mas** *also* **-ma•ta** \-mə-tə\ : a benign or malignant tumor esp. of the female genital tract held to be derived from the mesonephros

me•so•neph•ros \ˌme-zə-ˈne-frəs, ˌmē-, -sə-, -ˌfräs\ *n, pl* **-neph•roi** \-ˈne-ˌfrȯi\ : either member of the second and midmost of the three paired vertebrate renal organs that functions in adult fishes and amphibians but functions only in the embryo of reptiles, birds, and mammals in which it is replaced by a metanephros in the adult — called also *Wolffian body;* compare PRONEPHROS

me•sor•chi•um \mə-ˈzȯr-kē-əm\ *n, pl* **-chia** \-kē-ə\ : the fold of peritoneum that attaches the testis to the dorsal wall in the fetus

me•so•rec•tum \ˌme-zə-ˈrek-təm, ˌmē-, -sə-\ *n, pl* **-tums** *or* **-ta** \-tə\ : the mesentery that supports the rectum

mes•orid•a•zine \ˌme-zō-ˈri-də-ˌzēn, ˌmē-, -sō-\ *n* : a phenothiazine tranquilizer $C_{21}H_{26}N_2OS_2$ used formerly esp. to treat schizophrenia and anxiety

me•so•sal•pinx \ˌme-zō-ˈsal-(ˌ)piŋks, ˌmē-, -sō-\ *n, pl* **-sal•pin•ges** \-sal-ˈpin-(ˌ)jēz\ : a fold of the broad ligament investing and supporting the fallopian tube

me•so•sig•moid \-ˈsig-ˌmȯid\ *n* : the mesentery of the sigmoid part of the descending colon

me•so•ster•num \ˌme-zə-ˈstər-nəm, ˌmē-, -sə-\ *n, pl* **-ster•na** \-nə\ : GLADIOLUS

me•so•ten•don \-ˈten-dən\ *n* : a fold of synovial membrane connecting a tendon to its synovial sheath

me•so•the•li•o•ma \ˌme-zə-ˌthē-lē-ˈō-mə, ˌmē-, -sə-\ *n, pl* **-mas** *also* **-ma•ta** \-mə-tə\ : a tumor derived from mesothelial tissue (as that lining the peritoneum or pleura)

me•so•the•li•um \-ˈthē-lē-əm\ *n, pl* **-lia** \-lē-ə\ : epithelium derived from mesoderm that lines the body cavity of a vertebrate embryo and gives rise to epithelia (as of the peritoneum, pericardium, and pleurae), striated muscle, heart muscle, and several minor structures — **me•so•the•li•al** \-lē-əl\ *adj*

mes•ovar•i•um \-ˈvar-ē-əm\ *n, pl* **-ovar•ia** \-ē-ə\ : the mesentery uniting the ovary with the body wall

mes•ox•a•lyl•urea \-ˌäk-sə-li-ˈlu̇r-ē-ə, -ˌlil-ˈyu̇r-\ *n* : ALLOXAN

mes•sen•ger \ˈmes-ᵊn-jər\ *n* **1** : a substance (as a hormone) that mediates a biological effect — see FIRST MESSENGER, SECOND MESSENGER **2** : MESSENGER RNA

messenger RNA *n* : an RNA produced by transcription that carries the code for a particular protein from the nuclear DNA to a ribosome in the cytoplasm and acts as a template for the formation of that protein — called also *mRNA;* compare TRANSFER RNA

mes•ter•o•lone \me-ˈster-ə-ˌlōn\ *n* : an androgen $C_{20}H_{32}O_2$ used in the treatment of hypogonadism

Mes•ti•non \ˈmes-tə-ˌnän\ *trademark* — used for a preparation of the bromide of pyridostigmine

mes•tra•nol \ˈmes-trə-ˌnȯl, -ˌnōl\ *n* : a synthetic estrogen $C_{21}H_{26}O_2$ used in birth control pills — see ENOVID, ORTHO-NOVUM

mes•y•late \ˈme-si-ˌlāt\ *n* : a salt or ester of an acid CH_4O_3S used esp. in pharmaceutical preparations — see ERGOLOID MESYLATES

met \ˈmet, ˌem-(ˌ)ē-ˈtē\ *n, often all cap* : a unit of measure of the rate at which the body expends energy that is based on the energy expenditure while sitting at rest and is equal to 3.5 milliliters of oxygen per kilogram of body weight per minute — called also *metabolic equivalent*

Met *abbr* methionine

meta- *or* **met-** *prefix* **1** : situated behind or beyond ⟨*met*encephalon⟩ **2** : change in : transformation of ⟨*meta*plasia⟩

meta–ana•ly•sis \ˌme-tə-ə-ˈna-lə-səs\ *n* : a quantitative statistical analysis of several separate but similar experiments or studies in order to test the pooled data for statistical significance

met•a•bol•ic \ˌme-tə-ˈbä-lik\ *adj* **1** : of, relating to, or based on metabolism **2** : VEGETATIVE 1a(2) — used esp. of a cell nucleus that is not dividing — **met•a•bol•i•cal•ly** *adv*

metabolic acidosis *n* : acidosis resulting from excess acid due to abnormal metabolism, excessive acid intake, or renal retention or from excessive loss of bicarbonate (as in diarrhea)

metabolic alkalosis *n* : alkalosis resulting from excessive alkali intake or excessive acid loss (as from vomiting)

metabolic equivalent *n* : MET
metabolic pathway *n* : PATHWAY 2
metabolic rate *n* : metabolism per unit time esp. as estimated by food consumption, energy released as heat, or oxygen used in metabolic processes — see BASAL METABOLIC RATE
metabolic syndrome *n* : a syndrome marked by the presence of usu. three or more of a group of factors (as high blood pressure, abdominal obesity, high triglyceride levels, low HDL levels, and high fasting levels of blood sugar) that are linked to an increased risk of cardiovascular disease and type 2 diabetes — called also *insulin resistance syndrome, syndrome X*
me•tab•o•lism \mə-ˈta-bə-ˌli-zəm\ *n* **1** : the sum of the processes in the buildup and destruction of protoplasm; *specif* : the chemical changes in living cells by which energy is provided for vital processes and activities and new material is assimilated — see ANABOLISM, CATABOLISM **2** : the sum of the processes by which a particular substance is handled (as by assimilation and incorporation or by detoxification and excretion) in the living body
me•tab•o•lite \-ˌlīt\ *n* **1** : a product of metabolism: **a** : a metabolic waste usu. more or less toxic to the organism producing it : EXCRETION **b** : a product of one metabolic process that is essential to another such process in the same organism **c** : a metabolic waste of one organism that is markedly toxic to another : ANTIBIOTIC **2** : a substance essential to the metabolism of a particular organism or to a particular metabolic process
me•tab•o•lize \-ˌlīz\ *vb* **-lized; -liz•ing** : to subject to metabolism — **me•tab•o•liz•able** \mə-ˌta-bə-ˈlī-zə-bəl\ *adj*
me•tab•o•tro•pic \mə-ˌta-bə-ˈtrō-pik, -ˈträ\ *adj* : relating to or being a receptor for glutamate that when complexed with G protein triggers increased production of certain intracellular messengers
[1]**meta•car•pal** \ˌme-tə-ˈkär-pəl\ *adj* : of, relating to, or being the metacarpus or a metacarpal
[2]**metacarpal** *n* : any bone of the metacarpus of the human hand or the front foot in quadrupeds
meta•car•po•pha•lan•ge•al \ˌme-tə-ˌkär-pō-ˌfā-lən-ˈjē-əl, -ˌfa-, -fə-ˈlan-jē-\ *adj* : of, relating to, or involving both the metacarpus and the phalanges
meta•car•pus \-ˈkär-pəs\ *n* : the part of the human hand or the front foot in quadrupeds between the carpus and the phalanges that contains five more or less elongated bones when all the digits are present (as in humans) but is modified in many animals by the loss or reduction of some bones or the fusing of adjacent bones
meta•cen•tric \ˌme-tə-ˈsen-trik\ *adj* : having the centromere medially situated so that the two chromosomal arms are of roughly equal length — compare ACROCENTRIC, TELOCENTRIC — **metacentric** *n*
meta•cer•car•ia \ˌme-tə-(ˌ)sər-ˈkar-ē-ə\ *n, pl* **-i•ae** \-ē-ˌē\ : a tailless encysted late larva of a digenetic trematode that is usu. the form which is infective for the definitive host — **meta•cer•car•i•al** \-ē-əl\ *adj*
meta•ces•tode \-ˈses-ˌtōd\ *n* : a stage of a tapeworm occurring in an intermediate host : a larval tapeworm
metachromatic leukodystrophy *n* : a genetic neurodegenerative disorder that is inherited as an autosomal recessive trait and is marked by the accumulation of sulfatides resulting in the loss of myelin in the central nervous system and leading to progressive deterioration of cognitive and motor functioning
me•tach•ro•nous \mə-ˈta-krə-nəs\ *adj* : occurring or starting at different times ⟨~ cancers⟩
meta•cre•sol \ˌme-tə-ˈkrē-ˌsȯl, -ˌsōl\ *n* : an isomer of cresol that has antiseptic properties
Meta•gon•i•mus \-ˈgä-nə-məs\ *n* : a genus of intestinal flukes (family Heterophyidae) including a parasite (*M. yokogawai*) of humans, dogs, and cats in eastern Asia contracted by eating raw fish containing larva
Meta•hy•drin \-ˈhī-drin\ *trademark* — used for a preparation of trichlormethiazide
metall- *or* **metallo-** *comb form* : containing a metal atom or ion in the molecule ⟨*metallo*porphyrin⟩
me•tal•lo•en•zyme \mə-ˌta-lō-ˈen-ˌzīm\ *n* : an enzyme consisting of a protein linked with a specific metal
met•al•loid \ˈmet-ᵊl-ˌȯid\ *n* : an element (as boron, silicon, or arsenic) intermediate in properties between the typical metals and nonmetals
me•tal•lo•por•phy•rin \-ˈpȯr-fə-rən\ *n* : a compound (as heme) formed from a porphyrin and a metal ion
me•tal•lo•pro•tein \-ˈprō-ˌtēn, -ˈprōt-ē-ən\ *n* : a conjugated protein in which the prosthetic group is a metal
me•tal•lo•thio•ne•in \-ˌthī-ə-ˈnē-ən\ *n* : any of various metal-binding proteins involved in the metabolism of copper and zinc in body tissue (as of the liver) and in the binding of toxic metals (as cadmium)
meta•mere \ˈme-tə-ˌmir\ *n* : any of a linear series of primitively similar segments into which the body of a higher invertebrate or vertebrate is divisible : SOMITE — **meta•mer•ic** \ˌme-tə-ˈmer-ik\ *adj*
meta•mor•pho•sis \ˌme-tə-ˈmȯr-fə-səs\ *n, pl* **-pho•ses** \-ˌsēz\ : change of physical form, structure, or substance
Met•a•mu•cil \ˌme-tə-ˈmyüs-ᵊl\ *trademark* — used for a laxative preparation of a hydrophilic mucilloid from the husk of psyllium seed

meta·my·elo·cyte \ˌme-tə-ˈmī-ə-lə-ˌsīt\ *n* : any of the most immature granulocytes present in normal blood that are distinguished by typical cytoplasmic granulation in combination with a simple kidney-shaped nucleus

meta·neph·ric \ˌme-tə-ˈne-frik\ *adj* : of or relating to the metanephros

meta·neph·rine \-ˈne-ˌfrēn\ *n* : a catabolite of epinephrine that is found in the urine and some tissues

meta·neph·ro·gen·ic \-ˌne-frə-ˈje-nik\ *adj* : giving rise to the metanephroi

meta·neph·ros \-ˈne-frəs, -ˌfräs\ *n, pl* **-neph·roi** \-ˈne-ˌfrȯi\ : either member of the final and most caudal pair of the three successive pairs of vertebrate renal organs that functions as a permanent adult kidney in reptiles, birds, and mammals but is not present at all in lower forms — compare MESONEPHROS, PRONEPHROS

meta·phase \ˈme-tə-ˌfāz\ *n* : the stage of mitosis and meiosis in which the chromosomes become arranged in the equatorial plane of the spindle

metaphase plate *n* : a section in the equatorial plane of the metaphase spindle having the chromosomes oriented upon it

me·taph·y·se·al *also* **me·taph·y·si·al** \mə-ˌta-fə-ˈsē-əl, -ˈzē-, ˌme-tə-ˈfi-zē-əl\ *adj* : of or relating to a metaphysis

me·taph·y·sis \mə-ˈta-fə-səs\ *n, pl* **-y·ses** \-ˌsēz\ : the transitional zone at which the diaphysis and epiphysis of a bone come together

meta·pla·sia \ˌme-tə-ˈplā-zhə, -zhē-ə\ *n* **1** : transformation of one tissue into another ⟨~ of cartilage into bone⟩ **2** : abnormal replacement of cells of one type by cells of another — **meta·plas·tic** \-ˈplas-tik\ *adj*

meta·pro·ter·e·nol \-prō-ˈter-ə-ˈnȯl, -ˌnōl\ *n* : a beta-adrenergic bronchodilator that is administered in the form of its sulfate $(C_{11}H_{17}NO_3)_2 \cdot H_2SO_4$ in the treatment of bronchial asthma and reversible bronchospasm associated with bronchitis and emphysema — called also *orciprenaline*

meta·ram·i·nol \ˌme-tə-ˈra-mə-ˌnȯl, -ˌnōl\ *n* : a vasoconstrictor used in the form of its bitartrate $C_9H_{13}NO_2 \cdot C_4H_6O_6$ esp. to raise or maintain blood pressure

met·ar·te·ri·ole \ˌmet-ˌär-ˈtir-ē-ˌōl\ *n* : any of the delicate blood vessels that branch from the smallest arterioles and connect with the capillary bed — called also *precapillary*

me·tas·ta·sis \mə-ˈtas-tə-səs\ *n, pl* **-ta·ses** \-ˌsēz\ **1 a** : change of position, state, or form **b** : the spread of a disease-producing agent (as cancer cells or bacteria) or disease from the initial or primary site of occurrence to another part of the body; *also* : the process by which such spreading occurs **2** : a secondary malignant tumor resulting from metastasis

me·tas·ta·size \mə-ˈtas-tə-ˌsīz\ *vb* **-sized; -siz·ing** : to spread by metastasis ⟨colon cancer *metastasized* to the liver⟩

met·a·sta·tic \ˌme-tə-ˈsta-tik\ *adj* **1** : of, relating to, or caused by metastasis ⟨~ carcinoma⟩ ⟨~ spread⟩ **2** : tending to metastasize ⟨~ breast cancer⟩ — **met·a·stat·i·cal·ly** \-ti-k(ə-)lē\ *adv*

Meta·stron·gy·lus \ˌme-tə-ˈsträn-jə-ləs\ *n* : a genus of nematode worms (family Metastrongylidae) that are parasitic esp. in the lungs of mammals

[1]**meta·tar·sal** \ˌme-tə-ˈtär-səl\ *adj* : of, relating to, or being the part of the human foot or of the hind foot in quadrupeds between the tarsus and the phalanges that in humans comprises five elongated bones which form the front of the instep and ball of the foot

[2]**metatarsal** *n* : a metatarsal bone

meta·tar·sal·gia \-ˌtär-ˈsal-jə, -jē-ə\ *n* : a cramping burning pain below and between the metatarsal bones where they join the toe bones — see MORTON'S TOE

meta·tar·sec·to·my \-ˌtär-ˈsek-tə-mē\ *n, pl* **-mies** : surgical removal of the metatarsus or a metatarsal bone

meta·tar·so·pha·lan·ge·al joint \-ˌtär-sō-ˌfā-lən-ˈjē-əl-, -ˌfa-, -fə-ˈlan-jē-\ *n* : any of the joints between the metatarsals and the phalanges

meta·tar·sus \ˌme-tə-ˈtär-səs\ *n* : the part of the human foot or of the hind foot in quadrupeds that is between the tarsus and phalanges, contains when all the digits are present (as in humans) five more or less elongated bones but is modified in many animals with loss or reduction of some bones or fusing of others, and in humans forms the instep

meta·thal·a·mus \-ˈtha-lə-məs\ *n, pl* **-mi** \-ˌmī\ : the part of the diencephalon on each side that comprises the lateral and medial geniculate bodies

met·ax·a·lone \mə-ˈtak-sə-ˌlōn\ *n* : a drug $C_{12}H_{15}NO_3$ used as a skeletal muscle relaxant — see SKELAXIN

meta·zo·an \ˌme-tə-ˈzō-ən\ *n* : any of a group (Metazoa) that comprises all animals having the body composed of cells differentiated into tissues and organs and usu. a digestive cavity — **metazoan** *adj*

met·en·ceph·a·lon \ˌmet-ˌen-ˈse-fə-ˌlän, -lən\ *n* : the anterior segment of the developing vertebrate hindbrain or the corresponding part of the adult brain composed of the cerebellum and pons — **met·en·ce·phal·ic** \-ˌen-sə-ˈfa-lik\ *adj*

Met–en·keph·a·lin \ˌme-ten-ˈke-fə-lin\ *n* : METHIONINE-ENKEPHALIN

me·te·or·ism \ˈmē-tē-ə-ˌri-zəm\ *n* : gaseous distension of the stomach or intestine : TYMPANITES

me·ter \ˈmē-tər\ *n* : the base unit of length in the International System of Units that is equal to the distance traveled by light in a vacuum in $^1/_{299,792,458}$ second or to about 39.37 inches

-meter *n comb form* : instrument or means for measuring ⟨calori*meter*⟩

metered–dose inhaler *n* : a pocket-sized handheld inhaler that delivers a standardized dose of medication for bronchodilation — abbr. *MDI*

meter–kilogram–second *adj* : MKS

met•for•min \met-ˈfȯr-mən\ *n* : an antidiabetic drug used in the form of its hydrochloride $C_4H_{11}N_5 \cdot HCl$ esp. to treat type 2 diabetes in patients unresponsive to or intolerant of approved sulfonylurea drugs — see GLUCOPHAGE, GLUCOVANCE, INVOKAMET, JANUMET, JENTADUETO, KOMBIGLYZE

meth \ˈmeth\ *n* : METHAMPHETAMINE

meth- *or* **metho-** *comb form* : methyl ⟨*meth*amphetamine⟩

metha•cho•line \ˌme-thə-ˈkō-ˌlēn\ *n* : a parasympathomimetic drug administered in the form of its crystalline chloride $C_8H_{18}ClNO_2$ esp. to diagnose hypersensitivity of the bronchial air passages (as in asthma) — see MECHOLYL, PROVOCHOLINE

metha•cy•cline \ˌme-thə-ˈsī-ˌklēn\ *n* : a semisynthetic tetracycline $C_{22}H_{22}N_2O_8$ with longer duration of action than most other tetracyclines and used in the treatment of gonorrhea esp. in penicillin-sensitive subjects

meth•a•done \ˈme-thə-ˌdōn\ *also* **meth•a•don** \-ˌdän\ *n* : a synthetic addictive narcotic drug used esp. in the form of its hydrochloride $C_{21}H_{27}NO \cdot HCl$ for the relief of pain and as a substitute narcotic in the treatment of heroin addiction — called also *amidone*

met•haem•al•bu•min, met•hae•mo•glo•bin, met•hae•mo•glo•bi•nae•mia *chiefly Brit var of* METHEMALBUMIN, METHEMOGLOBIN, METHEMOGLOBINEMIA

meth•am•phet•amine \ˌme-tham-ˈfe-tə-ˌmēn, -thəm-, -mən\ *n* : an amine $C_{10}H_{15}N$ that is used medically in the form of its hydrochloride $C_{10}H_{15}N \cdot HCl$ esp. to treat attention deficit disorder and obesity and that is often abused illicitly as a stimulant — called also *meth, methedrine, methylamphetamine, speed*

meth•an•dro•sten•o•lone \ˌme-ˌthan-drō-ˈste-nə-ˌlōn\ *n* : an anabolic steroid $C_{20}H_{28}O_2$

meth•ane \ˈme-ˌthān\ *n* : a colorless odorless flammable gaseous hydrocarbon CH_4 that is lighter than air, forms explosive mixtures with air or oxygen, and occurs naturally as a by-product of the decomposition of organic matter by anaerobic bacteria

meth•a•nol \ˈme-thə-ˌnȯl, -ˌnōl\ *n* : a volatile pungent flammable poisonous liquid alcohol CH_3OH used esp. as a solvent, antifreeze, or denaturant for ethanol — called also *methyl alcohol, wood alcohol*

meth•an•the•line \me-ˈthan-thə-ˌlēn, -lən\ *n* : an anticholinergic drug usu. administered in the form of its crystalline bromide $C_{21}H_{26}BrNO_3$ in the treatment of peptic ulcers

meth•a•pyr•i•lene \-ˈpir-ə-ˌlēn\ *n* : an antihistamine drug $C_{14}H_{19}N_3S$ formerly used as a mild sedative in proprietary sleep-inducing drugs

meth•aqua•lone \me-ˈtha-kwə-ˌlōn\ *n* : a sedative and hypnotic nonbarbiturate drug $C_{16}H_{14}N_2O$ that is habit-forming — see QUAALUDE

meth•ar•bi•tal \me-ˈthär-bə-ˌtȯl, -ˌtäl\ *n* : an anticonvulsant barbiturate $C_9H_{14}N_2O_3$

meth•a•zol•amide \ˌme-thə-ˈzō-lə-ˌmīd\ *n* : a sulfonamide $C_5H_8N_4O_3S_2$ that inhibits the production of carbonic anhydrase, reduces intraocular pressure, and is used in the treatment of glaucoma — see NEPTAZANE

meth•dil•a•zine \meth-ˈdi-lə-ˌzēn, -ˈdī-lə-ˌzīn\ *n* : a phenothiazine antihistamine used in the form of its hydrochloride $C_{18}H_{20}N_2S \cdot HCl$ as an antipruritic

meth•e•drine \ˈme-thə-drən, -ˌdrēn\ *n* : METHAMPHETAMINE

met•hem•al•bu•min \ˌmet-ˌhē-mal-ˈbyü-mən\ *n* : an albumin complex with hematin found in plasma during diseases (as blackwater fever) associated with extensive hemolysis

met•he•mo•glo•bin \(ˌ)met-ˈhē-mə-ˌglō-bin\ *n* : a soluble brown crystalline basic blood pigment that is found in normal blood in much smaller amounts than hemoglobin, that is formed from blood, hemoglobin, or oxyhemoglobin by oxidation, and that differs from hemoglobin in containing ferric iron and in being unable to combine reversibly with molecular oxygen — called also *ferrihemoglobin*

met•he•mo•glo•bi•ne•mia \ˌmet-ˌhē-mə-ˌglō-bə-ˈnē-mē-ə\ *n* : the presence of methemoglobin in the blood due to conversion of part of the hemoglobin to this inactive form

me•the•na•mine \mə-ˈthē-nə-ˌmēn, -mən\ *n* : a crystalline compound used esp. in the form of its mandelate $C_6H_{12}N_4 \cdot C_8H_8O_3$ as a urinary antiseptic esp. to treat bacteriuria associated with cystitis and pyelitis — called also *hexamethylenetetramine, hexamine;* see MANDELAMINE

me•the•no•lone \mə-ˈthē-nə-lōn, me-ˈthe-\ *n* : a hormone $C_{20}H_{30}O_2$ that is an anabolic steroid

Meth•er•gine \ˈme-thər-jən\ *trademark* — used for a preparation of the maleate of methylergonovine

meth•i•cil•lin \ˌme-thə-ˈsi-lən\ *n* : a semisynthetic penicillin $C_{17}H_{19}N_2O_6NaS$ that is esp. effective against beta-lactamase producing staphylococci

me•thi•ma•zole \me-ˈthī-mə-ˌzōl, mə-\ *n* : a drug $C_4H_6N_2S$ used to inhibit activity of the thyroid gland

meth•io•dal sodium \mə-ˈthī-ə-ˌdal-\ *n* : a crystalline salt CH_2ISO_3Na used as a radiopaque contrast medium in intravenous urography

me·thi·o·nine \mə-ˈthī-ə-ˌnēn\ *n* : a crystalline sulfur-containing essential amino acid $C_5H_{11}NO_2S$ that occurs in the L-form as a constituent of many proteins (as casein and egg albumin) and that is used as a dietary supplement and in the treatment of fatty infiltration of the liver

methionine–en·keph·a·lin \-en-ˈkə-fə-lin\ *n* : a pentapeptide having a terminal methionine residue that is one of the two enkephalins occurring naturally in the brain — called also *Met-enkephalin*

meth·is·a·zone \me-ˈthi-sə-ˌzōn\ *n* : an antiviral drug $C_{10}H_{10}N_4OS$ formerly used to prevent smallpox

me·thix·ene \me-ˈthik-ˌsēn\ *n* : an anticholinergic drug $C_{20}H_{23}NS$ used as an antispasmodic to treat functional bowel hypermotility and spasm

metho- — see METH-

meth·o·car·ba·mol \ˌme-thə-ˈkär-bə-ˌmȯl\ *n* : a skeletal muscle relaxant drug $C_{11}H_{15}NO_5$

meth·o·hex·i·tal \ˌme-thə-ˈhek-sə-ˌtȯl, -ˌtal\ *n* : a barbiturate with a short period of action usu. used in the form of its sodium salt $C_{14}H_{17}N_2NaO_3$ as an intravenous general anesthetic

meth·o·hex·i·tone \-ˌtōn\ *n, Brit* : METHOHEXITAL

meth·o·trex·ate \-ˈtrek-ˌsāt\ *n* : a toxic drug $C_{20}H_{22}N_8O_5$ that is an analog of folic acid and is used to treat certain cancers, severe psoriasis, and rheumatoid arthritis — called also *amethopterin*

meth·o·tri·mep·ra·zine \-ˌtrī-ˈme-prə-ˌzēn\ *n* : a nonnarcotic analgesic and tranquilizer $C_{19}H_{24}N_2OS$ — see LEVOPROME

me·thox·amine \me-ˈthäk-sə-ˌmēn, -mən\ *n* : a sympathomimetic amine used in the form of its hydrochloride $C_{11}H_{17}NO_3 \cdot HCl$ esp. to raise or maintain blood pressure (as during surgery) by its vasoconstrictor effects

me·thox·sa·len \me-ˈthäk-sə-lən\ *n* : a drug $C_{12}H_8O_4$ used to increase the production of melanin in the skin upon exposure to ultraviolet light and in the treatment of vitiligo — called also *8-methoxsalen, xanthotoxin*

me·thoxy·flu·rane \me-ˌthäk-sē-ˈflu̇r-ˌān\ *n* : a potent inhalational general anesthetic $C_3H_4Cl_2F_2O$ withdrawn from the U.S. market because of its link to liver and kidney damage

8–meth·oxy·psor·a·len \ˈāt-ˌme-ˌthäk-sē-ˈsȯr-ə-lən\ *n* : METHOXSALEN

meth·sco·pol·amine \ˌmeth-skō-ˈpä-lə-ˌmēn, -mən\ *n* : an anticholinergic derivative of scopolamine that is usu. used in the form of its bromide $C_{18}H_{24}BrNO_4$ for its inhibitory effect on gastric secretion and gastrointestinal motility esp. in the treatment of peptic ulcer and gastric disorders — see PAMINE

meth·sux·i·mide \-ˈsək-si-ˌmīd\ *n* : an anticonvulsant drug $C_{12}H_{13}NO_2$ used esp. in the control of absence seizures

meth·y·clo·thi·azide \ˌme-thē-ˌklō-ˈthī-ə-ˌzīd\ *n* : a thiazide drug $C_9H_{11}Cl_2N_3O_4S_2$ used as a diuretic and antihypertensive agent

meth·yl \ˈme-thəl, *Brit also* ˈmē-ˌthīl\ *n* : an alkyl group CH_3 that is derived from methane by removal of one hydrogen atom

meth·yl·al \ˈme-thə-ˌlal\ *n* : a volatile flammable liquid $C_3H_8O_2$ used as a hypnotic and anesthetic

methyl alcohol *n* : METHANOL

me·thyl·am·phet·amine \ˌme-thəl-ˌam-ˈfe-tə-ˌmēn\ *n* : METHAMPHETAMINE

methylated spirit *n* : ethyl alcohol denatured with methanol — often used in pl. with a sing. verb

meth·yl·ation \ˌme-thə-ˈlā-shən\ *n* : introduction of the methyl group into a chemical compound; *esp* : DNA METHYLATION — **meth·yl·ate** \ˈme-thə-ˌlāt\ *vb*—

meth·yl·ben·ze·tho·ni·um chloride \ˌme-thəl-ˌben-zə-ˌthō-nē-əm-\ *n* : a quaternary ammonium salt $C_{28}H_{44}ClNO_2$ used as a bactericide and antiseptic esp. to treat diaper rash — called also *methylbenzethonium*

methyl bromide *n* : a poisonous gaseous compound CH_3Br

meth·yl·cel·lu·lose \ˌme-thəl-ˈsel-yə-ˌlōs, -ˌlōz\ *n* : any of various gummy products of cellulose methylation that swell in water and are used as bulk laxatives

meth·yl·cho·lan·threne \-kə-ˈlan-ˌthrēn\ *n* : a potent carcinogenic hydrocarbon $C_{21}H_{16}$ obtained from certain bile acids and cholesterol as well as synthetically

***N*–meth·yl–D–as·par·tate** \ˈen-ˌme-thəl-ˌdē-ə-ˈspär-ˌtāt\ *n* : NMDA

meth·yl·do·pa \-ˈdō-pə\ *n* : an antihypertensive drug $C_{10}H_{13}NO_4$

meth·y·lene blue \ˈme-thə-ˌlēn-, -lən-\ *n* : a basic thiazine dye $C_{16}H_{18}ClN_3S \cdot 3H_2O$ used in the treatment of methemoglobinemia and as an antidote in cyanide poisoning

meth·y·lene·di·oxy·am·phet·amine \ˌme-thə-ˌlēn-dī-ˌäk-sē-am-ˈfe-tə-ˌmēn\ *also* **3,4–methylenedioxyamphetamine** \ˌthrē-ˌfōr-\ *n* : MDA

meth·y·lene·di·oxy·meth·am·phet·amine \-ˌme-tham-ˈfe-tə-ˌmēn\ *also* **3,4–methylenedioxymethamphetamine** *n* : ECSTASY 2

meth·y·lene·di·oxy·py·ro·val·e·rone \ˌme-thə-ˌlēn-(ˌ)dī-ˌäk-sē-ˌpī-rō-ˈva-lə-ˌrōn\ *also* **3,4–methylenedioxypyrovalerone** *n* : MDPV

meth·yl·er·go·no·vine \ˌme-thəl-ˌər-gə-ˈnō-ˌvēn\ *n* : an oxytocic drug that is usu. administered in the form of its maleate $C_{20}H_{25}N_3O_2 \cdot C_4H_4O_4$ and is used similarly to ergonovine — see METHERGINE

meth·yl·glu·ca·mine \-ˈglü-kə-ˌmēn\ *n* : MEGLUMINE

meth·yl·hex·ane·amine \ˌme-thəl-ˌhek-sā-ˈna-mēn\ *n* : an amine base $C_7H_{17}N$ used as a local vasoconstrictor of nasal mucosa in the treatment of nasal congestion

meth·yl iso·cy·a·nate \-ˌī-sō-ˈsī-ə-ˌnāt\ *n* : an extremely toxic chemical CH_3NCO that is used esp. in the manufacture of pesticides and was the cause of numerous deaths and injuries in a leak at a chemical plant in Bhopal, India, in 1984 — abbr. *MIC*

meth·yl·ma·lon·ic acid \ˌme-thəl-mə-ˈlä-nik-\ *n* : a structural isomer of succinic acid present in minute amounts in healthy human urine but excreted in large quantities in the urine of individuals with a vitamin B_{12} deficiency

methylmalonic aciduria *n* : a metabolic defect which is controlled by an autosomal recessive gene and in which methylmalonic acid is not converted to succinic acid with chronic metabolic acidosis resulting

meth·yl mer·cap·tan \ˈme-thəl-mər-ˈkap-ˌtan\ *n* : a pungent gas CH_4S produced in the intestine by the decomposition of certain proteins and responsible for the characteristic odor of fetor hepaticus

meth·yl·mer·cury \ˌme-thəl-ˈmər-kyə-rē\ *n, pl* **-cu·ries** : any of various toxic compounds of mercury containing the complex $CH_3Hg–$ that often occur as pollutants formed as industrial by-products or pesticide residues, tend to accumulate in living organisms (as fish) esp. in higher levels of a food chain, are rapidly and easily absorbed through the human intestinal wall, and cause neurological dysfunction in humans — see MINAMATA DISEASE

meth·yl·mor·phine \ˌme-thəl-ˈmȯr-ˌfēn\ *n* : CODEINE

meth·yl·para·ben \ˌme-thəl-ˈpar-ə-ˌben\ *n* : a crystalline compound $C_8H_8O_3$ used as an antifungal preservative (as in pharmaceutical ointments and cosmetic creams)

methyl parathion *n* : a potent synthetic organophosphate insecticide $C_8H_{10}NO_5PS$ that is more toxic than parathion

meth·yl·phe·ni·date \ˌme-thəl-ˈfe-nə-ˌdāt, -ˈfē-\ *n* : a mild stimulant of the central nervous system that is administered orally in the form of its hydrochloride $C_{14}H_{19}NO_2 \cdot HCl$ to treat narcolepsy and attention deficit disorder — see CONCERTA, QUILLIVANT, RITALIN

meth·yl·pred·nis·o·lone \-pred-ˈni-sə-ˌlōn\ *n* : a glucocorticoid $C_{22}H_{30}O_5$ that is a derivative of prednisolone and is used as an anti-inflammatory agent; *also* : any of several of its salts used similarly — see MEDROL

methyl salicylate *n* : a liquid ester $C_8H_8O_3$ that is obtained from the leaves of a wintergreen (*Gaultheria procumbens*) or the bark of a birch (*Betula lenta*), but is usu. made synthetically, and that is used as a flavoring and a counterirritant — see OIL OF WINTERGREEN

methylsulfate — see PENTAPIPERIUM METHYLSULFATE

meth·yl·tes·tos·ter·one \-te-ˈstäs-tə-ˌrōn\ *n* : a synthetic androgen $C_{20}H_{30}O_2$ taken orally esp. to treat male testosterone deficiency

meth·yl·thio·ura·cil \-ˌthī-ō-ˈyu̇r-ə-ˌsil\ *n* : a crystalline compound $C_5H_6N_2OS$ used in the suppression of hyperactivity of the thyroid

α-meth·yl·ty·ro·sine \ˌal-fə-ˌme-thəl-ˈtī-rə-ˌsēn\ *n* : a compound $C_{10}H_{13}NO_3$ that inhibits the synthesis of catecholamines but not of serotonin

meth·yl·xan·thine \ˌme-thəl-ˈzan-ˌthēn\ *n* : a methylated xanthine derivative (as caffeine, theobromine, or theophylline)

meth·y·pry·lon \ˌme-thə-ˈprī-ˌlän\ *n* : a sedative and hypnotic drug $C_{10}H_{17}NO_2$

meth·y·ser·gide \ˌme-thə-ˈsər-ˌjīd\ *n* : a serotonin antagonist used in the form of its maleate $C_{21}H_{27}N_3O_2 \cdot C_4H_4O_4$ esp. in the treatment and prevention of migraine headaches

met·o·clo·pra·mide \ˌme-tə-ˈklō-prə-ˌmīd\ *n* : an antiemetic drug used in the form of its hydrated hydrochloride $C_{14}H_{22}ClN_3O_2 \cdot HCl \cdot H_2O$

met·o·cur·ine iodide \ˌme-tə-ˈkyu̇r-ˌēn-\ *n* : a crystalline iodine-containing powder $C_{40}H_{48}I_2N_2O_6$ that is derived from the dextrorotatory form of tubocurarine and is a potent skeletal muscle relaxant — called also *metocurine*

me·to·la·zone \me-ˈtō-lə-ˌzōn\ *n* : a diuretic and antihypertensive drug $C_{16}H_{16}ClN_3O_3S$

me·top·ic \me-ˈtä-pik\ *adj* : of or relating to the forehead : FRONTAL; *esp* : of, relating to, or being a suture uniting the frontal bones in the fetus and sometimes persistent after birth

met·o·pim·a·zine \ˌme-tə-ˈpi-mə-ˌzēn\ *n* : an antiemetic drug $C_{22}H_{27}N_3O_3S_2$

Met·o·pir·one \ˌme-tə-ˈpir-ˌōn\ *trademark* — used for a preparation of metyrapone

met·o·pon \ˈme-tə-ˌpän\ *n* : a narcotic drug that is derived from morphine and is used in the form of the hydrochloride $C_{18}H_{21}NO_3 \cdot HCl$ to relieve pain

met·o·pro·lol \me-ˈtō-prə-ˌlȯl, -ˌlōl\ *n* : a beta-blocker $C_{15}H_{25}NO_3$ used in the form of its tartrate $(C_{15}H_{25}NO_3)_2 \cdot C_4H_6O_6$ or succinate $(C_{15}H_{25}NO_3)_2 \cdot C_4H_6O_4$ esp. to treat hypertension, angina pectoris, and congestive heart failure — see LOPRESSOR, TOPROL

metr- *or* **metro-** *comb form* : uterus ⟨*metr*itis⟩

-me·tra \ˈmē-trə\ *n comb form* : a (specified) condition of the uterus ⟨hemato*metra*⟩

Met·ra·zol \ˈme-trə-ˌzȯl, -ˌzōl\ *n* : a preparation of pentylenetetrazol — formerly a U.S. registered trademark

me•tre *chiefly Brit var of* METER

met•ric \ˈme-trik\ *adj* : of, relating to, or using the metric system — **met•ri•cal•ly** *adv*

-met•ric \ˈme-trik\ *or* **-met•ri•cal** \ˈme-tri-kəl\ *adj comb form* **1** : of, employing, or obtained by (such) a meter ⟨calori*metric*⟩ **2** : of or relating to (such) an art, process, or science of measuring ⟨psycho*metric*⟩

metric system *n* : a decimal system of weights and measures based on the meter and on the kilogram — compare CGS, MKS

me•tri•tis \mə-ˈtrī-təs\ *n* : inflammation of the uterus

-me•tri•um \ˈmē-trē-əm\ *n comb form, pl* **-me•tria** : part or layer of the uterus ⟨endo*metrium*⟩

me•triz•a•mide \me-ˈtri-za-ˌmīd\ *n* : a radiopaque medium $C_{18}H_{22}I_3N_3O_8$

met•ri•zo•ate sodium \ˌme-tri-ˈzō-āt-\ *n* : a radiopaque medium $C_{12}H_{10}I_3N_2NaO_4$ — see ISOPAQUE

met•ro•ni•da•zole \ˌme-trə-ˈnī-də-ˌzōl\ *n* : an antiprotozoal and antibacterial drug $C_6H_9N_3O_3$ used esp. to treat vaginal trichomoniasis, amebiasis, and infections by anaerobic bacteria

met•ro•nom•ic \ˌme-trə-ˈnä-mik\ *adj* : of, relating to, or being a drug or regimen of drugs administered in low doses at regular intervals over an extended period of time ⟨∼ chemotherapy⟩

me•tror•rha•gia \ˌmē-trə-ˈrā-jə, -jē-ə, -zhə; -ˈrä-\ *n* : irregular uterine bleeding esp. between menstrual periods — compare MENORRHAGIA — **me•tror•rhag•ic** \-ˈra-jik\ *adj*

-me•try \mə-trē\ *n comb form, pl* **-me•tries** : art, process, or science of measuring (something specified) ⟨audi*ometry*⟩

me•tu•re•depa \mə-ˌtür-ə-ˈde-pə, ˌme-tyə-rə-\ *n* : an antineoplastic drug $C_{11}H_{22}N_3O_3P$

me•tyr•a•pone \mə-ˈtir-ə-ˌpōn, -ˈtīr-\ *n* : a metabolic hormone $C_{14}H_{14}N_2O$ that inhibits biosynthesis of cortisol and corticosterone and is used to test for normal functioning of the pituitary gland — see METOPIRONE

Met•zen•baum scissors \ˈmet-sən-ˌbau̇m-\ *n* : surgical scissors having curved blades with blunt ends

Metzenbaum, Myron Firth (1876–1944), American surgeon.

Mev•a•cor \ˈme-və-ˌkȯr\ *trademark* — used for a preparation of lovastatin

me•ze•re•um \mə-ˈzir-ē-əm\ *n* : the dried bark of various European shrubs (genus *Daphne* and esp. *D. mezereum* of the family Thymelaeaceae) used externally as a vesicant and irritant

mg *abbr* milligram

Mg *symbol* magnesium

MH *abbr* mental health

MHC *abbr* major histocompatibility complex

MHPG \ˌem-ˌāch-ˌpē-ˈjē\ *n* : a metabolite of norepinephrine that is reported for some patients to fall to lower levels during periods of depression

MI *abbr* **1** mitral incompetence; mitral insufficiency **2** myocardial infarction

mi•an•ser•in \mī-ˈan-sər-in\ *n* : a drug administered in the form of its hydrochloride $C_{18}H_{20}N_2{\cdot}HCl$ esp. as an antidepressant

MIC *abbr* **1** methyl isocyanate **2** minimal inhibitory concentration; minimum inhibitory concentration

Mi•car•dis \mī-ˈkär-dəs\ *trademark* — used for a preparation of telmisartan

Mi•ca•tin \ˈmī-kə-ˌtin\ *trademark* — used for a preparation of the nitrate of miconazole

mice *pl of* MOUSE

mi•con•a•zole \mī-ˈkä-nə-ˌzōl\ *n* : an antifungal agent administered esp. in the form of its nitrate $C_{18}H_{14}Cl_4N_2O{\cdot}HNO_3$ — see MICATIN

micr- *or* **micro-** *comb form* **1 a** : small : minute ⟨*micro*aneurysm⟩ **b** : used for or involving minute quantities or variations ⟨*micro*analysis⟩ **2 a** : using microscopy ⟨*micro*dissection⟩ : used in microscopy ⟨*micro*needle⟩ **b** : revealed by or having its structure discernible only by microscopical examination ⟨*micro*organism⟩ **3** : abnormally small ⟨*micro*cyte⟩

micra *pl of* MICRON

mi•cren•ceph•a•ly \ˌmī-ˌkren-ˈse-fə-lē\ *n, pl* **-lies** : the condition of having an abnormally small brain

mi•cro•ab•scess \ˈmī-krō-ˌab-ses\ *n* : a very small abscess

mi•cro•ad•e•no•ma \ˌmī-krō-ˌad-ᵊn-ˈō-mə\ *n, pl* **-mas** *also* **-ma•ta** \-mə-tə\ : a very small adenoma

mi•cro•ag•gre•gate \-ˈa-gri-gət\ *n* : an aggregate of microscopic particles (as of fibrin) formed esp. in stored blood

mi•cro•al•bu•min•uria \-al-ˌbyü-mə-ˈnu̇r-ē-ə, -ˈnyu̇r-\ *n* : albuminuria characterized by a relatively low rate of urinary excretion of albumin typically between 30 and 300 milligrams per 24-hour period — compare MACROALBUMINURIA

mi•cro•anat•o•my \-ə-ˈna-tə-mē\ *n, pl* **-mies** : HISTOLOGY — **mi•cro•ana•tom•i•cal** \-ˌa-nə-ˈtä-mi-kəl\ *adj*

mi•cro•an•eu•rysm *also* **mi•cro•an•eu•rism** \-ˈa-nyə-ˌri-zəm\ *n* : a saccular enlargement of the venous end of a retinal capillary associated esp. with diabetic retinopathy — **mi•cro•an•eu•rys•mal** \-ˌa-nyə-ˈriz-məl\ *adj*

mi•cro•an•gi•og•ra•phy \-ˌan-jē-ˈä-grə-fē\ *n, pl* **-phies** : minutely detailed angiography — **mi•cro•an•gio•graph•ic** \-ˌan-jē-ə-ˈgra-fik\ *adj*

mi•cro•an•gi•op•a•thy \-ˈä-pə-thē\ *n, pl* **-thies** : a disease of very fine blood vessels ⟨thrombotic ∼⟩ — **mi•cro•an•gio•path•ic** \-ˌan-jē-ə-ˈpa-thik\ *adj*

mi•cro•ar•ray \-ə-ˈrā\ *n* : a supporting material (as a glass slide) onto which numerous molecules or molecular fragments usu. of DNA or protein are attached in a regular pattern for use in biochemical or genetic analysis

mi·cro·ar·te·ri·og·ra·phy \-ˌär-ˌtir-ē-ˈä-grə-fē\ *n, pl* **-phies** : minutely detailed arteriography

mi·crobe \ˈmī-ˌkrōb\ *n* : MICROORGANISM, GERM — used esp. of pathogenic bacteria

mi·cro·bi·al \mī-ˈkrō-bē-əl\ *adj* : of, relating to, caused by, or being microbes — **mi·cro·bi·al·ly** \-ē\ *adv*

mi·cro·bic \mī-ˈkrō-bik\ *adj* : MICROBIAL

mi·cro·bi·cide \mī-ˈkrō-bə-ˌsīd\ *n* : an agent that destroys microbes — **mi·cro·bi·ci·dal** \mī-ˌkrō-bə-ˈsīd-ᵊl\ *adj*

mi·cro·bi·ol·o·gy \ˌmī-krō-bī-ˈä-lə-jē\ *n, pl* **-gies** : a branch of biology dealing esp. with microorganisms (as bacteria and protozoa) — **mi·cro·bi·o·log·i·cal** \ˈmī-krō-ˌbī-ə-ˈlä-ji-kəl\ *also* **mi·cro·bi·o·log·ic** \-ˈlä-jik\ *adj* — **mi·cro·bi·o·log·i·cal·ly** *adv* — **mi·cro·bi·ol·o·gist** \-jist\ *n*

mi·cro·bi·ome \ˌmī-krō-ˈbī-ˌōm\ *n* **1** : the collection of microorganisms (as bacteria and fungi) living in or on the human body **2** : the collective genomes of microorganisms inhabiting the human body

mi·cro·body \ˈmī-krō-ˌbä-dē\ *n, pl* **-bod·ies** : PEROXISOME

mi·cro·cal·ci·fi·ca·tion \-ˌkal-sə-fə-ˈkā-shən\ *n* : a tiny abnormal deposit of calcium salts typically in the breast that is often benign but may be an indicator of breast cancer esp. when appearing in compact clusters or a linear or branching pattern

mi·cro·cap·sule \ˈmī-krō-ˌkap-səl, -(ˌ)sül\ *n* : a tiny capsule containing material (as a medicine) that is released when the capsule is broken, melted, or dissolved

[1]**mi·cro·ce·phal·ic** \ˌmī-krō-sə-ˈfa-lik\ *adj* : having a small head; *specif* : having an abnormally small head

[2]**microcephalic** *n* : an individual with an abnormally small head

mi·cro·ceph·a·lus \-ˈse-fə-ləs\ *n, pl* **-li** \-ˌlī\ : MICROCEPHALY

mi·cro·ceph·a·ly \-ˈse-fə-lē\ *n, pl* **-lies** : abnormal smallness of the head often associated with developmental delays, impaired cognitive functioning, poor coordination, hearing and vision deficits, and seizures

mi·cro·cir·cu·la·tion \-ˌsər-kyə-ˈlā-shən\ *n* : blood circulation in the microvascular system; *also* : the microvascular system itself — **mi·cro·cir·cu·la·to·ry** \-ˈsər-kyə-lə-ˌtōr-ē\ *adj*

mi·cro·coc·cus \ˌmī-krō-ˈkä-kəs\ *n* **1** *cap* : a genus of nonmotile spherical bacteria (family Micrococcaceae) that occur in tetrads or irregular clusters and include nonpathogenic forms found on the skin **2** *pl* **-coc·ci** \-ˈkä-ˌkī, -ˈkäk-ˌsī\ : a small spherical bacterium; *esp* : any bacterium of the genus *Micrococcus* — **mi·cro·coc·cal** \ˌmī-krō-ˈkä-kəl\ *adj*

mi·cro·cul·ture \ˈmī-krō-ˌkəl-chər\ *n* : a microscopic culture of cells or organisms — **mi·cro·cul·tur·al** \ˌmī-krō-ˈkəlch-(ə-)rəl\ *adj*

mi·cro·cu·rie \ˈmī-krō-ˌkyu̇r-ē, ˌmī-krō-kyu̇-ˈrē\ *n* : a unit of quantity or of radioactivity equal to one millionth of a curie

mi·cro·cyte \ˈmī-krə-ˌsīt\ *n* : an abnormally small red blood cell present esp. in some anemias

mi·cro·cyt·ic \ˌmī-krə-ˈsi-tik\ *adj* : of, relating to, being, or characterized by the presence of microcytes

microcytic anemia *n* : an anemia characterized by the presence of microcytes in the blood

mi·cro·cy·to·sis \-sī-ˈtō-səs\ *n, pl* **-to·ses** \-ˌsēz\ : decrease in the size of red blood cells

mi·cro·cy·to·tox·ic·i·ty test \-ˌsī-tō-ˌtäk-ˈsi-sə-tē\ *n* : a procedure using microscopic quantities of materials (as complement and lymphocytes in cell-mediated immunity) to determine cytotoxicity (as to cancer cells or cells of transplanted tissue) — called also *microcytotoxicity assay*

mi·cro·derm·abra·sion \ˌmī-krō-ˌdər-mə-ˈbrā-zhən\ *n* : a cosmetic procedure for the skin that involves the mechanical abrasion and removal of all or part of the stratum corneum and is used to rejuvenate the skin and to treat skin blemishes or imperfections (as scars or wrinkles)

mi·cro·dis·sec·tion \ˌmī-krō-di-ˈsek-shən, -dī-\ *n* : dissection under the microscope; *specif* : dissection of cells and tissues by means of fine needles that are precisely manipulated by levers — **mi·cro·dis·sect·ed** \-ˈsek-təd\ *adj*

mi·cro·dose \ˈmī-krō-ˌdōs\ *n* : an extremely small dose

mi·cro·do·sim·e·try \ˌmī-krō-dō-ˈsi-mə-trē\ *n, pl* **-tries** : dosimetry involving microdoses of radiation or minute amounts of radioactive materials

mi·cro·drop \ˈmī-krō-ˌdräp\ *n* : a very small drop or minute droplet (as 0.1 to 0.01 of a drop)

mi·cro·drop·let \-ˌdrä-plət\ *n* : MICRODROP

mi·cro·elec·trode \ˌmī-krō-i-ˈlek-ˌtrōd\ *n* : a minute electrode; *esp* : one that is inserted in a living biological cell or tissue in studying its electrical characteristics

mi·cro·elec·tro·pho·re·sis \-ˌlek-trə-fə-ˈrē-səs\ *n, pl* **-re·ses** \-ˌsēz\ : electrophoresis in which the movement of single particles is observed in a microscope — **mi·cro·elec·tro·pho·ret·ic** \-ˈre-tik\ *adj* — **mi·cro·elec·tro·pho·ret·i·cal·ly** *adv*

mi·cro·el·e·ment \ˌmī-krō-ˈe-lə-mənt\ *n* : TRACE ELEMENT

mi·cro·em·bo·lism \-ˈem-bə-ˌli-zəm\ *n* : a small embolism (as one consisting of an aggregation of platelets) that blocks an arteriole or the terminal part of an artery

mi•cro•em•bo•lus \-ˈem-bə-ləs\ *n, pl* **-li** \-ˌlī\ : an extremely small embolus

mi•cro•en•cap•su•late \-in-ˈkap-sə-ˌlāt\ *vb* **-lat•ed; -lat•ing** : to enclose in a microcapsule — **mi•cro•en•cap•su•la•tion** \-in-ˌkap-sə-ˈlā-shən\ *n*

mi•cro•en•vi•ron•ment \-in-ˈvī-rən-mənt, -ˈvī-ərn-\ *n* : a small usu. distinctly specialized and effectively isolated habitat or environment (as of a nerve cell) — **mi•cro•en•vi•ron•men•tal** \-ˌvī-rən-ˈment-ᵊl\ *adj*

mi•cro•fi•bril \-ˈfī-brəl, -ˈfi-\ *n* : an extremely fine fibril — **mi•cro•fi•bril•lar** \-brə-lər\ *adj*

mi•cro•fil•a•ment \ˌmī-krō-ˈfi-lə-mənt\ *n* : any of the minute actin-containing protein filaments that are widely distributed in the cytoplasm of eukaryotic cells, help maintain their structural framework, and play a role in the movement of cell components — **mi•cro•fil•a•men•tous** \-ˌfi-lə-ˈmen-təs\ *adj*

mi•cro•fil•a•rae•mia *chiefly Brit var of* MICROFILAREMIA

mi•cro•fil•a•re•mia \-ˌfi-lə-ˈrē-mē-ə\ *n* : the presence of microfilariae in the blood of one affected with some forms of filariasis

mi•cro•fi•lar•ia \ˌmī-krō-fə-ˈlar-ē-ə\ *n, pl* **-i•ae** \-ē-ē\ : a minute larval filaria — **mi•cro•fi•lar•i•al** \-ē-əl\ *adj*

mi•cro•flo•ra \ˌmī-krə-ˈflōr-ə\ *n* : a small or strictly localized flora ⟨intestinal ~⟩ — **mi•cro•flo•ral** \-əl\ *adj*

mi•cro•flu•o•rom•e•try \-ˌflü-ˈrä-mə-trē\ *n, pl* **-tries** : the detection and measurement of the fluorescence produced by minute quantities of materials (as in cells) — **mi•cro•flu•o•rom•e•ter** \-ˈrä-mə-tər\ *n* — **mi•cro•flu•o•ro•met•ric** \-rə-ˈme-trik\ *adj*

mi•cro•frac•ture \ˌmī-krō-ˈfrak-chər, -shər\ *n* **1** : a small or minute fracture in a material (as bone) **2** : arthroscopic knee surgery for the repair of damaged articular cartilage that involves removal of loose and calcified cartilage and the drilling of small holes in the bone beneath for blood and bone marrow to pass through and form a clot which eventually develops into replacement fibrocartilage

mi•cro•ga•mete \-ˈga-ˌmēt, -gə-ˈmēt\ *n* : the smaller and usu. male gamete of an organism producing two types of gametes — compare MACROGAMETE

mi•crog•lia \mī-ˈkrä-glē-ə\ *n* : glia consisting of small cells with few processes that are scattered throughout the central nervous system, that are of mesodermal origin and are thought to be derived from fetal monocytes, and that have a phagocytic function as part of the mononuclear phagocyte system — **mi•crog•li•al** \-glē-əl\ *adj*

β_2–mi•cro•glob•u•lin \ˌbā-tə-ˌtü-ˌmī-krō-ˈglä-byə-lən\ *n* : a beta globulin of low molecular weight that is present at a low level in plasma, is normally excreted in the urine, comprises the light chain in certain histocompatibility antigens, and occurs at elevated levels in blood serum or urine in some pathological conditions (as tubulointerstitial disease)

mi•cro•glos•sia \ˌmī-krō-ˈglä-sē-ə, -ˈglȯ-\ *n* : abnormal smallness of the tongue

mi•cro•gna•thia \ˌmī-krō-ˈnā-thē-ə, -ˈna-, ˌmī-ˌkräg-\ *n* : abnormal smallness of one or both jaws

mi•cro•gram \ˈmī-krə-ˌgram\ *n* : one millionth of a gram

mi•cro•graph \-ˌgraf\ *n* : a graphic reproduction (as a photograph) of the image of an object formed by a microscope — **micrograph** *vb*

mi•cro•graph•ia \ˌmī-krō-ˈgraf-ē-ə\ *n* : abnormally small handwriting or handwriting that becomes progressively smaller that is characteristic esp. of Parkinson's disease

mi•cro•hab•i•tat \ˌmī-krō-ˈha-bə-ˌtat\ *n* : the microenvironment in which an organism lives

mi•cro•he•mat•o•crit \-hi-ˈma-tə-ˌkrit\ *n* **1** : a procedure for determining the ratio of the volume of packed red blood cells to the volume of whole blood by centrifuging a minute quantity of blood in a capillary tube coated with heparin **2** : a hematocrit value obtained by microhematocrit

mi•cro•in•farct \-in-ˈfärkt\ *n* : a very small infarct

mi•cro•in•jec•tion \ˌmī-krō-in-ˈjek-shən\ *n* : injection under the microscope; *specif* : injection esp. by a micropipette into a tissue or single cell — **mi•cro•in•ject** \-in-ˈjekt\ *vb*

mi•cro•in•va•sive \-in-ˈvā-siv\ *adj* : of, relating to, or marked by very slight invasion into adjacent tissues by malignant cells of a carcinoma in situ — **mi•cro•in•va•sion** \-ˈvā-zhən\ *n*

mi•cro•ion•to•pho•re•sis \-(ˌ)ī-ˌän-tə-fə-ˈrē-səs\ *n, pl* **-re•ses** \-ˌsēz\ : a process for observing or recording the effect of an ionized substance on nerve cells that involves inserting a double micropipette into the brain close to a nerve cell, injecting an ionized fluid through one barrel of the pipette, and using a concentrated saline solution in the other tube as an electrical conductor to pick up and transmit back to an oscilloscope any change in neural activity — **mi•cro•ion•to•pho•ret•ic** \-ˈre-tik\ *adj*

mi•cro•li•ter \ˌmī-krō-ˈlē-tər\ *n* : a unit of capacity equal to one millionth of a liter

mi•cro•lith \ˈmī-krō-ˌlith\ *n* : a microscopic calculus or concretion

mi•cro•li•thi•a•sis \ˌmī-krō-li-ˈthī-ə-səs\ *n, pl* **-a•ses** \-ˌsēz\ : the formation or presence of microliths or gravel

mi•cro•ma•nip•u•la•tion \ˌmī-krō-mə-ˌni-pyə-ˈlā-shən\ *n* : the technique or practice of manipulating cells or tissues (as by microdissection or microinjection) — **mi•cro•ma•nip•u•late** \-ˈni-pyə-ˌlāt\ *vb* — **mi•cro•ma•nip•u•la•tor** \-ˈni-pyə-ˌlā-tər\ *n*

mi•cro•mas•tia \-ˈmas-tē-ə\ *n* : postpubertal immaturity and abnormal smallness of the breasts

mi•cro•me•lia \-ˈmē-lē-ə\ *n* : a condition characterized by abnormally small and imperfectly developed extremities — **mi•cro•me•lic** \-ˈmē-lik\ *adj*

mi•cro•me•tas•ta•sis \ˌmī-krō-mə-ˈtas-tə-səs\ *n, pl* **-ta•ses** \-ˌsēz\ : the spread of cancer cells from a primary site and the formation of microscopic tumors at secondary sites; *also* : one of the microscopic tumors resulting from micrometastasis — **mi•cro•met•a•stat•ic** \-ˌme-tə-ˈsta-tik\ *adj*

mi•cro•me•ter \ˈmī-krō-ˌmē-tər\ *n* : MICRON

mi•cro•mi•cro•cu•rie \ˌmī-krō-ˈmī-krō-ˌkyu̇r-ē\ *n* : one millionth of a microcurie

mi•cro•mol•e•cule \-ˈmä-lə-ˌkyül\ *n* : a molecule (as of an amino acid or a fatty acid) of relatively low molecular weight — compare MACROMOLECULE — **mi•cro•mo•lec•u•lar** \-mə-ˈle-kyə-lər\ *adj*

mi•cro•mono•spo•ra \-ˌmä-nə-ˈspȯr-ə\ *n* **1** *cap* : a genus of actinomycetes that includes several antibiotic-producing forms (as *M. purpurea,* the source of gentamicin) **2** *pl* **-rae** \-rē\ : any bacterium of the genus *Micromonospora*

mi•cron \ˈmī-ˌkrän\ *n* : a unit of length equal to one millionth of a meter — called also *micrometer, mu*

Mi•cro•nase \ˈmī-krō-ˌnās\ *trademark* — used for a preparation of glyburide

mi•cro•nee•dle \ˈmī-krō-ˌnēd-ᵊl\ *n* : a needle for micromanipulation

mi•cro•nod•u•lar \ˌmī-krō-ˈnä-jə-lər\ *adj* : characterized by the presence of extremely small nodules

mi•cro•nu•tri•ent \-ˈnü-trē-ənt, -ˈnyü-\ *n* : a chemical element or substance (as calcium or vitamin C) that is essential in minute amounts to growth and health — see TRACE ELEMENT; compare MACRONUTRIENT

mi•cro•or•gan•ism \-ˈȯr-gə-ˌni-zəm\ *n* : an organism of microscopic or submicroscopic size — **mi•cro•or•gan•is•mal** \-ˌȯr-gə-ˈniz-məl\ *adj*

mi•cro•par•a•site \ˌmī-krō-ˈpar-ə-ˌsīt\ *n* : a parasitic microorganism — **mi•cro•par•a•sit•ic** \-ˌpar-ə-ˈsi-tik\ *adj*

mi•cro•pe•nis \-ˈpē-nəs\ *n, pl* **-pe•nes** \-(ˌ)nēz\ *or* **-pe•nis•es** : MICROPHALLUS

mi•cro•per•fu•sion \-pər-ˈfyü-zhən\ *n* : an act or instance of forcing a fluid through a small organ or tissue by way of a tubule or blood vessel — **mi•cro•per•fused** \-ˈfyüzd\ *adj*

mi•cro•phage \ˈmī-krə-ˌfāj\ *n* : a small phagocyte

mi•cro•pha•kia \ˌmī-krō-ˈfā-kē-ə\ *n* : abnormal smallness of the lens of the eye

mi•cro•phal•lus \-ˈfa-ləs\ *n* : smallness of the penis esp. to an abnormal degree — called also *micropenis*

mi•cro•phon•ic \ˌmī-krō-ˈfä-nik\ *n* : COCHLEAR MICROPHONIC — **microphonic** *adj*

mi•cro•pho•to•graph \-ˈfō-tə-ˌgraf\ *n* : PHOTOMICROGRAPH — **mi•cro•pho•tog•ra•phy** \-fə-ˈtä-grə-fē\ *n*

mi•croph•thal•mia \ˌmī-ˌkräf-ˈthal-mē-ə\ *n* : abnormal smallness of the eye usu. occurring as a congenital anomaly

mi•croph•thal•mic \-ˈthal-mik\ *adj* : exhibiting microphthalmia : having small eyes

mi•croph•thal•mos \-məs, -ˌmäs\ *or* **mi•croph•thal•mus** \-ˈthal-məs\ *n, pl* **-moi** \-ˌmȯi\ *or* **-mi** \-ˌmī, -ˌmē\ : MICROPHTHALMIA

mi•cro•pi•pette *also* **mi•cro•pi•pet** \ˌmī-krō-pī-ˈpet\ *n* **1** : a pipette for the measurement of minute volumes **2** : a small and extremely fine-pointed pipette used in making microinjections — **micropipette** *vb*

mi•cro•po•rous \ˈmī-krō-ˌpōr-əs\ *adj* : marked by very small pores or channels with diameters in the micron or nanometer range ⟨~ membranes⟩

mi•crop•sia \mī-ˈkräp-sē-ə\ *also* **mi•crop•sy** \ˈmī-ˌkräp-sē\ *n, pl* **-sias** *also* **-sies** : a condition of abnormal visual perception in which objects appear to be smaller than they are in reality

mi•cro•punc•ture \ˌmī-krō-ˈpəŋk-chər\ *n* : an extremely small puncture (as of a nephron); *also* : an act of making such a puncture

mi•cro•pyle \ˈmī-krə-ˌpīl\ *n* : a differentiated area of surface in an egg through which a sperm enters — **mi•cro•py•lar** \ˌmī-krə-ˈpī-lər\ *adj*

mi•cro•ra•dio•gram \ˌmī-krō-ˈrā-dē-ə-ˌgram\ *n* : MICRORADIOGRAPH

mi•cro•ra•dio•graph \-ˌgraf\ *n* : an X-ray photograph prepared by microradiography

mi•cro•ra•di•og•ra•phy \-ˌrā-dē-ˈä-grə-fē\ *n, pl* **-phies** : radiography in which an X-ray photograph is prepared showing minute internal structure — **mi•cro•ra•dio•graph•ic** \-ˌrā-dē-ə-ˈgra-fik\ *adj*

mi•cro•RNA \ˌmī-krō-ˌär-en-ˈā\ *n* : a short segment of RNA that suppresses gene expression by binding to complementary segments of messenger RNA and interfering with protein formation — called also *miRNA*

mi•cro•sat•el•lite \-ˈsa-tᵊl-ˌīt\ *n* : any of numerous short segments of DNA that are distributed throughout the genome, that consist of repeated sequences of usu. two to five nucleotides, and that are often useful markers in studies of genetic linkage because they tend to vary from one individual to another — compare MINISATELLITE

mi•cro•scis•sors \ˈmī-krō-ˌsi-zərz\ *n sing or pl* : extremely small scissors for use in microsurgery

mi•cro•scope \ˈmī-krə-ˌskōp\ *n* **1** : an optical instrument consisting of a lens or combination of lenses for making enlarged images of minute objects; *esp*

: COMPOUND MICROSCOPE — see LIGHT MICROSCOPE, PHASE-CONTRAST MICROSCOPE, POLARIZING MICROSCOPE **2** : a non-optical instrument (as one using radiations other than light) for making enlarged images of minute objects — see ELECTRON MICROSCOPE, SCANNING ELECTRON MICROSCOPE

mi•cro•scop•ic \ˌmī-krə-ˈskä-pik\ *also* **mi•cro•scop•i•cal** \-pi-kəl\ *adj* **1** : of, relating to, or conducted with the microscope or microscopy **2** : so small or fine as to be invisible or indistinguishable without the use of a microscope — compare MACROSCOPIC, SUBMICROSCOPIC — **mi•cro•scop•i•cal•ly** *adv*

microscopic anatomy *n* : HISTOLOGY

mi•cros•co•py \mī-ˈkräs-kə-pē\ *n, pl* **-pies** : the use of or investigation with the microscope — **mi•cros•co•pist** \-pist\ *n*

mi•cro•sec•ond \ˈmī-krō-ˌse-kənd, -kənt\ *n* : one millionth of a second

mi•cro•sec•tion \-ˌsek-shən\ *n* : a thin section (as of tissue) prepared for microscopic examination — **microsection** *vb*

mi•cro•some \ˈmī-krə-ˌsōm\ *n* **1** : any of various minute cellular structures (as a ribosome) **2** : a particle in a particulate fraction that is obtained by heavy centrifugation of broken cells and consists of various amounts of ribosomes, fragmented endoplasmic reticulum, and mitochondrial cristae — **mi•cro•som•al** \ˌmī-krə-ˈsō-məl\ *adj*

mi•cro•so•mia \ˌmī-krə-ˈsō-mē-ə\ *n* : abnormal smallness of the body

mi•cro•sphe•ro•cy•to•sis \-ˌsfir-ō-sī-ˈtō-səs, -ˌsfer-\ *n, pl* **-to•ses** \-ˈtō-ˌsēz\ : spherocytosis esp. when marked by very small spherocytes

mi•cro•spo•rid•i•an \ˌmī-krō-spə-ˈri-dē-ən\ *n* : any of an order (Microsporidia) of spore-forming parasitic protozoans that typically invade and destroy host cells and include some (as of the genera *Enterocytozoon* and *Nosema*) that cause infections in immunocompromised humans — **microsporidian** *adj*

mi•cro•spo•rid•i•o•sis \-spə-ˌri-dē-ˈō-səs\ *n, pl* **-o•ses** \-ˌsēz\ : infestation with or disease caused by microsporidian protozoans

mi•cros•po•rum \mī-ˈkräs-pə-rəm\ *n* **1** *cap* : a genus of fungi (family Moniliaceae) producing both small single-celled spores and large multicellular spores and including several that cause ringworm, tinea capitis, and tinea corporis **2** *pl* **-ra** : any fungus of the genus *Microsporum*

mi•cro•struc•ture \ˈmī-krō-ˌstrək-chər\ *n* : microscopic structure (as of a cell) — **mi•cro•struc•tur•al** \ˌmī-krō-ˈstrək-chə-rəl, -ˈstrək-shrəl\ *adj*

mi•cro•sur•gery \ˌmī-krō-ˈsər-jə-rē\ *n, pl* **-ger•ies** : minute dissection or manipulation (as by a micromanipulator or laser beam) of living structures or tissue — **mi•cro•sur•geon** \ˈmī-krō-ˌsər-jən\ *n* — **mi•cro•sur•gi•cal** \ˌmī-krō-ˈsər-ji-kəl\ *adj* — **mi•cro•sur•gi•cal•ly** *adv*

mi•cro•sy•ringe \-sə-ˈrinj\ *n* : a hypodermic syringe equipped for the precise measurement and injection of minute quantities of fluid

mi•cro•tech•nique \ˌmī-krō-tek-ˈnēk\ *also* **mi•cro•tech•nic** \ˈmī-krō-ˌtek-nik, ˌmī-krō-tek-ˈnēk\ *n* : any of various methods of handling and preparing material for microscopic observation and study

mi•cro•throm•bus \-ˈthräm-bəs\ *n, pl* **-bi** \-ˌbī\ : a very small thrombus

mi•cro•tia \mī-ˈkrō-shə, -shē-ə\ *n* : abnormal smallness of the external ear — **mi•crot•ic** \mī-ˈkrä-tik\ *adj*

mi•cro•tome \ˈmī-krə-ˌtōm\ *n* : an instrument for cutting sections (as of organic tissues) for microscopic examination — **microtome** *vb*

mi•cro•trau•ma \ˈmī-krō-ˌtrau̇-mə, -ˌtrȯ-\ *n* : a very slight injury or lesion

mi•cro•tu•bule \ˌmī-krō-ˈtü-ˌbyül, -ˈtyü-\ *n* : any of the minute tubules in eukaryotic cytoplasm that are composed of tubulin and form an important component of the cytoskeleton, mitotic spindle, cilia, and flagella — **mi•cro•tu•bu•lar** \-byə-lər\ *adj*

mi•cro•unit \ˈmī-krō-ˌyü-nət\ *n* : one millionth of a standard unit and esp. an international unit ⟨∼*s* of insulin⟩

mi•cro•vas•cu•lar \-ˈvas-kyə-lər\ *adj* : of, relating to, or constituting the part of the circulatory system made up of minute vessels (as venules or capillaries) that average less than 0.3 millimeters in diameter — **mi•cro•vas•cu•la•ture** \-lə-ˌchu̇r, -ˌtyu̇r\ *n*

mi•cro•ves•i•cle \-ˈve-si-kəl\ *n* : a very small vesicle

mi•cro•ves•sel \-ˈve-səl\ *n* : a blood vessel (as a capillary or arteriole) of the microcirculatory system

mi•cro•vil•lus \-ˈvi-ləs\ *n, pl* **-vil•li** \-ˌlī\ : a microscopic projection of a tissue, cell, or cell organelle; *esp* : any of the fingerlike outward projections of some cell surfaces — **mi•cro•vil•lar** \-ˈvi-lər\ *adj* — **mi•cro•vil•lous** \-ˈvi-ləs\ *adj*

mi•cro•wave \ˈmī-krō-ˌwāv\ *n, often attrib* : a comparatively short electromagnetic wave; *esp* : one between about 1 millimeter and 1 meter in wavelength

microwave sickness *n* : a condition of impaired health reported esp. in the Russian medical literature that is held to be caused by prolonged exposure to low-intensity microwave radiation

Mi•cru•rus \mī-ˈkru̇r-əs\ *n* : a genus of small venomous elapid snakes comprising the American coral snakes

mic•tu•ri•tion \ˌmik-chə-ˈri-shən, ˌmik-tyu̇-\ *n* : URINATION — **mic•tu•rate** \ˈmik-chə-ˌrāt, -tyu̇-\ *vb*

MID *abbr* minimal infective dose

mid•ax•il•lary line \ˌmid-ˈak-sə-ˌler-ē-\ *n* : an imaginary line through the axilla parallel to the long axis of the body and midway between its ventral and dorsal surfaces

mid·azo·lam \mi-ˈdā-zō-ˌlam\ *n* : a benzodiazepine tranquilizer that is administered in the form of its hydrochloride $C_{18}H_{13}ClFN_3 \cdot HCl$ esp. to produce sedation before a medical procedure or surgery

mid·brain \ˈmid-ˌbrān\ *n* : the middle of the three primary divisions of the developing vertebrate brain or the corresponding part of the adult brain that includes a ventral part containing the cerebral peduncles and a dorsal tectum containing the corpora quadrigemina and that surrounds the aqueduct of Sylvius connecting the third and fourth ventricles — called also *mesencephalon*

mid·cla·vic·u·lar line \-kla-ˈvi-kyə-lər-, -klə-\ *n* : an imaginary line that is parallel to the long axis of the body and passes through the midpoint of the clavicle on the ventral surface of the body

middle age *n* : the period of life from about 45 to about 64 years of age — **mid·dle–aged** \ˌmid-ᵊl-ˈājd\ *adj* — **mid·dle–ag·er** \-ˈā-jər\ *n*

middle cerebellar peduncle *n* : CEREBELLAR PEDUNCLE b

middle cerebral artery *n* : CEREBRAL ARTERY b

middle concha *n* : NASAL CONCHA b

middle constrictor *n* : a fan-shaped muscle of the pharynx that arises from the ceratohyal and thyrohyal of the hyoid bone and from the stylohyoid ligament, inserts into the median line at the back of the pharynx, and acts to constrict part of the pharynx in swallowing — called also *constrictor pharyngis medius, middle pharyngeal constrictor muscle;* compare INFERIOR CONSTRICTOR, SUPERIOR CONSTRICTOR

middle ear *n* : the intermediate portion of the ear of higher vertebrates consisting typically of a small air-filled membrane-lined chamber in the temporal bone continuous with the nasopharynx through the eustachian tube, separated from the external ear by the tympanic membrane and from the inner ear by fenestrae, and containing a chain of three ossicles that extends from the tympanic membrane to the oval window and transmits vibrations to the inner ear — called also *tympanic cavity;* compare INCUS, MALLEUS, STAPES

Middle East respiratory syndrome *n* : MERS

middle finger *n* : the midmost of the five digits of the hand

middle hemorrhoidal artery *n* : RECTAL ARTERY b

middle hemorrhoidal vein *n* : RECTAL VEIN b

middle meatus *n* : a curved anteroposterior passage in each nasal cavity that is situated below the middle nasal concha and extends along the entire superior border of the inferior nasal concha — compare INFERIOR MEATUS, SUPERIOR MEATUS

middle meningeal artery *n* : a branch of the first portion of the maxillary artery that is the largest artery supplying the dura mater, enters the cranium through the foramen spinosum, and divides into anterior and posterior branches in a groove in the greater wing of the sphenoid bone

middle nasal concha *n* : NASAL CONCHA b

middle peduncle *n* : CEREBELLAR PEDUNCLE b

middle pharyngeal constrictor muscle *n* : MIDDLE CONSTRICTOR

middle rectal artery *n* : RECTAL ARTERY b

middle rectal vein *n* : RECTAL VEIN b

middle sacral artery *n* : a small artery that arises from the back of the abdominal part of the aorta just before it forks into the two common iliac arteries and that descends near the midline in front of the fourth and fifth lumbar vertebrae, the sacrum, and the coccyx to the glomus coccygeum

middle temporal artery *n* : TEMPORAL ARTERY 2b

middle temporal gyrus *n* : TEMPORAL GYRUS b

middle temporal vein *n* : TEMPORAL VEIN a (2)

middle turbinate *n* : NASAL CONCHA b

middle turbinate bone *also* **middle turbinated bone** *n* : NASAL CONCHA b

mid·dor·sal \(ˌ)mid-ˈdȯr-səl\ *adj* : of, relating to, or situated in the middle part or median line of the back ⟨the ~ region⟩

mid·epi·gas·tric \-ˌe-pi-ˈgas-trik\ *adj* : of, relating to, or located in the middle of the epigastric region of the abdomen ⟨~ tenderness⟩

mid·face \ˈmid-ˌfās\ *n* : the middle of the face including the nose and its associated bony structures — **mid·fa·cial** \ˌmid-ˈfā-shəl\ *adj*

mid·for·ceps \-ˈfȯr-səps, -ˌseps\ *n* : a procedure for delivery of an infant by the use of forceps after engagement has occurred but before the head has reached the lower part of the birth canal — compare HIGH FORCEPS, LOW FORCEPS

midge \ˈmij\ *n* : any of numerous tiny dipteran flies (esp. families Ceratopogonidae, Cecidomyiidae, and Chironomidae) including many which inflict painful bites and some which are vectors or intermediate hosts of parasites of humans and other vertebrates — see BITING MIDGE

midg·et \ˈmi-jət\ *n, sometimes offensive* : a person of unusually small size

mid·gut \ˈmid-ˌgət\ *n* : the middle part of the digestive tract of a vertebrate embryo that in humans gives rise to the more distal part of the duodenum and to the jejunum, ileum, cecum and appendix, ascending colon, and much of the transverse colon

mid•life \(ˌ)mid-ˈlīf\ *n* : MIDDLE AGE

midlife crisis *n* : a period of emotional turmoil in middle age caused by the realization that one is no longer young and characterized esp. by a strong desire for change

mid•line \ˈmid-ˌlīn, ˌmid-ˈlīn\ *n* : a median line; *esp* : the median line or median plane of the body or some part of the body

mid•preg•nan•cy \(ˌ)mid-ˈpreg-nən-sē\ *n, pl* **-cies** : the middle period of a term of pregnancy

mid•riff \ˈmi-ˌdrif\ *n* **1** : DIAPHRAGM 1 **2** : the mid-region of the human torso

mid•sag•it•tal \(ˌ)mid-ˈsa-jət-ᵊl\ *adj* : median and sagittal

midsagittal plane *n* : the median vertical longitudinal plane that divides a bilaterally symmetrical animal into right and left halves — called also *median plane*

mid•sec•tion \ˈmid-ˌsek-shən\ *n* : a section midway between the extremes; *esp* : MIDRIFF 2

mid•stream \ˌmid-ˈstrēm\ *adj* : of, relating to, or being urine passed during the middle of an act of urination and not at the beginning or end ⟨a ~ specimen⟩

mid•tar•sal \-ˈtär-səl\ *adj* : of, relating to, or being the articulation between the two rows of tarsal bones

midtarsal amputation *n* : amputation of the forepart of the foot through the midtarsal joint

mid•tri•mes•ter \-(ˌ)trī-ˈmes-tər\ *adj* : of, performed during, or occurring during the fourth through sixth months of human pregnancy

mid•ven•tral \-ˈven-trəl\ *adj* : of, relating to, or being the middle of the ventral surface — **mid•ven•tral•ly** *adv*

mid•wife \ˈmid-ˌwīf\ *n* : one who assists women in childbirth — see NURSE-MIDWIFE

mid•wife•ry \ˌmid-ˈwi-fə-rē, -ˈwī-; ˈmid-ˌwī-\ *n, pl* **-ries** : the art or act of assisting at childbirth; *also* : OBSTETRICS — see NURSE-MIDWIFERY

mi•fep•ris•tone \mɪ-ˈfe-pri-ˌstōn\ *n* : a drug $C_{29}H_{35}NO_2$ taken orally to induce abortion esp. early in pregnancy by blocking the body's use of progesterone — called also *RU-486*

mig•li•tol \ˈmi-glə-ˌtȯl\ *n* : an antidiabetic drug $C_8H_{17}NO_5$ that is taken orally as a tablet in the treatment of type 2 diabetes and acts to slow the absorption of glucose in the small intestine — see GLYSET

mi•graine \ˈmī-ˌgrān\ *n* **1** : a condition marked by recurring usu. moderate to severe headache with throbbing pain that usu. lasts from four hours to three days, typically begins on one side of the head but may spread to both sides, is often accompanied by nausea, vomiting, and sensitivity to light or sound, is sometimes preceded by an aura and is often followed by sleep, that tends to occur in more than one member of a family, and that is of uncertain origin though attacks appear to be associated with dilation of intracranial blood vessels and release of inflammatory substances (as serotonin) **2** : an episode or attack of migraine ⟨suffers from ~*s*⟩ — called also *sick headache* — **mi•grain•ous** \-ˌgrā-nəs\ *adj*

mi•grain•eur \ˌmē-gre-ˈnər\ *n* : a person who experiences migraines

mi•grain•oid \ˈmī-ˌgrā-ˌnȯid, mī-ˈgrā-\ *adj* : resembling migraine

migrans — see ERYTHEMA CHRONICUM MIGRANS, LARVAL MIGRANS, LARVA MIGRANS

migrantes — see LARVA MIGRANS

mi•grate \ˈmī-ˌgrāt, mī-ˈ\ *vb* **mi•grat•ed; mi•grat•ing** : to move from one place to another: as **a** : to move from one site to another in a host organism esp. as part of a life cycle **b** *of an atom or group* : to shift position within a molecule — **mi•gra•tion** \mī-ˈgrā-shən\ *n* — **mi•gra•to•ry** \ˈmī-grə-ˌtōr-ē\ *adj*

migration inhibitory factor *n* : a lymphokine which inhibits the migration of macrophages away from the site of interaction between lymphocytes and antigens

mi•ka•my•cin \ˌmī-kə-ˈmī-sən\ *n* : an antibiotic complex isolated from a bacterium of the genus *Streptomyces* (*S. mitakaensis*)

Mi•ku•licz resection \ˈme-kü-ˌlich-\ *n* : an operation for removal of part of the intestine and esp. the colon that involves bringing the diseased portion out of the body, closing the wound around the two parts of the loop which have been sutured together, and cutting off the diseased part leaving a double opening which is later joined by crushing the common wall and closed from the exterior

Mikulicz–Ra•dec•ki \-ra-ˈdet-skē\, **Johann von (1850–1905)**, Polish surgeon.

Mi•ku•licz's disease \-ˌli-chəz-\ *n* : abnormal enlargement of the lacrimal and salivary glands

Mikulicz's syndrome *n* : Mikulicz's disease esp. when occurring as a complication of another disease (as leukemia or sarcoidosis)

mild \ˈmīld\ *adj* **1** : moderate in action or effect ⟨a ~ drug⟩ **2** : not severe

mil•dew \ˈmil-ˌdü, -ˌdyü\ *n* **1** : a superficial usu. whitish growth produced esp. on organic matter or living plants by fungi (as of the families Erysiphaceae and Peronosporaceae) **2** : a fungus producing mildew

mild silver protein *n* : SILVER PROTEIN a

mil•i•ar•ia \ˌmi-lē-ˈar-ē-ə\ *n* : an inflammatory disorder of the skin characterized by redness, eruption, burning or itching, and the release of sweat in abnormal ways (as by the eruption of vesicles) due to blockage of the ducts of the sweat glands; *esp* : PRICKLY HEAT — **mil•i•ar•i•al** \-əl\ *adj*

miliaria crys•tal•li•na \-ˌkris-tə-ˈlē-nə\ *n* : SUDAMINA

mil•i•ary \ˈmi-lē-ˌer-ē\ *adj* **1** : resembling or suggesting a small seed or many small seeds ⟨a ~ aneurysm⟩ ⟨~ tubercles⟩ **2** : characterized by the formation of numerous small lesions ⟨~ pneumonia⟩

miliary tuberculosis *n* : acute tuberculosis in which minute tubercles are formed in one or more organs of the body by tubercle bacilli usu. spread by way of the blood

mi•lieu \mēl-ˈyə(r), -ˈyü; ˈmēl-ˌyü, mē-ˈlyœ\ *n, pl* **milieus** *or* **mi•lieux** *same or* -ˈyə(r)z, -ˈyüz; -ˌyüz, -ˈlyœz\ : ENVIRONMENT

milieu therapy *n* : psychotherapy involving manipulation of the environment of a patient for therapeutic purposes

mil•i•um \ˈmi-lē-əm\ *n, pl* **mil•ia** \-lē-ə\ : a small pearly firm noninflammatory elevation of the skin (as of the face) due to retention of keratin in an oil gland duct blocked by a thin layer of epithelium — called also *whitehead;* compare BLACKHEAD 1

[1]**milk** \ˈmilk\ *n* **1** : a fluid secreted by the mammary glands of females for the nourishment of their young **2 a** : milk from an animal and esp. a cow used as food by people **b** : a food product produced from seeds or fruit that resembles and is used similarly to cow's milk ⟨soy ~⟩

[2]**milk** *vb* : to draw off the milk of

milk•er's nodules \ˈmil-kərz-\ *n* : a mild virus infection characterized by reddish-blue nodules on the hands, arms, face, or neck acquired by direct contact with the udders of cows infected with pseudocowpox

milk fever *n* **1** : a febrile disorder following childbirth **2** : a disease of newly lactating cows, sheep, or goats caused by excessive drain on the body's mineral reserves — called also *parturient paresis*

milk leg *n* : postpartum thrombophlebitis of a femoral vein — called also *phlegmasia alba dolens*

Milk•man's syndrome \ˈmilk-mənz-\ *n* : an abnormal condition marked by porous bone and spontaneous often symmetrical fractures

Milkman, Louis Arthur (1895–1951), American radiologist.

milk of bismuth *n* : a thick white suspension in water of the hydroxide of bismuth and bismuth subcarbonate used esp. to treat diarrhea

milk of magnesia *n* : a milk-white suspension of magnesium hydroxide in water used as an antacid and laxative — called also *magnesia magma*

milk sickness *n* : an acute disease characterized by weakness, vomiting, and constipation and caused by eating dairy products or meat from cattle affected with trembles

milk sugar *n* : LACTOSE

milk thistle *n* **1** : a tall purple-flowered thistle (*Silybum marianum*) that is the source of silymarin **2** : an extract of milk thistle and esp. its seeds : SILYMARIN

milk tooth *n* : a temporary tooth of a young mammal; *esp* : one of the human dentition including four incisors, two canines, and four molars in each jaw which fall out during childhood and are replaced by the permanent teeth — called also *baby tooth, deciduous tooth, primary tooth*

Mil•ler–Ab•bott tube \ˈmi-lər-ˈa-bət-\ *n* : a double-lumen balloon-tipped rubber tube used for the purpose of decompression in treating intestinal obstruction

Miller, Thomas Grier (1886–1981), and **Abbott, William Osler (1902–1943),** American physicians.

milli- *comb form* : thousandth — used esp. in terms belonging to the metric system ⟨*milli*rad⟩

mil•li•bar \ˈmi-lə-ˌbär\ *n* : a unit of atmospheric pressure equal to a/qppp bar or 1000 dynes per square centimeter

mil•li•cu•rie \ˌmi-lə-ˈkyu̇r-(ˌ)ē, -kyu̇-ˈrē\ *n* : one thousandth of a curie — abbr. *mCi*

mil•li•gram \ˈmi-lə-ˌgram\ *n* : one thousandth of a gram — abbr. *mg*

mil•li•li•ter \-ˌlē-tər\ *n* : one thousandth of a liter — abbr. *ml*

mil•li•me•ter \-ˌmē-tər\ *n* : one thousandth of a meter — abbr. *mm*

mil•li•mi•cron \ˌmi-lə-ˈmī-ˌkrän\ *n* : NANOMETER

mil•li•os•mol *or* **mil•li•os•mole** \ˌmi-lē-ˈäz-ˌmōl, -ˈäs-\ *n* : one thousandth of an osmol

mil•li•pede \ˈmi-lə-ˌpēd\ *n* : any of a class (Diplopoda) of arthropods having usu. a cylindrical segmented body, two pairs of legs on most segments, and including some forms that secrete toxic substances causing skin irritation but that unlike centipedes possess no poison fangs

mil•li•rad \-ˌrad\ *n* : one thousandth of a rad — abbr. *mrad*

mil•li•rem \-ˌrem\ *n* : one thousandth of a rem — abbr. *mrem*

mil•li•roent•gen \ˌmi-lə-ˈrent-gən, -ˈrənt-, -jən; -ˈren-chən, -ˈrən-\ *n* : one thousandth of a roentgen — abbr. *mR*

mil•li•unit \ˈmi-lə-ˌyü-nət\ *n* : one thousandth of a standard unit and esp. of an international unit

mil•ri•none \ˈmil-rə-ˌnōn\ *n* : an inotropic vasodilator used in the form of its lactate $C_{12}H_9N_3O \cdot C_3H_6O_3$ esp. in short-term intravenous therapy for congestive heart failure

Mil•roy's disease \ˈmil-ˌrȯiz-\ *n* : a hereditary lymphedema esp. of the legs

Milroy, William Forsyth (1855–1942), American physician.

Mil•town \ˈmil-ˌtau̇n\ *trademark* — used for a preparation of meprobamate

Mil•wau•kee brace \mil-ˈwȯ-kē-, -ˈwä-\ *n* : an orthopedic brace that extends from the pelvis to the neck and is used esp. to treat scoliosis

mi•met•ic \mə-ˈme-tik, mī-\ *adj* : simulating the action or effect of — usu. used in combination ⟨sympatho*mimetic* drugs⟩

mim•ic \ˈmi-mik\ *vb* **mim•icked** \-mikt\; **mim•ick•ing** : to imitate or resemble closely: as **a** : to imitate the symptoms of **b** : to produce an effect and esp. a physiological effect similar to — **mimic** *n* — **mim•ic•ry** \ˈmi-mi-krē\ *n*

min *abbr* minim

Min•a•mata disease \ˌmi-nə-ˈmä-tə-\ *n* : a toxic neuropathy caused by the ingestion of methylmercury compounds (as in contaminated seafood) and characterized by impairment of cerebral functions, constriction of the visual field, and progressive weakening of muscles

Mi•nas•trin \mi-ˈna-strən\ *trademark* — used for a preparation of ethinyl estradiol and the acetate of norethindrone

mind \ˈmīnd\ *n* **1** : the element or complex of elements in an individual that feels, perceives, thinks, wills, and esp. reasons **2** : the conscious mental events and capabilities in an organism **3** : the organized conscious and unconscious adaptive mental activity of an organism

mind–altering *adj* : PSYCHOACTIVE

mind–set \ˈmīnd-ˌset\ *n* : a mental inclination, tendency, or habit

[1]**min•er•al** \ˈmi-nə-rəl\ *n* : a solid homogeneous crystalline chemical element or compound that results from the inorganic processes of nature

[2]**mineral** *adj* **1** : of or relating to minerals; *also* : INORGANIC **2** : impregnated with mineral substances

min•er•al•ize \ˈmi-nə-rə-ˌlīz\ *vb* **-ized; -iz•ing** : to impregnate or supply with minerals or an inorganic compound — **min•er•al•i•za•tion** \ˌmi-nə-rəl-ə-ˈzā-shən\ *n*

min•er•al•o•cor•ti•coid \ˌmi-nə-rə-lō-ˈkȯr-tə-ˌkȯid\ *n* : a corticosteroid (as aldosterone) that affects chiefly the electrolyte and fluid balance in the body — compare GLUCOCORTICOID

mineral oil *n* : a transparent oily liquid obtained usu. by distilling petroleum and used in medicine esp. for treating constipation

min•er's asthma \ˈmī-nərz-\ *n* : PNEUMOCONIOSIS

miner's elbow *n* : bursitis of the elbow that tends to occur in miners who work in small tunnels and rest their weight on their elbows

miner's phthisis *n* : an occupational respiratory disease (as pneumoconiosis or anthracosilicosis) of miners

mini•lap•a•rot•o•my \ˌmi-nē-ˌla-pə-ˈrä-tə-mē\ *n, pl* **-mies** : a ligation of the Fallopian tubes performed through a small incision in the abdominal wall

min•im \ˈmi-nəm\ *n* : either of two units of capacity equal to 1/60 fluid dram: **a** : a U.S. unit of liquid capacity equivalent to 0.003760 cubic inch or 0.061610 milliliter **b** : a British unit of liquid capacity and dry measure equivalent to 0.003612 cubic inch or 0.059194 milliliter

minimae — see VENAE CORDIS MINIMAE

min•i•mal \ˈmi-nə-məl\ *adj* : relating to or being a minimum : constituting the least possible with respect to size, number, degree, or certain stated conditions ⟨side effects were ~⟩ ⟨~ hearing loss⟩

minimal brain dysfunction *n* : ATTENTION DEFICIT DISORDER — abbr. *MBD*

minimal change disease *n* : a kidney disease that is marked by renal tissue which appears normal when examined by light microscope but shows minimal pathological changes when examined by electron microscope, that is the most common cause of nephrotic syndrome in children, and that is typically idiopathic but may sometimes be associated with an identifiable cause (as NSAID use)

minimal infective dose *n* : the smallest quantity of infective material that regularly produces infection — abbr. *MID*

minimal inhibitory concentration *n* : the smallest concentration of an antibiotic that regularly inhibits growth of a bacterium in vitro — abbr. *MIC*

minimally invasive *adj, of a surgical procedure* : involving entry into the living body through a relatively small incision ⟨*minimally invasive* spine surgery with limited tissue damage⟩ ⟨*minimally invasive* arthroscopic rotator cuff repair⟩

minimi — see ABDUCTOR DIGITI MINIMI, EXTENSOR DIGITI MINIMI, FLEXOR DIGITI MINIMI BREVIS, GLUTEUS MINIMUS, OPPONENS DIGITI MINIMI

min•i•mum \ˈmi-nə-məm\ *n, pl* **-i•ma** \-mə\ *or* **-i•mums** **1** : the least quantity assignable, admissible, or possible **2** : the lowest degree or amount of variation (as of temperature) reached or recorded — **minimum** *adj*

minimum dose *n* : the smallest dose of a medicine or drug that will produce an effect

minimum inhibitory concentration *n* : MINIMAL INHIBITORY CONCENTRATION

minimum lethal dose *n* : the smallest dose experimentally found to kill any one animal of a test group

minimus — see GLUTEUS MINIMUS

mini•pill \ˈmi-nē-ˌpill\ *n* : a birth control pill that contains a very low dose of a progestogen and esp. norethindrone but no estrogen and is intended to minimize side effects

Mini•press \-ˌpres\ *trademark* — used for a preparation of the hydrochloride of prazosin

mini•sat•el•lite \-ˈsa-tᵊl-ˌīt\ *n* : any of numerous DNA segments located mainly near the ends of chromosomes that consist of repeating sequences of at least five but usu. not more than 100 nucleotides and that are useful in DNA fingerprinting — compare MICROSATELLITE

mini•stroke \-ˌstrōk\ *n* : TRANSIENT ISCHEMIC ATTACK

Min•ne•so•ta Mul•ti•pha•sic Personality Inventory \ˌmi-nə-ˈsō-tə-ˌməl-ti-ˈfā-zik-, -ˌməl-ˌtī-\ *n* : a test of personal and social adjustment based on a complex scaling of the answers to an elaborate true or false test

Mi•no•cin \mi-ˈnō-sin\ *trademark* — used for a preparation of the hydrochloride of minocycline

min•o•cy•cline \ˌmi-nō-ˈsī-klēn\ *n* : a broad-spectrum tetracycline antibiotic administered in the form of its hydrochloride $C_{23}H_{27}N_3O_7 \cdot HCl$

[1]**mi•nor** \ˈmī-nər\ *adj* : not serious or involving risk to life ⟨~ illness⟩ ⟨a ~ operation⟩ — compare MAJOR

[2]**minor** *n* : a person of either sex under the age of legal qualification for adult rights and responsibilities

minora — see LABIA MINORA

minor surgery *n* : surgery involving little risk to the life of the patient; *specif* : an operation on the superficial structures of the body or a manipulative procedure that does not involve a serious risk — compare MAJOR SURGERY

min•ox•i•dil \mi-ˈnäk-sə-ˌdil\ *n* : a peripheral vasodilator $C_9H_{15}N_5O$ used orally to treat hypertension and topically in a propylene glycol solution to promote hair regrowth in male-pattern baldness — see LONITEN, ROGAINE

minute volume *n* : CARDIAC OUTPUT

mi•o•sis *also* **my•o•sis** \mī-ˈō-səs, mē-\ *n, pl* **mi•o•ses** *also* **my•o•ses** \-ˌsēz\ : excessive smallness or contraction of the pupil of the eye

[1]**mi•ot•ic** *also* **my•ot•ic** \-ˈä-tik\ *n* : an agent that causes miosis

[2]**miotic** *also* **my•ot•ic** *adj* : relating to or characterized by miosis

mir•a•beg•ron \ˌmir-ə-ˈbeg-ˌrän\ *n* : a beta-agonist $C_{21}H_{24}N_4O_2S$ that relaxes the detrusor musculature of the bladder and is taken orally to treat the symptoms (as urinary incontinence and urgency) associated with an overactive bladder — SEE MYRBETRIQ

mi•ra•cid•i•um \ˌmir-ə-ˈsi-dē-əm, ˌmī-rə-\ *n, pl* **-cid•ia** \-dē-ə\ : the free-swimming ciliated first larva of a digenetic trematode that develops into a sporocyst after penetrating a suitable intermediate host — **mi•ra•cid•i•al** \-dē-əl\ *adj*

mir•a•cil D \ˈmir-ə-ˌsil-ˈdē\ *n* : LUCANTHONE

mir•a•cle drug \ˈmir-ə-kəl-\ *n* : a drug usu. newly discovered that elicits a dramatic response in a patient's condition — called also *wonder drug*

mi•rage \mə-ˈräzh\ *n* : an optical effect that is sometimes seen at sea, in the desert, or over a hot pavement, that may have the appearance of a pool of water or a mirror in which distant objects are seen inverted, and that is caused by the bending or reflection of rays of light by a layer of heated air of varying density

Mir•cera \mər-ˈser-ə\ *trademark* — used for a preparation of epoetin

Mi•rena \mi-ˈre-nə\ *trademark* — used for a T-shaped intrauterine device containing levonorgestrol

mi•rex \ˈmī-ˌreks\ *n* : an organochlorine insecticide $C_{10}Cl_{12}$ formerly used esp. against ants that is a suspected carcinogen

miRNA \ˌem-ˌī-ˌär-ˌen-ˈā\ *n* : MICRORNA

mirror writing *n* : backward writing resembling in slant and order of letters the reflection of ordinary writing in a mirror

mir•taz•a•pine \mir-ˈta-zə-ˌpēn\ *n* : an antidepressant drug $C_{17}H_{19}N_3$ taken orally esp. to treat major depressive disorder — see REMERON

Mir•va•so \mər-ˈvā-sō\ *trademark* — used for a topical gel containing brimonidine

MIS *abbr* Müllerian inhibiting substance

mis- *prefix* : badly : wrongly ⟨*mis*diagnose⟩

mis•ad•min•i•stra•tion \ˌmis-əd-ˌmi-nə-ˈstrā-shən, -(ˌ)ad-\ *n* : the act, process, or an instance of administering poorly or wrongly ⟨~ of radiation therapy⟩

mis•car•riage \mis-ˈkar-ij\ *n* : spontaneous expulsion of a human fetus before it is viable and esp. between the 12th and 28th weeks of gestation — compare ABORTION 1a — **mis•car•ry** \(ˌ)mis-ˈkar-ē\ *vb*

mis•di•ag•nose \(ˌ)mis-ˈdī-ig-ˌnōs, -ˌnōz\ *vb* **-nosed; -nos•ing** : to diagnose incorrectly — **mis•di•ag•no•sis** \(ˌ)mis-ˌdī-ig-ˈnō-səs\ *n*

mi•sog•y•nist \mə-ˈsä-jə-nist\ *n* : one who hates women — **misogynist** *adj* — **mi•sog•y•ny** \mə-ˈsä-jə-nē\ *n*

mi•so•pros•tol \ˌmī-sō-ˈpräs-ˌtōl, -ˌtȯl\ *n* : a prostaglandin analog $C_{22}H_{38}O_5$ used to prevent stomach ulcers associated with NSAID use and to induce abortion in conjunction with mifepristone

missed abortion \ˈmist-\ *n* : an intrauterine death of a fetus that is not followed by its immediate expulsion

missed labor *n* : a retention of a fetus in the uterus beyond the normal period of pregnancy

[1]**mis•sense** \ˈmis-ˌsens\ *adj* : relating to or being a genetic mutation involving alteration of one or more codons so that different amino acids are determined — compare ANTISENSE, NONSENSE

[2]**missense** *n* : missense genetic mutation

missionary position *n* : a coital position in which the female lies on her back with the male on top and with his face opposite hers

mit- *or* **mito-** *comb form* **1** : thread ⟨*mito*chondrion⟩ **2** : mitosis ⟨*mito*genesis⟩

mite \ˈmīt\ *n* : any of numerous small to very minute acarid arachnids that include parasites of insects and vertebrates some of which are important disease vectors, parasites of plants, pests of various stored products, and free-living aquatic and terrestrial forms — see ITCH MITE

mith·ra·my·cin \ˌmi-thrə-ˈmīs-ᵊn\ *n* : PLICAMYCIN

mith·ri·da·tism \ˌmi-thrə-ˈdā-ˌti-zəm\ *n* : tolerance to a poison acquired by taking gradually increased doses of it

Mith·ra·da·tes VI Eu·pa·tor \ˌmi-thrə-ˈdā-tēz-ˈsiks-ˈyü-pə-ˌtȯr\, (*d* 63 BC), king of Pontus.

mi·ti·cide \ˈmī-tə-ˌsīd\ *n* : an agent used to kill mites — **mi·ti·cid·al** \ˌmī-tə-ˈsīd-ᵊl\ *adj*

mitochondrial DNA *n* : an extranuclear double-stranded DNA found exclusively in mitochondria that in most eukaryotes is a circular molecule and is maternally inherited — called also *mtDNA*

mi·to·chon·dri·on \ˌmī-tə-ˈkän-drē-ən\ *n, pl* **-dria** \-drē-ə\ : any of various round or long cellular organelles of most eukaryotes that are found outside the nucleus, produce energy for the cell through cellular respiration, and are rich in fats, proteins, and enzymes — **mi·to·chon·dri·al** \-drē-əl\ *adj* — **mi·to·chon·dri·al·ly** *adv*

mi·to·gen \ˈmī-tə-jən\ *n* : a substance that induces mitosis

mi·to·gen·e·sis \ˌmī-tə-ˈje-nə-səs\ *n, pl* **-e·ses** \-ˌsēz\ : the production of cell mitosis

mi·to·gen·ic \-ˈje-nik\ *adj* : of, producing, or stimulating mitosis

mi·to·my·cin \ˌmī-tə-ˈmīs-ᵊn\ *n* **1** : a complex of antibiotic substances which is produced by a Japanese bacterium of the genus *Streptomyces* (*S. caespitosus*) **2** : a component $C_{15}H_{18}N_4O_5$ of mitomycin that inhibits DNA synthesis and is used as an antineoplastic in the palliative treatment of some carcinomas — called also *mitomycin C*

mi·to·sis \mī-ˈtō-səs\ *n, pl* **-to·ses** \-ˌsēz\ **1** : a process that takes place in the nucleus of a dividing cell, involves typically a series of steps consisting of prophase, metaphase, anaphase, and telophase, and results in the formation of two new nuclei each having the same number of chromosomes as the parent nucleus — compare MEIOSIS **2** : cell division in which mitosis occurs — **mi·tot·ic** \-ˈtä-tik\ *adj* — **mi·tot·i·cal·ly** *adv*

mitotic index *n* : the number of cells per thousand cells actively dividing at a particular time

mi·to·xan·trone \ˌmī-tō-ˈzan-ˌtrōn\ *n* : an antineoplastic drug that is used in the form of its dihydrochloride $C_{22}H_{28}N_4O_6 \cdot 2HCl$ either alone or in combination in the treatment of some leukemias and carcinomas

mi·tral \ˈmī-trəl\ *adj* : of, relating to, being, or adjoining a mitral valve or orifice

mitral cell *n* : any of the pyramidal cells of the olfactory bulb about which terminate numerous fibers from the olfactory cells of the nasal mucosa

mitral insufficiency *n* : inability of the mitral valve to close perfectly permitting blood to flow back into the atrium and leading to varying degrees of heart failure — called also *mitral incompetence*

mitral orifice *n* : the left atrioventricular orifice

mitral regurgitation *n* : backward flow of blood into the atrium due to mitral insufficiency

mitral stenosis *n* : a condition usu. the result of disease in which the mitral valve is abnormally narrow

mitral valve *n* : a valve in the heart consisting of two triangular flaps which allow only unidirectional blood flow from the left atrium to the left ventricle — called also *bicuspid valve, left atrioventricular valve*

mitral valve prolapse *n* : a valvular heart disorder in which one or both mitral valve flaps close incompletely during systole usu. producing either a click or murmur and sometimes mitral regurgitation and which is often a benign symptomless condition but may be marked by varied symptoms (as chest pain, fatigue, or palpitations) — abbr. *MVP;* called also *Barlow's syndrome*

mit·tel·schmerz \ˈmi-tᵊl-ˌshmertz\ *n* : abdominal pain occurring between the menstrual periods and usu. considered to be associated with ovulation

mixed \ˈmikst\ *adj* **1** : combining features or exhibiting symptoms of more than one condition or disease ⟨a ~ tumor⟩ **2** : producing more than one kind of secretion ⟨~ salivary glands⟩

mixed connective tissue disease *n* : a syndrome characterized by symptoms of various rheumatic diseases (as systemic lupus erythematosus, scleroderma, and polymyositis) and by high concentrations of antibodies to extractable nuclear antigens

mixed dementia *n* : dementia involving both Alzheimer's disease and vascular dementia

mixed glioma *n* : a brain tumor (as an oligoastrocytoma) comprised of more than one type of glial tissue

mixed nerve *n* : a nerve containing both sensory and motor fibers

mix·ture \ˈmiks-chər\ *n* : a product of mixing: as **a** : a portion of matter consisting of two or more components in varying proportions that retain their own properties **b** : an aqueous liquid medicine; *specif* : a preparation in which insoluble substances are suspended in watery fluids by the addition of a viscid material (as gum, sugar, or glycerol)

mks \ˌem-ˌkā-ˈes\ *adj, often cap M&K&S* : of, relating to, or being a system of units based on the meter, the kilogram, and the second ⟨~ system⟩ ⟨~ units⟩

ml *abbr* milliliter

MLD *abbr* **1** median lethal dose **2** minimum lethal dose

M line \ˈem-ˌlīn\ *n* : a thin dark line across the center of the H zone of a striated muscle fiber — called also *M band*

MLT *abbr* medical laboratory technician

mm *abbr* millimeter

mm Hg \ˌmi-lə-ˌmē-tər-əv-ˈmər-kyə-rē\ *n* : a unit of pressure equal to the pressure exerted by a column of mercury 1 millimeter high at 0°C and under the acceleration of gravity and nearly equivalent to 1 torr ⟨blood pressure was 110/70 *mm Hg*⟩

M–mode \ˈem-ˌmōd\ *adj* : of, relating to, or being an ultrasonographic technique that is used for studying the movement of internal body structures

MMPI *abbr* Minnesota Multiphasic Personality Inventory

MMR *abbr* measles-mumps-rubella (vaccine)

Mn *symbol* manganese

MN *abbr* master of nursing

-m•ne•sia \m-ˈnē-zhə\ *n comb form* : a (specified) type or condition of memory ⟨par*amnesia*⟩

Mo *symbol* molybdenum

MO *abbr* medical officer

Mo•bic \ˈmo-bik\ *trademark* — used for a preparation of meloxicam

mo•bile \ˈmō-bəl, -ˌbīl\ *adj* **1** : capable of moving or being moved about readily **2** : characterized by an extreme degree of fluidity — **mo•bil•i•ty** \mō-ˈbi-lə-tē\ *n*

mo•bi•lize \ˈmō-bə-ˌlīz\ *vb* **-lized; -liz•ing** **1** : to put into movement or circulation : make mobile; *specif* : to release (something stored in the body) for body use **2** : to assemble (as resources) and make ready for use **3** : to separate (an organ or part) from associated structures so as to make more accessible for operative procedures **4** : to develop to a state of acute activity — **mo•bi•li•za•tion** \ˌmō-bə-lə-ˈzā-shən\ *n*

Mö•bius syndrome *or* **Moe•bius syn•drome** \ˈmu̇-bē-əs-, ˈmœ-\ *n* : congenital bilateral paralysis of the facial muscles associated with other neurological disorders

Möbius, Paul Julius (1853–1907), German neurologist.

moc•ca•sin \ˈmä-kə-sən\ *n* **1** : WATER MOCCASIN **2** : a snake (as of the genus *Natrix*) resembling a water moccasin

mo•dal•i•ty \mō-ˈda-lə-tē\ *n, pl* **-ties** **1** : one of the main avenues of sensation (as vision) **2 a** : a usu. physical therapeutic agency **b** : an apparatus for applying a modality

¹mod•el \ˈmäd-ᵊl\ *n* **1 a** : a pattern of something to be made **b** : a cast of a tooth or oral cavity **2** : something (as a similar object or a construct) used to help visualize or explore something else (as the living human body) that cannot be directly observed or experimented on — see ANIMAL MODEL

²model *vb* **mod•eled** *or* **mod•elled; mod•el•ing** *or* **mod•el•ling** : to produce (as by computer) a representation or simulation of

mod•er•ate \ˈmä-də-rət\ *adj* **1** : avoiding extremes of behavior : observing reasonable limits ⟨a ~ drinker⟩ **2** : not severe in effect ⟨~ pain⟩

modified radical mastectomy *n* : a mastectomy that is similar to a radical mastectomy but does not include removal of the pectoral muscles

mod•i•fi•er \ˈmä-də-ˌfī-ər\ *n* **1** : one that modifies **2** : a gene that modifies the effect of another

mod•i•fy \ˈmä-də-ˌfī\ *vb* **-fied; -fy•ing** : to make a change in ⟨~ behavior by the use of drugs⟩ — **mod•i•fi•ca•tion** \ˌmä-də-fə-ˈkā-shən\ *n*

mo•di•o•lar \mə-ˈdī-ə-lər\ *adj* : of or relating to the modiolus of the ear

mo•di•o•lus \mə-ˈdī-ə-ləs\ *n, pl* **-li** \-ˌlī\ : a central bony column in the cochlea of the ear

MODS *abbr* multiple organ dysfunction syndrome

mod•u•late \ˈmä-jə-ˌlāt\ *vb* **-lat•ed; -lat•ing** : to adjust to or keep in proper measure or proportion ⟨~ an immune response⟩ ⟨~ cell activity⟩ — **mod•u•la•tion** \ˌmä-jə-ˈlā-shən\ *n* — **mod•u•la•tor** \ˈmä-jə-ˌlā-tər\ *n* — **mod•u•la•to•ry** \-lə-ˌtōr-ē\ *adj*

MODY *abbr* maturity-onset diabetes of the young

Moebius syndrome *var of* MÖBIUS SYNDROME

mo•ex•i•pril \mō-ˈek-sə-ˌpril\ *n* : an ACE inhibitor used in the form of its hydrochloride $C_{27}H_{34}N_2O_7{\cdot}HCl$ to treat hypertension — see UNIVASC

Mohs surgery \ˈmōz-\ *n* : a surgical technique for the removal of skin cancers (as basal cell carcinoma) in which tissue is progressively removed to a depth and width at which the tissue is microscopically free of cancer — called also *Mohs micrographic surgery, Mohs technique*

Mohs, Frederic Edward (1910–2002), American surgeon.

moist \ˈmȯist\ *adj* **1** : slightly or moderately wet **2 a** : marked by a discharge or exudation of liquid ⟨~ eczema⟩ **b** : suggestive of the presence of liquid — used of sounds heard in auscultation ⟨~ rales⟩

moist gangrene *n* : gangrene that develops in the presence of combined arterial and venous obstruction, is usu. accompanied by an infection, and is characterized by a watery discharge usu. of foul odor

mol•al \ˈmō-ləl\ *adj* : of, relating to, or containing a mole of solute per 1000 grams of solvent ⟨a ~ solution⟩ — **mo•lal•i•ty** \mō-ˈla-lə-tē\ *n*

[1]**mo•lar** \ˈmō-lər\ *n* : a tooth with a rounded or flattened surface adapted for grinding; *specif* : one of the mammalian teeth behind the incisors and canines sometimes including the premolars but more exactly restricted to the three posterior pairs in each human jaw on each side which are not preceded by milk teeth

[2]**molar** *adj* **1 a** : pulverizing by friction ⟨~ teeth⟩ **b** : of, relating to, or located near the molar teeth ⟨~ gland⟩ **2** : of, relating to, possessing the qualities of, or characterized by a hydatidiform mole ⟨~ pregnancy⟩

[3]**molar** *adj* **1** : of or relating to a mole of a substance ⟨the ~ volume of a gas⟩ **2** : containing one mole of solute in one liter of solution — **mo•lar•i•ty** \mō-ˈlar-ə-tē\ *n*

[1]**mold** \ˈmōld\ *n* : a cavity in which a fluid or malleable substance is shaped

[2]**mold** *vb* : to give shape to esp. in a mold

[3]**mold** *vb* : to become moldy

[4]**mold** *n* **1** : a superficial often woolly growth produced esp. on damp or decaying organic matter or on living organisms by a fungus (as of the order Mucorales) **2** : a fungus that produces mold

mold•ing \ˈmōl-diŋ\ *n* : the shaping of the fetal head to allow it to pass through the birth canal during birth

moldy \ˈmōl-dē\ *adj* **mold•i•er; -est** : covered with a mold-producing fungus ⟨~ bread⟩

[1]**mole** \ˈmōl\ *n* : a pigmented spot, mark, or small permanent protuberance on the human body; *esp* : NEVUS

[2]**mole** *n* : an abnormal mass in the uterus: **a** : a blood clot containing a degenerated fetus and its membranes **b** : HYDATIDIFORM MOLE

[3]**mole** *also* **mol** \ˈmōl\ *n* : the base unit in the International System of Units for the amount of pure substance that contains the same number of elementary entities as there are atoms in exactly 12 grams of the isotope carbon 12

mo•lec•u•lar \mə-ˈle-kyə-lər\ *adj* : of, relating to, consisting of, or produced by molecules — **mo•lec•u•lar•ly** *adv*

molecular biology *n* : a branch of biology dealing with the study and understanding of biological activity and processes at the molecular level and esp. the molecular basis of gene function and protein synthesis — **molecular biologist** *n*

molecular formula *n* : a chemical formula that gives the total number of atoms of each element in a molecule ⟨the *molecular formula* of water is H_2O⟩ — see STRUCTURAL FORMULA

molecular genetics *n pl* : a branch of genetics dealing with the structure and activity of genetic material at the molecular level — **molecular geneticist** *n*

molecular weight *n* : the mass of a molecule that may be calculated as the sum of the atomic weights of its constituent atoms

mol•e•cule \ˈmä-li-ˌkyül\ *n* : the smallest particle of a substance that retains all the properties of the substance and is composed of one or more atoms

mole•skin \ˈmōl-ˌskin\ *n* : adhesive padding (as for blisters) typically made of a heavy, durable, cotton fabric with a soft nap on one side

mol•in•done \mō-ˈlin-ˌdōn\ *n* : an antipsychotic drug used in the form of its hydrochloride $C_{16}H_{24}N_2O_2 \cdot HCl$ esp. in the treatment of schizophrenia

Moll's gland \ˈmälz\ *n* : GLAND OF MOLL

mol•lus•cum \mə-ˈləs-kəm\ *n, pl* **-ca** \-kə\ : any of several skin diseases marked by soft pulpy nodules; *esp* : MOLLUSCUM CONTAGIOSUM

molluscum body *n* : any of the rounded cytoplasmic bodies found in the central opening of the nodules characteristic of molluscum contagiosum

molluscum con•ta•gi•o•sum \-kən-ˌtā-jē-ˈō-səm\ *n, pl* **mollusca con•ta•gi•o•sa** \-sə\ : a mild chronic disease of the skin caused by a poxvirus (species *Molluscum contagiosum virus* of the genus *Molluscipoxvirus*) and characterized by the formation of small nodules with a central opening and contents resembling curd

mol•lusk *or* **mol•lusc** \ˈmä-ləsk\ *n* : any of a phylum (Mollusca) of invertebrate animals (as snails) with a soft unsegmented body usu. enclosed in a calcareous shell — **mol•lus•can** *also* **mol•lus•kan** \mə-ˈles-kən, mä-\ *adj*

Mol•ly \ˈmä-lē\ *n* : the illicit drug ecstasy esp. when in a powdered or crystalline form contained in a capsule

molt \ˈmōlt\ *vb* : to shed hair, feathers, shell, horns, or an outer layer periodically — **molt** *n*

mo•lyb•de•num \mə-ˈlib-də-nəm\ *n* : a metallic element that is a trace element in plant and animal metabolism — symbol *Mo;* see ELEMENT table

mo•met•a•sone \mō-ˈme-tə-ˌsōn\ *n* : a synthetic corticosteroid $C_{27}H_{30}Cl_2O_6$ that is used as a topical cream or ointment to treat inflammatory and pruritic dermatoses, as a nasal spray to relieve symptoms of allergic rhinitis, or as an inhalational aerosol or powder to treat asthma — called also *mometasone fu•ro•ate* \-ˈfyu̇r-ə-ˌwāt\; see ASMANEX, DULERA, ELOCON, NASONEX

mon- *or* **mono-** *comb form* **1** : one : single ⟨*mono*filament⟩ **2** : affecting a single part ⟨*mono*plegia⟩

monarticular *var of* MONOARTICULAR

mon•au•ral \(ˌ)mä-ˈnȯr-əl\ *adj* : of, relating to, affecting, or designed for use with one ear ⟨~ hearing aid systems⟩ — **mon•au•ral•ly** *adv*

Möncke•berg's sclerosis \ˈmu̇ŋ-kə-ˌbərgz-, ˈmeŋ-\ *n* : arteriosclerosis characterized by the formation of calcium deposits in the mediae of esp. the peripheral arteries

Möncke•berg \ˈmœŋ-kə-ˌberk\, **Johann Georg (1877–1925)**, German pathologist.

mo•nen•sin \mō-ˈnen-sən\ *n* : an antibiotic $C_{36}H_{62}O_{11}$ obtained from a bacterium of the genus *Streptomyces* (*S. cinnamonensis*) and used as an antiprotozoal, antibacterial, and antifungal agent and as an additive to cattle feed

mo•ne•ran \mə-ˈnir-ən\ *n* : PROKARYOTE — **moneran** *adj*

mon•es•trous \(ˌ)mä-ˈnes-trəs\ *adj* : experiencing estrus once each year or breeding season

mon•gol \ˈmäŋ-gəl; ˈmän-ˌgōl, ˈmäŋ-\ *n, often cap, dated, now usu offensive* : a person affected with Down syndrome

mon•go•lian \män-ˈgōl-yən, mäŋ-, -ˈgō-lē-ən\ *adj, often cap, dated, now usu offensive* : of, relating to, or affected with Down syndrome

Mongolian spot *n* : a bluish pigmented area near the base of the spine that is present at birth esp. in Asian, southern European, American Indian, and black infants and that usu. disappears during childhood

mon•gol•ism \ˈmäŋ-gə-ˌli-zəm\ *n dated, now usu offensive* : DOWN SYNDROME

mon•gol•oid \ˈmäŋ-gə-ˌlȯid\ *adj, often cap, dated, now usu offensive* : of, relating to, or affected with Down syndrome — **mongoloid** *n, often cap, dated, now usu offensive*

mo•nie•zia \ˌmä-nē-ˈe-zē-ə\ *n* **1** *cap* : a genus of tapeworms (family Anoplocephalidae) parasitizing the intestine of various ruminants **2** : any tapeworm of the genus *Moniezia*

Moniez \mȯn-ˈyā\, **Romain–Louis (1852–1936)**, French parasitologist.

mo•nil•e•thrix \mə-ˈni-lə-ˌthriks\ *n, pl* **mon•i•let•ri•ches** \ˌmä-nə-ˈle-trə-ˌkēz\ : a hereditary disease of the hair that is typically inherited as an autosomal dominant trait in which each strand of hair has a beaded appearance due to periodic narrowing of the hair shaft and that is marked chiefly by fragile brittle hair and patchy alopecia

mo•nil•ia \mə-ˈni-lē-ə\ *n, pl* **monilias** *or* **monilia** *also* **mo•nil•i•ae** \-lē-ˌē\ **1** : any fungus of the genus *Candida* **2** *pl monilias* : CANDIDIASIS

Mo•nil•ia \mə-ˈni-lē-ə\ *n, syn of* CANDIDA

mo•nil•i•al \mə-ˈni-lē-əl\ *adj* : of, relating to, or caused by a fungus of the genus *Candida* ⟨~ vaginitis⟩

mo•ni•li•a•sis \ˌmō-nə-ˈlī-ə-səs, ˌmä-\ *n, pl* **-a•ses** \-ˌsēz\ : CANDIDIASIS

mo•nil•iid \mə-ˈni-lē-əd\ *n* : a secondary commonly generalized dermatitis resulting from hypersensitivity developed in response to a primary focus of infection with a fungus of the genus *Candida*

[1]**mon•i•tor** \ˈmä-nə-tər\ *n* : one that monitors; *esp* : a device for observing or measuring a biologically important condition or function ⟨a heart ~⟩

[2]**monitor** *vb* **1** : to watch, observe, or check closely or continuously ⟨~ a patient's vital signs⟩ **2** : to test for intensity of radiations esp. if due to radioactivity

mon•key•pox \ˈməŋ-kē-ˌpäks\ *n* : a rare virus disease esp. of central and western Africa that is caused by a poxvirus of the genus *Orthopoxvirus* (species *Monkeypox virus*), occurs chiefly in wild rodents and primates, and when transmitted to humans resembles smallpox but is milder

mono \ˈmä-(ˌ)nō\ *n* : INFECTIOUS MONONUCLEOSIS

mono- — see MON-

monoacetate — see RESORCINOL MONOACETATE

mono•am•ine \ˌmä-nō-ə-ˈmēn, -ˈa-ˌmēn\ *n* : an amine RNH_2 that has one organic substituent attached to the nitrogen atom; *esp* : one (as serotonin) that is functionally important in neural transmission

monoamine oxidase *n* : an enzyme that deaminates monoamines oxidatively and that functions in the nervous system by breaking down monoamine neurotransmitters oxidatively

monoamine oxidase inhibitor *n* : any of various antidepressant drugs which increase the concentration of monoamines in the brain by inhibiting the action of monoamine oxidase

mono•am•in•er•gic \ˌmä-nō-ˌa-mə-ˈnər-jik\ *adj* : liberating or involving monoamines (as serotonin or norepinephrine) in neural transmission ⟨~ neurons⟩ ⟨~ mechanisms⟩

mono•ar•tic•u•lar \ˌmä-nō-är-ˈti-kyə-lər\ *also* **mon•ar•tic•u•lar** \ˌmä-när-\ *adj* : affecting only one joint of the body ⟨~ arthritis⟩ — compare OLIGOARTICULAR, POLYARTICULAR

mono•bac•tam \ˌmä-nō-ˈbak-tam\ *n* : any of the class of beta-lactam antibiotics (as aztreonam) containing one ring in their molecular structure

mono•ben•zone \ˌmä-nō-ˈben-ˌzōn\ *n* : a drug $C_{13}H_{12}O_2$ applied topically as a melanin inhibitor in the treatment of hyperpigmentation

mono•blast \ˈmä-nō-ˌblast\ *n* : a motile cell of the spleen and bone marrow that gives rise to the monocyte of the circulating blood

mono•cho•ri•on•ic \ˌmä-nō-ˌkōr-ē-ˈä-nik\ *also* **mono•cho•ri•al** \-ˈkō-rē-əl\ *adj, of twins* : sharing or developed with a common chorion

mono•chro•ma•cy \-ˈkrō-mə-sē\ *n, pl* **-cies** : MONOCHROMATISM

mono•chro•mat \ˈmä-nō-krō-ˌmat, ˌmä-ˈ\ *n* : a person who is completely color-blind

mono•chro•mat•ic \ˌmä-nō-krō-ˈma-tik\ *adj* **1** : having or consisting of one color or hue **2** : consisting of radiation of a single wavelength or of a very small range of wavelengths **3** : of, relating to, or exhibiting monochromatism

mono•chro•ma•tism \-ˈkrō-mə-ˌti-zəm\ *n* : complete color blindness in which all colors appear as shades of gray — called also *monochromacy*

mon•o•cle \ˈmä-ni-kəl\ *n* : an eyeglass for one eye

[1]**mono•clo•nal** \ˌmä-nō-ˈklōn-ᵊl\ *adj* : produced by, being, or composed of cells derived from a single cell ⟨a ~ tumor⟩; *esp* : relating to or being an antibody derived from a single cell in large quantities for use against a specific antigen (as a cancer cell)

[2]**monoclonal** *n* : a monoclonal antibody

monoclonal gammopathy *n* : any of various disorders marked by proliferation of a single clone of antibody-producing lymphoid cells resulting in an abnormal increase of a monoclonal antibody in the blood serum and urine and that include both benign or asymptomatic conditions and neoplastic conditions (as multiple myeloma) — called also *plasma cell dyscrasia;* see M PROTEIN 2

mono•crot•ic \-ˈkrä-tik\ *adj, of the pulse* : having a simple beat and forming a smooth single-crested curve on a sphygmogram — compare DICROTIC 1

mon•oc•u•lar \mä-ˈnä-kyə-lər, mə-\ *adj* **1** : of, involving, or affecting a single eye ⟨a ~ cataract⟩ **2** : suitable for use with only one eye ⟨a ~ microscope⟩ — **mon•oc•u•lar•ly** *adv*

mono•cyte \ˈmä-nə-ˌsīt\ *n* : a large white blood cell with finely granulated chromatin dispersed throughout the nucleus that is formed in the bone marrow, enters the blood, and migrates into the connective tissue where it differentiates into a macrophage — **mono•cyt•ic** \ˌmä-nə-ˈsi-tik\ *adj*

monocytic leukemia *n* : leukemia characterized by the presence of large numbers of monocytes in the circulating blood

mono•cy•to•sis \ˌmä-nō-sī-ˈtō-səs\ *n, pl* **-to•ses** \-ˌsēz\ : an abnormal increase in the number of monocytes in the circulating blood — compare GRANULOCYTOSIS, LYMPHOCYTOSIS

mono•fac•to•ri•al \-fak-ˈtōr-ē-əl\ *adj* : MONOGENIC

mono•fil•a•ment \-ˈfi-lə-mənt\ *n* : a single untwisted synthetic filament (as of nylon) used to make surgical sutures

mo•nog•a•my \mə-ˈnä-gə-mē\ *n, pl* **-mies** : the state or custom of being married to one person at a time or of having only one mate at a time — **mo•nog•a•mist** \-mist\ *n* — **mo•nog•a•mous** \-məs\ *adj*

mono•gen•ic \-ˈje-nik, -ˈjē-\ *adj* : of, relating to, or controlled by a single gene and esp. by either of an allelic pair — **mono•gen•i•cal•ly** *adv*

mono•graph \ˈmä-nə-ˌgraf\ *n* **1** : a learned detailed treatise covering a small area of a field of learning **2** : a description (as in the *U.S. Pharmacopeia*) of the name, chemical formula, and uniform method for determining the strength and purity of a drug — **monograph** *vb*

mono•iodo•ty•ro•sine \ˌmä-nō-ī-ˌō-də-ˈtī-rə-ˌsēn, -ī-ˌä-\ *n* : an iodine-containing tyrosine $C_9H_{10}INO_3$ that is produced in the thyroid gland and that combines with diiodotyrosine to form triiodothyronine

mono•lay•er \ˈmä-nō-ˌlā-ər\ *n* : a single continuous layer or film that is one cell or molecule in thickness

mono•ma•nia \ˌmä-nō-ˈmā-nē-ə, -nyə\ *n* : mental illness esp. when limited in expression to one idea or area of thought — **mono•ma•ni•a•cal** \-mə-ˈnī-ə-kəl\ *adj*

mono•ma•ni•ac \-nē-ˌak\ *n* : an individual affected by monomania

mono•me•lic \-ˈmē-lik\ *adj* : relating to or affecting only one limb

mono•mer \ˈmä-nə-mər\ *n* : a chemical compound that can undergo polymerization — **mo•no•mer•ic** \ˌmä-nə-ˈmer-ik, ˌmō-\ *adj*

mono•neu•ri•tis \ˌmä-nō-nu̇-ˈrī-təs, -nyu̇-\ *n, pl* **-rit•i•des** \-ˈri-tə-ˌdēz\ *or* **-ri•tis•es** : neuritis of a single nerve

mononeuritis mul•ti•plex \-ˈməl-ti-ˌpleks\ *n* : neuritis that affects several separate nerves — called also *mononeuropathy multiplex*

mono•neu•rop•a•thy \-nu̇-ˈrä-pə-thē, -nyu̇-\ *n, pl* **-thies** : a nerve disease affecting only a single nerve

[1]**mono•nu•cle•ar** \ˌmä-nō-ˈnü-klē-ər, -ˈnyü-\ *adj* : having only one nucleus

[2]**mononuclear** *n* : a mononuclear cell; *esp* : MONOCYTE

mononuclear phagocyte system *n* : a system of cells comprising all free and fixed phagocytes and esp. macrophages together with their ancestral cells including monocytes and their precursors in the bone marrow — compare RETICULOENDOTHELIAL SYSTEM

mono•nu•cle•at•ed \-ˈnü-klē-ˌā-təd, -ˈnyü-\ *also* **mono•nu•cle•ate** \-klē-ət, -ˌāt\ *adj* : MONONUCLEAR

mono•nu•cle•o•sis \-ˌnü-klē-ˈō-səs, -ˌnyü-\ *n* : an abnormal increase of mononuclear white blood cells in the blood; *specif* : INFECTIOUS MONONUCLEOSIS

mono•nu•cle•o•tide \-ˈnü-klē-ə-ˌtīd, -ˈnyü-\ *n* : a nucleotide that is derived from one molecule each of a nitrogenous base, a sugar, and a phosphoric acid

mono·pha·sic \-ˈfā-zik\ *adj* **1** : having a single phase; *specif* : relating to or being a record of a nerve impulse that is negative or positive but not both ⟨a ~ action potential⟩ — compare DIPHASIC b, POLYPHASIC 1 **2** : having a single period of activity followed by a period of rest in each 24-hour period

mono·phos·phate \-ˈfäs-ˌfāt\ *n* : a phosphate containing a single phosphate group

mono·ple·gia \-ˈplē-jə, -jē-ə\ *n* : paralysis affecting a single limb, body part, or group of muscles — **mono·ple·gic** \-jik\ *adj*

mono·ploid \ˈmä-nō-ˌplȯid\ *adj* : HAPLOID

mono·po·lar \ˌmä-nō-ˈpō-lər\ *adj* : UNIPOLAR

Mon·o·pril \ˈmä-nə-ˌpril\ *trademark* — used for a preparation of fosinopril

mon·or·chid \mä-ˈnȯr-kəd\ *n* : an individual who has only one testis or only one descended into the scrotum — compare CRYPTORCHID — **monorchid** *adj*

mon·or·chid·ism \-kə-ˌdi-zəm\ *also* **mon·or·chism** \mä-ˈnȯr-ˌki-zəm\ *n* : the quality or state of being monorchid — compare CRYPTORCHIDISM

mono·sac·cha·ride \ˌmä-nō-ˈsa-kə-ˌrīd\ *n* : a sugar not decomposable to simpler sugars by hydrolysis — called also *simple sugar*

mono·so·di·um glu·ta·mate \ˌmä-nō-ˈsō-dē-əm-ˈglü-tə-ˌmāt\ *n* : a crystalline salt $C_5H_8NO_4Na$ used to enhance the flavor of food and medicinally to reduce ammonia levels in blood and tissues in ammoniacal azotemia (as in hepatic insufficiency) — abbr. *MSG;* called also *sodium glutamate;* see CHINESE RESTAURANT SYNDROME

monosodium urate *n* : a salt of uric acid that precipitates out in cartilage as tophi in gout

mono·some \ˈmä-nō-ˌsōm\ *n* **1** : a chromosome lacking a synaptic mate; *esp* : an unpaired X chromosome **2** : a single ribosome

mono·so·mic \ˌmä-nə-ˈsō-mik\ *adj* : having one less than the diploid number of chromosomes — **mono·so·my** \ˈmä-nə-ˌsō-mē\ *n*

mono·spe·cif·ic \ˌmä-nō-spə-ˈsi-fik\ *adj* : specific for a single antigen or receptor site on an antigen — **mono·spec·i·fic·i·ty** \-ˌspe-sə-ˈfi-sə-tē\ *n*

mono·sper·mic \-ˈspər-mik\ *adj* : involving or resulting from a single sperm cell ⟨~ fertilization⟩

mono·sper·my \ˈmä-nō-ˌspər-mē\ *n, pl* **-mies** : the entry of a single fertilizing sperm into an egg — compare POLYSPERMY

mon·os·tot·ic \ˌmä-ˌnäs-ˈtä-tik\ *adj* : relating to or affecting a single bone

mono·symp·tom·at·ic \ˌmä-nō-ˌsimp-tə-ˈma-tik\ *adj* : exhibiting or manifested by a single principal symptom

mono·syn·ap·tic \-sə-ˈnap-tik\ *adj* : having or involving a single neural synapse — **mono·syn·ap·ti·cal·ly** *adv*

mono·ther·a·py \ˌmä-nə-ˈther-ə-pē\ *n, pl* **-pies** : the use of a single drug to treat a particular disorder or disease

mono·un·sat·u·rate \-ˌən-ˈsa-chə-rət\ *n* : a monounsaturated oil or fatty acid

mono·un·sat·u·rat·ed \-ˌən-ˈsa-chə-ˌrā-təd\ *adj, of an oil, fat, or fatty acid* : containing one double or triple bond per molecule — compare POLYUNSATURATED

mono·va·lent \ˌmä-nə-ˈvā-lənt\ *adj* **1** : having a chemical valence of one **2** : containing antibodies specific for or antigens of a single strain of a microorganism ⟨a ~ vaccine⟩

mon·ovu·lar \(ˌ)mä-ˈnä-vyə-lər, -ˈnō-\ *adj* : MONOZYGOTIC ⟨~ twins⟩

mon·ox·ide \mə-ˈnäk-ˌsīd\ *n* : an oxide containing one atom of oxygen per molecule — see CARBON MONOXIDE

mono·zy·got·ic \ˌmä-nō-zī-ˈgä-tik\ *adj* : derived from a single egg ⟨~ twins⟩ — **mono·zy·gos·i·ty** \-ˈgä-sə-tē\ *n* — **mono·zy·gote** \-ˈzī-ˌgōt\ *n*

mono·zy·gous \ˌmä-nō-ˈzī-gəs, (ˌ)mä-ˈnä-zə-gəs\ *adj* : MONOZYGOTIC

mons \ˈmänz\ *n, pl* **mon·tes** \ˈmän-ˌtēz\ : a body part or area raised above or demarcated from surrounding structures (as the papilla of mucosa through which the ureter enters the bladder)

mons pubis *n, pl* **montes pubis** : a rounded eminence of fatty tissue upon the pubic symphysis esp. of the human female — see MONS VENERIS

mon·ster \ˈmän-stər\ *n* : an animal or plant displaying a major developmental abnormality in form or structure

mon·stros·i·ty \män-ˈsträ-sə-tē\ *n, pl* **-ties** **1** : a malformation of a plant or animal **2** : the quality or state of deviating greatly from the natural form or character — **mon·strous** \ˈmän-strəs\ *adj*

mons ve·ne·ris \-ˈve-nə-rəs\ *n, pl* **montes veneris** : the mons pubis of a female

Mon·teg·gia fracture \män-ˈte-jə-\ *or* **Mon·teg·gia's fracture** \-ˈte-jəz-\ *n* : a fracture in the proximal part of the ulna with dislocation of the head of the radius

Monteggia, Giovanni Battista (1762–1815), Italian surgeon.

mon·te·lu·kast \ˌmän-tə-ˈlü-ˌkast\ *n* : a leukotriene antagonist used orally in the form of its sodium salt $C_{35}H_{35}ClNNaO_3S$ to treat asthma or to relieve the symptoms of seasonal allergic rhinitis — see SINGULAIR

Mon·te·zu·ma's revenge \ˌmän-tə-ˈzü-məz-\ *n* : traveler's diarrhea esp. when contracted in Mexico

Montezuma II (1466–1520), Aztec emperor of Mexico.

Mont·gom·ery's gland \(ˌ)mənt-ˈgəm-rēz-, mänt-ˈgäm-\ *n* : an apocrine gland in the areola of the mammary gland

Montgomery, William Fetherston (1797–1859), British obstetrician.

month·lies \ˈmənth-lēz\ *n pl* : a menstrual period

mon·tic·u·lus \män-ˈtik-yə-ləs\ *n* : the median dorsal ridge of the cerebellum formed by the vermis

mood \ˈmüd\ *n* : a conscious state of mind or predominant emotion : affective state : FEELING 3

mood disorder *n* : any of several psychological disorders characterized by abnormalities of emotional state and including esp. major depressive disorder, dysthymia, and bipolar disorder — called also *affective disorder*

moon \ˈmün\ *n* : LUNULA a

moon blindness *n* : a recurrent inflammation of the eye of the horse — called also *periodic ophthalmia*

moon face *n* : the full rounded facies characteristic esp. of Cushing's syndrome and typically associated with deposition of fat — called also *moon facies*

Moon's molar *or* **Moon molar** *n* : a first molar tooth which has become dome-shaped due to malformation by congenital syphilis; *also* : MULBERRY MOLAR

Moon, Henry (1845–1892), British surgeon.

MOPP \ˌem-(ˌ)ō-(ˌ)pē-ˈpē\ *n* : a drug regimen that includes mechlorethamine, vincristine, procarbazine, and prednisone and is used in the treatment of some forms of cancer (as Hodgkin's lymphoma)

Mor·ax–Ax·en·feld bacillus \ˈmȯr-äks-ˈäk-sən-ˌfeld-\ *n* : a rod-shaped bacterium of the genus *Moraxella* (*M. lacunata*) that causes Morax-Axenfeld conjunctivitis

Morax, Victor (1866–1935), French ophthalmologist.

Axenfeld, Karl Theodor Paul Polykarpos (1867–1930), German ophthalmologist.

Morax–Axenfeld conjunctivitis *n* : a chronic conjunctivitis caused by a rod-shaped bacterium of the genus *Moraxella* (*M. lacunata*) and now occurring rarely but formerly more prevalent in persons living under poor hygienic conditions

Mor·ax·el·la \ˌmȯr-ak-ˈse-lə\ *n* : a genus of short rod-shaped gram-negative bacteria that is placed in either of two families (Moraxellaceae or Neisseriaceae) and includes the causative agent (*M. lacunata*) of Morax-Axenfeld conjunctivitis

mor·bid \ˈmȯr-bəd\ *adj* **1 a** : of, relating to, or characteristic of disease **b** : affected with or induced by disease ⟨a ~ condition⟩ **c** : productive of disease ⟨~ substances⟩ **2** : abnormally susceptible to or characterized by gloomy or unwholesome feelings

mor·bid·i·ty \mȯr-ˈbi-də-tē\ *n, pl* **-ties 1** : a diseased state or symptom : ill health; *also* : a complication or undesirable side effect following surgery or medical treatment **2** : the incidence of disease : the rate of illness (as in a specified population); *also* : the incidence of complications or undesirable side effects following surgery or medical treatment

mor·bil·li \mȯr-ˈbi-ˌlī\ *n pl* : MEASLES 1

mor·bil·li·form \mȯr-ˈbi-lə-ˌfȯrm\ *adj* : resembling the eruption of measles ⟨a ~ pruritic rash⟩

mor·bil·li·vi·rus \-ˌvī-rəs\ *n* **1** *cap* : a genus of paramyxoviruses that includes the causative agents of canine distemper, measles, and rinderpest **2** : any virus of the genus *Morbillivirus*

mor·bus \ˈmȯr-bəs\ *n, pl* **mor·bi** \-ˌbī\ : DISEASE — see CHOLERA MORBUS

mor·cel·la·tion \mȯr-sə-ˈlā-shən\ *n* : division and removal in small pieces (as of a tumor)

mor·gan \ˈmȯr-gən\ *n* : a unit of inferred distance between genes on a chromosome that is used in constructing genetic maps and is equal to the distance for which the frequency of crossing-over between specific pairs of genes is 100 percent

Morgan, Thomas Hunt (1866–1945), American geneticist.

morgue \ˈmȯrg\ *n* : a place where the bodies of dead persons are kept temporarily pending identification or release for burial or autopsy

mor·i·bund \ˈmȯr-ə-(ˌ)bənd, ˈmär-\ *adj* : being in the state of dying : approaching death

mo·ric·i·zine \mə-ˈri-sə-ˌzēn\ *n* : an antiarrhythmic drug used in the form of its hydrochloride $C_{22}H_{25}N_3O_4S{\cdot}HCl$ esp. in the treatment of life-threatening ventricular arrhythmias

morning–after pill *n* : an oral drug typically containing high doses of estrogen taken up to usu. three days after unprotected sexual intercourse that interferes with pregnancy by inhibiting ovulation or by blocking implantation of a fertilized egg in the human uterus

morning breath *n* : halitosis upon awakening from sleep that is caused by the buildup of bacteria in the mouth due to decreased saliva production

morning sickness *n* : nausea and vomiting that occurs typically in the morning esp. during the earlier months of pregnancy

mo·ron \ˈmōr-ˌän\ *n, dated, now offensive* : a person affected with mild intellectual disability

Moro reflex \ˈmȯr-ō-\ *n* : a reflex reaction of infants upon being startled (as by a loud noise or a bright light) that is characterized by extension of the arms and legs away from the body and to the side and then by drawing them together as if in an embrace

Moro, Ernst (1874–1951), German pediatrician.

Moro test *n* : a diagnostic skin test formerly used to detect infection or past infection by the tubercle bacillus and involving the rubbing of an ointment containing tuberculin directly on the skin with the appearance of reddish papules after one or two days indicating a positive result

morph- *or* **morpho-** *comb form* : form : shape : structure : type ⟨*morpho*logy⟩

-morph \ˌmȯrf\ *n comb form* : one having (such) a form ⟨ecto*morph*⟩

mor·phea \mȯr-ˈfē-ə\ *n, pl* **mor·phe·ae** \-ˈfē-ˌē\ : localized scleroderma

mor·phia \ˈmȯr-fē-ə\ *n* : MORPHINE

-mor·phic \ˈmȯr-fik\ *adj comb form* : having (such) a form ⟨endo*morphic*⟩

mor·phine \ˈmȯr-ˌfēn\ *n* : a bitter crystalline addictive narcotic base $C_{17}H_{19}NO_3$ that is the principal alkaloid of opium and is used in the form of its hydrated sulfate $(C_{17}H_{19}NO_3)_2 \cdot H_2SO_4 \cdot 5H_2O$ or hydrated hydrochloride $C_{17}H_{19}NO_3 \cdot HCl \cdot 3H_2O$ as an analgesic and sedative

mor·phin·ism \ˈmȯr-ˌfē-ˌni-zəm, -fə-\ *n* : a disordered condition of health produced by habitual use of morphine

mor·phi·no·mi·met·ic \ˌmȯr-fē-nə-mə-ˈme-tik, -fə-, -mī-\ *adj* : resembling opiates in their affinity for opiate receptors in the brain

-mor·phism \ˈmȯr-ˌfi-zəm\ *n comb form* : quality or state of having (such) a form ⟨poly*morphism*⟩

mor·pho·dif·fer·en·ti·a·tion \ˌmȯr-fō-ˌdi-fə-ˌren-chē-ˈā-shən\ *n* : structure or organ differentiation (as in tooth development)

mor·phoea *Brit var of* MORPHEA

mor·pho·gen \ˈmȯr-fə-jən, -ˌjen\ *n* : a diffusible chemical substance that exerts control over morphogenesis esp. by forming a gradient in concentration

mor·pho·gen·e·sis \ˌmȯr-fə-ˈje-nə-səs\ *n, pl* **-e·ses** \-ˌsēz\ : the development of normal form or structure esp. as controlled by the growth, differentiation, and movement of cells and tissues — **mor·pho·ge·net·ic** \-jə-ˈne-tik\ *also* **mor·pho·gen·ic** \-ˈje-nik\ *adj* — **mor·pho·ge·net·i·cal·ly** \-jə-ˈne-ti-k(ə-)lē\ *adv*

mor·pho·log·i·cal \ˌmȯr-fə-ˈlä-ji-kəl\ *also* **mor·pho·log·ic** \-ˈlä-jik\ *adj* : of, relating to, or concerned with form or structure — **mor·pho·log·i·cal·ly** *adv*

mor·phol·o·gy \mȯr-ˈfä-lə-jē\ *n, pl* **-gies** **1** : a branch of biology that deals with the form and structure of animals and plants esp. apart from their functions **2** : the form and structure of an organism or any of its parts — **mor·phol·o·gist** \-jist\ *n*

-mor·phous \ˈmȯr-fəs\ *adj comb form* : having (such) a form ⟨poly*morphous*⟩

-mor·phy \ˌmȯr-fē\ *n comb form, pl* **-mor·phies** : quality or state of having (such) a form ⟨meso*morphy*⟩

Mor·quio's disease \ˈmȯr-kē-ˌōz-\ *n* : a mucopolysaccharidosis that is inherited as an autosomal recessive trait and is characterized by excretion of keratan sulfate in the urine, dwarfism, a short neck, protruding sternum, kyphosis, scoliosis, a flat nose, prominent upper jaw, and a waddling gait

Morquio, Luis (1867–1935), Uruguayan physician.

mor·rhu·ate sodium \ˈmȯr-ə-ˌwāt-\ *n* : a granular mixture of the salts of fatty acids obtained from cod-liver oil that is administered in solution intravenously as a sclerosing agent esp. in the treatment of varicose veins

mor·tal \ˈmȯrt-ᵊl\ *adj* **1** : having caused or being about to cause death : FATAL ⟨a ~ injury⟩ **2** : of, relating to, or connected with death

mor·tal·i·ty \mȯr-ˈta-lə-tē\ *n, pl* **-ties** **1** : the quality or state of being mortal **2 a** : the number of deaths in a given time or place **b** : the proportion of deaths to population : DEATH RATE — called also *mortality rate;* compare FERTILITY 2, MORBIDITY 2

mor·tar \ˈmȯr-tər\ *n* : a strong vessel in which material is pounded or rubbed with a pestle

mor·ti·cian \mȯr-ˈti-shən\ *n* : UNDERTAKER

mor·ti·fi·ca·tion \ˌmȯr-tə-fə-ˈkā-shən\ *n* : local death of tissue in the animal body : NECROSIS, GANGRENE

mortis — see ALGOR MORTIS, RIGOR MORTIS

Mor·ton's neuroma \ˌmȯr-tᵊnz-\ *n* : a neuroma formed in conjunction with Morton's toe

Morton, Thomas George (1835–1903), American surgeon.

Morton's toe *n* : metatarsalgia that is caused by compression of a branch of the plantar nerve between the heads of the metatarsal bones — called also *Morton's disease, Morton's foot*

mor·tu·ary \ˈmȯr-chə-ˌwer-ē\ *n, pl* **-aries** : a place in which dead bodies are kept and prepared for burial or cremation

mor·u·la \ˈmȯr-yu̇-lə, ˈmär-\ *n, pl* **-lae** \-ˌlē, -ˌlī\ : a globular solid mass of blastomeres formed by cleavage of a zygote that typically precedes the blastula — compare GASTRULA — **mor·u·la·tion** \ˌmȯr-yu̇-ˈlā-shən, ˌmär-\ *n*

[1]**mo·sa·ic** \mō-ˈzā-ik\ *n* : an organism or one of its parts composed of cells of more than one genotype : CHIMERA

[2]**mosaic** *adj* **1** : exhibiting mosaicism **2** : DETERMINATE — **mo·sa·i·cal·ly** *adv*

mo·sa·icism \mō-ˈzā-ə-ˌsi-zəm\ *n* : the condition of possessing cells of two or more different genetic constitutions

mos·qui·to \mə-ˈskē-tō\ *n, pl* **-toes** *also* **-tos** : any of a family (Culicidae) of dipteran flies with females that have a set of needlelike organs in the proboscis adapted to puncture the skin of animals and to suck their blood and that are in some cases vectors of serious diseases — see AEDES, ANOPHELES, CULEX

mosquito forceps *n* : a very small surgical forceps — called also *mosquito clamp*

mossy fiber *n* : any of the complexly branched axons that innervate the granule cells of the cerebellar cortex

mother cell *n* : a cell that gives rise to other cells usu. of a different sort

mo•tile \ˈmōt-ᵊl, ˈmō-ˌtīl\ *adj* : exhibiting or capable of movement

mo•til•in \mō-ˈti-lən\ *n* : a polypeptide hormone secreted by the small intestine that increases gastrointestinal motility and stimulates the production of pepsin

mo•til•i•ty \mō-ˈti-lə-tē\ *n, pl* **-ties** : the quality or state of being motile : CONTRACTILITY ⟨gastrointestinal ~⟩

mo•tion \ˈmō-shən\ *n* **1** : an act, process, or instance of changing place : MOVEMENT **2 a** : an evacuation of the bowels **b** : the matter evacuated — often used in pl. ⟨blood in the ~*s*⟩

motion sickness *n* : sickness induced by motion (as in travel by air, car, or ship) and characterized by nausea

mo•ti•vate \ˈmō-tə-ˌvāt\ *vb* **-vat•ed; -vat•ing** : to provide with a motive or serve as a motive for — **mo•ti•va•tion** \ˌmō-tə-ˈvā-shən\ *n* — **mo•ti•va•tion•al** \-shnəl, -shən-ᵊl\ *adj* — **mo•ti•va•tion•al•ly** *adv*

mo•tive \ˈmō-tiv\ *n* : something (as a need or desire) that causes a person to act

moto- *comb form* : motion : motor ⟨*moto*neuron⟩

mo•to•neu•ron \ˌmō-tō-ˈnü-ˌrän, -ˈnyü-\ *n* : MOTOR NEURON — **mo•to•neu•ro•nal** \-ˈnu̇r-ən-ᵊl, -ˈnyu̇r-; -nü-ˈrōn-, -nyu̇-\ *adj*

mo•tor \ˈmō-tər\ *adj* **1** : causing or imparting motion **2** : of, relating to, or being a motor neuron or a nerve containing motor neurons ⟨~ fibers⟩ **3** : of, relating to, concerned with, or involving muscular movement

motor aphasia *n* : the inability to speak or to organize the muscular movements of speech — called also *Broca's aphasia*

motor area *n* : any of various areas of cerebral cortex believed to be associated with the initiation, coordination, and transmission of motor impulses to lower centers; *specif* : a region immediately anterior to the central sulcus having an unusually thick zone of cortical gray matter and communicating with lower centers chiefly through the corticospinal tracts — see PRECENTRAL GYRUS

motor center *n* : a nervous center that controls or modifies (as by inhibiting or reinforcing) a motor impulse

motor cortex *n* : the cortex of a motor area; *also* : the motor areas as a functional whole

motor end plate *n* : the terminal arborization of a motor axon on a muscle fiber

mo•tor•ic \mō-ˈtȯr-ik, -ˈtär-\ *adj* : MOTOR 3 — **mo•tor•i•cal•ly** *adv*

motor neuron *n* : a neuron that passes from the central nervous system or a ganglion toward or to a muscle and conducts a nerve impulse that causes movement — called also *motoneuron;* compare INTERNEURON, SENSORY NEURON

motor paralysis *n* : paralysis of the voluntary muscles

motor protein *n* : a protein (as dynein, kinesin, or myosin) that moves itself along a filament or polymeric molecule using energy generated by the hydrolysis of ATP

motor root *n* : a nerve root containing only motor fibers; *specif* : VENTRAL ROOT — compare SENSORY ROOT

motor unit *n* : a motor neuron together with the muscle fibers on which it acts

Mo•trin \ˈmō-trən\ *trademark* — used for a preparation of ibuprofen

mottled enamel *n* : spotted tooth enamel typically caused by drinking water containing excessive fluorides during the time teeth are calcifying

mou•lage \mü-ˈläzh\ *n* : a mold of a lesion or defect used as a guide in applying medical treatment (as in radiotherapy) or in performing reconstructive surgery esp. on the face

mould, mould•ing, mouldy *chiefly Brit var of* MOLD, MOLDING, MOLDY

moult *chiefly Brit var of* MOLT

mount \ˈmau̇nt\ *n* **1** : a glass slide with its accessories on which objects are placed for examination with a microscope **2** : a specimen mounted on a slide for microscopic examination — **mount** *vb*

mountain fever *n* : any of various febrile diseases occurring in mountainous regions

mountain sickness *n* : altitude sickness experienced esp. above 8000 to 10,000 feet (about 2500 to 3000 meters) and caused by insufficient oxygen in the air; *esp* : ACUTE MOUNTAIN SICKNESS

mouse \ˈmau̇s\ *n, pl* **mice** \ˈmīs\ **1** : any of numerous small rodents (as of the genus *Mus*) with pointed snout, rather small ears, elongated body, and slender hairless or sparsely haired tail **2** : a dark-colored swelling caused by a blow; *specif* : BLACK EYE

mouse•pox \ˈmau̇s-ˌpäks\ *n* : a highly contagious disease of mice that is caused by a poxvirus of the genus *Orthopoxvirus* (species *Ectromelia virus*) — called also *ectromelia*

mouth \ˈmau̇th\ *n, pl* **mouths** \ˈmau̇t͟hz\ : the natural opening through which food passes into the animal body and which in vertebrates is typically bounded externally by the lips and internally by the pharynx and encloses the tongue, gums, and teeth

mouth breather *n* : a person who breathes mostly through the mouth rather than the nose

mouth–to–mouth *adj* : of, relating to, or being a method of artificial respiration in which the rescuer's mouth is placed tightly over the victim's mouth in order to force air into the victim's lungs by blowing forcefully enough every few seconds to inflate them ⟨~ resuscitation⟩
mouth·wash \ˈmau̇th-ˌwȯsh, -ˌwäsh\ *n* : a liquid preparation (as an antiseptic solution) for cleansing the mouth and teeth — called also *collutorium*
move \ˈmüv\ *vb* **moved; mov·ing 1** : to go or pass from one place to another **2** *of the bowels* : to eject fecal matter : EVACUATE
move·ment \ˈmüv-mənt\ *n* **1** : the act or process of moving **2 a** : an act of voiding the bowels : BOWEL MOVEMENT **b** : matter expelled from the bowels at one passage : STOOL
moxa \ˈmäk-sə\ *n* : a soft woolly mass prepared from the ground young leaves of an aromatic Eurasian plant (genus *Artemesia*, esp. *A. vulgaris*) that is used in traditional Asian medicine typically in the form of sticks or cones which are ignited and placed on or close to the skin or used to heat acupuncture needles
moxa·lac·tam \ˌmäk-sə-ˈlak-ˌtam\ *n* : a cephalosporin antibiotic administered parenterally in the form of its disodium salt $C_{20}H_{18}N_6Na_2O_9S$
mox·i·bus·tion \ˌmäk-si-ˈbəs-chən\ *n* : the therapeutic use of moxa
MPC *abbr* maximum permissible concentration
MPD *abbr* multiple personality disorder
MPH *abbr* master of public health
M phase \ˈem-ˌfāz\ *n* : the period in the cell cycle during which cell division takes place — compare G_1 PHASE, G_2 PHASE, S PHASE
M protein *n* **1** : an antigenic protein of Group A streptococci that is found on the cell wall extending into the surrounding capsule and confers streptococcal virulence by protecting the cell from phagocytotic action — called also *M substance* **2** : a monoclonal antibody that is produced by plasma cells abnormally proliferating from a single clone and that is characteristic of monoclonal gammopathy
MPTP \ˌem-ˌpē-ˌtē-ˈpē\ *n* [1-*m*ethyl-4-*p*henyl-1,2,3,6-*t*etrahydro*p*yridine] : a neurotoxin $C_{12}H_{15}N$ that destroys dopamine-producing neurons of the substantia nigra and causes symptoms (as tremors and rigidity) similar to those of Parkinson's disease
mR *abbr* milliroentgen
MR *abbr* magnetic resonance
MRA *abbr* magnetic resonance angiogram; magnetic resonance angiography
mrad *abbr* millirad
Mrad *abbr* megarad
MR angiography \ˈem-ˈär-\ *n* : MAGNETIC RESONANCE ANGIOGRAPHY
mrem *abbr* millirem
MRI \ˌem-ˌär-ˈī\ *n* : MAGNETIC RESONANCE IMAGING; *also* : the procedure in which magnetic resonance imaging is used
MRKH syndrome \ˌem-ˌär-ˌkā-ˈāch-\ *n* : MAYER-ROKITANSKY-KÜSTER-HAUSER SYNDROME
mRNA \ˌem-(ˌ)är-(ˌ)en-ˈā\ *n* : MESSENGER RNA
MRS *abbr* magnetic resonance spectroscopy
MRSA \ˌem-ˌär-ˌes-ˈā, ˈmər-sə\ *n* [*m*ethicillin-*r*esistant *S*taphylococcus *a*ureus] : any of several strains of a bacterium (*Staphylococcus aureus*) that are resistant to methicillin and related antibiotics (as penicillin) and often live harmlessly on the skin and mucous membranes but may cause usu. mild infections of the skin or sometimes more severe infections (as of the blood or bone) esp. in hospitalized or immunocompromised individuals — see CA-MRSA
MS *abbr* multiple sclerosis
MSA *abbr* multiple system atrophy
MSG *abbr* monosodium glutamate
MSH *abbr* melanocyte-stimulating hormone
MSN *abbr* master of science in nursing
M substance \ˈem-ˌ\ *n* : M PROTEIN 1
MSW *abbr* master of social work
Mt *symbol* meitnerium
MT *abbr* medical technologist
mtDNA \ˌem-ˈtē-ˌdē-ˌen-ˈā\ *n* : MITOCHONDRIAL DNA
mu \ˈmyü, ˈmü\ *n, pl* **mu** : MICRON
muc- *or* **muci-** *or* **muco-** *comb form* **1** : mucus ⟨*muc*in⟩ ⟨*muco*protein⟩ **2** : mucous and ⟨*muco*purulent⟩
mu·cate \ˈmyü-ˌkāt\ *n* : a salt of a crystalline acid $C_6H_{10}O_8$ esp. when formed by combination with a drug that is an organic base and used as a vehicle for administration of the drug
mu·ci·lage \ˈmyü-sə-lij\ *n* **1** : a gelatinous substance of various plants (as legumes or seaweeds) that contains protein and polysaccharides and is similar to plant gums **2** : an aqueous usu. viscid solution (as of a gum) used in pharmacy as an excipient and in medicine as a demulcent — **mu·ci·lag·i·nous** \ˌmyü-sə-ˈla-jə-nəs\ *adj*
mu·cil·loid \ˈmyü-sə-ˌlȯid\ *n* : a mucilaginous substance
mu·cin \ˈmyüs-ᵊn\ *n* : any of a group of mucoproteins that are found in various human and animal secretions and tissues (as in saliva, the lining of the stomach, and the skin) and that are white or yellowish powders when dry and viscid when moist
mu·cin·o·gen \myü-ˈsi-nə-jən, -ˌjen\ *n* : any of various substances which undergo conversion into mucins
mu·ci·nous \ˈmyüs-ᵊn-əs\ *adj* : of, relating to, resembling, or containing mucin ⟨~ fluid⟩ ⟨~ carcinoma⟩
muco- — see MUC-
mu·co·buc·cal fold \ˌmyü-kō-ˈbə-kəl-\ *n* : the fold formed by the oral mucosa

where it passes from the mandible or maxilla to the cheek

mu·co·cele \ˈmyü-kə-ˌsēl\ *n* : a swelling like a sac that is due to distension of a hollow organ or cavity with mucus ⟨a ~ of the appendix⟩; *specif* : a dilated lacrimal sac

mu·co·cil·i·ary \ˌmyü-kō-ˈsi-lē-ˌer-ē\ *adj* : of, relating to, or involving cilia of the mucous membranes of the respiratory system

mu·co·cu·ta·ne·ous \ˌmyü-kō-kyu̇-ˈtā-nē-əs\ *adj* : made up of or involving both typical skin and mucous membrane ⟨~ candidiasis⟩

mucocutaneous lymph node disease *n* : KAWASAKI DISEASE

mucocutaneous lymph node syndrome *n* : KAWASAKI DISEASE

mu·co·epi·der·moid \ˌmyü-kō-ˌe-pə-ˈdər-ˌmoid\ *adj* : of, relating to, or consisting of both mucous and squamous epithelial cells; *esp* : being a tumor of the salivary glands made up of mucous and epithelial elements ⟨~ carcinoma⟩

mu·co·gin·gi·val \-ˈjin-jə-vəl\ *adj* : of, relating to, or being the junction between the oral mucosa and the gingiva ⟨the ~ line⟩

[1]mu·coid \ˈmyü-ˌkoid\ *adj* : resembling mucus

[2]mucoid *n* : MUCOPROTEIN

mu·co·lip·i·do·sis \ˌmyü-kō-ˌli-pə-ˈdō-səs\ *n, pl* **-do·ses** \-ˌsēz\ : any of several metabolic disorders that are marked by the accumulation of glycosaminoglycans and lipids in tissues and by lysosomal enzymes which are produced in deficient amounts or which fail to be incorporated into lysosomes, that are inherited as autosomal recessive traits, and that have characteristics (as intellectual disability) resembling Hurler syndrome

mu·co·lyt·ic \ˌmyü-kə-ˈli-tik\ *adj* : hydrolyzing glycosaminoglycans : tending to break down or lower the viscosity of mucin-containing body secretions or components

Mu·co·myst \ˈmyü-kə-ˌmist\ *trademark* — used for a preparation of acetylcysteine

mu·co·pep·tide \ˌmyü-kō-ˈpep-ˌtīd\ *n* : PEPTIDOGLYCAN

mu·co·peri·os·te·um \-ˌper-ē-ˈäs-tē-əm\ *n* : a periosteum backed with mucous membrane (as that of the palatine surface of the mouth) — **mu·co·peri·os·te·al** \-ˈäs-tē-əl\ *adj*

mu·co·poly·sac·cha·ride \ˌmyü-kō-ˌpä-li-ˈsa-kə-ˌrīd\ *n* : GLYCOSAMINOGLYCAN

mu·co·poly·sac·cha·ri·do·sis \-ˌsa-kə-rī-ˈdō-səs\ *n, pl* **-do·ses** \-ˌsēz\ : any of a group of inherited disorders (as Hunter's syndrome and Hurler syndrome) of glycosaminoglycan metabolism that are characterized by the accumulation of glycosaminoglycans in the tissues and their excretion in the urine — called also *gargoylism, lipochondrodystrophy*

mu·co·pro·tein \ˌmyü-kə-ˈprō-ˌtēn\ *n* : any of a group of various complex conjugated proteins (as mucins) that contain glycosaminoglycans (as chondroitin sulfate) combined with amino acid units or polypeptides and that occur in body fluids and tissues — called also *mucoid;* compare GLYCOPROTEIN

mu·co·pu·ru·lent \-ˈpyu̇r-yə-lənt\ *adj* : containing both mucus and pus ⟨a ~ discharge⟩

mu·co·pus \ˈmyü-kō-ˌpəs\ *n* : mucus mixed with pus

mu·cor \ˈmyü-ˌkȯr\ *n* **1** *cap* : a genus (family Mucoraceae) of molds including several (as *M. corymbifer*) causing infections in humans and animals **2** : any mold of the genus *Mucor*

mu·cor·my·co·sis \ˌmyü-kər-mī-ˈkō-səs\ *n, pl* **-co·ses** \-ˌsēz\ : mycosis caused by fungi of the genus *Mucor* usu. primarily involving the lungs and invading other tissues by means of metastatic lesions — **mu·cor·my·cot·ic** \-ˈkä-tik\ *adj*

mu·co·sa \myü-ˈkō-zə\ *n, pl* **-sae** \-(ˌ)zē, -ˌzī\ *or* **-sas** : MUCOUS MEMBRANE — **mu·co·sal** \-zəl\ *adj*

mucosae — see MUSCULARIS MUCOSAE

mucosal disease *n* : a usu. fatal form of bovine viral diarrhea marked esp. by high fever, diarrhea, and ulcers of the digestive tract mucosa; *broadly* : BOVINE VIRAL DIARRHEA

mu·co·si·tis \ˌmyü-kə-ˈsī-təs\ *n* : inflammation of a mucous membrane

mu·co·stat·ic \ˌmyü-kə-ˈsta-tik\ *adj* **1** : of, relating to, or representing the mucosal tissues of the jaws as they are in a state of rest **2** : stopping the secretion of mucus

mu·cous \ˈmyü-kəs\ *adj* **1** : covered with or as if with mucus ⟨a ~ surface⟩ **2** : of, relating to, or resembling mucus ⟨a ~ secretion⟩ **3** : secreting or containing mucus ⟨~ glands⟩

mucous cell *n* : a cell that secretes mucus

mucous colitis *n* : IRRITABLE BOWEL SYNDROME; *esp* : irritable bowel syndrome characterized by the passage of unusually large amounts of mucus

mucous membrane *n* : a moist membranous layer rich in mucous glands that lines body passages and cavities (as of the digestive, respiratory, and genitourinary tracts) which connect directly or indirectly with the exterior, that functions in protection, support, nutrient absorption, and secretion of mucus, enzymes, and salts, and that is composed of epithelium supported below by the lamina propria and sometimes muscularis mucosae — called also *mucosa;* compare SEROUS MEMBRANE

mu·co·vis·ci·do·sis \ˌmyü-kō-ˌvi-sə-ˈdō-səs\ *n, pl* **-do·ses** \-ˌsēz\ : CYSTIC FIBROSIS

mu•cus \ˈmyü-kəs\ *n* : a viscid slippery secretion that is usu. rich in mucins and is produced by mucous membranes which it moistens and protects

mud bath *n* : an immersion of all or part of the body in mud for relaxation or therapeutic purposes

mud fever *n* **1** : a chapped inflamed condition of the skin of the legs and belly of a horse due to irritation from mud or drying resulting from washing off mud spatters and closely related or identical in nature to grease heel **2** : a mild leptospirosis that occurs chiefly in European agricultural and other workers in wet soil, is caused by infection with a spirochete of the genus *Leptospira* (*L. interrogans*) present in native field mice, and is marked by fever and headache without accompanying jaundice

Muel•le•ri•us \myü-ˈlir-ē-əs\ *n* : a genus of lungworms (family Metastrongylidae) including one (*M. capillaris*) that infects the lungs of sheep and goats

Mül•ler \ˈmue-ler\, **Fritz (Johann Friedrich Theodor) (1822–1897),** German zoologist.

MUFA \ˈməfə, ˈm(y)ü-\ *n* : a monounsaturated fatty acid

mulberry molar *n* : a first molar tooth whose occlusal surface is pitted due to congenital syphilis with nodules replacing the cusps — see MOON'S MOLAR

Mül•ler cell *or* **Muller cell** \ˈmyü-lər-, ˈmi-, ˈmə-\ *n* : any of the glial fibers that extend through the entire thickness of the retina and act as a support for the other structures — called also *fiber of Müller, sustentacular fiber of Müller*

Mül•ler \ˈmue-lər, ˈmyü-\, **Heinrich (1820–1864),** German anatomist.

Mül•le•ri•an agenesis \myü-ˈlir-ē-ən-, mi-, mə-\ *or* **Mul•le•ri•an agenesis** *n* : MAYER-ROKITANSKY-KÜSTER-HAUSER SYNDROME

Mül•ler \ˈmue-lər, ˈmyü-\, **Johannes Peter (1801–1858),** German physiologist and anatomist.

Müllerian duct *or* **Mul•le•ri•an duct** *n* : either of a pair of embryonic ducts parallel to the Wolffian ducts and giving rise in the female to the fallopian tubes, uterus, cervix, and upper portion of the vagina — called also *paramesonephric duct*

J. P. Müller — see MÜLLERIAN AGENESIS

Müllerian inhibiting substance *or* **Mullerian inhibiting substance** *n* : a glycoprotein hormone produced by the Sertoli cells of the male testis during fetal development that causes regression and atrophy of the Müllerian ducts : ANTI-MULLERIAN HORMONE — abbr. *MIS*

J. P. Müller — see MÜLLERIAN AGENESIS

Müllerian tubercle *or* **Mullerian tubercle** *n* : an elevation on the wall of the embryonic urogenital sinus where the Müllerian ducts enter

J. P. Müller — see MÜLLERIAN AGENESIS

¹mult•an•gu•lar \ˌməl-ˈtaŋ-gyə-lər\ *adj* : having many angles ⟨a ~ bone⟩

²multangular *n* : a multangular bone — see TRAPEZIUM, TRAPEZOID

multi- *comb form* **1 a** : many : multiple : much ⟨*multi*neuronal⟩ **b** : consisting of, containing, or having more than two ⟨*multi*nucleate⟩ **c** : more than one ⟨*multi*parous⟩ **2** : affecting many parts ⟨*multi*glandular⟩

mul•ti•an•gu•lar \ˌməl-tē-ˈaŋ-gyə-lər, ˌməl-ˌtī-\ *adj* : MULTANGULAR

mul•ti•cel•lu•lar \-ˈsel-yə-lər\ *adj* : having or consisting of many cells — **mul•ti•cel•lu•lar•i•ty** \-ˌsel-yə-ˈlar-ə-tē\ *n*

mul•ti•cen•ter \-ˈsen-tər\ *adj* : involving more than one medical or research institution ⟨a ~ study⟩

mul•ti•cen•tric \-ˈsen-trik\ *adj* : having multiple centers of origin ⟨a ~ tumor⟩

mul•ti•ceps \ˈməl-tə-ˌseps\ *n* **1** *cap* : a genus of taeniid tapeworms that have a coenurus larva and are now usu. placed in the genus *Taenia* **2** : COENURUS

mul•ti•clo•nal \ˌməl-tē-ˈklō-nəl, -ˌtī-\ *adj* : POLYCLONAL

mul•ti•cus•pid \-ˈkəs-pəd\ *adj* : having several cusps ⟨a ~ tooth⟩

mul•ti•cys•tic \-ˈsis-tik\ *adj* : POLYCYSTIC

mul•ti•dose \ˈməl-tē-ˌdōs, -ˌtī-\ *adj* : utilizing or containing more than one dose

mul•ti•drug \-ˌdrəg\ *adj* : utilizing or relating to more than one drug ⟨~ therapy⟩

mul•ti•en•zyme \ˌməl-te-ˈen-ˌzīm, -ˌtī-\ *adj* : composed of or involving two or more enzymes that function in a biosynthetic pathway ⟨a ~ complex⟩

mul•ti•fac•to•ri•al \-fak-ˈtōr-ē-əl\ *adj* **1** : having characters or a mode of inheritance dependent on a number of genes at different loci **2** *or* **mul•ti•fac•tor** \-ˈfak-tər\ : having, involving, or produced by a variety of elements or causes ⟨a ~ study⟩ ⟨a ~ etiology⟩ — **mul•ti•fac•to•ri•al•ly** *adv*

mul•tif•i•dus \ˌməl-ˈti-fə-dəs\ *n, pl* **-di** \-ˌdī\ : a muscle of the fifth and deepest layer of the back filling up the groove on each side of the spinous processes of the vertebrae from the sacrum to the skull and consisting of many fasciculi that pass upward and inward to the spinous processes and help to erect and rotate the spine

mul•ti•fo•cal \ˌməl-tē-ˈfō-kəl\ *adj* **1** : having more than one focal length ⟨~ lenses⟩ **2** : arising from or occurring in more than one focus or location ⟨~ seizures⟩

multifocal leukoencephalopathy — see PROGRESSIVE MULTIFOCAL LEUKOENCEPHALOPATHY

mul·ti·form \ˈməl-ti-ˌfȯrm\ *adj* : having or occurring in many forms

multiforme — see ERYTHEMA MULTIFORME, GLIOBLASTOMA MULTIFORME

mul·ti·gene \ˌməl-tē-ˈjēn, -ˌtī-\ *adj* : relating to or determined by a group of genes which were orig. copies of the same gene but evolved by mutation to become different from each other

mul·ti·gen·ic \-ˈje-nik, -ˈjē-\ *adj* : MULTIFACTORIAL 1

mul·ti·glan·du·lar \-ˈglan-jə-lər\ *adj* : POLYGLANDULAR

mul·ti·grav·i·da \-ˈgra-vi-də\ *n, pl* **-dae** \-ˌdē\ *also* **-das** : a woman who has been pregnant more than once — compare MULTIPARA

mul·ti–han·di·capped \ˌməl-tē-ˈhan-di-ˌkapt, -ˌtī-\ *adj* : having or affected by more than one disability; *also* : of, relating to, serving, or designed for individuals with more than one disability

mul·ti–hos·pi·tal \-ˈhäs-ˌpit-ᵊl\ *adj* : relating to, consisting of, or involving more than one hospital

multi–infarct dementia *n* : irreversible vascular dementia of gradual progression that results from a series of small strokes in which cerebral infarction occurs

mul·ti·lobed \-ˈlōbd\ *adj* : having two or more lobes

mul·ti·loc·u·lar \-ˈlä-kyə-lər\ *adj* : having or divided into many small chambers or vesicles ⟨a ~ cyst⟩

mul·ti·mam·mate rat \-ˈma-ˌmāt-\ *n* : any of several African rodents (genus *Mastomys*) that are vectors of disease (as Lassa fever) and are used in medical research — called also *multimammate mouse*

mul·ti·mo·dal \-ˈmōd-ᵊl\ *adj* : relating to, having, or utilizing more than one mode or modality (as of stimulation or treatment)

mul·ti·neu·ro·nal \-ˈnu̇r-ən-ᵊl, -ˈnyu̇r-; -nu̇-ˈrōn-, -nyu̇-\ *adj* : made up of or involving more than one neuron

mul·ti·nod·u·lar \-ˈnä-jə-lər\ *adj* : having many nodules ⟨~ goiter⟩

mul·ti·nu·cle·ate \-ˈnü-klē-ət, -ˈnyü-\ *or* **mul·ti·nu·cle·at·ed** \-klē-ˌā-təd\ *adj* : having more than two nuclei

mul·ti–or·gan \-ˈȯr-gən\ *adj* : of, involving, or affecting more than one organ ⟨~ failure⟩

mul·ti–or·gas·mic \-ȯr-ˈgaz-mik\ *adj* : capable of having more than one orgasm during a single period of sexual activity; *also* : of, relating to, or characterized by multiple orgasms ⟨~ sex⟩

mul·tip·a·ra \ˌməl-ˈti-pə-rə\ *n* : a woman who has borne more than one child — compare MULTIGRAVIDA

mul·ti·par·i·ty \ˌməl-ti-ˈpar-ə-tē\ *n, pl* **-ties** **1** : the production of two or more young at a birth **2** : the condition of having borne a number of children

mul·tip·a·rous \ˌməl-ˈti-pər-əs\ *adj* **1** : producing many or more than one at a birth **2** : having experienced one or more previous childbirths — compare PRIMIPAROUS

Multiphasic — see MINNESOTA MULTIPHASIC PERSONALITY INVENTORY

mul·ti·ple \ˈməl-tə-pəl\ *adj* **1** : consisting of, including, or involving more than one ⟨~ births⟩ **2** : affecting many parts of the body at once

multiple allele *n* : an allele of a genetic locus having more than two allelic forms within a population

multiple factor *n* : POLYGENE

multiple myeloma *n* : a disease of bone marrow that is characterized by the presence of numerous myelomas in various bones of the body — called also *myelomatosis*

multiple organ dysfunction syndrome *n* : progressive dysfunction of two or more major organ systems in a critically ill patient that makes it impossible to maintain homeostasis without medical intervention and that is typically a complication of sepsis and is a major factor in predicting mortality — abbr. *MODS*

multiple personality disorder *n* : a dissociative disorder that is characterized by the presence of two or more distinct and complex identities or personality states each of which becomes dominant and controls behavior from time to time to the exclusion of the others — called also *alternating personality, dissociative identity disorder, multiple personality*

multiple sclerosis *n* : a demyelinating disease marked by patches of hardened tissue in the brain or the spinal cord and associated esp. with partial or complete paralysis and jerking muscle tremor

multiple system atrophy *n* : any of several progressive neurodegenerative diseases that are of unknown cause, have an onset usu. during middle age and are characterized by a combination of symptoms (as orthostatic hypotension, urinary incontinence, rigidity, and loss of balance) indicative of autonomic dysfunction, parkinsonism, and cerebellar ataxia — abbr. MSA; see SHY-DRAGER SYNDROME

multiplex — see ARTHROGRYPOSIS MULTIPLEX CONGENITA, MONONEURITIS MULTIPLEX, PARAMYOCLONUS MULTIPLEX

mul·ti·po·lar \ˌməl-tē-ˈpō-lər, -ˌtī-\ *adj* **1** : having several poles ⟨~ mitoses⟩ **2** : having several dendrites ⟨~ neurons⟩ — **mul·ti·po·lar·i·ty** \-pō-ˈlar-ə-tē\ *n*

mul·tip·o·tent \ˌməl-ˈti-pə-tənt\ *adj* : having the potential of becoming any of several mature cell types ⟨~ stem cells⟩

mul·ti·po·ten·tial \ˌməl-tē-pə-ˈten-chəl, -ˌtī-\ *adj* : MULTIPOTENT

mul·ti·re·sis·tant \-ri-ˈzis-tənt\ *adj* : biologically resistant to several toxic agents ⟨~ strains of bacteria⟩

mul·ti·spe·cial·ty \-ˈspe-shəl-tē\ *adj* : providing service in or staffed by members of several medical specialties ⟨~ health centers⟩

mul·ti·syn·ap·tic \-sə-ˈnap-tik\ *adj* : relating to or consisting of more than one synapse ⟨~ pathways⟩

mul·ti·sys·tem \-ˈsis-təm\ *also* **mul·ti·sys·te·mic** \-sis-ˈte-mik\ *adj* : relating to, involving, or affecting more than one body system ⟨~ organ failure⟩

[1]**mul·ti·va·lent** \-ˈvā-lənt\ *adj* **1** : represented more than twice in the somatic chromosome number ⟨~ chromosomes⟩ **2** : POLYVALENT

[2]**multivalent** *n* : a multivalent group of chromosomes

mul·ti·ve·sic·u·lar \-və-ˈsi-kyə-lər, -ve-\ *adj* : having, containing, or composed of many vesicles ⟨a ~ cyst⟩

multivesicular body *n* : a lysosome that is a membranous sac containing numerous small endocytic vesicles

mul·ti·ves·sel \-ˈve-səl\ *adj* : affecting more than one blood vessel ⟨~ coronary artery disease⟩

[1]**mul·ti·vi·ta·min** \-ˈvī-tə-mən, -ˈvi-\ *adj* : containing several vitamins and esp. all known to be essential to health

[2]**multivitamin** *n* : a multivitamin preparation

mum·mi·fy \ˈmə-mi-ˌfī\ *vb* **-fied; -fy·ing** : to dry up and shrivel like a mummy ⟨a *mummified* fetus⟩ — **mum·mi·fi·ca·tion** \ˌmə-mi-fə-ˈkā-shən\ *n*

mumps \ˈməmps\ *n sing or pl* : an acute contagious virus disease caused by a paramyxovirus of the genus *Rubulavirus* (species *Mumps virus*) and marked by fever and by swelling esp. of the parotid gland — called also *epidemic parotitis*

Mun·chau·sen syndrome \ˈmən-ˌchau̇-zən-\ *or* **Mun·chau·sen's syndrome** \-zənz-\ *n* : a psychological disorder characterized by the feigning of the symptoms of a disease or injury in order to undergo diagnostic tests, hospitalization, or medical or surgical treatment

Münch·hau·sen \ˈmuenk-ˌhau̇-zən\, **Karl Friedrich Hieronymous, Freiherr von (1720–1797)**, German soldier.

Munchausen syndrome by proxy *also* **Munchausen's syndrome by proxy** *n* : a psychological disorder in which a parent and typically a mother harms her child (as by poisoning), falsifies the child's medical history, or tampers with the child's medical specimens in order to create a situation that requires or seems to require medical attention

mu·pir·o·cin \myü-ˈpir-ō-sən\ *n* : an antibacterial drug $C_{26}H_{44}O_9$ or its hydrated calcium salt $(C_{26}H_{43}O_9)_2Ca \cdot 2H_2O$ that is derived from a bacterium of the genus *Pseudomonas* (*P. fluorescens*) and is used esp. in the topical treatment of impetigo caused by bacteria of the genera *Streptococcus* (*S. pyogenes*) and *Staphylococcus* (*S. aureus*) — see BACTROBAN, CENTANY

mu·ral \ˈmyu̇r-əl\ *adj* : attached to and limited to a wall or a cavity ⟨a ~ thrombus⟩ ⟨~ abscesses⟩

mu·ram·i·dase \myu̇-ˈra-mə-ˌdās, -ˌdāz\ *n* : LYSOZYME

mu·rein \ˈmyu̇r-ē-ən, ˈmyu̇r-ˌēn\ *n* : PEPTIDOGLYCAN

mu·ri·at·ic acid \ˌmyu̇r-ē-ˈa-tik-\ *n* : HYDROCHLORIC ACID

mu·rid \ˈmyu̇r-id\ *n* : any of a large family (Muridae) of relatively small rodents including various Old World forms (as the house mouse and the common rats) — **murid** *adj*

[1]**mu·rine** \ˈmyu̇r-ˌīn\ *adj* **1 a** : of or relating to the genus *Mus* or its subfamily (Murinae) that includes the common household rats and mice **b** : of, relating to, or produced by the house mouse ⟨a ~ odor⟩ **2** : affecting or transmitted by rats or mice ⟨~ rickettsial diseases⟩

[2]**murine** *n* : a murine animal

murine leukemia virus *n* : a retrovirus (species *Murine leukemia virus* of the genus *Gammaretrovirus*) that includes several strains producing leukemia in mice — see FRIEND VIRUS

murine typhus *n* : a mild febrile disease that is marked by headache and rash, is caused by a bacterium of the genus *Rickettsia* (*R. typhi*), is widespread in nature in rodents, and is transmitted to humans by a flea — called also *endemic typhus*

mur·mur \ˈmər-mər\ *n* : an atypical sound of the heart indicating a functional or structural abnormality — called also *heart murmur*

Mur·ray Val·ley encephalitis \ˈmər-ē-ˈva-lē-\ *n* : an encephalitis endemic in northern Australia and Papua New Guinea that is caused by a virus of the genus *Flavivirus* (species *Murray Valley encephalitis virus*) transmitted by mosquitoes (esp. *Culex annulirostris*) and that is often asymptomatic but may cause serious potentially fatal disease

Mus \ˈməs\ *n* : a genus of rodents (family Muridae) that includes the house mouse (*M. musculus*)

Mus·ca \ˈməs-kə\ *n* : a genus of flies (family Muscidae) including the common housefly (*M. domestica*)

mus·cae vo·li·tan·tes \ˈməs-ˌkē-ˌvä-lə-ˈtan-ˌtēz, ˈmə-ˌsē-\ *n pl* : spots before the eyes due to cells and cell fragments in the vitreous humor and lens — compare FLOATER

mus·ca·rine \ˈməs-kə-ˌrēn\ *n* : a toxic ammonium base $[C_9H_{20}NO_2]^+$ that is biochemically related to acetylcholine, was orig. extracted from fly agaric but also occurs in other mushrooms (as of the genus *Inocybe*), and when ingested produces symptoms of parasympathetic nervous system stimulation (as excessive salivation, lacrimation, bronchial secretion, diarrhea, miosis, and bradycardia)

mus·ca·rin·ic \ˌməs-kə-ˈri-nik\ *adj* : relating to, resembling, producing, or mediating the parasympathetic effects (as a slowed heart rate and increased activity of smooth muscle) produced by muscarine ⟨~ receptors⟩ — compare NICOTINIC

mus·cle \ˈmə-səl\ *n, often attrib* **1 :** a body tissue consisting of long cells that contract when stimulated and produce motion — see CARDIAC MUSCLE, SMOOTH MUSCLE, STRIATED MUSCLE **2 :** an organ that is essentially a mass of muscle tissue attached at either end to a fixed point and that by contracting moves or checks the movement of a body part — see AGONIST 1, ANTAGONIST a, SYNERGIST 2

mus·cle–bound \ˈmə-səl-ˌbau̇nd\ *adj* : having some of the muscles tense and enlarged and of impaired elasticity sometimes as a result of excessive exercise

muscle dysmorphia *n* : pathological preoccupation with the perceived smallness or weakness of one's body and musculature often leading to excessive exercise, steroid abuse, or eating disorders — called also *bigorexia, reverse anorexia*

muscle fiber *n* : any of the elongated cells characteristic of muscle

muscle sense *n* : the part of kinesthesia mediated by end organs located in muscles

muscle spasm *n* : persistent involuntary hypertonicity of one or more muscles usu. of central origin and commonly associated with pain and excessive irritability

muscle spindle *n* : a sensory end organ in a muscle that is sensitive to stretch in the muscle, consists of small striated muscle fibers richly supplied with nerve fibers, and is enclosed in a connective tissue sheath — called also *stretch receptor*

muscle tone *n* : TONUS 2

muscul- *or* **musculo-** *comb form* **1** : muscle ⟨*muscul*ar⟩ **2 :** muscular and ⟨*musculo*skeletal⟩

mus·cu·lar \ˈməs-kyə-lər\ *adj* **1 a :** of, relating to, or constituting muscle **b** : of, relating to, or performed by the muscles **2 :** having well-developed musculature — **mus·cu·lar·ly** *adv*

muscular coat *n* : an outer layer of smooth muscle surrounding a hollow or tubular organ (as the bladder, esophagus, large intestine, small intestine, stomach, ureter, uterus, and vagina) that often consists of an inner layer of circular fibers serving to narrow the lumen of the organ and an outer layer of longitudinal fibers serving to shorten its length — called also *muscularis externa, tunica muscularis*

muscular dystrophy *n* : any of a group of hereditary diseases characterized by progressive wasting of muscles — see BECKER MUSCULAR DYSTROPHY, DUCHENNE MUSCULAR DYSTROPHY

mus·cu·la·ris \ˌməs-kyə-ˈlar-is\ *n* **1** : the smooth muscular layer of the wall of various more or less contractile organs (as the bladder) **2 :** the thin layer of smooth muscle that forms part of a mucous membrane

muscularis ex·ter·na \-eks-ˈtər-nə\ *n* : MUSCULAR COAT

muscularis mu·co·sae \-myü-ˈkō-sē\ *also* **muscularis mu·co·sa** \-sə\ *n* : MUSCULARIS 2

mus·cu·lar·i·ty \ˌməs-kyə-ˈlar-ə-tē\ *n, pl* **-ties :** the quality or state of being muscular

mus·cu·la·ture \ˈməs-kyə-lə-ˌchu̇r, -chər, -ˌtyu̇r\ *n* : the muscles of all or a part of the body

mus·cu·li pec·ti·na·ti \ˈməs-kyə-ˌlī-ˌpek-ti-ˈnā-ˌtī\ *n pl* : small muscular ridges on the inner wall of the auricular appendage of the left and the right atria of the heart

musculo- — see MUSCUL-

mus·cu·lo·cu·ta·ne·ous \ˌməs-kyə-lō-kyu̇-ˈtā-nē-əs\ *adj* : of, relating to, supplying, or consisting of both muscle and skin ⟨~ flaps⟩

musculocutaneous nerve *n* **1 :** a large branch of the brachial plexus supplying various parts of the upper arm (as flexor muscles) and forearm (as the skin) **2 :** SUPERFICIAL PERONEAL NERVE

mus·cu·lo·fas·cial \-ˈfa-shəl, -shē-əl\ *adj* : relating to or consisting of both muscular and fascial tissue

mus·cu·lo·fi·brous \-ˈfī-brəs\ *adj* : relating to or consisting of both muscular and fibrous connective tissue

mus·cu·lo·mem·bra·nous \-ˈmem-brə-nəs\ *adj* : relating to or consisting of both muscle and membrane

mus·cu·lo·phren·ic artery \-ˈfre-nik-\ *n* : a branch of the internal mammary artery that gives off branches to the seventh, eighth, and ninth intercostal spaces as anterior intercostal arteries, to the pericardium, to the diaphragm, and to the abdominal muscles

musculorum — see DYSTONIA MUSCULORUM DEFORMANS

mus·cu·lo·skel·e·tal \ˌməs-kyə-lō-ˈske-lət-ᵊl\ *adj* : of, relating to, or involving both musculature and skeleton

mus·cu·lo·ten·di·nous \-ˈten-də-nəs\ *adj* : of, relating to, or affecting muscular and tendinous tissue

musculotendinous cuff *n* : ROTATOR CUFF

mus·cu·lus \ˈməs-kyə-ləs\ *n, pl* **-li** \-ˌlī\ : MUSCLE

mush·room \ˈməsh-ˌrüm, -ˌru̇m\ *n* **1** : an enlarged complex fleshy fruiting body of a fungus (as a basidiomycete) that arises from an underground mycelium and consists typically of a stem bearing a spore-bearing structure; *esp* : one that is edible — compare TOADSTOOL **2** : FUNGUS 1

mu·si·co·gen·ic \ˌmyü-zi-kō-ˈje-nik\ *adj* : of, relating to, or being epileptic seizures precipitated by music

music therapy *n* : therapy based on engagement in musical activities : the therapeutic use of music (as to reduce anxiety or improve cognitive functioning) that typically involves listening to music, singing, playing musical instruments, or composing music — **music therapist** *n*

mussel poisoning *n* : a toxic reaction and esp. paralytic shellfish poisoning following the consumption of mussels

mus·tard \ˈməs-tərd\ *n* **1** : a pungent yellow powder of the seeds of any of several herbs (*Brassica nigra*, *B. hirta*, or *B. juncea* of the family Cruciferae syn. Brassicaceae, the mustard family) used as a condiment or in medicine as a stimulant and diuretic, an emetic, and a counterirritant **2 a** : MUSTARD GAS **b** : NITROGEN MUSTARD

mustard gas *n* : an irritant oily liquid $C_4H_8Cl_2S$ used esp. as a chemical weapon that causes blistering, attacks the eyes and lungs, and is a systemic poison — called also *sulfur mustard*

mustard oil *n* **1** : a colorless to pale yellow pungent irritating essential oil that is obtained by distillation from mustard seeds, that consists largely of allyl isothiocyanate, and that is used esp. in liniments and medicinal plasters **2** : ALLYL ISOTHIOCYANATE

mustard plaster *n* : a counterirritant and rubefacient plaster containing powdered mustard — called also *mustard paper*

mu·ta·gen \ˈmyü-tə-jən\ *n* : a substance (as a chemical or various radiations) that tends to increase the frequency or extent of mutation

mu·ta·gen·e·sis \ˌmyü-tə-ˈje-nə-səs\ *n, pl* **-e·ses** \-ˌsēz\ : the occurrence or induction of mutation — **mu·ta·gen·ic** \-ˈje-nik\ *adj* — **mu·ta·ge·nic·i·ty** \-jə-ˈni-sə-tē\ *n*

mu·ta·gen·ize \ˈmyü-tə-jə-ˌnīz\ *vb* **-ized; -iz·ing** : MUTATE

[1]**mu·tant** \ˈmyüt-ᵊnt\ *adj* : of, relating to, or produced by mutation

[2]**mutant** *n* : a mutant individual

mu·ta·tion \myü-ˈtā-shən\ *n* **1** : a relatively permanent change in hereditary material involving either a change in chromosome structure or number or a change in the nucleotide sequence of a gene's codons; *also* : the process of producing a mutation **2** : an individual, strain, or trait resulting from mutation — **mu·tate** \ˈmyü-ˌtāt, myü-ˈ\ *vb* — **mu·ta·tion·al** \-shə-nəl\ *adj* — **mu·ta·tion·al·ly** *adv*

[1]**mute** \ˈmyüt\ *adj* **mut·er; mut·est** : unable to speak : lacking the power of speech — **mute·ness** *n*

[2]**mute** *n* : a person who cannot or does not speak

mu·ti·late \ˈmyüt-ᵊl-ˌāt\ *vb* **-lat·ed; -lat·ing** : to cut off or permanently destroy a limb or essential part of; *also* : CASTRATE — **mu·ti·la·tion** \ˌmyüt-ᵊl-ˈā-shən\ *n*

mut·ism \ˈmyü-ˌti-zəm\ *n* : the condition of being mute whether from physical, functional, or psychological cause — see SELECTIVE MUTISM

muz·zle \ˈmə-zəl\ *n* **1** : the projecting jaws and nose of an animal **2** : a fastening or covering for the mouth of an animal used to prevent eating or biting

MVP *abbr* mitral valve prolapse

my- *or* **myo-** *comb form* **1 a** : muscle ⟨*my*asthenia⟩ ⟨*myo*globin⟩ **b** : muscular and ⟨*myo*neural⟩ **2** : myoma and ⟨*myo*edema⟩

my·al·gia \mī-ˈal-jē, -jē-ə\ *n* : pain in one or more muscles — **my·al·gic** \-jik\ *adj*

myalgic encephalomyelitis *n, chiefly Brit* : CHRONIC FATIGUE SYNDROME

My·am·bu·tol \mī-ˈam-byu̇-ˌtȯl, -ˌtōl\ *trademark* — used for a preparation of the dihydrochloride of ethambutol

my·an·e·sin \mī-ˈa-nə-sən\ *n* : MEPHENESIN

my·as·the·nia \ˌmī-əs-ˈthē-nē-ə\ *n* : muscular debility; *also* : MYASTHENIA GRAVIS — **my·as·then·ic** \-ˈthe-nik\ *adj*

myasthenia gra·vis \-ˈgra-vis, -ˈgrä-\ *n* : a disease characterized by progressive weakness of voluntary muscles without atrophy or sensory disturbance and caused by an autoimmune attack on acetylcholine receptors at neuromuscular junctions

my·a·to·nia \ˌmī-ə-ˈtō-nē-ə\ *n* : lack of muscle tone : muscular flabbiness

myc- *or* **myco-** *comb form* : fungus or fungus-like bacterium ⟨*myc*elium⟩ ⟨*myco*logy⟩ ⟨*myc*osis⟩

my·ce·li·um \mī-ˈsē-lē-əm\ *n, pl* **-lia** \-lē-ə\ : the mass of interwoven filaments that forms esp. the vegetative body of a fungus and is often submerged in another body (as of soil or organic matter or the tissues of a host); *also* : a similar mass of filaments formed by some bacteria (as of the genus *Streptomyces*) — **my·ce·li·al** \-lē-əl\ *adj*

-my·ces \ˈmī-ˌsēz\ *n comb form* : fungus — used esp. in taxonomic names of fungi and certain bacteria resembling fungi and in their corresponding vernacular names ⟨Strepto*myces*⟩

mycet- *or* **myceto-** *comb form* : fungus ⟨*mycet*oma⟩

-my·cete \ˈmī-ˌsēt, ˌmī-ˈsēt\ *n comb form* : fungus ⟨actino*mycete*⟩

my·ce·tis·mus \ˌmī-sə-ˈtiz-məs\ *n, pl* **-mi** \-ˌmī\ : mushroom poisoning

my·ce·to·ma \ˌmī-sə-ˈtō-mə\ *n, pl* **-mas** *also* **-ma·ta** \-mə-tə\ **1** : a condition marked by invasion of the deep subcutaneous tissues with fungi or actinomycetes: **a** : MADUROMYCOSIS **b** : NOCARDIOSIS **2** : a tumorous mass occurring in mycetoma — **my•ce•to•ma•tous** \-mə-təs\ *adj*

-my•cin \ˈmīs-ᵊn\ *n comb form* : substance obtained from a fungus-like bacterium ⟨erythro*mycin*⟩

my•co•bac•te•ri•o•sis \ˌmī-kō-bak-ˌtir-ē-ˈō-səs\ *n, pl* **-o•ses** \-ˌsēz\ : a disease caused by bacteria of the genus *Mycobacterium*

my•co•bac•te•ri•um \-bak-ˈtir-ē-əm\ *n* **1** *cap* : a genus of nonmotile acid-fast aerobic bacteria (family Mycobacteriaceae) that include the causative agents of tuberculosis (*M. tuberculosis*) and leprosy (*M. leprae*) as well as numerous purely saprophytic forms **2** *pl* **-ria** : any bacterium of the genus *Mycobacterium* or a closely related genus — **my•co•bac•te•ri•al** \-ē-əl\ *adj*

Mycobacterium avi•um complex \-ˈā-vē-əm-\ *n* : two bacteria of the genus *Mycobacterium* (*M. avium* and *M. intracellulare*) that account for most mycobacterial infections in humans other than tuberculosis, that usu. affect the lungs, and that may cause disseminated disease in immunosuppressed conditions (as AIDS)

Mycobacterium avium–in•tra•cel•lu•la•re complex \-ˌin-trə-ˌsel-yə-ˈlär-ē-\ *n* : MYCOBACTERIUM AVIUM COMPLEX

my•col•o•gy \mī-ˈkä-lə-jē\ *n, pl* **-gies 1** : a branch of biology dealing with fungi **2** : fungal life — **my•co•log•i•cal** \ˌmī-kə-ˈlä-ji-kəl\ *adj* — **my•col•o•gist** \mī-ˈkä-lə-jist\ *n*

my•co•my•cin \ˌmī-kə-ˈmīs-ᵊn\ *n* : an antibiotic acid $C_{13}H_{10}O_2$ obtained from an actinomycete of the genus *Nocardia* (*N. acidophilus*)

my•co•phe•no•lic acid \ˌmī-kō-fi-ˈnō-lik-, -ˈnä-\ *n* : a crystalline antibiotic $C_{17}H_{20}O_6$ obtained from fungi of the genus *Penicillium*

my•co•plas•ma \ˌmī-kō-ˈplaz-mə\ *n* **1** *cap* : a genus of minute pleomorphic gram-negative chiefly nonmotile bacteria (family Mycoplasmataceae) that are mostly parasitic usu. in mammals — see PLEUROPNEUMONIA 2 **2** *pl* **-mas** *also* **-ma•ta** \-mə-tə\ : any bacterium of the genus *Mycoplasma* or of the family (Mycoplasmataceae) to which it belongs — called also *pleuropneumonia-like organism, PPLO* — **my•co•plas•mal** \-məl\ *adj*

my•co•sis \mī-ˈkō-səs\ *n, pl* **my•co•ses** \-ˌsēz\ : infection with or disease caused by a fungus

mycosis fun•goi•des \-fəŋ-ˈgȯi-ˌdēz\ *n* : cutaneous T-cell lymphoma characterized by a chronic patchy red scaly irregular and often eczematous dermatitis that progresses over a period of years to form elevated plaques and then tumors

my•co•stat \ˈmī-kə-ˌstat\ *n* : an agent that inhibits the growth of molds — **my•co•stat•ic** \ˌmī-kə-ˈsta-tik\ *adj*

My•co•stat•in \-ˈsta-tən\ *trademark* — used for a preparation of nystatin

my•cot•ic \mī-ˈkä-tik\ *adj* : of, relating to, or characterized by mycosis

my•co•tox•ic \ˌmī-kō-ˈtäk-sik\ *adj* : of, relating to, or caused by a mycotoxin — **my•co•tox•ic•i•ty** \-täk-ˈsi-sə-tē\ *n*

my•co•tox•i•co•sis \ˌmī-kō-ˌtäk-sə-ˈkō-səs\ *n, pl* **-co•ses** \-ˈkō-ˌsēz\ : poisoning caused by a mycotoxin

my•co•tox•in \-ˈtäk-sən\ *n* : a poisonous substance produced by a fungus and esp. a mold — see AFLATOXIN

My•dri•a•cyl \mə-ˈdrī-ə-ˌsil\ *trademark* — used for a preparation of tropicamide

my•dri•a•sis \mə-ˈdrī-ə-səs\ *n, pl* **-a•ses** \-ˌsēz\ : excessive or prolonged dilation of the pupil of the eye

¹**myd•ri•at•ic** \ˌmi-drē-ˈa-tik\ *adj* : causing or involving dilation of the pupil of the eye

²**mydriatic** *n* : a drug that produces dilation of the pupil of the eye

my•ec•to•my \mī-ˈek-tə-mē\ *n, pl* **-mies** : surgical excision of part of a muscle

myel- *or* **myelo-** *comb form* : marrow: as **a** : bone marrow ⟨*myelo*cyte⟩ **b** : spinal cord ⟨*myelo*dysplasia⟩

my•el•en•ceph•a•lon \ˌmī-ə-len-ˈse-fə-ˌlän, -lən\ *n* : the posterior part of the developing vertebrate hindbrain or the corresponding part of the adult brain composed of the medulla oblongata — **my•el•en•ce•phal•ic** \-ˌlen-sə-ˈfa-lik\ *adj*

-my•e•lia \ˌmī-ˈē-lē-ə\ *n comb form* : a (specified) condition of the spinal cord ⟨hemato*myelia*⟩ ⟨syringo*myelia*⟩

my•elin \ˈmī-ə-lən\ *n* : a soft white material of lipid and protein that is secreted by oligodendrocytes and Schwann cells and forms a thick sheath about axons — see MYELIN SHEATH — **my•elin•ic** \ˌmī-ə-ˈli-nik\ *adj*

my•elin•at•ed \ˈmī-ə-lə-ˌnā-təd\ *adj* : having a myelin sheath

my•e•li•na•tion \ˌmī-ə-lə-ˈnā-shən\ *n* **1** : the process of acquiring a myelin sheath **2** : the condition of being myelinated

myelin basic protein *n* : a protein that is a constituent of myelin and is often found in higher than normal amounts in the cerebrospinal fluid of people affected with some demyelinating disease (as multiple sclerosis)

my•e•lin•i•za•tion \ˌmī-ə-ˌli-nə-ˈzā-shən\ *n* : MYELINATION

my•eli•nol•y•sis \-ˈnä-lə-səs\ *n* : DEMYELINATION — see CENTRAL PONTINE MYELINOLYSIS

myelin sheath *n* : the insulating covering that surrounds an axon with multiple spiral layers of myelin, that is discontinuous at the nodes of Ranvier, and that increases the speed at which a nerve impulse can travel along an axon

my•eli•tis \ˌmī-ə-ˈlī-təs\ *n, pl* **my•elit•i•des** \-ˈli-tə-ˌdēz\ : inflammation of the spinal cord or of the bone marrow — **my•elit•ic** \-ˈli-tik\ *adj*

my•elo•blast \ˈmī-ə-lə-ˌblast\ *n* : a large mononuclear nongranular bone marrow cell; *esp* : one that is a precursor of a myelocyte — **my•elo•blas•tic** \ˌmī-ə-lə-ˈblas-tik\ *adj*

myeloblastic leukemia *n* : MYELOGENOUS LEUKEMIA

my•elo•blas•to•sis \ˌmī-ə-lō-blas-ˈtō-səs\ *n, pl* **-to•ses** \-ˌsēz\ : the presence of an abnormally large number of myeloblasts in the tissues, organs, or circulating blood

my•elo•cele \ˈmī-ə-lə-ˌsēl\ *n* : spina bifida in which the neural tissue of the spinal cord is exposed

my•elo•cyte \ˈmī-ə-lə-ˌsīt\ *n* : a bone marrow cell; *esp* : a motile cell with cytoplasmic granules that gives rise to the blood granulocytes and occurs abnormally in the circulating blood (as in myelogenous leukemia) — **my•elo•cyt•ic** \ˌmī-ə-lə-ˈsi-tik\ *adj*

myelocytic leukemia *n* : MYELOGENOUS LEUKEMIA

my•elo•cy•to•ma \-sī-ˈtō-mə\ *n, pl* **-mas** *also* **-ma•ta** \-mə-tə\ : a tumor esp. of fowl in which the typical cellular element is a myelocyte or a cell of similar differentiation

my•elo•cy•to•sis \-sī-ˈtō-səs\ *n, pl* **-to•ses** \-ˌsēz\ : the presence of excess numbers of myelocytes esp. in the blood or bone marrow

my•elo•dys•pla•sia \-dis-ˈplā-zhə, -zhē-ə\ *n* **1** : a developmental anomaly of the spinal cord **2** : MYELODYSPLASTIC SYNDROME — **my•elo•dys•plas•tic** \-ˈplas-tik\ *adj*

myelodysplastic syndrome *n* : any of a group of bone marrow disorders that are marked esp. by an abnormal reduction in one or more types of circulating blood cells due to defective growth and maturation of blood-forming cells in the bone marrow and that sometimes progress to acute myelogenous leukemia — called also *myelodysplasia, preleukemia*

my•elo•fi•bro•sis \ˌmī-ə-lō-fī-ˈbrō-səs\ *n, pl* **-bro•ses** \-ˌsēz\ : an anemic condition in which bone marrow becomes fibrotic and the liver and spleen usu. exhibit a development of blood cell precursors — **my•elo•fi•brot•ic** \-ˈbrä-tik\ *adj*

my•elog•e•nous \ˌmī-ə-ˈlä-jə-nəs\ *also* **my•elo•gen•ic** \ˌmī-ə-lə-ˈje-nik\ *adj* : of, relating to, originating in, or produced by the bone marrow

myelogenous leukemia *n* : leukemia characterized by proliferation of myeloid tissue (as of the bone marrow and spleen) and an abnormal increase in the number of granulocytes, myelocytes, and myeloblasts in the circulating blood — called also *granulocytic leukemia, myeloblastic leukemia, myelocytic leukemia, myeloid leukemia;* see ACUTE MYELOGENOUS LEUKEMIA, ACUTE NONLYMPHOCYTIC LEUKEMIA, CHRONIC MYELOGENOUS LEUKEMIA

my•elo•gram \ˈmī-ə-lə-ˌgram\ *n* **1** : a differential study of the cellular elements present in bone marrow usu. made on material obtained by sternal biopsy **2** : a radiograph of the spinal cord made by myelography

my•elo•graph•ic \ˌmī-ə-lə-ˈgra-fik\ *adj* : of, relating to, or made by means of a myelogram or myelography — **my•elo•graph•i•cal•ly** *adv*

my•elog•ra•phy \ˌmī-ə-ˈlä-grə-fē\ *n, pl* **-phies** : radiographic visualization of the spinal cord after injection of a contrast medium into the spinal subarachnoid space

my•eloid \ˈmī-ə-ˌlȯid\ *adj* **1** : of or relating to the spinal cord **2** : of, relating to, or resembling bone marrow

myeloid leukemia *n* : MYELOGENOUS LEUKEMIA

my•elo•li•po•ma \ˌmī-ə-lō-lī-ˈpō-mə, -li-\ *n, pl* **-mas** *also* **-ma•ta** \-mə-tə\ : a benign tumor esp. of the adrenal glands that consists of fat and hematopoietic tissue

my•elo•ma \ˌmī-ə-ˈlō-mə\ *n, pl* **-mas** *also* **-ma•ta** \-mə-tə\ : a primary tumor of the bone marrow formed of any one of the bone marrow cells (as myelocytes or plasma cells) and usu. involving several different bones at the same time — see MULTIPLE MYELOMA

my•elo•ma•to•sis \ˌmī-ə-lō-mə-ˈtō-səs\ *n, pl* **-to•ses** \-ˌsēz\ : MULTIPLE MYELOMA

my•elo•me•nin•go•cele \ˌmī-ə-lō-mə-ˈniŋ-gə-ˌsēl, -mə-ˈnin-jə-\ *n* : spina bifida in which neural tissue and the investing meninges protrude from the spinal column forming a sac under the skin

my•elo•mono•cyt•ic \-ˌmä-nə-ˈsi-tik\ *adj* : relating to or being a blood cell that has the characteristics of both monocytes and granulocytes

myelomonocytic leukemia *n* : a kind of monocytic leukemia in which the cells resemble granulocytes

my•elop•a•thy \ˌmī-ə-ˈlä-pə-thē\ *n, pl* **-thies** : any disease or disorder of the spinal cord or bone marrow — **my•elo•path•ic** \ˌmī-ə-lō-ˈpa-thik\ *adj*

my•elo•phthi•sic anemia \ˌmī-ə-lō-ˈti-zik-, -ˈtī-sik-\ *n* : anemia in which the blood-forming elements of the bone marrow are unable to reproduce normal blood cells and which is commonly caused by specific toxins or by overgrowth of tumor cells

my•elo•poi•e•sis \ˌmī-ə-lō-(ˌ)pȯi-ˈē-səs\ *n, pl* **-poi•e•ses** \-ˈē-ˌsēz\ **1** : production of marrow or marrow cells **2** : production of blood cells in bone marrow; *esp* : formation of blood granulocytes — **my•elo•poi•et•ic** \-(ˌ)pȯi-ˈe-tik\ *adj*

my•elo•pro•lif•er•a•tive \ˈmī-ə-lō-prə-ˈli-fə-ˌrā-tiv, -rə-\ *adj* : of, relating to, or being a disorder (as leukemia) marked by excessive proliferation of bone marrow elements and esp. blood cell precursors

my·elo·sis \ˌmī-ə-ˈlō-səs\ *n, pl* **-elo·ses** \-ˌsēz\ **1** : the proliferation of marrow tissue to produce the changes in cell distribution typical of myelogenous leukemia **2** : MYELOGENOUS LEUKEMIA

my·elo·sup·pres·sion \ˌmī-ə-lō-sə-ˈpre-shən\ *n* : suppression of the bone marrow's production of blood cells and platelets — **my·elo·sup·pres·sive** \-sə-ˈpre-siv\ *adj*

my·elot·o·my \ˌmī-ə-ˈlä-tə-mē\ *n, pl* **-mies** : surgical incision of the spinal cord; *esp* : section of crossing nerve fibers at the midline of the spinal cord and esp. of sensory fibers for the relief of intractable pain

my·elo·tox·ic \ˌmī-ə-lō-ˈtäk-sik\ *adj* : destructive to bone marrow or any of its elements ⟨a ~ agent⟩ — **my·elo·tox·ic·i·ty** \-täk-ˈsi-sə-tē\ *n*

my·en·ter·ic \ˌmī-ən-ˈter-ik\ *adj* : of or relating to the muscular coat of the intestinal wall

myenteric plexus *n* : a network of nerve fibers and ganglia between the longitudinal and circular muscle layers of the intestine — called also *Auerbach's plexus;* compare MEISSNER'S PLEXUS

myenteric plexus of Auerbach *n* : MYENTERIC PLEXUS

myenteric reflex *n* : a reflex that is responsible for the wave of peristalsis moving along the intestine and that involves contraction of the digestive tube above and relaxation below the place where it is stimulated by an accumulated mass of food

my·ia·sis \mī-ˈī-ə-səs, mē-\ *n, pl* **my·ia·ses** \-ˌsēz\ : infestation with fly maggots

myl- *or* **mylo-** *comb form* : molar ⟨*mylo*hyoid⟩

My·lan·ta \mī-ˈlan-tə\ *trademark* — used for an antacid and antiflatulent preparation of aluminum hydroxide, magnesium hydroxide, and simethicone

Myl·e·ran \ˈmi-lə-ˌran\ *trademark* — used for a preparation of busulfan

My·li·con \ˈmī-lə-ˌkän\ *trademark* — used for a preparation of simethicone

my·lo·hy·oid \ˌmī-lō-ˈhī-ˌȯid\ *adj* : of, indicating, or adjoining the mylohyoid muscle

my·lo·hy·oi·de·us \-hī-ˈȯi-dē-əs\ *n, pl* **-dei** \-dē-ˌī\ : MYLOHYOID MUSCLE

mylohyoid line *n* : a ridge on the inner side of the bone of the lower jaw giving attachment to the mylohyoid muscle and to the superior constrictor of the pharynx — called also *mylohyoid ridge*

mylohyoid muscle *n* : a flat triangular muscle on each side of the mouth that is located above the anterior belly of the digastric muscle, extends from the inner surface of the mandible to the hyoid bone, and with its mate on the opposite side forms the floor of the mouth — called also *mylohyoid, mylohyoideus*

myo- — see MY-

myo·blast \ˈmī-ə-ˌblast\ *n* : an undifferentiated cell capable of giving rise to muscle cells

myo·blas·to·ma \ˌmī-ə-(ˌ)blas-ˈtō-mə\ *n, pl* **-mas** *also* **-ma·ta** \-mə-tə\ : a tumor that is composed of cells resembling primitive myoblasts and is associated with striated muscle

myo·car·di·al \ˌmī-ə-ˈkär-dē-əl\ *adj* : of, relating to, or involving the myocardium — **myo·car·di·al·ly** *adv*

myocardial infarction *n* : HEART ATTACK

myocardial insufficiency *n* : inability of the myocardium to perform its function : HEART FAILURE

myo·car·di·op·a·thy \-ˌkär-dē-ˈä-pə-thē\ *n, pl* **-thies** : disease of the myocardium

myo·car·di·tis \ˌmī-ə-(ˌ)kär-ˈdī-təs\ *n* : inflammation of the myocardium

myo·car·di·um \ˌmī-ə-ˈkär-dē-əm\ *n, pl* **-dia** \-dē-ə\ : the middle muscular layer of the heart wall

Myo·chry·sine \ˌmī-ō-ˈkrī-ˌsēn, -sən\ *trademark* — used for a preparation of gold sodium thiomalate

myo·clo·nia \ˌmī-ə-ˈklō-nē-ə\ *n* : MYOCLONUS

myo·clon·ic \-ˈklä-nik\ *adj* : of, relating to, characterized by, or being myoclonus ⟨~ seizures⟩

myoclonic epilepsy *n* : epilepsy marked by myoclonic seizures: as **a** : JUVENILE MYOCLONIC EPILEPSY **b** : LAFORA DISEASE

my·oc·lo·nus \ˌmī-ˈä-klə-nəs\ *n* : irregular involuntary contraction of a muscle usu. resulting from functional disorder of controlling motor neurons; *also* : a condition characterized by myoclonus

myoclonus epilepsy *n* : MYOCLONIC EPILEPSY

myo·cyte \ˈmī-ə-ˌsīt\ *n* : a contractile cell; *specif* : a muscle cell

myo·ede·ma \ˌmī-ō-i-ˈdē-mə\ *n, pl* **-mas** *also* **-ma·ta** \-mə-tə\ : the formation of a lump in a muscle when struck a slight blow that occurs in states of exhaustion or in certain diseases

myo·elec·tric \ˌmī-ō-i-ˈlek-trik\ *also* **myo·elec·tri·cal** \-tri-kəl\ *adj* : of, relating to, or utilizing electricity generated by muscle

myo·epi·the·li·al \-ˌe-pə-ˈthē-lē-əl\ *adj* : of, relating to, or being large contractile cells of epithelial origin which are located at the base of the secretory cells of various glands (as the salivary and mammary glands)

myo·epi·the·li·o·ma \-ˌe-pə-ˌthē-lē-ˈō-mə\ *n, pl* **-mas** *also* **-ma·ta** \-mə-tə\

: a tumor arising from myoepithelial cells esp. of the sweat glands

myo·epi·the·li·um \-ˌe-pə-ˈthē-lē-əm\ *n, pl* **-lia** : tissue made up of myoepithelial cells

myo·fas·cial \-ˈfa-shəl, -shē-əl\ *adj* : of or relating to the fasciae of muscles

myo·fi·ber \ˈmī-ō-ˌfī-bər\ *n* : MUSCLE FIBER

myo·fi·bre *chiefly Brit var of* MYOFIBER

myo·fi·bril \ˌmī-ō-ˈfī-brəl, -ˈfi-\ *n* : one of the longitudinal parallel contractile elements of a muscle cell that are composed of myosin and actin — **myo·fi·bril·lar** \-brə-lər\ *adj*

myo·fi·bro·blast \-ˈfī-brə-ˌblast, -ˈfi-\ *n* : a fibroblast that has developed some of the functional and structural characteristics (as the presence of myofilaments) of smooth muscle cells

myo·fil·a·ment \-ˈfi-lə-mənt\ *n* : one of the individual filaments of actin or myosin that make up a myofibril

myo·func·tion·al \-ˈfəŋk-shə-nəl\ *adj* : of, relating to, or concerned with muscle function esp. in the treatment of orthodontic problems

myo·gen·e·sis \ˌmī-ə-ˈje-nə-səs\ *n, pl* **-e·ses** \-ˌsēz\ : the development of muscle tissue

myo·gen·ic \ˌmī-ə-ˈje-nik\ *also* **my·og·e·nous** \mī-ˈä-jə-nəs\ *adj* **1** : originating in muscle ⟨~ pain⟩ **2** : taking place or functioning in ordered rhythmic fashion because of the inherent properties of cardiac muscle rather than specific neural stimuli ⟨a ~ heartbeat⟩ — compare NEUROGENIC 2b — **myo·ge·nic·i·ty** \-jə-ˈni-sə-tē\ *n*

myo·glo·bin \ˌmī-ə-ˈglō-bən, ˈmī-ə-ˌ\ *n* : a red iron-containing protein pigment in muscles that is similar to hemoglobin

myo·glo·bin·uria \-ˌglō-bi-ˈnu̇r-ē-ə, -ˈnyu̇r-\ *n* : the presence of myoglobin in the urine

myo·gram \ˈmī-ə-ˌgram\ *n* : a graphic representation of the phenomena (as intensity) of muscular contractions

myo·graph \-ˌgraf\ *n* : an apparatus for producing myograms

my·oid \ˈmī-ˌȯid\ *adj* : resembling muscle

myo·ino·si·tol \ˌmī-ō-i-ˈnō-sə-ˌtȯl, -ˌtōl\ *n* : a biologically active inositol that is a component of many phospholipids — called also *mesoinositol*

myo·in·ti·mal \-ˈin-tə-məl\ *adj* : of, relating to, or being the smooth muscle cells of the intima of a blood vessel

myom- *or* **myomo-** *comb form* : myoma ⟨*myom*ectomy⟩

my·o·ma \mī-ˈō-mə\ *n, pl* **-mas** *also* **-ma·ta** \-mə-tə\ : a tumor consisting of muscle tissue

myo·mec·to·my \ˌmī-ə-ˈmek-tə-mē\ *n, pl* **-mies** : surgical excision of a myoma or fibroid

myo·me·tri·tis \-mə-ˈtrī-təs\ *n* : inflammation of the uterine myometrium

myo·me·tri·um \ˌmī-ə-ˈmē-trē-əm\ *n* : the muscular layer of the wall of the uterus — **myo·me·tri·al** \-ˈmē-trē-əl\ *adj*

myo·ne·cro·sis \-nə-ˈkrō-səs, -ne-\ *n, pl* **-cro·ses** \-ˌsēz\ : necrosis of muscle

myo·neu·ral \ˌmī-ə-ˈnu̇r-əl, -ˈnyu̇r-\ *adj* : of, relating to, or connecting muscles and nerves ⟨~ effects⟩

myoneural junction *n* : NEUROMUSCULAR JUNCTION

myo·path·ic \ˌmī-ə-ˈpa-thik\ *adj* **1** : involving abnormality of the muscles ⟨~ syndrome⟩ **2** : of or relating to myopathy ⟨~ dystrophy⟩

my·op·a·thy \mī-ˈä-pə-thē\ *n, pl* **-thies** : a disorder of muscle tissue or muscles

my·ope \ˈmī-ˌōp\ *n* : a myopic person — called also *myopic*

myo·peri·car·di·tis \ˌmī-ō-ˌper-ə-ˌkär-ˈdī-təs\ *n, pl* **-dit·i·des** \-ˈdi-tə-ˌdēz\ : inflammation of both the myocardium and pericardium

my·o·pia \mī-ˈō-pē-ə\ *n* : a condition in which the visual images come to a focus in front of the retina of the eye because of defects in the refractive media of the eye or of abnormal length of the eyeball resulting esp. in defective vision of distant objects — called also *nearsightedness;* compare ASTIGMATISM 2, EMMETROPIA

[1]**my·o·pic** \-ˈō-pik, -ˈä-\ *adj* : affected by myopia : of, relating to, or exhibiting myopia — **my·o·pi·cal·ly** *adv*

[2]**myopic** *n* : MYOPE

myo·plasm \ˈmī-ə-ˌpla-zəm\ *n* : the contractile portion of muscle tissue — compare SARCOPLASM — **myo·plas·mic** \ˌmī-ə-ˈplaz-mik\ *adj*

[1]**myo·re·lax·ant** \ˌmī-ō-ri-ˈlak-sənt\ *n* : a drug that causes relaxation of muscle

[2]**myorelaxant** *adj* : relating to or causing relaxation of muscle ⟨~ effects⟩ — **myo·re·lax·ation** \-ˌrē-ˌlak-ˈsā-shən, -ri-ˌlak-\ *n*

myo·sar·co·ma \-sär-ˈkō-mə\ *n, pl* **-mas** *also* **-ma·ta** \-mə-tə\ : a sarcomatous myoma

my·o·sin \ˈmī-ə-sən\ *n* : a fibrous globulin of muscle that can split ATP and that reacts with actin to form actomyosin

myosis *var of* MIOSIS

myo·si·tis \ˌmī-ə-ˈsī-təs\ *n* : muscular discomfort or pain

myositis os·sif·i·cans \-ä-ˈsi-fə-ˌkanz\ *n* : myositis accompanied by ossification of muscle tissue or bony deposits in the muscles

myo·stat·in \ˌmī-ə-ˈsta-tᵊn\ *n* : a protein found mainly in skeletal muscle that is a transforming growth factor acting to restrain the growth of muscles

myo·tat·ic reflex \ˌmī-ə-ˈta-tik-\ *n* : STRETCH REFLEX

myotic *var of* MIOTIC

myo·tome \ˈmī-ə-ˌtōm\ *n* **1** : the portion of an embryonic somite from which skeletal musculature is produced **2** : an instrument for myotomy — **myo·to·mal** \ˌmī-ə-ˈtō-məl\ *adj*

my·ot·o·my \mī-ˈä-tə-mē\ *n, pl* **-mies** : incision or division of a muscle

myo•to•nia \ˌmī-ə-ˈtō-nē-ə\ *n* : tonic spasm of one or more muscles; *also* : a condition characterized by such spasms — **myo•ton•ic** \-ˈtä-nik\ *adj*

myotonia con•gen•i•ta \-kän-ˈje-nə-tə\ *n* : an inherited condition that is characterized by delay in the ability to relax muscles after forceful contractions but not by wasting of muscle — called also *Thomsen's disease*

myotonia dys•tro•phi•ca \-dis-ˈträ-fi-kə, -ˈtrō-\ *n* : MYOTONIC DYSTROPHY

myotonic dystrophy *n* : an inherited condition characterized by delay in the ability to relax muscles after forceful contraction, wasting of muscles, the formation of cataracts, premature baldness, atrophy of the gonads, endocrine and cardiac abnormalities, and often intellectual disability — abbr. *DM;* called also *myotonic muscular dystrophy*

my•ot•o•nus \mī-ˈä-tə-nəs\ *n* : sustained spasm of a muscle or muscle group

myo•tox•ic \ˌmī-ō-ˈtäk-sik\ *adj* : having or being a toxic effect on muscle — **myo•tox•ic•i•ty** \-täk-ˈsi-sə-tē\ *n*

myo•trop•ic \ˌmī-ə-ˈträ-pik, -ˈtrō-\ *adj* : affecting or tending to invade muscles ⟨a ~ infection⟩

myo•tube \ˈmī-ə-ˌtüb, -ˌtyüb\ *n* : a developmental stage of a muscle fiber

Myr•bet•riq \mir-ˈbe-trik\ *trademark* — used for a preparation of mirabegron

myring- *or* **myringo-** *comb form* : tympanic membrane ⟨*myringo*tomy⟩

my•rin•go•plas•ty \mə-ˈriŋ-gə-ˌplas-tē\ *n, pl* **-ties** : a surgical operation for the repair of perforations in the tympanic membrane

myr•in•got•o•my \ˌmir-ən-ˈgä-tə-mē\ *n, pl* **-mies** : incision of the tympanic membrane — called also *tympanotomy*

my•ris•tate \mi-ˈris-ˌtāt\ — see ISOPROPYL MYRISTATE

myx- *or* **myxo-** *comb form* **1** : mucus ⟨*myx*oma⟩ **2** : myxoma ⟨*myxo*sarcoma⟩

myx•ede•ma \ˌmik-sə-ˈdē-mə\ *n* : severe hypothyroidism characterized by firm inelastic edema, dry skin and hair, and loss of mental and physical vigor — **myx•ede•ma•tous** \-ˈde-mə-təs, -ˈdē-\ *adj*

myx•oid \ˈmik-ˌsȯid\ *adj* : resembling mucus

myx•o•ma \mik-ˈsō-mə\ *n, pl* **-mas** *also* **-ma•ta** \-mə-tə\ : a soft tumor made up of gelatinous connective tissue resembling that found in the umbilical cord — **myx•o•ma•tous** \-mə-təs\ *adj*

myx•o•ma•to•sis \ˌmik-ˌsō-mə-ˈtō-səs\ *n, pl* **-to•ses** \-ˌsēz\ : a condition characterized by the presence of myxomas in the body; *specif* : a severe disease of rabbits that is caused by a poxvirus (species *Myxoma virus* of the genus *Leporipoxvirus*), is transmitted by mosquitoes, biting flies, and direct contact, and has been used in the biological control of wild rabbit populations

myxo•sar•co•ma \-sär-ˈkō-mə\ *n, pl* **-mas** *also* **-ma•ta** \-mə-tə\ : a sarcoma with myxomatous elements

myxo•vi•rus \ˈmik-sə-ˌvī-rəs\ *n* : any of the viruses classified as orthomyxoviruses and paramyxoviruses that were formerly included in a single now rejected family (Myxoviridae) — **myxo•vi•ral** \ˌmik-sə-ˈvī-rəl\ *adj*

N

n \ˈen\ *n, pl* **n's** *or* **ns** \ˈenz\ : the haploid or gametic number of chromosomes — compare X

N *symbol* nitrogen — usu. italicized when used as a prefix ⟨*N*-allylnormorphine⟩

Na *symbol* sodium

NA *abbr* **1** Narcotics Anonymous **2** Nomina Anatomica **3** nurse's aide

na·bo·thi·an cyst \nə-ˈbō-thē-ən-\ *n* : a mucous gland of the uterine cervix esp. when occluded and dilated — called also *nabothian follicle*

Na·both \ˈnä-ˌbȯt\, **Martin (1675–1721),** German anatomist and physician.

NAD \ˌen-(ˌ)ā-ˈdē\ *n* : a coenzyme $C_{21}H_{27}N_7O_{14}P_2$ of numerous dehydrogenases that occurs in most cells and plays an important role in all phases of intermediary metabolism as an oxidizing agent or when in the reduced form as a reducing agent for various metabolites — called also *nicotinamide adenine dinucleotide, diphosphopyridine nucleotide*

NADH \ˌen-(ˌ)ā-(ˌ)dē-ˈāch\ *n* : the reduced form of NAD

na·do·lol \nā-ˈdō-ˌlȯl, -ˌlōl\ *n* : a beta-blocker $C_{17}H_{27}NO_4$ taken orally in the treatment of hypertension and angina pectoris

NADP \ˌen-(ˌ)ā-(ˌ)dē-ˈpē\ *n* : a coenzyme $C_{21}H_{28}N_7O_{17}P_3$ of numerous dehydrogenases (as that acting on glucose-6-phosphate) that occurs esp. in red blood cells and plays a role in intermediary metabolism similar to NAD but acting often on different metabolites — called also *nicotinamide adenine dinucleotide phosphate, TPN, triphosphopyridine nucleotide*

NADPH \ˌen-(ˌ)ā-(ˌ)dē-(ˌ)pē-ˈāch\ *n* : the reduced form of NADP

Nae·gle·ria \nā-ˈglir-ē-ə\ *n* : a genus of protozoans occurring esp. in stagnant water and including one (*N. fowleri*) causing meningoencephalitis

nae·void, nae·vus *chiefly Brit var of* NEVOID, NEVUS

naf·cil·lin \naf-ˈsi-lən\ *n* : a semisynthetic penicillin that is resistant to beta-lactamase and is used esp. in the form of its hydrated sodium salt $C_{21}H_{21}N_2NaO_5S{\cdot}H_2O$ as an antibiotic

naf·ox·i·dine \na-ˈfäk-sə-ˌdēn\ *n* : an antiestrogen administered in the form of its hydrochloride $C_{29}H_{31}NO_2{\cdot}HCl$

na·ga·na *also* **n'ga·na** \nə-ˈgä-nə\ *n* : a fatal disease of domestic animals in tropical Africa caused by a protozoan of the genus *Trypanosoma* and transmitted by tsetse and other biting flies; *broadly* : trypanosomiasis of domestic animals

nail \ˈnāl\ *n* **1** : a horny sheath of thickened and condensed epithelial stratum lucidum that grows out from a vascular matrix of dermis and protects the upper surface of the end of each finger and toe — called also *nail plate* **2** : a rod (as of metal) used to fix the parts of a broken bone in normal relation ⟨a medullary ~⟩

nail bed *n* : the vascular epidermis upon which most of the fingernail or toenail rests that has a longitudinally ridged surface often visible through the nail; *also* : MATRIX 1b

nail–biting *n* : habitual biting at the fingernails usu. being symptomatic of emotional tensions and frustrations

nail fold *n* : the fold of the dermis at the margin of a fingernail or toenail

nail·ing \ˈnā-liŋ\ *n* : the act or process of fixing the parts of a broken bone by means of a nail

nail matrix *n* : MATRIX 1b

nail plate *n* : NAIL 1

na·ive *or* **na·ïve** \nä-ˈēv\ *adj* **na·iv·er; -est** **1** : not previously subjected to experimentation or a particular experimental situation ⟨~ laboratory rats⟩ **2** : not having previously used a particular drug (as marijuana) **3** : not having been exposed previously to an antigen ⟨~ T cells⟩

Na·ja \ˈnā-jə\ *n* : a genus of elapid snakes comprising the true cobras

na·ked \ˈnā-kəd\ *adj* : lacking some natural external covering (as of hair or myelin) — used of the animal body or one of its parts ⟨~ nerve endings⟩

na·li·dix·ic acid \ˌnā-lə-ˈdik-sik-\ *n* : an antibacterial agent $C_{12}H_{12}N_2O_3$ that is used esp. in the treatment of genitourinary infections — see NEGGRAM

Nal·line \ˈna-ˌlēn\ *n* : a preparation of nalorphine — formerly a U.S. registered trademark

na·lor·phine \na-ˈlȯr-ˌfēn\ *n* : a white crystalline compound $C_{19}H_{21}NO_3$ that is derived from morphine and is used as a respiratory stimulant to counteract poisoning by morphine and similar narcotic drugs — called also *N-allylnormorphine*

nal·ox·one \na-ˈläk-ˌsōn, ˈna-lək-ˌsōn\ *n* : a potent antagonist of narcotic drugs (as morphine and fentanyl) that is used esp. in the form of its hydrochloride $C_{19}H_{21}NO_4{\cdot}HCl$ to treat opioid dependence or overdose— see BUNAVAIL, EVZIO, NARCAN, SUBOXONE, ZUBSOLV

nal·trex·one \nal-ˈtrek-ˌsōn\ *n* : a synthetic opiate antagonist used in the form of its hydrochloride $C_{20}H_{23}NO_4{\cdot}HCl$ esp. to maintain detoxified opiate addicts in a drug-free state

Na·men·da \nə-ˈmen-də\ *trademark* — used for a preparation of memantine

Nam·zar·ic \nam-ˈzer-ik\ *trademark* — used for a preparation of memantine and donepezil

nan- *or* **nano-** *comb form* : dwarf ⟨*nano*cephalic⟩

nan•dro•lone \ˈnan-drə-ˌlōn\ *n* : a semisynthetic anabolic steroid $C_{18}H_{26}O_2$ derived from testosterone that is used in the form of its ester derivatives medically esp. to treat anemia associated with kidney disease and illicitly (as by athletes and bodybuilders) to build muscle mass — called also *19-nortestosterone*

na•nism \ˈna-ˌni-zəm, ˈnā-\ *n* : the condition of being abnormally or exceptionally small in stature : DWARFISM

nano- *comb form* : one billionth (10^{-9}) part of ⟨*nano*second⟩

nano•ce•phal•ic \ˌna-nō-si-ˈfa-lik\ *adj* : having an abnormally small head

nano•cu•rie \ˈna-nō-ˌkyu̇r-ē, -kyu̇-ˌrē\ *n* : one billionth of a curie

nano•gram \-ˌgram\ *n* : one billionth of a gram — abbr. *ng*

nano•me•ter \-ˌmē-tər\ *n* : one billionth of a meter — abbr. *nm*

nano•sec•ond \-ˌse-kənd, -kənt\ *n* : one billionth of a second — abbr. *ns, nsec*

nape \ˈnāp, ˈnap\ *n* : the back of the neck

na•phaz•o•line \nə-ˈfa-zə-ˌlēn\ *n* : a base used topically in the form of its hydrochloride $C_{14}H_{14}N_2{\cdot}HCl$ esp. to relieve nasal congestion and itching and redness of the eyes

naphthoate — see PAMAQUINE NAPHTHOATE

naph•tho•qui•none *also* **naph•tha•qui•none** \ˌnaf-thə-kwi-ˈnōn, -ˈkwi-ˌnōn\ *n* : any of three isomeric yellow to red crystalline compounds $C_{10}H_6O_2$; *esp* : one that occurs naturally in the form of derivatives (as vitamin K)

naph•thyl•amine \naf-ˈthi-lə-ˌmēn\ *n* : either of two isomeric crystalline bases $C_{10}H_9N$ that are used esp. in synthesizing dyes; *esp* : one (**β–naphthylamine**) with the amino group in the beta position that has been demonstrated to cause bladder cancer in individuals exposed to it while working in the dye industry

nap•kin \ˈnap-kən\ *n* : SANITARY NAPKIN

nap•ra•path \ˈna-prə-ˌpath\ *n* : a practitioner of naprapathy

na•prap•a•thy \nə-ˈpra-pə-thē\ *n, pl* **-thies** : a system of treatment by manipulation of connective tissue and adjoining structures (as ligaments, joints, and muscles) and by dietary measures that is held to facilitate the recuperative and regenerative processes of the body

Na•pro•syn \nə-ˈprōs-ᵊn\ *trademark* — used for a preparation of naproxen

na•prox•en \nə-ˈpräk-sᵊn\ *n* : an anti-inflammatory analgesic antipyretic drug $C_{14}H_{14}O_3$ used esp. to treat arthritis often in the form of its sodium salt $C_{14}H_{13}NaO_3$ — see ALEVE, NAPROSYN

nap•syl•ate \ˈnap-sə-ˌlāt\ *n* : a salt of either of two crystalline acids $C_{10}H_7SO_3H$

Naqua \ˈna-kwə\ *trademark* — used for a preparation of trichlormethiazide

nar•a•trip•tan \ˌner-ə-ˈtrip-ˌtan, -tən\ *n* : a triptan taken orally in the form of its hydrochloride $C_{17}H_{25}N_3O_2S{\cdot}HCl$ to treat migraine attacks — see AMERGE

narc- *or* **narco-** *comb form* **1** : numbness : stupor ⟨*narc*osis⟩ **2** : deep sleep ⟨*narco*lepsy⟩

Nar•can \ˈnär-ˌkan\ *trademark* — used for a preparation of naloxone

nar•cis•sism \ˈnär-sə-ˌsi-zəm\ *n* **1** : NARCISSISTIC PERSONALITY DISORDER **2** : love of or sexual desire for one's own body **3** : the state or stage of development in psychoanalytic theory in which there is considerable erotic interest in one's own body and ego and which in abnormal forms persists through fixation or reappears through regression — **nar•cis•sist** \-sist\ *n* — **nar•cis•sis•tic** \ˌnär-sə-ˈsis-tik\ *adj*

narcissistic personality disorder *n* : a personality disorder characterized esp. by an exaggerated sense of self-importance, persistent need for admiration, lack of empathy for others, excessive pride in achievements, and snobbish, disdainful, or patronizing attitudes

nar•co•anal•y•sis \ˌnär-kō-ə-ˈna-lə-səs\ *n, pl* **-y•ses** \-ˌsēz\ : psychotherapy that is performed under sedation for the recovery of repressed memories together with the emotion accompanying the experience

nar•co•lep•sy \ˈnär-kə-ˌlep-sē\ *n, pl* **-sies** : a condition characterized by brief attacks of deep sleep often occurring with cataplexy and hypnagogic hallucinations — compare HYPERSOMNIA 2

[1]**nar•co•lep•tic** \ˌnär-kə-ˈlep-tik\ *adj* : of, relating to, or affected with narcolepsy

[2]**narcoleptic** *n* : an individual who is subject to attacks of narcolepsy

nar•co•sis \när-ˈkō-səs\ *n, pl* **-co•ses** \-ˌsēz\ : a state of stupor, unconsciousness, or arrested activity produced by the influence of narcotics or other chemicals or physical agents — see NITROGEN NARCOSIS

nar•co•syn•the•sis \ˌnär-kō-ˈsin-thə-səs\ *n, pl* **-the•ses** \-ˌsēz\ : NARCOANALYSIS

[1]**nar•cot•ic** \när-ˈkä-tik\ *n* **1** : a drug (as codeine, methadone, or morphine) that in moderate doses dulls the senses, relieves pain, and induces profound sleep but in excessive doses causes stupor, coma, or convulsions **2** : a drug (as marijuana or LSD) subject to restriction similar to that of addictive narcotics whether physiologically addictive and narcotic or not

[2]**narcotic** *adj* **1** : having the properties of or yielding a narcotic **2** : of, induced by, or concerned with narcotics **3** : of, involving, or intended for narcotic addicts

nar•co•ti•za•tion \ˌnär-kə-tə-ˈzā-shən\ *n* : the act or process of inducing narcosis

nar•co•tize \ˈnär-kə-ˌtīz\ *vb* **-tized; -tiz•ing** **1** : to treat with or subject to a narcotic **2** : to put into a state of narcosis

Nar•dil \ˈnär-ˌdil\ *trademark* — used for a preparation of phenelzine

na•ris \ˈnar-əs\ *n, pl* **na•res** \-ˌēz\ : either of the pair of openings of the nose

narrow–angle glaucoma *n* : ANGLE-CLOSURE GLAUCOMA

narrow–spectrum *adj* : effective against only a limited range of organisms — compare BROAD-SPECTRUM

nas- *or* **naso-** *also* **nasi-** *comb form* **1** : nose : nasal ⟨*naso*pharyngoscope⟩ **2** : nasal and ⟨*naso*tracheal⟩

Na•sa•cort \ˈnā-zə-ˌkȯrt\ *trademark* — used for a preparation of triamcinolone

¹na•sal \ˈnā-zəl\ *n* : a nasal part (as a bone)

²nasal *adj* : of or relating to the nose — **na•sal•ly** *adv*

nasal bone *n* : either of two bones of the skull of vertebrates above the fishes that lie in front of the frontal bones and in humans are oblong in shape forming by their junction the bridge of the nose and partly covering the nasal cavity

nasal cavity *n* : the vaulted chamber that lies between the floor of the cranium and the roof of the mouth extending from the external nares to the pharynx, being enclosed by bone or cartilage and usu. incompletely divided into lateral halves by the septum of the nose, and having its walls lined with mucous membrane that is rich in venous plexuses and ciliated in the lower part which forms the beginning of the respiratory passage and warms and filters the inhaled air and that is modified as sensory epithelium in the upper olfactory part

nasal concha *n* : any of three thin bony plates on the lateral wall of the nasal fossa on each side with or without their covering of mucous membrane: **a** : a separate curved bony plate that is the largest of the three and separates the inferior and middle meatuses of the nose — called also *inferior concha, inferior nasal concha, inferior turbinate, inferior turbinate bone* **b** : the lower of two thin bony processes of the ethmoid bone on the lateral wall of each nasal fossa that separates the superior and middle meatuses of the nose — called also *middle concha, middle nasal concha, middle turbinate, middle turbinate bone* **c** : the upper of two thin bony processes of the ethmoid bone on the lateral wall of each nasal fossa that forms the upper boundary of the superior meatus of the nose — called also *superior concha, superior nasal concha, superior turbinate, superior turbinate bone*

nasal fossa *n* : either lateral half of the nasal cavity

na•sa•lis \nā-ˈzā-ləs, -ˈsā-\ *n* : a small muscle on each side of the nose that constricts the nasal aperture

nasal nerve *n* : NASOCILIARY NERVE

nasal notch *n* : the rough surface on the anterior lower border of the frontal bone between the orbits which articulates with the nasal bones and the maxillae

nasal process *n* : FRONTAL PROCESS 1

nasal septum *n* : the bony and cartilaginous partition between the nasal passages

nasal spine *n* : any of several median bony processes adjacent to the nasal passages: as **a** : ANTERIOR NASAL SPINE **b** : POSTERIOR NASAL SPINE

nasi — see ALA NASI, LEVATOR LABII SUPERIORIS ALAEQUE NASI

nasi- — see NAS-

na•si•on \ˈnā-zē-ˌän\ *n* : the middle point of the nasofrontal suture

naso- — see NAS-

na•so•al•ve•o•lar \ˌnā-zō-al-ˈvē-ə-lər\ *adj* : of, relating to, or affecting the nose and one or more maxillary alveoli ⟨a ~ cyst⟩

na•so•cil•i•ary \ˌnā-zō-ˈsi-lē-ˌer-ē\ *adj* : nasal and ciliary

nasociliary nerve *n* : a branch of the ophthalmic nerve distributed in part to the ciliary ganglion and in part to the mucous membrane and skin of the nose — called also *nasal nerve*

na•so•fron•tal \-ˈfrənt-ᵊl\ *adj* : of or relating to the nasal and frontal bones

nasofrontal suture *n* : the cranial suture between the nasal and frontal bones

na•so•gas•tric \-ˈgas-trik\ *adj* : of, relating to, being, or performed by intubation of the stomach by way of the nasal passages ⟨insert a ~ tube⟩

na•so•la•bi•al \-ˈlā-bē-əl\ *adj* : of, relating to, located between, or affecting the nose and the upper lip

na•so•lac•ri•mal *also* **na•so•lach•ry•mal** \-ˈla-krə-məl\ *adj* : of or relating to the lacrimal apparatus and nose

nasolacrimal duct *n* : a duct that transmits tears from the lacrimal sac to the inferior meatus of the nose

na•so•max•il•lary \-ˈmak-sə-ˌler-ē\ *adj* : of, relating to, or located between the nasal bone and the maxilla

Na•so•nex \ˈnā-zə-ˌneks\ *trademark* — used for a preparation of mometasone used intranasally

na•so•pal•a•tine \-ˈpa-lə-ˌtīn\ *adj* : of, relating to, or connecting the nose and the palate

nasopalatine nerve *n* : a parasympathetic and sensory nerve that arises in the pterygopalatine ganglion, passes through the sphenopalatine foramen, across the roof of the nasal cavity to the nasal septum, and obliquely downward to and through the incisive canal, and innervates esp. the glands and mucosa of the nasal septum and the anterior part of the hard palate

na•so•pha•ryn•geal \ˌnā-zō-fə-ˈrin-jəl, -jē-əl; -ˌfar-ən-ˈjē-əl\ *adj* : of, relating to, or affecting the nose and pharynx or the nasopharynx ⟨~ cancer⟩

nasopharyngeal tonsil *n* : PHARYNGEAL TONSIL

na•so•pha•ryn•go•scope \-fə-ˈriŋ-gə-ˌskōp\ *n* : an endoscope for visually examining the nasal passages and pharynx — **na•so•pha•ryn•go•scop•ic** \-fə-ˌriŋ-gə-ˈskä-pik\ *adj* — **na•so•phar•yn•gos•co•py** \-ˌfar-ən-ˈgäs-kə-pē\ *n*

na•so•phar•ynx \-ˈfar-iŋks\ *n, pl* **-pha•ryn•ges** \-fə-ˈrin-(ˌ)jēz\ *also* **-phar•ynx•es** : the upper part of the pharynx continuous with the nasal passages — compare LARYNGOPHARYNX

na•so•tra•che•al \-ˈtrā-kē-əl\ *adj* : of, relating to, being, or performed by means of intubation of the trachea by way of the nasal passage

na•tal \ˈnāt-ᵊl\ *adj* : of or relating to birth ⟨the ~ death rate⟩

na•tal•i•ty \nā-ˈta-lə-tē, nə-\ *n, pl* **-ties** : BIRTHRATE

na•tes \ˈnā-ˌtēz\ *n pl* : BUTTOCKS

National Formulary *n* : a periodically revised book of officially established and recognized drug names and standards — abbr. *NF*

na•tri•ure•sis \ˌnā-trē-yu̇-ˈrē-səs\ *n* : excessive loss of cations and esp. sodium in the urine — **na•tri•uret•ic** \-ˈre-tik\ *adj or n*

natural childbirth *n* : a system of managing childbirth in which the mother receives preparatory education in order to remain conscious during and assist in delivery with minimal or no use of drugs or anesthetics

natural family planning *n* : a method of birth control that involves abstention from sexual intercourse during the period of ovulation which is determined through observation and measurement of bodily signs (as cervical mucus and body temperature)

natural food *n* : food that has undergone minimal processing and contains no preservatives or artificial additives (as synthetic flavorings)

natural history *n* : the natural development of something (as an organism or disease) over a period of time

natural immunity *n* : INNATE IMMUNITY

natural killer cell *n* : a large granular lymphocyte capable esp. of destroying tumor cells or virally infected cells without prior exposure to the target cell and without having it presented with or marked by a histocompatibility antigen — called also *NK cell*

na•tu•ro•path \ˈnā-chə-rə-ˌpath, nə-ˈtyu̇r-ə-\ *n* : a practitioner of naturopathy

na•tu•rop•a•thy \ˌnā-chə-ˈrä-pə-thē\ *n, pl* **-thies** : a system of treatment of disease that avoids drugs and surgery and emphasizes the use of natural agents (as air, water, and herbs) and physical means (as tissue manipulation and electrotherapy) — **na•tu•ro•path•ic** \ˌnā-chə-rə-ˈpa-thik, nə-ˌtyu̇r-ə-\ *adj*

nau•sea \ˈnȯ-zē-ə, -sē-ə; ˈnȯ-zhə, -shə\ *n* : a stomach distress with distaste for food and an urge to vomit

nau•se•ant \ˈnȯ-zhənt, -zhē-ənt, -shənt, -shē-ənt\ *adj* : inducing nausea : NAUSEATING

nau•se•ate \ˈnȯ-zē-ˌāt, -zhē-, -sē-, -shē-\ *vb* **-at•ed; -at•ing** : to affect or become affected with nausea

nau•seous \ˈnȯ-shəs, ˈnȯ-zē-əs\ *adj* **1** : causing nausea **2** : affected with nausea

Nav•ane \ˈna-ˌvān\ *trademark* — used for a preparation of thiothixene

na•vel \ˈnā-vəl\ *n* : a depression in the middle of the abdomen that marks the point of former attachment of the umbilical cord to the embryo — called also *umbilicus*

navel ill *n* : a serious septicemia of newborn animals caused by pus-producing bacteria entering the body through the umbilical cord or opening — called also *joint ill*

[1]**na•vic•u•lar** \nə-ˈvi-kyə-lər\ *n* : a boat-shaped bone: **a** : the one of the seven tarsal bones of the human foot that is situated on the big-toe side between the talus and the cuneiform bones — called also *scaphoid* **b** : SCAPHOID 2

[2]**navicular** *adj* **1** : resembling or having the shape of a boat ⟨~ cells⟩ **2** : of, relating to, or involving a navicular bone ⟨~ fractures⟩

navicular disease *n* : inflammation of the navicular bone and forefoot of the horse

navicular fossa *n* : the dilated terminal portion of the urethra in the glans penis

navicularis — see FOSSA NAVICULARIS

Nb *symbol* niobium

NBRT *abbr* National Board for Respiratory Therapy

NCI *abbr* National Cancer Institute

Nd *symbol* neodymium

ND *abbr* doctor of naturopathy

NDT *abbr* neurodevelopmental treatment

Ne *symbol* neon

ne- *or* **neo-** *comb form* **1 a** : new : recent ⟨*neo*natal⟩ **b** : chemically new — used for compounds isomeric with or otherwise related to an indicated compound ⟨*neo*stigmine⟩ **2** : new and abnormal ⟨*neo*plasm⟩

near point *n* : the point nearest the eye at which an object is accurately focused on the retina when the maximum degree of accommodation is employed — compare FAR POINT

near•sight•ed \ˈnir-ˌsī-təd\ *adj* : able to see near things more clearly than distant ones : MYOPIC — **near•sight•ed•ly** *adv*

near•sight•ed•ness *n* : MYOPIA

ne•biv•o•lol \ne-ˈbiv-ə-ˌlȯl\ *n* : a beta-blocker $C_{22}H_{25}F_2NO_4{\cdot}HCl$ used orally to treat high blood pressure — see BYSTOLIC

neb•u•li•za•tion \ˌne-byə-lə-ˈzā-shən\ *n* **1** : reduction of a medicinal solution to a fine spray **2** : treatment (as of asthma) by means of a fine spray — **neb•u•lize** \ˈne-byə-ˌlīz\ *vb*

neb•u•liz•er \-ˌlī-zər\ *n* : ATOMIZER; *specif* : an atomizer equipped to produce an extremely fine spray for deep penetration of the lungs

Ne•ca•tor \nə-ˈkā-tər\ *n* : a genus of hookworms including internal parasites of humans

neck \ˈnek\ *n* **1 a** : the usu. narrowed part of an animal that connects the head with the body; *specif* : the cervical region of a vertebrate **b** : the part of a tapeworm immediately behind the scolex from which new proglottids are produced **2** : a relatively narrow part suggestive of a neck: as **a** : a narrow part of a bone ⟨the ~ of the femur⟩ **b** : CERVIX 2 **c** : the part of a tooth between the crown and the root

necr- *or* **necro-** *comb form* **1 a** : those that are dead : the dead : corpses ⟨*necro*philia⟩ **b** : one that is dead : corpse ⟨*necro*psy⟩ **2** : death : conversion to dead tissue : atrophy ⟨*necro*sis⟩

nec•ro \ˈne-(ˌ)krō\ *n* : NECROTIC ENTERITIS a

nec•ro•bac•il•lo•sis \ˌne-krō-ˌba-sə-ˈlō-səs\ *n, pl* **-lo•ses** \-ˌsēz\ : a disease or infection (as bullnose or calf diphtheria) that is marked by inflammation and lesions and is caused by or associated with a bacterium of the genus *Fusobacterium* (*F. necrophorum*)

nec•ro•bi•o•sis \-bī-ˈō-səs\ *n, pl* **-o•ses** \-ˌsēz\ : death of a cell or group of cells within a tissue whether normal (as in various epithelial tissues) or part of a pathologic process — compare NECROSIS

necrobiosis li•poid•i•ca \-li-ˈpȯi-di-kə\ *n* : a disease of the skin that is characterized by the formation of multiple necrobiotic lesions esp. on the legs and that is often associated with diabetes mellitus

necrobiosis lipoidica dia•bet•i•co•rum \-ˌdī-ə-ˌbe-ti-ˈkȯr-əm\ *n* : NECROBIOSIS LIPOIDICA

nec•ro•bi•ot•ic \ˌne-krə-bī-ˈä-tik\ *adj* : of, relating to, or being in a state of necrobiosis

nec•ro•phile \ˈne-krə-ˌfīl\ *n* : one that is affected with necrophilia

nec•ro•phil•ia \ˌne-krə-ˈfi-lē-ə\ *n* : obsession with and usu. erotic interest in or stimulation by corpses

[1]**nec•ro•phil•i•ac** \-ˈfi-lē-ˌak\ *adj* : of, relating to, or affected with necrophilia

[2]**necrophiliac** *n* : NECROPHILE

nec•ro•phil•ic \-ˈfi-lik\ *adj* : NECROPHILIAC

[1]**nec•rop•sy** \ˈne-ˌkräp-sē\ *n, pl* **-sies** : AUTOPSY; *esp* : an autopsy performed on an animal

[2]**necropsy** *vb* **-sied; -sy•ing** : AUTOPSY

nec•rose \ˈne-ˌkrōs, -ˌkrōz, ne-ˈkrōz\ *vb* **nec•rosed; nec•ros•ing** : to undergo or cause to undergo necrosis

ne•cro•sis \nə-ˈkrō-sis, ne-\ *n, pl* **ne•cro•ses** \-ˌsēz\ : death of living tissue; *specif* : death of a portion of tissue differentially affected by local injury (as loss of blood supply, corrosion, burning, or the local lesion of a disease) — compare *necrobiosis*

nec•ro•sper•mia \ˌne-krə-ˈspər-mē-ə\ *n* : a condition in which the spermatozoa in seminal fluid are dead or motionless

ne•crot•ic \nə-ˈkrä-tik, ne-\ *adj* : affected with, characterized by, or producing necrosis ⟨a ~ gall bladder⟩

necrotic enteritis *n* : either of two often fatal infectious diseases marked esp. by intestinal inflammation and necrosis and by diarrhea: **a** : one affecting young swine and caused by a bacterium of the genus *Salmonella* (*S. choleraesuis*) — called also *necro* **b** : one affecting poultry and caused by a bacterium of the genus *Clostridium* (*C. perfringens*)

necrotic rhinitis *n* : BULLNOSE

nec•ro•tiz•ing \ˈne-krə-ˌtī-ziŋ\ *adj* : causing, associated with, or undergoing necrosis ⟨~ infections⟩

necrotizing angiitis *n* : NECROTIZING VASCULITIS

necrotizing fasciitis *n* : a severe infection of soft tissue that is caused by bacteria (as Group A streptococci or MRSA), that is marked by edema and necrosis of subcutaneous tissue with involvement of adjacent fascia and by painful red swollen skin over affected areas, and that usu. occurs as a complication of surgery, injury, or infection

necrotizing papillitis *n* : necrosis of the papillae of the kidney — called also *necrotizing renal papillitis*

necrotizing ulcerative gingivitis *n* : ACUTE NECROTIZING ULCERATIVE GINGIVITIS

necrotizing vasculitis *n* : an inflammatory condition of the blood vessels characterized by necrosis of vascular tissue — called also *necrotizing angiitis, systemic necrotizing vasculitis*

NED *abbr* no evidence of disease

ne•do•cro•mil \nə-ˈdä-krə-mil\ *n* : a disodium salt $C_{19}H_{15}NNa_2O_7$ that is administered as eye drops for the treatment of itching associated with allergic conjunctivitis and formerly as an aerosol for oral inhalation in the treatment of asthma — called also *nedocromil sodium*

[1]**nee•dle** \ˈnēd-ᵊl\ *n* **1** : a small slender usu. steel instrument designed to carry sutures when sewing tissues in surgery **2** : a slender hollow instrument for introducing material into or removing material from the body parenterally

[2]**needle** *vb* **nee•dled; nee•dling** : to puncture, operate on, or inject with a needle

needle biopsy *n* : any of several methods (as fine needle aspiration or core biopsy) for obtaining a sample of cells or tissue by inserting a hollow needle through the skin and withdrawing the sample from the tissue or organ to be examined

nee•dle•stick \ˈnēd-ᵊl-ˌstik\ *n* : an accidental puncture of the skin with an unsterile instrument (as a syringe) — called also *needlestick injury*

neg•a•tive \ˈne-gə-tiv\ *adj* **1** : marked by denial, prohibition, or refusal **2** : marked by features (as hostility or pessimism) that hinder or oppose constructive treatment or development **3** : being, relating to, or charged with electricity of which the electron is the elementary unit **4** : not affirming the presence of a condition, substance, or organism suspected to be present; *also* : having a test result indicating the absence esp. of a condition, substance, or organism ⟨she is HIV ~⟩ — **negative** *n* — **neg•a•tive•ly** *adv* — **neg•a•tiv•i•ty** \ˌne-gə-ˈti-və-tē\ *n*

negative feedback *n* : feedback that tends to stabilize a process by reducing its rate or output when its effects are too great

negative pressure *n* : pressure that is less than existing atmospheric pressure

negative reinforcement *n* : psychological reinforcement by removal of an unpleasant stimulus when a desired response occurs

negative transfer *n* : the impeding of learning or performance in a situation by the carry-over of learned responses from another situation — compare INTERFERENCE 2

neg•a•tiv•ism \ˈne-gə-ti-ˌvi-zəm\ *n* **1** : an attitude of mind marked by skepticism about nearly everything affirmed by others **2** : a tendency to refuse to do, to do the opposite of, or to do something at variance with what is asked — **neg•a•tiv•ist•ic** \ˌne-gə-ti-ˈvis-tik\ *adj*

Neg•Gram \ˈneg-ˌgram\ *trademark* — used for a preparation of nalidixic acid

Ne•gri body \ˈnā-grē-\ *n* : an inclusion body found in the nerve cells in rabies

Negri, Adelchi (1876–1912), Italian physician and pathologist.

Neis•se•ria \nī-ˈsir-ē-ə\ *n* : a genus (family Neisseriaceae) of parasitic bacteria that grow in pairs and occas. tetrads and include the gonococcus (*N. gonorrhoeae*) and meningococcus (*N. meningitidis*)

Neis•ser \ˈnī-sər\, **Albert Ludwig Sigesmund (1855–1916),** German dermatologist.

neis•se•ri•an \nī-ˈsir-ē-ən\ *or* **neis•se•ri•al** \-ē-əl\ *adj* : of, relating to, or caused by bacteria of the genus *Neisseria* ⟨~ infections⟩

nel•fin•a•vir \nel-ˈfi-nə-ˌvir\ *n* : a protease inhibitor that is administered in the form of its mesylate $C_{32}H_{45}N_3O_4S·CH_4O_3S$ in the treatment of HIV infection — see VIRACEPT

nemat- *or* **nemato-** *comb form* **1** : thread ⟨*nemato*cyst⟩ **2** : nematode ⟨*nemato*logy⟩

ne•ma•to•cide *or* **ne•ma•ti•cide** \ˈne-mə-tə-ˌsīd, ni-ˈma-tə-\ *n* : a substance or preparation used to destroy nematodes — **ne•ma•to•cid•al** *also* **ne•ma•ti•cid•al** \ˌne-mə-tə-ˈsīd-ᵊl, ni-ˌma-tə-\ *adj*

ne•ma•to•cyst \ˈne-mə-tə-ˌsist, ni-ˈma-tə-\ *n* : one of the minute stinging organelles of various coelenterates

nem•a•tode \ˈne-mə-ˌtōd\ *n* : any of a phylum (Nematoda) of elongated cylindrical worms parasitic in animals or plants or free-living in soil or water

Nem•a•to•di•rus \ˌne-mə-tə-ˈdī-rəs\ *n* : a genus of reddish strongylid nematode worms parasitic in the small intestine esp. of ruminants

nem•a•tol•o•gy \ˌne-mə-ˈtä-lə-jē\ *n, pl* **-gies** : a branch of zoology that deals with nematodes — **nem•a•tol•o•gist** \-jist\ *n*

Nem•bu•tal \ˈnem-byə-ˌtȯl\ *trademark* — used for the sodium salt of pentobarbital

neo- — see NE-

neo•ars•phen•a•mine \ˌnē-ō-ärs-ˈfe-nə-ˌmēn\ *n* : a yellow powder $C_{13}H_{13}As_2N_2NaO_4S$ similar to arsphenamine in structure and use — called also *neosalvarsan*

neo•cer•e•bel•lum \ˌnē-ō-ˌser-ə-ˈbe-ləm\ *n, pl* **-bellums** *or* **-bel•la** : the part of the cerebellum associated with the cerebral cortex in the integration of voluntary limb movements and comprising most of the cerebellar hemispheres and the superior vermis — compare PALEOCEREBELLUM — **neo•cer•e•bel•lar** \ˌnē-ō-ˌser-ə-ˈbel-ər\ *adj*

neo•cin•cho•phen \ˌnē-ō-ˈsiŋ-kə-ˌfen\ *n* : a white crystalline compound $C_{19}H_{17}NO_2$ used as an analgesic and in the treatment of gout

neo•cor•tex \ˌnē-ō-ˈkȯr-ˌteks\ *n, pl* **-cor•ti•ces** \-ˈkȯr-tə-ˌsēz\ *or* **-cortexes** : the dorsal region of the cerebral cortex that is unique to mammals — **neo•cor•ti•cal** \-ˈkȯr-ti-kəl\ *adj*

neo•dym•i•um \ˌnē-ō-ˈdi-mē-əm\ *n* : a yellow metallic element — symbol *Nd;* see ELEMENT table

[1]**neo–Freud•ian** \-ˈfrȯi-dē-ən\ *adj, often cap N* : of or relating to a school of psychoanalysis that differs from Freudian orthodoxy in emphasizing the importance of social and cultural factors in the development of an individual's personality

S. Freud — see FREUDIAN

[2]**neo–Freudian** *n, often cap N* : a member of or advocate of a neo-Freudian school of psychoanalysis

neo•in•ti•ma \-ˈin-tə-mə\ *n* : a new or thickened layer of arterial intima formed esp. on a prosthesis or in atherosclerosis by migration and proliferation of cells from the media — **neo·in·ti·mal** \-məl\ *adj*

ne·ol·o·gism \nē-ˈä-lə-ˌji-zəm\ *n* : a new word that is coined esp. by a person affected with schizophrenia, is meaningless except to the coiner, and is typically a combination of two existing words or a shortening or distortion of an existing word

neo·my·cin \ˌnē-ə-ˈmīs-ᵊn\ *n* : a broad-spectrum highly toxic mixture of antibiotics produced by a bacterium of the genus *Streptomyces* (*S. fradiae*) and used esp. to treat topical infections

ne·on \ˈnē-ˌän\ *n* : a colorless odorless primarily inert gaseous element — symbol *Ne;* see ELEMENT table

neo·na·tal \ˌnē-ō-ˈnāt-ᵊl\ *adj* : of, relating to, or affecting the newborn and esp. the human infant during the first month after birth — compare PRENATAL, POSTNATAL — **neo·na·tal·ly** *adv*

ne·o·nate \ˈnē-ə-ˌnāt\ *n* : a newborn infant; *esp* : an infant less than a month old

neo·na·tol·o·gist \ˌnē-ə-nā-ˈtä-lə-jist\ *n* : a specialist in neonatology

neo·na·tol·o·gy \-jē\ *n, pl* **-gies** : a branch of medicine concerned with the care, development, and diseases of newborn infants

neonatorum — see ICTERUS GRAVIS NEONATORUM, ICTERUS NEONATORUM, OPHTHALMIA NEONATORUM, SCLEREMA NEONATORUM

neo·pal·li·um \ˌnē-ō-ˈpa-lē-əm\ *n, pl* **-lia** \-lē-ə\ : the part of the cerebral cortex that develops from the area between the piriform lobe and the hippocampus, comprises the nonolfactory region of the cortex, and attains its maximum development in humans where it makes up the greater part of the cerebral hemisphere on each side — compare ARCHIPALLIUM

neo·pho·bia \ˌnē-ə-ˈfō-bē-ə\ *n* : dread of or aversion to novelty

neo·pla·sia \ˌnē-ə-ˈplā-zhə, -zhē-ə\ *n* **1** : the process of tumor formation **2** : a tumorous condition of the body — see PROSTATIC INTRAEPITHELIAL NEOPLASIA

neo·plasm \ˈnē-ə-ˌpla-zəm\ *n* : a new growth of tissue serving no physiological function : TUMOR

neo·plas·tic \ˌnē-ə-ˈplas-tik\ *adj* : of, relating to, or constituting a neoplasm or neoplasia — **neo·plas·ti·cal·ly** *adv*

Ne·or·al \nē-ˈȯr-əl\ *trademark* — used for a preparation of cyclosporine

neo·sal·var·san \ˌnē-ō-ˈsal-vər-ˌsan\ *n* : NEOARSPHENAMINE

neo·stig·mine \ˌnē-ə-ˈstig-ˌmēn\ *n* : an anticholinergic drug that is used in the form of its bromide $C_{12}H_{19}BrN_2O_2$ or a sulfate derivative $C_{13}H_{22}N_2O_6S$ esp. in the diagnosis and treatment of myasthenia gravis and in the treatment of urinary bladder or bowel atony — see PROSTIGMIN

neo·stri·a·tum \ˌnē-ō-(ˌ)strī-ˈā-təm\ *n, pl* **-tums** *or* **-ta** \-tə\ : the part of the corpus striatum consisting of the caudate nucleus and putamen — **neo·stri·a·tal** \-ˈāt-ᵊl\ *adj*

Neo–Sy·neph·rine \ˌnē-ō-si-ˈne-frən, -ˌfrēn\ *trademark* — used for a preparation of the hydrochloride of phenylephrine

neo·vas·cu·lar·i·za·tion \-ˌvas-kyə-lə-rə-ˈzā-shən\ *n* : vascularization esp. in abnormal quantity (as in some conditions of the retina) or in abnormal tissue (as a tumor) — **neo·vas·cu·lar** \ˌnē-ō-ˈvas-kyə-lər\ *adj* — **neo·vas·cu·lar·i·ty** \-ˌvas-kyə-ˈlar-ə-tē\ *n*

neph·e·lom·e·ter \ˌne-fə-ˈlä-mə-tər\ *n* : an instrument for measuring turbidity (as to determine the number of bacteria suspended in a fluid) — **neph·e·lo·met·ric** \ˌne-fə-lō-ˈme-trik\ *adj* — **neph·e·lom·e·try** \-ˈläm-ə-trē\ *n*

nephr- *or* **nephro-** *comb form* : kidney ⟨*nephr*ectomy⟩ ⟨*nephro*logy⟩

ne·phrec·to·my \ni-ˈfrek-tə-mē\ *n, pl* **-mies** : the surgical removal of a kidney — **ne·phrec·to·mize** \-ˌmīz\ *vb*

neph·ric \ˈne-frik\ *adj* : RENAL

ne·phrit·ic \ni-ˈfri-tik\ *adj* **1** : RENAL **2** : of, relating to, or affected with nephritis

ne·phri·tis \ni-ˈfrī-təs\ *n, pl* **ne·phrit·i·des** \-ˈfri-tə-ˌdēz\ : acute or chronic inflammation of the kidney affecting the structure (as of the glomerulus or parenchyma) and caused by infection, a degenerative process, or vascular disease — compare NEPHROSCLEROSIS, NEPHROSIS

neph·ri·to·gen·ic \ˌne-frə-tə-ˈje-nik, ni-ˌfri-tə-\ *adj* : causing nephritis

neph·ro·blas·to·ma \ˌne-frō-blas-ˈtō-mə\ *n, pl* **-mas** *also* **-ma·ta** \-mə-tə\ : WILMS' TUMOR

neph·ro·cal·ci·no·sis \ˌne-frō-ˌkal-si-ˈnō-səs\ *n, pl* **-no·ses** \-ˌsēz\ : a condition marked by calcification of the tubules of the kidney

neph·ro·gen·ic \ˌne-frə-ˈje-nik\ *adj* **1** : originating in the kidney : caused by factors originating in the kidney ⟨~ hypertension⟩ **2** : developing into or producing kidney tissue

nephrogenic diabetes insipidus *n* : diabetes insipidus that is caused by partial or complete failure of the kidneys to respond to vasopressin

neph·ro·gram \ˈne-frə-ˌgram\ *n* : an X-ray of the kidney

ne·phrog·ra·phy \ni-ˈfrä-grə-fē\ *n, pl* **-phies** : radiography of the kidney

-nephroi *pl of* -NEPHROS

neph·ro·li·thi·a·sis \ˌne-frō-li-ˈthī-ə-səs\ *n, pl* **-a·ses** \-ˌsēz\ : a condition marked by the presence of renal calculi

neph·ro·li·thot·o·my \-li-ˈthä-tə-mē\ *n, pl* **-mies** : the surgical operation of removing a calculus from the kidney

ne·phrol·o·gist \ni-ˈfrä-lə-jist\ *n* : a specialist in nephrology

ne·phrol·o·gy \ni-ˈfrä-lə-jē\ *n, pl* **-gies** : a medical specialty concerned with the kidneys and esp. with their structure, functions, or diseases

ne·phro·ma \ni-ˈfrō-mə\ *n, pl* **-mas** *also* **-ma·ta** \-mə-tə\ : a malignant tumor of the renal cortex

neph·ron \ˈne-ˌfrän\ *n* : a single excretory unit of the vertebrate kidney typically consisting of a renal corpuscle, renal tubule, collecting tubule, and vascular and supporting tissues and discharging urine into the collecting ducts

ne·phrop·a·thy \ni-ˈfrä-pə-thē\ *n, pl* **-thies** : an abnormal state of the kidney; *esp* : one associated with or secondary to some other pathological process — **neph·ro·path·ic** \ˌne-frə-ˈpa-thik\ *adj*

neph·ro·pexy \ˈne-frə-ˌpek-sē\ *n, pl* **-pex·ies** : surgical fixation of a floating kidney

neph·rop·to·sis \ˌne-ˌfräp-ˈtō-səs\ *n, pl* **-to·ses** \-ˌsēz\ : abnormal mobility of the kidney : floating kidney

ne·phror·rha·phy \ne-ˈfrȯr-ə-fē\ *n, pl* **-phies** **1** : the fixation of a floating kidney by suturing it to the posterior abdominal wall **2** : the suturing of a kidney wound

-neph·ros \ˈne-frəs, -ˌfräs\ *n comb form, pl* **-neph·roi** \ˈne-ˌfrȯi\ : kidney ⟨pro*nephros*⟩

neph·ro·scle·ro·sis \ˌne-frō-sklə-ˈrō-səs\ *n, pl* **-ro·ses** \-ˌsēz\ : hardening of the kidney; *specif* : a condition that is characterized by sclerosis of the renal arterioles with reduced blood flow and contraction of the kidney, that is associated usu. with hypertension, and that terminates in renal failure and uremia — compare NEPHRITIS — **neph·ro·scle·ro·tic** \-ˈrä-tik\ *adj*

neph·ro·scope \ˈne-frə-ˌskōp\ *n* : an endoscope used for inspecting and passing instruments into the interior of the kidney — **neph·ros·co·py** \ni-ˈfrä-skə-pē\ *n*

ne·phro·sis \ni-ˈfrō-səs\ *n, pl* **ne·phro·ses** \-ˌsēz\ : a noninflammatory disease of the kidneys chiefly affecting function of the nephrons; *esp* : NEPHROTIC SYNDROME — compare NEPHRITIS

ne·phros·to·gram \ni-ˈfräs-tə-ˌgram\ *n* : a radiograph of the renal pelvis after injection of a radiopaque substance through an opening formed by nephrostomy

ne·phros·to·my \ni-ˈfräs-tə-mē\ *n, pl* **-mies** : the surgical formation of an opening between a renal pelvis and the outside of the body

ne·phrot·ic \ni-ˈfrä-tik\ *adj* : of, relating to, affected by, or associated with nephrosis ⟨~ edema⟩ ⟨a ~ patient⟩

nephrotic syndrome *n* : an abnormal condition that is marked esp. by a deficiency of albumin in the blood and excess excretion of protein in the urine due to altered permeability of the glomerular basement membranes (as from membranous glomerulonephritis or diabetes)

neph·ro·to·mo·gram \ˌne-frō-ˈtō-mə-ˌgram\ *n* : a radiograph made by nephrotomography

neph·ro·to·mog·ra·phy \-tō-ˈmä-grə-fē\ *n, pl* **-phies** : tomographic visualization of the kidney usu. combined with intravenous nephrography — **neph·ro·to·mo·graph·ic** \-ˌtō-mə-ˈgra-fik\ *adj*

ne·phrot·o·my \ni-ˈfrä-tə-mē\ *n, pl* **-mies** : surgical incision of a kidney (as for the extraction of a calculus)

neph·ro·tox·ic \ˌne-frə-ˈtäk-sik\ *adj* : poisonous to the kidney ⟨~ drugs⟩; *also* : resulting from or marked by poisoning of the kidney ⟨~ effects⟩ — **neph·ro·tox·i·ci·ty** \-täk-ˈsi-sə-tē\ *n*

neph·ro·tox·in \-ˈtäk-sən\ *n* : a cytotoxin that is destructive to kidney cells

Nep·ta·zane \ˈnep-tə-ˌzān\ *trademark* — used for a preparation of methazolamide

nep·tu·ni·um \nep-ˈtü-nē-əm, -ˈtyü-\ *n* : a radioactive metallic element — symbol *Np;* see ELEMENT table

nerve \ˈnərv\ *n* **1** : any of the filamentous bands of nervous tissue that connect parts of the nervous system with the other organs, conduct nerve impulses, and are made up of axons and dendrites together with protective and supportive structures and that for the larger nerves have the fibers gathered into funiculi surrounded by a perineurium and the funiculi enclosed in a common epineurium **2** **nerves** *pl* : a state or condition of nervous agitation or irritability **3** : the sensitive pulp of a tooth

nerve agent *n* : a toxic usu. odorless organophosphate (as sarin) that disrupts the transmission of nerve impulses esp. by inhibiting acetylcholinesterase, is used as a chemical weapon in gaseous or liquid form, and typically causes runny nose, coughing, vomiting, muscle weakness or paralysis, convulsions, coma, and respiratory arrest leading to death : NERVE GAS

nerve block *n* **1** : an interruption of the passage of impulses through a nerve (as with pressure or narcotization) — called also *nerve blocking* **2** : BLOCK ANESTHESIA

nerve cell *n* **1** : a grayish or reddish granular cell with specialized processes that is the fundamental functional unit of nervous tissue : NEURON **2** : CELL BODY

nerve center *n* : CENTER

nerve cord *n* : the dorsal tubular cord of nervous tissue above the notochord that in vertebrates includes or develops an anterior enlargement comprising the brain and a more posterior part comprising the spinal cord with the two together making up the central nervous system

nerve deafness *n* : hearing loss or impairment resulting from injury to or loss of function of the organ of Corti or the auditory nerve — called also *perceptive deafness;* compare CENTRAL DEAFNESS, CONDUCTION DEAFNESS

nerve ending *n* : the structure in which the distal end of the axon of a nerve fiber terminates

nerve fiber *n* : any of the processes (as an axon or a dendrite) of a neuron

nerve gas *n* : an organophosphate chemical weapon that may be inhaled, absorbed through the skin, or ingested and interferes with normal nerve transmission : NERVE AGENT

nerve growth factor *n* : a protein that promotes development of the sensory and sympathetic nervous systems and is required for maintenance of sympathetic neurons — abbr. *NGF*

nerve impulse *n* : an electrical signal that travels along a nerve fiber in response to a stimulus and serves to transmit a record of sensation from a receptor or an instruction to act to an effector : the propagation of an action potential along the length of a neuron— called also *nervous impulse*

nerve of Her•ing \-ˈher-iŋ\ *n* : a nerve that arises from the main trunk of the glossopharyngeal nerve and runs along the internal carotid artery to supply afferent fibers esp. to the baroreceptors of the carotid sinus

Hering, Heinrich Ewald (1866–1948), German physiologist.

nerve sheath *n* : NEURILEMMA

nerve trunk *n* : a bundle of nerve fibers enclosed in a connective tissue sheath

nervi *pl of* NERVUS

nerv•ing \ˈnər-viŋ\ *n* : the removal of part of a nerve trunk in chronic inflammation in order to cure lameness (as of a horse) by destroying sensation in the parts supplied

nervosa — see ANOREXIA NERVOSA, PARS NERVOSA

ner•vous \ˈnər-vəs\ *adj* **1** : of, relating to, or composed of neurons ⟨the ~ layer of the eye⟩ **2 a** : of or relating to the nerves; *also* : originating in or affected by the nerves ⟨~ energy⟩ **b** : easily excited or irritated — **ner•vous•ly** *adv* — **ner•vous•ness** *n*

nervous breakdown *n* : an attack of mental or emotional disorder esp. when of sufficient severity to require hospitalization

nervous impulse *n* : NERVE IMPULSE

nervous system *n* : the bodily system that in vertebrates is made up of the brain and spinal cord, nerves, ganglia, and parts of the receptor organs and that receives and interprets stimuli and transmits impulses to the effector organs — see AUTONOMIC NERVOUS SYSTEM, CENTRAL NERVOUS SYSTEM, PERIPHERAL NERVOUS SYSTEM

ner•vus \ˈnər-vəs, ˈner-\ *n, pl* **ner•vi** \ˈnər-ˌvī, ˈner-ˌvē\ : NERVE 1

nervus er•i•gens \-ˈer-i-ˌjenz\ *n, pl* **nervi er•i•gen•tes** \-ˌer-i-ˈjen-(ˌ)tēz\ : PELVIC SPLANCHNIC NERVE

nervus in•ter•me•di•us \-ˌin-tər-ˈmē-dē-əs\ *n* : the branch of the facial nerve that contains sensory and parasympathetic fibers and that supplies the anterior tongue and parts of the palate and fauces — called also *glossopalatine nerve*

nervus ra•di•a•lis \-ˌrā-dē-ˈā-ləs\ *n, pl* **nervi ra•di•a•les** \-(ˌ)lēz\ : RADIAL NERVE

nervus ter•mi•na•lis \-ˌtər-mə-ˈnā-ləs\ *n, pl* **nervi ter•mi•na•les** \-(ˌ)lēz\ : a group of ganglionated nerve fibers that arise in the cerebral hemisphere near where the nerve tract leading from the olfactory bulb joins the temporal lobe and that pass anteriorly along this tract and the olfactory bulb through the cribriform plate to the nasal mucosa — called also *terminal nerve*

Nes•a•caine \ˈne-sə-ˌkān\ *trademark* — used for a preparation of chloroprocaine

neti pot \ˈne-tē-\ *n* : a usu. plastic or ceramic container that resembles a small teapot and has a spout which is inserted into a nostril to direct a cleansing saline solution into the nasal passages

net•tle \ˈnet-ᵊl\ *n* **1** : any plant of the genus *Urtica* **2** : any of various prickly or stinging plants other than one of the genus *Urtica*

nettle rash *n* : an eruption on the skin caused by or resembling the condition produced by stinging with nettles : HIVES

Neu•las•ta \nü-ˈlas-tə\ *trademark* — used for a preparation of pegfilgrastim

Neu•po•gen \ˈnü-pə-jən, ˈnyü-\ *trademark* — used for a preparation of filgrastim

neur- *or* **neuro-** *comb form* **1** : nerve ⟨*neural*⟩ ⟨*neurology*⟩ **2** : neural : neural and ⟨*neuromuscular*⟩

neu•ral \ˈnu̇r-əl, ˈnyu̇r-\ *adj* **1** : of, relating to, or affecting a nerve or the nervous system **2** : situated in the region of or on the same side of the body as the brain and spinal cord : DORSAL — compare HEMAL 2 — **neu•ral•ly** *adv*

neural arch *n* : the cartilaginous or bony arch enclosing the spinal cord on the dorsal side of a vertebra — called also *vertebral arch*

neural canal *n* **1** : VERTEBRAL CANAL **2** : the cavity or system of cavities in a vertebrate embryo that form the central canal of the spinal cord and the ventricles of the brain

neural crest *n* : the ridge of one of the folds forming the neural tube that gives rise to the spinal ganglia and various structures of the autonomic nervous system — called also *neural ridge;* compare NEURAL PLATE

neural fold *n* : the lateral longitudinal fold on each side of the neural plate that by folding over and fusing with the opposite fold gives rise to the neural tube

neu•ral•gia \nu̇-ˈral-jə, nyu̇-\ *n* : acute paroxysmal pain radiating along the course of one or more nerves usu. without demonstrable changes in the nerve structure — compare NEURITIS — **neu•ral•gic** \-jik\ *adj*

neural groove *n* : the median dorsal longitudinal groove formed in the vertebrate embryo by the neural plate after the appearance of the neural folds — called also *medullary groove*

neural lobe *n* : the expanded distal portion of the neurohypophysis — called also *infundibular process, pars nervosa*

neural plate *n* : a thickened plate of ectoderm along the dorsal midline of the early embryo that gives rise to the neural tube and crests

neural ridge *n* : NEURAL CREST

neural tube *n* : the hollow longitudinal dorsal tube that is formed by infolding and subsequent fusion of the opposite ectodermal folds in the vertebrate embryo and gives rise to the brain and spinal cord

neural tube defect *n* : any of various congenital defects (as anencephaly and spina bifida) caused by incomplete closure of the neural tube during the early stages of embryonic development

neur•amin•ic acid \ˌnu̇r-ə-ˈmi-nik-, ˌnyu̇r-\ *n* : an amino acid $C_9H_{17}NO_8$ that is essentially a carbohydrate and occurs in the form of acyl derivatives

neur•amin•i•dase \ˌnu̇r-ə-ˈmi-nə-ˌdās, ˌnyu̇r-, -ˌdāz\ *n* : a hydrolytic enzyme that occurs on the surface of the pneumococcus, the orthomyxoviruses, and some paramyxoviruses and that cleaves terminal acetylated neuraminic acids from sugar residues (as in glycoproteins and mucoproteins)

neuraminidase inhibitor *n* : any of a class of antiviral drugs (as oseltamivir or zanamivir) used for prophylaxis against or treatment of influenza A or B that inhibit the action of viral neuraminidase so that the release of newly formed viruses from infected cells is impeded

neur•aprax•ia \ˌnu̇r-ə-ˈprak-sē-ə, ˌnyu̇r-, -(ˌ)ā-ˈ\ *n* : an injury to a nerve that interrupts conduction causing temporary paralysis but not degeneration and that is followed by a complete and rapid recovery

neur•as•the•nia \ˌnu̇r-əs-ˈthē-nē-ə, ˌnyu̇r-\ *n* : a condition that is characterized esp. by physical and mental exhaustion usu. with accompanying symptoms (as headaches, insomnia, and irritability), is of unknown cause but is often associated with depression or emotional stress, and is sometimes considered similar to or identical with chronic fatigue syndrome

[1]**neur•as•then•ic** \-ˈthe-nik\ *adj* : of, relating to, or having neurasthenia

[2]**neurasthenic** *n* : a person affected with neurasthenia

neur•ax•is \nu̇r-ˈak-səs, nyu̇r-\ *n, pl* **neur•ax•es** \-ˌsēz\ : CENTRAL NERVOUS SYSTEM

neu•rec•to•my \nu̇-ˈrek-tə-mē, nyu̇-\ *n, pl* **-mies** : the surgical excision of part of a nerve

neu•ri•lem•ma \ˌnu̇r-ə-ˈle-mə, ˌnyu̇r-\ *n* : the outer layer surrounding a Schwann cell of a myelinated axon — called also *nerve sheath, Schwann's sheath, sheath of Schwann* — **neu•ri•lem•mal** \-ˈle-məl\ *adj*

neu•ri•lem•mo•ma *or* **neu•ri•le•mo•ma** *or* **neu•ro•lem•mo•ma** \-lə-ˈmō-mə\ *n, pl* **-mas** *also* **-ma•ta** \-mə-tə\ : a tumor of the myelinated sheaths of nerve fibers that consist of Schwann cells in a matrix — called also *neurinoma, schwannoma*

neu•ri•no•ma \ˌnu̇r-ə-ˈnō-mə, ˌnyu̇r-\ *n, pl* **-mas** *also* **-ma•ta** \-mə-tə\ : NEURILEMMOMA

neu•rite \ˈn(y)u̇-ˌrīt\ *n* : AXON; *also* : DENDRITE

neu•ri•tis \nu̇-ˈrī-təs, nyu̇-\ *n, pl* **-rit•i•des** \-ˈri-tə-ˌdēz\ *or* **-ri•tis•es** : an inflammatory or degenerative lesion of a nerve marked esp. by pain, sensory disturbances, and impaired or lost reflexes — compare NEURALGIA — **neu•rit•ic** \-ˈri-tik\ *adj*

neu•ro \ˈnu̇-ˌrō, ˈnyu̇-\ *adj* : NEUROLOGICAL

neuro- — see NEUR-

neu•ro•ac•tive \ˌnu̇r-ō-ˈak-tiv, ˌnyu̇r-\ *adj* : stimulating neural tissue

neu•ro•anat•o•my \-ə-ˈna-tə-mē\ *n, pl* **-mies** : the anatomy of nervous tissue and the nervous system — **neu•ro•ana•tom•i•cal** \-ˌa-nə-ˈtä-mi-kəl\ *also* **neu•ro•ana•tom•ic** \-mik\ *adj* — **neu•ro•ana•tom•i•cal•ly** \-mi-k(ə-)lē\ *adv* — **neu•ro•anat•o•mist** \-ə-ˈna-tə-mist\ *n*

neu•ro•ar•throp•a•thy \-är-ˈthrä-pə-thē\ *n, pl* **-thies** : CHARCOT JOINT

neu•ro•be•hav•ior•al \-bi-ˈhā-vyə-rəl\ *adj* : of or relating to the relationship between the action of the nervous system and behavior

neu•ro•bio•feed•back \-ˌbī-ō-ˈfēd-ˌbak\ *n* : NEUROFEEDBACK

neu•ro•bi•ol•o•gy \-bī-ˈä-lə-jē\ *n, pl* **-gies** : a branch of biology that deals with the anatomy, physiology, and pathology of the nervous system — **neu•ro•bi•o•log•i•cal** \-ˌbī-ə-ˈlä-ji-kəl\ *also* **neu•ro•bi•o•log•ic** \-jik\ *adj* — **neu•ro•bi•o•log•i•cal•ly** \-ji-k(ə-)lē\ *adv* — **neu•ro•bi•ol•o•gist** \-bī-ˈä-lə-jist\ *n*

neu•ro•blast \ˈnu̇r-ə-ˌblast, ˈnyu̇r-\ *n* : a cellular precursor of a nerve cell; *esp* : an undifferentiated embryonic nerve cell — **neu•ro•blas•tic** \ˌnu̇r-ə-ˈblas-tik, ˌnyu̇r-\ *adj*

neu•ro•blas•to•ma \ˌnu̇r-ō-blas-ˈtō-mə, ˌnyu̇r-\ *n, pl* **-mas** *also* **-ma•ta** \-mə-tə\ : a malignant tumor formed of embryonic ganglion cells

neu•ro•bor•rel•i•o•sis \-bə-ˌre-lē-ˈō-səs\ *n, pl* **-o•ses** \-ˌsēz\ : disease of the central nervous system caused by infection with a spirochete of the genus *Borrelia; esp* : a late stage of Lyme disease typically involving the skin, joints, and central nervous system

neu•ro•car•dio•gen•ic syncope \-ˌkär-dē-(ˌ)ō-ˈje-nik-\ *n* : VASOVAGAL SYNCOPE

neu•ro•cen•trum \-ˈsen-trəm\ *n, pl* **-trums** *or* **-tra** \-trə\ : either of the two dorsal elements of a vertebra that unite to form a neural arch from which the vertebral spine is developed — **neu•ro•cen•tral** \-ˈsen-trəl\ *adj*

neu•ro•chem•is•try \-ˈke-mə-strē\ *n, pl* **-tries** **1** : the study of the chemical makeup and activities of nervous tissue **2** : chemical processes and phenomena related to the nervous system — **neu•ro•chem•i•cal** \-ˈke-mi-kəl\ *adj or n* — **neu•ro•chem•i•cal•ly** \-mi-k(ə-)lē\ *adv* — **neu•ro•chem•ist** \-mist\ *n*

neu•ro•cir•cu•la•to•ry \-ˈsər-kyə-lə-ˌtōr-ē\ *adj* : of or relating to the nervous and circulatory systems

neurocirculatory asthenia *n* : a condition marked by shortness of breath, fatigue, rapid pulse, and heart palpitation sometimes with extra beats that occurs chiefly with exertion and is not due to physical disease of the heart — called also *cardiac neurosis, effort syndrome, soldier's heart*

neu•ro•cog•ni•tive \-ˈkäg-nə-tiv\ *n* : of, relating to, or involving cognitive functioning and associated processes and structures of the central nervous system ⟨∼ deficits⟩

neu•ro•cra•ni•um \-ˈkrā-nē-əm\ *n, pl* **-ni•ums** *or* **-nia** \-nē-ə\ : the portion of the skull that encloses and protects the brain — **neu•ro•cra•ni•al** \-nē-əl\ *adj*

neu•ro•cu•ta•ne•ous \-kyu̇-ˈtā-nē-əs\ *adj* : of, relating to, or affecting the skin and nerves ⟨a ∼ syndrome⟩

neu•ro•cys•ti•cer•co•sis \-ˌsi-stə-(ˌ)sər-ˈkō-səs\ *n, pl* **-co•ses** \-ˌsēz\ : infection of the central nervous system with cysticerci of the pork tapeworm

neu•ro•cy•to•ma \-sī-ˈtō-mə\ *n, pl* **-mas** *also* **-ma•ta** \-mə-tə\ : any of various tumors of nerve tissue arising in the central or sympathetic nervous system

neu•ro•de•gen•er•a•tive \-di-ˈje-nə-rə-tiv, -ˌrā-\ *adj* : relating to or characterized by degeneration of nervous tissue — **neu•ro•de•gen•er•a•tion** \-ˌje-nə-ˈrā-shən\ *n*

neu•ro•der•ma•ti•tis \-ˌdər-mə-ˈtī-təs\ *n, pl* **-ti•tis•es** *or* **-tit•i•des** \-ˈti-tə-ˌdēz\ : chronic eczematous dermatitis arising from repeated rubbing or scratching of a real or imagined irritation of the skin — see LICHEN SIMPLEX CHRONICUS

neu•ro•de•vel•op•ment \-di-ˈve-ləp-mənt\ *n* : the development of the nervous system — **neu•ro•de•vel•op•ment•al** \-ˌve-ləp-ˈment-ᵊl\ *adj*

neu•ro•di•ag•nos•tic \-ˌdī-ig-ˈnäs-tik\ *adj* : of or relating to the diagnosis of diseases of the nervous system

neu•ro•dy•nam•ic \-dī-ˈna-mik\ *adj* : of, relating to, or involving communication between different parts of the nervous system — **neu•ro•dy•nam•ics** \-miks\ *n*

neu•ro•ec•to•derm \-ˈek-tə-ˌdərm\ *n* : embryonic ectoderm that gives rise to nervous tissue — **neu•ro•ec•to•der•mal** \-ˌek-tə-ˈdər-məl\ *adj*

neu•ro•ef•fec•tor \-i-ˈfek-tər, -ˌtȯr\ *adj* : of, relating to, or involving both neural and effector components

neu•ro•elec•tric \-i-ˈlek-trik\ *also* **neu•ro•elec•tri•cal** \-tri-kəl\ *adj* : of or relating to the electrical phenomena (as potentials or signals) generated by the nervous system

neu•ro•en•do•crine \-ˈen-də-krən, -ˌkrīn, -ˌkrēn\ *adj* **1** : of, relating to, or being a hormonal substance that influences the activity of nerves **2** : of, relating to, or functioning in neurosecretion

neu•ro•en•do•cri•nol•o•gy \-ˌen-də-kri-ˈnä-lə-jē, -(ˌ)krī-\ *n, pl* **-gies** : a branch of biology dealing with neurosecretion and the physiological interaction between the central nervous system and the endocrine system — **neu•ro•en•do•cri•no•log•i•cal** \-ˌkri-nəl-ˈäj-i-kəl, -ˌkrī-, -ˌkrē-\ *also* **neu•ro•en•do•cri•no•log•ic** \-nə-ˈlä-jik\ *adj* — **neu•ro•en•do•cri•nol•o•gist** \-ˈnä-lə-jist\ *n*

neu•ro•ep•i•the•li•al \ˌnu̇r-ō-ˌe-pə-ˈthē-lē-əl, ˌnyu̇r-\ *adj* **1** : of or relating to neuroepithelium **2** : having qualities of both neural and epithelial cells

neu•ro•epi•the•li•o•ma \-ˌthē-lē-ˈō-mə\ *n, pl* **-mas** *also* **-ma•ta** \-mə-tə\ : a neurocytoma or glioma esp. of the retina

neu•ro•epi•the•li•um \-ˈthē-lē-əm\ *n, pl* **-lia** \-lē-ə\ **1** : the part of the embryonic ectoderm that gives rise to the nervous system **2** : the modified epithelium of an organ of special sense

neuro•feed•back \-ˈfēd-ˌbak\ *n* : the technique of making brain activity perceptible to the senses (as by recording brain waves with an electroencephalograph and presenting them visually or audibly) in order to consciously alter such activity — called also *neurobiofeedback, neurotherapy*

neu•ro•fi•bril \ˌnu̇r-ō-ˈfī-brəl, ˌnyu̇r-, -ˈfi-\ *n* : a fine proteinaceous fibril found in cytoplasm (as of a neuron) and capable of conducting excitation — **neu•ro•fi•bril•lary** \-brə-ˌler-ē\ *also* **neu•ro•fi•bril•lar** \-brə-lər\ *adj*

neurofibrillary tangle *n* : a pathological accumulation of paired helical filaments composed of abnormally formed tau protein that is found chiefly in the cytoplasm of nerve cells of the brain and esp. the cerebral cortex and hippocampus and that occurs typically in Alzheimer's disease

neu•ro•fi•bro•ma \-fī-ˈbrō-mə\ *n, pl* **-mas** *also* **-ma•ta** \-mə-tə\ : a fibroma composed of nervous and connective tissue and produced by proliferation of Schwann cells

neu•ro•fi•bro•ma•to•sis \-fī-ˌbrō-mə-ˈtō-səs\ *n, pl* **-to•ses** \-ˌsēz\ **1** *also* **neurofibromatosis type 1** : a disorder inherited as an autosomal dominant trait and characterized by brown spots on the skin, neurofibromas of peripheral nerves, and deformities of subcutaneous tissues and bone — abbr. *NF;* called also *Recklinghausen's disease, von Recklinghausen's disease* **2** *also* **neurofibromatosis type 2** : a disorder inherited as an autosomal dominant trait and characterized by bilateral acoustic neuromas typically accompanied by other nonmalignant tumors of the central nervous system — abbr. *NF*

neu•ro•fi•bro•sar•co•ma \-ˌfī-brō-sär-ˈkō-mə\ *n, pl* **-mas** *also* **-ma•ta** \-mə-tə\ : a malignant neurofibroma

neu•ro•fil•a•ment \-ˈfi-lə-mənt\ *n* : a microscopic filament of protein that is found in the cytoplasm of neurons and that with neurotubules makes up the structure of neurofibrils — **neu•ro•fil•a•men•tous** \-ˌfi-lə-ˈmen-təs\ *adj*

neu•ro•gen•e•sis \ˌnu̇r-ə-ˈje-nə-səs, ˌnyu̇r-\ *n, pl* **-e•ses** \-ˌsēz\ : development of nerves, nervous tissue, or the nervous system

neu•ro•ge•net•ics \-jə-ˈne-tiks\ *n* : a branch of genetics dealing with the nervous system and esp. with its development

neu•ro•gen•ic \ˌnu̇r-ō-ˈje-nik, ˌnyu̇r-\ *also* **neu•rog•e•nous** \nu̇-ˈrä-jə-nəs, nyu̇-\ *adj* **1 a** : originating in nervous tissue ⟨a ~ tumor⟩ **b** : induced, controlled, or modified by nervous factors; *esp* : disordered because of abnormally altered neural relations ⟨the ~ kidney⟩ **2 a** : constituting the neural component of a bodily process ⟨~ factors in disease⟩ **b** : taking place or viewed as taking place in ordered rhythmic fashion under the control of a network of nerve cells scattered in the cardiac muscle ⟨a ~ heartbeat⟩ — compare MYOGENIC 2 — **neu•ro•gen•i•cal•ly** *adv*

neu•ro•glia \nu̇-ˈrō-glē-ə, nyu̇-, -ˈrä-; ˌnu̇r-ə-ˈglē-ə, ˌnyu̇r-, -ˈglī-\ *n* : GLIA — **neu•ro•gli•al** \-əl\ *adj*

neu•ro•his•tol•o•gy \ˌnu̇r-ō-hi-ˈstä-lə-jē, ˌnyu̇r-\ *n, pl* **-gies** : a branch of histology concerned with the nervous system — **neu•ro•his•to•log•i•cal** \-ˌhis-tə-ˈlä-ji-kəl\ *also* **neu•ro•his•to•log•ic** \-ˈlä-jik\ *adj* — **neu•ro•his•tol•o•gist** \-hi-ˈstä-lə-jist\ *n*

neu•ro•hor•mon•al \-hȯr-ˈmōn-ᵊl\ *adj* **1** : involving both neural and hormonal mechanisms **2** : of, relating to, or being a neurohormone

neu•ro•hor•mone \-ˈhȯr-ˌmōn\ *n* : a hormone (as norepinephrine) produced by or acting on nervous tissue

neu•ro•hu•mor \-ˈhyü-mər, -ˈyü-\ *n* : NEUROHORMONE; *esp* : NEUROTRANSMITTER — **neu•ro•hu•mor•al** \-mə-rəl\ *adj*

neu•ro•hy•po•phy•se•al *or* **neu•ro•hy•po•phy•si•al** \-(ˌ)hī-ˌpä-fə-ˈsē-əl, -ˌhī-pə-fə-, -ˈzē-; -ˌhī-pə-ˈfi-zē-əl\ *adj* : of, relating to, or secreted by the neurohypophysis ⟨~ hormones⟩

neu•ro•hy•poph•y•sis \-hī-ˈpä-fə-səs\ *n* : the portion of the pituitary gland that is derived from the embryonic brain, is composed of the infundibulum and neural lobe, and is concerned with the secretion of various hormones — called also *posterior pituitary gland;* compare ADENOHYPOPHYSIS

neu•ro•im•ag•ing \-ˈi-mə-jiŋ\ *n* : a clinical specialty concerned with producing images of the brain by noninvasive techniques (as computed tomography, magnetic resonance imaging, and positron-emission tomography); *also* : imaging of the brain by these techniques

neu•ro•im•mu•nol•o•gy \-ˌi-myə-ˈnä-lə-jē\ *n, pl* **-gies** : a branch of immunology that deals esp. with the interrelationships of the nervous system and immune responses and autoimmune disorders — **neu•ro•im•mu•no•log•i•cal** \-nə-ˈlä-ji-kəl\ *adj*

neurolemmoma *var of* NEURILEMMOMA

neu•ro•lept•an•al•ge•sia \-ˌlep-ˌtan-ᵊl-ˈjē-zhə, -zhē-ə, -zē-ə\ *also* **neu•ro•lep•to•an•al•ge•sia** \-ˌlep-tō-ˌan-ᵊl-\ *n* : joint administration of a tranquilizing drug and an analgesic esp. for relief of surgical pain — **neu•ro•lept•an•al•ge•sic** \-ˈjē-zik, -sik\ *adj*

neu•ro•lep•tic \-ˈlep-tik\ *n* : ANTIPSYCHOTIC

neu•ro•lin•guis•tics \-liŋ-ˈgwis-tiks\ *n* : the study of the relationships between the human nervous system and language esp. with respect to the correspondence between disorders of language and the nervous system — **neu•ro•lin•guis•tic** \-tik\ *adj*

neu•ro•log•i•cal \ˌnu̇r-ə-ˈlä-ji-kəl, ˌnyu̇r-\ *or* **neu•ro•log•ic** \-jik\ *adj* : of, relating to, or affecting the nervous system ⟨a ~ disorder⟩ ⟨~ tests⟩ — **neu•ro•log•i•cal•ly** *adv*

neu•rol•o•gist \nu̇-ˈrä-lə-jist, nyu̇-\ *n* : a person specializing in neurology; *esp* : a physician skilled in the diagnosis and treatment of disease of the nervous system

neu•rol•o•gy \-jē\ *n, pl* **-gies** : a branch of medicine concerned esp. with the structure, function, and diseases of the nervous system

neu•rol•y•sis \nu̇-ˈrä-lə-səs, nyu̇-\ *n, pl* **-y•ses** \-ˌsēz\ **1 a** : the breaking down of nervous tissue (as from disease or injury) **b** : destruction of nervous tissue (as by the use of chemicals or radio frequencies) to temporarily or permanently block nerve pathways esp. to relieve pain or spasticity **2** : the surgical operation of freeing a nerve from perineural adhesions — **neu•ro•lyt•ic** \ˌnu̇r-ə-ˈli-tik, ˌnyu̇r-\ *adj*

neu•ro•ma \nu̇-ˈrō-mə, nyu̇-\ *n, pl* **-mas** *also* **-ma•ta** \-mə-tə\ **1** : a tumor or mass growing from a nerve and usu. consisting of nerve fibers **2** : a mass of nerve tissue in an amputation stump resulting from abnormal regrowth of the stumps of severed nerves — called also *amputation neuroma*

neu•ro•mod•u•la•tor \ˌnu̇r-ō-ˈmä-jə-ˌlā-tər, ˌnyu̇r-\ *n* : something (as a polypeptide) that potentiates or inhibits the transmission of a nerve impulse but is not the actual means of transmission itself — **neu•ro•mod•u•la•to•ry** \-lə-ˌtōr-ē\ *adj*

neu•ro•mo•tor \-ˈmō-tər\ *adj* : relating to efferent nerve impulses

neu•ro•mus•cu•lar \-ˈməs-kyə-lər\ *adj* : of or relating to nerves and muscles; *esp* : jointly involving nervous and muscular elements ⟨~ disease⟩

neuromuscular junction *n* : the junction of an efferent nerve fiber and the muscle fiber plasma membrane — called also *myoneural junction*

neuromuscular spindle *n* : MUSCLE SPINDLE

neu•ro•my•eli•tis \ˌnu̇r-ō-ˌmī-ə-ˈlī-təs, ˌnyu̇r-\ *n* **1** : inflammation of the medullary substance of the nerves **2** : inflammation of both spinal cord and nerves

neu•ro•my•op•a•thy \-ˌmī-ˈä-pə-thē\ *n, pl* **-thies** : a disease of nerves and associated muscle tissue

neu•ron \ˈnü-ˌrän, ˈnyü-\ *also* **neu•rone** \-ˌrōn\ *n* : one of the cells that constitute nervous tissue, that have the property of transmitting and receiving nerve impulses, and that possess cytoplasmic processes which are highly differentiated frequently as multiple dendrites or usu. as solitary axons and which conduct impulses toward and away from the cell body : NERVE CELL 1 — **neu•ro•nal** \ˈnu̇-rən-ᵊl, ˈnyu̇-; nu̇-ˈrōn-ᵊl, nyu̇-\ *also* **neu•ron•ic** \nu̇-ˈrä-nik, nyu̇-\ *adj*

neu•ro•neu•ro•nal \ˌnu̇r-ō-ˈnu̇-rən-ᵊl, ˌnyu̇r-ō-ˈnyu̇-; ˌnu̇r-ō-nu̇-ˈrōn-ᵊl, ˌnyu̇r-ō-nyu̇-\ *adj* : between neurons or nerve fibers

neu•ron•i•tis \ˌnu̇r-ō-ˈnī-təs, ˌnyu̇r-\ *n* : inflammation of neurons; *esp* : neuritis involving nerve roots and neurons within the spinal cord

neu•ro•no•tro•pic \-ˈtrō-pik, -ˈträ-\ *adj* : having an affinity for neurons : NEUROTROPIC

Neu•ron•tin \ˈnu̇r-än-tin\ *trademark* — used for a preparation of gabapentin

neu•ro–on•col•o•gy \ˌn(y)u̇r-ō-än-ˈkä-lə-jē, -äŋ-\ *n* : a branch of medical science dealing with tumors of the nervous system — **neu•ro–on•co•log•i•cal** \-ˌäŋ-kə-ˈläj-i-kəl\ *also* **neu•ro–on•co•log•ic** \-ˌäŋ-kə-ˈläj-ik\ *adj* — **neu•ro–on•col•o•gist** \-än-ˈkäl-ə-jəst, -äŋ-\ *n*

neu•ro–oph•thal•mol•o•gy \-ˌäf-thəl-ˈmä-lə-jē, -ˌäp-\ *n, pl* **-gies** : the neurological study of the eye — **neu•ro–oph•thal•mo•log•ic** \-mə-ˈlä-jik\ *or* **neu•ro–oph•thal•mo•log•i•cal** \-ˈlä-ji-kəl\ *adj*

neuro–otology *var of* NEUROTOLOGY

neu•ro•par•a•lyt•ic \-ˌpar-ə-ˈli-tik\ *adj* : of, relating to, causing, or characterized by paralysis or loss of sensation due to a lesion in a nerve

neu•ro•path•ic \ˌnu̇r-ə-ˈpa-thik, ˌnyu̇r-\ *adj* : of, relating to, characterized by, or being a neuropathy ⟨~ pain⟩ ⟨~ disorders⟩ — **neu•ro•path•i•cal•ly** *adv*

neuropathic arthropathy *n* : CHARCOT JOINT

neu•ro•patho•gen•e•sis \-ˌpa-thə-ˈje-nə-səs\ *n, pl* **-e•ses** \-ˌsēz\ : the pathogenesis of a nervous disease

neu•ro•patho•gen•ic \-ˈje-nik\ *adj* : causing or capable of causing disease of nervous tissue ⟨~ viruses⟩

neu•ro•pa•thol•o•gist \ˌnu̇r-ō-pə-ˈthä-lə-jist, ˌnyu̇r-\ *n* : a specialist in neuropathology

neu•ro•pa•thol•o•gy \-pə-ˈthä-lə-jē, -pa-\ *n, pl* **-gies** : pathology of the nervous system — **neu•ro•path•o•log•ic** \-ˌpa-thə-ˈlä-jik\ *or* **neu•ro•path•o•log•i•cal** \-ji-kəl\ *adj* — **neu•ro•path•o•log•i•cal•ly** \-ji-k(ə-)lē\ *adv*

neu•rop•a•thy \nu̇-ˈrä-pə-thē, nyu̇-\ *n, pl* **-thies** : an abnormal and usu. degenerative state of the nervous system or nerves; *also* : a systemic condition that stems from a neuropathy

neu•ro•pep•tide \ˌnu̇r-ō-ˈpep-ˌtīd, ˌnyu̇r-\ *n* : an endogenous peptide (as an endorphin) that influences neural activity or functioning

neuropeptide Y *n* : a neurotransmitter that has a vasoconstrictive effect on blood vessels and is held to play a role in regulating eating behavior

neu•ro•phar•ma•ceu•ti•cal \-ˌfär-mə-ˈsü-ti-kəl\ *n* : a drug used to treat neuropsychiatric, neuropsychological, or nervous-system disorders (as depression or schizophrenia)

neu•ro•phar•ma•col•o•gist \-ˌfär-mə-ˈkä-lə-jist\ *n* : a specialist in neuropharmacology

neu•ro•phar•ma•col•o•gy \-ˌfär-mə-ˈkä-lə-jē\ *n, pl* **-gies** **1** : a branch of medical science dealing with the action of drugs on and in the nervous system **2** : the properties and reactions of a drug on and in the nervous system — **neu•ro•phar•ma•co•log•i•cal** \-kə-ˈlä-ji-kəl\ *also* **neu•ro•phar•ma•co•log•ic** \-jik\ *adj*

neu•ro•phy•sin \-ˈfī-sᵊn\ *n* : any of several brain hormones that bind with and carry either oxytocin or vasopressin

neu•ro•phys•i•ol•o•gist \-ˌfi-zē-ˈä-lə-jist\ *n* : a specialist in neurophysiology

neu•ro•phys•i•ol•o•gy \-ˌfi-zē-ˈä-lə-jē\ *n, pl* **-gies** : physiology of the nervous system — **neu•ro•phys•i•o•log•i•cal** \-zē-ə-ˈlä-ji-kəl\ *also* **neu•ro•phys•i•o•log•ic** \-jik\ *adj* — **neu•ro•phys•i•o•log•i•cal•ly** *adv*

neu•ro•pil \ˈnu̇r-ō-ˌpil, ˈnyu̇r-\ *also* **neu•ro•pile** \-ˌpīl\ *n* : a fibrous network of delicate unmyelinated nerve fibers found in concentrations of nervous tissue esp. in parts of the brain where it is highly developed — **neu•ro•pi•lar** \ˌnu̇r-ō-ˈpī-lər, ˌnyu̇r-\ *adj*

neu•ro•pro•tec•tant \ˌnu̇r-ō-prə-ˈtek-tənt, ˌnyu̇r-\ *n* : a neuroprotective drug that protects against or helps repair the damaging effects of a stroke

neu•ro•pro•tec•tive \ˌnu̇r-ō-prə-ˈtek-tiv\ *adj* : serving to protect nerve cells from injury or degeneration — **neu•ro•pro•tec•tion** \-shən\ *n*

neu•ro•psy•chi•a•trist \ˌnu̇r-ō-sə-ˈkī-ə-trist, ˌnyu̇r-, -sī-\ *n* : a specialist in neuropsychiatry

neu•ro•psy•chi•a•try \-sə-ˈkī-ə-trē, -sī-\ *n, pl* **-tries** : a branch of medicine concerned with both neurology and psychiatry — **neu•ro•psy•chi•at•ric** \-ˌsī-kē-ˈa-trik\ *adj* — **neu•ro•psy•chi•at•ri•cal•ly** *adv*

neu•ro•psy•chol•o•gist \-sī-ˈkä-lə-jist\ *n* : a specialist in neuropsychology

neu•ro•psy•chol•o•gy \-jē\ *n, pl* **-gies** : a science concerned with the integration of psychological observations on behavior and the mind with neurological observations on the brain and nervous system — **neu•ro•psy•cho•log•i•cal** \-ˌsī-kə-ˈlä-ji-kəl\ *adj* — **neu•ro•psy•cho•log•i•cal•ly** *adv*

neu•ro•psy•cho•phar•ma•col•o•gy \-ˌsī-kō-ˌfär-mə-ˈkä-lə-jē\ *n, pl* **-gies** : a branch of medical science combining neuropharmacology and psychopharmacology

neu•ro•ra•di•ol•o•gist \-ˌrā-dē-ˈä-lə-jist\ *n* : a specialist in neuroradiology

neu•ro•ra•di•ol•o•gy \-ˌrā-dē-ˈä-lə-jē\ *n, pl* **-gies** : radiology of the nervous system — **neu•ro•ra•dio•log•i•cal** \-dē-ə-ˈlä-ji-kəl\ *also* **neu•ro•ra•dio•log•ic** \-jik\ *adj*

neu•ro•ret•i•ni•tis \-ˌret-ᵊn-ˈī-təs\ *n, pl* **-nit•i•des** \-ˈni-tə-ˌdēz\ : inflammation of the optic nerve and the retina

neu•ror•rha•phy \nu̇-ˈrȯr-ə-fē, nyu̇-\ *n, pl* **-phies** : the surgical suturing of a divided nerve

neu•ro•sci•ence \ˌnu̇r-ō-ˈsī-əns, ˌnyu̇r-\ *n* : a branch (as neurophysiology) of biology that deals with the anatomy, physiology, biochemistry, or molecular biology of nerves and nervous tissue and esp. their relation to behavior and learning — **neu•ro•sci•en•ti•fic** \-ˌsī-ən-ˈti-fik\ *adj* — **neu•ro•sci•en•tist** \-ˈsī-ən-tist\ *n*

neu•ro•se•cre•tion \-si-ˈkrē-shən\ *n* **1** : the process of producing a secretion by neurons **2** : a secretion produced by neurosecretion — **neu•ro•se•cre•to•ry** \-ˈsē-krə-ˌtȯr-ē\ *adj*

neu•ro•sen•so•ry \-ˈsen-sə-rē\ *adj* : of or relating to afferent nerves

neu•ro•sis \nu̇-ˈrō-səs, nyu̇-\ *n, pl* **-ro•ses** \-ˌsēz\ : a mental and emotional disorder that affects only part of the personality, is accompanied by a less distorted perception of reality than in a psychosis, does not result in disturbance of the use of language, and is accompanied by various physical, physiological, and mental disturbances (as visceral symptoms, anxieties, or phobias)

neu•ro•stim•u•la•tor \ˌnu̇r-ō-ˈsti-myə-ˌlā-tər, ˌnyu̇r-\ *n* : a device that provides electrical stimulation to nerves

neu•ro•sur•geon \-ˈsər-jən\ *n* : a surgeon specializing in neurosurgery

neu•ro•sur•gery \-ˈsər-jə-rē\ *n, pl* **-gies** : surgery of nervous structures (as nerves, the brain, or the spinal cord) — **neu•ro•sur•gi•cal** \-ˈsər-ji-kəl\ *adj* — **neu•ro•sur•gi•cal•ly** *adv*

neu•ro•syph•i•lis \-ˈsi-fə-ləs\ *n* : syphilis of the central nervous system — **neu•ro•syph•i•lit•ic** \-ˌsi-fə-ˈli-tik\ *adj*

neu•ro•ten•di•nous spindle \-ˈten-di-nəs-\ *n* : GOLGI TENDON ORGAN

neu•ro•ten•sin \-ˈten-sən\ *n* : a protein composed of 13 amino acid residues that causes hypertension and vasodilation and is present in the brain

neu•ro•ther•a•py \-ˈther-ə-pē\ *n* : NEUROFEEDBACK

[1]**neu•rot•ic** \nu̇-ˈrä-tik, nyu̇-\ *adj* **1 a** : of, relating to, or involving the nerves ⟨a ~ disorder⟩ **b** : being a neurosis : NERVOUS **2** : affected with, relating to, or characterized by neurosis ⟨a ~ person⟩ — **neu•rot•i•cal•ly** *adv*

[2]**neurotic** *n* **1** : one affected with a neurosis **2** : an emotionally unstable individual

neu•rot•i•cism \-ˈrä-tə-ˌsi-zəm\ *n* : a neurotic character, condition, or trait

neu•ro•tol•o•gy \ˌnu̇r-ō-ˈtä-lə-jē, ˌnyu̇r-\ *or* **neu•ro–otol•o•gy** \-ō-ˈtä-lə-jē\ *n, pl* **-gies** : the neurological study of the ear — **neu•ro•to•log•ic** \-tə-ˈlä-jik\ *or* **neu•ro–oto•log•i•cal** \-ˌō-tə-ˈlä-ji-kəl\ *also* **neu•ro–oto•log•ic** \-ō-tə-ˈlä-jik\ *or* **neu•ro•to•log•ic•al** \-tə-ˈlä-ji-kəl\ *adj*

neu•rot•o•my \-ˈrä-tə-mē\ *n, pl* **-mies** **1** : the dissection or cutting of nerves **2** : the division of a nerve (as to relieve neuralgia)

neu•ro•tox•ic \ˌnu̇r-ō-ˈtäk-sik, ˌnyu̇r-\ *adj* : toxic to the nerves or nervous tissue — **neu•ro•tox•ic•i•ty** \-ˌtäk-ˈsi-sə-tē\ *n*

neu•ro•tox•i•col•o•gist \-ˌtäk-sə-ˈkä-lə-jist\ *n* : a specialist in the study of neurotoxins and their effects

neu•ro•tox•i•col•o•gy \-jē\ *n, pl* **-gies** : the study of neurotoxins and their effects — **neu•ro•tox•i•co•log•i•cal** \-kə-ˈlä-jə-kəl\ *adj*

neurotoxic shellfish poisoning *n* : shellfish poisoning that is characterized by neurological and gastrointestinal symptoms (as numbness and tingling, nausea, vomiting, diarrhea, and loss of muscle control) and is typically caused by a brevetoxin ingested in contaminated shellfish

neu•ro•tox•in \-ˈtäk-sən\ *n* : a poisonous substance (as tetrodotoxin or saxitoxin) that acts on the nervous system and disrupts the normal function of nerve cells

neu•ro•trans•mis•sion \-trans-ˈmi-shən, -tranz-\ *n* : the transmission of nerve impulses across a synapse

neu•ro•trans•mit•ter \-trans-ˈmi-tər, -tranz-; -ˈtrans-ˌmi-, -ˈtranz-\ *n* : a substance (as norepinephrine or acetylcholine) that transmits nerve impulses across a synapse — see FALSE NEUROTRANSMITTER

neu•ro•trau•ma \-ˈtrȯ-mə, -ˈtrau̇-\ *n* : injury to a nerve or to the nervous system

neu•ro•troph•ic \-ˈträ-fik, -ˈtrō-\ *adj* **1** : relating to or dependent on the influence of nerves on the nutrition of tissue **2** : NEUROTROPIC

neurotrophic factor *n* : any of a group of neuropeptides (as nerve growth factor) that regulate the growth, differentiation, and survival of neurons

neu•ro•tro•phin \-ˈtrō-fən\ *n* : NEUROTROPHIC FACTOR

neu•ro•trop•ic \-ˈträ-pik\ *adj* : having an affinity for or localizing selectively in nerve tissue ⟨~ viruses⟩ — compare PANTROPIC — **neu•rot•ro•pism** \nu̇-ˈrä-trə-ˌpi-zəm, nyu̇-\ *n*

neu•ro•tu•bule \ˌnu̇r-ō-ˈtü-ˌbyül, ˌnyu̇r-ō-ˈtyü-\ *n* : a microtubule occurring in a neuron — see NEUROFILAMENT

neu•ro•typ•i•cal \-ˈti-pi-kəl\ *adj* : not affected with a developmental disorder and esp. autism spectrum disorder : exhibiting or characteristic of typical neurological development — **neurotypical** *n*

neu•ro•vas•cu•lar \-ˈvas-kyə-lər\ *adj* : of, relating to, or involving both nerves and blood vessels

neu•ro•vi•rol•o•gy \-vī-ˈrä-lə-jē\ *n, pl* **-gies** : virology concerned with viral infections of the nervous system

neu•ro•vir•u•lence \-ˈvir-yə-ləns, -ˈvir-ə-\ *n* : the tendency or capacity of a microorganism to cause disease of the nervous system — **neu•ro•vir•u•lent** \-lənt\ *adj*

neu•ru•la \ˈnu̇r-yu̇-lə, ˈnyu̇r-, -ü-lə\ *n, pl* **-lae** \-ˌlē\ *or* **-las** : an early vertebrate embryo which follows the gastrula and in which nervous tissue begins to differentiate — **neu•ru•la•tion** \ˌnu̇r-yu̇-ˈlā-shən, ˌnyu̇r-, -u̇-ˈlā-\ *n*

[1]**neu•ter** \ˈnü-tər, ˈnyü-\ *n* : a spayed or castrated animal (as a cat)

[2]**neuter** *vb* : CASTRATE 1, ALTER

neu•tral \ˈnü-trəl, ˈnyü-\ *adj* **1** : not decided or pronounced as to characteristics **2** : neither acid nor basic : neither acid nor alkaline; *specif* : having a pH value of 7.0 **3** : not electrically charged

neutral fat *n* : TRIGLYCERIDE

neu•tral•ize \ˈnü-trə-ˌlīz, ˈnyü-\ *vb* **-ized; -iz•ing 1** : to make chemically neutral **2** : to counteract the activity or effect of : make ineffective **3** : to make electrically inert by combining equal positive and negative quantities — **neu•tral•i•za•tion** \ˌnü-trə-lə-ˈzā-shən, ˌnyü-\ *n*

neutro- *comb form* **1** : neutral ⟨*neutro*phil⟩ **2** : neutrophil ⟨*neutro*penia⟩

neu•tron \ˈnü-ˌträn, ˈnyü-\ *n* : an uncharged atomic particle that is nearly equal in mass to the proton

neu•tro•pe•nia \ˌnü-trə-ˈpē-nē-ə, ˌnyü-\ *n* : leukopenia in which the decrease in white blood cells is chiefly in neutrophils — **neu•tro•pe•nic** \-ˈpē-nik\ *adj*

[1]**neu•tro•phil** \ˈnü-trə-ˌfil, ˈnyü-\ *or* **neu•tro•phil•ic** \ˌnü-trə-ˈfi-lik, ˌnyü-\ *adj* : staining to the same degree with acid or basic dyes ⟨~ granulocytes⟩

[2]**neutrophil** *n* : a granulocyte that is the chief phagocytic white blood cell

neu•tro•phil•ia \ˌnü-trə-ˈfi-lē-ə, ˌnyü-\ *n* : leukocytosis in which the increase in white blood cells is chiefly in neutrophils

ne•vi•ra•pine \nə-ˈvir-ə-ˌpēn, -ˈvī-rə-\ *n* : a reverse transcriptase inhibitor $C_{15}H_{14}N_4O$ that is administered orally in combination with at least one other antiretroviral agent in the treatment of HIV-1 infection

ne•void \ˈnē-ˌvȯid\ *adj* : resembling a nevus ⟨a ~ melanoma⟩

ne•vus \ˈnē-vəs\ *n, pl* **ne•vi** \-ˌvī\ : a congenital or acquired usu. highly pigmented area on the skin that is either flat or raised : MOLE — see BLUE NEVUS, SPIDER NEVUS

nevus flam•me•us \-ˈfla-mē-əs\ *n* : PORT=WINE STAIN

[1]**new•born** \ˈnü-ˈbȯrn, ˈnyü-\ *adj* **1** : recently born ⟨a ~ infant⟩ **2** : affecting or relating to the newborn

[2]**new•born** \-ˌbȯrn\ *n, pl* **newborn** *or* **newborns** : a newborn infant : NEONATE

New•cas•tle disease \ˈnü-ˌka-səl-, ˈnyü-; nü-ˈka-səl-, ˌnyü-\ *n* : a contagious mild to fatal virus disease of birds and esp. the domestic chicken that is caused by a paramyxovirus (species *Newcastle disease virus* of the genus *Avulavirus*)

new drug *n* : a drug that has not been declared safe and effective by qualified experts under the conditions prescribed, recommended, or suggested in the label and that may be a new chemical formula or an established drug prescribed for use in a new way

New Latin *n* : Latin as used since the end of the medieval period esp. in scientific description and classification

new•ton \ˈnü-tən, ˈnyü-\ *n* : the unit of force in the metric system equal to the force required to impart an acceleration of one meter per second per second to a mass of one kilogram

Newton, Sir Isaac (1642–1727), British physicist and mathematician.

new variant Creutzfeldt–Jakob disease *n* : VARIANT CREUTZFELDT-JAKOB DISEASE — abbr. *nvCJD*

Nex•i•um \ˈnek-sē-əm\ *trademark* — used for a preparation of the magnesium salt of esomeprazole

Nex•pla•non \ˈnek-splə-ˌnän\ *trademark* — used for a subcutaneous contraceptive implant containing etonogestrel

NF *abbr* **1** National Formulary **2** neurofibromatosis

NFP *abbr* natural family planning

ng *abbr* nanogram

NG *abbr* nasogastric

n'gana *var of* NAGANA

NGF *abbr* nerve growth factor

NGU *abbr* nongonococcal urethritis

NHS *abbr* National Health Service

Ni *symbol* nickel

ni•a•cin \ˈnī-ə-sən\ *n* : a crystalline acid $C_6H_5NO_2$ of the vitamin B complex that occurs usu. in the form of a complex of niacinamide in various animal and plant parts (as blood, liver, yeast, bran, and legumes) and is used esp. to lower LDL and triglyceride levels in the blood and to treat pellagra — called also *nicotinic acid*

ni•a•cin•amide \ˌnī-ə-ˈsi-nə-ˌmīd\ *n* : a crystalline amide $C_6H_6N_2O$ of the vitamin B complex that is formed from and converted to niacin in the living organism, occurs naturally usu. as a constituent of coenzymes, and is used similarly to niacin — called also *nicotinamide*

ni•al•amide \nī-ˈa-lə-ˌmīd\ *n* : a synthetic antidepressant drug $C_{16}H_{18}N_4O_2$ that is an inhibitor of monoamine oxidase

Ni•a•span \ˈnī-ə-ˌspan\ *trademark* — used for a preparation of niacin in extended-release form

ni•car•di•pine \ˌnī-ˈkär-də-ˌpēn\ *n* : a calcium channel blocker administered orally in the form of its hydrochloride $C_{26}H_{29}N_3O_6{\cdot}HCl$ to treat angina pectoris and hypertension

nick \ˈnik\ *n* : a break in one strand of two-stranded DNA caused by a missing phosphodiester bond — **nick** *vb*

nick•el \ˈni-kəl\ *n* : a silver-white hard malleable ductile metallic element — symbol *Ni;* see ELEMENT table

nick•ing \ˈni-kiŋ\ *n* : localized constriction of a retinal vein by the pressure from an artery crossing it seen esp. in arterial hypertension

Nic•o•derm \ˈni-kə-ˌdərm\ *trademark* — used for a transdermal patch containing nicotine

Nic•o•rette \ˌni-kə-ˈret\ *trademark* — used for a gum or lozenge containing nicotine

nicotin- *or* **nicotino-** *comb form* **1** : nicotine ⟨*nicotin*ic⟩ **2** : nicotinic acid ⟨*nicotin*amide⟩

nic•o•tin•amide \ˌni-kə-ˈtē-nə-ˌmīd, -ˈti-\ *n* : NIACINAMIDE

nicotinamide adenine dinucleotide *n* : NAD

nicotinamide adenine dinucleotide phosphate *n* : NADP

nic•o•tine \ˈni-kə-ˌtēn\ *n* : a poisonous alkaloid $C_{10}H_{14}N_2$ that is the chief active principle of tobacco and is sometimes used in smoking cessation aids — see NICODERM, NICORETTE, NICOTROL

Ni•cot \nē-ˈkō\, **Jean (1530?–1600),** French diplomat.

nic•o•tin•ic \ˌni-kə-ˈtē-nik, -ˈti-\ *adj* : relating to, resembling, producing, or mediating the effects that are produced by acetylcholine liberated by nerve fibers at autonomic ganglia and at the neuromuscular junctions of voluntary muscle and that are mimicked by nicotine which increases activity in small doses and inhibits it in larger doses ⟨~ receptors⟩ — compare MUSCARINIC

nicotinic acid *n* : NIACIN

Nic•o•trol \ˈni-kə-ˌtrōl\ *trademark* — used for an oral inhalant or nasal spray containing nicotine

nictitans — see MEMBRANA NICTITANS

nic•ti•ta•ting membrane \ˈnik-tə-ˌtā-tiŋ-\ *n* : a thin membrane found in many vertebrate animals at the inner angle or beneath the lower lid of the eye and capable of extending across the eyeball — called also *membrana nictitans, third eyelid*

NICU *abbr* neonatal intensive care unit

ni•da•tion \nī-ˈdā-shən\ *n* **1** : the development of the epithelial membrane lining the inner surface of the uterus following menstruation **2** : IMPLANTATION b

NIDDK *abbr* National Institute of Diabetes and Digestive and Kidney Diseases

NIDDM *abbr* non-insulin-dependent diabetes mellitus

ni•dus \ˈnī-dəs\ *n, pl* **ni•di** \-ˌdī\ *or* **ni•dus•es** : a place where something originates or is fostered or develops; *specif* : the point of origin or focus of an infection or disease process

Nie•mann–Pick disease \ˈnē-ˌmän-ˈpik-\ *n* : a genetic disease that is marked by the accumulation of phospholipids (as sphingomyelin) in various tissues due to the deficient enzymatic breakdown of lipids in the body, that is typically characterized by enlargement of the spleen, liver, and lymph nodes and in the more severe forms by progressive neurological deterioration and death, and that is inherited as an autosomal recessive trait

Niemann, Albert (1880–1921), and **Pick, Ludwig (1868–1944),** German physicians.

ni·fed·i·pine \nī-ˈfe-də-ˌpēn\ *n* : a calcium channel blocker $C_{17}H_{18}N_2O_6$ that is a coronary vasodilator used esp. in the treatment of angina pectoris — see ADALAT, PROCARDIA

night blindness *n* : reduced visual capacity in faint light (as at night) — called also *nyctalopia* — **night–blind** \ˈnīt-ˌblīnd\ *adj*

night·mare \ˈnīt-ˌmar\ *n* : a frightening or distressing dream that usu. awakens the sleeper

night·shade \ˈnīt-ˌshād\ *n* **1** : any plant of the genus *Solanum* (family Solanaceae, the nightshade family) including some poisonous weeds and important crop plants (as the potato and eggplant) **2** : BELLADONNA 1

night sweat *n* : profuse sweating during sleep (as that associated with menopause or tuberculosis)

night terror *n* : a sudden awakening in dazed terror that occurs in children during slow-wave sleep, is often preceded by a sudden shrill cry uttered in sleep, and is not remembered when the child awakes — usu. used in pl.; called also *pavor nocturnus*

night vision *n* : ability to see in dim light (as provided by moon and stars)

ni·gra \ˈnī-grə\ *n* : SUBSTANTIA NIGRA — **ni·gral** \-grəl\ *adj*

nigricans — see ACANTHOSIS NIGRICANS

ni·gro·stri·a·tal \ˌnī-grō-strī-ˈāt-ᵊl\ *adj* : of, relating to, or joining the corpus striatum and the substantia nigra

NIH *abbr* National Institutes of Health

ni·hi·lism \ˈnī-ə-ˌli-zəm, ˈnē-, -hə-\ *n* **1** : NIHILISTIC DELUSION **2** : skepticism as to the value of a drug or method of treatment ⟨therapeutic ~⟩ — **ni·hi·lis·tic** \ˌnī-ə-ˈlis-tik, ˌnē-, -hə-\ *adj*

nihilistic delusion *n* : the belief that oneself, a part of one's body, or the real world does not exist or has been destroyed

nik·eth·amide \ni-ˈke-thə-ˌmīd\ *n* : a bitter viscous liquid or crystalline compound $C_{10}H_{14}N_2O$ used esp. formerly as a respiratory stimulant

NIMH *abbr* National Institute of Mental Health

ni·mo·di·pine \ni-ˈmō-də-ˌpēn\ *n* : a calcium channel blocker $C_{21}H_{26}N_2O_7$

ninth cranial nerve *n* : GLOSSOPHARYNGEAL NERVE

ni·o·bi·um \nī-ˈō-bē-əm\ *n* : a lustrous ductile metallic element — symbol *Nb;* see ELEMENT table

NIOSH *abbr* National Institute of Occupational Safety and Health

Ni·pah virus \ˈnē-pə-\ *n* : a paramyxovirus (species *Nipah virus* of the genus *Henipavirus*) that has caused epidemics of respiratory disease in pigs and an often fatal encephalitis in humans in Malaysia, Singapore, and Bangladesh

nip·ple \ˈni-pəl\ *n* **1** : the protuberance of a mammary gland upon which in the female the lactiferous ducts open and from which milk is drawn **2** : an artificial teat through which a bottle-fed infant nurses

Ni·pride \ˈnī-ˌprīd\ *n* : a preparation of sodium nitroprusside — formerly a U.S. registered trademark

ni·sin \ˈnī-sən\ *n* : a polypeptide antibiotic that is produced by a bacterium (*Lactococcus lactis* syn. *Streptococcus lactis*) and is used as a food preservative

Nis·sen fundoplication \ˈni-sᵊn-\ *n* : fundoplication in which the fundus of the stomach is wrapped completely around the lower end of the esophagus

Nissen, Rudolph (1896–1981), Swiss (German-born) surgeon.

Nissl bodies \ˈni-səl-\ *n pl* : discrete granular bodies of variable size that occur in the cell body and dendrites but not the axon of neurons and are composed of RNA and polyribosomes — called also *Nissl granules, tigroid substance*

Nissl, Franz (1860–1919), German neurologist.

Nissl substance *n* : the nucleoprotein material of Nissl bodies

nit \ˈnit\ *n* : the egg of a louse or other parasitic insect; *also* : the insect itself when young

ni·trate \ˈnī-ˌtrāt, -trət\ *n* : a salt or ester of nitric acid

ni·tric acid \ˈnī-trik-\ *n* : a corrosive liquid inorganic acid HNO_3

nitric oxide *n* : a poisonous colorless gas NO that occurs as a common air pollutant formed by the oxidation of atmospheric nitrogen and that is also formed by the oxidation of arginine in the body where it regulates numerous biological processes (as vasodilation and neurotransmission)

nitric oxide syn·thase \-ˈsin-ˌthās, -ˌthāz\ *n* : any of various enzymes that catalyze the oxidation of arginine to form nitric oxide and citrulline

ni·trite \ˈnī-ˌtrīt\ *n* : a salt or ester of nitrous acid

ni·tri·toid reaction \ˈnī-trə-ˌtȯid-\ *n* : an acute reaction sometimes occurring to certain drugs (as gold sodium thiomalate) and resembling poisoning by nitrite esp. in the presence of flushing, tachycardia, and faintness — called also *nitritoid crisis*

ni·tro \ˈnī-(ˌ)trō\ *n, pl* **nitros** : any of various nitrated products; *specif* : NITROGLYCERIN

Ni·tro–Dur \ˈnī-trō-ˌdər\ *trademark* — used for a preparation of nitroglycerin

ni·tro·fu·ran \ˌnī-trō-ˈfyu̇r-ˌan, -fyu̇-ˈran\ *n* : any of several compounds containing a nitro group that are used as bacteria-inhibiting agents

ni·tro·fu·ran·to·in \-fyu̇-ˈran-tō-in\ *n* : a nitrofuran derivative $C_8H_6N_4O_5$ that is a broad-spectrum antimicrobial agent used esp. in treating urinary tract infections

ni•tro•fu•ra•zone \-ˈfyu̇r-ə-ˌzōn\ *n* : a pale yellow crystalline compound $C_6H_6N_4O_4$ used topically as a bacteriostatic or bactericidal dressing (as for wounds and infections)

ni•tro•gen \ˈnī-trə-jən\ *n* : a nonmetallic element that in the free form is normally a colorless odorless tasteless inert gas containing two atoms per molecule and comprising 78 percent of the atmosphere and that in the combined form is a constituent of biologically important compounds (as proteins and nucleic acids) — symbol *N;* see ELEMENT table

nitrogen balance *n* : the difference between nitrogen intake and nitrogen excretion in the animal body such that a greater intake results in a positive balance and an increased excretion causes a negative balance

nitrogen base *or* **nitrogenous base** *n* : a nitrogen-containing molecule with basic properties; *esp* : one that is a purine or pyrimidine

nitrogen dioxide *n* : a poisonous strongly oxidizing reddish-brown gas NO_2

nitrogen mustard *n* : any of various toxic blistering compounds analogous to mustard gas but containing nitrogen instead of sulfur; *esp* : MECHLORETHAMINE

nitrogen narcosis *n* : a state of euphoria and confusion similar to alcohol intoxication which occurs when nitrogen in normal air enters the bloodstream at increased partial pressure (as in deepwater diving) — called also *rapture of the deep*

ni•trog•e•nous \nī-ˈträ-jə-nəs\ *adj* : of, relating to, or containing nitrogen in combined form (as in proteins)

ni•tro•glyc•er•in *or* **ni•tro•glyc•er•ine** \ˌnī-trə-ˈgli-sə-rən\ *n* : a heavy oily explosive poisonous liquid $C_3H_5N_3O_9$ used in medicine as a vasodilator (as in angina pectoris) — see NITRO-DUR, NITROSTAT

ni•tro•mer•sol \ˌnī-trō-ˈmər-ˌsȯl, -ˌsōl\ *n* : a brownish-yellow to yellow solid organic mercurial $C_7H_5HgNO_3$ used esp. formerly as an antiseptic and disinfectant

nitroprusside — see SODIUM NITROPRUSSIDE

ni•tro•sa•mine \nī-ˈtrō-sə-ˌmēn\ *n* : any of various neutral compounds which are characterized by the group NNO and of which some are powerful carcinogens

ni•tro•so•di•meth•yl•amine \nī-ˌtrō-sō-ˌdī-ˌme-thə-ˈla-ˌmēn, -ə-ˈmēn\ *n* : DIMETHYLNITROSAMINE

ni•tro•so•urea \-yu̇-ˈrē-ə\ *n* : any of a group of lipid-soluble antineoplastic drugs that function as alkylating agents with the ability to cross the blood-brain barrier — see CARMUSTINE

Ni•tro•stat \ˈnī-trə-ˌstat\ *trademark* — used for a preparation of nitroglycerin

ni•trous oxide \ˈnī-trəs-\ *n* : a colorless gas N_2O that when inhaled produces loss of sensibility to pain preceded by exhilaration and sometimes laughter and is used esp. as an anesthetic in dentistry — called also *laughing gas*

ni•zat•i•dine \nī-ˈza-tə-ˌdīn, -ˌdēn\ *n* : an H_2 antagonist $C_{12}H_{21}N_5O_2S_2$ that is taken orally to inhibit gastric acid secretion in the treatment of duodenal and gastric ulcers and gastroesophageal reflux disease— see AXID

Ni•zo•ral \ˈnī-zə-ˌral\ *trademark* — used for a preparation of ketoconazole

NK cell \ˌen-ˈkā-\ *n* : NATURAL KILLER CELL

nm *abbr* nanometer

NMDA \ˌen-ˌem-ˌdē-ˈā\ *n* : a synthetic amino acid $C_5H_9NO_4$ that binds selectively to glutamate receptors on neurons resulting in the opening of calcium channels — called also *N-methyl-D-aspartate*

NMR *abbr* nuclear magnetic resonance

NNK \ˌen-ˌen-ˈkā\ *n* : a nitrosamine $C_{10}H_{13}N_3O_2$ in tobacco smoke that is derived from nicotine and is a powerful carcinogen

No *symbol* nobelium

no•bel•i•um \nō-ˈbe-lē-əm\ *n* : a radioactive element produced artificially — symbol *No;* see ELEMENT table

No•bel \nō-ˈbel\, **Alfred Bernhard (1833–1896)**, Swedish inventor and philanthropist.

no•ble gas \ˈnō-bəl-\ *n* : any of a group of rare gases that include helium, neon, argon, krypton, xenon, and sometimes radon and that exhibit great stability and extremely low reaction rates — called also *inert gas*

no•car•dia \nō-ˈkär-dē-ə\ *n* **1** *cap* : a genus of aerobic actinomycetes (family Actinomycetaceae) that include various pathogens as well as some soil-dwelling saprophytes **2** : any actinomycete of the genus *Nocardia* — **no•car•di•al** \-əl\ *adj*

No•card \nȯ-ˈkär\, **Edmond–Isidore–Etienne (1850–1903),** French veterinarian and biologist.

no•car•di•o•sis \nō-ˌkär-dē-ˈō-səs\ *n, pl* **-o•ses** \-ˌsēz\ : actinomycosis caused by a bacteria of the genus *Nocardia* and characterized by production of spreading granulomatous lesions

no•ce•bo \nō-ˈsē-(ˌ)bō\ *n* : a harmless substance or treatment that when taken by or administered to a patient is associated with undesirable or harmful effects or worsening of symptoms due to negative expectations or the psychological condition of the patient

nocebo effect *n* : the development of adverse side effects or worsening in the condition of a patient that occurs in response to medical treatment but cannot be considered due to the specific treatment used

noci- *comb form* : pain ⟨*noci*ceptor⟩

no·ci·cep·tion \ˌnō-si-ˈsep-shən\ *n* : the perception of a painful or injurious stimulus — called also *nociperception*

no·ci·cep·tive \ˌnō-si-ˈsep-tiv\ *adj* **1** *of a stimulus* : causing pain or injury **2** : of, induced by, or responding to a nociceptive stimulus — used esp. of receptors or protective reflexes

no·ci·cep·tor \-ˈsep-tər\ *n* : a receptor for injurious or painful stimuli : a pain sense organ

no·ci·per·cep·tion \-pər-ˈsep-shən\ *n* : NOCICEPTION

no code *n* : an order not to revive or sustain a patient who experiences a life-threating event (as heart stoppage); *also* : a patient assigned a no code

noc·tu·ria \näk-ˈtu̇r-ē-ə, -ˈtyu̇r-\ *n* : urination at night esp. when excessive

noc·tur·nal \näk-ˈtərn-ᵊl\ *adj* **1** : of, relating to, or occurring at night ⟨~ myoclonus⟩ **2** : characterized by nocturnal activity

nocturnal emission *n* : an involuntary discharge of semen during sleep often accompanied by an erotic dream

nocturnus — see PAVOR NOCTURNUS

noc·u·ous \ˈnä-kyə-wəs\ *adj* : likely to cause injury ⟨a ~ stimulus⟩

nod·al \ˈnōd-ᵊl\ *adj* : being, relating to, or located at or near a node — **nod·al·ly** *adv*

node \ˈnōd\ *n* **1** : a pathological swelling or enlargement (as of a rheumatic joint) **2** : a body part resembling a knot; *esp* : a discrete mass of one kind of tissue enclosed in tissue of a different kind — see ATRIOVENTRICULAR NODE, LYMPH NODE

node–negative *adj* : being or having cancer that has not spread to nearby lymph nodes ⟨~ breast cancer⟩

node of Ran·vier \-ˈrän-vē-ˌā\ *n* : a small gap in the myelin sheath of a myelinated axon

Ran·vier \räⁿ-vyā\, **Louis–Antoine (1835–1922)**, French histologist.

nodosa — see PERIARTERITIS NODOSA, POLYARTERITIS NODOSA

no·dose ganglion \ˈnō-ˌdōs-\ *n* : INFERIOR GANGLION 2

nodosum — see ERYTHEMA NODOSUM

nod·u·lar \ˈnä-jə-lər\ *adj* : of, relating to, characterized by, or occurring in the form of nodules ⟨~ lesions⟩ — **nod·u·lar·i·ty** \ˌnä-jə-ˈlar-ə-tē\ *n*

nodular disease *n* : infestation with or disease caused by nodular worms of the genus *Oesophagostomum* — called also *nodule worm disease*

nodular worm *n* : any of several nematode worms of the genus *Oesophagostomum* that are parasitic in the large intestine of ruminants and swine — called also *nodule worm*

nod·ule \ˈnä-(ˌ)jül\ *n* : a small mass of rounded or irregular shape: as **a** : a small abnormal knobby bodily protuberance (as a tumorous growth or a calcification near an arthritic joint) **b** : the nodulus of the cerebellum

nod·u·lo·cys·tic \ˌnä-jə-lə-ˈsi-stik\ *adj* : characterized by the formation of nodules and cystic lesions ⟨~ acne⟩

nod·u·lus \ˈnä-jə-ləs\ *n, pl* **nod·u·li** \-ˌlī\ : NODULE; *esp* : a prominence on the inferior surface of the cerebellum forming the anterior end of the vermis

noire — see TACHE NOIRE

noise pollution *n* : environmental pollution consisting of annoying or harmful noise (as of cars or airplanes) — called also *sound pollution*

Nol·va·dex \ˈnäl-və-ˌdeks\ *trademark* — used for a preparation of the citrate of tamoxifen

no·ma \ˈnō-mə\ *n* : a spreading invasive gangrene chiefly of the lining of the cheek and lips that is usu. fatal and occurs most often in persons severely debilitated by disease or profound nutritional deficiency — see CANCRUM ORIS

no·men·cla·ture \ˈnō-mən-ˌklā-chər\ *n* : a system of terms used in a particular science; *esp* : an international system of standardized New Latin names used in biology for kinds and groups of kinds of animals and plants — see BINOMIAL NOMENCLATURE — **no·men·cla·tur·al** \ˌnō-mən-ˈklā-chə-rəl\ *adj*

No·mi·na An·a·tom·i·ca \ˈnä-mi-nə-ˌa-nə-ˈtä-mi-kə, ˈnō-\ *n* : the Latin anatomical nomenclature that was prepared by revising the Basle Nomina Anatomica, adopted in 1955 at the Sixth International Congress of Anatomists, and modified at subsequent Congresses — abbr. *NA*

nom·i·nal aphasia \ˈnä-mə-nᵊl-, ˈnäm-nəl-\ *n* : ANOMIC APHASIA

no·mo·to·pic \ˌnä-mə-ˈtō-pik, ˌnō-, -ˈtä-\ *adj* : occurring in the normal place

-n·o·my \n-ə-mē\ *n comb form, pl* **-n·o·mies** : system of laws or sum of knowledge regarding a (specified) field ⟨taxo*nomy*⟩

non- *prefix* : not : reverse of : absence of ⟨*non*allergic⟩

non·ab·sorb·able \ˌnän-əb-ˈsȯr-bə-bəl, -ˈzȯr-\ *adj* : not capable of being absorbed ⟨~ silk sutures⟩

non·ac·id \-ˈa-səd\ *adj* : not acid : being without acid properties

non·adap·tive \ˌnän-ə-ˈdap-tiv\ *adj* : not serving to adapt the individual to the environment ⟨~ traits⟩

non·ad·dict \-ˈa-dikt\ *n* : a person who is not addicted to a drug

non·ad·dict·ing \-ə-ˈdik-tiŋ\ *adj* : NONADDICTIVE

non·ad·dic·tive \-ə-ˈdik-tiv\ *adj* : not causing addiction ⟨~ painkillers⟩

non·al·le·lic \ˌnän-ə-ˈlē-lik, -ˈle-\ *adj* : not behaving as alleles toward one another ⟨~ genes⟩

non·al·ler·gen·ic \-ˌa-lər-ˈje-nik\ *adj* : not causing an allergic reaction

non·al·ler·gic \-ə-ˈlər-jik\ *adj* : not allergic; *also* : not caused by an allergic reaction ⟨~ rhinitis⟩

non·am·bu·la·tory \-ˈam-byə-lə-ˌtōr-ē\ *adj* : not able to walk about ⟨~ patients⟩

non–A, non–B hepatitis \ˌnän-ˈā-ˌnän-ˈbē-\ *n* : hepatitis clinically and immunologically similar to hepatitis A and hepatitis B but caused by different viruses; *esp* : HEPATITIS C

non·an·ti·bi·ot·ic \-ˌan-tē-bī-ˈä-tik, -ˌan-ˌtī-\ *adj* : not antibiotic

non·an·ti·gen·ic \-ˌan-ti-ˈje-nik\ *adj* : not antigenic ⟨~ materials⟩

non·ar·tic·u·lar \ˌnän-är-ˈti-kyə-lər\ *adj* : affecting or involving soft tissues (as muscles and connective tissues) rather than joints ⟨~ rheumatism⟩

non·as·so·cia·tive \-ə-ˈsō-shē-ˌā-tiv, -sē-ˌā-tiv, -shə-tiv\ *adj* : relating to or being learning (as habituation and sensitization) that is not associative learning

non·ato·pic \-(ˌ)ā-ˈtä-pik, -ˈtō-\ *adj* : not affected with atopy ⟨~ patients⟩

non·bac·te·ri·al \-bak-ˈtir-ē-əl\ *adj* : not of, relating to, caused by, or being bacteria ⟨~ pneumonia⟩

non·bar·bi·tu·rate \-bär-ˈbi-chə-rət, -ˌrāt\ *adj* : not derived from barbituric acid ⟨~ sedatives⟩

non·bi·o·log·i·cal \-ˌbī-ə-ˈlä-ji-kəl\ *adj* : not biological ⟨~ factors⟩

non·cal·ci·fied \-ˈkal-sə-ˌfīd\ *adj* : not calcified ⟨a ~ lesion⟩

non·ca·lo·ric \-kə-ˈlȯr-ik, -ˈlär-; -ˈka-lə-rik\ *adj* : free from or very low in calories ⟨~ beverages⟩

non·can·cer·ous \-ˈkan-sə-rəs\ *adj* : not affected with or being cancer : not cancerous ⟨~ tumors⟩ ⟨~ patients⟩

non·car·ci·no·gen·ic \-kär-ˌsi-nə-ˈje-nik, -ˌkärs-ᵊn-ə-\ *adj* : not causing cancer — **non·car·cin·o·gen** \-kär-ˈsi-nə-jən, -ˈkärs-ᵊn-ə-ˌjen\ *n*

non·car·di·ac \-ˈkär-dē-ˌak\ *adj* : not cardiac: as **a** : not affected with heart disease **b** : not relating to the heart or heart disease ⟨~ disorders⟩

non·ca·se·at·ing \-ˈkā-sē-ˌā-tiŋ\ *adj* : not exhibiting caseation ⟨~ granulomas⟩

non·cel·lu·lar \-ˈsel-yə-lər\ *adj* : not made up of or divided into cells

non·chro·mo·som·al \-ˌkrō-mə-ˈsō-məl\ *adj* **1** : not situated on a chromosome ⟨~ DNA⟩ **2** : not involving chromosomes ⟨~ mutations⟩

non·cod·ing \-ˈkō-diŋ\ *adj* : not specifying the genetic code ⟨~ introns⟩

non·co·ital \-ˈkō-ət-ᵊl, -kō-ˈēt-\ *adj* : not involving heterosexual copulation

non·com·e·do·gen·ic \-ˌkä-mə-dō-ˈje-nik\ *adj* : not tending to clog pores (as by the formation of blackheads)

non·com·mu·ni·ca·ble \-kə-ˈmyü-ni-kə-bəl\ *adj* : not capable of being communicated; *specif* : not transmissible by direct contact ⟨a ~ disease⟩

non·com·pli·ance \-kəm-ˈplī-əns\ *n* : failure or refusal to comply (as in the taking of prescribed medication) — **non·com·pli·ant** \-ənt\ *adj*

non com·pos men·tis \ˌnän-ˈkäm-pəs-ˈmen-təs, ˌnōn-\ *adj* : not of sound mind

non·con·scious \-ˈkän-chəs\ *adj* : not conscious

non·con·ta·gious \ˌnän-kən-ˈtā-jəs\ *adj* : not contagious ⟨a ~ disease⟩

non·con·trac·tile \-kən-ˈtrakt-ᵊl, -ˌīl\ *adj* : not contractile ⟨~ fibers⟩

non·con·vul·sive \-kən-ˈvəl-siv\ *adj* : not convulsive ⟨~ seizures⟩

non·cor·o·nary \-ˈkȯr-ə-ˌner-ē, -ˈkär-\ *adj* : not affecting, affected with disease of, or involving the coronary vessels of the heart ⟨~ patients⟩

non·cy·to·tox·ic \-ˌsī-tə-ˈtäk-sik\ *adj* : not toxic to cells ⟨~ drug doses⟩

non·de·form·ing \-di-ˈfȯr-miŋ\ *adj* : not causing deformation ⟨~ arthritis⟩

non·de·pressed \-di-ˈprest\ *adj* : not suffering from depression : not depressed ⟨~ adults⟩

[1]**non·di·a·bet·ic** \-ˌdī-ə-ˈbe-tik\ *adj* : not affected with diabetes ⟨~ persons⟩

[2]**nondiabetic** *n* : an individual not affected with diabetes

non·di·ag·nos·tic \-ˌdī-ig-ˈnäs-tik, -əg-\ *adj* : not diagnostic ⟨a ~ lung scan⟩

non·di·a·lyz·able \-ˌdī-ə-ˈlī-zə-bəl\ *adj* : not dialyzable

non·di·rec·tive \ˌnän-də-ˈrek-tiv, -(ˌ)dī-\ *adj* : of, relating to, or being psychotherapy, counseling, or interviewing in which the counselor refrains from interpretation or explanation but encourages the client (as by repeating phrases) to talk freely

non·dis·junc·tion \-dis-ˈjəŋk-shən\ *n* : failure of homologous chromosomes or sister chromatids to separate subsequent to metaphase in meiosis or mitosis so that one daughter cell has both and the other neither of the chromosomes

non·dis·sem·i·nat·ed \-di-ˈse-mə-ˌnā-təd\ *adj* : not disseminated ⟨~ lupus erythematosus⟩

non·di·vid·ing \-də-ˈvī-diŋ\ *adj* : not undergoing cell division ⟨~ cells⟩

non·drowsy \-ˈdrau̇-zē\ *adj* : not causing or accompanied by drowsiness

non·drug \(ˌ)nän-ˈdrəg\ *adj* : not relating to, being, or employing drugs

non·elas·tic \-i-ˈlas-tik\ *adj* : not elastic ⟨~ fibrous tissue⟩

non·emer·gen·cy \-i-ˈmər-jən-sē\ *adj* : not being or requiring emergency care ⟨~ surgery⟩ ⟨~ patients⟩

non·en·zy·mat·ic \-ˌen-zə-ˈma-tik\ *or* **non·en·zy·mic** \-en-ˈzī-mik\ *also* **non·en·zyme** \-ˈen-ˌzīm\ *adj* : not involving the action of enzymes

non·ero·sive \-i-ˈrō-siv, -ziv\ *adj* : not characterized by erosion of tissue

non·es·sen·tial \-i-ˈsen-chəl\ *adj* : being a substance synthesized by the body in sufficient quantity for normal health and growth ⟨a ∼ fatty acid⟩ — compare ESSENTIAL

nonessential amino acid *n* : any of various amino acids that are required for normal health and growth, that can be synthesized within the body or derived in the body from essential amino acids, and that include alanine, asparagine, aspartic acid, cystine, glutamic acid, glutamine, glycine, proline, serine, and tyrosine

non•fa•mil•ial \-fə-ˈmil-yəl\ *adj* : not familial ⟨∼ colon cancer⟩

non•fat \ˌnän-ˈfat\ *adj* : lacking fat solids : having fat solids removed ⟨∼ milk⟩

non•fa•tal \-ˈfāt-ᵊl\ *adj* : not fatal

non•fatty \-ˈfa-tē\ *adj* : not fatty : containing little or no fat ⟨a ∼ meal⟩ ⟨∼ tissue⟩

non•fe•brile \-ˈfe-ˌbrīl, -ˈfē-\ *adj* : not marked or affected by a fever ⟨∼ illnesses⟩ ⟨∼ patients⟩; *also* : not occurring with a fever ⟨∼ seizures⟩

non•flag•el•lat•ed \-ˈfla-jə-ˌlā-təd\ *adj* : not having flagella

non•func•tion•al \-ˈfəŋk-shə-nəl\ *adj* : not performing or able to perform a regular function ⟨a ∼ muscle⟩

non•ge•net•ic \-jə-ˈne-tik\ *adj* : not genetic ⟨∼ diseases⟩

non•glan•du•lar \-ˈglan-jə-lər\ *adj* : not glandular ⟨the ∼ mucosa⟩

non•gono•coc•cal \-ˌgä-nə-ˈkä-kəl\ *adj* : not caused by a gonococcus

nongonococcal urethritis *n* : urethritis caused by a microorganism other than a gonococcus; *esp* : urethritis that is sexually transmitted and is caused esp. by a bacterium of the genus *Chlamydia* (*C. trachomatis*) or of the genus *Ureaplasma* (*U. urealyticum*) — called also *nonspecific urethritis*

non•gran•u•lar \-ˈgra-nyə-lər\ *adj* : not granular; *specif* : lacking granules with an affinity for specific biological stains ⟨∼ white blood cells⟩

non•grav•id \-ˈgra-vid\ *adj* : not pregnant

non•heal•ing \-ˈhē-liŋ\ *adj* : not healing ⟨∼ ulcers⟩

non•heme \-ˈhēm\ *adj* : not containing or being iron that is bound in a porphyrin ring like that of heme

non•he•mo•lyt•ic \-ˌhē-mə-ˈli-tik\ *adj* : not causing or characterized by hemolysis ⟨a ∼ streptococcus⟩

non•hem•or•rhag•ic \-ˌhe-mə-ˈra-jik\ *adj* : not causing or associated with hemorrhage ⟨∼ shock⟩

non•he•red•i•tary \-hə-ˈre-də-ˌter-ē\ *adj* : not hereditary

non•her•i•ta•ble \-ˈher-ə-tə-bəl\ *adj* : not heritable ⟨∼ diseases⟩

non•his•tone \-ˈhis-ˌtōn\ *adj* : relating to or being any of the eukaryotic proteins (as DNA polymerase) that form complexes with DNA but are not considered histones

non–Hodg•kin lymphoma \-ˈhäj-kin-\ *or* **non–Hodg•kin's lymphoma** \-kinz-\ *n* : any of various malignant lymphomas (as Burkitt's lymphoma) that are not classified as Hodgkin's lymphoma, have malignant cells derived from B cells, T cells, or natural killer cells, and are characterized esp. by enlarged lymph nodes, fever, night sweats, fatigue, and weight loss — called also *non-Hodgkin's disease*

non•ho•mol•o•gous \-hō-ˈmä-lə-gəs, -hə-\ *adj* : being of unlike genetic constitution — used of chromosomes of one set containing nonallelic genes

non•hor•mo•nal \-hȯr-ˈmōn-ᵊl\ *adj* : not hormonal ⟨∼ therapies⟩

non•hos•pi•tal \-ˈhäs-ˌpit-ᵊl\ *adj* : not relating to, associated with, or occurring within a hospital ⟨∼ clinics⟩

non•hos•pi•tal•ized \-ˈhäs-ˌpit-ᵊl-ˌīzd\ *adj* : not hospitalized ⟨∼ patients⟩

non•iden•ti•cal \-(ˌ)ī-ˈden-ti-kəl\ *adj* : not identical; *esp* : FRATERNAL

non•im•mune \-i-ˈmyün\ *adj* **1** : not immune : lacking immunity ⟨∼ people⟩ **2** : not caused or mediated by the immune system ⟨drug-induced ∼ thromobocytopenia⟩

non•in•fect•ed \-in-ˈfek-təd\ *adj* : not having been subjected to infection

non•in•fec•tious \-in-ˈfek-shəs\ *adj* : not infectious ⟨∼ diseases⟩

non•in•fec•tive \-tiv\ *adj* : not infective ⟨∼ enteritis⟩

non•in•flam•ma•to•ry \-in-ˈfla-mə-ˌtōr-ē\ *adj* : not inflammatory

non•in•sti•tu•tion•al•ized \-ˌin-stə-ˈtü-shə-nə-ˌlīzd, -ˈtyü-\ *adj* : not institutionalized

non–insulin–dependent diabetes *n* : TYPE 2 DIABETES

non–insulin–dependent diabetes mellitus *n* : TYPE 2 DIABETES — abbr. *NIDDM*

non•in•va•sive \-in-ˈvā-siv, -ziv\ *adj* **1** : not tending to spread; *specif* : not tending to infiltrate and destroy healthy tissue ⟨∼ cancer of the bladder⟩ **2** : not being or involving an invasive medical procedure ⟨∼ imaging techniques that do not require the injection of dyes⟩ — **non•in•va•sive•ly** *adv* — **non•in•va•sive•ness** *n*

non•ir•ra•di•at•ed \-i-ˈrā-dē-ˌā-təd\ *adj* : not having been exposed to radiation

non•isch•emic \-is-ˈkē-mik\ *adj* : not marked by or resulting from ischemia ⟨∼ tissue⟩

non•ke•ra•ti•nized \-ˈker-ə-tə-ˌnīzd, -kə-ˈra-tᵊn-ˌīzd\ *adj* : not marked by the formation of or conversion to keratin or keratinous tissue ⟨∼ epithelium⟩

non•ke•tot•ic \-kē-ˈtä-tik\ *adj* : not associated with ketosis ⟨∼ coma⟩

non•liv•ing \-ˈli-viŋ\ *adj* : not having or characterized by life

non•lym•pho•cyt•ic \-ˌlim-fə-ˈsi-tik\ *adj* : not lymphocytic — see ACUTE NONLYMPHOCYTIC LEUKEMIA

non•lym•phoid \-ˈlim-ˌfȯid\ *adj* : not derived from or being lymphoid tissue ⟨∼ cells⟩; *also* : not composed of lymphoid cells ⟨a ∼ tumor⟩

non•ma•lig•nant \-mə-ˈlig-nənt\ *adj* : not malignant ⟨a ~ tumor⟩

non•med•ul•lat•ed \-ˈmed-ᵊl-ˌā-təd, -ˈme-jə-ˌlā-\ *adj* : UNMYELINATED

non•mel•a•no•ma \-ˌme-lə-ˈnō-mə\ *n, often attrib* : a tumor that is not a melanoma : cancer that does not begin in melanocytes⟨~ skin cancer⟩

non•met•al \-ˈmet-ᵊl\ *n* : a chemical element (as carbon) that lacks the characteristics of a metal — **non•me•tal•lic** \-mə-ˈta-lik\ *adj*

non•met•a•stat•ic \-ˌme-tə-ˈsta-tik\ *adj* : not metastatic ⟨~ tumors⟩

non•mi•cro•bi•al \-mī-ˈkrō-bē-əl\ *adj* : not microbial ⟨~ diseases⟩

non•mo•tile \-ˈmōt-ᵊl, -ˈmō-ˌtīl\ *adj* : not exhibiting or capable of movement ⟨~ gametes⟩

non•my•elin•at•ed \-ˈmī-ə-lə-ˌnā-təd\ *adj* : UNMYELINATED

non•my•eloid \-ˈmī-ə-ˌlȯid\ *adj* : not being, involving, or affecting bone marrow ⟨~ malignancies⟩

non•nar•cot•ic \-när-ˈkä-tik\ *adj* : not narcotic ⟨~ analgesics⟩

non•neo•plas•tic \-ˌnē-ə-ˈplas-tik\ *adj* : not being or not caused by neoplasms ⟨~ diseases⟩

non•ner•vous \-ˈnər-vəs\ *adj* : not nervous ⟨~ tissue⟩

non•neu•ro•nal \-ˈnu̇r-ə-nᵊl, -ˈnyu̇-, -nu̇-ˈrō-nᵊl, -nyu̇-\ *adj* : of, relating to, or being cells other than neurons

non•nu•cle•at•ed \-ˈnü-klē-ˌā-təd, -ˈnyü-\ *adj* : not nucleated ⟨~ cells⟩

non•nu•tri•tive \-ˈnü-trə-tiv, -ˈnyü-\ *adj* : not relating to or providing nutrition

non•obese \-ō-ˈbēs\ *adj* : not obese

non•ob•struc•tive \-əb-ˈstrək-tiv\ *adj* : not causing or characterized by obstruction (as of a bodily passage)

non•oc•clu•sive \-ə-ˈklü-siv\ *adj* : not causing or characterized by occlusion

non•of•fi•cial \-ə-ˈfi-shəl\ *adj* : not described in the current *U.S. Pharmacopeia* and *National Formulary* and never having been described therein — compare OFFICIAL

non•ol•fac•to•ry \-äl-ˈfak-tə-rē, -ōl-\ *adj* : not olfactory

non•op•er•a•tive \-ˈä-pə-rə-tiv, -ˌrā-\ *adj* : not involving an operation ⟨~ treatment⟩

non•or•gas•mic \-ȯr-ˈgaz-mik\ *adj* : not capable of experiencing orgasm

no•nox•y•nol–9 \nä-ˈnäk-sə-ˌnōl-ˈnīn, -ˌnȯl-\ *n* : a spermicide used in contraceptive products that consists of a mixture of compounds having the general formula $C_{15}H_{23}(OCH_2CH_2)_n$-OH with an average of nine ethylene oxide groups per molecule

non•par•a•sit•ic \-ˌpar-ə-ˈsi-tik\ *adj* : not parasitic; *esp* : not caused by parasites ⟨~ diseases⟩

non•patho•gen•ic \-ˌpa-thə-ˈje-nik\ *adj* : not capable of inducing disease

non•per•sis•tent \-pər-ˈsis-tənt\ *adj* : not persistent; *esp* : decomposed rapidly by environmental action ⟨~ insecticides⟩

non•phy•si•cian \-fə-ˈzi-shən\ *n* : a person who is not a legally qualified physician

non•pig•ment•ed \-ˈpig-mən-təd\ *adj* : not pigmented ⟨~ skin lesions⟩

non•poi•son•ous \-ˈpȯi-zə-nəs\ *adj* : not poisonous ⟨~ snakes⟩

non•po•lar \-ˈpō-lər\ *adj* : not polar; *esp* : consisting of molecules not having a dipole

non•pol•yp•o•sis \-ˌpä-li-ˈpō-səs\ *adj* : characterized by the absence of polyps ⟨hereditary ~ colorectal cancer⟩

non•preg•nant \-ˈpreg-nənt\ *adj* : not pregnant

non•pre•scrip•tion \-pri-ˈskrip-shən\ *adj* : available for purchase without a doctor's prescription ⟨~ drugs⟩

non•pro•duc•tive \-prə-ˈdək-tiv\ *adj, of a cough* : not effective in raising mucus or exudate from the respiratory tract : DRY 2

non•pro•gres•sor \-prə-ˈgre-sər\ *n* : LONG-TERM NONPROGRESSOR

non•pro•pri•etary \-prə-ˈprī-ə-ˌter-ē\ *adj* : not proprietary ⟨a drug's ~ name⟩

non•pro•tein \-ˈprō-ˌtēn\ *adj* : not being or derived from protein

non•psy•chi•at•ric \-ˌsī-kē-ˈa-trik\ *adj* : not psychiatric ⟨~ patients⟩

non•psy•chi•a•trist \-sə-ˈkī-ə-trist, -sī-\ *adj* : not specializing in psychiatry ⟨~ physicians⟩ — **nonpsychiatrist** *n*

non•psy•chot•ic \-sī-ˈkä-tik\ *adj* : not psychotic ⟨~ emotional disorders⟩

non•pul•sa•tile \-ˈpəl-sət-ᵊl, -sə-ˌtīl\ *adj* : not marked by or occurring in pulsations : occurring continuously ⟨~ blood flow⟩

non•ra•dio•ac•tive \-ˌrā-dē-ō-ˈak-tiv\ *adj* : not radioactive ⟨~ probes⟩

non•re•ac•tive \-rē-ˈak-tiv\ *adj* : not reactive; *esp* : not exhibiting a positive reaction in a particular laboratory test ⟨all of the serums were ~⟩

non–REM sleep \-ˌrem-\ *n* : SLOW-WAVE SLEEP

non•re•nal \-ˈrēn-ᵊl\ *adj* : not renal; *esp* : not resulting from dysfunction of the kidneys ⟨~ alkalosis⟩

non•rep•li•cat•ing \-ˈre-plə-ˌkā-tiŋ\ *adj* **1** : not undergoing or marked by replication ⟨a ~ virus⟩ ⟨~ DNA⟩ **2** : containing an inactivated pathogen (as a virus) incapable of replication ⟨~ vaccines⟩

non•re•spond•er \-ri-ˈspän-dər\ *n* : one (as a patient) that does not respond (as to medical treatment)

non•rheu•ma•toid \-ˈrü-mə-ˌtȯid\ *adj* : not relating to, affected with, or being rheumatoid arthritis

non•rhyth•mic \-ˈrith-mik\ *adj* : not rhythmic ⟨~ contractions⟩

[1]**non•schizo•phren•ic** \-ˌskit-sə-ˈfre-nik\ *adj* : not relating to, affected with, or being schizophrenia

[2]**nonschizophrenic** *n* : a nonschizophrenic individual

non•se•cre•tor \-si-ˈkrē-tər\ *n* : an individual of blood group A, B, or AB who does not secrete the antigens characteristic of these blood groups in bodily fluids (as saliva)

non·se·cre·to·ry \-ˈsē-krə-ˌtōr-ē\ *adj* : not secretory ⟨~ cells⟩

non·se·dat·ing \-si-ˈdā-tiŋ\ *adj* : not producing sedation ⟨~ antihistamines⟩

[1]**non·sed·a·tive** \-ˈse-də-tiv\ *adj* : NONSEDATING

[2]**nonsedative** *n* : a nonsedating drug

non·se·lec·tive \-sə-ˈlek-tiv\ *adj* : not selective; *esp* : not limited (as to a single body part or organism) in action or effect ⟨~ anti-infective agents⟩

non·self \ˌnän-ˈself\ *n* : material that is foreign to the body of an organism — **nonself** *adj*

[1]**non·sense** \ˈnän-ˌsens, -səns\ *n* : genetic information consisting of one or more codons that do not code for any amino acid and usu. cause termination of the molecular chain in protein synthesis — compare ANTISENSE, MISSENSE

[2]**nonsense** *adj* : consisting of one or more codons that are genetic nonsense ⟨~ mutations⟩

non·sen·si·tive \-ˈsen-sə-tiv\ *adj* : not sensitive ⟨~ skin⟩

non·sex·u·al \-ˈsek-shə-wəl\ *adj* : not sexual ⟨~ reproduction⟩

non–small cell lung cancer *n* : any carcinoma (as an adenocarcinoma or squamous cell carcinoma) of the lungs that is not a small-cell lung cancer — called also *non-small cell cancer, non-small cell carcinoma, non-small cell lung carcinoma;* see LARGE-CELL CARCINOMA

non·smok·er \-ˈsmō-kər\ *n* : a person who does not smoke tobacco

non·spe·cif·ic \-spi-ˈsi-fik\ *adj* : not specific: as **a** : not caused by a specific agent ⟨~ enteritis⟩ **b** : having a general purpose or effect — **non·spe·cif·i·cal·ly** *adv*

nonspecific urethritis *n* : NONGONOCOCCAL URETHRITIS

nonspecific vaginitis *n* : BACTERIAL VAGINOSIS

non·ste·roi·dal \-stə-ˈrȯid-ᵊl\ *also* **non·ste·roid** \-ˈstir-ˌȯid, -ˈster-\ *adj* : of, relating to, or being a compound and esp. a drug that is not a steroid — see NSAID — **nonsteroid** *n*

non·stress test \ˈnän-ˈstres-\ *n* : a test of fetal well-being that is performed by ultrasound monitoring of the increase in fetal heartbeat following fetal movement

nonstriated muscle *n* : SMOOTH MUSCLE

non·sug·ar \-ˈshu̇-gər\ *n* : a substance that is not a sugar; *esp* : AGLYCONE

non·sup·pu·ra·tive \-ˈsə-pyə-ˌrā-tiv\ *adj* : not characterized by or accompanied by suppuration

non·sur·gi·cal \-ˈsər-ji-kəl\ *adj* : not surgical ⟨~ hospital care⟩ — **non·sur·gi·cal·ly** *adv*

non·sys·tem·ic \-sis-ˈte-mik\ *adj* : not systemic ⟨~ infections⟩

non·tast·er \-ˈtā-stər\ *n* : a person unable to taste the chemical phenylthiocarbamide

non·ther·a·peu·tic \-ˌther-ə-ˈpyü-tik\ *adj* : not relating to or being therapy

non·throm·bo·cy·to·pe·nic \-ˌthräm-bə-ˌsī-tə-ˈpē-nik\ *adj* : not relating to, affected with, or associated with thrombocytopenia ⟨~ purpura⟩

non·tox·ic \-ˈtäk-sik\ *adj* **1** : not toxic ⟨~ chemicals⟩ **2** *of goiter* : not associated with hyperthyroidism

non·trau·mat·ic \-trə-ˈma-tik, -trȯ-, -trau̇-\ *adj* : not causing, caused by, or associated with trauma and esp. traumatic injury ⟨~ hemorrhage⟩

non·trop·i·cal sprue \-ˈträ-pi-kəl-\ *n* : CELIAC DISEASE

non·tu·ber·cu·lous \-tu̇-ˈbər-kyə-ləs, -tyu̇-\ *adj* : not causing, caused by, or affected with tuberculosis ⟨~ mycobacteria⟩

non·union \-ˈyün-yən\ *n* : failure of the fragments of a broken bone to knit together

non·vas·cu·lar \-ˈvas-kyə-lər\ *adj* : lacking blood vessels or a vascular system ⟨a ~ layer of the skin⟩

non·ven·om·ous \-ˈve-nə-məs\ *adj* : not venomous

non·vi·a·ble \-ˈvī-ə-bəl\ *adj* : not capable of living, growing, or developing and functioning successfully

no·o·tro·pic \ˌnō-ə-ˈtrō-pik, -ˈträ-\ *n* : a drug that promotes the enhancement of cognition and memory and the facilitation of learning — called also *smart drug* — **nootropic** *adj*

NOPHN *abbr* National Organization for Public Health Nursing

nor·adren·a·line *also* **nor·adren·a·lin** \ˌnȯr-ə-ˈdren-ᵊl-ən\ *n* : NOREPINEPHRINE

nor·ad·ren·er·gic \ˌnȯr-ˌa-drə-ˈnər-jik\ *adj* : liberating, activated by, or involving norepinephrine in the transmission of nerve impulses — compare ADRENERGIC 1, CHOLINERGIC 1

nor·el·ges·tro·min \ˌnȯr-el-ˈjes-trə-mən\ *n* : a synthetic progestogen $C_{21}H_{29}NO_2$ that is used in combination with ethinyl estradiol in a contraceptive transdermal patch — see ORTHO EVRA

nor·epi·neph·rine \ˌnȯr-ˌe-pə-ˈne-frən, -ˌfrēn\ *n* : a catecholamine $C_8H_{11}NO_3$ that is the chemical means of transmission across synapses in postganglionic neurons of the sympathetic nervous system and in some parts of the central nervous system, is a vasopressor hormone of the adrenal medulla, and is a precursor of epinephrine in its major biosynthetic pathway — called also *noradrenaline;* see LEVOPHED

nor·eth·in·drone \nȯ-ˈre-thən-ˌdrōn\ *n* : a synthetic progestational hormone $C_{20}H_{26}O_2$ used in birth control pills often in the form of its acetate $C_{22}H_{28}O_3$ — see LOESTRIN, MINASTRIN, ORTHO-NOVUM

nor·ethis·ter·one \ˌnȯr-ə-ˈthis-tə-ˌrōn\ *n, chiefly Brit* : NORETHINDRONE

nor·ethyn·o·drel \ˌnȯr-ə-ˈthi-nə-ˌdrəl\ *n* : a progesterone derivative $C_{20}H_{26}O_2$ used in birth control pills and in the treatment of endometriosis and hypermenorrhea — see ENOVID

nor·flox·a·cin \nȯr-ˈfläk-sə-ˌsin\ *n* : a fluoroquinolone $C_{16}H_{18}FN_3O_3$ used topically to treat conjunctivitis and orally to treat various bacterial infections (as of the urinary tract)

nor·ges·ti·mate \nȯr-ˈjes-tə-ˌmāt\ *n* : a synthetic progestogen $C_{23}H_{31}NO_3$ that is used in combination with an estrogen (as ethinyl estradiol) in birth control pills — see ORTHO TRI-CYCLEN

nor·ges·trel \nȯr-ˈjes-trel\ *n* : a synthetic progestogen $C_{21}H_{28}O_2$ having two optically active forms of which the biologically active levorotatory form is used in birth control pills — see LEVONORGESTREL

norm \ˈnȯrm\ *n* : an established standard or average: as **a** : a set standard of development or achievement usu. derived from the average or median achievement of a large group **b** : a pattern or trait taken to be typical in the behavior of a social group

norm- *or* **normo-** *comb form* : normal ⟨*normo*blast⟩ ⟨*normo*tensive⟩

[1]**nor·mal** \ˈnȯr-məl\ *adj* **1 a** : according with, constituting, or not deviating from a norm, rule, or principle **b** : conforming to a type, standard, or regular pattern **2** : occurring naturally and not because of disease, inoculation, or any experimental treatment ⟨~ immunity⟩ **3 a** : of, relating to, or characterized by average intelligence or development **b** : free from mental illness : mentally sound **c** : characterized by balanced well-integrated functioning of the organism as a whole — **nor·mal·ize** \ˈnȯr-mə-ˌlīz\ *vb* — **nor·mal·ly** \ˈnȯr-mə-lē\ *adv*

[2]**normal** *n* : a subject who is normal

nor·meta·neph·rine \ˌnȯr-ˌme-tə-ˈne-frən, -ˌfrēn\ *n* : a metabolite of norepinephrine $C_9H_{13}NO_3$ found esp. in the urine

nor·mo·ac·tive \ˌnȯr-mō-ˈak-tiv\ *adj* : normally active ⟨~ children⟩; *also* : indicating normal activity ⟨~ bowel sounds⟩

nor·mo·blast \ˈnȯr-mə-ˌblast\ *n* : an immature red blood cell containing hemoglobin and a pyknotic nucleus and normally present in bone marrow but appearing in the blood in many anemias — compare ERYTHROBLAST — **nor·mo·blas·tic** \ˌnȯr-mə-ˈblas-tik\ *adj*

nor·mo·cal·cae·mia *chiefly Brit var of* NORMOCALCEMIA

nor·mo·cal·ce·mia \ˌnȯr-mō-kal-ˈsē-mē-ə\ *n* : the presence of a normal concentration of calcium in the blood — **nor·mo·cal·ce·mic** \-mik\ *adj*

nor·mo·chro·mia \ˌnȯr-mə-ˈkrō-mē-ə\ *n* : the color of red blood cells that contain a normal amount of hemoglobin — **nor·mo·chro·mic** \-ˈkrō-mik\ *adj*

normochromic anemia *n* : an anemia marked by reduced numbers of normochromic red blood cells in the circulating blood

nor·mo·cyte \ˈnȯr-mə-ˌsīt\ *n* : a red blood cell that is normal in size and in hemoglobin content

nor·mo·cyt·ic \ˌnȯr-mə-ˈsi-tik\ *adj* : characterized by red blood cells that are normal in size and usu. also in hemoglobin content ⟨~ blood⟩

normocytic anemia *n* : an anemia marked by reduced numbers of normal red blood cells in the circulating blood

nor·mo·gly·ce·mia \ˌnȯr-mō-glī-ˈsē-mē-ə\ *n* : the presence of a normal concentration of glucose in the blood — **nor·mo·gly·ce·mic** \-mik\ *adj*

nor·mo·ka·le·mic \ˌnȯr-mō-kā-ˈlē-mik\ *adj* : having or characterized by a normal concentration of potassium in the blood ⟨~ patients⟩

nor·mo·ten·sive \ˌnȯr-mō-ˈten-siv\ *adj* : having normal blood pressure

nor·mo·ther·mia \-ˈthər-mē-ə\ *n* : normal body temperature — **nor·mo·ther·mic** \-mik\ *adj*

nor·mo·vo·lae·mia *chiefly Brit var of* NORMOVOLEMIA

nor·mo·vol·emia \ˌnȯr-mō-ˌvä-ˈlē-mē-ə\ *n* : a normal volume of blood in the body — called also *euvolemia* — **nor·mo·vol·emic** \-mik\ *adj*

nor·o·virus \ˌnȯr-ō-ˈvī-rəs\ *n* **1** *cap* : a genus of small single-stranded highly infectious RNA viruses that include a single species (species *Norwalk virus*) with various strains causing gastroenteritis **2** : any virus of the genus *Norovirus* — see NORWALK VIRUS

Nor·plant \ˈnōr-ˌplant\ *n* : a contraceptive implant of encapsulated levonorgestrel — formerly a U.S. registered trademark

Nor·pra·min \ˈnȯr-prə-mən\ *trademark* — used for a preparation of the hydrochloride of desipramine

Nor·rie disease *also* **Nor·rie's disease** \ˈnȯr-ē(z)-\ *n* : a rare congenital X-linked disease that affects males and is characterized esp. by retinal malformation and opacification of the vitreous body leading to blindness, by progressive mental deterioration, and by deafness

Norrie, Gordon (1855–1941), Danish ophthalmologist.

19–nor·tes·tos·ter·one \(ˌ)nīn-ˈtēn-ˌnȯr-te-ˈstäs-tə-ˌrōn\ *n* : NANDROLONE

North American blastomycosis *n* : blastomycosis that involves esp. the skin, lymph nodes, and lungs and is caused by infection with a fungus of the genus *Blastomyces* (*B. dermatitidis*) — called also *Gilchrist's disease*

Northern blot *n* : a blot consisting of a sheet of a cellulose derivative that contains spots of RNA for identification by a suitable molecular probe — compare SOUTHERN BLOT, WESTERN BLOT — **Northern blotting** *n*

northern cattle grub *n* : an immature form or adult of a warble fly of the genus *Hypoderma* (*H. bovis*) — called also *cattle grub*

northern fowl mite *n* : a parasitic mite (*Ornithonyssus sylviarum*) that is a pest of birds and esp. poultry

northern rat flea *n* : a common and widely distributed flea of the genus *Nosopsyllus* (*N. fasciatus*) that is parasitic on rats and transmits murine typhus and possibly plague

nor•trip•ty•line \nȯr-ˈtrip-tə-ˌlēn\ *n* : a tricyclic antidepressant administered in the form of its hydrochloride $C_{19}H_{21}N \cdot HCl$ — see AVENTYL

Nor•vasc \ˈnȯr-ˌvask\ *trademark* — used for a preparation of the salt of amlodipine

Nor•vir \ˈnȯr-ˌvir\ *trademark* — used for a preparation of ritonavir

Nor•walk virus \ˈnȯr-ˌwȯk-\ *n* : a highly infectious virus first identified as the causative agent of an outbreak of gastroenteritis in a school in Norwalk, Ohio in 1968 and later classified as a norovirus (species *Norwalk virus*) — called also *Norwalk agent*

Nor•way rat \ˈnȯr-wā-\ *n* : BROWN RAT

Nor•wood procedure \ˈnȯr-ˌwu̇d-\ *n* : a complex surgical procedure esp. for the palliative treatment of hypoplastic left heart syndrome — called also *Norwood operation*

Norwood, William I. (*b* 1941), American surgeon.

nos- *or* **noso-** *comb form* : disease ⟨*no*sology⟩

nose \ˈnōz\ *n* **1 a** : the part of the face that bears the nostrils and covers the anterior part of the nasal cavity; *broadly* : this part together with the nasal cavity **b** : the anterior part of the head above or projecting beyond the muzzle **2** : the sense of smell : OLFACTION **3** : OLFACTORY ORGAN

nose•bleed \-ˌblēd\ *n* : an attack of bleeding from the nose — called also *epistaxis*

nose botfly *n* : a botfly of the genus *Gasterophilus* (*G. haemorrhoidalis*) that is a parasite esp. of horses and mules — called also *nose fly*

nose job *n* : RHINOPLASTY

nose•piece \ˈnōz-ˌpēs\ *n* : the bridge of a pair of eyeglasses

nos•o•co•mi•al \ˌnä-sə-ˈkō-mē-əl\ *adj* : acquired or occurring in a hospital ⟨∼ infection⟩ — **nos•o•co•mi•al•ly** \-ē\ *adv*

no•sol•o•gy \nō-ˈsä-lə-jē, -ˈzä-\ *n, pl* **-gies 1** : a classification or list of diseases **2** : a branch of medical science that deals with classification of diseases — **no•so•log•i•cal** \ˌnō-sə-ˈlä-ji-kəl\ *or* **no•so•log•ic** \-jik\ *adj* — **no•so•log•i•cal•ly** *adv* — **no•sol•o•gist** \nō-ˈsä-lə-jist\ *n*

Nos•o•psyl•lus \ˌnä-sə-ˈsi-ləs\ *n* : a genus of fleas that includes the northern rat flea (*N. fasciatus*)

nos•tril \ˈnäs-trəl\ *n* **1** : either of the external nares; *broadly* : either of the nares with the adjoining passage on the same side of the nasal septum **2** : either fleshy lateral wall of the nose

nos•trum \ˈnäs-trəm\ *n* : a medicine of secret composition recommended by its preparer but usu. without scientific proof of its effectiveness

not- *or* **noto-** *comb form* : back : back part ⟨*noto*chord⟩

notch \ˈnäch\ *n* : a V-shaped indentation (as on a bone) — **notched** \ˈnächt\ *adj*

no•ti•fi•able \ˌnō-tə-ˈfī-ə-bəl\ *adj* : required by law to be reported to official health authorities ⟨a ∼ disease⟩

no•ti•fi•ca•tion \ˌnō-tə-fə-ˈkā-shən\ *n* : the act of reporting the occurrence of a communicable disease or of an individual affected with such a disease — **no•ti•fy** \ˈnō-tə-ˌfī\ *vb*

no•to•chord \ˈnō-tə-ˌkȯrd\ *n* : a longitudinal flexible rod of cells that in all vertebrates and some more primitive forms provides the supporting axis of the body, that is almost obliterated in the adult of higher vertebrates as the body develops, and that arises as an outgrowth from the dorsal lip of the blastopore extending forward between epiblast and hypoblast in the middorsal line — **no•to•chord•al** \ˌnō-tə-ˈkȯrd-ᵊl\ *adj*

No•to•ed•res \ˌnō-tō-ˈe-ˌdrēz\ *n* : a genus of mites (family Sarcoptidae) containing mange mites that attack various mammals and esp. cats and occas. infest humans usu. through contact with cats

nour•ish \ˈnər-ish\ *vb* : to furnish or sustain with nutriment

nour•ish•ing *adj* : giving nourishment : NUTRITIOUS

nour•ish•ment \ˈnər-ish-mənt\ *n* **1** : FOOD 1, NUTRIMENT **2** : the act of nourishing or the state of being nourished

no•vo•bi•o•cin \ˌnō-və-ˈbī-ə-sən\ *n* : a highly toxic antibiotic $C_{31}H_{36}N_2O_{11}$ used in some serious cases of staphylococcal and urinary tract infection

No•vo•cain \ˈnō-və-ˌkān\ *trademark* — used for a preparation of the hydrochloride of procaine

no•vo•caine \-ˌkān\ *n* : procaine in the form of its hydrochloride; *broadly* : a local anesthetic

No•vo•Log \ˈnō-vō-ˌlȯg, -ˌläg\ *trademark* — used for a preparation of insulin aspart

noxa \ˈnäk-sə\ *n, pl* **nox•ae** \-ˌsē, -sī\ : something that exerts a harmful effect on the body

nox•ious \ˈnäk-shəs\ *adj* : physically harmful or destructive to living beings

Np *symbol* neptunium

NP *abbr* **1** neuropsychiatric; neuropsychiatry **2** nurse practitioner

NPH insulin \ˌen-ˌpē-ˈāch-\ *n* [*n*eutral *p*rotamine of *H*agedorn] : ISOPHANE INSULIN

NPN *abbr* nonprotein nitrogen

NPO *abbr* [Latin *nil per os*] nothing by mouth

NR *abbr* no refill

NREM sleep \ˈen-ˌrem-\ *n* : SLOW-WAVE SLEEP

ns *abbr* nanosecond

NSAID \ˈen-ˌsed, -ˌsād\ *n* : a nonsteroidal anti-inflammatory drug (as ibuprofen)

nsec *abbr* nanosecond

NSU *abbr* nonspecific urethritis

NTD *abbr* neural tube defect

nu•chae \ˈnü-kē, ˈnyü-\ — see LIGAMENTUM NUCHAE

nu•chal \ˈnü-kəl, ˈnyü-\ *adj* : of, relating to, or lying in the region of the nape

nuchal line *n* : any of several ridges on the outside of the skull: as **a** : one on each side that extends laterally in a curve from the external occipital protuberance to the mastoid process of the temporal bone — called also *superior nuchal line* **b** : OCCIPITAL CREST a **c** : one on each side that extends laterally from the middle of the external occipital crest below and roughly parallel to the superior nuchal line — called also *inferior nuchal line*

nucle- *or* **nucleo-** *comb form* **1** : nucleus ⟨*nucleo*n⟩ ⟨*nucleo*plasm⟩ **2** : nucleic acid ⟨*nucleo*protein⟩

nu•cle•ar \ˈnü-klē-ər, ˈnyü-\ *adj* **1** : of, relating to, or constituting a nucleus **2** : of, relating to, or utilizing the atomic nucleus, atomic energy, the atomic bomb, or atomic power

nuclear family *n* : a family group that consists only of father, mother, and children — see EXTENDED FAMILY

nuclear fission *n* : FISSION 2

nuclear magnetic resonance *n* **1** : the magnetic resonance of an atomic nucleus **2** : chemical analysis that uses nuclear magnetic resonance esp. to study molecular structure — abbr. *NMR;* see MAGNETIC RESONANCE IMAGING

nuclear medicine *n* : a branch of medicine dealing with the use of radioactive materials in the diagnosis and treatment of disease

nuclear membrane *n* : a double membrane enclosing a cell nucleus and having its outer part continuous with the endoplasmic reticulum

nuclear sap *n* : NUCLEOPLASM

nu•cle•ase \ˈnü-klē-ˌās, ˈnyü-, -ˌāz\ *n* : any of various enzymes that promote hydrolysis of nucleic acids

nu•cle•at•ed \-ˌā-təd\ *or* **nu•cle•ate** \-klē-ət\ *adj* : having a nucleus or nuclei

nuclei *pl of* NUCLEUS

nu•cle•ic acid \nu̇-ˈklē-ik-, nyu̇-, -ˈklā-\ *n* : any of various acids (as an RNA or a DNA) composed of nucleotide chains

nu•cle•in \ˈnü-klē-in, ˈnyü-\ *n* **1** : NUCLEOPROTEIN **2** : NUCLEIC ACID

nucleo- — see NUCLE-

nu•cleo•cap•sid \ˌnü-klē-ō-ˈkap-səd, ˌnyü-\ *n* : the nucleic acid and surrounding protein coat of a virus

nu•cleo•cy•to•plas•mic \-ˌsī-tə-ˈplaz-mik\ *adj* : of or relating to the nucleus and cytoplasm

nu•cleo•his•tone \-ˈhis-ˌtōn\ *n* : a nucleoprotein in which the protein is a histone

nu•cle•oid \ˈnü-klē-ˌȯid, ˈnyü-\ *n* : the DNA-containing area of a prokaryotic cell (as a bacterium)

nucleol- *or* **nucleolo-** *comb form* : nucleolus ⟨*nucleol*ar⟩

nu•cle•o•lar \nü-ˈklē-ə-lər, nyü-, ˌnü-klē-ˈō-lər, ˌnyü-\ *adj* : of, relating to, or constituting a nucleolus

nucleolar organizer *n* : NUCLEOLUS ORGANIZER

nu•cle•o•lus \nü-ˈklē-ə-ləs, nyü-\ *n, pl* **-li** \-ˌlī\ : a spherical body of the nucleus of most eukaryotes that becomes enlarged during protein synthesis, is associated with a nucleolus organizer, and contains the DNA templates for ribosomal RNA

nucleolus organizer *n* : the specific part of a chromosome with which a nucleolus is associated esp. during its reorganization after nuclear division — called also *nucleolar organizer*

nu•cleo•plasm \ˈnü-klē-ə-ˌpla-zəm, ˈnyü-\ *n* : the fluid or semifluid portion of a cell nucleus

nu•cleo•pro•tein \ˌnü-klē-ō-ˈprō-ˌtēn, ˌnyü-\ *n* : a compound that consists of a protein (as a histone) conjugated with a nucleic acid (as a DNA) and that is the principal constituent of the hereditary material in chromosomes

nu•cle•o•side \ˈnü-klē-ə-ˌsīd, ˈnyü-\ *n* : a compound (as guanosine or adenosine) that consists of a purine or pyrimidine base combined with deoxyribose or ribose and is found esp. in DNA or RNA

nu•cleo•some \-ˌsōm\ *n* : any of the repeating globular subunits of chromatin that consist of a complex of DNA and histone — **nu•cleo•so•mal** \ˌnü-klē-ə-ˈsō-məl, ˌnyü-\ *adj*

nu•cle•o•tide \ˈnü-klē-ə-ˌtīd, ˈnyü-\ *n* : any of several compounds that consist of a ribose or deoxyribose sugar joined to a purine or pyrimidine base and to a phosphate group and that are the basic structural units of RNA and DNA

nu•cle•us \ˈnü-klē-əs, ˈnyü-\ *n, pl* **nu•clei** \-klē-ˌī\ *also* **nu•cle•us•es** **1** : a cellular organelle of eukaryotes that is essential to cell functions (as reproduction and protein synthesis), is composed of a fluid or semifluid portion and a nucleoprotein-rich network from which chromosomes and nucleoli arise, and is enclosed in a definite membrane **2** : a mass of gray matter or group of nerve cells in the central nervous system **3** : the positively charged central portion of an atom that comprises nearly all of the atomic mass and that consists of protons and usu. neutrons

nucleus ac•cum•bens \-ə-ˈkəm-bənz\ *n* : a nucleus forming the floor of the caudal part of the anterior prolongation of the lateral ventricle of the brain and receiving dopaminergic innervation from the ventral tegmental area as part of the mesolimbic pathway

nucleus am•big•u•us \-am-ˈbi-gyə-wəs\ *n* : an elongated nucleus in the medulla oblongata that is a continuation of a group of cells in the ventral horn of the spinal cord and gives rise to the motor fibers of the glossopharyngeal, vagus, and accessory nerves supplying striated muscle of the larynx and pharynx

nucleus ba•sa•lis \-bə-ˈsā-ləs\ *n* : the gray matter of the substantia innominata of the forebrain that consists mostly of cholinergic neurons

nucleus basalis of Mey•nert \-ˈmī-nert\ *n* : NUCLEUS BASALIS

Meynert, Theodor Hermann (1833–1892), Austrian psychiatrist and neurologist.

nucleus cu•ne•a•tus \-ˌkyü-nē-ˈā-təs\ *n* : the nucleus in the medulla oblongata in which the fibers of the fasciculus cuneatus terminate and synapse with a component of the medial lemniscus — called also *cuneate nucleus*

nucleus grac•i•lis \-ˈgra-sə-ləs\ *n* : a nucleus in the posterior part of the medulla oblongata in which the fibers of the fasciculus gracilis terminate

nucleus pul•po•sus \-ˌpəl-ˈpō-səs\ *n, pl* **nuclei pul•po•si** \-ˌsī\ : an elastic pulpy mass lying in the center of each intervertebral fibrocartilage

nu•clide \ˈnü-ˌklīd, ˈnyü-\ *n* : a species of atom characterized by the constitution of its nucleus and hence by the number of protons, the number of neutrons, and the energy content

null cell \ˈnəl-\ *n* : a lymphocyte in the blood that does not have on its surface the receptors typical of either mature B cells or T cells

nul•li•grav•i•da \ˌnə-lə-ˈgra-və-də\ *n, pl* **-dae** \-ˌdī, -ˌdē\ *also* **-das** : a woman who has never been pregnant

nul•lip•a•ra \ˌnə-ˈli-pə-rə\ *n, pl* **-ras** *or* **-rae** \-ˌrē\ : a woman who has never borne a child

nul•lip•a•rous \ˌnə-ˈli-pə-rəs\ *adj* : of, relating to, or being a female that has not borne offspring — **nul•li•par•i•ty** \ˌnə-lə-ˈpar-ə-tē\ *n*

numb \ˈnəm\ *adj* : devoid of sensation (as from the administration of anesthesia or exposure to cold) — **numb** *vb* — **numb•ness** *n*

num•mu•lar \ˈnə-myə-lər\ *adj* **1** : circular or oval in shape ⟨~ lesions⟩ **2** : characterized by circular or oval lesions or drops ⟨~ dermatitis⟩

[1]**nurse** \ˈnərs\ *n* **1** : a woman who suckles an infant not her own : WET NURSE **2** : a licensed health-care professional who practices independently or is supervised by a physician, surgeon, or dentist and who is skilled in promoting and maintaining health — see LICENSED PRACTICAL NURSE, LICENSED VOCATIONAL NURSE, REGISTERED NURSE

[2]**nurse** *vb* **nursed; nurs•ing** **1 a** : to nourish at the breast : SUCKLE **b** : to take nourishment from the breast : SUCK **2 a** : to care for and wait on (as an injured or infirm person) **b** : to attempt a cure of (as an ailment) by care and treatment

nurse–anes•the•tist \-ə-ˈnes-thə-tist\ *n* : a registered nurse who has completed two years of additional training in anesthesia and is qualified to serve as an anesthetist under the supervision of a physician

nurse clinician *n* : NURSE-PRACTITIONER

nurse–midwife *n, pl* **nurse–midwives** : a registered nurse with additional training as a midwife who is certified to deliver infants and provide prenatal and postpartum care, newborn care, and some routine care (as gynecological exams) of women — **nurse–midwifery** *n*

nurse practitioner *n* : a registered nurse who through advanced training is qualified to assume some of the duties and responsibilities formerly assumed only by a physician — abbr. *NP;* called also *nurse clinician*

nurs•ery \ˈnər-sə-rē\ *n, pl* **-er•ies** : the department of a hospital where newborn infants are cared for

nurse's aide *n* : a person who assists trained nurses in a hospital by performing general services (as giving baths or taking vital signs)

nurs•ing \ˈnər-siŋ\ *n* **1** : the profession of a nurse **2** : the duties of a nurse

nursing bottle *n* : a bottle with a nipple (as of rubber) used in supplying food to infants

nursing home *n* : a public or private residential facility providing a high level of long-term personal and nursing care for persons (as the aged or the chronically ill) who are unable to care for themselves properly

nur•tur•ance \ˈnər-chə-rəns\ *n* : affectionate care and attention — **nur•tur•ant** \-rənt\ *adj*

nu•tra•ceu•ti•cal *also* **nu•tri•ceu•ti•cal** \ˌnü-trə-ˈsü-ti-kəl, ˌnyü-\ *n* : a foodstuff (as a fortified food or a dietary supplement) that is held to provide health or medical benefits in addition to its basic nutritional value — called also *functional food*

Nu•tra•Sweet \ˈnü-trə-ˌswēt, ˈnyü-\ *trademark* — used for a preparation of aspartame

[1]**nu•tri•ent** \ˈnü-trē-ənt, ˈnyü-\ *adj* : furnishing nourishment

[2]**nutrient** *n* : a nutritive substance or ingredient

nu·tri·ment \ˈnü-trə-mənt, ˈnyü-\ *n* : something that nourishes or promotes growth, provides energy, repairs body tissues, and maintains life

nu·tri·tion \nu̇-ˈtri-shən, nyu̇-\ *n* **1** : the act or process of nourishing or being nourished; *specif* : the sum of the processes by which an animal or plant takes in and utilizes food substances **2** : FOOD 1, NOURISHMENT — **nu·tri·tion·al** \-ˈtri-shə-nəl\ *adj* — **nu·tri·tion·al·ly** *adv*

nutritional anemia *n* : anemia (as hypochromic anemia) that results from inadequate intake or assimilation of materials essential for the production of red blood cells and hemoglobin — called also *deficiency anemia*

nu·tri·tion·ist \-ˈtri-shə-nist\ *n* : a specialist in the study of nutrition

nu·tri·tious \nu̇-ˈtri-shəs, nyu̇-\ *adj* : providing nourishment

nu·tri·tive \ˈnü-trə-tiv, ˈnyü-\ *adj* **1** : of or relating to nutrition **2** : NOURISHING

nu·tri·ture \ˈnü-trə-ˌchu̇r, ˈnyü-, -chər\ *n* : bodily condition with respect to nutrition and esp. with respect to a given nutrient (as zinc)

Nu·va·Ring \ˈnü-və-ˌriŋ\ *trademark* — used for a contraceptive flexible ring containing ethinyl estradiol and etonogestrel that is inserted into the vagina

nux vom·i·ca \ˈnəks-ˈvä-mi-kə\ *n, pl* **nux vomica** **1** : the poisonous seed of an Asian tree of the genus *Strychnos* (*S. nux-vomica*) that contains the alkaloids strychnine and brucine **2** : a drug containing nux vomica

nvCJD *abbr* new variant Creutzfeldt-Jakob disease

nyc·ta·lo·pia \ˌnik-tə-ˈlō-pē-ə\ *n* : NIGHT BLINDNESS

ny·li·drin \ˈnī-li-drən\ *n* : a synthetic adrenergic drug that acts as a peripheral vasodilator and is usu. administered in the form of its hydrochloride $C_{19}H_{25}NO_2 \cdot HCl$

nymph \ˈnimf\ *n* **1** : any of various immature insects; *esp* : a larva of an insect that differs from the adult esp. in size and in its incompletely developed wings and genitalia **2** : a mite or tick in the first eight-legged form that immediately follows the last larval molt — **nymph·al** \ˈnim-fəl\ *adj*

nymph- *or* **nympho-** *also* **nymphi-** *comb form* : nymph : nymphae ⟨*nympho*mania⟩

nym·phae \ˈnim-(ˌ)fē\ *n pl* : LABIA MINORA

nym·pho \ˈnim-(ˌ)fō\ *n, pl* **nymphos** : NYMPHOMANIAC

nym·pho·ma·nia \ˌnim-fə-ˈmā-nē-ə, -nyə\ *n* : excessive sexual desire by a female — compare SATYRIASIS

[1]**nym·pho·ma·ni·ac** \-nē-ˌak\ *n* : one affected with nymphomania

[2]**nymphomaniac** *or* **nym·pho·ma·ni·a·cal** \-mə-ˈnī-ə-kəl\ *adj* : of, affected with, or characterized by nymphomania

nys·tag·mus \ni-ˈstag-məs\ *n* : involuntary usu. rapid movement of the eyeballs occurring normally with dizziness during and after bodily rotation or abnormally following head injury or as a symptom of disease

nys·ta·tin \ˈnis-tət-ən\ *n* : an antifungal agent that is derived from a soil actinomycete of the genus *Streptomyces* (*S. noursei*) and is used esp. in the treatment of candidiasis

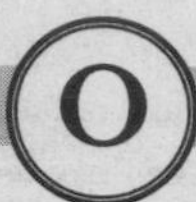

O \ˈō\ *n* : the one of the four ABO blood groups characterized by the absence of antigens designated by the letters A and B and by the presence of antibodies against these antigens

O *abbr* [Latin *octarius*] pint — used in writing prescriptions

O *symbol* oxygen

o- *or* **oo-** *comb form* : egg : ovum ⟨*oo*cyte⟩

OA *abbr* osteoarthritis

O antigen \ˈō-\ *n* : an antigen that occurs in the body of a gram-negative bacterial cell — compare H ANTIGEN

oat cell \ˈōt-\ *n* : any of the small round or oval cells with a high ratio of nuclear protoplasm to cytoplasm that resemble oat grains and are characteristic of small-cell lung cancer

oat–cell cancer *n* : SMALL-CELL LUNG CANCER

oat–cell carcinoma *n* : SMALL-CELL LUNG CANCER

oath — see HIPPOCRATIC OATH

OB *abbr* **1** obstetric **2** obstetrician **3** obstetrics

obese \ō-ˈbēs\ *adj* : having excessive body fat : affected by obesity

obe•si•ty \ō-ˈbē-sə-tē\ *n, pl* **-ties** : a condition that is characterized by excessive accumulation and storage of fat in the body and that in an adult is typically indicated by a body mass index of 30 or greater

obe•so•gen•ic \ə-ˌbē-sə-ˈje-nik, ō-\ *adj* : promoting excessive weight gain : producing obesity ⟨an ~ environment⟩

obex \ˈō-ˌbeks\ *n* : a thin triangular lamina of gray matter in the roof of the fourth ventricle of the brain

ob–gyn \ˌō-(ˌ)bē-ˈjin, -(ˌ)jē-(ˌ)wī-ˈen\ *n, pl* **ob–gyns** : a physician who specializes in obstetrics and gynecology

OB–GYN *abbr* obstetrics-gynecology

ob•jec•tive \əb-ˈjek-tiv, äb-\ *adj* **1** : of, relating to, or being an object, phenomenon, or condition in the realm of sensible experience independent of individual thought and perceptible by all observers ⟨~ reality⟩ **2** : perceptible to persons other than the affected individual ⟨an ~ symptom of disease⟩ — compare SUBJECTIVE 2b — **ob•jec•tive•ly** *adv*

ob•li•gate \ˈä-bli-gət, -ˌgāt\ *adj* **1** : restricted to one particularly characteristic mode of life or way of functioning **2** : biologically essential for survival — **ob•li•gate•ly** *adv*

oblig•a•to•ry \ə-ˈbli-gə-ˌtōr-ē, ä-\ *adj* : OBLIGATE 1

[1]**oblique** \ō-ˈblēk, ə-, -ˈblīk\ *adj* **1** : neither perpendicular nor parallel : being on an incline **2** : situated obliquely and having one end not inserted on bone ⟨~ muscles⟩ — **oblique•ly** *adv*

[2]**oblique** *n* : any of several oblique muscles: as **a** : either of two flat muscles on each side that form the middle and outer layers of the lateral walls of the abdomen and that act to compress the abdominal contents and to assist in expelling the contents of various visceral organs (as in urination and expiration): (1) : one that forms the outer layer of the lateral abdominal wall — called also *external oblique, obliquus externus abdominis* (2) : one situated under the external oblique in the lateral and ventral part of the abdominal wall — called also *internal oblique, obliquus internus abdominis* **b** (1) : a long thin extraocular muscle that arises just above the margin of the optic foramen, is inserted on the upper part of the eyeball, and moves the eye downward and laterally — called also *superior oblique, obliquus superior oculi* (2) : a short extraocular muscle that arises from the orbital surface of the maxilla, is inserted slightly in front of and below the superior oblique, and moves the eye upward and laterally — called also *inferior oblique, obliquus inferior oculi* **c** (1) : a muscle that arises from the superior surface of the transverse process of the atlas, passes medially upward to insert into the occipital bone, and functions to extend the head and bend it to the side — called also *obliquus capitis superior, obliquus superior* (2) : a muscle that arises from the apex of the spinous process of the axis, inserts into the transverse process of the atlas, and rotates the atlas turning the face in the same direction — called also *obliquus capitis inferior, obliquus inferior*

oblique fissure *n* : either of two fissures of the lungs of which the one on the left side of the body separates the superior lobe of the left lung from the inferior lobe and the one on the right separates the superior and middle lobes of the right lung from the inferior lobe

oblique popliteal ligament *n* : a strong broad flat fibrous ligament that passes obliquely across and strengthens the posterior part of the knee — compare ARCUATE POPLITEAL LIGAMENT

oblique vein of Mar•shall \-ˈmär-shəl\ *n* : OBLIQUE VEIN OF THE LEFT ATRIUM

Marshall, John (1818–1891), British anatomist and surgeon.

oblique vein of the left atrium *n* : a small vein that passes obliquely down the posterior surface of the left atrium and empties into the coronary sinus — called also *oblique vein, oblique vein of left atrium*

ob·li·quus \ō-ˈblī-kwəs\ *n, pl* **ob·li·qui** \-ˌkwī\ : OBLIQUE
obliquus cap·i·tis inferior \-ˈka-pə-təs-\ *n* : OBLIQUE c(2)
obliquus capitis superior *n* : OBLIQUE c(1)
obliquus ex·ter·nus ab·dom·i·nis \-ek-ˈstər-nəs-ab-ˈdä-mə-nəs\ *n* : OBLIQUE a(1)
obliquus inferior *n* : OBLIQUE c(2)
obliquus inferior oc·u·li \ˈä-kyü-ˌlī, -ˌlē\ *n* : OBLIQUE b(2)
obliquus in·ter·nus ab·dom·i·nis \-in-ˈtər-nəs-ab-ˈdä-mə-nəs\ *n* : OBLIQUE a(2)
obliquus superior *n* : OBLIQUE c(1)
obliquus superior oc·u·li \-ˈä-kyü-ˌlī, -ˌlē\ *n* : OBLIQUE b(1)
obliterans — see ARTERIOSCLEROSIS OBLITERANS, ENDARTERITIS OBLITERANS, THROMBOANGIITIS OBLITERANS
oblit·er·ate \ə-ˈbli-tə-ˌrāt, ō-\ *vb* **-at·ed; -at·ing** : to cause to disappear (as a bodily part or a scar) or collapse (as a duct conveying body fluid) — **oblit·er·a·tion** \-ˌbli-tə-ˈrā-shən\ *n* — **oblit·er·a·tive** \ə-ˈbli-tə-ˌrā-tiv, ō-, -rə-\ *adj*
obliterating endarteritis *n* : ENDARTERITIS OBLITERANS
ob·lon·ga·ta \ˌä-ˌblȯŋ-ˈgä-tə\ *n, pl* **-tas** *or* **-tae** \-ˌtē\ : MEDULLA OBLONGATA
OBS *abbr* **1** obstetrician **2** obstetrics
ob·ser·va·tion \ˌäb-sər-ˈvā-shən, -zər-\ *n* **1** : the noting of a fact or occurrence (as in nature) often involving the measurement of some magnitude with suitable instruments; *also* : a record so obtained **2** : close watch or examination (as to monitor or diagnose a condition) 〈postoperative ~〉
ob·sess \əb-ˈses, äb-\ *vb* **1** : to preoccupy intensely or abnormally **2** : to engage in obsessive thinking : become obsessed with an idea
ob·ses·sion \äb-ˈse-shən, əb-\ *n* : a persistent disturbing preoccupation with an often unreasonable idea or feeling; *also* : something that causes such preoccupation — compare COMPULSION, PHOBIA — **ob·ses·sion·al** \-ˈse-shə-nəl\ *adj*
obsessional neurosis *n* : an obsessive-compulsive disorder in which obsessive thinking predominates with little need to perform compulsive acts
[1]**ob·ses·sive** \äb-ˈse-siv, əb-\ *adj* : of, relating to, causing, or characterized by obsession : deriving from obsession 〈~ behavior〉 — **ob·ses·sive·ly** *adv* — **ob·ses·sive·ness** *n*
[2]**obsessive** *n* : an obsessive individual
[1]**obsessive–compulsive** *adj* : relating to or characterized by recurring obsessions and compulsions esp. as symptoms of an obsessive-compulsive disorder
[2]**obsessive–compulsive** *n* : an individual affected with an obsessive-compulsive disorder
obsessive–compulsive disorder *n* : an anxiety disorder characterized by recurrent obsessions or compulsions or both that cause significant distress, are time-consuming or interfere with normal daily functioning, and are recognized by the individual affected as excessive or unreasonable — abbr. *OCD;* called also *obsessive-compulsive neurosis, obsessive-compulsive reaction*
ob·stet·ric \əb-ˈste-trik, äb-\ *or* **ob·stet·ri·cal** \-tri-kəl\ *adj* : of, relating to, or associated with childbirth or obstetrics — **ob·stet·ri·cal·ly** *adv*
obstetric forceps *n* : a forceps for grasping the fetal head or other part to facilitate delivery in difficult labor
ob·ste·tri·cian \ˌäb-stə-ˈtri-shən\ *n* : a physician specializing in obstetrics
ob·stet·rics \əb-ˈste-triks, äb-\ *n sing or pl* : a branch of medical science that deals with birth and with its antecedents and sequelae
ob·sti·pa·tion \ˌäb-stə-ˈpā-shən\ *n* : severe and intractable constipation
ob·struct \əb-ˈstrəkt, äb-\ *vb* : to block or close up by an obstacle
ob·struc·tion \əb-ˈstrək-shən, äb-\ *n* **1 a** : an act of obstructing **b** : a condition of being clogged or blocked 〈intestinal ~〉 **2** : something that obstructs 〈an airway ~〉 — **ob·struc·tive** \-tiv\ *adj*
obstructive jaundice *n* : jaundice due to obstruction of the biliary passages
obstructive sleep apnea *n* : sleep apnea that is caused by recurring interruption of breathing during sleep due to obstruction usu. of the upper airway esp. by weak, redundant, or malformed pharyngeal tissues, that occurs chiefly in overweight middle-aged and elderly individuals, and that results in hypoxemia and frequent arousals during the night and in excessive sleepiness during the day — abbr. *OSA;* called also *obstructive apnea, obstructive sleep apnea syndrome*
ob·tund \äb-ˈtənd\ *vb* : to reduce the intensity or sensitivity of : make dull 〈agents that ~ pain〉 — **ob·tun·da·tion** \ˌäb-(ˌ)tən-ˈdā-shən\ *n*
ob·tu·ra·tor \ˈäb-tyə-ˌrā-tər, -tə-\ *n* **1 a** : either of two muscles arising from the obturator membrane and adjacent bony surfaces: (1) : OBTURATOR EXTERNUS (2) : OBTURATOR INTERNUS **b** : OBTURATOR NERVE **2 a** : a prosthetic device that closes or blocks up an opening (as a fissure in the palate) **b** : a device that blocks the opening of an instrument (as a sigmoidoscope) that is being introduced into the body
obturator artery *n* : an artery that arises from the internal iliac artery or one of its branches, passes out through the obturator canal, and divides into two branches which are distributed to the muscles and fasciae of the hip and thigh

obturator canal *n* : the small opening of the obturator foramen through which nerves and vessels pass

obturator ex·ter·nus \-ek-ˈstər-nəs\ *n* : a flat triangular muscle that arises esp. from the medial side of the obturator foramen and from the medial part of the obturator membrane, that inserts by a tendon into the trochanteric fossa of the femur, and that acts to rotate the thigh laterally

obturator foramen *n* : an opening that is situated between the ischium and pubis of the hip bone

obturator in·ter·nus \-in-ˈtər-nəs\ *n* : a muscle that arises from the margin of the obturator foramen and from the obturator membrane, that inserts into the greater trochanter of the femur, and that acts to rotate the thigh laterally when it is extended and to abduct it in the flexed position

obturator membrane *n* : a firm fibrous membrane covering most of the obturator foramen except for the obturator canal

obturator nerve *n* : a branch of the lumbar plexus that arises from the second, third, and fourth lumbar nerves and that supplies the hip and knee joints, the adductor muscles of the thigh, and the skin

obturator vein *n* : a tributary of the internal iliac vein that accompanies the obturator artery

occipit- *or* **occipito-** *comb form* : occipital and ⟨*occipito*temporal⟩

occipita *pl of* OCCIPUT

[1]**oc·cip·i·tal** \äk-ˈsi-pət-ᵊl\ *adj* : of, relating to, or located within or near the occiput or the occipital bone

[2]**occipital** *n* : OCCIPITAL BONE

occipital artery *n* : an artery that arises from the external carotid artery, ascends within the superficial fascia of the scalp, and supplies or gives off branches supplying structures and esp. muscles of the back of the neck and head

occipital bone *n* : a compound bone that forms the posterior part of the skull and surrounds the foramen magnum, bears the condyles for articulation with the atlas, is composed of four united elements, is much curved and roughly trapezoidal in outline, and ends in front of the foramen magnum in the basilar process

occipital condyle *n* : an articular surface on the occipital bone by which the skull articulates with the atlas

occipital crest *n* : either of the two ridges on the occipital bone: **a** : a median ridge on the outer surface of the occipital bone that with the external occipital protuberance gives attachment to the ligamentum nuchae — called also *external occipital crest, median nuchal line* **b** : a median ridge similarly situated on the inner surface of the occipital bone that bifurcates near the foramen magnum to give attachment to the falx cerebelli — called also *internal occipital crest*

occipital fontanel *n* : a triangular fontanel at the meeting of the sutures between the parietal and occipital bones

oc·cip·i·ta·lis \äk-ˌsi-pə-ˈtā-ləs\ *n* : the posterior belly of the occipitofrontalis that arises from the lateral two-thirds of the superior nuchal lines and from the mastoid part of the temporal bone, inserts into the galea aponeurotica, and acts to move the scalp

occipital lobe *n* : the posterior lobe of each cerebral hemisphere that bears the visual areas and has the form of a 3-sided pyramid

occipital nerve *n* : either of two nerves that arise mostly from the second cervical nerve: **a** : one that innervates the scalp at the top of the head — called also *greater occipital nerve* **b** : one that innervates the scalp esp. in the lateral area of the head behind the ear — called also *lesser occipital nerve*

occipital protuberance *n* : either of two prominences on the occipital bone: **a** : a prominence on the outer surface of the occipital bone midway between the upper border and the foramen magnum — called also *external occipital protuberance, inion* **b** : a prominence similarly situated on the inner surface of the occipital bone — called also *internal occipital protuberance*

occipital sinus *n* : a single or paired venous sinus that arises near the margin of the foramen magnum by the union of several small veins and empties into the confluence of sinuses or sometimes into one of the transverse sinuses

occipito- — see OCCIPIT-

oc·cip·i·to·fron·ta·lis \äk-ˌsi-pə-tō-frən-ˈtā-ləs\ *n* : a fibrous and muscular sheet on each side of the vertex of the skull that extends from the eyebrow to the occiput, that is composed of the frontalis muscle in front and the occipitalis muscle in back with the galea aponeurotica in between, and that acts to draw back the scalp to raise the eyebrow and wrinkle the forehead — called also *epicranius*

oc·cip·i·to·pa·ri·etal \-pə-ˈrī-ət-ᵊl\ *adj* : of or relating to the occipital and parietal bones of the skull

oc·cip·i·to·tem·po·ral \-ˈtem-pə-rəl\ *adj* : of, relating to, or distributed to the occipital and temporal lobes of a cerebral hemisphere ⟨the ~ cortex⟩

oc·ci·put \ˈäk-sə-(ˌ)pət\ *n, pl* **occiputs** *or* **oc·cip·i·ta** \äk-ˈsi-pə-tə\ : the back part of the head or skull

oc·clude \ə-ˈklüd, ä-\ *vb* **oc·clud·ed; oc·clud·ing** **1** : to close up or block off : OBSTRUCT **2** : to bring (upper and lower teeth) into occlusion **3** : SORB

occlus- *or* **occluso-** *comb form* : occlusion ⟨*occlus*al⟩

oc•clu•sal \ə-ˈklü-səl, ä-, -zəl\ *adj* : of, relating to, or being the grinding or biting surface of a tooth; *also* : of or relating to occlusion of the teeth ⟨~ abnormalities⟩ — **oc•clu•sal•ly** *adv*

occlusal disharmony *n* : a condition in which incorrect positioning of one or more teeth causes an abnormal increase in or change of direction of the force applied to one or more teeth when the upper and lower teeth are occluded

occlusal plane *n* : an imaginary plane formed by the occlusal surfaces of the teeth when the jaw is closed

oc•clu•sion \ə-ˈklü-zhən\ *n* **1** : the act of occluding or the state of being occluded : a shutting off or obstruction of something ⟨a coronary ~⟩; *esp* : a blocking of the central passage of one reflex by the passage of another **2 a** : the bringing of the opposing surfaces of the teeth of the two jaws into contact; *also* : the relation between the surfaces when in contact **b** : the transient approximation of the edges of a natural opening ⟨~ of the eyelids⟩ — **oc•clu•sive** \-siv\ *adj*

occlusive dressing *n* : a dressing that seals a wound to protect against infection

oc•cult \ə-ˈkəlt, ˈä-ˌkəlt\ *adj* : not manifest or detectable by clinical methods alone ⟨~ carcinoma⟩; *also* : not present in macroscopic amounts ⟨~ blood in a stool specimen⟩ ⟨fecal ~ blood testing⟩ — compare GROSS 2

occulta — see SPINA BIFIDA OCCULTA

oc•cu•pa•tion•al \ˌä-kyə-ˈpā-shə-nəl\ *adj* : relating to or being an occupational disease ⟨~ asthma⟩ — **oc•cu•pa•tion•al•ly** *adv*

occupational disease *n* : an illness caused by factors arising from one's occupation — called also *industrial disease*

occupational medicine *n* : a branch of medicine concerned with the prevention and treatment of occupational diseases

occupational therapist *n* : a person trained and licensed in the practice of occupational therapy

occupational therapy *n* : therapy based on engagement in meaningful activities of daily life (as self-care skills, education, work, or social interaction) esp. to enable or encourage participation in such activities despite impairments or limitations in physical or mental functioning

OCD *abbr* obsessive-compulsive disorder

och•ra•tox•in \ˌō-krə-ˈtäk-sən\ *n* : a mycotoxin produced by a fungus of the genus *Aspergillus* (*A. ochraceus*)

ochro•no•sis \ˌō-krə-ˈnō-səs\ *n, pl* **-no•ses** \-ˌsēz\ : a condition often associated with alkaptonuria and marked by pigment deposits in cartilages, ligaments, and tendons — **ochro•not•ic** \-ˈnä-tik\ *adj*

oc•treo•tide \äk-ˈtrē-ə-ˌtīd\ *n* : a long-acting synthetic analog of somatostatin that is administered esp. by subcutaneous injection in the form of its acetate $C_{49}H_{66}N_{10}O_{10}S_2$ and is used to treat acromegaly and to treat severe diarrhea associated with metastatic carcinoid tumors and vipomas

ocul- *or* **oculo-** *comb form* **1** : eye ⟨*oculo*motor⟩ **2** : ocular and ⟨*oculo*cutaneous⟩

oc•u•lar \ˈä-kyə-lər\ *adj* : of or relating to the eye ⟨~ muscles⟩ ⟨~ diseases⟩

oc•u•lar•ist \ˈä-kyə-lə-rist\ *n* : a person who makes and fits artificial eyes

oculi — see OBLIQUUS INFERIOR OCULI, OBLIQUUS SUPERIOR OCULI, ORBICULARIS OCULI, RECTUS OCULI

oc•u•list \ˈä-kyə-list\ *n* **1** : OPHTHALMOLOGIST **2** : OPTOMETRIST

oc•u•lo•ce•re•bro•re•nal syndrome \ˌä-kyə-lō-sə-ˌrē-brō-ˈrē-nᵊl-\ *n* : a rare disorder that is inherited as an X-linked recessive trait and is marked esp. by congenital cataracts, intellectual disability, generalized hypotonia, and dysfunction of the renal tubules — called also *Lowe syndrome*

oc•u•lo•cu•ta•ne•ous \ˌä-kyə-(ˌ)lō-kyu̇-ˈtā-nē-əs\ *adj* : relating to or affecting both the eyes and the skin

oc•u•lo•glan•du•lar \-ˌglan-jə-lər\ *adj* : affecting or producing symptoms in the eye and lymph nodes — see PARINAUD'S OCULOGLANDULAR SYNDROME

oc•u•lo•gy•ric crisis \ˌä-kyə-lō-ˈjī-rik-\ *n* : acute dystonia of the ocular muscles that is marked by involuntary intermittent or sustained deviation of the eyes in a usu. upward direction and is often an adverse reaction to certain medications (as antipsychotic or antiemetic drugs) but may be associated with certain medical conditions (as postencephalitic parkinsonism) — called also *oculogyric spasm*

oc•u•lo•mo•tor \ˌä-kyə-lə-ˈmō-tər\ *adj* **1** : moving or tending to move the eyeball **2** : of or relating to the oculomotor nerve

oculomotor nerve *n* : either nerve of the third pair of cranial nerves that are motor nerves with some associated autonomic fibers, arise from the midbrain, supply most muscles of the eye with motor fibers, and supply the ciliary body and iris with autonomic fibers by way of the ciliary ganglion — called also *third cranial nerve*

oculomotor nucleus *n* : a nucleus that is situated under the aqueduct of Sylvius rostral to the trochlear nucleus and is the source of the motor fibers of the oculomotor nerve

oc•u•lo•plas•ty \ˈä-kyə-lō-ˌplas-tē\ *n* : plastic surgery of the eye and adjacent parts (as the tear ducts or eyelids) — **oc•u•lo•plas•tic** \ˌä-kyə-lō-ˈplas-tik\ *adj*

od *abbr* [Latin *omnes dies*] every day — used in writing prescriptions

[1]**OD** \(ˌ)ō-ˈdē\ *n* **1 :** an overdose of a narcotic **2 :** one who has taken an OD

[2]**OD** *vb* **OD'd** *or* **ODed; OD'•ing; OD's :** to become ill or die of an OD

OD *abbr* **1** doctor of optometry **2** [Latin *oculus dexter*] right eye — used in writing prescriptions

ODD *abbr* oppositional defiant disorder

Od•di's sphincter \ˈä-dēz-\ *n* **:** SPHINCTER OF ODDI

odont- *or* **odonto-** *comb form* **:** tooth ⟨*odont*itis⟩ ⟨*odonto*blast⟩

odon•tal•gia \(ˌ)ō-ˌdän-ˈtal-jə, -jē-ə\ *n* **:** TOOTHACHE — **odon•tal•gic** \-jik\ *adj*

-odon•tia \ə-ˈdän-chə, -chē-ə\ *n comb form* **:** form, condition, or mode of treatment of the teeth ⟨orth*odontia*⟩

odon•ti•tis \-ˈtī-təs\ *n, pl* **odon•tit•i•des** \-ˈti-tə-ˌdēz\ **:** inflammation of a tooth

odon•to•blast \ō-ˈdän-tə-ˌblast\ *n* **:** one of the elongated radially arranged outer cells of the dental pulp that secrete dentin — **odon•to•blas•tic** \-ˌdän-tə-ˈblas-tik\ *adj*

odon•to•gen•e•sis \ō-ˌdän-tə-ˈje-nə-səs\ *n, pl* **-e•ses** \-ˌsēz\ **:** the formation and development of teeth

odon•to•gen•ic \ō-ˌdän-tə-ˈje-nik\ *adj* **1 :** forming or capable of forming teeth ⟨∼ tissues⟩ **2 :** containing or arising from odontogenic tissues ⟨∼ tumors⟩

odon•toid process \ō-ˈdän-ˌtȯid-\ *n* **:** DENS

odon•tol•o•gist \(ˌ)ō-ˌdän-ˈtä-lə-jist\ *n* **:** a specialist in odontology

odon•tol•o•gy \(ˌ)ō-ˌdän-ˈtä-lə-jē\ *n, pl* **-gies 1 :** a science dealing with the teeth, their structure and development, and their diseases **2 :** FORENSIC ODONTOLOGY — **odon•to•log•i•cal** \-ˌdänt-ᵊl-ˈä-ji-kəl\ *adj*

odon•to•ma \(ˌ)ō-ˌdän-ˈtō-mə\ *n, pl* **-mas** *also* **-ma•ta** \-mə-tə\ **:** a tumor originating from a tooth and containing dental tissue (as enamel)

odon•tome \ō-ˈdän-ˌtōm\ *n* **:** ODONTOMA

odor \ˈō-dər\ *n* **1 :** a quality of something that stimulates the olfactory organ **:** SMELL **2 :** a sensation resulting from adequate chemical stimulation of the olfactory organ ⟨a disagreeable ∼⟩ — **odored** *adj* — **odor•less** *adj*

odour *chiefly Brit var of* ODOR

-o•dyn•ia \ə-ˈdi-nē-ə\ *n comb form* **:** pain ⟨pleur*odynia*⟩

odyno•pha•gia \ō-ˌdi-nə-ˈfā-jə, -jē-ə\ *n* **:** pain produced by swallowing

oe•de•ma *chiefly Brit var of* EDEMA

oe•di•pal \ˈe-də-pəl, ˈē-\ *adj, often cap* **:** of, relating to, or resulting from the Oedipus complex — **oe•di•pal•ly** *adv, often cap*

[1]**Oe•di•pus** \-pəs\ *adj* **:** OEDIPAL

[2]**Oedipus** *n* **:** OEDIPUS COMPLEX

Oedipus complex *n* **:** the positive libidinal feelings of a child toward the parent of the opposite sex and hostile or jealous feelings toward the parent of the same sex that may be a source of adult personality disorder when unresolved — used esp. of the male child; see ELECTRA COMPLEX

oesophag- *or* **oesophago-** *chiefly Brit var of* ESOPHAG-

oe•soph•a•ge•al, oe•soph•a•gec•to•my, oe•soph•a•go•gas•trec•to•my, oe•soph•a•go•plas•ty, oe•soph•a•gus *chiefly Brit var of* ESOPHAGEAL, ESOPHAGECTOMY, ESOPHAGOGASTRECTOMY, ESOPHAGOPLASTY, ESOPHAGUS

oe•soph•a•go•sto•mi•a•sis *also* **esoph•a•go•sto•mi•a•sis** \i-ˌsä-fə-(ˌ)gō-stə-ˈmī-ə-səs\ *n, pl* **-a•ses** \-ˌsēz\ **:** infestation with or disease caused by nematode worms of the genus *Oesophagostomum* **:** NODULAR DISEASE

Oe•soph•a•gos•to•mum \i-ˌsä-fə-ˈgäs-tə-məm\ *n* **:** a genus of strongylid nematode worms comprising the nodular worms of ruminants and swine and other worms affecting primates including humans esp. in Africa

oestr- *or* **oestro-** *chiefly Brit var of* ESTR-

oes•tra•di•ol \ˌēs-trə-ˈdī-ˌȯl, -ˌōl\, **oes•tro•gen** \ˈē-strə-jən\, **oes•trus** \ˈē-strəs\ *chiefly Brit var of* ESTRADIOL, ESTROGEN, ESTRUS

Oes•trus \ˈes-trəs, ˈēs-\ *n* **:** a genus (family *Oestridae*) of dipteran flies including the sheep botfly (*O. ovis*)

of•fi•cial \ə-ˈfi-shəl\ *adj* **:** prescribed or recognized as authorized; *specif* **:** described by the *U.S. Pharmacopeia* or the *National Formulary* — compare NONOFFICIAL, UNOFFICIAL — **of•fi•cial•ly** *adv*

[1]**of•fi•ci•nal** \ə-ˈfis-ᵊn-əl, ȯ-, ä-; ˌȯ-fə-ˈsīn-ᵊl, ˌä-\ *adj* **1 a :** available without special preparation or compounding ⟨∼ medicine⟩ **b :** OFFICIAL 2 **c** *of a plant* **:** MEDICINAL ⟨∼ herbs⟩

[2]**officinal** *n* **:** an officinal drug, medicine, or plant

off–la•bel \ˌȯf-ˈlā-bəl\ *adj* **:** of, relating to, or being an approved drug legally prescribed or a medical device legally used by a physician for a purpose (as the treatment of children or of a certain disease or condition) for which it has not been specif. approved

off•spring \ˈȯf-ˌspriŋ\ *n, pl* **offspring** *also* **offsprings :** the progeny of an animal or plant

oflox•a•cin \ō-ˈfläk-sə-sən\ *n* **:** a fluoroquinolone $C_{18}H_{20}FN_3O_4$ that is a broad-spectrum antibacterial agent that is used in topical solution for otic or ophthalmic use or is administered orally or intravenously for other uses — see LEVOFLOXACIN

Ogil•vie's syndrome \ˈō-gəl-vēz-\ *n* **:** distension of the colon that is similar to that occurring as a consequence of bowel obstruction but in which no physical obstruction exists and that occurs esp. in seriously ill individuals and as a complication of abdominal surgery

Ogilvie, Sir William Heneage (1887–1971), British surgeon.

ohm \ˈōm\ *n* **:** a unit of electrical resistance equal to the resistance of a circuit in which a potential difference of one volt produces a current of one ampere

Ohm, Georg Simon (1789–1854), German physicist.

Ol *abbr* opportunistic infection

oil \ˈȯil\ *n* **1 :** any of numerous fatty combustible substances that are liquid or can be liquefied easily on warming, are soluble in ether but not in water, and leave a greasy stain on paper or cloth — see ESSENTIAL OIL, FATTY OIL, VOLATILE OIL **2 :** a substance (as a cosmetic preparation) of oily consistency — **oil** *adj*

oil gland *n* **:** a gland (as of the skin) that produces an oily secretion; *specif* **:** SEBACEOUS GLAND

oil of wintergreen *n* **:** a preparation of methyl salicylate obtained by distilling the leaves of wintergreen (*Gaultheria procumbens*) — called also *gaultheria oil, wintergreen oil*

oily \ˈȯi-lē\ *adj* **oil·i·er; -est 1 :** of, relating to, or consisting of oil **2 :** excessively high in naturally secreted oils ⟨~ hair⟩ ⟨~ skin⟩

oint·ment \ˈȯint-mənt\ *n* **:** a salve or unguent for application to the skin; *specif* **:** a semisolid medicinal preparation usu. having a base of fatty or greasy material

-ol \ˌȯl, ˌōl\ *n suffix* **:** chemical compound (as an alcohol or phenol) containing hydroxyl ⟨glycer*ol*⟩

OL *abbr* [Latin *oculus laevus*] left eye — used in writing prescriptions

olan·za·pine \ō-ˈlan-zə-ˌpēn\ *n* **:** an antipsychotic drug $C_{17}H_{20}H_4S$ used esp. in the short-term treatment of schizophrenia and acute manic episodes of bipolar disorder — see ZYPREXA

ole- *or* **oleo-** *also* **olei-** *comb form* **:** oil ⟨*ole*in⟩

olea *pl of* OLEUM

ole·an·der \ˈō-lē-ˌan-dər, ˌō-lē-ˈ\ *n* **:** a poisonous evergreen shrub (*Nerium oleander*) of the dogbane family (Apocynaceae) that contains the cardiac glycoside oleandrin

ole·an·do·my·cin \ˌō-lē-ˌan-də-ˈmīs-ᵊn\ *n* **:** an antibiotic $C_{35}H_{61}NO_{12}$ produced by a bacterium of the genus *Streptomyces* (*S. antibioticus*)

ole·an·drin \ˌō-lē-ˈan-drən\ *n* **:** a poisonous crystalline glycoside $C_{32}H_{48}O_9$ found in oleander leaves and resembling digitalis in its action

ole·ate \ˈō-lē-ˌāt\ *n* **1 :** a salt or ester of oleic acid **2 :** a liquid or semisolid preparation of a medicinal dissolved in an excess of oleic acid

olec·ra·non \ō-ˈle-krə-ˌnän\ *n* **:** the large process of the ulna that projects behind the elbow, forms the bony prominence of the elbow, and receives the insertion of the triceps muscle

olecranon fossa *n* **:** the fossa at the distal end of the humerus into which the olecranon fits when the arm is in full extension — compare CORONOID FOSSA

ole·ic acid \ō-ˈlē-ik-, -ˈlā-\ *n* **:** a monounsaturated fatty acid $C_{18}H_{34}O_2$ found in natural fats and oils

ole·in \ˈō-lē-ən\ *n* **:** an ester of glycerol and oleic acid

oleo- *see* OLE-

oleo·res·in \ˌō-lē-ō-ˈrez-ᵊn\ *n* **1 :** a natural plant product containing chiefly essential oil and resin **2 :** a preparation consisting essentially of oil holding resin in solution — **oleo·res·in·ous** \-ˈrez-ᵊn-əs\ *adj*

oleo·tho·rax \-ˈthōr-ˌaks\ *n, pl* **-tho·rax·es** *or* **-tho·ra·ces** \-ˈthōr-ə-ˌsēz\ **:** a state in which oil is present in the pleural cavity usu. as a result of injection — compare PNEUMOTHORAX

oles·tra \ō-ˈles-trə\ *n* **:** a noncaloric fat substitute that consists of sucrose esters resistant to absorption by the digestive system due to their large size

ole·um \ˈō-lē-əm\ *n, pl* **olea** \-lē-ə\ **:** OIL 1

ol·fac·tion \äl-ˈfak-shən, ōl-\ *n* **1 :** the sense of smell **2 :** the act or process of smelling

ol·fac·to·ry \äl-ˈfak-tə-rē, ōl-\ *adj* **:** of, relating to, or connected with the sense of smell

olfactory area *n* **1 :** the sensory area for olfaction lying in the parahippocampal gyrus **2 :** the area of nasal mucosa in which the olfactory organ is situated

olfactory bulb *n* **:** a bulbous anterior projection of the olfactory lobe that is the place of termination of the olfactory nerves

olfactory cell *n* **:** a sensory cell specialized for the reception of sensory stimuli caused by odors; *specif* **:** any of the spindle-shaped neurons in the nasal mucous membrane of vertebrates — see OLFACTORY ORGAN

olfactory cortex *n* **:** a group of cortical areas of the cerebrum that receive sensory input from the olfactory bulb via the olfactory tract and includes the piriform cortex and parts of the olfactory tubercle, amygdala, and entorhinal cortex

olfactory epithelium *n* **:** the nasal mucosa containing olfactory cells

olfactory gland *n* **:** any of the tubular and often branched glands occurring beneath the olfactory epithelium of the nose — called also *Bowman's gland, gland of Bowman*

olfactory glomerulus *n* **:** GLOMERULUS b

olfactory gyrus *n* **:** either a lateral or a medial gyrus on each side of the brain by which the olfactory tract on the corresponding side communicates with the olfactory area

olfactory lobe *n* **:** a lobe of the brain that rests on the lower surface of a temporal lobe and projects forward from the anterior lower part of each cerebral hemisphere and that consists of an olfactory bulb, an olfactory tract, and an olfactory trigone

olfactory nerve *n* : either of the pair of nerves that are the first cranial nerves, that serve to conduct sensory stimuli from the olfactory organ to the brain, and that arise from the olfactory cells and terminate in the olfactory bulb — called also *first cranial nerve*

olfactory organ *n* : an organ of chemical sense that receives stimuli interpreted as odors, that lies in the walls of the upper part of the nasal cavity, and that forms a mucous membrane continuous with the rest of the lining of the nasal cavity

olfactory pit *n* : a depression on the head of an embryo that becomes converted into a nasal passage

olfactory tract *n* : a tract of nerve fibers in the olfactory lobe on the inferior surface of the frontal lobe of the brain that passes from the olfactory bulb to the olfactory trigone

olfactory trigone *n* : a triangular area of gray matter on each side of the brain forming the junction of an olfactory tract with a cerebral hemisphere near the optic chiasma

olfactory tubercle *n* : a small area of gray matter behind the olfactory trigone that is innervated by dopaminergic neurons from the ventral tegmental area

olig- *or* **oligo-** *comb form* **1** : few <*oligo*peptide> **2** : deficiency : insufficiency <*olig*uria>

ol•i•gae•mia *chiefly Brit var of* OLIGEMIA

ol•i•ge•mia \ˌä-lə-ˈgē-mē-ə, -ˈjē-\ *n* : a condition in which the total volume of the blood is reduced — **ol•i•ge•mic** \-mik\ *adj*

oli•go•ar•tic•u•lar \ˌä-li-gō-är-ˈti-kyə-lər, ə-ˌli-gə-\ *adj* : affecting a few joints <~ arthritis> — compare MONOARTICULAR, POLYARTICULAR

ol•i•go•as•tro•cy•to•ma \-ˌa-strə-sī-ˈtō-mə\ *n, pl* **-mas** : a brain tumor that is composed of glial tissue containing both oligodendrocytes and astrocytes and that occurs chiefly in the frontal and temporal lobes of the cerebrum — see MIXED GLIOMA

oli•go•dac•tyl•ism \ˌä-li-gō-ˈdak-tə-ˌli-zəm, ə-ˌli-gō-\ *also* **oli•go•dac•tyly** \-lē\ *n, pl* **-tyl•isms** *also* **-tylies** : the presence of fewer than five digits on a hand or foot

oli•go•den•dro•cyte \-ˈden-drə-ˌsīt\ *n* : a glial cell resembling an astrocyte but smaller with few and slender processes having few branches and forming the myelin sheath around axons in the central nervous system

oli•go•den•drog•lia \ˌä-li-gō-den-ˈdrä-glē-ə, ˌō-li-, -ˈdrō-\ *n* : glia made up of oligodendrocytes — **oli•go•den•drog•li•al** \-lē-əl\ *adj*

oli•go•den•dro•gli•o•ma \-ˌden-drō-glī-ˈō-mə\ *n, pl* **-mas** *also* **-ma•ta** \-mə-tə\ : a tumor of the nervous system composed of oligodendroglia

oli•go•fruc•tose \-ˈfrək-ˌtōs, -ˈfrük-, -ˈfru̇k, -ˌtōz\ *n* : a short-chain polysaccharide produced by partial enzymatic hydrolysis of inulin and used similarly to inulin in processed foods

oli•go•hy•dram•ni•os \-ˌhī-ˈdram-nē-ˌäs\ *n* : deficiency of amniotic fluid sometimes resulting in an embryonic defect through adherence between embryo and amnion

oli•go•men•or•rhea \-ˌme-nə-ˈrē-ə\ *n* : abnormally infrequent or scanty menstrual flow

oli•go•men•or•rhoea *chiefly Brit var of* OLIGOMENORRHEA

oli•go•nu•cle•o•tide \-ˈnü-klē-ə-ˌtīd, -ˈnyü-\ *n* : a nucleic-acid chain usu. consisting of up to 20 nucleotides

oli•go•pep•tide \ˌä-li-gō-ˈpep-ˌtīd, ˌō-li-\ *n* : a protein fragment or molecule that usu. consists of less than 25 amino acid residues linked in a polypeptide chain

oli•go•phre•nia \-ˈfrē-nē-ə\ *n* : INTELLECTUAL DISABILITY

oli•go•sper•mia \-ˈspər-mē-ə\ *n* : deficiency of sperm in the semen — **oli•go•sper•mic** \-mik\ *adj*

ol•i•gu•ria \ˌä-lə-ˈgu̇r-ē-ə, -ˈgyu̇r-\ *n* : reduced excretion of urine — **ol•i•gur•ic** \-ik\ *adj*

ol•i•vary \ˈä-lə-ˌver-ē\ *adj* **1** : shaped like an olive **2** : of, relating to, situated near, or comprising one or more of the olives, inferior olives, or superior olives <the ~ complex>

olivary body *n* : OLIVE

olivary nucleus *n* **1** : INFERIOR OLIVE **2** : SUPERIOR OLIVE

ol•ive \ˈä-liv\ *n* : an oval eminence on each ventrolateral aspect of the medulla oblongata that contains the inferior olive of the same side — called also *olivary body*

olive oil *n* : a pale yellow to yellowish-green edible oil obtained from the pulp of olives that is high in monounsaturated fatty acids and is used chiefly as a salad oil and in cooking, in soaps, and as an emollient

ol•i•vo•cer•e•bel•lar tract \ˌä-li-vō-ˌser-ə-ˈbe-lər-\ *n* : a tract of fibers that arises in the olive on one side, crosses to the olive on the other, and enters the cerebellum by way of the inferior cerebellar peduncle

ol•i•vo•pon•to•cer•e•bel•lar atrophy \-ˌpän-tō-ˌser-ə-ˈbe-lər-\ *n* : an inherited disease esp. of mid to late life that is characterized by ataxia, hypotonia, dysarthria, and degeneration of the cerebellar cortex, middle cerebellar peduncles, and inferior olives — called also *olivopontocerebellar degeneration*

ol•i•vo•spi•nal tract \-ˈspīn-ᵊl-\ *n* : a tract of fibers on the peripheral aspect of the ventral side of the cervical part of the spinal cord that communicates with the inferior olive

ol·me·sar·tan \ˌäl-mə-ˈsär-ˌtan\ *n* : an angiotensin-receptor blocker $C_{29}H_{30}N_6O_6$ taken orally to treat hypertension — called also *olmesartan medox·o·mil* \-mə-ˈdäk-sə-ˌmil\; see AZOR, BENICAR, BENICAR HCT, TRIBENZOR

olo·pat·a·dine \ˌō-lō-ˈpat-ə-ˌdēn\ *n* : an antihistamine $C_{21}H_{23}NO_3{\cdot}HCl$ administered as eye drops to treat itching associated with allergic conjunctivitis — see PATADAY, PATANOL

ol·sal·a·zine \ōl-ˈsa-lə-ˌzēn\ *n* : a disodium salicylate salt $C_{14}H_8N_2Na_2O_6$ administered orally as an anti-inflammatory agent to treat ulcerative colitis — called also *olsalazine sodium*

-o·ma \ˈō-mə\ *n suffix, pl* **-o·mas** \-məz\ *also* **-o·ma·ta** \-mə-tə\ : tumor ⟨aden*oma*⟩ ⟨fibr*oma*⟩

oma·liz·u·mab \ˌō-mə-ˈliz-ə-ˌmab\ *n* : an immunosuppressive drug that is a recombinant monoclonal antibody administered by subcutaneous injection esp. in the treatment of asthma and chronic hives — see XOLAIR

ome·ga–6 \ō-ˈme-gə-ˈsiks, -ˈmā-\ *adj* : being or composed of polyunsaturated fatty acids in which the first double bond in the hydrocarbon chain occurs between the sixth and seventh carbon atoms from the end of the molecule most distant from the carboxylic acid group and which are found esp. in vegetable oils, nuts, beans, seeds, and grains — **omega–6** *n*

ome·ga–3 \-ˈthrē\ *adj* : being or composed of polyunsaturated fatty acids in which the first double bond in the hydrocarbon chain occurs between the third and fourth carbon atoms from the end of the molecule most distant from the carboxylic acid group and which are found esp. in fish (as tuna and salmon), fish oils, green leafy vegetables, and some vegetable oils — **omega–3** *n*

oment- *or* **omento-** *comb form* : omentum ⟨*oment*ectomy⟩ ⟨*omento*pexy⟩

omen·tec·to·my \ˌō-men-ˈtek-tə-mē\ *n, pl* **-mies** : excision or resection of all or part of an omentum — called also *epiploectomy*

omen·to·pexy \ō-ˈmen-tə-ˌpek-sē\ *n, pl* **-pex·ies** : the operation of suturing the omentum esp. to another organ

omen·to·plas·ty \-ˌplas-tē\ *n, pl* **-ties** : the use of a piece or flap of tissue from an omentum as a graft

omen·tor·rha·phy \ˌō-men-ˈtȯr-ə-fē\ *n, pl* **-phies** : surgical repair of an omentum by suturing

omen·tum \ō-ˈmen-təm\ *n, pl* **-ta** \-tə\ *or* **-tums** : a fold of peritoneum connecting or supporting abdominal structures (as the stomach or liver) — see GREATER OMENTUM, LESSER OMENTUM — **omen·tal** \-ˈment-ᵊl\ *adj*

omep·ra·zole \ō-ˈme-prə-ˌzōl\ *n* : a proton pump inhibitor $C_{17}H_{19}N_3O_3S$ taken orally to treat duodenal and gastric ulcers, gastroesophageal reflux disease, erosive esophagitis, and disorders (as Zollinger-Ellison syndrome) involving gastric acid hypersecretion — see PRILOSEC

Om·nar·is \ˌäm-ˈner-əs\ *trademark* — used for a nasal spray containing ciclesonide

omo·hy·oi·de·us \-hī-ˈȯi-dē-əs\ *n, pl* **-dei** \-dē-ˌī\ : OMOHYOID MUSCLE

omo·hy·oid muscle \ˌō-mō-ˈhī-ˌȯid-\ *n* : a muscle that arises from the upper border of the scapula, is inserted in the body of the hyoid bone, and acts to draw the hyoid bone in a caudal direction — called also *omohyoid*

omphal- *or* **omphalo-** *comb form* **1** : umbilicus ⟨*omphal*itis⟩ **2** : umbilical and ⟨*omphalo*mesenteric duct⟩

om·pha·lec·to·my \ˌäm-fə-ˈlek-tə-mē\ *n, pl* **-mies** : surgical excision of the navel — called also *umbilectomy*

om·phal·ic \(ˌ)äm-ˈfa-lik\ *adj* : of or relating to the navel

om·pha·li·tis \ˌäm-fə-ˈlī-təs\ *n, pl* **-lit·i·des** \-ˈli-tə-ˌdēz\ : inflammation of the navel

om·pha·lo·cele \äm-ˈfa-lə-ˌsēl, ˈäm-fə-lə-\ *n* : protrusion of abdominal contents through an opening at the navel occurring esp. as a congenital defect

om·pha·lo·mes·en·ter·ic duct \ˌäm-fə-lō-ˌmez-ᵊn-ˈter-ik-, -ˌmes-\ *n* : the duct by which the yolk sac or umbilical vesicle remains connected with the digestive tract of the vertebrate embryo — called also *vitelline duct, yolk stalk*

om·pha·lo·phle·bi·tis \-fli-ˈbī-təs\ *n, pl* **-bit·i·des** \-ˈbi-tə-ˌdēz\ : a condition (as navel ill) characterized by or resulting from inflammation and infection of the umbilical vein

onan·ism \ˈō-nə-ˌni-zəm\ *n* **1** : MASTURBATION **2** : COITUS INTERRUPTUS — **onan·is·tic** \ˌō-nə-ˈnis-tik\ *adj*

onan·ist \ˈō-nə-nist\ *n* : an individual that practices onanism

On·cho·cer·ca \ˌäŋ-kə-ˈsər-kə\ *n* : a genus of long slender filarial worms (family Dipetalonematidae) that are parasites of mammalian subcutaneous and connective tissues

on·cho·cer·ci·a·sis \ˌäŋ-kō-ˌsər-ˈkī-ə-səs\ *n, pl* **-a·ses** \-ˌsēz\ : infestation with or disease caused by filarial worms of the genus *Onchocerca; esp* : a human disease marked by subcutaneous nodules, dermatitis, and visual impairment and that is caused by a worm (*O. volvulus*) found in Africa and tropical America and transmitted by the bite of a female blackfly — called also *river blindness*

onco- *or* **oncho-** *comb form* **1** : tumor ⟨*onco*logy⟩ **2** : bulk : mass ⟨*onco*sphere⟩

on·co·cyte \ˈäŋ-kō-ˌsīt\ *n* : an acidophilic granular cell esp. of the parotid gland

on·co·cy·to·ma \ˌäŋ-kō-sī-ˈtō-mə\ *n, pl* **-mas** *also* **-ma·ta** \-mə-tə\ : a tumor (as of the parotid gland) consisting chiefly or entirely of oncocytes

on•co•fer•til•i•ty \-fər-ˈti-lə-tē\ *n* : a field of medicine concerned with minimizing the negative effects of cancer treatment on the reproductive system and fertility and with assisting individuals with reproductive impairments resulting from cancer therapy

on•co•fetal \-ˈfēt-ᵊl\ *adj* : of, relating to, or occurring in both tumorous and fetal tissues

on•co•gene \ˈäŋ-kō-ˌjēn\ *n* : a gene having the potential to cause a normal cell to become cancerous

on•co•gen•e•sis \ˌäŋ-kō-ˈje-nə-səs\ *n, pl* **-e•ses** \-ˌsēz\ : the induction or formation of tumors

on•co•gen•ic \-ˈje-nik\ *adj* **1** : relating to tumor formation **2** : tending to cause tumors ⟨an ∼ virus⟩ — **on•co•gen•i•cal•ly** *adv* — **on•co•ge•nic•i•ty** \-jə-ˈni-sə-tē\ *n*

on•col•o•gist \än-ˈkä-lə-jəst, äŋ-\ *n* : a specialist in oncology

on•col•o•gy \än-ˈkä-lə-jē, äŋ-\ *n, pl* **-gies** : the study of tumors and neoplastic diseases — **on•co•log•i•cal** \ˌäŋ-kə-ˈlä-ji-kəl\ *also* **on•co•log•ic** \-jik\ *adj*

on•col•y•sis \-ˈkä-lə-səs\ *n, pl* **-y•ses** \-ˌsēz\ : the destruction of tumor cells — **on•co•lyt•ic** \ˌäŋ-kə-ˈli-tik\ *adj* — **on•co•lyt•i•cal•ly** *adv*

on•co•pro•tein \ˌäŋ-kō-ˈprō-ˌtēn\ *n* : a protein that is coded for by a viral oncogene and that is involved in the regulation or synthesis of proteins linked to tumorigenic cell growth

on•cor•na•vi•rus \ˌäŋ-ˌkȯr-nə-ˈvī-rəs\ *n* : ONCOVIRUS

on•co•sphere *also* **on•cho•sphere** \ˈäŋ-kō-ˌsfir\ *n* : an embryo of a tapeworm (order Cyclophyllidea) that has six hooks

on•cot•ic pressure \(ˌ)äŋ-ˈkä-tik-, (ˌ)än-\ *n* : the pressure exerted by plasma proteins on the capillary wall

On•co•vin \ˈäŋ-kō-ˌvin\ *n* : a preparation of vincristine — formerly a U.S. registered trademark

on•co•vi•rus \ˈäŋ-kō-ˌvī-rəs\ *n* : any of various tumor-forming retroviruses

on•dan•se•tron \än-ˈdän-si-ˌträn\ *n* : an antiemetic drug administered orally or parenterally in the form of its hydrated hydrochloride $C_{18}H_{19}N_3O·HCl·2H_2O$ to prevent nausea and vomiting occurring esp. as a consequence of chemotherapy or surgery — see ZOFRAN

one–egg *adj* : MONOZYGOTIC ⟨∼ twins⟩

On•gly•za \än-ˈglī-zə\ *trademark* — used for a preparation of saxagliptin

on•lay \ˈȯn-ˌlā, ˈän-\ *n* **1** : a metal covering attached to a tooth to restore one or more of its surfaces **2** : a graft applied to the surface of a tissue (as bone)

on•set \ˈȯn-ˌset, ˈän-\ *n* : the initial existence or symptoms of a disease

ont- *or* **onto-** *comb form* : organism ⟨*onto*geny⟩

-ont \ˌänt\ *n comb form* : cell : organism ⟨schiz*ont*⟩

on•to•gen•e•sis \ˌän-tə-ˈje-nə-səs\ *n, pl* **-gen•e•ses** \-ˌsēz\ : ONTOGENY

on•to•ge•net•ic \-jə-ˈne-tik\ *adj* : of, relating to, or appearing in the course of ontogeny — **on•to•ge•net•i•cal•ly** *adv*

on•tog•e•ny \än-ˈtä-jə-nē\ *n, pl* **-nies** : the development or course of development of an individual organism — called also *ontogenesis;* compare PHYLOGENY 2

onych- *or* **onycho-** *comb form* : nail of the finger or toe ⟨*onycho*lysis⟩

on•ych•ec•to•my \ˌä-ni-ˈkek-tə-mē\ *n, pl* **-mies** : surgical excision of a fingernail or toenail

onych•ia \ō-ˈni-kē-ə\ *n* : inflammation of the matrix of a nail often leading to suppuration and loss of the nail

-o•nych•ia \ə-ˈni-kē-ə\ *n comb form* : condition of the nails of the fingers or toes ⟨leuk*onychia*⟩

-o•nych•i•um \ə-ˈni-kē-əm\ *n comb form* : fingernail : toenail : region of the fingernail or toenail ⟨ep*onychium*⟩

on•y•cho•gry•po•sis \ˌä-ni-kō-gri-ˈpō-səs\ *n, pl* **-po•ses** \-ˌsēz\ : an abnormal condition of the nails characterized by marked hypertrophy and increased curvature

on•y•chol•y•sis \ˌä-nə-ˈkä-lə-səs\ *n, pl* **-y•ses** \-ˌsēz\ : a loosening of a nail from the nail bed beginning at the free edge and proceeding to the root

on•y•cho•ma•de•sis \ˌä-ni-kō-mə-ˈdē-səs\ *n, pl* **-de•ses** \-ˌsēz\ : loosening and shedding of the nails

on•y•cho•my•co•sis \-mī-ˈkō-səs\ *n, pl* **-co•ses** \-ˌsēz\ : a fungal disease of the nails

on•y•cho•til•lo•ma•nia \ˌä-ni-kə-ˌti-lə-ˈmā-nē-ə\ *n* : an obsessive-compulsive disorder marked by the picking at or pulling out of one's fingernails or toenails

oo- — see O-

oo•cy•e•sis \ˌō-ə-sī-ˈē-səs\ *n, pl* **-e•ses** \-ˌsēz\ : extrauterine pregnancy in an ovary

oo•cyst \ˈō-ə-ˌsist\ *n* : ZYGOTE; *specif* : a sporozoan zygote undergoing sporogenous development

oo•cyte \ˈō-ə-ˌsīt\ *n* : an egg before maturation : a female gametocyte

oo•gen•e•sis \ˌō-ə-ˈje-nə-səs\ *n, pl* **-e•ses** \-ˌsēz\ : formation and maturation of the egg — called also *ovogenesis*

oo•go•ni•um \ˌō-ə-ˈgō-nē-əm\ *n* : a descendant of a primordial germ cell that gives rise to oocytes — **oo•go•ni•al** \-nē-əl\ *adj*

oophor- *or* **oophoro-** *comb form* : ovary ⟨*oophor*ectomy⟩

oo•pho•rec•to•my \ˌō-ə-fə-ˈrek-tə-mē\ *n, pl* **-mies** : the surgical removal of an ovary — called also *ovariectomy* — **oo•pho•rec•to•mize** \-ˌmīz\ *vb*

oo•pho•ri•tis \ˌō-ə-fə-ˈrī-təs\ *n* : inflammation of one or both ovaries

oophorus — see CUMULUS OOPHORUS

oo•plasm \ˈō-ə-ˌpla-zəm\ *n* : the cytoplasm of an egg — **oo•plas•mic** \-ˈplaz-mik\ *adj*

oo•tid \ˈō-ə-ˌtid\ *n* : an egg cell after meiosis — compare SPERMATID

opac•i•fi•ca•tion \ō-ˌpa-sə-fə-ˈkā-shən\ *n* : an act or the process of becoming or rendering opaque ⟨~ of the cornea⟩ — **opac•i•fy** \ō-ˈpa-sə-ˌfī\ *vb*

opac•i•ty \ō-ˈpa-sə-tē\ *n, pl* **-ties** **1** : the quality or state of a body that makes it impervious to the rays of light; *broadly* : the relative capacity of matter to obstruct by absorption or reflection the transmission of radiant energy **2** : an opaque spot in a normally transparent structure (as the lens of the eye)

opaque \ō-ˈpāk\ *adj* : exhibiting opacity : not allowing passage of radiant energy

OPD *abbr* outpatient department

[1]**open** \ˈō-pən\ *adj* **1 a** : not covered, enclosed, or scabbed over **b** : not involving or encouraging a covering (as by bandages or overgrowth of tissue) or enclosure ⟨~ treatment of burns⟩ **c** : relating to or being a compound fracture **d** : being an operation or surgical procedure in which an incision is made such that the tissues and organs are fully exposed — compare OPEN-HEART **2** : shedding the infective agent to the exterior ⟨~ tuberculosis⟩ — compare CLOSED 2 **3 a** : unobstructed by congestion or occlusion ⟨~ sinuses⟩ **b** : not constipated ⟨~ bowels⟩ **4** : using a minimum of physical restrictions and custodial restraints on the freedom of movement of the patients or inmates

[2]**open** *vb* **opened; open•ing** **1 a** : to make available for entry or passage by removing (as a cover) or clearing away (as an obstruction) **b** : to free (a body passage) of congestion or occlusion ⟨~ clogged arteries⟩ **2** : to make one or more openings in ⟨~*ed* the boil⟩

open–angle glaucoma *n* : a progressive form of glaucoma in which the drainage channel for the aqueous humor remains open but drainage is reduced leading to a gradual loss of vision with serious vision loss occurring only in advanced stages — compare ANGLE-CLOSURE GLAUCOMA

open chain *n* : an arrangement of atoms represented in a structural formula by a chain whose ends are not joined so as to form a ring

open–heart *adj* : of, relating to, or performed on a heart temporarily stopped and relieved of circulatory function and surgically opened for repair of defects or damage ⟨~ surgery⟩

open–label *adj* : being or relating to a clinical trial in which the treatment given to each subject is not concealed from either the researchers or the subject — compare DOUBLE-BLIND, SINGLE-BLIND

open reduction *n* : realignment of a fractured bone after incision into the fracture site

op•er•a•ble \ˈä-pə-rə-bəl\ *adj* **1** : fit, possible, or desirable to use **2** : likely to result in a favorable outcome upon surgical treatment — **op•er•a•bil•i•ty** \ˌä-pə-rə-ˈbi-lə-tē\ *n*

[1]**op•er•ant** \ˈä-pə-rənt\ *adj* : of, relating to, or being an operant or operant conditioning ⟨~ behavior⟩ — **op•er•ant•ly** *adv*

[2]**operant** *n* : behavior that operates on the environment to produce rewarding and reinforcing effects

operant conditioning *n* : conditioning in which the desired behavior or increasingly closer approximations to it are followed by a rewarding or reinforcing stimulus — compare CLASSICAL CONDITIONING

op•er•ate \ˈä-pə-ˌrāt\ *vb* **-at•ed; -at•ing** : to perform surgery

op•er•at•ing *adj* : of, relating to, or used for operations ⟨an ~ room⟩

op•er•a•tion \ˌä-pə-ˈrā-shən\ *n* : a procedure performed on a living body usu. with instruments for the repair of damage or the restoration of health and esp. one that involves incision, excision, or suturing

op•er•a•tive \ˈä-pə-rə-tiv, -ˌrā-\ *adj* : of, relating to, involving, or resulting from an operation ⟨~ treatment⟩

op•er•a•tor \ˈä-pə-ˌrā-tər\ *n* **1** : one who performs surgical operations **2** : a binding site in a DNA chain at which a genetic repressor binds to inhibit the initiation of transcription of messenger RNA by one or more nearby structural genes — called also *operator gene;* compare OPERON

op•er•a•to•ry \ˈä-pə-rə-ˌtōr-ē\ *n, pl* **-ries** : a working space (as of a dentist or surgeon) : SURGERY

oper•cu•lum \ō-ˈpər-kyə-ləm\ *n, pl* **-la** \-lə\ *also* **-lums** : any of several parts of the cerebrum bordering the sylvian fissure and concealing the insula

op•er•on \ˈä-pə-ˌrän\ *n* : a group of closely linked genes that produces a single messenger RNA molecule in transcription and that consists of structural genes and regulating elements (as an operator and promoter)

ophthalm- *or* **ophthalmo-** *comb form* : eye ⟨*ophthalmo*logy⟩ : eyeball ⟨*ophthalmo*dynamometry⟩

oph•thal•mia \äf-ˈthal-mē-ə, äp-\ *n* : inflammation of the conjunctiva or the eyeball

-oph•thal•mia \ˌäf-ˈthal-mē-ə, ˌäp-\ *n comb form* : condition of having (such) eyes ⟨micr*ophthalmia*⟩

ophthalmia neo•na•to•rum \-ˌnē-ə-nə-ˈtōr-əm\ *n* : acute inflammation of the eyes of a newborn from infection during passage through the birth canal

oph•thal•mic \äf-ˈthal-mik, äp-\ *adj* **1** : of, relating to, or situated near the eye **2** : supplying or draining the eye or structures in the region of the eye

ophthalmic artery *n* : a branch of the internal carotid artery following the optic nerve through the optic foramen into the orbit and supplying the eye and adjacent structures

ophthalmic nerve *n* : the one of the three major branches or divisions of the trigeminal nerve that supply sensory fibers to the lacrimal gland, eyelids, ciliary muscle, nose, forehead, and adjoining parts — called also *ophthalmic, ophthalmic division;* compare MANDIBULAR NERVE, MAXILLARY NERVE

ophthalmic vein *n* : either of two veins that pass from the orbit: **a** : one that begins at the inner angle of the orbit and empties into the cavernous sinus — called also *superior ophthalmic vein* **b** : one that drains a venous network in the floor and medial wall of the orbit and divides into two parts of which one joins the pterygoid plexus of veins and the other empties into the cavernous sinus — called also *inferior ophthalmic vein*

ophthalmo- — see OPHTHALM-

oph·thal·mo·dy·na·mom·e·try \äf-ˌthal-mō-ˌdī-nə-ˈmä-mə-trē, äp-\ *n, pl* **-tries** : measurement of the arterial blood pressure in the retina

oph·thal·mol·o·gist \ˌäf-thəl-ˈmä-lə-jist, ˌäp-, -ˌthal-\ *n* : a physician who specializes in ophthalmology — compare OPTICIAN 2, OPTOMETRIST

oph·thal·mol·o·gy \-jē\ *n, pl* **-gies** : a branch of medical science dealing with the structure, functions, and diseases of the eye — **oph·thal·mo·log·ic** \-mə-ˈlä-jik\ *or* **oph·thal·mo·log·i·cal** \-ji-kəl\ *adj* — **oph·thal·mo·log·i·cal·ly** *adv*

oph·thal·mom·e·ter \-ˈmä-mə-tər\ *n* : an instrument for measuring the eye; *specif* : KERATOMETER

oph·thal·mo·ple·gia \-ˈplē-jə, -jē-ə\ *n* : paralysis of some or all of the muscles of the eye — **oph·thal·mo·ple·gic** \-jik\ *adj*

oph·thal·mo·scope \äf-ˈthal-mə-ˌskōp\ *n* : an instrument for viewing the interior of the eye consisting of a concave mirror with a hole in the center through which the observer examines the eye, a source of light that is reflected into the eye by the mirror, and lenses in the mirror which can be rotated into the opening in the mirror — **oph·thal·mo·scop·ic** \äf-ˌthal-mə-ˈskä-pik\ *adj*

oph·thal·mos·co·py \ˌäf-thal-ˈmäs-kə-pē\ *n, pl* **-pies** : examination of the eye with an ophthalmoscope

-o·pia \ˈō-pē-ə\ *n comb form* **1** : condition of having (such) vision ⟨diplo*pia*⟩ **2** : condition of having (such) a visual defect ⟨hyper*opia*⟩

[1]**opi·ate** \ˈō-pē-ət, -ˌāt\ *n* **1** : a drug (as morphine or codeine) containing or derived from opium and tending to induce sleep and to alleviate pain; *broadly* : NARCOTIC 1 **2** : OPIOID 1 — not used technically

[2]**opiate** *adj* **1** : of, relating to, or being opium or an opium derivative **2** : of, relating to, binding, or being an opiate ⟨~ receptors⟩

opin·ion \ə-ˈpin-yən\ *n* : a formal expression of judgment or advice by an expert ⟨wanted a second ~⟩

[1]**opi·oid** \ˈō-pē-ˌȯid\ *adj* **1** : possessing some properties characteristic of opiate narcotics but not derived from opium **2** : of, involving, or induced by an opioid

[2]**opioid** *n* **1** : any of a group of endogenous neural polypeptides (as an endorphin or enkephalin) that bind esp. to opiate receptors and mimic some of the pharmacological properties of opiates — called also *opioid peptide* **2 a** : a synthetic drug (as methadone) possessing narcotic properties similar to opiates but not derived from opium **b** : OPIATE 1 — not used technically

opisth- *or* **opistho-** *comb form* : dorsal : posterior ⟨*opistho*tonos⟩

opis·thor·chi·a·sis \ə-ˌpis-ˌthȯr-ˈkī-ə-səs\ *n* : infestation with or disease caused by trematode worms of the genus *Opisthorchis*

Op·is·thor·chis \ˌä-pəs-ˈthȯr-kəs\ *n* : a genus of digenetic trematode worms (family Opisthorchiidae) including two (*O. felineus* and *O. viverrini*) that are liver parasites acquired esp. by eating raw or undercooked infected freshwater fish

op·is·thot·o·nos \ˌä-pəs-ˈthät-ᵊn-əs\ *n* : a condition of spasm of the muscles of the back, causing the head and lower limbs to bend backward and the trunk to arch forward

opi·um \ˈō-pē-əm\ *n* : a highly addictive stimulant narcotic that consists of the dried milky juice from the seed capsules of the opium poppy, was formerly used in medicine to soothe pain, and is smoked illicitly as an intoxicant

opium poppy *n* : an annual Eurasian poppy (*Papaver somniferum*) that is the source of opium

op·po·nens \ə-ˈpō-ˌnenz\ *n, pl* **-nen·tes** \ˌä-pə-ˈnen-(ˌ)tēz\ *or* **-nens** : any of several muscles of the hand or foot that tend to draw one of the lateral digits across the palm or sole toward the others

opponens dig·i·ti min·i·mi \-ˈdi-jə-ˌtī-ˈmi-nə-ˌmī\ *n* : a triangular muscle of the hand that arises from the hamate and adjacent flexor retinaculum, is inserted along the ulnar side of the metacarpal of the little finger, and functions to abduct, flex, and rotate the fifth metacarpal in opposing the little finger and thumb

opponens pol·li·cis \-ˈpä-lə-səs\ *n* : a small triangular muscle of the hand that is located below the abductor pollicis brevis, arises from the trapezium and the flexor retinaculum of the hand, is inserted along the radial side of the metacarpal of the thumb, and functions to abduct, flex, and rotate the metacarpal of the thumb in opposing the thumb and fingers

op·po·nent \ə-ˈpō-nənt\ *n* **:** a muscle that opposes or counteracts and limits the action of another

op·por·tun·ist \ˌä-pər-ˈtü-nist, -ˈtyü-\ *n* **:** an opportunistic microorganism

op·por·tu·nist·ic \-tü-ˈnis-tik, -tyü-\ *adj* **1 :** of, relating to, or being a microorganism that is usu. harmless but can become pathogenic when the host's resistance to disease is impaired **2 :** of, relating to, or being an infection or disease caused by an opportunistic organism

op·pos·able \ə-ˈpō-zə-bəl\ *adj* **:** capable of being placed against one or more of the remaining digits of a hand or foot ⟨an ~ thumb⟩

oppositional defiant disorder *n* **:** a disruptive behavior pattern of childhood and adolescence characterized by defiant, disobedient, and hostile behavior esp. toward adults in positions of authority — abbr. *ODD*

-op·sia \ˈäp-sē-ə\ *n comb form, pl* **-op·sias :** vision of a (specified) kind or condition ⟨hemian*opsia*⟩

op·sin \ˈäp-sən\ *n* **:** any of various colorless proteins that in combination with retinal or a related prosthetic group form a visual pigment (as rhodopsin) in a reaction which is reversed by light

op·so·nin \ˈäp-sə-nən\ *n* **:** any of various proteins (as complement or antibodies) that bind to foreign particles and microorganisms (as bacteria) making them more susceptible to the action of phagocytes — **op·son·ic** \äp-ˈsä-nik\ *adj*

op·son·iza·tion \ˌäp-sə-nə-ˈzā-shən, -ˌnī-ˈzā-\ *n* **:** the process of modifying (as a bacterium) by the action of opsonins — **op·son·ize** \ˈäp-sə-ˌnīz\ *vb*

-op·sy \ˌäp-sē, əp-\ *n comb form, pl* **-op·sies :** examination ⟨bi*opsy*⟩ ⟨necr*opsy*⟩

opt *abbr* optician

¹op·tic \ˈäp-tik\ *adj* **1 :** of or relating to vision ⟨~ phenomena⟩ **2 a :** of or relating to the eye **:** OCULAR **b :** affecting the eye or an optic structure

²optic *n* **:** any of the elements (as lenses or mirrors) of an optical instrument or system — usu. used in pl.

op·ti·cal \ˈäp-ti-kəl\ *adj* **1 :** of or relating to the science of optics **2 a :** of or relating to vision **:** VISUAL **b :** using the properties of light to aid vision **3 :** of, relating to, or utilizing light ⟨~ microscopy⟩ — **op·ti·cal·ly** *adv*

optical activity *n* **:** ability of a chemical substance to rotate the plane of vibration of polarized light to the right or left

optical axis *n* **:** a straight line perpendicular to the front of the cornea of the eye and extending through the center of the pupil — called also *optic axis*

optical illusion *n* **:** visual perception of a real object in such a way as to misinterpret its actual nature

optically active *adj* **:** capable of rotating the plane of vibration of polarized light to the right or left **:** either dextrorotatory or levorotatory — used of compounds, molecules, or atoms

optic atrophy *n* **:** degeneration of the optic nerve

optic axis *n* **:** OPTICAL AXIS

optic canal *n* **:** OPTIC FORAMEN

optic chiasma *n* **:** the X-shaped partial decussation on the undersurface of the hypothalamus through which the optic nerves are continuous with the brain — called also *optic chiasm*

optic cup *n* **:** the optic vesicle after invaginating to form a 2-layered cup from which the retina and pigmented layer of the eye will develop — called also *eyecup*

optic disk *n* **:** BLIND SPOT

optic foramen *n* **:** the passage through the orbit of the eye in the lesser wing of the sphenoid bone that is traversed by the optic nerve and ophthalmic artery — called also *optic canal;* see CHIASMATIC GROOVE

op·ti·cian \äp-ˈti-shən\ *n* **1 :** a maker of or dealer in optical items and instruments **2 :** a person who reads prescriptions for visual correction, orders lenses, and dispenses eyeglasses and contact lenses — compare OPHTHALMOLOGIST, OPTOMETRIST

op·ti·cian·ry \-rē\ *n, pl* **-ries :** the profession or practice of an optician

optic lobe *n* **:** SUPERIOR COLLICULUS

optic nerve *n* **:** either of the pair of sensory nerves that comprise the second pair of cranial nerves, arise from the ventral part of the diencephalon, form an optic chiasma before passing to the eye and spreading over the anterior surface of the retina, and conduct visual stimuli to the brain — called also *second cranial nerve*

op·tics \ˈäp-tiks\ *n sing or pl* **1 :** a science that deals with the nature and properties of light **2 :** optical properties

optic stalk *n* **:** the constricted part of the optic vesicle by which it remains continuous with the embryonic forebrain

optic tectum *n* **:** SUPERIOR COLLICULUS

optic tract *n* **:** the portion of each optic nerve between the optic chiasma and the diencephalon proper

optic vesicle *n* **:** an evagination of each lateral wall of the embryonic vertebrate forebrain from which the nervous structures of the eye develop

opto- *comb form* **1 :** vision ⟨*opto*metry⟩ **2 :** optic **:** optic and ⟨*opto*kinetic⟩

op·to·ki·net·ic \ˌäp-tō-kə-ˈne-tik, -kī-\ *adj* **:** of, relating to, or involving movements of the eyes ⟨~ nystagmus⟩

op·tom·e·trist \äp-ˈtä-mə-trist\ *n* : a specialist licensed to practice optometry — compare OPHTHALMOLOGIST, OPTICIAN 2

op·tom·e·try \-trē\ *n, pl* **-tries** : the health-care profession concerned esp. with examining the eye for defects and faults of refraction, with prescribing corrective lenses or eye exercises, with diagnosing diseases of the eye, and with treating such diseases or referring them for treatment — **op·to·met·ric** \ˌäp-tə-ˈme-trik\ *adj*

OPV *abbr* oral polio vaccine

OR *abbr* operating room

ora *pl of* ²OS

orad \ˈōr-ˌad\ *adv* : toward the mouth or oral region

orae serratae *pl of* ORA SERRATA

oral \ˈōr-əl, ˈär-\ *adj* **1 a** : of, relating to, or involving the mouth : BUCCAL ⟨the ~ mucous membrane⟩ **b** : given or taken through or by way of the mouth ⟨an ~ vaccine⟩ **c** : acting on the mouth **2 a** : of, relating to, or characterized by the first stage of psychosexual development in psychoanalytic theory during which libidinal gratification is derived from intake (as of food), by sucking, and later by biting **b** : of, relating to, or characterized by personality traits of passive dependence and aggressiveness — compare ANAL 2, GENITAL 3, PHALLIC 2 — **oral·ly** *adv*

oral cavity *n* : the cavity of the mouth; *esp* : the part of the mouth behind the gums and teeth that is bounded above by the hard and soft palates and below by the tongue and by the mucous membrane connecting it with the inner part of the mandible

oral contraceptive *n* : BIRTH CONTROL PILL

oral contraceptive pill *n* : BIRTH CONTROL PILL

oral hairy leukoplakia *n* : HAIRY LEUKOPLAKIA

oral sex *n* : oral stimulation of the genitals : CUNNILINGUS : FELLATIO

oral surgeon *n* : a specialist in oral surgery

oral surgery *n* **1** : a branch of dentistry that deals with the diagnosis and treatment of oral conditions requiring surgical intervention **2** : a branch of surgery that deals with conditions of the jaws and mouth structures requiring surgery

oral suspension *n* : a suspension consisting of undissolved particles of one or more medicinal agents mixed with a liquid vehicle for oral administration

ora ser·ra·ta \ˌōr-ə-sə-ˈrä-tə, -ˈrā-\ *n, pl* **orae ser·ra·tae** \ˌōr-ē-sə-ˈrā-tē\ : the dentate border of the retina

or·bi·cu·lar·is oculi \ōr-ˌbi-kyə-ˈlar-əs-ˈä-kyü-ˌlī,-ˌlē\ *n, pl* **or·bi·cu·lar·es oc·uli** \-ˈlar-(ˌ)ēz-\ : the muscle encircling the opening of the orbit and functioning to close the eyelids

orbicularis oris \-ˈōr-əs\ *n, pl* **orbiculares oris** : a muscle made up of several layers of fibers passing in different directions that encircles the mouth and controls most movements of the lips

or·bic·u·lus cil·i·ar·is \ȯr-ˈbi-kyə-ləs-ˌsi-lē-ˈer-əs\ *n* : PARS PLANA

or·bit \ˈȯr-bət\ *n* : the bony cavity perforated for the passage of nerves and blood vessels that occupies the lateral front of the skull immediately beneath the frontal bone on each side and encloses and protects the eye and its appendages — called also *eye socket, orbital cavity* — **or·bit·al** \-ᵊl\ *adj*

orbital fissure *n* : either of two openings transmitting nerves and blood vessels to or from the orbit: **a** : one situated superiorly between the greater wing and the lesser wing of the sphenoid bone — called also *superior orbital fissure, supraorbital fissure* **b** : one situated inferiorly between the greater wing of the sphenoid bone and the maxilla — called also *inferior orbital fissure, infraorbital fissure, sphenomaxillary fissure*

orbital plate *n* **1** : the part of the frontal bone forming most of the top of the orbit **2** : a thin plate of bone forming the lateral wall enclosing the ethmoidal air cells and forming part of the side of the orbit next to the nose

or·bi·to·fron·tal \ˌȯr-bi-tə-ˈfrən-tᵊl\ *adj* : located in, supplying, or being the part of the cerebral cortex in the basal region of the frontal lobe near the orbit ⟨the ~ cortex⟩

or·bi·tot·o·my \ˌȯr-bə-ˈtä-tə-mē\ *n, pl* **-mies** : surgical incision of the orbit

or·bi·vi·rus \ˈȯr-bi-ˌvī-rəs\ *n* **1** *cap* : a genus of reoviruses having a genome composed of usu. 10 segments of double-stranded RNA and including the causative agents of African horse sickness and bluetongue **2** : any virus of the genus *Orbivirus*

or·chi·dec·to·my \ˌȯr-kə-ˈdek-tə-mē\ *n, pl* **-mies** : ORCHIECTOMY

-or·chi·dism \ˈȯr-kə-ˌdi-zəm\ *also* **-or·chism** \ˈȯr-ˌki-zəm\ *n comb form* : a (specified) form or condition of the testes ⟨crypt*orchidism*⟩

or·chi·do·pexy \ˈȯr-kə-dō-ˌpek-sē\ *n, pl* **-pex·ies** : surgical fixation of a testis — called also *orchiopexy*

or·chi·ec·to·my \ˌȯr-kē-ˈek-tə-mē\ *n, pl* **-mies** : surgical excision of a testis or of both testes — called also *orchidectomy*

or·chi·o·pexy \ˈȯr-kē-ō-ˌpek-sē\ *n, pl* **-pex·ies** : ORCHIDOPEXY

or·chi·tis \ȯr-ˈkī-təs\ *n* : inflammation of a testis — **or·chit·ic** \ȯr-ˈki-tik\ *adj*

or·ci·pren·a·line \ˌȯr-sə-ˈpre-nə-ˌlēn\ *n, Brit* : METAPROTERENOL

¹**or·der** \ˈȯr-dər\ *vb* **or·dered; or·der·ing** : to give a prescription for : PRESCRIBE ⟨the doctor ~*ed* bed rest⟩

[2]**order** *n* **:** a category of taxonomic classification ranking above the family and below the class

or·der·ly \-lē\ *n, pl* **-lies :** a hospital attendant who does routine or heavy work (as cleaning, carrying supplies, or moving patients)

Oren·cia \ō-ˈren-sē-ə\ *trademark* — used for a preparation of abatacept

Oret·ic \ȯr-ˈe-tik\ *n* **:** a preparation of hydrochlorothiazide — formerly a U.S. trademark

-o·rex·ia \ə-ˈrek-sē-ə, ə-ˈrek-shə\ *n comb form* **:** appetite ⟨an*orexia*⟩

orex·in \ə-ˈrek-sən\ *n* **:** either of two neuropeptides that are produced in the hypothalamus and play a role in regulating wakefulness and food intake — called also *hypocretin*

or·gan \ˈȯr-gən\ *n* **:** a differentiated structure (as a heart or kidney) consisting of cells and tissues and performing some specific function in an organism

organ- *or* **organo-** *comb form* **1 :** organ ⟨*organ*elle⟩ ⟨*organo*genesis⟩ **2 :** organic ⟨*organo*phosphorus⟩

or·gan·elle \ˌȯr-gə-ˈnel\ *n* **:** a specialized cellular part (as a mitochondrion or nucleus) that has a specific function and is considered analogous to an organ

or·gan·ic \ȯr-ˈga-nik\ *adj* **1 a :** of, relating to, or arising in a bodily organ **b :** affecting the structure of the organism ⟨an ~ disease⟩ — compare FUNCTIONAL 1b **2 a :** of, relating to, or derived from living organisms **b** (1) **:** of, relating to, or containing carbon compounds (2) **:** relating to, being, or dealt with by a branch of chemistry concerned with the carbon compounds of living beings and most other carbon compounds — **or·gan·i·cal·ly** *adv*

organic brain syndrome *n* **:** any mental dysfunction (as delirium or senile dementia) resulting from physical changes in brain structure and characterized esp. by impaired cognition — called also *organic brain disorder, organic mental syndrome*

or·gan·ism \ˈȯr-gə-ˌni-zəm\ *n* **:** an individual constituted to carry on the activities of life by means of organs separate in function but mutually dependent **:** a living being — **or·gan·is·mic** \ˌȯr-gə-ˈniz-mik\ *also* **or·gan·is·mal** \-məl\ *adj* — **or·gan·is·mi·cal·ly** *adv*

or·ga·ni·za·tion \ˌȯr-gə-nə-ˈzā-shən\ *n* **:** the formation of fibrous tissue from a clot or exudate by invasion of connective tissue cells and capillaries from adjoining tissues — **or·ga·nize** \ˈȯr-gə-ˌnīz\ *vb*

or·ga·niz·er \ˈȯr-gə-ˌnī-zər\ *n* **:** a region of a developing embryo (as part of the dorsal lip of the blastopore) or a substance produced by such a region that is capable of inducing a specific type of development in undifferentiated tissue — called also *inductor*

organo- — see ORGAN-

or·gano·chlo·rine \ȯr-ˌga-nə-ˈklōr-ˌēn, -ən\ *adj* **:** of, relating to, or being a chlorinated hydrocarbon and esp. one used as a pesticide (as aldrin, DDT, or dieldrin) — **organochlorine** *n*

organ of Cor·ti \-ˈkȯr-tē\ *n* **:** a complex epithelial structure in the cochlea that in mammals is the chief part of the ear by which sound is directly perceived

Corti, Alfonso Giacomo Gaspare (1822–1876), Italian anatomist.

organ of Ro·sen·mül·ler \-ˈrō-zən-ˌmyü-lər\ *n* **:** EPOOPHORON

Rosenmüller, Johann Christian (1771–1820), German anatomist.

or·gan·o·gen·e·sis \ˌȯr-gə-nō-ˈje-nə-səs, ȯr-ˌga-nə-\ *n, pl* **-e·ses** \-ˌsēz\ **:** the origin and development of bodily organs — **or·gan·o·ge·net·ic** \-jə-ˈne-tik\ *adj*

or·gan·oid \ˈȯr-gə-ˌnȯid\ *adj* **:** resembling an organ in structural appearance or qualities — used esp. of abnormal masses (as tumors)

or·gan·o·lep·tic \ˌȯr-gə-nō-ˈlep-tik, ȯr-ˌga-nə-\ *adj* **1 :** being, affecting, or relating to qualities (as taste, color, and odor) of a substance (as a food) that stimulate the sense organs **2 :** involving use of the sense organs

or·gan·ol·o·gy \ˌȯr-gə-ˈnä-lə-jē\ *n, pl* **-gies :** the study of the organs of plants and animals

or·ga·no·meg·a·ly \ˌȯr-gə-nō-ˈme-gə-lē\ *n, pl* **-lies :** abnormal enlargement of the viscera — called also *visceromegaly*

or·gano·mer·cu·ri·al \ȯr-ˌga-nō-(ˌ)mər-ˈkyu̇r-ē-əl\ *n* **:** an organic compound or a pharmaceutical preparation containing mercury — **organomercurial** *adj*

or·gano·phos·phate \ȯr-ˌga-nə-ˈfäs-ˌfāt\ *n* **:** an organophosphorus pesticide — **organophosphate** *adj*

or·gano·phos·pho·rus \-ˈfäs-fə-rəs\ *also* **or·gano·phos·pho·rous** \-fäs-ˈfōr-əs\ *adj* **:** of, relating to, or being a phosphorus-containing organic pesticide (as malathion) that acts by inhibiting cholinesterase — **organophosphorus** *n*

or·gasm \ˈȯr-ˌga-zəm\ *n* **:** the climax of sexual excitement that is usu. accompanied by ejaculation of semen in the male and by vaginal contractions in the female — **orgasm** *vb* — **or·gas·mic** \ȯr-ˈgaz-mik\ *also* **or·gas·tic** \-ˈgas-tik\ *adj*

ori- *comb form* **:** mouth ⟨*ori*fice⟩

ori·ent \ˈōr-ē-ˌent\ *vb* **:** to acquaint with or adjust according to the existing situation or environment

oriental rat flea *n* **:** a flea of the genus *Xenopsylla* (*X. cheopis*) that is widely distributed on rodents and is a vector of plague

oriental sore *n* **:** a skin disease caused by a protozoan of the genus *Leishmania* (*L. tropica*) that is marked by persistent granulomatous and ulcerating lesions and occurs widely in Asia and in tropical regions — called also *Baghdad boil*

ori•en•ta•tion \ˌōr-ē-ən-ˈtā-shən, -ˌen-\ *n* **1 a** : the act or process of orienting or of being oriented **b** : the state of being oriented **2** : a usu. general or lasting direction of thought, inclination, or interest — see SEXUAL ORIENTATION **3** : change of position by organs, organelles, or organisms in response to external stimulus **4** : awareness of the existing situation with reference to time, place, and identity of persons — **ori•en•ta•tion•al** \-shə-nəl\ *adj*

oriented *adj* : having psychological orientation ⟨an alert and ~ patient⟩

or•i•fice \ˈȯr-ə-fəs, ˈär-\ *n* : an opening through which something may pass — **or•i•fi•cial** \ˌȯr-ə-ˈfi-shəl, ˌär-\ *adj*

or•i•gin \ˈȯr-ə-jən, ˈär-\ *n* **1** : the point at which something begins or rises or from which it derives **2** : the more fixed, central, or larger attachment of a muscle — compare INSERTION 1

oris — see CANCRUM ORIS, LEVATOR ANGULI ORIS, ORBICULARIS ORIS

or•li•stat \ˈȯr-li-ˌstat\ *n* : a drug $C_{29}H_{53}NO_5$ that prevents the digestion of fat by inhibiting the activity of gastrointestinal lipases and is taken orally to treat obesity — see ALLI, XENICAL

Or•mond's disease \ˈȯr-ˌmändz-\ *n* : RETROPERITONEAL FIBROSIS

Ormond, John Kelso (1886–1978), American urologist.

or•ni•thine \ˈȯr-nə-ˌthēn\ *n* : a crystalline amino acid $C_5H_{12}N_2O_2$ that functions esp. in urea production

ornithine car•ba•moyl•trans•fer•ase \-ˌkär-bə-ˌmȯil-ˈtrans-fər-ˌās\ *n* : ORNITHINE TRANSCARBAMYLASE

ornithine trans•car•ba•moy•lase \-ˌtrans-ˌkär-bə-ˈmȯi-ˌlās\ *n* : ORNITHINE TRANSCARBAMYLASE

ornithine trans•car•ba•myl•ase \-ˈmi-ˌlās\ *n* : an enzyme of hepatic mitochondria that catalyzes the conversion of ornithine to citrulline as part of urea formation and that when deficient in the body results in hyperammonemia, vomiting, coma, seizures, and sometimes death

Or•ni•thod•o•ros \ˌȯr-nə-ˈthä-də-rəs\ *n* : a genus of ticks (family Argasidae) including some that are vectors of relapsing fever and Q fever

or•ni•tho•sis \ˌȯr-nə-ˈthō-səs\ *n, pl* **-tho•ses** \-ˌsēz\ : PSITTACOSIS; *esp* : psittacosis of birds (as turkeys and pigeons) not in the family (Psittacidae) containing the parrots

oro- *comb form* **1** : mouth ⟨*oro*pharynx⟩ **2** : oral and ⟨*oro*facial⟩

oro•an•tral \ˌōr-ō-ˈan-trəl\ *adj* : of, relating to, or connecting the mouth and the maxillary sinus

oro•fa•cial \-ˈfā-shəl\ *adj* : of or relating to the mouth and face

oro•gas•tric \-ˈgas-trik\ *adj* : traversing or affecting the digestive tract from the mouth to the stomach

oro•man•dib•u•lar \-man-ˈdi-byə-lər\ *adj* : of or affecting the mouth and mandible

oro•na•sal \-ˈnā-zəl\ *adj* : of or relating to the mouth and nose; *esp* : connecting the mouth and the nasal cavity

oro•pha•ryn•geal \-ˌfar-ən-ˈjē-əl, -fə-ˈrin-jəl, -jē-əl\ *adj* **1** : of or relating to the oropharynx **2** : of or relating to the mouth and pharynx

oropharyngeal airway *n* : a tube used to provide free passage of air between the mouth and pharynx of an unconscious person

oro•phar•ynx \-ˈfar-iŋks\ *n, pl* **-pha•ryn•ges** \-fə-ˈrin-(ˌ)jēz\ *also* **-phar•ynx•es** : the part of the pharynx that is below the soft palate and above the epiglottis and is continuous with the mouth

oro•so•mu•coid \ˌȯr-ə-sō-ˈmyü-ˌkȯid\ *n* : a plasma glycoprotein believed to be associated with inflammation

oro•tra•che•al \ˌōr-ō-ˈtrā-kē-əl\ *adj* : relating to or being intubation of the trachea by way of the mouth

Oroya fever \ȯr-ˈȯi-ə-\ *n* : the acute first stage of bartonellosis characterized by high fever and severe anemia

orphan disease *n* : a disease which affects a relatively small number of individuals and for which no drug therapy has been developed because the small market would make the research and the drug unprofitable

orphan drug *n* : a drug that is not developed or marketed because its extremely limited use (as in the treatment of a rare disease) makes it unprofitable

or•phen•a•drine \ȯr-ˈfe-nə-drən, -ˌdrēn\ *n* : a drug used in the form of its citrate $C_{18}H_{23}NO{\cdot}C_6H_8O_7$ or hydrochloride $C_{18}H_{23}NO{\cdot}HCl$ as a muscle relaxant and antispasmodic

ORS *abbr* oral rehydration salts; oral rehydration solution

orth- *or* **ortho-** *comb form* : correct : corrective ⟨*ortho*dontia⟩

Or•tho•bun•ya•vi•rus \ˌȯrthə-ˈbən-yə-ˌvī-rəs\ *n* : a genus of bunyaviruses that are transmitted by arthropods (esp. mosquitoes and ticks) and include the causative virus of La Crosse encephalitis

orth•odon•tia \ˌȯr-thə-ˈdän-chə, -chē-ə\ *n* **1** : ORTHODONTICS **2** : dental appliances (as braces) used in orthodontic treatment

orth•odon•tics \-ˈdän-tiks\ *n* **1** : a branch of dentistry dealing with irregularities of the teeth and their correction (as by means of braces) **2** : the treatment provided by an orthodontist — **orth•odon•tic** \-tik\ *adj* — **or•tho•don•ti•cal•ly** *adv*

or•tho•don•tist \ˌȯr-thə-ˈdän-tist\ *n* : a specialist in orthodontics

orthodox sleep *n* : SLOW-WAVE SLEEP

or•tho•drom•ic \ˌȯr-thə-ˈdrä-mik\ *adj* **1** : proceeding or conducting in a normal direction — used esp. of a nerve impulse or fiber **2 :** characterized by orthodromic conduction

Or•tho Ev•ra \ˈȯr-thō-ˈev-rə\ *trademark* — used for a contraceptive transdermal patch containing norelgestromin and ethinyl estradiol

or•thog•nath•ic \ˌȯr-thag-ˈna-thik, -ˌthäg-\ *adj* : correcting deformities of the jaw and the associated malocclusion ⟨∼ surgery⟩

or•tho•myxo•vi•rus \ˌȯr-thō-ˈmik-sə-ˌvī-rəs\ *n* : any of a family (*Orthomyxoviridae*) of single-stranded RNA viruses that have a spherical or filamentous virion with numerous surface glycoprotein projections and include the causative agents of influenza — see INFLUENZA VIRUS

Or•tho–No•vum \ˌȯr-thō-ˈnō-vəm\ *trademark* — used for a preparation of norethindrone and either ethinyl estradiol or mestranol

or•tho•pae•dic, or•tho•pae•dics, or•tho•pae•dist *chiefly Brit var of* ORTHOPEDIC, ORTHOPEDICS, ORTHOPEDIST

or•tho•pe•dic \ˌȯr-thə-ˈpē-dik\ *adj* **1** : of, relating to, or employed in orthopedics **2 :** marked by or affected with a deformity, disorder, or injury of the skeleton and associated structures — **or•tho•pe•di•cal•ly** *adv*

or•tho•pe•dics \-ˈpē-diks\ *n sing or pl* : a branch of medicine concerned with the correction or prevention of deformities, disorders, or injuries of the skeleton and associated structures (as tendons and ligaments)

or•tho•pe•dist \-ˈpē-dist\ *n* : a specialist in orthopedics

or•tho•phos•pho•ric acid \ˌȯr-thə-ˌfäs-ˈfȯr-ik-, -ˈfär-; -ˈfäs-fə-rik-\ *n* : PHOSPHORIC ACID 1

or•thop•nea \ȯr-ˈthäp-nē-ə, ˌȯr-ˌthap-ˈnē-ə\ *n* : difficulty in breathing that occurs when lying down and is relieved upon changing to an upright position (as in congestive heart failure) — **or•thop•ne•ic** \-ik\ *adj*

or•thop•noea *chiefly Brit var of* ORTHOPNEA

or•tho•pox•vi•rus \ˈȯr-thō-päks-ˌvī-rəs\ *n* **1** *cap* : a genus of brick-shaped poxviruses that hybridize extensively within the genus and that include the vaccinia virus and the causative agents of cowpox, monkeypox, mousepox, and smallpox **2 :** any virus of the genus *Orthopoxvirus*

or•tho•psy•chi•a•trist \ˌȯr-thə-sə-ˈkī-ə-trəst, -(ˌ)sī-\ *n* : a specialist in orthopsychiatry

or•tho•psy•chi•a•try \-sə-ˈkī-ə-trē, -(ˌ)sī-\ *n, pl* **-tries** : prophylactic psychiatry concerned esp. with incipient mental and behavioral disorders in youth — **or•tho•psy•chi•at•ric** \-ˌsī-kē-ˈa-trik\ *adj*

or•thop•tics \ȯr-ˈthäp-tiks\ *n sing or pl* : the treatment or the art of treating defective visual habits, defects of binocular vision, and muscle imbalance (as strabismus) by reeducation of visual habits, exercise, and visual training — **or•thop•tic** \-tik\ *adj*

or•thop•tist \-tist\ *n* : a person specializing in orthoptics

or•tho•sis \ȯr-ˈthō-səs\ *n, pl* **or•tho•ses** \-ˌsēz\ : ORTHOTIC

or•tho•stat•ic \ˌȯr-thə-ˈsta-tik\ *adj* : of, relating to, or caused by erect posture ⟨∼ hypotension⟩

orthostatic albuminuria *n* : albuminuria that occurs only when a person is in an upright position

[1]**or•thot•ic** \ȯr-ˈthä-tik\ *adj* **1** : of or relating to orthotics **2 :** designed for the support of weak or ineffective joints or muscles ⟨∼ devices⟩

[2]**orthotic** *n* : a device (as a brace or splint) for supporting, immobilizing, or treating muscles, joints, or skeletal parts which are weak, ineffective, or injured — called also *orthosis*

or•thot•ics \-tiks\ *n* : a branch of mechanical and medical science that deals with the support and bracing of weak or ineffective joints or muscles

or•thot•ist \-tist\ *n* : a person specializing in orthotics

or•tho•top•ic \ˌȯr-thə-ˈtä-pik\ *adj* : of or relating to the grafting of tissue in a natural position ⟨∼ transplant⟩ — **or•tho•top•i•cal•ly** *adv*

Or•tho Tri–Cy•clen \ˌȯr-thō-ˌtrī-ˈsī-klən\ *trademark* — used for a preparation of norgestimate and ethinyl estradiol

or•tho•vol•tage \ˈȯr-thō-ˌvōl-tij\ *n* : X-ray voltage of about 150 to 500 kilovolts

[1]**os** \ˈäs\ *n, pl* **os•sa** \ˈä-sə\ : BONE

[2]**os** \ˈōs\ *n, pl* **ora** \ˈōr-ə\ : ORIFICE — see EXTERNAL OS, INTERNAL OS, PER OS

Os *symbol* osmium

OS *abbr* [Latin *oculus sinister*] left eye — used in writing prescriptions

OSA *abbr* obstructive sleep apnea

os cal•cis \-ˈkal-səs\ *n, pl* **ossa calcis** : CALCANEUS

os•cil•late \ˈä-sə-ˌlāt\ *vb* **-lat•ed; -lat•ing** **1** : to swing backward and forward like a pendulum **2 :** to move or travel back and forth between two points — **os•cil•la•tion** \ˌä-sə-ˈlā-shən\ *n* — **os•cil•la•tor** \ˈä-sə-ˌlā-tər\ *n* — **os•cil•la•to•ry** \ˈä-sə-lə-ˌtōr-ē\ *adj*

os•cil•lo•scope \ä-ˈsi-lə-ˌskōp, ə-\ *n* : an instrument in which the variations in a fluctuating electrical quantity appear temporarily as a visible waveform on the fluorescent screen of a cathode-ray tube — called also *cathode-ray oscilloscope* — **os•cil•lo•scop•ic** \ä-ˌsi-lə-ˈskä-pik, ˌä-sə-lə-\ *adj*

os cox•ae \-ˈkäk-ˌsē\ *n, pl* **ossa coxae** : HIP BONE

-ose \ˌōs\ *n suffix* : carbohydrate; *esp* : sugar ⟨fruct*ose*⟩ ⟨pent*ose*⟩

osel•tam•i•vir \ˌō-ˌsel-ˈta-mə-ˌvir\ *n* : a neuraminidase inhibitor administered orally in the form of its phosphate $C_{16}H_{28}N_2O_4{\cdot}H_3PO_4$ in the treatment and prevention of influenza A and B — see TAMIFLU

Os•good–Schlat•ter's disease \ˈäz-ˌgu̇d-ˈshlä-tərz-\ *n* : an osteochondritis of the tuberosity of the tibia that occurs esp. among adolescent males

Osgood, Robert Bayley (1873–1956), American orthopedic surgeon.

Schlatter, Carl (1864–1934), Swiss surgeon.

-o•side \ə-ˌsīd\ *n suffix* : glycoside or similar compound ⟨ganglio*side*⟩

-o•sis \ˈō-səs\ *n suffix, pl* **-o•ses** \ˈō-ˌsēz\ *or* **-o•sis•es 1 a** : action : process : condition ⟨hypn*osis*⟩ **b** : abnormal or diseased condition ⟨leuk*osis*⟩ **2** : increase : formation ⟨leukocyt*osis*⟩

Os•ler's maneuver *or* **Os•ler maneuver** \ˈäs-lər(z)-\ *n* : a sphygmomanometric procedure of disputed usefulness in detecting false cases of hypertension in the elderly that involves inflating the cuff above the systolic blood pressure and that is held to indicate pseudohypertension if the arteries remain palpable presumably due to inelasticity and sclerosis

W. Osler — see RENDU-OSLER-WEBER DISEASE

os•mic acid \ˈäz-mik-\ *n* : OSMIUM TETROXIDE

os•mi•um \ˈäz-mē-əm\ *n* : a hard brittle blue-gray or blue-black metallic element — symbol *Os;* see ELEMENT table

osmium tetroxide *n* : a crystalline compound OsO_4 that is an oxide of osmium used as a biological fixative and stain

osmo- *comb form* : osmosis : osmotic ⟨*osmo*regulation⟩

os•mol *or* **os•mole** \ˈäz-ˌmōl, ˈäs-\ *n* : a standard unit of osmotic pressure based on a one molal concentration of an ion in a solution

os•mo•lal•i•ty \ˌäz-mō-ˈla-lə-tē, ˌäs-\ *n, pl* **-ties** : the concentration of an osmotic solution esp. when measured in osmols or milliosmols per 1000 grams of solvent — **os•mo•lal** \äz-ˈmō-ləl, äs-\ *adj*

os•mo•lar•i•ty \ˌäz-mō-ˈlar-ə-tē, ˌäs-\ *n, pl* **-ties** : the concentration of an osmotic solution esp. when measured in osmols or milliosmols per liter of solution — **os•mo•lar** \äz-ˈmō-lər, äs-\ *adj*

os•mo•re•cep•tor \ˌäz-mō-ri-ˈsep-tər\ *n* : any of a group of cells sensitive to plasma osmolality that are held to exist in the brain and to regulate water balance in the body by controlling thirst and the release of vasopressin

os•mo•reg•u•la•to•ry \-ˈre-gyə-lə-ˌtōr-ē\ *adj* : of, relating to, or concerned with the maintenance of constant osmotic pressure — **os•mo•reg•u•la•tion** \ˌäz-mō-ˌre-gyə-ˈlā-shən, ˌäs-\ *n*

os•mo•sis \äz-ˈmō-səs, äs-\ *n, pl* **os•mo•ses** \-ˌsēz\ : movement of a solvent through a semipermeable membrane (as of a living cell) into a solution of higher solute concentration that tends to equalize the concentrations of solute on the two sides of the membrane — **os•mot•ic** \-ˈmä-tik\ *adj* — **os•mot•i•cal•ly** *adv*

osmotic pressure *n* : the pressure produced by or associated with osmosis and dependent on molar concentration and absolute temperature: as **a** : the maximum pressure that develops in a solution separated from a solvent by a membrane permeable only to the solvent **b** : the pressure that must be applied to a solution to just prevent osmosis

ossa *pl of* [1]os

ossea — see LEONTIASIS OSSEA

os•seo•in•te•gra•tion \ˌä-sē-ōˌin-tə-ˈgrā-shən\ *n* : the firm anchoring of a surgical implant (as in dentistry or in bone surgery) by the growth of bone around it without fibrous tissue formation at the interface — **os•seo•in•te•grat•ed** \-ˈin-tə-ˌgrā-təd\ *adj*

os•se•ous \ˈä-sē-əs\ *adj* : of, relating to, or composed of bone — **os•se•ous•ly** *adv*

osseous labyrinth *n* : BONY LABYRINTH

ossi- *comb form* : bone ⟨*ossi*fy⟩

os•si•cle \ˈä-si-kəl\ *n* : a small bone or bony structure; *esp* : any of three small bones of the middle ear including the malleus, incus, and stapes — **os•sic•u•lar** \ä-ˈsi-kyə-lər\ *adj*

ossificans — see MYOSITIS OSSIFICANS

os•si•fi•ca•tion \ˌä-sə-fə-ˈkā-shən\ *n* **1 a** : the process of bone formation usu. beginning at particular centers in each prospective bone and involving the activities of special osteoblasts that segregate and deposit inorganic bone substance about themselves **b** : an instance of this process **2 a** : the condition of being altered into a hard bony substance ⟨∼ of the muscular tissue⟩ **b** : a mass or particle of ossified tissue : a calcareous deposit in the tissues ⟨∼*s* in the aortic wall⟩ — **os•si•fy** \ˈä-sə-ˌfī\ *vb*

ossium — see FRAGILITAS OSSIUM

oste- *or* **osteo-** *comb form* : bone ⟨*os*teal⟩ ⟨*osteo*myelitis⟩

os•te•al \ˈäs-tē-əl\ *adj* : of, relating to, or resembling bone; *also* : affecting or involving bone or the skeleton

os•tec•to•my \äs-ˈtek-tə-mē\ *n, pl* **-mies** : surgical removal of all or part of a bone

os•te•itis \ˌäs-tē-ˈī-təs\ *n, pl* **-it•i•des** \-ˈi-tə-ˌdēz\ : inflammation of bone — called also *ostitis* — **os•te•it•ic** \-ˈi-tik\ *adj*

osteitis de•for•mans \-di-ˈfȯr-ˌmanz\ *n* : PAGET'S DISEASE 2

osteitis fi•bro•sa \-fī-ˈbrō-sə\ *n* : a disease of bone that is characterized by fibrous degeneration of the bone and the formation of cystic cavities and that results in deformities of the affected bones and sometimes in fracture — called also *osteodystrophia fibrosa*

osteitis fibrosa cys·ti·ca \-ˈsis-tə-kə\ *n* : OSTEITIS FIBROSA

osteitis fibrosa cystica gen·er·al·is·ta \-ˌje-nə-rə-ˈlis-tə\ *n* : OSTEITIS FIBROSA

os·teo·ar·thri·tis \ˌäs-tē-ō-är-ˈthrī-təs\ *n, pl* **-thrit·i·des** \-ˈthri-tə-ˌdēz\ : a common form of arthritis typically with onset during middle or old age that is characterized by progressive degenerative changes in the cartilage of one or more joints (as of the knees, hips, and hands) accompanied by thickening and overgrowth of adjacent bone and that is marked symptomatically chiefly by stiffness, swelling, pain, deformation of joints, and loss of range of motion — abbr. *OA;* called also *degenerative arthritis, degenerative joint disease, hypertrophic arthritis;* compare RHEUMATOID ARTHRITIS — **os·teo·ar·thrit·ic** \-ˈthri-tik\ *adj*

os·teo·ar·throp·a·thy \-är-ˈthrä-pə-thē\ *n, pl* **-thies** : a disease of joints or bones; *specif* : HYPERTROPHIC OSTEOARTHROPATHY

os·teo·ar·thro·sis \-är-ˈthrō-sis\ *n* : OSTEOARTHRITIS — **os·teo·ar·throt·ic** \-ˈthrä-tik\ *adj*

os·teo·ar·tic·u·lar \-är-ˈti-kyə-lər\ *adj* : relating to, involving, or affecting bones and joints ⟨~ diseases⟩

os·teo·blast \ˈäs-tē-ə-ˌblast\ *n* : a bone-forming cell

os·teo·blas·tic \ˌäs-tē-ə-ˈblas-tik\ *adj* **1** : relating to or involving the formation of bone **2** : composed of or being osteoblasts

os·teo·blas·to·ma \-bla-ˈstō-mə\ *n, pl* **-mas** *also* **-ma·ta** \-mə-tə\ : a benign tumor of bone

os·teo·cal·cin \-ˈkal-sən\ *n* : a protein produced by osteoblasts that is found in the extracellular matrix of bone and in the serum of circulating blood and when present at excessive levels in serum may be indicative of various disorders (as postmenopausal osteoporosis) of bone metabolism

os·teo·car·ti·lag·i·nous \-ˌkärt-ᵊl-ˈa jə-nəs\ *adj* : relating to or composed of bone and cartilage ⟨an ~ nodule⟩

osteochondr- *or* **osteochondro-** *comb form* : bone and cartilage ⟨*osteochondritis*⟩

os·teo·chon·dral \-ˈkän-drəl\ *adj* : relating to or composed of bone and cartilage

os·teo·chon·dri·tis \-ˌkän-ˈdrī-təs\ *n* : inflammation of bone and cartilage

osteochondritis dis·se·cans \-ˈdi-sə-ˌkanz\ *n* : partial or complete detachment of a fragment of bone and cartilage at a joint

os·teo·chon·dro·dys·pla·sia \-ˌkän-drō-ˌdis-ˈplā-zhə, -zhē-ə\ *n* : abnormal growth or development of cartilage and bone

os·teo·chon·dro·ma \-ˌkän-ˈdrō-mə\ *n, pl* **-mas** *also* **-ma·ta** \-mə-tə\ : a benign tumor containing both bone and cartilage and usu. occurring near the end of a long bone

os·teo·chon·dro·sis \-ˌkän-ˈdrō-səs\ *n, pl* **-dro·ses** \-ˌsēz\ : a disease esp. of children and young animals in which an ossification center esp. in the epiphyses of long bones undergoes degeneration followed by calcification — **os·teo·chon·drot·ic** \-ˈdrä-tik\ *adj*

os·teo·clast \ˈäs-tē-ə-ˌklast\ *n* : any of the large multinucleate cells closely associated with areas of bone resorption (as in a healing fracture) — **os·teo·clas·tic** \ˌäs-tē-ə-ˈklas-tik\ *adj*

os·teo·clas·to·ma \ˌäs-tē-ō-kla-ˈstō-mə\ *n, pl* **-mas** *also* **-ma·ta** \-mə-tə\ : GIANT-CELL TUMOR

os·teo·cyte \ˈäs-tē-ə-ˌsīt\ *n* : a cell that is characteristic of adult bone, is derived from an osteoblast, and occupies a lacuna of the bone matrix

os·teo·dys·tro·phia fi·bro·sa \ˌäs-tē-ō-di-ˈstrō-fē-ə-fī-ˈbrō-sə\ *n* : OSTEITIS FIBROSA

os·teo·dys·tro·phy \-ˈdis-trə-fē\ *n, pl* **-phies** : defective ossification of bone usu. associated with disturbed calcium and phosphorus metabolism

os·teo·gen·e·sis \ˌäs-tē-ə-ˈje-nə-səs\ *n, pl* **-e·ses** \-ˌsēz\ : development and formation of bone

osteogenesis im·per·fec·ta \-ˌim-pər-ˈfek-tə\ *n* : a hereditary disease caused by defective or deficient collagen production and marked by extreme brittleness of the long bones and a bluish color of the whites of the eyes — called also *brittle bone disease, brittle bones, fragilitas ossium, osteopsathyrosis*

osteogenesis imperfecta con·gen·i·ta \-kən-ˈje-nə-tə\ *n* : a severe and often fatal form of osteogenesis imperfecta characterized by usu. multiple fractures in utero

osteogenesis imperfecta tar·da \-ˈtär-də\ *n* : a less severe form of osteogenesis imperfecta which is not apparent at birth

os·teo·gen·ic \ˌäs-tē-ə-ˈje-nik\ *also* **os·teo·ge·net·ic** \-jə-ˈne-tik\ *adj* **1** : of, relating to, or functioning in osteogenesis; *esp* : producing bone **2** : originating in bone

osteogenic sarcoma *n* : OSTEOSARCOMA

[1]**os·te·oid** \ˈäs-tē-ˌȯid\ *adj* : resembling bone ⟨~ tissue⟩

[2]**osteoid** *n* : uncalcified bone matrix

osteoid osteoma *n* : a small benign painful tumor of bony tissue occurring esp. in the extremities of children and young adults

os·te·ol·o·gy \ˌäs-tē-ˈä-lə-jē\ *n, pl* **-gies** **1** : a branch of anatomy dealing with the bones **2** : the bony structure of an organism — **os·te·o·log·i·cal**

\ˌäs-tē-ə-ˈlä-ji-kəl\ *adj* — **os•te•ol•o•gist** \ˌäs-tē-ˈä-lə-jist\ *n*

os•te•ol•y•sis \ˌäs-tē-ˈä-lə-səs\ *n, pl* **-y•ses** \-ˌsēz\ : dissolution of bone esp. when associated with resorption — **os•te•o•lyt•ic** \ˌäs-tē-ə-ˈli-tik\ *adj*

os•te•o•ma \ˌäs-tē-ˈō-mə\ *n, pl* **-mas** *also* **-ma•ta** \-mə-tə\ : a benign tumor composed of bone tissue

os•teo•ma•la•cia \ˌäs-tē-ō-mə-ˈlā-shə, -shē-ə\ *n* : a disease of adults that is characterized by softening of the bones and is analogous to rickets in the young — **os•teo•ma•la•cic** \-ˈlā-sik\ *adj*

os•teo•my•eli•tis \-ˌmī-ə-ˈlī-təs\ *n, pl* **-elit•i•des** \-ə-ˈli-tə-ˌdēz\ : an infectious usu. painful inflammatory disease of bone that is often of bacterial origin and may result in death of bony tissue — **os•teo•my•elit•ic** \-ˈli-tik\ *adj*

os•te•on \ˈäs-tē-ˌän\ *n* : HAVERSIAN SYSTEM — **os•te•on•al** \ˌäs-tē-ˈän-ᵊl, -ˈōn-\ *adj*

os•teo•ne•cro•sis \ˌäs-tē-ō-nə-ˈkrō-səs\ *n, pl* **-cro•ses** \-ˌsēz\ : necrosis of bone; *esp* : AVASCULAR NECROSIS

os•teo•path \ˈäs-tē-ə-ˌpath\ *n* : a practitioner of osteopathy

os•te•op•a•thy \ˌäs-tē-ˈä-pə-thē\ *n, pl* **-thies** **1** : a disease of bone **2** : a system of medical practice based on a theory that diseases are due chiefly to loss of structural integrity which can be restored by manipulation of the parts supplemented by therapeutic measures (as use of medicine or surgery) — **os•teo•path•ic** \ˌäs-tē-ə-ˈpa-thik\ *adj* — **os•teo•path•i•cal•ly** *adv*

os•teo•pe•nia \ˌäs-tē-ō-ˈpē-nē-ə\ *n* : reduction in bone volume to below normal levels esp. due to inadequate replacement of bone lost to normal lysis — **os•teo•pe•nic** \-nik\ *adj*

os•teo•pe•tro•sis \-pə-ˈtrō-səs\ *n, pl* **-tro•ses** \-ˌsēz\ : a rare hereditary disease characterized by extreme density and hardness and abnormal fragility of the bones with partial or complete obliteration of the marrow cavities — called also *Albers-Schönberg disease* — **os•teo•pe•trot•ic** \-pə-ˈträ-tik\ *adj*

os•teo•phyte \ˈäs-tē-ə-ˌfīt\ *n* : an abnormal bony outgrowth or projection (as near a joint affected by osteoarthritis) : BONE SPUR — **os•teo•phyt•ic** \ˌäs-tē-ə-ˈfi-tik\ *adj*

os•teo•plas•tic \ˌäs-tē-ə-ˈplas-tik\ *adj* : of, relating to, or being osteoplasty

osteoplastic flap *n* : a surgically excised portion of the skull folded back on a hinge of skin to expose the underlying tissues (as in a craniotomy)

os•teo•plas•ty \ˈäs-tē-ə-ˌplas-tē\ *n, pl* **-ties** : plastic surgery on bone; *esp* : replacement of lost bone tissue or reconstruction of defective bony parts

os•teo•poi•ki•lo•sis \ˌäs-tē-ō-ˌpȯi-kə-ˈlō-səs\ *n* : an asymptomatic hereditary bone disorder characterized by numerous sclerotic foci giving bones a mottled or spotted appearance

os•teo•po•ro•sis \ˌäs-tē-ō-pə-ˈrō-səs\ *n, pl* **-ro•ses** \-ˌsēz\ : a condition that affects esp. older women and is characterized by decrease in bone mass with decreased density and enlargement of bone spaces producing porosity and fragility — **os•teo•po•rot•ic** \-ˈrä-tik\ *adj*

os•te•op•sath•y•ro•sis \ˌäs-tē-äp-ˌsa-thə-ˈrō-səs\ *n, pl* **-ro•ses** \-ˌsēz\ : OSTEOGENESIS IMPERFECTA

os•teo•ra•dio•ne•cro•sis \ˌäs-tē-ō-ˌrā-dē-ō-nə-ˈkrō-səs\ *n, pl* **-cro•ses** \-ˌsēz\ : necrosis of bone following irradiation

os•teo•sar•co•ma \-sär-ˈkō-mə\ *n, pl* **-mas** *also* **-ma•ta** \-mə-tə\ : a sarcoma derived from bone or containing bone tissue — called also *osteogenic sarcoma*

os•teo•scle•ro•sis \-sklə-ˈrō-səs\ *n, pl* **-ro•ses** \-ˌsēz\ : abnormal hardening of bone or of bone marrow — **os•teo•scle•rot•ic** \-ˈrä-tik\ *adj*

os•teo•syn•the•sis \-ˈsin-thə-səs\ *n, pl* **-the•ses** \-ˌsēz\ : the operation of uniting the ends of a fractured bone by mechanical means (as a wire)

os•te•o•tome \ˈäs-tē-ə-ˌtōm\ *n* : a chisel without a bevel used for cutting bone

os•te•ot•o•my \ˌäs-tē-ˈä-tə-mē\ *n, pl* **-mies** : a surgical operation in which a bone is divided or a piece of bone is excised (as to correct a deformity)

Os•ter•ta•gia \ˌäs-tər-ˈtā-jə, -jē-ə\ *n* : a genus of nematode worms (family Trichostrongylidae) parasitic in the stomach of ruminants

os•ti•tis \ˌäs-ˈtī-təs\ *n* : OSTEITIS

os•ti•um \ˈäs-tē-əm\ *n, pl* **os•tia** \-tē-ə\ : a mouthlike opening in a bodily part (as a fallopian tube or a blood vessel) — **os•ti•al** \ˈäs-tē-əl\ *adj*

os•to•mate \ˈäs-tə-ˌmāt\ *n* : a person who has undergone an ostomy

os•to•my \ˈäs-tə-mē\ *n, pl* **-mies** : an operation (as a colostomy, ileostomy, or urostomy) to create an artificial passage for bodily elimination

-os•to•sis \äs-ˈtō-səs\ *n comb form, pl* **-os•to•ses** \-ˌsēz\ *or* **-os•to•sis•es** : ossification of a (specified) part or to a (specified) degree ⟨hyper*ostosis*⟩

OT *abbr* **1** occupational therapist **2** occupational therapy

ot- *or* **oto-** *comb form* **1** : ear ⟨*ot*itis⟩ **2** : ear and ⟨*oto*laryngology⟩

otal•gia \ō-ˈtal-jə, -jē-ə\ *n* : EARACHE

other–directed *adj* : directed in thought and action primarily by external norms rather than by one's own scale of values — compare INNER-DIRECTED

otic \ˈō-tik\ *adj* : of, relating to, or located in the region of the ear

[1]**-ot•ic** \ˈä-tik\ *adj suffix* **1 a** : of, relating to, or characterized by a (specified) action, process, or condition ⟨symbi*otic*⟩ **b** : having an abnormal or diseased condition of a (specified) kind ⟨epizo*otic*⟩ **2** : showing an increase or a formation of ⟨leukocyt*otic*⟩

²-otic \ˈō-tik\ *adj comb form* : having (such) a relationship to the ear ⟨dich*otic*⟩

otic ganglion *n* : a small parasympathetic ganglion that is associated with the mandibular nerve and sends postganglionic fibers to the parotid gland by way of the auriculotemporal nerve

oti•tis \ō-ˈtī-təs\ *n, pl* **otit•i•des** \ō-ˈti-tə-ˌdēz\ : inflammation of the ear — **otit•ic** \-ˈti-tik\ *adj*

otitis ex•ter•na \-ek-ˈstər-nə\ *n* : inflammation of the external auditory canal; *esp* : SWIMMER'S EAR — called also *external otitis media*

otitis in•ter•na \-in-ˈtər-nə\ *n* : inflammation of the inner ear; *specif* : LABYRINTHITIS

otitis me•dia \-ˈmē-dē-ə\ *n* : inflammation of the middle ear marked by pain, fever, dizziness, and abnormalities of hearing; *esp* : ACUTE OTITIS MEDIA — see AERO-OTITIS MEDIA, SEROUS OTITIS MEDIA

oto- — see OT-

Oto•bi•us \ō-ˈtō-bē-əs\ *n* : a genus of ticks (family Argasidae) that includes the spinose ear tick (*O. megnini*)

oto•co•nia \ˌō-tə-ˈkō-nē-ə\ *n pl* : small crystals of calcium carbonate in the saccule and utricle of the ear that under the influence of acceleration in a straight line cause stimulation of the hair cells by their movement relative to the gelatinous supporting substrate containing the embedded cilia of the hair cells — called also *statoconia*

Oto•dec•tes \ˌō-tə-ˈdek-ˌtēz\ *n* : a genus of mites that includes one (*O. cynotis*) causing otodectic mange — **oto•dec•tic** \-ˈdek-tik\ *adj*

otodectic mange *n* : ear mange caused by a mite (*O. cynotis*) of the genus *Otodectes*

oto•lar•yn•gol•o•gist \ˌō-tō-ˌlar-ən-ˈgä-lə-jist\ *n* : a specialist in otolaryngology — called also *otorhinolaryngologist*

oto•lar•yn•gol•o•gy \-jē\ *n, pl* **-gies** : a medical specialty concerned esp. with the ear, nose, and throat — called also *otorhinolaryngology* — **oto•lar•yn•go•log•i•cal** \-ˌlar-ən-gə-ˈlä-ji-kəl\ *adj*

oto•lith \ˈōt-ᵊl-ˌith\ *n* : a calcareous concretion in the internal ear composed of masses of otoconia — called also *statolith* — **oto•lith•ic** \ˌōt-ᵊl-ˈi-thik\ *adj*

otol•o•gist \ō-ˈtä-lə-jist\ *n* : a specialist in otology

otol•o•gy \-jē\ *n, pl* **-gies** : a science that deals with the ear and its diseases — **oto•log•ic** \ˌō-tə-ˈlä-jik\ *also* **oto•log•i•cal** \-ˈlä-ji-kəl\ *adj* — **oto•log•i•cal•ly** *adv*

oto•my•co•sis \ˌō-tō-mī-ˈkō-səs\ *n, pl* **-co•ses** \-ˌsēz\ : disease of the ear produced by the growth of fungi in the external auditory canal

oto•plas•ty \ˈō-tə-ˌplas-tē\ *n, pl* **-ties** : plastic surgery of the external ear

oto•rhi•no•lar•yn•gol•o•gist \ˌō-tō-ˌrī-nō-ˌlar-ən-ˈgä-lə-jist\ *n* : OTOLARYNGOLOGIST

oto•rhi•no•lar•yn•gol•o•gy \-jē\ *n, pl* **-gies** : OTOLARYNGOLOGY — **oto•rhi•no•lar•yn•go•log•i•cal** \-gə-ˈlä-ji-kəl\ *adj*

otor•rhea \ˌō-tə-ˈrē-ə\ *n* : a discharge from the external ear

otor•rhoea *chiefly Brit var of* OTORRHEA

oto•scle•ro•sis \ˌō-tō-sklə-ˈrō-səs\ *n, pl* **-ro•ses** \-ˌsēz\ : growth of spongy bone in the inner ear where it gradually obstructs the oval window or round window or both and causes progressively increasing deafness — **oto•scle•rot•ic** \-sklə-ˈrä-tik\ *adj*

oto•scope \ˈō-tə-ˌskōp\ *n* : an instrument fitted with lighting and magnifying lens systems and used to facilitate visual examination of the auditory canal and ear drum — **oto•scop•ic** \ˌō-tə-ˈskä-pik\ *adj* — **otos•co•py** \ō-ˈtäs-kə-pē\ *n*

oto•tox•ic \ˌō-tə-ˈtäk-sik\ *adj* : producing, involving, or being adverse effects on organs or nerves involved in hearing or balance — **oto•tox•ic•i•ty** \-täk-ˈsi-sə-tē\ *n*

OTR *abbr* registered occupational therapist

oua•bain \wä-ˈbā-ən, ˈwä-ˌbān\ *n* : a poisonous glycoside $C_{29}H_{44}O_{12}$ used medically like digitalis

ounce \ˈau̇ns\ *n* **1 a** : a unit of weight equal to 1/12 troy pound or 31.103 grams **b** : a unit of weight equal to 1/16 avoirdupois pound or 28.350 grams **2** : FLUID OUNCE

out•break \ˈau̇t-ˌbrāk\ *n* : a sudden rise in the incidence of a disease ⟨an ~ of measles⟩

out•er•course \ˈau̇-tər-ˌkōrs\ *n* : physical sexual activity between individuals that typically includes stimulation of the genitalia but does not involve penetration of the vagina or anus with the penis

outer ear *n* : the outer visible portion of the ear that collects and directs sound waves toward the tympanic membrane by way of a canal which extends inward through the temporal bone

out•growth \ˈau̇t-ˌgrōth\ *n* **1** : the process of growing out **2** : something that grows directly out of something else ⟨an ~ of hair⟩ ⟨a bony ~⟩

out•let \ˈau̇t-ˌlet, -lət\ *n* **1** : an opening or a place through which something is let out ⟨the pelvic ~⟩ **2** : a means of release or satisfaction for an emotion or impulse

outlet forceps *n* : LOW FORCEPS

out–of–body *adj* : relating to or involving a feeling of separation from one's body and of being able to view oneself and others from an external perspective ⟨an ~ experience⟩

out•pa•tient \ˈau̇t-ˌpā-shənt\ *n* : a patient who is not hospitalized overnight but who visits a hospital, clinic, or associated facility for diagnosis or treatment — compare INPATIENT

out·pock·et·ing \ˈau̇t-ˌpä-kə-tiŋ\ *n* : EVAGINATION
out·pouch·ing \-ˌpau̇-chiŋ\ *n* : EVAGINATION
out·put \ˈau̇t-ˌpu̇t\ *n* : the amount of energy or matter discharged usu. within a specified time by a bodily system or organ ⟨renal ~⟩ ⟨urinary ~⟩ — see CARDIAC OUTPUT
ov- *or* **ovi-** *or* **ovo-** *comb form* : egg ⟨*ovi*cide⟩ : ovum ⟨*ovi*duct⟩
ova *pl of* OVUM
ovale — see FORAMEN OVALE
ova·le malaria \ō-ˈvā-lē-\ *n* : a relatively mild form of malaria caused by a protozoan of the genus *Plasmodium* (*P. ovale*) that is characterized by tertian chills and febrile paroxysms and that usu. ends spontaneously
ovalis — see FENESTRA OVALIS, FOSSA OVALIS
oval window *n* : an oval opening between the middle ear and the vestibule having the base of the stapes or columella attached to its membrane — called also *fenestra ovalis, fenestra vestibuli*
ovari- *or* **ovario-** *also* **ovar-** *comb form* **1** : ovary ⟨*ovari*ectomy⟩ ⟨*ovari*otomy⟩ **2** : ovary and ⟨*ovario*hysterectomy⟩
ovar·i·an \ō-ˈvar-ē-ən\ *also* **ovar·i·al** \-ē-əl\ *adj* : of, relating to, affecting, or involving an ovary
ovarian artery *n* : either of two arteries in the female that arise from the aorta below the renal arteries with one on each side and are distributed to the ovaries with branches supplying the ureters, the fallopian tubes, the labia majora, and the groin
ovarian follicle *n* : FOLLICLE 3
ovarian ligament *n* : LIGAMENT OF THE OVARY
ovarian vein *n* : either of two veins in the female with one on each side that drain a venous plexus in the broad ligament of the same side and empty on the right into the inferior vena cava and on the left into the left renal vein
ovari·ec·to·my \ō-ˌvar-ē-ˈek-tə-mē\ *n, pl* **-mies** : OOPHORECTOMY — **ovari·ec·to·mize** \ō-ˌvar-ē-ˈek-tə-ˌmīz\ *vb*
ovar·io·hys·ter·ec·to·my \ō-ˌvar-ē-ō-ˌhis-tə-ˈrek-tə-mē\ *n, pl* **-mies** : surgical removal of the ovaries and the uterus
ovar·i·ot·o·my \ō-ˌvar-ē-ˈä-tə-mē\ *n, pl* **-mies** **1** : surgical incision of an ovary **2** : OOPHORECTOMY
ova·ry \ˈō-və-rē\ *n, pl* **-ries** : one of the typically paired essential female reproductive organs that produce eggs and female sex hormones, that occur in the adult human as oval flattened bodies about one and a half inches (four centimeters) long suspended from the dorsal surface of the broad ligament of either side, that arise from the mesonephros, and that consist of a vascular fibrous stroma enclosing developing egg cells
over·achiev·er \ˌō-vər-ə-ˈchē-vər\ *n* : one who achieves success over and above the standard or expected level esp. at an early age — **over·achieve** *vb*
over·ac·tive \ˌō-vər-ˈak-tiv\ *adj* : excessively or abnormally active — **over·ac·tiv·i·ty** \-ˌak-ˈti-və-tē\ *n*
over·bite \ˈō-vər-ˌbīt\ *n* : the projection of the upper anterior teeth over the lower when the jaws are in the position they occupy in occlusion
over·breathe \ˌō-vər-ˈbrēth\ *vb* **-breathed; -breath·ing** : HYPERVENTILATE
over·com·pen·sa·tion \-ˌkäm-pən-ˈsā-shən, -ˌpen-\ *n* : excessive compensation; *specif* : excessive reaction to a feeling of inferiority, guilt, or inadequacy leading to an exaggerated attempt to overcome the feeling — **over·com·pen·sate** \-ˈkäm-pən-ˌsāt\ *vb*
over·di·ag·no·sis \-ˌdī-ig-ˈnō-səs, -əg-\ *n, pl* **-no·ses** \-ˌsēz\ : the diagnosis of a condition or disease more often than it is actually present — **over·di·ag·nose** \-ˈdī-ig-ˌnōs, -əg-\ *vb*
over·dis·ten·sion *or* **over·dis·ten·tion** \-dis-ˈten-chən\ *n* : excessive distension ⟨~ of the alveoli⟩ — **over·dis·tend·ed** \-dis-ˈten-dəd\ *adj*
over·dose \ˈō-vər-ˌdōs\ *n* : too great a dose (as of a therapeutic agent); *also* : a lethal or toxic amount (as of a drug) — **over·dos·age** \ˌō-vər-ˈdō-sij\ *n* — **over·dose** \ˌō-vər-ˈdōs\ *vb*
over·eat \ˌō-vər-ˈēt\ *vb* **over·ate** \-ˈāt\; **over·eat·en** \-ˈēt-ᵊn\; **over·eat·ing** : to eat to excess — **over·eat·er** *n*
overeating disease *n* : ENTEROTOXEMIA
over·ex·ert \-ig-ˈzərt\ *vb* : to exert (oneself) too much — **over·ex·er·tion** \-ˈzər-shən\ *n*
over·ex·pose \ˌō-vər-ik-ˈspōz\ *vb* **-posed; -pos·ing** : to expose excessively ⟨skin *overexposed* to sunlight⟩ — **over·ex·po·sure** \-ˈspō-zhər\ *n*
over·ex·pres·sion \-ik-ˈspre-shən\ *n* : excessive expression of a gene (as that caused by increasing the frequency of transcription) — **over·ex·press** \-ik-ˈspres\ *vb*
over·ex·tend \-ik-ˈstend\ *vb* : to extend too far ⟨~ the back⟩ — **over·ex·ten·sion** \-ik-ˈsten-chən\ *n*
over·fa·tigue \-fə-ˈtēg\ *n* : excessive fatigue esp. when carried beyond the recuperative capacity of the individual
over·feed \-ˈfēd\ *vb* **-fed** \-ˈfed\; **-feed·ing** : to feed or eat to excess
over·growth \ˈō-vər-ˌgrōth\ *n* **1 a** : excessive growth or increase in numbers **b** : HYPERTROPHY, HYPERPLASIA **2** : something (as cells or tissue) grown over something else
over·hang \ˈō-vər-ˌhaŋ\ *n* : a portion of a filling that extends beyond the normal contour of a tooth
over·hy·dra·tion \ˌō-vər-hī-ˈdrā-shən\ *n* : a condition in which the body contains an excessive amount of fluids

over·jet \ˈō-vər-ˌjet\ *n* : displacement of the mandibular teeth sideways when the jaws are held in the position they occupy in occlusion
over·med·i·cate \-ˈme-di-ˌkāt\ *vb* **-cat·ed; -cat·ing** : to administer too much medication to : prescribe too much medication for — **over·med·i·ca·tion** \-ˌme-di-ˈkā-shən\ *n*
over·nu·tri·tion \ˌō-vər-nü-ˈtri-shən, -nyü-\ *n* : excessive food intake esp. when viewed as a factor in pathology
over·pre·scribe \-pri-ˈskrīb\ *vb* **-scribed; -scrib·ing** : to prescribe excessive or unnecessary medication — **over·pre·scrip·tion** \-pri-ˈskrip-shən\ *n*
over·pro·na·tion \-prō-ˈnā-shən\ *n* : excessive pronation of the foot in walking or running — **over·pro·nate** \-ˈprō-ˌnāt\ *vb*
over·se·da·tion \-si-ˈdā-shən\ *n* : excessive sedation
over·shot \ˈō-vər-ˌshät\ *adj* **1** : having the upper jaw extending beyond the lower **2** : projecting beyond the lower jaw
over·stim·u·la·tion \ˌō-vər-ˌsti-myə-ˈlā-shən\ *n* : excessive stimulation — **over·stim·u·late** \-ˈsti-myə-ˌlāt\ *vb*
overt \ō-ˈvərt, ˈō-ˌvərt\ *adj* : open to view : readily perceived
over–the–count·er *adj* : sold lawfully without prescription ⟨~ painkillers⟩
over·ven·ti·la·tion \ˌō-vər-ˌvent-ᵊl-ˈā-shən\ *n* : HYPERVENTILATION
over·weight \-ˈwāt\ *adj* : weighing in excess of the normal for one's age, height, and build ⟨~ adults typically have a body mass index of 25 to 29.9⟩ — **overweight** *n*
over·work \-ˈwərk\ *vb* : to cause to work too hard, too long, or to exhaustion
ovi- — see OV-
ovi·cide \ˈō-və-ˌsīd\ *n* : an agent that kills eggs; *esp* : an insecticide effective against the egg stage — **ovi·cid·al** \ˌō-və-ˈsīd-ᵊl\ *adj*
ovi·du·cal \ˌō-və-ˈdü-kəl, -ˈdyü-\ *adj* : OVIDUCTAL
ovi·duct \ˈō-və-ˌdəkt\ *n* : a tube that serves exclusively or esp. for the passage of eggs from an ovary
ovi·duc·tal \ˌō-və-ˈdəkt-ᵊl\ *adj* : of, relating to, or affecting an oviduct
ovine \ˈō-ˌvīn\ *adj* : of, relating to, or resembling sheep ⟨~ diseases⟩
ovine progressive pneumonia *n* : a progressive usu. fatal disease of sheep caused by a retrovirus of the genus *Lentivirus* (species *Visna/maedi virus*) — see MAEDI, VISNA
ovip·a·rous \ō-ˈvi-pə-rəs\ *adj* : producing eggs that develop and hatch outside the maternal body — compare OVOVIVIPAROUS, VIVIPAROUS — **ovi·par·i·ty** \ˌō-və-ˈpar-ə-tē\ *n*
ovi·pos·it \ˈō-və-ˌpä-zət, ˌō-və-ˈ\ *vb* : to lay eggs — used esp. of insects — **ovi·po·si·tion** \ˌō-və-pə-ˈzi-shən\ *n* — **ovi·po·si·tion·al** \-ˈzi-shə-nəl\ *adj*
ovi·pos·i·tor \ˈō-və-ˌpä-zə-tər, ˌō-və-ˈ\ *n* : a specialized organ (as of an insect) for depositing eggs
ovo- — see OV-
ovo·gen·e·sis \ˌō-və-ˈje-nə-səs\ *n, pl* **-e·ses** \-ˌsēz\ : OOGENESIS
ovoid \ˈō-ˌvȯid\ *adj* : shaped like an egg ⟨an ~ tumor⟩
ovo–lacto vegetarian *n* : LACTO-OVO VEGETARIAN
ovo·mu·coid \-ˈmyü-ˌkȯid\ *n* : a mucoprotein present in egg white
ovo·plasm \ˈō-və-ˌpla-zəm\ *n* : the cytoplasm of an unfertilized egg
ovo·tes·tis \ˌō-vō-ˈtes-təs\ *n, pl* **-tes·tes** \-ˌtēz\ : a gonad containing both ovarian and testicular tissue
ovo·vi·tel·lin \-vī-ˈte-lən\ *n* : VITELLIN
ovo·vi·vip·a·rous \ˌō-vō-ˌvī-ˈvi-pə-rəs\ *adj* : producing eggs that develop within the maternal body — compare OVIPAROUS, VIVIPAROUS — **ovo·vi·vi·par·i·ty** \-ˌvī-və-ˈpar-ə-tē, -ˌvi-\ *n*
ovu·lar \ˈä-vyə-lər, ˈō-\ *adj* : of or relating to an ovule or ovum
ovu·la·tion \ˌä-vyə-ˈlā-shən, ˌō-\ *n* : the discharge of a mature ovum from the ovary — **ovu·late** \ˈä-vyə-ˌlāt\ *vb* — **ovu·la·to·ry** \ˈä-vyə-lə-ˌtōr-ē, ˈō-\ *adj*
ovule \ˈä-ˌvyül, ˈō-\ *n* **1** : an outgrowth of the ovary of a seed plant that after fertilization develops into a seed **2** : a small egg; *esp* : one in an early stage of growth
ovum \ˈō-vəm\ *n, pl* **ova** \-və\ : a female gamete : MACROGAMETE; *esp* : a mature egg that has undergone reduction, is ready for fertilization, and takes the form of a relatively large inactive gamete providing a comparatively great amount of reserve material and contributing most of the cytoplasm of the zygote
ox·a·cil·lin \ˌäk-sə-ˈsi-lən\ *n* : a semisynthetic penicillin administered in the form of its hydrated sodium salt $C_{19}H_{18}N_3NaO_5S{\cdot}H_2O$ to treat infections caused by penicillin-resistant staphylococci
[1]**ox·a·late** \ˈäk-sə-ˌlāt\ *n* : a salt or ester of oxalic acid
[2]**oxalate** *vb* **-lat·ed; -lat·ing** : to add an oxalate to (blood or plasma) to prevent coagulation
ox·al·ic acid \(ˌ)äk-ˈsa-lik-\ *n* : a poisonous strong acid $(COOH)_2$ or $H_2C_2O_4$ that occurs in various plants as oxalates
ox·a·lo·ace·tic acid \ˌäk-sə-lō-ə-ˈsē-tik-\ *also* **ox·al·ace·tic acid** \ˌäk-sə-lə-ˈsē-tik-\ *n* : a crystalline acid $C_4H_4O_5$ that is formed by reversible oxidation of malic acid (as in carbohydrate metabolism via the Krebs cycle) and in reversible transamination reactions (as from aspartic acid)
ox·a·lo·sis \ˌäk-sə-ˈlō-səs\ *n* : an abnormal condition characterized by hyperoxaluria and the formation of calcium oxalate deposits in tissues
ox·an·a·mide \äk-ˈsa-nə-ˌmīd\ *n* : a tranquilizing drug $C_8H_{15}NO_2$

ox·an·dro·lone \äk-ˈsan-drə-ˌlōn\ *n* : an anabolic steroid $C_{19}H_{30}O_3$ administered orally esp. to promote weight gain (as after chronic infection) and to relieve bone pain in osteoporosis

ox·a·pro·zin \ˌäk-sə-ˈprō-zən\ *n* : an NSAID $C_{18}H_{15}NO_3$ administered orally to treat osteoarthritis and rheumatoid arthritis — see DAYPRO

ox·az·e·pam \äk-ˈsa-zə-ˌpam\ *n* : a benzodiazepine tranquilizer $C_{15}H_{11}ClN_2O_2$

ox·a·zol·i·dine \ˌäk-sə-ˈzō-lə-ˌdēn, -ˈzä-\ *n* : the heterocyclic compound C_3H_7NO; *also* : an anticonvulsant derivative (as trimethadione) of this compound

ox·i·dase \ˈäk-sə-ˌdās, -ˌdāz\ *n* : any of various enzymes that catalyze oxidations; *esp* : one able to react directly with molecular oxygen

ox·i·da·tion \ˌäk-sə-ˈdā-shən\ *n* **1** : the act or process of oxidizing **2** : the state or result of being oxidized — **ox·i·da·tive** \ˈäk-sə-ˌdā-tiv\ *adj* — **ox·i·da·tive·ly** *adv*

oxidation–reduction *n* : a chemical reaction in which one or more electrons are transferred from one atom or molecule to another — called also *redox*

oxidative phosphorylation *n* : the synthesis of ATP by phosphorylation of ADP for which energy is obtained by electron transport and which takes place in the mitochondria during aerobic respiration

oxidative stress *n* : physiological stress on the body that is caused by the cumulative damage done by free radicals inadequately neutralized by antioxidants and that is held to be associated with aging

ox·ide \ˈäk-ˌsīd\ *n* : a binary compound of oxygen with an element or chemical group

ox·i·dize \ˈäk-sə-ˌdīz\ *vb* **-dized; -diz·ing 1** : to combine with oxygen **2** : to dehydrogenate esp. by the action of oxygen **3** : to change (a compound) by increasing the proportion of the part tending to attract electrons or change (an element or ion) from a lower to a higher positive valence : remove one or more electrons from (an atom, ion, or molecule) — **ox·i·diz·able** \ˌäk-sə-ˈdī-zə-bəl\ *adj*

oxidized cellulose *n* : an acid degradation product of cellulose that is used esp. as an absorbable hemostatic agent (as in surgery)

oxidizing agent *n* : a substance that oxidizes something esp. chemically (as by accepting electrons) — compare REDUCING AGENT

ox·i·do·re·duc·tase \ˌäk-sə-dō-ri-ˈdək-ˌtās, -ˌtāz\ *n* : an enzyme that catalyzes an oxidation-reduction reaction

ox·im·e·ter \äk-ˈsi-mə-tər\ *n* : an instrument for measuring continuously the degree of oxygen saturation of the circulating blood — **ox·i·met·ric** \ˌäk-sə-ˈme-trik\ *adj* — **ox·im·e·try** \äk-ˈsi-mə-trē\ *n*

oxo·phen·ar·sine \ˌäk-sə-fe-ˈnär-ˌsēn, -sən\ *n* : an arsenical formerly used in the form of its hydrochloride $C_6H_6AsNO_2{\cdot}HCl$ to treat syphilis

oxo·trem·o·rine \ˌäk-sō-ˈtre-mə-ˌrēn, -rən\ *n* : a cholinergic agent $C_{12}H_{18}N_2O$ that induces tremors

ox·pren·o·lol \ˌäks-ˈpre-nə-ˌlȯl\ *n* : a beta-adrenergic blocking agent used in the form of the hydrochloride $C_{15}H_{23}NO_3{\cdot}HCl$ as a coronary vasodilator

ox·tri·phyl·line \ˌäks-ˌtri-ˈfi-ˌlēn, -ˈtri-fə-ˌlēn\ *n* : the choline salt $C_{12}H_{21}N_5O_3$ of theophylline used chiefly as a bronchodilator

ox warble *n* : the maggot of a cattle grub

oxy \ˈäk-sē\ *adj* : containing oxygen or additional oxygen — often used in combination ⟨*oxy*hemoglobin⟩

oxy- *comb form* **1** : sharp : pointed : acute ⟨*oxy*cephaly⟩ **2** : quick ⟨*oxy*tocic⟩ **3** : acid ⟨*oxy*ntic⟩

oxy·ben·zone \ˌäk-sē-ˈben-ˌzōn\ *n* : a sunscreen $C_{14}H_{12}O_3$ that absorbs UVB and some UVA radiation

oxy·bu·ty·nin \ˌäk-sē-ˈbyü-tᵊn-ən\ *n* : an antispasmodic and anticholinergic drug $C_{22}H_{31}NO_3$ administered transdermally as a skin patch or orally in the form of its hydrochloride $C_{22}H_{31}NO_3{\cdot}HCl$ to relax the smooth muscles of the bladder in the treatment of urge incontinence, frequent urination, and urinary urgency

oxy·bu·tyr·ic acid \-byü-ˈtir-ik-\ *n* : HYDROXYBUTYRIC ACID

oxy·ceph·a·ly \-ˈse-fə-lē\ *n, pl* **-lies** : congenital deformity of the skull due to early synostosis of the parietal and occipital bones with compensating growth in the region of the anterior fontanel resulting in a pointed or pyramidal skull — called also *acrocephaly, turricephaly* — **oxy·ce·phal·ic** \-si-ˈfa-lik\ *adj*

oxy·chlo·ro·sene \-ˈklōr-ə-ˌsēn\ *n* : a topical antiseptic $C_{20}H_{34}O_3S{\cdot}HOCl$

oxy·co·done \-ˈkō-ˌdōn\ *n* : a narcotic analgesic used esp. in the form of its hydrochloride $C_{18}H_{21}NO_4{\cdot}HCl$ to relieve moderate to severe pain— see OXYCONTIN, PERCOCET, PERCODAN

Oxy·Con·tin \-ˈkän-tin\ *trademark* — used for a preparation of the hydrochloride of oxycodone

ox·y·gen \ˈäk-si-jən\ *n* : a colorless tasteless odorless gaseous element that constitutes 21 percent of the atmosphere, is active in physiological processes, and is involved esp. in combustion processes — symbol *O*; see ELEMENT table

ox·y·gen·ate \ˈäk-si-jə-ˌnāt, äk-ˈsi-jə-\ *vb* **-at·ed; -at·ing** : to impregnate, combine, or supply with oxygen ⟨*oxygenated* blood⟩ — **ox·y·gen·ation** \ˌäk-si-jə-ˈnā-shən, äk-ˌsi-jə-\ *n*

ox•y•gen•ator \'äk-si-jə-ˌnā-tər, äk-'si-jə-\ *n* : one that oxygenates; *specif* : an apparatus that oxygenates the blood extracorporeally (as during open-heart surgery)

oxygen capacity *n* : the amount of oxygen which a quantity of blood is able to absorb

oxygen debt *n* : a cumulative deficit of oxygen available for oxidative metabolism that develops during periods of intense bodily activity and must be made good when the body returns to rest

oxygen mask *n* : a device worn over the nose and mouth through which oxygen is supplied from a storage tank

oxygen tent *n* : a canopy which can be placed over a bedridden person and within which a flow of oxygen can be maintained

oxy•he•mo•glo•bin \ˌäk-si-'hē-mə-ˌglō-bən\ *n* : hemoglobin loosely combined with oxygen that it releases to the tissues

oxy•me•taz•o•line \-mə-'ta-zə-ˌlēn\ *n* : a sympathomimetic drug with vasoconstrictive activity that is used in the form of its hydrochloride $C_{16}H_{24}N_2O·HCl$ chiefly as a topical nasal decongestant

oxy•mor•phone \-'mȯr-ˌfōn\ *n* : a semisynthetic opioid analgesic with pharmacological action similar to morphine that is used in the form of its hydrochloride $C_{17}H_{19}NO_4·HCl$

oxy•myo•glo•bin \ˌäk-si-'mī-ə-ˌglō-bən\ *n* : a pigment formed by the combination of myoglobin with oxygen

ox•yn•tic \äk-'sin-tik\ *adj* : secreting acid — used esp. of the parietal cells of the gastric glands

oxy•phen•bu•ta•zone \ˌäk-sē-ˌfen-'byü-tə-ˌzōn\ *n* : a phenylbutazone derivative $C_{19}H_{20}N_2O_3$ having anti-inflammatory, analgesic, and antipyretic effects

oxy•phen•cy•cli•mine \-'sī-klə-ˌmēn\ *n* : an anticholinergic drug with actions similar to atropine usu. used in the form of its hydrochloride $C_{20}H_{28}N_2O_3·HCl$ as an antispasmodic esp. in the treatment of peptic ulcer

oxy•quin•o•line \-'kwin-ᵊl-ˌēn\ *n* : 8-HYDROXYQUINOLINE

Oxy•spi•ru•ra \ˌäk-si-ˌspī-'rür-ə\ *n* : a genus of nematode worms (family Thelaziidae) comprising the eye worms of birds and esp. poultry

oxy•tet•ra•cy•cline \-ˌte-trə-'sī-ˌklēn\ *n* : a broad-spectrum antibiotic $C_{22}H_{24}N_2O_9$ produced by a soil actinomycete of the genus *Streptomyces* (*S. rimosus*) — see TERRAMYCIN

[1]**oxy•to•cic** \ˌäk-si-'tō-sik\ *adj* : hastening childbirth; *also* : inducing contraction of uterine smooth muscle

[2]**oxytocic** *n* : a substance that stimulates contraction of uterine smooth muscle or hastens childbirth

oxy•to•cin \-'tōs-ᵊn\ *n* **1** : a hormone $C_{43}H_{66}N_{12}O_{12}S_2$ secreted by the posterior lobe of the pituitary gland that stimulates esp. the contraction of uterine muscle and the secretion of milk **2** : a synthetic version of oxytocin used esp. to initiate or increase uterine contractions (as in the induction of labor) — see PITOCIN

oxy•uri•a•sis \ˌäk-si-yü-'rī-ə-səs\ *n, pl* **-a•ses** \-ˌsēz\ : infestation with or disease caused by pinworms (as of the genera *Enterobius* and *Oxyuris*)

oxy•urid \ˌäk-sē-'yür-əd\ *n* : any of a family (Oxyuridae) of nematode worms that are chiefly parasites of the vertebrate intestinal tract — see PINWORM — **oxyurid** *adj*

oxy•uris \-'yür-əs\ *n* **1** *cap* : a genus of parasitic nematodes (family Oxyuridae) **2** : any nematode worm of the genus *Oxyuris* or a related genus (as *Enterobius*) : PINWORM

oz *abbr* ounce; ounces

oze•na \ō-'zē-nə\ *n* : a chronic disease of the nose accompanied by a fetid discharge and marked by atrophic changes in the nasal structures

ozone \'ō-ˌzōn\ *n* : a very reactive form of oxygen containing three atoms per molecule that is a bluish irritating gas of pungent odor, that is a major air pollutant in the lower atmosphere but a beneficial component of the upper atmosphere, and that is used for oxidizing, bleaching, disinfecting, and deodorizing

P

P *abbr* **1** parental **2** pressure **3** pulse
P *symbol* phosphorus
p- *abbr* para- ⟨*p*-dichlorobenzene⟩
Pa *symbol* protactinium
PA \ˌpē-ˈā\ *n* : PHYSICIAN ASSISTANT
PA *abbr* pernicious anemia
PABA \ˈpa-bə, ˌpē-ˌā-ˈbē-ˌā\ *n* : PARA-AMINOBENZOIC ACID
pab·u·lum \ˈpa-byə-ləm\ *n* : FOOD; *esp* : a suspension or solution of nutrients in a state suitable for absorption
PA–C *abbr* physician assistant, certified
pac·chi·o·ni·an body \ˌpa-kē-ˈō-nē-ən-\ *n* : ARACHNOID GRANULATION
Pac·chi·o·ni \ˌpä-kē-ˈō-nē\, **Antonio (1665–1726)**, Italian anatomist.
pace·mak·er \ˈpās-ˌmā-kər\ *n* **1** : a group of cells or a body part (as the sinoatrial node of the heart) that serves to establish and maintain a rhythmic activity **2** : an electrical device for stimulating or steadying the heartbeat or reestablishing the rhythm of an arrested heart — called also *pacer*
pace·mak·ing \-mā-kiŋ\ *n* : the act or process of serving as a pacemaker
pac·er \ˈpā-sər\ *n* : PACEMAKER 2
pachy- *comb form* : thick ⟨*pachy*tene⟩
pachy·gy·ria \ˌpa-kē-ˈjī-rē-ə\ *n* : mild to moderate lissencephaly marked by a cerebral cortex with only a few broad, flat convolutions : incomplete lissencephaly — compare AGYRIA
pachy·men·in·gi·tis \ˌpa-kē-ˌme-nən-ˈjī-təs\ *n, pl* **-git·i·des** \-ˈji-tə-ˌdēz\ : inflammation of the dura mater
pachy·me·ninx \-ˈmē-niŋks, -ˈme-\ *n, pl* **-me·nin·ges** \-mə-ˈnin-(ˌ)jēz\ : DURA MATER
pachy·o·nych·ia \ˌpa-kē-ō-ˈni-kē-ə\ *n* : extreme usu. congenital thickness of the nails
pachy·tene \ˈpa-ki-ˌtēn\ *n* : the stage of meiotic prophase which immediately follows the zygotene and in which the paired chromosomes are thickened and visibly divided into chromatids — **pachytene** *adj*
pac·i·fi·er \ˈpa-sə-ˌfī-ər\ *n* **1** : a usu. nipple-shaped device for babies to suck or bite on **2** : TRANQUILIZER
pac·ing \ˈpā-siŋ\ *n* : the act or process of regulating or changing the timing or intensity of cardiac contractions (as by an artificial pacemaker)
Pa·cin·i·an corpuscle \pə-ˈsi-nē-ən-\ *also* **Pa·ci·ni's corpuscle** \pə-ˈchē-nēz-\ *n* : a pressure-sensitive mechanoreceptor that is an oval capsule terminating some sensory nerve fibers esp. in the skin (as of the hands and feet)
Pacini, Filippo (1812–1883), Italian anatomist.
[1]**pack** \ˈpak\ *n* **1** : a container shielded with lead or mercury for holding radium in large quantities esp. for therapeutic application **2 a** : absorbent material saturated with water or other liquid for therapeutic application to the body or a body part — see COLD PACK, HOT PACK; compare ICE PACK **b** : a folded square or compress of gauze or other absorbent material used esp. to maintain a clear field in surgery, to plug cavities, to check bleeding by compression, or to apply medication
[2]**pack** *vb* : to cover or surround with a pack; *specif* : to envelop (a patient) in a wet or dry sheet or blanket
packed cell volume *n* : HEMATOCRIT 2 — abbr. *PCV*
packed red blood cells *n pl* : a concentrated preparation of red blood cells that is obtained from whole blood by removing the plasma (as by centrifugation) and is used in transfusion
pack·ing \ˈpa-kiŋ\ *n* **1** : the therapeutic application of a pack **2** : the material used in packing
pac·li·tax·el \ˌpa-kli-ˈtak-səl\ *n* : an antineoplastic agent $C_{47}H_{51}NO_{14}$ orig. derived from the bark of a yew tree (*Taxus brevifolia* of the family Taxaceae) of the western U.S. and Canada but now typically derived as a semisynthetic product of the English yew (*T. baccata*) and used esp. to treat ovarian cancer — see TAXOL
$PaCO_2$ *abbr* partial pressure of arterial carbon dioxide
PACU *abbr* postanesthesia care unit
pad \ˈpad\ *n* **1** : a usu. square or rectangular piece of often folded typically absorbent material (as gauze) fixed in place over some part of the body as a dressing or other protective covering **2** : a part of the body or of an appendage that resembles or is suggestive of a cushion : a thick fleshy resilient part: as **a** : the sole of the foot or underside of the toes of an animal (as a dog) that is typically thickened so as to form a cushion **b** : the underside of the extremities of the fingers; *esp* : the ball of the thumb
PAD *abbr* peripheral arterial disease
pad·dle \ˈpa-dᵊl\ *n* : a flat electrode that is the part of a defibrillator placed on the chest of a patient and through which a shock of electricity is discharged — called also *paddle electrode*
pad·i·mate O \ˈpa-di-ˌmāt-ˈō\ *n* : a sunscreen $C_{17}H_{27}NO_2$ effective against UVB radiation
paed- *or* **paedo-** *chiefly Brit var of* PED-
pae·di·a·trics, pae·do·don·tics, pae·do·phil·ia *chiefly Brit var of* PEDIATRICS, PEDODONTICS, PEDOPHILIA
PAF *abbr* platelet-activating factor
Pag·et's disease \ˈpa-jəts-\ *n* **1** : a rare form of breast cancer initially manifested as a scaly red rash on the

nipple and areola **2** : a chronic bone disease characterized by one or more enlarged weak bones (as of the pelvis, spine, or skull) with bowing of the long bones, deformation of the flat bones, abnormal fractures, and often pain — called also *osteitis deformans, Paget's disease of bone*

Pag•et \'pa-jət\, **Sir James (1814–1899),** British surgeon.

pa•go•pha•gia \ˌpā-gə-'fā-jə, -jē-ə\ *n* : the compulsive eating of ice that is a symptom of iron deficiency

-pa•gus \pə-gəs\ *n comb form, pl* **-pa•gi** \pə-ˌjī, -ˌgī\ : congenitally united twins with a (specified) type of fixation ⟨cranio*pagus*⟩

PAH \ˌpē-(ˌ)ā-'āch\ *n* : POLYCYCLIC AROMATIC HYDROCARBON

PAH *abbr* **1** para-aminohippurate; para-aminohippuric acid **2** polynuclear aromatic hydrocarbon

[1]**pain** \'pān\ *n* **1 a** : a usu. localized physical suffering associated with bodily disorder (as a disease or an injury); *also* : a basic bodily sensation that is induced by a noxious stimulus, is received by naked nerve endings, is characterized by physical discomfort (as pricking, throbbing, or aching), and typically leads to evasive action **b** : acute mental or emotional suffering or distress **2 pains** *pl* : the protracted series of involuntary contractions of the uterine musculature that constitute the major factor in parturient labor and that are often accompanied by considerable pain — **pain•ful** \-fəl\ *adj* — **pain•ful•ly** *adv* — **pain•less** \-ləs\ *adj* — **pain•less•ly** *adv*

[2]**pain** *vb* : to cause or experience pain

pain•kill•er \-ˌki-lər\ *n* : something (as a drug) that relieves pain — **pain•kill•ing** *adj*

pain spot *n* : one of many small localized areas of the skin that respond to stimulation (as by pricking or burning) by giving a sensation of pain

paint•er's colic \'pān-tərz-\ *n* : intestinal colic associated with obstinate constipation due to chronic lead poisoning

paired–associate learning *n* : the learning of items (as syllables, digits, or words) in pairs so that one member of the pair evokes recall of the other — compare ASSOCIATIVE LEARNING

palae- *or* **palaeo-** *chiefly Brit var of* PALE-

pal•aeo•cer•e•bel•lum, pal•aeo•pa•thol•ogy *chiefly Brit var of* PALEOCEREBELLUM, PALEOPATHOLOGY

pal•a•tal \'pa-lət-ᵊl\ *adj* : of, relating to, forming, or affecting the palate — **pal•a•tal•ly** *adv*

palatal bar *n* : a connector extending across the roof of the mouth to join the parts of a maxillary partial denture

palatal process *n* : PALATINE PROCESS

pal•ate \'pa-lət\ *n* : the roof of the mouth separating the mouth from the nasal cavity — see HARD PALATE, SOFT PALATE

palati — see TENSOR PALATI

[1]**pal•a•tine** \'pa-lə-ˌtīn\ *adj* : of, relating to, or lying near the palate

[2]**palatine** *n* : PALATINE BONE

palatine aponeurosis *n* : a thin fibrous lamella attached to the posterior part of the hard palate that supports the soft palate, includes the tendon of the tensor veli palatini, and supports the other muscles of the palate

palatine artery *n* **1** : either of two arteries of each side of the face: **a** : an inferior artery that arises from the facial artery and divides into two branches of which one supplies the soft palate and the palatine glands and the other supplies esp. the tonsils and the eustachian tube — called also *ascending palatine artery* **b** : a superior artery that arises from the maxillary artery and sends branches to the soft palate, the palatine glands, the mucous membrane of the hard palate, and the gums — called also *greater palatine artery* **2** : any of the branches of the palatine arteries

palatine bone *n* : a bone of extremely irregular form on each side of the skull that is situated in the posterior part of the nasal cavity between the maxilla and the pterygoid process of the sphenoid bone and that consists of a horizontal plate which joins the bone of the opposite side and forms the back part of the hard palate and a vertical plate which is extended into three processes and helps to form the floor of the orbit, the outer wall of the nasal cavity, and several adjoining parts — called also *palatine*

palatine foramen *n* : any of several foramina in the palatine bone giving passage to the palatine vessels and nerves — see GREATER PALATINE FORAMEN

palatine gland *n* : any of numerous small mucous glands in the palate opening into the mouth

palatine nerve *n* : any of several nerves arising from the pterygopalatine ganglion and supplying the roof of the mouth, parts of the nose, and adjoining parts

palatine process *n* : a process of the maxilla that projects medially, articulates posteriorly with the palatine bone, and forms with the corresponding process on the other side the anterior three-fourths of the hard palate — called also *palatal process*

palatine suture *n* : either of two sutures in the hard palate: **a** : a transverse suture lying between the horizontal plates of the palatine bones and the maxillae **b** : a median suture lying between the maxillae in front and continued posteriorly between the palatine bones

palatine tonsil *n* : TONSIL 1a

palatini — see LEVATOR VELI PALATINI, TENSOR VELI PALATINI

palato- *comb form* **1** : palate : of the palate ⟨*palato*plasty⟩ **2** : palatal and ⟨*palato*glossal arch⟩

pal·a·to·glos·sal arch \ˌpa-lə-tō-ˈglä-səl-, -ˌglȯ-\ *n* : the more anterior of the two ridges of soft tissue at the back of the mouth on each side that curves downward from the uvula to the side of the base of the tongue forming a recess for the palatine tonsil as it diverges from the palatopharyngeal arch and that is composed of part of the palatoglossus with its covering of mucous membrane — called also *anterior pillar of the fauces, glossopalatine arch*

pal·a·to·glos·sus \-ˈglä-səs, -ˈglȯ-\ *n, pl* **-glos·si** \-(ˌ)sī\ : a thin muscle that arises from the soft palate on each side, contributes to the structure of the palatoglossal arch, and is inserted into the side and dorsum of the tongue — called also *glossopalatinus*

pal·a·to·pha·ryn·geal arch \-ˌfar-ən-ˈjē-əl-; -fə-ˈrin-jəl-, -jē-əl-\ *n* : the more posterior of the two ridges of soft tissue at the back of the mouth on each side that curves downward from the uvula to the side of the pharynx forming a recess for the palatine tonsil as it diverges from the palatoglossal arch and that is composed of part of the palatopharyngeus with its covering of mucous membrane — called also *pharyngopalatine arch, posterior pillar of the fauces*

pal·a·to·pha·ryn·ge·us \-ˌfar-ən-ˈjē-əs; -fə-ˈrin-jəs, -jē-əs\ *n* : a longitudinal muscle of the pharynx that arises from the soft palate, contributes to the structure of the palatopharyngeal arch, and is inserted into the thyroid cartilage and the wall of the pharynx

pal·a·to·plas·ty \ˈpa-lə-tə-ˌplas-tē\ *n, pl* **-ties** : a plastic operation for repair of the palate (as in cleft palate)

pale \ˈpāl\ *adj* **pal·er; pal·est** : deficient in color or intensity of color ⟨a ~ face⟩ — **pale·ness** \-nəs\ *n*

pale- *or* **paleo-** *comb form* : early : old ⟨*paleo*pathology⟩

pa·leo·cer·e·bel·lum \ˌpā-lē-ō-ˌser-ə-ˈbe-ləm\ *n, pl* **-bel·lums** *or* **-bel·la** \-ˈbe-lə\ : the part of the cerebellum concerned with maintenance of normal postural relationships and made up chiefly of the anterior lobe of the vermis and of the pyramid — compare NEOCEREBELLUM

pa·leo·pa·thol·o·gy \ˌpā-lē-ō-pə-ˈthä-lə-jē\ *n, pl* **-gies** : a branch of pathology concerned with diseases of former times as determined esp. from fossil or other remains — **pa·leo·pa·thol·o·gist** \-jist\ *n*

pali- *comb form* : pathological state characterized by repetition of a (specified) act ⟨*pali*lalia⟩

pali·la·lia \ˌpa-lə-ˈlā-lē-ə\ *n* : a speech defect marked by abnormal repetition of syllables, words, or phrases

pal·in·drome \ˈpa-lən-ˌdrōm\ *n* : a palindromic sequence of DNA

pal·in·dro·mic \ˌpa-lən-ˈdrō-mik\ *adj* **1** : RECURRENT ⟨~ rheumatism⟩ **2** : of, relating to, or consisting of a double-stranded sequence of DNA in which the order of the nucleotides is the same on each side but running in opposite directions

pal·i·sade worm \ˌpa-lə-ˈsād-\ *n* : BLOODWORM

pal·la·di·um \pə-ˈlā-dē-əm\ *n* : a silver-white malleable metallic element — symbol *Pd;* see ELEMENT table

pal·li·ate \ˈpa-lē-ˌāt\ *vb* **-at·ed; -at·ing** : to reduce the intensity or severity of (a disease); *also* : to ease (symptoms) without curing the underlying disease — **pal·li·a·tion** \ˌpa-lē-ˈā-shən\ *n*

[1]**pal·lia·tive** \ˈpa-lē-ˌā-tiv, ˈpal-yə-\ *adj* : reducing the severity of a disease or condition without curing it : providing palliative care ⟨~ treatment⟩

[2]**palliative** *n* : something that reduces the severity of a disease or condition without curing it

palliative care *n* : medical and related care provided to a patient with a serious life-threatening or terminal illness that is not intended to provide curative treatment but rather to manage symptoms, relieve pain and discomfort, improve quality of life, and meet the emotional, social, and spiritual needs of the patient

pal·li·dal \ˈpa-ləd-ᵊl\ *adj* : of, relating to, or involving the globus pallidus

pal·li·dum \ˈpa-lə-dəm\ *n* : GLOBUS PALLIDUS

pallidus — see GLOBUS PALLIDUS

pal·li·um \ˈpa-lē-əm\ *n, pl* **-lia** \-lē-ə\ *or* **-li·ums** : CEREBRAL CORTEX

pal·lor \ˈpa-lər\ *n* : deficiency of color esp. of the face : PALENESS

palm \ˈpälm, ˈpäm\ *n* : the somewhat concave part of the hand between the bases of the fingers and the wrist — **pal·mar** \ˈpal-mər, ˈpäl-, ˈpä-\ *adj*

palmar aponeurosis *n* : an aponeurosis of the palm of the hand that consists of a superficial longitudinal layer continuous with the tendon of the palmaris longus and of a deeper transverse layer — called also *palmar fascia*

palmar arch *n* : either of two loops of blood vessels in the palm of the hand: **a** : a deeply situated transverse artery that is composed of the terminal part of the radial artery joined to a branch of the ulnar artery and that supplies principally the deep muscles of the hand, thumb, and index finger — called also *deep palmar arch* **b** : a superficial arch that is the continuation of the ulnar artery which anastomoses with a branch derived from the radial artery and that sends branches mostly to the fingers — called also *superficial palmar arch*

palmar fascia *n* : PALMAR APONEUROSIS

palmar interosseus *n* : any of three small muscles of the palmar surface of the hand each of which arises from, extends along, and inserts on the side of the second, fourth, or fifth finger facing the middle finger and which acts to adduct its finger toward the middle finger, flex its metacarpophalangeal joint, and extend its distal two phalanges — called also *interosseus palmaris, palmar interosseous muscle*

pal•mar•is \pal-ˈmar-əs\ *n, pl* **pal•mar•es** \-ˌēz\ : either of two muscles of the palm of the hand: **a** : PALMARIS BREVIS **b** : PALMARIS LONGUS

palmaris brev•is \-ˈbrev-əs\ *n* : a short transverse superficial muscle of the ulnar side of the palm of the hand that arises from the flexor retinaculum and palmar aponeurosis, inserts into the skin on the ulnar edge of the palm, and functions to tense and stabilize the palm (as in catching a ball)

palmaris lon•gus \-ˈlȯŋ-gəs\ *n* : a superficial muscle of the forearm lying on the medial side of the flexor carpi radialis that arises esp. from the medial epicondyle of the humerus, inserts esp. into the palmar aponeurosis, and acts to flex the hand

pal•mit•ic acid \(ˌ)pal-ˈmi-tik-, (ˌ)päl-, (ˌ)pä-\ *n* : a waxy crystalline saturated fatty acid $C_{16}H_{32}O_2$ occurring free or in the form of esters (as glycerides) in most fats and fatty oils and in several essential oils and waxes

pal•mo•plan•tar \ˌpal-mō-ˈplan-tər, ˌpäl-, ˌpä-\ *adj* : of, relating to, or affecting both the palms of the hands and the soles of the feet ⟨~ psoriasis⟩

pal•pa•ble \ˈpal-pə-bəl\ *adj* : capable of being touched or felt; *esp* : capable of being examined by palpation

pal•pa•tion \pal-ˈpā-shən\ *n* **1** : an act of touching or feeling **2** : physical examination in medical diagnosis by pressure of the hand or fingers to the surface of the body esp. to determine the condition (as of size or consistency) of an underlying part or organ ⟨~ of the liver⟩ — compare INSPECTION — **pal•pate** \ˈpal-ˌpāt\ *vb* — **pal•pa•to•ry** \ˈpal-pə-ˌtōr-ē\ *adj*

pal•pe•bra \ˈpal-pə-brə, pal-ˈpē-brə\ *n, pl* **pal•pe•brae** \-brē\ : EYELID — **pal•pe•bral** \pal-ˈpē-brəl\ *adj*

palpebrae — see LEVATOR PALPEBRAE SUPERIORIS

palpebral fissure *n* : the space between the margins of the eyelids — called also *rima palpebrarum*

palpebrarum — see RIMA PALPEBRARUM, XANTHELASMA PALPEBRARUM

pal•pi•tate \ˈpal-pə-ˌtāt\ *vb* **-tat•ed; -tat•ing** : to beat rapidly, irregularly, or forcibly — used esp. of the heart

pal•pi•ta•tion \ˌpal-pə-ˈtā-shən\ *n* : a rapid pulsation; *esp* : an abnormally rapid or irregular beating of the heart (as that caused by panic, arrhythmia, or strenuous physical exercise)

pal•sied \ˈpȯl-zēd\ *adj* : affected with palsy ⟨hands weak and ~⟩

pal•sy \ˈpȯl-zē\ *n, pl* **pal•sies** **1** : PARALYSIS — used chiefly in combination ⟨oculomotor ~⟩; see BELL'S PALSY, CEREBRAL PALSY **2** : a condition that is characterized by uncontrollable tremor or quivering of the body or one or more of its parts — not used technically

pal•u•drine \ˈpa-lə-drən\ *n* : PROGUANIL

L–PAM \ˈel-ˌpam\ *n* : MELPHALAN

2–PAM \ˌtü-ˌpē-ˌā-ˈem\ *n* : PRALIDOXIME

pam•a•quine \ˈpa-mə-ˌkwin, -ˌkwēn\ *n* : a toxic antimalarial drug $C_{19}H_{29}N_3O$; *also* : PAMAQUINE NAPHTHOATE

pamaquine naph•tho•ate \-ˈnaf-thə-ˌwāt\ *n* : an insoluble salt $C_{42}H_{45}N_3O_7$ of pamaquine

pam•id•ro•nate \ˌpa-mi-ˈdrō-ˌnāt\ *n* : a disodium bisphosphonate bone-resorption inhibitor $C_3H_9NNa_2O_7P_2$ administered as an intravenous infusion esp. in the treatment of Paget's disease of bone and of hypercalcemia associated with malignancy — called also *pamidronate disodium*

Pam•ine \ˈpa-ˌmēn\ *trademark* — used for a preparation of the bromide salt of methscopolamine

pam•o•ate \ˈpa-mə-ˌwāt\ *n* : any of various salts or esters of an acid $C_{23}H_{16}O_6$ — see HYDROXYZINE

pam•pin•i•form plexus \pam-ˈpi-nə-ˌfȯrm-\ *n* : a venous plexus that is associated with each testicular vein in the male and each ovarian vein in the female — called also *pampiniform venous plexus*

PAN *abbr* peroxyacetyl nitrate

pan- *comb form* : whole : general ⟨*pan*carditis⟩ ⟨*pan*leukopenia⟩

Panadol \ˈpa-nə-ˌdȯl\ *trademark* — used for a preparation of acetaminophen

pan•car•di•tis \ˌpan-kär-ˈdī-təs\ *n* : general inflammation of the heart

Pan•coast's syndrome \ˈpan-ˌkōsts-\ *n* : a complex of symptoms associated with Pancoast's tumor which includes Horner's syndrome and neuralgia of the arm resulting from pressure on the brachial plexus

Pancoast, Henry Khunrath (1875–1939), American radiologist.

Pancoast's tumor *or* **Pancoast tumor** *n* : a malignant tumor formed at the upper extremity of the lung

pan•cre•as \ˈpaŋ-krē-əs, ˈpan-\ *n, pl* **-cre•as•es** *also* **-cre•ata** \pan-ˈkrē-ə-tə\ : a large lobulated gland that in humans lies in front of the upper lumbar vertebrae and behind the stomach and is somewhat hammer-shaped and firmly attached anteriorly to the curve of the duodenum with which it communicates through one or more pancreatic ducts and that consists of (1) tubular acini secreting digestive enzymes which pass to the intestine and function in the breakdown of proteins, fats, and carbohydrates; (2) modified acinar cells that form islets of Langerhans between the tubules and secrete the hormones insulin and glucagon; and (3) a firm connective-tissue capsule that extends supportive strands into the organ

pancreat- *or* **pancreato-** *comb form* **1** : pancreas : pancreatic ⟨*pancreat*ectomy⟩ ⟨*pancreat*in⟩ **2** : pancreas and ⟨*pancreato*duodenectomy⟩

pan•cre•atec•to•my \ˌpaŋ-krē-ə-ˈtek-tə-mē, ˌpan-\ *n, pl* **-mies** : surgical excision of all or part of the pancreas — **pan•cre•atec•to•mized** \ˌpaŋ-krē-ə-ˈtek-tə-ˌmīzd, ˌpan-\ *adj*

pan•cre•at•ic \ˌpaŋ-krē-ˈa-tik, ˌpan-\ *adj* : of, relating to, or produced in the pancreas ⟨∼ amylase⟩

pancreatic cholera *n* : VERNER-MORRISON SYNDROME

pancreatic duct *n* : a duct connecting the pancreas with the intestine: **a** : the chief duct of the pancreas that runs from left to right through the body of the gland, passes out its neck, and empties into the duodenum either through an opening shared with the common bile duct or through one close to it — called also *duct of Wirsung, Wirsung's duct* **b** : ACCESSORY PANCREATIC DUCT

pancreatic juice *n* : a clear alkaline secretion of pancreatic digestive enzymes (as trypsin and lipase) that flows into the duodenum

pancreatico- *comb form* : pancreatic : pancreatic and ⟨*pancreatico*duodenal⟩

pan•cre•at•i•co•du•o•de•nal \ˌpaŋ-krē-ˌa-ti-(ˌ)kō-ˌdü-ə-ˈdē-nəl, ˌpan-, -ˌdyü-; dù-ˈäd-ᵊn-əl, -dyù-\ *adj* : of or relating to the pancreas and the duodenum

pancreaticoduodenal artery *n* : either of two arteries that supply the pancreas and duodenum forming an anastomosis giving off numerous branches to these parts: **a** : one arising from the superior mesenteric artery — called also *inferior pancreaticoduodenal artery* **b** : one arising from the gastroduodenal artery — called also *superior pancreaticoduodenal artery*

pancreaticoduodenal vein *n* : any of several veins that drain the pancreas and duodenum accompanying the inferior and superior pancreaticoduodenal arteries

pan•cre•at•i•co•du•o•de•nec•to•my \-ˌdü-ə-ˌdē-ˈnek-tə-mē, -ˌdyü-; -dù-ˌä-də-ˈnek-tə-mē, -dyù-\ *n, pl* **-mies** : partial or complete excision of the pancreas and the duodenum — called also *pancreatoduodenectomy*

pan•cre•at•i•co•du•o•de•nos•to•my \-ˈnäs-tə-mē\ *n, pl* **-mies** : surgical formation of an artificial opening connecting the pancreas to the duodenum

pan•cre•at•i•co•je•ju•nos•to•my \-ji-ˌjü-ˈnäs-tə-mē, -ˌje-jü-\ *n, pl* **-mies** : surgical formation of an artificial passage connecting the pancreas to the jejunum

pan•cre•atin \pan-ˈkrē-ə-tən; ˈpaŋ-krē-, ˈpan-\ *n* : a mixture of enzymes from the pancreatic juice; *also* : a preparation containing such a mixture obtained from the pancreas of the domestic swine or ox and used as a digestant

pan•cre•ati•tis \ˌpaŋ-krē-ə-ˈtī-təs, ˌpan-\ *n, pl* **-atit•i•des** \-ˈti-tə-ˌdēz\ : inflammation of the pancreas

pancreato- — see PANCREAT-

pan•cre•at•o•bil•i•ary \ˌpan-krē-ə-tō-ˈbi-lē-ˌer-ē\ *adj* : of, relating to, or affecting the pancreas and the bile ducts and gallbladder ⟨∼ disease⟩

pan•cre•a•to•du•o•de•nec•to•my \ˈpan-krē-ə-tō-ˌdü-ə-ˌdē-ˈnek-tə-mē, -ˌdyü-; -dù-ˌäd-ə-ˈnek-tə-mē, -dyù-\ *n, pl* **-mies** : PANCREATICODUODENECTOMY

pan•creo•zy•min \ˌpan-krē-ō-ˈzī-mən\ *n* : CHOLECYSTOKININ

pan•cu•ro•ni•um bromide \ˌpan-kyə-ˈrō-nē-əm-\ *n* : a neuromuscular blocking agent $C_{35}H_{60}Br_2N_2O_4$ used as a skeletal muscle relaxant — called also *pancuronium*

pan•cy•to•pe•nia \ˌpan-ˌsī-tə-ˈpē-nē-ə\ *n* : an abnormal reduction in the number of red blood cells, white blood cells, and blood platelets in the blood; *also* : a disorder (as aplastic anemia) characterized by such a reduction — **pan•cy•to•pe•nic** \-ˈpē-nik\ *adj*

[1]**pan•dem•ic** \pan-ˈde-mik\ *adj* : occurring over a wide geographic area and affecting an exceptionally high proportion of the population ⟨∼ malaria⟩

[2]**pandemic** *n* : a pandemic outbreak of a disease

pan•en•ceph•a•li•tis \ˌpan-in-ˌse-fə-ˈlī-təs\ *n, pl* **-lit•i•des** \-ˈli-tə-ˌdēz\ : inflammation of the brain affecting both white and gray matter — see SUBACUTE SCLEROSING PANENCEPHALITIS

pan•en•do•scope \-ˈen-də-ˌskōp\ *n* : a cystoscope fitted with an obliquely forward telescopic system that permits wide-angle viewing of the interior of the urinary bladder — **pan•en•do•scop•ic** \-ˌen-də-ˈskä-pik\ *adj* — **pan•en•dos•co•py** \-en-ˈdäs-kə-pē\ *n*

Pa•neth cell \ˈpä-net-\ *n* : any of the granular epithelial cells with large acidophilic nuclei occurring at the base of the crypts of Lieberkühn in the small intestine and appendix

Paneth, Josef (1857–1890), Austrian physiologist.

pang \ˈpaŋ\ *n* : a brief piercing spasm of pain — see BIRTH PANG, HUNGER PANGS

pan•hy•po•pi•tu•ita•rism \(ˌ)pan-ˌhī-pō-pə-ˈtü-ə-tə-ˌri-zəm, -ˈtyü-\ *n* : generalized secretory deficiency of the anterior lobe of the pituitary gland; *also* : a disorder (as Simmonds' disease) characterized by such deficiency

— **pan·hy·po·pi·tu·itary** \-ˈtü-ə-ˌter-ē, -ˈtyü-\ *adj*

pan·hys·ter·ec·to·my \(ˌ)pan-ˌhis-tə-ˈrek-tə-mē\ *n, pl* **-mies** : surgical excision of the uterus and uterine cervix — called also *total hysterectomy*

pan·ic \ˈpa-nik\ *n* **1** : a sudden overpowering fright; *also* : acute extreme anxiety **2** : a sudden unreasoning terror often accompanied by mass flight — **panic** *vb*

panic attack *n* : an episode of intense fear or apprehension that is of sudden onset and may occur for no apparent reason or as a reaction to an identifiable triggering stimulus (as a stressful event); *specif* : one that is accompanied by usu. four or more bodily or cognitive symptoms (as heart palpitations, dizziness, shortness of breath, or feelings of unreality) and that typically peaks within 10 minutes of onset

panic disorder *n* : an anxiety disorder characterized by recurrent unexpected panic attacks followed by a month or more of worry about their recurrence, implications, or consequences or by a change in behavior related to the panic attacks

pan·leu·ko·pe·nia \ˌpan-ˌlü-kə-ˈpē-nē-ə\ *n* : an acute usu. fatal epizootic disease esp. of cats that is caused by a virus of the genus *Parvovirus* (species *Feline panleukopenia virus*) and is characterized by fever, diarrhea and dehydration, and extensive destruction of white blood cells — called also *cat distemper, cat fever, feline distemper, feline enteritis, feline panleukopenia*

pan·nic·u·li·tis \pə-ˌni-kyə-ˈlī-təs\ *n* **1** : inflammation of the subcutaneous layer of fat **2** : a syndrome characterized by recurring fever and usu. painful inflammatory and necrotic nodules in the subcutaneous tissues esp. of the thighs, abdomen, or buttocks — called also *relapsing febrile nodular nonsuppurative panniculitis, Weber-Christian disease*

pan·nic·u·lus \pə-ˈni-kyə-ləs\ *n, pl* **-u·li** \-ˌlī\ : a sheet or layer of tissue; *esp* : PANNICULUS ADIPOSUS

panniculus ad·i·po·sus \-ˌa-də-ˈpō-səs\ *n* : any superficial fascia bearing deposits of fat

pan·nus \ˈpa-nəs\ *n, pl* **pan·ni** \-ˌnī\ **1** : a vascular tissue causing a superficial opacity of the cornea and occurring esp. in trachoma **2** : a sheet of inflammatory granulation tissue that spreads from the synovial membrane and invades the joint in rheumatoid arthritis ultimately leading to fibrous ankylosis

pan·oph·thal·mi·tis \(ˌ)pan-ˌäf-thəl-ˈmī-təs, -ˌäp-\ *n* : inflammation involving all the tissues of the eyeball

pan·sys·tol·ic \(ˌ)pan-sis-ˈtä-lik\ *adj* : persisting throughout systole ⟨a ~ heart murmur⟩

pant \ˈpant\ *vb* : to breathe quickly, spasmodically, or in a labored manner

pan·to·caine \ˈpan-tə-ˌkān\ *n* : TETRACAINE

pan·to·pra·zole \pan-ˈtō-prə-ˌzōl\ *n* : a benzimidazole derivative that inhibits gastric acid secretion and is used in the form of its sodium salt $C_{16}H_{14}F_2N_3NaO_4S$ to treat erosive esophagitis and disorders (as Zollinger-Ellison syndrome) involving gastric acid hypersecretion — see PROTONIX

pan·to·the·nate \ˌpan-tə-ˈthe-ˌnāt, pan-ˈtä-thə-ˌnāt\ *n* : a salt or ester of pantothenic acid — see CALCIUM PANTOTHENATE

pan·to·then·ic acid \ˌpan-tə-ˈthe-nik-\ *n* : a viscous oily acid $C_9H_{17}NO_5$ of the vitamin B complex found in all living tissues

pan·trop·ic \(ˌ)pan-ˈträ-pik\ *adj* : affecting various tissues without showing special affinity for one of them ⟨a ~ virus⟩ — compare NEUROTROPIC

pa·pa·in \pə-ˈpā-ən, -ˈpī-\ *n* : a protease in the juice of the green fruit of the papaya (*Carica papaya* of the family Caricaceae) used chiefly as a tenderizer for meat and in medicine as a digestant and as a topical agent in the debridement of necrotic tissue

Pa·pa·ni·co·laou smear \ˌpä-pə-ˈnē-kə-ˌlau̇-, ˌpa-pə-ˈni-kə-\ *n* : PAP SMEAR

Papanicolaou, George Nicholas (1883–1962), American anatomist and cytologist.

Papanicolaou test *n* : PAP SMEAR

Pa·pa·ver \pə-ˈpa-vər, -ˈpā-\ *n* : a genus (family Papaveraceae) of chiefly bristly hairy herbs that contains the opium poppy (*P. somniferum*)

pa·pav·er·ine \pə-ˈpa-və-ˌrēn, -rən\ *n* : a crystalline alkaloid that is used in the form of its hydrochloride $C_{20}H_{21}NO_4{\cdot}HCl$ esp. as a vasodilator because of its ability to relax smooth muscle

papill- *or* **papillo-** *comb form* **1** : papilla ⟨*papill*itis⟩ **2** : papillary ⟨*papill*oma⟩

pa·pil·la \pə-ˈpi-lə\ *n, pl* **pa·pil·lae** \-ˈpi-(ˌ)lē, -ˌlī\ : a small projecting body part similar to a nipple in form: as **a** : a vascular process of connective tissue extending into and nourishing the root of a hair or developing tooth **b** : any of the vascular protuberances of the dermal layer of the skin extending into the epidermal layer and often containing tactile corpuscles **c** : RENAL PAPILLA **d** : any of the small protuberances on the upper surface of the tongue — see CIRCUMVALLATE PAPILLA, FILIFORM PAPILLA, FUNGIFORM PAPILLA, INTERDENTAL PAPILLA

papilla of Vater *n* : AMPULLA OF VATER

pap·il·lary \ˈpa-pə-ˌler-ē\ *adj* : of, relating to, or resembling a papilla : PAPILLOSE

papillary carcinoma *n* : a carcinoma characterized by a papillary structure

papillary layer *n* : the superficial layer of the dermis raised into papillae that fit into corresponding depressions on the inner surface of the epidermis

papillary muscle *n* : one of the small muscular columns attached at one end to the chordae tendineae and at the other to the wall of the ventricle and that maintain tension on the chordae tendineae as the ventricle contracts

pap•il•late \ˈpa-pə-ˌlāt, pə-ˈpi-lət\ *adj* : covered with or bearing papillae

pap•il•lec•to•my \ˌpa-pə-ˈlek-tə-mē\ *n, pl* **-mies** : the surgical removal of a papilla

pap•il•le•de•ma \ˌpa-pə-lə-ˈdē-mə\ *n* : swelling and protrusion of the blind spot of the eye caused by edema — called also *choked disk*

pap•il•li•tis \ˌpa-pə-ˈlī-təs\ *n* : inflammation of a papilla; *esp* : inflammation of the optic disk — see NECROTIZING PAPILLITIS

pap•il•lo•ma \ˌpa-pə-ˈlō-mə\ *n, pl* **-mas** *also* **-ma•ta** \-mə-tə\ : a benign tumor (as a wart or condyloma) resulting from an overgrowth of epithelial tissue on papillae of vascularized connective tissue (as of the skin) — see PAPILLOMAVIRUS

pap•il•lo•ma•to•sis \-ˌlō-mə-ˈtō-səs\ *n, pl* **-to•ses** \-ˌsēz\ : a condition marked by the presence of numerous papillomas

pap•il•lo•ma•tous \-ˈlō-mə-təs\ *adj* **1** : resembling or being a papilloma ⟨a ~ lesion⟩ **2** : marked or characterized by papillomas ⟨~ dermatitis⟩

pap•il•lo•ma•vi•rus \ˌpa-pə-ˈlō-mə-ˌvī-rəs\ *n* : any of a family (*Papillomaviridae*) of viruses that contain a single molecule of circular double-stranded DNA and cause papillomas in mammals — see HUMAN PAPILLOMAVIRUS

pap•il•lose \ˈpa-pə-ˌlōs\ *adj* : covered with, resembling, or bearing papillae

pa•po•va•vi•rus \pə-ˈpō-və-ˌvī-rəs\ *n* : any of a former family (Papovaviridae) that included the papillomaviruses and polyomaviruses

pap•pa•ta•ci fever *also* **pa•pa•ta•ci fever** \ˌpä-pə-ˈtä-chē-\ *or* **pa•pa•ta•si fever** \-ˈtä-sē-\ *n* : SANDFLY FEVER

Pap smear \ˈpap-\ *n* : a method or a test based on it for the early detection of cancer esp. of the uterine cervix that involves staining exfoliated cells by a special technique which differentiates diseased tissue — called also *Papanicolaou smear, Papanicolaou test, Pap test*

G. N. Papanicolaou — see PAPANICOLAOU SMEAR

pap•u•la \ˈpa-pyə-lə\ *n, pl* **pap•u•lae** \-ˌlē\ **1** : PAPULE **2** : a small papilla

pap•u•lar \ˈpa-pyə-lər\ *adj* : consisting of or characterized by papules

pap•u•la•tion \ˌpa-pyə-ˈlā-shən\ *n* **1** : a stage in some eruptive conditions marked by the formation of papules **2** : the formation of papules

pap•ule \ˈpa-(ˌ)pyül\ *n* : a small solid usu. conical elevation of the skin caused by inflammation, accumulated secretion, or hypertrophy of tissue elements

papulo- *comb form* : characterized by papules and ⟨*papulo*vesicular⟩

pap•u•lo•pus•tu•lar \ˌpa-pyə-lō-ˈpəs-chə-lər, -ˈpəs-tyü-\ *adj* : consisting of both papules and pustules ⟨~ acne⟩

pap•u•lo•sis \ˌpa-pyə-ˈlō-səs\ *n* : the condition of having papular lesions

pap•u•lo•ve•sic•u•lar \ˌpa-pyə-lō-və-ˈsi-kyə-lər\ *adj* : marked by the presence of both papules and vesicles

pap•y•ra•ceous \ˌpa-pə-ˈrā-shəs\ *adj* : of, relating to, or being the flattened remains of one of twin fetuses which has died in the uterus and been compressed by the growth of the other

para \ˈpar-ə\ *n, pl* **par•as** *or* **par•ae** \ˈpar-ˌē\ : a woman delivered of a specified number of children — used in combination with a term or figure to indicate the number ⟨multi*para*⟩ ⟨a 36-year-old *para* 5⟩; compare GRAVIDA

para- \ˌpar-ə, ˈpar-ə\ *or* **par-** *prefix* **1** : beside : alongside of : beyond : aside from ⟨*para*thyroid⟩ ⟨*par*enteral⟩ **2 a** : closely related to ⟨*par*aldehyde⟩ **b** : involving substitution at or characterized by two opposite positions in the benzene ring that are separated by two carbon atoms ⟨*para*dichlorobenzene⟩ — abbr. *p-* **3 a** : faulty : abnormal ⟨*par*esthesia⟩ **b** : associated in a subsidiary or accessory capacity ⟨*para*medical⟩ **c** : closely resembling : almost ⟨*para*typhoid⟩

para–ami•no•ben•zo•ic acid \ˈpar-ə-ə-ˌmē-nō-ˌben-ˈzō-ik-, ˈpar-ə-ˌa-mə-(ˌ)nō-\ *n* : a colorless aminobenzoic acid derivative that is a growth factor of the vitamin B complex and is used as a sunscreen — called also *PABA*

para–ami•no•hip•pu•rate \-ˈhi-pyə-ˌrāt\ *n* : a salt of para-aminohippuric acid

para–ami•no•hip•pu•ric acid \-hi-ˈpyu̇r-ik-\ *n* : a crystalline acid administered intravenously in the form of its sodium salt $C_9H_9N_2NaO_3$ in testing kidney function

para–ami•no•sal•i•cyl•ic acid \-ˌsal-ə-ˈsi-lik-\ *n* : the white crystalline isomer of aminosalicylic acid that is made synthetically and is used in the treatment of tuberculosis

para–aor•tic \ˌpar-ə-ā-ˈȯr-tik\ *adj* : close to the aorta ⟨~ lymph nodes⟩

para–api•cal \-ˈā-pi-kəl, -ˈa-\ *adj* : close to the apex of the heart

para•ben \ˈpar-ə-ben\ *n* : either of two antifungal agents used as preservatives in foods and pharmaceuticals: **a** : METHYLPARABEN **b** : PROPYLPARABEN

para•bi•o•sis \ˌpar-ə-(ˌ)bī-ˈō-səs, -bē-\ *n, pl* **-o•ses** \-ˌsēz\ : the anatomical and physiological union of two organisms either natural or artificially produced — **para•bi•ot•ic** \-ˈä-tik\ *adj* — **para•bi•ot•i•cal•ly** *adv*

para•cen•te•sis \ˌpar-ə-(ˌ)sen-ˈtē-səs\ *n, pl* **-te•ses** \-ˌsēz\ : a surgical puncture of a cavity of the body (as with a trocar or aspirator) usu. to draw off any abnormal effusion

para·cen·tral \ˌpar-ə-ˈsen-trəl\ *adj* : lying near a center or central part

para·cen·tric \-ˈsen-trik\ *adj* : being an inversion that occurs in a single arm of one chromosome and does not involve the chromomere — compare PERICENTRIC

para·cer·vi·cal \-ˈsər-və-kəl\ *adj* **1** : located or administered next to the uterine cervix ⟨~ injection⟩ **2** : of, relating to, or occurring in the neck and esp. the back part of the neck

para·cet·a·mol \ˌpar-ə-ˈsē-tə-ˌmȯl\ *n, Brit* : ACETAMINOPHEN

para·chlo·ro·phe·nol \-ˌklōr-ə-ˈfē-ˌnōl, -ˌnȯl, -fi-ˈnōl\ *n* : a chlorinated phenol C_6H_5ClO used as a germicide

para·chol·era \-ˈkä-lə-rə\ *n* : a disease clinically resembling Asiatic cholera but caused by a different vibrio

Para·coc·cid·i·oi·des \ˌpar-ə-(ˌ)käk-ˌsi-dē-ˈȯi-ˌdēz\ *n* : a genus of imperfect fungi that includes the causative agent (*P. brasiliensis*) of South American blastomycosis

para·coc·cid·i·oi·do·my·co·sis \-(ˌ)käk-ˌsi-dē-ˌȯi-dō-(ˌ)mī-ˈkō-sis\ *n, pl* **-co·ses** \-ˌsēz\ : SOUTH AMERICAN BLASTOMYCOSIS

para·co·lic \-ˈkō-lik, -ˈkä-\ *adj* : adjacent to the colon ⟨~ lymph nodes⟩

paracolic gutter *n* : either of two grooves formed by the peritoneum and lying respectively lateral to the ascending and descending colons

para·crine \ˈpar-ə-krən\ *adj* : of, relating to, promoted by, or being a substance secreted by a cell and acting on adjacent cells — see AUTOCRINE

par·acu·sis \ˌpar-ə-ˈkyü-səs, -ˈkü-\ *n, pl* **-acu·ses** \-ˌsēz\ : a disorder in the sense of hearing

para·den·tal \-ˈdent-ᵊl\ *adj* : adjacent to a tooth ⟨~ infections⟩

para·di·chlo·ro·ben·zene *also* **p-dichlorobenzene** \ˌpar-ə-ˌdī-ˌklōr-ə-ˈben-ˌzēn, -ˌben-ˈ\ *n* : a white crystalline compound $C_6H_4Cl_2$ used chiefly as a moth repellent and deodorizer — called also *PDB*

para·did·y·mis \-ˈdi-də-məs\ *n, pl* **-y·mi·des** \-mə-ˌdēz\ : a group of coiled tubules situated in front of the lower end of the spermatic cord above the enlarged upper extremity of the epididymis and considered to be a remnant of tubes of the mesonephros

par·a·dox·i·cal \ˌpar-ə-ˈdäk-si-kəl\ *also* **par·a·dox·ic** \-sik\ *adj* : not being the normal or usual kind ⟨~ embolisms⟩

paradoxical sleep *n* : REM SLEEP

paradoxus — see PULSUS PARADOXUS

para·esoph·a·ge·al \-i-ˌsä-fə-ˈjē-əl\ *adj* : adjacent to the esophagus; *esp* : relating to or being a hiatal hernia in which the connection between the esophagus and the stomach remains in its normal location but part or all of the stomach herniates through the hiatus into the thorax

par·aes·the·sia *chiefly Brit var of* PARESTHESIA

par·af·fin \ˈpar-ə-fən\ *n* **1** : a waxy crystalline substance that is a complex mixture of hydrocarbons and is used in pharmaceuticals and cosmetics **2** : ALKANE

para·fol·lic·u·lar \ˌpar-ə-fə-ˈli-kyə-lər\ *adj* : located in the vicinity of or surrounding a follicle ⟨~ thyroid cells⟩

para·for·mal·de·hyde \-fȯr-ˈmal-də-ˌhīd, -fər-\ *n* : a white powder $(CH_2O)_x$ consisting of a polymer of formaldehyde used esp. as a fungicide

para·fo·vea \-ˈfō-vē-ə\ *n, pl* **-fo·ve·ae** \-ˈfō-vē-ˌē, -vē-ˌī\ : the area surrounding the fovea and containing both rods and cones — **para·fo·ve·al** \-ˈfō-vē-əl\ *adj*

para·gan·gli·o·ma \-ˌgaŋ-glē-ˈō-mə\ *n, pl* **-mas** *also* **-ma·ta** \-mə-tə\ : a ganglioma derived from chromaffin cells — compare PHEOCHROMOCYTOMA

para·gan·gli·on \-ˈgaŋ-glē-ən\ *n, pl* **-glia** \-glē-ə\ : one of numerous collections of chromaffin cells associated with ganglia and plexuses of the sympathetic nervous system and similar in structure to the medulla of the adrenal glands — **para·gan·gli·on·ic** \-ˌgaŋ-glē-ˈä-nik\ *adj*

par·a·gon·i·mi·a·sis \ˌpar-ə-ˌgä-nə-ˈmī-ə-səs\ *n, pl* **-a·ses** \-ˌsēz\ : infestation with or disease caused by a lung fluke of the genus *Paragonimus* (*P. westermanii*) that invades the lung

Par·a·gon·i·mus \ˌpar-ə-ˈgä-nə-məs\ *n* : a genus of digenetic trematodes (family Troglotrematidae) comprising forms normally parasitic in the lungs of mammals including humans

para·gran·u·lo·ma \-ˌgra-nyə-ˈlō-mə\ *n, pl* **-mas** *also* **-ma·ta** \-mə-tə\ **1** : a granuloma esp. of the lymph glands that is characterized by inflammation and replacement of the normal cell structure by an infiltrate **2** : a benign form of Hodgkin's lymphoma in which paragranulomas of the lymph glands are a symptom — called also *Hodgkin's paragranuloma*

para·hip·po·cam·pal gyrus \-ˌhi-pə-ˈkam-pəl-\ *n* : a convolution on the inferior surface of the cerebral cortex of the temporal lobe that borders the hippocampus and contains elements of both the archipallium and neopallium — called also *hippocampal convolution, hippocampal gyrus*

para·in·flu·en·za \ˌpar-ə-ˌin-flü-ˈen-zə\ *n* : PARAINFLUENZA VIRUS; *also* : a respiratory illness caused by a parainfluenza virus

parainfluenza virus *n* : any of several paramyxoviruses (genera *Respirovirus* and *Rubulavirus*) that are a frequent cause of infections (as croup) of the lower respiratory tract esp. in infants and children

para·ker·a·to·sis \ˌpar-ə-ˌker-ə-ˈtō-səs\ *n, pl* **-to·ses** \-ˌsēz\ : an abnormality of the horny layer of the skin resulting in a disturbance in the process of keratinization

par·al·de·hyde \pa-ˈral-də-ˌhīd, pə-\ *n* : a colorless liquid polymer $C_6H_{12}O_3$ derived from acetaldehyde and used esp. as an anticonvulsant, hypnotic, and sedative

pa·ral·y·sis \pə-ˈra-lə-səs\ *n, pl* **-y·ses** \-ˌsēz\ : complete or partial loss of function esp. when involving the power of motion or of sensation in any part of the body — see HEMIPLEGIA, PARAPLEGIA, PARESIS 1

paralysis agi·tans \-ˈa-jə-ˌtanz\ *n* : PARKINSON'S DISEASE

[1]**par·a·lyt·ic** \ˌpar-ə-ˈli-tik\ *adj* **1** : affected with or characterized by paralysis **2** : of, relating to, or resembling paralysis

[2]**paralytic** *n* : one affected with paralysis

paralytica — see DEMENTIA PARALYTICA

paralytic dementia *n* : GENERAL PARESIS

paralytic ileus *n* : ILEUS

paralytic rabies *n* : rabies in which paralysis is the predominant symptom and that is characterized by muscle weakness typically beginning in the bitten extremity and spreading to the rest of the body often in an ascending pattern — called also *dumb rabies;* compare FURIOUS RABIES

paralytic shellfish poisoning *n* : shellfish poisoning that is characterized by numbness and tingling, nausea, vomiting, abdominal cramping, muscle weakness, and sometimes paralysis which may lead to respiratory failure and death and that is typically caused by a saxitoxin ingested in contaminated shellfish

par·a·lyze \ˈpar-ə-ˌlīz\ *vb* **-lyzed; -lyz·ing** : to affect with paralysis — **par·a·ly·za·tion** \ˌpar-ə-lə-ˈzā-shən\ *n*

para·me·di·an \ˌpar-ə-ˈmē-dē-ən\ *adj* : situated adjacent to the midline

para·med·ic \ˌpar-ə-ˈme-dik\ *also* **para·med·i·cal** \-di-kəl\ *n* **1** : a person who works in a health field in an auxiliary capacity to a physician (as by giving injections and taking X-rays) **2** : a specially trained medical technician certified to provide a wide range of emergency medical services (as defibrillation and the intravenous administration of drugs) before or during transport to the hospital — compare EMT

para·med·i·cal \ˌpar-ə-ˈme-di-kəl\ *also* **para·med·ic** \-dik\ *adj* : concerned with supplementing the work of highly trained medical professionals

para·me·so·neph·ric duct \-ˌme-zə-ˈne-frik-, -ˌmē-, -sə-\ *n* : MÜLLERIAN DUCT

para·metha·di·one \-ˌme-thə-ˈdī-ˌōn\ *n* : a liquid compound $C_7H_{11}NO_3$ that is a derivative of trimethadione and is sometimes used in the treatment of absence seizures

para·meth·a·sone \-ˈme-thə-ˌzōn\ *n* : a glucocorticoid used for its anti-inflammatory and anti-allergy actions esp. in the form of its acetate $C_{24}H_{31}FO_6$

para·me·tri·tis \-mə-ˈtrī-təs\ *n* : inflammation of the parametrium

para·me·tri·um \-ˈmē-trē-əm\ *n, pl* **-tria** \-trē-ə\ : the connective tissue and fat adjacent to the uterus

par·am·ne·sia \ˌpar-ˌam-ˈnē-zhə, -əm-\ *n* : a disorder of memory: as **a** : a condition in which the proper meaning of words cannot be remembered **b** : the illusion of remembering scenes and events when experienced for the first time — called also *déjà vu;* compare JAMAIS VU

para·mo·lar \ˌpar-ə-ˈmō-lər\ *adj* : of, relating to, or being a supernumerary tooth esp. on the buccal side of a permanent molar or a cusp or tubercle located esp. on the buccal aspect of a molar and representing such a tooth

par·am·y·loid·osis \ˌpar-ˌa-mə-ˌlȯi-ˈdō-səs\ *n, pl* **-oses** \-ˌsēz\ : amyloidosis characterized by the accumulation of an atypical form of amyloid in the tissues

para·my·oc·lo·nus mul·ti·plex \ˌpar-ə-ˌmī-ˈä-klə-nəs-ˈməl-tə-ˌpleks\ *n* : a myoclonus characterized by tremors in corresponding muscles on the two sides

para·myo·to·nia \ˌpar-ə-ˌmī-ə-ˈtō-nē-ə\ *n* : an abnormal state characterized by tonic muscle spasm

para·myxo·vi·rus \ˌpar-ə-ˈmik-sə-ˌvī-rəs\ *n* : any of a family (*Paramyxoviridae*) of single-stranded RNA viruses that have a helical nucleocapsid and lipid-containing envelope and that include the parainfluenza viruses, respiratory syncytial virus, and the causative agents of canine distemper, measles, mumps, Newcastle disease, and rinderpest — see MORBILLIVIRUS, RUBULAVIRUS; compare MYXOVIRUS

para·na·sal \-ˈnā-zəl\ *adj* : adjacent to the nasal cavities; *esp* : of, relating to, or affecting the paranasal sinuses

paranasal sinus *n* : any of various sinuses (as the maxillary sinus and frontal sinus) in the bones of the face and head that are lined with mucous membrane derived from and continuous with the lining of the nasal cavity

para·neo·plas·tic \ˌpar-ə-ˌnē-ə-ˈplas-tik\ *adj* : caused by or resulting from the presence of cancer in the body but not the physical presence of cancerous tissue in the part or organ affected

para·noia \ˌpar-ə-ˈnȯi-ə\ *n* **1** : a psychosis characterized by systematized delusions of persecution or grandeur usu. without hallucinations **2** : a tendency on the part of an individual or group toward excessive or irrational suspiciousness and distrustfulness of others

¹para·noi·ac \-ˈnȯi-ˌak, -ˈnȯi-ik\ *also* **para·no·ic** \-ˈnō-ik\ *adj* : of, relating to, affected with, or characteristic of paranoia or paranoid schizophrenia

²paranoiac *also* **paranoic** *n* : PARANOID

¹para·noid \ˈpar-ə-ˌnȯid\ *also* **para·noi·dal** \ˌpar-ə-ˈnȯid-ᵊl\ *adj* **1** : characterized by or resembling paranoia or paranoid schizophrenia **2** : characterized by suspiciousness, persecutory trends, or megalomania

²paranoid *n* : one affected with paranoia or paranoid schizophrenia — called also *paranoiac*

paranoid personality disorder *n* : a personality disorder characterized by a pervasive pattern of distrust and suspicion of others resulting in a tendency to attribute the motives of others to malevolence

paranoid schizophrenia *n* : schizophrenia characterized esp. by delusions of persecution, grandiosity, or jealousy and by hallucinations (as hearing voices) chiefly of an auditory nature

paranoid schizophrenic *n* : a person affected with paranoid schizophrenia

para·nor·mal \ˌpar-ə-ˈnȯr-məl\ *adj* : not understandable in terms of known scientific laws and phenomena — **para·nor·mal·ly** *adv*

para·ol·fac·to·ry \ˌpar-ə-äl-ˈfak-tə-rē, -ōl-\ *n* : a small area of the cerebral cortex situated on the medial side of the frontal lobe below the corpus callosum and considered part of the limbic system

para·ox·on \-ˈäk-ˌsän\ *n* : a phosphate ester $C_{10}H_{14}NO_6P$ that is formed from parathion in the body and that is a potent anticholinesterase

para·pa·re·sis \ˌpar-ə-pə-ˈrē-səs, ˌpar-ə-ˈpar-ə-səs\ *n, pl* **-re·ses** \-ˌsēz\ : partial paralysis affecting the lower limbs — **para·pa·ret·ic** \-pə-ˈre-tik\ *adj*

para·per·tus·sis \-(ˌ)pər-ˈtə-sis\ *n* : a human respiratory disease closely resembling whooping cough but milder and less often fatal and caused by a different bacterium of the genus *Bordetella* (*B. parapertussis*)

para·pha·ryn·geal space \-ˌfar-ən-ˈjē-əl-, -fə-ˈrin-jəl-, -jē-əl-\ *n* : a space bounded medially by the superior constrictor of the pharynx, laterally by the medial pterygoid muscle, posteriorly by the cervical vertebrae, and below by the muscles arising from the styloid process

par·a·pha·sia \-ˈfā-zhə, -zhē-ə\ *n* : aphasia in which the patient uses wrong words or uses words or sounds in senseless combinations — **par·a·pha·sic** \-ˈfā-zik\ *adj*

para·phen·yl·ene·di·amine \-ˌfen-ᵊl-ˌēn-ˈdī-ə-ˌmēn\ *n* : a benzene derivative C_6H_8N used esp. in dyeing hair and sometimes causing an allergic reaction

para·phil·ia \-ˈfi-lē-ə\ *n* : a pattern of recurring sexually arousing mental imagery or behavior that involves unusual and esp. socially unacceptable sexual practices (as sadism, masochism, fetishism, or pedophilia)

¹para·phil·iac \-ˈfi-lē-ˌak\ *adj* : of, relating to, or characterized by paraphilia

²paraphiliac *n* : a person who engages in paraphilia

para·phi·mo·sis \-fī-ˈmō-səs, -fi-\ *n, pl* **-mo·ses** \-ˌsēz\ : a condition in which the foreskin is retracted behind the glans penis and cannot be brought back to its original position

para·phre·nia \-ˈfrē-nē-ə\ *n* **1** : the group of paranoid disorders **2** : any of the paranoid disorders; *also* : SCHIZOPHRENIA — **para·phren·ic** \-ˈfre-nik\ *adj*

para·ple·gia \ˌpar-ə-ˈplē-jə, -jē-ə\ *n* : partial or complete paralysis of the lower half of the body with the involvement of both legs that is usu. due to injury or disease of the spinal cord in the thoracic or lumbar region

¹para·ple·gic \-ˈplē-jik\ *adj* : of, relating to, or affected with paraplegia

²paraplegic *n* : an individual affected with paraplegia

para·prax·is \-ˈprak-səs\ *n, pl* **-prax·es** \-ˈprak-ˌsēz\ : a faulty act (as a Freudian slip) of purposeful behavior

para·pro·tein \-ˈprō-ˌtēn\ *n* : any of various abnormal serum globulins with unique physical and electrophoretic characteristics

para·pro·tein·emia \-ˌprō-tē-ˈnē-mē-ə, -ˌprō-tē-ə-ˈnē-\ *n* : the presence of a paraprotein in the blood

para·pso·ri·a·sis \-sə-ˈrī-ə-səs\ *n, pl* **-a·ses** \-ˌsēz\ : a rare skin disease characterized by red scaly patches similar to those of psoriasis but causing no sensations of pain or itch

para·psy·chol·o·gy \ˌpar-ə-(ˌ)sī-ˈkä-lə-jē\ *n, pl* **-gies** : a field of study concerned with the investigation of evidence for paranormal psychological phenomena (as telepathy, clairvoyance, and psychokinesis) — **para·psych·o·log·i·cal** \-ˌsī-kə-ˈlä-ji-kəl\ *adj* — **para·psy·chol·o·gist** \-sī-ˈkä-lə-jist, -sə-\ *n*

para·quat \ˈpar-ə-ˌkwät\ *n* : an herbicide containing a salt of a cation $[C_{12}H_{14}N_2]^{2+}$ that is extremely toxic to the liver, kidneys, and lungs if ingested

para·re·nal \ˌpar-ə-ˈrēn-ᵊl\ *adj* : adjacent to the kidney

para·ros·an·i·line \ˌpar-ə-ˌrō-ˈzan-ᵊl-ən\ *n* : a white crystalline base $C_{19}H_{19}N_3O$ that is the parent compound of many dyes; *also* : its red chloride used esp. as a biological stain

para·sag·it·tal \-ˈsa-jət-ᵊl\ *adj* : situated alongside of or adjacent to a sagittal location or a sagittal plane

Par·as·ca·ris \(ˌ)par-ˈas-kə-rəs\ *n* : a genus of nematode worms (family Ascaridae) including a large roundworm (*P. equorum*) that is parasitic in horses

parasit- *or* **parasito-** *also* **parasiti-** *comb form* : parasite ⟨*parasit*emia⟩

para·sit·ae·mia *chiefly Brit var of* PARASITEMIA

par·a·site \ˈpar-ə-ˌsīt\ *n* : an organism living in, with, or on another organism in parasitism

par·a·sit·emia \ˌpar-ə-ˌsī-ˈtē-mē-ə\ *n* : a condition in which parasites are present in the blood — used esp. to indicate the presence of parasites without clinical symptoms

par·a·sit·ic \ˌpar-ə-ˈsi-tik\ *also* **par·a·sit·i·cal** \-ti-kəl\ *adj* **1** : relating to or having the habit of a parasite : living on another organism **2** : caused by or resulting from the effects of parasites — **par·a·sit·i·cal·ly** *adv*

par·a·sit·i·cide \-ˈsi-tə-ˌsīd\ *n* : an agent that is destructive to parasites — **par·a·sit·i·cid·al** \-ˌsi-tə-ˈsīd-ᵊl\ *adj*

par·a·sit·ism \ˈpar-ə-sə-ˌti-zəm, -ˌsī-\ *n* **1** : an intimate association between organisms of two or more kinds; *esp* : one in which a parasite obtains benefits from a host which it usu. injures **2** : PARASITOSIS

par·a·sit·ize \-sə-ˌtīz, -ˌsī-\ *vb* **-ized; -iz·ing** : to infest or live on or with as a parasite — **par·a·sit·iza·tion** \ˌpar-ə-sə-tə-ˈzā-shən, -ˌsī-\ *n*

parasito- — see PARASIT-

par·a·si·tol·o·gist \-ˈtä-lə-jist\ *n* : a specialist in parasitology; *esp* : one who deals with the worm parasites of animals

par·a·si·tol·o·gy \ˌpar-ə-sə-ˈtä-lə-jē, -ˌsī-\ *n, pl* **-gies** : a branch of biology dealing with parasites and parasitism esp. among animals — **par·a·si·to·log·i·cal** \-ˌsit-ᵊl-ˈä-ji-kəl, -ˌsīt-\ *also* **par·a·si·to·log·ic** \-jik\ *adj* — **par·a·si·to·log·i·cal·ly** *adv*

par·a·sit·o·sis \-sə-ˈtō-səs, -ˌsī-\ *n, pl* **-o·ses** \-ˌsēz\ : infestation with or disease caused by parasites

para·som·nia \-ˈsäm-nē-ə\ *n* : any of various disorders of sleep characterized by abnormal behavioral or physiological activity (such as sleepwalking or night terrors) during sleep or in the transitional stage between sleep and wakefulness

para·spe·cif·ic \-spi-ˈsi-fik\ *adj* : having or being curative actions or properties in addition to the specific one considered medically useful

para·spi·nal \-ˈspīn-ᵊl\ *adj* : adjacent to the spinal column ⟨~ muscles⟩

para·ster·nal \-ˈstər-nəl\ *adj* : adjacent to the sternum — **para·ster·nal·ly** *adv*

¹**para·sym·pa·thet·ic** \ˌpar-ə-ˌsim-pə-ˈthe-tik\ *adj* : of, relating to, being, or acting on the parasympathetic nervous system ⟨~ drugs⟩

²**parasympathetic** *n* **1** : a parasympathetic nerve **2** : PARASYMPATHETIC NERVOUS SYSTEM

parasympathetic nervous system *n* : the part of the autonomic nervous system that contains chiefly cholinergic fibers, that tends to induce secretion, to increase the tone and contractility of smooth muscle, and to slow the heart rate, and that consists of a cranial part and a sacral part — called also *parasympathetic system;* compare SYMPATHETIC NERVOUS SYSTEM

¹**para·sym·pa·tho·lyt·ic** \ˌpar-ə-ˈsim-pə-thō-ˈli-tik\ *adj* : tending to oppose the physiological results of parasympathetic nervous activity or of parasympathomimetic drugs — compare SYMPATHOLYTIC

²**parasympatholytic** *n* : a parasympatholytic substance

¹**para·sym·pa·tho·mi·met·ic** \ˌpar-ə-ˈsim-pə-(ˌ)thō-mī-ˈme-tik, -mə-\ *adj* : simulating parasympathetic nervous action in physiological effect — compare SYMPATHOMIMETIC

²**parasympathomimetic** *n* : a parasympathomimetic agent (as a drug)

para·sys·to·le \-ˈsis-tə-(ˌ)lē\ *n* : an irregularity in cardiac rhythm caused by an ectopic pacemaker in addition to the normal one

para·tax·ic \ˌpar-ə-ˈtak-sik\ *adj* : relating to or being thinking in which a cause and effect relationship is attributed to events occurring at about the same time but having no logical relationship

para·ten·on \ˌpar-ə-ˈte-nən, -(ˌ)nän\ *n* : the areolar tissue filling the space between a tendon and its sheath

para·thi·on \ˌpar-ə-ˈthī-ən, -ˌän\ *n* : an extremely toxic sulfur-containing insecticide $C_{10}H_{14}NO_5PS$

par·a·thor·mone \ˌpar-ə-ˈthȯr-ˌmōn\ *n* : PARATHYROID HORMONE

¹**para·thy·roid** \-ˈthī-ˌrȯid\ *n* : PARATHYROID GLAND

²**parathyroid** *adj* **1** : adjacent to a thyroid gland **2** : of, relating to, or produced by the parathyroid glands

para·thy·roid·ec·to·my \-ˌthī-ˌrȯi-ˈdek-tə-mē\ *n, pl* **-mies** : partial or complete excision of the parathyroid glands — **para·thy·roid·ec·to·mized** \-ˌmīzd\ *adj*

parathyroid gland *n* : any of usu. four small endocrine glands that are adjacent to or embedded in the thyroid gland, are composed of irregularly arranged secretory epithelial cells lying in a stroma rich in capillaries, and produce parathyroid hormone

parathyroid hormone *n* : a hormone of the parathyroid gland that regulates the metabolism of calcium and phosphorus in the body — abbr. *PTH;* called also *parathormone*

para·thy·ro·trop·ic \ˌpar-ə-ˌthī-rō-ˈträ-pik\ *adj* : acting on or stimulating the parathyroid glands ⟨a ~ hormone⟩

para·tra·che·al \-ˈtrā-kē-əl\ *adj* : adjacent to the trachea

para·tu·ber·cu·lo·sis \-tu̇-ˌbər-kyə-ˈlō-səs, -tyu̇-\ *n, pl* **-lo·ses** \-ˌsēz\ : JOHNE'S DISEASE

¹**para·ty·phoid** \ˌpar-ə-ˈtī-ˌfȯid, -(ˌ)tī-ˈ\ *adj* **1** : resembling typhoid fever **2** : of or relating to paratyphoid or its causative bacteria ⟨~ infection⟩

²**paratyphoid** *n* : any of numerous salmonelloses (as necrotic enteritis) re-

sembling typhoid fever and commonly contracted by eating contaminated food — called also *paratyphoid fever*

para·um·bil·i·cal \-ˌəm-ˈbi-li-kəl\ *adj* : adjacent to the navel ⟨~ pain⟩

para·ure·thral \-yu̇-ˈrē-thrəl\ *adj* : adjacent to the urethra

paraurethral gland *n* : any of several small glands that open into the female urethra near its opening and are homologous to glandular tissue in the prostate gland in the male — called also *Skene's gland*

para·vac·cin·ia \-vak-ˈsi-nē-ə\ *n* **1** : MILKER'S NODULES **2** : PSEUDOCOWPOX

para·ven·tric·u·lar nucleus \-ven-ˈtri-kyə-lər-, -vən-\ *n* : a discrete band of neurons in the anterior part of the hypothalamus that produce vasopressin and esp. oxytocin and that innervate the neurohypophysis

para·ver·te·bral \-(ˌ)vər-ˈtē-brəl, -ˈvər-tə-\ *adj* : situated, occurring, or performed beside or adjacent to the spinal column ⟨~ sympathectomy⟩

Par·co·pa \pär-ˈkō-pə\ *trademark* — used for a preparation of carbidopa and L-dopa

par·e·go·ric \ˌpar-ə-ˈgōr-ik, -ˈgär-\ *n* : camphorated tincture of opium used esp. to relieve pain

par·ei·do·lia \ˌper-ˌī-ˈdōl-ē-ə, -ˈdōl-yə\ *n* : the tendency to perceive a specific often meaningful image in a random or ambiguous visual pattern — compare APOPHENIA

pa·ren·chy·ma \pə-ˈreŋ-kə-mə\ *n* : the essential and distinctive tissue of an organ or an abnormal growth as distinguished from its supportive framework

pa·ren·chy·mal \pə-ˈreŋ-kə-məl, ˌpar-ən-ˈkī-məl\ *adj* : PARENCHYMATOUS

par·en·chy·ma·tous \ˌpar-ən-ˈkī-mə-təs, -ˈki-\ *adj* : of, relating to, made up of, or affecting parenchyma

par·ent \ˈpar-ənt\ *n* **1** : one that begets or brings forth offspring **2** : the material or source from which something is derived — **parent** *adj* — **pa·ren·tal** \pə-ˈrent-ᵊl\ *adj*

parental generation *n* : a generation that supplies the parents of a subsequent generation; *esp* : P_1 GENERATION — see FILIAL GENERATION

[1]**par·en·ter·al** \pə-ˈren-tə-rəl\ *adj* : situated or occurring outside the digestive tract; *esp* : introduced or administered otherwise than by way of the digestive tract ⟨enteric versus ~ nutrition⟩ — **par·en·ter·al·ly** *adv*

[2]**parenteral** *n* : an agent intended for parenteral administration

par·ent·ing \ˈpar-ənt-iŋ\ *n* : the raising of a child by his or her parents

pa·re·sis \pə-ˈrē-səs, ˈpar-ə-səs\ *n, pl* **pa·re·ses** \-ˌsēz\ **1** : slight or partial paralysis **2** : GENERAL PARESIS

par·es·the·sia \ˌpar-es-ˈthē-zhə, -zhē-ə\ *n* : a sensation of pricking, tingling, or creeping on the skin having no objective cause and usu. associated with injury or irritation of a sensory nerve or nerve root — **par·es·thet·ic** \-ˈthe-tik\ *adj*

paresthetica — see MERALGIA PARESTHETICA

[1]**pa·ret·ic** \pə-ˈre-tik\ *adj* : of, relating to, or affected with paresis

[2]**paretic** *n* : a person affected with paresis

par·gy·line \ˈpär-jə-ˌlēn\ *n* : a monoamine oxidase inhibitor used in the form of its hydrochloride $C_{11}H_{13}N·HCl$ esp. as an antihypertensive

par·i·es \ˈpar-ē-ˌēz\ *n, pl* **pa·ri·etes** \pə-ˈrī-ə-ˌtēz\ : the wall of a cavity or hollow organ — usu. used in pl.

[1]**pa·ri·etal** \pə-ˈrī-ət-ᵊl\ *adj* **1** : of or relating to the walls of a part or cavity — compare VISCERAL **2** : of, relating to, or located in the upper posterior part of the head; *specif* : relating to the parietal bones

[2]**parietal** *n* : a parietal part (as a bone)

parietal bone *n* : either of a pair of membrane bones of the roof of the skull between the frontal and occipital bones that are large and quadrilateral in outline, meet in the sagittal suture, and form much of the top and sides of the cranium

parietal cell *n* : any of the large oval cells of the gastric mucous membrane that secrete hydrochloric acid and lie between the chief cells and the basement membrane

parietal emissary vein *n* : a vein that passes from the superior sagittal sinus inside the skull through a foramen in the parietal bone to connect with veins of the scalp

parietalis — see DECIDUA PARIETALIS

parietal lobe *n* : the middle division of each cerebral hemisphere that is situated behind the central sulcus, above the sylvian fissure, and in front of the parieto-occipital sulcus and that contains an area concerned with bodily sensations

parietal pericardium *n* : the tough thickened membranous outer layer of the pericardium that is attached to the central part of the diaphragm and the posterior part of the sternum — compare EPICARDIUM

parietal peritoneum *n* : the part of the peritoneum that lines the abdominal wall — compare VISCERAL PERITONEUM

parieto- *comb form* : parietal and ⟨*parieto*temporal⟩

pa·ri·e·to–oc·cip·i·tal \pə-ˌrī-ə-tō-äk-ˈsi-pət-ᵊl\ *adj* : of, relating to, or situated between the parietal and occipital bones or lobes

parieto–occipital sulcus *n* : a fissure near the posterior end of each cerebral hemisphere separating the parietal and occipital lobes — called also *parieto-occipital fissure*

pa·ri·e·to·tem·po·ral \-ˈtem-pə-rəl\ *adj* : of or relating to the parietal and temporal bones or lobes

Par•i•naud's oc•u•lo•glan•du•lar syn•drome \ˌpar-i-ˈnōz-ˌä-kyə-lō-ˈglan-jə-lər-\ *n* : conjunctivitis that is often unilateral, is usu. characterized by dense local infiltration by lymphoid tissue with tenderness and swelling of the preauricular lymph nodes, and is usu. associated with a bacterial infection (as in cat scratch disease and tularemia) — called also *Parinaud's conjunctivitis*

Parinaud, Henri (1844–1905), French ophthalmologist.

Parinaud's syndrome *n* : paralysis of the upward movements of the two eyes that is associated esp. with a lesion or compression of the superior colliculi of the midbrain

Par•is green \ˈpar-əs-\ *n* : a very poisonous copper-based bright green powder $Cu(C_2H_3O_2)_2 \cdot 3Cu(AsO_2)_2$ that is used as an insecticide and pigment

par•i•ty \ˈpar-ə-tē\ *n, pl* **-ties** **1** : the state or fact of having borne offspring **2** : the number of times a female has given birth counting multiple births as one and usu. including stillbirths — compare GRAVIDITY 2

[1]**par•kin•so•nian** \ˌpär-kən-ˈsō-nē-ən, -nyən\ *adj* **1** : of or similar to that of parkinsonism ⟨~ symptoms⟩ **2** : affected with parkinsonism and esp. Parkinson's disease ⟨~ patients⟩

Par•kin•son \ˈpär-kən-sən\, **James (1755–1824),** British surgeon.

[2]**parkinsonian** *n* : an individual affected with parkinsonism and esp. Parkinson's disease

parkinsonian syndrome *n* **1** : PARKINSON'S DISEASE **2** : PARKINSONISM 2

par•kin•son•ism \ˈpär-kən-sə-ˌni-zəm\ *n* **1** : PARKINSON'S DISEASE **2** : any of several neurological disorders that are characterized by symptoms (as muscle rigidity, slowness of movement, and impaired balance) similar to those of Parkinson's disease but have an attributable cause (as drugs, toxins, or brain injury) resulting in low levels or blocked activity of dopamine — called also *parkinsonian syndrome, Parkinson's syndrome*

Par•kin•son's disease \ˈpär-kən-sənz-\ *also* **Parkinson disease** *n* : a chronic progressive neurological disease chiefly of later life that is linked to decreased dopamine production in the substantia nigra, is marked by tremor of resting muscles, rigidity, slowness of movement, impaired balance, and a shuffling gait, and is of unknown causes — called also *paralysis agitans, parkinsonian syndrome, parkinsonism, Parkinson's, Parkinson's syndrome*

Parkinson's syndrome *n* **1** : PARKINSON'S DISEASE **2** : PARKINSONISM 2

par•odon•tal \ˌpar-ə-ˈdänt-ᵊl\ *adj* : PERIODONTAL 2 — **par•odon•tal•ly** *adv*

par•o•mo•my•cin \ˌpar-ə-mō-ˈmīs-ᵊn\ *n* : a broad-spectrum antibiotic that is obtained from a bacterium of the genus *Streptomyces* (*S. rimosus paromomycinus*) and is usu. used in the form of its sulfate $C_{23}H_{45}H_5O_{14} \cdot H_2SO_4$ to treat intestinal amebiasis

par•o•nych•ia \ˌpar-ə-ˈni-kē-ə\ *n* : inflammation of the tissues adjacent to the nail of a finger or toe usu. accompanied by infection and pus formation — compare FELON, WHITLOW 1

par•oöph•o•ron \ˌpar-ō-ˈä-fə-ˌrän\ *n* : a group of rudimentary tubules in the broad ligament between the epoophoron and the uterus that constitutes a remnant of the lower part of the mesonephros in the female

par•os•mia \ˌpar-ˈäz-mē-ə\ *n* : a distortion of the sense of smell

[1]**pa•rot•id** \pə-ˈrä-təd\ *adj* : of, relating to, being, produced by, or located near the parotid gland

[2]**parotid** *n* : PAROTID GLAND

parotid duct *n* : the duct of the parotid gland opening on the inner surface of the cheek opposite the second upper molar tooth — called also *Stensen's duct*

parotid gland *n* : a serous salivary gland that is situated on each side of the face below and in front of the ear, in humans is the largest of the salivary glands, and communicates with the mouth by the parotid duct

par•o•ti•tis \ˌpar-ə-ˈtī-təs\ *n* **1** : inflammation and swelling of one or both parotid glands or other salivary glands (as in mumps) **2** : MUMPS

par•ous \ˈpar-əs\ *adj* **1** : having produced offspring **2** : of or characteristic of the parous female

-p•a•rous \p-ə-rəs\ *adj comb form* : giving birth to : producing ⟨multi*parous*⟩

par•o•var•i•um \ˌpar-ō-ˈvar-ē-əm\ *n* : EPOOPHORON — **par•o•var•i•an** \-ē-ən\ *adj*

par•ox•e•tine \par-ˈäk-sə-ˌtēn\ *n* : a drug that functions as an SSRI and is taken orally in the form of its hydrochloride $C_{19}H_{20}FNO_3 \cdot HCl$ or mesylate $C_{19}H_{20}FNO_3 \cdot CH_4O_3S$ to treat depression, anxiety, panic disorder, and obsessive-compulsive disorder and to relieve symptoms (as hot flashes) of menopause — see BRISDELLE, PAXIL, PEXEVA

par•ox•ysm \ˈpar-ək-ˌsi-zəm, pə-ˈräk-\ *n* **1** : a sudden attack or spasm (as of a disease) **2** : a sudden recurrence of symptoms or an intensification of existing symptoms — **par•ox•ys•mal** \ˌpar-ək-ˈsiz-məl, pə-ˌräk-\ *adj*

paroxysmal dyspnea *n* : CARDIAC ASTHMA

paroxysmal nocturnal hemoglobinuria *n* : a form of hemolytic anemia that is characterized by an abnormally strong response to the action of complement, by acute episodes of hemolysis esp. at night with hemoglobinuria noted upon urination after awakening, venous occlusion, and often leukopenia and thrombocytopenia — abbr. *PNH*

paroxysmal tachycardia *n* : tachycardia that begins and ends abruptly and that is initiated by a premature supraventricular beat originating in the atrium or in the atrioventricular node or bundle of His or by a premature ventricular beat

par•rot fever \ˈpar-ət-\ *n* : PSITTACOSIS

pars \ˈpärs\ *n, pl* **par•tes** \ˈpär-(ˌ)tēz\ : an anatomical part

pars com•pac•ta \-käm-ˈpak-tə\ *n* : the large dorsal part of gray matter of the substantia nigra that is next to the tegmentum

pars dis•ta•lis \-di-ˈstā-ləs\ *n* : the anterior part of the adenohypophysis that is the major secretory part of the gland

pars in•ter•me•dia \-ˌin-tər-ˈmē-dē-ə\ *n* : a thin slip of tissue fused with the neurohypophysis and representing the remains of the posterior wall of Rathke's pouch

pars ner•vo•sa \-nər-ˈvō-sə\ *n* : NEURAL LOBE

Par•sol \ˈpär-ˌsōl\ *trademark* — used for a preparation of avobenzone

pars pla•na \ˈpärs-ˈplā-nə\ *n* : the posterior part of the ciliary body extending from the pars plicata to the ora serrata — called also *ciliary ring, orbiculus ciliaris*

pars pli•ca•ta \-ˌplī-ˈkā-tə\, *n* : the anterior part of the ciliary body that contains the ciliary muscle and ciliary processes

pars re•tic•u•la•ta \-ri-ˌtik-yə-ˈlä-tə, -ˈlā-\ *n* : the ventral part of gray matter of the substantia nigra continuous with the globus pallidus

pars tu•ber•a•lis \-ˌtü-bə-ˈrā-ləs, -ˌtyü-\ *n* : a thin plate of cells that is an extension of the adenohypophysis on the ventral or anterior aspect of the infundibulum

partes *pl of* PARS

parthen- *or* **partheno-** *comb form* : virgin : without fertilization ⟨*parthenogenesis*⟩

par•the•no•gen•e•sis \ˌpär-thə-nō-ˈje-nə-səs\ *n, pl* **-e•ses** \-ˌsēz\ : reproduction by development of an unfertilized usu. female gamete that occurs esp. among lower plants and invertebrate animals — **par•the•no•ge•net•ic** \-jə-ˈne-tik\ *also* **par•the•no•gen•ic** \-ˈje-nik\ *adj*

partial–birth abortion *n* : DILATION AND EXTRACTION

par•tial denture \ˈpär-shəl-\ *n* : a usu. removable artificial replacement of one or more teeth

partial epilepsy *n* : FOCAL EPILEPSY

partial mastectomy *n* : a mastectomy in which only a tumor and a wedge of surrounding healthy tissue are removed

partial pressure *n* : the pressure exerted by a (specified) component in a mixture of gases

partial seizure *n* : a seizure that originates in a localized part of the cerebral cortex, that involves motor, sensory, autonomic, or psychic symptoms (as twitching of muscles, localized numbness, auras, and sometimes loss of consciousness), and that may progress to a generalized seizure — called also *focal seizure;* compare GENERALIZED SEIZURE

[1]**par•tic•u•late** \pär-ˈti-kyə-lət\ *adj* : of, relating to, or existing in the form of minute separate particles

[2]**particulate** *n* : a particulate substance

particulate inheritance *n* : MENDELIAN INHERITANCE

[1]**par•tu•ri•ent** \pär-ˈtu̇r-ē-ənt, -ˈtyu̇r-\ *adj* **1** : bringing forth or about to bring forth young **2** : of or relating to parturition ⟨~ pangs⟩ **3** : typical of parturition ⟨the ~ uterus⟩

[2]**parturient** *n* : a parturient individual

parturient paresis *n* : MILK FEVER 2

par•tu•ri•tion \ˌpär-tə-ˈri-shən, ˌpär-chə-, ˌpär-tyu̇-\ *n* : the action or process of giving birth to offspring : CHILDBIRTH — **par•tu•ri•tion•al** \-shə-nəl\ *adj*

pa•ru•lis \pə-ˈrü-ləs\ *n, pl* **-li•des** \-lə-ˌdēz\ : an abscess in the gum : GUMBOIL

par•um•bil•i•cal vein \ˌpar-ˌəm-ˈbi-li-kəl-\ *n* : any of several small veins that connect the veins of the anterior abdominal wall with the portal vein and the internal and common iliac veins

parv- *or* **parvi-** *also* **parvo-** *comb form* : small ⟨*parvo*virus⟩

par•vo \ˈpär-ˌvō\ *n* : PARVOVIRUS 2

par•vo•cel•lu•lar *also* **par•vi•cel•lu•lar** \ˌpär-və-ˈsel-yə-lər\ *adj* : of, relating to, or being small cell bodies — compare MAGNOCELLULAR

par•vo•vi•rus \ˈpär-vō-ˌvī-rəs\ *n* **1 a** *cap* : a genus of single-stranded DNA viruses (family *Parvoviridae*) including the causative agents of panleukopenia in cats and fifth disease in humans **b** : any virus of the genus *Parvovirus* or the family (*Parvoviridae*) to which the genus belongs **2** : a highly contagious febrile disease of dogs that is caused by a parvovirus (species *Canine parvovirus* of the genus *Parvovirus*), is spread esp. by contact with infected feces, and is marked by loss of appetite, lethargy, often bloody diarrhea and vomiting, and sometimes death — called also *parvo*

PAS \ˌpē-(ˌ)ā-ˈes\ *adj* : PERIODIC ACID-SCHIFF

PAS *abbr* para-aminosalicylic acid

PASA *abbr* para-aminosalicylic acid

pass \ˈpas\ *vb* : to emit or discharge from a bodily part and esp. from the bowels : EVACUATE 2, VOID

[1]**pas•sage** \ˈpa-sij\ *n* **1** : the action or process of passing from one place, condition, or stage to another **2** : an anatomical channel ⟨the nasal ~*s*⟩ **3** : a movement or an evacuation of the bowels **4 a** : an act or action of passing something or undergoing a passing ⟨~ of a catheter through the urethra⟩ **b** : incubation of a pathogen (as a virus) in a tissue culture, a developing egg, or a living organism to in-

crease the amount of pathogen or to alter its characteristics

[2]**passage** *vb* **pas•saged; pas•sag•ing** : to subject to passage

pas•sive \ˈpa-siv\ *adj* **1 a** (1) : lethargic or lacking in energy or will (2) : tending not to take an active or dominant part **b** : induced by an outside agency ⟨~ exercise of a paralyzed leg⟩ **2 a** : of, relating to, or characterized by a state of chemical inactivity **b** : not involving expenditure of chemical energy ⟨~ transport across a cell membrane⟩ **3** : producing passive immunity ⟨~ immunotherapy⟩ — **pas•sive•ly** *adv* — **pas•sive•ness** *n*

[1]**passive–aggressive** *adj* : being, marked by, or displaying behavior characterized by expression of negative feelings, resentment, and aggression in an unassertive way (as through procrastination, stubbornness, and unwillingness to communicate) — **passive–aggressively** *adv*

[2]**passive–aggressive** *n* : a passive-aggressive individual

passive congestion *n* : congestion caused by obstruction to the return flow of venous blood — called also *passive hyperemia*

passive immunity *n* : short-acting immunity acquired by transfer of antibodies (as by injection of gamma globulin) — compare ACQUIRED IMMUNITY, ACTIVE IMMUNITY, INNATE IMMUNITY — **passive immunization** *n*

passive smoke *n* : SECONDHAND SMOKE

passive smoking *n* : the involuntary inhalation of tobacco smoke (as from another's cigarette) esp. by a nonsmoker — **passive smoker** *n*

passive transfer *n* : a local transfer of skin sensitivity from an allergic to a normal individual by injection of the allergic individual's serum that is used esp. for identifying specific allergens when a high degree of sensitivity is suspected — called also *Prausnitz-Küstner reaction*

pas•siv•i•ty \pa-ˈsi-və-tē\ *n, pl* **-ties** : the quality or state of being passive or submissive

pass out *vb* : to lose consciousness

paste \ˈpāst\ *n* : a soft plastic mixture or composition; *esp* : an external medicament that has a stiffer consistency than an ointment and is less greasy because of its higher percentage of powdered ingredients

pas•tern \ˈpas-tərn\ *n* : a part of the foot of an equine extending from the fetlock to the top of the hoof

pas•teu•rel•la \ˌpas-tə-ˈre-lə\ *n* **1** *cap* : a genus of gram-negative facultatively anaerobic nonmotile rod bacteria (family Pasteurellaceae) including pathogens esp. of domestic animals — see HEMORRHAGIC SEPTICEMIA, YERSINIA **2** *pl* **-las** *or* **-lae** \-ˌlī\ : any bacterium of the genus *Pasteurella*

Pas•teur \pa-ˈstər, -ˈstœr\, **Louis (1822–1895)**, French chemist and bacteriologist.

pas•teu•rel•lo•sis \ˌpas-tə-rə-ˈlō-səs\ *n, pl* **-lo•ses** \-ˌsēz\ : infection with or disease caused by bacteria of the genus *Pasteurella*

pas•teur•i•za•tion \ˌpas-chə-rə-ˈzā-shən, ˌpas-tə-\ *n* **1** : partial sterilization of a substance and esp. a liquid (as milk) at a temperature and for a period of exposure that destroys pathogenic microorganisms **2** : partial sterilization of perishable food products (as fruit or poultry) with radiation — **pas•teur•ize** \ˈpas-chə-ˌrīz, ˈpas-tə-\ *vb*

Pasteur treatment *n* : a method of aborting rabies by stimulating production of antibodies through successive inoculations with attenuated virus of gradually increasing strength

pas•tille \pas-ˈtēl\ *also* **pas•til** \ˈpast-ᵊl\ *n* : LOZENGE

PAT *abbr* paroxysmal atrial tachycardia

Pat•a•day \ˈpat-ə-ˌdā\ *trademark* — used for a preparation of olopatadine

Pat•a•nol \ˈpat-ə-ˌnȯl\ *trademark* — used for a preparation of olopatadine

Pa•tau syndrome \pä-ˈtau̇-\ *or* **Patau's syndrome** \-ˈtau̇z-\ *n* : TRISOMY 13

Patau, Klaus (*fl* 1960), American (German-born) geneticist.

patch \ˈpach\ *n* **1 a** : a piece of material used medically usu. to cover a wound or repair a defect — see PATCH GRAFT **b** : a usu. disk-shaped piece of material that is worn on the skin and contains a substance (as a drug) that is absorbed at a constant rate through the skin and into the bloodstream ⟨a nicotine ~⟩ — called also *skin patch* **c** : a shield worn over the socket of an injured or missing eye **2** : a circumscribed region of tissue (as on the skin or in a section from an organ) that differs from the normal color or composition — **patch** *vb* — **patchy** \ˈpa-chē\ *adj*

patch graft *n* : a graft of living or synthetic material used to repair a defect in a blood vessel

patch test *n* : a test for determining allergic sensitivity that is made by applying to the unbroken skin small pads soaked with the allergen to be tested and that indicates sensitivity when irritation develops at the point of application — compare INTRADERMAL TEST, PRICK TEST, SCRATCH TEST

pa•tel•la \pə-ˈte-lə\ *n, pl* **-lae** \-ˈte-(ˌ)lē, -ˌlī\ *or* **-las** : a thick flat triangular movable bone that forms the anterior point of the knee, protects the front of the knee joint, and increases the leverage of the quadriceps — called also *kneecap* — **pa•tel•lar** \-lər\ *adj*

patellar ligament *n* : PATELLAR TENDON

patellar reflex *n* : KNEE JERK

patellar tendinitis *also* **patellar tendonitis** *n* : injury to the patellar tendon that is marked esp. by pain or tenderness in the area immediately below the front of the knee and that typically involves microscopic tearing of the patellar tendon often accompanied by inflammation or tissue degeneration — called also *apicitis, jumper's knee, patellar tendinopathy*

patellar tendon *n* : the part of the tendon of the quadriceps that extends from the patella to the tibia — called also *patellar ligament*

pat•el•lec•to•my \ˌpa-tə-ˈlek-tə-mē\ *n, pl* **-mies** : surgical excision of the patella

pa•tel•lo•fem•o•ral \pə-ˌte-lō-ˈfe-mə-rəl\ *adj* : of or relating to the patella and femur ⟨the ~ articulation⟩

pa•ten•cy \ˈpat-ᵊn-sē, ˈpāt-\ *n, pl* **-cies** : the quality or state of being open or unobstructed

pa•tent \ˈpat-ᵊnt\ *adj* **1** : protected by a trademark or a trade name so as to establish proprietary rights analogous to those conveyed by a patent : PROPRIETARY ⟨~ drugs⟩ **2** \ˈpāt-\ : affording free passage : being open and unobstructed

pa•tent ductus arteriosus \ˈpāt-ᵊnt-\ *n* : an abnormal condition in which the ductus arteriosus fails to close after birth

pat•ent medicine \ˈpat-ᵊnt-\ *n* : a packaged nonprescription drug which is protected by a trademark and whose contents are incompletely disclosed; *also* : any drug that is a proprietary

pa•ter•ni•ty test \pə-ˈtər-nə-tē-\ *n* : a test esp. of DNA or genetic traits to determine whether a given man could be the biological father of a given child — **paternity testing** *n*

path \ˈpath\ *n, pl* **paths** \ˈpat͟hz, ˈpaths\ : PATHWAY 1

path *abbr* pathological; pathology

path- *or* **patho-** *comb form* **1** : pathological ⟨*patho*biology⟩ **2** : pathological state : disease ⟨*patho*gen⟩

-path \ˌpath\ *n comb form* **1** : practitioner of a (specified) system of medicine that emphasizes one aspect of disease or its treatment ⟨naturo*path*⟩ **2** : one affected with a disorder (of such a part or system) ⟨psycho*path*⟩

-path•ia \ˈpa-thē-ə\ *n comb form* : -PATHY 2 ⟨hyper*pathia*⟩

-path•ic \ˈpa-thik\ *adj comb form* **1** : feeling or affected in a (specified) way ⟨tele*pathic*⟩ **2** : affected by disease of a (specified) part or kind ⟨myo*pathic*⟩ **3** : relating to therapy based on a (specified) unitary theory of disease or its treatment ⟨homeo*pathic*⟩

Path•i•lon \ˈpa-thə-ˌlän\ *n* : a preparation of tridihexethyl chloride — formerly a U.S. registered trademark

patho•bi•ol•o•gy \ˌpa-thō-bī-ˈä-lə-jē\ *n, pl* **-gies** : PATHOLOGY 1, 2

patho•gen \ˈpa-thə-jən\ *n* : a specific causative agent (as a bacterium or virus) of disease

patho•gen•e•sis \ˌpa-thə-ˈje-nə-səs\ *n, pl* **-e•ses** \-ˌsēz\ : the origination and development of a disease

patho•ge•net•ic \-jə-ˈne-tik\ *adj* **1** : of or relating to pathogenesis **2** : PATHOGENIC 2

patho•gen•ic \-ˈje-nik\ *adj* **1** : PATHOGENETIC 1 **2** : causing or capable of causing disease ⟨~ microorganisms⟩ — **pa•tho•gen•i•cal•ly** *adv*

patho•ge•nic•i•ty \-jə-ˈni-sə-tē\ *n, pl* **-ties** : the quality or state of being pathogenic : degree of pathogenic capacity

path•og•nom•ic \ˌpa-thəg-ˈnä-mik, -thə-\ *adj* : PATHOGNOMONIC

pa•tho•gno•mon•ic \ˌpa-thəg-nō-ˈmä-nik, -thə-\ *adj* : distinctively characteristic of a particular disease or condition

pathol *abbr* pathological; pathologist; pathology

patho•log•i•cal \ˌpa-thə-ˈlä-ji-kəl\ *also* **patho•log•ic** \-jik\ *adj* **1** : of or relating to pathology ⟨a ~ laboratory⟩ **2** : altered or caused by disease ⟨~ tissue⟩; *also* : indicative of disease ⟨~ lesions⟩ — **patho•log•i•cal•ly** *adv*

pathological fracture *n* : a fracture of a bone weakened by disease

pathological liar *n* : a person who lies compulsively usu. for no external gain or benefit and often with detrimental consequences

pa•thol•o•gist \pə-ˈthä-lə-jist, pa-\ *n* : a specialist in pathology; *specif* : a physician who interprets and diagnoses the changes caused by disease in tissues and body fluids

pa•thol•o•gy \-jē\ *n, pl* **-gies** **1** : the study of the essential nature of diseases and esp. of the structural and functional changes produced by them **2** : the anatomic and physiological deviations from the normal that constitute disease or characterize a particular disease **3** : a treatise on or compilation of abnormalities

patho•mor•phol•o•gy \ˌpa-thō-mȯr-ˈfä-lə-jē\ *n, pl* **-gies** : morphology of abnormal conditions — **patho•mor•pho•log•i•cal** \-ˌmȯr-fə-ˈlä-ji-kəl\ *or* **patho•mor•pho•log•ic** \-jik\ *adj*

patho•phys•i•ol•o•gy \-ˌfi-zē-ˈä-lə-jē\ *n, pl* **-gies** : the physiology of abnormal states; *specif* : the functional changes that accompany a particular syndrome or disease — **patho•phys•i•o•log•i•cal** \-ˌfi-zē-ə-ˈlä-ji-kəl\ *or* **patho•phys•i•o•log•ic** \-jik\ *adj*

path•way \ˈpath-ˌwā\ *n* **1** : a line of communication over interconnecting neurons extending from one organ or center to another; *also* : a network of interconnecting neurons along which a nerve impulse travels **2** : the sequence of usu. enzyme-catalyzed reactions by which one substance is converted into another

-pa•thy \pə-thē\ *n comb form, pl* **-pathies** **1** : feeling ⟨a*pathy*⟩ ⟨tele*pathy*⟩ **2** : disease of a (specified) part or kind ⟨myo*pathy*⟩ **3** : therapy or system of therapy based on a (specified) unitary theory of disease or its treatment ⟨homeo*pathy*⟩

pa·tient \ˈpā-shənt\ *n* **1** : a sick individual esp. when awaiting or under the care and treatment of a physician or surgeon **2** : a client for medical service (as of a physician or dentist)

pat·tern \ˈpa-tərn\ *n* **1** : a model for making a mold used to form a casting **2** : a reliable sample of traits, acts, tendencies, or other observable characteristics of a person, group, or institution ⟨∼*s* of behavior⟩ **3** : an established mode of behavior or cluster of mental attitudes, beliefs, and values that are held in common by members of a group

pat·tern·ing *n* : physical therapy esp. for neurological impairment based on a theory holding that repeated manipulation of body parts to simulate normal motor developmental activity (as crawling or walking) promotes neurological development or repair

pat·u·lin \ˈpa-chə-lən\ *n* : a very toxic colorless antibiotic $C_7H_6O_4$ produced by several molds (as *Aspergillus clavatus* and *Penicillium patulum*)

pat·u·lous \ˈpa-chə-ləs\ *adj* : spread widely apart : wide open or distended

Paul–Bun·nell test \ˈpȯl-ˈbə-nəl-\ *n* : a test for heterophile antibodies used in the diagnosis of infectious mononucleosis — called also *Paul-Bunnell reaction*

Paul, John Rodman (1893–1971), and **Bunnell, Walls Willard (1902–1965),** American physicians.

pa·vil·ion \pə-ˈvil-yən\ *n* : a more or less detached part of a hospital devoted to a special use

Pav·lov·ian \pav-ˈlō-vē-ən, -ˈlō-; -ˈlȯ-fē-\ *adj* : of or relating to Ivan Pavlov or to his work and theories

Pav·lov \ˈpav-lȯf\, **Ivan Petrovich (1849–1936),** Russian physiologist.

pav·or noc·tur·nus \ˈpa-ˌvȯr-näk-ˈtər-nəs\ *n* : NIGHT TERRORS

Pax·il \ˈpak-səl\ *trademark* — used for a preparation of the hydrochloride of paroxetine

Pb *symbol* lead

PBA *abbr* pseudobulbar affect

PBB \ˌpē-(ˌ)bē-ˈbē\ *n* : POLYBROMINATED BIPHENYL

PBL *abbr* peripheral blood lymphocyte

PBMC *abbr* peripheral blood mononuclear cell

PC *abbr* **1** [Latin *post cibos*] after meals — used in writing prescriptions **2** professional corporation

PCB \ˌpē-(ˌ)sē-ˈbē\ *n* : POLYCHLORINATED BIPHENYL

pCi *abbr* picocurie

PCI *abbr* percutaneous coronary intervention

PCL \ˌpē-ˌsē-ˈel\ *n* : POSTERIOR CRUCIATE LIGAMENT

PCOS *abbr* polycystic ovary syndrome

PCP \ˌpē-(ˌ)sē-ˈpē\ *n* **1** : PHENCYCLIDINE **2** : a health-care professional and esp. a physician who is authorized (as by an HMO) to provide primary care

PCP *abbr* Pneumocystis carinii pneumonia

PCR *abbr* polymerase chain reaction

PCV *abbr* packed cell volume

PCWP *abbr* pulmonary capillary wedge pressure

Pd *symbol* palladium

PD *abbr* **1** Parkinson's disease **2** peritoneal dialysis

PDB \ˌpē-(ˌ)dē-ˈbē\ *n* : PARADICHLOROBENZENE

PDD *abbr* pervasive developmental disorder

PDGF *abbr* platelet-derived growth factor

PDR *abbr Physicians' Desk Reference*

PE *abbr* **1** physical examination **2** pulmonary embolism

peak flow meter *n* : a device that measures the maximum rate of air flow out of the lungs during forced expiration and that is used esp. for monitoring lung capacity of individuals with asthma (as to indicate bronchial narrowing) — called also *peak expiratory flow meter*

pearl \ˈpərl\ *n* **1** : PERLE **2** : one of the rounded concentric masses of squamous epithelial cells characteristic of certain tumors **3** : a miliary leproma of the iris **4** : a rounded abnormal mass of enamel on a tooth

peau d'o·range \ˌpō-ˌdȯr-ˈänj\ *n* : thickened dimpled skin that resembles the rind of an orange and is often associated with some forms of breast cancer

pec \ˈpek\ *n* : PECTORALIS — usu. used in pl.

pec·tin \ˈpek-tən\ *n* **1** : any of various water-soluble substances that bind adjacent cell walls in plant tissues and yield a gel which is the basis of fruit jellies **2** : a product containing mostly pectin and used chiefly in making jelly and other foods, in pharmaceutical products esp. for the control of diarrhea, and in cosmetics

pectinati — see MUSCULI PECTINATI

pec·tin·e·al line \pek-ˈti-nē-əl-\ *n* : a ridge on the posterior surface of the femur that runs downward from the lesser trochanter and gives attachment to the pectineus

pec·tin·e·us \pek-ˈti-nē-əs\ *n, pl* **-tin·ei** \-nē-ˌī, -nē-ˌē\ : a flat quadrangular muscle of the upper front and inner aspect of the thigh that arises mostly from the iliopectineal line of the pubis and is inserted along the pectineal line of the femur

¹pec·to·ral \ˈpek-tə-rəl\ *n* **1** : a pectoral part or organ; *esp* : PECTORALIS **2** : a medicinal substance for treating diseases of the respiratory tract

²pectoral *adj* **1** : of, relating to, or occurring in or on the chest ⟨∼ arch⟩ **2** : relating to or good for diseases of the respiratory tract ⟨a ∼ syrup⟩

pectoral girdle *n* : SHOULDER GIRDLE

pec·to·ra·lis \ˌpek-tə-ˈrā-ləs\ *n, pl* **-ra·les** \-ˌlēz\ : either of the muscles that connect the ventral walls of the chest with the bones of the upper arm and shoulder of which in humans there are two on each side: **a** : a larger one that arises from the clavicle, the sternum, the cartilages of most or all of the ribs, and the aponeurosis of the external oblique muscle and is inserted by a strong flat tendon into the posterior bicipital ridge of the humerus — called also *pectoralis major* **b** : a smaller one that lies beneath the larger, arises from the third, fourth, and fifth ribs, and is inserted by a flat tendon into the coracoid process of the scapula — called also *pectoralis minor*

pectoralis major *n* : PECTORALIS a

pectoralis minor *n* : PECTORALIS b

pectoralis muscle *n* : PECTORALIS

pectoral muscle *n* : PECTORALIS

pectoral nerve *n* : either of two nerves that arise from the brachial plexus on each side or from the nerve trunks forming it and that supply the pectoral muscles: **a** : one lateral to the axillary artery — called also *lateral pectoral nerve, superior pectoral nerve* **b** : one medial to the axillary artery — called also *inferior pectoral nerve, medial pectoral nerve*

pec·to·ril·o·quy \ˌpek-tə-ˈri-lə-kwē\ *n, pl* **-quies** : the sound of words heard through the chest wall and usu. indicating a cavity or consolidation of lung tissue — compare BRONCHOPHONY

pectoris — see ANGINA PECTORIS

pec·tus ex·ca·va·tum \ˈpek-təs-ˌek-skə-ˈvā-təm\ *n* : FUNNEL CHEST

PED \ˌpē-ˌē-ˈdē\ *abbr or n* : a performance enhancing drug : a substance (as an anabolic steroid) used illicitly esp. to improve athletic performance

ped- *or* **pedo-** *comb form* : child : children ⟨*ped*iatrics⟩

ped·al \ˈped-ᵊl, ˈpēd-\ *adj* : of or relating to the foot

pe·di·at·ric \ˌpē-dē-ˈa-trik\ *adj* **1** : of, relating to, or specializing in pediatrics or its practice ⟨a ~ nurse⟩ **2** : of, relating to, affecting, or being an infant, child, or adolescent ⟨~ patients⟩ ⟨~ trauma⟩

pe·di·a·tri·cian \ˌpē-dē-ə-ˈtri-shən\ *n* : a specialist in pediatrics

pe·di·at·rics \ˌpē-dē-ˈa-triks\ *n* : a branch of medicine dealing with the development, care, and diseases of infants, children, and adolescents

ped·i·cle \ˈpe-di-kəl\ *n* : a basal attachment: as **a** : the basal part of each side of the neural arch of a vertebra connecting the laminae with the centrum **b** : the narrow basal part by which various organs (as kidney or spleen) are continuous with other body structures **c** : the narrow base of a tumor **d** : the part of a pedicle flap left attached to the original site — **ped·i·cled** \-kəld\ *adj*

pedicle flap *n* : a flap which is left attached to the original site by a narrow base of tissue to provide a blood supply during grafting — called also *pedicle graft*

pe·dic·u·li·cide \pi-ˈdi-kyə-lə-ˌsīd\ *n* : an agent for destroying lice

pe·dic·u·lo·sis \pi-ˌdi-kyə-ˈlō-səs\ *n, pl* **-lo·ses** \-ˌsēz\ : infestation with lice

pediculosis cap·i·tis \-ˈka-pi-təs\ *n* : infestation of the scalp by head lice

pediculosis cor·po·ris \-ˈkȯr-pə-rəs\ *n* : infestation by body lice

pediculosis pubis *n* : infestation by pubic lice

pe·dic·u·lus \pi-ˈdi-kyə-ləs\ *n* **1** *cap* : a genus of lice (family Pediculidae) that includes the body louse (*P. humanus humanus*) and head louse (*P. humanus capitis*) infesting humans **2** *pl* **pe·dic·u·li** \-ˌlī\ *or* **pediculus** : any louse of the genus *Pediculus*

pedis — see DORSALIS PEDIS ARTERY, TINEA PEDIS

pedo- — see PED-

pe·do·don·tics \ˌpē-də-ˈdän-tiks\ *n* : a branch of dentistry that is concerned with the dental care of children — **pe·do·don·tic** *adj*

pe·do·don·tist \ˌpē-də-ˈdän-tist\ *n* : a specialist in pedodontics

pe·do·phile \ˈpe-də-ˌfīl, ˈpē-\ *n* : an individual affected with pedophilia

pe·do·phil·ia \ˌpe-də-ˈfi-lē-ə, ˌpē-\ *n* : sexual perversion in which children are the preferred sexual object; *specif* : a psychiatric disorder in which an adult has sexual fantasies about or engages in sexual acts with a prepubescent child — **pe·do·phil·i·ac** \ˌpe-də-ˈfi-lē-ˌak, ˌpē-\ *or* **pe·do·phil·ic** \-ˈfi-lik\ *adj*

ped·or·thics \pə-ˈdȯr-thiks\ *n* : the art and practice of designing, making, and fitting therapeutic shoes for relieving painful or disabling conditions of the feet — **ped·or·thic** \-thik\ *adj*

ped·or·thist \pə-ˈdȯr-thist\ *n* : a specialist in pedorthics

pe·dun·cle \ˈpē-ˌdəŋ-kəl, pi-ˈ\ *n* **1** : a band of white matter joining different parts of the brain — see CEREBELLAR PEDUNCLE, CEREBRAL PEDUNCLE **2** : a narrow stalk by which a tumor or polyp is attached — **pe·dun·cu·lar** \pi-ˈdəŋ-kyə-lər\ *adj*

pe·dun·cu·lat·ed \pi-ˈdəŋ-kyə-ˌlā-təd\ *also* **pe·dun·cu·late** \-lət\ *adj* : having, growing on, or being attached by a peduncle ⟨a ~ tumor⟩

pe·dun·cu·lot·o·my \pi-ˌdəŋ-kyə-ˈlä-tə-mē\ *n, pl* **-mies** : surgical incision of a cerebral peduncle for relief of involuntary movements

pe·dun·cu·lus ce·re·bel·la·ris inferior \pi-ˌdəŋ-kyə-ləs-ˌser-ə-be-ˈler-əs-\ *n* : CEREBELLAR PEDUNCLE c

pedunculus cerebellaris me·di·us \-ˈmē-dē-əs\ *n* : CEREBELLAR PEDUNCLE b

pedunculus cerebellaris superior *n* : CEREBELLAR PEDUNCLE a

peel *n* : CHEMICAL PEEL

PEEP *abbr* positive end-expiratory pressure

peep•er \ˈpē-pər\ *n* : VOYEUR

Peep•ing Tom \ˌpē-piŋ-ˈtäm\ *n* : VOYEUR

peer review organization *n* : any of a group of organizations staffed by local practicing physicians that evaluate the quality, necessity, cost, and adherence to professional standards of medical care provided to Medicare patients as a prerequisite for payment of the medical services by Medicare — abbr. *PRO*

PEG *abbr* **1** percutaneous endoscopic gastrostomy **2** polyethylene glycol

Peg•a•none \ˈpe-gə-ˌnōn\ *trademark* — used for a preparation of ethotoin

peg•fil•gras•tim \ˌpeg-fil-ˈgras-təm\ *n* : a form of filgrastim administered by injection esp. to stimulate production of neutrophils following chemotherapy — see NEULASTA

pe•li•o•sis hep•a•tis \ˌpe-lē-ˈō-səs-ˈhep-ə-təs, ˌpē-\ *n* : an abnormal condition characterized by the occurrence of numerous small blood-filled cystic lesions throughout the liver

Pel•i•zae•us–Merz•bach•er disease \ˌpe-lēt-ˈsā-əs-ˈmerts-ˌbä-kər-\ *n* : a progressive disease of the central nervous system that is a leukodystrophy marked by myelin degeneration resulting in deterioration of cognitive and motor functioning and that is inherited as an X-linked recessive trait

Pelizaeus, Friedrich (1850–1917) and **Merzbacher, Ludwig (1875–1942),** German neurologists.

pel•la•gra \pə-ˈla-grə, -ˈlā-, -ˈlä-\ *n* : a disease marked by dermatitis, gastrointestinal disorders, mental disturbance, and memory loss and associated with a diet deficient in niacin and protein — compare KWASHIORKOR — **pel•la•grous** \-grəs\ *adj*

pellagra–preventive factor *n* : NIACIN

pel•la•grin \-grən\ *n* : one that is affected with pellagra

pel•let \ˈpe-lət\ *n* : a usu. small rounded or spherical body; *specif* : a small cylindrical or ovoid compressed mass (as of a hormone) that is implanted subcutaneously for slow absorption into bodily tissues

pel•li•cle \ˈpe-li-kəl\ *n* : a thin skin or film: as **a** : an outer membrane of some protozoans **b** : a thin layer of salivary glycoproteins coating the surface of the teeth

pellucida — see SEPTUM PELLUCIDUM, ZONA PELLUCIDA

pel•oid \ˈpe-ˌlȯid\ *n* : mud prepared and used for therapeutic purposes

pel•ta•tin \pel-ˈtā-tən\ *n* : either of two lactones that occur as glycosides in the rootstock of the mayapple (*Podophyllum peltatum*) and have some antineoplastic activity

pelv- *or* **pelvi-** *or* **pelvo-** *comb form* : pelvis ⟨*pelv*ic⟩ ⟨*pelvi*metry⟩

pelves *pl of* PELVIS

¹pel•vic \ˈpel-vik\ *adj* : of, relating to, or located in or near the pelvis

²pelvic *n* : a pelvic part

pelvic bone *n* : HIP BONE

pelvic brim *n* : the bony ridge in the cavity of the pelvis that marks the boundary between the false pelvis and the true pelvis

pelvic cavity *n* : the cavity of the pelvis comprising in humans a broad upper and a more contracted lower part — compare FALSE PELVIS, TRUE PELVIS

pelvic colon *n* : SIGMOID COLON

pelvic diaphragm *n* : the muscular floor of the pelvis

pelvic fascia *n* : the fascia lining the pelvic cavity

pelvic girdle *n* : the bony or cartilaginous arch that supports the hind limbs of a vertebrate and that in humans consists of paired hip bones articulating solidly with the sacrum dorsally and with one another at the pubic symphysis

pelvic inflammatory disease *n* : infection of the female reproductive tract (as the fallopian tubes and ovaries) that results from microorganisms (as *Neisseria gonorrhea* or *Chlamydia trachomatis*) transmitted esp. during sexual intercourse but also by other means (as during surgery, abortion, or childbirth), is marked esp. by lower abdominal pain, an abnormal vaginal discharge, and fever, and is a leading cause of infertility in women — abbr. *PID*

pelvic outlet *n* : the irregular bony opening bounded by the lower border of the pelvis and closed by muscle and other soft tissues through which the terminal parts of the excretory, reproductive, and digestive systems pass to communicate with the surface of the body

pelvic plexus *n* : a plexus of the autonomic nervous system that is formed by the hypogastric plexus, by branches from the sacral part of the sympathetic chain, and by the visceral branches of the second, third, and fourth sacral nerves and that is distributed to the viscera of the pelvic region

pelvic splanchnic nerve *n* : any of the groups of parasympathetic fibers that originate with cells in the second, third, and fourth sacral segments of the spinal cord, pass through the inferior portion of the hypogastric plexus, and supply the descending colon, rectum, anus, bladder, prostate gland, and external genitalia — called also *nervus erigens*

pel•vim•e•ter \pel-ˈvi-mə-tər\ *n* : an instrument for measuring the dimensions of the pelvis

pel•vim•e•try \pel-ˈvi-mə-trē\ *n, pl* **-tries** : measurement of the pelvis (as by X-ray examination)

pel•vis \ˈpel-vəs\ *n, pl* **pel•vis•es** \-və-səz\ *or* **pel•ves** \-ˌvēz\ **1** : a basin-shaped structure in the skeleton of many vertebrates that in humans is composed of the two hip bones bounding it on each side and in front while the sacrum and coccyx complete it behind **2** : PELVIC CAVITY **3** : RENAL PELVIS

pelvo- — see PELV-

pem•e•trex•ed \ˌpem-ə-ˈtrek-ˌsed\ *n* : an antineoplastic drug that is an antagonist of folic acid and is administered by injection in the form of its hydrated disodium salt $C_{20}H_{19}N_5Na_2O_6 \cdot 7H_2O$ to treat pleural mesothelioma — see ALIMTA

pem•o•line \ˈpe-mə-ˌlēn\ *n* : a synthetic drug $C_9H_8N_2O_2$ that is a mild stimulant of the central nervous system and has been used to treat attention deficit disorder and narcolepsy

[1]**pem•phi•goid** \ˈpem-fə-ˌgȯid\ *adj* : resembling pemphigus

[2]**pemphigoid** *n* : any of several diseases that resemble pemphigus; *esp* : BULLOUS PEMPHIGOID

pem•phi•gus \ˈpem-fi-gəs, pem-ˈfī-gəs\ *n, pl* **-gus•es** *or* **-gi** \-ˌjī\ : any of several diseases characterized by the formation of successive eruptions of large blisters on apparently normal skin and mucous membranes often in association with sensations of itching or burning

pemphigus er•y•the•ma•to•sus \-ˌer-i-ˌthē-mə-ˈtō-səs\ *n* : a relatively benign form of chronic pemphigus that is characterized by the eruption esp. on the face and trunk of lesions resembling those which occur in systemic lupus erythematosus

pemphigus fo•li•a•ce•us \-ˌfō-lē-ˈā-s(h)ē-əs\ *n* : an uncommon form of chronic pemphigus characterized by superficial blisters of the skin and rarely mucous membranes which rupture to produce scaly crusted lesions

pemphigus vul•gar•is \-vəl-ˈgar-əs\ *n* : a severe and often fatal form of chronic pemphigus

pen \ˈpen\ *n* : a medical device for injecting drugs that resembles a fountain pen, contains a cartridge filled with usu. several doses of medication, and when designed for multiple injections has a needle that is replaced after each use

Pen•brit•in \pen-ˈbri-tən\ *n* : a preparation of ampicillin — formerly a U.S. registered trademark

pen•ci•clo•vir \ˌpen-ˈsī-klō-ˌvir\ *n* : an antiviral drug $C_{10}H_{15}N_5O_3$ that is applied topically esp. to treat recurrent herpes labialis

pen•cil \ˈpen-səl\ *n* : a small medicated or cosmetic roll or stick for local applications ⟨a menthol ~⟩

pen•du•lar nystagmus \ˈpen-jə-lər-\ *n* : nystagmus marked by rhythmic side-to-side or up-and-down movements of constant speed

pe•nec•to•my \pē-ˈnek-tə-mē\ *n, pl* **-mies** : surgical removal of the penis

penes *pl of* PENIS

pen•e•trance \ˈpe-nə-trəns\ *n* : the proportion of individuals of a particular genotype that express its phenotypic effect in a given environment — compare EXPRESSIVITY

pen•e•trate \ˈpe-nə-ˌtrāt\ *vb* **-trat•ed; -trat•ing 1** : to pass, extend, pierce, or diffuse into or through something **2** : to insert the penis into the vagina of in copulation — **pen•e•tra•tion** \ˌpe-nə-ˈtrā-shən\ *n*

pen•flur•i•dol \ˌpen-ˈflu̇r-i-ˌdȯl\ *n* : a tranquilizing drug $C_{28}H_{27}ClF_5NO$

-pe•nia \ˈpē-nē-ə\ *n comb form* : deficiency of ⟨eosino*penia*⟩

pen•i•cil•la•mine \ˌpe-nə-ˈsi-lə-ˌmēn\ *n* : an amino acid $C_5H_{11}NO_2S$ that is obtained from penicillins and is used esp. to treat cystinuria, rheumatoid arthritis, and metal poisoning (as by copper or lead)

pen•i•cil•lic acid \ˌpe-nə-ˈsi-lik-\ *n* : a crystalline antibiotic $C_8H_{10}O_4$ produced by several molds of the genera *Penicillium* and *Aspergillus*

pen•i•cil•lin \ˌpe-nə-ˈsi-lən\ *n* **1** : a mixture of relatively nontoxic antibiotic acids produced esp. by molds of the genus *Penicillium* (as *P. notatum* or *P. chrysogenum*) and having a powerful bacteriostatic effect against chiefly gram-positive bacteria (as staphylococci, gonococci, and pneumococci) **2** : any of numerous often hygroscopic and unstable acids (as penicillin G, penicillin O, and penicillin V) that are components of the penicillin mixture **3** : a salt or ester of a penicillin acid or a mixture of such salts or esters

pen•i•cil•lin•ase \-ˈsi-lə-ˌnās, -ˌnāz\ *n* : BETA-LACTAMASE; *specif* : a beta-lactamase that inactivates penicillin

penicillin F \-ˈef\ *n* : a penicillin $C_{14}H_{20}N_2O_4S$ that was the first of the penicillins isolated in Great Britain

penicillin G \-ˈjē\ *n* : the penicillin $C_{16}H_{18}N_2O_4S$ that constitutes the principal or sole component of most commercial preparations and is used chiefly in the form of stable salts (as the sodium salt $C_{16}H_{17}N_2NaO_4S$ or the potassium salt $C_{16}H_{17}KN_2O_4S$) — called also *benzylpenicillin;* see PENICILLIN G BENZATHINE, PENICILLIN G PROCAINE

penicillin G benzathine *n* : an aqueous suspension of a relatively insoluble salt of penicillin G that is absorbed slowly following intramuscular injection to provide a low but persistent level of penicillin G in the blood — called also *benzathine penicillin G*

penicillin G procaine *n* : an aqueous suspension of penicillin G and procaine that is absorbed slowly following intramuscular injection to provide a low but persistent level of penicillin

G in the blood — called also *procaine penicillin G*

penicillin O \-ˈō\ *n* : a penicillin $C_{13}H_{18}N_2O_4S_2$ that is similar to penicillin G in antibiotic activity

penicillin V \-ˈvē\ *n* : a crystalline acid that is used in the form of its potassium salt $C_{16}H_{17}KN_2O_2S$ and has antibacterial action similar to penicillin G and is more resistant to inactivation by gastric acids — called also *phenoxymethyl penicillin*

pen•i•cil•li•o•sis \ˌpe-nə-ˌsi-lē-ˈō-səs\ *n, pl* **-o•ses** \-ˌsēz\ : infection with or disease caused by molds of the genus *Penicillium*

pen•i•cil•li•um \ˌpe-nə-ˈsi-lē-əm\ *n* **1** *cap* : a genus of fungi (as the blue molds) that have been grouped with the imperfect fungi but are now often placed with the ascomycetes and that are found chiefly on moist nonliving organic matter (as decaying fruit) and including molds useful in economic fermentation and the production of antibiotics **2** *pl* **-lia** \-lē-ə\ : any mold of the genus *Penicillium*

pen•i•cil•lo•yl–poly•ly•sine \ˌpe-nə-ˈsi-lō-ˌil-ˌpä-li-ˈlī-ˌsēn\ *n* : a preparation of a penicillic acid and polylysine which is used in a skin test to determine hypersensitivity to penicillin

pen•i•cil•lus \ˌpe-nə-ˈsi-ləs\ *n, pl* **-li** \-ˌlī\ : one of the small straight arteries of the red pulp of the spleen

pe•nile \ˈpē-ˌnīl\ *adj* : of, relating to, or affecting the penis ⟨~ cancer⟩

pe•nis \ˈpē-nəs\ *n, pl* **pe•nes** \ˈpē-(ˌ)nēz\ *or* **pe•nis•es** : a male erectile copulatory organ that in most mammals including humans usu. functions as the channel by which urine and semen are discharged from the body and is typically a cylindrical organ that is suspended from the pubic arch, contains a pair of large lateral corpora cavernosa and a smaller ventromedial corpus cavernosum containing the urethra, and has a terminal glans enclosing the ends of the corpora cavernosa, covered by mucous membrane, and sheathed by a foreskin continuous with the skin covering the body of the organ

penis envy *n* : the supposed coveting of the penis by a young human female which is held in Freudian psychoanalytic theory to lead to feelings of inferiority and defensive or compensatory behavior

Pen•lac \ˈpen-ˌlak\ *trademark* — used for a preparation of ciclopirox

pen•nate \ˈpe-ˌnāt\ *adj* : having a structure like that of a feather; *esp* : being a muscle in which fibers extend obliquely from either side of a central tendon

pen•ni•form \ˈpe-ni-ˌfȯrm\ *adj* : PENNATE

pe•no•scro•tal \ˌpē-nō-ˈskrōt-ᵊl\ *adj* : of or relating to the penis and scrotum

penoscrotal raphe *n* : the ridge on the surface of the scrotum that divides it into two lateral halves and is continued forward on the underside of the penis and backward along the midline of the perineum to the anus

Pen•rose drain \ˈpen-ˌrōz-\ *n* : CIGARETTE DRAIN

Penrose, Charles Bingham (1862–1925), American gynecologist.

pen•ta•chlo•ro•phe•nol \ˌpen-tə-ˌklōr-ə-ˈfē-ˌnōl, -fi-ˈ\ *n* : a crystalline compound C_6Cl_5OH used esp. as a wood preservative, insecticide, and fungicide

pen•ta•eryth•ri•tol tet•ra•ni•trate \-i-ˈri-thrə-ˌtȯl-ˌte-trə-ˈnī-ˌtrāt, -ˌtōl-\ *n* : a crystalline ester $C_5H_8N_4O_{12}$ used in the treatment of angina pectoris

pen•ta•gas•trin \ˌpen-tə-ˈgas-trən\ *n* : a pentapeptide $C_{37}H_{49}N_7O_9S$ that stimulates gastric acid secretion

pen•ta•me•tho•ni•um \ˌpen-tə-me-ˈthō-nē-əm\ *n* : an organic ion $[C_{11}H_{28}N_2]^{2+}$ used in the form of its salts (as the bromide and iodide) for its ganglionic blocking activity in the treatment of hypertension

pent•am•i•dine \pen-ˈta-mə-ˌdēn, -dən\ *n* : a drug used chiefly in the form of its salt $C_{23}H_{36}N_4O_{10}S_2$ to treat protozoal infections (as leishmaniasis) and to prevent Pneumocystis carinii pneumonia in HIV-infected individuals

pen•ta•pep•tide \ˌpen-tə-ˈpep-ˌtīd\ *n* : a polypeptide that contains five amino acid residues

pen•ta•pip•eride methylsulfate \ˌpen-tə-ˈpi-pər-ˌīd-\ *n* : PENTAPIPERIUM METHYLSULFATE

pen•ta•pi•per•i•um meth•yl•sul•fate \ˌpen-tə-pī-ˈper-ē-əm-ˌme-thəl-ˈsəl-ˌfāt\ *n* : a synthetic quaternary ammonium anticholinergic and antisecretory agent $C_{20}H_{33}NO_6S$ used esp. in the treatment of peptic ulcer

pen•ta•quine \ˈpen-tə-ˌkwēn\ *n* : an antimalarial drug used esp. in the form of its pale yellow crystalline phosphate $C_{18}H_{27}N_3O{\cdot}H_3PO_4$

pen•taz•o•cine \pen-ˈta-zə-ˌsēn\ *n* : a synthetic analgesic drug $C_{19}H_{27}NO$ that is less addictive than morphine — see TALWIN

pen•to•bar•bi•tal \ˌpen-tə-ˈbär-bə-ˌtȯl\ *n* : a barbiturate used esp. in the form of its sodium salt $C_{11}H_{17}N_2NaO_3$ or calcium salt $(C_{11}H_{17}N_2O_3)_2Ca$ as a sedative, hypnotic, and antispasmodic

pen•to•bar•bi•tone \-ˌtōn\ *n, Brit* : PENTOBARBITAL

pen•to•lin•i•um tartrate \ˌpen-tə-ˈli-nē-əm-\ *n* : a ganglionic blocking agent $C_{23}H_{42}N_2O_{12}$ used as an antihypertensive drug

pen•tose \ˈpen-ˌtōs, -ˌtōz\ *n* : a monosaccharide $C_5H_{10}O_5$ that contains five carbon atoms in a molecule

pen•tos•uria \ˌpen-tō-ˈsu̇r-ē-ə, -ˈsyu̇r-\ *n* : the excretion of pentoses in the urine; *specif* : a rare hereditary anomaly characterized by regular excretion of pentoses

Pen•to•thal \ˈpen-tə-ˌthȯl\ *trademark* — used for a preparation of thiopental

pent·ox·i·fyl·line \ˌpen-ˌtäk-ˈsi-fə-ˌlēn\ *n* : a methylxanthine derivative $C_{13}H_{18}N_4O_3$ that reduces blood viscosity, increases microcirculatory blood flow, and is used to treat intermittent claudication resulting from occlusive arterial disease — see TRENTAL

pen·tyl·ene·tet·ra·zol \ˌpen-ti-ˌlēn-ˈte-trə-ˌzȯl, -ˌzōl\ *n* : a white crystalline drug $C_6H_{10}N_4$ used as a respiratory and circulatory stimulant and for producing a state of convulsion in treating certain mental illnesses — called also *leptazol;* see METRAZOL

pe·num·bra \pə-ˈnəm-brə\ *n, pl* **-brae** \-(ˌ)brē, -(ˌ)brī\ *or* **-bras** : a blurred area in a radiograph at the edge of an anatomical structure — **pe·num·bral** \-brəl\ *adj*

Pep·cid \ˈpep-səd\ *trademark* — used for a preparation of famotidine

pep pill *n* : any of various stimulant drugs (as amphetamine) in pill or tablet form

-pep·sia \ˈpep-shə, ˈpep-sē-ə\ *n comb form* : digestion ⟨dys*pepsia*⟩

pep·sin \ˈpep-sən\ *n* **1** : a crystallizable protease that in an acid medium digests most proteins to polypeptides, that is secreted by glands in the mucous membrane of the stomach, and that in combination with dilute hydrochloric acid is the chief active principle of gastric juice **2** : a preparation containing pepsin obtained from the stomach esp. of the hog and used esp. as a digestant

pep·sin·o·gen \pep-ˈsi-nə-jən\ *n* : a granular zymogen of the gastric glands that is readily converted into pepsin in a slightly acid medium

pept- *or* **pepto-** *comb form* : protein fragment or derivative ⟨*pept*ide⟩

pep·tic \ˈpep-tik\ *adj* **1** : relating to or promoting digestion : DIGESTIVE **2** : of, relating to, producing, or caused by pepsin ⟨~ digestion⟩

peptic ulcer *n* : an ulcer in the wall of the stomach or duodenum resulting from the digestive action of the gastric juice on the mucous membrane when the latter is rendered susceptible to its action (as from infection with the bacterium *Helicobacter pylori* or the chronic use of NSAIDs)

pep·ti·dase \ˈpep-tə-ˌdās, -ˌdāz\ *n* : an enzyme that hydrolyzes simple peptides or their derivatives

pep·tide \ˈpep-ˌtīd\ *n* : any of various amides that are derived from two or more amino acids by combination of the amino group of one acid with the carboxyl group of another and are usu. obtained by partial hydrolysis of proteins — **pep·tid·ic** \pep-ˈti-dik\ *adj*

peptide bond *n* : the chemical bond between carbon and nitrogen in a peptide linkage

peptide linkage *n* : the group CONH that unites the amino acid residues in a peptide

pep·tid·er·gic \ˌpep-tī-ˈdər-jik\ *adj* : being, relating to, releasing, or activated by neurotransmitters that are short peptide chains ⟨~ neurons⟩

pep·ti·do·gly·can \ˌpep-tə-dō-ˈglī-ˌkan\ *n* : a polymer that is composed of polysaccharide and peptide chains and is found esp. in bacterial cell walls — called also *mucopeptide, murein*

Pep·to–Bis·mol \ˌpep-tō-ˈbiz-ˌmȯl\ *trademark* — used for a preparation of bismuth subsalicylate

pep·tone \ˈpep-ˌtōn\ *n* **1** : any of various protein derivatives that are formed by the partial hydrolysis of proteins (as by enzymes of the gastric and pancreatic juices or by acids or alkalies) **2** : a water-soluble product containing peptones and other protein derivatives that is obtained by digesting protein with an enzyme (as pepsin or trypsin) and is used chiefly in nutrient media in bacteriology

per \ˈpər\ *prep* : by the means or agency of : by way of : through ⟨blood ~ rectum⟩ — see PER OS

per·acute \ˌpər-ə-ˈkyüt\ *adj* : very acute and violent

per·ceive \pər-ˈsēv\ *vb* **per·ceived; per·ceiv·ing** : to become aware of through the senses — **per·ceiv·able** \-ˈsē-və-bəl\ *adj*

per·cept \ˈpər-ˌsept\ *n* : an impression of an object obtained by use of the senses : SENSE-DATUM

per·cep·ti·ble \pər-ˈsep-tə-bəl\ *adj* : capable of being perceived esp. by the senses — **per·cep·ti·bly** \-blē\ *adv*

per·cep·tion \pər-ˈsep-shən\ *n* : awareness of the elements of environment through physical sensation ⟨color ~⟩ — compare SENSATION 1a

per·cep·tive \pər-ˈsep-tiv\ *adj* : responsive to sensory stimulus ⟨a ~ eye⟩ — **per·cep·tive·ly** *adv*

perceptive deafness *n* : NERVE DEAFNESS

per·cep·tu·al \(ˌ)pər-ˈsep-chə-wəl, -shə-\ *adj* : of, relating to, or involving perception esp. in relation to immediate sensory experience ⟨auditory ~ deficits⟩ — **per·cep·tu·al·ly** *adv*

Per·co·cet \ˈpər-kō-ˌset\ *trademark* — used for a preparation of acetaminophen and the hydrochloride of oxycodone

Per·co·dan \ˈpər-kə-ˌdan\ *trademark* — used for a preparation of aspirin and the hydrochloride of oxycodone

per·co·late \ˈpər-kə-ˌlāt, -lət\ *n* : a product of percolation

per·co·la·tion \ˌpər-kə-ˈlā-shən\ *n* **1** : the slow passage of a liquid through a filtering medium **2** : a method of extraction or purification by means of filtration **3** : the process of extracting the soluble constituents of a powdered drug by passage of a liquid through it — **per·co·late** \ˈpər-kə-ˌlāt\ *vb* — **per·co·la·tor** \-ˌlā-tər\ *n*

per·cus·sion \pər-ˈkə-shən\ *n* **1** : the act or technique of tapping the surface of a body part to learn the condition of the parts beneath by the resulting sound **2** : massage consisting of the striking of a body part with light rapid blows — called also *tapotement* — **per•cuss** \pər-ˈkəs\ *vb*

per•cu•ta•ne•ous \ˌpər-kyu̇-ˈtā-nē-əs\ *adj* : effected or performed through the skin ⟨~ absorption⟩ — **per•cu•ta•ne•ous•ly** *adv*

percutaneous coronary intervention *n* : balloon angioplasty of a coronary artery : PERCUTANEOUS TRANSLUMINAL CORONARY ANGIOPLASTY; *broadly* : any procedure that is performed to widen the lumen of an obstructed coronary artery and involves passing a catheter through the skin and into a blood vessel (as of the groin) to the site of obstruction so the blockage can be compressed (as by use of a balloon catheter often followed by placement of a stent) or removed (as by atherectomy) — abbr. *PCI*

percutaneous endoscopic gastrostomy *n* : an endoscopic surgical procedure for placement of a feeding tube directly into the stomach through a small opening created in the skin and abdominal wall — abbr. *PEG*

percutaneous transluminal angioplasty *n* : a cardiovascular procedure that is performed to widen the lumen of a partially or fully occluded blood vessel (as the femoral or coronary artery) narrowed or blocked typically by atherosclerotic plaque and that involves passing a balloon catheter through the skin and into a blood vessel (as of the groin or arm) to be guided to the site of the obstruction where the tip of the catheter is expanded by inflation to compress and flatten the plaque; *esp* : PERCUTANEOUS TRANSLUMINAL CORONARY ANGIOPLASTY — abbr. *PTA*

percutaneous transluminal coronary angioplasty *n* : percutaneous transluminal angioplasty of a coronary artery : BALLOON ANGIOPLASTY; *also* : PERCUTANEOUS CORONARY INTERVENTION — abbr. *PTCA*

Per•di•em \pər-ˈdē-ˌem\ *trademark* — used for a laxative preparation of psyllium seed husks and senna

pe•ren•ni•al \pə-ˈre-nē-əl\ *adj* : present at all seasons of the year ⟨~ rhinitis⟩

per•fo•rate \ˈpər-fə-ˌrāt\ *vb* **-rat•ed; -rat•ing** : to enter, penetrate, or make a hole through ⟨an ulcer ~*s* the duodenal wall⟩

per•fo•rat•ed \-ˌrā-təd\ *adj* : characterized by perforation ⟨a ~ eardrum⟩

per•fo•ra•tion \ˌpər-fə-ˈrā-shən\ *n* **1** : the act or process of perforating; *specif* : the penetration of a body part through accident or disease **2 a** : a rupture in a body part caused esp. by accident or disease **b** : a natural opening in an organ or body part

per•fo•ra•tor \ˈpər-fə-ˌrā-tər\ *n* : one that perforates: as **a** : an instrument used to perforate tissue (as bone) **b** : a nerve or blood vessel forming a connection between a deep system and a superficial one

Per•for•o•mist \pər-ˈfȯr-ə-mist\ *trademark* — used for a preparation of formoterol for oral inhalation

per•fus•ate \(ˌ)pər-ˈfyü-ˌzāt, -zət\ *n* : a fluid (as a solution pumped through the heart) that is perfused

per•fuse \(ˌ)pər-ˈfyüz\ *vb* **-fused; -fus•ing 1** : SUFFUSE **2 a** : to cause to flow or spread : DIFFUSE **b** : to force a fluid through (an organ or tissue) esp. by way of the blood vessels

per•fu•sion \-ˈfyü-zhən\ *n* : an act or instance of perfusing; *specif* : the pumping of a fluid through an organ or tissue

per•fu•sion•ist \pər-ˈfyü-zhə-nist\ *n* : a certified medical technician responsible for extracorporeal oxygenation of the blood during open-heart surgery and for the operation and maintenance of equipment (as a heart-lung machine) controlling it

per•go•lide \ˈpər-gə-ˌlīd\ *n* : an agonist of dopamine receptors $C_{19}H_{26}N_2S \cdot CH_4O_3S$ formerly used esp. to treat Parkinson's disease

per•hex•i•line \ˌpər-ˈhek-sə-ˌlēn\ *n* : a drug $C_{19}H_{35}N$ used as a coronary vasodilator

peri- *prefix* **1** : near : around ⟨*peri*menopausal⟩ **2** : enclosing : surrounding ⟨*peri*neurium⟩

peri•anal \ˌper-ē-ˈān-ᵊl\ *adj* : of, relating to, occurring in, or being the tissues surrounding the anus

peri•aor•tic \-ā-ˈȯr-tik\ *adj* : of, relating to, occurring in, or being the tissues surrounding the aorta

peri•api•cal \-ˈā-pi-kəl, -ˈa-\ *adj* : of, relating to, occurring in, affecting, or being the tissues surrounding the apex of the root of a tooth

peri•aq•ue•duc•tal \-ˌa-kwə-ˈdəkt-ᵊl\ *adj* : of, relating to, or being the gray matter which surrounds the aqueduct of Sylvius

peri•ar•te•ri•al \-är-ˈtir-ē-əl\ *adj* : of, relating to, occurring in, or being the tissues surrounding an artery

peri•ar•te•ri•o•lar \-är-ˌtir-ē-ˈō-lər\ *adj* : of, relating to, occurring in, or being the tissues surrounding an arteriole

peri•ar•ter•i•tis no•do•sa \ˌper-ē-ˌär-tə-ˈrī-təs-nō-ˈdō-sə\ *n* : POLYARTERITIS NODOSA

peri•ar•thri•tis \-är-ˈthrī-təs\ *n, pl* **-thrit•i•des** \-ˈthri-tə-ˌdēz\ : inflammation of the structures (as the muscles, tendons, and bursa of the shoulder) around a joint

peri•ar•tic•u•lar \-är-ˈti-kyə-lər\ *adj* : of, relating to, occurring in, or being the tissues surrounding a joint

peri•bron•chi•al \ˌper-ə-ˈbräŋ-kē-əl\ *adj* : of, relating to, occurring in, affecting, or being the tissues surrounding a bronchus ⟨a ~ growth⟩

peri•cap•il•lary \-ˈka-pə-ˌler-ē\ *adj* : of, relating to, occurring in, or being the tissues surrounding a capillary

pericardi- *or* **pericardio-** *or* **pericardo-** *comb form* **1** : pericardium ⟨*pericar*diectomy⟩ **2** : pericardial and ⟨*pericar-dio*phrenic artery⟩

peri•car•di•al \ˌper-ə-ˈkär-dē-əl\ *adj* : of, relating to, or affecting the pericardium; *also* : situated around the heart

pericardial cavity *n* : the fluid-filled space between the two layers of the pericardium

pericardial fluid *n* : the serous fluid that fills the pericardial cavity and protects the heart from friction

pericardial friction rub *n* : the auscultatory sound produced by the rubbing together of inflamed pericardial membranes in pericarditis — called also *pericardial rub*

peri•car•di•ec•to•my \ˌper-ə-ˌkär-dē-ˈek-tə-mē\ *n, pl* **-mies** : surgical excision of the pericardium

peri•car•dio•cen•te•sis \ˌper-ə-ˌkär-dē-ō-(ˌ)sen-ˈtē-səs\ *n, pl* **-te•ses** \-ˌsēz\ : surgical puncture of the pericardium esp. to aspirate pericardial fluid

peri•car•dio•phren•ic artery \ˌper-ə-ˌkär-dē-ə-ˈfre-nik-\ *n* : a branch of the internal mammary artery that descends through the thorax accompanying the phrenic nerve between the pleura and the pericardium to the diaphragm

peri•car•di•os•to•my \ˌper-ə-ˌkär-dē-ˈäs-tə-mē\ *n, pl* **-mies** : surgical formation of an opening into the pericardium

peri•car•di•ot•o•my \-ˈä-tə-mē\ *n, pl* **-mies** : surgical incision of the pericardium

peri•car•di•tis \-ˌkär-ˈdī-təs\ *n, pl* **-dit•i•des** \-ˈdi-tə-ˌdēz\ : inflammation of the pericardium — see ADHESIVE PERICARDITIS

peri•car•di•um \ˌper-ə-ˈkär-dē-əm\ *n, pl* **-dia** \-dē-ə\ : the conical sac of serous membrane that encloses the heart and the roots of the great blood vessels of vertebrates and consists of an outer fibrous coat that loosely invests the heart and is prolonged on the outer surface of the great vessels except the inferior vena cava and a double inner serous coat of which one layer is closely adherent to the heart while the other lines the inner surface of the outer coat with the intervening space being filled with pericardial fluid

pericardo- — see PERICARDI-

peri•cel•lu•lar \-ˈsel-yə-lər\ *adj* : of, relating to, occurring in, or being the tissues surrounding a cell

peri•ce•men•ti•tis \-ˌsē-ˌmen-ˈtī-təs\ *n* : PERIODONTITIS

peri•ce•men•tum \-si-ˈmen-təm\ *n* : PERIODONTAL LIGAMENT

peri•cen•tric \-ˈsen-trik\ *adj* : of, relating to, or involving the centromere of a chromosome ⟨~ inversion⟩ — compare PARACENTRIC

peri•chol•an•gi•tis \-ˌkō-ˌlan-ˈjī-təs, -ˌkä-\ *n* : inflammation of the tissues surrounding the bile ducts

peri•chon•dri•tis \-ˌkän-ˈdrī-təs\ *n* : inflammation of a perichondrium

peri•chon•dri•um \ˌper-ə-ˈkän-drē-əm\ *n, pl* **-dria** \-drē-ə\ : the membrane of fibrous connective tissue that invests cartilage except at joints — **peri-chon•dri•al** \-drē-əl\ *adj*

Peri–Co•lace \ˌper-ə-ˈkō-ˌlās\ *trademark* — used for a preparation containing senna-derived glucosides and the sodium salt of docusate

peri•co•ro•nal \ˌper-ə-ˈkȯr-ən-ᵊl, -ˈkär-; -kə-ˈrōn-ᵊl\ *adj* : occurring about or surrounding the crown of a tooth

peri•cor•o•ni•tis \-ˌkȯr-ə-ˈnī-təs, -ˌkär-\ *n, pl* **-nit•i•des** \-ˈni-tə-ˌdēz\ : inflammation of the gum about the crown of a partially erupted tooth

peri•cyte \ˈper-ə-ˌsīt\ *n* : a cell of the connective tissue about capillaries or other small blood vessels

peri•du•ral \ˌper-i-ˈdu̇r-əl, -ˈdyu̇r-\ *adj* : occurring or applied about the dura mater

peridural anesthesia *n* : EPIDURAL ANESTHESIA

peri•fo•cal \ˌper-ə-ˈfō-kəl\ *adj* : of, relating to, occurring in, or being the tissues surrounding a focus (as of infection) — **peri•fo•cal•ly** *adv*

peri•fol•lic•u•lar \ˌper-ə-fə-ˈli-kyə-lər, -fä-\ *adj* : of, relating to, occurring in, or being the tissues surrounding a follicle

peri•hep•a•ti•tis \-ˌhe-pə-ˈtī-təs\ *n, pl* **-tit•i•des** \-ˈti-tə-ˌdēz\ : inflammation of the peritoneal capsule of the liver

peri•kary•on \-ˈkar-ē-ˌän, -ən\ *n, pl* **-karya** \-ē-ə\ : CELL BODY — **peri-kary•al** \-ē-əl\ *adj*

peri•lymph \ˈper-ə-ˌlimf\ *n* : the fluid between the membranous and bony labyrinths of the ear

peri•lym•phat•ic \ˌper-ə-lim-ˈfa-tik\ *adj* : relating to or containing perilymph

peri•men•o•pause \-ˈme-nə-ˌpȯz, -ˈmē-\ *n* : the period around the onset of menopause that is often marked by various physical signs (as hot flashes and menstrual irregularity) — **peri•men•o-paus•al** \-ˌme-nə-ˈpȯ-zəl, -ˌmē-\ *adj*

pe•rim•e•ter \pə-ˈri-mə-tər\ *n* : an instrument for examining the discriminative powers of different parts of the retina

peri•me•tri•um \ˌper-ə-ˈmē-trē-əm\ *n, pl* **-tria** \-trē-ə\ : the peritoneum covering the fundus and ventral and dorsal aspects of the uterus

pe•rim•e•try \pə-ˈri-mə-trē\ *n, pl* **-tries** : examination of the eye by means of a perimeter — **peri•met•ric** \ˌper-ə-ˈme-trik\ *adj*

peri•mor•tem \ˌper-ə-ˈmȯr-təm\ *adj* : taking place at or around the time of death ⟨~ injury⟩ ⟨~ cesarean delivery⟩

peri•my•si•um \ˌper-ə-ˈmi-zhē-əm, -zē-\ *n, pl* **-sia** \-zhē-ə, -zē-ə\ : the connective-tissue sheath that surrounds a muscle and forms sheaths for the bundles of muscle fibers — **peri·my·si·al** \-əl\ *adj*

peri·na·tal \-ˈnāt-ᵊl\ *adj* : occurring in, concerned with, or being in the period around the time of birth ⟨~ mortality⟩ — **peri·na·tal·ly** *adv*

peri·na·tol·o·gist \ˌper-ə-ˌnā-ˈtä-lə-jist\ *n* : a specialist in perinatology

peri·na·tol·o·gy \-ˌnā-ˈtä-lə-jē\ *n, pl* **-gies** : a branch of medicine concerned with perinatal care

per·in·do·pril \pə-ˈrin-də-ˌpril\ *n* : an ACE inhibitor used in the form of its amine salt $C_{19}H_{32}N_2O_5 \cdot C_4H_{11}N$ to treat essential hypertension

per·i·ne·al \ˌper-ə-ˈnē-əl\ *adj* : of or relating to the perineum

perineal artery *n* : a branch of the internal pudendal artery that supplies the skin of the external genitalia and the superficial parts of the perineum

perineal body *n* : a mass of muscle and fascia that separates the lower end of the vagina and the rectum in the female and the urethra and the rectum in the male

perinei — see TRANSVERSUS PERINEI SUPERFICIALIS

perineo- *comb form* : perineum ⟨*perineo*tomy⟩

per·i·ne·o·plas·ty \ˌper-i-ˈnē-ō-ˌplas-tē\ *n, pl* **-ties** : plastic surgery of the perineum

per·i·ne·or·rha·phy \ˌper-ə-nē-ˈȯr-ə-fē\ *n, pl* **-phies** : suture of the perineum usu. to repair a laceration occurring during labor

peri·ne·ot·o·my \ˌper-ə-nē-ˈä-tə-mē\ *n, pl* **-mies** : surgical incision of the perineum

peri·neph·ric \ˌper-ə-ˈne-frik\ *adj* : PERIRENAL ⟨a ~ abscess⟩

per·i·ne·um \ˌper-ə-ˈnē-əm\ *n, pl* **-nea** \-ˈnē-ə\ : an area of tissue that marks externally the approximate boundary of the pelvic outlet and gives passage to the urogenital ducts and rectum; *also* : the area between the anus and the posterior part of the external genitalia esp. in the female

peri·neu·ral \ˌper-ə-ˈnu̇r-əl, -ˈnyu̇r-\ *adj* : occurring about or surrounding nervous tissue or a nerve

peri·neu·ri·al \-ˈnu̇r-ē-əl, -ˈnyu̇r-\ *adj* **1** : of or relating to the perineurium **2** : PERINEURAL

peri·neu·ri·um \ˌper-ə-ˈnu̇r-ē-əm, -ˈnyu̇r-\ *n, pl* **-ria** \-ē-ə\ : the sheath of connective tissue that surrounds a bundle of nerve fibers

peri·nu·cle·ar \-ˈnü-klē-ər, -ˈnyü-\ *adj* : situated around or surrounding the nucleus of a cell ⟨~ structures⟩

peri·oc·u·lar \ˌper-ē-ˈä-kyə-lər\ *adj* : surrounding the eyeball but within the orbit ⟨~ space⟩

pe·ri·od \ˈpir-ē-əd\ *n* **1 a** : a portion of time determined by some recurring phenomenon **b** : a single cyclic occurrence of menstruation **2** : a chronological division

pe·ri·od·ic \ˌpir-ē-ˈä-dik\ *adj* : occurring or recurring at regular intervals

per·iod·ic acid \ˌpər-(ˌ)ī-ˈä-dik-\ *n* : any of the strongly oxidizing iodine-containing acids (as H_5IO_6 or HIO_4)

periodic acid–Schiff \-ˈshif\ *adj* : relating to, being, or involving a reaction testing for polysaccharides and related substances in which tissue sections are treated with periodic acid and then Schiff's reagent with a reddish-violet color indicating a positive test

periodic breathing *n* : abnormal breathing characterized by an irregular respiratory rhythm; *esp* : CHEYNE-STOKES RESPIRATION

periodic ophthalmia *n* : MOON BLINDNESS

periodic table *n* : an arrangement of chemical elements based on their atomic numbers

peri·odon·tal \ˌper-ē-ō-ˈdänt-ᵊl\ *adj* **1** : investing or surrounding a tooth **2** : of or affecting the periodontium ⟨~ infection⟩ — **peri·odon·tal·ly** *adv*

periodontal disease *n* : any disease (as gingivitis or periodontis) affecting the periodontium

periodontal ligament *n* : the fibrous connective-tissue layer covering the cementum of a tooth and holding it in place in the jawbone — called also *pericementum, periodontal membrane*

peri·odon·tics \ˌper-ə-ˈdän-tiks\ *n* : a branch of dentistry that deals with diseases of the supporting and investing structures of the teeth including the gums, cementum, periodontal ligaments, and alveolar bone — called also *periodontology*

peri·odon·tist \-ˈdän-tist\ *n* : a specialist in periodontics — called also *periodontologist*

peri·odon·ti·tis \ˌper-ē-(ˌ)ō-ˌdän-ˈtī-təs\ *n* : inflammation of the periodontium and esp. chronic inflammation that typically follows untreated gingivitis and that results in progressive destruction of the periodontal ligament and resorption of alveolar bone with loosening or loss of teeth — called also *pericementitis*

peri·odon·tium \ˌper-ē-ō-ˈdän-chē-əm, -chəm\ *n, pl* **-tia** \-chē-ə, -chə\ : the supporting structures of the teeth including the cementum, the periodontal ligament, the bone of the alveolar process, and the gums

peri·odon·to·cla·sia \-ō-ˌdän-tə-ˈklā-zhə, -zhē-ə\ *n* : any periodontal disease characterized by destruction of the periodontium

peri·odon·tol·o·gist \ˌper-ē-ō-ˌdän-ˈtä-lə-jist\ *n* : PERIODONTIST

peri·odon·tol·o·gy \-ˌdän-ˈtä-lə-jē\ *n, pl* **-gies** : PERIODONTICS

peri·odon·to·sis \ˌper-ē-ō-ˌdän-ˈtō-səs\ *n, pl* **-to·ses** \-ˌsēz\ : a degenerative disease of the periodontium orig.

thought to lack accompanying inflammation

peri·onych·i·um \ˌper-ē-ō-ˈnik-ē-əm\ *n, pl* **-ia** \-ē-ə\ : the tissue bordering the sides of a fingernail or toenail

peri·op·er·a·tive \ˌper-ē-ˈä-pə-rə-tiv, -ˌrā-\ *adj* : relating to, occurring in, or being the period around the time of a surgical operation ⟨~ morbidity⟩

peri·oral \-ˈōr-əl, -ˈär-\ *adj* : of, relating to, occurring in, or being the tissues around the mouth

peri·or·bit·al \-ˈȯr-bət-ᵊl\ *adj* : of, relating to, occurring in, or being the tissues surrounding or lining the orbit of the eye ⟨~ edema⟩

periost- *or* **perioste-** *or* **periosteo-** *comb form* : periosteum ⟨*periost*itis⟩

peri·os·te·al \ˌper-ē-ˈäs-tē-əl\ *adj* **1** : situated around or produced external to bone **2** : of, relating to, or involving the periosteum ⟨~ cells⟩

periosteal elevator *n* : a surgical instrument used to separate the periosteum from bone

peri·os·te·um \ˌper-ē-ˈäs-tē-əm\ *n, pl* **-tea** \-tē-ə\ : the membrane of connective tissue that closely invests all bones except at the articular surfaces

peri·os·ti·tis \-ˌäs-ˈtī-təs\ *n* : inflammation of the periosteum

peri·pan·cre·at·ic \ˌper-ə-ˌpaŋ-krē-ˈa-tik, -ˌpan-\ *adj* : of, relating to, occurring in, or being the tissue surrounding the pancreas

peri·par·tum \-ˈpär-təm\ *adj* : occurring in or being the period preceding or following childbirth ⟨~ cardiomyopathy⟩

pe·riph·er·al \pə-ˈri-fə-rəl\ *adj* **1** : of, relating to, involving, forming, or located near a periphery or surface part (as of the body) **2** : of, relating to, affecting, or being part of the peripheral nervous system ⟨~ nerves⟩ **3** : of, relating to, or being the outer part of the visual field ⟨good ~ vision⟩ **4** : of, relating to, or being blood in the systemic circulation ⟨~ blood⟩ — **pe·riph·er·al·ly** *adv*

peripheral arterial disease *n* : damage to or dysfunction of the arteries outside the heart resulting in reduced blood flow; *esp* : narrowing or obstruction (as from atherosclerosis) of an artery (as the iliac artery or femoral artery) supplying the legs that is marked chiefly by intermittent claudication and by numbness and tingling in the legs

peripheral nervous system *n* : the part of the nervous system that is outside the central nervous system and comprises the cranial nerves excepting the optic nerve, the spinal nerves, and the autonomic nervous system

peripheral neuropathy *n* : a disease or degenerative state (as polyneuropathy) of the peripheral nerves in which motor, sensory, or vasomotor nerve fibers may be affected and which is marked by muscle weakness and atrophy, pain, and numbness

peripheral vascular disease *n* : vascular disease (as Raynaud's disease and Buerger's disease) affecting blood vessels and esp. those supplying the extremities

peripheral vascular resistance *n* : vascular resistance to the flow of blood in peripheral arterial vessels that is typically a function of the internal vessel diameter, vessel length, and blood viscosity — called also *peripheral resistance*

Peri·pla·ne·ta \ˌper-ē-plə-ˈnē-tə\ *n* : a genus of large cockroaches that includes the American cockroach

peri·plas·mic \ˌper-ə-ˈplaz-mik\ *adj* : of, relating to, occurring in, or being the space between the cell wall and the cell membrane

peri·por·tal \ˌper-ə-ˈpōrt-ᵊl\ *adj* : of, relating to, occurring in, or being the tissues surrounding a portal vein

peri·pro·ce·dur·al \-prə-ˈsē-jə-rəl\ *adj* : occurring soon before, during, or soon after the performance of a medical procedure ⟨~ mortality⟩

peri·rec·tal \-ˈrek-tᵊl\ *adj* : of, relating to, occurring in, or being the tissues surrounding the rectum

peri·re·nal \-ˈrēn-ᵊl\ *adj* : of, relating to, occurring in, or being the tissues surrounding the kidney ⟨~ abscesses⟩

peri·si·nu·soi·dal \-ˌsī-nə-ˈsȯid-ᵊl, -nyə-\ *adj* : of, relating to, or occurring in the tissue surrounding one or more sinusoids ⟨~ fibrosis⟩

peri·stal·sis \ˌper-ə-ˈstȯl-səs, -ˈstäl-, -ˈstal-\ *n, pl* **-stal·ses** \-ˌsēz\ : successive waves of involuntary contraction passing along the walls of a hollow muscular structure (as the esophagus or intestine) and forcing the contents onward — **peri·stal·tic** \-tik\ *adj*

peri·ten·di·ni·tis \ˌper-ə-ˌten-də-ˈnī-təs\ *n* : inflammation of the tissues around a tendon

periton- *or* **peritone-** *or* **peritoneo-** *comb form* **1** : peritoneum ⟨*peritoni*tis⟩ **2** : peritoneal and ⟨*peritoneo*venous shunt⟩

peri·to·nae·um *chiefly Brit var of* PERITONEUM

peri·to·ne·al \ˌper-ə-tə-ˈnē-əl\ *adj* : of, relating to, or affecting the peritoneum — **peri·to·ne·al·ly** *adv*

peritoneal cavity *n* : a space formed when the parietal and visceral layers of the peritoneum spread apart

peritoneal dialysis *n* : DIALYSIS 2b

peri·to·neo·scope \ˌper-ə-tə-ˈnē-ə-ˌskōp\ *n* : LAPAROSCOPE — **peri·to·neo·scop·ic** \-ˌnē-ə-ˈskä-pik\ *adj*

peri·to·ne·os·co·py \ˌper-ə-ˌtō-nē-ˈäs-kə-pē\ *n, pl* **-pies** : LAPAROSCOPY 1

peri·to·neo·ve·nous shunt \ˌper-ə-tə-ˌnē-ō-ˈvē-nəs-\ *n* : a shunt between the peritoneum and the jugular vein for relief of peritoneal ascites

peri·to·ne·um \ˌper-ə-tə-ˈnē-əm\ *n, pl* **-ne·ums** *or* **-nea** \-ˈnē-ə\ : the smooth transparent serous membrane that lines the cavity of the abdomen, is folded inward over the abdominal and pelvic viscera, and consists of an outer layer closely adherent to the walls of the abdomen and an inner layer that folds to invest the viscera — see PARIETAL PERITONEUM, VISCERAL PERITONEUM; compare MESENTERY 1

peri•to•ni•tis \ˌper-ə-tə-ˈnī-təs\ *n* : inflammation of the peritoneum

peri•ton•sil•lar abscess \ˌper-ə-ˈtän-sə-lər-\ *n* : QUINSY

peri•tu•bu•lar \ˌper-ə-ˈtü-byə-lər, -ˈtyü-\ *adj* : being adjacent to or surrounding a tubule

peritubular capillary *n* : any of a network of capillaries surrounding the renal tubules

peri•um•bi•li•cal \ˌper-ē-ˌəm-ˈbi-li-kəl\ *adj* : situated or occurring adjacent to the navel ⟨~ pain⟩

peri•un•gual \-ˈəŋ-gwəl, -ˈən-\ *adj* : situated or occurring around a fingernail or toenail

peri•ure•thral \-yu̇-ˈrē-thrəl\ *adj* : of, relating to, occurring in, or being the tissues surrounding the urethra

peri•vas•cu•lar \ˌper-ə-ˈvas-kyə-lər\ *adj* : of, relating to, occurring in, or being the tissues surrounding a blood vessel

peri•vas•cu•li•tis \-ˌvas-kyə-ˈlī-təs\ *n* : inflammation of a perivascular sheath ⟨~ in the retina⟩

peri•ve•nous \ˌper-ə-ˈvē-nəs\ *adj* : of, relating to, occurring in, or being the tissues surrounding a vein

peri•ven•tric•u•lar \-ven-ˈtri-kyə-lər\ *adj* : situated or occurring around a ventricle esp. of the brain

peri•vi•tel•line space \ˌper-ə-vī-ˈte-lən-, -ˌlēn-, -ˌlīn-\ *n* : the fluid-filled space between the fertilization membrane and the ovum after the entry of a sperm into the egg

per•i•win•kle \ˈper-i-ˌwiŋ-kəl\ *n* : any of several evergreen plants of the dogbane family (Apocynaceae); *esp* : ROSY PERIWINKLE

perle \ˈpərl\ *n* **1** : a soft gelatin capsule for enclosing volatile or unpleasant tasting liquids intended to be swallowed **2** : a fragile glass vial that contains a liquid (as amyl nitrite) and that is intended to be crushed and the vapor inhaled

per•lèche \per-ˈlesh\ *n* : a superficial inflammatory condition of the angles of the mouth often with fissure formation that is caused esp. by infection or avitaminosis

per•ma•nent \ˈpər-mə-nənt\ *adj* : of, relating to, or being a permanent tooth ⟨~ dentition⟩

permanent tooth *n* : one of the second set of teeth of a mammal that follow the milk teeth, typically persist into old age, and in humans are 32 in number including 4 incisors, 2 canines, and 10 premolars and molars in each jaw

per•me•able \ˈpər-mē-ə-bəl\ *adj* : capable of being permeated; *esp* : having pores or openings that permit liquids or gases to pass through — **per•me•abil•i•ty** \ˌpər-mē-ə-ˈbi-lə-tē\ *n*

per•me•ate \ˈpər-mē-ˌāt\ *vb* **-at•ed; -at•ing** : to diffuse through or penetrate something — **per•me•ation** \ˌpər-mē-ˈā-shən\ *n*

per•mis•sive \pər-ˈmi-siv\ *adj* : supporting genetic replication (as of a virus)

Per•mi•til \ˈpər-mə-ˌtil\ *trademark* — used for a preparation of fluphenazine

per•ni•cious \pər-ˈni-shəs\ *adj* : highly injurious or destructive : tending to a fatal issue : DEADLY ⟨~ disease⟩

pernicious anemia *n* : a severe hyperchromic anemia marked by a progressive decrease in number and increase in size and hemoglobin content of the red blood cells and by pallor, weakness, and gastrointestinal and nervous disturbances and associated with reduced ability to absorb vitamin B_{12} due to the absence of intrinsic factor — called also *addisonian anemia*

per•nio \ˈpər-nē-ˌō\ *n, pl* **per•ni•o•nes** \ˌpər-nē-ˈō-(ˌ)nēz\ : CHILBLAIN

pe•ro•me•lia \ˌpē-rə-ˈmē-lē-ə\ *n* : congenital malformation of the limbs

pe•ro•ne•al \ˌper-ō-ˈnē-əl, pə-ˈrō-nē-\ *adj* **1** : of, relating to, or located near the fibula **2** : relating to or involving a peroneal part

peroneal artery *n* : a deeply seated artery running along the back part of the fibular side of the leg to the heel, arising from the posterior tibial artery, and ending in branches near the ankle

peroneal muscle *n* : PERONEUS

peroneal muscular atrophy *n* : CHARCOT-MARIE-TOOTH DISEASE — called also *peroneal atrophy*

peroneal nerve *n* : COMMON PERONEAL NERVE — see DEEP PERONEAL NERVE, SUPERFICIAL PERONEAL NERVE

peroneal retinaculum *n* : either of two bands of fascia that support and bind in place the tendons of the peroneus longus and peroneus brevis muscles as they pass along the lateral aspect of the ankle: **a** : one that is situated more superiorly — called also *superior peroneal retinaculum* **b** : one that is situated more inferiorly — called also *inferior peroneal retinaculum*

peroneal vein *n* : any of several veins that drain the muscles in the lateral and posterior parts of the leg, accompany the peroneal artery, and empty into the posterior tibial veins about two-thirds of the way up the leg

per•o•ne•us \ˌper-ə-ˈnē-əs\ *n, pl* **-nei** \-ˈnē-ˌī\ : any of three muscles of the lower leg: **a** : PERONEUS BREVIS **b** : PERONEUS LONGUS **c** : PERONEUS TERTIUS

peroneus brev•is \-ˈbre-vis\ *n* : a peroneus muscle that arises esp. from the side of the lower part of the fibula, ends in a tendon that inserts on the tuberosity at the base of the fifth metatarsal bone, and assists in everting and pronating the foot

peroneus lon•gus \-ˈlȯŋ-gəs\ *n* : a peroneus muscle that arises esp. from the head and side of the fibula, ends in a long tendon that inserts on the side of the first metatarsal bone and the cuneiform bone on the medial side, and aids in everting and pronating the foot

peroneus ter•ti•us \-ˈtər-shē-əs\ *n* : a branch of the extensor digitorum longus muscle that arises esp. from the lower portion of the fibula, inserts on the dorsal surface of the base of the fifth metatarsal bone, and flexes the foot dorsally and assists in everting it

per•oral \(ˌ)pər-ˈōr-əl, per-, -ˈär-\ *adj* : done, occurring, or obtained through or by way of the mouth ⟨~ infection⟩ — **per•oral•ly** *adv*

per os \ˌpər-ˈōs\ *adv* : by way of the mouth ⟨infection *per os*⟩

pe•ro•sis \pə-ˈrō-səs\ *n, pl* **pe•ro•ses** \-ˌsēz\ : a disorder of poultry that is characterized by leg deformity and is caused by a deficiency of vitamins or minerals in the diet — called also *hock disease, slipped tendon*

per•ox•i•dase \pə-ˈräk-sə-ˌdās, -ˌdāz\ *n* : an enzyme that catalyzes the oxidation of various substances by peroxides

per•ox•ide \pə-ˈräk-ˌsīd\ *n* : a compound (as hydrogen peroxide) in which oxygen is visualized as joined to oxygen

per•ox•i•some \pə-ˈräk-sə-ˌsōm\ *n* : a cytoplasmic cell organelle containing enzymes (as catalase) which act esp. in the production and decomposition of hydrogen peroxide — called also *microbody* — **per•ox•i•som•al** \-ˌräk-sə-ˈsō-məl\ *adj*

per•oxy•ace•tyl nitrate \pə-ˌräk-sē-ə-ˈsēt-ᵊl-\ *n* : a toxic compound $C_2H_3O_5N$ that is found esp. in smog and is irritating to the eyes and upper respiratory tract — abbr. *PAN*

per•pen•dic•u•lar plate \ˌpər-pən-ˈdi-kyə-lər-\ *n* **1** : a flattened bony lamina of the ethmoid bone that is the largest bony part assisting in forming the nasal septum **2** : a long thin vertical bony plate forming part of the palatine bone — compare HORIZONTAL PLATE

per•phen•a•zine \(ˌ)pər-ˈfe-nə-ˌzēn\ *n* : a phenothiazine tranquilizer $C_{21}H_{26}ClN_3OS$ that is used to control symptoms (as anxiety, agitation, and delusions) of psychotic conditions

per•rec•tal \ˌpər-ˈrekt-ᵊl\ *adj* : done or occurring through or by way of the rectum ⟨~ administration⟩ — **per•rec•tal•ly** *adv*

per rectum *adv* : by way of the rectum ⟨a solution injected *per rectum*⟩

Per•san•tine \pər-ˈsan-ˌtēn\ *trademark* — used for a preparation of dipyridamole

persecution complex *n* : the feeling of being persecuted esp. without basis in reality

per•se•cu•to•ry \ˈpər-sə-kyü-ˌtōr-ē, pər-ˈse-kyə-\ *adj* : of, relating to, or being feelings of persecution : PARANOID

per•sev•er•a•tion \pər-ˌse-və-ˈrā-shən\ *n* : continual involuntary repetition of a mental act usu. exhibited by speech or by some other form of overt behavior — **per•sev•er•ate** \pər-ˈse-və-ˌrāt\ *vb* — **per•sev•er•a•tive** \pər-ˈse-və-ˌrā-tiv\ *adj*

per•sis•tent \pər-ˈsis-tənt\ *adj* **1** : existing or continuing for a long time: as **a** : effective in the open for an appreciable time usu. through slow formation of a vapor ⟨mustard gas is ~⟩ **b** : degraded only slowly by the environment ⟨~ pesticides⟩ **c** : remaining infective for a relatively long time in a vector after an initial period of incubation ⟨~ viruses⟩ **2** : continuing to exist despite interference or treatment ⟨a ~ cough⟩ ⟨has been in a ~ vegetative state for two years⟩

per•so•na \pər-ˈsō-nə, -ˌnä\ *n, pl* **personas** : an individual's social facade or front that esp. in the analytic psychology of C.G. Jung reflects the role in life the individual is playing — compare ANIMA

per•son•al•i•ty \ˌpər-sə-ˈna-lə-tē\ *n, pl* **-ties** **1** : the complex of characteristics that distinguishes an individual esp. in relationships with others **2 a** : the totality of an individual's behavioral and emotional tendencies **b** : the organization of the individual's distinguishing character traits, attitudes, or habits

personality disorder *n* : a psychopathological condition or group of conditions in which an individual's entire life pattern is considered deviant or nonadaptive although the individual shows neither neurotic symptoms nor psychotic disorganization

personality inventory *n* : any of several tests that attempt to characterize the personality of an individual by objective scoring of replies to a large number of questions concerning the individual's behavior and attitudes — see MINNESOTA MULTIPHASIC PERSONALITY INVENTORY

personality test *n* : any of several tests that consist of standardized tasks designed to determine various aspects of the personality or the emotional status of the individual examined

per•spi•ra•tion \ˌpər-spə-ˈrā-shən\ *n* **1** : the act or process of perspiring **2** : a saline fluid that is secreted by the sweat glands, that consists chiefly of water containing sodium chloride and other salts, nitrogenous substances (as urea), carbon dioxide, and other solutes, and that serves both as a means of excretion and as a regulator of body temperature through the cooling effect of its evaporation — **per•spire** \pər-ˈspīr\ *vb*

per·spi·ra·to·ry \pər-ˈspī-rə-ˌtōr-ē, ˈpər-spə-rə-\ *adj* : of, relating to, secreting, or inducing perspiration

per·sua·sion \pər-ˈswā-zhən\ *n* : a method of treating neuroses consisting essentially in rational conversation and reeducation

per·tech·ne·tate \pər-ˈtek-nə-ˌtāt\ *n* : an anion $[TcO_4]^-$ of technetium used esp. in the form of its sodium salt as a radiopharmaceutical in medical diagnostic scanning (as of the thyroid)

Per·thes disease \ˈpər-ˌtēz-\ *n* : LEGG-CALVÉ-PERTHES DISEASE

Per·to·frane \ˈpər-tə-ˌfrān\ *n* : a preparation of desipramine — formerly a U.S. registered trademark

per·tus·sis \pər-ˈtə-səs\ *n* : WHOOPING COUGH

peruana — see VERRUGA PERUANA

Peru balsam *n* : BALSAM OF PERU

Peruvian balsam *n* : BALSAM OF PERU

per·va·sive developmental disorder \pər-ˈvā-siv-, -ziv-\ *n* : AUTISM SPECTRUM DISORDER — abbr. *PDD*

per·ver·sion \pər-ˈvər-zhən, -shən\ *n* **1** : the action of perverting or the condition of being perverted **2** : an aberrant sexual practice or interest esp. when habitual — **per·verse** \pər-ˈvərs\ *adj*

[1]**per·vert** \pər-ˈvərt\ *vb* : to cause to engage in perversion or to become perverted

[2]**per·vert** \ˈpər-ˌvərt\ *n* : one given to some form of sexual perversion

perverted *adj* : marked by abnormality or perversion

pes an·se·ri·nus \ˈpez-ˌan-sə-ˈrī-nəs\ *n* : the combined tendinous insertion on the medial aspect of the tuberosity of the tibia of the sartorius, gracilis, and semitendinosus muscles

pes ca·vus \-ˈkā-vəs\ *n* : a foot deformity characterized by an abnormally high arch

pes·sa·ry \ˈpe-sə-rē\ *n, pl* **-ries** **1** : a vaginal suppository **2** : a device worn in the vagina to support the uterus, remedy a malposition, or prevent conception

pest \ˈpest\ *n* **1** : an epidemic disease associated with high mortality; *specif* : PLAGUE 2 **2** : something resembling a pest in destructiveness; *esp* : a plant or animal detrimental to humans or human concerns

pes·ti·cide \ˈpes-tə-ˌsīd\ *n* : an agent used to destroy pests — **pes·ti·ci·dal** \ˌpes-tə-ˈsīd-ᵊl\ *adj*

pes·tif·er·ous \pes-ˈti-fə-rəs\ *adj* **1** : carrying or propagating infection : PESTILENTIAL ⟨a ∼ insect⟩ **2** : infected with a pestilential disease

pes·ti·lence \ˈpes-tə-ləns\ *n* : a contagious or infectious epidemic disease that is virulent and devastating; *specif* : BUBONIC PLAGUE — **pes·ti·len·tial** \ˌpes-tə-ˈlen-chəl\ *adj*

pes·tis \ˈpes-təs\ *n* : PLAGUE 2

pes·ti·vir·us \ˈpes-tə-ˌvī-rəs\ *n* **1** *cap* : a genus of flaviviruses that includes the causative agents of bovine viral diarrhea and hog cholera and are transmitted by direct or indirect contact esp. with bodily secretions **2** : any virus of the genus *Pestivirus*

pes·tle \ˈpe-səl, ˈpes-təl\ *n* : a usu. club-shaped implement for pounding or grinding substances in a mortar

PET *abbr* positron-emission tomography

$PetCO_2$ *abbr* partial pressure of end-tidal carbon dioxide

pe·te·chia \pə-ˈtē-kē-ə\ *n, pl* **-chi·ae** \-kē-ˌī\ : a minute reddish or purplish spot containing blood that appears in skin or mucous membrane as a result of localized hemorrhage — **pe·te·chi·al** \-kē-əl\ *adj* — **pe·te·chi·a·tion** \pə-ˌtē-kē-ˈā-shən\ *n*

peth·i·dine \ˈpe-thə-ˌdēn, -dən\ *n, chiefly Brit* : MEPERIDINE

pe·tit mal \ˈpe-tē-ˌmal, -ˌmäl\ *n* **1** *or* **petit mal epilepsy** : epilepsy characterized by absence seizures : ABSENCE EPILEPSY; *also* : CHILDHOOD ABSENCE EPILEPSY **2** *or* **petit mal seizure** : ABSENCE SEIZURE

pe·tri dish \ˈpē-trē-\ *n* : a small shallow dish of thin glass or plastic with a loose cover used esp. for cultures in bacteriology

Pe·tri \ˈpā-trē\, **Julius Richard (1852–1921)**, German bacteriologist.

pe·tris·sage \ˌpā-tri-ˈsäzh\ *n* : massage in which the muscles are kneaded

pet·ro·la·tum \ˌpe-trə-ˈlā-təm, -ˈlä-\ *n* : PETROLEUM JELLY

pe·tro·leum jelly \pə-ˈtrō-lē-əm-ˈje-lē\ *n* : a neutral unctuous odorless tasteless substance obtained from petroleum and used esp. in ointments and dressings

pe·tro·sal \pə-ˈtrō-səl\ *n* : PETROSAL BONE

petrosal bone *n* : the petrous portion of the human temporal bone

petrosal ganglion *n* : INFERIOR GANGLION 1

petrosal nerve *n* : any of several small nerves passing through foramina in the petrous portion of the temporal bone: as **a** : DEEP PETROSAL NERVE **b** : GREATER PETROSAL NERVE **c** : LESSER PETROSAL NERVE

petrosal sinus *n* : either of two venous sinuses on each side of the base of the brain: **a** : a small superior sinus that connects the cavernous and transverse sinuses of the same side — called also *superior petrosal sinus* **b** : a larger inferior sinus that extends from the posterior inferior end of the cavernous sinus through the jugular foramen to join the internal jugular vein of the same side — called also *inferior petrosal sinus*

pe·tro·tym·pan·ic fissure \ˌpe-trō-tim-ˈpa-nik-, ˌpē-trō-\ *n* : a narrow transverse slit dividing the glenoid fossa of the temporal bone — called also *Glaserian fissure*

pe•trous \ˈpe-trəs, ˈpē-\ *adj* : of, relating to, or constituting the exceptionally hard and dense portion of the human temporal bone that contains the internal auditory organs and is a pyramidal process wedged in at the base of the skull between the sphenoid and occipital bones

PET scan \ˈpet-\ *n* : a sectional view of the body constructed by positron-emission tomography — **PET scanning** *n*

PET scanner *n* : a medical instrument consisting of integrated X-ray and computing equipment and used for positron-emission tomography

Peutz–Je•ghers syndrome \ˈpœts-ˈjā-gərz-\ *n* : a familial polyposis inherited as an autosomal dominant trait and characterized by numerous polyps in the stomach, small intestine, and colon and by melanin-containing spots on the skin and mucous membranes esp. of the lips and gums

Peutz, J. L. A. (1886–1957), Dutch physician.

Jeghers, Harold (1904–1990), American physician.

Pex•e•va \pek-ˈsē-və\ *trademark* — used for a preparation of the mesylate of paroxetine

-pexy \ˌpek-sē\ *n comb form, pl* **-pex•ies** : fixation : making fast ⟨gastro*pexy*⟩

Pey•er's patch \ˈpī-ərz-\ *n* : any of numerous large oval patches of closely aggregated nodules of lymphoid tissue in the walls of the small intestines esp. in the ileum that partially or entirely disappear in advanced life and in typhoid fever become the seat of ulcers which may perforate the intestines — called also *Peyer's gland*

Peyer, Johann Conrad (1653–1712), Swiss physician and anatomist.

pey•o•te \pā-ˈō-tē\ *also* **pey•otl** \-ˈōt-ᵊl\ *n* **1** : a hallucinogenic drug containing mescaline that is derived from peyote buttons **2** : a small spineless cactus (*Lophophora williamsii*) of the southwestern U.S. and Mexico — called also *mescal*

peyote button *n* : one of the dried disk-shaped tops of the peyote cactus — called also *mescal button*

Pey•ro•nie's disease \ˌpā-rə-ˈnēz-, pā-ˈrō-nēz-\ *n* : the formation of fibrous plaques in one or both corpora cavernosa of the penis resulting in distortion or deflection of the erect organ

La Peyronie \lä-pā-rȯ-ˈnē\, **François Gigot de (1678–1747),** French surgeon.

Pfan•nen•stiel incision \ˈpfä-nən-ˌs(h)tēl-\ *also* **Pfan•nen•stiel's incision** \-s(h)tēlz-\ *n* : a long horizontal abdominal incision made below the line of the pubic hair and above the mons veneris down to and through the sheath of the rectus abdominus muscles but not the muscles themselves which are separated in the direction of their fibers — called also *bikini incision*

Pfannenstiel, Hermann Johann (1862–1909), German gynecologist.

Pfie•ster•ia \fē-ˈstir-ē-ə\ *n* : a genus of dinoflagellates including one (*Pfiesteria piscicida*) found in waters esp. along the U.S. Atlantic coast that produces a toxin which causes skin lesions in fish and may cause symptoms (as skin lesions and memory loss) in humans exposed to the toxin

p53 \ˌpē-ˌfif-tē-ˈthrē\ *n* : a tumor suppressor gene that in a defective form tends to be associated with a high risk of certain cancers (as of the colon, lung, and breast)

pg *abbr* picogram

PG *abbr* prostaglandin

PGA *abbr* pteroylglutamic acid

PGR *abbr* psychogalvanic reaction; psychogalvanic reflex; psychogalvanic response

PGY *abbr* postgraduate year

pH \ˌpē-ˈāch\ *n* : a measure of acidity and alkalinity of a solution that is a number on a scale whose values run from 0 to 14 with 7 representing neutrality, numbers less than 7 increasing acidity, and numbers greater than 7 increasing alkalinity

PHA *abbr* phytohemagglutinin

phac- *or* **phaco-** *comb form* : lens ⟨*phaco*emulsification⟩

phaco•emul•si•fi•ca•tion \ˌfa-kō-i-ˌməl-sə-fə-ˈkā-shən\ *n* : a cataract operation in which the diseased lens is reduced to a liquid by ultrasonic vibrations and drained out of the eye — **phaco•emul•si•fi•er** \-ˈməl-sə-ˌfī- ər\ *n*

phaco•ma•to•sis \ˌfa-kō-mə-ˈtō-səs\ *n, pl* **-to•ses** \-ˌsēz\ : any of a group of hereditary or congenital diseases (as neurofibromatosis) affecting the central nervous system and characterized by the development of hamartomas

phaeo•chro•mo•cy•to•ma *Brit var of* PHEOCHROMOCYTOMA

phag- *or* **phago-** *comb form* : eating : feeding ⟨*phag*edena⟩

phage \ˈfāj, ˈfäzh\ *n* : BACTERIOPHAGE

-phage \ˌfāj, fäzh\ *n comb form* : one that eats ⟨bacterio*phage*⟩

phag•e•de•na \ˌfa-jə-ˈdē-nə\ *n* : rapidly spreading destructive ulceration of soft tissue — **phag•e•de•nic** \-ˈde-nik, -ˈdē-\ *adj*

phage lambda *n* : BACTERIOPHAGE LAMBDA

-pha•gia \ˈfā-jə, -jē-ə\ *n comb form* : -PHAGY ⟨dys*phagia*⟩

phago•cyte \ˈfa-gə-ˌsīt\ *n* : a cell (as a macrophage or neutrophil) that engulfs and consumes foreign material (as microorganisms) and debris (as dead tissue cells) — **phago•cyt•ic** \ˌfa-gə-ˈsi-tik\ *adj*

phago•cy•tize \ˈfa-gō-ˌsə-ˌtīz, -ˌsī-\ *vb* **-tized; -tiz•ing** : PHAGOCYTOSE

phago•cy•tose \ˌfa-gō-ˈsī-ˌtōs, -ˌtōz\ *vb* **-tosed; -tos•ing** : to consume by phagocytosis — **phago•cy•tos•able** \ˌfa-gə-sī-ˈtō-zə-bəl, -sə-, -ˌtōs-\ *adj*

phago·cy·to·sis \ˌfa-gə-sī-ˈtō-səs, -sə-\ *n, pl* **-to·ses** \-ˌsēz\ : the engulfing and usu. the destruction of particulate matter by phagocytes — **phago·cy·tot·ic** \-ˈtä-tik\ *adj*

phago·some \ˈfa-gə-ˌsōm\ *n* : a membrane-bound vesicle that encloses particulate matter taken into the cell by phagocytosis

-pha·gous \fə-gəs\ *adj comb form* : feeding esp. on a (specified) kind of food ⟨hemato*phagous*⟩

-ph·a·gy \f-ə-jē\ *n comb form, pl* **-phagies** : eating : eating of a (specified) type or substance ⟨geo*phagy*⟩

phak- *or* **phako-** — see PHAC-

pha·lan·ge·al \ˌfā-lən-ˈjē-əl, ˌfa-; fə-ˈlan-jē-, fā-\ *adj* : of or relating to a phalanx or the phalanges

pha·lan·gec·to·my \ˌfā-lən-ˈjek-tə-mē, ˌfa-\ *n, pl* **-mies** : surgical excision of a phalanx of a finger or toe

pha·lanx \ˈfā-ˌlaŋks\ *n, pl* **pha·lan·ges** \fə-ˈlan-(ˌ)jēz, fā-\ : any of the digital bones of the hand or foot distal to the metacarpus or metatarsus that in humans are three to each finger and toe with the exception of the thumb and big toe which have only two each

phall- *or* **phallo-** *comb form* : penis ⟨*phallo*plasty⟩

phal·lic \ˈfa-lik\ *adj* **1** : of, relating to, or resembling a penis **2** : of, relating to, or characterized by the stage of psychosexual development in psychoanalytic theory during which a child becomes interested in his or her own sexual organs — compare ANAL 2, GENITAL 3, ORAL 2

phal·loi·din \fa-ˈlȯid-ᵊn\ *also* **phal·loi·dine** \fa-ˈlȯid-ᵊn, ˈfa-lȯi-ˌdēn\ *n* : a very toxic crystalline peptide $C_{35}H_{46}N_8O_{10}S{\cdot}H_2O$ obtained from the death cap mushroom

phal·lo·plas·ty \ˈfa-lō-ˌplas-tē\ *n, pl* **-ties** : plastic surgery of the penis or scrotum

phal·lus \ˈfa-ləs\ *n, pl* **phal·li** \ˈfa-ˌlī, -ˌlē\ *or* **phal·lus·es** **1** : PENIS **2** : the first embryonic rudiment of the penis or clitoris

phan·ero·zo·ite \ˌfa-nə-rō-ˈzō-ˌīt\ *n* : an exoerythrocytic malaria parasite found late in the course of an infection — **phan·ero·zo·it·ic** \-zō-ˈi-tik\ *adj*

phan·tasm \ˈfan-ˌta-zəm\ *n* **1** : a figment of the imagination or disordered mind **2** : an apparition of a living or dead person

phantasy *var of* FANTASY

phan·tom \ˈfan-təm\ *n* **1** : a model of the body or one of its parts **2** : a body of material resembling a body or bodily part in mass, composition, and dimensions and used to measure absorption of radiations

phantom limb *n* : an often painful sensation of the presence of a limb that has been amputated — called also *phantom pain, phantom sensations*

phantom tumor *n* : a swelling (as of the abdomen) suggesting a tumor

Phar. D. *abbr* doctor of pharmacy

pharm *abbr* pharmaceutical; pharmacist; pharmacy

phar·ma \fär-mə\ *n* : a pharmaceutical company; *also* : large pharmaceutical companies as a group

[1]**phar·ma·ceu·ti·cal** \ˌfär-mə-ˈsü-ti-kəl\ *also* **phar·ma·ceu·tic** \-tik\ *adj* : of, relating to, or engaged in pharmacy or the manufacture and sale of pharmaceuticals ⟨a ~ company⟩ — **phar·ma·ceu·ti·cal·ly** *adv*

[2]**pharmaceutical** *also* **pharmaceutic** *n* : a medicinal drug

phar·ma·ceu·tics \-tiks\ *n* : the science of preparing, using, or dispensing medicines : PHARMACY

phar·ma·cist \ˈfär-mə-sist\ *n* : a person licensed to engage in pharmacy

pharmaco- *comb form* : medicine : drug ⟨*pharmaco*logy⟩

phar·ma·co·dy·nam·ics \ˌfär-mə-kō-dī-ˈna-miks, -də-\ *n* : a branch of pharmacology dealing with the reactions between drugs and living systems — **phar·ma·co·dy·nam·ic** \-mik\ *adj* — **phar·ma·co·dy·nam·i·cal·ly** *adv*

phar·ma·co·ge·net·ics \-jə-ˈne-tiks\ *n* : the study of how genetic differences among individuals cause varied responses to a drug — **phar·ma·co·ge·net·ic** \-tik\ *adj*

phar·ma·co·ge·no·mics \-jē-ˈnō-miks\ *n* : the science concerned with understanding how genetic differences among individuals cause varied responses to the same drug and with developing drug therapies to compensate for these differences — **phar·ma·co·ge·no·mic** \-mik\ *adj*

phar·ma·cog·no·sist \ˌfär-mə-ˈkäg-nə-sist\ *n* : a specialist in pharmacognosy

phar·ma·cog·no·sy \ˌfär-mə-ˈkäg-nə-sē\ *n, pl* **-sies** : a branch of pharmacology dealing esp. with the composition, use, and development of medicinal substances of biological origin — **phar·ma·cog·nos·tic** \-ˌkäg-ˈnäs-tik\ *or* **phar·ma·cog·nos·ti·cal** \-ti-kəl\ *adj*

phar·ma·co·ki·net·ics \-kō-kə-ˈne-tiks, -kō-kī-\ *n* **1** : the study of the bodily absorption, distribution, metabolism, and excretion of drugs **2** : the characteristic interactions of a drug and the body in terms of its absorption, distribution, metabolism, and excretion — **phar·ma·co·ki·net·ic** \-tik\ *adj*

phar·ma·col·o·gist \ˌfär-mə-ˈkä-lə-jist\ *n* : a specialist in pharmacology

phar·ma·col·o·gy \ˌfär-mə-ˈkä-lə-jē\ *n, pl* **-gies** **1** : the science of drugs including their origin, composition, pharmacokinetics, therapeutic use, and toxicology **2** : the properties and reactions of drugs esp. with relation to their therapeutic value — **phar·ma·co·log·i·cal** \-kə-ˈlä-ji-kəl\ *also* **phar·ma·co·log·ic** \-jik\ *adj* — **phar·ma·co·log·i·cal·ly** *adv*

phar·ma·co·poe·ia *or* **phar·ma·co·pe·ia** \ˌfär-mə-kə-ˈpē-ə\ *n* **1** : a book describing drugs, chemicals, and medicinal preparations; *esp* : one issued by an officially recognized authority and serving as a standard **2** : a collection or stock of drugs — **phar·ma·co·poe·ial** *or* **phar·ma·co·pe·ial** \-əl\ *adj*

phar·ma·co·ther·a·peu·tic \-ˌther-ə-ˈpyü-tik\ *adj* : of or relating to pharmacotherapeutics or pharmacotherapy ⟨a ~ agent⟩

phar·ma·co·ther·a·peu·tics \-tiks\ *n sing or pl* : the study of the therapeutic uses and effects of drugs

phar·ma·co·ther·a·py \ˌfär-mə-kō-ˈther-ə-pē\ *n, pl* **-pies** : the treatment of disease and esp. mental illness with drugs

phar·ma·co·vig·i·lance \-ˈvi-jə-lən(t)s\ *n* : the monitoring, evaluation, and prevention of adverse effects associated with the administration of medicines

phar·ma·cy \ˈfär-mə-sē\ *n, pl* **-cies** **1** : the art, practice, or profession of preparing, preserving, compounding, and dispensing medical drugs **2 a** : a place where medicines are compounded or dispensed **b** : DRUGSTORE **3** : PHARMACOPOEIA 2

Pharm. D. *abbr* doctor of pharmacy

pharyng- *or* **pharyngo-** *comb form* **1** : pharynx ⟨*pharyng*itis⟩ **2** : pharyngeal and ⟨*pharyngo*esophageal⟩

pha·ryn·geal \ˌfar-ən-ˈjē-əl; fə-ˈrin-jəl, -jē-əl\ *adj* **1** : relating to or located in the region of the pharynx **2 a** : innervating the pharynx esp. by contributing to the formation of the pharyngeal plexus ⟨the ~ branch of the vagus nerve⟩ **b** : supplying or draining the pharynx ⟨the ~ branch of the maxillary artery⟩

pharyngeal aponeurosis *n* : the middle or fibrous coat of the walls of the pharynx

pharyngeal arch *n* : BRANCHIAL ARCH

pharyngeal cavity *n* : the cavity of the pharynx that consists of a part continuous anteriorly with the nasal cavity by way of the nasopharynx, a part opening into the oral cavity by way of the isthmus of the fauces, and a part continuous posteriorly with the esophagus and opening into the larynx by way of the epiglottis

pharyngeal cleft *n* : BRANCHIAL CLEFT

pharyngeal plexus *n* : a plexus formed by branches of the glossopharyngeal, vagus, and sympathetic nerves supplying the muscles and mucous membrane of the pharynx and adjoining parts

pharyngeal pouch *n* : any of a series of evaginations of ectoderm on either side of the pharynx that meet the corresponding external furrows and give rise to the branchial clefts of the vertebrate embryo

pharyngeal tonsil *n* : a mass of lymphoid tissue at the back of the pharynx between the eustachian tubes that is usu. best developed in young children, is commonly atrophied in the adult, and is markedly subject to hypertrophy and adenoid formation esp. in children — called also *nasopharyngeal tonsil*

phar·yn·gec·to·my \ˌfar-ən-ˈjek-tə-mē\ *n, pl* **-mies** : surgical removal of a part of the pharynx

pharyngis — see CONSTRICTOR PHARYNGIS INFERIOR, CONSTRICTOR PHARYNGIS MEDIUS, CONSTRICTOR PHARYNGIS SUPERIOR

phar·yn·gi·tis \ˌfar-ən-ˈjī-təs\ *n, pl* **-git·i·des** \-ˈji-tə-ˌdēz\ : inflammation of the pharynx (as from bacterial infection)

pharyngo- — see PHARYNG-

pha·ryn·go·con·junc·ti·val fever \fə-ˌriŋ-gō-ˌkän-ˌjəŋk-ˈtī-vəl-\ *n* : an acute epidemic illness caused by various adenoviruses of the genus *Mastadenovirus* (esp. serotypes of species *Human adenovirus B, Human adenovirus C,* and *Human adenovirus E*) that usu. affects children of school age and is typically characterized by fever, pharyngitis, and conjunctivitis

pha·ryn·go–epi·glot·tic fold \fə-ˌriŋ-gō-ˌe-pə-ˈglä-tik-\ *n* : either of two folds of mucous membrane extending from the base of the tongue to the epiglottis with one on each side of the midline

pha·ryn·go·esoph·a·ge·al \-i-ˌsä-fə-ˈjē-əl\ *adj* : of or relating to the pharynx and the esophagus

pharyngoesophageal diverticulum *n* : ZENKER'S DIVERTICULUM

pha·ryn·go·lar·yn·gec·to·my \fə-ˌriŋ-gō-ˌlar-ən-ˈjek-tə-mē\ *n, pl* **-mies** : surgical excision of the hypopharynx and larynx

pha·ryn·go·pal·a·tine arch \-ˈpa-lə-ˌtīn-\ *n* : PALATOPHARYNGEAL ARCH

pha·ryn·go·plas·ty \fə-ˈriŋ-gō-ˌplas-tē\ *n, pl* **-ties** : plastic surgery performed on the pharynx

phar·yn·gos·to·my \ˌfar-iŋ-ˈgäs-tə-mē\ *n, pl* **-mies** : surgical formation of an artificial opening into the pharynx

phar·yn·got·o·my \ˌfar-iŋ-ˈgä-tə-mē\ *n, pl* **-mies** : surgical incision into the pharynx

pha·ryn·go·ton·sil·li·tis \fə-ˌriŋ-gō-ˌtän-sə-ˈlī-təs\ *n* : inflammation of the pharynx and the tonsils

pha·ryn·go·tym·pan·ic tube \-tim-ˈpa-nik-\ *n* : EUSTACHIAN TUBE

phar·ynx \ˈfar-iŋks\ *n, pl* **pha·ryn·ges** \fə-ˈrin-(ˌ)jēz\ *also* **phar·ynx·es** : the part of the digestive and respiratory tracts situated between the cavity of the mouth and the esophagus and in humans being a conical musculomembranous tube about four and a half inches (11.43 centimeters) long that is continuous above with the mouth and nasal passages, communicates through the eustachian tubes with the ears, and extends downward past the opening into the larynx to the lower border of the cricoid cartilage where it is continuous with the esophagus — see LARYNGOPHARYNX, NASOPHARYNX, OROPHARYNX

phase \ˈfāz\ *n* **1** : a particular appearance or state in a regularly recurring cycle of changes **2** : a distinguishable part in a course, development, or cycle ⟨the early ∼*s* of a disease⟩ **3** : a point or stage in the period of a periodic motion or process (as a light wave or a vibration) in relation to an arbitrary reference or starting point in the period **4** : a homogeneous, physically distinct, and mechanically separable portion of matter present in a nonhomogeneous physicochemical system; *esp* : one of the fundamental states of matter usu. considered to include the solid, liquid, and gaseous forms

phase–contrast microscope *n* : a microscope that translates differences in phase of the light transmitted through or reflected by the object into differences of intensity in the image — **phase–contrast microscopy** *n*

-pha•sia \ˈfā-zhə, -zhē-ə\ *also* **-pha•sy** \fə-sē\ *n comb form, pl* **-phasias** *also* **-phasies** : speech disorder (of a specified type) ⟨dys*phasia*⟩

PhD \ˌpē-(ˌ)āch-ˈdē\ *abbr or n* **1** : an earned academic degree conferring the rank and title of doctor of philosophy **2** : a person who has a doctor of philosophy

Phe *abbr* phenylalanine

phe•na•caine \ˈfē-nə-ˌkān, ˈfe-\ *n* : a crystalline base that has been used as a local anesthetic in the form of its hydrochloride $C_{18}H_{22}N_2O_2·HCl$

phen•ac•e•tin \fi-ˈnas-ə-tən\ *n* : a compound $C_{10}H_{13}NO_2$ formerly used to ease pain or fever but now withdrawn from use because of its link to high blood pressure, heart attacks, cancer, and kidney disease — called also *acetophenetidin*

phe•naz•o•cine \fi-ˈna-zə-ˌsēn\ *n* : a drug $C_{22}H_{27}NO$ related to morphine that has greater pain-relieving and slighter narcotic effect

phen•a•zone \ˈfe-nə-ˌzōn\ *n* : ANTIPYRINE

phen•cy•cli•dine \ˌfen-ˈsi-klə-ˌdēn, -ˈsī-, -dən\ *n* : a piperidine derivative used chiefly in the form of its hydrochloride $C_{17}H_{25}N·HCl$ esp. as a veterinary anesthetic and sometimes illicitly as a psychedelic drug to induce vivid mental imagery — called also *angel dust, PCP*

phen•el•zine \ˈfen-ᵊl-ˌzēn\ *n* : a monoamine oxidase inhibitor $C_8H_{12}N_2$ that suppresses REM sleep and is used esp. as an antidepressant drug — see NARDIL

Phen•er•gan \fe-ˈnər-ˌgan\ *trademark* — used for a preparation of the hydrochloride of promethazine

phe•neth•i•cil•lin \fi-ˌne-thə-ˈsi-lən\ *n* : a semisynthetic penicillin administered orally in the form of its potassium salt $C_{17}H_{19}KN_2O_5S$ and used esp. in the treatment of less severe infections caused by bacteria that do not produce beta-lactamase

phen•eth•yl alcohol \fe-ˈne-thəl-\ *n* : PHENYLETHYL ALCOHOL

phen•eth•yl•amine *var of* PHENYLETHYLAMINE

phen-fen \ˈfen-ˌfen\ *n* : FEN-PHEN

phen•for•min \fen-ˈfȯr-mən\ *n* : a compound $C_{10}H_{15}N_5$ formerly used to treat diabetes but now withdrawn from use because of its link to life-threatening lactic acidosis

phen•in•di•one \ˌfen-in-ˈdī-ˌōn\ *n* : an anticoagulant drug $C_{15}H_{10}O_2$

phen•ip•ra•zine \fe-ˈni-prə-ˌzēn\ *n* : a monoamine oxidase inhibitor $C_9H_{14}N_2$

phen•ir•amine \fe-ˈnir-ə-ˌmēn, -mən\ *n* : a drug used in the form of its maleate $C_{16}H_{20}N_2·C_4H_4O_4$ as an antihistamine

phen•met•ra•zine \fen-ˈme-trə-ˌzēn\ *n* : a sympathomimetic stimulant used in the form of its hydrochloride $C_{11}H_{15}NO·HCl$ as an appetite suppressant — see PRELUDIN

phe•no•barb \ˈfē-nō-ˌbärb\ *n* : PHENOBARBITAL; *also* : a pill containing phenobarbital

phe•no•bar•bi•tal \ˌfē-nō-ˈbär-bə-ˌtȯl\ *n* : a crystalline barbiturate $C_{12}H_{12}N_2O_3$ that is used orally or is administered by injection in the form of its sodium salt $C_{12}H_{11}N_2NaO_3$ as a hypnotic and sedative — see LUMINAL

phe•no•bar•bi•tone \-bə-ˌtōn\ *n, chiefly Brit* : PHENOBARBITAL

phe•no•copy \ˈfē-nə-ˌkä-pē\ *n, pl* **-copies** : a phenotypic variation that is caused by unusual environmental conditions and resembles the normal expression of a genotype other than its own

phe•nol \ˈfē-ˌnōl, -ˌnȯl, fi-ˈ\ *n* **1** : a corrosive poisonous crystalline acidic compound C_6H_5OH present in coal tar that is used in the manufacture of some pharmaceuticals and as a topical anesthetic in dilute solution — called also *carbolic, carbolic acid* **2** : any of various acidic compounds analogous to phenol — **phe•no•lic** \fi-ˈnō-lik, -ˈnä-\ *adj*

phe•nol•phtha•lein \ˌfēn-ᵊl-ˈtha-lē-ən, -ˈtha-ˌlēn, -ˈthā-\ *n* : a white or yellowish-white crystalline compound $C_{20}H_{14}O_4$ used in analysis as an indicator because its solution is brilliant red in alkalies and is decolorized by acids and in medicine as a laxative

phenol red *n* : PHENOLSULFONPHTHALEIN

phe•nol•sul•fon•phtha•lein \ˌfēn-ᵊl-ˌsəl-fän-ˈtha-lē-ən, -ˈtha-ˌlēn, -ˈthā-\ *n* : a red crystalline compound $C_{19}H_{14}O_5S$ used chiefly as a test of kidney function and as an acid-base indicator

phenolsulfonphthalein test *n* : a test in which phenolsulfonphthalein is administered by injection and urine samples are subsequently taken at regular intervals to measure the rate at which it is excreted by the kidneys

phe·nom·e·non \fi-ˈnä-mə-ˌnän, -nən\ *n, pl* **-na** \-nə, -ˌnä\ **1 :** an observable fact or event **2 a :** an object or aspect known through the senses rather than by thought or intuition **b :** a fact or event of scientific interest susceptible of scientific description and explanation

phe·no·thi·azine \ˌfē-nō-ˈthī-ə-ˌzēn\ *n* **1 :** a greenish-yellow crystalline compound $C_{12}H_9NS$ used as an anthelmintic and insecticide esp. in veterinary practice **2 :** any of various phenothiazine derivatives (as chlorpromazine) that are used as tranquilizing agents esp. in the treatment of schizophrenia

phe·no·type \ˈfē-nə-ˌtīp\ *n* **:** the observable properties of an organism that are produced by the interaction of the genotype and the environment — compare GENOTYPE — **phe·no·typ·ic** \ˌfē-nə-ˈti-pik\ *also* **phe·no·typ·i·cal** \-pi-kəl\ *adj* — **phe·no·typ·i·cal·ly** *adv*

phe·noxy·ben·za·mine \fi-ˌnäk-sē-ˈben-zə-ˌmēn\ *n* **:** a drug that blocks the activity of alpha-receptors and is used in the form of its hydrochloride $C_{18}H_{22}ClNO{\cdot}HCl$ esp. to treat hypertension and sweating due to pheochromocytoma

phe·noxy·meth·yl penicillin \-ˈmeth-ᵊl-\ *n* **:** PENICILLIN V

phen·pro·cou·mon \ˌfen-prō-ˈkü-ˌmän\ *n* **:** an anticoagulant drug $C_{18}H_{16}O_3$

phen·sux·i·mide \ˌfen-ˈsək-si-ˌmīd\ *n* **:** an anticonvulsant drug $C_{11}H_{11}NO_2$ sometimes used in the treatment of absence seizures

phen·ter·mine \ˈfen-tər-ˌmēn\ *n* **:** an anorectic drug administered in the form of its hydrochloride $C_{10}H_{15}N{\cdot}HCl$ to treat obesity

phen·tol·amine \fen-ˈtä-lə-ˌmēn, -mən\ *n* **:** a drug that blocks the activity of alpha-receptors and is administered by injection in the form of its mesylate $C_{17}H_{19}N_3O{\cdot}CH_4O_3S$ esp. in the diagnosis and treatment of hypertension due to pheochromocytoma — see REGITINE

phe·nyl \ˈfen-ᵊl, ˈfēn-\ *n* **:** a monovalent chemical group C_6H_5 derived from benzene — often used in combination ⟨*phenyl*alanine⟩

phe·nyl·al·a·nine \ˌfen-ᵊl-ˈa-lə-ˌnēn, ˌfēn-\ *n* **:** an essential amino acid $C_9H_{11}NO_2$ that is obtained in its levorotatory L-form by the hydrolysis of proteins (as lactalbumin), that is essential in human nutrition, and that is converted in the normal body to tyrosine — abbr. *Phe;* see PHENYLKETONURIA, PHENYLPYRUVIC ACID

phenylalanine mustard *or* **L-phenylalanine mustard** \ˈel-\ *n* **:** MELPHALAN

phen·yl·bu·ta·zone \ˌfen-ᵊl-ˈbyü-tə-ˌzōn\ *n* **:** a drug $C_{19}H_{20}N_2O_2$ that is used for its analgesic and anti-inflammatory properties esp. in the treatment of arthritis, gout, and bursitis — see BUTAZOLIDIN

phen·yl·eph·rine \ˌfen-ᵊl-ˈe-ˌfrēn, -frən\ *n* **:** a sympathomimetic agent with vasoconstrictive properties that is used in the form of its hydrochloride $C_9H_{13}NO_2{\cdot}HCl$ esp. as a nasal decongestant and mydriatic and to raise blood pressure — see ACTIFED, NEO-SYNEPHRINE

phe·nyl·eth·yl alcohol \ˌfen-ᵊl-ˈeth-ᵊl-, ˌfēn-\ *n* **:** a fragrant liquid alcohol $C_8H_{10}O$ that is used as an antibacterial preservative esp. in ophthalmic solutions with limited effectiveness

phe·nyl·eth·yl·amine \ˌfen-ᵊl-ˌeth-ᵊl-ˈa-ˌmēn, ˌfēn-\ *or* **phen·eth·yl·amine** \ˌfen-ˌeth-əl-ˈam-ˌēn\ *n* **:** a neurotransmitter $C_8H_{11}N$ that is an amine resembling amphetamine in structure and pharmacological properties; *also* **:** any of its derivatives

phe·nyl·ke·ton·uria \ˌfen-ᵊl-ˌkē-tə-ˈnu̇r-ē-ə, ˌfēn-, -ˈnyu̇r-\ *n* **:** a metabolic disorder that is caused by an enzyme deficiency resulting in the accumulation of phenylalanine and its metabolites (as phenylpyruvic acid) in the blood and their excess excretion in the urine, that is inherited as an autosomal recessive trait, and that causes usu. severe intellectual disability, seizures, eczema, and abnormal body odor unless phenylalanine is restricted from the diet beginning at birth — abbr. *PKU*

[1]**phe·nyl·ke·ton·uric** \-ˈnu̇r-ik, -ˈnyu̇r-\ *n* **:** a person affected with phenylketonuria

[2]**phenylketonuric** *adj* **:** of, relating to, or affected with phenylketonuria ⟨~ siblings⟩

phen·yl·mer·cu·ric \ˌfen-ᵊl-mər-ˈkyu̇r-ik\ *adj* **:** being a salt containing the positively charged ion $[C_6H_5Hg]^+$

phenylmercuric acetate *n* **:** a crystalline salt $C_8H_8HgO_2$ used chiefly as a fungicide and herbicide

phenylmercuric nitrate *n* **:** a crystalline basic salt that is a mixture of $C_6H_5HgNO_3$ and C_6H_5HgOH and that is used chiefly as a fungicide and antiseptic

phen·yl·pro·pa·nol·amine \ˌfen-ᵊl-ˌprō-pə-ˈnō-lə-ˌmēn, -ˈnō-; -nō-ˈla-ˌmēn\ *n* **:** a sympathomimetic drug that has been used in the form of its hydrochloride $C_9H_{13}NO{\cdot}HCl$ esp. as a nasal decongestant and appetite suppressant but has been largely withdrawn from use because of its link to hemorrhagic stroke — abbr. *PPA*

phe·nyl·py·ru·vic acid \ˌfen-ᵊl-pī-ˈrü-vik-, ˌfēn-\ *n* **:** a crystalline keto acid $C_9H_8O_3$ found in the urine as a metabolic product of phenylalanine esp. in phenylketonuria

phenyl salicylate *n* **:** a crystalline ester $C_{13}H_{10}O_3$ used as a sunscreen to absorb ultraviolet light and also as an analgesic and antipyretic — called also *salol*

phen·yl·thio·car·ba·mide \ˌfen-ᵊl-ˌthī-ō-ˈkär-bə-ˌmīd\ *n* : a compound $C_7H_8N_2S$ that is extremely bitter or tasteless depending on the presence or absence of a single dominant gene in the taster — called also *PTC*

phen·yl·thio·urea \-ˌthī-ō-yu̇-ˈrē-ə\ *n* : PHENYLTHIOCARBAMIDE

phe·nyt·o·in \fə-ˈni-tə-wən\ *n* : an anticonvulsant used often in the form of its sodium salt $C_{15}H_{11}N_2NaO_2$ to prevent or treat seizures — called also *diphenylhydantoin;* see DILANTIN

pheo·chro·mo·cy·to·ma \ˌfē-ə-ˌkrō-mə-sə-ˈtō-mə, -sī-\ *n, pl* **-mas** *also* **-ma·ta** \-mə-tə\ : a tumor that is derived from chromaffin cells and is usu. associated with paroxysmal or sustained hypertension

phe·re·sis \fə-ˈrē-səs\ *n, pl* **phe·re·ses** \-ˌsēz\ : APHERESIS

pher·o·mone \ˈfer-ə-ˌmōn\ *n* : a chemical substance that is produced by an animal and serves esp. as a stimulus to other individuals of the same species for one or more behavioral responses — **pher·o·mon·al** \ˌfer-ə-ˈmōn-ᵊl\ *adj*

PhG *abbr* graduate in pharmacy

phi·al \ˈfīl\ *n* : VIAL

Phi·a·loph·o·ra \ˌfī-ə-ˈlä-fə-rə\ *n* : a genus of imperfect fungi (family Dematiaceae) of which some forms are important in human mycotic infections (as chromoblastomycosis)

¹-phil \ˌfil\ *or* **-phile** \ˌfīl\ *n comb form* : lover : one having an affinity for or a strong attraction to ⟨acido*phil*⟩

²-phil *or* **-phile** *adj comb form* : loving : having a fondness or affinity for ⟨he*mophile*⟩

Philadelphia chromosome *n* : an abnormally short chromosome 22 that is found in the hematopoietic cells of persons affected with chronic myelogenous leukemia and lacks the major part of its long arm which has usu. undergone translocation to chromosome 9

-phil·ia \ˈfi-lē-ə\ *n comb form* **1** : tendency toward ⟨hemo*philia*⟩ **2** : abnormal appetite or liking for ⟨necro*philia*⟩

-phil·i·ac \ˈfi-lē-ˌak\ *n comb form* **1** : one having a tendency toward ⟨hemo*philiac*⟩ **2** : one having an abnormal appetite or liking for ⟨copro*philiac*⟩

-phil·ic \ˈfi-lik\ *adj comb form* : having an affinity for : loving ⟨acido*philic*⟩

phil·trum \ˈfil-trəm\ *n, pl* **phil·tra** \-trə\ : the vertical groove on the median line of the upper lip

phi·mo·sis \fī-ˈmō-səs, fi-\ *n, pl* **phi·mo·ses** \-ˌsēz\ : tightness or constriction of the orifice of the foreskin arising either congenitally or postnatally (as from balanoposthitis) and preventing retraction of the foreskin over the glans

phi phenomenon \ˈfī-\ *n* : apparent motion resulting from an orderly sequence of stimuli (as lights flashed in rapid succession a short distance apart on a sign) without any actual motion being presented to the eye

phleb- *or* **phlebo-** *comb form* : vein ⟨*phleb*itis⟩

phle·bi·tis \fli-ˈbī-təs\ *n, pl* **phle·bit·i·des** \-ˈbi-tə-ˌdēz\ : inflammation of a vein — **phle·bit·ic** \-ˈbi-tik\ *adj*

phle·bo·gram \ˈflē-bə-ˌgram\ *n* **1** : a tracing made with a sphygmograph that records the pulse in a vein **2** : a radiograph of a vein after injection of a radiopaque medium

phle·bo·graph \-ˌgraf\ *n* : a sphygmograph adapted for recording the venous pulse

phle·bog·ra·phy \fli-ˈbä-grə-fē\ *n, pl* **-phies** : the process of making phlebograms — **phle·bo·graph·ic** \ˌflē-bə-ˈgra-fik\ *adj*

phle·bo·lith \ˈflē-bə-ˌlith\ *n* : a calculus in a vein usu. resulting from the calcification of an old thrombus

phle·bol·o·gist \fli-ˈbä-lə-jist\ *n* : a specialist in phlebology

phle·bol·o·gy \fli-ˈbä-lə-jē\ *n, pl* **-gies** : a branch of medicine concerned with the veins

phle·bo·throm·bo·sis \ˌflē-bō-thräm-ˈbō-səs\ *n, pl* **-bo·ses** \-ˌsēz\ : venous thrombosis accompanied by little or no inflammation — compare THROMBOPHLEBITIS

phle·bot·o·mist \fli-ˈbä-tə-mist\ *n* : one who practices phlebotomy

phle·bot·o·mize \fli-ˈbä-tə-ˌmīz\ *vb* **-mized; -miz·ing** : to draw blood from : BLEED

phle·bot·o·mus \fli-ˈbä-tə-məs\ *n* **1** *cap* : a genus of small bloodsucking sand flies (family Psychodidae) including one (*P. papatasii*) that transmits sandfly fever and leishmaniasis **2** *pl* **-mi** \-ˌmī\ *also* **-mus·es** : any sand fly of the genus *Phlebotomus*

phlebotomus fever *n* : SANDFLY FEVER

phle·bot·o·my \fli-ˈbä-tə-mē\ *n, pl* **-mies** : the letting of blood (as by venipuncture) for transfusion, apheresis, diagnostic testing, or experimental procedures and widely used in the past to treat many types of disease but now limited to the treatment of only a few specific conditions (as hemochromatosis and polycythemia vera) — called also *venesection, venotomy*

Phle·bo·vi·rus \ˈflē-bə-ˌvī-rəs\ *n* : a genus of bunyaviruses including the causative agents of Rift Valley fever and sandfly fever

phlegm \ˈflem\ *n* : viscid mucus secreted in abnormal quantity in the respiratory passages

phleg·ma·sia \fleg-ˈmā-zhə, -zhē-ə\ *n, pl* **-siae** \-zhē, -zhē-ˌē\ : INFLAMMATION

phlegmasia al·ba do·lens \-ˈal-bə-ˈdō-ˌlenz\ *n* : MILK LEG

phlegmasia ce·ru·lea dolens \-sə-ˈrü-lē-ə-\ *n* : severe thrombophlebitis with extreme pain, edema, cyanosis, and possible ischemic necrosis

phleg·mon \ˈfleg-ˌmän\ *n* : purulent inflammation and infiltration of connective tissue — compare ABSCESS — **phleg·mon·ous** \ˈfleg-mə-nəs\ *adj*

phlor·e·tin \ˈflȯr-ət-ən, flə-ˈrēt-ᵊn\ *n* : a crystalline phenolic ketone $C_{15}H_{14}O_5$ that is a potent inhibitor of transport systems for sugars and anions

phlo·ri·zin *or* **phlo·rhi·zin** \ˈflōr-ə-zən, flə-ˈrīz-ᵊn\ *or* **phlo·rid·zin** \ˈflōr-əd-zən, flə-ˈrid-zən\ *n* : a glucoside $C_{21}H_{24}O_{10}$ used esp. in producing experimental diabetes in animals

phlyc·ten·u·lar \flik-ˈten-yə-lər\ *adj* : marked by or associated with phlyctenules ⟨~ conjunctivitis⟩

phlyc·te·nule \flik-ˈten-(ˌ)yül; ˈflik-tə-ˌnül, -ˌnyül\ *n* : a small vesicle or pustule; *esp* : one on the conjunctiva or cornea of the eye

PHN *abbr* public health nurse

-phobe \ˌfōb\ *n comb form* : one fearing or averse to (something specified) ⟨chromo*phobe*⟩

pho·bia \ˈfō-bē-ə\ *n* : an exaggerated and often disabling fear usu. inexplicable to the subject and having sometimes a logical but usu. an illogical or symbolic object, class of objects, or situation — compare COMPULSION, OBSESSION

-pho·bia \ˈfō-bē-ə\ *n comb form* **1** : abnormal fear of ⟨acro*phobia*⟩ **2** : intolerance or aversion for ⟨photo*phobia*⟩

pho·bi·ac \ˈfō-bē-ˌak\ *n* : PHOBIC

[1]**pho·bic** \ˈfō-bik\ *adj* : of, relating to, affected with, marked by, involving, or constituting a phobia ⟨~ disorders⟩ ⟨~ patients⟩

[2]**phobic** *n* : one who exhibits a phobia

-pho·bic \ˈfō-bik\ *or* **-ph·o·bous** \f-ə-bəs\ *adj comb form* **1** : having an aversion for or fear of ⟨agora*phobic*⟩ **2** : lacking affinity for ⟨hydro*phobic*⟩

phobic reaction *n* : a psychoneurosis in which the principal symptom is a phobia

pho·co·me·lia \ˌfō-kə-ˈmē-lē-ə\ *n* : a congenital deformity in which the limbs are extremely shortened so that the feet and hands arise close to the trunk — **pho·co·me·lic** \-ˈmē-lik\ *adj*

pho·com·e·lus \fō-ˈkä-mə-ləs\ *n, pl* **-li** \-ˌlī\ : an individual exhibiting phocomelia

phon \ˈfän\ *n* : the unit of loudness on a scale beginning at zero for the faintest audible sound and corresponding to the decibel scale of sound intensity with the number of phons of a given sound being equal to the decibels of a pure 1000-hertz tone judged by the average listener to be equal in loudness to the given sound

phon- *or* **phono-** *comb form* : sound : voice : speech : tone ⟨*phon*ation⟩

pho·na·tion \fō-ˈnā-shən\ *n* : the production of vocal sounds and esp. speech — **pho·nate** \ˈfō-ˌnāt\ *vb*

-pho·nia \ˈfō-nē-ə, ˈfōn-yə\ *or* **-pho·ny** \fə-nē\ *n comb form, pl* **-phonias** *or* **-phonies** : speech disorder (of a specified type esp. relating to phonation) ⟨dys*phonia*⟩

pho·no·car·dio·gram \ˌfō-nə-ˈkär-dē-ə-ˌgram\ *n* : a graphic record of heart sounds made by means of a phonocardiograph

pho·no·car·dio·graph \-ˌgraf\ *n* : an instrument used for producing a graphic record of heart sounds

pho·no·car·di·og·ra·phy \-ˌkär-dē-ˈä-grə-fē\ *n, pl* **-phies** : the recording of heart sounds by means of a phonocardiograph — **pho·no·car·dio·graph·ic** \-ˌkär-dē-ə-ˈgra-fik\ *adj*

pho·no·pho·bia \ˌfō-nə-ˈfō-bē-ə\ *n* **1** : pathological fear of sound or of speaking aloud **2** : an intolerance or hypersensitivity to sound

phor·bol \ˈfȯr-ˌbȯl, -ˌbōl\ *n* : an alcohol $C_{20}H_{28}O_6$ that is the parent compound of tumor-promoting esters occurring in croton oil

-pho·re·sis \fə-ˈrē-səs\ *n comb form, pl* **-pho·re·ses** \-ˌsēz\ : transmission ⟨electro*phoresis*⟩

pho·ria \ˈfō-rē-ə\ *n* : any of various tendencies of the lines of vision to deviate from the normal when binocular fusion of the retinal images is prevented

-pho·ria \ˈfor-ē-ə\ *n comb form* : bearing : state : tendency ⟨eu*phoria*⟩

-phor·ic \ˈfōr-ik\ *adj comb form* : having (such) a bearing or tendency ⟨thanato*phoric*⟩

Phor·mia \ˈfȯr-mē-ə\ *n* : a genus of dipteran flies (family Calliphoridae) including one (*P. regina*) causing myiasis in sheep

phos- *comb form* : light ⟨*phos*phene⟩

phos·gene \ˈfäz-ˌjēn\ *n* : a colorless gas $COCl_2$ of unpleasant odor that is a severe respiratory irritant and has been used in chemical warfare

phosph- *or* **phospho-** *comb form* : phosphoric acid : phosphate ⟨*phospho*lipid⟩

phos·pha·gen \ˈfäs-fə-jən, -ˌjen\ *n* : any of several phosphate compounds (as phosphocreatine) occurring esp. in muscle and releasing energy on hydrolysis of the phosphate

phos·pha·tase \ˈfäs-fə-ˌtās, -ˌtāz\ *n* : an enzyme that accelerates the hydrolysis and synthesis of organic esters of phosphoric acid and the transfer of phosphate groups to other compounds: **a** : ALKALINE PHOSPHATASE **b** : ACID PHOSPHATASE

phos·phate \ˈfäs-ˌfāt\ *n* **1 a** : a salt or ester of a phosphoric acid **b** : the negatively charged ion PO_4^{3-} having a chemical valence of three and derived from phosphoric acid H_3PO_4 **2** : an organic compound of phosphoric acid in which the acid group is bound to nitrogen or a carboxyl group in a way that permits useful energy to be released (as in metabolism)

phos·pha·tide \ˈfäs-fə-ˌtīd\ *n* : PHOSPHOLIPID

phos·pha·tid·ic acid \ˌfäs-fə-ˈti-dik-\ *n* : any of several acids $(RCOO)_2$-$C_3H_5OPO_3H_2$ that are formed from phosphatides and yield on hydrolysis two fatty-acid molecules RCOOH and one molecule each of glycerol and phosphoric acid

phos·pha·ti·dyl·cho·line \ˌfäs-fə-ˌtīd-ᵊl-ˈkō-ˌlēn, (ˌ)fäs-ˌfa-təd-ᵊl-\ *n* : LECITHIN

phos·pha·ti·dyl·eth·a·nol·amine \-ˌe-thə-ˈnä-lə-ˌmēn, -ˈnō-\ *n* : any of a group of phospholipids that occur esp. in blood plasma and in the white matter of the central nervous system — called also *cephalin*

phos·pha·ti·dyl·ser·ine \-ˈser-ˌēn\ *n* : a phospholipid found in mammalian cells

phos·pha·tu·ria \ˌfäs-fə-ˈtu̇r-ē-ə, -ˈtyu̇r-\ *n* : the excretion of excessive amounts of phosphate in the urine

phos·phene \ˈfäs-ˌfēn\ *n* : a sensation of light produced by stimulation of the retina (as by pressure on the eyeball when the lid is closed)

phospho- — see PHOSPH-

phos·pho·cre·atine \ˌfäs-(ˌ)fō-ˈkrē-ə-ˌtēn\ *n* : a compound $C_4H_{10}N_3O_5P$ of creatine and phosphoric acid that is found esp. in vertebrate muscle where it is an energy source for muscle contraction — called also *creatine phosphate*

phos·pho·di·es·ter·ase \-dī-ˈes-tə-ˌrās, -ˌrāz\ *n* : a phosphatase that acts on compounds (as some nucleotides) having two ester groups to hydrolyze only one of the groups

phos·pho·di·es·ter bond \-dī-ˈes-tər-\ *n* : a covalent bond in RNA or DNA that holds a polynucleotide chain together by joining a phosphate group at position 5 in the pentose sugar of one nucleotide to the hydroxyl group at position 3 in the pentose sugar of the next nucleotide — called also *phosphodiester linkage*

phos·pho·enol·pyr·uvate \ˈfäs-ˌfō-ə-ˌnȯl-pī-ˈrü-ˌvāt, -nōl-, -ˌpir-ˈyü-\ *n* : a salt or ester of phosphoenolpyruvic acid

phos·pho·enol·pyr·uvic acid \-pī-ˈrü-vik-, -ˌpir-ˈyü-vik-\ *n* : a phosphate $H_2C{=}C(OPO_3H_2)COOH$ formed as an intermediate in carbohydrate metabolism

phos·pho·fruc·to·ki·nase \ˌfäs-(ˌ)fō-ˌfrək-tō-ˈkī-ˌnās, -ˌfrük-, -ˌfru̇k-, -ˌnāz\ *n* : an enzyme that functions in carbohydrate metabolism and esp. in glycolysis by catalyzing the transfer of a second phosphate (as from ATP) to fructose

phos·pho·glu·co·mu·tase \-ˌglü-kō-ˈmyü-ˌtās, -ˌtāz\ *n* : an enzyme that catalyzes the reversible isomerization of glucose-1-phosphate to glucose-6-phosphate

phos·pho·glu·co·nate \-ˈglü-kə-ˌnāt\ *n* : a compound formed by dehydrogenation of glucose-6-phosphate as the first step in a glucose degradation pathway alternative to the Krebs cycle

phosphogluconate dehydrogenase *n* : an enzyme that catalyzes the oxidative decarboxylation of phosphogluconate with the generation of NADPH

phos·pho·glyc·er·al·de·hyde \-ˌgli-sə-ˈral-də-ˌhīd\ *n* : a phosphate of glyceraldehyde $C_3H_5O_3(H_2PO_3)$ that is formed esp. in anaerobic metabolism of carbohydrates by the splitting of a diphosphate of fructose

phos·pho·ino·si·tide \-i-ˈnō-sə-ˌtīd\ *n* : any of a group of inositol-containing derivatives of phosphatidic acid that do not contain nitrogen and are found in the brain

phos·pho·ki·nase \ˌfäs-fō-ˈkī-ˌnās, -ˌnāz\ *n* : KINASE

phos·pho·li·pase \-ˈlī-ˌpās, -ˌpāz\ *n* : any of several enzymes that hydrolyze lecithins or phosphatidylethanolamines — called also *lecithinase*

phos·pho·lip·id \-ˈli-pəd\ *n* : any of various phosphorus-containing lipids (as lecithins and phosphatidylethanolamines) that are derived from glycerol and are major constituents of the membranes of cells and intracellular organelles and vesicles — called also *phosphatide*

phos·pho·lip·in \-ˈli-pən\ *n* : PHOSPHOLIPID

phos·pho·mono·es·ter·ase \-ˌmä-nō-ˈes-tə-ˌrās, -ˌrāz\ *n* : a phosphatase that acts on esters (as glucose phosphate) containing only a single ester group

phos·pho·pro·tein \ˌfäs-fō-ˈprō-ˌtēn\ *n* : any of various proteins (as casein) that contain combined phosphoric acid

phosphor- *or* **phosphoro-** *comb form* : phosphoric acid ⟨*phosphoro*lysis⟩

phos·pho·ri·bo·syl·py·ro·phos·phate \ˌfäs-fō-ˌrī-bə-ˌsil-ˌpī-rō-ˈfäs-ˌfāt\ *n* : a substance that is formed enzymatically from ATP and the phosphate of ribose and that plays a fundamental role in nucleotide synthesis

phosphoribosyltransferase — see HYPOXANTHINE-GUANINE PHOSPHORIBOSYLTRANSFERASE

phos·pho·ric \fäs-ˈfȯr-ik, -ˈfär-; ˈfäs-fə-rik\ *adj* : of, relating to, or containing phosphorus esp. with a valence higher than in phosphorous compounds

phosphoric acid *n* **1** : a syrupy or deliquescent acid H_3PO_4 — called also *orthophosphoric acid* **2** : a compound consisting of phosphate groups linked directly to each other by oxygen

phos·pho·rol·y·sis \ˌfäs-fə-ˈrä-lə-səs\ *n, pl* **-y·ses** \-ˌsēz\ : a reversible reaction analogous to hydrolysis in which phosphoric acid functions in a manner similar to that of water with the formation of a phosphate (as glucose-1-phosphate in the breakdown of liver glycogen) — **phos•pho•ro•lyt•ic** \-rō-ˈli-tik\ *adj*

phos•pho•rous \ˈfäs-fə-rəs, fäs-ˈfōr-əs\ *adj* : of, relating to, or containing phosphorus esp. with a valence lower than in phosphoric compounds

phos•pho•rus \ˈfäs-fə-rəs\ *n, often attrib* : a nonmetallic element that occurs widely in combined form esp. as inorganic phosphates in minerals, soils, natural waters, bones, and teeth and as organic phosphates in all living cells — symbol *P;* see ELEMENT table

phosphorus 32 *n* : a heavy radioactive isotope of phosphorus having a mass number of 32 and a half-life of 14.3 days that is produced in nuclear reactors and used chiefly in tracer studies (as in biology and in chemical analysis) and in medical diagnosis (as in location of tumors) — symbol P^{32} or ^{32}P

phos•phor•y•lase \fäs-ˈfȯr-ə-ˌlāz\ *n* : any of a group of enzymes that catalyze phosphorolysis with the formation of organic phosphates (as glucose-1-phosphate in the breakdown and synthesis of glycogen)

phos•phor•y•la•tion \ˌfäs-ˌfȯr-ə-ˈlā-shən\ *n* : the process by which a chemical compound takes up or combines with phosphoric acid or a phosphorus-containing group; *esp* : the enzymatic conversion of carbohydrates into their phosphoric esters in metabolic processes — **phos•phor•y•late** \fäs-ˈfȯr-ə-ˌlāt\ *vb* — **phos•phor•y•la•tive** \fäs-ˌfȯr-ə-ˈlā-tiv\ *adj*

phos•pho•ryl•cho•line \ˌfäs-fə-ˌril-ˈkō-ˌlēn\ *n* : a hapten used medicinally in the form of its chloride $C_5H_{15}ClNO_4P$ to treat hepatobiliary dysfunction

phos•pho•trans•fer•ase \ˌfäs-fō-ˈtrans-(ˌ)fər-ˌās, -ˌāz\ *n* : any of several enzymes that catalyze the transfer of phosphorus-containing groups from one compound to another

phos•sy jaw \ˈfä-sē-\ *n* : a jawbone destroyed by chronic phosphorus poisoning

phot- *or* **photo-** *comb form* : light : radiant energy ⟨*photo*dermatitis⟩

pho•tic \ˈfō-tik\ *adj* : of, relating to, or involving light esp. in relation to organisms — **pho•ti•cal•ly** *adv*

pho•to•ac•ti•va•tion \ˌfō-tō-ˌak-tə-ˈvā-shən\ *n* : the process of activating a substance by means of radiant energy and esp. light — **pho•to•ac•ti•vate** \-ˈak-tə-ˌvāt\ *vb*

pho•to•ac•tive \-ˈak-tiv\ *adj* : physically or chemically responsive to radiant energy and esp. to light — **pho•to•ac•tiv•i•ty** \-ak-ˈti-və-tē\ *n*

pho•to•ag•ing \ˌfō-tō-ˈā-jiŋ\ *n* : the cumulative detrimental effects (as wrinkles or dark spots) on skin that result from long-term exposure to sunlight and esp. ultraviolet light — **pho•to•aged** \-ˈājd\ *adj*

pho•to•al•ler•gic \ˌfō-tō-ə-ˈlər-jik\ *adj* : of, relating to, caused by, or affected with a photoallergy ⟨~ dermatitis⟩

pho•to•al•ler•gy \-ˈa-lər-jē\ *n, pl* **-gies** : an allergic sensitivity to light

pho•to•bi•ol•o•gy \-(ˌ)bī-ˈä-lə-jē\ *n, pl* **-gies** : a branch of biology that deals with the effects of radiant energy (as light) on living things — **pho•to•bi•ol•o•gist** \ˌfō-tō-(ˌ)bī-ˈä-lə-jist\ *n*

pho•to•chem•i•cal \ˌfō-tō-ˈke-mi-kəl\ *adj* : of, relating to, or resulting from the chemical action of radiant energy and esp. light ⟨~ smog⟩

pho•to•che•mo•ther•a•py \-ˌkē-mō-ˈther-ə-pē\ *n, pl* **-pies** : treatment esp. for psoriasis in which administration of a photosensitizing drug (as psoralen) is followed by exposure to ultraviolet radiation or sunlight

[1]**pho•to•chro•mic** \ˌfō-tə-ˈkrō-mik\ *adj* **1** : capable of changing color on exposure to radiant energy (as light) ⟨eyeglasses with ~ lenses⟩ **2** : of, relating to, or utilizing the change of color shown by a photochromic substance ⟨a ~ process⟩ — **pho•to•chro•mism** \-ˌmi-zəm\ *n*

[2]**photochromic** *n* : a photochromic substance — usu. used in pl.

pho•to•co•ag•u•la•tion \-kō-ˌa-gyə-ˈlā-shən\ *n* : a surgical process of coagulating tissue by means of a precisely oriented high-energy light source (as a laser beam) — **pho•to•co•ag•u•la•tor** \-kō-ˈa-gyə-ˌlā-tər\ *n*

pho•to•con•vul•sive \ˌfō-tō-kən-ˈvəl-siv\ *adj* : of, relating to, being, or marked by an abnormal electroencephalographic response to a flickering light

pho•to•dam•age \-ˈda-mij\ *n* : damage (as to skin or DNA) caused by exposure to ultraviolet radiation — **pho•to•dam•aged** \-mijd\ *adj*

pho•to•der•ma•ti•tis \-ˌdər-mə-ˈtī-təs\ *n, pl* **-ti•tis•es** *or* **-tit•i•des** \-ˈti-tə-ˌdēz\ : any dermatitis caused or precipitated by exposure to light

pho•to•der•ma•to•sis \-ˌdər-mə-ˈtō-səs\ *n, pl* **-to•ses** \-ˌsēz\ : any dermatosis produced by exposure to light

pho•to•dy•nam•ic \-dī-ˈna-mik\ *adj* : of, relating to, or having the property of intensifying or inducing a toxic reaction to light (as the destruction of cancer cells stained with a light-sensitive dye) in a living system ⟨~ therapy⟩

pho•to•flu•o•rog•ra•phy \-(ˌ)flu̇-ə-ˈrä-grə-fē\ *n, pl* **-phies** : the photography of the image produced on a fluorescent screen by X-rays — **pho•to•flu•o•ro•graph•ic** \-ˌflu̇r-ə-ˈgra-fik\ *adj*

Pho•to•frin \ˈfō-tə-frin\ *trademark* — used for a preparation of porfimer sodium

pho•to•gen•ic \ˌfō-tə-ˈje-nik\ *adj* **1** : produced or precipitated by light ⟨~ dermatitis⟩ **2** : producing or generating light ⟨~ bacteria⟩

pho·to·ker·a·ti·tis \ˌfō-tō-ˌker-ə-ˈti-təs\ *n, pl* **-tit·i·des** \-ˈti-tə-ˌdēz\ : keratitis of the cornea caused by exposure to ultraviolet radiation

pho·tom·e·ter \fō-ˈtä-mə-tər\ *n* : an instrument for measuring the intensity of light

pho·to·mi·cro·graph \ˌfō-tə-ˈmī-krə-ˌgraf\ *n* : a photograph of a microscopic image — called also *microphotograph* — **pho·to·mi·cro·graph·ic** \-ˌmī-krə-ˈgra-fik\ *adj* — **pho·to·mi·cro·graph·i·cal·ly** *adv* — **pho·to·mi·crog·ra·phy** \-mī-ˈkrä- grə-fē\ *n*

pho·ton \ˈfō-ˌtän\ *n* **1** : a unit of intensity of light at the retina equal to the illumination received per square millimeter of a pupillary area from a surface having a brightness of one candela per square meter — called also *troland* **2** : a quantum of electromagnetic radiation — **pho·ton·ic** \fō-ˈtä-nik\ *adj*

pho·to·patch test \ˈfō-tō-ˌpach-\ *n* : a test of the capability of a particular substance to photosensitize a particular human skin in which the substance is applied to the skin under a patch and the area is irradiated with ultraviolet light

pho·to·phe·re·sis \ˌfō-to-fə-ˈrē-səs\ *n* : an immunomodulating therapy used esp. to treat cutaneous T-cell lymphomas that involves treating blood with a photoactive drug (as methoxsalen), obtaining a fraction rich in white blood cells, exposing the fraction to damaging ultraviolet radiation, and returning it to the body where it stimulates a therapeutic immunological response

pho·to·pho·bia \ˌfō-tə-ˈfō-bē-ə\ *n* **1** : intolerance to light; *esp* : painful sensitiveness to strong light **2** : an abnormal fear of light — **pho·to·pho·bic** \-ˈfō-bik\ *adj*

phot·oph·thal·mia \ˌfōt-ˌäf-ˈthal-mē-ə, -ˌäp-\ *n* : inflammation of the eye and esp. of the cornea and conjunctiva caused by exposure to light of short wavelength (as ultraviolet light)

phot·opic \fōt-ˈō-pik, -ˈä-\ *adj* : relating to or being vision in bright light with light-adapted eyes that is mediated by the cones of the retina

pho·to·pig·ment \ˈfō-tō-ˌpig-mənt\ *n* : a pigment (as a compound in the retina) that undergoes a physical or chemical change under the action of light

pho·top·sia \fō-ˈtäp-sē-ə\ *n* : the perception of light (as luminous rays or flashes) that is purely subjective and accompanies a pathological condition esp. of the retina or brain

pho·to·re·cep·tor \ˌfō-tō-ri-ˈsep-tər\ *n* : a receptor for light stimuli

pho·to·re·frac·tive keratectomy \-ri-ˌfrak-tiv-\ *n* : surgical ablation of part of the corneal surface using an excimer laser in order to correct for myopia — abbr. *PRK;* compare RADIAL KERATOTOMY

pho·to·scan \ˈfō-tō-ˌskan\ *n* : a photographic representation of variation in tissue state (as of the kidney) determined by gamma ray emission from an injected radioactive substance — **photoscan** *vb*

pho·to·sen·si·tive \ˌfō-tō-ˈsen-sə-tiv\ *adj* **1** : sensitive or sensitized to the action of radiant energy **2** : being or caused by an abnormal reaction to sunlight ⟨~ rashes⟩ — **pho·to·sen·si·tiv·i·ty** \-ˌsen-sə-ˈti-və-tē\ *n*

pho·to·sen·si·tize \-ˈsen-sə-ˌtīz\ *vb* **-tized; -tiz·ing** : to make sensitive to the influence of radiant energy and esp. light — **pho·to·sen·si·ti·za·tion** \-ˌsen-sə-tə-ˈzā-shən\ *n* — **pho·to·sen·si·tiz·er** *n*

pho·to·syn·the·sis \-ˈsin-thə-səs\ *n, pl* **-the·ses** \-ˌsēz\ : the formation of carbohydrates from carbon dioxide and a source of hydrogen (as water) in chlorophyll-containing cells (as of green plants) exposed to light — **pho·to·syn·the·size** \-ˌsīz\ *vb* — **pho·to·syn·thet·ic** \-sin-ˈthe-tik\ *adj*

pho·to·ther·a·py \-ˈther-ə-pē\ *n, pl* **-pies** : the application of light for therapeutic purposes

pho·to·tox·ic \ˌfō-tō-ˈtäk-sik\ *adj* **1** : rendering the skin susceptible to damage (as sunburn or blisters) upon exposure to light and esp. ultraviolet light ⟨~ antibiotics⟩ **2** : induced by a phototoxic substance ⟨a ~ response⟩ — **pho·to·tox·ic·i·ty** \-täk-ˈsi-sə-tē\ *n*

PHR *abbr* personal health record

phren- *or* **phreno-** *comb form* **1** : mind ⟨*phreno*logy⟩ **2** : diaphragm ⟨*phren*ic⟩

phren·em·phrax·is \ˌfren-ˌem-ˈfrak-səs\ *n, pl* **-phrax·es** \-ˌsēz\ : crushing of the phrenic nerve for therapeutic purposes

phreni- *comb form* : phrenic nerve ⟨*phreni*cotomy⟩

-phre·nia \ˈfrē-nē-ə, ˈfre-\ *n comb form* : disordered condition of mental functions ⟨hebe*phrenia*⟩

[1]**phren·ic** \ˈfre-nik\ *adj* : of or relating to the diaphragm

[2]**phrenic** *n* : PHRENIC NERVE

phrenic artery *n* : any of the several arteries supplying the diaphragm: **a** : either of two arising from the thoracic aorta and distributed over the upper surface of the diaphragm — called also *superior phrenic artery* **b** : either of two that arise from the abdominal aorta and that supply the underside of the diaphragm and the adrenal glands — called also *inferior phrenic artery*

phren·i·cec·to·my \ˌfre-nə-ˈsek-tə-mē\ *n, pl* **-mies** : surgical removal of part of a phrenic nerve to secure collapse of a diseased lung by paralyzing the diaphragm on one side — compare PHRENICOTOMY

phrenic nerve *n* : a nerve on each side of the body that arises chiefly from the fourth cervical nerve, passes down through the thorax to the diaphragm, and supplies or gives off branches supplying esp. the pericardium, pleura, and diaphragm — called also *phrenic*

phren•i•cot•o•my \ˌfre-ni-ˈkä-tə-mē\ *n, pl* **-mies** : surgical division of a phrenic nerve to secure collapse of a diseased lung by paralyzing the diaphragm on one side — compare PHRENICECTOMY

phrenic vein *n* : any of the veins that drain the diaphragm and accompany the phrenic arteries: **a** : one that accompanies the pericardiophrenic artery and usu. empties into the internal mammary vein — called also *superior phrenic vein* **b** : any of two or three veins which follow the course of the inferior phrenic arteries and of which the one on the right empties into the inferior vena cava and the one or two on the left empty into the left renal or suprarenal vein or the inferior vena cava — called also *inferior phrenic vein*

phreno- — see PHREN-

phre•nol•o•gy \fri-ˈnä-lə-jē\ *n, pl* **-gies** : the former study of the conformation of the skull based on the belief that it is indicative of mental attributes

phry•no•der•ma \ˌfrī-nə-ˈdər-mə\ *n* : a rough dry skin eruption marked by keratosis and usu. associated with vitamin A deficiency

PHS *abbr* Public Health Service

phthal•yl•sul•fa•thi•a•zole \ˌtha-ˌlil-ˌsəl-fə-ˈthī-ə-ˌzōl\ *n* : a sulfonamide $C_{17}H_{13}N_3O_5S_2$ used in the treatment of intestinal infections

phthi•ri•a•sis \thə-ˈrī-ə-səs, thī-\ *n, pl* **-a•ses** \-ˌsēz\ : PEDICULOSIS; *esp* : infestation with pubic lice

Phthir•i•us \ˈthir-ē-əs\ *n* : a genus of lice (family Pediculidae) containing the pubic louse (*P. pubis*)

Phthi•rus \ˈthī-rəs\ *n, syn of* PHTHIRIUS

phthi•sic \ˈti-zik, ˈtī-sik\ *n* : PHTHISIS — **phthisic** *or* **phthi•si•cal** \ˈti-zi-kəl, ˈtī-si-\ *adj*

phthisio- *comb form* : phthisis ⟨*phthisio*logy⟩

phthis•i•ol•o•gy \ˌti-zē-ˈä-lə-je, ˌthi-\ *n, pl* **-gies** : the care, treatment, and study of tuberculosis — **phthis•i•ol•o•gist** \-jist\ *n*

phthi•sis \ˈtī-səs, ˈthī, ˈti-, ˈthi-\ *n, pl* **phthi•ses** \-ˌsēz\ : a progressively wasting or consumptive condition; *esp* : pulmonary tuberculosis

phthisis bul•bi \-ˈbəl-ˌbī\ *n* : wasting and shrinkage of the eyeball following destructive diseases of the eye (as panophthalmitis)

phy•co•my•cete \ˌfī-kō-ˈmī-ˌsēt, -ˌmī-ˈsēt\ *n* : any of a group of lower fungi that are often grouped in a class (Phycomycetes) or separated into two subdivisions (Mastigomycotina and Zygomycotina)

phy•co•my•co•sis \-ˌmī-ˈkō-səs\ *n, pl* **-co•ses** \-ˈkō-ˌsēz\ : any mycosis caused by a phycomycete (as of the genera *Rhizopus* and *Mucor*)

phyl- *or* **phylo-** *comb form* : tribe : race : phylum ⟨*phylo*geny⟩

phyl•lode \ˈfi-ˌlōd\ *adj* : having a cross section that resembles a leaf ⟨~ tumors of the breast⟩

phyl•lo•qui•none \ˌfi-lō-kwi-ˈnōn, -ˈkwi-ˌnōn\ *n* : VITAMIN K 1a

phy•log•e•ny \fi-ˈlä-jə-nē\ *n, pl* **-nies** **1** : the evolutionary history of a kind of organism **2** : the evolution of a genetically related group of organisms as distinguished from the development of the individual organism — compare ONTOGENY — **phy•lo•ge•net•ic** \ˌfī-lō-jə-ˈne-tik\ *adj* — **phy•lo•ge•net•i•cal•ly** *adv*

phy•lum \ˈfī-ləm\ *n, pl* **phy•la** \-lə\ : a major group of animals or in some classifications plants sharing one or more fundamental characteristics that set them apart from all other animals and plants

phys *abbr* **1** physical **2** physician **3** physiological

phy•sa•lia \fī-ˈsā-lē-ə\ *n* **1** *cap* : a genus of large oceanic siphonophores (family Physaliidae) including the Portuguese man-of-wars **2** : any siphonophore of the genus *Physalia*

Phy•sa•lop•tera \ˌfī-sə-ˈläp-tə-rə, ˌfi-\ *n* : a large genus of nematode worms (family Physalopteridae) parasitic in the digestive tract of various vertebrates including humans

physes *pl of* PHYSIS

physi- *or* **physio-** *comb form* **1** : physical ⟨*physio*therapy⟩ **2** : physiological : physiological and ⟨*physio*pathologic⟩

phys•iat•rics \ˌfi-zē-ˈa-triks\ *n* : PHYSICAL MEDICINE AND REHABILITATION

phys•iat•rist \ˌfi-zē-ˈa-trist\ *n* : a physician who specializes in physical medicine and rehabilitation

phys•iat•ry \ˌfi-zē-ˈa-trē, fə-ˈzī-ə-trē\ *n* : PHYSICAL MEDICINE AND REHABILITATION

¹phys•ic \ˈfi-zik\ *n* **1 a** : the art or practice of healing disease **b** : the practice or profession of medicine **2** : a medicinal agent or preparation; *esp* : PURGATIVE

²physic *vb* **phys•icked; phys•ick•ing** : to treat with or administer medicine to; *esp* : PURGE

¹phys•i•cal \ˈfi-zi-kəl\ *adj* **1** : having material existence : perceptible esp. through the senses and subject to the laws of nature **2** : of or relating to the body — **phys•i•cal•ly** *adv*

²physical *n* : PHYSICAL EXAMINATION

physical examination *n* : an examination of the bodily functions and condition of an individual

physical medicine and rehabilitation *n* : a medical specialty concerned with the prevention, diagnosis, treatment, and management of disabling diseases, disorders, and injuries typically of a musculoskeletal, cardiovascular, neuromuscular, or neurological nature by physical means (as by the use of electromyography, electrotherapy, therapeutic exercise, or pharmaceutical pain control) — called also *physiatrics, physiatry, physical medicine*

physical sign *n* : an indication of bodily condition that can be directly perceived

physical therapist *n* : a person trained and licensed to practice physical therapy — called also *physiotherapist*

physical therapy *n* : therapy for the preservation, enhancement, or restoration of movement and physical function impaired or threatened by disability, injury, or disease that utilizes therapeutic exercise, physical modalities (as massage and electrotherapy), assistive devices, and patient education and training — called also *physiotherapy*

phy•si•cian \fə-ˈzi-shən\ *n* : a skilled health-care professional trained and licensed to practice medicine; *specif* : a doctor of medicine or osteopathy

physician assistant *also* **physician's assistant** *n* : a specially trained person who is certified to provide basic medical services (as the diagnosis and treatment of common ailments) usu. under the supervision of a licensed physician — called also *PA*

physician–assisted suicide *n* : suicide by a patient facilitated by means or information (as a drug prescription or indication of lethal dosage) provided by a physician

phys•i•co•chem•i•cal \ˌfi-zi-kō-ˈke-mi-kəl\ *adj* : being physical and chemical — **phys•i•co•chem•i•cal•ly** *adv*

physio- — see PHYSI-

phys•i•o•log•i•cal \ˌfi-zē-ə-ˈlä-ji-kəl\ *or* **phys•i•o•log•ic** \-jik\ *adj* **1** : of or relating to physiology **2** : characteristic of or appropriate to an organism's healthy or normal functioning **3** : differing in, involving, or affecting physiological factors ⟨a ~ strain of bacteria⟩ — **phys•i•o•log•i•cal•ly** *adv*

physiological chemistry *n* : a branch of science dealing with the chemical aspects of physiological and biological systems : BIOCHEMISTRY

physiological dead space *n* : the total dead space in the entire respiratory system including the alveoli — compare ANATOMICAL DEAD SPACE

physiological psychology *n* : PSYCHOPHYSIOLOGY

physiological saline *n* : a solution of a salt or salts that is essentially isotonic with tissue fluids or blood; *esp* : an approximately 0.9 percent solution of sodium chloride — called also *physiological saline solution, physiological salt solution*

phys•i•ol•o•gy \ˌfi-zē-ˈä-lə-jē\ *n, pl* **-gies** **1** : a branch of biology that deals with the functions and activities of life or of living matter (as organs, tissues, or cells) and of the physical and chemical phenomena involved — compare ANATOMY 1 **2** : the organic processes and phenomena of an organism or any of its parts or of a particular bodily process **3** : a treatise on physiology — **phys•i•ol•o•gist** \-jist\ *n*

phys•io•pa•thol•o•gy \ˌfi-zē-ō-pə-ˈthä-lə-jē, -pa-\ *n, pl* **-gies** : a branch of biology or medicine that combines physiology and pathology esp. in the study of altered bodily function in disease — **phys•io•path•o•log•ic** \-ˌpa-thə-ˈlä-jik\ *or* **phys•io•path•o•log•i•cal** \-ji-kəl\ *adj*

phys•io•ther•a•peu•tic \ˌfi-zē-ō-ˌther-ə-ˈpyü-tik\ *adj* : of or relating to physical therapy

phys•io•ther•a•pist \-ˈther-ə-pist\ *n* : PHYSICAL THERAPIST

phys•io•ther•a•py \ˌfi-zē-ō-ˈther-ə-pē\ *n, pl* **-pies** : PHYSICAL THERAPY

phy•sique \fi-ˈzēk\ *n* : the form or structure of a person's body : bodily makeup ⟨a muscular ~⟩

phy•sis \ˈfī-səs\ *n, pl* **phy•ses** \-ˌsēz\ : GROWTH PLATE

Phy•so•ceph•a•lus \ˌfī-sə-ˈse-fə-ləs\ *n* : a genus of nematode worms (family Thelaziidae) including an internal parasite (*P. sexalatus*) of swine

phy•so•stig•mine \ˌfī-sə-ˈstig-ˌmēn\ *n* : a crystalline alkaloid that is an anticholinesterase obtained from an African vine (*Physostigma venenosum*) of the legume family (Leguminosae) and is used parenterally in the form of its salicylate $C_{15}H_{21}N_3O_2 \cdot C_7H_6O_3$ esp. to reverse the toxic effects of an anticholinergic agent (as atropine) and topically in the form of its sulfate $(C_{15}H_{21}N_3O_2)_2 \cdot H_2SO_3$ as a miotic in the treatment of glaucoma — called also *eserine*

phyt- *or* **phyto-** *comb form* : plant ⟨*phyto*toxin⟩

phy•tan•ic acid \fī-ˈta-nik-\ *n* : a fatty acid that accumulates in the blood and tissues of patients affected with Refsum's disease

-phyte \ˌfīt\ *n comb form* **1** : plant having a (specified) characteristic or habitat ⟨sapro*phyte*⟩ **2** : pathological growth ⟨osteo*phyte*⟩

phy•tic acid \ˌfī-tik-\ *n* : an acid $C_6H_{18}P_6O_{24}$ that occurs in cereal grains and that when ingested interferes with the intestinal absorption of various minerals (as calcium and magnesium)

phy•to•be•zoar \ˌfī-tō-ˈbē-ˌzōr\ *n* : a concretion formed in the stomach or intestine and composed chiefly of undigested compacted vegetable fiber

phy•to•chem•i•cal \-ˈke-mi-kəl\ *n* : a chemical compound (as a carotenoid or phytosterol) occurring naturally in plants; *esp* : PHYTONUTRIENT

phy•to•es•tro•gen \-ˈes-trə-jən\ *n* : a chemical compound (as genistein) that occurs naturally in plants and has estrogenic properties

phy•to•hem•ag•glu•ti•nin \ˌfī-tō-ˌhē-mə-ˈglüt-ᵊn-ən\ *n* : a proteinaceous hemagglutinin of plant origin used esp. to induce mitosis (as in lymphocytes) — abbr. *PHA*

phy·to·na·di·one \ˌfī-tō-nə-ˈdī-ˌōn\ *n* : VITAMIN K 1a

phy·to·nu·tri·ent \-ˈnü-trē-ənt, -ˈnyü-\ *n* : a bioactive plant-derived compound (as resveratrol or sulforaphane) associated with positive health effects

phy·to·pho·to·der·ma·ti·tis \ˌfī-tō-ˌfō-tō-ˌdər-mə-ˈtī-təs\ *n, pl* **-ti·tis·es** *or* **-tit·i·des** \-ˈti-tə-ˌdēz\ : an inflammatory reaction of skin that has been exposed to sunlight and esp. UVA radiation after being made hypersensitive by contact with any of various plants or plant parts and esp. those (as limes and celery) with high levels of psoralens and that is typically characterized by a burning sensation, blisters, and erythema followed by hyperpigmentation

phy·tos·ter·ol \fī-ˈtäs-tə-ˌrȯl, -ˌrōl\ *n* : any of various sterols derived from plants

phy·to·ther·a·py \ˌfī-tō-ˈther-ə-pē\ *n, pl* **-pies** : the use of vegetable drugs in medicine

phy·to·tox·in \-ˈtäk-sən\ *n* : a toxin (as ricin) produced by a plant

pia \ˈpī-ə, ˈpē-ə\ *n* : PIA MATER

pia–arach·noid \ˌpī-ə-ə-ˈrak-ˌnȯid, ˌpē-\ *n* : LEPTOMENINGES

Pia·get·ian \ˌpē-ə-ˈje-tē-ən\ *adj* : of, relating to, or dealing with Jean Piaget or his writings, theories, or methods esp. with respect to child development

Pia·get \pē-ä-ˈzhā\, **Jean (1896–1980),** Swiss psychologist.

pi·al \ˈpī-əl, ˈpē-\ *adj* : of or relating to the pia mater ⟨a ∼ artery⟩

pia ma·ter \-ˈmā-tər\ *n* : the delicate and highly vascular membrane of connective tissue investing the brain and spinal cord, lying internal to the arachnoid and dura mater, dipping down between the convolutions of the brain, and sending an ingrowth into the anterior fissure of the spinal cord — called also *pia*

pi·an \pē-ˈan, ˈpyän\ *n* : YAWS

pi·blok·to \pi-ˈbläk-(ˌ)tō\ *or* **pi·blok·toq** \pi-ˈbläk-(ˌ)tōk\ *n* : a condition among the Inuit that is characterized by attacks of disturbed behavior (as screaming and crying) and that occurs chiefly in winter

pi·ca \ˈpī-kə\ *n* : an abnormal craving for and eating of substances (as chalk, ashes, or bones) not normally eaten that occurs in nutritional deficiency states (as aphosphorosis) in humans or animals or in some forms of mental disorder — compare GEOPHAGY

¹Pick's disease \ˈpiks-\ *n* : a dementia marked by progressive impairment of intellect and judgment and transitory aphasia, caused by progressive atrophic changes of the cerebral cortex, and usu. beginning in late middle age

Pick \ˈpik\, **Arnold (1851–1924),** Czechoslovakian psychiatrist and neurologist.

²Pick's disease *n* : pericarditis with adherent pericardium resulting in circulatory disturbances with edema and ascites

Pick, Friedel (1867–1926), Czechoslovakian physician.

Pick·wick·ian syndrome \pik-ˈwi-kē-ən-\ *n* : obesity accompanied by somnolence and lethargy, hypoventilation, hypoxia, and secondary polycythemia

pico- *comb form* **1** : one trillionth (10^{-12}) part of ⟨*pico*gram⟩ **2** : very small ⟨*pi*-*co*rnavirus⟩

pi·co·cu·rie \ˌpē-kō-ˈkyu̇r-ē, -kyu̇-ˈrē\ *n* : one trillionth of a curie — abbr. *pCi*

pi·co·gram \ˈpē-kō-ˌgram\ *n* : one trillionth of a gram — abbr. *pg*

pi·co·li·nate \pi-ˈkä-lə-ˌnāt\ *n* : a salt of picolinic acid

pic·o·lin·ic acid \ˌpik-ə-ˈli-nik-\ *n* : a crystalline acid $C_6H_5NO_2$ isomeric with niacin

pi·cor·na·vi·rus \pē-ˌkȯr-nə-ˈvī-rəs\ *n* : any of a family (*Picornaviridae*) of small single-stranded RNA viruses that include the causative agents of encephalomyocarditis, hepatitis A, polio, foot-and-mouth disease, and hand, foot and mouth disease — see COXSACKIEVIRUS, ECHOVIRUS, ENTEROVIRUS, RHINOVIRUS

pic·ric acid \ˈpi-krik-\ *n* : a bitter toxic explosive yellow crystalline acid $C_6H_3N_3O_7$ — called also *trinitrophenol*

pic·ro·tox·in \ˌpi-krō-ˈtäk-sən\ *n* : a poisonous bitter stimulant and convulsant substance $C_{30}H_{34}O_{13}$ obtained esp. from the berry of a southeast Asian vine (*Anamirta cocculus* of the family Menispermaceae) and administered intravenously as an antidote for barbiturate poisoning

PID *abbr* pelvic inflammatory disease

pie·dra \pē-ˈā-drə\ *n* : a fungus disease of the hair marked by the formation of small stony nodules along the hair shafts

Pierre Ro·bin syndrome \ˌpyer-rȯ-ˈbeⁿ-\ *n* : a congenital defect of the face characterized by micrognathia, abnormal smallness of the tongue, cleft palate, absence of the gag reflex, and sometimes accompanied by bilateral eye defects, glaucoma, or retinal detachment

Robin, Pierre (1867–1950), French pediatrician.

pi·geon breast \ˈpi-jən-\ *n* : a rachitic deformity of the chest marked by sharp projection of the sternum — **pi·geon–breast·ed** \-ˈbres-təd\ *adj*

pigeon chest *n* : PIGEON BREAST

pigeon–toed \-ˈtōd\ *adj* : having the toes turned in toward the midline of the body

pig·ment \ˈpig-mənt\ *n* : a coloring matter in animals and plants esp. in a cell or tissue; *also* : any of various related colorless substances — **pig·men·tary** \ˈpig-mən-ˌter-ē\ *adj*

pigmentary retinopathy *n* : RETINITIS PIGMENTOSA

pig·men·ta·tion \ˌpig-mən-ˈtā-shən, -ˌmen-\ *n* : coloration with or deposition of pigment; *esp* : an excessive deposition of bodily pigment

pigment cell *n* : a cell containing a deposition of coloring matter

pig·ment·ed \ˈpig-ˌmen-təd\ *adj* : colored by a deposit of pigment

pigmentosa — see RETINITIS PIGMENTOSA

pigmentosum — see XERODERMA PIGMENTOSUM

pig·weed \ˈpig-ˌwēd\ *n* : any of several plants of the genus *Amaranthus* (as *A. retroflexus* and *A. hybridus*) with pollen that acts as a hay fever allergen

pil *abbr* [Latin *pilula*] pill — used in writing prescriptions

pil- *or* **pili-** *or* **pilo-** *comb form* : hair ⟨*pilo*motor⟩

pilaris — see KERATOSIS PILARIS, PITYRIASIS RUBRA PILARIS

Pi·la·tes \pə-ˈlä-tēz\ *n* : an exercise regimen typically performed with the use of specialized apparatus and designed to improve the overall condition of the body

pile \ˈpīl\ *n* **1** : a single hemorrhoid **2 piles** *pl* : HEMORRHOIDS; *also* : the condition of one affected with hemorrhoids

pili *pl of* PILUS

pili — see ARRECTOR PILI MUSCLE

pill \ˈpil\ *n* **1** : a usu. medicinal or dietary preparation in a small rounded mass to be swallowed whole **2** *often cap* : BIRTH CONTROL PILL — usu. used with *the*

pil·lar \ˈpi-lər\ *n* : a body part likened to a pillar or column (as the margin of the external inguinal ring); *specif* : PILLAR OF THE FAUCES

pillar of the fauces *n* : either of two curved folds on each side that bound the fauces and enclose the tonsil — see PALATOGLOSSAL ARCH, PALATOPHARYNGEAL ARCH

pi·lo·car·pine \ˌpī-lə-ˈkär-ˌpēn\ *n* : a miotic alkaloid that is obtained from the dried crushed leaves of two So. American shrubs (*Pilocarpus jaborandi* and *P. microphyllus*) of the rue family (Rutaceae) and is used chiefly in the form of its hydrochloride $C_{11}H_{16}N_2O_2{\cdot}HCl$ or nitrate $C_{11}H_{16}N_2O_2{\cdot}HNO_3$ esp. in the treatment of glaucoma and xerostomia

pi·lo·erec·tion \ˌpī-lō-i-ˈrek-shən\ *n* : involuntary erection or bristling of hairs due to a sympathetic reflex usu. triggered by cold, shock, or fright or due to a sympathomimetic agent

pi·lo·mo·tor \ˌpī-lə-ˈmō-tər\ *adj* : moving or tending to cause movement of the hairs of the skin ⟨~ nerves⟩

pi·lo·ni·dal \ˌpī-lə-ˈnīd-ᵊl\ *adj* **1** : containing hair nested in a cyst — used of congenitally anomalous cysts in the sacrococcygeal area that often become infected and discharge through a channel near the anus **2** : of, relating to, involving, or for use on pilonidal cysts, tracts, or sinuses

pi·lo·se·ba·ceous \ˌpī-lō-si-ˈbā-shəs\ *adj* : of or relating to hair and the sebaceous glands

pi·lus \ˈpī-ləs\ *n, pl* **pi·li** \-ˌlī\ : a hair or a structure (as on the surface of a bacterial cell) resembling a hair

pi·mar·i·cin \pi-ˈmar-ə-sən\ *n* : an antifungal antibiotic $C_{34}H_{49}NO_{14}$ derived from a bacterium of the genus *Streptomyces*

pim·o·zide \ˈpi-mə-ˌzīd\ *n* : a tranquilizer $C_{28}H_{29}F_2N_3O$

pim·ple \ˈpim-pəl\ *n* **1** : a small inflamed elevation of the skin : PAPULE; *esp* : PUSTULE **2** : a swelling or protuberance like a pimple — **pim·pled** \-pəld\ *adj* — **pim·ply** *adj*

pin \ˈpin\ *n* **1** : a metal rod driven into or through a fractured bone to immobilize it **2** : a metal rod driven into the root of a reconstructed tooth to provide support for a crown or into the jaw to provide support for an artificial tooth — **pin** *vb*

PIN *abbr* prostatic intraepithelial neoplasia

pinch \ˈpinch\ *vb* : to squeeze or compress (as part of the body) usu. in a painful or discomforting way ⟨a ~*ed* nerve caused by entrapment⟩

pin·do·lol \ˈpin-də-ˌlȯl, -ˌlōl\ *n* : a beta-blocker $C_{14}H_{20}N_2O_2$ used in the treatment of hypertension

[1]**pi·ne·al** \ˈpi-nē-əl, ˈpī-, pī-ˈ\ *adj* : of, relating to, or being the pineal gland

[2]**pineal** *n* : PINEAL GLAND

pi·ne·al·ec·to·my \ˌpi-nē-ə-ˈlek-tə-mē, pī-ˌnē-, ˌpī-\ *n, pl* **-mies** : surgical removal of the pineal gland — **pi·ne·a·lec·to·mize** \ˌpi-nē-ə-ˈlek-tə-ˌmīz\ *vb*

pineal gland *n* : a small body that arises from the roof of the third ventricle and is enclosed by the pia mater and that functions primarily as an endocrine gland that produces melatonin — called also *pineal, pineal body, pineal organ*

pin·e·a·lo·cyte \ˈpi-nē-ə-lō-ˌsīt\ *n* : the parenchymatous epithelioid cell of the pineal gland that has prominent nucleoli and long processes ending in bulbous expansions

pin·e·a·lo·ma \ˌpi-nē-ə-ˈlō-mə\ *n, pl* **-mas** *also* **-ma·ta** \-mə-tə\ : a tumor (as a germinoma) of the pineal gland or pineal region

pineal organ *n* : PINEAL GLAND

pine–needle oil *n* : a colorless or yellowish bitter essential oil obtained from the needles of various pines (as *Pinus sylvestris* or *P. mugo*) and used in medicine chiefly as an inhalant in treating bronchitis

pine tar *n* : tar obtained from the wood of pine trees (genus *Pinus* and esp. *P. palustris* of the family Pinaceae) and used in soaps and in the treatment of skin diseases

pink disease \ˈpiŋk-\ *n* : ACRODYNIA

pink eye \ˈpiŋ-ˌkī\ *n* : CONJUNCTIVITIS; *esp* : contagious conjunctivitis typically caused by a virus or bacterium

pink spot *n* : the appearance of pulp through the attenuated hard tissue of the crown of a tooth affected with resorption of dentin

pin•na \ˈpi-nə\ *n, pl* **pin•nae** \ˈpi-ˌnē, -ˌnī\ *or* **pinnas** : the largely cartilaginous projecting portion of the external ear — **pin•nal** \ˈpin-ᵊl\ *adj*

pi•no•cy•to•sis \ˌpi-nə-sə-ˈtō-səs, ˌpī-, -ˌsī-\ *n, pl* **-to•ses** \-ˌsēz\ : the uptake of fluid by a cell by invagination and pinching off of the cell membrane — **pi•no•cy•tot•ic** \-ˈtä-tik\ *or* **pi•no•cyt•ic** \-ˈsī-tik\ *adj*

pins and needles *n pl* : a pricking tingling sensation in a limb growing numb or recovering from numbness

pint \ˈpīnt\ *n* : any of various measures of liquid capacity equal to one-half quart: as **a** : a U.S. measure equal to 16 fluid ounces, 473.176 milliliters, or 28.875 cubic inches **b** : a British measure equal to 20 fluid ounces, 568.26 milliliters, or 34.678 cubic inches

pin•ta \ˈpin-tə, -ˌtä\ *n* : a chronic skin disease that is endemic in tropical America, that occurs successively as an initial papule, a generalized eruption, and a patchy loss of pigment, and that is caused by a spirochete of the genus *Treponema* (*T. carateum*) morphologically indistinguishable from the causative agent of syphilis — called also *mal del pinto*

pin•tid \ˈpin-təd\ *n* : one of many initially reddish, then brown, slate blue, or black patches on the skin characteristic of the second stage of pinta

pin•worm \ˈpin-ˌwərm\ *n* : any of numerous small oxyurid nematode worms that have the tail of the female prolonged into a sharp point and infest the intestines and esp. the cecum of various vertebrates; *esp* : a worm of the genus *Enterobius* (*E. vermicularis*) that is parasitic in humans

pi•o•glit•a•zone \ˌpī-ə-ˈgli-tə-ˌzōn\ *n* : a drug administered in the form of its hydrochloride $C_{19}H_{20}N_2O_3S{\cdot}HCl$ to treat type 2 diabetes by decreasing insulin resistance — see ACTOS

pi•per•a•zine \pī-ˈper-ə-ˌzēn\ *n* : a crystalline heterocyclic base $C_4H_{10}N_2$ used esp. as an anthelmintic

pi•per•i•dine \pī-ˈper-ə-ˌdēn\ *n* : a liquid heterocyclic base $C_5H_{11}N$ that has a peppery ammoniacal odor

pi•per•o•caine \pī-ˈper-ə-ˌkān\ *n* : a compound derived from piperidine and benzoic acid that has been used in the form of its hydrochloride $C_{16}H_{23}NO_2{\cdot}HCl$ as a local anesthetic

pi•per•o•nyl bu•tox•ide \pī-ˈper-ə-ˌnil-byü-ˈtäk-ˌsīd, -nəl-\ *n* : an insecticide $C_{19}H_{30}O_5$; *also* : an oily liquid containing this compound that is used chiefly as a synergist (as for pyrethrum insecticides)

pip•er•ox•an \ˌpi-pə-ˈräk-ˌsan\ *n* : an adrenolytic drug that has been used in the form of its crystalline hydrochloride $C_{14}H_{19}NO_2{\cdot}HCl$ to diagnose pheochromocytoma

pi•pette *also* **pi•pet** \pī-ˈpet\ *n* : a small piece of apparatus which typically consists of a narrow tube into which fluid is drawn by suction (as for dispensing or measurement) and retained by closing the upper end — **pipette** *also* **pipet** *vb*

pir•ac•e•tam \ˌpī-ˈra-sə-ˌtam\ *n* : an amine $C_6H_{10}N_2O_2$ that has been used as a nootropic

pir•i•form *or* **pyr•i•form** \ˈpir-ə-ˌfȯrm\ *adj* **1** : having the form of a pear **2** : of, relating to, or being the part of the cerebral cortex of the piriform lobe that receives primary input from the olfactory bulb ⟨the ~ cortex⟩

piriform aperture *n* : the anterior opening of the nasal cavities in the skull

piriform area *n* : PIRIFORM LOBE

piriform fossa *n* : PIRIFORM RECESS

pir•i•for•mis *or* **pyr•i•for•mis** \ˌpir-ə-ˈfȯr-mis\ *n* : a muscle that arises from the front of the sacrum, passes out of the pelvis through the greater sciatic foramen, is inserted into the upper border of the greater trochanter of the femur, and rotates the thigh laterally

piriformis syndrome *n* : sciatica that is caused by compression or irritation of the sciatic nerve by the piriformis muscle and is characterized by pain, tingling, and numbness in the buttocks often extending down the leg

piriform lobe *n* : the lateral olfactory gyrus and the parahippocampal gyrus taken together

piriform recess *n* : a small cavity or pocket between the lateral walls of the pharynx on each side and the upper part of the larynx — called also *piriform fossa, piriform sinus*

Pi•ro•goff's amputation \ˌpir-ə-ˈgȯfs-\ *or* **Pi•ro•goff amputation** \-ˈgȯf-\ *n* : amputation of the foot through the articulation of the ankle with retention of part of the calcaneus — compare SYME'S AMPUTATION

Pirogoff, Nikolai Ivanovich (1810–1881), Russian surgeon.

piro•plasm \ˈpir-ə-ˌpla-zəm\ *or* **piro•plas•ma** \ˌpir-ə-ˈplaz-mə\ *n, pl* **piro•plasms** *or* **piro•plas•ma•ta** \ˌpir-ə-ˈplaz-mə-tə\ : BABESIA 2

Piro•plas•ma \ˌpir-ə-ˈplaz-mə\ *n, syn of* BABESIA

piro•plas•mo•sis \ˌpir-ə-ˌplaz-ˈmō-səs\ *n, pl* **-mo•ses** \-ˌsēz\ : infection with or disease that is caused by protozoans of a family (Babesiidae) and esp. of the genus *Babesia* and that includes Texas fever and equine piroplasmosis

pi•rox•i•cam \pi-ˈräk-sə-ˌkam\ *n* : a nonsteroidal anti-inflammatory drug

$C_{15}H_{13}N_3O_4S$ that is used to treat rheumatic diseases (as osteoarthritis)

Pir•quet test \pir-ˈkā-\ *n* : a tuberculin test made by applying a drop of tuberculin to a scarified spot on the skin — called also *Pirquet reaction*

Pir•quet von Ce•se•na•ti•co \pir-ˈkā-fȯn-ˌchā-se-ˈnä-ti-kō\, **Clemens Peter (1874–1929)**, Austrian physician.

pi•si•form \ˈpī-sə-ˌfȯrm\ *n* : a bone on the little-finger side of the carpus that articulates with the triquetral bone — called also *pisiform bone*

pit \ˈpit\ *n* : a hollow or indentation esp. in a surface of an organism: as **a** : a natural hollow in the surface of the body **b** : one of the indented scars left in the skin by a pustular disease : POCKMARK **c** : a usu. developmental imperfection in the enamel of a tooth that takes the form of a small pointed depression — **pit** *vb*

pi•tav•a•stat•in \pi-ˈta-və-ˌsta-tᵊn\ *n* : a statin $C_{50}H_{46}CaF_2N_2O_8$ taken orally to lower LDL and triglyceride levels and increase HDL levels — see LIVALO

pitch \ˈpich\ *n* : the property of a sound and esp. a musical tone that is determined by the frequency of the waves producing it : highness or lowness of sound

pitch•blende \ˈpich-ˌblend\ *n* : a brown to black mineral that has a distinctive luster and contains radium

Pi•to•cin \pi-ˈtō-sən\ *trademark* — used for a preparation of oxytocin

pi•tot tube \ˌpē-ˈtō-\ *n, often cap P* : a device that consists of a tube that is used with a manometer to measure the velocity of fluid flow (as in a blood vessel)

Pitot, Henri (1695–1771), French hydraulic engineer.

Pi•tres•sin \pi-ˈtres-ᵊn\ *trademark* — used for a preparation of vasopressin

pitting *n* **1** : the action or process of forming pits (as in acned skin or a tooth) **2** : the formation of a depression or indentation in living tissue that is produced by pressure with a finger or blunt instrument and disappears slowly following release of the pressure in some forms of edema

pitting edema *n* : edema in which pitting results in a depression in the edematous tissue which disappears only slowly

pi•tu•i•cyte \pə-ˈtü-ə-ˌsīt, -ˈtyü-\ *n* : one of the pigmented more or less fusiform cells of the stalk and posterior lobe of the pituitary gland that are derived from glial cells

¹pi•tu•i•tary \pə-ˈtü-ə-ˌter-ē, -ˈtyü-\ *adj* **1** : of or relating to the pituitary gland **2** : caused or characterized by secretory disturbances of the pituitary gland ⟨a ~ dwarf⟩

²pituitary *n, pl* **-tar•ies** **1** : PITUITARY GLAND **2** : the cleaned, dried, and powdered posterior lobe of the pituitary gland of cattle that is used in the treatment of uterine atony and hemorrhage, shock, and intestinal paresis

pituitary ba•soph•i•lism \-bā-ˈsä-fə-ˌli-zəm\ *n* : CUSHING'S DISEASE

pituitary gland *n* : a small oval endocrine organ that is attached to the infundibulum of the brain and occupies the sella turcica, that consists of an epithelial anterior lobe derived from a diverticulum of the oral cavity and joined to a posterior lobe of nervous origin by a pars intermedia, and that produces various hormones which directly or indirectly affect most basic bodily functions and include substances exerting a controlling and regulating influence on other endocrine organs, controlling growth and development, or modifying the contraction of smooth muscle, renal function, and reproduction — called also *hypophysis, pituitary body;* see ADENOHYPOPHYSIS, NEUROHYPOPHYSIS

pituitary portal system *n* : a portal system supplying blood to the anterior lobe of the pituitary gland through veins connecting the capillaries of the median eminence of the hypothalamus with those of the anterior lobe

pit viper *n* : any of various mostly New World venomous snakes (subfamily Crotalinae of the family Viperidae) including the rattlesnake, copperhead, and water moccasin that have a small depression on each side of the head and hollow perforated fangs

pit•y•ri•a•sis \ˌpi-tə-ˈrī-ə-səs\ *n, pl* **pit•y•ri•a•ses** \-ˌsēz\ **1** : any of several skin diseases marked by the formation and desquamation of fine scales **2** : a disease of domestic animals marked by dry epithelial scales or scurf

pityriasis li•che•noi•des et var•i•o•li•for•mis acu•ta \-ˌlī-kə-ˈnȯi-ˌdēz-et-ˌvar-ē-ˌō-lə-ˈfȯr-mis-ə-ˈkyü-tə, -ˈkü-\ *n* : a disease of unknown cause that is characterized by the sudden appearance of polymorphous lesions (as papules, purpuric vesicles, crusts, or ulcerations) resembling chicken pox but tending to persist from a month to as long as years — called also *PLEVA*

pityriasis ro•sea \-ˈrō-zē-ə\ *n* : an acute benign and self-limited skin eruption of unknown cause that consists of dry, scaly, oval, pinkish or fawn-colored papules, usu. lasts six to eight weeks, and affects esp. the trunk, arms, and thighs

pityriasis ru•bra pi•lar•is \-ˈrü-brə-pi-ˈlar-əs\ *n* : chronic dermatitis characterized by the formation of papular horny plugs in the hair follicles and pinkish macules which tend to spread and become scaly plaques

pityriasis versicolor *n* : TINEA VERSICOLOR

Pit•y•ros•po•rum \ˌpi-tə-ˈräs-pə-rəm\ *n, syn of* MALASSEZIA

piv•ot \ˈpi-vət\ *n* : a usu. metallic pin holding an artificial crown to the root of a tooth

pivot joint *n* : an anatomical articulation that consists of a bony pivot in a ring of bone and ligament (as that of the dens and atlas) and that permits rotatory movement only — called also *trochoid*

pivot tooth *n* : an artificial crown attached to the root of a tooth by a usu. metallic pin — called also *pivot crown*

PK \ˌpē-ˈkā\ *n* : PSYCHOKINESIS

PKC *abbr* protein kinase C

PKU *abbr* phenylketonuria

pla•ce•bo \plə-ˈsē-(ˌ)bō\ *n, pl* **-bos** **1** : a usu. pharmacologically inert preparation prescribed more for the mental relief of the patient than for its actual effect on a disorder **2** : an inert or innocuous substance used esp. in controlled experiments testing the efficacy of another substance (as a drug)

placebo effect *n* : improvement in the condition of a patient that occurs in response to treatment but cannot be considered due to the specific treatment used

pla•cen•ta \plə-ˈsen-tə\ *n, pl* **-centas** *or* **-cen•tae** \-ˈsen-(ˌ)tē\ : the vascular organ that unites the fetus to the maternal uterus and mediates its metabolic exchanges through a more or less intimate association of uterine mucosal with chorionic and usu. allantoic tissues permitting exchange of material by diffusion between the maternal and fetal vascular systems but without direct contact between maternal and fetal blood and typically involving the interlocking of fingerlike vascular chorionic villi with corresponding modified areas of the uterine mucosa — see ABRUPTIO PLACENTAE — **pla•cen•tal** \-təl\ *adj*

placental barrier *n* : a semipermeable membrane made up of placental tissues and limiting the kind and amount of material exchanged between mother and fetus

placentalis — see DECIDUA PLACENTALIS

placental lactogen *n* : a hormone secreted by the syncytiotrophoblast that inhibits production of maternal insulin during pregnancy — called also *chorionic somatomammotropin*

placenta pre•via \-ˈprē-vē-ə\ *n, pl* **placentae pre•vi•ae** \-vē-ˌē\ : an abnormal implantation of the placenta at or near the internal opening of the uterine cervix so that it tends to precede the child at birth usu. causing severe maternal hemorrhage

plac•en•ti•tis \ˌplas-ᵊn-ˈtī-təs\ *n, pl* **-tit•i•des** \-ˈti-tə-ˌdēz\ : inflammation of the placenta

plac•en•tog•ra•phy \ˌplas-ᵊn-ˈtä-grə-fē\ *n, pl* **-phies** : radiographic visualization of the placenta after injection of a radiopaque medium

Plac•i•dyl \ˈpla-sə-ˌdil\ *trademark* — used for a preparation of ethchlorvynol

pla•gi•o•ceph•a•ly \ˌplā-jē-ō-ˈse-fə-lē\ *n, pl* **-lies** : a malformation of the head marked by an oblique slant to the main axis of the skull and usu. caused by closure of half of the coronal suture

plague \ˈplāg\ *n* **1** : an epidemic disease causing a high rate of mortality : PESTILENCE ⟨a ~ of cholera⟩ **2** : a virulent contagious febrile disease that is caused by a bacterium of the genus *Yersinia* (*Y. pestis* syn. *Pasteurella pestis*), that occurs in bubonic, pneumonic, and septicemic forms, and that is usu. transmitted from rats to humans by the bite of infected fleas (as in bubonic plague) or directly from person to person (as in pneumonic plague) — called also *black death*

plana — see PARS PLANA

Plan B *trademark* — used for a preparation of levonorgestrel intended to prevent pregnancy following unprotected intercourse or contraceptive failure

plane \ˈplān\ *n* **1 a** : a surface that contains at least three points not all in a straight line and is such that a line drawn through any two points in it lies wholly in the surface **b** : an imaginary plane used to identify parts of the body or a part of the skull — see FRANKFORT HORIZONTAL PLANE, MIDSAGITTAL PLANE **2** : a stage in surgical anesthesia ⟨a light ~ of anesthesia⟩

plane joint *n* : GLIDING JOINT

plane of polarization *n* : the plane in which electromagnetic radiation vibrates when it is polarized so as to vibrate in a single plane

plane wart *n* : FLAT WART

pla•ni•gram \ˈplā-nə-ˌgram, ˈpla-\ *n* : TOMOGRAM

pla•nig•ra•phy \plə-ˈni-grə-fē\ *n, pl* **-phies** : TOMOGRAPHY

Planned Par•ent•hood \ˈpland-ˈpar-ᵊnt-ˌhu̇d\ *service mark* — used for services and materials promoting the accessibility of effective means of voluntary fertility control

Pla•nor•bis \plə-ˈnȯr-bis\ *n* : a genus of snails (family Planorbidae) that includes several intermediate hosts for schistosomes infecting humans

plantae — see QUADRATUS PLANTAE

plan•ta•go \plan-ˈtā-(ˌ)gō\ *n* **1** *cap* : a large genus of weeds (family Plantaginaceae) including several (*P. psyllium*, *P. indica*, and *P. ovata*) that have indigestible and mucilaginous seeds used as a mild cathartic — see PSYLLIUM SEED **2** : PLANTAIN

plantago seed *n* : PSYLLIUM SEED

plan•tain \ˈplant-ᵊn\ *n* : any plant of the genus *Plantago*

plan·tar \ˈplan-tər, -ˌtär\ *adj* : of, relating to, or typical of the sole of the foot ⟨the ~ aspect of the foot⟩

plantar arch *n* : an arterial arch in the sole of the foot formed by the lateral plantar artery and a branch of the dorsalis pedis artery

plantar artery *n* : either of the two terminal branches into which the posterior tibial artery divides: **a** : one that is larger and passes laterally and then medially to join with a branch of the dorsalis pedis artery to form the plantar arch — called also *lateral plantar artery* **b** : one that is smaller and follows a more medial course as it passes distally supplying or giving off branches which supply the plantar part of the foot and the toes — called also *medial plantar artery*

plantar cal·ca·neo·na·vic·u·lar ligament \-(ˌ)kal-ˌkā-nē-ō-nə-ˈvi-kyə-lər-\ *n* : an elastic ligament of the sole of the foot that connects the calcaneus and navicular bone and supports the head of the talus — called also *spring ligament*

plantar fascia *n* : a very strong dense fibrous membrane of the sole of the foot that lies beneath the skin and superficial layer of fat and binds together the deeper structures

plantar fasciitis *n* : inflammation involving the plantar fascia of the foot esp. in the area of its attachment to the calcaneus that is marked esp. by heel or arch pain

plantar flexion *n* : movement of the foot in which the foot or toes flex downward toward the sole — compare DORSIFLEXION

plantar interosseus *n* : any of three small muscles of the plantar aspect of the foot each of which lies along the plantar side of one of the third, fourth, and fifth toes facing the second toe and acts to flex the proximal phalanx and extend the distal phalanges of its toe and to adduct its toe toward the second toe — called also *interosseus plantaris, plantar interosseus muscle*

plan·tar·is \plan-ˈtar-əs\ *n, pl* **plan·tar·es** \-ˈtar-ˌēz\ : a small muscle of the calf of the leg that arises from the lower end of the femur and the posterior ligament of the knee joint, is inserted with the Achilles tendon by a very long slender tendon into the calcaneus, and weakly flexes the leg at the knee and the foot at the ankle — see PLANTAR INTEROSSEUS, VERRUCA PLANTARIS

plantar nerve *n* : either of two nerves of the foot that are the two terminal branches into which the tibial nerve divides: **a** : a smaller one that supplies most of the deeper muscles of the foot and the skin on the lateral part of the sole and on the fifth toe as well as on the lateral part of the fourth toe — called also *lateral plantar nerve* **b** : a larger one that accompanies the medial plantar artery and supplies a number of muscles of the medial part of the foot, the skin on the medial two-thirds of the sole, and the skin on the first to fourth toes — called also *medial plantar nerve*

plantar reflex *n* : a reflex movement of flexing the foot and toes that after the first year is the normal response to tickling of the sole — compare BABINSKI REFLEX

plantar vein *n* : either of two veins that accompany the plantar arteries: **a** : one accompanying the lateral plantar artery — called also *lateral plantar vein* **b** : one accompanying the medial plantar artery — called also *medial plantar vein*

plantar wart *n* : a wart on the sole of the foot — called also *verruca plantaris*

plan·ter's wart \ˈplan-tərz-\ *n* : PLANTAR WART

plan·ti·grade \ˈplan-tə-ˌgrād\ *adj* : walking on the sole with the heel touching the ground — **plantigrade** *n*

pla·num \ˈplā-nəm\ *n, pl* **pla·na** \-nə\ : a flat surface of bone esp. of the skull

planum tem·po·ra·le \-ˌtem-pə-ˈra-lē\ *n* : an area of the cerebral cortex between Heschl's gyrus and the sylvian fissure that is involved in speech and is usu. larger in the cerebral hemisphere on the left side of the brain

planus — see LICHEN PLANUS

plaque \ˈplak\ *n* **1 a** : a localized abnormal patch on a body part or surface and esp. on the skin ⟨psoriatic ~⟩ **b** : a sticky usu. colorless film on teeth that is formed by and harbors bacteria **c** : an atherosclerotic lesion **d** : a histopathologic lesion of brain tissue that is characteristic of Alzheimer's disease and consists of a dense proteinaceous core composed primarily of beta-amyloid that is often surrounded and infiltrated by a cluster of degenerating axons and dendrites **2** : a visibly distinct and esp. a clear or opaque area in a bacterial culture produced by damage to or destruction of cells by a virus

Plaque·nil \ˈpla-kə-ˌnil\ *trademark* — used for a preparation of the sulfate of hydroxychloroquine

-pla·sia \ˈplā-zhə, -zhē-ə\ *or* **-pla·sy** \ˌplā-sē, -plə-sē\ *n comb form, pl* **-pla·sias** *or* **-plasies** : development : formation ⟨dys*plasia*⟩

plasm- *or* **plasmo-** *comb form* : plasma ⟨*plasm*apheresis⟩

-plasm \ˌpla-zəm\ *n comb form* : formative or formed material (as of a cell or tissue) ⟨cyto*plasm*⟩ ⟨endo*plasm*⟩

plas·ma \ˈplaz-mə\ *n* : the fluid part esp. of blood, lymph, or milk that is distinguished from suspended material — see BLOOD PLASMA

plasma cell *n* : a lymphocyte that is a mature antibody-secreting B cell

plasma cell dyscrasia *n* : MONOCLONAL GAMMOPATHY

plas•ma•cy•toid \ˌplaz-mə-ˈsī-ˌtȯid\ *adj* : resembling or derived from a plasma cell

plas•ma•cy•to•ma *also* **plas•mo•cy•to•ma** \ˌplaz-mə-sī-ˈtō-mə\ *n, pl* **-mas** *also* **-ma•ta** \-mə-tə\ : a myeloma composed of plasma cells

plas•ma•cy•to•sis \ˌplaz-mə-sī-ˈtō-səs\ *n, pl* **-to•ses** \-ˌsēz\ : the presence of abnormal numbers of plasma cells in the blood

plas•ma•lem•ma \ˌplaz-mə-ˈle-mə\ *n* : PLASMA MEMBRANE

plas•mal•o•gen \plaz-ˈma-lə-jən, -ˌjen\ *n* : any of a group of phospholipids in which a fatty acid group is replaced by a fatty aldehyde and which include lecithins and phosphatidylethanolamines

plasma membrane *n* : a semipermeable limiting layer of cell protoplasm consisting of a fluid phospholipid bilayer with intercalated proteins — called also *cell membrane, plasmalemma*

plas•ma•pher•e•sis \ˌplaz-mə-fə-ˈrē-səs, -ˈfer-ə-səs\ *n, pl* **-e•ses** \-ˌsēz\ : apheresis used to remove blood plasma (as in the treatment of myasthenia gravis or in the collection of blood plasma for use in transfusion)

plasma thromboplastin an•te•ced•ent \-ˌan-tə-ˈsēd-ᵊnt\ *n* : a clotting factor whose absence is associated with a form of hemophilia — abbr. *PTA;* called also *factor XI*

plasma thromboplastin component *n* : FACTOR IX — abbr. *PTC*

plas•mat•ic \plaz-ˈma-tik\ *adj* : of, relating to, or occurring in plasma esp. of blood ⟨~ fibrils⟩

plas•mid \ˈplaz-mid\ *n* : an extrachromosomal ring of DNA that replicates independently and is found esp. in bacteria — compare EPISOME

plas•min \-min\ *n* : a proteolytic enzyme that dissolves the fibrin of blood clots

plas•min•o•gen \plaz-ˈmi-nə-jən\ *n* : the precursor of plasmin that is found in blood plasma and serum — called also *profibrinolysin*

plasminogen activator *n* : any of a group of substances (as urokinase) that convert plasminogen to plasmin — see TISSUE PLASMINOGEN ACTIVATOR

plasmo- — see PLASM-

plas•mo•di•al \plaz-ˈmō-dē-əl\ *adj* : of, relating to, or resembling a plasmodium

plas•mo•di•um \plaz-ˈmō-dē-əm\ *n* **1** *cap* : a genus of sporozoans (family Plasmodiidae) that includes all the malaria parasites affecting humans **2** *pl* **-dia** : any individual malaria parasite

-plast \ˌplast\ *n comb form* : organized particle or granule : cell ⟨chloro*plast*⟩

plas•ter \ˈplas-tər\ *n* : a medicated or protective dressing that consists of a film (as of cloth or plastic) spread with a usu. medicated substance

plaster cast *n* : a rigid dressing of gauze impregnated with plaster of paris

plaster of par•is \-ˈpar-is\ *n* : a white powdery slightly hydrated calcium sulfate $CaSO_4{\cdot}{}^1/_2H_2O$ or $2CaSO_4{\cdot}H_2O$ that forms a quick-setting paste with water and is used in medicine chiefly in casts and for surgical bandages

plas•tic \ˈplas-tik\ *adj* **1** : capable of being deformed continuously and permanently in any direction without breaking or tearing **2 a** : capable of growth, repair, or differentiation ⟨a ~ tissue⟩ **b** : relating to, characterized by, or exhibiting neural plasticity **3** : of, relating to, or involving plastic surgery ⟨~ repair⟩

-plas•tic \ˈplas-tik\ *adj comb form* **1** : developing : forming ⟨thrombo*plastic*⟩ **2** : of or relating to (something designated by a term ending in *-plasia, -plasm*, or *-plasty*) ⟨neo*plastic*⟩

plas•tic•i•ty \pla-ˈsti-sə-tē\ *n, pl* **-ties** **1** : the quality or state of being plastic; *esp* : capacity for being molded or altered **2** : the ability to retain a shape attained by pressure deformation **3** : the capacity of organisms with the same genotype to vary in developmental pattern, in phenotype, or in behavior according to varying environmental conditions **4** : the capacity for continuous alteration of the neural pathways and synapses of the living brain and nervous system in response to experience or injury

plastic surgeon *n* : a specialist in plastic surgery

plastic surgery *n* : a branch of surgery concerned with the repair, restoration, or improvement of lost, injured, defective, or misshapen parts of the body chiefly by transfer of tissue; *also* : an operation performed for such a purpose

plas•ty \ˈplas-tē\ *n, pl* **plas•ties** : a surgical procedure for the repair, restoration, or replacement (as by a prosthesis) of a part of the body

-plas•ty \ˌplas-tē\ *n comb form, pl* **-plas•ties** : plastic surgery ⟨osteo*plasty*⟩

-plasy — see -PLASIA

plat- — see PLATY-

[1]**plate** \ˈplāt\ *n* **1** : a flat thin piece or lamina (as of bone) that is part of the body **2 a** : a flat glass dish used chiefly for culturing microorganisms; *esp* : PETRI DISH **b** : a culture or culture medium contained in such a dish **3** : a supporting or reinforcing element: as **a** : the part of a denture that fits in the mouth; *broadly* : DENTURE **b** : a thin flat narrow piece of metal (as stainless steel) that is used to repair a bone defect or fracture

[2]**plate** *vb* **plat•ed; plat•ing** **1** : to inoculate and culture (microorganisms or cells) on a plate; *also* : to distribute (an inoculum) on a plate or plates for cultivation **2** : to repair (as a fractured bone) with metal plates

pla•teau \pla-ˈtō\ *n, pl* **plateaus** *also* **pla•teaux** \-ˈtōz\ : a relatively flat elevated area — see TIBIAL PLATEAU

plate•let \ˈplāt-lət\ *n* : a minute colorless anucleate disklike body of mammalian blood that is derived from fragments of megakaryocyte cytoplasm, that is released from the bone marrow into the blood, and that assists in blood clotting by adhering to other platelets and to damaged epithelium — called also *blood platelet, thrombocyte*

platelet–activating factor *n* : phospholipid that is produced esp. by mast cells and basophils, causes the aggregation of platelets and the release of platelet substances (as histamine or serotonin), and is a mediator of inflammation (as in asthma) — abbr. *PAF*

platelet–derived growth factor *n* : a mitogenic growth factor that is found esp. in platelets, consists of two polypeptide chains linked by bonds containing two sulfur atoms each, stimulates cell proliferation (as in connective tissue, smooth muscle, and glia), and plays a role in wound healing — abbr. *PDGF*

plate•let•phe•re•sis \ˌplāt-lət-ˈfer-ə-səs, -fə-ˈrē-səs\ *n, pl* **-re•ses** \-ˌsēz\ : apheresis used to remove blood platelets (as in the treatment of thrombocytosis or in the collection of platelets for use in transfusion)

plat•ing \ˈplāt-iŋ\ *n* **1** : the spreading of a sample of cells or microorganisms on a nutrient medium in a petri dish **2** : the immobilization of a fractured bone by securing a metal plate to it

Plat•i•nol \ˈpla-tə-ˌnȯl, -ˌnōl\ *trademark* — used for a preparation of cisplatin

plat•i•num \ˈplat-ᵊn-əm\ *n* : a grayish-white ductile malleable metallic element used esp. as a catalyst and in alloys (as in dentistry) — symbol *Pt;* see ELEMENT table

platy- *also* **plat-** *comb form* : flat : broad ⟨*platy*pelloid⟩

platy•ba•sia \ˌpla-ti-ˈbā-sē-ə\ *n* : a developmental deformity of the base of the skull in which the lower occiput is pushed by the upper cervical spine into the cranial fossa

platy•hel•minth \ˌpla-ti-ˈhel-ˌminth\ *n* : FLATWORM — **platy•hel•min•thic** \-ˌhel-ˈmin-thik, -tik\ *adj*

platy•pel•loid \-ˈpe-ˌlȯid\ *adj, of the pelvis* : broad and flat — compare ANDROID 1, ANTHROPOID, GYNECOID 1

pla•tys•ma \plə-ˈtiz-mə\ *n, pl* **-ma•ta** \-mə-tə\ *also* **-mas** : a broad thin layer of muscle that is situated on each side of the neck immediately under the superficial fascia belonging to the group of facial muscles, that is innervated by the facial nerve, and that draws the lower lip and the corner of the mouth to the side and down and when moved forcefully expands the neck and draws its skin upward

Plav•ix \ˈplav-iks\ *trademark* — used for a preparation of the bisulfate of clopidogrel

play therapy *n* : psychotherapy in which a child is encouraged to reveal feelings and conflicts in play rather than by verbalization

pleasure principle *n* : a tendency for individual behavior to be directed toward immediate satisfaction of instinctual drives and immediate relief from pain or discomfort — compare REALITY PRINCIPLE

pled•get \ˈple-jət\ *n* : a compress or small flat mass usu. of gauze or absorbent cotton that is laid over a wound or into a cavity to apply medication, exclude air, retain dressings, or absorb the matter discharged

-ple•gia \ˈplē-jə, -jē-ə\ *n comb form* : paralysis ⟨di*plegia*⟩

pleio•tro•pic \ˌplī-ə-ˈtrō-pik, -ˈträ-\ *adj* : producing more than one genetic effect; *specif* : having multiple phenotypic expressions ⟨a ~ gene⟩ — **plei•ot•ro•py** \plī-ˈä-trə-pē\ *n*

pleo•cy•to•sis \ˌplē-ō-ˌsī-ˈtō-səs\ *n, pl* **-to•ses** \-ˌsēz\ : an abnormal increase in the number of cells (as lymphocytes) in the cerebrospinal fluid

pleo•mor•phic \ˌplē-ə-ˈmȯr-fik\ *also* **pleio•mor•phic** \ˌplī-ə-\ *adj* : able to assume different forms : POLYMORPHIC ⟨a benign ~ salivary adenoma of mixed cell type⟩ — **pleo•mor•phism** \ˌplē-ə-ˈmȯr-ˌfi-zəm\ *n*

ple•op•tics \plē-ˈäp-tiks\ *n* : a system of treating amblyopia by retraining visual habits using guided exercises — **ple•op•tic** \-tik\ *adj*

pleth•o•ra \ˈple-thə-rə\ *n* : a bodily condition characterized by an excess of blood and marked by turgescence and a florid complexion — **ple•tho•ric** \plə-ˈthȯr-ik, ple-, -ˈthär-; ˈple-thə-rik\ *adj*

ple•thys•mo•gram \ple-ˈthiz-mə-ˌgram, plə-\ *n* : a tracing made by a plethysmograph

ple•thys•mo•graph \-ˌgraf\ *n* : an instrument for determining and registering variations in the size of an organ or limb resulting from changes in the amount of blood present or passing through it — **ple•thys•mo•graph•ic** \-ˌthiz-mə-ˈgra-fik\ *adj* — **ple•thys•mo•graph•i•cal•ly** *adv* — **pleth•ys•mog•ra•phy** \ˌple-thiz-ˈmä-grə-fē\ *n*

pleur- *or* **pleuro-** *comb form* **1** : pleura ⟨*pleuro*pneumonia⟩ **2** : pleura and ⟨*pleuro*peritoneal⟩

pleu•ra \ˈplu̇r-ə\ *n, pl* **pleu•rae** \ˈplu̇r-ē\ *or* **pleuras** : either of a pair of two-walled sacs of serous membrane each of which lines one lateral half of the thorax, has an inner layer closely adherent to the corresponding lung, is reflected at the root of the lung to form a parietal layer that adheres to the walls of the thorax, the pericardium, the upper surface of the diaphragm, and adjacent parts, and contains a small amount of serous fluid that minimizes the friction of respiratory movements

pleu·ral \ˈplu̇r-əl\ *adj* : of or relating to the pleura or the sides of the thorax

pleural cavity *n* : the space that is formed when the two layers of the pleura spread apart — called also *pleural space*

pleural effusion *n* **1** : an exudation of fluid from the blood or lymph into a pleural cavity **2** : an exudate in a pleural cavity

pleu·rec·to·my \plu̇-ˈrek-tə-mē\ *n, pl* **-mies** : surgical excision of part of the pleura

pleu·ri·sy \ˈplu̇r-ə-sē\ *n, pl* **-sies** : inflammation of the pleura that is typically characterized by sudden onset, painful and difficult respiration, cough, and exudation of fluid or fibrinous material into the pleural cavity — **pleu·rit·ic** \plü-ˈri-tik\ *adj*

pleu·ri·tis \plü-ˈrī-təs\ *n, pl* **pleu·rit·i·des** \-ˈri-tə-ˌdēz\ : PLEURISY

pleu·rod·e·sis \plu̇-ˈrä-də-səs\ *n* : obliteration of the pleural cavity by inducing adherence of the visceral and parietal pleural layers (as by the use of sclerosing agents or surgical abrasion) esp. to treat pleural effusion, pneumothorax, and chylothorax

pleu·ro·dyn·ia \ˌplu̇r-ə-ˈdi-nē-ə\ *n* **1** : a sharp pain in the side usu. located in the intercostal muscles and believed to arise from inflammation of fibrous tissue **2** : EPIDEMIC PLEURODYNIA

pleu·ro·peri·car·di·tis \ˌplu̇r-ō-ˌper-ə-ˌkär-ˈdī-təs\ *n, pl* **-dit·i·des** \-ˈdi-tə-ˌdēz\ : inflammation of the pleura and the pericardium

pleu·ro·peri·to·ne·al \-ˌper-ə-tə-ˈnē-əl\ *adj* : of or relating to the pleura and the peritoneum

pleu·ro·pneu·mo·nia \ˌplu̇r-ō-nu̇-ˈmō-nyə, -nyu̇-\ *n* **1** : pleurisy accompanied by pneumonia **2** : a highly contagious pneumonia usu. associated with pleurisy of cattle, goats, and sheep that is caused by a bacterium of the genus *Mycoplasma* (esp. *M. mycoides*) **3** : a contagious often fatal respiratory disease esp. of young pigs that is caused by a bacterium of the genus *Actinobacillus* (*A. pleuropneumoniae*) **4** : pleurisy of horses that is often accompanied by pneumonia and is caused by various bacteria

pleuropneumonia–like organism *n* : MYCOPLASMA 2

pleu·ro·pul·mo·nary \ˌplu̇r-ō-ˈpu̇l-mə-ˌner-ē, -ˈpəl-\ *adj* : of or relating to the pleura and the lungs

pleu·ros·co·py \plu̇r-ˈä-skə-pē\ *n, pl* **-pies** : THORACOSCOPY — **pleu·ro·scop·ic** \ˌplu̇r-ə-ˈskä-pik\ *adj*

PLEVA \ˈplā-və\ *n* : PITYRIASIS LICHENOIDES ET VARIOLIFORMIS ACUTA

plex·ec·to·my \plek-ˈsek-tə-mē\ *n, pl* **-mies** : surgical removal of a plexus

plexi·form \ˈplek-sə-ˌfȯrm\ *adj* : of, relating to, or having the form or characteristics of a plexus ⟨~ networks⟩

plexiform layer *n* : either of two reticular layers of the retina consisting of nerve cell processes and situated between layers of ganglion cells and cell bodies

plex·im·e·ter \plek-ˈsi-mə-tər\ *n* : a small hard flat plate (as of ivory) placed in contact with the body to receive the blow in percussion

plex·op·a·thy \plek-ˈsä-pə-thē\ *n, pl* **-thies** : an injured or diseased condition of a plexus and esp. a nerve plexus

plex·or \ˈplek-sər\ *n* : a small hammer with a rubber head used in medical percussion

plex·us \ˈplek-səs\ *n, pl* **plex·us·es** : a network of anastomosing or interlacing blood vessels or nerves

pli·ca \ˈplī-kə\ *n, pl* **pli·cae** \-ˌkē, -ˌsē\ : a fold or folded part; *esp* : a groove or fold of skin

plicae cir·cu·la·res \-ˌsər-kyə-ˈlar-(ˌ)ēz\ *n pl* : the numerous permanent crescentic folds of mucous membrane found in the small intestine esp. in the lower part of the duodenum and the jejunum — called also *valvulae conniventes*

plica fim·bri·a·ta \-ˌfim-brē-ˈā-tə\ *n, pl* **plicae fim·bri·a·tae** \-ˈā-tē\ : a fold resembling a fringe on the under surface of the tongue on either side of the frenulum

pli·ca·my·cin \ˌplī-kə-ˈmīs-ᵊn\ *n* : an antineoplastic agent $C_{52}H_{76}O_{24}$ produced by three bacteria of the genus *Streptomyces* (*S. argillaceus*, *S. tanashiensis*, and *S. plicatus*) and administered intravenously esp. in the treatment of malignant tumors of the testes or in the treatment of hypercalcemia and hypercalciuria associated with advanced neoplastic disease — called also *mithramycin*

plica semi·lu·na·ris \-ˌse-mi-ˌlü-ˈnar-əs\ *n, pl* **plicae semi·lu·na·res** \-(ˌ)ēz\ : the vertical fold of conjunctiva that occupies the canthus of the eye nearer the nose

pli·ca·tion \plī-ˈkā-shən\ *n* **1** : the tightening of stretched or weakened bodily tissues or channels by folding the excess in tucks and suturing **2** : the folding of one part on and the fastening of it to another (as areas of the bowel freed from adhesions and left without normal serosal covering) — **pli·cate** \ˈplī-ˌkāt\ *vb*

-ploid \ˌplȯid\ *adj comb form* : having or being a chromosome number that bears (such) a relationship to or is (so many) times the basic chromosome number characteristic of a given plant or animal group ⟨poly*ploid*⟩

ploi•dy \ˈplȯi-dē\ *n, pl* **ploi•dies** : degree of repetition of the basic number of chromosomes

plom•bage \ˌpləm-ˈbäzh\ *n* : the practice of inserting an inert material into the thoracic cavity to exert sustained pressure on the lungs and induce their collapse that formerly was used as a treatment for pulmonary tuberculosis

PLSS *abbr* portable life-support system

plug \ˈpləg\ *n* **1** : an obstructing mass of material in a bodily vessel or opening (as of the cervix or a skin lesion) **2** : a filling for a hollow tooth — **plugged** \ˈpləgd\ *adj*

plug•ger \ˈplə-gər\ *n* : a dental instrument used for packing, condensing, and consolidating filling material in a tooth cavity

plum•bism \ˈpləm-ˌbi-zəm\ *n* : LEAD POISONING; *esp* : chronic lead poisoning

Plum•mer–Vin•son syndrome \ˈplə-mər-ˈvin-sən-\ *n* : a condition that is marked esp. by the growth of a mucous membrane across the esophageal lumen, by difficulty in swallowing, and by hypochromic anemia and that is usu. considered to be due to an iron deficiency

Plummer, Henry Stanley (1874–1936), American physician.

Vinson, Porter Paisley (1890–1959), American surgeon.

plu•ri•po•ten•cy \ˌplu̇r-ə-ˈpōt-ᵊn-sē\ *n, pl* **-cies** : PLURIPOTENTIALITY

plu•rip•o•tent \plu̇-ˈri-pə-tənt\ *adj* **1** : not fixed as to developmental potentialities; *esp* : capable of differentiating into one of many cell types ⟨~ stem cells⟩ **2** : capable of having more than one effect ⟨~ activity⟩

plu•ri•po•ten•tial \ˌplu̇r-ə-pə-ˈten-chəl\ *adj* : PLURIPOTENT

plu•ri•po•ten•ti•al•i•ty \-pə-ˌten-chē-ˈa-lə-tē\ *n, pl* **-ties** : the quality or state of being pluripotent

plu•to•ni•um \plü-ˈtō-nē-əm\ *n* : a radioactive metallic element similar chemically to uranium that undergoes slow disintegration with the emission of an alpha particle to form uranium 235 — symbol *Pu;* see ELEMENT table

pm *abbr* premolar

Pm *symbol* promethium

PM *abbr* **1** [Latin *post meridiem*] after noon **2** postmortem

PMDD *abbr* premenstrual dysphoric disorder

PMN *abbr* polymorphonuclear leukocyte; polymorphonuclear neutrophil

PMNL *abbr* polymorphonuclear leukocyte

PMS \ˌpē-ˌem-ˈes\ *n* : PREMENSTRUAL SYNDROME

PN *abbr* psychoneurotic

-pnea \p-nē-ə\ *n comb form* : breath : breathing ⟨*apnea*⟩

pneum- *or* **pneumo-** *comb form* **1** : air : gas ⟨*pneumo*thorax⟩ **2** : lung ⟨*pneumo*coniosis⟩ : pulmonary and ⟨*pneumo*gastric⟩ **3** : respiration ⟨*pneumo*graph⟩ **4** : pneumonia ⟨*pneumo*coccus⟩

pneumat- *or* **pneumato-** *comb form* : air : vapor : gas ⟨*pneumat*osis⟩

pneu•mat•ic \nu̇-ˈma-tik, nyu̇-\ *adj* : of, relating to, or using gas (as air): as **a** : moved or worked by air pressure **b** : adapted for holding or inflated with compressed air **c** : having air-filled cavities ⟨~ bone⟩ — **pneu•mat•i•cal•ly** *adv*

pneu•ma•ti•za•tion \ˌnü-mə-tə-ˈzā-shən, ˌnyü-\ *n* : the presence or development of air-filled cavities in a bone ⟨~ of the temporal bone⟩ — **pneu•ma•tized** \ˈnü-mə-ˌtīzd, ˈnyü-\ *adj*

pneu•ma•to•cele \ˈnü-mə-tō-ˌsēl, ˈnyü-; nyü-ˈma-tə-, nü-\ *n* : a gas-filled cavity or sac occurring esp. in the lung

pneu•ma•to•sis \ˌnü-mə-ˈtō-səs, ˌnyü-\ *n, pl* **-to•ses** \-ˌsēz\ : the presence of air or gas in abnormal places in the body

pneu•ma•tu•ria \ˌnü-mə-ˈtu̇r-ē-ə, ˌnyü-\ *n* : passage of gas in the urine

pneu•mo•ba•cil•lus \ˌnü-mō-bə-ˈsi-ləs, ˌnyü\ *n, pl* **-cil•li** \-ˌlī\ : a bacterium of the genus *Klebsiella* (*K. pneumoniae*) associated with inflammatory conditions of the respiratory tract (as pneumonia)

pneu•mo•coc•cae•mia *chiefly Brit var of* PNEUMOCOCCEMIA

pneu•mo•coc•cal \ˌnü-mə-ˈkä-kəl, ˌnyü-\ *adj* : of, relating to, caused by, or derived from pneumococci ⟨~ pneumonia⟩ ⟨a ~ vaccine⟩

pneu•mo•coc•ce•mia \ˌnü-mə-ˌkäk-ˈsē-mē-ə, ˌnyü-\ *n* : the presence of pneumococci in the circulating blood

pneu•mo•coc•cus \ˌnü-mə-ˈkä-kəs, ˌnyü-\ *n, pl* **-coc•ci** \-ˈkä-ˌkī, -ˈkäk-ˌsī\ : a bacterium of the genus *Streptococcus* (*S. pneumoniae*) that causes an acute pneumonia involving one or more lobes of the lung

pneu•mo•co•lon \ˌnü-mə-ˈkō-lən, ˌnyü-\ *n* : the presence of air in the colon

pneu•mo•co•ni•o•sis \ˌnü-mō-ˌkō-nē-ˈō-səs, ˌnyü-\ *n, pl* **-o•ses** \-ˌsēz\ : a disease of the lungs caused by the habitual inhalation of irritants (as mineral or metallic particles) — called also *miner's asthma, pneumonoconiosis;* see BLACK LUNG, SILICOSIS

pneu•mo•cys•tic pneumonia \ˌnü-mə-ˈsis-tik-, ˌnyü-\ *n* : PNEUMOCYSTIS CARINII PNEUMONIA

Pneu•mo•cys•tis \ˌnü-mə-ˈsis-təs, ˌnyü-\ *n* **1** : a genus of ascomycetous fungi that were formerly classified as protozoans and include one (*P. carinii* syn. *P. jiroveci*) causing pneumonia esp. in immunocompromised individuals **2** : PNEUMOCYSTIS CARINII PNEUMONIA

Pneumocystis ca•ri•nii pneumonia \-kə-ˈrī-nē-ˌē-\ *n* : a pneumonia chiefly affecting immunocompromised individuals that is caused by a fungus of the genus *Pneumocystis* (*P. carinii*

syn. *P. jiroveci*), that attacks esp. the interstitial and alveolar tissues of the lungs, and that is characterized esp. by a nonproductive cough, shortness of breath, and fever — abbr. *PCP;* called also *pneumocystic pneumonia, Pneumocystis carinii pneumonitis, Pneumocystis pneumonia*

pneu•mo•cys•tog•ra•phy \ˌnü-mə-ˌsi-ˈstä-grə-fē, ˌnyü-\ *n, pl* **-phies** : radiography of the urinary bladder after it has been injected with air

pneu•mo•cyte \ˈnü-mə-ˌsīt, ˈnyü-\ *n* : any of the specialized cells that occur in the alveoli of the lungs

pneu•mo•en•ceph•a•li•tis \ˌnü-mō-in-ˌse-fə-ˈlī-təs, ˌnyü-\ *n, pl* **-lit•i•des** \-ˈli-tə-ˌdēz\ : NEWCASTLE DISEASE

pneu•mo•en•ceph•a•lo•gram \-in-ˈse-fə-lə-ˌgram\ *n* : a radiograph made by pneumoencephalography

pneu•mo•en•ceph•a•lo•graph \-ˌgraf\ *n* : PNEUMOENCEPHALOGRAM

pneu•mo•en•ceph•a•log•ra•phy \-in-ˌse-fə-ˈlä-grə-fē\ *n, pl* **-phies** : radiography of the brain after the injection of air into the ventricles — **pneu•mo•en•ceph•a•lo•graph•ic** \-in-ˌse-fə-lə-ˈgra-fik\ *adj*

pneu•mo•en•ter•i•tis \-ˌen-tə-ˈrī-təs\ *n, pl* **-en•ter•it•i•des** \-ˈri-tə-ˌdēz\ *or* **-en•ter•i•tis•es** : pneumonia combined with enteritis

pneu•mo•gas•tric nerve \ˌnü-mə-ˈgas-trik-, ˌnyü-\ *n* : VAGUS NERVE

pneu•mo•gram \ˈnü-mə-ˌgram, ˈnyü-\ *n* : a record of respiratory movements obtained by pneumography

pneu•mo•graph \ˈnü-mə-ˌgraf, ˈnyü-\ *n* : an instrument for recording the thoracic movements or volume change during respiration

pneu•mog•ra•phy \nü-ˈmä-grə-fē, nyü-\ *n, pl* **-phies** **1** : a description of the lungs **2** : radiography after the injection of air into a body cavity **3** : the process of making a pneumogram — **pneu•mo•graph•ic** \ˌnü-mə-ˈgra-fik, ˌnyü-\ *adj*

pneu•mol•y•sis \-ˈmä-lə-səs\ *n, pl* **-y•ses** \-ˌsēz\ : PNEUMONOLYSIS

pneu•mo•me•di•as•ti•num \ˌnü-mō-ˌmē-dē-ə-ˈstī-nəm, ˌnyü-\ *n, pl* **-ti•na** \-nə\ **1** : an abnormal state characterized by the presence of gas (as air) in the mediastinum **2** : the induction of pneumomediastinum as an aid to radiography

pneu•mo•my•co•sis \-mī-ˈkō-səs\ *n, pl* **-co•ses** \-ˌsēz\ : a fungus disease of the lungs; *esp* : aspergillosis in poultry

pneumon- *or* **pneumono-** *comb form* : lung ⟨*pneumon*ectomy⟩

pneu•mo•nec•to•my \ˌnü-mə-ˈnek-tə-mē, ˌnyü-\ *n, pl* **-mies** : surgical excision of an entire lung or of one or more lobes of a lung — compare SEGMENTAL RESECTION

pneu•mo•nia \nu̇-ˈmō-nyə, nyu̇-\ *n* : an acute disease that is marked by inflammation of lung tissue accompanied by infiltration of alveoli and often bronchioles with white blood cells (as neutrophils) and fibrinous exudate, is characterized by fever, chills, cough, difficulty in breathing, fatigue, chest pain, and reduced lung expansion, and is typically caused by an infectious agent (as a bacterium, virus, or fungus) — see BRONCHOPNEUMONIA, LOBAR PNEUMONIA, PNEUMOCYSTIS CARINII PNEUMONIA, PRIMARY ATYPICAL PNEUMONIA

pneu•mon•ic \nu̇-ˈmä-nik, nyu̇-\ *adj* **1** : of, relating to, or affecting the lungs : PULMONARY **2** : of, relating to, or affected with pneumonia

pneumonic plague *n* : plague of an extremely virulent form that is caused by a bacterium of the genus *Yersinia* (*Y. pestis* syn. *Pasteurella pestis*), involves chiefly the lungs, and usu. is transmitted from person to person by droplet infection — compare BUBONIC PLAGUE

pneu•mo•ni•tis \ˌnü-mə-ˈnī-təs, ˌnyü-\ *n, pl* **-nit•i•des** \-ˈni-tə-ˌdēz\ **1** : acute or chronic inflammation of the lungs that is characterized esp. by cough, shortness of breath, fatigue, and fever, may result in the development of fibrotic scar tissue when chronic or untreated, and is often distinguished from pneumonia by having a causative agent (as mold, toxic chemicals, or radiation) which is noninfectious; *broadly* : PNEUMONIA **2** : FELINE PNEUMONITIS

pneu•mo•no•cen•te•sis \ˌnü-mə-(ˌ)nō-sen-ˈtē-səs, ˌnyü-\ *n, pl* **-te•ses** \-ˌsēz\ : surgical puncture of a lung for aspiration

pneu•mo•no•co•ni•o•sis \-ˌkō-nē-ˈō-səs\ *n, pl* **-o•ses** \-ˌsēz\ : PNEUMOCONIOSIS

pneu•mo•nol•y•sis \ˌnü-mə-ˈnä-lə-səs, ˌnyü-\ *n, pl* **-y•ses** \-ˌsēz\ : either of two surgical procedures to permit collapse of a lung: **a** : separation of the parietal pleura from the fascia of the chest wall **b** : separation of the visceral and parietal layers of the pleura — called also *intrapleural pneumonolysis*

pneu•mo•nos•to•my \ˌnü-mə-ˈnäs-tə-mē, ˌnyü-\ *n, pl* **-mies** : surgical formation of an artificial opening (as for drainage of an abscess) into a lung

Pneu•mo•nys•sus \ˌnü-mə-ˈni-səs, ˌnyü-\ *n* : a genus of mites (family Halarachnidae) that live in the air passages of mammals and include one (*P. caninum*) found in dogs

pneu•mop•a•thy \nü-ˈmä-pə-thē, nyü-\ *n, pl* **-thies** : any disease of the lungs

pneu•mo•peri•car•di•um \ˌnü-mō-ˌper-ə-ˈkär-dē-əm, ˌnyü-\ *n, pl* **-dia** \-dē-ə\ : an abnormal state characterized by the presence of gas (as air) in the pericardium

pneu•mo•peri•to•ne•um \-ˌper-ə-tə-ˈnē-əm\ *n, pl* **-ne•ums** *or* **-nea** \-ˈnē-ə\ **1** : an abnormal state characterized by the presence of gas (as air) in the peritoneal cavity **2** : the induction of pneumoperitoneum as a therapeutic measure or as an aid to radiography

pneu·mo·pyo·peri·car·di·um \-ˌpī-ə-ˌper-ə-ˈkär-dē-əm\ *n* : PYOPNEUMOPERICARDIUM

pneu·mo·scle·ro·sis \-sklə-ˈrō-səs\ *n, pl* **-ro·ses** \-ˌsēz\ : fibrosis of the lungs

pneu·mo·tacho·gram \ˌnü-mō-ˈtak-ə-ˌgram, ˌnyü-\ *n* : a record of the velocity of the respiratory function obtained by use of a pneumotachograph

pneu·mo·tacho·graph \-ˌgraf\ *n* : a device or apparatus for measuring the rate of the respiratory function

pneu·mo·tax·ic center \ˌnü-mə-ˈtak-sik-, ˌnyü-\ *n* : a neural center in the upper part of the pons that provides inhibitory impulses on inspiration and thereby prevents overdistension of the lungs and helps to maintain alternately recurrent inspiration and expiration

pneu·mo·tho·rax \-ˈthōr-ˌaks\ *n, pl* **-tho·rax·es** *or* **-tho·ra·ces** \-ˈthōr-ə-ˌsēz\ : a condition in which air or other gas is present in the pleural cavity and which occurs spontaneously as a result of disease or injury of lung tissue, rupture of air-filled pulmonary cysts, or puncture of the chest wall or is induced as a therapeutic measure to collapse the lung — see TENSION PNEUMOTHORAX; compare OLEOTHORAX

pneu·mo·tro·pic \-ˈtrō-pik, -ˈträ-\ *adj* : turning, directed toward, or having an affinity for lung tissues — used esp. of infective agents

PNF *abbr* proprioceptive neuromuscular facilitation

PNH *abbr* paroxysmal nocturnal hemoglobinuria

-pnoea *chiefly Brit var of* -PNEA

po *abbr* per os — used esp. in writing prescriptions

Po *symbol* polonium

pock \ˈpäk\ *n* : a pustule in an eruptive disease (as smallpox)

pock·et \ˈpä-kət\ *n* : a small cavity or space; *esp* : an abnormal cavity formed in diseased tissue ⟨a gingival ~⟩ — **pocketing** *n*

pock·mark \ˈpäk-ˌmärk\ *n* : a mark, pit, or depressed scar caused by smallpox or acne — **pock·marked** *adj*

POD *abbr* postoperative day

pod- *or* **podo-** *comb form* **1** : foot ⟨*po*diatry⟩ **2** : hoof ⟨*podo*dermatitis⟩

po·dag·ra \pə-ˈda-grə\ *n* **1** : GOUT **2** : a painful condition of the big toe caused by gout

po·dal·ic \pō-ˈda-lik\ *adj* : of, relating to, or by means of the feet; *specif* : being an obstetric version in which the fetus is turned so that the feet emerge first in delivery

po·di·a·try \pə-ˈdī-ə-trē, pō-\ *n, pl* **-tries** : the medical care and treatment of the human foot — called also *chiropody* — **po·di·at·ric** \ˌpō-dē-ˈa-trik\ *adj* — **po·di·a·trist** \pə-ˈdī-ə-trist\ *n*

podo·der·ma·ti·tis \ˌpä-dō-ˌdər-mə-ˈtī-təs\ *n, pl* **-ti·tis·es** *or* **-tit·i·des** \-ˈti-tə-ˌdēz\ : a condition (as foot rot) characterized by inflammation of the dermal tissue underlying the horny layers of a hoof

podo·phyl·lin \ˌpä-də-ˈfi-lən\ *n* : a resin obtained from podophyllum and used in medicine as a caustic

podo·phyl·lo·tox·in \ˌpä-də-ˌfi-lə-ˈtäk-sən\ *n* : a crystalline polycyclic compound $C_{22}H_{22}O_8$ constituting one of the active principles of podophyllum and podophyllin

podo·phyl·lum \-ˈfi-ləm\ *n* **1** *cap* : a genus of herbs (family Berberidaceae) that have poisonous rootstocks and large fleshy sometimes edible berries **2** *pl* **-phyl·li** \-ˈfi-ˌlī\ *or* **-phyllums** : the dried rhizome and rootlet of the mayapple (*Podophyllum peltatum*) that is used as a caustic or as a source of the more effective podophyllin

podophyllum resin *n* : PODOPHYLLIN

po·go·ni·on \pə-ˈgō-nē-ən\ *n* : the most projecting median point on the anterior surface of the chin

-poi·e·sis \(ˌ)pȯi-ˈē-səs\ *n comb form, pl* **-poi·e·ses** \-ˈē-ˌsēz\ : production : formation ⟨lympho*poiesis*⟩

-poi·et·ic \(ˌ)pȯi-ˈe-tik\ *adj comb form* : productive : formative ⟨lympho*poietic*⟩

poi·kilo·cyte \ˈpȯi-ki-lə-ˌsīt, (ˌ)pȯi-ˈki-\ *n* : an abnormally formed red blood cell characteristic of various anemias

poi·kilo·cy·to·sis \ˌpȯi-ki-lō-sī-ˈtō-səs\ *n, pl* **-to·ses** \-ˌsēz\ : a condition characterized by the presence of poikilocytes in the blood

poi·ki·lo·der·ma \ˌpȯi-kə-lə-ˈdər-mə\ *n, pl* **-mas** *or* **-ma·ta** \-mə-tə\ : any of several disorders characterized by patchy discoloration of the skin

poi·ki·lo·ther·mic \-ˈthər-mik\ *adj* : COLD-BLOODED

[1]**point** \ˈpȯint\ *n* **1** : a narrowly localized place or area **2** : the terminal usu. sharp or narrowly rounded part of something

[2]**point** *vb, of an abscess* : to become distended with pus prior to breaking

pointer — see HIP POINTER

point mutation *n* : a gene mutation involving the substitution, addition, or deletion of a single nucleotide base

point–of–service *adj* : of, relating to, or being a health-care insurance plan that allows enrollees to seek care from a physician affiliated with the service provider at a fixed co-payment or to choose a nonaffiliated physician and pay a larger share of the cost — abbr. *POS*

Poi·seuille's law \pwä-ˈzœiz-\ *n* : a statement in physics that relates the velocity of flow of a fluid (as blood) through a narrow tube (as a blood vessel or a catheter) to the pressure and viscosity of the fluid and the length and radius of the tube

Poiseuille, Jean–Léonard–Marie (1797–1869), French physiologist and physician.

[1]poi•son \ˈpȯiz-ᵊn\ *n* **1 :** a substance that through its chemical action usu. kills, injures, or impairs an organism **2 :** a substance that inhibits the activity of another substance or the course of a reaction or process

[2]poison *vb* **poi•soned; poi•son•ing 1 :** to injure or kill with poison **2 :** to treat, taint, or impregnate with poison

[3]poison *adj* **1 :** POISONOUS ⟨a ~ plant⟩ **2 :** impregnated with poison ⟨a ~ arrow⟩

poison dog•wood \-ˈdȯg-ˌwu̇d\ *n* **:** POISON SUMAC

poison gas *n* **:** a poisonous gas or a liquid or a solid giving off poisonous vapors designed (as in chemical warfare) to kill, injure, or disable by inhalation or contact

poison hemlock *n* **:** a large poisonous herb (*Conium maculatum*) of the carrot family (Umbelliferae) with finely divided leaves and white flowers — compare WATER HEMLOCK

poison ivy *n* **1 a :** a climbing plant of the genus *Toxicodendron* (*T. radicans* syn. *Rhus radicans*) that is esp. common in the eastern and central U.S., that has leaves in groups of three and white berries, and that produces an acutely irritating oil causing a usu. intensely itching skin rash **b :** any of several plants closely related to poison ivy; *esp* **:** POISON OAK 1b **2 :** a skin rash produced by poison ivy

poison oak *n* **1 :** any of several plants related to poison ivy and producing an oil with similar irritating properties: as **a :** a bushy plant (*Toxicodendron diversilobum* syn. *Rhus diversiloba*) of the Pacific coast **b :** a bushy plant (*T. toxicarium* syn. *R. toxicodendron*) chiefly of the southeastern U.S. **2 :** POISON IVY 1a **3 :** a skin rash produced by poison oak

poi•son•ous \ˈpȯiz-ᵊn-əs\ *adj* **1 :** having the properties or effects of poison <~ chemicals> **2 :** producing a toxic substance that causes injury or death when absorbed or ingested <~ frogs>; *also* **:** VENOMOUS

poison su•mac \-ˈshü-ˌmak, -ˈsü-\ *n* **:** a swamp shrub of the genus *Toxicodendron* (*T. vernix* syn. *Rhus vernix*) chiefly of the eastern U.S. and Canada that has greenish-white berries and produces an irritating oil — called also *poison dogwood*

poi•son•wood \ˈpȯiz-ᵊn-ˌwu̇d\ *n* **:** a caustic or poisonous tree (*Metopium toxiferum*) of the cashew family (Anacardiaceae) that is native to Florida and the West Indies and has compound leaves, clusters of greenish flowers, and orange-yellow fruits

poke•weed \ˈpōk-ˌwēd\ *n* **:** a poisonous American perennial herb (*Phytolacca americana* of the family Phytolaccaceae) from which is obtained a mitogen that has been used to stimulate lymphocyte proliferation

po•lar \ˈpō-lər\ *adj* **1 :** of or relating to one or more poles (as of a spherical body) **2 :** exhibiting polarity; *esp* **:** having a dipole or characterized by molecules having dipoles ⟨a ~ solvent⟩ **3 :** being at opposite ends of a spectrum of symptoms or manifestations ⟨~ types of leprosy⟩

polar body *n* **:** a cell that separates from an oocyte during meiosis: **a :** one containing a nucleus produced in the first meiotic division — called also *first polar body* **b :** one containing a nucleus produced in the second meiotic division — called also *second polar body*

po•lar•i•ty \pō-ˈlar-ə-tē, pə-\ *n, pl* **-ties 1 :** the quality or condition inherent in a body that exhibits contrasting properties or powers in contrasting parts or directions **2 :** attraction toward a particular object or in a specific direction **3 :** the particular state either positive or negative with reference to the two poles or to electrification

po•lar•ize \ˈpō-lə-ˌrīz\ *vb* **-ized; -iz•ing 1 :** to vibrate or cause (as light waves) to vibrate in a definite pattern **2 :** to give physical polarity to — **po•lar•i•za•tion** \ˌpō-lə-rə-ˈzā-shən\ *n*

polarizing microscope *n* **:** a microscope equipped to produce polarized light for examination of a specimen

pole \ˈpōl\ *n* **1 a :** either of the two terminals of an electric cell or battery **b :** one of two or more regions in a magnetized body at which the magnetism is concentrated **2 :** either of two morphologically or physiologically differentiated areas at opposite ends of an axis in an organism, organ, or cell

poli- *or* **polio-** *comb form* **:** of or relating to the gray matter of the brain or spinal cord ⟨*polio*myelitis⟩

pol•i•clin•ic \ˈpä-lē-ˌkli-nik\ *n* **:** a dispensary or department of a hospital at which outpatients are treated — compare POLYCLINIC

pol•i•co•sa•nol *also* **poly•co•sa•nol** \ˌpä-lē-ˈkō-sə-ˌnȯl\ *n* **:** a mixture of alcohols derived chiefly from the waxy coating of sugarcane and used esp. as a dietary supplement to lower cholesterol levels

po•lio \ˈpō-lē-ˌō\ *n* **:** an infectious disease esp. of young children that is caused by the poliovirus, often causes no symptoms or a mild to moderate illness marked by headache, fever, sore throat, vomiting, diarrhea, and fatigue, and when affecting the central nervous system causes temporary or permanent muscle weakness or flaccid paralysis of muscles esp. of the legs and may become life-threatening when paralysis affects muscles involved in breathing and swallowing — called also *infantile paralysis, poliomyelitis;* see POST-POLIO SYNDROME

po•lio•dys•tro•phy \ˌpō-lē-ō-ˈdis-trə-fē\ *n, pl* **-phies :** atrophy of the gray matter esp. of the cerebrum

po•lio•en•ceph•a•li•tis \ˌpō-lē-(ˌ)ō-in-ˌse-fə-ˈlī-təs\ *n, pl* **-lit•i•des** \-ˈli-tə-ˌdēz\

: inflammation of the gray matter of the brain

po•lio•en•ceph•alo•my•eli•tis \-in-ˌse-fə-lō-ˌmī-ə-ˈlī-təs\ *n, pl* **-elit•i•des** \-ˈli-tə-ˌdēz\ : inflammation of the gray matter of the brain and the spinal cord

po•lio•my•eli•tis \ˌpō-lē-(ˌ)ō-ˌmī-ə-ˈlī-təs\ *n, pl* **-elit•i•des** \-ˈli-tə-ˌdēz\ : POLIO — **po•lio•my•elit•ic** \-ˈli-tik\ *adj*

po•li•o•sis \ˌpō-lē-ˈō-səs\ *n, pl* **-o•ses** \-ˌsēz\ : loss of color from the hair

polio vaccine *n* : a vaccine intended to confer immunity to polio — see SABIN VACCINE, SALK VACCINE

po•lio•vi•rus \ˈpō-lē-(ˌ)ō-ˌvī-rəs\ *n* : a picornavirus of the genus *Enterovirus* (species *Poliovirus*) occurring in three distinct serotypes that cause polio

po•litz•er bag \ˈpō-lit-sər-, ˈpä-\ *n* : a soft rubber bulb used to inflate the middle ear by increasing air pressure in the nasopharynx

Politzer, Ádam (1835–1920), Austrian otologist.

pol•len \ˈpä-lən\ *n* : a mass of male spores in a seed plant appearing usu. as a fine dust

pol•lex \ˈpä-ˌleks\ *n, pl* **pol•li•ces** \ˈpä-lə-ˌsēz\ : the first digit of the forelimb : THUMB

pollicis — see ABDUCTOR POLLICIS BREVIS, ABDUCTOR POLLICIS LONGUS, ADDUCTOR POLLICIS, EXTENSOR POLLICIS BREVIS, EXTENSOR POLLICIS LONGUS, FLEXOR POLLICIS BREVIS, FLEXOR POLLICIS LONGUS, OPPONENS POLLICIS, PRINCEPS POLLICIS

pol•li•ci•za•tion \ˌpä-lə-sə-ˈzā-shən\ *n* : the reconstruction or replacement of the thumb esp. from part of the index finger

pol•li•no•sis *or* **pol•le•no•sis** \ˌpä-lə-ˈnō-səs\ *n, pl* **-no•ses** \-ˌsēz\ : HAY FEVER

po•lo•ni•um \pə-ˈlō-nē-əm\ *n* : a radioactive metallic element that emits an alpha particle to form an isotope of lead — symbol *Po;* see ELEMENT table

poly- *comb form* **1** : many : several : much : MULTI- ⟨*poly*arthritis⟩ **2** : excessive : abnormal : HYPER- ⟨*poly*dactyly⟩

poly(A) \ˌpä-lē-ˈā\ *n* : RNA or a segment of RNA that is composed of a polynucleotide chain consisting entirely of adenine-containing nucleotides and that codes for polylysine when functioning as messenger RNA in protein synthesis — called also *polyadenylate, polyadenylic acid*

poly•acryl•amide \ˌpä-lē-ə-ˈkri-lə-ˌmīd\ *n* : a polymer $(-CH_2CHCONH_2-)_x$ derived from acrylic acid

polyacrylamide gel *n* : hydrated polyacrylamide that is used esp. to provide a medium for the suspension of a substance to be subjected to gel electrophoresis

poly•ad•e•nyl•ate \ˌpä-lē-ˌad-ᵊn-ˈi-ˌlāt\ *n* : POLY(A) — **poly•ad•e•nyl•at•ed** \-ˌā-təd\ *adj* — **poly•aden•y•la•tion** \-ə-de-nə-lā-shən\ *n*

poly•ad•e•nyl•ic acid \-ˈi-lik-\ *n* : POLY(A)

poly•ar•ter•i•tis \ˌpä-lē-ˌär-tə-ˈrī-təs\ *n* : POLYARTERITIS NODOSA

polyarteritis nodosa *n* : an acute inflammatory disease involving all layers of the arterial wall and characterized by degeneration, necrosis, exudation, and the formation of inflammatory nodules along the outer layer — called also *periarteritis nodosa*

poly•ar•thral•gia \-är-ˈthral-jē-ə\ *n* : pain in two or more joints

poly•ar•thri•tis \-är-ˈthrī-təs\ *n, pl* **-thrit•i•des** \-ˈthri-tə-ˌdēz\ : arthritis involving two or more joints

poly•ar•tic•u•lar \-är-ˈti-kyə-lər\ *adj* : having or affecting many joints ⟨~ arthritis⟩ — compare MONOARTICULAR, OLIGOARTICULAR

poly•bro•mi•nat•ed biphenyl \ˌpä-lē-ˈbrō-mə-ˌnā-təd-\ *n* : any of several compounds that are similar to polychlorinated biphenyls in environmental toxicity and in structure except that various hydrogen atoms are replaced by bromine rather than chlorine — called also *PBB*

poly(C) \ˌpä-lē-ˈsē\ *n* : POLYCYTIDYLIC ACID

poly•chlo•ri•nat•ed biphenyl \ˌpä-lē-ˈklōr-ə-ˌnā-təd-\ *n* : any of several compounds that are produced by replacing hydrogen atoms in biphenyl with chlorine, have various industrial applications, and are toxic environmental pollutants which tend to accumulate in animal tissues — called also *PCB*

poly•chon•dri•tis \-kän-ˈdrī-təs\ *n* : inflammation of cartilage at multiple sites in the body — see RELAPSING POLYCHONDRITIS

poly•chro•ma•sia \-krō-ˈmā-zhə, -zhē-ə\ *n* : the quality of being polychromatic; *specif* : POLYCHROMATOPHILIA

poly•chro•mat•ic \-krō-ˈma-tik\ *adj* **1** : showing a variety or a change of colors **2** *of a cell or tissue* : exhibiting polychromatophilia

[1]**poly•chro•ma•to•phil** \-krō-ˈma-tə-ˌfil, -ˈkrō-mə-tə-\ *n* : a young or degenerated red blood cell staining with both acid and basic dyes

[2]**polychromatophil** *adj* : exhibiting polychromatophilia; *esp* : staining with both acid and basic dyes

poly•chro•mato•phil•ia \-krō-ˌma-tə-ˈfi-lē-ə\ *n* : the quality of being stainable with more than one type of stain and esp. with both acid and basic dyes — **poly•chro•mato•phil•ic** \-krō-ˌma-tə-ˈfi-lik\ *adj*

poly•clin•ic \ˌpä-lē-ˈkli-nik\ *n* : a clinic or hospital treating diseases of many sorts — compare POLICLINIC

poly•clo•nal \ˌpä-lē-ˈklōn-ᵊl\ *adj* : produced by or being cells derived from two or more cells of different ancestry or genetic constitution ⟨~ antibody synthesis⟩

polycosanol *var of* POLICOSANOL
poly·cy·clic \ˌpä-lē-ˈsī-klik, -ˈsi-\ *adj* : having more than one cyclic component; *esp* : having two or more usu. fused rings in a molecule
polycyclic aromatic hydrocarbon *n* : any of a class of hydrocarbon molecules with multiple carbon rings that include numerous carcinogenic substances and environmental pollutants — called also *PAH, polynuclear aromatic hydrocarbon*
poly·cys·tic \-ˈsis-tik\ *adj* : having or involving more than one cyst
polycystic kidney disease *n* : either of two hereditary diseases characterized by gradually enlarging bilateral cysts of the kidney which lead to reduced renal functioning: **a** : a disease that is inherited as an autosomal dominant trait, is usu. asymptomatic until middle age, and is marked by side or back pain, hematuria, urinary tract infections, and nephrolithiasis **b** : a disease that is inherited as an autosomal recessive trait, usu. affects infants or children, and results in renal failure
polycystic ovary syndrome *n* : a variable disorder that is marked esp. by amenorrhea, hirsutism, obesity, infertility, and ovarian enlargement and is usu. initiated by an elevated level of luteinizing hormone, androgen, or estrogen which results in an abnormal cycle of gonadotropin release by the pituitary gland — called also *polycystic ovarian disease, polycystic ovarian syndrome, polycystic ovary disease, Stein-Leventhal syndrome*
poly·cy·thae·mia, poly·cy·thae·mic *chiefly Brit var of* POLYCYTHEMIA, POLYCYTHEMIC
poly·cy·the·mia \-(ˌ)sī-ˈthē-mē-ə\ *n* : a condition marked by an abnormal increase in the number of circulating red blood cells; *esp* : POLYCYTHEMIA VERA
polycythemia ve·ra \-ˈvir-ə\ *n* : chronic polycythemia that is a myeloproliferative disorder of unknown cause characterized by an increase in total blood volume and viscosity and typically accompanied by nosebleed, headache, dizziness, weakness, itchy skin, reddish complexion, distension of the circulatory vessels, and splenomegaly — called also *erythremia, Vaquez's disease*
poly·cy·the·mic \ˌpä-lē-(ˌ)sī-ˈthē-mik\ *adj* : relating to or involving polycythemia or polycythemia vera
poly·cyt·i·dyl·ic acid \-ˌsi-tə-ˈdi-lik-\ *n* : RNA or a segment of RNA that is composed of a polynucleotide chain consisting entirely of cytosine-containing nucleotides and that codes for a polypeptide chain consisting of proline residues when functioning as messenger RNA in protein synthesis — called also *poly(C)*; see POLY I:C
poly·dac·tyl \-ˈdak-tᵊl\ *adj* : characterized by polydactyly; *also* : being a gene that determines polydactyly
poly·dac·tyl·ia \-dak-ˈti-lē-ə\ *n* : POLYDACTYLY
poly·dac·tyl·ism \-ˈdakt-ᵊl-ˌi-zəm\ *n* : POLYDACTYLY
poly·dac·ty·ly \-ˈdak-tə-lē\ *n, pl* **-lies** : the condition of having more than the normal number of toes or fingers
poly·dip·sia \-ˈdip-sē-ə\ *n* : excessive or abnormal thirst — **poly·dip·sic** \-sik\ *adj*
poly·drug \ˈpä-lē-ˈdrəg\ *adj* : of, relating to, or being the abuse of more than one drug esp. when illicit; *also* : engaging in polydrug abuse
poly·em·bry·o·ny \ˌpä-lē-ˈem-brē-ə-nē, -(ˌ)em-ˈbrī-\ *n, pl* **-nies** : the production of two or more embryos from one ovule or egg
poly·en·do·crine \-ˈen-də-krən, -ˌkrīn, -ˌkrēn\ *adj* : relating to or affecting more than one endocrine gland
poly·eth·yl·ene gly·col \ˌpäl-ē-ˈeth-ə-ˌlēn-ˈglī-ˌkȯl, -ˌkōl\ *n* : any of a series of polymers that vary from viscous liquids to white solids and are used in medicine esp. as laxatives and as bases for pharmaceutical ointments and cosmetic creams — abbr. *PEG*
poly·gene \ˈpä-lē-ˌjēn\ *n* : any of a group of nonallelic genes that collectively control the inheritance of a quantitative character or modify the expression of a qualitative character — called also *multiple factor*
poly·ge·nic \ˌpä-lē-ˈjē-nik, -ˈje-\ *adj* : of, relating to, or resulting from polygenes : MULTIFACTORIAL
poly·glan·du·lar \-ˈglan-jə-lər\ *adj* : of, relating to, or involving several glands
poly·graph \ˈpä-lē-ˌgraf\ *n* : an instrument for simultaneously recording variations of several different pulsations (as of the pulse, blood pressure, and respiration) — see LIE DETECTOR — **poly·graph·ic** \ˌpä-lē-ˈgra-fik\ *adj*
poly·hy·dram·ni·os \ˌpä-lē-hī-ˈdram-nē-ˌäs\ *n* : HYDRAMNIOS
poly I:C \ˌpä-lē-ˌī-ˈsē\ *n* : a synthetic 2-stranded RNA composed of one strand of polyinosinic acid and one strand of polycytidylic acid that induces interferon formation and has been used experimentally as an anticancer and antiviral agent — called also *poly I·poly C*
poly·ino·sin·ic acid \ˌpä-lē-ˌi-nə-ˈsi-nik-, -ˌī-nə-\ *n* : RNA or a segment of RNA that is composed of a polynucleotide chain consisting entirely of inosinic acid residues — see POLY I:C
poly I·poly C \ˌpä-lē-ˈī-ˌpä-lē-ˈsē\ *n* : POLY I:C
poly·ke·tide \ˌpä-lē-ˈkē-ˌtīd\ *n* : any of a large class of diverse compounds that are characterized by more than two CO groups connected by single intervening carbon atoms, that are produced esp. by certain bacteria and fungi, and that

include various substances (as erythromycin and lovastatin) having antibiotic, anticancer, cholesterol-lowering, or immunosuppressive effects

poly·ly·sine \ˌpä-lē-ˈlī-ˌsēn\ *n* : a protein whose polypeptide chain consists entirely of lysine residues

poly·mer \ˈpä-lə-mər\ *n* : a chemical compound or mixture of compounds formed by polymerization and consisting essentially of repeating structural units — **poly·mer·ic** \ˌpä-lə-ˈmer-ik\ *adj* — **po·ly·mer·ism** \pə-ˈli-mə-ˌri-zəm, ˈpä-lə-mə-\ *n*

poly·mer·ase \-mə-ˌrās, -ˌrāz\ *n* : any of several enzymes that catalyze the formation of DNA or RNA from precursor substances in the presence of preexisting DNA or RNA acting as a template

polymerase chain reaction *n* : an in vitro technique for rapidly synthesizing large quantities of a given DNA segment that involves separating the DNA into its two complementary strands, binding a primer to each single strand at the end of the given DNA segment where synthesis will start, using DNA polymerase to synthesize two-stranded DNA from each single strand, and repeating the process — abbr. *PCR*

po·ly·mer·i·za·tion \pə-ˌli-mə-rə-ˈzā-shən, ˌpä-lə-mə-rə-\ *n* : a chemical reaction in which two or more small molecules combine to form larger molecules that contain repeating structural units of the original molecules — compare ASSOCIATION 3 — **po·ly·mer·ize** \pə-ˈli-mə-ˌrīz, ˈpä-lə-mə-\ *vb*

poly·meth·yl meth·ac·ry·late \ˌpä-lē-ˈme-thəl-me-ˈtha-krə-ˌlāt\ *n* : a thermoplastic polymeric resin that is used esp. in hard contact lenses and in prostheses to replace bone

poly·mi·cro·bi·al \ˌpä-lē-mī-ˈkrō-bē-əl\ *adj* : of, relating to, or caused by several types of microorganisms

poly·mod·al \ˌpä-lē-ˈmō-dᵊl\ *adj* : responding to several different forms of sensory stimulation

poly·morph \ˈpä-lē-ˌmȯrf\ *n* **1** : a polymorphic organism; *also* : one of the several forms of such an organism **2** : POLYMORPHONUCLEAR LEUKOCYTE

poly·mor·phic \ˌpä-lē-ˈmȯr-fik\ *adj* : of, relating to, or having polymorphism — **poly·mor·phi·cal·ly** \-fi-k(ə-)lē\ *adv*

polymorphic light eruption *n* : POLYMORPHOUS LIGHT ERUPTION

poly·mor·phism \-ˈmȯr-ˌfi-zəm\ *n* : the quality or state of existing in or assuming different forms: as **a** : existence of a species in several forms independent of the variations of sex **b** : existence of a gene in several allelic forms; *also* : a variation in a specific DNA sequence **c** : existence of a molecule (as an enzyme) in several forms in a single species

[1]**poly·mor·pho·nu·cle·ar** \-ˌmȯr-fō-ˈnü-klē-ər, -ˈnyü-\ *adj, of a cell* : having the nucleus complexly lobed and often of varied form; *esp* : of, relating to, or being a polymorphonuclear leukocyte ⟨~ neutrophils⟩

[2]**polymorphonuclear** *n* : POLYMORPHONUCLEAR LEUKOCYTE

polymorphonuclear leukocyte *n* : a mature white blood cell having a complexly lobed nucleus and granulocytic cytoplasm and including the neutrophils, basophils, and eosinophils; *esp* : NEUTROPHIL

poly·mor·phous \-ˈmȯr-fəs\ *adj* : having, assuming, or occurring in various forms — **poly·mor·phous·ly** *adv*

polymorphous light eruption *n* : photodermatosis that is marked esp. by red papules or blisters often accompanied by itching or a burning sensation

poly·my·al·gia \ˌpä-li-mī-ˈal-jē-ə\ *n* : myalgia affecting several muscle groups; *specif* : POLYMYALGIA RHEUMATICA

polymyalgia rheu·mat·i·ca \-rü-ˈma-ti-kə\ *n* : a disorder of the elderly characterized by muscular pain and stiffness in the shoulders and neck and in the pelvic area

poly·myo·si·tis \-ˌmī-ə-ˈsī-təs\ *n* : inflammation of several muscles at once; *specif* : an inflammatory muscle disease of unknown cause that affects skeletal muscles and is marked esp. by pain and weakness of muscles (as of the shoulder or hip) closest to the trunk — see DERMATOMYOSITIS

poly·myx·in \ˌpä-lē-ˈmik-sən\ *n* : any of several toxic antibiotics obtained from a soil bacterium of the genus *Bacillus* (*B. polymyxa*) and active against gram-negative bacteria

polymyxin B *n* : the least toxic of the polymyxins used in the form of its sulfate chiefly in the treatment of some localized, gastrointestinal, or systemic infections

polymyxin E *n* : COLISTIN

poly·neu·ri·tis \ˌpä-lē-nu̇-ˈrī-təs, -nyu̇-\ *n, pl* **-rit·i·des** \-ˈri-tə-ˌdēz\ *or* **-ri·tis·es** : neuritis of several peripheral nerves at the same time — see GUILLAIN-BARRÉ SYNDROME — **poly·neu·rit·ic** \-ˈri-tik\ *adj*

poly·neu·ro·pa·thy \-nu̇-ˈrä-pə-thē, -nyu̇-\ *n, pl* **-thies** : a disease of nerves; *esp* : a noninflammatory degenerative disease of nerves usu. caused by toxins (as of lead)

poly·nu·cle·ar \-ˈnü-klē-ər, -ˈnyü-\ *adj* : chemically polycyclic esp. with respect to the benzene ring

polynuclear aromatic hydrocarbon *n* : POLYCYCLIC AROMATIC HYDROCARBON

poly·nu·cle·o·tide \-ˈnü-klē-ə-ˌtīd, -ˈnyü-\ *n* : a polymeric chain of nucleotides

poly·oma·vi·rus \ˌpä-lē-ˈō-mə-ˌvī-rəs\ *n* **1** *cap* : a genus of double-stranded DNA viruses (family *Polyomaviridae*) that induce tumors usu. in specific mammals and that include simian virus 40 and the causative agent of progressive multifocal leukoencephalopathy **2** : any virus of the genus *Polyomavirus* or of the family (*Polyomaviridae*) to which it belongs

poly•opia \ˌpä-lē-ˈō-pē-ə\ *n* : perception of more than one image of a single object esp. with one eye

poly•os•tot•ic \ˌpä-lē-ä-ˈstä-tik\ *adj* : involving or relating to many bones

pol•yp \ˈpä-ləp\ *n* : a projecting mass of swollen and hypertrophied or tumorous membrane

pol•yp•ec•to•my \ˌpä-li-ˈpek-tə-mē\ *n, pl* **-mies** : the surgical excision of a polyp

poly•pep•tide \ˌpä-lē-ˈpep-ˌtīd\ *n* : a molecular chain of amino acids — **poly•pep•tid•ic** \-(ˌ)pep-ˈti-dik\ *adj*

poly•pha•gia \-ˈfa-jə, -jē-ə\ *n* : excessive appetite or eating — compare HYPERPHAGIA

poly•phar•ma•cy \-ˈfär-mə-sē\ *n, pl* **-cies** : the practice of administering many different medicines esp. concurrently for the treatment of the same disease; *also* : the concurrent use of multiple medications by a patient to treat usu. coexisting conditions and which may result in adverse drug interactions

poly•pha•sic \-ˈfā-zik\ *adj* **1** : of, relating to, or having more than one phase — compare DIPHASIC b, MONOPHASIC 1 **2** : having several periods of activity interrupted by intervening periods of rest in each 24 hours ⟨an infant is essentially ~⟩

poly•phe•nol \ˌpä-li-ˈfē-ˌnōl, -ˌnȯl\ *n* : a phenol containing more than one hydroxyl group in a molecule; *esp* : an antioxidant phytochemical that tends to prevent or neutralize the damaging effects of free radicals — **poly•phe•no•lic** \-fi-ˈnō-lik, -ˈnä-\ *adj*

poly•ploid \ˈpä-lē-ˌplȯid\ *adj* : having or being a chromosome number that is a multiple greater than two of the monoploid number — **poly•ploi•dy** \-ˌplȯi-dē\ *n*

po•lyp•nea \pä-ˈlip-nē-ə, pə-\ *n* : rapid or panting respiration — **po•lyp•ne•ic** \-nē-ik\ *adj*

po•lyp•noea *chiefly Brit var of* POLYPNEA

pol•yp•oid \ˈpä-lə-ˌpȯid\ *adj* **1** : resembling a polyp ⟨a ~ intestinal growth⟩ **2** : marked by the formation of lesions suggesting polyps ⟨~ disease⟩

pol•yp•o•sis \ˌpä-li-ˈpō-səs\ *n, pl* **-o•ses** \-ˌsēz\ : a condition characterized by the presence of numerous polyps — see FAMILIAL ADENOMATOUS POLYPOSIS

poly•ra•dic•u•lo•neu•rop•a•thy \ˌpä-lirə-ˌdi-kyə-lō-nu̇-ˈrä-pə-thē, -nyu̇-\ *n, pl* **-thies** : an inflammatory disorder (as Guillain-Barré syndrome) affecting peripheral nerves and the nerve roots of the spinal nerves and marked by demyelination or axon degeneration

poly•ri•bo•some \ˌpä-lē-ˈrī-bə-ˌsōm\ *n* : a cluster of ribosomes linked together by a molecule of messenger RNA and forming the site of protein synthesis — called also *polysome* — **poly•ri•bo•som•al** \-ˌrī-bə-ˈsō-məl\ *adj*

poly•sac•cha•ride \-ˈsa-kə-ˌrīd\ *n* : a carbohydrate that can be decomposed by hydrolysis into two or more molecules of monosaccharides; *esp* : one (as cellulose, starch, or glycogen) containing many monosaccharide units and marked by complexity — called also *glycan*

poly•se•ro•si•tis \-ˌsir-ə-ˈsī-təs\ *n* : inflammation of several serous membranes (as the pleura, pericardium, and peritoneum) at the same time

poly•some \ˈpä-lē-ˌsōm\ *n* : POLYRIBOSOME

poly•som•no•gram \ˌpä-lē-ˈsäm-nə-ˌgram\ *n* : a record of physiological variables during sleep obtained by polysomnography

poly•som•no•graph \ˌpä-lē-ˈsäm-nə-ˌgraf\ *n* : a polygraph used for polysomnography

poly•som•nog•ra•phy \ˌpä-lē-ˌsäm-ˈnä-grə-fē\ *n, pl* **-phies** : the technique or process of using a polygraph to make a continuous record during sleep of multiple physiological variables (as breathing, heart rate, and muscle activity) — **poly•som•nog•ra•pher** \-ˌsäm-ˈnä-grə-fər\ *n* — **poly•som•no•graph•ic** \-nə-ˈgra-fik\ *adj*

poly•sor•bate \ˌpä-lē-ˈsȯr-ˌbāt\ *n* : any of several emulsifiers used in the preparation of some pharmaceuticals and foods — see TWEEN

poly•sper•my \ˈpä-lē-ˌspər-mē\ *n, pl* **-mies** : the entrance of several spermatozoa into one egg — compare MONOSPERMY — **poly•sper•mic** \ˌpä-lē-ˈspər-mik\ *adj*

poly•sub•stance \ˌpä-lē-ˈsəb-stəns\ *n, often attrib* : a group of substances used often indiscriminately by a substance abuser

poly•syn•ap•tic \ˌpä-lē-sə-ˈnap-tik\ *adj* : involving two or more synapses in the central nervous system — **poly•syn•ap•ti•cal•ly** *adv*

poly•tene \ˈpä-lē-ˌtēn\ *adj* : relating to, being, or having chromosomes each of which consists of many strands with the corresponding chromomeres in contact — **poly•te•ny** \-ˌtē-nē\ *n*

poly•tet•ra•flu•o•ro•eth•yl•ene \ˌpä-lē-ˌte-trə-ˌflu̇r-ō-ˈe-thə-ˌlēn\ *n* : a polymer $(CF_2{-}CF_2)_n$ that is a resin used to fabricate prostheses — abbr. *PTFE;* see TEFLON

poly•the•lia \ˌpä-lē-ˈthē-lē-ə\ *n* : the condition of having more than the normal number of nipples

poly•thi•a•zide \-ˈthī-ə-ˌzīd, -zəd\ *n* : an antihypertensive and diuretic drug $C_{11}H_{13}ClF_3N_3O_4S_3$ — see RENESE

poly(U) \ˌpä-lē-ˈyü\ *n* : POLYURIDYLIC ACID

poly•un•sat•u•rate \ˌpä-lē-ˌən-ˈsa-chə-rət\ *n* : a polyunsaturated oil or fatty acid

poly·un·sat·u·rat·ed \-ˌən-ˈsa-chə-ˌrā-təd\ *adj, of an oil, fat, or fatty acid* : having in each molecule many chemical bonds in which two or three pairs of electrons are shared by two atoms — compare MONOUNSATURATED

poly·uria \-ˈyu̇r-ē-ə\ *n* : excessive secretion of urine

poly·uri·dyl·ic acid \-ˌyu̇r-ə-ˌdi-lik-\ *n* : RNA or a segment of RNA that is composed of a polynucleotide chain consisting entirely of uracil-containing nucleotides and that codes for a polypeptide chain consisting of phenylalanine residues when functioning as messenger RNA in protein synthesis — called also *poly(U)*

poly·va·lent \ˌpä-lē-ˈvā-lənt\ *adj* : effective against, sensitive toward, or counteracting more than one exciting agent (as a toxin or antigen) ⟨a ~ vaccine⟩ — **poly·va·lence** \-ləns\ *n*

poly·vi·nyl·pyr·rol·i·done \-ˌvīn-ᵊl-pi-ˈrä-lə-ˌdōn\ *n* : a water-soluble chemically inert polymer $(C_6H_9NO)_n$ used in medicine as a vehicle for drugs (as iodine) and esp. formerly as a plasma expander — called also *povidone*

Pom·pe disease \ˌpäm-ˈpā-\ *or* **Pom·pe's disease** \ˌpäm-ˈpāz\ *n* : an inherited glycogen storage disease that results from an enzyme deficiency, is characterized by abnormal accumulation of glycogen esp. in the liver, heart, and muscle, has a severe fatal form with onset during infancy and a slowly progressive form with onset during childhood or adulthood, and is inherited as an autosomal recessive trait — called also *acid maltase deficiency*

Pompe, Johann Cassianius (*fl* 1932), Dutch physician.

pom·pho·lyx \ˈpäm-fə-ˌliks\ *n* : a skin disease marked by an eruption of vesicles esp. on the palms and soles

pon·der·al index \ˈpän-də-rəl-\ *n* : a measure of relative body mass expressed as the ratio of the cube root of body weight to height multiplied by 100

P_1 generation \ˈpē-ˈwən-\ *n* : a generation consisting of stocks which are usu. homozygous for one or more traits and from which the parents used in the first cross of a genetic experiment are selected — compare F_1 GENERATION

pons \ˈpänz\ *n, pl* **pon·tes** \ˈpän-ˌtēz\ : a broad mass of chiefly transverse nerve fibers in the mammalian brain stem lying ventral to the cerebellum at the anterior end of the medulla oblongata

pons Va·ro·lii \-və-ˈrō-lē-ˌī, -lē-ˌē\ *n, pl* **pontes Varolii** : PONS

Va·ro·lio \vä-ˈrō-lē-ō\, **Costanzo (1543–1575),** Italian anatomist.

Pon·ti·ac fever \ˈpän-tē-ˌak-\ *n* : an illness caused by a bacterium of the genus *Legionella* (*L. pneumophila*) that is a less severe form of Legionnaires' disease in which pneumonia does not develop

pon·tic \ˈpän-tik\ *n* : an artificial tooth on a dental bridge

pon·tile \ˈpän-ˌtīl, -təl\ *adj* : PONTINE

pon·tine \ˈpän-ˌtīn\ *adj* : of or relating to the pons ⟨a study of ~ lesions⟩

pontine flexure *n* : a flexure of the embryonic hindbrain that serves to delimit the developing cerebellum and medulla oblongata

pontine nucleus *n* : any of various large groups of nerve cells in the basal part of the pons that receive fibers from the cerebral cortex and send fibers to the cerebellum by way of the middle cerebellar peduncles

pontis — see BRACHIUM PONTIS

Pon·to·caine \ˈpän-tə-ˌkān\ *trademark* — used for a preparation of the hydrochloride of tetracaine

[1]**pool** \ˈpül\ *vb, of blood* : to accumulate or become static (as in the veins of a bodily part) ⟨blood ~*ed* in his legs⟩

[2]**pool** *n* : a readily available supply: as **a** : the whole quantity of a particular material present in the body and available for function or the satisfying of metabolic demands — see GENE POOL **b** : a body product (as blood) collected from many donors and stored for later use

pop·li·te·al \ˌpä-plə-ˈtē-əl, päp-ˈli-tē-\ *adj* : of or relating to the back part of the leg behind the knee joint

popliteal artery *n* : the continuation of the femoral artery that after passing through the thigh crosses the popliteal space and soon divides into the anterior and posterior tibial arteries

popliteal fossa *n* : POPLITEAL SPACE

popliteal ligament — see ARCUATE POPLITEAL LIGAMENT, OBLIQUE POPLITEAL LIGAMENT

popliteal nerve — see LATERAL POPLITEAL NERVE, MEDIAL POPLITEAL NERVE

popliteal space *n* : a lozenge-shaped space at the back of the knee joint — called also *popliteal fossa*

popliteal vein *n* : a vein formed by the union of the anterior and posterior tibial veins and ascending through the popliteal space to the thigh where it becomes the femoral vein

pop·li·te·us \pä-plə-ˈtē-əs, päp-ˈli-tē-əs\ *n, pl* **-li·tei** \-tē-ˌī\ : a flat muscle that originates from the lateral condyle of the femur, forms part of the floor of the popliteal space, and functions to flex the leg and rotate the femur medially

pop·per \ˈpä-pər\ *n, slang* : a vial of amyl nitrite or butyl nitrite esp. when used illicitly as an aphrodisiac

pop·py \ˈpä-pē\ *n, pl* **poppies** : any herb of the genus *Papaver* (family Papaveraceae); *esp* : OPIUM POPPY

pop·u·la·tion \ˌpä-pyə-ˈlā-shən\ *n* **1** : the organisms inhabiting a particular locality **2** : a group of individual persons, objects, or items from which samples are taken for statistical measurement

population genetics *n* : a branch of genetics concerned with gene and genotype frequencies in populations — see HARDY-WEINBERG LAW

por•ce•lain \ˈpōr-sə-lən\ *n* : a hard, fine-grained, nonporous, and usu. translucent and white ceramic ware that has many uses in dentistry

por•cine \ˈpȯr-ˌsīn\ *adj* : of or derived from swine ⟨~ heterografts⟩

pore \ˈpōr\ *n* : a minute opening esp. in an animal or plant; *esp* : one by which matter passes through a membrane

-pore \ˌpōr\ *n comb form* : opening ⟨blasto*pore*⟩

por•en•ceph•a•ly \ˌpȯr-in-ˈse-fə-lē\ *n, pl* **-lies** : the presence of cavities in the brain — **por•en•ce•phal•ic** \-ˌen-sə-ˈfa-lik\ *adj*

por•fi•mer sodium \ˈpȯr-fə-mər-\ *n* : a photosensitizing mixture of porphyrin polymers that is administered by intravenous injection to induce photosensitivity in tumor cells (as of esophageal carcinoma) before subjecting them to laser light in photodynamic therapy — see PHOTOFRIN

pork tapeworm \ˈpȯrk-\ *n* : a tapeworm of the genus *Taenia* (*T. solium*) that infests the human intestine as an adult, has a cysticercus larva that typically develops in swine, and is contracted by humans through ingestion of the larva in raw or imperfectly cooked pork

po•ro•ceph•a•li•a•sis \ˌpō-rō-ˌse-fə-ˈlī-ə-səs\ *n, pl* **-a•ses** \-ˌsēz\ : infestation with or disease caused by a tongue worm of the genus *Porocephalus*

Po•ro•ceph•a•lus \-ˈse-fə-ləs\ *n* : a genus of tongue worms (family Porocephalidae) occurring as adults in the lungs of reptiles and as young in various vertebrates including humans

po•ro•ker•a•to•sis \-ˌker-ə-ˈtō-səs\ *n* : any of several often inherited skin disorders characterized by proliferation of atypical keratinocytes and marked by the presence of usu. circular atrophic skin lesions which are surrounded by a ridgelike horny border

po•ro•sis \pə-ˈrō-səs\ *n, pl* **po•ro•ses** \-ˌsēz\ *or* **porosises** : a condition (as of a bone) characterized by porosity; *specif* : rarefaction (as of bone) with increased translucency to X-rays

po•ros•i•ty \pə-ˈrä-sə-tē, pō-, pȯ-\ *n, pl* **-ties** **1 a** : the quality or state of being porous **b** : the ratio of the volume of interstices of a material to the volume of its mass **2** : PORE

po•rot•ic \pə-ˈrä-tik\ *adj* : exhibiting or marked by porous structure or osteoporosis ⟨~ bone⟩

po•rous \ˈpōr-əs\ *adj* **1** : possessing or full of pores ⟨~ bones⟩ **2** : permeable to fluids

por•pho•bi•lin•o•gen \ˌpȯr-fō-bī-ˈli-nə-jən\ *n* : an acid $C_{10}H_{14}N_2O_4$ having two carboxyl groups per molecule that is derived from pyrrole and is found in the urine in acute porphyria

por•phyr•ia \pȯr-ˈfir-ē-ə\ *n* : any of several usu. hereditary abnormalities of porphyrin metabolism characterized by excretion of excess porphyrins in the urine

porphyria cu•ta•nea tar•da \-kyu̇-ˈtā-nē-ə-ˈtär-də\ *n* : a common porphyria that is marked by an excess of uroporphyrin caused by an enzyme deficiency chiefly of the liver and that is characterized esp. by skin lesions upon exposure to light, scarring, hyperpigmentation, and hypertrichosis

por•phy•rin \ˈpȯr-fə-rən\ *n* : any of various compounds with a structure that consists essentially of four pyrrole rings joined by four =CH– groups; *esp* : one (as hemoglobin) containing a central metal atom and usu. having biological activity

por•phy•rin•uria \ˌpȯr-fə-rə-ˈnu̇r-ē-ə, -ˈnyu̇r-\ *n* : the presence of porphyrin in the urine

port \ˈpȯrt\ *n* : an opening, passage, or channel through which something can be introduced into the body: as **a** : a small medical device (as of plastic or titanium) that is implanted below the skin, is attached to a catheter typically inserted into a blood vessel, and has a small opening through which a needle can be inserted to administer fluids or drugs or withdraw blood **b** : an incision (as one made between intercostal spaces) for passing a medical instrument (as an endoscope) into the body

por•ta \ˈpȯr-tə\ *n, pl* **por•tae** \-ˌtē\ : an opening in a bodily part where the blood vessels, nerves, or ducts leave and enter : HILUM

por•ta•ca•val \ˌpȯr-tə-ˈkā-vəl\ *adj* : extending from the portal vein to the vena cava ⟨~ anastomosis⟩

portacaval shunt *n* : a surgical shunt by which the portal vein is made to empty into the inferior vena cava in order to bypass a damaged liver

porta hep•a•tis \-ˈhe-pə-təs\ *n* : the fissure running transversely on the underside of the liver where most of the vessels enter or leave — called also *transverse fissure*

¹por•tal \ˈpȯrt-ᵊl\ *n* : a communicating part or area of an organism: as **a** : PORTAL VEIN **b** : the point at which something enters the body

²portal *adj* **1** : of or relating to the porta hepatis **2** : of, relating to, or being a portal vein or a portal system

portal cirrhosis *n* : LAENNEC'S CIRRHOSIS

portal hypertension *n* : hypertension in the hepatic portal system caused by venous obstruction or occlusion that produces splenomegaly and ascites in its later stages

portal system *n* : a system of veins that begins and ends in capillaries — see HEPATIC PORTAL SYSTEM, PITUITARY PORTAL SYSTEM

portal vein *n* : a large vein that is formed by fusion of other veins, that terminates in a capillary network, and that delivers blood to some area of the body other than the heart; *esp* : HEPATIC PORTAL VEIN

por•tio \ˈpȯr-shē-ˌō, ˈpȯr-tē-ˌō\ *n, pl* **-ti•o•nes** \ˌpȯr-shē-ˈō-ˌnēz\ : a part, segment, or branch (as of an organ or nerve) ⟨the visible ~ of the cervix⟩

por•to•sys•tem•ic \ˌpȯr-tō-sis-ˈte-mik\ *adj* : connecting the hepatic portal system and the venous part of the systemic circulation ⟨a ~ shunt⟩

Por•tu•guese man–of–war \ˈpȯr-chə-ˌgēz-ˌman-əv-ˈwȯr\ *n, pl* **Portuguese man–of–wars** *also* **Portuguese men–of–war** : any siphonophore of the genus *Physalia* including tropical and subtropical oceanic forms having a large crested bladderlike float and long tentacles capable of inflicting a painful sting

port–wine stain \ˈpȯrt-ˌwīn-\ *n* : a reddish-purple superficial hemangioma of the skin commonly occurring as a birthmark — called also *nevus flammeus, port-wine mark*

POS *abbr* point-of-service

[1]**po•si•tion** \pə-ˈzi-shən\ *n* : a particular arrangement or location; *specif* : an arrangement of the parts of the body considered particularly desirable for some medical or surgical procedure ⟨knee-chest ~⟩ ⟨prone ~⟩ — **po•si•tion•al** \pə-ˈzi-shə-nəl\ *adj*

[2]**position** *vb* : to put in proper position

pos•i•tive \ˈpä-zə-tiv\ *adj* **1** : being, relating to, or charged with electricity of which the proton is the elementary unit **2** : affirming the presence of that sought or suspected to be present ⟨a ~ test for blood⟩ — **positive** *n* — **pos•i•tive•ly** *adv* — **pos•i•tive•ness** *n*

positive electron *n* : POSITRON

positive end–expiratory pressure *n* : a technique of assisting breathing by increasing the air pressure in the lungs and air passages near the end of expiration so that an increased amount of air remains in the lungs following expiration — abbr. *PEEP*

positive pressure *n* : pressure that is greater than atmospheric pressure

pos•i•tron \ˈpä-zə-ˌträn\ *n* : a positively charged particle having the same mass and magnitude of charge as the electron

positron–emission tomography *n* : tomography in which an in vivo, noninvasive, cross-sectional image of regional metabolism is obtained by a usu. color-coded cathode-ray tube representation of the distribution of gamma radiation given off in the collision of electrons in cells with positrons emitted by radionuclides incorporated into metabolic substances — abbr. *PET*

post- *prefix* **1** : after : later than ⟨*post*operative⟩ ⟨*post*coronary⟩ **2** : behind : posterior to ⟨*post*auricular⟩

post•abor•tion \ˌpōst-ə-ˈbȯr-shən\ *adj* : occurring after an abortion

post•ab•sorp•tive \-əb-ˈsȯrp-tiv\ *adj* : being in or typical of the period following absorption of nutrients from the digestive tract

post•ad•o•les•cence \-ˌad-ᵊl-ˈes-ᵊns\ *n* : the period following adolescence and preceding adulthood — **post•ad•o•les•cent** \-ᵊnt\ *adj or n*

post•an•es•the•sia \-ˌa-nəs-ˈthē-zhə\ *adj* : POSTANESTHETIC

postanesthesia care unit *n* : RECOVERY ROOM

post•an•es•thet•ic \-ˈthe-tik\ *adj* : occurring in, used in, or being the period following administration of an anesthetic ⟨~ encephalopathy⟩

post•an•ox•ic \-a-ˈnäk-sik\ *adj* : occurring or being after a period of anoxia

post•au•ric•u•lar \-ȯ-ˈri-kyə-lər\ *adj* : located or occurring behind the auricle of the ear ⟨a ~ incision⟩

post•ax•i•al \-ˈak-sē-əl\ *adj* : of or relating to the ulnar side of the vertebrate forelimb or the fibular side of the hind limb; *also* : of or relating to the side of an animal or side of one of its limbs that is posterior to the axis of its body or limbs

post•cap•il•lary \-ˈka-pə-ˌler-ē\ *adj* : of, relating to, affecting, or being a venule of the circulatory system

post•car•di•ot•o•my \-ˌkär-dē-ˈä-tə-mē\ *adj* : occurring or being in the period following open-heart surgery

post•cen•tral \-ˈsen-trəl\ *adj* : located behind a center or central structure; *esp* : located behind the central sulcus of the cerebral cortex

postcentral gyrus *n* : a gyrus of the parietal lobe located just posterior to the central sulcus, lying parallel to the precentral gyrus of the temporal lobe, and comprising the somatosensory cortex

post•cho•le•cys•tec•to•my syndrome \-ˌkō-lə-(ˌ)sis-ˈtek-tə-mē-\ *n* : persistent pain and associated symptoms (as indigestion and nausea) following a cholecystectomy

post•co•i•tal \-ˈkō-ət-ᵊl, -ˈēt-ᵊl; -ˈkȯit-ᵊl\ *adj* : occurring, existing, or being administered after coitus

post•cor•o•nary \-ˈkȯr-ə-ˌner-ē, -ˈkär-\ *adj* **1** : relating to, occurring in, or being the period following a heart attack ⟨~ exercise⟩ **2** : having suffered a heart attack ⟨a ~ patient⟩

post•dam \ˌpōst-ˈdam\ *n* : a posterior extension of a full denture to accomplish a complete seal between denture and tissues

post•en•ceph•a•lit•ic \-in-ˌse-fə-ˈli-tik\ *adj* : occurring after and presumably as a result of encephalitis <~ parkinsonism>

[1]**pos·te·ri·or** \pō-ˈstir-ē-ər, pä-\ *adj* : situated behind: as **a** : situated at or toward the hind part of the body : CAUDAL **b** : DORSAL — used of human anatomy in which the upright posture makes dorsal and caudal identical

[2]**pos·te·ri·or** \pä-ˈstir-ē-ər, pō-\ *n* : the posterior bodily parts; *esp* : BUTTOCKS

posterior auricular artery *n* : a small branch of the external carotid artery that supplies or gives off branches supplying the back of the ear and the adjacent region of the scalp, the middle ear, tympanic membrane, and mastoid cells — called also *posterior auricular*

posterior auricular vein *n* : a vein formed from venous tributaries in the region behind the ear that joins with the posterior facial vein to form the external jugular vein

posterior brachial cutaneous nerve *n* : a branch of the radial nerve that arises on the medial side of the arm in the axilla and supplies the skin on the dorsal surface almost to the olecranon

posterior cerebral artery *n* : CEREBRAL ARTERY c

posterior chamber *n* : a narrow space in the eye that is behind the peripheral part of the iris and in front of the suspensory ligament of the lens and the ciliary processes and that is filled with aqueous humor— compare ANTERIOR CHAMBER

posterior column *n* : DORSAL HORN

posterior commissure *n* : a bundle of white matter crossing from one side of the brain to the other just rostral to the superior colliculi and above the opening of the aqueduct of Sylvius into the third ventricle

posterior communicating artery *n* : COMMUNICATING ARTERY b

posterior cord *n* : a cord of nerve tissue that is formed from the posterior divisions of the three trunks of the brachial plexus and that divides into the axillary and radial nerves — compare LATERAL CORD, MEDIAL CORD

posterior cricoarytenoid *n* : CRICOARYTENOID 2

posterior cruciate ligament *n* : a cruciate ligament of each knee that attaches the back of the tibia with the front of the femur and functions esp. to limit the backward motion of the tibia — called also *PCL*

posterior elastic lamina *n* : DESCEMET'S MEMBRANE

posterior facial vein *n* : a vein that is formed in the upper part of the parotid gland behind the mandible by the union of several tributaries and joins with the posterior auricular vein to form the external jugular vein

posterior femoral cutaneous nerve *n* : a nerve that arises from the sacral plexus and is distributed to the skin of the perineum and of the back of the thigh and leg — compare LATERAL FEMORAL CUTANEOUS NERVE

posterior funiculus *n* : a longitudinal division on each side of the spinal cord comprising white matter between the dorsal root and the posterior median sulcus — compare LATERAL FUNICULUS, VENTRAL FUNICULUS

posterior gray column *n* : DORSAL HORN

posterior horn *n* **1** : DORSAL HORN **2** : the cornu of the lateral ventricle of each cerebral hemisphere that curves backward into the occipital lobe — compare ANTERIOR HORN 2, INFERIOR HORN

posterior humeral circumflex artery *n* : an artery that branches from the axillary artery in the shoulder, curves around the back of the humerus, and is distributed esp. to the deltoid muscle and shoulder joint — compare ANTERIOR HUMERAL CIRCUMFLEX ARTERY

posterior inferior cerebellar artery *n* : an artery that usu. branches from the vertebral artery and supplies much of the medulla oblongata, the inferior portion of the cerebellum, and part of the floor of the fourth ventricle

posterior inferior iliac spine *n* : a projection on the posterior margin of the ilium that is situated below the posterior superior iliac spine and is separated from it by a notch — called also *posterior inferior spine*

posterior intercostal artery *n* : INTERCOSTAL ARTERY b

posterior lobe *n* **1** : NEUROHYPOPHYSIS **2** : the part of the cerebellum between the primary fissure and the flocculonodular lobe

pos·te·ri·or·ly *adv* : in a posterior direction

posterior malleolus *n* : MALLEOLUS c

posterior median septum *n* : a sheet of glial tissue in the midsagittal plane of the spinal cord that partitions the posterior part of the spinal cord into right and left halves

posterior median sulcus *n* : a shallow groove along the midline of the posterior part of the spinal cord that separates the two posterior funiculi

posterior naris *n* : CHOANA

posterior nasal spine *n* : the nasal spine that is formed by the union of processes of the two palatine bones

posterior pillar of the fauces *n* : PALATOPHARYNGEAL ARCH

posterior pituitary *n* **1** : NEUROHYPOPHYSIS **2** : an extract of the neurohypophysis of domesticated animals for medicinal use — called also *posterior pituitary extract*

posterior pituitary gland *n* : NEUROHYPOPHYSIS

posterior root *n* : DORSAL ROOT

posterior sacrococcygeal muscle *n* : SACROCOCCYGEUS DORSALIS

posterior spinal artery *n* : SPINAL ARTERY b

posterior spinocerebellar tract *n* : SPINOCEREBELLAR TRACT a

posterior superior alveolar artery *n* : a branch of the maxillary artery that supplies the upper molar and bicuspid teeth

posterior superior alveolar vein *n* : any of several tributaries of the pterygoid plexus that drain the upper posterior teeth and gums

posterior superior iliac spine *n* : a projection at the posterior end of the iliac crest — called also *posterior superior spine*

posterior synechia *n* : SYNECHIA b

posterior temporal artery *n* : TEMPORAL ARTERY 3c

posterior tibial artery *n* : TIBIAL ARTERY a

posterior tibial vein *n* : TIBIAL VEIN a

posterior triangle *n* : a triangular region that is a landmark in the neck and has its apex above at the occipital bone — compare ANTERIOR TRIANGLE

posterior ulnar recurrent artery *n* : ULNAR RECURRENT ARTERY b

posterior vein of the left ventricle *n* : a vein that ascends on the surface of the left ventricle facing the diaphragm and that usu. empties into the coronary sinus — called also *posterior vein*

posterior vitreous detachment *n* : VITREOUS DETACHMENT

postero- *comb form* : posterior and ⟨*postero*anterior⟩ ⟨*postero*lateral⟩

pos•tero•an•te•ri•or \ˌpäs-tə-rō-an-ˈtir-ē-ər\ *adj* : involving or produced in a direction from the back toward the front (as of the body or an organ)

pos•tero•lat•er•al \ˌpäs-tə-rō-ˈla-tə-rəl\ *adj* : posterior and lateral in position or direction ⟨the ~ aspect of the leg⟩ — **pos•tero•lat•er•al•ly** *adv*

pos•tero•me•di•al \-ˈmē-dē-əl\ *adj* : located on or near the dorsal midline of the body or a body part

post•ex•po•sure \ˌpōst-ik-ˈspō-zhər\ *adj* : occurring after exposure (as to a virus) — **postexposure** *adv*

[1]**post•fer•til•i•za•tion** \-ˌfər-tᵊl-ə-ˈzā-shən\ *adj* : occurring in the period following fertilization

[2]**postfertilization** *adv* : after fertilization ⟨occurred 48 hours ~⟩

post•gan•gli•on•ic \-ˌgaŋ-glē-ˈä-nik\ *adj* : distal to a ganglion; *specif* : of, relating to, or being an axon arising from a cell body within an autonomic ganglion — compare PREGANGLIONIC

post•gas•trec•to•my \-ga-ˈstrek-tə-mē\ *adj* : occurring in, being in, or characteristic of the period following a gastrectomy

postgastrectomy syndrome *n* : dumping syndrome following a gastrectomy

post•hem•or•rhag•ic \-ˌhe-mə-ˈra-jik\ *adj* : occurring after and as the result of a hemorrhage ⟨~ shock⟩

post•he•pat•ic \-hi-ˈpa-tik\ *adj* : occurring or located behind the liver

post•hep•a•tit•ic \-ˌhe-pə-ˈti-tik\ *adj* : occurring after and esp. as a result of hepatitis ⟨~ cirrhosis⟩

post•her•pet•ic \-hər-ˈpe-tik\ *adj* : occurring after and esp. as a result of herpes ⟨~ scars⟩

pos•thi•tis \(ˌ)päs-ˈthī-təs\ *n, pl* **pos•thit•i•des** \-ˈthi-tə-ˌdēz\ : inflammation of the prepuce

post•hyp•not•ic \ˌpōst-hip-ˈnä-tik\ *adj* : of, relating to, or characteristic of the period following a hypnotic trance during which the subject will still carry out suggestions made by the operator during the trance state

post•ic•tal \-ˈikt-ᵊl\ *adj* : occurring after a sudden attack (as of epilepsy)

posticus — see TIBIALIS POSTICUS

post•im•mu•ni•za•tion \-ˌi-myə-nə-ˈzā-shən\ *adj* : occurring or existing after immunization ⟨~ symptoms⟩

post•in•farc•tion \-in-ˈfärk-shən\ *adj* **1** : occurring after and esp. as a result of myocardial infarction ⟨~ ventricular septal defect⟩ **2** : having suffered myocardial infarction

post•in•fec•tion \-in-ˈfek-shən\ *adj* : relating to, occurring in, or being the period following infection : POSTINFECTIOUS — **postinfection** *adv*

post•in•fec•tious \-in-ˈfek-shəs\ : relating to or occurring in the period following infection : caused by a previous infection ⟨~ syndromes⟩

post•in•jec•tion \-in-ˈjek-shən\ *adj* : occurring or existing in the period following injection ⟨~ pain⟩ — **postinjection** *adv*

post•ir•ra•di•a•tion \-i-ˌrā-dē-ˈā-shən\ *adj* : occurring after irradiation — **postirradiation** *adv*

post•isch•emic \-is-ˈkē-mik\ *adj* : occurring after and esp. as a result of ischemia ⟨~ renal failure⟩

post•junc•tion•al \-ˈjəŋk-shə-nəl\ *adj* : of, relating to, occurring on, or located on the muscle fiber side of a neuromuscular junction

post•mas•tec•to•my \-ma-ˈstek-tə-mē\ *adj* **1** : occurring after and esp. as a result of a mastectomy **2** : having undergone mastectomy

post•ma•ture \-mə-ˈchůr, -ˈtyůr, -ˈtůr\ *adj* : remaining in the uterus for longer than the normal period of gestation ⟨a ~ fetus⟩

post•meno•paus•al \ˌpōst-ˌme-nə-ˈpȯ-zəl\ *adj* **1** : having undergone menopause ⟨~ women⟩ **2** : occurring after menopause ⟨~ osteoporosis⟩ — **post•meno•paus•al•ly** *adv*

[1]**post•mor•tem** \-ˈmȯr-təm\ *adj* : done, occurring, or collected after death ⟨~ tissue specimens⟩

[2]**postmortem** *n* : AUTOPSY

post–mortem *adv* : after death

postmortem examination *n* : AUTOPSY

postmortem lividity *n* : LIVOR MORTIS

post·na·sal \-ˈnā-zəl\ *adj* : lying or occurring posterior to the nose

postnasal drip *n* : flow of mucous secretion from the posterior part of the nasal cavity onto the wall of the pharynx occurring usu. as a chronic accompaniment of an allergic state or a viral infection

post·na·tal \-ˈnāt-ᵊl\ *adj* : occurring or being after birth; *specif* : of or relating to an infant immediately after birth ⟨~ care⟩ — compare NEONATAL, PRENATAL — **post·na·tal·ly** *adv*

post·ne·crot·ic cirrhosis \-nə-ˈkrä-tik-\ *n* : cirrhosis of the liver following widespread necrosis of liver cells esp. as a result of hepatitis

post·neo·na·tal \-ˌnē-ō-ˈnāt-ᵊl\ *adj* : of, relating to, or affecting the infant usu. from the end of the first month to a year after birth ⟨~ mortality⟩

post·nor·mal \-ˈnȯr-məl\ *adj* : having, characterized by, or resulting from a position (as of the mandible) that is distal to the normal position ⟨~ occlusion⟩ — compare PRENORMAL — **post·nor·mal·i·ty** \-nȯr-ˈma-lə-tē\ *n*

post–op \ˈpōst-ˈäp\ *adj* : POSTOPERATIVE — **post–op** *adv*

post·op·er·a·tive \ˌpōst-ˈä-pə-rə-tiv\ *adj* **1** : relating to, occurring in, or being the period following a surgical operation ⟨~ care⟩ **2** : having undergone a surgical operation ⟨a ~ patient⟩ — **post·op·er·a·tive·ly** *adv*

post·or·bit·al \-ˈȯr-bət-ᵊl\ *adj* : situated or occurring behind the orbit of the eye

post·ovu·la·to·ry \-ˈä-vyə-lə-ˌtōr-ē, -ˈō-\ *adj* : occurring, being, or used in the period following ovulation

post·par·tum \-ˈpär-təm\ *adj* **1** : occurring in or being the period following childbirth ⟨~ depression⟩ **2** : being in the postpartum period ⟨~ mothers⟩ — **postpartum** *adv*

post·phle·bit·ic \-flə-ˈbi-tik\ *adj* : occurring after and esp. as the result of phlebitis ⟨~ edema⟩

postphlebitic syndrome *n* : CHRONIC VENOUS INSUFFICIENCY

post·pi·tu·i·tary \-pə-ˈtü-ə-ˌter-ē, -ˈtyü-\ *adj* : arising in or derived from the posterior lobe of the pituitary gland

post–po·lio \-ˈpō-lē-ˌō\ *adj* : recovered from polio; *also* : affected with post-polio syndrome

post–polio syndrome *n* : a condition that affects former polio patients long after recovery from the disease and that is characterized by muscle weakness, joint and muscle pain, and fatigue

post·pran·di·al \-ˈpran-dē-əl\ *adj* : occurring after a meal ⟨~ hypoglycemia⟩ — **post·pran·di·al·ly** *adv*

post·pu·ber·tal \-ˈpyü-bərt-ᵊl\ *adj* : occurring after puberty

post·pu·bes·cent \-pyü-ˈbes-ᵊnt\ *adj* : occurring or being in the period following puberty : POSTPUBERTAL

post·ra·di·a·tion \-ˌrā-dē-ˈā-shən\ *adj* : occurring after exposure to radiation

postrema — see AREA POSTREMA

post–res·i·den·cy \-ˈrez-ə-dən-sē\ *adj* : occurring or obtained in the period following medical residency ⟨~ training⟩

post·sple·nec·to·my \-spli-ˈnek-tə-mē\ *adj* : occurring after and esp. as a result of a splenectomy ⟨~ sepsis⟩

post·stroke \-ˈstrōk\ *adj* : occurring in or being in the period following a stroke ⟨~ depression⟩ ⟨a ~ patient⟩

post·sur·gi·cal \-ˈsər-ji-kəl\ *adj* : POSTOPERATIVE ⟨~ swelling⟩

post·syn·ap·tic \ˌpōst-sə-ˈnap-tik\ *adj* **1** : occurring after synapsis ⟨a ~ chromosome⟩ **2** : relating to, occurring in, or being part of a neuron that receives a nerve impulse after it has crossed a synapse ⟨~ dopamine receptors⟩ — **post·syn·ap·ti·cal·ly** *adv*

post·tran·scrip·tion·al \-trans-ˈkrip-shə-nəl\ *adj* : occurring, acting, or existing after genetic transcription — **post·tran·scrip·tion·al·ly** *adv*

post·trans·fu·sion \-trans-ˈfyü-zhən\ *adj* **1** : caused by transfused blood ⟨~ hepatitis⟩ **2** : occurring after blood transfusion ⟨~ shock⟩

post·trans·la·tion·al \-trans-ˈlā-shə-nəl, -shən-ᵊl\ *adj* : occurring or existing after genetic translation — **post·trans·la·tion·al·ly** *adv*

post·trans·plant \-ˈtrans-ˌplant\ *adj* : occurring or being in the period following transplant surgery

post·trans·plan·ta·tion \-ˌtrans-ˌplan-ˈtā-shən\ *adj* : POSTTRANSPLANT

post–trau·mat·ic \ˌpōst-trə-ˈma-tik, -trȯ-, -trau̇-\ *adj* : occurring after or as a result of trauma ⟨~ epilepsy⟩

post–traumatic stress disorder *n* : a psychological reaction that occurs after experiencing a highly stressing event (as wartime combat, physical violence, or a natural disaster) outside the range of normal human experience and that is usu. characterized by depression, anxiety, flashbacks, recurrent nightmares, and avoidance of reminders of the event — abbr. *PTSD;* called also *delayed-stress disorder, delayed-stress syndrome, post-traumatic stress syndrome;* compare COMBAT FATIGUE

post·treat·ment \-ˈtrēt-mənt\ *adj* : relating to, typical of, or occurring in the period following treatment ⟨~ examinations⟩ — **posttreatment** *adv*

pos·tur·al \ˈpäs-chə-rəl\ *adj* : of, relating to, or involving posture; *also* : ORTHOSTATIC ⟨~ hypotension⟩

postural drainage *n* : drainage of the lungs by placing the patient in an inverted position so that fluids are drawn by gravity toward the trachea

pos·ture \ˈpäs-chər\ *n* : the position or bearing of the body whether characteristic or assumed for a special purpose ⟨erect ~⟩

post·vac·ci·nal \-ˈvak-sən-ᵊl\ *adj* : POSTVACCINATION

post·vac·ci·na·tion \-ˌvak-sə-ˈnā-shən\ *adj* : occurring after and esp. as a result of vaccination ⟨~ dermatosis⟩

post·wean·ing \-ˈwē-niŋ\ *adj* : relating to, occurring in, or being the period following weaning

pot \ˈpät\ *n* : MARIJUANA

po·ta·ble \ˈpō-tə-bəl\ *adj* : suitable for drinking ⟨~ water⟩

po·tas·si·um \pə-ˈta-sē-əm\ *n* : a silver-white soft low-melting metallic element that occurs abundantly in nature esp. combined in minerals — symbol *K;* see ELEMENT table

potassium alum *n* : ALUM

potassium aluminum sulfate *n* : ALUM

potassium an·ti·mo·nyl·tar·trate \-ˌan-tə-mə-ˌnil-ˈtär-ˌtrāt, -ˌnēl-\ *n* : TARTAR EMETIC

potassium bicarbonate *n* : a crystalline water-soluble salt $KHCO_3$ that is sometimes used as an antacid and urinary alkalizer and to treat potassium deficiency — see KLOR-CON

potassium bromide *n* : a crystalline salt KBr that is used as a sedative

potassium chlorate *n* : a crystalline salt $KClO_3$ used esp. in veterinary medicine as a mild astringent

potassium chloride *n* : a crystalline salt KCl that is used esp. in the treatment of potassium deficiency — see K-DUR, KLOR-CON

potassium citrate *n* : a crystalline salt $K_3C_6H_5O_7$ used chiefly as a systemic and urinary alkalizer and in the treatment of hypokalemia

potassium cyanide *n* : a very poisonous crystalline salt KCN

potassium hydroxide *n* : a white solid KOH that dissolves in water to form a strongly alkaline liquid and that is used as a powerful caustic and in the making of pharmaceuticals

potassium iodide *n* : a crystalline salt KI that is very soluble in water and is used medically chiefly in the treatment of hyperthyroidism, to block thyroidal uptake of radioactive iodine, and as an expectorant

potassium nitrate *n* : a crystalline salt KNO_3 that is a strong oxidizing agent and has been used in medicine chiefly as a diuretic — called also *saltpeter*

potassium perchlorate *n* : a crystalline salt $KClO_4$ that is sometimes used as a thyroid inhibitor

potassium permanganate *n* : a dark purple salt $KMnO_4$ used as a disinfectant

potassium phosphate *n* : any of various phosphates of potassium; *esp* : a salt K_2HPO_4 used as a saline cathartic

potassium sodium tartrate *n* : ROCHELLE SALT

potassium thiocyanate *n* : a crystalline salt KSCN that has been used as an antihypertensive agent

pot·bel·ly \ˈpät-ˌbe-lē\ *n, pl* **-lies** : an enlarged, swollen, or protruding abdomen; *also* : a condition characterized by such an abdomen that is symptomatic of disease or malnourishment

po·ten·cy \ˈpōt-ᵊn-sē\ *n, pl* **-cies** : the quality or state of being potent: as **a** : chemical or medicinal strength or efficacy ⟨a drug's ~⟩ **b** : the ability to copulate — usu. used of the male **c** : initial inherent capacity for development of a particular kind

po·tent \ˈpōt-ᵊnt\ *adj* **1** : having force or power **2** : chemically or medicinally effective ⟨a ~ vaccine⟩ **3** : able to copulate — usu. used of the male — **po·tent·ly** *adv*

[1]**po·ten·tial** \pə-ˈten-chəl\ *adj* : existing in possibility : capable of development into actuality — **po·ten·tial·ly** *adv*

[2]**potential** *n* **1** : something that can develop or become actual **2 a** : any of various functions from which the intensity or the velocity at any point in a field may be readily calculated; *specif* : ELECTRICAL POTENTIAL **b** : POTENTIAL DIFFERENCE

potential difference *n* : the difference in electrical potential between two points that represents the work involved or the energy released in the transfer of a unit quantity of electricity from one point to the other

po·ten·ti·ate \pə-ˈten-chē-ˌāt\ *vb* **-at·ed; -at·ing** : to make effective or active or more effective or more active; *also* : to augment the activity of (as a drug) synergistically — **po·ten·ti·a·tion** \-ˌten-chē-ˈā-shən\ *n* — **po·ten·ti·a·tor** \-ˈten-chē-ˌā-tər\ *n*

Po·to·mac horse fever \pə-ˈtō-mək-\ *n* : an often fatal febrile disease of horses that is caused by a rickettsial bacterium (*Neorickettsia risticii* syn. *Ehrlichia risticii*) — called also *Potomac fever*

Pott's disease \ˈpäts-\ *n* : tuberculosis of the spine with destruction of bone resulting in curvature of the spine and occas. in paralysis of the lower extremities

Pott, Percivall (1714–1788), British surgeon.

Pott's fracture *n* : a fracture of the lower part of the fibula often accompanied with injury to the tibial articulation so that the foot is dislocated outward

potty training *n* : TOILET TRAINING — **potty train** *vb*

pouch \ˈpau̇ch\ *n* : an anatomical structure resembling a bag or pocket

pouch of Doug·las \-ˈdə-gləs\ *n* : a deep peritoneal recess between the uterus and the upper vaginal wall anteriorly and the rectum posteriorly — called also *cul-de-sac, cul-de-sac of Douglas, Douglas's cul-de-sac, Douglas's pouch*

Douglas, James (1675–1742), British anatomist.

poul·tice \ˈpōl-təs\ *n* : a soft usu. heated and sometimes medicated mass spread on cloth and applied to sores or other lesions to supply moist warmth, relieve pain, or act as a counterirritant or antiseptic — called also *cataplasm* — **poultice** *vb*

pound \ˈpau̇nd\ *n, pl* **pounds** *also* **pound** : any of various units of mass and weight; *specif* : a unit now in general use among English-speaking peoples equal to 16 avoirdupois ounces or 7000 grains or 0.4536 kilogram — called also *avoirdupois pound*

Pou•part's ligament \pü-ˈpärz-\ *n* : INGUINAL LIGAMENT

Poupart, François (1661–1709), French surgeon and naturalist.

po•vi•done \ˈpō-və-ˌdōn\ *n* : POLYVINYLPYRROLIDONE

povidone–iodine *n* : a solution of polyvinylpyrrolidone and iodine that is applied topically as a broad-spectrum antibacterial agent — see BETADINE

pow•der \ˈpau̇-dər\ *n* : a product in the form of discrete usu. fine particles; *specif* : a medicine or medicated preparation in the form of a powder

pow•er \ˈpau̇-ər\ *n* : MAGNIFICATION

pox \ˈpäks\ *n, pl* **pox** *or* **pox•es** **1** : a virus disease (as chicken pox) characterized by pustules or eruptions **2** *archaic* : SMALLPOX **3** : SYPHILIS

pox•vi•rus \ˈpäks-ˌvī-rəs\ *n* : any of a family (*Poxviridae*) of large brick-shaped or ovoid double-stranded DNA viruses that include the vaccinia virus, the orthopoxviruses, and the causative agents of fowl pox, molluscum contagiosum, myxomatosis of rabbits, sheep pox, sore mouth of sheep, and swinepox

PPA *abbr* phenylpropanolamine

ppb *abbr* parts per billion

PPD *abbr* purified protein derivative

PPI *abbr* proton pump inhibitor

PPLO \ˌpē-(ˌ)pē-(ˌ)el-ˈō\ *n, pl* **PPLO** : MYCOPLASMA

ppm *abbr* parts per million

PPO \ˌpē-(ˌ)pē-ˈō\ *n, pl* **PPOs** : an organization providing health care that gives economic incentives to the individual purchaser of a health-care contract to patronize certain physicians, laboratories, and hospitals which agree to supervision and reduced fees — called also *preferred provider organization;* compare HMO

Pr *symbol* praseodymium

practical nurse *n* : a nurse who cares for the sick professionally without having the training or experience required of a registered nurse; *esp* : LICENSED PRACTICAL NURSE

prac•tice *also* **prac•tise** \ˈprak-təs\ *n* **1** : the continuous exercise of a profession **2** : a professional business; *esp* : one constituting an incorporeal property ⟨the doctor sold his ~ and retired⟩ — **practice** *also* **practise** *vb*

prac•ti•tio•ner \prak-ˈti-shə-nər\ *n* : one who practices a profession and esp. medicine

prac•to•lol \ˈprak-tə-ˌlȯl\ *n* : a beta-blocker $C_{14}H_{22}N_2O_3$ used in the control of arrhythmia

Pra•daxa \prə-ˈdak-sə\ *trademark* — used for a preparation of dabigatran

Pra•der–Wil•li syndrome \ˈprä-dər-ˈvi-lē-\ *n* : a genetic disorder characterized by short stature, intellectual disability, hypotonia, abnormally small hands and feet, hypogonadism, and uncontrolled appetite leading to extreme obesity

Prader, Andrea (1919–2001) and **Willi, Heinrich (1900–1971),** Swiss pediatricians.

praecox — see DEMENTIA PRAECOX, EJACULATIO PRAECOX

pral•i•dox•ime \ˌpra-li-ˈdäk-ˌsēm\ *n* : a substance that restores the reactivity of cholinesterase and is used in the form of its chloride $C_7H_9ClN_2O$ to counteract phosphorylation (as by an organophosphate pesticide) — called also *2-PAM, pralidoxime chloride;* see PROTOPAM

pram•i•pex•ole \ˌpra-mi-ˈpek-ˌsōl\ *n* : a dopamine agonist administered in the form of its dihydrochloride $C_{10}H_{17}N_3S{\cdot}2HCl$ to treat the symptoms of Parkinson's disease

pram•lin•tide \ˈpram-lin-ˌtīd\ *n* : a synthetic amylin analog that is administered by injection in the form of its acetate $C_{171}H_{267}N_{51}O_{53}S_2{\cdot}C_2H_4O_2$ and is used with insulin therapy to lower blood sugar levels in patients with type 1 and type 2 diabetes— see SYMLIN

pran•di•al \ˈpran-dē-əl\ *adj* : of or relating to a meal

Pran•din \ˈpran-din\ *trademark* — used for a preparation of repaglinide

pra•seo•dym•i•um \ˌprā-zē-ō-ˈdi-mē-əm, ˌprā-sē-\ *n* : a yellowish-white trivalent metallic element — symbol *Pr;* see ELEMENT table

pra•su•grel \ˈprä-su̇-ˌgrel\ *n* : a drug that inhibits the activation and aggregation of platelets and is administered orally in the form of its hydrochloride $C_{20}H_{20}FNO_3S{\cdot}HCl$ to reduce the risk of a cardiovascular event (as a heart attack or stent blockage) caused by blood clot formation — see EFFIENT

Praus•nitz–Küst•ner reaction \ˈprau̇s-nits-ˈkœst-nər-\ *n* : PASSIVE TRANSFER

Prausnitz, Carl Willy (1876–1963), German bacteriologist.

Küstner, Heinz (1897–1963), German gynecologist.

Prav•a•chol \ˈpra-və-ˌkōl\ *trademark* — used for a preparation of pravastatin

prav•a•stat•in \ˈpra-və-ˌsta-tᵊn\ *n* : a statin $C_{23}H_{35}NaO_7$ that is administered orally to treat hypercholesterolemia — called also *pravastatin sodium;* see PRAVACHOL

-prax•ia \ˈprak-sē-ə\ *n comb form* : performance of movements ⟨a*praxia*⟩

pra•ze•pam \ˈprä-zə-ˌpam\ *n* : a benzodiazepine derivative $C_{19}H_{17}ClN_2O$ used as a tranquilizer

praz·i·quan·tel \ˌpra-zi-ˈkwän-ˌtel\ *n* : an anthelmintic drug $C_{19}H_{24}N_2O_2$ used esp. in the treatment of schistosomiasis and infection by liver flukes — see BILTRICIDE

pra·zo·sin \ˈprä-zə-ˌsin\ *n* : an antihypertensive peripheral vasodilator usu. used in the form of its hydrochloride $C_{19}H_{21}N_5O_4{\cdot}HCl$ — see MINIPRESS

pre- *prefix* **1** : earlier than : prior to : before ⟨*pre*natal⟩ ⟨*pre*cancerous⟩ **2** : in front of : before ⟨*pre*molar⟩

pre·ad·mis·sion \ˌprē-əd-ˈmi-shən\ *adj* : occurring in or relating to the period prior to admission (as to a hospital)

pre·ad·o·les·cence \ˌprē-ˌad-ᵊl-ˈes-ᵊns\ *n* : the period of human development just preceding adolescence; *specif* : the period between the approximate ages of 9 and 12 — **pre·ad·o·les·cent** \-ˌad-ᵊl-ˈes-ᵊnt\ *adj or n*

pre·adult \-ə-ˈdəlt, -ˈa-ˌdəlt\ *adj* : occurring or existing prior to adulthood

pre·al·bu·min \-al-ˈbyü-mən, -ˈal-ˌbyü-\ *n* : TRANSTHYRETIN

[1]**pre·an·es·thet·ic** \-ˌa-nəs-ˈthe-tik\ *adj* : used or occurring before administration of an anesthetic ⟨~ medication⟩

[2]**preanesthetic** *n* : a substance used to induce an initial light state of anesthesia

pre·au·ric·u·lar \-ȯ-ˈri-kyə-lər\ *adj* : situated or occurring anterior to the auricle of the ear ⟨~ lymph nodes⟩

pre·ax·i·al \-ˈak-sē-əl\ *adj* : situated in front of an axis of the body

pre·bi·ot·ic \-bī-ˈät-ik\ *n* : a substance and esp. a carbohydrate (as inulin) that is nearly or wholly indigestible and that when consumed (as in food) promotes the growth of beneficial bacteria in the digestive tract — compare PROBIOTIC

pre·can·cer \-ˈkan-sər\ *n* : a precancerous lesion or condition

pre·can·cer·ous \-ˈkan-sə-rəs\ *adj* : tending to become cancerous : PREMALIGNANT

[1]**pre·cap·il·lary** \-ˈka-pə-ˌler-ē\ *adj* : being on the arterial side of and immediately adjacent to a capillary

[2]**precapillary** *n, pl* **-lar·ies** : METARTERIOLE

precapillary sphincter *n* : a sphincter of smooth muscle tissue located at the arterial end of a capillary and serving to control blood flow to the tissues

pre·cen·tral \-ˈsen-trəl\ *adj* : situated in front of the central sulcus of the brain

precentral gyrus *n* : the gyrus containing the motor area immediately anterior to the central sulcus

pre·cep·tee \ˌprē-ˌsep-ˈtē\ *n* : a person who works for and studies under a preceptor ⟨a ~ in urology⟩

pre·cep·tor \pri-ˈsep-tər, ˈprē-ˌ\ *n* : a practicing physician who gives personal instruction, training, and supervision to a medical student or young physician

pre·cep·tor·ship \pri-ˈsep-tər-ˌship, ˈprē-ˌ\ *n* : the state of being a preceptee : a period of training under a preceptor

[1]**pre·cip·i·tate** \pri-ˈsi-pə-ˌtāt\ *vb* **-tat·ed; -tat·ing** **1** : to bring about esp. abruptly **2 a** : to separate or cause to separate from solution or suspension **b** : to cause (vapor) to condense and fall or deposit

[2]**pre·cip·i·tate** \pri-ˈsi-pə-tət, -ˌtāt\ *n* : a substance separated from a solution or suspension by chemical or physical change usu. as an insoluble amorphous or crystalline solid

precipitated chalk *n* : precipitated calcium carbonate used esp. as an ingredient of toothpastes and tooth powders for its polishing qualities

precipitated sulfur *n* : sulfur obtained as a pale yellowish or grayish powder by precipitation and used chiefly in treating skin diseases

pre·cip·i·ta·tion \pri-ˌsi-pə-ˈtā-shən\ *n* **1 a** : the process of forming a precipitate from a solution **b** : the process of precipitating or removing solid or liquid particles from a smoke or gas by electrical means **2** : PRECIPITATE

pre·cip·i·tin \pri-ˈsi-pə-tən\ *n* : any of various antibodies which form insoluble precipitates with specific antigens

precipitin test *n* : a serological test using precipitins to detect the presence of a specific antigen; *specif* : a test used in criminology for determining the human or other source of a bloodstain

pre·clin·i·cal \ˌprē-ˈkli-ni-kəl\ *adj* **1 a** : of, relating to, concerned with, or being the period preceding clinical manifestations ⟨the ~ stage of diabetes mellitus⟩ **b** : occurring prior to a clinical trial ⟨~ animal testing⟩ **2** : of, relating to, or being the period in medical or dental education preceding the clinical study of medicine or dentistry

pre·co·cious \pri-ˈkō-shəs\ *adj* **1** : exceptionally early in development or occurrence ⟨~ puberty⟩ **2** : exhibiting mature qualities at an unusually early age — **pre·co·cious·ly** *adv* — **pre·co·cious·ness** *n* — **pre·coc·i·ty** \pri-ˈkä-sə-tē\ *n*

pre·cog·ni·tion \ˌprē-(ˌ)käg-ˈni-shən\ *n* : clairvoyance relating to an event or state not yet experienced — compare PSYCHOKINESIS, TELEKINESIS — **pre·cog·ni·tive** \-ˈkäg-nə-tiv\ *adj*

pre·co·i·tal \-ˈkō-ət-ᵊl, -kō-ˈēt-\ *adj* : used or occurring before coitus

pre·co·ma \-ˈkō-mə\ *n* : a stuporous condition preceding coma ⟨diabetic ~⟩

pre·con·cep·tion \-kən-ˈsep-shən\ *adj* : occurring prior to conception

[1]**pre·con·scious** \ˌprē-ˈkän-chəs\ *adj* : not present in consciousness but capable of being recalled without en-

countering any inner resistance or repression — **pre·con·scious·ly** *adv*

[2]**preconscious** *n* : the preconscious part of the psyche esp. in psychoanalysis

pre·cor·dial \-ˈkȯr-dē-əl, -ˈkȯr-jəl\ *adj* **1** : situated or occurring in front of the heart **2** : of or relating to the precordium

pre·cor·di·um \-ˈkȯr-dē-əm\ *n, pl* **-dia** \-dē-ə\ : the part of the ventral surface of the body overlying the heart and stomach and comprising the epigastrium and the lower median part of the thorax

pre·cu·ne·us \-ˈkyü-nē-əs\ *n, pl* **-nei** \-nē-ˌī\ : a somewhat rectangular convolution bounding the mesial aspect of the parietal lobe of the cerebrum and lying immediately in front of the cuneus

pre·cur·sor \pri-ˈkər-sər, ˈprē-ˌ\ *n* **1** : one that precedes and indicates the onset of another **2** : a substance, cell, or cellular component from which another substance, cell, or cellular component is formed esp. by natural processes

pre·den·tin \ˌprē-ˈdent-ᵊn\ *or* **pre·den·tine** \-ˈden-ˌtēn, -den-ˈ\ *n* : immature uncalcified dentin consisting chiefly of fibrils

pre·di·a·be·tes \ˌprē-ˌdī-ə-ˈbē-tēz, -ˈbē-təs\ *n* : a usu. symptomless condition that is marked by somewhat elevated levels of blood sugar and that often progresses to type 2 diabetes

[1]**pre·di·a·bet·ic** \-ˈbe-tik\ *n* : a prediabetic individual

[2]**prediabetic** *adj* : of, relating to, or affected with prediabetes ⟨~ patients⟩

pre·dic·tor \pri-ˈdik-tər\ *n* : a preliminary symptom or indication (as of the development of a disease)

pre·di·ges·tion \ˌprē-dī-ˈjes-chən, -də-\ *n* : artificial or natural partial digestion of food — **pre·di·gest** \-ˈjest\ *vb*

pre·dis·pose \ˌprē-di-ˈspōz\ *vb* **-posed; -pos·ing** : to make susceptible — **pre·dis·po·si·tion** \ˌprē-ˌdis-pə-ˈzi-shən\ *n*

pred·nis·o·lone \pred-ˈni-sə-ˌlōn\ *n* : a glucocorticoid $C_{21}H_{28}O_5$ used often in the form of an ester or methyl derivative esp. as an anti-inflammatory drug in the treatment of arthritis

pred·ni·sone \ˈpred-nə-ˌsōn, -ˌzōn\ *n* : a glucocorticoid $C_{21}H_{26}O_5$ that is used as an anti-inflammatory agent, as an antineoplastic agent, and as an immunosuppressant

pre·drug \ˌprē-ˈdrəg\ *adj* : existing or occurring prior to the administration of a drug ⟨~ baseline values⟩

pre·eclamp·sia \ˌprē-i-ˈklamp-sē-ə\ *n* : a serious condition developing in late pregnancy that is characterized by a sudden rise in blood pressure, excessive weight gain, generalized edema, proteinuria, severe headache, and visual disturbances and that may result in eclampsia if untreated — compare ECLAMPSIA a, TOXEMIA OF PREGNANCY

[1]**pre·eclamp·tic** \-tik\ *adj* : relating to or affected with preeclampsia ⟨a ~ patient⟩

[2]**preeclamptic** *n* : a woman affected with preeclampsia

pree·mie *also* **pre·mie** \ˈprē-mē\ *n* : a baby born prematurely

pre·erup·tive \ˌprē-i-ˈrəp-tiv\ *adj* : occurring or existing prior to an eruption ⟨a ~ tooth position⟩

pre·ex·ci·ta·tion \-ˌek-ˌsī-ˈtā-shən, -sə-\ *n* : premature activation of part or all of the cardiac ventricle by an electrical impulse from the atrium that typically is conducted along an anomalous pathway (as muscle fibers on the heart surface) bypassing the atrioventricular node, that may produce arrhythmias, and that is characteristic of Lown-Ganong-Levine syndrome and Wolff-Parkinson-White syndrome — **pre·ex·cit·ed** \-ik-ˈsī-təd\ *adj*

pre·ex·po·sure \-ik-ˈspō-zhər\ *adj* : of, relating to, occurring in, or being the period preceding exposure (as to a stimulus or a pathogen)

preferred provider organization *n* : PPO

pre·fron·tal \ˌprē-ˈfrənt-ᵊl\ *adj* **1** : situated or occurring anterior to a frontal structure ⟨a ~ bone⟩ **2** : of, relating to, or constituting the prefrontal lobe or prefrontal cortex of the brain

prefrontal cortex *n* : the gray matter of the anterior part of the frontal lobe that is highly developed in humans and plays a role in the regulation of complex cognitive, emotional, and behavioral functioning

prefrontal lobe *n* : the anterior part of the frontal lobe that is bounded posteriorly by the ascending frontal convolution, is made up chiefly of association areas, and mediates various inhibitory controls

prefrontal lobotomy *n* : lobotomy of the white matter in the frontal lobe of the brain — called also *frontal lobotomy*

pre·gab·a·lin \prē-ˈga-bə-lən\ *n* : an anticonvulsant drug $C_8H_{17}NO_2$ that is taken orally for the relief of pain associated esp. with fibromyalgia, diabetic peripheral neuropathy, and postherpetic neuralgia and as an adjunctive therapy in the treatment of partial seizures — see LYRICA

pre·gan·gli·on·ic \ˌprē-ˌgaŋ-glē-ˈä-nik\ *adj* : anterior or proximal to a ganglion; *specif* : being, affecting, involving, or relating to a usu. myelinated efferent nerve fiber arising from a cell body in the central nervous system and terminating in an autonomic ganglion — compare POSTGANGLIONIC

pre·gen·i·tal \-ˈjen-ət-ᵊl\ *adj* : of, relating to, or characteristic of the oral, anal, and phallic phases of psychosexual development

preg·nan·cy \ˈpreg-nən-sē\ *n, pl* **-cies** **1** : the condition of being pregnant **2** : an instance of being pregnant

pregnancy disease *n* : a form of ketosis affecting pregnant ewes

pregnancy test *n* : a physiological test to determine the existence of pregnancy in an individual

preg•nane \ˈpreg-ˌnān\ *n* : a crystalline steroid $C_{21}H_{36}$ that is the parent compound of the corticosteroid and progestational hormones

preg•nane•di•ol \ˌpreg-ˌnān-ˈdī-ˌȯl\ *n* : a crystalline biologically inactive derivative $C_{21}H_{36}O_2$ of pregnane found esp. in the urine of pregnant women

preg•nant \ˈpreg-nənt\ *adj* : containing a developing embryo, fetus, or unborn offspring within the body : GESTATING : GRAVID

preg•nen•o•lone \preg-ˈnen-ᵊl-ˌōn\ *n* : a steroid ketone $C_{21}H_{32}O_2$ that is formed by the oxidation of steroids (as cholesterol) and yields progesterone on dehydrogenation

pre•he•pat•ic \ˌprē-hi-ˈpat-ik\ *adj* : existing or occurring before the liver; *specif* : of, relating to, or occurring in the hepatic portal system ⟨~ blood⟩

pre•hos•pi•tal \ˌprē-ˈhäs-(ˌ)pit-ᵊl\ *adj* : occurring before or during transportation (as of a trauma victim) to a hospital ⟨~ emergency care⟩

pre•hy•per•ten•sion \-ˌhī-pər-ˈten-chən\ *n* : slightly to moderately elevated arterial blood pressure that in adults is usu. indicated by a systolic blood pressure of 120 to 139 mm Hg or a diastolic blood pressure of 80 to 89 mm Hg and that is considered a risk factor for hypertension — **pre•hy•per•ten•sive** \-ˈhī-pər-ˌten-siv\ *adj*

pre•im•mu•ni•za•tion \-ˌi-myə-nə-ˈzā-shən\ *adj* : existing or occurring in the period before immunization

pre•im•plan•ta•tion \-ˌim-ˌplan-ˈtā-shən\ *adj* : of, involving, or being an embryo before uterine implantation

pre•in•cu•ba•tion \ˌprē-ˌiŋ-kyə-ˈbā-shən\ *n* : incubation (as of a cell or culture) prior to a treatment or process — **pre•in•cu•bate** \-ˈiŋ-kyə-ˌbāt\ *vb*

pre•in•va•sive \-in-ˈvā-siv\ *adj* : not yet having become invasive — used of malignant cells or lesions remaining in their original focus

pre•leu•ke•mia \-lü-ˈkē-mē-ə\ *n* : MYELODYSPLASTIC SYNDROME — **pre•leu•ke•mic** \-mik\ *adj*

pre•load \ˌprē-ˈlōd\ *n* : the stretched condition of the heart muscle at the end of diastole just before contraction

Pre•lu•din \pri-ˈlüd-ᵊn\ *n* : a preparation of the hydrochloride of phenmetrazine — formerly a U.S. registered trademark

pre•ma•lig•nant \ˌprē-mə-ˈlig-nənt\ *adj* : tending to become malignant : PRECANCEROUS ⟨~ cells⟩ ⟨a ~ condition⟩ — **pre•ma•lig•nan•cy** \-ˈlig-nən-sē\ *n*

Prem•a•rin \ˈpre-mə-rən\ *trademark* — used for a preparation of conjugated estrogens

¹pre•ma•ture \ˌprē-mə-ˈchu̇r, -ˈtyu̇r, -ˈtu̇r-\ *adj* : happening, arriving, existing, or performed before the proper, usual, or intended time ⟨~ puberty⟩ ⟨~ aging⟩; *esp* : born after a gestation period of less than 37 weeks ⟨~ babies⟩ — **pre•ma•ture•ly** *adv*

²premature *n* : PREEMIE

premature beat *n* : EXTRASYSTOLE

premature birth *n* : birth of a baby after a gestation period of less than 37 weeks — called also *premature delivery*

premature ejaculation *n* : ejaculation of semen that occurs prior to or immediately after penetration of the vagina by the penis — called also *ejaculatio praecox*

premature ejaculator *n* : a man who experiences premature ejaculation

pre•ma•tu•ri•ty \ˌprē-mə-ˈtu̇r-ə-tē, -ˈtyu̇r-, -ˈchu̇r-\ *n, pl* **-ties** : the condition of an infant born viable but before 37 weeks of gestation

pre•max•il•la \ˌprē-mak-ˈsi-lə\ *n, pl* **-lae** \-ˌlē\ : either member of a pair of bones of the upper jaw situated between and in front of the maxillae that in humans form the median anterior part of the superior maxillary bones

pre•max•il•lary \-ˈmak-sə-ˌler-ē\ *adj* **1** : situated in front of the maxillary bones **2** : relating to or being the premaxillae

¹pre•med \ˌprē-ˈmed\ *n* : a premedical student or course of study

²premed *adj* : PREMEDICAL

pre•med•i•cal \-ˈme-di-kəl\ *adj* : preceding and preparing for the professional study of medicine

pre•med•i•ca•tion \-ˌme-də-ˈkā-shən\ *n* : preliminary medication; *esp* : medication to induce a relaxed state preparatory to the administration of an anesthetic — **pre•med•i•cate** \-ˈme-də-ˌkāt\ *vb*

pre•mei•ot•ic \ˌprē-mī-ˈä-tik\ *adj* : of, occurring in, or typical of a stage prior to meiosis ⟨~ DNA synthesis⟩

pre•me•nar•chal \ˌprē-me-ˈnär-kəl\ *or* **pre•me•nar•che•al** \-kē-əl\ *adj* : of, relating to, or being in the period of life of a female before the first menstrual period occurs

pre•meno•paus•al \-ˌme-nə-ˈpȯ-zəl, -ˌmē-\ *adj* : of, relating to, or being in the period preceding menopause and esp. the perimenopausal period

pre•meno•pause \-ˈme-nə-ˌpȯz, -ˈmē-\ *n* : the premenopausal period of a woman's life; *esp* : PERIMENOPAUSE

pre•men•stru•al \-ˈmen-strə-wəl\ *adj* : of, relating to, occurring, or being in the period just preceding menstruation — **pre•men•stru•al•ly** *adv*

premenstrual dysphoric disorder *n* : severe premenstrual syndrome characterized by symptoms (as depression, anxiety, cyclical mood shifts, and lethargy) that markedly interfere with normal daily functioning — abbr. *PMDD*

premenstrual syndrome *n* : a varying constellation of symptoms manifested by some women prior to menstruation that may include emotional instability, irritability, insomnia, fatigue, anxiety, depression, headache, edema, and abdominal pain — called also *PMS*

premenstrual tension *n* : tension occurring as a part of the premenstrual syndrome

pre•men•stru•um \-ˈmen-strə-wəm\ *n, pl* **-stru•ums** *or* **-strua** \-strə-wə\ : the period or physiological state that immediately precedes menstruation

premie *var of* PREEMIE

[1]**pre•mo•lar** \ˌprē-ˈmō-lər\ *adj* : situated in front of or preceding the molar teeth; *esp* : being or relating to those teeth in front of the true molars and behind the canines

[2]**premolar** *n* : a premolar tooth that in humans is one of two in each side of each jaw — called also *bicuspid*

pre•mon•i•to•ry \pri-ˈmä-nə-ˌtōr-ē\ *adj* : giving warning ⟨a ~ symptom⟩

pre•mor•bid \ˌprē-ˈmȯr-bəd\ *adj* : occurring or existing before the occurrence of physical disease or emotional illness ⟨~ personality⟩

pre•mor•tem \-ˈmȯrt-ᵊm\ *adj* : existing or taking place immediately before death — **premortem** *adv*

pre•mo•tor \-ˈmō-tər\ *adj* : of, relating to, or being the area of the cortex of the frontal lobe lying immediately in front of the motor area of the precentral gyrus

Prem•phase \ˈprem–ˌfāz\ *trademark* — used for a preparation of conjugated estrogens and medroxyprogesterone acetate taken by mouth

Prem•pro \ˈprem-ˌprō\ *trademark* — used for a preparation of conjugated estrogens and medroxyprogesterone acetate taken by mouth

pre•my•cot•ic \ˌprē-mī-ˈkä-tik\ *adj* : of, relating to, or being the earliest and nonspecific stage of eczematoid eruptions of mycosis fungoides

pre•na•tal \-ˈnāt-ᵊl\ *adj* **1** : occurring, existing, or performed before birth ⟨~ care⟩ ⟨the ~ period⟩ ⟨~ testing⟩ **2** : providing or receiving prenatal medical care ⟨a ~ clinic⟩ ⟨a ~ patient⟩ — called also *antenatal;* compare NEONATAL, POSTNATAL — **pre•na•tal•ly** *adv*

pre•neo•plas•tic \-ˌnē-ə-ˈplas-tik\ *adj* : existing or occurring prior to the formation of a neoplasm ⟨~ cells⟩

pre•nor•mal \-ˈnȯr-məl\ *adj* : having, characterized by, or resulting from a position (as of the mandible) that is proximal to the normal position — compare POSTNORMAL — **pre•nor•mal•i•ty** \-nȯr-ˈma-lə-tē\ *n*

pre•op \ˈprē-ˌäp\ *adj* : PREOPERATIVE

pre•op•er•a•tive \ˌprē-ˈä-pə-rə-tiv, -ˌrāt-\ *adj* **1** : occurring, performed, or administered before and usu. close to a surgical operation ⟨~ care⟩ **2** : having not yet undergone a surgical operation ⟨~ patients⟩ — **pre•op•er•a•tive•ly** *adv*

pre•op•tic \-ˈäp-tik\ *adj* : situated in front of an optic part or region

preoptic area *n* : a region of the brain that is situated immediately below the anterior commissure, above the optic chiasma, and anterior to the hypothalamus and that regulates certain autonomic activities often with the hypothalamus

preoptic nucleus *n* : any of several groups of nerve cells located in the preoptic area esp. in the lateral and the medial portions

preoptic region *n* : PREOPTIC AREA

pre•ovu•la•to•ry \ˌprē-ˈä-vyə-lə-ˌtōr-ē, -ˈō-\ *adj* : occurring in, being in, existing in, or typical of the period immediately preceding ovulation ⟨~ ovarian follicles⟩

[1]**prep** \ˈprep\ *n* : the act or an instance of preparing a patient for a surgical operation

[2]**prep** *vb* **prepped; prep•ping** : to prepare for a surgical operation or examination ⟨nurses *prepped* the patient⟩

prep•a•ra•tion \ˌpre-pə-ˈrā-shən\ *n* : a medicinal substance made ready for use ⟨a ~ for colds⟩

prepared chalk *n* : finely ground calcium carbonate that is freed of most of its impurities and used esp. in dentistry for polishing

pre•par•tum \ˌprē-ˈpär-təm\ *adj* : ANTEPARTUM

pre•pa•tel•lar bursa \-pə-ˈte-lər-\ *n* : a synovial bursa situated between the patella and the skin

pre•pa•tent period \-ˈpāt-ᵊnt-\ *n* : the period between infection with a parasite and the demonstration of the parasite in the body

pre•po•ten•cy \-ˈpōt-ᵊn-sē\ *n, pl* **-cies** : unusual ability of an individual or strain to transmit its characters to offspring because of homozygosity for numerous dominant genes — **pre•po•tent** \-ˈpōt-ᵊnt\ *adj*

pre•pran•di•al \-ˈpran-dē-əl\ *adj* : of, relating to, or suitable for the time just before a meal ⟨~ blood glucose⟩

pre•preg•nan•cy \-ˈpreg-nən-sē\ *adj* : existing or occurring prior to pregnancy ⟨~ obesity⟩

pre•psy•chot•ic \-sī-ˈkä-tik\ *adj* : preceding or predisposing to psychosis : possessing recognizable features prognostic of psychosis

pre•pu•ber•al \-ˈpyü-bə-rəl\ *adj* : PREPUBERTAL

pre•pu•ber•tal \-ˈpyü-bərt-ᵊl\ *adj* : of, relating to, occurring in, or being in the period immediately preceding puberty — **pre•pu•ber•ty** \-bər-tē\ *n*

pre•pu•bes•cent \-pyü-ˈbes-ᵊnt\ *adj* : PREPUBERTAL

pre•puce \ˈprē-ˌpyüs\ *n* : FORESKIN; *also* : a similar fold investing the clitoris

pre·pu·tial \prē-ˈpyü-shəl\ *adj* : of, relating to, or being a prepuce

preputial gland *n* : any of the small glands at the base of the glans penis that secrete smegma — called also *gland of Tyson, Tyson's gland*

pre·pu·tium cli·tor·i·dis \prē-ˈpyü-shəm-kli-ˈtȯr-ə-dəs\ *n* : the prepuce which invests the clitoris

pre·py·lo·ric \ˌprē-pī-ˈlōr-ik\ *adj* : situated or occurring anterior to the pylorus ⟨∼ ulcers⟩

pre·re·nal \-ˈrēn-ᵊl\ *adj* : occurring in the circulatory system before the kidney is reached ⟨∼ disorders⟩

prerenal azotemia *n* : uremia caused by extrarenal factors

pre·rep·li·cat·ive \ˌprē-ˈre-pli-ˌkā-tiv\ *adj* : relating to or being the G_1 phase of the cell cycle

pre·ret·i·nal \-ˈret-ᵊn-əl\ *adj* : situated or occurring anterior to the retina

pre·sa·cral \-ˈsa-krəl, -ˈsā-\ *adj* **1** : done or effected by way of the anterior aspect of the sacrum ⟨∼ nerve block⟩ **2** : located anterior to the sacrum ⟨the ∼ region⟩

presby- *or* **presbyo-** *comb form* : old age ⟨*presby*opia⟩

pres·by·cu·sis \ˌprez-bi-ˈkyü-səs, ˌpres-\ *n, pl* **-cu·ses** \-ˌsēz\ : a lessening of hearing acuteness resulting from degenerative changes in the ear that occur esp. in old age

pres·by·ope \ˈprez-bē-ˌōp; ˈpres-\ *n* : one affected with presbyopia

pres·by·opia \ˌprez-bē-ˈō-pē-ə, ˌpres-\ *n* : a visual condition which becomes apparent esp. in middle age and in which loss of elasticity of the lens of the eye causes defective accommodation and inability to focus sharply for near vision — **pres·by·opic** \-ˈō-pik, -ˈä-\ *adj*

pre·scribe \pri-ˈskrīb\ *vb* **pre·scribed; pre·scrib·ing** : to designate the use of as a remedy ⟨∼ a drug⟩

pre·scrip·tion \pri-ˈskrip-shən\ *n* **1** : a written direction for the preparation, compounding, and administration of a medicine **2** : a prescribed remedy **3** : a written formula for the grinding of corrective lenses for eyeglasses **4** : a written direction for the application of physical therapy measures (as directed exercise or electrotherapy) in cases of injury or disability

prescription drug *n* : a drug that can be obtained only by means of a physician's prescription

pre·se·nile \ˌprē-ˈsē-ˌnīl\ *adj* **1** : of, relating to, occurring in, or being the period immediately preceding the development of senility ⟨∼ depression⟩ **2** : prematurely displaying symptoms of senile dementia

presenile dementia *n* : dementia beginning in middle age and progressing rapidly

pre·sen·il·in \prē-ˌse-ˈni-lən\ *n* : any of several proteins of cell membranes that are believed to contribute to the development of Alzheimer's disease

pre·sent \pri-ˈzent\ *vb* **1 a** : to show or manifest ⟨patients who ∼ symptoms of malaria⟩ **b** : to become manifest ⟨Lyme disease often ∼*s* with erythema migrans, fatigue, fever, and chills⟩ **c** : to come forward as a patient ⟨he ∼*ed* with fever and abdominal pain⟩ **2** : to become directed toward the opening of the uterus — used of a fetus or a part of a fetus

pre·sen·ta·tion \ˌprē-ˌzen-ˈtā-shən, ˌprez-ᵊn-\ *n* **1** : the position in which the fetus lies in the uterus in labor with respect to the mouth of the uterus ⟨face ∼⟩ **2** : appearance in conscious experience either as a sensory product or as a memory image **3** : a presenting symptom or group of symptoms **4** : a formal oral report of a patient's medical history

pre·sent·ing \pri-ˈzen-tiŋ\ *adj* : of, relating to, or being a symptom, condition, or sign which is observed or detected upon initial examination of a patient or which the patient discloses to the physician ⟨∼ symptoms⟩

pre·ser·va·tive \pri-ˈzər-və-tiv\ *n* : something that preserves or has the power of preserving; *specif* : an additive used to protect against decay, discoloration, or spoilage ⟨a food ∼⟩

pre·sphe·noid \ˌprē-ˈsfē-ˌnȯid\ *n* : a bone or cartilage usu. united with the basisphenoid in the adult and in humans forming the anterior part of the body of the sphenoid — **presphenoid** *also* **pre·sphe·noi·dal** \-sfi-ˈnȯid-ᵊl\ *adj*

pres·sor \ˈpre-ˌsȯr, -sər\ *adj* : raising or tending to raise blood pressure ⟨∼ substances⟩; *also* : involving or producing an effect of vasoconstriction

pres·so·re·cep·tor \ˌpre-sō-ri-ˈsep-tər\ *n* : BARORECEPTOR

pres·sure \ˈpre-shər\ *n* **1** : the application of force to something by something else in direct contact with it : COMPRESSION **2** : ATMOSPHERIC PRESSURE **3** : a touch sensation aroused by moderate compression of the skin

pressure bandage *n* : a thick pad of gauze or other material placed over a wound and attached firmly so that it will exert pressure — called also *pressure dressing*

pressure point *n* **1** : a region of the body in which the distribution of soft and skeletal parts is such that a static position (as of a part in a cast or of a bedridden person) tends to cause circulatory deficiency and necrosis due to local compression of blood vessels — compare BEDSORE **2** : a discrete point on the body to which pressure is applied (as in acupressure or reflexology) for therapeutic purposes **3** : a point on the body where a blood vessel (as the brachial artery) can be compressed against an underlying bone to slow blood flow and control bleeding

pressure sore *n* : BEDSORE

pressure suit *n* : an inflatable suit for high-altitude or space flight to protect the body from low pressure

pre·sump·tive \pri-ˈzəmp-tiv\ *adj* **1** : expected to develop in a particular direction under normal conditions **2** : being the embryonic precursor of ⟨∼ neural tissue⟩

pre·sur·gi·cal \ˌprē-ˈsər-ji-kəl\ *adj* : occurring before, performed before, or preliminary to surgery ⟨∼ care⟩

pre·symp·to·mat·ic \-ˌsimp-tə-ˈma-tik\ *adj* : relating to, being, or occurring before symptoms appear ⟨∼ diagnosis of a hereditary disease⟩

pre·syn·ap·tic \-sə-ˈnap-tik\ *adj* : of, occurring in, or being part of a neuron by which a nerve impulse is conveyed to a synapse ⟨a ∼ neuron⟩ ⟨∼ inhibition⟩ — **pre·syn·ap·ti·cal·ly** *adv*

pre·sys·tol·ic \-sis-ˈtä-lik\ *adj* : of, relating to, or occurring just before cardiac systole ⟨a ∼ murmur⟩

pre·tec·tal \-ˈtekt-ᵊl\ *adj* : occurring in or being the transitional zone of the brain stem between the midbrain and the diencephalon that is associated esp. with the analysis and distribution of light impulses

pre·term \-ˈtərm\ *adj* : of, relating to, being, or born by premature birth ⟨∼ infants⟩ ⟨∼ labor⟩

pre·ter·mi·nal \-ˈtər-mə-nəl\ *adj* **1** : occurring or being in the period prior to death ⟨∼ cancer⟩ ⟨a ∼ patient⟩ **2** : situated or occurring anterior to an end (as of a nerve) ⟨∼ axons⟩

pre·tib·i·al \-ˈti-bē-əl\ *adj* : lying or occurring anterior to the tibia

pretibial fever *n* : a rare infectious disease that is characterized by an eruption in the pretibial region, headache, backache, malaise, chills, and fever and that is caused by a spirochete of the genus *Leptospira* (*L. interrogans autumnalis*)

pretibial myxedema *n* : myxedema characterized primarily by a mucoid edema in the pretibial area

pre·trans·plant \-ˈtran(t)s-ˌplant\ *adj* : occurring or being in the period before transplant surgery ⟨∼ hospitalization⟩

pre·trans·plan·ta·tion \-ˌtran(t)s-ˌplan-ˈtā-shən\ *adj* : PRETRANSPLANT

pre·treat·ment \ˌprē-ˈtrēt-mənt\ *n* : preliminary or preparatory treatment — **pre·treat** \-ˈtrēt\ *vb* — **pretreatment** *adj*

Prev·a·cid \ˈpre-və-ˌsid\ *trademark* — used for a preparation of lansoprazole

prev·a·lence \ˈpre-və-ləns\ *n* : the percentage of a population that is affected with a particular disease at a given time — compare INCIDENCE

pre·ven·ta·tive \pri-ˈven-tə-tiv\ *adj or n* : PREVENTIVE ⟨a ∼ drug⟩

¹pre·ven·tive \pri-ˈven-tiv\ *n* : something (as a drug) used to prevent disease

²preventive *adj* : devoted to or concerned with the prevention of disease

preventive medicine *n* : a branch of medical science dealing with methods (as vaccination) of preventing the occurrence of disease

pre·ver·te·bral \ˌprē-ˈvər-tə-brəl, -(ˌ)vər-ˈtē-brəl\ *adj* : situated or occurring anterior to a vertebra or the spinal column ⟨∼ muscles⟩

pre·ves·i·cal space \ˌprē-ˈve-si-kəl-\ *n* : RETROPUBIC SPACE

previa — see PLACENTA PREVIA

pre·vi·able \-ˈvī-ə-bəl\ *adj* : not sufficiently developed to survive outside the uterus ⟨a ∼ fetus⟩

pre·vil·lous \-ˈvi-ləs\ *adj* : relating to, being in, or being the stage of embryonic development before the formation of villi ⟨a ∼ human embryo⟩

Prez·co·bix \ˈprez-kə-ˌbiks\ *trademark* — used for a preparation of cobicistat and darunavir

Pre·zis·ta \prə-ˈzis-tə\ *trademark* — used for a preparation of darunavir

pri·a·pism \ˈprī-ə-ˌpi-zəm\ *n* : an abnormal, more or less persistent, and often painful erection of the penis; *esp* : one caused by disease rather than sexual desire

Price–Jones curve \ˈprīs-ˈjōnz-\ *n* : a graph of the frequency distribution of the diameters of red blood cells in a sample that has been smeared, stained, and magnified for direct observation and counting

Price–Jones, Cecil (1863–1943), British hematologist.

prick·le cell \ˈpri-kəl-\ *n* : a cell of the stratum spinosum of the skin having numerous intercellular bridges which give the separated cells a prickly appearance in microscopic preparations

prickle cell layer *n* : STRATUM SPINOSUM

prick·ly heat \ˈpri-klē-\ *n* : a noncontagious cutaneous eruption of red pimples with intense itching and tingling caused by inflammation around the sweat ducts — called also *heat rash;* see MILIARIA

prick test *n* : a test for allergic susceptibility made by placing a drop of the allergy-producing substance on the skin and making breaks in the skin by lightly pricking the surface — compare INTRADERMAL TEST, PATCH TEST, SCRATCH TEST

pril·o·caine \ˈpri-lə-ˌkān\ *n* : a local anesthetic related to lidocaine and used in the form of its hydrochloride $C_{13}H_{20}N_2O{\cdot}HCl$ as a nerve block for pain esp. in surgery and dentistry

Pril·o·sec \ˈpri-lə-ˌsek\ *trademark* — used for a preparation of omeprazole

pri·mal scream therapy \ˈprī-məl-\ *n* : psychotherapy in which the patient recalls and reenacts a particularly disturbing past experience usu. occurring early in life and expresses normally repressed anger or frustration esp. through spontaneous and unrestrained screams, hysteria, or violence

— called also *primal scream, primal therapy*

pri•ma•quine \ˈprī-mə-ˌkwēn, ˈpri-, -kwin\ *n* : an antimalarial drug used in the form of its diphosphate $C_{15}H_{21}N_3O·2H_3PO_4$

pri•ma•ry \ˈprī-ˌmer-ē, ˈprī-mə-rē\ *adj* **1 a** (1) : first in order of time or development (2) : relating to or being the milk teeth and esp. the 20 milk teeth in the human set **b** (1) : arising spontaneously : IDIOPATHIC ⟨~ insomnia⟩ (2) : being an initial tumor or site esp. of cancer **c** : providing primary care ⟨a ~ physician⟩ **2** : belonging to the first group or order in successive divisions, combinations, or ramifications ⟨~ nerves⟩ **3** : of, relating to, or being the amino acid sequence in proteins — compare SECONDARY 3, TERTIARY 2

primary aldosteronism *n* : aldosteronism caused by an adrenal tumor — called also *Conn's syndrome*

primary amenorrhea *n* : amenorrhea in which menstruation has not yet occurred by age 16

primary atypical pneumonia *n* : any of a group of pneumonias (as Q fever and psittacosis) caused esp. by a virus, mycoplasma, rickettsia, or chlamydia

primary care *n* : health care provided by a medical professional (as a general practitioner or a pediatrician) with whom a patient has initial contact and by whom the patient may be referred to a specialist for further treatment — often used attributively ⟨*primary care* physicians⟩; called also *primary health care;* compare SECONDARY CARE, TERTIARY CARE

primary fissure *n* : a fissure of the cerebellum that is situated between the culmen and declive and that marks the boundary between the anterior lobe and the posterior lobe

primary health care *n* : PRIMARY CARE

primary host *n* : DEFINITIVE HOST

primary hypertension *n* : ESSENTIAL HYPERTENSION

primary oocyte *n* : a diploid oocyte that has not yet undergone meiosis

primary spermatocyte *n* : a diploid spermatocyte that has not yet undergone meiosis

primary syphilis *n* : the first stage of syphilis that is marked by the development of a chancre and the spread of the causative spirochete in the tissues of the body

primary thrombocythemia *n* : THROMBOCYTHEMIA

primary tooth *n* : MILK TOOTH

pri•mate \ˈprī-ˌmāt\ *n* : any of an order (Primates) of mammals including humans, apes, monkeys, lemurs, and living and extinct related forms

prime mover \ˈprīm-\ *n* : AGONIST 1

prim•er \ˈprī-mər\ *n* : a molecule (as a short strand of RNA or DNA) whose presence is required for formation of another molecule (as a longer chain of DNA)

pri•mi•done \ˈprī-mə-ˌdōn\ *n* : an anticonvulsant phenobarbital derivative $C_{12}H_{14}N_2O_2$ used esp. to control epileptic seizures

pri•mi•grav•id \ˌprī-mə-ˈgra-vid\ *adj* : pregnant for the first time

pri•mi•grav•i•da \-ˈgra-vi-də\ *n, pl* **-i•das** *or* **-i•dae** \-ˌdē\ : an individual pregnant for the first time

pri•mip•a•ra \prī-ˈmi-pə-rə\ *n, pl* **-ras** *or* **-rae** \-ˌrē\ **1** : an individual bearing a first offspring **2** : an individual that has borne only one offspring

pri•mip•a•rous \-rəs\ *adj* : of, relating to, or being a primipara : bearing young for the first time — compare MULTIPAROUS 2

prim•i•tive \ˈpri-mə-tiv\ *adj* **1** : closely approximating an early ancestral type : little evolved **2** : belonging to or characteristic of an early stage of development ⟨~ cells⟩

primitive streak *n* : an elongated band of cells that forms along the axis of an embryo early in gastrulation by the movement of lateral cells toward the axis and that develops a groove along its midline through which cells move to the interior of the embryo to form the mesoderm

pri•mor•di•al \prī-ˈmȯr-dē-əl\ *adj* : earliest formed in the growth of an individual or organ : PRIMITIVE

pri•mor•di•um \-dē-əm\ *n, pl* **-dia** \-dē-ə\ : the rudiment or commencement of a part or organ : ANLAGE

prin•ceps pol•li•cis \ˈprin-ˌseps-ˈpä-lə-səs\ *n* : a branch of the radial artery that passes along the ulnar side of the first metacarpal and divides into branches running along the palmar side of the thumb

prin•ci•ple \ˈprin-sə-pəl\ *n* : an ingredient (as a chemical) that exhibits or imparts a characteristic quality ⟨the active ~ of a drug⟩

Prin•i•vil \ˈpri-nə-ˌvil\ *trademark* — used for a preparation of lisinopril

P–R interval \ˌpē-ˈär-\ *n* : the interval between the beginning of the P wave and the beginning of the QRS complex of an electrocardiogram that represents the time between the beginning of the contraction of the atria and the beginning of the contraction of the ventricles

Prinz•met•al's angina \ˈprinz-ˌmet^əlz-\ *n* : angina pectoris of a variant form that is characterized by chest pain during rest and by an elevated ST segment during pain and that is typically caused by an obstructive lesion in the coronary artery

Prinzmetal, Myron (1908–1987), American cardiologist.

pri•on \ˈprē-ˌän\ *n* : any of various infectious proteins that are abnormal forms of normal cellular proteins, that proliferate by inducing the normal protein to convert to the abnormal form, and that in mammals include pathogenic forms which arise sporadically, as a result of genetic mutation, or by transmission (as by ingestion of infected tissue) and which upon accumulation in the brain cause a prion disease

prion disease *n* : any of a group of spongiform encephalopathies that are caused and transmitted by prions and that include bovine spongiform encephalopathy, Creutzfeldt-Jakob disease, fatal familial insomnia, Gerstmann-Sträussler-Scheinker syndrome, kuru, scrapie, and variant Creutzfeldt-Jakob disease — called also *transmissible spongiform encephalopathy*

Pris•tiq \pri-ˈstēk\ *trademark* — used for a preparation of desvenlafaxine

pri•vate \ˈprī-vət\ *adj* **1** : of, relating to, or receiving hospital service in which the patient has more privileges than a semiprivate or ward patient **2** : of, relating to, or being private practice ⟨a ~ practitioner⟩

private–duty *adj* : caring for a single patient either in the home or in a hospital ⟨a ~ nurse⟩

private practice *n* **1** : practice of a profession (as medicine) independently and not as an employee **2** : the patients depending on and using the services of a physician in private practice

privileged communication *n* : a communication between parties to a confidential relation (as between physician and patient) such that the recipient cannot be legally compelled to disclose it as a witness

PRK *abbr* photorefractive keratectomy

PRL *abbr* prolactin

prn *abbr* [Latin *pro re nata*] as needed; as the circumstances require — used in writing prescriptions

PRO *abbr* peer review organization

pro- *prefix* **1 a** : PRE- 1 ⟨*pro*estrus⟩ **b** : rudimentary : PROT- ⟨*pro*nucleus⟩ **c** : being a precursor of ⟨*pro*insulin⟩ **2** : front : anterior ⟨*pro*nephros⟩ **3** : projecting ⟨*pro*gnathous⟩

pro•ac•cel•er•in \ˌprō-ak-ˈse-lə-rən\ *n* : FACTOR V

pro•ac•tive \-ˈak-tiv\ *adj* : relating to, caused by, or being interference between previous learning and the recall or performance of later learning ⟨~ inhibition of memory⟩

pro•band \ˈprō-ˌband\ *n* : an individual affected with a disorder who is the first subject in a study (as of a genetic character in a family lineage) — called also *propositus*

Pro–Ban•thine \ˌprō-ˈban-ˌthēn\ *n* : a preparation of propantheline bromide — formerly a U.S. registered trademark

probe \ˈprōb\ *n* **1** : a surgical instrument that consists typically of a light slender fairly flexible pointed metal instrument like a small rod that is used typically for locating a foreign body, for exploring a wound or suppurative tract by prodding or piercing, or for penetrating and exploring bodily passages and cavities **2** : a device (as an ultrasound generator) or a substance (as radioactively labeled DNA) used to obtain specific information for diagnostic or experimental purposes — **probe** *vb*

pro•ben•e•cid \prō-ˈbe-nə-səd\ *n* : a drug $C_{13}H_{19}NO_4S$ that acts on renal tubular function and is used to increase the concentration of some drugs (as penicillin) in the blood by inhibiting their excretion and to increase the excretion of urates in gout

pro•bi•ot•ic \prō-bī-ˈä-tik\ *n* : a product or preparation (as a dietary supplement or food) containing live microorganisms (as lactobacilli or bifidobacteria) that when consumed maintains or restores beneficial bacteria to the digestive tract; *also* : a microorganism in such a preparation — compare PREBIOTIC — **probiotic** *adj*

pro•bos•cis \prə-ˈbä-səs, -ˈbäs-kəs\ *n, pl* **-bos•cis•es** *also* **-bos•ci•des** \-ˈbä-sə-ˌdēz\ : any of various elongated or extensible tubular organs or processes of the oral region of an invertebrate

pro•bu•col \ˈprō-byə-ˌkȯl\ *n* : an antioxidant drug $C_{31}H_{48}O_2S_2$ that is used to reduce levels of serum cholesterol

pro•cain•amide \prō-ˈkā-nə-ˌmīd, -məd; -ˌkā-ˈna-məd\ *n* : a base of an amide related to procaine that is used in the form of its hydrochloride $C_{13}H_{21}N_3O{\cdot}HCl$ as a cardiac depressant esp. in the treatment of ventricular and atrial arrhythmias — see PRONESTYL

pro•caine \ˈprō-ˌkān\ *n* : a basic ester $C_{13}H_{20}N_2O_2$ of para-aminobenzoic acid used in the form of its hydrochloride $C_{13}H_{20}N_2O_2{\cdot}HCl$ as a local anesthetic — see NOVOCAIN, NOVOCAINE

procaine penicillin G *n* : PENICILLIN G PROCAINE

pro•car•ba•zine \prō-ˈkär-bə-ˌzēn, -zən\ *n* : an antineoplastic drug that is a monoamine oxidase inhibitor and is used in the form of its hydrochloride $C_{12}H_{19}N_3O{\cdot}HCl$ esp. in the palliative treatment of Hodgkin's lymphoma

Pro•car•dia \prō-ˈkär-dē-ə\ *trademark* — used for a preparation of nifedipine

procaryote *var of* PROKARYOTE

pro•ce•dure \prə-ˈsē-jər\ *n* **1** : a particular way of accomplishing something or of acting **2** : a step in a procedure; *esp* : a series of steps followed in a regular definite order

pro•ce•rus \prō-ˈsir-əs\ *n, pl* **-ri** \-ˌrī\ *or* **-rus•es** : a facial muscle that arises from the nasal bone and a cartilage in the side of the nose and that inserts into the skin of the forehead between the eyebrows

pro·cess \ˈprä-ˌses, ˈprō-, -səs\ *n* **1 a** : a natural progressively continuing operation or development marked by a series of gradual changes that succeed one another in a relatively fixed way and lead toward a particular result or end ⟨the ~ of growth⟩ **b** : a natural continuing activity or function ⟨such life ~*es* as breathing⟩ **2** : a part of the mass of an organism or organic structure that projects outward from the main mass ⟨a bone ~⟩

pro·ces·sus \prō-ˈse-səs\ *n, pl* **proces·sus** : PROCESS 2

processus vag·i·na·lis \-ˌva-jə-ˈnā-ləs\ *n* : a pouch of peritoneum that is carried into the scrotum by the descent of the testicle and which in the scrotum forms the tunica vaginalis

pro·chlor·per·azine \ˌprō-ˌklȯr-ˈper-ə-ˌzēn\ *n* : a drug $C_{20}H_{24}ClN_3S$ that is a phenothiazine derivative having antiemetic and antipsychotic properties — see COMPAZINE

pro·ci·den·tia \ˌprō-sə-ˈden-chə, ˌprä-, -chē-ə\ *n* : PROLAPSE; *esp* : severe prolapse of the uterus in which the cervix projects from the vaginal opening

proc·li·na·tion \ˌprä-klə-ˈnā-shən\ *n* : the condition of being inclined forward ⟨~ of the upper incisors⟩

[1]**pro·co·ag·u·lant** \ˌprō-kō-ˈa-gyə-lənt\ *n* : a procoagulant substance

[2]**procoagulant** *adj* : promoting the coagulation of blood ⟨~ activity⟩

pro·col·la·gen \-ˈkä-lə-jən\ *n* : a molecular precursor of collagen

pro·con·ver·tin \-kən-ˈvərt-ᵊn\ *n* : FACTOR VII

pro·cre·ate \ˈprō-krē-ˌāt\ *vb* **-at·ed; -at·ing** : to beget or bring forth offspring : PROPAGATE, REPRODUCE — **pro·cre·ation** \ˌprō-krē-ˈā-shən\ *n* — **pro·cre·ative** \ˈprō-krē-ˌā-tiv\ *adj*

Pro·crit \ˈprō-ˌkrit\ *trademark* — used for a preparation of epoetin

proct- *or* **procto-** *comb form* **1 a** : rectum ⟨*procto*scope⟩ **b** : rectum and ⟨*procto*sigmoidectomy⟩ **2** : anus and rectum ⟨*procto*logy⟩

proct·al·gia fu·gax \ˌpräk-ˈtal-jə-ˈfyü-ˌgaks, -jē-ə-\ *n* : a condition characterized by the intermittent occurrence of sudden sharp pain in the rectal area

proc·tec·to·my \präk-ˈtek-tə-mē\ *n, pl* **-mies** : surgical excision of the rectum

proc·ti·tis \präk-ˈtī-təs\ *n* : inflammation of the anus and rectum

proc·toc·ly·sis \präk-ˈtä-klə-səs\ *n, pl* **-ly·ses** \-ˌsēz\ : slow injection of large quantities of a fluid (as a solution of salt) into the rectum in supplementing the liquid intake of the body

proc·to·co·li·tis \ˌpräk-tō-kə-ˈlī-təs\ *n* : inflammation of the rectum and colon

proc·tol·o·gy \präk-ˈtä-lə-jē\ *n, pl* **-gies** : a branch of medicine dealing with the structure and diseases of the anus, rectum, and sigmoid colon — **proc·to·log·ic** \ˌpräk-tə-ˈlä-jik\ *or* **proc·to·log·i·cal** \-ji-kəl\ *adj* — **proc·tol·o·gist** \-jist\ *n*

proc·to·pexy \ˈpräk-tə-ˌpek-sē\ *n, pl* **-pex·ies** : the suturing of the rectum to an adjacent structure (as the sacrum)

proc·to·plas·ty \ˈpräk-tə-ˌplas-tē\ *n, pl* **-ties** : plastic surgery of the rectum and anus

proc·to·scope \ˈpräk-tə-ˌskōp\ *n* : an instrument used for dilating and visually inspecting the rectum — **proc·to·scop·ic** \ˌpräk-tə-ˈskä-pik\ *adj* — **proc·to·scop·i·cal·ly** *adv* — **proc·tos·co·py** \präk-ˈtäs-kə-pē\ *n*

proc·to·sig·moid·ec·to·my \ˌpräk-tō-ˌsig-mȯi-ˈdek-tə-mē\ *n, pl* **-mies** : complete or partial surgical excision of the rectum and sigmoid colon

proc·to·sig·moid·itis \-ˌsig-mȯi-ˈdī-təs\ *n* : inflammation of the rectum and sigmoid colon

proc·to·sig·moid·o·scope \-sig-ˈmȯi-də-ˌskōp\ *n* : SIGMOIDOSCOPE

proc·to·sig·moid·os·co·py \-ˌsig-ˌmȯi-ˈdäs-kə-pē\ *n, pl* **-pies** : SIGMOIDOSCOPY — **proc·to·sig·moid·o·scop·ic** \-ˌmȯi-də-ˈskä-pik\ *adj*

proc·tot·o·my \präk-ˈtä-tə-mē\ *n, pl* **-mies** : surgical incision into the rectum

prod·ro·ma \ˈprä-drə-mə\ *n, pl* **-mas** *or* **-ma·ta** \prō-ˈdrō-mə-tə\ : PRODROME

pro·drome \ˈprō-ˌdrōm\ *n* : a premonitory symptom of disease — **pro·dro·mal** \ˌprō-ˈdrō-məl\ *also* **pro·dro·mic** \-mik\ *adj*

pro·drug \ˈprō-ˌdrəg\ *n* : a pharmacologically inactive substance that is the modified form of a pharmacologically active drug to which it is converted (as by enzymatic action) in the body

pro·duc·tive \prə-ˈdək-tiv, prō-\ *adj* : raising mucus or sputum (as from the bronchi) ⟨a ~ cough⟩

pro·en·zyme \ˌprō-ˈen-ˌzīm\ *n* : ZYMOGEN

pro·eryth·ro·blast \-i-ˈri-thrə-ˌblast\ *n* : a hemocytoblast that gives rise to erythroblasts

pro·es·trus \-ˈes-trəs\ *n* : a preparatory period immediately preceding estrus and characterized by growth of graafian follicles, increased estrogenic activity, and alteration of uterine and vaginal mucosa

professional corporation *n* : a corporation organized by one or more licensed individuals (as a doctor or dentist) esp. for the purpose of providing professional services and obtaining tax advantages — abbr. *PC*

pro·fi·bri·no·ly·sin \ˌprō-ˌfī-brə-nə-ˈlīsᵊn\ *n* : PLASMINOGEN

pro·file \ˈprō-ˌfīl\ *n* **1** : a set of data exhibiting the significant features of something and often obtained by multiple tests **2** : a graphic representation of the extent to which an individual or group exhibits traits or abilities as determined by tests or ratings ⟨a personality ~⟩

pro·fla·vine \ˌprō-ˈflā-ˌvēn\ *also* **pro·fla·vin** \-vin\ *n* : a yellow crystalline mutagenic acridine dye $C_{13}H_{11}N_3$;

also : the orange to brownish-red hygroscopic crystalline sulfate used as an antiseptic esp. for wounds

pro·found·ly \prə-ˈfau̇nd-lē, prō-\ *adv* **1** : totally or completely 〈~ deaf persons〉 **2** : to the greatest possible degree 〈~ hypothermic patients〉

pro·fun·da artery \prə-ˈfən-də-\ *n* **1** : DEEP BRACHIAL ARTERY **2** : DEEP FEMORAL ARTERY

profunda fem·o·ris \-ˈfe-mə-rəs\ *n* : DEEP FEMORAL ARTERY

profunda femoris artery *n* : DEEP FEMORAL ARTERY

profundus — see FLEXOR DIGITORUM PROFUNDUS

pro·gen·i·tor \prō-ˈje-nə-tər, prə-\ *n* **1** : an ancestor of an individual in a direct line of descent along which some or all of the ancestral genes could theoretically have passed **2** : a biologically ancestral form

prog·e·ny \ˈprä-jə-nē\ *n, pl* **-nies** : offspring of animals or plants

pro·ge·ria \prō-ˈjir-ē-ə\ *n* : a rare genetic disorder of childhood marked by slowed physical growth and characteristic signs (as baldness, wrinkled skin, and atherosclerosis) of rapid aging with death usu. occurring during puberty

pro·ges·ta·tion·al \ˌprō-ˌjes-ˈtā-shə-nəl\ *adj* : preceding pregnancy or gestation; *esp* : of, relating to, inducing, or constituting the modifications of the female mammalian system associated with ovulation and corpus luteum formation 〈~ hormones〉

pro·ges·ter·one \prō-ˈjes-tə-ˌrōn\ *n* : a female steroid sex hormone $C_{21}H_{30}O_2$ that is secreted by the corpus luteum to prepare the endometrium for implantation and later by the placenta during pregnancy to prevent rejection of the developing embryo or fetus; *also* : a synthetic steroid resembling progesterone in action

pro·ges·tin \prō-ˈjes-tən\ *n* : PROGESTERONE; *esp* : a synthetic progesterone (as levonorgestrel)

pro·ges·to·gen *also* **pro·ges·ta·gen** \-ˈjes-tə-jən\ *n* : a naturally occurring or synthetic progestational steroid — **pro·ges·to·gen·ic** *also* **pro·ges·ta·gen·ic** \prə-ˌjes-tə-ˈje-nik\ *adj*

pro·glot·tid \ˌprō-ˈglä-tid\ *n* : a segment of a tapeworm containing both male and female reproductive organs

pro·glot·tis \-ˈglä-tis\ *n, pl* **-glot·ti·des** \-ˈglä-tə-ˌdēz\ : PROGLOTTID

prog·na·thic \präg-ˈna-thik, -ˈnā-\ *adj* : PROGNATHOUS

prog·na·thous \ˈpräg-nə-thəs\ *adj* : being or having an upper or lower jaw that projects abnormally forward — **prog·na·thism** \ˈpräg-nə-ˌthi-zəm, präg-ˈnā-\ *n*

prog·no·sis \präg-ˈnō-səs\ *n, pl* **-no·ses** \-ˌsēz\ **1** : the act or art of foretelling the course of a disease **2** : the prospect of survival and recovery from a disease as anticipated from the usual course of that disease or indicated by special features of the case — **prog·nos·tic** \präg-ˈnäs-tik\ *adj*

prog·nos·ti·cate \präg-ˈnäs-tə-ˌkāt\ *vb* **-cat·ed; -cat·ing** : to make a prognosis about the probable outcome of — **prog·nos·ti·ca·tion** \-ˌnäs-tə-ˈkā-shən\ *n*

programmed cell death *n* : APOPTOSIS

pro·gres·sive \prə-ˈgre-siv\ *adj* **1** : increasing in extent or severity 〈a ~ disease〉 **2** : of, relating to, or being a multifocal lens with a gradual transition between focal lengths 〈~ bifocals〉 — **pro·gres·sive·ly** *adv*

progressive multifocal leukoencephalopathy *n* : a progressive and often fatal demyelinating disease of the central nervous system that typically affects immunocompromised individuals, is characterized esp. by muscle weakness and loss of coordination with impairments in speech, vision, and cognitive function, that commonly progresses to paralysis, and is caused by reactivation of a latent virus of the genus *Polyomavirus* (species *JC polyomavirus*)

progressive supranuclear palsy *n* : an uncommon neurological disorder that is of unknown etiology, typically occurs from late middle age onward, and is marked by loss of voluntary vertical eye movement, muscular rigidity and dystonia of the neck and trunk, pseudobulbar paralysis, bradykinesia, and dementia — called also *supranuclear palsy*

pro·guan·il \ˌprō-ˈgwän-ᵊl\ *n* : an antimalarial drug used in the form of its hydrochloride $C_{11}H_{16}ClN_5{\cdot}HCl$ — called also *chloroguanide;* see MALARONE

pro·hor·mone \ˌprō-ˈhȯr-ˌmōn\ *n* : a physiologically inactive precursor of a hormone

pro–in·flam·ma·to·ry \-in-ˈfla-mə-ˌtȯr-ē\ *adj* : promoting inflammation : capable of causing inflammation

pro·in·su·lin \-ˈin-sə-lən\ *n* : a single-chain pancreatic polypeptide precursor of insulin that gives rise to the double chain of insulin by loss of the middle part of the molecule

pro·ject \prə-ˈjekt\ *vb* **1** : to attribute or assign (something in one's own mind or a personal characteristic) to a person, group, or object **2** : to connect by sending nerve fibers or processes

pro·jec·tile vomiting \prə-ˈjek-təl-, -ˌtīl-\ *n* : vomiting that is sudden, usu. without nausea, and so sufficiently vigorous that the vomit is forcefully projected to a distance

pro·jec·tion \prə-ˈjek-shən\ *n* **1 a** : the act of referring a mental image constructed by the brain from bits of data collected by the sense organs to the actual source of stimulation outside the body **b** : the attribution of one's own ideas, feelings, or attitudes to other people or to objects; *esp* : the externalization of blame, guilt, or responsibility as a defense against anxiety **2**

: the functional correspondence and connection of parts of the cerebral cortex with other parts of the organism

projection area *n* : an area of the cerebral cortex having connection through projection fibers with subcortical centers that in turn are linked with peripheral sense or motor organs

projection fiber *n* : a nerve fiber connecting some part of the cerebral cortex with lower sensory or motor centers — compare ASSOCIATION FIBER

pro•jec•tive \prə-ˈjek-tiv\ *adj* : of, relating to, or being a technique, device, or test (as the Rorschach test) designed to analyze the psychodynamic constitution of an individual by presenting unstructured or ambiguous material (as blots of ink, pictures, and sentence elements) that will elicit interpretive responses revealing personality structure

pro•kary•ote *also* **pro•cary•ote** \ˌprō-ˈkar-ē-ˌōt\ *n* : a typically unicellular organism (as a bacterium) that lacks a distinct nucleus and membrane-bound organelles — compare EUKARYOTE — **pro•kary•ot•ic** *also* **pro•cary•ot•ic** \-ˌkar-ē-ˈä-tik\ *adj*

pro•ki•net•ic \ˌprō-kə-ˈne-tik, -kī-\ *adj* : stimulating motility of the esophageal and gastrointestinal muscles — **prokinetic** *n*

pro•lac•tin \prō-ˈlak-tən\ *n* : a protein hormone of the adenohypophysis of the pituitary gland that induces and maintains lactation in the postpartum mammalian female — abbr. *PRL;* called also *luteotropic hormone, luteotropin, mammotropin*

pro•la•min *or* **pro•la•mine** \ˈprō-lə-mən, -ˌmēn\ *n* : any of various simple proteins that are found esp. in the seeds of grasses and are soluble in alcohol

pro•lapse \prō-ˈlaps, ˈprō-ˌ\ *n* : the falling down or slipping of a body part from its usual position or relations ⟨uterine ~⟩ — **pro•lapse** \prō-ˈlaps\ *vb*

Pro•lia \ˈprō-lē-ə\ *trademark* — used for a preparation of denosumab

proliferans — see RETINITIS PROLIFERANS

pro•lif•er•a•tion \prə-ˌli-fə-ˈrā-shən\ *n* **1 a** : rapid and repeated production of new parts or of offspring (as in a mass of cells by a rapid succession of cell divisions) **b** : a growth so formed **2** : the action, process, or result of increasing by proliferation — **pro•lif•er•ate** \-ˈli-fə-ˌrāt\ *vb* — **pro•lif•er•a•tive** \-ˈli-fə-ˌrā-tiv\ *adj*

proligerus — see DISCUS PROLIGERUS

pro•line \ˈprō-ˌlēn\ *n* : an amino acid $C_5H_9NO_2$ that can be synthesized by animals from glutamate

Pro•lix•in \prō-ˈlik-sən\ *trademark* — used for a preparation of fluphenazine

pro•lo•ther•a•py \ˌprō-lō-ˈther-ə-pē\ *n* : an alternative therapy for treating musculoskeletal pain that involves injecting an irritant substance (as dextrose) into a ligament or tendon to promote the growth of new tissue

pro•mas•ti•gote \prō-ˈmas-ti-ˌgōt\ *n* : a protozoan (family Trypanosomatidae and esp. genus *Leishmania*) that is in a flagellated usu. extracellular stage characterized by a single anterior flagellum and no undulating membrane — **promastigote** *adj*

pro•ma•zine \ˈprō-mə-ˌzēn\ *n* : a tranquilizer derived from phenothiazine that is used in the form of its hydrochloride $C_{17}H_{20}N_2S{\cdot}HCl$ similarly to chlorpromazine — see SPARINE

pro•mega•kary•o•cyte \ˌprō-ˌme-gə-ˈkar-ē-ō-ˌsīt\ *n* : a cell in an intermediate stage of development between a megakaryoblast and a megakaryocyte

pro•meth•a•zine \prō-ˈme-thə-ˌzēn\ *n* : an antihistamine drug derived from phenothiazine and used chiefly in the form of its hydrochloride $C_{17}H_{20}N_2S{\cdot}HCl$ — see PHENERGAN

pro•meth•es•trol \-me-ˈthes-ˌtrȯl\ *n* : a synthetic estrogen $C_{20}H_{26}O_2$

pro•me•thi•um \prə-ˈmē-thē-əm\ *n* : a radioactive metallic element obtained as a fission product of uranium or from neutron-irradiated neodymium — symbol *Pm;* see ELEMENT table

prom•i•nence \ˈprä-mə-nəns\ *n* : an elevation or projection on an anatomical structure (as a bone)

prominens — see VERTEBRA PROMINENS

pro•mis•cu•ous \prə-ˈmis-kyə-wəs\ *adj* : not restricted to one sexual partner — **pro•mis•cu•i•ty** \ˌprä-məs-ˈkyü-ə-tē, prə-ˌmis-\ *n*

pro•mono•cyte \prə-ˈmä-nə-ˌsīt\ *n* : a cell in an intermediate stage of development between a monoblast and a monocyte

prom•on•to•ry \ˈprä-mən-ˌtōr-ē\ *n, pl* **-ries** : a bodily prominence: as **a** : the angle of the ventral side of the sacrum where it joins the vertebra **b** : a prominence on the inner wall of the tympanum of the ear

pro•mot•er \prə-ˈmō-tər\ *n* **1** : a substance that in very small amounts is able to increase the activity of a catalyst **2** : a binding site in a DNA chain at which RNA polymerase binds to initiate transcription of messenger RNA by one or more nearby structural genes **3** : a chemical believed to promote carcinogenicity or mutagenicity

pro•my•elo•cyte \prō-ˈmī-ə-lə-ˌsīt\ *n* : a cell in bone marrow that is in an intermediate stage of development between a myeloblast and a myelocyte and has the characteristic granulations but lacks the specific staining reactions of a mature granulocyte of the blood — **pro•my•elo•cyt•ic** \-ˌmī-ə-lə-ˈsi-tik\ *adj*

promyelocytic leukemia *n* : a leukemia in which the predominant blood cell type is the promyelocyte

pro•na•tion \prō-ˈnā-shən\ *n* : rotation of an anatomical part towards the midline: as **a** : rotation of the hand and forearm so that the palm faces backwards or downwards **b** : rotation of the medial bones in the midtarsal region of the foot inward and downward so that in walking the foot tends to come down on its inner margin — **pro•nate** \ˈprō-ˌnāt\ *vb*

pro•na•tor \ˈprō-ˌnā-tər\ *n* : a muscle that produces pronation

pronator qua•dra•tus \-kwä-ˈdrā-təs\ *n* : a deep muscle of the forearm passing transversely from the ulna to the radius and serving to pronate the forearm

pronator te•res \-ˈtir-ˌēz\ *n* : a muscle of the forearm arising from the medial epicondyle of the humerus and the coronoid process of the ulna, inserting into the lateral surface of the middle third of the radius, and serving to pronate and flex the forearm

prone \ˈprōn\ *adj* : having the front or ventral surface downward; *esp* : lying facedown — **prone** *adv*

pro•neph•ros \prō-ˈne-frəs, -ˌfräs\ *n, pl* **-neph•roi** \-ˈne-ˌfrȯi\ : either member of the first and most anterior pair of the three paired vertebrate renal organs present but nonfunctional in embryos of reptiles, birds, and mammals — compare MESONEPHROS, METANEPHROS — **pro•neph•ric** \prō-ˈne-frik\ *adj*

Pro•nes•tyl \prō-ˈnes-til\ *trademark* — used for a preparation of the hydrochloride of procainamide

pron•to•sil \ˈprän-tə-ˌsil\ *n* : any of three sulfonamide drugs: **a** : a red azo dye $C_{12}H_{13}N_5O_2S$ that was the first sulfa drug tested clinically **b** : SULFANILAMIDE **c** : AZOSULFAMIDE

pro•nu•cle•us \prō-ˈnü-klē-əs, -ˈnyü-\ *n, pl* **-clei** \-klē-ˌī\ *also* **-cle•us•es** : the haploid nucleus of a male or female gamete (as an egg or sperm) up to the time of fusion with that of another gamete in fertilization — **pro•nu•cle•ar** \-klē-ər\ *adj*

prop•a•gate \ˈprä-pə-ˌgāt\ *vb* **-gat•ed; -gat•ing** **1** : to reproduce or cause to reproduce sexually or asexually **2** : to cause to spread or to be transmitted — **prop•a•ga•tion** \ˌprä-pə-ˈgā-shən\ *n* — **prop•a•ga•tive** \ˈprä-pə-ˌgā-tiv\ *adj*

pro•pam•i•dine \prō-ˈpa-mə-ˌdēn, -dən\ *n* : an antiseptic drug $C_{17}H_{20}N_4O_2$

pro•pan•o•lol \prō-ˈpa-nə-ˌlȯl, -ˌlōl\ *n* : PROPRANOLOL

pro•pan•the•line bromide \prō-ˈpan-thə-ˌlēn-\ *n* : an anticholinergic drug $C_{23}H_{30}BrNO_3$ used esp. in the treatment of peptic ulcer — called also *propantheline;* see PRO-BANTHINE

pro•par•a•caine \prō-ˈpar-ə-ˌkān\ *n* : a drug used in the form of its hydrochloride $C_{16}H_{26}N_2O_3{\cdot}HCl$ as a topical anesthetic

Pro•pe•cia \prō-ˈpē-shə\ *trademark* — used for a preparation of finasteride

pro•per•din \prō-ˈpərd-ᵊn\ *n* : a blood serum protein that participates in the activation of complement in a pathway which does not involve the presence of antibodies

pro•peri•to•ne•al \prō-ˌper-ə-tə-ˈnē-əl\ *adj* : lying between the parietal peritoneum and the ventral musculature of the body cavity ⟨~ fat⟩

pro•phage \ˈprō-ˌfāj, -ˌfäzh\ *n* : an intracellular form of a bacteriophage in which it is harmless to the host, is usu. integrated into the hereditary material of the host, and reproduces when the host does

pro•phase \-ˌfāz\ *n* **1** : the initial stage of mitosis and of the mitotic division of meiosis characterized by the condensation of chromosomes consisting of two chromatids, disappearance of the nucleolus and nuclear membrane, and formation of the mitotic spindle **2** : the initial stage of the first division of meiosis in which the chromosomes become visible, homologous pairs of chromosomes undergo synapsis and crossing-over, chiasmata appear, chromosomes condense with homologues visible as tetrads, and the nuclear membrane and nucleolus disappear — see DIAKINESIS, DIPLOTENE, LEPTOTENE, PACHYTENE, ZYGOTENE — **pro•pha•sic** \prō-ˈfā-zik\ *adj*

[1]**pro•phy•lac•tic** \ˌprō-fə-ˈlak-tik, ˌprä-\ *adj* **1** : guarding from or preventing the spread or occurrence of disease or infection ⟨~ therapy⟩ **2** : tending to prevent or ward off : PREVENTIVE — **pro•phy•lac•ti•cal•ly** *adv*

[2]**prophylactic** *n* : something (as a drug) that is prophylactic; *esp* : a device and esp. a condom for preventing venereal infection or conception

pro•phy•lax•is \-ˈlak-səs\ *n, pl* **-lax•es** \-ˈlak-ˌsēz\ : measures designed to preserve health and prevent the spread of disease : protective or preventive treatment

pro•pio•lac•tone \ˌprō-pē-ō-ˈlak-ˌtōn\ *or* **β-pro•pio•lac•tone** \ˌbā-tə-\ *n* : a liquid disinfectant $C_3H_4O_2$

pro•pi•o•ma•zine \ˌprō-pē-ˈō-mə-ˌzēn\ *n* : a phenothiazine used esp. in the form of its hydrochloride $C_{20}H_{24}N_2OS{\cdot}HCl$ as a sedative

pro•pi•o•nate \ˈprō-pē-ə-ˌnāt\ *n* : a salt or ester of propionic acid

pro•pi•oni•bac•te•ri•um \ˌprō-pē-ˌä-nə-bak-ˈtir-ē-əm\ *n* **1** *cap* : a genus of gram-positive nonmotile usu. anaerobic bacteria (family Propionibacteriaceae) including forms found esp. on human skin and in dairy products **2** *pl* **-ria** \-ē-ə\ : any bacterium of the genus *Propionibacterium*

pro•pi•on•ic acid \ˌprō-pē-ˈä-nik-\ *n* : a liquid sharp-odored fatty acid $C_3H_6O_2$

pro•po•fol \ˈprō-pō-ˌfōl\ *n* : a sedating and hypnotic agent $C_{12}H_{18}O$ administered intravenously to induce and maintain anesthesia or sedation

pro•pos•i•ta \prō-ˈpä-zə-tə\ *n, pl* **-i•tae** \-ˌtē\ : a female proband

pro•pos•i•tus \prō-ˈpä-zə-təs\ *n, pl* **-i•ti** \-ˌtī\ : PROBAND

pro•poxy•phene \prō-ˈpäk-sə-ˌfēn\ *n* : a narcotic analgesic structurally related to methadone but less addicting that is administered in the form of its hydrochloride $C_{22}H_{29}NO_2 \cdot HCl$ or hydrated napsylate $C_{22}H_{29}NO_2 \cdot C_{10}H_8SO_3 \cdot H_2O$ — called also *dextropropoxyphene;* see DARVOCET-N, DARVON

pro•pran•o•lol \prō-ˈpra-nə-ˌlȯl, -ˌlōl\ *n* : a beta-blocker used in the form of its hydrochloride $C_{16}H_{21}NO_2 \cdot HCl$ esp. in the treatment of hypertension, cardiac arrhythmias, and angina pectoris and in the prevention of migraine headache — called also *propanolol;* see INDERAL, INNOPRAN

propria — see LAMINA PROPRIA, SUBSTANTIA PROPRIA, TUNICA PROPRIA

¹pro•pri•e•tary \prə-ˈprī-ə-ˌter-ē\ *n, pl* **-tar•ies** : something that is used, produced, or marketed under exclusive legal right of the inventor or maker; *specif* : a drug (as a patent medicine) that is protected by secrecy, patent, or copyright against free competition as to name, product, composition, or process of manufacture

²proprietary *adj* **1** : used, made, or marketed by one having the exclusive legal right ⟨a ~ drug⟩ **2** : privately owned and managed and run as a profit-making organization ⟨a ~ clinic⟩

pro•prio•cep•tion \ˌprō-prē-ō-ˈsep-shən\ *n* : the reception of stimuli produced within the organism — **pro•prio•cep•tive** \-ˈsep-tiv\ *adj*

proprioceptive neuromuscular facilitation *n* : a method of stretching muscles to maximize their flexibility that is often performed with a partner or trainer and that involves a series of contractions and relaxations with enforced stretching during the relaxation phase — abbr. *PNF*

pro•prio•cep•tor \-ˈsep-tər\ *n* : a sensory receptor located deep in the tissues (as in skeletal or heart muscle) that functions in proprioception

pro•prio•spi•nal \-ˈspīn-ᵊl\ *adj* : distinctively or exclusively spinal ⟨a ~ neuron⟩

proprius — see EXTENSOR DIGITI QUINTI PROPRIUS, EXTENSOR INDICIS PROPRIUS

pro•pto•sis \präp-ˈtō-səs, prō-ˈtō-\ *n, pl* **-pto•ses** \-ˌsēz\ : forward projection or displacement esp. of the eyeball

pro•pyl•ene glycol \ˈprō-pə-ˌlēn-\ *n* : a sweet viscous liquid $C_3H_8O_2$ used esp. as an antifreeze and solvent, in brake fluids, and as a food preservative

pro•pyl gallate \ˈprō-pəl-\ *n* : a white crystalline antioxidant $C_{10}H_{12}O_5$ that is used as a preservative

pro•pyl•hex•e•drine \ˌprō-pəl-ˈhek-sə-ˌdrēn\ *n* : a sympathomimetic drug $C_{10}H_{21}N$ used chiefly as a nasal decongestant

pro•pyl•par•a•ben \-ˈpar-ə-ˌben\ *n* : an ester $C_{10}H_{12}O_3$ used as a preservative in pharmaceutical preparations

pro•pyl•thio•ura•cil \-ˌthī-ō-ˈyu̇r-ə-ˌsil\ *n* : a crystalline compound $C_7H_{10}N_2OS$ used as an antithyroid drug in the treatment of goiter

pro•re•nin \prō-ˈrē-nən, -ˈre-\ *n* : the precursor of the kidney enzyme renin

pros- *prefix* : in front ⟨*pros*encephalon⟩

Pros•car \ˈpräs-ˌkär\ *trademark* — used for a preparation of finasteride

pro•sec•tor \prō-ˈsek-tər\ *n* : a person who makes dissections for anatomic demonstrations

pros•en•ceph•a•lon \ˌprä-ˌsen-ˈse-fə-ˌlän, -lən\ *n* : FOREBRAIN

prosop- *or* **prosopo-** *comb form* : face ⟨*prosop*agnosia⟩

pros•op•ag•no•sia \ˌprä-sə-pag-ˈnō-zhə\ *n* : a form of visual agnosia characterized by an inability to recognize faces

pro•spec•tive \prə-ˈspek-tiv\ *adj* : relating to or being a study (as of the incidence of disease) that starts with the present condition of a population of individuals and follows them into the future — compare RETROSPECTIVE

pros•ta•cy•clin \ˌpräs-tə-ˈsī-klən\ *n* : a prostaglandin that is a metabolite of arachidonic acid, inhibits aggregation of platelets, and dilates blood vessels

pros•ta•glan•din \ˌpräs-tə-ˈglan-dən\ *n* : any of various oxygenated unsaturated cyclic fatty acids of animals that have a variety of hormonelike actions (as in controlling blood pressure or smooth muscle contraction)

prostaglandin E₁ \-ˈē-ˈwən\ *n* : ALPROSTADIL

prostat- *or* **prostato-** *comb form* : prostate gland ⟨*prostat*itis⟩

prostatae — see LEVATOR PROSTATAE

pros•tate \ˈpräs-ˌtāt\ *n* : PROSTATE GLAND

pros•ta•tec•to•my \ˌpräs-tə-ˈtek-tə-mē\ *n, pl* **-mies** : surgical removal or resection of the prostate gland

prostate gland *n* : a firm partly muscular partly glandular body that is situated about the base of the mammalian male urethra and secretes an alkaline viscid fluid which is a major constituent of semen — called also *prostate*

prostate–specific antigen *n* : a protease that is secreted by the epithelial cells of the prostate and is used in the diagnosis of prostate cancer since its concentration in the blood serum tends to be proportional to the clinical stage of the disease — abbr. *PSA*

pros•tat•ic \prä-ˈsta-tik\ *adj* : of, relating to, or affecting the prostate gland

prostatic intraepithelial neoplasia *n* : the formation of atypical epithelial cells in the prostate gland that are believed to be early precursors of adenocarcinoma — abbr. *PIN*

prostatic urethra *n* : the part of the male urethra from the base of the prostate gland where the urethra begins as the outlet of the bladder to the point where it emerges from the apex of the prostate gland

prostatic utricle *n* : a small blind pouch that projects from the wall of the prostatic urethra into the prostate gland

pros•ta•tism \ˈpräs-tə-ˌti-zəm\ *n* : disease of the prostate gland; *esp* : a disorder resulting from obstruction of the bladder neck by an enlarged prostate gland

pros•ta•ti•tis \ˌpräs-tə-ˈtī-təs\ *n* : inflammation of the prostate gland

pros•the•sis \präs-ˈthē-səs, ˈpräs-thə-\ *n, pl* **-the•ses** \-ˌsēz\ : an artificial device to replace a missing part of the body ⟨a dental ~⟩

pros•thet•ic \präs-ˈthe-tik\ *adj* **1** : of, relating to, or being a prosthesis ⟨a ~ device⟩; *also* : of or relating to prosthetics ⟨~ research⟩ **2** : of, relating to, or constituting a nonprotein group of a conjugated protein — **pros•thet•i•cal•ly** *adv*

prosthetic dentistry *n* : PROSTHODONTICS

pros•thet•ics \-tiks\ *n sing or pl* : the surgical and dental specialty concerned with the design, construction, and fitting of prostheses

prosthetic valve endocarditis *n* : endocarditis caused by or involving a surgically implanted prosthetic heart valve — abbr. *PVE*

pros•the•tist \ˈpräs-thə-tist\ *n* : a specialist in prosthetics

pros•thi•on \ˈpräs-thē-ˌän\ *n* : a point on the alveolar arch midway between the median upper incisor teeth

prosth•odon•tics \ˌpräs-thə-ˈdän-tiks\ *n sing or pl* : the dental specialty concerned with the making of artificial replacements for missing parts of the mouth and jaw — called also *prosthetic dentistry* — **prosth•odon•tic** \-tik\ *adj*

prosth•odon•tist \-ˈdän-tist\ *n* : a specialist in prosthodontics

Pro•stig•min \prō-ˈstig-mən\ *trademark* — used for a preparation of neostigmine

[1]**pros•trate** \ˈpräs-ˌtrāt\ *adj* : completely overcome ⟨was ~ from the heat⟩

[2]**prostrate** *vb* **pros•trat•ed; pros•trat•ing** : to put into a state of extreme bodily exhaustion ⟨*prostrated* by fever⟩

pros•tra•tion \prä-ˈstrā-shən\ *n* : complete physical or mental exhaustion — see HEAT EXHAUSTION

prot•ac•tin•i•um \ˌprō-ˌtak-ˈti-nē-əm\ *n* : a shiny metallic radioelement — symbol *Pa;* see ELEMENT table

prot•amine \ˈprō-tə-ˌmēn\ *n* : any of various strongly basic proteins of relatively low molecular weight that are rich in arginine and are found associated esp. with DNA in place of histone in the sperm cells of various animals (as fish)

protamine zinc insulin *n* : a suspension of insulin and salts of protamine and zinc in a buffered aqueous solution that is used for subcutaneous injection and has a slow onset and long duration — abbr. *PZI*

prot•anom•a•ly \ˌprō-tə-ˈnä-mə-lē\ *n, pl* **-lies** : deficient color vision in which an abnormally large proportion of red is required to match the spectrum — compare DEUTERANOMALY, TRICHROMAT — **prot•anom•a•lous** \-ləs\ *adj*

pro•ta•nope \ˈprō-tə-ˌnōp\ *n* : an individual affected with protanopia

prot•an•opia \ˌprō-tə-ˈnō-pē-ə\ *n* : a dichromatism in which the spectrum is seen in tones of yellow and blue with confusion of red and green and reduced sensitivity to monochromatic lights from the red end of the spectrum

prote- *or* **proteo-** *comb form* : protein ⟨*proteo*lysis⟩

pro•te•ase \ˈprō-tē-ˌās, -ˌāz\ *n* : any of numerous enzymes that hydrolyze proteins and are classified according to the most prominent functional group (as serine or cysteine) at the active site — called also *proteinase*

protease inhibitor *n* : a substance that inhibits the action of a protease; *specif* : any of various drugs (as indinavir or saquinavir) that inhibit the action of HIV protease so that cleavage of viral proteins into mature infectious particles is prevented and that are used esp. in combination with other antiretroviral agents in the treatment of HIV infection

[1]**pro•tec•tive** \prə-ˈtek-tiv\ *adj* : serving to protect the body or one of its parts from disease or injury

[2]**protective** *n* : a protective agent (as a medicine or a dressing)

pro•tein \ˈprō-ˌtēn\ *n, often attrib* **1** : any of numerous naturally occurring extremely complex substances that consist of amino acid residues joined by peptide bonds, contain the elements carbon, hydrogen, nitrogen, oxygen, usu. sulfur, and occas. other elements (as phosphorus or iron), and include many essential biological compounds (as enzymes, hormones, or antibodies) **2** : the total nitrogenous material in plant or animal substances; *esp* : CRUDE PROTEIN

pro•tein•aceous \ˌprō-tə-ˈnā-shəs, -ˌtē-\ *adj* : of, relating to, resembling, or being protein

pro•tein•ase \ˈprō-tə-ˌnās, -ˌtē-, -ˌnāz\ *n* : PROTEASE

protein C *n* : a vitamin K-dependent proteolytic glycoprotein synthesized in the liver that circulates in the blood plasma in an inactive form and when activated forms a complex with protein S to cleave factors V and VIII and inhibit the formation of thrombin

protein kinase *n* : any of a class of allosteric enzymes that possess a catalytic subunit which transfers a phosphate from ATP to one or more amino acid residues in a protein's side chain resulting in a conformational change affecting protein function and that include many which are activated by the binding of a second messenger (as cyclic AMP)

protein kinase C *n* : any of a group of isoenzymes of protein kinase that modify the conformation and activity of various intracellular proteins by catalyzing the phosphorylation of specific serine or threonine amino acid residues — abbr. *PKC*

pro•tein•o•sis \ˌprō-ˌtē-ˈnō-səs\ *n, pl* **-o•ses** \-ˌsēz\ *or* **-o•sis•es** : the accumulation of abnormal amounts of protein in bodily tissues — see PULMONARY ALVEOLAR PROTEINOSIS

protein S *n* : a vitamin K-dependent glycoprotein synthesized in the liver that circulates in the blood plasma and in its free form functions as a cofactor to facilitate the action of activated protein C

pro•tein•uria \ˌprō-tə-ˈnu̇r-ē-ə, -ˌtē-, -ˈnyu̇r-\ *n* : the presence of excess protein in the urine — **pro•tein•uric** \-ˈnu̇r-ik, -ˈnyu̇r-\ *adj*

pro•teo•gly•can \ˌprō-tē-ə-ˈglī-ˌkan\ *n* : any of a class of glycoproteins of high molecular weight that are found in the extracellular matrix of connective tissue

pro•teo•lip•id \-ˈli-pəd\ *n* : any of a class of proteins that have a high lipid content and are soluble in lipids and insoluble in water

pro•te•ol•y•sis \ˌprō-tē-ˈä-lə-səs\ *n, pl* **-y•ses** \-ˌsēz\ : the hydrolysis of proteins or peptides with formation of simpler and soluble products (as in digestion) — **pro•teo•lyt•ic** \ˌprō-tē-ə-ˈli-tik\ *adj* — **pro•teo•lyt•i•cal•ly** *adv*

pro•te•ome \ˈprō-tē-ˌōm\ *n* : the complement of proteins expressed in a cell, tissue, or organism by a genome

pro•te•o•mics \ˌprō-tē-ˈō-miks\ *n* : a branch of biotechnology concerned with applying the techniques of molecular biology, biochemistry, and genetics to analyzing the structure, function, and interactions of the proteins produced by the genes of a particular cell, tissue, or organism, with organizing the information in databases, and with applications of the data — compare GENOMICS — **pro•te•o•mic** \-mik\ *adj*

pro•te•us \ˈprō-tē-əs\ *n* **1** *cap* : a genus of aerobic usu. motile enterobacteria that are often found in decaying organic matter and include a common causative agent (*P. mirabilis*) of urinary tract infections **2** *pl* **-tei** \-ˌī\ : any bacterium of the genus *Proteus*

pro•throm•bin \prō-ˈthräm-bən\ *n* : a plasma protein produced in the liver in the presence of vitamin K and converted into thrombin by the action of various activators (as thromboplastin) in the clotting of blood — **pro•throm•bic** \-bik\ *adj*

prothrombin time *n* : the time required for a particular specimen of prothrombin to induce blood-plasma clotting under standardized conditions in comparison with a time of between 11.5 and 12 seconds for normal human blood

pro•ti•re•lin \prō-ˈtī-rə-lən\ *n* : THYROTROPIN-RELEASING HORMONE

pro•tist \ˈprō-ˌtist\ *n* : any of a diverse taxonomic group and esp. a kingdom (Protista syn. Protoctista) of eukaryotic organisms that are unicellular and sometimes colonial or less often multicellular and that typically include the protozoans, most algae, and often some fungi (as slime molds) — **pro•tis•tan** \prō-ˈtis-tən\ *adj or n*

pro•to•col \ˈprō-tə-ˌkȯl, -ˌkäl\ *n* **1** : an official account of a proceeding; *esp* : the notes or records relating to a case, an experiment, or an autopsy **2** : a detailed plan of a scientific or medical experiment, treatment, or procedure

pro•to•di•as•to•le \ˌprō-tō-dī-ˈas-tə-lē\ *n* **1** : the period just before aortic valve closure **2** : the period just after aortic valve closure — **pro•to•di•a•stol•ic** \-ˌdī-ə-ˈstä-lik\ *adj*

pro•ton \ˈprō-ˌtän\ *n* : an elementary particle that is identical with the nucleus of the hydrogen atom, that along with neutrons is a constituent of all other atomic nuclei, that carries a positive charge numerically equal to the charge of an electron, and that has a mass of 1.673×10^{-24} gram — **pro•ton•ic** \prō-ˈtä-nik\ *adj*

Pro•to•nix \ˈprō-tə-ˌniks\ *trademark* — used for a preparation of the sodium salt of pantoprazole

proton pump *n* : a molecular mechanism that transports hydrogen ions across cell membranes — called also *acid pump*

proton pump inhibitor *n* : any of a group of drugs (as omeprazole and rabeprazole) that inhibit the activity of proton pumps and are used to inhibit gastric acid secretion in the treatment of ulcers and gastroesophageal reflux disease — abbr. *PPI*

pro•to–on•co•gene \ˌprō-tō-ˈäŋ-kə-ˌjēn\ *n* : a gene having the potential for change into an active oncogene

Pro•to•pam \ˈprō-tə-ˌpam\ *trademark* — used for a preparation of pralidoxime

pro•to•path•ic \ˌprō-tə-ˈpa-thik\ *adj* : of, relating to, being, or mediating cutaneous sensory reception that is responsive only to rather gross stimuli — compare EPICRITIC

pro•to•plasm \ˈprō-tə-ˌpla-zəm\ *n* **1** : the organized colloidal complex of organic and inorganic substances (as proteins and water) that constitutes esp. the living nucleus, cytoplasm, and mitochondria of the cell **2** : CYTOPLASM — **pro•to•plas•mic** \ˌprō-tə-ˈplaz-mik\ *adj*

pro•to•plast \ˈprō-tə-ˌplast\ *n* : the nucleus, cytoplasm, and plasma membrane of a cell as distinguished from inert walls and inclusions

pro•to•por•phyr•ia \ˌprō-tō-pȯr-ˈfir-ē-ə\ *n* : the presence of protoporphyrin in the blood — see ERYTHROPOIETIC PROTOPORPHYRIA

pro•to•por•phy•rin \ˌprō-tō-ˈpȯr-fə-rən\ *n* : a purple porphyrin acid $C_{34}H_{34}N_4O_4$ obtained from hemin or heme by removal of bound iron

Pro•to•stron•gy•lus \-ˈsträn-jə-ləs\ *n* : a genus of lungworms (family Metastrongylidae) including one (*P. rufescens*) parasitic esp. in sheep and goats

Pro•to•the•ca \ˌprō-tə-ˈthē-kə\ *n* : a genus of unicellular algae including two (*P. zopfii* and *P. wickerhamii*) that cause mastitis in cows and sometimes localized infection in humans

pro•to•the•co•sis \-thē-ˈkō-səs\ *n, pl* **-co•ses** \-ˌsēz\ : an infection produced by an alga of the genus *Prototheca*

protozoa *pl of* PROTOZOON

pro•to•zo•a•ci•dal \ˌprō-tə-ˌzō-ə-ˈsīd-ᵊl\ *adj* : destroying protozoans

pro•to•zo•al \ˌprō-tə-ˈzō-əl\ *adj* : of or relating to protozoans

pro•to•zo•an \-ˈzō-ən\ *n* : any of a phylum or subkingdom (Protozoa) of chiefly motile unicellular protists (as amoebas, trypanosomes, sporozoans, and paramecia) that are represented in almost every kind of habitat and include some pathogenic parasites of humans and domestic animals — **protozoan** *adj*

pro•to•zo•ol•o•gy \-zō-ˈä-lə-jē\ *n, pl* **-gies** : a branch of zoology dealing with protozoans — **pro•to•zo•ol•o•gist** \-jist\ *n*

pro•to•zo•on \ˌprō-tə-ˈzō-ˌän\ *n, pl* **pro•to•zoa** : PROTOZOAN

pro•tract \prō-ˈtrakt\ *vb* : to extend forward or outward — compare RETRACT

pro•trac•tion \-ˈtrak-shən\ *n* **1** : the act of moving an anatomical part forward **2** : the state of being protracted; *esp* : protrusion of the jaws

pro•trip•ty•line \prō-ˈtrip-tə-ˌlēn\ *n* : a tricyclic antidepressant drug $C_{19}H_{21}N$ — see VIVACTIL

pro•trude \prō-ˈtrüd\ *vb* **pro•trud•ed; pro•trud•ing** : to project or cause to project : jut out — **pro•tru•sion** \prō-ˈtrü-zhən\ *n*

pro•tru•sive \-ˈtrü-siv, -ziv\ *adj* **1** : thrusting forward **2** : PROTUBERANT

pro•tu•ber•ance \prō-ˈtü-bə-rəns, -ˈtyü-\ *n* **1** : something that is protuberant ⟨a bony ~⟩ **2** : the quality or state of being protuberant

protuberans — see DERMATOFIBROSARCOMA PROTUBERANS

pro•tu•ber•ant \-rənt\ *adj* : bulging beyond the surrounding or adjacent surface ⟨a ~ joint⟩ ⟨~ eyes⟩

proud flesh *n* : an excessive growth of granulation tissue (as in an ulcer)

Pro•ven•til \prō-ˈven-til\ *trademark* — used for a preparation of the sulfate of albuterol

Pro•vera \prō-ˈver-ə\ *trademark* — used for a preparation of medroxyprogesterone acetate taken by mouth

pro•vi•rus \-ˈvī-rəs\ *n* : a form of a virus that is integrated into the genetic material of a host cell and by replicating with it can be transmitted from one cell generation to the next without causing lysis — **pro•vi•ral** \prō-ˈvī-rəl\ *adj*

pro•vi•ta•min \-ˈvī-tə-mən\ *n* : a precursor of a vitamin convertible into the vitamin in an organism

provitamin A *n* : a provitamin of vitamin A; *esp* : CAROTENE

Pro•vo•cho•line \ˌprō-və-ˈkō-ˌlēn\ *trademark* — used for a preparation of the chloride of methacholine

pro•voke \prə-ˈvōk\ *vb* **pro•voked; pro•vok•ing** : to call forth or induce (a physical reaction) — **prov•o•ca•tion** \ˌprä-və-ˈkā-shən\ *n* — **pro•voc•a•tive** \prə-ˈvä-kə-tiv\ *adj*

prox•e•mics \präk-ˈsē-miks\ *n sing or pl* : the study of the nature, degree, and effect of the spatial separation individuals naturally maintain (as in various social and interpersonal situations) and of how this separation relates to environmental and cultural factors — **prox•e•mic** \-mik\ *adj*

prox•i•mad \ˈpräk-sə-ˌmad\ *adv* : PROXIMALLY

prox•i•mal \ˈpräk-sə-məl\ *adj* **1 a** : situated next to or near the point of attachment or origin or a central point; *esp* : located toward the center of the body ⟨the ~ end of a bone⟩ — compare DISTAL 1a **b** : of, relating to, or being the mesial and distal surfaces of a tooth **2** : sensory rather than physical or social ⟨~ stimuli⟩ — compare DISTAL 2 — **prox•i•mal•ly** *adv*

proximal convoluted tubule *n* : the convoluted portion of the vertebrate nephron that lies between Bowman's capsule and the loop of Henle and functions esp. in the resorption of sugar, sodium and chloride ions, and water from the glomerular filtrate — called also *proximal tubule*

proximal radioulnar joint *n* : a pivot joint between the upper end of the radius and the ring formed by the radial notch of the ulna and its annular ligament that permits rotation of the proximal head of the radius

proximal tubule *n* : PROXIMAL CONVOLUTED TUBULE

prox•i•mate cause \ˈpräk-sə-mət-\ *n* : a cause that directly or with no intervening agency produces an effect

Pro•zac \ˈprō-ˌzak\ *trademark* — used for a preparation of the hydrochloride of fluoxetine

PrP *abbr* prion protein

pru•rig•i•nous \prü-ˈri-jə-nəs\ *adj* : resembling, caused by, affected with, or being prurigo ⟨~ dermatosis⟩

pru•ri•go \prü-ˈrī-(ˌ)gō\ *n* : a chronic inflammatory skin disease marked by a general eruption of small itching papules

pru•rit•ic \prü-ˈri-tik\ *adj* : of, relating to, or marked by itching

pru•ri•tus \prü-ˈrī-təs\ *n* : localized or generalized itching due to irritation of sensory nerve endings : ITCH

pruritus ani \-ˈā-ˌnī\ *n* : pruritus of the anal region

pruritus vul•vae \-ˈvəl-vē\ *n* : pruritus of the vulva

Prus•sian blue \ˈprə-shən-ˈblü\ *n* : a dark blue iron-containing dye $Fe_4[Fe(CN)_6]_3{\cdot}xH_2O$ used as a test for ferric iron

prus•sic acid \ˈprə-sik-\ *n* : HYDROCYANIC ACID

PSA *abbr* prostate-specific antigen

psal•te•ri•um \sȯl-ˈtir-ē-əm\ *n, pl* **-ria** \-ē-ə\ : HIPPOCAMPAL COMMISSURE

psam•mo•ma \sa-ˈmō-mə\ *n, pl* **-mas** *also* **-ma•ta** \-mə-tə\ : a hard fibrous tumor of the meninges of the brain and spinal cord containing calcareous matter — **psam•mo•ma•tous** \sa-ˈmō-mə-təs, -ˈmä-\ *adj*

pseud- *or* **pseudo-** *comb form* : false : spurious ⟨*pseud*arthrosis⟩

pseud•ar•thro•sis \ˌsüd-är-ˈthrō-səs\ *also* **pseu•do•ar•thro•sis** \ˌsü-dō-\ *n, pl* **-thro•ses** \-ˈthrō-ˌsēz\ : an abnormal union formed by fibrous tissue between parts of a bone that has fractured usu. spontaneously due to congenital weakness — called also *false joint*

pseu•do•an•eu•rysm \ˌsü-dō-ˈan-yə-ˌrizəm\ *n* : a vascular abnormality (as a bulging of the aorta) that resembles an aneurysm in radiography

pseu•do•bul•bar \-ˈbəl-bər\ *adj* : simulating that (as bulbar paralysis) which is caused by lesions of the medulla oblongata ⟨~ paralysis⟩

pseudobulbar affect *n* : a condition marked by episodes of uncontrollable crying or laughing which is inappropriate or of disproportionate intensity and that is associated with various neurological disorders (as multiple sclerosis, traumatic brain injury and stroke) — abbr. *PBA*

pseu•do•cho•lin•es•ter•ase \-ˌkō-lə-ˈnes-tə-ˌrās, -ˌrāz\ *n* : BUTYRYLCHOLINESTERASE

pseu•do•cow•pox \-ˈkau̇-ˌpäks\ *n* : a common infection of the teats and udders of cows that is marked by the formation of often painful lesions and scabs and is caused by a double-stranded DNA virus (species *Pseudocowpox virus* of the genus *Parapoxvirus*) — called also *false cowpox;* see MILKER'S NODULES

pseu•do•cy•e•sis \-sī-ˈē-səs\ *n, pl* **-e•ses** \-ˌsēz\ : a psychosomatic state that occurs without conception and is marked by some of the physical symptoms (as cessation of menses, enlargement of the abdomen, and apparent fetal movements) and changes in hormonal balance of pregnancy

pseu•do•cyst \ˈsü-dō-ˌsist\ *n* : a cluster of toxoplasmas in an enucleate host cell

pseu•do•de•men•tia \ˌsü-dō-di-ˈmen-chə\ *n* : a condition that outwardly resembles the cognitive impairment of dementia but does not result from neurodegeneration and that typically has a psychological cause (as depression)

pseu•do•ephed•rine \-i-ˈfe-drən\ *n* : an alkaloid $C_{10}H_{15}NO$ that is isomeric with ephedrine and is used chiefly in the form of its hydrochloride $C_{10}H_{15}NO{\cdot}HCl$ or sulfate $(C_{10}H_{15}NO)_2{\cdot}H_2SO_4$ esp. to relieve nasal congestion

pseu•do•gout \-ˈgau̇t\ *n* : an arthritic condition which resembles gout but is characterized by the deposition of crystalline salts other than urates in and around the joints

pseu•do•her•maph•ro•dite \-(ˌ)hər-ˈma-frə-ˌdīt\ *n* : an individual exhibiting pseudohermaphroditism — **pseu•do•her•maph•ro•dit•ic** \-(ˌ)hər-ˌma-frə-ˈdi-tik\ *adj*

pseu•do•her•maph•ro•dit•ism \-rə-ˌdī-ˌti-zəm\ *n* : the condition (as that occurring in androgen insensitivity syndrome) of having the gonads and karyotype of one sex and external genitalia that is of the other sex or is ambiguous

pseu•do•hy•per•ten•sion \-ˌhī-pər-ˈten-chən\ *n* : a condition esp. of some elderly, diabetic, and uremic individuals in which an erroneously high blood pressure reading is given by sphygmomanometry usu. due to loss of flexibility of the arterial walls

pseu•do•hy•per•tro•phic \ˌsü-dō-ˌhī-pər-ˈtrō-fik\ *adj* : falsely hypertrophic; *specif* : being a form of muscular dystrophy in which the muscles become swollen with deposits of fat and fibrous tissue — **pseu•do•hy•per•tro•phy** \-hī-ˈpər-trə-fē\ *n*

pseu•do•hy•po•para•thy•roid•ism \-ˌhī-pō-ˌpar-ə-ˈthī-ˌrȯi-ˌdi-zəm\ *n* : a usu. inherited disorder that clinically resembles hypoparathyroidism but results from the body's inability to respond normally to parathyroid hormone rather than from a deficiency of the hormone itself

pseu•do•mem•brane \ˌsü-dō-ˈmem-ˌbrān\ *n* : FALSE MEMBRANE

pseu•do•mem•bra•nous \-ˈmem-brə-nəs\ *adj* : characterized by the presence or formation of a false membrane ⟨~ colitis⟩

pseu•do•mo•nad \-ˈmō-ˌnad, -nəd\ *n* : any bacterium of the genus *Pseudomonas*

pseu•do•mo•nal \-ˈmō-nəl\ *adj* : of, relating to, or caused by bacteria of the genus *Pseudomonas* ⟨~ infection⟩

pseu•do•mo•nas \ˌsü-dō-ˈmō-nəs, sü-ˈdä-mə-nəs\ *n* **1** *cap* : a genus of gram-negative rod-shaped motile bacteria (family Pseudomonadaceae) including some that are saprophytes or plant or animal pathogens — see BURKHOLDERIA **2** *pl* **pseu·do·mo·na·des** \ˌsü-dō-ˈmō-nə-ˌdēz, -ˈmä-\ : PSEUDOMONAD

pseu·do·neu·rot·ic \-nu̇-ˈrä-tik, -nyu̇-\ *adj* : having or characterized by neurotic symptoms which mask an underlying psychosis ⟨∼ schizophrenia⟩

pseu·do·pa·ral·y·sis \-pə-ˈra-lə-səs\ *n, pl* **-y·ses** \-ˌsēz\ : apparent lack or loss of muscular power (as that produced by pain) that is not accompanied by true paralysis

pseu·do·par·kin·son·ism \-ˈpär-kən-sə-ˌni-zəm\ *n* : a condition (as one induced by a drug) characterized by symptoms like those of parkinsonism

pseu·do·phyl·lid·ean \ˌsü-dō-fi-ˈli-dē-ən\ *n* : any of an order (Pseudophyllidea) of tapeworms (as the fish tapeworm of humans) including numerous parasitcs of fish-eating vertebrates — **pseudophyllidean** *adj*

pseu·do·pod \ˈsü-də-ˌpäd\ *n* **1** : PSEUDOPODIUM **2 a** : a slender extension from the edge of a wheal at the site of injection of an allergen **b** : one of the slender processes of some tumor cells extending out from the main mass of a tumor

pseu·do·po·di·um \ˌsü-də-ˈpō-dē-əm\ *n, pl* **-dia** \-dē-ə\ : a temporary protrusion or retractile process of the cytoplasm of a cell (as an amoeba or a white blood cell) that functions esp. as an organ of locomotion or in taking up food or other particulate matter

pseu·do·pol·yp \ˈsü-dō-ˌpä-ləp\ *n* : a projecting mass of hypertrophied mucous membrane (as in the colon) resulting from local inflammation

pseu·do·preg·nan·cy \ˌsü-dō-ˈpreg-nən-sē\ *n, pl* **-cies** : a condition which resembles pregnancy: as **a** : PSEUDOCYESIS **b** : an anestrous state resembling pregnancy that occurs in various mammals usu. after an infertile copulation — **pseu·do·preg·nant** \-nənt\ *adj*

pseu·do·ra·bies \-ˌrā-bēz\ *n* : an acute febrile virus disease of domestic animals (as cattle and swine) that is caused by a herpesvirus of the genus *Varicellovirus* (species *Suid herpesvirus 1*) and is marked by cutaneous irritation and intense itching followed by encephalomyelitis and pharyngeal paralysis and commonly terminating in death within 48 hours — called also *mad itch*

pseu·do·sar·co·ma·tous \ˌsü-dō-sär-ˈkō-mə-təs\ *adj* : resembling but not being a true sarcoma ⟨a ∼ polyp⟩

pseu·do·strat·i·fied \-ˈstra-tə-ˌfīd\ *adj* : of, relating to, or being an epithelium consisting of closely packed cells which appear to be arranged in layers but are in fact attached to the basement membrane — **pseu·do·strat·i·fi·ca·tion** \-ˌstra-tə-fə-ˈkā-shən\ *n*

pseu·do·tu·ber·cle \-ˈtü-bər-kəl, -ˈtyü-\ *n* : a nodule or granuloma resembling a tubercle of tuberculosis but due to other causes

pseu·do·tu·ber·cu·lo·sis \-tu̇-ˌbər-kyə-ˈlō-səs, -tyu̇-\ *n, pl* **-lo·ses** \-ˌsēz\ **1** : any of several diseases that are characterized by the formation of granulomas resembling tubercular nodules and are caused by a bacterium (as *Yersinia pseudotuberculosis*) other than the tubercle bacillus **2** : CASEOUS LYMPHADENITIS

pseu·do·tu·mor \-ˈtü-mər, -ˈtyü-\ *n* : an abnormality (as a temporary swelling) that resembles a tumor — **pseu·do·tu·mor·al** \-mə-rəl\ *adj*

pseudotumor cer·e·bri \-ˈser-ə-ˌbrī\ *n* : IDIOPATHIC INTRACRANIAL HYPERTENSION

pseu·do·uri·dine \-ˈyu̇r-ə-ˌdēn\ *n* : a nucleoside $C_9H_{12}O_6N_2$ that is a uracil derivative incorporated as a structural component into transfer RNA

pseu·do·xan·tho·ma elas·ti·cum \ˌsü-dō-zan-ˈthō-mə-i-ˈlas-ti-kəm\ *n* : a chronic degenerative disease of elastic tissues that is marked by the occurrence of small yellowish papules and plaques on areas of abnormally loose skin

[1]**psi** \ˈsī\ *adj* : relating to, concerned with, or being parapsychological psychic events or powers

[2]**psi** *n* : psi events or phenomena

psi·lo·cin \ˈsī-lə-sən\ *n* : a hallucinogenic tertiary amine $C_{12}H_{16}N_2O$ obtained from a basidiomycetous fungus (*Psilocybe mexicana*)

psi·lo·cy·bin \ˌsī-lə-ˈsī-bən\ *n* : a hallucinogenic indole $C_{12}H_{17}N_2O_4P$ obtained from a basidiomycetous fungus (*Psilocybe mexicana* or *P. cubensis* syn. *Stropharia cubensis*)

psit·ta·co·sis \ˌsi-tə-ˈkō-səs\ *n, pl* **-co·ses** \-ˌsēz\ : an infectious disease of birds that is caused by a bacterium (*Chlamydia psittaci* syn. *Chlamydophila psittaci*), is marked by diarrhea and wasting, and is transmissible to humans in whom it usu. occurs as an atypical pneumonia accompanied by high fever — called also *parrot fever;* compare ORNITHOSIS — **psit·ta·co·tic** \-ˈkä-tik, -ˈkō-\ *adj*

pso·as \ˈsō-əs\ *n, pl* **pso·ai** \ˈsō-ˌī\ *or* **pso·ae** \-ˌē\ : either of two internal muscles of the loin: **a** : PSOAS MAJOR **b** : PSOAS MINOR

psoas major *n* : the larger of the two psoas muscles that arises from the anterolateral surfaces of the lumbar vertebrae, passes beneath the inguinal ligament to insert with the iliacus into the lesser trochanter of the femur, and serves esp. to flex the thigh

psoas minor *n* : the smaller of the two psoas muscles that arises from the last dorsal and first lumbar vertebrae and inserts into the brim of the pelvis, that functions to flex the trunk and the lumbar spinal column, and that is often absent

psoas muscle *n* : PSOAS

pso•ra•len \ˈsȯr-ə-lən\ *n* : a substance $C_{11}H_6O_3$ found in some plants that photosensitizes mammalian skin and is used in conjunction with ultraviolet light to treat psoriasis; *also* : any of various derivatives of psoralen having similar properties — see PUVA

pso•ri•a•si•form \sə-ˈrī-ə-si-ˌfȯrm\ *adj* : resembling psoriasis or a psoriatic lesion

pso•ri•a•sis \sə-ˈrī-ə-səs\ *n, pl* **-a•ses** \-ˌsēz\ : a chronic skin disease characterized by circumscribed red patches covered with white scales — **pso•ri•at•ic** \ˌsȯr-ē-ˈa-tik\ *adj*

psoriatic arthritis *n* : a severe form of arthritis accompanied by inflammation, psoriasis of the skin or nails, and a negative test for rheumatoid factor — called also *psoriatic arthropathy*

Pso•rop•tes \sə-ˈräp-(ˌ)tēz\ *n* : a genus of parasitic mites (family Psoroptidae) that cause inflammatory skin diseases (as mange)

pso•rop•tic \sə-ˈräp-tik\ *adj* : of, relating to, caused by, or being mites of the genus *Psoroptes* ⟨~ mange⟩

PSRO *abbr* professional standards review organization

PSVT *abbr* paroxysmal supraventricular tachycardia

psych *abbr* psychology

psych- *or* **psycho-** *comb form* **1** : mind : mental processes and activities ⟨*psycho*dynamic⟩ ⟨*psycho*logy⟩ **2** : psychological methods ⟨*psycho*therapy⟩ **3** : brain ⟨*psycho*surgery⟩ **4** : mental and ⟨*psycho*somatic⟩

psych•as•the•nia \ˌsī-kəs-ˈthē-nē-ə\ *n* : a neurotic state characterized esp. by phobias, obsessions, or compulsions that one knows are irrational

psy•che \ˈsī-(ˌ)kē\ *n* : the specialized cognitive, conative, and affective aspects of a psychosomatic unity : MIND; *specif* : the totality of the id, ego, and superego including both conscious and unconscious components

[1]**psy•che•del•ic** \ˌsī-kə-ˈde-lik\ *n* : a psychedelic drug (as LSD)

[2]**psychedelic** *adj* **1** : of, relating to, or being drugs (as LSD) capable of producing abnormal psychic effects (as hallucinations) and sometimes psychotic states **2** : produced by or associated with the use of psychedelic drugs — **psy•che•del•i•cal•ly** *adv*

psy•chi•at•ric \ˌsī-kē-ˈa-trik\ *adj* **1** : relating to or employed in psychiatry ⟨~ disorders⟩ **2** : engaged in the practice of psychiatry : dealing with cases of mental illness ⟨~ nursing⟩ — **psy•chi•at•ri•cal•ly** *adv*

psy•chi•a•trist \sə-ˈkī-ə-trist, sī-\ *n* : a physician specializing in psychiatry

psy•chi•a•try \-trē\ *n, pl* **-tries** : a branch of medicine that deals with the science and practice of treating mental, emotional, or behavioral disorders esp. as originating in endogenous causes or resulting from faulty interpersonal relationships

[1]**psy•chic** \ˈsī-kik\ *also* **psy•chi•cal** \-ki-kəl\ *adj* **1** : of or relating to the psyche : PSYCHOGENIC **2** : sensitive to nonphysical or supernatural forces and influences — **psy•chi•cal•ly** *adv*

[2]**psychic** *n* : a person apparently sensitive to nonphysical forces

psychic energizer *n* : ANTIDEPRESSANT

psychic energy *n* : the force driving and sustaining mental activity

psy•cho \ˈsī-(ˌ)kō\ *n, pl* **psychos** : a deranged or psychopathic individual — not used technically — **psycho** *adj*

psycho- — see PSYCH-

psy•cho•acous•tics \ˌsī-kō-ə-ˈkü-stiks\ *n* : a branch of science dealing with hearing, the sensations produced by sounds, and the problems of communication — **psy•cho•acous•tic** \-stik\ *adj*

psy•cho•ac•tive \ˌsī-kō-ˈak-tiv\ *adj* : affecting the mind or behavior ⟨~ drugs⟩

psy•cho•anal•y•sis \ˌsī-kō-ə-ˈna-lə-səs\ *n, pl* **-y•ses** \-ˌsēz\ **1** : a method of analyzing psychic phenomena and treating mental and emotional disorders that is based on the concepts and theories of Sigmund Freud, that emphasizes the importance of free association and dream analysis, and that involves treatment sessions during which the patient is encouraged to talk freely about personal experiences and esp. about early childhood and dreams **2** : a body of empirical findings and a set of theories on human motivation, behavior, and personality development that developed esp. with the aid of psychoanalysis **3** : a school of psychology, psychiatry, and psychotherapy founded by Sigmund Freud and rooted in and applying psychoanalysis — **psy•cho•an•a•lyt•ic** \-ˌan-ᵊl-ˈi-tik\ *also* **psy•cho•an•a•lyt•i•cal** \-ti-kəl\ *adj* — **psy•cho•an•a•lyt•i•cal•ly** *adv* — **psy•cho•an•a•lyze** \-ˈan-ᵊl-ˌīz\ *vb*

psy•cho•an•a•lyst \-ˈan-ᵊl-ist\ *n* : one who practices or adheres to the principles of psychoanalysis; *specif* : a psychotherapist trained at an established psychoanalytic institute

psy•cho•bi•ol•o•gy \-bī-ˈä-lə-jē\ *n, pl* **-gies** : the study of mental functioning and behavior in relation to other biological processes — **psy•cho•bi•o•log•i•cal** \-ˌbī-ə-ˈlä-ji-kəl\ *also* **psy•cho•bi•o•log•ic** \-jik\ *adj* — **psy•cho•bi•ol•o•gist** \-bī-ˈä-lə-jist\ *n*

psy•cho•di•ag•nos•tics \-ˌdī-ig-ˈnäs-tiks\ *n* : a branch of psychology concerned with the use of tests in the evaluation of personality and the determination of factors underlying human behavior — **psy•cho•di•ag•nos•tic** \-tik\ *adj*

psy•cho•dra•ma \ˌsī-kō-ˈdrä-mə, -ˈdra-\ *n* : an extemporized dramatization designed to afford catharsis and social relearning for one or more of the participants from whose life history the plot is abstracted — **psy•cho•dra•mat•ic** \-kō-drə-ˈma-tik\ *adj*

psy•cho•dy•nam•ics \ˌsī-kō-dī-ˈna-miks, -də-\ *n sing or pl* **1** : the psychology of mental or emotional forces or processes developing esp. in early childhood and their effects on behavior and mental states **2** : explanation or interpretation (as of behavior or mental states) in terms of mental or emotional forces or processes **3** : motivational forces acting esp. at the unconscious level — **psy•cho•dy•nam•ic** \-mik\ *adj* — **psy•cho•dy•nam•i•cal•ly** *adv*

psy•cho•ed•u•ca•tion•al \-ˌe-jə-ˈkā-shə-nəl\ *adj* : of or relating to the psychological aspects of education; *specif* : relating to or used in the education of children with behavioral disorders or learning disabilities

psy•cho•gal•van•ic reflex \-gal-ˈva-nik-\ *n* : a momentary decrease in the apparent electrical resistance of the skin resulting from activity of the sweat glands in response to mental or emotional stimulation — called also *psychogalvanic reaction, psychogalvanic response*

psy•cho•gen•e•sis \ˌsī-kō-ˈje-nə-səs\ *n, pl* **-e•ses** \-ˌsēz\ **1** : the origin and development of mental functions, traits, or states **2** : development from mental as distinguished from physical origins

psy•cho•gen•ic \-ˈje-nik\ *adj* : originating in the mind : attributable to psychological or emotional factors ⟨a ~ movement disorder⟩ — **psy•cho•gen•i•cal•ly** *adv*

psy•cho•ge•ri•at•rics \-ˌjer-ē-ˈa-triks, -ˌjir-\ *n* : a branch of psychiatry concerned with behavioral and emotional disorders among the elderly — **psy•cho•ge•ri•at•ric** \-trik\ *adj*

psy•cho•ki•ne•sis \-kə-ˈnē-səs, -kī-\ *n, pl* **-ne•ses** \-ˌsēz\ : movement of physical objects by the mind without use of physical means — called also *PK;* compare PRECOGNITION, TELEKINESIS — **psy•cho•ki•net•ic** \-ˈne-tik\ *adj*

psy•cho•ki•net•ics \-kə-ˈne-tiks, -kī-\ *n* : a branch of parapsychology that deals with psychokinesis

psychol *abbr* psychologist; psychology

psy•cho•lin•guis•tics \ˌsī-kō-liŋ-ˈgwis-tiks\ *n* : the study of the mental faculties involved in the perception, production, and acquisition of language — **psy•cho•lin•guist** \-ˈliŋ-gwist\ *n* — **psy•cho•lin•guis•tic** \-liŋ-ˈgwis-tik\ *adj*

psy•cho•log•i•cal \ˌsī-kə-ˈlä-ji-kəl\ *also* **psy•cho•log•ic** \-jik\ *adj* **1 a** : relating to, characteristic of, directed toward, influencing, arising in, or acting through the mind esp. in its affective or cognitive functions ⟨~ phenomena⟩ **b** : directed toward the will or toward the mind specif. in its conative function ⟨~ warfare⟩ **2** : relating to, concerned with, deriving from, or used in psychology ⟨~ tests⟩ ⟨a ~ clinic⟩ — **psy•cho•log•i•cal•ly** *adv*

psy•chol•o•gist \sī-ˈkä-lə-jist\ *n* : a specialist in psychology

psy•chol•o•gize \-ˌjīz\ *vb* **-gized; -giz•ing** : to explain, interpret, or speculate in psychological terms

psy•chol•o•gy \-jē\ *n, pl* **-gies** **1** : the science of mind and behavior **2 a** : the mental or behavioral characteristics typical of an individual or group or a particular form of behavior ⟨mob ~⟩ **b** : the study of mind and behavior in relation to a particular field of knowledge or activity ⟨the ~ of learning⟩ **3** : a theory, system, or branch of psychology ⟨Freudian ~⟩

psy•cho•met•ric \ˌsī-kə-ˈme-trik\ *adj* : of or relating to psychometrics — **psy•cho•met•ri•cal•ly** *adv*

psy•cho•me•tri•cian \-mə-ˈtri-shən\ *n* **1** : a person (as a clinical psychologist) who is skilled in the administration and interpretation of objective psychological tests **2** : a psychologist who devises, constructs, and standardizes psychometric tests

psy•cho•met•rics \-ˈme-triks\ *n* **1** : a branch of clinical or applied psychology dealing with the use and application of mental measurement **2** : the technique of mental measurements : the use of quantitative devices for assessing psychological trends

psy•chom•e•trist \sī-ˈkä-mə-trist\ *n* : PSYCHOMETRICIAN

psy•chom•e•try \sī-ˈkä-mə-trē\ *n, pl* **-tries** : PSYCHOMETRICS

psy•cho•mo•tor \ˌsī-kō-ˈmō-tər\ *adj* **1** : of or relating to motor action directly proceeding from mental activity **2** : of or relating to temporal lobe epilepsy ⟨~ seizures⟩

psychomotor epilepsy *n* : TEMPORAL LOBE EPILEPSY

psy•cho•neu•ro•im•mu•nol•o•gy \-ˌnu̇r-ō-ˌi-myü-ˈnä-lə-jē, -ˌnyu̇r-\ *n* : a field of medicine that deals with the influence of emotional states (as stress) and nervous system activity on immune function esp. in relation to their role in affecting the onset and progression of disease — **psy•cho•neu•ro•im•mu•nol•o•gist** \-jəst\ *n*

psy•cho•neu•ro•sis \ˌsī-kō-nu̇-ˈrō-səs, -nyu̇-\ *n, pl* **-ro•ses** \-ˌsēz\ : NEUROSIS; *esp* : a neurosis based on emotional conflict in which an impulse that has been blocked seeks expression in a disguised response or symptom

¹psy•cho•neu•rot•ic \-ˈrä-tik\ *adj* : of, relating to, being, or affected with a psychoneurosis ⟨a ~ disorder⟩

²psychoneurotic *n* : a psychoneurotic individual

psy•cho•path \ˈsī-kō-ˌpath\ *n* : a person having an egocentric and antisocial personality marked by a lack of remorse for one's actions, an absence of empathy for others, and often criminal tendencies

psy·cho·path·ic \ˌsī-kō-ˈpa-thik\ *adj* : of, relating to, or marked by psychopathy — **psy·cho·path·i·cal·ly** *adv*

psychopathic personality disorder *n, esp formerly* : ANTISOCIAL PERSONALITY DISORDER

psy·cho·pa·thol·o·gist \-pə-ˈthä-lə-jist, -pa-\ *n* : a specialist in psychopathology

psy·cho·pa·thol·o·gy \ˌsī-kō-pə-ˈthä-lə-jē, -pa-\ *n, pl* **-gies** **1** : the study of psychological and behavioral dysfunction occurring in mental illness or in social disorganization **2** : disordered psychological and behavioral functioning (as in mental illness) — **psy·cho·patho·log·i·cal** \-ˌpa-thə-ˈlä-ji-kəl\ *also* **psy·cho·patho·log·ic** \-jik\ *adj* — **psy·cho·patho·log·i·cal·ly** *adv*

psy·chop·a·thy \sī-ˈkä-pə-thē\ *n, pl* **-thies** : mental disorder esp. when marked by egocentric and antisocial activity, a lack of remorse for one's actions, an absence of empathy for others, and often criminal tendencies

psy·cho·phar·ma·ceu·ti·cal \ˌsī-kō-ˌfär-mə-ˈsü-ti-kəl\ *n* : a drug having an effect on the mental state of the user

psy·cho·phar·ma·col·o·gy \ˌsī-kō-ˌfär-mə-ˈkä-lə-jē\ *n, pl* **-gies** : the study of the effect of drugs on the mind and behavior — **psy·cho·phar·ma·co·log·i·cal** \-ˌfär-mə-kə-ˈlä-ji-kəl\ *also* **psy·cho·phar·ma·co·log·ic** \-ˈlä-jik\ *adj* — **psy·cho·phar·ma·col·o·gist** \-ˌfär-mə-ˈkä-lə-jist\ *n*

psy·cho·phys·ics \-ˈfi-ziks\ *n* : a branch of psychology concerned with the effect of physical processes (as intensity of stimulation) on mental processes and esp. sensations of an organism — **psy·cho·phys·i·cal** \ˌsī-kō-ˈfi-zi-kəl\ *adj* — **psy·cho·phys·i·cal·ly** *adv* — **psy·cho·phys·i·cist** \-ˈfi-zə-sist\ *n*

psy·cho·phys·i·o·log·i·cal \ˌsī-kō-ˌfi-zē-ə-ˈlä-ji-kəl\ *also* **psy·cho·phys·i·o·log·ic** \-jik\ *adj* **1** : of or relating to psychophysiology **2** : combining or involving mental and bodily processes

psy·cho·phys·i·ol·o·gy \-ˌfi-zē-ˈä-lə-jē\ *n, pl* **-gies** : a branch of psychology that deals with the effects of normal and pathological physiological processes on mental functioning — called also *physiological psychology* — **psy·cho·phys·i·ol·o·gist** \-jist\ *n*

psy·cho·sex·u·al \ˌsī-kō-ˈsek-shə-wəl\ *adj* **1** : of or relating to the mental, emotional, and behavioral aspects of sexual development **2** : of or relating to mental or emotional attitudes concerning sexual activity **3** : of or relating to the psychophysiology of sex

psy·cho·sis \sī-ˈkō-səs\ *n, pl* **-cho·ses** \-ˌsēz\ : a serious mental illness (as schizophrenia) characterized by defective or lost contact with reality often with hallucinations or delusions

psy·cho·so·cial \ˌsī-kō-ˈsō-shəl\ *adj* **1** : involving both psychological and social aspects **2** : relating social conditions to mental health ⟨~ medicine⟩ — **psy·cho·so·cial·ly** *adv*

psy·cho·so·mat·ic \ˌsī-kō-sə-ˈma-tik\ *adj* **1** : of, relating to, or involving both mind and body **2 a** : of, relating to, involving, or concerned with bodily symptoms caused by mental or emotional disturbance **b** : exhibiting psychosomatic symptoms — **psy·cho·so·mat·i·cal·ly** *adv*

psy·cho·so·mat·ics \-tiks\ *n* : a branch of medical science dealing with interrelationships between the mind or emotions and the body and esp. with the relation of psychological conflict to somatic symptomatology

psy·cho·stim·u·lant \-ˈstim-yə-lənt\ *n* : a substance (as dextroamphetamine) that has mood-enhancing and stimulant properties

psy·cho·sur·geon \-ˈsər-jən\ *n* : a surgeon specializing in psychosurgery

psy·cho·sur·gery \-ˈsər-jə-rē\ *n, pl* **-ger·ies** : cerebral surgery employed in treating psychic symptoms — **psy·cho·sur·gi·cal** \-ˈsər-ji-kəl\ *adj*

psy·cho·syn·the·sis \ˌsī-kō-ˈsin-thə-səs\ *n, pl* **-the·ses** \-ˌsēz\ : a form of psychotherapy combining psychoanalytic techniques with meditation and exercise

psy·cho·ther·a·peu·tics \-tiks\ *n sing or pl* : PSYCHOTHERAPY

psy·cho·ther·a·pist \-ˈther-ə-pist\ *n* : an individual (as a clinical psychologist or psychiatric social worker) who is a practitioner of psychotherapy

psy·cho·ther·a·py \ˌsī-kō-ˈther-ə-pē\ *n, pl* **-pies** **1** : treatment of mental or emotional disorder or maladjustment by psychological means esp. involving verbal communication (as in psychoanalysis, nondirective psychotherapy, reeducation, or hypnosis) **2** : any alteration in an individual's interpersonal environment, relationships, or life situation brought about esp. by a qualified therapist and intended to have the effect of alleviating symptoms of mental or emotional disturbance — **psy·cho·ther·a·peu·tic** \-ˌther-ə-ˈpyü-tik\ *adj* — **psy·cho·ther·a·peu·ti·cal·ly** *adv*

[1]**psy·chot·ic** \sī-ˈkä-tik\ *adj* : of, relating to, marked by, or affected with psychosis — **psy·chot·i·cal·ly** *adv*

[2]**psychotic** *n* : a psychotic individual

[1]**psy·choto·mi·met·ic** \sī-ˌkä-tō-mə-ˈme-tik, -mī-\ *adj* : of, relating to, involving, or inducing psychotic alteration of behavior and personality ⟨~ drugs⟩ — **psy·choto·mi·met·i·cal·ly** *adv*

[2]**psychotomimetic** *n* : a psychotomimetic agent (as a drug)

[1]**psy·cho·tro·pic** \ˌsī-kə-ˈtrō-pik\ *adj* : acting on the mind ⟨~ drugs⟩

[2]**psychotropic** *n* : a psychotropic substance (as a drug)

psyl·li·um \ˈsi-lē-əm\ *n* **1** : FLEAWORT **2** : PSYLLIUM SEED; *also* : the husks of psyllium seed

psyllium seed *n* : the seed of a fleawort (esp. *Plantago psyllium*) that has the property of swelling and becoming gelatinous when moist and is used as a mild laxative — called also *plantago seed, psyllium;* see METAMUCIL

pt *abbr* **1** patient **2** pint

Pt *symbol* platinum

PT *abbr* **1** physical therapist **2** physical therapy

PTA *abbr* **1** percutaneous transluminal angioplasty **2** plasma thromboplastin antecedent

PTC \ˌpē-(ˌ)tē-ˈsē\ *n* : PHENYLTHIOCARBAMIDE

PTC *abbr* plasma thromboplastin component

PTCA *abbr* percutaneous transluminal coronary angioplasty

pter·o·yl·glu·tam·ic acid \ˌter-ō-il-glü-ˈta-mik-\ *n* : FOLIC ACID — abbr. *PGA*

pteryg- *or* **pterygo-** *comb form* : pterygoid and ⟨*pterygo*maxillary⟩

pte·ryg·i·um \te-ˈri-jē-əm\ *n, pl* **-iums** *or* **-ia** \-jē-ə\ **1** : a triangular fleshy mass of thickened conjunctiva occurring usu. at the inner side of the eyeball, covering part of the cornea, and causing a disturbance of vision **2** : a forward growth of the cuticle over the nail

[1]**pter·y·goid** \ˈter-ə-ˌgȯid\ *adj* : of, relating to, being, or lying in the region of the inferior part of the sphenoid bone

[2]**pterygoid** *n* : a pterygoid part (as a pterygoid muscle or nerve)

pterygoid canal *n* : an anteroposterior canal in the base of each medial pterygoid plate of the sphenoid bone that gives passage to the Vidian artery and the Vidian nerve — called also *Vidian canal*

pter·y·goi·de·us \ˌter-ə-ˈgȯi-dē-əs\ *n, pl* **-dei** \-dē-ˌī\ : PTERYGOID MUSCLE

pterygoid fossa *n* : a V-shaped depression on the posterior part of each pterygoid process that contains the medial pterygoid muscle and the tensor veli palatini

pterygoid hamulus *n* : a hook-shaped process forming the inferior extremity of each medial pterygoid plate of the sphenoid bone and providing a support around which the tendon of the tensor veli palatini moves

pterygoid muscle *n* : either of two muscles extending from the sphenoid bone to the lower jaw: **a** : a muscle that arises from the greater wing of the sphenoid bone and from the outer surface of the lateral pterygoid plate, is inserted into the condyle of the mandible and the articular disk of the temporomandibular joint, and acts as an antagonist of the masseter, temporalis, and medial pterygoid muscles — called also *external pterygoid muscle, lateral pterygoid muscle* **b** : a muscle that arises from the inner surface of the lateral pterygoid plate and from the palatine and maxillary bones, is inserted into the ramus and the gonial angle, cooperates with the masseter and temporalis in elevating the lower jaw, and controls certain lateral and rotary movements of the jaw — called also *internal pterygoid muscle, medial pterygoid muscle*

pterygoid nerve *n* : either of two branches of the mandibular nerve: **a** : one that is distributed to the lateral pterygoid muscle — called also *lateral pterygoid nerve* **b** : one that is distributed to the medial pterygoid muscle, tensor tympani, and tensor veli palatini — called also *medial pterygoid nerve*

pterygoid plate *n* : either of two vertical plates making up a pterygoid process of the sphenoid bone: **a** : a broad thin plate that forms the lateral part of the pterygoid process and gives attachment to the lateral pterygoid muscle on its lateral surface and to the medial pterygoid muscle on its medial surface — called also *lateral pterygoid plate* **b** : a long narrow plate that forms the medial part of the pterygoid process and terminates in the pterygoid hamulus — called also *medial pterygoid plate*

pterygoid plexus *n* : a plexus of veins draining the region of the pterygoid muscles and emptying chiefly into the facial vein by way of the deep facial vein and into the maxillary vein

pterygoid process *n* : a process that extends downward from each side of the sphenoid bone, that consists of the medial and lateral pterygoid plates which are fused above anteriorly and separated below by a fissure whose edges articulate with a process of the palatine bone, and that contains on its posterior aspect the pterygoid and scaphoid fossae which give attachment to muscles

pter·y·go·man·dib·u·lar raphe \ˌter-ə-gō-man-ˈdi-byə-lər-\ *n* : a fibrous seam that descends from the pterygoid hamulus of the medial pterygoid plate to the mylohyoid line of the mandible and that separates and gives rise to the superior constrictor of the pharynx and the buccinator

pter·y·go·max·il·lary \ˌter-ə-gō-ˈmak-sə-ˌler-ē\ *adj* : of, relating to, or connecting the pterygoid process of the sphenoid bone and the maxilla

pterygomaxillary fissure *n* : a vertical gap between the lateral pterygoid plate of the pterygoid process and the maxilla that gives passage to part of the maxillary artery and vein

pter·y·go·pal·a·tine fossa \ˌter-ə-gō-ˈpa-lə-ˌtīn-\ *n* : a small triangular space beneath the apex of the orbit that contains among other structures the pterygopalatine ganglion — called also *pterygomaxillary fossa*

pterygopalatine ganglion *n* : an autonomic ganglion of the maxillary nerve that is situated in the pterygopalatine fossa and that receives preganglionic parasympathetic fibers from the facial nerve and sends postganglionic fibers to the nasal mucosa, palate, pharynx, and orbit — called also *Meckel's ganglion, sphenopalatine ganglion*

PTFE *abbr* polytetrafluoroethylene

PTH *abbr* parathyroid hormone

Pthir·us \ˈthir-əs\ *n, syn of* PHTHIRUS

pto·maine \ˈtō-ˌmān, tō-ˈ\ *n* : any of various organic bases formed by the action of putrefactive bacteria on nitrogenous matter and including some which are poisonous

ptomaine poisoning *n* : food poisoning caused by bacteria or bacterial products — not used technically

pto·sis \ˈtō-səs\ *n, pl* **pto·ses** \-ˌsēz\ : a sagging or prolapse of an organ or part; *esp* : a drooping of the upper eyelid (as from paralysis of the oculomotor nerve) — **ptot·ic** \ˈtä-tik\ *adj*

PTSD *abbr* post-traumatic stress disorder

ptyal- *or* **ptyalo-** *comb form* : saliva ⟨*ptyalism*⟩

pty·a·lin \ˈtī-ə-lən\ *n* : an amylase found in saliva that converts starch into sugar

pty·a·lism \-ˌli-zəm\ *n* : HYPERSALIVATION, SIALORRHEA

-p·ty·sis \p-tə-səs\ *n comb form, pl* **-pty·ses** \p-tə-ˌsēz\ : spewing : expectoration ⟨hemo*ptysis*⟩

Pu *symbol* plutonium

pub·ar·che \ˈpyü-ˌbär-kē\ *n* : the beginning of puberty marked by the first growth of pubic hair

pu·ber·al \ˈpyü-bər-əl\ *adj* : PUBERTAL

pu·ber·tal \ˈpyü-bərt-ᵊl\ *adj* : of, relating to, or occurring in puberty

pu·ber·ty \ˈpyü-bər-tē\ *n, pl* **-ties** **1** : the condition of being or the period of becoming first capable of reproducing sexually marked by maturing of the genital organs, development of secondary sex characteristics, and in humans and the higher primates by the first occurrence of menstruation in the female **2** : the age at which puberty occurs being typically between 13 and 16 years in boys and 11 and 14 in girls

¹pu·bes \ˈpyü-(ˌ)bēz\ *n, pl* **pubes** **1** : the hair that appears on the lower part of the hypogastric region at puberty — called also *pubic hair* **2** : the lower part of the hypogastric region : the pubic region

²pubes *pl of* PUBIS

pu·bes·cent \pyü-ˈbes-ᵊnt\ *adj* **1** : arriving at or having reached puberty **2** : of or relating to puberty

pu·bic \ˈpyü-bik\ *adj* : of, relating to, or situated in or near the region of the pubes or the pubis

pubic arch *n* : the notch formed by the inferior rami of the two conjoined pubic bones as they diverge from the midline

pubic bone *n* : PUBIS

pubic crest *n* : the border of a pubis between its pubic tubercle and the pubic symphysis

pubic hair *n* : PUBES 1

pubic louse *n* : a sucking louse of the genus *Phthirius* (*P. pubis*) infesting the pubic region of the human body — called also *crab louse*

pubic symphysis *n* : the rather rigid articulation of the two pubic bones in the midline of the lower anterior part of the abdomen — called also *symphysis pubis*

pubic tubercle *n* : a rounded eminence on the upper margin of each pubis near the pubic symphysis

pu·bis \ˈpyü-bəs\ *n, pl* **pu·bes** \-(ˌ)bēz\ : the ventral and anterior of the three principal bones composing either half of the pelvis that in humans consists of two rami diverging posteriorly from the region of the pubic symphysis with the superior ramus extending to the acetabulum of which it forms a part and uniting there with the ilium and ischium and the inferior ramus extending below the obturator foramen where it unites with the ischium — called also *pubic bone*

public health *n* : the art and science dealing with the protection and improvement of community health by organized community effort and including preventive medicine and sanitary and social science

public health nurse *n* : VISITING NURSE

pu·bo·cap·su·lar ligament \ˌpyü-bō-ˈkap-sə-lər-\ *n* : PUBOFEMORAL LIGAMENT

pu·bo·coc·cy·geus \-käk-ˈsi-jəs, -jē-əs\ *n, pl* **-cy·gei** \-ˈsi-jē-ˌī\ : the inferior subdivision of the levator ani that arises from the dorsal surface of the pubis, that inserts esp. into the coccyx, and that acts to help support the pelvic viscera, to draw the lower end of the rectum toward the pubis, and to constrict the rectum and in the female the vagina — compare ILIOCOCCYGEUS — **pu·bo·coc·cy·geal** \ˌpyü-bō-käk-ˈsi-jəl, -jē-əl\ *adj*

pu·bo·fem·o·ral ligament \ˌpyü-bō-ˈfe-mə-rəl-\ *n* : a ligament of the hip joint that extends from the superior ramus of the pubis to the capsule of the hip joint near the neck of the femur and that acts to prevent excessive extension and abduction of the thigh

pu·bo·pros·tat·ic ligament \ˌpyü-bō-präs-ˈta-tik-\ *n* : any of three strands of pelvic fascia in the male that correspond to the pubovesical ligament in the female and that support the prostate gland and indirectly the bladder

pu·bo·rec·ta·lis \ˌpyü-bō-rek-ˈtā-ləs\ *n* : a band of muscle fibers that is part of the pubococcygeus and acts to hold the rectum and anal canal at right angles to each other except during defecation

pu·bo·vag·i·na·lis \ˌpyü-bō-ˌva-jə-ˈnā-ləs\ *n* : the most medial and anterior fasciculi of the pubococcygeal part of the levator ani in the female that correspond to the levator prostatae in the male, pass along the sides of the vagina, insert into the coccyx, and act to constrict the vagina

pu•bo•ves•i•cal ligament \ˌpyü-bō-ˈve-si-kəl-\ *n* : any of three strands of pelvic fascia in the female that correspond to the puboprostatic ligament in the male and that support the bladder

¹pu•den•dal \pyu̇-ˈdend-ᵊl\ *adj* : of, relating to, occurring in, or lying in the region of the external genital organs

²pudendal *n* : a pudendal anatomical part (as the pudendal nerve)

pudendal artery — see EXTERNAL PUDENDAL ARTERY, INTERNAL PUDENDAL ARTERY

pudendal nerve *n* : a nerve that arises from the second, third, and fourth sacral nerves and that supplies the external genitalia, the skin of the perineum, and the anal sphincters

pudendal vein — see INTERNAL PUDENDAL VEIN

pu•den•dum \pyu̇-ˈden-dəm\ *n, pl* **-da** \-də\ : the external genital organs of a human; *esp* : the external genitalia of a woman : VULVA — usu. used in pl.

pu•er•ile \ˈpyu̇-ər-əl, -ˌīl\ *adj* **1** : marked by or suggesting childishness and immaturity **2** : being respiration that is like that of a child in being louder than normal ⟨~ breathing⟩

pu•er•per•al \pyü-ˈər-pə-rəl\ *adj* : of, relating to, or occurring during childbirth or the period immediately following ⟨~ infection⟩

puerperal fever *n* : an abnormal condition that results from infection (as by streptococci) of the placental site following delivery or abortion and is characterized in mild form by fever of not over 100.4°F (38.0°C) but may progress to a localized endometritis or spread through the uterine wall and develop into peritonitis or pass into the bloodstream and produce sepsis — called also *childbed fever, puerperal sepsis*

pu•er•pe•ri•um \ˌpyü-ər-ˈpir-ē-əm\ *n, pl* **-ria** \-ē-ə\ : the period between childbirth and the return of the uterus to its normal size

PUFA \ˈpə-fə\ *n* : a polyunsaturated fatty acid

puff•er *n* : PUFFER FISH

puffer fish *n* : any of a family (Tetraodontidae) of chiefly tropical marine fishes that when threatened can distend themselves to a large roundish form and most of which are highly poisonous — called also *blowfish, globefish;* see FUGU

Pu•lex \ˈpyü-ˌleks\ *n* : a genus of fleas (family Pulicidae) including one (*P. irritans*) that regularly attacks humans

¹pull \ˈpu̇l\ *vb* **1** : EXTRACT 1 **2** : to strain or stretch abnormally ⟨~ a muscle⟩

²pull *n* : an injury resulting from abnormal straining or stretching esp. of a muscle — see GROIN PULL

pul•lo•rum disease \pə-ˈlōr-əm-\ *n* : salmonellosis esp. of the domestic chicken caused by a bacterium of the genus *Salmonella* (*S. pullorum*) — called also *pullorum*

Pul•mi•cort \ˈpu̇l-mə-ˌkȯrt\ *trademark* — used for a preparation of budesonide for oral inhalation

pulmon- *also* **pulmoni-** *or* **pulmono-** *comb form* : lung ⟨*pulmono*logist⟩

pulmonale, pulmonalia — see COR PULMONALE

pul•mo•nary \ˈpu̇l-mə-ˌner-ē, ˈpəl-\ *adj* : relating to, functioning like, associated with, or carried on by the lungs

pulmonary adenomatosis *n* : JAAGSIEKTE

pulmonary alveolar proteinosis *n* : a chronic disease of the lungs characterized by the filling of the alveoli with proteinaceous material and by the progressive loss of lung function

pulmonary artery *n* : an arterial trunk or either of its two main branches that carry venous blood to the lungs: **a** : a large arterial trunk that arises from the conus arteriosus of the right ventricle and branches into the right and left pulmonary arteries — called also *pulmonary trunk* **b** : a branch of the pulmonary trunk that passes to the right lung where it divides into branches — called also *right pulmonary artery* **c** : a branch of the pulmonary trunk that passes to the left lung where it divides into branches — called also *left pulmonary artery*

pulmonary capillary wedge pressure *n* : WEDGE PRESSURE — abbr. *PCWP*

pulmonary circulation *n* : the passage of venous blood from the right atrium of the heart through the right ventricle and pulmonary arteries to the lungs where it is oxygenated and its return via the pulmonary veins to enter the left auricle and participate in the systemic circulation

pulmonary edema *n* : abnormal accumulation of fluid in the lungs

pulmonary embolism *n* : obstruction of a pulmonary artery or one of its branches that is usu. produced by a blood clot which has originated in a vein of the leg or pelvis and traveled to the lungs and that is marked by labored breathing, chest pain, fainting, rapid heart rate, cyanosis, shock, and sometimes death — abbr. *PE*

pulmonary ligament *n* : a supporting fold of pleura that extends from the lower part of the lung to the pericardium

pulmonary plexus *n* : either of two nerve plexuses associated with each lung that lie on the dorsal and ventral aspects of the bronchi of each lung

pulmonary stenosis *n* : abnormal narrowing of the orifice between the pulmonary artery and the right ventricle

pulmonary trunk *n* : PULMONARY ARTERY a

pulmonary valve *n* : a valve consisting of three semilunar cusps separating the pulmonary trunk from the right ventricle

pulmonary vein *n* : any of usu. four veins comprising two from each lung that return oxygenated blood from the lungs to the superior part of the left atrium

pulmonary wedge pressure *n* : WEDGE PRESSURE

pulmoni- *or* **pulmono-** — see PULMON-

pul•mon•ic \pu̇l-ˈmä-nik, ˌpəl-\ *adj* : PULMONARY ⟨~ lesions⟩

pulmonic stenosis *n* : PULMONARY STENOSIS

pul•mo•nol•o•gist \ˌpu̇l-mə-ˈnä-lə-jist, ˌpəl-\ *n* : a specialist in pulmonology

pul•mo•nol•o•gy \-jē\ *n, pl* **-gies** : a branch of medicine concerned with the anatomy, physiology, and pathology of the lungs

pulp \ˈpəlp\ *n* : a mass of soft tissue: as **a** : DENTAL PULP **b** : the characteristic somewhat spongy tissue of the spleen **c** : the fleshy portion of the fingertip — **pulp•al** \ˈpəl-pəl\ *adj* — **pulp•less** *adj*

pulp canal *n* : ROOT CANAL 1

pulp cavity *n* : the central cavity of a tooth containing the dental pulp and made up of the root canal and the pulp chamber

pulp chamber *n* : the part of the pulp cavity lying in the crown of a tooth

pulp•ec•to•my \ˌpəl-ˈpek-tə-mē\ *n, pl* **-mies** : the removal of the pulp of a tooth

pulp•i•tis \ˌpəl-ˈpī-təs\ *n, pl* **pulp•it•i•des** \-ˈpi-tə-ˌdēz\ : inflammation of the pulp of a tooth

pulposi, pulposus — see NUCLEUS PULPOSUS

pulp•ot•o•my \ˌpəl-ˈpä-tə-mē\ *n, pl* **-mies** : removal in a dental procedure of the coronal portion of the pulp of a tooth in such a manner that the pulp of the root remains intact and viable

pulp stone *n* : a lump of calcified tissue within the dental pulp — called also *denticle*

pulpy kidney \ˈpəl-pē-\ *n* : a destructive enterotoxemia of lambs caused by a bacterium of the genus *Clostridium* (*C. perfringens*) — called also *pulpy kidney disease*

pul•sate \ˈpəl-ˌsāt\ *vb* **pul•sat•ed; pul•sat•ing** : to exhibit a pulse or pulsation ⟨a *pulsating* artery⟩

pul•sa•tion \ˌpəl-ˈsā-shən\ *n* : rhythmic throbbing or vibrating (as of an artery); *also* : a single beat or throb — **pul•sa•tile** \ˈpəl-sət-ᵊl, -sə-ˌtīl\ *adj*

pulse \ˈpəls\ *n* **1 a** : a regularly recurrent wave of distension in arteries that results from the progress through an artery of blood injected into the arterial system at each contraction of the ventricles of the heart **b** : the palpable beat resulting from such pulse as detected in a superficial artery (as the radial artery); *also* : the number of such beats in a specified period of time (as one minute) ⟨a resting ~ of 70⟩ **2** : PULSATION **3** : a dose of a substance esp. when applied over a short period of time ⟨~*s* of intravenous methylprednisolone⟩ — **pulse** *vb* — **pulse•less** \ˈpəls-ləs\ *adj*

pulse–chase *adj* : involving the exposure of cells to a substrate bearing a radioactive label for a predetermined time followed by exposure to a high concentration of unlabeled substrate in order to stop uptake of the labeled substrate and follow its metabolic course

pulsed–field gel electrophoresis *n* : gel electrophoresis that is used esp. to separate large fragments of DNA and that involves changing the direction of the electric current periodically in order to minimize overlap of the separated molecules due to diffusion — called also *pulsed-field electrophoresis*

pulsed light *n* : high intensity white light that is emitted in a series of flashes of brief duration (as 10 to 20 milliseconds in length) ⟨*pulsed light* therapy to treat rosacea⟩

pulse–la•bel \ˈpəls-ˌlā-bəl\ *vb* **-la•beled** *or* **-la•belled; -la•bel•ing** *or* **-la•bel•ling** : to cause a pulse of a radiolabeled atom or substance to become incorporated into (as a molecule or cell component) ⟨~*ed* DNA⟩

pulseless disease *n* : TAKAYASU'S ARTERITIS

pulse oximeter *n* : a device that measures the oxygen saturation of arterial blood in an individual by utilizing a sensor attached typically to a finger, toe, or ear to determine the percentage of oxyhemoglobin in blood pulsating through a network of capillaries — **pulse oximetry** *n*

pulse pressure *n* : the pressure that is characteristic of the arterial pulse and represents the difference between diastolic and systolic pressures of the heart cycle

pulse rate *n* : the rate of the arterial pulse usu. observed at the wrist and stated in beats per minute

pul•sus alternans \ˈpəl-səs-\ *n* : alternation of strong and weak beats of the arterial pulse due to alternate strong and weak ventricular contractions

pulsus par•a•dox•us \-ˌpar-ə-ˈdäk-səs\ *n* : a pulse that weakens abnormally during inspiration and is symptomatic of various abnormalities (as pericarditis)

pulv *abbr* [Latin *pulvis*] powder — used in writing prescriptions

pul·vi·nar \ˌpəl-ˈvī-nər\ *n* **:** a rounded prominence on the back of the thalamus

Pul·vule \ˈpəl-ˌvyül\ *trademark* — used for a gelatin-based medicinal capsule

¹pump \ˈpəmp\ *n* **1 :** a device that raises, transfers, or compresses fluids or that attenuates gases esp. by suction or pressure or both **2 :** HEART **3 :** an act or the process of pumping **4 :** a mechanism by which atoms, ions, or molecules are transported across cell membranes — see PROTON PUMP, SODIUM PUMP

²pump *vb* **1 :** to raise (as water) with a pump **2 :** to draw fluid from with a pump **3 :** to transport (as ions) against a concentration gradient by the expenditure of energy

punch biopsy \ˈpənch-\ *n* **:** a biopsy in which a small round sample of tissue (as skin) is obtained by using an instrument with a circular blade

punch–drunk \ˈpənch-ˌdrəŋk\ *adj* **:** suffering from brain injury from repeated blows to the head **:** exhibiting chronic traumatic encephalopathy

punch–drunk syndrome *n* **:** CHRONIC TRAUMATIC ENCEPHALOPATHY

puncta *pl of* PUNCTUM

punctata — see KERATITIS PUNCTATA

punc·tate \ˈpəŋk-ˌtāt\ *adj* **:** characterized by dots or points ⟨~ skin lesions⟩

punc·tum \ˈpəŋk-təm\ *n, pl* **punc·ta** \-tə\ **:** a small area marked off from a surrounding surface — see LACRIMAL PUNCTUM

¹punc·ture \ˈpəŋk-chər\ *n* **1 :** an act of puncturing **2 :** a hole, wound, or perforation made by puncturing

²puncture *vb* **punc·tured; punc·tur·ing :** to pierce with or as if with a pointed instrument or object

pu·pa \ˈpyü-pə\ *n, pl* **pu·pae** \-(ˌ)pē, -ˌpī\ *or* **pupas :** an intermediate usu. quiescent stage of certain insects (as moths and beetles) that occurs between the larva and the adult and is characterized by internal changes by which larval structures are replaced by those typical of the adult — **pu·pal** \ˈpyü-pəl\ *adj*

pu·pil \ˈpyü-pəl\ *n* **:** the contractile usu. round aperture in the iris of the eye — **pu·pil·lary** *also* **pu·pi·lary** \ˈpyü-pə-ˌler-ē\ *adj*

pupillae — see SPHINCTER PUPILLAE

pupillary reflex *n* **:** the contraction of the pupil in response to light entering the eye

pupillo- *comb form* **:** pupil ⟨*pupillo*meter⟩

pu·pil·log·ra·phy \ˌpyü-pə-ˈlä-grə-fē\ *n, pl* **-phies :** the measurement of the reactions of the pupil

pu·pil·lom·e·ter \ˌpyü-pə-ˈlä-mə-tər\ *n* **:** an instrument for measuring the diameter of the pupil of the eye — **pu·pil·lom·e·try** \-mə-trē\ *n*

pur·ga·tion \ˌpər-ˈgā-shən\ *n* **1 :** the act of purging; *specif* **:** vigorous evacuation of the bowels (as from the action of a cathartic) **2 :** administration of or treatment with a purgative

¹pur·ga·tive \ˈpər-gə-tiv\ *adj* **:** purging or tending to purge **:** CATHARTIC — **pur·ga·tive·ly** *adv*

²purgative *n* **:** a purging medicine **:** CATHARTIC

¹purge \ˈpərj\ *vb* **purged; purg·ing :** to have or cause strong and usu. repeated emptying of the bowels

²purge *n* **1 :** something that purges; *esp* **:** PURGATIVE **2 :** an act or instance of purging

purified protein derivative *n* **:** a purified preparation of tuberculin used in skin tests (as the Mantoux test) to detect tubercle bacillus infection — abbr. *PPD*

pu·rine \ˈpyu̇r-ˌēn\ *n* **1 :** a crystalline base $C_5H_4N_4$ that is the parent of compounds of the uric-acid group **2 :** a derivative of purine; *esp* **:** a base (as adenine or guanine) that is a constituent of DNA or RNA

purine base *n* **:** any of a group of crystalline bases comprising purine and bases derived from it (as adenine) some of which are components of nucleosides and nucleotides

Pur·kin·je cell \pər-ˈkin-jē-\ *n* **:** any of numerous nerve cells that occupy the middle layer of the cerebellar cortex and are characterized by a large globe-shaped body with massive dendrites directed outward and a single slender axon directed inward — called also *Purkinje neuron*

Pur·ky·ně *or* **Purkinje** \ˈpu̇r-kin-ye, -yā\, **Jan Evangelista (1787–1869),** Bohemian physiologist.

Purkinje fiber *n* **:** any of the modified cardiac muscle fibers with few nuclei, granulated central cytoplasm, and sparse peripheral striations that make up Purkinje's network

Purkinje's network *n* **:** a network of intracardiac conducting tissue made up of syncytial Purkinje fibers that lie in the myocardium and constitute the bundle of His and other conducting tracts which spread out from the sinoatrial node — called also *Purkinje's system, Purkinje's tissue*

pu·ro·my·cin \ˌpyu̇r-ə-ˈmīs-ᵊn\ *n* **:** an antibiotic $C_{22}H_{29}N_7O_5$ that is obtained from an actinomycete (*Streptomyces alboniger*) and is a potent inhibitor of protein synthesis

pur·pu·ra \ˈpər-pu̇-rə, -pyu̇-\ *n* **:** any of several hemorrhagic states characterized by patches of purplish discoloration resulting from extravasation of blood into the skin and mucous membranes — see THROMBOCYTOPENIC PURPURA — **pur·pu·ric** \ˌpər-ˈpyu̇r-ik\ *adj*

purpura ful·mi·nans \-ˈfu̇l-mə-ˌnanz, -ˈfəl-\ *n* **:** purpura of an often severe progressive form esp. of children that is characterized by widespread necrosis of the skin and that occurs chiefly in conjunction with acute infection (as by meningococci) esp. as a manifestation of disseminated intravascular coagulation and that in neonates is typically associated with deficiency of protein C or protein S

purpura hem•or•rhag•i•ca \-ˌhe-mə-ˈra-jə-kə\ *n* : THROMBOCYTOPENIC PURPURA

purse–string suture *n* : a surgical suture passed as a running stitch in and out along the edge of a circular wound in such a way that when the ends of the suture are drawn tight the wound is closed like a purse

pu•ru•lence \ˈpyu̇r-ə-ləns, ˈpyu̇r-yə-\ *n* : the quality or state of being purulent; *also* : PUS

pu•ru•lent \-lənt\ *adj* **1** : containing, consisting of, or being pus **2** : accompanied by suppuration

pus \ˈpəs\ *n* : a thick opaque usu. yellowish-white fluid matter that is formed as part of an inflammatory response typically associated with an infection and is composed of exudate chiefly containing dead white blood cells, tissue debris, and pathogenic microorganisms (as bacteria) — **pus•sy** \ˈpə-sē\ *adj*

pus•tu•lar \ˈpəs-chə-lər, ˈpəs-tyə-\ *adj* **1** : of, relating to, or resembling pustules ⟨~ eruptions⟩ **2** : covered with pustules

pus•tule \ˈpəs-(ˌ)chül, -(ˌ)tyül, -(ˌ)tül\ *n* **1** : a small circumscribed elevation of the skin containing pus and having an inflamed base **2** : a small often distinctively colored elevation or spot resembling a blister or pimple

pu•ta•men \pyü-ˈtā-mən\ *n, pl* **pu•tam•i•na** \-ˈta-mə-nə\ : an outer reddish layer of gray matter in the lentiform nucleus

pu•tre•fac•tion \ˌpyü-trə-ˈfak-shən\ *n* **1** : the decomposition of organic matter; *esp* : the typically anaerobic splitting of proteins by bacteria and fungi with the formation of foul-smelling incompletely oxidized products **2** : the state of being putrefied — **pu•tre•fac•tive** \-tiv\ *adj* — **pu•tre•fy** \ˈpyü-trə-ˌfī\ *vb*

pu•tres•cine \pyü-ˈtre-ˌsēn\ *n* : a crystalline slightly poisonous ptomaine $C_4H_{12}N_2$ that is formed by decarboxylation of ornithine, occurs widely but in small amounts in living things, and is found esp. in putrid flesh

pu•trid \ˈpyü-trəd\ *adj* **1** : being in a state of putrefaction **2** : of, relating to, or characteristic of putrefaction

PUVA \ˌpē-ˌyü-ˌvē-ˈā\ *n* [*p*soralen *u*ltra*v*iolet *A*] : treatment for psoriasis that involves the administration of psoralen to photosensitize the skin followed by exposure to UVA radiation

PVD *abbr* peripheral vascular disease

PVE *abbr* prosthetic valve endocarditis

PVP *abbr* polyvinylpyrrolidone

PVS *abbr* persistent vegetative state

PWA \ˌpē-ˌdə-bəl-ˌyü-ˈā\ *n* : a person affected with AIDS

P wave \ˈpē-ˌwāv\ *n* : a deflection in an electrocardiographic tracing that represents atrial activity of the heart — compare QRS COMPLEX, T WAVE

Px *abbr* **1** pneumothorax **2** prognosis

py- *or* **pyo-** *comb form* : pus ⟨*py*emia⟩

py•ae•mia *chiefly Brit var of* PYEMIA

py•ar•thro•sis \ˌpī-är-ˈthrō-səs\ *n, pl* **-thro•ses** \-ˌsēz\ : the formation or presence of pus within a joint

pycn- *or* **pycno-** — see PYKN-

pycnic, pycnosis *var of* PYKNIC, PYKNOSIS

pyc•no•dys•os•to•sis *or* **pyk•no•dys•os•to•sis** \ˌpik-nō-ˌdis-ä-ˈstō-səs\ *n, pl* **-to•ses** \-ˌsēz\ : a rare genetic condition inherited as an autosomal recessive trait and characterized esp. by short stature, fragile bones, shortness of the fingers and toes, failure of the anterior fontanel to close properly, and a receding chin

pyel- *or* **pyelo-** *comb form* : renal pelvis ⟨*pyelo*graphy⟩

py•eli•tis \ˌpī-ə-ˈlī-təs\ *n* : inflammation of the lining of the renal pelvis

py•elo•gram \ˈpī-ə-lə-ˌgram\ *n* : a radiograph made by pyelography

py•elog•ra•phy \ˌpī-ə-ˈlä-grə-fē\ *n, pl* **-phies** : radiographic visualization of the renal pelvis after injection of a radiopaque substance through the ureter or into a vein — see RETROGRADE PYELOGRAPHY — **py•elo•graph•ic** \ˌpī-ə-lə-ˈgra-fik\ *adj*

py•elo•li•thot•o•my \ˌpī-ə-lō-li-ˈthä-tə-mē\ *n, pl* **-mies** : surgical incision of the renal pelvis of a kidney for removal of a kidney stone

py•elo•ne•phri•tis \ˌpī-ə-lō-ni-ˈfrī-təs\ *n, pl* **-phrit•i•des** \-ˈfri-tə-ˌdēz\ : inflammation of both the parenchyma of a kidney and the lining of its renal pelvis esp. due to bacterial infection — **py•elo•ne•phrit•ic** \-ˈfri-tik\ *adj*

py•elo•plas•ty \ˈpī-ə-lə-ˌplas-tē\ *n, pl* **-ties** : plastic surgery of the renal pelvis of a kidney

py•emia \pī-ˈē-mē-ə\ *n* : septicemia accompanied by multiple abscesses and secondary toxemic symptoms and caused by pus-forming microorganisms (as the bacterium *Staphylococcus aureus*) — **py•emic** \-mik\ *adj*

Py•emo•tes \ˌpī-ə-ˈmō-tēz\ *n* : a genus of mites that includes one (*P. ventricosus*) causing grain itch in humans

py•gop•a•gus \pī-ˈgä-pə-gəs\ *n, pl* **-gi** \-ˌgī, -ˌjī\ : conjoined twins united in the sacral region

pykn- *or* **pykno-** *also* **pycn-** *or* **pycno-** *comb form* **1** : close : compact : dense : bulky ⟨*pykn*ic⟩ **2** : marked by short stature or shortness of digits ⟨*pycno*dysostosis⟩

[1]**pyk•nic** *also* **pyc•nic** \ˈpik-nik\ *adj* : characterized by shortness of stature, broadness of girth, and powerful muscularity : ENDOMORPHIC 2

²pyknic *also* **pycnic** *n* : a person of pyknic build

pyknodysostosis *var of* PYCNODYSOSTOSIS

pyk·no·lep·sy \ˈpik-nə-ˌlep-sē\ *n, pl* **-sies** : a condition marked by epileptiform attacks resembling those of petit mal epilepsy

pyk·no·sis *also* **pyc·no·sis** \pik-ˈnō-səs\ *n, pl* **pyk·no·ses** *also* **pyc·no·ses** : a degenerative condition of a cell nucleus marked by clumping of the chromosomes, hyperchromatism, and shrinking of the nucleus — **pyk·not·ic** *also* **pyc·not·ic** \-ˈnä-tik\ *adj*

pyl- *or* **pyle-** *or* **pylo-** *comb form* : portal vein ⟨*pyle*phlebitis⟩

py·le·phle·bi·tis \ˌpī-lə-fli-ˈbī-təs\ *n, pl* **-bit·i·des** \-ˈbi-tə-ˌdēz\ : inflammation of the renal portal vein usu. secondary to intestinal disease and with suppuration

py·lon \ˈpī-ˌlän, -lən\ *n* : a simple temporary artificial leg

pylor- *or* **pyloro-** *comb form* : pylorus ⟨*pyloro*plasty⟩

py·lo·ric \pī-ˈlōr-ik, pə-\ *adj* : of or relating to the pylorus; *also* : of, relating to, or situated in or near the posterior part of the stomach

pyloric glands *n pl* : the short coiled tubular glands of the mucous coat of the stomach occurring chiefly near the pyloric end

pyloric sphincter *n* : the circular fold of mucous membrane containing a ring of muscle fibers that closes the pylorus — called also *pyloric valve*

pyloric stenosis *n* : narrowing of the pyloric opening (as from congenital malformation)

py·lo·ro·my·ot·o·my \pī-ˌlōr-ō-mī-ˈä-tə-mē, pə-ˌlōr-ə-\ *n, pl* **-mies** : surgical incision of the muscle fibers of the pyloric sphincter for relief of stenosis caused by muscular hypertrophy

py·lo·ro·plas·ty \pī-ˈlōr-ə-ˌplas-tē\ *n, pl* **-ties** : plastic surgery on the pylorus (as to enlarge a stricture)

py·lo·ro·spasm \pī-ˈlōr-ə-ˌspa-zəm\ *n* : spasm of the pyloric sphincter often marked by pain and vomiting

py·lo·rus \pī-ˈlōr-əs, pə-\ *n, pl* **py·lo·ri** \-ˈlōr-ˌī, -(ˌ)ē\ : the opening from the stomach into the intestine — see PYLORIC SPHINCTER

pyo- — see PY-

pyo·der·ma \ˌpī-ə-ˈdər-mə\ *n* : a bacterial skin inflammation marked by pus-filled lesions

pyoderma gan·gre·no·sum \-ˌgaŋ-gri-ˈnō-səm\ *n* : a chronic noninfectious condition that is marked by the formation of purplish nodules and pustules which tend to coalesce and form ulcers and that is associated with various underlying systemic or malignant diseases (as ulcerative colitis, rheumatoid arthritis, or leukemia)

pyo·gen·ic \ˌpī-ə-ˈje-nik\ *adj* : producing pus ⟨~ bacteria⟩; *also* : marked by pus production ⟨~ meningitis⟩

pyo·me·tra \ˌpī-ə-ˈmē-trə\ *n* : an accumulation of pus in the uterine cavity

pyo·myo·si·tis \ˌpī-ō-ˌmī-ə-ˈsī-təs\ *n* : infiltrative bacterial inflammation of muscles leading to the formation of abscesses

pyo·ne·phro·sis \-ni-ˈfrō-səs\ *n, pl* **-phro·ses** \-ˌsēz\ : a collection of pus in the kidney

pyo·pneu·mo·peri·car·di·um \-ˌn(y)ü-mō-ˌper-ə-ˈkär-dē-əm\ *n* : the presence of pus and air in the pericardium — called also *pneumopyopericardium*

py·or·rhea \ˌpī-ə-ˈrē-ə\ *n* **1** : a discharge of pus **2** : an advanced form of chronic periodontitis marked esp. by the discharge of pus from the alveoli — **py·or·rhe·ic** \-ˈrē-ik\ *adj*

py·or·rhoea *chiefly Brit var of* PYORRHEA

pyo·sal·pinx \ˌpī-ō-ˈsal-(ˌ)piŋks\ *n, pl* **-sal·pin·ges** \-sal-ˈpin-(ˌ)jēz\ : a collection of pus in an oviduct

pyo·tho·rax \-ˈthōr-ˌaks\ *n, pl* **-tho·rax·es** *or* **-tho·ra·ces** \-ˈthōr-ə-(ˌ)sēz\ : EMPYEMA

pyr- *or* **pyro-** *comb form* **1** : fire : heat ⟨*pyro*mania⟩ **2** : fever ⟨*pyro*gen⟩

pyr·a·mid \ˈpir-ə-ˌmid\ *n* **1** : a polyhedron having for its base a polygon and for faces triangles with a common vertex **2** : an anatomical structure resembling a pyramid: as **a** : RENAL PYRAMID **b** : either of two large bundles of motor fibers from the cerebral cortex that reach the medulla oblongata and are continuous with the corticospinal tracts of the spinal cord **c** : a conical projection making up the central part of the inferior vermis of the cerebellum — **py·ram·i·dal** \pə-ˈra-məd-ᵊl\ *adj*

pyramidal cell *n* : any of numerous large multipolar pyramid-shaped cells in the cerebral cortex

pyramidal decussation *n* : the crossing of fibers of the corticospinal tracts from one side of the central nervous system to the other near the junction of the medulla and the spinal cord — called also *decussation of the pyramids*

py·ram·i·da·lis \pə-ˌra-mə-ˈdā-ləs\ *n, pl* **-da·les** \-(ˌ)lēz\ *or* **-dalises** : a small triangular muscle of the lower front part of the abdomen that is situated in front of and in the same sheath with the rectus and functions to tense the linea alba

pyramidal tract *n* : CORTICOSPINAL TRACT

py·ram·i·dot·o·my \pə-ˌra-mə-ˈdä-tə-mē\ *n, pl* **-mies** : a surgical procedure in which a corticospinal tract is severed (as for relief of parkinsonism)

pyr·a·mis \ˈpir-ə-məs\ *n, pl* **py·ram·i·des** \pə-ˈra-mə-ˌdēz\ : PYRAMID 2

py·ran·tel \pə-ˈran-ˌtel\ *n* : an anthelmintic drug used in the form of its pamoate $C_{11}H_{14}N_2S \cdot C_{23}H_{16}O_6$ or tartrate $C_{11}H_{14}N_2S \cdot C_4H_6O_6$

pyr•a•zin•amide \ˌpir-ə-ˈzi-nə-ˌmīd, -məd\ *n* : a tuberculostatic drug $C_5H_5N_3O$

py•re•thrin \pī-ˈrē-thrən, -ˈre-\ *n* : either of two oily liquid esters $C_{21}H_{28}O_3$ and $C_{22}H_{28}O_5$ that have insecticidal properties and are the active components of pyrethrum

py•re•thrum \pī-ˈrē-thrəm, -ˈre-\ *n* : an insecticide made from the dried heads of any of several Old World chrysanthemums (genus *Chrysanthemum* of the family Compositae)

py•rex•ia \pī-ˈrek-sē-ə\ *n* : abnormal elevation of body temperature : FEVER — **py•rex•i•al** \-sē-əl\ *adj*

py•rex•ic \-sik\ *adj* : PYREXIAL

pyr•i•dine \ˈpir-ə-ˌdēn\ *n* : a toxic water-soluble flammable liquid base C_5H_5N of pungent odor

pyridine nucleotide *n* : a nucleotide characterized by a pyridine derivative as a nitrogen base; *esp* : NAD

pyr•i•do•stig•mine \ˌpir-ə-dō-ˈstig-ˌmēn\ *n* : a drug that is an anticholinesterase administered in the form of its bromide $C_9H_{13}BrN_2O_2$ esp. in the treatment of myasthenia gravis — called also *pyridostigmine bromide;* see MESTINON

pyr•i•dox•al \ˌpir-ə-ˈdäk-ˌsal\ *n* : a crystalline aldehyde $C_8H_9NO_3$ of the vitamin B_6 group that in the form of its phosphate is active as a coenzyme

pyr•i•dox•amine \ˌpir-ə-ˈdäk-sə-ˌmēn\ *n* : an amine $C_8H_{12}N_2O_2$ of the vitamin B_6 group that in the form of its phosphate is active as a coenzyme

pyr•i•dox•ine \ˌpir-ə-ˈdäk-ˌsēn, -sən\ *n* : a crystalline phenolic alcohol $C_8H_{11}NO_3$ of the vitamin B_6 group found esp. in cereals and convertible in the body into pyridoxal and pyridoxamine

pyridoxine hydrochloride *n* : the hydrochloride salt $C_8H_{11}NO_3 \cdot HCl$ of pyridoxine that is used therapeutically (as in the treatment of pyridoxine deficiency)

pyriform, pyriformis *var of* PIRIFORM, PIRIFORMIS

py•ril•amine \pī-ˈri-lə-ˌmēn\ *n* : an oily liquid base $C_{17}H_{23}N_3O$ or its bitter crystalline maleate $C_{21}H_{27}N_3O_5$ used as an antihistamine drug in the treatment of various allergies

py•ri•meth•amine \ˌpī-rə-ˈme-thə-ˌmēn\ *n* : a folic acid antagonist $C_{12}H_{13}ClN_4$ that is used in the treatment of toxoplasmosis and in the prevention and treatment of malaria — see DARAPRIM

py•rim•i•dine \pī-ˈri-mə-ˌdēn, pə-\ *n* **1** : a weakly basic organic compound $C_4H_2N_2$ of penetrating odor that is composed of a single six-membered ring having four carbon atoms with nitrogen atoms in positions one and three **2** : a derivative of pyrimidine having its characteristic ring structure; *esp* : a base (as cytosine, thymine, or uracil) that is a constituent of DNA or RNA

pyrithione zinc *n* : ZINC PYRITHIONE

pyro- — see PYR-

py•ro•gal•lic acid \ˌpī-rō-ˈga-lik-\ *n* : PYROGALLOL

py•ro•gal•lol \-ˈga-ˌlȯl, -ˈgȯ-, -ˌlōl\ *n* : a poisonous crystalline phenol $C_6H_6O_3$ formerly used as a topical antimicrobial (as in the treatment of psoriasis)

py•ro•gen \ˈpī-rə-jən\ *n* : a fever-producing substance

py•ro•gen•ic \ˌpī-rō-ˈje-nik\ *adj* : producing or produced by fever — **py•ro•ge•nic•i•ty** \-jə-ˈni-sə-tē\ *n*

py•ro•ma•nia \ˌpī-rō-ˈmā-nē-ə, -nyə\ *n* : an irresistible impulse to start fires — **py•ro•ma•ni•a•cal** \-mə-ˈnī-ə-kəl\ *adj*

py•ro•ma•ni•ac \-nē-ˌak\ *n* : an individual affected with pyromania

py•ro•sis \pī-ˈrō-səs\ *n* : HEARTBURN

py•rox•y•lin \pī-ˈräk-sə-lin\ *n* : a flammable mixture of nitrates of cellulose — see COLLODION

pyr•role \ˈpir-ˌōl\ *n* : a toxic liquid heterocyclic compound C_4H_5N that has a ring consisting of four carbon atoms and one nitrogen atom and that is the parent compound of many biologically important substances (as bile pigments, porphyrins, and chlorophyll); *broadly* : a derivative of pyrrole

py•ru•vate \pī-ˈrü-ˌvāt\ *n* : a salt or ester of pyruvic acid

pyruvate kinase *n* : an enzyme that functions in glycolysis by catalyzing esp. the transfer of phosphate from phosphoenolpyruvate to ADP forming pyruvate and ATP

py•ru•vic acid \pī-ˈrü-vik-\ *n* : a 3-carbon acid $C_3H_4O_3$ that is an intermediate in carbohydrate metabolism and can be formed either from glucose after phosphorylation or from glycogen by glycolysis

py•uria \pī-ˈyu̇r-ē-ə\ *n* : the presence of pus in the urine; *also* : a condition (as pyelonephritis) characterized by pus in the urine

PZI *abbr* protamine zinc insulin

Q

qd *abbr* [Latin *quaque die*] every day — used in writing prescriptions

Q fever *n* : a disease that is characterized by high fever, chills, muscular pains, headache, and sometimes pneumonia, that is caused by a gram-negative bacterium of the genus *Coxiella* (*C. burnetii*) of which domestic animals serve as reservoirs, and that is transmitted to humans esp. by inhalation of infective airborne bacteria (as in contaminated dust)

qh *or* **qhr** *abbr* [Latin *quaque hora*] every hour — used in writing prescriptions often with a number indicating the hours between doses ⟨*q*4*h* means every 4 hours⟩

qhs *abbr* [Latin *quaque hora somni*] every night at bedtime — used in writing prescriptions

qid *abbr* [Latin *quater in die*] four times a day — used in writing prescriptions

qi•gong \ˈchē-ˈgu̇ŋ\ *n, often cap* : an ancient Chinese healing art involving meditation, controlled breathing, and movement exercises designed to improve physical and mental well-being and prevent disease — called also *chi kung, ch'i kung*

QNASL \ˈkyü-ˈnā-zəl\ *trademark* — used for a preparation of the dipropionate of beclomethasone administered as a nasal aerosol

QRS \ˌkyü-(ˌ)är-ˈes\ *n* : QRS COMPLEX

QRS complex *n* : the series of deflections in an electrocardiogram that represent electrical activity generated by ventricular depolarization prior to contraction of the ventricles — compare P WAVE, T WAVE

qt *abbr* quart

QT interval \ˌkyü-ˈtē-\ *n* : the interval from the beginning of the QRS complex to the end of the T wave on an electrocardiogram representing ventricular depolarization and repolarization and indicating the time during which ventricular contraction and subsequent relaxation occurs — see LONG QT SYNDROME

quaa•lude \ˈkwā-ˌlüd\ *n* : a tablet or capsule of methaqualone

quack \ˈkwak\ *n* : an ignorant or dishonest practitioner of medicine — **quack** *adj* — **quack•ery** \ˈkwa-kə-rē\ *n*

quad \ˈkwäd\ *n* : QUADRICEPS — usu. used in pl.

quad•rant \ˈkwä-drənt\ *n* : any of the four more or less equivalent segments into which an anatomic structure may be divided by vertical and horizontal partitioning through its midpoint ⟨pain in the lower right ∼ of the abdomen⟩

quad•rant•ec•to•my \ˌkwä-drən-ˈtek-tə-mē\ *n* : a partial mastectomy involving excision of a tumor along with the involved quadrant of the breast including the skin and underlying fascia — compare LUMPECTOMY

quad•rate lobe \ˈkwä-ˌdrāt-\ *n* : a small lobe of the liver on the underside of the right lobe to the left of the fissure for the gallbladder

qua•dra•tus fem•o•ris \kwä-ˈdrā-təs-ˈfe-mə-rəs\ *n* : a small flat muscle of the gluteal region that arises from the ischial tuberosity, inserts into the greater trochanter and adjacent region of the femur, and serves to rotate the thigh laterally

quadratus la•bii su•pe•ri•or•is \-ˈlā-bē-ˌī-su̇-ˌpir-ē-ˈȯr-əs\ *n* : LEVATOR LABII SUPERIORIS

quadratus lum•bor•um \-ləm-ˈbȯr-əm\ *n* : a quadrilateral-shaped muscle of the abdomen that arises from the iliac crest and the iliolumbar ligament, inserts into the lowest rib and the upper four lumbar vertebrae, and functions esp. to flex the trunk laterally

quadratus plan•tae \-ˈplan-ˌtē\ *n* : a muscle of the sole of the foot that arises by two heads from the calcaneus, inserts into the lateral side of the tendons of the flexor digitorum longus, and aids in flexing the toes

quad•ri•ceps \ˈkwä-drə-ˌseps\ *n* : a large extensor muscle of the front of the thigh divided above into four parts which include the rectus femoris, vastus lateralis, vastus intermedius, and vastus medialis, and which unite in a single tendon to enclose the patella as a sesamoid bone at the knee and insert as the patellar tendon into the tuberosity of the tibia — called also *quadriceps muscle*

quadriceps fem•o•ris \-ˈfe-mə-rəs\ *n* : QUADRICEPS

quadrigemina — see CORPORA QUADRIGEMINA

quad•ri•pa•re•sis \ˌkwä-drə-pə-ˈrē-səs\ *n, pl* **-re•ses** \-ˌsēz\ : muscle weakness affecting all four limbs — called also *tetraparesis*

quad•ri•pa•ret•ic \-pə-ˈre-tik\ *adj* : of, relating to, or affected with quadriparesis ⟨a ∼ patient⟩

quad•ri•ple•gia \ˌkwä-drə-ˈplē-jə, -jē-ə\ *n* : partial or complete paralysis of both the arms and legs that is usu. due to injury or disease of the spinal cord in the region of the neck — called also *tetraplegia*

[1]**quad•ri•ple•gic** \ˌkwä-drə-ˈplē-jik\ *adj* : of, relating to, or affected with quadriplegia ⟨∼ patients⟩

[2]**quadriplegic** *n* : one affected with quadriplegia

quad•ru•ped \ˈkwä-drə-ˌped\ *n* : an animal having four feet — **qua•dru•pe•dal** \kwä-ˈdrü-pəd-ᵊl, ˌkwä-drə-ˈped-\ *adj*

qua•dru•plet \kwä-ˈdrə-plət, -ˈdrü-; ˈkwä-drə-\ *n* **1** : one of four offspring born at one birth **2 quadruplets** *pl* : a group of four offspring born at one birth

quads *pl of* QUAD

qual•i•ty \ˈkwä-lə-tē\ *n, pl* **-ties** : the character of an X-ray beam that determines its penetrating power and is dependent upon its wavelength distribution

quantitative character *n* : an inherited character that is expressed phenotypically in all degrees of variation between one often indefinite extreme and another : a character determined by polygenes

quantitative inheritance *n* : genetic inheritance of a character (as human skin color) controlled by polygenes

quan•tum \ˈkwän-təm\ *n, pl* **quan•ta** \ˈkwän-tə\ **1** : one of the very small increments or parcels into which many forms of energy are subdivided **2** : one of the small molecular packets of a neurotransmitter (as acetylcholine) released into the synaptic cleft in the transmission of a nerve impulse across a synapse — **quan•tal** \-təl\ *adj*

quar•an•tine \ˈkwȯr-ən-ˌtēn, ˈkwär-\ *n* **1 a** : a term during which a ship arriving in port and suspected of carrying contagious disease is held in isolation from the shore **b** : a regulation placing a ship in quarantine **c** : a place where a ship is detained during quarantine **2 a** : a restraint upon the activities or communication of persons or the transport of goods designed to prevent the spread of disease or pests **b** : a place in which those under quarantine are kept — **quar•an•tin•able** *adj* — **quarantine** *vb*

quart \ˈkwȯrt\ *n* **1** : a British unit of liquid or dry capacity equal to $^1/_4$ gallon or 69.355 cubic inches or 1.136 liters **2** : a U.S. unit of liquid capacity equal to $^1/_4$ gallon or 57.75 cubic inches or 0.946 liters

quar•tan \ˈkwȯrt-ᵊn\ *adj* : recurring at approximately 72-hour intervals <~ chills and fever> — compare TERTIAN

quartan malaria *n* : MALARIAE MALARIA

quartz \ˈkwȯrts\ *n* : a silica-containing mineral SiO_2

quas•sia \ˈkwä-shə, -shē-ə, -sē-ə\ *n* : a drug derived from the heartwood and bark of various tropical trees (family Simaroubaceae) and used esp. as a remedy for roundworms

qua•ter•na•ry \ˈkwä-tər-ˌner-ē, kwə-ˈtər-nə-rē\ *adj* : consisting of, containing, or being an atom bonded to four other atoms

quaternary ammonium compound *n* : any of numerous strong bases and their salts derived from ammonium by replacement of the hydrogen atoms with organic radicals and important esp. as surface-active agents, disinfectants, and drugs

que•bra•cho \kā-ˈbrä-(ˌ)chō, ki-\ *n* : a tree (*Aspidosperma quebracho*) of the dogbane family (Apocynaceae) which occurs in Argentina and Chile and whose dried bark has been used medicinally esp. to relieve dyspnea

Queck•en•stedt test \ˈkvek-ᵊn-ˌshtet-\ *n* : a test for spinal blockage of the subarachnoid space in which manual pressure is applied to the jugular vein to elevate venous pressure, which indicates the absence of a block when there is a simultaneous increase in cerebrospinal fluid pressure, and which indicates the presence of a block when cerebrospinal fluid pressure remains the same or almost the same — called also *Queckenstedt sign*

Queckenstedt, Hans Heinrich Georg (1876–1918), German physician.

quer•ce•tin \ˈkwər-sə-tən\ *n* : a yellow crystalline pigment $C_{15}H_{10}O_7$ occurring usu. in the form of glycosides in various plants

Quete•let index \ke-tə-ˈlā-\ *or* **Quete•let's index** \-ˈlāz-\ *n* : BODY MASS INDEX

Qué•te•let \kā-tə-lā\, **Lambert Adolphe Jacques (1796–1874),** Belgian astronomer and statistician.

que•ti•a•pine \kwe-ˈtī-ə-ˌpēn\ *n* : an antipsychotic drug taken orally in the form of its fumarate $(C_{21}H_{25}N_3O_2S)_2 \cdot C_4H_4O_4$ esp. to treat schizophrenia and bipolar disorder — called also *quetiapine fumarate;* see SEROQUEL

quick \ˈkwik\ *n* : a painfully sensitive spot or area of flesh (as that underlying a fingernail or toenail)

quick•en \ˈkwi-kən\ *vb* **quick•ened; quick•en•ing** : to reach the stage of gestation at which fetal motion is felt

quickening *n* : the first motion of a fetus in the uterus felt by the mother usu. somewhat before the middle of the period of gestation

quick•sil•ver \ˈkwik-ˌsil-vər\ *n* : MERCURY 1

qui•es•cent \kwī-ˈes-ᵊnt, kwē-\ *adj* **1** : being in a state of arrest <~ tuberculosis> **2** : causing no symptoms <~ gallstones> — **qui•es•cence** \-ᵊns\ *n*

Quil•li•vant \ˈkwi-lə-vənt\ *trademark* — used for a preparation of the hydrochloride of methylphenidate

quin- *or* **quino-** *comb form* **1** : quina : cinchona bark <*quin*ine> <*quino*line> **2** : quinoline <*quin*ethazone>

qui•na \ˈkē-nə\ *n* : CINCHONA 2, 3

quin•a•crine \ˈkwi-nə-ˌkrēn\ *n* : an antimalarial drug derived from acridine and used esp. in the form of its dihydrochloride $C_{23}H_{30}ClN_3O \cdot 2HCl \cdot 2H_2O$ — called also *mepacrine;* see ATABRINE

quin•al•bar•bi•tone \ˌkwi-nal-ˈbär-bi-ˌtōn\ *n, chiefly Brit* : SECOBARBITAL

quin•a•pril \ˈkwi-nə-ˌpril\ *n* : an ACE inhibitor used orally in the form of its hydrochloride $C_{25}H_{30}N_2O_5 \cdot HCl$ either alone or in combination with a thiazide diuretic to treat hypertension — see ACCUPRIL

Quin·cke's disease \ˈkviŋ-kəz-\ *n* : ANGIOEDEMA

Quincke, Heinrich Irenaeus (1842–1922), German physician.

Quincke's edema *n* : ANGIOEDEMA

quin·eth·a·zone \ˌkwi-ˈne-thə-ˌzōn\ *n* : a diuretic $C_{10}H_{12}ClN_3O_3S$ used in the treatment of edema and hypertension

quin·i·dine \ˈkwi-nə-ˌdēn, -dən\ *n* : a dextrorotatory stereoisomer of quinine found in some species of cinchona and used chiefly in the form of its hydrated sulfate $(C_{20}H_{24}N_2O_2)_2 \cdot H_2SO_4 \cdot 2H_2O$ to treat irregularities of cardiac rhythm and sometimes in place of quinine as an antimalarial

qui·nine \ˈkwī-ˌnīn, ˈkwi-, -ˌnēn\ *n* **1** : a bitter crystalline alkaloid $C_{20}H_{24}N_2O_2$ obtained from cinchona bark that is administered orally in the form of its salts (as the hydrated sulfate $(C_{20}H_{24}N_2O_2)_2 \cdot H_2SO_4 \cdot 2H_2O$) as an antimalarial

quin·o·line \ˈkwin-ᵊl-ˌēn\ *n* **1** : a pungent oily nitrogenous base C_9H_7N that is the parent compound of many alkaloids, drugs, and dyes **2** : a derivative of quinoline

quin·o·lone \ˈkwi-nə-ˌlōn\ *n* : any of a class of synthetic antibacterial drugs that are derivatives of quinolines and inhibit the replication of bacterial DNA; *esp* : FLUOROQUINOLONE

qui·none \kwi-ˈnōn, ˈkwi-ˌ\ *n* **1** : either of two isomeric cyclic crystalline compounds $C_6H_4O_2$ that are irritating to the skin and mucous membranes **2** : any of various usu. yellow, orange, or red compounds structurally related to the quinones and including several that are biologically important as coenzymes, hydrogen acceptors, or vitamins

quin·sy \ˈkwin-zē\ *n, pl* **quin·sies** : an abscess in the connective tissue around a tonsil usu. resulting from bacterial infection and often accompanied by fever, pain, and swelling — called also *peritonsillar abscess*

quint \ˈkwint\ *n* : QUINTUPLET

quinti — see EXTENSOR DIGITI QUINTI PROPRIUS

quin·tu·plet \kwin-ˈtə-plət, -ˈtü-, -ˈtyü-; ˈkwin-tə-\ *n* **1** : one of five children or offspring born at one birth **2 quintuplets** *pl* : a group of five such offspring

qui·nu·cli·di·nyl ben·zi·late \kwi-ˈnü-klə-ˌdēn-ᵊl-ˈben-zə-ˌlāt, -ˈnyü-\ *n* : BZ

quit·tor \ˈkwi-tər\ *n* : a purulent inflammation of the cartilage of the lower leg and foot of horses

quo·tid·i·an \kwō-ˈti-dē-ən\ *adj* : occurring every day ⟨~ fever⟩

quo·tient \ˈkwō-shənt\ *n* : the numerical ratio usu. multiplied by 100 between a test score and a measurement on which that score might be expected largely to depend

qv *abbr* [Latin *quantum vis*] as much as you will — used in writing prescriptions

Qvar \ˈkyü-ˌvär\ *trademark* — used for a preparation of the dipropionate of beclomethasone for oral inhalation

Q wave \ˈkyü-ˌ\ *n* : the short initial downward stroke of the QRS complex in an electrocardiogram formed during the beginning of ventricular depolarization

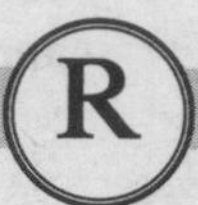

r *abbr* roentgen

R *symbol* chemical group and esp. an organic chemical group

Ra *symbol* radium

RA *abbr* rheumatoid arthritis

rabbit fever *n* : TULAREMIA

ra•bep•ra•zole \rə-ˈbe-prə-ˌzōl\ *n* : a proton pump inhibitor taken orally in the form of its sodium salt $C_{18}H_{20}NaN_3O_3S$ esp. to treat gastroesophageal reflux disease, duodenal ulcers, and disorders (as Zollinger-Ellison syndrome) involving gastric acid hypersecretion — see ACIPHEX

ra•bid \ˈra-bəd\ *adj* : affected with rabies ⟨a ~ dog⟩

ra•bies \ˈrā-bēz\ *n, pl* **rabies** : an acute virus disease of the central nervous system of warm-blooded animals that is caused by a rhabdovirus (species *Rabies virus* of the genus *Lyssavirus*) transmitted in infected saliva usu. through the bite of a rabid animal and that is typically characterized by fatigue, headache, fever, and general discomfort progressing to increased salivation, excitability, confusion, muscle weakness and spasms, hallucinations, abnormal behavior, paralysis, coma, and death when untreated — called also *hydrophobia*

race \ˈrās\ *n* **1** : an actually or potentially interbreeding group within a species; *also* : a taxonomic category (as a subspecies) representing such a group **2** : a category of humankind that shares certain distinctive physical traits

ra•ce•mic \rā-ˈsē-mik, rə-\ *adj* : of, relating to, or constituting a compound or mixture that is composed of equal amounts of dextrorotatory and levorotatory forms of the same compound and is not optically active

ra•ce•mose \ˈra-sə-ˌmōs; rā-ˈsē-, rə-\ *adj* : having or growing in a form like that of a cluster of grapes ⟨~ glands⟩

rachi- *or* **rachio-** *comb form* : spine ⟨*rachi*schisis⟩

ra•chis•chi•sis \rə-ˈkis-kə-səs\ *n, pl* **-chi•ses** \-kə-ˌsēz\ : a congenital abnormality (as spina bifida) characterized by a cleft of the spinal column

ra•chit•ic \rə-ˈki-tik\ *adj* : of, relating to, or affected by rickets ⟨~ lesions⟩

rachitic rosary *n* : BEADING

ra•chi•tis \rə-ˈkī-təs\ *n, pl* **-chit•i•des** \-ˈki-tə-ˌdēz\ : RICKETS

rad \ˈrad\ *n* : a unit of absorbed dose of ionizing radiation equal to an energy of 100 ergs per gram of irradiated material

rad *abbr* [Latin *radix*] root — used in writing prescriptions

radi- — see RADIO-

[1]**ra•di•al** \ˈrā-dē-əl\ *adj* **1** : arranged or having parts arranged like rays **2** : of, relating to, or situated near the radius or the thumb side of the hand or forearm **3** : developing uniformly around a central axis ⟨~ cleavage of an egg⟩ — **ra•di•al•ly** *adv*

[2]**radial** *n* : a body part (as an artery) lying near or following the course of the radius

radial artery *n* : the smaller of the two branches into which the brachial artery divides just below the bend of the elbow and which passes along the radial side of the forearm to the wrist then winds backward around the outer side of the carpus and enters the palm between the first and second metacarpal bones to form the deep palmar arch

radial collateral ligament *n* **1** : a triangular ligament of the elbow that connects the lateral epicondyle with the lateral side of the annular ligament and helps to stabilize the elbow joint — called also *lateral collateral ligament;* compare ULNAR COLLATERAL LIGAMENT 1 **2** : a ligament of the wrist on the thumb side that connects the distal end of the radius of the arm with the trapezium and scaphoid bones and helps to stabilize the wrist joint — compare ULNAR COLLATERAL LIGAMENT 2 **3** : a ligament of the outer middle joint of the thumb that connects the head of the metacarpal bone with the adjacent phalanx — compare ULNAR COLLATERAL LIGAMENT 3

radialis — see EXTENSOR CARPI RADIALIS BREVIS, EXTENSOR CARPI RADIALIS LONGUS, FLEXOR CARPI RADIALIS, NERVUS RADIALIS

radial keratotomy *n* : a surgical operation on the cornea for the correction of myopia that involves flattening the cornea by making a series of incisions in a radial pattern resembling the spokes of a wheel — abbr. *RK;* compare PHOTOREFRACTIVE KERATECTOMY

radial nerve *n* : a large nerve that arises from the posterior cord of the brachial plexus and passes spirally down the humerus to the front of the lateral epicondyle where it divides into a superficial branch distributed to the skin of the back of the hand and arm and a deep branch to the underlying extensor muscles — called also *nervus radialis*

radial notch *n* : a narrow depression on the lateral side of the coronoid process of the ulna that articulates with the head of the radius and gives attachment to the annular ligament of the radius

radial tuberosity *n* : an oval eminence on the medial side of the radius distal to the neck where the tendon of the biceps brachii muscle inserts

radial vein *n* : any of several deep veins of the forearm that unite at the elbow with the ulnar veins to form the brachial veins

ra·di·ant energy \ˈrā-dē-ənt-\ *n* : energy traveling as electromagnetic waves

radiata — see CORONA RADIATA

ra·di·ate \ˈrā-dē-ˌāt\ *vb* **-at·ed; -at·ing 1** : to issue in or as if in rays : spread from a central point **2** : IRRADIATE

ra·di·ate ligament \ˈrā-dē-ət-, -ˌāt-\ *n* : a branching ligament uniting the front of the head of a rib with the bodies of the two vertebrae and the intervertebral disk between them — called also *stellate ligament*

ra·di·a·tion \ˌrā-dē-ˈā-shən\ *n* **1** : energy radiated in the form of waves or particles **2 a** : the action or process of radiating **b** (1) : the process of emitting radiant energy in the form of waves or particles (2) : the combined processes of emission, transmission, and absorption of radiant energy **3** : a tract of nerve fibers within the brain; *esp* : one concerned with the distribution of impulses arising from sensory stimuli to the relevant coordinating centers and nuclei

radiation sickness *n* : sickness that results from exposure to radiation and is commonly marked by fatigue, nausea, vomiting, loss of teeth and hair, and in more severe cases by damage to blood-forming tissue with decrease in red and white blood cells and with bleeding — called also *radiation syndrome*

radiation therapist *n* : RADIOTHERAPIST

radiation therapy *n* : RADIOTHERAPY

[1]rad·i·cal \ˈra-di-kəl\ *adj* **1** : designed to remove the root of a disease or all diseased tissue ⟨~ surgery⟩ **2** : involving complete removal of an organ ⟨~ prostatectomy⟩ — compare CONSERVATIVE — **rad·i·cal·ly** *adv*

[2]radical *n* : FREE RADICAL; *also* : a group of atoms bonded together that is considered an entity in various kinds of reactions

radical hysterectomy *n* : the surgical removal of the uterus, parametrium, and uterine cervix along with the partial removal of the pelvic lymph nodes that is typically performed to treat cervical or endometrial cancer — see WERTHEIM OPERATION

radical mastectomy *n* : a mastectomy in which the breast tissue, associated skin, nipple, areola, axillary lymph nodes, and pectoral muscles are removed — called also *Halsted radical mastectomy;* compare MODIFIED RADICAL MASTECTOMY, TOTAL MASTECTOMY

ra·dic·u·lar \rə-ˈdi-kyə-lər, ra-\ *adj* **1** : of, relating to, or involving a nerve root **2** : of, relating to, or occurring at the root of a tooth ⟨a ~ cyst⟩

ra·dic·u·li·tis \rə-ˌdi-kyə-ˈlī-təs\ *n* : inflammation of a nerve root

ra·dic·u·lop·a·thy \-ˈlä-pə-thē\ *n, pl* **-thies** : irritation of or injury to a nerve root (as from being compressed) that typically causes pain, numbness, or weakness in the part of the body which is supplied with nerves from that root

radii *pl of* RADIUS

radio- *also* **radi-** *comb form* **1** : radiant energy : radiation ⟨*radio*active⟩ ⟨*radi*opaque⟩ **2** : radioactive ⟨*radio*element⟩ **3** : radium : X-rays ⟨*radio*therapy⟩ **4** : radioactive isotopes esp. as produced artificially ⟨*radio*cobalt⟩

ra·dio·ac·tiv·i·ty \ˌrā-dē-ō-ak-ˈti-və-tē\ *n, pl* **-ties** : the property possessed by some elements (as uranium) or isotopes (as carbon 14) of spontaneously emitting alpha or beta rays and sometimes also gamma rays by the disintegration of their atomic nuclei — **ra·dio·ac·tive** \-ˈak-tiv\ *adj* — **ra·dio·ac·tive·ly** *adv*

ra·dio·al·ler·go·sor·bent \ˌrā-dē-ō-ə-ˌlər-gō-ˈsȯr-bənt\ *adj* : relating to, involving, or being a radioallergosorbent test ⟨~ testing⟩

radioallergosorbent test *n* : a radioimmunoassay for specific antibodies of immunoglobulin class IgE in which an insoluble matrix containing allergenic antigens is reacted with a sample of antibody-containing serum and then reacted again with antihuman antibodies against individual IgE antibodies to make specific determinations — abbr. *RAST*

ra·dio·as·say \ˌrā-dē-ō-ˈa-ˌsā, -a-ˈsā\ *n* : an assay based on examination of the sample in terms of radiation components

ra·dio·au·to·gram \-ˈȯ-tə-ˌgram\ *n* : AUTORADIOGRAPH

ra·dio·au·to·graph \-ˈȯ-tə-ˌgraf\ *n* : AUTORADIOGRAPH — **radioautograph** *vb* — **ra·dio·au·to·graph·ic** \-ˌȯ-tə-ˈgra-fik\ *adj* — **ra·dio·au·tog·ra·phy** \-ȯ-ˈtä-grə-fē\ *n*

ra·dio·bi·ol·o·gy \ˌrā-dē-ō-bī-ˈä-lə-jē\ *n, pl* **-gies** : a branch of biology dealing with the effects of radiation or radioactive materials on biological systems — **ra·dio·bi·o·log·i·cal** \-ˌbī-ə-ˈlä-ji-kəl\ *also* **ra·dio·bi·o·log·ic** \-jik\ *adj* — **ra·dio·bi·o·log·i·cal·ly** *adv* — **ra·dio·bi·ol·o·gist** \-bī-ˈä-lə-jist\ *n*

ra·dio·chro·mato·gram \-krō-ˈma-tə-ˌgram\ *n* : a chromatogram revealing one or more radioactive substances

ra·dio·chro·ma·tog·ra·phy \-ˌkrō-mə-ˈtä-grə-fē\ *n, pl* **-phies** : the process of making a quantitative or qualitative determination of a radioisotope-labeled substance by measuring the radioactivity of the appropriate zone or spot in the chromatogram — **ra·dio·chro·ma·to·graph·ic** \-krə-ˌma-tə-ˈgra-fik, -ˌkrō-mə-\ *adj*

ra·dio·co·balt \-ˈkō-ˌbȯlt\ *n* : radioactive cobalt; *esp* : COBALT 60

ra·dio·con·trast \-ˈkän-ˌtrast\ *adj* : relating to or being a radioactive contrast medium

ra•dio•den•si•ty \-ˈden-sə-tē\ *n, pl* **-ties** : RADIOPACITY

ra•dio•der•ma•ti•tis \-ˌdər-mə-ˈtī-təs\ *n, pl* **-ti•tis•es** *or* **-tit•i•des** \-ˈti-tə-ˌdēz\ : dermatitis resulting from overexposure to sources of radiant energy (as X-rays or radium)

ra•dio•di•ag•no•sis \-ˌdī-ig-ˈnō-səs\ *n, pl* **-no•ses** \-ˌsēz\ : diagnosis by means of radiology — compare RADIOTHERAPY

ra•dio•el•e•ment \-ˈe-lə-mənt\ *n* : a radioactive element whether formed naturally or produced artificially

ra•dio•en•zy•mat•ic \-ˌen-zə-ˈma-tik\ *adj* : of, relating to, or produced by a radioactive enzyme

radio frequency *n, pl* **-cies** : any of the electromagnetic wave frequencies that lie in the range extending from below 3000 hertz to about 300 billion hertz and that include the frequencies used for communications signals (as for radio and television broadcasting and cell-phone transmissions) or radar signals — **radiofrequency** *adj*

ra•dio•gen•ic \ˌrā-dē-ō-ˈje-nik\ *adj* : produced or caused by radioactivity

ra•dio•gram \ˈrā-dē-ō-ˌgram\ *n* : RADIOGRAPH

ra•dio•graph \-ˌgraf\ *n* : an X-ray or gamma-ray photograph — **radiograph** *vb* — **ra•dio•graph•ic** \ˌrā-dē-ō-ˈgra-fik\ *adj*

ra•di•og•ra•pher \ˌrā-dē-ˈä-grə-fər\ *n* : a person who makes radiographs; *specif* : an X-ray technician

ra•di•og•ra•phy \ˌrā-dē-ˈä-grə-fē\ *n, pl* **-phies** : the art, act, or process of making radiographs

ra•dio•im•mu•no•as•say \ˌrā-dē-ō-i-myə-nō-ˈa-ˌsā, -i-ˌmyü-, -a-ˈsā\ *n* : immunoassay of a substance (as insulin) that has been radiolabeled — abbr. *RIA* — **ra•dio•im•mu•no•as•say•able** *adj*

ra•dio•im•mu•no•elec•tro•pho•re•sis \-i-ˌlek-trə-fə-ˈrē-səs\ *n, pl* **-re•ses** \-ˌsēz\ : immunoelectrophoresis in which the substances separated in the electrophoretic system are identified by radioactive labels on antigens or antibodies

ra•dio•im•mu•no•log•i•cal \-ˌi-myə-nə-ˈlä-ji-kəl\ *also* **ra•dio•im•mu•no•log•ic** \-ˈlä-jik\ *adj* : of, relating to, or involving a radioimmunoassay

ra•dio•io•dide \-ˈī-ə-ˌdīd\ *n* : an iodide containing radioactive iodine

ra•dio•io•din•ate \-ˈī-ə-də-ˌnāt\ *vb* **-at•ed; -at•ing** : to treat or label with radioactive iodine — **ra•dio•io•din•ation** \-ˌī-ə-də-ˈnā-shən\ *n*

ra•dio•io•dine \-ˈī-ə-ˌdīn, -dən, -ˌdēn\ *n* : radioactive iodine; *esp* : IODINE-131

ra•dio•iron \-ˈī(-ə)rn\ *n* : radioactive iron; *esp* : a heavy isotope having the mass number 59 that is produced in nuclear reactors or cyclotrons and is used in biochemical tracer studies

ra•dio•iso•tope \ˌrā-dē-ō-ˈī-sə-ˌtōp\ *n* : a radioactive isotope — **ra•dio•iso•to•pic** \-ˌī-sə-ˈtä-pik, -ˈtō-\ *adj*

radio knife *n* : ELECTRIC SCALPEL

ra•dio•la•bel \-ˈlā-bəl\ *vb* **-la•beled** *or* **-la•belled; -la•bel•ing** *or* **-la•bel•ling** : to label with a radioactive atom or substance — **radiolabel** *n*

ra•di•ol•o•gist \ˌrā-dē-ˈä-lə-jist\ *n* : a physician specializing in the use of radiant energy for diagnostic and therapeutic purposes

ra•di•ol•o•gy \-jē\ *n, pl* **-gies** **1** : the science of radioactive substances and high-energy radiations **2** : a branch of medicine concerned with the use of radiant energy (as X-rays or ultrasound) in the diagnosis and treatment of disease — **ra•di•o•log•i•cal** \ˌrā-dē-ə-ˈlä-ji-kəl\ *or* **ra•di•o•log•ic** \-jik\ *adj* — **ra•dio•log•i•cal•ly** *adv*

ra•dio•lu•cent \ˌrā-dē-ō-ˈlüs-ᵊnt\ *adj* : partly or wholly permeable to radiation and esp. X-rays — compare RADIOPAQUE — **ra•dio•lu•cen•cy** \-ˈlüs-ᵊn-sē\ *n*

ra•dio•mi•met•ic \-mə-ˈme-tik, -mī-\ *adj* : producing effects similar to those of radiation ⟨~ agents⟩

ra•dio•ne•cro•sis \-nə-ˈkrō-səs, -ne-\ *n, pl* **-cro•ses** \-ˌsēz\ : ulceration or destruction of tissue resulting from irradiation — **ra•dio•ne•crot•ic** \-ˈkrä-tik\ *adj*

ra•dio•nu•clide \-ˈnü-ˌklīd, -ˈnyü-\ *n* : a radioactive nuclide

ra•di•opac•i•ty \ˌrā-dē-ō-ˈpa-sə-tē\ *n, pl* **-ties** : the quality or state of being radiopaque

ra•di•opaque \-ō-ˈpāk\ *adj* : being opaque to radiation and esp. X-rays — compare RADIOLUCENT

ra•dio•phar•ma•ceu•ti•cal \ˌrā-dē-ō-ˌfär-mə-ˈsü-ti-kəl\ *n* : a radioactive drug used for diagnostic or therapeutic purposes — **radiopharmaceutical** *adj*

ra•dio•phar•ma•cy \-ˈfär-mə-sē\ *n, pl* **-cies** : a branch of pharmacy concerned with radiopharmaceuticals; *also* : a pharmacy that supplies radiopharmaceuticals — **ra•dio•phar•ma•cist** \-sist\ *n*

ra•dio•phos•pho•rus \-ˈfäs-fə-rəs\ *n* : radioactive phosphorus; *esp* : PHOSPHORUS 32

ra•dio•pro•tec•tive \-prə-ˈtek-tiv\ *adj* : serving to protect or aiding in protecting against the injurious effect of radiations ⟨~ drugs⟩ — **ra•dio•pro•tec•tion** \-ˈtek-shən\ *n*

ra•dio•pro•tec•tor \-ˈtek-tər\ *also* **ra•dio•pro•tec•tor•ant** \-ˈtek-tə-rənt\ *n* : a radioprotective chemical agent

ra•dio•re•cep•tor assay \-ri-ˈsep-tər-\ *n* : an assay for a substance and esp. a hormone in which a mixture of the test sample and a known amount of the radiolabeled substance under test is exposed to a measured quantity of receptors for the substance and the amount in the test sample is determined from the proportion of receptors occupied by radiolabeled molecules of the substance

ra·dio·re·sis·tant \-ri-ˈzis-tənt\ *adj* : resistant to the effects of radiant energy ⟨~ cancer cells⟩ — **ra·dio·re·sis·tance** \-təns\ *n*

ra·dio·sen·si·tive \ˌrā-dē-ō-ˈsen-sə-tiv\ *adj* : sensitive to the effects of radiant energy ⟨~ cancer cells⟩ — **ra·dio·sen·si·tiv·i·ty** \-ˌsen-sə-ˈti-və-tē\ *n*

ra·dio·sen·si·tiz·er \-ˈsen-sə-ˌtī-zər\ *n* : a substance or condition capable of increasing the radiosensitivity of a cell or tissue — **ra·dio·sen·si·ti·za·tion** \-ˌsen-sə-tə-ˈzā-shən\ *n* — **ra·dio·sen·si·tiz·ing** \-ˈsen-sə-ˌtī-ziŋ\ *adj*

ra·dio·so·di·um \-ˈsō-dē-əm\ *n* : radioactive sodium; *esp* : a heavy isotope having the mass number 24 that is produced in nuclear reactors and is used in the form of a salt (as sodium chloride) chiefly in biochemical tracer studies

ra·dio·stron·tium \-ˈsträn-chē-əm, -chəm, -tē-əm\ *n* : radioactive strontium; *esp* : STRONTIUM 90

ra·dio·sur·gery \-ˈsər-jə-rē\ *n, pl* **-ger·ies** : STEREOTACTIC RADIOSURGERY — **ra·dio·sur·gi·cal** \-ˈsər-ji-kəl\ *adj*

ra·dio·te·lem·e·try \-tə-ˈle-mə-trē\ *n, pl* **-tries** **1** : TELEMETRY **2** : BIOTELEMETRY — **ra·dio·tele·met·ric** \-ˌte-lə-ˈme-trik\ *adj*

ra·dio·ther·a·py \ˌrā-dē-ō-ˈther-ə-pē\ *n, pl* **-pies** : the treatment of disease by means of radiation (as X-rays) — called also *radiation therapy;* compare RADIODIAGNOSIS — **ra·dio·ther·a·peut·ic** \-ˌther-ə-ˈpyü-tik\ *adj* — **ra·dio·ther·a·pist** \-ˈther-ə-pist\ *n*

ra·dio·tox·ic·i·ty \-täk-ˈsi-sə-tē\ *n, pl* **-ties** : the toxicity of radioactive substances

ra·dio·trac·er \ˈrā-dē-ō-ˌtrā-sər\ *n* : a radioactive tracer

ra·dio·ul·nar \ˌrā-dē-ō-ˈəl-nər\ *adj* : of, relating to, or connecting the radius and ulna

radioulnar joint *n* : any of three joints connecting the radius and ulna at their proximal and distal ends and along their shafts — see DISTAL RADIOULNAR JOINT

radio wave *n* : an electromagnetic wave with radio frequency

ra·di·um \ˈrā-dē-əm\ *n, often attrib* : an intensely radioactive shining white metallic element that emits alpha particles and gamma rays to form radon and is used in the treatment of cancer — symbol *Ra;* see ELEMENT table

ra·di·us \ˈrā-dē-əs\ *n, pl* **ra·dii** \-dē-ˌī\ *also* **ra·di·us·es** : the bone on the thumb side of the forearm that is articulated with the ulna at both ends so as to permit partial rotation about that bone, that bears on its inner aspect somewhat distal to the head a prominence for the insertion of the biceps tendon, and that has the lower end broadened for articulation with the proximal bones of the carpus so that rotation of the radius involves also that of the hand

ra·don \ˈrā-dän\ *n* : a heavy radioactive gaseous element of the group of inert gases formed by disintegration of radium and used similarly to radium in medicine — symbol *Rn;* see ELEMENT table

rag·weed \ˈrag-ˌwēd\ *n* : any of various chiefly No. American weedy herbaceous plants comprising the genus *Ambrosia* and producing highly allergenic pollen: as **a** : a common annual (*A. artemisiifolia*) with finely divided foliage **b** : a coarse annual (*A. trifida*) with some or all of the leaves usu. deeply 3-cleft or 5-cleft — called also *great ragweed*

Rail·lie·ti·na \ˌrāl-yə-ˈtī-nə\ *n* : a large genus of tapeworms (family Davaineidae of the order Cyclophyllidea) that includes parasites esp. of birds and rodents

Rail·liet \rī-ˈyā\, **Louis–Joseph Alcide (1852–1930),** French veterinarian.

rain·bow \ˈrān-ˌbō\ *n, slang* : a combination of the sodium derivatives of amobarbital and secobarbital in a blue and red capsule

rale \ˈral, ˈräl\ *n* : an abnormal sound heard accompanying the normal respiratory sounds on auscultation of the chest — compare RATTLE, RHONCHUS

ral·ox·i·fene \ˌra-ˈläk-sə-ˌfēn\ *n* : a selective estrogen receptor modulator used orally in the form of its hydrochloride $C_{28}H_{27}NO_4S{\cdot}HCl$ to prevent and treat postmenopausal osteoporosis and to reduce the risk of developing invasive breast cancer — see EVISTA

ral·teg·ra·vir \ˌral-ˈteg-rə-ˌvir\ *n* : an antiretroviral drug $C_{20}H_{20}FKN_6O_5$ that inhibits an enzyme necessary for viral replication and is administered orally typically with other antiretroviral drugs in the treatment of HIV infection — see ISENTRESS

ram·i·fi·ca·tion \ˌra-mə-fə-ˈkā-shən\ *n* **1** : the act or process of branching; *specif* : the mode of arrangement of branches **2** : a branch or offshoot from a main stock or channel ⟨the ~ of an artery⟩; *also* : the resulting branched structure — **ram·i·fy** \ˈra-mə-ˌfī\ *vb*

ra·mip·ril \rə-ˈmi-prəl\ *n* : an ACE inhibitor $C_{23}H_{32}N_2O_5$ taken orally esp. to treat hypertension and congestive heart failure — see ALTACE

ra·mus \ˈrā-məs\ *n, pl* **ra·mi** \-ˌmī\ : a projecting part, elongated process, or branch: as **a** : the posterior more or less vertical part of the lower jaw on each side which articulates with the skull **b** (1) : the upper more cranial branch of the pubis that extends from the pubic symphysis to the body of the pubis at the acetabulum and forms the cranial part of the obturator foramen — called also *superior ramus* (2) : the thin flat lower branch of the pubis that extends from the pubic symphysis to unite with the ramus of the ischium in forming the inferior rim of the obturator foramen — called also *inferior ramus* **c** : a branch of the ischium that extends down and forward from the ischial tuberosity to unite with the inferior ramus of the pubis in forming the inferior rim of the obturator foramen — called also *inferior ramus* **d** : a branch of a nerve — see RAMUS COMMUNICANS

ramus com•mu•ni•cans \-kə-ˈmyü-nə-ˌkanz\ *n, pl* **rami com•mu•ni•can•tes** \-kə-ˌmyü-nə-ˈkan-ˌtēz\ : any of the bundles of nerve fibers connecting a sympathetic ganglion with a spinal nerve and being divided into two kinds: **a** : one consisting of myelinated preganglionic fibers — called also *white ramus, white ramus communicans* **b** : one consisting of unmyelinated postganglionic fibers — called also *gray ramus*

ran *past of* RUN

randomized controlled trial *n* : a clinical trial in which the subjects are randomly distributed into groups which are either subjected to the experimental procedure (as use of a drug) or which serve as controls — called also *randomized clinical trial*

Ra•nexa \ra-ˈnek-sə\ *trademark* — used for a preparation of ranolazine

rang *past of* RING

ran•i•biz•u•mab \ˌra-nə-ˈbi-zü-ˌmab\ *n* : an antiangiogenic drug that is a genetically engineered monoclonal antibody administered by injection into the eye esp. to treat age-related macular degeneration and diabetic retinopathy — see LUCENTIS

ra•nit•i•dine \ra-ˈni-tə-ˌdēn\ *n* : an antihistamine used in the form of its hydrochloride $C_{13}H_{22}N_4O_3S{\cdot}HCl$ to inhibit gastric acid secretion (as in the treatment of duodenal ulcers or Zollinger-Ellison syndrome) — see ZANTAC

ra•no•la•zine \rə-ˈnō-lə-ˌzēn\ *n* : a drug $C_{24}H_{33}N_3O_4$ taken orally in the treatment of angina pectoris — see RANEXA

ran•u•la \ˈran-yə-lə\ *n* : a cyst formed under the tongue by obstruction of a gland duct

Rap•a•mune \ˈrap-ə-ˌmyün\ *trademark* — used for a preparation of sirolimus

rap•a•my•cin \ˌra-pə-ˈmī-sᵊn\ *n* : SIROLIMUS

rape \ˈrāp\ *n* : unlawful sexual activity and usu. sexual intercourse carried out forcibly or under threat of injury against the will usu. of a female or with a person who is beneath a certain age or incapable of valid consent — compare SEXUAL ASSAULT, STATUTORY RAPE — **rape** *vb*

ra•phe \ˈrā-fē\ *n* : the seamlike union of the two lateral halves of a part or organ (as of the tongue, perineum, or scrotum) having externally a ridge or furrow and internally usu. a fibrous connective tissue septum

raphe nucleus *n* : any of several groups of nerve cells situated along or near the median plane of the tegmentum of the midbrain

rapid eye movement *n* : a rapid movement of the eyes associated esp. with REM sleep — called also *REM*

rapid eye movement sleep *n* : REM SLEEP

rapid plasma reagin test *n* : a flocculation test for syphilis employing the antigen used in the VDRL test with charcoal particles added so that the flocculation can be seen without the aid of a microscope — called also *RPR card test*

rap•port \ra-ˈpȯr, rə-\ *n* : harmonious accord or relation that fosters cooperation, communication, or trust ⟨~ between a patient and psychotherapist⟩

rapture of the deep *n* : NITROGEN NARCOSIS

rap•tus \ˈrap-təs\ *n* : a pathological paroxysm of activity giving vent to impulse or tension (as in an act of violence)

rar•efy *also* **rar•i•fy** \ˈrar-ə-ˌfī\ *vb* **-efied** *also* **-i•fied; -efy•ing** *also* **-i•fy•ing** : to make or become rare, thin, porous, or less dense : to expand without the addition of matter — **rar•efac•tion** \ˌrar-ə-ˈfak-shən\ *n*

ras \ˈras\ *n, often attrib* [*ra*t *s*arcoma] : any of a family of genes that undergo mutation to oncogenes and esp. to some commonly linked to human cancers (as of the colon, lung, and pancreas) ⟨~ oncogenes⟩

rash \ˈrash\ *n* : an eruption on the body typically with little or no elevation above the surface

RAST *abbr* radioallergosorbent test

rat \ˈrat\ *n* : any of the numerous rodents (family Muridae) of *Rattus* and related genera that include forms (as the brown rat and the black rat) which live in and about human habitations and are destructive pests and vectors of various diseases (as bubonic plague)

rat–bite fever *n* : either of two febrile human diseases usu. transmitted by the bite of a rat: **a** : a disease that is marked by irregular relapsing fever with chills and nausea or vomiting, rashes on the arms, legs, hands, and feet, and muscular pain and arthritis and that is caused by a bacterium of the genus *Streptobacillus* (*S. moniliformis*) **b** : a disease that is marked by recurrent fever and chills, inflammation of the bite wound, and muscular pain, rash, and enlargement of the lymph nodes esp. in the region where the bite occurred and that is caused by a bacterium of the genus *Spirillum* (*S. minor* syn. *S. minus*) — called also *sodoku*

rate \ˈrāt\ *n* **1** : a fixed ratio between two things **2** : a quantity, amount, or degree of something measured per unit of something else — see DEATH RATE, HEART RATE, METABOLIC RATE, PULSE RATE, SEDIMENTATION RATE

rat flea *n* : any of various fleas that occur on rats: as **a** : NORTHERN RAT FLEA **b** : ORIENTAL RAT FLEA

Rath·ke's pouch \ˈrät-kəz-\ *n* : a pouch of ectoderm that grows out from the upper surface of the embryonic stomodeum and gives rise to the adenohypophysis of the pituitary gland — called also *Rathke's pocket*

Rathke, Martin Heinrich (1793–1860), German anatomist.

rat·i·cide \ˈra-tə-ˌsīd\ *n* : a substance used to kill rats

ra·tio \ˈrā-(ˌ)shō, -shē-ˌō\ *n, pl* **ra·tios** : the relationship in quantity, amount, or size between two or more things — see SEX RATIO

ra·tion \ˈra-shən, ˈrā-\ *n* : a food allowance for one day — **ration** *vb*

ra·tio·nal–emo·tive therapy \ˈra-shə-nᵊl-i-ˈmō-tiv-\ *n* : cognitive therapy based on a theory of Albert Ellis that a patient can be taught to effect emotional well-being by changing negative and irrational thoughts to positive and rational ones

ra·tio·nal·ize \ˈra-shə-nə-ˌlīz\ *vb* **-ized; -iz·ing** : to attribute (one's actions) to rational and creditable motives without analysis of true and esp. unconscious motives; *also* : to provide plausible but untrue reasons for conduct — **ra·tio·nal·i·za·tion** \ˌra-shə-nə-lə-ˈzā-shən\ *n*

rational therapy *n* : RATIONAL-EMOTIVE THERAPY

rat louse *n* : a sucking louse (*Polyplax spinulosa*) that is a parasite of rats and transmits murine typhus from rat to rat

rat mite *n* : a mite (*Ornithonyssus bacoti*) that feeds on rodents but may cause dermatitis in and transmit typhus to humans

rat·tle \ˈrat-ᵊl\ *n* : a throat noise caused by air passing through mucus; *specif* : DEATH RATTLE — compare RALE, RHONCHUS

rat·tle·box \-ˌbäks\ *n* : CROTALARIA 2; *esp* : one (*Crotalaria spectabilis*) that is highly toxic to farm animals

rat·tle·snake \-ˌsnāk\ *n* : any of the American pit vipers that have a series of horny interlocking joints at the end of the tail which make a sharp rattling sound when vibrated and that comprise the genera *Sistrurus* and *Crotalus* — see DIAMONDBACK RATTLESNAKE, TIGER RATTLESNAKE, TIMBER RATTLESNAKE

Rat·tus \ˈra-təs\ *n* : a genus of rodents (family Muridae) that comprise the common rats

Rau·dix·in \rau̇-ˈdiks-ən, rȯ-\ *trademark* — used for a preparation of reserpine

rau·wol·fia \rau̇-ˈwu̇l-fē-ə, rȯ-\ *n* **1** : any of a genus (*Rauvolfia* syn. *Rauwolfia*) of tropical trees and shrubs of the dogbane family (Apocynaceae) that yield medicinal alkaloids (as reserpine) **2** : the dried root or an extract from the root of a rauwolfia (esp. *Rauvolfia serpentina* of Asia) used chiefly in the treatment of hypertension

Rauwolf, Leonhard (1535–1596), German botanist.

ray·less goldenrod \ˈrā-ləs-\ *n* : a shrubby or herbaceous plant (*Haplopappus heterophyllus* syn. *Isocoma wrightii* of the family Compositae) that causes trembles in cattle

Ray·naud's disease \rā-ˈnōz-\ *n* : a vascular disorder marked by recurrent spasm of the capillaries and esp. those of the fingers and toes upon exposure to cold, characterized by pallor, cyanosis and redness in succession, usu. accompanied by pain, and in severe cases progressing to local gangrene — called also *Raynaud's*

Raynaud, Maurice (1834–1881), French physician.

Raynaud's phenomenon *n* : the symptoms associated with Raynaud's disease — called also *Raynaud's syndrome*

Rb *symbol* rubidium

RBC *abbr* **1** red blood cells **2** red blood count

RBE *abbr* relative biological effectiveness

rBGH *abbr* recombinant bovine growth hormone

RBRVS *abbr* resource-based relative value scale

rBST *abbr* recombinant bovine somatotropin

RCT *abbr* randomized clinical trial; randomized controlled trial

rd *abbr* rutherford

RD *abbr* registered dietitian

RDA *abbr* recommended daily allowance; recommended dietary allowance

RDH *abbr* registered dental hygienist

RDS *abbr* respiratory distress syndrome

Re *symbol* rhenium

re·ab·sorb \ˌrē-əb-ˈsȯrb, -ˈzȯrb\ *vb* : to take up (something previously secreted or emitted) ⟨sugars ~*ed* in the kidney⟩; *also* : RESORB — **re·ab·sorp·tion** \-ˈsȯrp-shən, -ˈzȯrp-\ *n*

re·act \rē-ˈakt\ *vb* **1** : to respond to a stimulus **2** : to undergo or cause to undergo chemical reaction

re·ac·tion \rē-ˈak-shən\ *n* **1** : the act or process or an instance of reacting **2** : bodily response to or activity aroused by a stimulus: **a** : an action induced by vital resistance to another action; *esp* : the response of tissues to a foreign substance (as an antigen or infective agent) **b** : depression or exhaustion due to excessive exertion or stimulation **c** : abnormally heightened activity succeeding depression or shock **d** : a mental or emotional disorder forming an individual's response to his or her life situation **3 a** (1) : chemical transformation or change : the interaction of chemical entities (2) : the state resulting from such a reaction **b** : a process involving change in atomic nuclei

reaction formation *n* : a psychological defense mechanism in which one form of behavior substitutes for or conceals a diametrically opposed repressed impulse in order to protect against it

reaction time *n* : the time elapsing between the beginning of the application of a stimulus and the beginning of an organism's reaction to it

re•ac•ti•vate \rē-ˈak-tə-ˌvāt\ *vb* **-vat•ed; -vat•ing** : to cause to be again active or more active: as **a** : to cause (as a repressed complex) to reappear in consciousness or behavior **b** : to cause (a quiescent disease) to become active again in an individual — **re•ac•ti•va•tion** \-ˌak-tə-ˈvā-shən\ *n*

re•ac•tive \rē-ˈak-tiv\ *adj* **1 a** : of, relating to, or marked by reaction ⟨~ symptoms⟩ **b** : capable of reacting chemically **2 a** : readily responsive to a stimulus **b** : occurring as a result of stress or emotional upset esp. from factors outside the organism ⟨~ depression⟩ — **re•ac•tiv•i•ty** \rē-ˌak-ˈti-və-tē\ *n*

reactive arthritis *n* : acute arthritis that sometimes develops following a bacterial infection (as with the bacteria of the genera *Shigella, Salmonella,* or *Chlamydia*) and may be accompanied by conjunctivitis or urethritis

reactive attachment disorder *n* : ATTACHMENT DISORDER

re•ac•tor \rē-ˈak-tər\ *n* **1** : one that reacts: as **a** : a chemical reagent **b** : an individual reacting to a stimulus **c** : an individual reacting positively to a foreign substance (as in a test for disease) **2** : a device for the controlled release of nuclear energy

re•agent \rē-ˈā-jənt\ *n* : a substance used (as in detecting a component or in preparing a product) because of its chemical or biological activity

re•agin \rē-ˈā-jən, -gən\ *n* **1** : a substance that is in the blood of individuals with syphilis and is responsible for positive serological reactions for syphilis **2** : an antibody (as IgE in humans) that mediates hypersensitive allergic reactions of rapid onset — **re•agin•ic** \ˌrē-ə-ˈji-nik, -ˈgi-\ *adj*

reality principle *n* : the tendency to defer immediate instinctual gratification so as to achieve longer-range goals or so as to meet external demands — compare PLEASURE PRINCIPLE

reality testing *n* : the psychological process in which acts are explored and their outcomes determined so that the individual will be aware of these consequences when the stimulus to act in a given fashion recurs

ream•er \ˈrē-mər\ *n* : an instrument used in dentistry to enlarge and clean out a root canal

re•am•pu•ta•tion \ˌrē-ˌam-pyə-ˈtā-shən\ *n* : the second of two amputations performed upon the same member

re•anas•to•mo•sis \ˌrē-ə-ˌnas-tə-ˈmō-səs\ *n, pl* **-mo•ses** \-ˌsēz\ : the reuniting (as by surgery or healing) of a divided vessel

re•at•tach \ˌrē-ə-ˈtach\ *vb* : to attach again ⟨~ a severed finger⟩ — **re•at•tach•ment** \-mənt\ *n*

re•base \rē-ˈbās\ *vb* **re•based; re•bas•ing** : to modify the base of (a denture) after an initial period of wear in order to produce a good fit

re•bleed \ˈrē-ˌblēd\ *vb* **re•bled** \-ˌbled\; **re•bleed•ing 1** : to bleed or hemorrhage again ⟨identify patients at risk of ~*ing*⟩ **2** *of a hemorrhage* : to occur again — **rebleed** *n*

re•bound \ˈrē-ˌbau̇nd, ri-ˈ\ *n* : a return to a previous state or condition following removal of a stimulus or cessation of treatment

rebound tenderness *n* : a sensation of pain felt when pressure (as to the abdomen) is suddenly removed

re•breathe \ˌrē-ˈbrēth\ *vb* **re•breathed; re•breath•ing 1** : to breathe (as reconstituted air) again **2** : to inhale previously exhaled air or gases

re•cal•ci•fi•ca•tion \ˌrē-ˌkal-sə-fə-ˈkā-shən\ *n* : the restoration of calcium or calcium compounds to decalcified tissue (as bone or blood) — **re•cal•ci•fied** \-ˈkal-sə-ˌfīd\ *adj*

recalcification time *n* : a measure of the time taken for clot formation in recalcified blood

re•cal•ci•trant \ri-ˈkal-sə-trənt\ *adj* : not responsive to treatment ⟨~ warts⟩

re•call \ri-ˈkȯl, ˈrē-ˌ\ *n* : remembrance of what has been previously learned or experienced — **re•call** \ri-ˈkȯl\ *vb*

re•can•a•li•za•tion \ˌrē-ˌkan-ᵊl-ə-ˈzā-shən\ *n* : the process of restoring flow to or reuniting an interrupted channel of a bodily tube (as an artery or vas deferens) — **re•can•a•lize** \-kə-ˈna-ˌlīz, -ˈkan-ᵊl-ˌīz\ *vb*

re•cep•tive \ri-ˈsep-tiv\ *adj* **1** : open and responsive to ideas, impressions, or suggestions **2 a** *of a sensory end organ* : fit to receive and transmit stimuli **b** : SENSORY 1 — **re•cep•tive•ness** *n* — **re•cep•tiv•i•ty** \ˌrē-ˌsep-ˈti-və-tē, ri-\ *n*

re•cep•tor \ri-ˈsep-tər\ *n* **1** : a cell or group of cells that receives stimuli : SENSE ORGAN **2** : a chemical group or molecule (as a protein) on the cell surface or in the cell interior that has an affinity for a specific chemical group, molecule, or virus **3 :** a cellular entity (as a beta-receptor) that is a postulated intermediary between a chemical agent (as a neurohormone) acting on nervous tissue and the physiological or pharmacological response

re•cess \ˈrē-ˌses, ri-ˈ\ *n* **:** an anatomical depression or cleft **:** FOSSA

re•ces•sion \ri-ˈse-shən\ *n* **:** pathological withdrawal of tissue from its normal position ⟨advanced gum ~⟩

[1]**re•ces•sive** \ri-ˈse-siv\ *adj* **1 :** producing little or no phenotypic effect when occurring in heterozygous condition with a contrasting allele ⟨~ genes⟩ **2 :** expressed only when the determining gene is in the homozygous condition ⟨~ traits⟩ — **re•ces•sive•ly** *adv* — **re•ces•sive•ness** *n*

[2]**recessive** *n* **1 :** a recessive character or gene **2 :** an organism possessing one or more recessive characters

re•cid•i•vism \ri-ˈsi-də-ˌvi-zəm\ *n* **:** a tendency to relapse into a previous condition or mode of behavior ⟨~ among former cigarette smokers⟩ — **re•cid•i•vist** \-vist\ *n*

re•cip•i•ent \ri-ˈsi-pē-ənt\ *n* **:** one who receives biological material (as blood or an organ) from a donor

reciprocal inhibition *n* **1 :** RECIPROCAL INNERVATION **2 :** behavior therapy in which the patient is exposed to anxiety-producing stimuli while in a controlled state of relaxation so that the anxiety response is gradually inhibited

reciprocal innervation *n* **:** innervation so that the contraction of a muscle or set of muscles (as of a joint) is accompanied by the simultaneous inhibition of an antagonistic muscle or set of muscles

reciprocal translocation *n* **:** exchange of parts between nonhomologous chromosomes

Reck•ling•hau•sen's disease \ˈre-kliŋ-ˌhau̇-zənz-\ *n* **:** NEUROFIBROMATOSIS 1

Recklinghausen, Friedrich Daniel von (1833–1910), German pathologist.

rec•og•ni•tion \ˌre-kəg-ˈni-shən\ *n* **:** the form of memory that consists in knowing or feeling that a present object has been met before

[1]**re•com•bi•nant** \ˌrē-ˈkäm-bə-nənt\ *adj* **1 :** relating to or exhibiting genetic recombination **2 a :** relating to or containing genetically engineered DNA **b :** produced by genetic engineering ⟨~ bovine growth hormone⟩

[2]**recombinant** *n* **:** an individual exhibiting recombination

recombinant DNA *n* **:** genetically engineered DNA usu. incorporating DNA from more than one species of organism

re•com•bi•na•tion \ˌrē-ˌkäm-bə-ˈnā-shən\ *n* **:** the formation by the processes of crossing-over and independent assortment of new combinations of genes in progeny that did not occur in the parents — **re•com•bi•na•tion•al** *adj*

recommended daily allowance *n, often cap R&D&A* **:** the amount of a nutriment (as a vitamin or mineral) that is recommended for daily consumption by the Food and Nutrition Board of the National Academy of Sciences — abbr. *RDA;* called also *recommended dietary allowance*

re•com•pres•sion \ˌrē-kəm-ˈpre-shən\ *n* **:** a renewed heightening of atmospheric pressure esp. as treatment for decompression sickness

re•con•sti•tute \rē-ˈkän-stə-ˌtüt, -ˌtyüt\ *vb* **-tut•ed; -tut•ing :** to constitute again or anew; *esp* **:** to restore to a former condition by adding liquid ⟨*reconstituted* blood⟩ — **re•con•sti•tu•tion** \-ˌkän-stə-ˈtü-shən, -ˈtyü-\ *n*

re•con•struc•tion \ˌrē-kən-ˈstrək-shən\ *n* **:** repair of an organ or part by reconstructive surgery ⟨breast ~⟩ — **re•con•struct** \ˌrē-kən-ˈstrəkt\ *vb* — **re•con•struc•tive** \-ˈstrək-tiv\ *adj*

reconstructive surgery *n* **:** surgery to restore function or normal appearance by remaking defective organs or parts

re•cov•er \ri-ˈkə-vər\ *vb* **re•cov•ered; re•cov•er•ing :** to regain a normal position or condition (as of health) — **re•cov•er•able** \ri-ˈkə-və-rə-bəl\ *adj*

recovered memory *n* **:** a forgotten memory of a traumatic event (as sexual abuse) experienced typically during childhood and recalled many years later that is sometimes held to be an invalid or false remembrance generated by outside influence

re•cov•ery \ri-ˈkə-və-rē\ *n, pl* **-er•ies :** the act of regaining or returning toward a normal or healthy state

recovery room *n* **:** a hospital room which is equipped with apparatus for meeting postoperative emergencies and in which surgical patients are kept during the immediate postoperative period for care and recovery from anesthesia — abbr. *RR*

rec•re•a•tion•al drug \ˌre-krē-ˈā-shə-nəl-\ *n* **:** a drug (as cocaine, marijuana, or methamphetamine) used without medical justification for its psychoactive effects often in the belief that occasional use of such a substance is not habit-forming or addictive

recreational therapy *n* **:** therapy based on engagement in recreational activities (as sports or music) esp. to enhance the functioning, independence, and well-being of individuals affected with a disabling condition — **recreational therapist** *n*

re•cru•des•cence \ˌrē-krü-ˈdes-ᵊns\ *n* **:** increased severity of a disease after a remission; *also* **:** recurrence of a disease after a brief intermission — **re·cru·desce** \ˌrē-krü-ˈdes\ *vb* — **re·cru·des·cent** \-ˈdes-ᵊnt\ *adj*

re·cruit·ment \ri-ˈkrüt-mənt\ *n* **1** : the increase in intensity of a reflex when the initiating stimulus is prolonged without alteration of intensity due to the activation of increasing numbers of motor neurons **2** : an abnormally rapid increase in the sensation of loudness with increasing sound intensity that occurs in deafness of neural origin

rect- *or* **recto-** *comb form* **1** : rectum ⟨*rect*al⟩ **2** : rectal and ⟨*recto*vaginal⟩

recta *pl of* RECTUM

recta — see VASA RECTA

rec·tal \ˈrekt-ᵊl\ *adj* : relating to, affecting, or being near the rectum ⟨~ bleeding⟩ — **rec·tal·ly** *adv*

rectal artery *n* : any of three arteries supplying esp. the rectum: **a** : one arising from the internal pudendal artery and supplying the lower part of the rectum and the perineal region — called also *inferior hemorrhoidal artery, inferior rectal artery* **b** : one arising from the internal iliac artery and supplying the middle part of the rectum — called also *middle hemorrhoidal artery, middle rectal artery* **c** : one that is a continuation of the inferior mesenteric artery and that supplies the upper part of the rectum — called also *superior hemorrhoidal artery, superior rectal artery*

rectal vein *n* : any of three veins that receive blood from the rectal venous plexus: **a** : one draining the lower part of the rectal venous plexus and emptying into the internal pudendal vein — called also *inferior hemorrhoidal vein, inferior rectal vein* **b** : one draining the bladder, prostate, and seminal vesicle by way of the middle part of the rectal venous plexus and emptying into the internal iliac vein — called also *middle hemorrhoidal vein, middle rectal vein* **c** : one draining the upper part of the rectal venous plexus and forming the first part of the inferior mesenteric vein — called also *superior hemorrhoidal vein, superior rectal vein*

rectal venous plexus *n* : a plexus of veins that surrounds the rectum and empties esp. into the rectal veins — called also *rectal plexus*

recti *pl of* RECTUS

recto- — see RECT-

rec·to·cele \ˈrek-tə-ˌsēl\ *n* : herniation of the rectum through a defect in the intervening fascia into the vagina

rec·to·sig·moid \ˌrek-tō-ˈsig-ˌmȯid\ *n* : the distal part of the sigmoid colon and the proximal part of the rectum

rec·to·uter·ine pouch \ˌrek-tō-ˈyü-tə-ˌrīn-, -rən-\ *n* : a sac between the rectum and the uterus that is formed by a folding of the peritoneum — compare RECTOVESICAL POUCH

rec·to·vag·i·nal \-ˈvaj-ən-ᵊl\ *adj* : of, relating to, or connecting the rectum and the vagina ⟨a ~ fistula⟩

rec·to·ves·i·cal fascia \ˌrek-tō-ˈve-si-kəl-\ *n* : a membrane derived from the pelvic fascia and investing the rectum, bladder, and adjacent parts

rectovesical pouch *n* : a sac between the rectum and the urinary bladder in males that is formed by a folding of the peritoneum — compare RECTOUTERINE POUCH

rec·tum \ˈrek-təm\ *n, pl* **rectums** *or* **rec·ta** \-tə\ : the terminal part of the intestine from the sigmoid colon to the anus

rec·tus \ˈrek-təs\ *n, pl* **rec·ti** \-ˌtī\ **1** : any of several straight muscles (as the rectus femoris) **2** : any of four extraocular muscles of the eyeball that arise from the border of the optic foramen and run forward to insert into the sclera of the eyeball: **a** : one that inserts into the superior aspect of the sclera — called also *rectus superior, superior rectus* **b** : one that inserts into the lateral aspect of the sclera — called also *lateral rectus, rectus lateralis* **c** : one that inserts into the medial aspect of the sclera — called also *medial rectus, rectus medialis* **d** : one that inserts into the inferior aspect of the sclera — called also *inferior rectus, rectus inferior*

rectus ab·do·mi·nis \-ab-ˈdä-mə-nəs\ *n* : a long flat muscle on either side of the linea alba extending along the whole length of the front of the abdomen, arising from the pubic crest and symphysis, inserted into the cartilages of the fifth, sixth, and seventh ribs, and acting to flex the spinal column, tense the anterior wall of the abdomen, and assist in compressing the contents of the abdomen

rectus ca·pi·tis posterior major \-ˈka-pə-təs-\ *n* : a muscle on each side of the back of the neck that arises from the spinous process of the axis, inserts into the lateral aspect of the inferior nuchal line and the adjacent inferior area of the occipital bone, and acts to extend and rotate the head

rectus capitis posterior minor *n* : a muscle on each side of the back of the neck that arises from the posterior arch of the atlas, inserts esp. into the medial aspect of the inferior nuchal line, and acts to extend the head

rectus fe·mo·ris \-ˈfe-mə-rəs\ *n* : a division of the quadriceps muscle lying in the anterior middle region of the thigh, arising from the ilium by two heads, inserted into the tuberosity of the tibia by a narrow flattened tendon, and acting to flex the thigh at the hip and with the rest of the quadriceps to extend the leg at the knee

rectus inferior *n* : RECTUS 2d

rectus lat·e·ra·lis \-ˌla-tə-ˈrā-ləs, -ˈra-\ *n* : RECTUS 2b

rectus me•di•a•lis \-ˌmē-dē-ˈā-ləs, -ˈa-\ *n* : RECTUS 2c
rectus oc•u•li \-ˈä-kyu̇-ˌlī, -ˌlē\ *n* : RECTUS 2
rectus superior *n* : RECTUS 2a
re•cum•bent \ri-ˈkəm-bənt\ *adj* : lying down ⟨a patient ~ on a stretcher⟩ — **re•cum•ben•cy** \-bən-sē\ *n*
re•cu•per•a•tion \rē-ˌkü-pə-ˈrā-shən, -ˌkyü-\ *n* : restoration to health or strength — **re•cu•per•ate** \ri-ˈkü-pə-ˌrāt\ *vb*
re•cu•per•a•tive \-ˈkü-pə-ˌrā-tiv, -ˈkyü-\ *adj* **1** : of or relating to recuperation ⟨~ powers⟩ **2** : aiding in recuperation : RESTORATIVE
re•cur•rence \ri-ˈkər-əns\ *n* **1** : return of symptoms of a disease after a remission **2** : reappearance of a tumor after previous removal — **re•cur** \ri-ˈkər\ *vb*
re•cur•rent \-ˈkər-ənt\ *adj* **1** : running or turning back in a direction opposite to a former course — used of various nerves and branches of vessels in the arms and legs **2** : returning or happening time after time ⟨~ pain⟩ — **re•cur•rent•ly** *adv*
recurrent fever *n* : RELAPSING FEVER
recurrent laryngeal nerve *n* : LARYNGEAL NERVE b — called also *recurrent laryngeal*
red alga \ˈred-\ *n* : any of a division (Rhodophyta) of chiefly marine algae with mostly red pigmentation
red–blind *adj* : affected with protanopia
red blindness *n* : PROTANOPIA
red blood cell *n* : any of the hemoglobin-containing cells that carry oxygen to the tissues and are responsible for the red color of blood — called also *erythrocyte, red blood corpuscle, red cell, red corpuscle;* compare WHITE BLOOD CELL
red blood count *n* : a blood count of the red blood cells — abbr. *RBC*
red bone marrow *n* : BONE MARROW b
red bug \-ˌbəg\ *n, Southern & Midland* : CHIGGER 2
red cell *n* : RED BLOOD CELL
red corpuscle *n* : RED BLOOD CELL
red devils *n pl, slang* : REDS
red–green color blindness *n* : deficiency of color vision ranging from imperfect perception of red and green to an ability to see only tones of yellow, blue, and gray — called also *red-green blindness*
re•dia \ˈrē-dē-ə\ *n, pl* **re•di•ae** \-dē-ˌē\ *also* **re•di•as** : a larva produced within the sporocyst of many trematodes that produces another generation of larvae like itself or develops into a cercaria — **re•di•al** \-dē-əl\ *adj*
red•in•te•gra•tion \ri-ˌdin-tə-ˈgrā-shən, re-\ *n* **1** : revival of the whole of a previous mental state when a phase of it recurs **2** : arousal of any response by a part of the complex of stimuli that orig. aroused that response — **red•in•te•gra•tive** \-ˈdin-tə-ˌgrā-tiv\ *adj*
red marrow *n* : BONE MARROW b
red nucleus *n* : a nucleus of gray matter in the tegmentum of the midbrain on each side of the middle line that receives fibers from the cerebellum of the opposite side by way of the superior cerebellar peduncle and gives rise to fibers of the rubrospinal tract of the opposite side
red•out \ˈred-ˌau̇t\ *n* : a condition in which centripetal acceleration (as that created when an aircraft abruptly enters a dive) drives blood to the head and causes reddening of the visual field and headache — compare BLACKOUT, GRAYOUT
re•dox \ˈrē-ˌdäks\ *n* : OXIDATION-REDUCTION — **redox** *adj*
red pulp *n* : a parenchymatous tissue of the spleen that consists of loose plates or cords infiltrated with red blood cells — compare WHITE PULP
reds *n pl, slang* : red drug capsules containing the sodium salt of secobarbital — called also *red devils*
red tide *n* : seawater discolored by the presence of large numbers of dinoflagellates (as of the genera *Karenia, Gymnodinium,* and *Alexandrium*) which typically produce toxins poisonous esp. to many forms of vertebrate marine life and to humans who consume contaminated shellfish — see BREVETOXIN, SAXITOXIN
re•duce \ri-ˈdüs, -ˈdyüs\ *vb* **re•duced; re•duc•ing** **1** : to correct (as a fracture or a herniated mass) by bringing displaced or broken parts back into their normal positions **2 a** : to combine with or subject to the action of hydrogen **b** (1) : to change (an element or ion) from a higher to a lower oxidation state (2) : to add one or more electrons to (an atom or ion or molecule) **3** : to lose weight by dieting — **re•duc•ible** \-ˈdü-sə-bəl, -ˈdyü-\ *adj*
reducing *adj* : causing or facilitating reduction
reducing agent *n* : a substance (as hydrogen) that donates electrons or a share in its electrons to another substance — compare OXIDIZING AGENT
reducing sugar *n* : a sugar (as glucose or lactose) that is capable of reducing a mild oxidizing agent (as Fehling solution) — see BENEDICT'S TEST
re•duc•tase \ri-ˈdək-ˌtās, -ˌtāz\ *n* : an enzyme that catalyzes chemical reduction
re•duc•tion \ri-ˈdək-shən\ *n* **1** : the replacement or realignment of a body part in normal position or restoration of a bodily condition to normal **2** : the process of reducing by chemical or electrochemical means **3** : MEIOSIS; *specif* : production of the gametic chromosome number in the first meiotic division
reduction division *n* : the usu. first division of meiosis in which chromosome reduction occurs; *also* : MEIOSIS

re·dun·dant \ri-ˈdən-dənt\ *adj* : characterized by or containing an excess or superfluous amount

re·du·pli·ca·tion \ri-ˌdü-pli-ˈkā-shən, ˌrē-, -ˌdyü-\ *n* : an act or instance of doubling ⟨∼ of the chromosomes⟩

red water *n* : any of several cattle diseases characterized by hematuria; *esp* : any of several babesioses (as Texas fever) in which hemoglobin released by the destruction of red blood cells appears in the urine

red worm *n* : BLOODWORM

Reed–Stern·berg cell \ˈrēd-ˈstərn-bərg-\ *n* : a binucleate or multinucleate acidophilic giant cell of B cell origin found in the tissues in Hodgkin's lymphoma

Reed, Dorothy (1874–1964), American pathologist.

Sternberg, Carl (1872–1935), Austrian pathologist.

re·ed·u·ca·tion \ˌrē-ˌe-jə-ˈkā-shən\ *n* **1** : training in the use of muscles in new functions or of prosthetic devices in old functions in order to replace or restore lost functions ⟨neuromuscular ∼⟩ **2** : training to develop new behaviors (as habits) to replace others that are considered undesirable — **re·ed·u·cate** \-ˈe-jə-ˌkāt\ *vb*

reef·er \ˈrē-fər\ *n* : a marijuana cigarette; *also* : MARIJUANA 2

re·en·try \ˌrē-ˈen-trē\ *n, pl* **-tries** : a cardiac mechanism that is held to explain certain abnormal heart actions (as tachycardia) and that involves the transmission of a wave of depolarization along an alternate pathway when the original pathway is blocked with return of the impulse along the blocked pathway when the alternate pathway is refractory and then transmission along the open pathway resulting in an abnormality

re·ep·i·the·li·al·i·za·tion \ˌrē-ˌe-pə-ˌthē-lē-ə-li-ˈzā-shən\ *n* : restoration of epithelium over a denuded area (as a burn site) by natural growth or plastic surgery

re·fer \ri-ˈfər\ *vb* **re·ferred; re·fer·ring 1** : to regard as coming from or localized in a certain portion of the body or of space **2** : to send or direct for diagnosis or treatment

re·fer·able *also* **re·fer·rable** \ˈre-fə-rə-bəl, ri-ˈfər-ə-\ *adj* : capable of being considered in relation to something else ⟨complaints ∼ to the upper left abdominal quadrant⟩

ref·er·ence \ˈre-frəns, -fə-rəns\ *adj* : of known potency and used as a standard in the biological assay of a sample of the same drug of unknown strength

reference — see IDEA OF REFERENCE

re·fer·ral \ri-ˈfər-əl\ *n* **1** : the process of directing or redirecting (as a medical case or a patient) to an appropriate specialist or agency for definitive treatment **2** : one that is referred

referred pain *n* : a pain subjectively localized in one region though due to irritation in another region

[1]**re·fill** \ˌrē-ˈfil\ *vb* : to fill (a prescription) a second or subsequent time — **re·fill·able** *adj*

[2]**re·fill** \ˈrē-ˌfil\ *n* : a prescription compounded and dispensed for a second or subsequent time without an order from the physician

re·flect \ri-ˈflekt\ *vb* **1** : to bend or fold back : impart a backward curve, bend, or fold to **2** : to push or lay aside (as tissue or an organ) during surgery in order to gain access to the part to be operated on **3** : to throw back light or sound — **re·flec·tion** \ri-ˈflek-shən\ *n*

[1]**re·flex** \ˈrē-ˌfleks\ *n* **1** : an automatic and often inborn response to a stimulus that involves a nerve impulse passing inward from a receptor to the spinal cord and thence outward to an effector (as a muscle or gland) without reaching the level of consciousness and often without passing to the brain ⟨the knee-jerk ∼⟩ **2** : the process that culminates in a reflex and comprises reception, transmission, and reaction **3 reflexes** *pl* : the power of acting or responding with adequate speed

[2]**reflex** *adj* **1** : bent, turned, or directed back : REFLECTED **2** : of, relating to, or produced by a reflex without intervention of consciousness

reflex arc *n* : the complete nervous path that is involved in a reflex

re·flex·ion *Brit var of* REFLECTION

re·flex·ive \ri-ˈflek-siv\ *adj* : characterized by habitual and unthinking behavior; *also* : relating to or consisting of a reflex

re·flex·ly *adv* : in a reflex manner : by means of reflexes

re·flexo·gen·ic \ri-ˌflek-sə-ˈje-nik\ *adj* **1** : causing or being the point of origin of reflexes ⟨a ∼ zone⟩ **2** : originating reflexly

re·flex·ol·o·gy \ˌrē-ˌflek-ˈsä-lə-jē\ *n, pl* **-gies 1** : the study and interpretation of behavior in terms of simple and complex reflexes **2** : massage of the feet or hands based on the belief that pressure applied to specific points on these extremities benefits other parts of the body — **re·flex·ol·o·gist** \-jist\ *n*

reflex sympathetic dystrophy *n* : a painful disorder that usu. follows a localized injury, that is marked by burning pain, swelling, and motor and sensory disturbances esp. of an extremity, and that is often considered a type of regional pain syndrome in which peripheral nerve injury has not been identified — abbr. *RSD;* see SHOULDER-HAND SYNDROME

re·flux \ˈrē-ˌfləks\ *n* **1** : a flowing back : REGURGITATION ⟨∼ of gastric acid⟩ ⟨mitral valve ∼⟩ **2** : GASTROESOPHAGEAL REFLUX — **reflux** *adj* — **reflux** *vb*

re·frac·tile \ri-ˈfrak-təl, -ˌtīl\ *adj* : REFRACTIVE ⟨~ cells⟩

re·frac·tion \ri-ˈfrak-shən\ *n* **1** : the deflection from a straight path undergone by a light ray or a wave of energy in passing obliquely from one medium (as air) into another (as glass) in which its velocity is different **2 a** : the refractive power of the eye **b** : the act or technique of determining ocular refraction and identifying abnormalities as a basis for the prescription of corrective lenses — **re·fract** \ri-ˈfrakt\ *vb*

re·frac·tion·ist \-shə-nist\ *n* : a person (as an optometrist) skilled esp. in the determination of errors of refraction in the eye

re·frac·tive \ri-ˈfrak-tiv\ *adj* **1** : having power to refract ⟨a ~ lens⟩ **2** : relating to or due to refraction — **re·frac·tive·ly** *adv*

refractive index *n* : INDEX OF REFRACTION

re·frac·to·ri·ness \ri-ˈfrak-tə-rē-nəs\ *n* : the insensitivity to further immediate stimulation that develops in irritable and esp. nervous tissue as a result of intense or prolonged stimulation

re·frac·to·ry \ri-ˈfrak-tə-rē\ *adj* **1** : resistant to treatment or cure ⟨a ~ fulminant lesion⟩ **2** : unresponsive to stimulus **3** : resistant or not responding to an infectious agent : IMMUNE

refractory period *n* : the brief period immediately following the response esp. of a muscle or nerve before it recovers the capacity to make a second response — called also *refractory phase;* see ABSOLUTE REFRACTORY PERIOD, RELATIVE REFRACTORY PERIOD

re·frac·ture \ˌrē-ˈfrak-chər\ *vb* **-tured; -tur·ing** : to break along the line of a previous fracture — **refracture** *n*

Ref·sum's disease \ˈref-səmz-\ *n* : an autosomal recessive lipidosis characterized by faulty metabolism of phytanic acid resulting in its accumulation in the blood, retinitis pigmentosa, ataxia, deafness, and intellectual disability

Refsum, Sigvold Bernhard (1907–1991), Norwegian physician.

re·gen·er·a·tion \ri-ˌje-nə-ˈrā-shən, ˌrē-\ *n* : the renewal, regrowth, or restoration of a body or a bodily part, tissue, or substance after injury or as a normal bodily process ⟨continual ~ of epithelial cells⟩ — compare REGULATION 2a — **re·gen·er·ate** \ri-ˈje-nə-ˌrāt\ *vb* — **re·gen·er·a·tive** \ri-ˈje-nə-ˌrā-tiv, -rə-\ *adj*

regenerative medicine *n* : a branch of medicine concerned with therapies that regenerate or replace injured, diseased, or defective cells, tissues, or organs to restore or establish function or structure

re·gime \rā-ˈzhēm, ri-ˈjēm\ *n* : REGIMEN

reg·i·men \ˈre-jə-mən\ *n* : a systematic plan (as of diet, therapy, or medication) esp. when designed to improve and maintain the health of a patient

re·gion \ˈrē-jən\ *n* **1** : any of the major subdivisions into which the body or one of its parts is divisible **2** : an indefinite area surrounding a specified body part ⟨pain in the ~ of the heart⟩

re·gion·al \ˈrēj-ən-ᵊl\ *adj* : of, relating to, or affecting a particular bodily region : LOCALIZED

regional anatomy *n* : a branch of anatomy dealing with regions of the body esp. with reference to diagnosis and treatment of disease or injury — called also *topographic anatomy*

regional anesthesia *n* : anesthesia of a region of the body accomplished by a series of encircling injections of an anesthetic — compare BLOCK ANESTHESIA

regional enteritis *n* : CROHN'S DISEASE

regional ileitis *n* : CROHN'S DISEASE

reg·is·tered \ˈre-ji-stərd\ *adj* : qualified by formal, official, or legal certification or authentication

registered nurse *n* : a graduate trained nurse who has been licensed by a state authority after passing qualifying examinations for registration — called also *RN*

reg·is·trar \ˈre-ji-ˌsträr\ *n* **1** : an admitting officer at a hospital **2** *Brit* : RESIDENT

reg·is·try \ˈre-ji-strē\ *n, pl* **-tries** **1** : a place where data, records, or laboratory samples are kept and usu. are made available for research or comparative study ⟨a cancer ~⟩ **2** : an establishment at which nurses available for employment are listed and through which they are hired

Reg·i·tine \ˈre-ji-ˌtēn\ *n* : a preparation of the mesylate of phentolamine — formerly a U.S. registered trademark

re·gres·sion \ri-ˈgre-shən\ *n* : a trend or shift toward a lower, less severe, or less perfect state: as **a** : progressive decline (as in size or severity) of a manifestation of disease ⟨tumor ~⟩ **b** (1) : a gradual loss of differentiation and function by a body part esp. as a physiological change accompanying aging ⟨menopausal ~ of the ovaries⟩ (2) : gradual loss (as in old age) of memories and acquired skills **c** : reversion to an earlier mental or behavioral level or to an earlier stage of psychosexual development (as in response to stress or to suggestion) — **re·gress** \ri-ˈgres\ *vb* — **re·gres·sive** \ri-ˈgre-siv\ *adj*

re·grow \ˌrē-ˈgrō\ *vb* **re·grew** \-ˈgrü\; **re·grown** \-ˈgrōn\; **re·grow·ing** : to continue growth after interruption or injury — **re·growth** \-ˈgrōth\ *n*

reg·u·lar \ˈre-gyə-lər\ *adj* : conforming to what is usual or normal: as **a** : recurring or functioning at fixed or normal intervals ⟨~ bowel movements> **b** : having menstrual periods or bowel movements at normal intervals — **reg·u·lar·i·ty** \ˌre-gyə-ˈlar-ə-tē\ *n* — **reg·u·lar·ly** *adv*

reg·u·la·tion \ˌre-gyə-ˈlā-shən, -gə-\ *n* **1** : the act of fixing or adjusting the time, amount, degree, or rate of something; *also* : the resulting state or condition **2 a** : the process of redistributing material (as in an embryo) to restore a damaged or lost part independent of new tissue growth — compare REGENERATION **b** : the mechanism by which an early embryo maintains normal development **3** : the control of the kind and rate of cellular processes by controlling the activity of individual genes — **reg·u·late** \-ˌlāt\ *vb* — **reg·u·la·tory** \-lə-ˌtōr-ē\ *adj*

reg·u·la·tive \ˈre-gyə-ˌlā-tiv, -lə\ *adj* : INDETERMINATE <~ eggs>

reg·u·la·tor \ˈre-gyə-ˌlā-tər\ *n* : REGULATORY GENE

regulatory gene *or* **regulator gene** *n* : a gene that regulates the expression of one or more structural genes by controlling the production of a protein (as a genetic repressor) which regulates their rate of transcription

re·gur·gi·tant \rē-ˈgər-jə-tənt\ *adj* : characterized by, allowing, or being a backward flow (as of blood) <~ cardiac valves>

re·gur·gi·ta·tion \rē-ˌgər-jə-ˈtā-shən\ *n* **1** : an act of bringing swallowed food back up into the mouth **2** : the backward flow of blood through a defective heart valve — see AORTIC REGURGITATION, MITRAL REGURGITATION — **re·gur·gi·tate** \rə-ˈgər-jə-ˌtāt\ *vb*

re·hab \ˈrē-ˌhab\ *n, often attrib* : REHABILITATION; *esp* : a program for rehabilitating esp. drug or alcohol abusers

re·ha·bil·i·tant \ˌrē-hə-ˈbi-lə-tənt, ˌrē-ə-\ *n* : an individual undergoing rehabilitation

re·ha·bil·i·ta·tion \ˌrē-hə-ˌbi-lə-ˈtā-shən, ˌrē-ə-\ *n, often attrib* **1 a** : the physical restoration of a sick or disabled person by therapeutic measures and reeducation **b** : the process of restoring an individual (as a drug addict) to a useful and constructive place in society through some form of vocational, correctional, or therapeutic retraining **2** : the result of rehabilitation : the state of undergoing or of having undergone rehabilitation — **re·ha·bil·i·tate** \-ˈbi-lə-ˌtāt\ *vb* — **re·ha·bil·i·ta·tive** \-ˈbi-lə-ˌtā-tiv\ *adj*

re·hears·al \ri-ˈhər-səl\ *n* **1** : a method for improving memory by mentally or verbally repeating over and over the information to be remembered **2** : the repeated mental review of a desired action or behavioral response

Reh·fuss tube \ˈrā-fəs-\ *n* : a flexible tube that is used esp. for withdrawing gastric juice from the stomach for analysis

Rehfuss, Martin Emil (1887–1964), American physician.

re·hy·drate \rē-ˈhī-ˌdrāt\ *vb* **-drat·ed; -drat·ing** : to restore fluid to (something dehydrated); *esp* : to restore body fluid lost in dehydration to <~ a patient> — **re·hy·dra·tion** \ˌrē-ˌhī-ˈdrā-shən\ *n*

Rei·ki \ˈrā-ˌkē\ *n* : a system of hands-on touching based on the belief that such touching by an experienced practitioner produces beneficial effects by strengthening and normalizing certain vital energy fields held to exist within the body

re·im·plan·ta·tion \ˌrē-ˌim-ˌplan-ˈtā-shən\ *n* **1** : the restoration of a bodily tissue or part (as a tooth) to the site from which it was removed **2** : the implantation of a fertilized egg in the uterus after it has been removed from the body and fertilized in vitro — **re·im·plant** \-im-ˈplant\ *vb*

re·in·farc·tion \ˌrē-in-ˈfärk-shən\ *n* : an infarction occurring subsequent to a previous infarction

re·in·fec·tion \ˌrē-in-ˈfek-shən\ *n* : infection following recovery from or superimposed on a previous infection of the same type

re·in·force·ment \ˌrē-ən-ˈfōrs-mənt\ *n* : the action of causing a subject (as a student or an experimental animal) to learn to give or to increase the frequency of a desired response that in classical conditioning involves the repeated presentation of an unconditioned stimulus (as the sight of food) paired with a conditioned stimulus (as the sound of a bell) and that in operant conditioning involves the use of a reward following a correct response or a punishment following an incorrect response; *also* : the reward, punishment, or unconditioned stimulus used in reinforcement — **re·in·force** \-ˈfōrs\ *vb*

re·in·forc·er \-ˈfōr-sər\ *n* : a stimulus (as a reward or removal of an electric shock) that increases the probability of a desired response in operant conditioning by being applied or removed following the desired response

re·in·fuse \ˌrē-in-ˈfyüz\ *vb* **-fused; -fus·ing** : to return (as blood or lymphocytes) to the body by infusion after having been previously withdrawn — **re·in·fu·sion** \-ˈfyü-zhən\ *n*

re·in·jec·tion \ˌrē-in-ˈjek-shən\ *n* : an injection made subsequent to a previous injection — **re·in·ject** \-ˈjekt\ *vb*

re·in·ner·va·tion \ˌrē-ˌi-nər-ˈvā-shən, -in-ˌər-\ *n* : restoration of function esp. to a denervated muscle by supplying it with nerves by regrowth or by grafting — **re·in·ner·vate** \-i-ˈnər-ˌvāt, -ˈi-nər-\ *vb*

re·in·oc·u·la·tion \ˌrē-i-ˌnä-kyə-ˈlā-shən\ *n* : inoculation a second or subsequent time with the same organism as the original inoculation — **re·in·oc·u·late** \-ˈnä-kyə-ˌlāt\ *vb*

re·in·te·gra·tion \rē-ˌin-tə-ˈgrā-shən\ *n* : repeated and renewed integration (as of the personality and mental activity after mental illness) — **re·in·te·grate** \-ˈin-tə-ˌgrāt\ *vb*

Reiss·ner's membrane \ˈrīs-nərz-\ *n* : VESTIBULAR MEMBRANE

Reissner, Ernst (1824–1878), German anatomist.

Rei·ter's syndrome \ˈrī-tərz-\ *or* **Reiter syndrome** *n, esp formerly* : REACTIVE ARTHRITIS — called also *Reiter's disease*

Reiter, Hans Conrad Julius (1881–1969), German bacteriologist.

re·jec·tion \ri-ˈjek-shən\ *n* **1** : the action of rebuffing, repelling, refusing to hear, or withholding love from another esp. by communicating negative feelings toward and a wish to be free of the other person **2** : an immune response in which foreign tissue (as of a skin graft or transplanted organ) is attacked by immune system components (as antibodies, T cells, and macrophages) of the recipient organism — **re·ject** \-ˈjekt\ *vb* — **re·jec·tive** \-ˈjek-tiv\ *adj*

re·lapse \ri-ˈlaps, ˈrē-ˌ\ *n* : a recurrence of illness; *esp* : a recurrence of symptoms of a disease after a period of improvement ⟨a ~ after a year-long remission⟩ — **re·lapse** \ri-ˈlaps\ *vb*

relapsing febrile nodular non·sup·pu·ra·tive panniculitis \-ˌnän-ˈsə-pyə-rə-tiv-, -ˌrā-\ *n* : PANNICULITIS 2

relapsing fever *n* : a variable acute infectious disease that is marked by sudden recurring episodes of high fever which usu. last from three to seven days, are typically accompanied by myalgia, arthralgia, headache, nausea, and chills, and often end in a crisis stage marked by a spike in fever followed by an afebrile period and that is caused by a spirochete of the genus *Borrelia* (as *B. hermsii, B. parkerii,* or *B. recurrentis*) which circulates in the blood and is transmitted by the bite of a body louse (*Pediculus humanus humanus*) or a tick of the genus *Ornithodoros*

relapsing polychondritis *n* : a connective tissue disease esp. of cartilage that is characterized usu. by recurrent progressively destructive episodes of tissue inflammation (as of the ears, nose, larynx, and trachea)

re·late \ri-ˈlāt\ *vb* **re·lat·ed; re·lat·ing** : to have meaningful social relationships : interact realistically ⟨an inability to ~ to other people⟩

re·la·tion \ri-ˈlā-shən\ *n* **1** : the attitude or stance which two or more persons or groups assume toward one another ⟨race ~*s*⟩ **2 a** : the state of being mutually or reciprocally interested (as in social matters) **b rela·tions** *pl* : SEXUAL INTERCOURSE — **re·la·tion·al** \-shə-nəl\ *adj*

re·la·tion·ship \-shən-ˌship\ *n* **1** : the state of being related or interrelated ⟨the ~ between diet and health⟩ **2 a** : a state of affairs existing between those having relations or dealings ⟨doctor-patient ~*s*⟩ **b** : an emotional attachment between individuals

relative biological effectiveness *n* : the relative capacity of a particular ionizing radiation to produce a response in a biological system — abbr. *RBE*

relative humidity *n* : the ratio of the amount of water vapor actually present in the air to the greatest amount possible at the same temperature — compare ABSOLUTE HUMIDITY

relative refractory period *n* : the period shortly after the firing of a nerve fiber when partial repolarization has occurred and a greater than normal stimulus can stimulate a second response — called also *relative refractory phase;* compare ABSOLUTE REFRACTORY PERIOD

re·lax \ri-ˈlaks\ *vb* **1** : to slacken or make less tense or rigid ⟨alternately contracting and ~*ing* their muscles⟩ **2** : to relieve from nervous tension **3** *of a muscle or muscle fiber* : to return to an inactive or resting state; *esp* : to become inactive and lengthen **4** : to relieve from constipation — **re·lax·a·tion** \ˌrē-ˌlak-ˈsā-shən, ri-ˌlak-\ *n*

re·lax·ant \ri-ˈlak-sənt\ *n* : a substance (as a drug) that relaxes; *specif* : one that relieves muscular tension — **relaxant** *adj*

re·lax·in \ri-ˈlak-sən\ *n* : a polypeptide sex hormone of the corpus luteum that facilitates birth by causing relaxation of the pelvic ligaments

re·leas·er \ri-ˈlē-sər\ *n* : a stimulus that serves as the initiator of complex reflex behavior

releasing factor *n* : HYPOTHALAMIC RELEASING FACTOR

Re·len·za \rə-ˈlen-zə\ *trademark* — used for a preparation of zanamivir

re·lief \ri-ˈlēf\ *n* : removal or lightening of something oppressive or distressing ⟨~ of pain⟩

re·lieve \ri-ˈlēv\ *vb* **re·lieved; re·liev·ing** **1** : to bring about the removal or alleviation of (pain or discomfort) **2** : to emit the contents of the bladder or bowels of (oneself) — **re·liev·er** *n*

Rel·pax \ˈrel-ˌpaks\ *trademark* — used for a preparation of eletriptan

rem \ˈrem\ *n* : the dosage of an ionizing radiation that will cause the same biological effect as one roentgen of X-ray or gamma-ray dosage — compare REP

REM \ˈrem\ *n* : RAPID EYE MOVEMENT

re·me·di·a·ble \ri-ˈmē-dē-ə-bəl\ *adj* : capable of being remedied

re•me•di•al \ri-ˈmē-dē-əl\ *adj* : affording a remedy : intended as a remedy ⟨~ surgery⟩

re•me•di•a•tion \ri-ˌmē-dē-ˈā-shən\ *n* : the act or process of remedying

rem•e•dy \ˈre-mə-dē\ *n, pl* **-dies** : a medicine, application, or treatment that relieves or cures a disease — **remedy** *vb*

Rem•e•ron \ˈre-mə-ˌrän\ *trademark* — used for a preparation of mirtazapine

Rem•i•cade \ˈrem-i-ˌkād\ *trademark* — used for a preparation of infliximab

re•min•er•al•i•za•tion \ˌrē-ˌmi-nə-rə-lə-ˈzā-shən\ *n* : the restoring of minerals to demineralized structures or substances ⟨~ of bone⟩ — **re•min•er•al•ize** \-ˈmi-nə-rə-ˌlīz\ *vb*

re•mis•sion \ri-ˈmi-shən\ *n* : a state or period during which the symptoms of a disease are abated

re•mit \ri-ˈmit\ *vb* **re•mit•ted; re•mit•ting** : to abate symptoms for a period : go into or be in remission

re•mit•tent \ri-ˈmit-ᵊnt\ *adj* : marked by alternating periods of abatement and increase of symptoms ⟨~ fever⟩

REM latency *n* : the time span between the start of sleeping and the start of REM sleep

re•mod•el•ing \rē-ˈmä-dᵊl-iŋ\ *n, of living tissue* : the process of undergoing structural reorganization, alteration, or renewal ⟨ventricular ~⟩; *esp* : the continuous process of bone resorption and formation that involves the activity of osteoclasts and osteoblasts — **re•mod•el** \-ˈmä-dᵊl\ *vb*

REM sleep *n* : a state of sleep that recurs cyclically several times during a normal period of sleep and that is characterized by increased neuronal activity of the forebrain and midbrain, by depressed muscle tone, and esp. in humans by dreaming, rapid eye movements, and vascular congestion of the sex organs — called also *paradoxical sleep, rapid eye movement sleep;* compare SLOW-WAVE SLEEP

Ren•a•gel \ˈren-ə-ˌjel\ *trademark* — used for a preparation of the hydrochloride of sevelamer

re•nal \ˈrēn-ᵊl\ *adj* : relating to, involving, affecting, or located in the region of the kidneys : NEPHRIC

renal artery *n* : either of two branches of the abdominal aorta of which each supplies one of the kidneys and gives off smaller branches to the ureter, adrenal gland, and adjoining structures

renal calculus *n* : KIDNEY STONE

renal cast *n* : a cast of a renal tubule consisting of granular, hyaline, albuminoid, or other material formed in and discharged from the kidney in renal disease

renal clearance *n* : CLEARANCE

renal colic *n* : the severe pain produced by the passage of a calculus from the kidney through the ureter

renal column *n* : COLUMN OF BERTIN

renal corpuscle *n* : the part of a nephron that consists of Bowman's capsule with its included glomerulus — called also *Malpighian body, Malpighian corpuscle*

renal diabetes *n* : RENAL GLYCOSURIA

renal glycosuria *n* : excretion of glucose associated with increased permeability of the kidneys without increased sugar concentration in the blood

renal hypertension *n* : hypertension that is associated with disease of the kidneys and is caused by kidney damage or malfunctioning

renal osteodystrophy *n* : a painful rachitic condition of abnormal bone growth that is associated with chronic acidosis, hypocalcemia, hyperplasia of the parathyroid glands, and hyperphosphatemia caused by chronic renal insufficiency — called also *renal rickets*

renal papilla *n* : the apex of a renal pyramid which projects into the lumen of a calyx of the kidney and through which collecting ducts discharge urine

renal pelvis *n* : a funnel-shaped structure in each kidney that is formed at one end by the expanded upper portion of the ureter lying in the renal sinus and at the other end by the union of the calyxes of the kidney

renal plexus *n* : a plexus of the autonomic nervous system that arises esp. from the celiac plexus, surrounds the renal artery, and accompanies it into the kidney which it innervates

renal pyramid *n* : any of the conical masses that form the medullary substance of the kidney, project as the renal papillae into the renal pelvis, and are made up of bundles of straight uriniferous tubules opening at the apex of the conical mass — called also *Malpighian pyramid*

renal rickets *n* : RENAL OSTEODYSTROPHY

renal sinus *n* : the main cavity of the kidney that is an expansion behind the hilum and contains the renal pelvis, calyxes, and the major renal vessels

renal syndrome — see HEMORRHAGIC FEVER WITH RENAL SYNDROME

renal threshold *n* : the concentration level up to which a substance (as glucose) in the blood is prevented from passing through the kidneys into the urine

renal tubular acidosis *n* : decreased ability of the kidneys to excrete hydrogen ions that is associated with a defect in the renal tubules without a defect in the glomeruli and that results in the production of urine deficient in acidity

renal tubule *n* : the part of a nephron that leads away from a glomerulus, that is made up of a proximal convoluted tubule, loop of Henle, and distal convoluted tubule, and that empties into a collecting duct

renal vein *n* : a short thick vein that is formed in each kidney by the convergence of the interlobar veins, leaves the kidney through the hilum, and empties into the inferior vena cava

Ren·du–Os·ler–Web·er disease \ˌrän-ˈdü-ˈäs-lər-ˈwe-bər-, ˌrän-ˈdyü-\ *n* : HEREDITARY HEMORRHAGIC TELANGIECTASIA — called also *Rendu-Osler-Weber syndrome*

Ren·du \rän-ˈdü̅\, **Henry–Jules–Louis–Marie (1844–1902),** French physician.

Osler, Sir William (1849–1919), American physician.

F. P. Weber — see WEBER-CHRISTIAN DISEASE

Ren·ese \ˈre-ˌnēz\ *trademark* — used for a preparation of polythiazide

reni- *or* **reno-** *comb form* **1** : kidney ⟨*reni*form⟩ **2** : renal and ⟨*reno*vascular⟩

re·ni·form \ˈrē-nə-ˌfȯrm, ˈre-\ *adj* : suggesting a kidney in outline

re·nin \ˈrē-nən, ˈre-\ *n* : a proteolytic enzyme of the blood that is produced and secreted by the juxtaglomerular cells of the kidney and hydrolyzes angiotensinogen to angiotensin I

ren·nin \ˈre-nən\ *n* : an enzyme that coagulates milk, occurs esp. with pepsin in the gastric juice of young animals, and is used chiefly in making cheese

re·no·gram \ˈrē-nə-ˌgram\ *n* : a radiographic scan made by renography; *broadly* : RENOGRAPHY

re·nog·ra·phy \rē-ˈnä-grə-fē\ *n, pl* **-phies** : the radiographic visualization of the kidneys and ureters after administration of a radiolabeled substance — **re·no·graph·ic** \ˌrē-nə-ˈgra-fik\ *adj*

re·no·vas·cu·lar \ˌrē-nō-ˈvas-kyə-lər\ *adj* : of, relating to, or involving the blood vessels of the kidneys ⟨~ hypertension⟩

Ren·shaw cell \ˈren-ˌshȯ-\ *n* : an interneuron in the ventral horn of gray matter of the spinal cord that has an inhibitory effect on motor neurons

Renshaw, Birdsey (1911–1948), American neurologist.

Ren·vela \ren-ˈvel-ə\ *trademark* — used for a preparation of the carbonate of sevelamer

re·oc·clu·sion \ˌrē-ə-ˈklü-zhən\ *n* : the reoccurrence of occlusion in an artery after it has been treated (as by balloon angioplasty) with apparent success — **re·oc·clude** \-ə-ˈklüd\ *vb*

re·op·er·a·tion \ˌrē-ˌä-pə-ˈrā-shən\ *n* : an operation to correct a condition not corrected by a previous operation or to correct the complications of a previous operation — **re·op·er·ate** \-ˈä-pə-ˌrāt\ *vb*

Reo·Pro \rē-ō-ˌprō\ *trademark* — used for a preparation of abciximab

reo·vi·rus \ˌrē-ō-ˈvī-rəs\ *n* : any of a family (*Reoviridae*) of double-stranded RNA viruses that include the rotaviruses and the causative agents of bluetongue and Colorado tick fever — **reo·vi·ral** \-rəl\ *adj*

rep \ˈrep\ *n, pl* **rep** *or* **reps** : the dosage of an ionizing radiation that will develop the same amount of energy upon absorption in human tissues as one roentgen of X-ray or gamma-ray exposure — compare REM

rep *abbr* [Latin *repetatur*] let it be repeated — used in writing prescriptions

re·pag·li·nide \ri-ˈpa-glə-ˌnīd\ *n* : a drug $C_{27}H_{36}N_2O_4$ that stimulates insulin release and is taken orally to treat type 2 diabetes — see PRANDIN

re·peat \ri-ˈpēt, ˈrē-ˌ\ *n* : a genetic duplication in which the duplicated parts are adjacent to each other along the chromosome

re·per·fu·sion \ˌrē-pər-ˈfyü-zhən\ *n* : restoration of the flow of blood to a previously ischemic tissue or organ (as the heart) ⟨~ following heart attack⟩ — **re·per·fuse** \-ˈfyüz\ *vb*

repetition compulsion *n* : an irresistible tendency to repeat an emotional experience or to return to a previous psychological state

repetitive strain injury *n* : any of various musculoskeletal disorders (as carpal tunnel syndrome or tendinitis) that are caused by cumulative damage to muscles, tendons, ligaments, nerves, or joints (as of the hand or arm) from highly repetitive movements and that are characterized esp. by pain, weakness, and loss of feeling — called also *cumulative trauma disorder, repetitive motion injury, repetitive stress injury, repetitive stress syndrome, RSI*

replacement therapy *n* : therapy involving the supplying of something (as hormones or blood) lacking from or lost to the system — see ESTROGEN REPLACEMENT THERAPY, HORMONE REPLACEMENT THERAPY

re·plan·ta·tion \ˌrē-(ˌ)plan-ˈtā-shən\ *n* : reattachment or reinsertion of a bodily part (as a limb or tooth) after separation from the body — **re·plant** \rē-ˈplant\ *vb*

rep·li·case \ˈre-pli-ˌkās, -ˌkāz\ *n* : a polymerase that promotes synthesis of a particular RNA in the presence of a template of RNA — called also *RNA replicase, RNA synthetase*

rep·li·ca·tion \ˌre-plə-ˈkā-shən\ *n* **1** : the action or process of reproducing or duplicating ⟨~ of DNA⟩ **2** : performance of an experiment or procedure more than once — **rep·li·cate** \ˈre-pli-ˌkāt\ *vb* — **rep·li·cate** \-kət\ *n* — **rep·li·ca·tive** \ˈre-pli-ˌkā-tiv\ *adj*

rep·li·con \ˈre-pli-ˌkän\ *n* : a linear or circular section of DNA or RNA which replicates sequentially as a unit

re·po·lar·i·za·tion \ˌrē-pō-lə-rə-ˈzā-shən\ *n* : restoration of the difference in charge between the inside and outside of the plasma membrane of a muscle fiber or cell following depolarization — **re·po·lar·ize** \-ˈpō-lə-ˌrīz\ *vb*

re·port·able \ri-ˈpōr-tə-bəl\ *adj* : required by law to be reported ⟨~ diseases⟩

re·po·si·tion \ˌrē-pə-ˈzi-shən\ *vb* : to return to or place in a normal or proper position ⟨~ a dislocated shoulder⟩

re·pos·i·to·ry \ri-ˈpä-zə-ˌtōr-ē\ *adj, of a drug* : designed to act over a prolonged period ⟨~ penicillin⟩

re·press \ri-ˈpres\ *vb* **1** : to exclude from consciousness ⟨~ conflicts⟩ **2** : to inactivate (a gene or formation of a gene product) by allosteric combination at a DNA binding site

re·pressed \ri-ˈprest\ *adj* : subjected to or marked by repression ⟨~ anger⟩

re·press·ible \ri-ˈpre-sə-bəl\ *adj* : capable of being repressed

re·pres·sion \ri-ˈpre-shən\ *n* **1** : the action or process of repressing ⟨gene ~⟩ **2 a** : a process by which unacceptable desires or impulses are excluded from consciousness and left to operate in the unconscious — compare SUPPRESSION c **b** : an item so excluded

re·pres·sive \ri-ˈpre-siv\ *adj* : tending to repress or to cause repression

re·pres·sor \ri-ˈpre-sər\ *n* : one that represses; *esp* : a protein that is determined by a regulatory gene, binds to a genetic operator, and inhibits the initiation of transcription of messenger RNA

re·pro·duce \ˌrē-prə-ˈdüs, -ˈdyüs\ *vb* **-duced; -duc·ing 1** : to produce (new individuals of the same kind) by a sexual or asexual process **2** : to achieve (an original result or score) again or anew by repeating an experiment or test

re·pro·duc·tion \ˌrē-prə-ˈdək-shən\ *n* : the act or process of reproducing; *specif* : the process by which plants and animals give rise to offspring — **re·pro·duc·tive** \ˌrē-prə-ˈdək-tiv\ *adj* — **re·pro·duc·tive·ly** *adv*

reproductive system *n* : the system of organs and parts which function in reproduction consisting in the male esp. of the testes, penis, seminal vesicles, prostate, and urethra and in the female esp. of the ovaries, fallopian tubes, uterus, vagina, and vulva

RES *abbr* reticuloendothelial system

res·cin·na·mine \re-ˈsi-nə-ˌmēn, -mən\ *n* : an antihypertensive, tranquilizing, and sedative drug $C_{35}H_{42}N_2O_9$

re·sect \ri-ˈsekt\ *vb* : to perform resection on ⟨~ an ulcer⟩ — **re·sect·abil·i·ty** \ri-ˌsek-tə-ˈbi-lə-tē\ *n* — **re·sect·able** \ri-ˈsek-tə-bəl\ *adj*

re·sec·tion \ri-ˈsek-shən\ *n* : the surgical removal of part of an organ or structure ⟨~ of the lower bowel⟩

re·sec·to·scope \ri-ˈsek-tə-ˌskōp\ *n* : an instrument consisting of a tubular fenestrated sheath with a sliding knife within it that is used for surgery within cavities (as of the prostate through the urethra)

re·ser·pine \ri-ˈsər-ˌpēn, ˈre-sər-pən\ *n* : an alkaloid $C_{33}H_{40}N_2O_9$ extracted esp. from the root of rauwolfias and used in the treatment of hypertension, mental illness, and tension states — see RAUDIXIN, SERPASIL

reservatus — see COITUS RESERVATUS

re·serve \ri-ˈzərv\ *n* **1** : something stored or kept available for future use or need ⟨oxygen ~⟩ — see CARDIAC RESERVE **2** : the capacity of a solution to neutralize alkali or acid when its reaction is shifted from one hydrogen-ion concentration to another — **reserve** *adj*

res·er·voir \ˈre-zər-ˌvwär, -ˌvwȯr\ *n* **1** : a space (as the cavity of a glandular acinus) in which a body fluid is stored **2** : an organism in which a parasite that is pathogenic for some other species lives and multiplies without damaging its host; *also* : a noneconomic organism within which a pathogen of economic or medical importance flourishes without regard to its pathogenicity for the reservoir ⟨rats are ~*s* of plague⟩ — compare CARRIER

reservoir host *n* : RESERVOIR 2

res·i·den·cy \ˈre-zəd-ən-sē\ *n, pl* **-cies** : a period of advanced medical training and education that normally follows graduation from medical school and licensing to practice medicine and that consists of supervised practice of a specialty in a hospital and in its outpatient department and instruction from specialists on the hospital staff

res·i·dent \ˈre-zə-dənt\ *n* : a physician serving a residency

res·i·den·tial \ˌre-zə-ˈden-shəl\ *adj* : provided to patients residing in a facility ⟨~ drug treatment⟩

[1]**re·sid·u·al** \ri-ˈzi-jə-wəl\ *adj* **1** : of, relating to, or being something that remains: as **a** : remaining after a disease or operation ⟨~ paralysis⟩ **b** : remaining in a body cavity after maximum normal expulsion has occurred ⟨~ urine⟩ — see RESIDUAL VOLUME **2 a** : leaving a residue that remains effective for some time after application ⟨~ insecticides⟩ **b** : of or relating to a residual insecticide

[2]**residual** *n* **1** : an internal aftereffect of experience or activity that influences later behavior **2** : a residual abnormality (as a scar or limp)

residual air *n* : RESIDUAL VOLUME

residual volume *n* : the volume of air still remaining in the lungs after the most forcible expiration possible and amounting usu. to 60 to 100 cubic inches (980 to 1640 cubic centimeters) — called also *residual air;* compare SUPPLEMENTAL AIR

res•i•due \ˈre-zə-ˌdü, -ˌdyü\ *n* : something that remains after a part is taken, separated, or designated; *specif* : a constituent structural unit of a usu. complex molecule ⟨amino acid ~*s* in a protein⟩

res•in \ˈrez-ᵊn\ *n* : any of various substances obtained from the gum or sap of some trees and used esp. in various varnishes and plastics and in medicine; *also* : a comparable synthetic product — **res•in•ous** \ˈrez-ᵊn-əs\ *adj*

re•sis•tance \ri-ˈzis-təns\ *n* **1 a** : the inherent ability of an organism to resist harmful influences (as infection) **b** : the capacity of a species or strain of microorganism to survive exposure to a toxic agent (as a drug) formerly effective against it **2 a** : the opposition offered by a body to the passage through it of a steady electric current **b** : opposition or impediment to the flow of a fluid (as blood or respiratory gases) through one or more passages — see VASCULAR RESISTANCE **3** : a psychological defense mechanism wherein a psychoanalysis patient rejects, denies, or otherwise opposes therapeutic efforts by the analyst — **re•sis•tant** \-tənt\ *adj*

re•so•cial•i•za•tion \ˌrē-ˌsō-shə-lə-ˈzā-shən\ *n* : readjustment of an individual to life in society

res•o•lu•tion \ˌre-zə-ˈlü-shən\ *n* **1** : the separating of a chemical compound or mixture into its constituents **2** : the process or capability of making distinguishable the individual parts of an object, closely adjacent optical images, or sources of light **3** : the subsidence of a pathological state (as inflammation) — **re•solve** \ri-ˈzälv, -ˈzȯlv\ *vb*

res•o•nance \ˈrez-ᵊn-əns\ *n* **1** : a quality imparted to voiced sounds by vibration in anatomical resonating chambers or cavities (as the mouth or the nasal cavity) **2** : the sound elicited on percussion of the chest **3** : the enhancement of an atomic, nuclear, or particle reaction or a scattering event by excitation of internal motion in the system **b** : MAGNETIC RESONANCE

re•sorb \rē-ˈsȯrb, -ˈzȯrb\ *vb* : to break down and assimilate the components of (as bone) ⟨~*ed* bone⟩ — **re•sorb•a•ble** \-ə-bəl\ *adj*

res•or•cin \rə-ˈzȯrs-ᵊn\ *n* : RESORCINOL

res•or•cin•ol \-ˌȯl, -ˌōl\ *n* : a crystalline phenol $C_6H_6O_2$ used in medicine as a fungicidal, bactericidal, and keratolytic agent

resorcinol monoacetate *n* : a liquid compound $C_8H_8O_3$ that slowly liberates resorcinol and that is used esp. to treat diseases of the scalp

re•sorp•tion \rē-ˈsȯrp-shən, -ˈzȯrp-\ *n* : the action or process of resorbing something — **re•sorp•tive** \-tiv\ *adj*

re•spi•ra•ble \ˈres-pə-rə-bəl, ri-ˈspī-rə-\ *adj* : fit for breathing; *also* : capable of being taken in by breathing

res•pi•ra•tion \ˌres-pə-ˈrā-shən\ *n* **1 a** : the movement of respiratory gases (as oxygen and carbon dioxide) into and out of the lungs **b** : a single complete act of breathing ⟨30 ~*s* per minute⟩ **2** : the physical and chemical processes by which an organism supplies its cells and tissues with the oxygen needed for metabolism and relieves them of the carbon dioxide formed in energy-producing reactions **3** : CELLULAR RESPIRATION

res•pi•ra•tor \ˈres-pə-ˌrā-tər\ *n* **1** : a device (as a gas mask) worn over the mouth or nose to protect the respiratory system by filtering out dangerous substances (as dust or fumes) **2** : a device for maintaining artificial respiration — called also *ventilator*

res•pi•ra•to•ry \ˈres-pə-rə-ˌtōr-ē, ri-ˈspī-rə-\ *adj* **1** : of or relating to respiration ⟨~ diseases⟩ **2** : serving for or functioning in respiration ⟨~ organs⟩

respiratory acidosis *n* : acidosis caused by excessive retention of carbon dioxide due to a respiratory abnormality (as obstructive lung disease)

respiratory alkalosis *n* : alkalosis that is caused by excessive elimination of carbon dioxide due to a respiratory abnormality (as hyperventilation)

respiratory center *n* : a region in the medulla oblongata that regulates respiratory movements

respiratory chain *n* : the metabolic pathway along which electron transport occurs in cellular respiration; *also* : the series of enzymes involved in this pathway

respiratory distress syndrome *n* : a respiratory disorder occurring in newborn premature infants that is characterized by deficiency of the surfactant coating the inner surface of the lungs resulting in failure of the lungs to expand and contract properly during breathing — abbr. *RDS;* called also *hyaline membrane disease;* see ACUTE RESPIRATORY DISTRESS SYNDROME

respiratory pigment *n* : any of various permanently or intermittently colored conjugated proteins and esp. hemoglobin that function in the transfer of oxygen in cellular respiration

respiratory quotient *n* : the ratio of the volume of carbon dioxide given off in respiration to that of the oxygen consumed — abbr. *RQ*

respiratory syncytial virus *n* : a paramyxovirus (species *Human respiratory syncytial virus* of the genus *Pneumovirus*) that forms syncytia in tissue culture and is responsible for severe respiratory diseases (as bronchopneumonia and bronchiolitis) in children and esp. in infants — abbr. *RSV*

respiratory system *n* : a system of organs functioning in respiration and consisting esp. of the nose, nasal passages, nasopharynx, larynx, trachea, bronchi, and lungs — called also *respiratory tract;* see LOWER RESPIRATORY TRACT, UPPER RESPIRATORY TRACT

respiratory therapist *n* : a specialist in respiratory therapy

respiratory therapy *n* : therapy concerned with the maintenance or improvement of respiratory functioning

respiratory tract *n* : RESPIRATORY SYSTEM

respiratory tree *n* : the trachea, bronchi, and bronchioles

re•spire \ri-ˈspīr\ *vb* **re•spired; re•spir•ing** **1** : BREATHE; *specif* : to inhale and exhale air successively **2** *of a cell or tissue* : to take up oxygen and produce carbon dioxide through oxidation

res•pi•rom•e•ter \ˌres-pə-ˈrä-mə-tər\ *n* : an instrument for studying the character and extent of respiration — **res•pi•ro•met•ric** \ˌres-pə-rō-ˈme-trik\ *adj* — **res•pi•rom•e•try** \ˌres-pə-ˈrä-mə-trē\ *n*

re•spond \ri-ˈspänd\ *vb* **1** : to react in response **2** : to show favorable reaction ⟨~ to chemotherapy⟩

re•spon•dent \ri-ˈspän-dənt\ *adj* : relating to or being behavior or responses to a stimulus that are followed by a reward ⟨~ conditioning⟩

re•spond•er \ri-ˈspän-dər\ *n* : one that responds (as to treatment)

re•sponse \ri-ˈspäns\ *n* : the activity or inhibition of previous activity of an organism or any of its parts resulting from stimulation ⟨a conditioned ~⟩

re•spon•sive \ri-ˈspän-siv\ *adj* : making a response; *esp* : responding to treatment — **re•spon•sive•ness** *n*

rest \ˈrest\ *n* **1** : a state of repose or sleep; *also* : a state of inactivity or motionlessness — see BED REST **2** : the part of a partial denture that rests on an abutment tooth, distributes stresses, and holds the clasp in position **3** : a firm cushion used to raise or support a portion of the body during surgery ⟨a kidney ~⟩ — **rest** *vb*

Re•sta•sis \rə-ˈstā-səs\ *trademark* — used for a topical ophthalmic preparation containing cyclosporine

re•ste•no•sis \ˌres-tə-ˈnō-səs\ *n, pl* **-no•ses** \-ˌsēz\ : the reoccurrence of stenosis in a blood vessel or heart valve following apparently successful treatment (as by balloon angioplasty)

rest home *n* : an establishment that provides housing and general care for the aged or the convalescent

res•ti•form body \ˈres-tə-ˌfȯrm-\ *n* : CEREBELLAR PEDUNCLE c

rest•ing *adj* **1** : not physiologically active **2** : occurring in or performed on a subject at rest ⟨a ~ tremor⟩

resting cell *n* : a living cell with a nucleus that is not undergoing division (as by mitosis)

resting potential *n* : the membrane potential of a cell that is not exhibiting the activity resulting from a stimulus — compare ACTION POTENTIAL

resting stage *n* : INTERPHASE

rest•less \ˈrest-ləs\ *adj* **1** : deprived of rest or sleep **2** : providing no rest

restless legs syndrome *n* : a neurological disorder of uncertain pathophysiology that is characterized by aching, burning, crawling, or creeping sensations of the legs that occur esp. at night usu. when lying down (as before sleep) — called also *restless legs*

res•to•ra•tion \ˌres-tə-ˈrā-shən\ *n* : the act of restoring or the condition of being restored: as **a** : a returning to a normal or healthy condition **b** : the replacing of missing teeth or crowns; *also* : a dental replacement (as a denture) used for restoration — **re•stor•ative** \ri-ˈstōr-ə-tiv\ *adj or n*

re•store \ri-ˈstōr\ *vb* **re•stored; re•stor•ing** : to bring back to or put back into a former or original state

Res•to•ril \ˈres-tə-ˌril\ *trademark* — used for a preparation of temazepam

re•straint \ri-ˈstrānt\ *n* : a device (as a straitjacket) that restricts movement

re•stric•tion \ri-ˈstrik-shən\ *n, often attrib* : the breaking of double-stranded DNA into fragments by restriction enzymes ⟨~ sites⟩

restriction endonuclease *n* : RESTRICTION ENZYME

restriction enzyme *n* : any of various enzymes that break DNA into fragments at specific sites in the interior of the molecule and are often used as tools in molecular analysis

restriction fragment *n* : a segment of DNA produced by the action of a restriction enzyme on a molecule of DNA

restriction fragment length polymorphism *n* : variation in the length of a restriction fragment produced by a specific restriction enzyme acting on DNA from different individuals that usu. results from a genetic mutation (as an insertion or deletion) and that may be used as a genetic marker — called also *RFLP*

rest seat *n* : an area on the surface of a tooth that is specially prepared (as by grinding) for the attachment of a dental rest

re•sus•ci•ta•tion \ri-ˌsə-sə-ˈtā-shən, rē-\ *n* : the act of reviving from apparent death or from unconsciousness — see CARDIOPULMONARY RESUSCITATION — **re•sus•ci•tate** \-ˈsə-sə-ˌtāt\ *vb* — **re•sus•ci•ta•tive** \ri-ˈsə-sə-ˌtā-tiv\ *adj*

re•sus•ci•ta•tor \ri-ˈsə-sə-ˌtā-tər\ *n* : an apparatus used to restore respiration (as of a partially asphyxiated person)

res•ver•a•trol \rez-ˈvir-ə-ˌtrȯl\ *n* : a compound $C_{14}H_{12}O_3$ found esp. in the skin of grapes and certain grape-derived products (as red wine) that has been linked to a reduced risk of coronary artery disease and cancer

re•tain•er \ri-ˈtā-nər\ *n* **1** : the part of a dental replacement (as a bridge) by which it is made fast to adjacent natural teeth **2** : a dental appliance used to hold teeth in their correct position esp. following orthodontic treatment

re•tar•da•tion \ˌrē-ˌtär-ˈdā-shən, ri-\ *n* **1 a** : an abnormal slowness of thought or action ⟨psychomotor ~⟩ **b** *now often offensive* : INTELLECTUAL DISABILITY **2** : slowness in development or progress ⟨fetal growth ~⟩

re•tard•ed \ri-ˈtär-dəd\ *adj, dated, now usu offensive* : slow or limited in intellectual or emotional development : affected by intellectual disability

retch \ˈrech\ *vb* : to make an effort to vomit; *also* : VOMIT — **retch** *n*

re•te \ˈrē-tē, ˈrā-\ *n, pl* **re•tia** \-tē-ə\ **1** : a network esp. of blood vessels or nerves : PLEXUS **2** : an anatomical part resembling or including a network

re•ten•tion \ri-ˈten-chən\ *n* **1** : the act of retaining: as **a** : abnormal retaining of a fluid or secretion in a body cavity ⟨~ of urine⟩ **b** : the holding in place of a tooth or dental replacement by means of a retainer **2** : a preservation of the aftereffects of experience and learning that makes recall or recognition possible

re•ten•tive \ri-ˈten-tiv\ *adj* : tending to retain: as **a** : having a good memory ⟨a ~ mind⟩ **b** : of, relating to, or being a dental retainer

rete peg *n* : any of the inwardly directed prolongations of the epidermal Malpighian layer that mesh with the dermal papillae of the skin

rete testis *n, pl* **retia tes•ti•um** \-ˈtes-tē-əm\ : the network of tubules in the mediastinum testis

retia *pl of* RETE

reticul- *or* **reticulo-** *comb form* : reticulum ⟨*reticulo*cyte⟩

reticula *pl of* RETICULUM

re•tic•u•lar \ri-ˈti-kyə-lər\ *adj* : of, relating to, or forming a network

reticular activating system *n* : a part of the reticular formation that extends from the brain stem to the midbrain and thalamus with connections distributed throughout the cerebral cortex and that controls the degree of activity of the central nervous system (as in maintaining sleep and wakefulness)

reticular cell *n* : RETICULUM CELL; *esp* : RETICULOCYTE

reticular fiber *n* : any of the thin branching fibers of connective tissue that form an intricate interstitial network ramifying through other tissues and organs

reticular formation *n* : a mass of nerve cells and fibers situated primarily in the brain stem and functioning upon stimulation esp. in arousal of the organism — called also *reticular substance*

reticularis — see LIVEDO RETICULARIS, ZONA RETICULARIS

reticular lamina *n* : a thin extracellular layer that sometimes lies below the basal lamina, is composed chiefly of collagenous fibers, and serves to anchor the basal lamina to underlying connective tissue

reticular layer *n* : the deeper layer of the dermis formed of interlacing fasciculi of white fibrous tissue

reticular tissue *n* : RETICULUM a

re•tic•u•late body \ri-ˈti-kyə-lət-\ *n* : a chlamydial cell of a spherical intracellular form that is larger than an elementary body and reproduces by binary fission

re•tic•u•lin \ri-ˈti-kyə-lən\ *n* : a protein substance similar to collagen that is a constituent of reticular tissue

re•tic•u•lo•cyte \ri-ˈti-kyə-lō-ˌsīt\ *n* : an immature red blood cell that appears esp. during regeneration of lost blood and that has a fine basophilic reticulum formed of the remains of ribosomes — **re•tic•u•lo•cyt•ic** \ri-ˌti-kyə-lō-ˈsi-tik\ *adj*

re•tic•u•lo•cy•to•pe•nia \ri-ˌti-kyə-lō-ˌsī-tə-ˈpē-nē-ə\ *n* : an abnormal decrease in the number of reticulocytes in the blood

re•tic•u•lo•cy•to•sis \-ˌsī-ˈtō-səs\ *n, pl* **-to•ses** \-ˌsēz\ : an increase in the number of reticulocytes in the blood

re•tic•u•lo•en•do•the•li•al \ri-ˌti-kyə-lō-ˌen-də-ˈthē-lē-əl\ *adj* : of, relating to, or being the reticuloendothelial system ⟨~ tissue⟩ ⟨~ cells⟩

reticuloendothelial system *n* : MONONUCLEAR PHAGOCYTE SYSTEM; *broadly* : the mononuclear phagocyte system plus certain other cells now known to be pinocytic or only weakly phagocytic

re•tic•u•lo•en•do•the•li•o•sis \-ˌthē-lē-ˈō-səs\ *n, pl* **-o•ses** \-ˌsēz\ : any of several disorders characterized by proliferation of phagocytic cells (as macrophages) — called also *reticulosis*

re•tic•u•lo•sar•co•ma \-sär-ˈkō-mə\ *n, pl* **-mas** *or* **-ma•ta** \-mə-tə\ : HISTIOCYTIC LYMPHOMA

re•tic•u•lo•sis \ri-ˌti-kyə-ˈlō-səs\ *n, pl* **-lo•ses** \-ˌsēz\ : RETICULOENDOTHELIOSIS

re•tic•u•lo•spi•nal tract \ri-ˌti-kyə-lō-ˈspī-nᵊl-\ *n* : a tract of nerve fibers that originates in the reticular formation of the pons and medulla oblongata and descends to the spinal cord

re•tic•u•lum \ri-ˈti-kyə-ləm\ *n, pl* **-la** \-lə\ : a reticular structure: as **a** : the network of interstitial tissue composed of reticular fibers — called also *reticular tissue* **b** : the network often visible in fixed protoplasm both of the cell body and the nucleus of many cells

reticulum cell *n* : any of the branched anastomosing cells of the mononuclear phagocyte system that form the reticular fibers

reticulum cell sarcoma *n* : HISTIOCYTIC LYMPHOMA

retin- *or* **retino-** *comb form* : retina ⟨*retin*itis⟩ ⟨*retino*scopy⟩

ret•i•na \ˈret-ᵊn-ə\ *n, pl* **retinas** *also* **ret•i•nae** \-ᵊn-ˌē\ : the sensory membrane that lines most of the large posterior chamber of the eye, is composed of several layers including one containing the rods and cones, and functions as the immediate instrument of vision by receiving the image formed by the lens and converting it into chemical and nervous signals which reach the brain by way of the optic nerve

Ret•in–A \ˌret-ᵊn-ˈā\ *trademark* — used for a preparation of tretinoin

ret•i•nac•u•lar \ˌre-tᵊn-ˈak-yə-lər\ *adj* : of, relating to, or being a retinaculum

ret•i•nac•u•lum \ˌret-ᵊn-ˈa-kyə-ləm\ *n, pl* **-la** \-lə\ : a connecting or retaining band esp. of fibrous tissue — see EXTENSOR RETINACULUM, FLEXOR RETINACULUM, INFERIOR EXTENSOR RETINACULUM, INFERIOR PERONEAL RETINACULUM, PERONEAL RETINACULUM, SUPERIOR EXTENSOR RETINACULUM, SUPERIOR PERONEAL RETINACULUM

[1]**ret•i•nal** \ˈret-ᵊn-əl\ *adj* : of, relating to, involving, or being a retina ⟨∼ rods⟩

[2]**ret•i•nal** \ˈret-ᵊn-ˌal, -ˌȯl\ *n* : a yellowish to orange aldehyde $C_{20}H_{28}O$ derived from vitamin A that in combination with proteins forms the visual pigments of the retinal rods and cones — called also *retinene, retinene$_1$, vitamin A aldehyde*

retinal artery — see CENTRAL ARTERY OF THE RETINA

retinal detachment *n* : a condition of the eye in which the retina has separated from the choroid — called also *detached retina, detachment of the retina*

retinal disparity *n* : the slight difference in the two retinal images due to the angle from which each eye views an object

retinal vein — see CENTRAL RETINAL VEIN

ret•i•nene \ˈret-ᵊn-ˌēn\ *n* : either of two aldehydes derived from vitamin A: **a** : RETINAL **b** : an orange-red crystalline compound $C_{20}H_{26}O$ related to vitamin A_2

retinene$_1$ \-ˈwən\ *n* : RETINAL

retinene$_2$ \-ˈtü\ *n* : RETINENE b

ret•i•ni•tis \ˌret-ᵊn-ˈī-təs\ *n, pl* **-nit•i•des** \-ˈi-tə-ˌdēz\ : inflammation of the retina

retinitis pig•men•to•sa \-ˌpig-mən-ˈtō-sə, -(ˌ)men-, -zə\ *n* : any of several hereditary progressive degenerative diseases of the eye marked by night blindness in the early stages, atrophy and pigment changes in the retina, constriction of the visual field, and eventual blindness — abbr. *RP;* called also *pigmentary retinopathy*

retinitis pro•lif•er•ans \-prə-ˈli-fə-ˌranz\ *n* : neovascularization of the retina associated esp. with diabetic retinopathy

retino- — see RETIN-

ret•i•no•blas•to•ma \ˌret-ᵊn-ō-ˌblas-ˈtō-mə\ *n, pl* **-mas** *also* **-ma•ta** \-mə-tə\ : a hereditary malignant tumor of the retina that develops during childhood, is derived from retinal germ cells, and is associated with a chromosomal abnormality

ret•i•no•cho•roid•i•tis \-ˌkōr-ˌȯi-ˈdī-təs\ *n* : inflammation of the retina and the choroid

ret•i•no•ic acid \ˌret-ᵊn-ˈō-ik-\ *n* : either of two isomers of an acid $C_{20}H_{28}O_2$ derived from vitamin A and used esp. in the treatment of acne: **a** *or* **all-trans-retinoic acid** : TRETINOIN **b** *or* **13-cis-retinoic acid** : ISOTRETINOIN

ret•i•noid \ˈret-ᵊn-ˌȯid\ *n* : any of various synthetic or naturally occurring analogs of vitamin A — **retinoid** *adj*

ret•i•nol \ˈret-ᵊn-ˌȯl, -ˌōl\ *n* : VITAMIN A a

retinol palmitate *n* : RETINYL PALMITATE

ret•i•nop•a•thy \ˌret-ᵊn-ˈä-pə-thē\ *n, pl* **-thies** : any of various noninflammatory disorders of the retina including some that cause blindness ⟨diabetic ∼⟩

retinopathy of prematurity *n* : an ocular disorder of premature infants that is characterized by the presence of an opaque fibrous membrane behind the lens of each eye — abbr. *ROP;* called also *retrolental fibroplasia*

ret•i•no•scope \ˈret-ᵊn-ə-ˌskōp\ *n* : an apparatus used in retinoscopy

ret•i•nos•co•py \ˌret-ᵊn-ˈäs-kə-pē\ *n, pl* **-pies** : a method of determining the state of refraction of the eye by illuminating the retina with a mirror and observing the direction of movement of the retinal illumination and adjacent shadow when the mirror is turned

ret•i•no•tec•tal \ˌret-ᵊn-ō-ˈtek-təl\ *adj* : of, relating to, or being the nerve fibers connecting the retina and the tectum of the midbrain ⟨∼ pathways⟩

ret•i•nyl pal•mi•tate \ˈre-tᵊn-əl-ˈpal-mə-ˌtāt, -ˈpä(l)m-ə-\ *n* : a light yellow to red oil $C_{36}H_{60}O_2$ that is a derivative of vitamin A — called also *retinol palmitate, vitamin A palmitate*

re•tract \ri-ˈtrakt\ *vb* **1** : to draw back or in ⟨∼ the lower jaw⟩ — compare PROTRACT **2** : to use a retractor

re•trac•tion \ri-ˈtrak-shən\ *n* : an act or instance of retracting; *specif* : backward or inward movement of an organ or part

re•trac•tor \ri-ˈtrak-tər\ *n* : one that retracts: as **a** : any of various surgical instruments for holding tissues away from the field of operation **b** : a muscle that draws in an organ or part

retro- *prefix* **1** : backward : back ⟨*retro*flexion⟩ **2** : situated behind ⟨*retro*pubic⟩

ret•ro•bul•bar \ˌre-trō-ˈbəl-bər, -ˌbär\ *adj* : situated, occurring, or administered behind the eyeball ⟨a ~ injection⟩

retrobulbar neuritis *n* : inflammation of the part of the optic nerve lying immediately behind the eyeball

ret•ro•cli•na•tion \-kli-ˈnā-shən\ *n* : the condition of being inclined backward

ret•ro•flex•ion \ˌre-trō-ˈflek-shən\ *n* : the state of being bent back; *specif* : the bending back of the body of the uterus upon the cervix — compare RETROVERSION

ret•ro•gnath•ia \-ˈna-thē-ə\ *n* : RETROGNATHISM

ret•ro•gnath•ism \ˌre-trō-ˈna-ˌthi-zəm\ *n* : a condition characterized by recession of one or both of the jaws

ret•ro•grade \ˈre-trō-ˌgrād\ *adj* **1** : characterized by retrogression **2** : occurring or performed in a direction opposite to the normal or forward direction of conduction or flow: as **a** : occurring along nerve cell processes toward the cell body ⟨~ axonal transport⟩ **b** : occurring opposite to the normal direction or path of blood circulation ⟨~ blood flow⟩ — compare ANTEROGRADE 1 **3** : affecting memories of a period prior to a precipitating event (as brain injury or disease) ⟨~ amnesia⟩ — compare ANTEROGRADE 2 — **ret•ro•grade•ly** *adv*

retrograde pyelogram *n* : a radiograph of the kidney made by retrograde pyelography

retrograde pyelography *n* : pyelography performed by injection of radiopaque material through the ureter

ret•ro•gres•sion \ˌre-trō-ˈgre-shən\ *n* : a reversal in development or condition: as **a** : return to a former and less complex level of development or organization **b** : subsidence or decline of symptoms or manifestations of a disease — **ret•ro•gres•sive** \-ˈgre-siv\ *adj*

ret•ro•len•tal fibroplasia \ˌre-trō-ˈlent-ᵊl-\ *n* : RETINOPATHY OF PREMATURITY

ret•ro•mo•lar \-ˈmō-lər\ *adj* : situated or occurring behind the last molar

ret•ro•per•i•to•ne•al \-ˌper-ə-tə-ˈnē-əl\ *adj* : situated or occurring behind the peritoneum ⟨~ bleeding⟩ ⟨a ~ tumor⟩ — **ret•ro•per•i•to•ne•al•ly** *adv*

retroperitoneal fibrosis *n* : proliferation of fibrous tissue behind the peritoneum often leading to blockage of the ureters — called also *Ormond's disease*

retroperitoneal space *n* : RETROPERITONEUM

ret•ro•per•i•to•ne•um \-ˌper-ə-tə-ˈnē-əm\ *n, pl* **-ne•ums** *or* **-nea** \-ˈnē-ə\ : the space between the peritoneum and the posterior abdominal wall that contains esp. the kidneys and associated structures, the pancreas, and part of the aorta and inferior vena cava

ret•ro•pha•ryn•geal \-ˌfar-ən-ˈjē-əl, -fə-ˈrin-jəl, -jē-əl\ *adj* : situated or occurring behind the pharynx

ret•ro•pu•bic \ˌre-trō-ˈpyü-bik\ *adj* **1** : situated or occurring behind the pubis **2** : performed by way of the retropubic space ⟨~ prostatectomy⟩

retropubic space *n* : the potential space occurring between the pubic symphysis and the urinary bladder

ret•ro•rec•tal \-ˈrekt-ᵊl\ *adj* : situated or occurring behind the rectum

ret•ro•spec•tive \-ˈspek-tiv\ *adj* : relating to or being a study (as of a disease) that starts with the present condition of a population of individuals and collects data about their past history to explain their present condition — compare PROSPECTIVE

ret•ro•ster•nal \-ˈstər-nəl\ *adj* : situated or occurring behind the sternum

ret•ro•ver•sion \-ˈvər-zhən, -shən\ *n* : the bending backward of the uterus and cervix out of the normal axis so that the fundus points toward the sacrum and the cervix toward the pubic symphysis — compare RETROFLEXION

Ret•ro•vir \ˈre-trō-ˌvir\ *trademark* — used for a preparation of AZT

ret•ro•vi•rol•o•gy \ˌre-trō-vī-ˈrä-lə-jē\ *n, pl* **-gies** : a branch of virology concerned with the study of retroviruses — **ret•ro•vi•rol•o•gist** \-jist\ *n*

ret•ro•vi•rus \ˈre-trō-ˌvī-rəs\ *n* : any of a family (*Retroviridae*) of single-stranded RNA viruses that produce reverse transcriptase by means of which DNA is synthesized using their RNA as a template and incorporated into the genome of infected cells, that are often tumorigenic, and that include the lentiviruses (as HIV), HTLV-I, and Rous sarcoma virus — called also *RNA tumor virus* — **ret•ro•vi•ral** \-ˌvī-rəl\ *adj* — **ret•ro•vi•ral•ly** \-ē\ *adv*

re•tru•sion \ri-ˈtrü-zhən\ *n* : backward displacement; *specif* : a condition in which a tooth or the jaw is posterior to its proper occlusal position — **re•trude** \-ˈtrüd\ *vb* — **re•tru•sive** \-ˈtrü-siv\ *adj*

Rett syndrome *or* **Rett's syndrome** \ˌret(s)-\ *n* : a progressive neurodevelopmental genetic disorder that affects females usu. during infancy, that is characterized by cognitive and psychomotor deterioration, slowed head and brain growth, stereotyped hand movements, seizures, and intellectual disability

Rett, Andreas (1924–1997), Austrian physician.

reuniens — see DUCTUS REUNIENS

re•up•take \rē-ˈəp-ˌtāk\ *n* : the reabsorption by a neuron of a neurotransmitter following the transmission of a nerve impulse across a synapse

re•vac•ci•na•tion \rē-ˌvak-sə-ˈnā-shən\ *n* : vaccination administered some period after an initial vaccination esp. to strengthen or renew immunity — **re•vac•ci•nate** \-ˈvak-sə-ˌnāt\ *vb*

re•vas•cu•lar•iza•tion \rē-ˌvas-kyə-lə-rə-ˈzā-shən\ *n* : a surgical procedure for the provision of a new, augmented, or restored blood supply to a body part or organ ⟨myocardial ~⟩

Re•va•tio \ri-ˈvā-shē-ō\ *trademark* — used for a preparation of sildenafil

reverse anorexia *n* : MUSCLE DYSMORPHIA

reverse genetics *n* : genetics that is concerned with genetic material whose nucleotide sequence is known and that analyzes its contribution to the phenotype of the organism by modifying the nucleotide sequence and observing the resulting change in phenotype — **reverse–genetic** *adj*

reverse transcriptase *n* : a polymerase esp. of retroviruses that catalyzes the formation of DNA using RNA as a template

reverse transcriptase inhibitor *n* : a drug (as AZT) that inhibits the activity of retroviral reverse transcriptase

reverse transcription *n* : the process of synthesizing DNA using RNA as a template and reverse transcriptase as a catalyst

re•vers•ible \ri-ˈvər-sə-bəl\ *adj* **1** : capable of going through a series of actions (as changes) either backward or forward **2** : capable of being corrected or undone : not permanent or irrevocable — **re•vers•ibly** *adv*

re•ver•sion \ri-ˈvər-zhən, -shən\ *n* **1** : an act or the process of returning (as to a former condition) **2** : a return toward an ancestral type or condition : reappearance of an ancestral character — **re•vert** \ri-ˈvərt\ *vb*

revision surgery *n* : surgery performed to replace or compensate for a failed implant (as in a hip replacement) or to correct undesirable sequelae (as scar tissue) of previous surgery

re•vive \ri-ˈvīv\ *vb* **re•vived; re•viv•ing** **1** : to return or restore to consciousness or life **2** : to restore from a depressed, inactive, or unused state — **re•viv•able** \-ˈvī-və-bəl\ *adj*

re•ward \ri-ˈwȯrd\ *n* : a stimulus (as food) that serves to reinforce a desired response — **reward** *vb*

Rey•a•taz \ˈrā-ə-ˌtaz\ *trademark* — used for a preparation of atazanavir

Reye's syndrome \ˈrīz-, ˈrāz-\ *also* **Reye syndrome** \ˈrī-, ˈrā-\ *n* : an often fatal encephalopathy esp. of childhood characterized by fever, vomiting, fatty infiltration of the liver, and swelling of the kidneys and brain

Reye, Ralph Douglas Kenneth (1912–1977), Australian pathologist.

Rf *symbol* rutherfordium

RF *abbr* rheumatic fever

R factor \ˈär-\ *n* : a group of genes present in some bacteria that provide a basis for resistance to antibiotics and can be transferred from cell to cell by conjugation

RFLP \ˌär-(ˌ)ef-(ˌ)el-ˈpē\ *n* : RESTRICTION FRAGMENT LENGTH POLYMORPHISM

Rg *symbol* roentgenium

Rh \ˌär-ˈāch\ *adj* : of, relating to, or being an Rh factor ⟨~ antigens⟩

Rh *symbol* rhodium

rhabd- *or* **rhabdo-** *comb form* : rodlike structure ⟨*rhabdo*virus⟩

rhab•do•my•ol•y•sis \ˌrab-dō-mī-ˈä-lə-səs\ *n, pl* **-y•ses** \-ˌsēz\ : the destruction or degeneration of skeletal muscle tissue (as from traumatic injury, excessive exertion, or stroke) that is accompanied by the release of muscle cell contents (as myoglobin and potassium) into the bloodstream resulting in hypovolemia, hyperkalemia, and sometimes acute renal failure

rhab•do•my•o•ma \ˌrab-dō-mī-ˈō-mə\ *n, pl* **-mas** *also* **-ma•ta** \-mə-tə\ : a benign tumor composed of striated muscle fibers ⟨a cardiac ~⟩

rhab•do•myo•sar•co•ma \ˌrab-(ˌ)dō-ˌmī-ə-sär-ˈkō-mə\ *n, pl* **-mas** *also* **-ma•ta** \-mə-tə\ : a malignant tumor composed of striated muscle fibers

rhab•do•virus \-ˌvī-rəs\ *n* : any of a family (*Rhabdoviridae*) of single-stranded RNA viruses that are rod- or bullet-shaped, are found in plants and animals, and include the causative agents of rabies and vesicular stomatitis

rhachitis *var of* RACHITIS

rhag•a•des \ˈra-gə-ˌdēz\ *n pl* : linear cracks or fissures in the skin occurring esp. at the angles of the mouth or about the anus

rhaphe *var of* RAPHE

Rh disease *n* : ERYTHROBLASTOSIS FETALIS

rhe•ni•um \ˈrē-nē-əm\ *n* : a rare heavy metallic element — symbol *Re;* see ELEMENT table

rheo- *comb form* : flow : current ⟨*rheo*base⟩

rheo•base \ˈrē-ō-ˌbās\ *n* : the minimal electrical current required to excite a tissue (as nerve or muscle) given an indefinitely long time during which the current is applied — compare CHRONAXIE

rhe•sus factor \ˈrē-səs-\ *n* : RH FACTOR

rheum \ˈrüm\ *n* : a watery discharge from the mucous membranes esp. of the eyes or nose; *also* : a condition (as a cold) marked by such discharge — **rheumy** \ˈrü-mē\ *adj*

[1]**rheu•mat•ic** \ru̇-ˈma-tik\ *adj* : of, relating to, characteristic of, or affected with rheumatism ⟨~ pain⟩

[2]**rheumatic** *n* : a person affected with rheumatism

rheumatica — see POLYMYALGIA RHEUMATICA

rheumatic disease *n* : any of several diseases (as rheumatic fever or fibrositis) characterized by inflammation and pain in muscles or joints : RHEUMATISM

rheumatic fever *n* : an acute often recurrent disease that occurs chiefly in children and young adults following group A streptococcal infection of the upper respiratory tract (as in strep throat) and is characterized by fever, inflammation, pain, and swelling in and around the joints, inflammatory involvement of the pericardium and valves of the heart, and often the formation of small nodules chiefly in the subcutaneous tissues and the heart

rheumatic heart disease *n* : active or inactive disease of the heart that results from rheumatic fever and is characterized by inflammatory changes in the myocardium or scarring of the valves causing reduced functional capacity of the heart

rheu•ma•tism \ˈrü-mə-ˌti-zəm, ˈru̇-mə-\ *n* **1** : any of various conditions characterized by inflammation or pain in muscles, joints, or fibrous tissue ⟨muscular ~⟩ **2** : RHEUMATOID ARTHRITIS

rheu•ma•toid \-ˌtȯid\ *adj* : characteristic of or affected with rheumatoid arthritis

rheumatoid arthritis *n* : a usu. chronic disease that is considered an autoimmune disease and is characterized esp. by pain, stiffness, inflammation, swelling, and sometimes destruction of joints — abbr. *RA;* compare OSTEOARTHRITIS

rheumatoid factor *n* : an autoantibody of high molecular weight that reacts against immunoglobulins of the class IgG and is often present in rheumatoid arthritis

rheumatoid spondylitis *n* : ANKYLOSING SPONDYLITIS

rheu•ma•tol•o•gist \ˌrü-mə-ˈtä-lə-jist, ˌru̇-\ *n* : a specialist in rheumatology

rheu•ma•tol•o•gy \-jē\ *n, pl* **-gies** : a medical science dealing with rheumatic diseases — **rheu•ma•to•log•ic** \-tə-ˈlä-jik\ *or* **rheu•ma•to•log•i•cal** \-ji-kəl\ *adj*

Rh factor \ˌär-ˈāch-\ *n* : a genetically determined protein on the red blood cells of some people that is one of the substances used to classify human blood as to compatibility for transfusion and that when present in a fetus but not in the mother causes a serious immunogenic reaction in which the mother produces antibodies that cross the placenta and attack the red blood cells of the fetus — called also *rhesus factor*

rhin- *or* **rhino-** *comb form* **1 a** : nose ⟨*rhin*itis⟩ **b** : nose and ⟨*rhino*tracheitis⟩ **2** : nasal ⟨*rhino*virus⟩

rhi•nal \ˈrīn-ᵊl\ *adj* : of or relating to the nose : NASAL

rhin•en•ceph•a•lon \ˌrī-(ˌ)nen-ˈse-fə-ˌlän, -lən\ *n, pl* **-la** \-lə\ : the anterior inferior part of the forebrain that is chiefly concerned with olfaction and that is considered to include the olfactory bulb together with the forebrain olfactory structures receiving fibers directly from it and often esp. formerly the limbic system which is now known to be concerned with emotional states and affect — called also *smell brain* — **rhin•en•ce•pha•lic** \ˌrī-ˌnen-sə-ˈfa-lik\ *adj*

rhi•ni•tis \rī-ˈnī-təs\ *n, pl* **-nit•i•des** \-ˈni-tə-ˌdēz\ : inflammation of the mucous membrane of the nose marked esp. by rhinorrhea, nasal congestion and itching, and sneezing; *also* : any of various conditions characterized by rhinitis — see ALLERGIC RHINITIS, RHINITIS MEDICAMENTOSA, VASOMOTOR RHINITIS

rhinitis me•dic•a•men•to•sa \-mə-ˌdi-kə-men-ˈtō-sə\ *n* : an increase in the severity or duration of rhinitis that results from prolonged use of decongestant nasal spray

Rhi•no•cort Aqua \ˈrī-nō-ˌkȯrt-ˈak-wə, -ˈäk-\ *trademark* — used for a preparation of budesonide administered as a nasal spray

rhi•no•log•ic \ˌrī-nə-ˈlä-jik\ *or* **rhi•no•log•i•cal** \-ji-kəl\ *adj* : of or relating to the nose ⟨~ disease⟩

rhi•nol•o•gist \rī-ˈnä-lə-jist\ *n* : a physician who specializes in rhinology

rhi•nol•o•gy \-jē\ *n, pl* **-gies** : a branch of medicine that deals with the nose and its diseases

rhi•no•phar•yn•gi•tis \ˌrī-nō-ˌfar-ən-ˈjī-təs\ *n, pl* **-git•i•des** \-ˈji-tə-ˌdēz\ : inflammation of the mucous membrane of the nose and pharynx

rhi•no•phy•ma \-ˈfī-mə\ *n, pl* **-mas** *or* **-ma•ta** \-mə-tə\ : a nodular swelling and congestion of the nose in an advanced stage of rosacea

rhi•no•plas•ty \ˈrī-nō-ˌplas-tē\ *n, pl* **-ties** : plastic surgery on the nose usu. for cosmetic purposes — called also *nose job* — **rhi•no•plas•tic** \ˌrī-nō-ˈplas-tik\ *adj*

rhi•no•pneu•mo•ni•tis \ˌrī-nō-ˌnü-mə-ˈnī-təs, -ˌnyü-\ *n* : an acute febrile respiratory disease of horses that is caused by two herpesviruses of the genus *Varicellovirus* (species *Equid herpesvirus 1* and *Equid herpesvirus 4*) and is characterized esp. by rhinopharyngitis and tracheobronchitis

rhi•nor•rhea \ˌrī-nə-ˈrē-ə\ *n* : excessive mucous secretion from the nose

rhi•nor•rhoea *chiefly Brit var of* RHINORRHEA

rhi•no•scle•ro•ma \ˌrī-nō-sklə-ˈrō-mə\ *n* : a chronic inflammatory disease of the mucosa of the respiratory tract and esp. the nasal cavity that is caused by infection with a bacterium of the genus *Klebsiella* (*K. rhinoscleromatis*) and is marked by granulomatous swelling with the formation of rubbery nodules followed by sclerosis of tissue

rhi•no•scope \ˈrī-nə-ˌskōp\ *n* : an instrument (as an endoscope) for examining the cavities and passages of the nose

rhi•nos•co•py \rī-ˈnäs-kə-pē\ *n, pl* **-pies** : examination of the nasal passages — **rhi•no•scop•ic** \ˌrī-nə-ˈskä-pik\ *adj*

rhi•no•si•nus•itis \ˌrī-nō-ˌsī-nə-ˈsī-təs, -nyə-\ *n* : inflammation of the mucous membranes of the nose and one or more paranasal sinuses

rhi•no•spo•rid•i•o•sis \ˌrī-nō-spə-ˌri-dē-ˈō-səs\ *n, pl* **-o•ses** \-ˌsēz\ : a fungal disease of the external mucous membranes (as of the nose) that is characterized by the formation of pinkish-red, friable, sessile, or pedunculated polyps and is caused by an ascomycetous fungus (*Rhinosporidium seeberi*)

rhi•not•o•my \rī-ˈnä-tə-mē\ *n, pl* **-mies** : surgical incision of the nose

rhi•no•tra•che•itis \ˌrī-nō-ˌtrā-kē-ˈī-təs\ *n* : inflammation of the nasal cavities and trachea; *esp* : a disease of the upper respiratory system in cats and esp. young kittens that is characterized by sneezing, conjunctivitis with discharge, and nasal discharges — see INFECTIOUS BOVINE RHINOTRACHEITIS

rhi•no•vi•rus \ˌrī-nō-ˈvī-rəs\ *n* **1** *cap* : a genus of picornaviruses including two species (*Human rhinovirus A* and *Human rhinovirus B*) having numerous serotypes causing respiratory infections (as the common cold) in humans **2** : any virus of the genus *Rhinovirus*

Rhipi•ceph•a•lus \ˌri-pə-ˈse-fə-ləs\ *n* : a genus of ixodid ticks that are parasitic on many mammals and some birds and include vectors of serious diseases (as east coast fever)

rhi•zo•me•lic \ˌrī-zə-ˈmē-lik\ *adj* : of or relating to the hip and shoulder joints

rhi•zot•o•my \rī-ˈzä-tə-mē\ *n, pl* **-mies** : the operation of cutting the anterior or posterior spinal nerve roots

Rh–neg•a•tive \ˌär-ˌāch-ˈne-gə-tiv\ *adj* : lacking Rh factor in the blood

rhod- *or* **rhodo-** *comb form* : rose : red ⟨*rhod*opsin⟩

rho•di•um \ˈrō-dē-əm\ *n* : a white hard ductile metallic element — symbol *Rh;* see ELEMENT table

rho•dop•sin \rō-ˈdäp-sən\ *n* : a red photosensitive pigment in the retinal rods that is important in vision in dim light, is quickly bleached by light to a mixture of opsin and retinal, and is regenerated in the dark — called also *visual purple*

Rho•do•tor•u•la \ˌrō-də-ˈtȯr-yə-lə\ *n* : a genus of yeasts (family Cryptococcaceae) including one (*R. rubra* syn. *R. mucilaginosa*) sometimes present in the blood or involved in endocarditis prob. as a secondary infection

rhomb•en•ceph•a•lon \ˌräm-(ˌ)ben-ˈse-fə-ˌlän, -lən\ *n, pl* **-la** \-lə\ : HINDBRAIN — **rhomb•en•ce•phal•ic** \-sə-ˈfa-lik\ *adj*

rhom•boi•de•us \räm-ˈbȯi-dē-əs\ *n, pl* **-dei** \-dē-ˌī\ : either of two muscles that lie beneath the trapezius muscle and connect the spinous processes of various vertebrae with the medial border of the scapula: **a** : RHOMBOIDEUS MINOR **b** : RHOMBOIDEUS MAJOR

rhomboideus major *n* : a muscle arising from the spinous processes of the second through fifth thoracic vertebrae, inserted into the vertebral border of the scapula, and acting to adduct and laterally rotate the scapula — called also *rhomboid major*

rhomboideus minor *n* : a muscle arising from the inferior part of the ligamentum nuchae and from the spinous processes of the seventh cervical and first thoracic vertebrae, inserted into the vertebral border of the scapula at the base of the bony process terminating in the acromion, and acting to adduct and laterally rotate the scapula — called also *rhomboid minor*

rhomboid fossa *n* : the floor of the fourth ventricle of the brain formed by the dorsal surfaces of the pons and medulla oblongata

rhomboid major *n* : RHOMBOIDEUS MAJOR

rhomboid minor *n* : RHOMBOIDEUS MINOR

rhon•chus \ˈräŋ-kəs\ *n, pl* **rhon•chi** \ˈräŋ-ˌkī\ : a whistling or snoring sound heard on auscultation of the chest when the air channels are partly obstructed — compare RALE, RATTLE

rho•ta•cism \ˈrō-tə-ˌsi-zəm\ *n* : a defective pronunciation of *r*; *esp* : substitution of some other sound for that of *r*

Rh–pos•i•tive \ˌär-ˌāch-ˈpä-zə-tiv\ *adj* : containing Rh factor in the red blood cells

rhus \ˈrüs\ *n* **1** *cap* : a genus of shrubs and trees of the cashew family (Anacardiaceae) native to temperate and warm regions — see TOXICODENDRON **2** *pl* **rhuses** *or* **rhus** : any shrub or tree of the genus *Rhus* : SUMAC

rhus dermatitis *n* : dermatitis caused by contact with various plants (as poison ivy) of the genus *Rhus* or *Toxicodendron*

rhythm \ˈri-t͟həm\ *n* **1** : a regularly recurrent quantitative change in a variable biological process: as **a** : the pattern of recurrence of the cardiac cycle ⟨an irregular ∼⟩ **b** : the recurring pattern of physical and functional changes associated with the mammalian and esp. human sexual cycle **2** : RHYTHM METHOD — **rhyth•mic** \ˈrit͟h-mik\ *or* **rhyth•mi•cal** \-mi-kəl\ *adj* — **rhyth•mi•cal•ly** *adv* — **rhyth•mic•i•ty** \rit͟h-ˈmi-sə-tē\ *n*

rhythm method *n* : a method of birth control involving abstinence during the period in which ovulation is most likely to occur

rhyt•i•dec•to•my \ˌri-tə-ˈdek-tə-mē\ *n, pl* **-mies** : FACELIFT

RIA *abbr* radioimmunoassay

rib \ˈrib\ *n* : any of the paired curved bony or partly cartilaginous rods that stiffen the lateral walls of the body and protect the viscera and that in humans normally include 12 pairs of which all are articulated with the spinal column at the dorsal end and the first 10 are connected also at the ventral end with the sternum by costal cartilages — see FALSE RIB, FLOATING RIB, TRUE RIB

rib- *or* **ribo-** *comb form* : related to ribose ⟨*ribo*flavin⟩

ri•ba•vi•rin \ˌrī-bə-ˈvī-rən\ *n* : a synthetic broad-spectrum antiviral drug $C_8H_{12}N_4O_5$ that is a nucleoside resembling guanosine

rib cage *n* : the bony enclosing wall of the chest consisting chiefly of the ribs and the structures connecting them — called also *thoracic cage*

ri•bo•fla•vin \ˌrī-bə-ˈflā-vən, ˈrī-bə-ˌ\ *also* **ri•bo•fla•vine** \-ˌvēn\ *n* : a yellow crystalline compound $C_{17}H_{20}N_4O_6$ that is a growth-promoting member of the vitamin B complex and occurs both free (as in milk) and combined (as in liver) — called also *lactoflavin, vitamin B_2*

riboflavin phosphate *or* **riboflavin 5'–phosphate** \-ˈfīv-ˈprīm-\ *n* : FMN

ri•bo•nu•cle•ase \ˌrī-bō-ˈnü-klē-ˌās, -ˈnyü-, -ˌāz\ *n* : an enzyme that catalyzes the hydrolysis of RNA — called also *RNase*

ri•bo•nu•cle•ic acid \ˌrī-bō-nu̇-ˌklē-ik-, -nyu̇-, -ˌklā-\ *n* : RNA

ri•bo•nu•cleo•pro•tein \-ˌnü-klē-ō-ˈprō-ˌtēn, -ˌnyü-\ *n* : a nucleoprotein that contains RNA

ri•bo•nu•cle•o•side \-ˈnü-klē-ə-ˌsīd, -ˈnyü-\ *n* : a nucleoside that contains ribose

ri•bo•nu•cle•o•tide \-ˌtīd\ *n* : a nucleotide that contains ribose and occurs esp. as a constituent of RNA

ri•bose \ˈrī-ˌbōs, -ˌbōz\ *n* : a pentose $C_5H_{10}O_5$ found esp. in the levorotatory D-form as a constituent of a number of nucleosides (as adenosine, cytidine, and guanosine) esp. in RNA

ribosomal RNA *n* : RNA that is a fundamental structural element of ribosomes — called also *rRNA*

ri•bo•some \ˈrī-bə-ˌsōm\ *n* : any of the RNA- and protein-rich cytoplasmic organelles that are sites of protein synthesis — **ri•bo•som•al** \ˌrī-bə-ˈsō-məl\ *adj*

ri•bo•zyme \-ˌzīm\ *n* : a molecule of RNA that functions as an enzyme (as by catalyzing the cleavage of other RNA molecules)

RICE *abbr* rest, ice, compression, elevation — used esp. for the initial treatment of many usu. minor sports-related injuries (as sprains)

rice–water stool *n* : a watery stool containing white flecks of mucus, epithelial cells, and bacteria that is characteristic of severe forms of diarrhea (as in Asiatic cholera)

ri•cin \ˈrīs-ᵊn, ˈris-\ *n* : a poisonous protein in the castor bean

rick•ets \ˈri-kəts\ *n* : a deficiency disease that affects the young during the period of skeletal growth, is characterized esp. by soft and deformed bones, and is caused by failure to assimilate and use calcium and phosphorus normally due to inadequate sunlight or vitamin D — called also *rachitis;* see OSTEOMALACIA

rick•etts•ae•mia *chiefly Brit var of* RICKETTSEMIA

rick•etts•emia \ˌri-kət-ˈsē-mē-ə\ *n* : an abnormal presence of rickettsiae in the blood

Rick•etts, Howard Taylor (1871–1910), American pathologist.

rick•ett•sia \ri-ˈket-sē-ə\ *n* **1** *cap* : a genus of rod-shaped, coccoid, or diplococcus-shaped bacteria (family Rickettsiaceae) that are transmitted by biting arthropods (as lice or ticks) and cause a number of serious diseases (as Rocky Mountain spotted fever and typhus) **2** *pl* **-si•ae** \-sē-ˌē\ *also* **-sias** *or* **-sia** : any bacterium of the genus *Rickettsia* or of the order (Rickettsiales) to which it belongs — **rick•ett•si•al** \-sē-əl\ *adj*

rick•ett•si•al•pox \ri-ˌket-sē-əl-ˈpäks\ *n* : a disease characterized by fever, chills, headache, backache, and a spotty rash and caused by a bacterium of the genus *Rickettsia* (*R. akari*) transmitted to humans by the bite of a mite of the genus *Allodermanyssus* (*A. sanguineus*) living on rodents (as the house mouse)

rick•ett•si•o•sis \ri-ˌket-sē-ˈō-səs\ *n, pl* **-o•ses** \-ˌsēz\ : infection with or disease caused by a rickettsia

Ri•dau•ra \ri-ˈdȯr-ə\ *trademark* — used for a preparation of auranofin

Rie•del's disease \ˈrēd-ᵊlz-\ *n* : chronic thyroiditis in which the thyroid gland becomes hard and stony and firmly attached to surrounding tissues

Riedel, Bernhard Moritz Karl Ludwig (1846–1916), German surgeon.

Riedel's struma *n* : RIEDEL'S DISEASE

rif•a•bu•tin \ˈri-fə-ˌbyü-tᵊn\ *n* : a semisynthetic antibacterial drug $C_{46}H_{62}N_4O_{11}$ used esp. to prevent and treat infection with bacteria of the Mycobacterium avium complex

ri•fam•pin \rī-ˈfam-pən\ *or* **ri•fam•pi•cin** \rī-ˈfam-pə-sən\ *n* : a semisynthetic antibiotic $C_{43}H_{58}N_4O_{12}$ that is used esp. in the treatment of tuberculosis and to treat asymptomatic carriers of meningococci

rif•a•my•cin \ˌri-fə-ˈmīs-ᵊn\ *n* : any of several antibiotics that are derived from a soil bacterium (*Amycolatopsis mediterranei* syn. *Streptomyces mediterranei*)

Rift Valley fever *n* : an acute usu. epizootic mosquito-borne disease of domestic animals (as sheep and cattle) chiefly of eastern and southern Africa that is caused by a bunyavirus of the genus *Phlebovirus* (species *Rift Valley fever virus*), is marked esp. by fever, abortion, death of newborns, diarrhea, and jaundice, and is sometimes transmitted to humans usu. in a milder form marked by flu-like symptoms

right atrioventricular valve *n* : TRICUSPID VALVE

right brain *n* : the right cerebral hemisphere of the human brain esp. when viewed in terms of its predominant thought processes (as creativity and intuitive thinking) — **right–brained** *adj*

right colic flexure *n* : HEPATIC FLEXURE

right–eyed *adj* : using the right eye in preference (as in using a monocular microscope)

right gastric artery *n* : an artery that arises from the hepatic artery, passes to the left along the lesser curvature of the stomach while giving off a number of branches, and eventually joins a branch of the left gastric artery

right gastroepiploic artery *n* : GASTROEPIPLOIC ARTERY a

right–hand•ed \-ˈhan-dəd\ *adj* **1** : using the right hand habitually or more easily than the left **2** : relating to, designed for, or done with the right hand **3** : having the same direction or course as the movement of the hands of a watch viewed from in front **4** : DEXTROROTATORY — **right–handed** *adv* — **right–hand•ed•ness** *n*

right heart *n* : the right atrium and ventricle : the half of the heart that receives blood from the systemic circulation and passes it into the pulmonary arteries

right lymphatic duct *n* : a short vessel that receives lymph from the right side of the head, neck, and thorax, the right arm, right lung, right side of the heart, and convex surface of the liver and that discharges it into the right subclavian vein at its junction with the right internal jugular vein

right pulmonary artery *n* : PULMONARY ARTERY b

right subcostal vein *n* : SUBCOSTAL VEIN a

ri•gid•i•ty \rə-ˈji-də-tē\ *n, pl* **-ties** : the quality or state of being stiff or devoid of or deficient in flexibility: as **a** : abnormal stiffness of muscle **b** : emotional inflexibility and resistance to change — **rig•id** \ˈri-jəd\ *adj*

rigidus — see HALLUX RIGIDUS

rig•or \ˈri-gər\ *n* **1 a** : CHILL 1 **b** : a tremor caused by a chill **2 a** : rigidity or torpor of organs or tissue that prevents response to stimuli **b** : RIGOR MORTIS

rig•or mor•tis \ˈri-gər-ˈmȯr-təs\ *n* : temporary rigidity of muscles occurring after death

Ri•ley–Day syndrome \ˈrī-lē-ˈdā-\ *n* : FAMILIAL DYSAUTONOMIA

Riley, Conrad Milton (1913–2005), and **Day, Richard Lawrence (1905–1989),** American pediatricians.

ril•pi•vir•ine \ˌril-pə-ˈvir-ˌēn\ *n* : a reverse transcriptase inhibitor administered orally in the form of its hydrochloride $C_{22}H_{18}N_6·HCl$ in conjunction with other antiretroviral agents in the treatment of HIV infection — see COMPLERA, EDURANT

ri•ma \ˈrī-mə\ *n, pl* **ri•mae** \-ˌmē\ : an anatomical fissure or cleft

rima glot•ti•dis \-ˈglä-tə-dəs\ *n* : the passage in the glottis between the true vocal cords

ri•man•ta•dine \rə-ˈman-tə-ˌdēn\ *n* : a synthetic antiviral drug that is chemically related to amantadine and is administered orally in the form of its hydrochloride $C_{12}H_{21}N·HCl$ to prevent and treat influenza

rima pal•pe•bra•rum \-ˌpal-pē-ˈbrer-əm\ *n* : PALPEBRAL FISSURE

rin•der•pest \ˈrin-dər-ˌpest\ *n* : an infectious disease of ruminants (as cattle) that is caused by a paramyxovirus of the genus *Morbillivirus* (species *Rinderpest virus*), is marked by high mortality in epidemics, and has been eradicated globally by widespread vaccination

[1]**ring** \ˈriŋ\ *n* **1 a** : a circular band **b** : an anatomical structure having a circular opening : ANNULUS **2** : an arrangement of atoms represented in formulas or models in a cyclic manner as a closed chain

[2]**ring** *vb* **rang** \ˈraŋ\; **rung** \ˈrəŋ\; **ring•ing** : to have the sensation of being filled with a humming sound ⟨his ears *rang*⟩

ring•bone \-ˌbōn\ *n* : osteoarthritis of a horse's foot that usu. produces lameness

Ring•er's fluid \ˈriŋ-ərz-\ *n* : RINGER'S SOLUTION

Ringer, Sidney (1835–1910), British physiologist.

Ringer's lactate *or* **Ringer's lactate solution** *n* : LACTATED RINGER'S SOLUTION

Ring•er's solution \ˈriŋ-ərz-\ *also* **Ring•er solution** \ˈriŋ-ər-\ *n* : a sterile aqueous solution of calcium chloride, sodium chloride, and potassium chloride that provides a medium essentially isotonic to many animal tissues and that is used esp. to replenish fluids and electrolytes by intravenous infusion or to irrigate tissues by topical application — compare LACTATED RINGER'S SOLUTION

ring•hals \ˈriŋ-ˌhals\ *n* : a venomous African elapid snake (*Haemachatus haemachatus*) that rarely bites but when threatened spits a venom that is harmless to intact skin but may cause severe damage to eyes upon contact

ring•worm \ˈriŋ-ˌwərm\ *n* : any of several contagious diseases of the skin, hair, or nails of humans and domestic animals caused by fungi (as of the genus *Trichophyton*) and characterized by ring-shaped discolored patches on the skin that are covered with vesicles and scales — called also *tinea*

Rin•ne's test \ˈri-nəs-\ *or* **Rin•ne test** \ˈri-nə-\ *n* : a test for determining a subject's ability to hear a vibrating tuning fork when it is held next to the ear and when it is placed on the mastoid process with diminished hearing acuity through air and somewhat heightened hearing acuity through bone being symptomatic of conduction deafness

Rinne, Heinrich Adolf R. (1819–1868), German otologist.

ris•ed•ro•nate \ri-ˈse-drə-ˌnāt\ *n* : a sodium bisphosphonate salt $C_7H_{10}NNaO_7P_2$ taken orally to inhibit bone resorption esp. in the prevention or treatment of osteoporosis in postmenopausal women — called also *risedronate sodium;* see ACTONEL, ATELVIA

risk \ˈrisk\ *n* **1** : possibility of loss, injury, disease, or death ⟨hypertension increases the ∼ of stroke⟩ **2** : a person considered in terms of the possible bad effects of a particular course of treatment ⟨a poor surgical ∼⟩ — **at risk** : in a state or condition marked by a high level of risk or susceptibility ⟨patients *at risk* of developing infections⟩

risk factor *n* : something that increases risk or susceptibility ⟨poorly controlled hypertension is a *risk factor* for coronary heart disease⟩

ri•so•ri•us \ri-ˈsōr-ē-əs, -ˈzōr-\ *n, pl* **-rii** \-ē-ˌī\ : a narrow band of muscle fibers arising from the fascia over the masseter muscle, inserted into the tissues at the corner of the mouth, and acting to retract the angle of the mouth

Ris•per•dal \ˈris-pər-ˌdal\ *trademark* — used for a preparation of risperidone

ris•per•i•done \ri-ˈsper-ə-ˌdōn\ *n* : an antipsychotic drug $C_{28}H_{27}FN_4O_2$ used esp. to treat schizophrenia, acute manic episodes of bipolar disorder, and irritability associated with autism — see RISPERDAL

ris•to•ce•tin \ˌris-tə-ˈsēt-ᵊn\ *n* : either of two antibiotics or a mixture of both produced by an actinomycete of the genus *Nocardia* (*N. lurida*)

ri•sus sar•do•ni•cus \ˈrī-səs-ˌsär-ˈdä-ni-kəs, ˈrē-\ *n* : a facial expression characterized by raised eyebrows and grinning distortion of the face resulting from spasm of facial muscles esp. in tetanus

Rit•a•lin \ˈri-tə-lən\ *trademark* — used for a preparation of the hydrochloride of methylphenidate

rit•o•drine \ˈri-tə-ˌdrēn, -drən\ *n* : a drug administered intravenously in the form of its hydrochloride $C_{17}H_{21}NO_3{\cdot}HCl$ as a smooth muscle relaxant esp. to inhibit premature labor

ri•to•na•vir \ˌrī-ˈtō-nə-ˌvir\ *n* : an antiviral protease inhibitor $C_{37}H_{48}N_6O_5S_2$ administered orally to treat HIV infection and AIDS — see NORVIR

Rit•ter's disease \ˈri-tərz-\ *n* : STAPHYLOCOCCAL SCALDED SKIN SYNDROME

Ritter von Rittershain, Gottfried (1820–1883), German physician.

rit•u•al \ˈri-chə-wəl\ *n* : any act or practice regularly repeated in a set precise manner for relief of anxiety ⟨obsessive-compulsive ∼*s*⟩

Ri•tux•an \rī-ˈtək-sən\ *trademark* — used for a preparation of rituximab

ri•tux•i•mab \ri-ˈtək-si-ˌmab\ *n* : a drug that is a genetically engineered monoclonal antibody administered by intravenous injection esp. to treat non-Hodgkin lymphoma and chronic lymphocytic leukemia — see RITUXAN

riv•a•rox•a•ban \ˌri-və-ˈräk-sə-ˌban\ *n* : a drug $C_{19}H_{18}ClN_3O_5S$ that inhibits blood clot formation and is taken orally esp. to prevent and treat deep vein thrombosis and pulmonary embolism and to reduce the risk of stroke related to atrial fibrillation — see XARELTO

riv•a•stig•mine \ˌri-və-ˈstig-ˌmēn\ *n* : a drug $C_{14}H_{22}N_2O_2$ that is administered transdermally as a skin patch or is taken orally in the form of its tartrate $C_{14}H_{22}N_2O_2{\cdot}C_4H_6O_6$ to treat dementia associated with Alzheimer's disease and Parkinson's disease by inhibiting the action of cholinesterase — see EXELON

river blindness *n* : ONCHOCERCIASIS

RK *abbr* radial keratotomy

RLF *abbr* retrolental fibroplasia

RLQ *abbr* right lower quadrant (abdomen)

RLS *abbr* restless legs syndrome

Rn *symbol* radon

RN \ˌär-ˈen\ *n* : REGISTERED NURSE

RNA \ˌär-(ˌ)en-ˈā\ *n* : any of various nucleic acids that contain ribose and uracil as structural components and are associated with the control of cellular chemical activities — called also *ribonucleic acid;* see MESSENGER RNA, RIBOSOMAL RNA, TRANSFER RNA

RNAi *n* : RNA INTERFERENCE

RNA interference *n* : a posttranscriptional genetic mechanism which suppresses gene expression and in which double-stranded RNA cleaved into small fragments initiates the degradation of a complementary messenger RNA sequence; *also* : a technique (as the introduction of double-stranded RNA into an organism) that artificially induces RNA interference and is used for studying or regulating gene expression

RNA polymerase *n* : any of a group of enzymes that promote the synthesis of RNA using DNA or RNA as a template

RNA replicase *n* : REPLICASE

RNase *or* **RNAase** \ˌär-ˌen-ˈā-ˌās, -ˈā-ˌāz\ *n* : RIBONUCLEASE

RNA syn•the•tase \-ˈsin-thə-ˌtās, -ˌtāz\ *n* : REPLICASE
RNA tumor virus *n* : RETROVIRUS
RNA virus *n* : a virus (as a retrovirus) whose genome consists of RNA
roach \ˈrōch\ *n* : COCKROACH
road rash *n* : mild to severe skin abrasion resulting from a fall (as from a bicycle or motorcycle) which usu. involves sliding on a hard, rough surface
roar•ing \ˈrōr-iŋ\ *n* : noisy inhalation in a horse caused by paralysis and muscular atrophy of part of the larynx
Rob•ert•so•ni•an \ˌrä-bərt-ˈsō-nē-ən\ *adj* : relating to or being a reciprocal translocation that takes place between two acrocentric chromosomes and that yields one nonfunctional chromosome having two short arms and one functional chromosome having two long arms of which one arm is derived from each parent chromosome
Rob•ert•son \ˈrä-bərt-sən\, **William Rees Brebner (1881–1941)**, American biologist.
Ro•bi•nul \ˈrō-bi-ˌnu̇l\ *trademark* — used for a preparation of glycopyrrolate
Ro•cha•li•maea \ˌrō-kə-li-ˈmē-ə\ *n, syn of* BARTONELLA
Ro•chelle salt \rō-ˈshel-\ *n* : a crystalline salt $C_4H_4KNaO_6 \cdot 4H_2O$ that is a mild purgative — called also *potassium sodium tartrate, Seignette salt, sodium potassium tartrate*
rock \ˈräk\ *n* **1** : a small crystallized mass of crack cocaine **2** : CRACK — called also *rock cocaine*
Rocky Mountain spotted fever *n* : an acute bacterial disease that is characterized by chills, fever, prostration, pains in muscles and joints, and a red purple eruption and that is caused by a bacterium of the genus *Rickettsia* (*R. rickettsii*) usu. transmitted by ixodid ticks and esp. by the American dog tick and Rocky Mountain wood tick
Rocky Mountain wood tick *n* : a widely distributed wood tick of the genus *Dermacentor* (*D. andersoni*) of western No. America that is a vector of Rocky Mountain spotted fever and sometimes causes tick paralysis
rod \ˈräd\ *n* **1** : any of the long rod-shaped photosensitive receptors in the retina responsive to faint light — compare CONE 1 **2** : a bacterium shaped like a rod
ro•dent \ˈrōd-ᵊnt\ *n* : any of an order (Rodentia) of relatively small mammals (as a mouse or a rat) that have in both jaws a single pair of incisors with a chisel-shaped edge — **rodent** *adj*
ro•den•ti•cide \rō-ˈden-tə-ˌsīd\ *n* : an agent that kills, repels, or controls rodents
rodent ulcer *n* : a chronic persistent ulcer of the exposed skin and esp. of the face that is destructive locally, spreads slowly, and is usu. a carcinoma derived from basal cells
rod•like \ˈräd-ˌlīk\ *adj* : resembling a rod ⟨~ bacteria⟩
rod of Cor•ti \-ˈkȯr-tē\ *n* : any of the minute modified epithelial elements that rise from the basilar membrane of the organ of Corti in two spirally arranged rows so that the free ends of the members incline toward and interlock with corresponding members of the opposite row and enclose the tunnel of Corti
A. G. G. Corti — see ORGAN OF CORTI
[1]**roent•gen** *also* **rönt•gen** \ˈrent-gən, ˈrənt-, -jən, -shən\ *adj* : of, relating to, or using X-rays
Rönt•gen *or* **Roent•gen** \ˈrœnt-gən\, **Wilhelm Conrad (1845–1923)**, German physicist.
[2]**roentgen** *also* **röntgen** *n* : the international unit of x-radiation or gamma radiation equal to the amount of radiation that produces in one cubic centimeter of dry air at 0°C (32°F) and standard atmospheric pressure ionization of either sign equal to one electrostatic unit of charge
roent•gen•i•um \rent-ˈge-nē-əm, rənt-, -ˈje-\ *n* : a short-lived radioactive element that is artificially produced — symbol *Rg;* see ELEMENT table
roent•gen•o•gram \ˈrent-gə-nə-ˌgram, ˈrənt-, -jə-, -shə-\ *n* : RADIOGRAPH
roent•gen•og•ra•phy \ˌrent-gə-ˈnä-grə-fē, ˌrənt-, -jə-, -shə-\ *n, pl* **-phies** : RADIOGRAPHY — **roent•gen•o•graph•ic** \-nə-ˈgra-fik\ *adj* — **roent•gen•o•graph•i•cal•ly** *adv*
roent•gen•ol•o•gist \-ˈnä-lə-jist\ *n* : RADIOLOGIST
roent•gen•ol•o•gy \-ˈnä-lə-jē\ *n, pl* **-gies** : RADIOLOGY 2 — **roent•gen•o•log•ic** \-nə-ˈlä-jik\ *or* **roent•gen•o•log•i•cal** \-ji-kəl\ *adj* — **roent•gen•o•log•i•cal•ly** *adv*
roent•gen•os•co•py \-ˈnäs-kə-pē\ *n, pl* **-pies** : observation or examination by means of a fluoroscope : FLUOROSCOPY — **roent•gen•o•scop•ic** \-nə-ˈskä-pik\ *adj*
roentgen ray *n* : X-RAY 1
ro•fe•cox•ib \ˌrō-fe-ˈkäk-sib\ *n* : a COX-2 inhibitor $C_{17}H_{14}O_4S$ used to relieve the signs and symptoms of osteoarthritis and rheumatoid arthritis, to manage acute pain in adults, and to treat primary dysmenorrhea but withdrawn from sale by the manufacturer because of its link to cardiovascular events (as heart attack and stroke) — see VIOXX
Ro•gaine \ˈrō-ˌgān\ *trademark* — used for a preparation of minoxidil
Rog•er•ian \rä-ˈjer-ē-ən\ *adj* : of or relating to the system of therapy or the theory of personality of Carl Rogers
Rog•ers \ˈrä-jərz\, **Carl Ransom (1902–1987)**, American psychologist.

Ro•hyp•nol \rō-ˈhip-ˌnȯl\ *n* : a preparation of flunitrazepam — formerly a U.S. registered trademark

Ro•lan•dic area \rō-ˈlan-dik-\ *n* : the motor area of the cerebral cortex lying just anterior to the central sulcus and comprising part of the precentral gyrus

L. Rolando — see FISSURE OF ROLANDO

Rolandic fissure *n* : CENTRAL SULCUS

role *also* **rôle** \ˈrōl\ *n* : a socially prescribed pattern of behavior usu. determined by an individual's status in a particular society

role model *n* : a person whose behavior in a particular role is imitated by others

role–play \ˈrōl-ˌplā\ *vb* **1** : ACT OUT 1 **2** : to play a role

rolf \ˈrȯlf, ˈrälf\ *vb, often cap* : to practice Rolfing on

Rolf, Ida P. (1896–1979), American biochemist and physiotherapist.

Rolf•ing \ˈrȯl-fiŋ, ˈräl-\ *service mark* — used for the practice of manipulating the body's deep connective tissues for structural alignment

ro•li•tet•ra•cy•cline \ˌrō-li-ˌte-trə-ˈsī-ˌklēn\ *n* : a semisynthetic broad-spectrum tetracycline antibiotic $C_{27}H_{33}N_3O_8$ usu. administered intravenously or intramuscularly

roller — see TONGUE ROLLER

roll•er bandage \ˈrō-lər-\ *n* : a long rolled bandage

Rom•berg's sign \ˈräm-ˌbərgz-\ *or* **Rom•berg sign** \-ˌbərg-\ *n* : a diagnostic sign of tabes dorsalis and other diseases of the nervous system consisting of a swaying of the body when the feet are placed close together and the eyes are closed

Romberg, Moritz Heinrich (1795–1873), German pathologist.

Romberg's test *or* **Romberg test** *n* : a test for the presence of Romberg's sign by placing the feet close together and closing the eyes

ron•geur \rōⁿ-ˈzhər\ *n* : a heavy-duty forceps for removing small pieces of bone or tough tissue

ron•nel \ˈrän-ᵊl\ *n* : an organophosphate $C_8H_8Cl_3O_3PS$ that is used esp. as a systemic insecticide to protect cattle from pests

röntgen *var of* ROENTGEN

roof \ˈrüf, ˈru̇f\ *n, pl* **roofs** \ˈrüfs, ˈru̇fs, ˈrüvz, ˈru̇vz\ **1** : the vaulted upper boundary of the mouth supported largely by the palatine bones and limited anteriorly by the dental lamina and posteriorly by the uvula and upper part of the fauces **2** : a covering structure of any of various parts of the body other than the mouth ⟨∼ of the skull⟩

roof•ie \ˈrü-fē\ *n, pl* **roof•ies** *slang* : a tablet of flunitrazepam used illicitly

room•ing–in \ˈrü-miŋ-ˈin, ˈru̇-\ *n* : an arrangement whereby a newborn infant is kept in the mother's hospital room instead of in a nursery

room temperature *n* : a temperature of from 59° to 77°F (15° to 25°C) that is suitable for human occupancy

root \ˈrüt, ˈru̇t\ *n* **1** : the part of a tooth within the socket; *also* : any of the processes into which the root of a tooth is often divided **2** : the enlarged basal part of a hair within the skin — called also *hair root* **3** : the proximal end of a nerve; *esp* : one or more bundles of nerve fibers joining the cranial and spinal nerves with their respective nuclei and columns of gray matter — see DORSAL ROOT, VENTRAL ROOT **4** : the part of an organ or physical structure by which it is attached to the body ⟨the ∼ of the tongue⟩ — **root•less** \-ləs\ *adj*

root canal *n* **1** : the part of the pulp cavity lying in the root of a tooth — called also *pulp canal* **2** : a dental operation to save a tooth by removing the contents of its root canal and filling the cavity with a protective substance (as gutta-percha)

root•ed \ˈrü-təd, ˈru̇-\ *adj* **1** : having such or so many roots ⟨single-*rooted* premolars⟩ **2** : having a contracted root nearly closing the pulp cavity and preventing further growth

root•let \ˈrüt-lət, ˈru̇t-\ *n* : a small root; *also* : one of the ultimate divisions of a nerve root

root planing *n* : the scraping of a bacteria-impregnated layer of cementum from the surface of a tooth root to prevent or treat periodontitis

ROP *abbr* retinopathy of prematurity

Ror•schach \ˈrȯr-ˌshäk\ *adj* : of, relating to, used in connection with, or resulting from the Rorschach test

Rorschach test *n* : a projective personality test that uses a subject's interpretation of 10 standard black or colored inkblot designs to assess personality traits and emotional tendencies — called also *Rorschach, Rorschach inkblot test*

Rorschach, Hermann (1884–1922), Swiss psychiatrist.

ro•sa•cea \rō-ˈzā-shə, -shē-ə\ *n* : a chronic inflammatory skin disorder typically involving the nose, cheeks, forehead, and chin that is characterized esp. by redness, flushing, telangiectasia, inflamed lesions, burning sensation, and sometimes eye dryness and irritation and thickening of tissues esp. of the nose — called also *acne rosacea*

rosary pea *n* **1** : a tropical leguminous twining herb (*Abrus precatorius*) that bears jequirity beans and has a root used as a substitute for licorice **2** : JEQUIRITY BEAN 1

rosea — see PITYRIASIS ROSEA

rose ben•gal \-ben-ˈgȯl, -beŋ-\ *n* : either of two bluish-red acid dyes that are derivatives of fluorescein

rose bengal test *n* : a test of liver function by determining the time taken for an injected quantity of rose bengal to be absorbed from the bloodstream

rose cold *n* : ROSE FEVER

rose fever *n* : hay fever occurring in the spring or early summer

ro•se•o•la \ˌrō-zē-ˈō-lə, rō-ˈzē-ə-lə\ *n* : a rose-colored eruption in spots or a disease marked by such an eruption; *esp* : ROSEOLA INFANTUM — **ro•se•o•lar** \-lər\ *adj*

roseola in•fan•tum \-in-ˈfan-təm\ *n* : a mild virus disease of infants and children that is characterized by fever lasting three days followed by an eruption of rose-colored spots and is caused by a herpesvirus (species *Human herpesvirus 6* of the genus *Roseolovirus*) — called also *exanthema subitum, exanthem subitum*

ro•sette \rō-ˈzet\ *n* : a rose-shaped cluster of cells

ro•si•glit•a•zone \ˌrō-sə-ˈgli-tə-ˌzōn\ *n* : a drug that is taken orally in the form of its maleate $C_{18}H_{19}N_3O_3S{\cdot}C_4H_4O_4$ to treat type 2 diabetes by decreasing insulin resistance — see AVANDIA

ros•tral \ˈräs-trəl, ˈrȯs-\ *adj* **1** : of or relating to a rostrum **2** : situated toward the oral or nasal region: as **a** *of a part of the spinal cord* : SUPERIOR 1 **b** *of a part of the brain* : anterior or ventral ⟨the ~ pons⟩ — **ros•tral•ly** *adv*

ros•trum \ˈräs-trəm, ˈrȯs-\ *n, pl* **ros•trums** *or* **ros•tra** \-trə\ : a bodily part or process suggesting a bird's bill: as **a** : the reflected anterior portion of the corpus callosum below the genu **b** : the interior median spine of the body of the basisphenoid bone articulating with the vomer

ro•su•va•stat•in \rō-ˈsü-və-ˌsta-tᵊn\ *n* : a statin that is administered orally in the form of its calcium salt $(C_{22}H_{27}FN_3O_6S)_2Ca$ esp. to treat hypercholesterolemia — see CRESTOR

rosy periwinkle *n* : an Old World tropical shrub (*Catharanthus roseus* syn. *Vinca rosea*) of the dogbane family (Apocynaceae) that is the source of several antineoplastic drugs (as vinblastine and vincristine) — called also *Madagascar periwinkle, periwinkle*

¹rot \ˈrät\ *vb* **rot•ted; rot•ting** : to undergo decomposition from the action of bacteria or fungi

²rot *n* **1** : the process of rotting : the state of being rotten **2** : any of several parasitic diseases esp. of sheep marked by necrosis and wasting

ro•ta•tor \ˈrō-ˌtā-tər, rō-ˈ\ *n, pl* **rotators** *or* **ro•ta•to•res** \ˌrō-tə-ˈtōr-ēz\ : a muscle that partially rotates a part on its axis; *specif* : any of several small muscles in the dorsal region of the spine arising from the upper and back part of a transverse process and inserted into the lamina of the vertebra above

rotator cuff \-ˌkəf\ *n* : a supporting and strengthening structure of the shoulder joint that is made up of part of its capsule blended with tendons of the subscapularis, infraspinatus, supraspinatus, and teres minor muscles as they pass to the capsule or across it to insert on the humerus — called also *musculotendinous cuff*

ro•ta•vi•rus \ˈrō-tə-ˌvī-rəs\ *n* **1** *cap* : a genus of reoviruses that are causative agents of gastroenteritis, that include one (species *Rotavirus A*) causing epidemics of severe and sometimes fatal diarrhea in infants and young children worldwide, and that have a virion with a three-layered protein capsid lacking an outer lipid envelope **2** : any virus of the genus *Rotavirus* — **ro•ta•vi•ral** \-rəl\ *adj*

ro•te•none \ˈrōt-ᵊn-ˌōn\ *n* : a crystalline insecticide $C_{23}H_{22}O_6$ that is of low toxicity for warm-blooded animals and is used esp. in home gardens

rotunda — see FENESTRA ROTUNDA

rotundum — see FORAMEN ROTUNDUM

Rou•get cell \rü-ˈzhā-\ *n* : any of numerous branching cells adhering to the endothelium of capillaries and regarded as a contractile element in the capillary wall

Rouget, Charles–Marie–Benjamin (1824–1904), French physiologist and anatomist.

rough \ˈrəf\ *adj* : having a broken, uneven, or bumpy surface; *specif* : forming or being rough colonies usu. made up of organisms that form chains or filaments and tend to marked decrease in capsule formation and virulence — used of dissociated strains of bacteria; compare SMOOTH

rough•age \ˈrə-fij\ *n* : FIBER 2; *also* : food (as bran) containing much indigestible material acting as fiber

rough endoplasmic reticulum *n* : endoplasmic reticulum that is studded with ribosomes

rou•leau \rü-ˈlō\ *n, pl* **rou•leaux** *same or* -ˈlōz\ *or* **rouleaus** : a group of red blood corpuscles resembling a stack of coins

round \ˈrau̇nd\ *vb* : to go on rounds

round cell *n* : a small lymphocyte or a closely related cell esp. occurring in an area of chronic infection or as the typical cell of some sarcomas

round ligament *n* **1** : a fibrous cord resulting from the obliteration of the umbilical vein of the fetus and passing from the navel to the notch in the anterior border of the liver and along the undersurface of that organ **2** : either of a pair of rounded cords arising from each side of the uterus and traceable through the inguinal canal to the tissue of the labia majora into which they merge

rounds *n pl* : a series of professional calls on hospital patients made by a doctor or nurse — see GRAND ROUNDS

round–shouldered *adj* : having the shoulders stooping or rounded

round window *n* : a round opening between the middle ear and the cochlea that is closed over by a membrane — called also *fenestra cochleae, fenestra rotunda*

round•worm \ˈrau̇nd-ˌwərm\ *n* : NEMATODE; *also* : a related round-bodied unsegmented worm (as an acanthocephalan) as distinguished from a flatworm

roup \ˈrüp, ˈrau̇p\ *n* : TRICHOMONIASIS c

Rous sarcoma \ˈrau̇s-\ *n* : a readily transplantable malignant fibrosarcoma of chickens that is caused by the Rous sarcoma virus

Rous, Francis Peyton (1879–1970), American pathologist.

Rous sarcoma virus *n* : a retrovirus (species *Rous sarcoma virus* of the genus *Alpharetrovirus*) that contains an oncogene causing Rous sarcoma

route \ˈrüt, ˈrau̇t\ *n* : a method of transmitting a disease or of administering a remedy

Roux–en–Y gastric bypass \ˌrü-ˌen-ˈwī-, ˌrü-ˌän-ˌē-ˈgrek-\ *n* : a gastric bypass surgical procedure in the treatment of severe obesity that involves partitioning off part of the upper stomach to form a small pouch, dividing the jejunum into upper and lower parts, and forming a Y-shaped anastomosis by attaching the free end of the lower part of the jejunum to a new outlet on the upper stomach pouch and attaching the free end of what was the upper jejunum to a new opening on the small intestine — called also *Roux-en-Y*

Roux \ˈrü\, **César (1857–1934),** Swiss surgeon.

RP *abbr* retinitis pigmentosa

RPh *abbr* registered pharmacist

RPR card test \ˌär-ˌpē-ˌär-ˈkärd-\ *n* : RAPID PLASMA REAGIN TEST

RPT *abbr* registered physical therapist

RQ *abbr* respiratory quotient

RR *abbr* recovery room

RRA *abbr* registered records administrator

-r•rha•gia \ˈrā-jə, ˈrä-, -jē-ə, -zhə, -zhē-ə\ *n comb form* : abnormal or excessive discharge or flow ⟨metro*rrhagia*⟩ — **-r•rha•gic** \ˈra-jik\ *adj comb form*

-r•rha•phy \r-ə-fē\ *n comb form, pl* **-r•rha•phies** : suture : sewing ⟨nephro*rrhaphy*⟩

-r•rhea \ˈrē-ə\ *n comb form* : flow : discharge ⟨logo*rrhea*⟩ ⟨leuko*rrhea*⟩

-r•rhex•is \ˈrek-səs\ *n comb form, pl* **-r•rhex•es** \ˈrek-ˌsēz\ : rupture ⟨erythrocyto*rrhexis*⟩

-r•rhoea *chiefly Brit var of* -RRHEA

RRL *abbr* registered records librarian

rRNA \ˈär-ˌär-ˌen-ˈā\ *n* : RIBOSOMAL RNA

RRT *abbr* registered respiratory therapist

RSD *abbr* reflex sympathetic dystrophy

RSI \ˌär-ˌes-ˈī\ *n* : repetitive strain injury

RS–T segment \ˌär-ˌes-ˈtē-\ *n* : ST SEGMENT

RSV *abbr* **1** respiratory syncytial virus **2** Rous sarcoma virus

RT *abbr* **1** reaction time **2** recreational therapy **3** respiratory therapist

Ru *symbol* ruthenium

rub \ˈrəb\ *n* **1** : the application of friction with pressure ⟨an alcohol ~⟩ **2** : a sound heard in auscultation that is produced by the friction of one structure moving against another

rub•ber \ˈrə-bər\ *n* : CONDOM 1

rubber dam *n* : a thin sheet of rubber that is stretched around a tooth to keep it dry during dental work or is used in strips to provide drainage in surgical wounds

rubbing alcohol *n* : a cooling and soothing liquid for external application that contains approximately 70 percent denatured ethanol or isopropyl alcohol

[1]**ru•be•fa•cient** \ˌrü-bə-ˈfā-shənt\ *adj* : causing redness of the skin

[2]**rubefacient** *n* : a substance (as capsaicin) for external application that produces redness of the skin

ru•bel•la \rü-ˈbe-lə\ *n* : GERMAN MEASLES — see MATERNAL RUBELLA

ru•be•o•la \ˌrü-bē-ˈō-lə, rü-ˈbē-ə-lə\ *n* : MEASLES 1a — **ru•be•o•lar** \-lər\ *adj*

ru•be•o•sis \ˌrü-bē-ˈō-səs\ *n, pl* **-o•ses** \-ˈō-ˌsēz\ *or* **-osises** : a condition characterized by abnormal redness; *esp* : RUBEOSIS IRIDIS

rubeosis iri•dis \-ˈī-rə-dəs\ *n* : abnormal redness of the iris resulting from neovascularization and often associated with diabetes

ru•bid•i•um \rü-ˈbi-dē-əm\ *n* : a soft silvery metallic element — symbol *Rb;* see ELEMENT table

Ru•bin test \ˈrü-bən-\ *n* : a test to determine the patency or occlusion of the fallopian tubes by insufflating them with carbon dioxide

Rubin, Isidor Clinton (1883–1958), American gynecologist.

Ru•bi•vi•rus \ˌrü-bə-ˈvī-rəs\ *n* : a genus of togaviruses that consists of a single species (*Rubella virus*) that is the causative agent of German measles

ru•bor \ˈrü-ˌbȯr\ *n* : redness of the skin (as from inflammation)

rubra — see PITYRIASIS RUBRA PILARIS

ru•bri•cyte \ˈrü-bri-ˌsīt\ *n* : an immature red blood cell that has a nucleus, is about half the size of developing red blood cells in preceding stages, and has cytoplasm that stains erratically blue, purplish, and gray due to the presence of hemoglobin : a polychromatic normoblast

ru•bro•spi•nal \ˌrü-brō-ˈspī-nəl\ *adj* **1** : of, relating to, or connecting the red nucleus and the spinal cord **2** : of, relating to, or constituting a tract of crossed nerve fibers passing from the red nucleus to the spinal cord and relaying impulses from the cerebellum and corpora striata to the motor neurons of the spinal cord

Ru·bu·la·vi·rus \ˌrü-byə-lə-ˈvī-rəs\ *n* : a genus of paramyxoviruses that includes two of the parainfluenza viruses and the causative agent of mumps

ru·di·ment \ˈrü-də-mənt\ *n* : an incompletely developed organ or part; *esp* : an organ or part just beginning to develop : ANLAGE

ru·di·men·ta·ry \ˌrü-də-ˈmen-tə-rē\ *adj* : very imperfectly developed or represented only by a vestige

Ruf·fi·ni's corpuscle \rü-ˈfē-nēz-\ *or* **Ruf·fi·ni corpuscle** \-nē-\ *n* : any of numerous oval sensory end organs occurring in the subcutaneous tissue of the fingers — called also *Ruffini's brush, Ruffini's end organ*

Ruffini, Angelo (1864–1929), Italian histologist and embryologist.

RU–486 \ˌär-(ˌ)yü-ˌfōr-ˌā-tē-ˈsiks\ *n* : MIFEPRISTONE

ru·ga \ˈrü-gə\ *n, pl* **ru·gae** \-ˌgī, -ˌgē, -ˌjē\ : an anatomical fold or wrinkle esp. of the viscera — usu. used in pl. ⟨the *rugae* of an empty stomach⟩

ru·mi·nant \ˈrü-mə-nənt\ *adj* : of or relating to two suborders (Ruminantia and Tylopoda) of even-toed hoofed mammals (as sheep and oxen) that chew the cud and have a complex 3- or 4-chambered stomach — **ruminant** *n*

ru·mi·na·tion \ˌrü-mə-ˈnā-shən\ *n* **1** : the act or process of regurgitating and chewing again previously swallowed food **2** : obsessive thinking about an idea, situation, or choice esp. when it interferes with normal mental functioning; *specif* : a focusing of one's attention on negative or distressing thoughts or feelings that when excessive or prolonged may lead to or exacerbate an episode of depression — **ru·mi·nate** \ˈrü-mə-ˌnāt\ *vb*

rump \ˈrəmp\ *n* **1** : the upper rounded part of the hindquarters of a quadruped mammal **2** : the seat of the body : BUTTOCKS

Rum·pel–Leede test \ˈrüm-pel-ˈlēd-\ *n* : a test in which the increased bleeding tendency characteristic of various disorders (as scarlet fever and thrombocytopenia) is indicated by the formation of multiple petechiae on the forearm following application of a tourniquet to the upper arm

Rumpel, Theodor (1862–1923), German physician.

Leede, Carl Stockbridge (1882–1964), American physician.

run \ˈrən\ *vb* **ran** \ˈran\; **run; run·ning** : to discharge fluid (as pus or serum) ⟨a *running* sore⟩ — **run a fever** *or* **run a temperature** : to have a fever

rung *past part of* RING

runner's high *n* : a feeling of euphoria that is experienced by some individuals engaged in strenuous running and that is held to be associated with the release of endorphins by the brain

runner's knee *n* : pain in the region of the knee esp. when related to running that may have a simple anatomical basis (as tightness of a muscle) or may be a symptom of iliotibial band syndrome or an indication of chondromalacia patellae

run·ny \ˈrə-nē\ *adj* : secreting a thin flow of mucus ⟨a ~ nose⟩

runs \ˈrənz\ *n sing or pl* : DIARRHEA — used with *the*

ru·pia \ˈrü-pē-ə\ *n* : an eruption occurring esp. in tertiary syphilis consisting of vesicles having an inflamed base and filled with serous purulent or bloody fluid which dries up and forms large blackish conical crusts — **ru·pi·al** \-əl\ *adj*

rup·ture \ˈrəp-chər\ *n* **1** : the tearing apart of a tissue ⟨~ of an intervertebral disk⟩ **2** : HERNIA — **rupture** *vb*

RUQ *abbr* right upper quadrant (abdomen)

rush \ˈrəsh\ *n* **1** : a rapid and extensive wave of peristalsis along the walls of the intestine ⟨peristaltic ~⟩ **2** : the immediate pleasurable feeling produced by a drug (as heroin or amphetamine) — called also *flash*

Russian spring–summer encephalitis *n* : a tick-borne encephalitis of Europe and Asia caused by a strain (Far Eastern subtype) of the tick-borne encephalitis virus and transmitted by ticks of the genus *Ixodes*

ru·the·ni·um \rü-ˈthē-nē-əm\ *n* : a hard brittle grayish rare metallic element — symbol *Ru;* see ELEMENT table

ruth·er·ford \ˈrə-t͟hər-fərd\ *n* : a unit strength of a radioactive source corresponding to one million disintegrations per second — abbr. *rd*

Rutherford, Ernest (Baron Rutherford of Nelson) (1871–1937), British physicist.

ruth·er·ford·ium \ˌrə-t͟hər-ˈfȯr-dē-əm\ *n* : a short-lived radioactive element that is artificially produced — symbol *Rf;* see ELEMENT table

ru·tin \ˈrüt-ᵊn\ *n* : a yellow crystalline glycoside $C_{27}H_{30}O_{16}$ that occurs in various plants (as tobacco) and that is used chiefly for strengthening capillary blood vessels (as in cases of hypertension and radiation injury)

R wave \ˈär-ˌwāv\ *n* : the positive upward deflection in the QRS complex of an electrocardiogram that follows the Q wave

Rx \ˌär-ˈeks\ *n* : a medical prescription

Ry·tary \rī-ˈtär-ē\ *trademark* — used for a preparation containing carbidopa and L-dopa

S

S *abbr* **1** sacral — used esp. with a number from 1 to 5 to indicate a vertebra or segment of the spinal cord in the sacral region **2** signa — used to introduce the signature in writing a prescription **3** subject **4** svedberg
S *symbol* sulfur
sa *abbr* [Latin *secundum artem*] according to art — used in writing prescriptions
S–A *abbr* sinoatrial
sa•bal \ˈsā-ˌbal\ *n* : SAW PALMETTO
sa•ber shin \ˈsā-bər-\ *n* : a tibia that has a pronounced anterior convexity caused by disease (as congenital syphilis or rickets)
Sa•bin vaccine \ˈsā-bin-\ *n* : a polio vaccine that is taken by mouth and contains the three serotypes of poliovirus in a weakened live state — called also *Sabin oral vaccine;* compare SALK VACCINE
Sabin, Albert Bruce (1906–1993), American immunologist.
sac \ˈsak\ *n* : a soft-walled anatomical cavity usu. having a narrow opening or none at all and often containing a special fluid ⟨a synovial ~⟩ — see AIR SAC, AMNIOTIC SAC, LACRIMAL SAC
sac•cade \sa-ˈkäd\ *n* : a small rapid jerky movement of the eye esp. as it jumps from fixation on one point to another (as in reading) — **sac•cad•ic** \-ˈkä-dik\ *adj*
sacchar- *or* **sacchari-** *or* **saccharo-** *comb form* : sugar ⟨*sacchar*ide⟩
sac•cha•rase \ˈsa-kə-ˌrās, -ˌrāz\ *n* : INVERTASE
sac•cha•ride \ˈsa-kə-ˌrīd, -rid\ *n* : a simple sugar, combination of sugars, or polymerized sugar
sac•cha•rin \ˈsa-kə-rin\ *n* : a crystalline compound $C_7H_5NO_3S$ that is unrelated to the carbohydrates, is many times sweeter than sucrose, and is used as a calorie-free sweetener
sac•cha•ro•my•ces \ˌsa-kə-rō-ˈmī-(ˌ)sēz\ *n* **1** *cap* : a genus of usu. unicellular yeasts (family Saccharomycetaceae) distinguished by their sparse or absent mycelium and by their facility in reproducing asexually by budding **2** *pl* **saccharomyces** : any yeast of the genus *Saccharomyces*
sac•cu•lar \ˈsa-kyə-lər\ *adj* : resembling a sac ⟨a ~ aneurysm⟩
sac•cu•lat•ed \-ˌlā-təd\ *also* **sac•cu•late** \-ˌlāt, -lət\ *adj* : having or formed of a series of saccular expansions
sac•cu•la•tion \ˌsa-kyə-ˈlā-shən\ *n* **1** : the quality or state of being sacculated **2** : the process of developing or segmenting into sacculated structures **3** : a sac or sacculated structure; *esp* : one of a linear series of such structures ⟨the ~*s* of the colon⟩
sac•cule \ˈsa-(ˌ)kyül\ *n* : a little sac; *specif* : the smaller chamber of the membranous labyrinth of the ear that contains the macula sacculi
sac•cu•lus \ˈsa-kyə-ləs\ *n, pl* **-li** \-ˌlī, -ˌlē\ : SACCULE
sac•like \ˈsak-ˌlīk\ *adj* : having the form of or suggesting a sac
sacr- *or* **sacro-** *comb form* **1** : sacrum ⟨*sacr*al⟩ **2** : sacral and ⟨*sacro*iliac⟩
sacra *pl of* SACRUM
[1]**sa•cral** \ˈsa-krəl, ˈsā-\ *adj* : of, relating to, or lying near the sacrum
[2]**sacral** *n* : a sacral vertebra or sacral nerve
sacral artery — see LATERAL SACRAL ARTERY, MIDDLE SACRAL ARTERY
sacral canal *n* : the part of the vertebral canal lying in the sacrum
sacral cornu *n* : a rounded process on each side of the fifth sacral vertebra
sacral crest *n* : any of several crests or tubercles on the sacrum: as **a** : one on the midline of the dorsal surface — called also *median sacral crest* **b** : any of a series of tubercles on each side of the dorsal surface lateral to the sacral foramina that represent the transverse processes of the sacral vertebrae and serve as attachments for ligaments — called also *lateral sacral crest*
sacral foramen *n* : any of 16 openings in the sacrum of which there are four on each side of the dorsal surface giving passage to the posterior branches of the sacral nerves and four on each side of the pelvic surface giving passage to the anterior branches of the sacral nerves
sacral hiatus *n* : the opening into the vertebral canal in the midline of the dorsal surface of the sacrum between the laminae of the fifth sacral vertebra
sa•cral•i•za•tion \ˌsā-krə-lə-ˈzā-shən\ *n* : a congenital anomaly in which the fifth lumbar vertebra is fused to the sacrum in varying degrees
sacral nerve *n* : any of the spinal nerves of the sacral region of which there are five pairs and which have anterior and posterior branches passing out through the sacral foramina
sacral plexus *n* : a nerve plexus that lies against the posterior and lateral walls of the pelvis, is formed by the union of the lumbosacral trunk and the first, second, and third sacral nerves, and continues into the thigh as the sciatic nerve
sacral promontory *n* : the inwardly projecting anterior part of the body of the first sacral vertebra
sacral vein — see LATERAL SACRAL VEIN, MEDIAN SACRAL VEIN
sacral vertebra *n* : any of the five fused vertebrae that make up the sacrum
sacro- — see SACR-

sa•cro•coc•cy•geal \ˌsā-krō-käk-ˈsi-jəl, ˌsa-, -jē-əl\ *adj* : of, relating to, affecting, or performed by way of the region of the sacrum and coccyx

sa•cro•coc•cy•geus dor•sa•lis \-käk-ˈsi-jē-əs-ˌdȯr-ˈsā-ləs\ *n* : an inconstant muscle that sometimes extends from the dorsal part of the sacrum to the coccyx — called also *posterior sacrococcygeal muscle*

sacrococcygeus ven•tra•lis \-ven-ˈtrā-ləs\ *n* : an inconstant muscle that sometimes extends from the ventral surface of the lower sacral vertebrae to the coccyx — called also *anterior sacrococcygeal muscle*

[1]**sa•cro•il•i•ac** \ˌsa-krō-ˈi-lē-ˌak, ˌsā-\ *adj* : of, relating to, affecting, or being the region of the joint between the sacrum and the ilium ⟨~ distress⟩

[2]**sacroiliac** *n* : SACROILIAC JOINT

sacroiliac joint *n* : the joint or articulation between the sacrum and ilium — called also *sacroiliac, sacroiliac articulation*

sa•cro•il•i•i•tis \ˌsā-krō-ˌi-lē-ˈī-təs, ˌsa-\ *n* : inflammation of the sacroiliac joint or region

sa•cro•spi•na•lis \ˌsā-krō-spī-ˈnā-ləs, ˌsa-krō-spī-ˈna-ləs\ *n* : a muscle that extends the length of the back and neck, that arises from the iliac crest, the sacrum, and the lumbar and two lower thoracic vertebrae, and that splits in the upper lumbar region into the iliocostalis muscles, the longissimus muscles, and the spinalis muscles — called also *erector spinae*

sa•cro•spi•nous ligament \ˌsā-krō-ˈspī-nəs-, ˌsa-\ *n* : a ligament on each side of the body that is attached by a broad base to the lateral margins of the sacrum and coccyx and passes to the ischial spine and that closes off the greater sciatic notch to form the greater sciatic foramen and with the sacrotuberous ligament closes off the lesser sciatic notch to form the lesser sciatic foramen

sa•cro•tu•ber•ous ligament \ˌsā-krō-ˈtü-bə-rəs-, ˌsa-, -ˈtyü-\ *n* : a thin fan-shaped ligament on each side of the body that is attached above to the posterior superior and posterior inferior iliac spines and to the sacrum and coccyx, that passes obliquely downward to insert into the inner margin of the ischial tuberosity, and that with the sacrospinous ligament closes off the lesser sciatic notch to form the lesser sciatic foramen

sa•cro•uter•ine ligament \-ˈyü-tə-ˌrīn-, -rən-\ *n* : UTEROSACRAL LIGAMENT

sa•crum \ˈsa-krəm, ˈsā-\ *n, pl* **sa•cra** \ˈsa-krə, ˈsā-\ : the part of the spinal column that is directly connected with or forms a part of the pelvis by articulation with the ilia and that in humans forms the dorsal wall of the pelvis and consists of five fused vertebrae diminishing in size to the apex at the lower end which bears the coccyx

SAD *abbr* seasonal affective disorder

sad•dle \ˈsad-ᵊl\ *n* : the part of a partial denture that carries an artificial tooth and has connectors for adjacent teeth attached to its ends

sad•dle•bag \ˈsa-dᵊl-ˌbag\ *n* : a bulge of lumpy fat in the outer area of the upper thighs

saddle block anesthesia *n* : spinal anesthesia confined to the perineum, the buttocks, and the inner aspect of the thighs — called also *saddle block*

saddle joint *n* : a joint (as the carpometacarpal joint of the thumb) with saddle-shaped articular surfaces that are convex in one direction and concave in another and that permit movements in all directions except axial rotation

sad•dle•nose \ˈsad-ᵊl-ˌnōz\ *n* : a nose marked by depression of the bridge resulting from injury or disease

sa•dism \ˈsā-ˌdiz-əm, ˈsa-\ *n* : a sexual perversion in which gratification is obtained by the infliction of physical or mental pain on others (as on a love object) — compare ALGOLAGNIA, MASOCHISM — **sa•dis•tic** \sə-ˈdis-tik, sā-, sa-\ *adj* — **sa•dis•ti•cal•ly** *adv*

Sade \ˈsäd\, **Marquis de (Comte Donatien–Alphonse–François) (1740–1814),** French soldier and writer.

sa•dist \ˈsā-dist, ˈsa-\ *n* : an individual who practices sadism

sa•do•mas•och•ism \ˌsā-(ˌ)dō-ˈma-sə-ˌki-zəm, ˌsa-, -zə-ˌki-\ *n* : the derivation of pleasure from the infliction of physical or mental pain either on others or on oneself — **sa•do•mas•och•ist•ic** \-ˌma-sə-ˈkist-ik\ *also* **sadomasochist** *adj*

L. von Sacher–Masoch — see MASOCHISM

sa•do•mas•och•ist \-kist\ *n* : an individual who practices sadomasochism

safe \ˈsāf\ *adj* **saf•er; saf•est** : not causing harm or injury; *esp* : having a low incidence of adverse reactions and significant side effects when adequate instructions for use are given and having a low potential for harm under conditions of widespread availability — **safe•ty** \ˈsāf-tē\ *n*

safe period *n* : a portion of the menstrual cycle of the human female during which conception is least likely to occur and which usu. includes several days immediately before and after the menstrual period and the period itself

safe sex *n* : sexual activity and esp. sexual intercourse in which various measures (as the use of latex condoms or the practice of monogamy) are taken to avoid disease (as AIDS) transmitted by sexual contact — called also *safer sex*

sag•it•tal \ˈsa-jət-ᵊl\ *adj* **1** : of, relating to, or being the sagittal suture of the skull **2** : of, relating to, situated in, or being the median plane of the body or any plane parallel to it ⟨a ~ section⟩ — **sag·it·tal·ly** *adv*

sagittal plane *n* : MIDSAGITTAL PLANE; *also* : any plane parallel to a midsagittal plane : a parasagittal plane

sagittal sinus *n* : either of two venous sinuses of the dura mater: **a** : one passing backward in the convex attached superior margin of the falx cerebri and ending at the internal occipital protuberance by fusion with the transverse sinus — called also *superior sagittal sinus* **b** : one lying in the posterior two thirds of the concave free inferior margin of the falx cerebri and ending posteriorly by joining the great cerebral vein to form the straight sinus — called also *inferior sagittal sinus*

sagittal suture *n* : the deeply serrated articulation between the two parietal bones in the median plane of the top of the head

sa·go spleen \ˈsā-(ˌ)gō-\ *n* : a spleen which is affected with amyloid degeneration and in which the amyloid is deposited in the Malpighian corpuscles which appear in cross section as gray translucent bodies

sagrada — see CASCARA SAGRADA

Saint An·tho·ny's fire \ˌsānt-ˈan-thə-nēz-\ *n* : any of several inflammations or gangrenous conditions (as erysipelas or ergotism) of the skin

Anthony, Saint (*ca* 250–350), Egyptian monk.

Saint–John's–wort \ˌsānt-ˈjänz-ˌwərt, -ˌwȯrt\ *n* **1** : any of a genus (*Hypericum* of the family Guttiferae) of yellow-flowered herbs and shrubs; *esp* : one (*H. perforatum*) causing photosensitization in sheep, cattle, horses, and goats when ingested **2** *usu* **Saint John's wort** : the dried aerial parts of a Saint-John's-wort (*Hypericum perforatum*) that are held to relieve depression and are used in herbal remedies and dietary supplements

John the Baptist, Saint (*fl* first century AD), Jewish prophet.

Saint Lou·is encephalitis \ˌsānt-ˈlü-is-\ *n* : a No. American encephalitis that is caused by a virus of the genus *Flavivirus* (species *Saint Louis encephalitis virus*) transmitted by several mosquitoes of the genus *Culex*

Saint Vi·tus' dance \-ˈvī-təs-\ *also* **Saint Vitus's dance** \-ˈvī-tə-səz-\ *n* : CHOREA; *esp* : SYDENHAM'S CHOREA

Vitus, Saint (*d ca* 300), Italian martyr.

sal·abra·sion \ˌsa-lə-ˈbrā-zhən\ *n* : a method of removing tattoos from skin in which moist gauze pads saturated with sodium chloride are used to abrade the tattooed area by rubbing

sal am·mo·ni·ac \ˌsal-ə-ˈmō-nē-ˌak\ *n* : AMMONIUM CHLORIDE

sal·bu·ta·mol \sal-ˈbyü-tə-ˌmȯl, -ˌmōl\ *n* : ALBUTEROL

salicyl- *or* **salicylo-** *comb form* : related to salicylic acid ⟨*salicyl*amide⟩

sal·i·cyl·amide \ˌsa-lə-ˈsi-lə-ˌmīd\ *n* : the crystalline amide $C_7H_7NO_2$ of salicylic acid used chiefly as an analgesic, antipyretic, and antirheumatic

sal·i·cyl·an·il·ide \ˌsa-lə-sə-ˈlan-ᵊl-īd\ *n* : a fungicidal agent $C_{13}H_{11}NO_2$ used esp. in the external treatment of tinea capitis caused by a fungus of the genus *Microsporum* (*M. audouini*)

sa·lic·y·late \sə-ˈli-sə-ˌlāt\ *n* : a salt or ester of salicylic acid; *also* : SALICYLIC ACID

sal·i·cyl·azo·sul·fa·pyr·i·dine \ˌsa-lə-si-ˌlā-zō-ˌsəl-fə-ˈpir-ə-ˌdēn\ *n* : SULFASALAZINE

sal·i·cyl·ic acid \ˌsa-lə-ˈsi-lik-\ *n* : a crystalline phenolic acid $C_7H_6O_3$ that is used esp. in making pharmaceuticals and dyes, as an antiseptic and disinfectant esp. in treating skin diseases, and in the form of salts and other derivatives as an analgesic and antipyretic — see ASPIRIN

sal·i·cyl·ism \ˈsa-lə-si-ˌli-zəm\ *n* : a toxic condition produced by the excessive intake of salicylic acid or salicylates and marked by ringing in the ears, nausea, and vomiting

¹sa·line \ˈsā-ˌlēn, -ˌlīn\ *adj* **1** : consisting of or containing salt ⟨a ~ solution⟩ **2** : of, relating to, or resembling salt : SALTY ⟨a ~ taste⟩ **3** : consisting of or relating to the salts esp. of lithium, sodium, potassium, and magnesium ⟨a ~ cathartic⟩ **4** : relating to or being abortion induced by the injection of a highly concentrated saline solution into the amniotic sac ⟨~ amniocentesis⟩ — **sa·lin·i·ty** \sā-ˈlin-ət-ē, sə-\ *n*

²saline *n* **1 a** : a metallic salt; *esp* : a salt of potassium, sodium, or magnesium with a cathartic action **b** : an aqueous solution of one or more such salts **2** : a saline solution used in physiology; *esp* : PHYSIOLOGICAL SALINE

sa·li·va \sə-ˈlī-və\ *n* : a slightly alkaline secretion of water, mucin, protein, salts, and often a starch-splitting enzyme (as ptyalin) that is secreted into the mouth by salivary glands, lubricates ingested food, and often begins the breakdown of starches

saliva ejector *n* : a narrow tubular device providing suction to draw saliva, blood, and debris from the mouth of a dental patient in order to maintain a clear operative field

sal·i·vary \ˈsa-lə-ˌver-ē\ *adj* : of or relating to saliva or the glands that secrete it; *esp* : producing or carrying saliva

salivary gland *n* : any of various glands that discharge a fluid secretion and esp. saliva into the mouth cavity and that in humans comprise large compound racemose glands including the parotid glands, the sublingual glands, and the submandibular glands

sal·i·va·tion \ˌsa-lə-ˈvā-shən\ *n* : the act or process of producing a flow of saliva; *esp* : excessive secretion of saliva often accompanied by soreness of the mouth and gums — **sal·i·vate** \ˈsa-lə-ˌvāt\ *vb*

sal·i·va·to·ry \ˈsa-lə-və-ˌtōr-ē\ *adj* : inducing salivation

Salk vaccine \ˈsȯk-, ˈsȯlk-\ *n* : a polio vaccine that is administered by intramuscular injection and contains the three serotypes of poliovirus inactivated by treatment with formaldehyde — compare SABIN VACCINE

Salk, Jonas Edward (1914–1995), American immunologist.

sal·met·er·ol \sal-ˈme-tə-ˌrȯl, -ˌrōl\ *n* : a bronchodilator administered by oral inhalation in the form of a salt $C_{25}H_{37}NO_4 \cdot C_{11}H_8O_3$ to treat bronchospasm associated esp. with asthma and chronic obstructive pulmonary disease — see ADVAIR

sal·mo·nel·la \ˌsal-mə-ˈne-lə\ *n* **1** *cap* : a genus of aerobic gram-negative rod-shaped usu. motile enterobacteria that are pathogenic for humans and other warm-blooded animals and cause food poisoning, acute gastrointestinal inflammation, typhoid fever, or septicemia **2** *pl* **-nel·lae** \-ˈne-lē\ *or* **-nellas** *or* **-nella** : any bacterium of the genus *Salmonella*

Salm·on \ˈsa-mən\, **Daniel Elmer (1850–1914),** American veterinarian.

sal·mo·nel·lo·sis \ˌsal-mə-ˌne-ˈlō-səs\ *n, pl* **-lo·ses** \-ˌsēz\ : infection with or disease caused by bacteria of the genus *Salmonella* typically marked by gastroenteritis but often complicated by septicemia, meningitis, endocarditis, and various focal lesions (as in the kidneys)

salmon poisoning *n* : a highly fatal febrile disease of dogs and other canines that resembles canine distemper and is caused by a rickettsial bacterium (*Neorickettsia helminthoeca*) transmitted by encysted larvae of a fluke (*Nanophyetus salmincola*) ingested with the raw flesh of infested salmon, trout, or salamanders

sal·ol \ˈsa-ˌlȯl, -ˌōl\ *n* : PHENYL SALICYLATE

salping- *or* **salpingo-** *comb form* **1** : fallopian tube ⟨*salpingo*plasty⟩ **2** : eustachian tube ⟨*salpingo*pharyngeus⟩

sal·pin·gec·to·my \ˌsal-pən-ˈjek-tə-mē\ *n, pl* **-mies** : surgical excision of a fallopian tube

sal·pin·gi·tis \ˌsal-pən-ˈjī-təs\ *n, pl* **-giti·des** \-ˈji-tə-ˌdēz\ : inflammation of a fallopian or eustachian tube

salpingitis isth·mi·ca no·do·sa \-ˈis-mə-kə-nə-ˈdō-sə\ *n* : salpingitis of the fallopian tubes marked by nodular thickening of the muscular coat

sal·pin·gog·ra·phy \ˌsal-piŋ-ˈgä-grə-fē\ *n, pl* **-phies** : visualization of a fallopian tube by radiography following injection of an opaque medium

sal·pin·gol·y·sis \ˌsal-piŋ-ˈgä-lə-səs\ *n, pl* **-y·ses** : surgical correction of adhesions in a fallopian tube

sal·pin·go–oo·pho·rec·to·my \sal-ˌpiŋ-gō-ˌō-ə-fə-ˈrek-tə-mē\ *n, pl* **-mies** : surgical excision of a fallopian tube and an ovary

sal·pin·go–oo·pho·ri·tis \-ˌō-ə-fə-ˈrī-təs\ *n* : inflammation of a fallopian tube and an ovary

sal·pin·go·pha·ryn·ge·us \-fə-ˈrin-jē-əs\ *n* : a muscle of the pharynx that arises from the inferior part of the eustachian tube near its opening and passes downward to join the posterior part of the palatopharyngeus

sal·pin·go·plas·ty \sal-ˈpiŋ-gə-ˌplas-tē\ *n, pl* **-ties** : plastic surgery of a fallopian tube

sal·pin·gos·to·my \ˌsal-piŋ-ˈgäs-tə-mē\ *n, pl* **-mies** : a surgical opening of a fallopian tube (as to establish patency)

¹salt \ˈsȯlt\ *n* **1 a** : a crystalline compound NaCl that is the chloride of sodium, is abundant in nature, and is used esp. to season or preserve food — called also *sodium chloride* **b** : any of numerous compounds that result from replacement of part or all of the acid hydrogen of an acid by a metal or a group acting like a metal : an ionic crystalline compound **2 salts** *pl* **a** : a mineral or saline mixture (as Epsom salts) used as an aperient or cathartic **b** : SMELLING SALTS — **salty** \ˈsȯl-tē\ *adj*

²salt *adj* **1** : SALINE **2** : being or inducing the one of the four basic taste sensations that is suggestive of seawater — compare BITTER, SOUR, SWEET

sal·ta·to·ry \ˈsal-tə-ˌtōr-ē, ˈsȯl-\ *adj* : proceeding by leaps rather than by gradual transitions ⟨~ conduction of nerve impulses⟩

salt·pe·ter \ˈsȯlt-ˈpē-tər\ *n* **1** : POTASSIUM NITRATE **2** : SODIUM NITRATE

¹sal·uret·ic \ˌsal-yə-ˈre-tik\ *adj* : facilitating the urinary excretion of salt and esp. of sodium ion ⟨a ~ drug⟩

²saluretic *n* : a saluretic agent

sal·vage \ˈsal-vij\ *vb* **sal·vaged; sal·vag·ing** : to save (an organ, tissue, or patient) by preventive or therapeutic measures ⟨*salvaged* lung tissue⟩ — **salvage** *n*

sal·var·san \ˈsal-vər-ˌsan\ *n* : ARSPHENAMINE

salve \ˈsav, ˈsäv, ˈsalv, ˈsälv\ *n* : an unctuous adhesive substance for application to wounds or sores

sal vo·la·ti·le \ˌsal-və-ˈlat-ᵊl-ē\ *n* **1** : AMMONIUM CARBONATE **2** : SMELLING SALTS

sa·mar·i·um \sə-ˈmar-ē-əm\ *n* : a pale gray lustrous metallic element — symbol *Sm;* see ELEMENT table

SAMe \ˈsa-mē\ *n* : *S*-adenosylmethionine esp. when used as a dietary supplement (as to relieve depression or arthritic pain and inflammation)

san·a·to·ri·um \ˌsa-nə-ˈtōr-ē-əm\ *n, pl* **-riums** *or* **-ria** \-ē-ə\ **1** : an establishment that provides therapy combined with a regimen (as of diet and exercise) for treatment or rehabilitation **2 a** : an institution for rest and recuperation (as of convalescents) **b** : an establishment for the treatment of the chronically ill ⟨a tuberculosis ~⟩

sand \ˈsand\ *n* : gritty particles in various body tissues or fluids

sand crack *n* : a fissure in the wall of a horse's hoof often causing lameness

sand flea *n* : CHIGOE 1

sand fly *n* : any of various small biting dipteran flies (families Psychodidae, Simuliidae, and Ceratopogonidae); *esp* : any fly of the genus *Phlebotomus*

sand·fly fever \ˈsand-ˌflī-\ *n* : a virus disease of brief duration that is characterized by fever, headache, pain in the eyes, malaise, and leukopenia and is caused by a bunyavirus of the genus *Phlebovirus* (esp. species *Sandfly fever Naples virus* and species *Sandfly fever Sicilian virus*) transmitted by the bite of a sand fly of the genus *Phlebotomus* (esp. *P. papatasii*) — called also *pappataci fever, phlebotomus fever*

Sand·hoff–Jatz·ke·witz disease \-ˈjats-kə-ˌvits-\ *n* : SANDHOFF'S DISEASE

Sand·hoff's disease \ˈsand-ˌhȯfs-\ *or* **Sand·hoff disease** \-ˌhȯf-\ *n* : a hereditary disorder of lipid metabolism that is closely related to or is a variant of Tay-Sachs disease, typically affects individuals of non-Jewish ancestry, and is characterized by great reduction in or absence of both hexosaminidase A and hexosaminidase B

Sandhoff, K., An·dreae \än-ˈdrā-e\, **U.**, and **Jatzkewitz, H.**, German medical scientists.

Sand·im·mune \ˈsand-i-ˌmyün\ *trademark* — used for a preparation of cyclosporine administered orally or by intravenous injection

sane \ˈsān\ *adj* **san·er; san·est 1** : free from hurt or disease : HEALTHY **2** : mentally sound; *esp* : able to anticipate and appraise the effect of one's actions **3** : proceeding from a sound mind ⟨~ behavior⟩ — **sane·ly** *adv*

san·guin·eous \saŋ-ˈgwi-nē əs, san-\ *adj* : of, relating to, or containing blood

san·gui·nous \ˈsaŋ-gwə-nəs\ *adj* : SANGUINEOUS

san·i·tar·i·an \ˌsa-nə-ˈter-ē-ən\ *n* : a specialist in sanitary science and public health ⟨a milk ~⟩

san·i·tar·i·um \ˌsa-nə-ˈter-ē-əm\ *n, pl* **-i·ums** *or* **-ia** \-ē-ə\ : SANATORIUM

san·i·tary \ˈsa-nə-ˌter-ē\ *adj* **1** : of or relating to health ⟨~ measures⟩ **2** : of, relating to, or used in the disposal esp. of domestic waterborne waste **3** : characterized by or readily kept in cleanliness ⟨~ food handling⟩ — **san·i·tari·ly** \ˌsa-nə-ˈter-ə-lē\ *adv*

sanitary napkin *n* : a disposable absorbent pad used (as during menstruation) to absorb the flow from the uterus — called also *sanitary pad*

san·i·ta·tion \ˌsa-nə-ˈtā-shən\ *n* **1** : the act or process of making sanitary **2** : the promotion of hygiene and prevention of disease by maintenance of sanitary conditions ⟨mouth ~⟩

san·i·tize \ˈsa-nə-ˌtīz\ *vb* **-tized; -tiz·ing** : to make sanitary (as by cleaning or sterilizing) — **san·i·ti·za·tion** \ˌsa-nə-tə-ˈzā-shən\ *n*

san·i·to·ri·um \ˌsa-nə-ˈtōr-ē-əm\ *n, pl* **-ri·ums** *or* **-ria** \-ē-ə\ : SANATORIUM

san·i·ty \ˈsa-nə-tē\ *n, pl* **-ties** : the quality or state of being sane; *esp* : soundness or health of mind

San Joa·quin fever \ˌsan-ˌwä-ˈkēn-\ *n* : COCCIDIOIDOMYCOSIS

San Joaquin valley fever *n* : COCCIDIOIDOMYCOSIS

S–A node \ˌes-ˈā-\ *n* : SINOATRIAL NODE

santa — see YERBA SANTA

sap — see CELL SAP, NUCLEAR SAP

sa·phe·no·fem·o·ral \sə-ˌfē-nō-ˈfe-mə-rəl\ *adj* : of or relating to the saphenous and the femoral veins

sa·phe·nous \sə-ˈfē-nəs, ˈsa-fə-nəs\ *adj* : of, relating to, associated with, or being either of the saphenous veins

saphenous nerve *n* : a nerve that is the largest and longest branch of the femoral nerve and supplies the skin over the medial side of the leg

saphenous opening *n* : a passage for the great saphenous vein in the fascia lata of the thigh — called also *fossa ovalis*

saphenous vein *n* : either of two chiefly superficial veins of the leg: **a** : one originating in the foot and passing up the medial side of the leg and through the saphenous opening to join the femoral vein — called also *great saphenous vein, long saphenous vein* **b** : one originating similarly and passing up the back of the leg to join the popliteal vein at the knee — called also *short saphenous vein, small saphenous vein*

sa·pon·i·fi·ca·tion \sə-ˌpä-nə-fə-ˈkā-shən\ *n* **1** : the hydrolysis of a fat by an alkali with the formation of a soap and glycerol **2** : the hydrolysis esp. by an alkali of an ester into the corresponding alcohol and acid; *broadly* : HYDROLYSIS — **sa·pon·i·fy** \sə-ˈpä-nə-ˌfī\ *vb*

sapr- *or* **sapro-** *comb form* : dead or decaying organic matter ⟨*sapro*phyte⟩

sap·ro·phyte \ˈsa-prə-ˌfīt\ *n* : a saprophytic organism

sap·ro·phyt·ic \ˌsa-prə-ˈfi-tik\ *adj* : obtaining food by absorbing dissolved organic material; *esp* : obtaining nourishment from the products of organic breakdown and decay ⟨~ fungi⟩ — **sap·ro·phyt·i·cal·ly** *adv*

sap·ro·zo·ic \-ˈzō-ik\ *adj* : SAPROPHYTIC — used of animals (as protozoans)

sa·quin·a·vir \sə-ˈkwi-nə-ˌvir\ *n* : a protease inhibitor $C_{38}H_{50}N_6O_5$ or its mesylate $C_{38}H_{50}N_6O_5 \cdot CH_4O_3S$ administered orally often in combination with other antiretroviral drugs to treat HIV infection

sar·al·a·sin \sä-ˈra-lə-sən\ *n* : an antihypertensive polypeptide used esp. in the form of its hydrated acetate $C_{42}H_{65}N_{13}O_{10}·nC_2H_4O_2·nH_2O$ to treat and diagnose hypertension

sarc- *or* **sarco-** *comb form* **1** : flesh ⟨*sarc*oid⟩ **2** : striated muscle ⟨*sarco*lemma⟩

sar·co·cyst \ˈsär-kə-ˌsist\ *n* : the large intramuscular cyst of a protozoan of the genus *Sarcocystis*

Sar·co·cys·tis \ˌsär-kə-ˈsis-təs\ *n* : a genus of sporozoan protozoans (order Sarcosporidia) that form cysts in vertebrate muscle

sar·co·cys·to·sis \-sis-ˈtō-səs\ *n* : infestation with or disease caused by sporozoan protozoans of the genus *Sarcocystis* — called also *sarcosporidiosis*

[1]**sar·coid** \ˈsär-ˌkȯid\ *adj* : of, relating to, resembling, or being sarcoid or sarcoidosis ⟨~ fibroblastic tissue⟩

[2]**sarcoid** *n* **1** : any of various diseases characterized esp. by the formation of nodules in the skin **2** : a nodule characteristic of sarcoid or of sarcoidosis

sar·coid·o·sis \ˌsär-ˌkȯi-ˈdō-səs\ *n, pl* **-o·ses** \-ˌsēz\ : a chronic disease of unknown cause that is characterized by the formation of nodules resembling true tubercles esp. in the lymph nodes, lungs, bones, and skin — called also *Boeck's sarcoid*

sar·co·lem·ma \ˌsär-kə-ˈle-mə\ *n* : the thin transparent homogeneous sheath enclosing a striated muscle fiber — **sar·co·lem·mal** \-məl\ *adj*

sar·co·ly·sin \ˌsär-kə-ˈlī-sən\ *or* **sar·co·ly·sine** \-sēn\ *also* **L–sar·co·ly·sin** \ˈel-\ *or* **L–sar·co·ly·sine** *n* : MELPHALAN

sar·co·ma \sär-ˈkō-mə\ *n, pl* **-mas** *also* **-ma·ta** \-mə-tə\ : a malignant tumor arising in tissue of mesodermal origin (as connective tissue, bone, cartilage, or striated muscle) that spreads by extension into neighboring tissue or by way of the bloodstream — compare CARCINOMA

sarcoma bot·ry·oi·des \-ˌbä-trē-ˈȯi-ˌdēz\ *n* : a malignant tumor of striated muscle that resembles a bunch of grapes and occurs esp. in the urogenital tract of young children

sar·co·ma·to·sis \(ˌ)sär-ˌkō-mə-ˈtō-səs\ *n, pl* **-to·ses** \-ˌsēz\ : a disease characterized by the presence and spread of sarcomas

sar·co·ma·tous \sär-ˈkō-mə-təs\ *adj* : of, relating to, or resembling sarcoma

sar·co·mere \ˈsär-kə-ˌmir\ *n* : any of the repeating structural units of striated muscle fibrils — **sar·co·mer·ic** \ˌsär-kə-ˈmer-ik\ *adj*

sar·co·pe·nia \ˌsär-kō-ˈpē-nē-ə\ *n* : reduction in skeletal muscle mass due to aging

Sar·coph·a·ga \sär-ˈkä-fə-gə\ *n* : a genus of dipteran flies (family Sarcophagidae) comprising typical flesh flies

sar·co·plasm \ˈsär-kə-ˌpla-zəm\ *n* : the cytoplasm of a striated muscle fiber — compare MYOPLASM — **sar·co·plas·mic** \ˌsär-kə-ˈplaz-mik\ *adj*

sarcoplasmic reticulum *n* : the endoplasmic reticulum of cardiac muscle and skeletal striated muscle fiber that functions esp. as a storage and release area for calcium

Sar·cop·tes \sär-ˈkäp-(ˌ)tēz\ *n* : a genus of whitish itch mites (family Sarcoptidae)

sar·cop·tic \sär-ˈkäp-tik\ *adj* : of, relating to, caused by, or being itch mites of the genus *Sarcoptes*

sarcoptic mange *n* : mange caused by mites of the genus *Sarcoptes* that burrow in the skin esp. of the head and face — compare CHORIOPTIC MANGE, DEMODECTIC MANGE

sar·co·sine \ˈsär-kə-ˌsēn, -sən\ *n* : a sweetish crystalline amino acid $C_3H_7NO_2$ formed by the decomposition of creatine or made synthetically

sar·co·some \ˈsär-kə-ˌsōm\ *n* : a mitochondrion of a striated muscle fiber — **sar·co·som·al** \ˌsär-kə-ˈsō-məl\ *adj*

sar·co·spo·rid·i·o·sis \ˌsär-kō-spə-ˌri-dē-ˈō-səs\ *n, pl* **-o·ses** \-ˌsēz\ : SARCOCYSTOSIS

sardonicus — see RISUS SARDONICUS

sar·gram·o·stim \sär-ˈgra-məs-təm\ *n* : a granulocyte-macrophage colony-stimulating factor produced by recombinant DNA technology that is used esp. following autologous bone marrow transplantation to accelerate the division and differentiation of the transplanted bone marrow cells

sa·rin \ˈsär-ən, zä-ˈrēn\ *n* : an extremely toxic chemical warfare agent $C_4H_{10}FO_2P$ — called also *GB*

SARS \ˈsärz\ *n* : a severe respiratory illness that is transmitted esp. by contact with infectious material (as respiratory droplets or body fluids), is caused by a coronavirus (species *Severe acute respiratory syndrome-related coronavirus* of the genus *Betacoronavirus*), and is characterized by fever, headache, body aches, a dry cough, hypoxia, and usu. pneumonia — called also *severe acute respiratory syndrome*

sar·to·ri·us \sär-ˈtōr-ē-əs\ *n, pl* **-rii** \-ē-ˌī\ : a muscle that arises from the anterior superior iliac spine, crosses the front of the thigh obliquely to insert on the upper part of the inner surface of the tibia, is the longest muscle in the human body, and acts to flex, abduct, and rotate the thigh laterally at the hip joint and to flex the leg at the knee joint and to rotate it medially in a way that enables one to sit with the heel of one leg on the knee of the opposite leg

sas·sa·fras \ˈsa-sə-ˌfras\ *n* **1** : a tall eastern No. American tree (*Sassafras albidum*) of the laurel family (Lauraceae) with mucilaginous twigs and leaves **2** : the carcinogenic dried root bark of the sassafras formerly used as a diaphoretic and flavoring agent

sat·el·lite \ˈsat-ᵊl-ˌīt\ *n* **1 :** a short segment separated from the main body of a chromosome by a constriction **2 :** a bodily structure lying near or associated with another (as a vein accompanying an artery) **3 :** a smaller lesion accompanying a main one and situated nearby — **satellite** *adj*

satellite cell *n* **1 :** a cell surrounding a ganglion cell **2 :** a stem cell that lies adjacent to a skeletal muscle fiber and plays a role in muscle growth, repair, and regeneration

satellite DNA *n* **:** a fraction of a eukaryotic organism's DNA that differs in density from most of its DNA as determined by centrifugation, that apparently consists of short repetitive nucleotide sequences, that does not undergo transcription, and that is often found esp. in centromeric regions

sat·el·lit·osis \ˌsat-ᵊl-ī-ˈtō-səs\ *n, pl* **-o·ses** \-ˌsēz\ **:** the usu. abnormal clustering of one type of cell around another; *esp* **:** the clustering of glial cells around neurons in the brain that is associated with certain pathological states (as oligodendroglioma)

sa·ti·ety \sə-ˈtī-ə-tē\ *n, pl* **-ties :** the quality or state of being fed or gratified to or beyond capacity

[1]**sat·u·rate** \ˈsa-chə-ˌrāt\ *vb* **-rat·ed; -rat·ing 1 :** to treat, furnish, or charge with something to the point where no more can be absorbed, dissolved, or retained **2 :** to cause to combine until there is no further tendency to combine

[2]**sat·u·rate** \-rət\ *n* **:** a saturated chemical compound

sat·u·rat·ed \ˈsa-chə-ˌrā-təd\ *adj* **1 :** being a solution that is unable to absorb or dissolve any more of a solute at a given temperature and pressure **2 :** being an organic compound having no double or triple bonds between carbon atoms

sat·u·ra·tion \ˌsa-chə-ˈrā-shən\ *n* **1 :** the act of saturating **:** the state of being saturated **2 :** conversion of an unsaturated to a saturated chemical compound (as by hydrogenation) **3 :** a state of maximum impregnation; *esp* **:** the presence in air of the most water possible under existent pressure and temperature **4 :** the one of the three psychological dimensions of color perception that is related to the purity of the color and that decreases as the amount of white present in the stimulus increases — called also *intensity;* compare BRIGHTNESS, HUE

sat·ur·nine \ˈsa-tər-ˌnīn\ *adj* **1 :** of or relating to lead **2 :** of, relating to, or produced by the absorption of lead into the system ⟨~ poisoning⟩

sat·urn·ism \ˈsa-tər-ˌni-zəm\ *n* **:** LEAD POISONING

sa·ty·ri·a·sis \ˌsā-tə-ˈrī-ə-səs, ˌsa-\ *n, pl* **-a·ses** \-ˌsēz\ **:** excessive or abnormal sexual desire in the male — compare NYMPHOMANIA

sau·cer·ize \ˈsȯ-sər-ˌīz\ *vb* **-ized; -iz·ing :** to form a shallow depression by excavation of tissue to promote granulation and healing of (a wound) — **sau·cer·iza·tion** \ˌsȯ-sər-ə-ˈzā-shən\ *n*

sau·na \ˈsau̇-nə, ˈsȯ-nə\ *n* **1 :** a Finnish steam bath in which the steam is provided by water thrown on hot stones; *also* **:** a bathhouse or room used for such a bath **2 :** a dry heat bath; *also* **:** a room or cabinet used for such a bath

sa·vant \sə-ˈvänt\ *n* **:** a person affected with a developmental disorder (as autism or intellectual disability) who exhibits exceptional skill or brilliance in some limited field (as mathematics or music); *esp* **:** AUTISTIC SAVANT

saw \ˈsȯ\ *n* **:** a hand or power tool used to cut hard material (as bone) and equipped usu. with a toothed blade or disk

saw pal·met·to \-pal-ˈme-tō\ *n* **:** a preparation derived from the berrylike fruit of a shrubby palm (*Serenoa repens*) of the southeastern U.S. that is held to have a therapeutic effect on the prostate gland and is used in herbal remedies and dietary supplements — called also *sabal*

sax·a·glip·tin \ˌsak-sə-ˈglip-tən\ *n* **:** a hypoglycemic drug taken orally in the form of its hydrate $C_{18}H_{25}N_3O_2{\cdot}H_2O$ to treat type 2 diabetes — see KOMBIGLYZE, ONGLYZA

saxi·tox·in \ˌsak-sə-ˈtäk-sən\ *n* **:** a potent nonprotein neurotoxin $C_{10}H_{17}N_7O_4{\cdot}2HCl$ that originates esp. in dinoflagellates (as of the genera *Alexandrium*, *Gymnodinium*, and *Pyrodinium*) found in red tides and causes paralytic shellfish poisoning when ingested in contaminated shellfish

Sb *symbol* [Latin *stibium*] antimony

SBP *abbr* systolic blood pressure

SBS *abbr* sick building syndrome

Sc *symbol* scandium

SCA *abbr* **1** sickle cell anemia **2** spinocerebellar ataxia **3** sudden cardiac arrest

scab \ˈskab\ *n* **1 :** scabies of domestic animals **2 :** a hardened covering of dried secretions (as blood, serum, or pus) that forms over a wound — called also *crust* — **scab** *vb* — **scab·by** \ˈska-bē\ *adj*

scabby mouth *n* **:** SORE MOUTH 1

sca·bi·cide \ˈskā-bə-ˌsīd\ *n* **:** a drug that destroys the itch mite causing scabies

sca·bies \ˈskā-bēz\ *n, pl* **scabies :** contagious itch or mange esp. with exudative crusts that is caused by parasitic mites and esp. by a mite of the genus *Sarcoptes* (*S. scabiei*) — **sca·bi·et·ic** \ˌskā-bē-ˈe-tik\ *adj*

scab mite *n* **:** any of several small mites that cause mange, scabies, or scab; *esp* **:** one of the genus *Psoroptes*

sca·la \ˈskā-lə\ *n, pl* **sca·lae** \-ˌlē\ **:** any of the three spirally arranged canals into which the bony canal of the cochlea is partitioned by the vestibular and basilar membranes and which comprise the cochlear duct, scala tympani, and scala vestibuli

scala me•dia \-ˈmē-dē-ə\ *n, pl* **scalae me•di•ae** \-dē-ˌē\ : COCHLEAR DUCT

scala tym•pa•ni \-ˈtim-pə-ˌnī, -ˌnē\ *n, pl* **scalae tym•pa•no•rum** \-ˌtim-pə-ˈnōr-əm\ : the lymph-filled spirally arranged canal in the bony canal of the cochlea that is separated from the cochlear duct by the basilar membrane, communicates at its upper end with the scala vestibuli, and abuts at its lower end upon the membrane that separates the round window from the middle ear

scala ves•tib•u•li \-ve-ˈsti-byə-ˌlī\ *n, pl* **scalae ves•tib•ulo•rum** \-ve-ˌsti-byə-ˈlō-rəm\ : the lymph-filled spirally arranged canal in the bony canal of the cochlea that is separated from the cochlear duct below by the vestibular membrane, is connected with the oval window, and receives vibrations from the stapes

[1]scald \ˈskȯld\ *vb* : to burn with hot liquid or steam ⟨~*ed* skin⟩

[2]scald *n* : an injury to the body caused by scalding

scalded–skin syndrome *n* : TOXIC EPIDERMAL NECROLYSIS — see STAPHYLOCOCCAL SCALDED SKIN SYNDROME

[1]scale \ˈskāl\ *n* **1** : a small thin dry lamina shed (as in many skin diseases) from the skin **2** : a film of tartar encrusting the teeth

[2]scale *vb* **scaled; scal•ing 1** : to take off or come off in thin layers or scales ⟨~ tartar from the teeth⟩ **2** : to shed scales or fragmentary surface matter : EXFOLIATE ⟨*scaling* skin⟩

[3]scale *n* **1** : a series of marks or points at known intervals used to measure distances (as the height of the mercury in a thermometer) **2** : a graduated series or scheme of rank or order **3** : a graded series of tests or of performances used in rating individual intelligence or achievement

sca•lene \ˈskā-ˌlēn, skā-ˈ\ *n* : SCALENUS — called also *scalene muscle*

sca•le•not•o•my \ˌskā-lə-ˈnä-tə-mē\ *n, pl* **-mies** : surgical severing of one or more scalenus muscles near their insertion on the ribs

sca•le•nus \skā-ˈlē-nəs\ *n, pl* **sca•le•ni** \-ˌnī\ : any of usu. three deeply situated muscles on each side of the neck of which each extends from the transverse processes of two or more cervical vertebrae to the first or second rib: **a** : one arising from the transverse processes of the third to sixth cervical vertebrae, inserting on the scalene tubercle of the first rib, and functioning to bend the neck forward and laterally and to rotate it to the side — called also *scalenus anterior, scalenus anticus* **b** : one arising from the transverse processes of the lower six cervical vertebrae, inserting on the upper surface of the first rib, and functioning similarly to the scalenus anterior — called also *scalenus medius* **c** : one arising from the transverse processes of the fourth to sixth cervical vertebrae, inserting on the outer surface of the second rib, and functioning to raise the second rib and to bend and slightly rotate the neck — called also *scalenus posterior*

scalenus anterior *n* : SCALENUS a

scalenus an•ti•cus \-an-ˈtī-kəs\ *n* : SCALENUS a

scalenus anticus syndrome *n* : a complex of symptoms including pain and numbness in the region of the shoulder, arm, and neck that is caused by compression of the brachial plexus or subclavian artery or both by the scalenus anticus muscle

scalenus me•di•us \-ˈmē-dē-əs\ *n* : SCALENUS b

scalenus posterior *n* : SCALENUS c

scal•er \ˈskā-lər\ *n* : any of various dental instruments for removing tartar from teeth

scalp \ˈskalp\ *n* : the part of the integument of the head usu. covered with hair in both sexes

scal•pel \ˈskal-pəl\ *n* : a small straight thin-bladed knife used esp. in surgery

scalp ringworm *n* : TINEA CAPITIS

scaly \ˈskā-lē\ *adj* **scal•i•er; -est** : covered with or composed of scale or scales ⟨~ skin⟩ — **scal•i•ness** *n*

[1]scan \ˈskan\ *vb* **scanned; scan•ning 1 a** : to examine esp. systematically with a sensing device (as a beam of radiation) **b** : to pass an electron beam over and convert (an image) into variations of electrical properties (as voltage) that convey information electronically **2** : to make a scan of (as the human body) in order to detect the presence or localization of radioactive material

[2]scan *n* **1** : the act or process of scanning **2 a** : a depiction (as a photograph) of the distribution of a radioactive material in something (as a bodily organ) **b** : an image of a bodily part produced (as by computer) by combining ultrasonic or radiographic data obtained from several angles or sections

scan•di•um \ˈskan-dē-əm\ *n* : a white metallic element — symbol *Sc;* see ELEMENT table

scan•ner \ˈska-nər\ *n* : a device for making scans of a living body — see CT SCANNER, PET SCANNER

scanning electron micrograph *n* : a micrograph made by scanning electron microscopy

scanning electron microscope *n* : an electron microscope in which a beam of focused electrons moves across the object with the secondary electrons produced by the object and the electrons scattered by the object being collected to form a three-dimensional image on a display screen — called also *scanning microscope* — **scan·ning electron microscopy** *n*

scanning speech *n* : speech characterized by regularly recurring pauses between words or syllables

Scan·zo·ni maneuver \skänt-ˈsō-nē-\ *also* **Scan·zo·ni's maneuver** \-nēz-\ *n* : rotation of an abnormally positioned fetus by means of forceps with subsequent reapplication of forceps for delivery

Scanzoni, Friedrich Wilhelm (1821–1891), German obstetrician.

scaph- *or* **scapho-** *comb form* : scaphoid ⟨*scapho*cephaly⟩

sca·pha \ˈska-fə\ *n* : an elongated depression of the ear that separates the helix and antihelix

scaph·o·ceph·a·ly \ˌska-fō-ˈse-fə-lē\ *n, pl* **-lies** : a congenital deformity of the skull in which the vault is narrow, elongated, and boat-shaped because of premature ossification of the sagittal suture

¹scaph·oid \ˈska-ˌfȯid\ *adj* **1** : shaped like a boat : NAVICULAR **2** : characterized by concavity ⟨a ∼ abdomen⟩

²scaphoid *n* **1** : NAVICULAR a **2** : the largest carpal bone of the proximal row of the wrist that occupies the most lateral position on the thumb side — called also *navicular*

scaphoid bone *n* : SCAPHOID

scaphoid fossa *n* : a shallow oval depression that is situated above the pterygoid fossa on the pterygoid process of the sphenoid bone and that provides attachment for the origin of the tensor veli palatini muscle

scapul- *or* **scapulo-** *comb form* : scapular and ⟨*scapulo*humeral⟩

scap·u·la \ˈska-pyə-lə\ *n, pl* **-lae** \-ˌlē, -ˌlī\ *or* **-las** : either of a pair of large essentially flat and triangular bones lying one in each dorsolateral part of the thorax, being the principal bone of the corresponding half of the shoulder girdle, providing articulation for the humerus, and articulating with the corresponding clavicle — called also *shoulder blade*

scapulae — see LEVATOR SCAPULAE

scap·u·lar \ˈska-pyə-lər\ *adj* : of, relating to, or affecting the shoulder or scapula ⟨a ∼ fracture⟩

scapular notch *n* : a semicircular notch on the superior border of the scapula next to the coracoid process that gives passage to the suprascapular nerve and is converted to a foramen by the suprascapular ligament

scap·u·lo·hu·mer·al \ˌska-pyə-lō-ˈhyü-mə-rəl\ *adj* : of or relating to the scapula and the humerus

scap·u·lo·tho·rac·ic \ˌska-pyə-lō-thə-ˈra-sik\ *adj* : of or relating to the scapula and the thorax ⟨∼ pain⟩

scar \ˈskär\ *n* **1** : a mark left (as in the skin) by the healing of injured tissue **2** : a lasting emotional injury — **scar** *vb*

scar·i·fy \ˈskar-ə-ˌfī\ *vb* **-fied; -fy·ing** : to make scratches or small cuts in (as the skin) ⟨∼ an area for vaccination⟩ — **scar·i·fi·ca·tion** \ˌskar-ə-fə-ˈkā-shən\ *n*

scar·la·ti·na \ˌskär-lə-ˈtē-nə\ *n* : SCARLET FEVER — **scar·la·ti·nal** \-ˈtēn-ᵊl\ *adj*

scar·la·ti·ni·form \-ˈtē-nə-ˌfȯrm\ *adj* : resembling the rash of scarlet fever

scar·let fever \ˈskär-lət-\ *n* : an acute contagious febrile disease caused by Group A bacteria of the genus *Streptococcus* (esp. various strains of *S. pyogenes*) and characterized by inflammation of the nose, throat, and mouth, generalized toxemia, and a red rash — called also *scarlatina*

scarlet red *n* : SUDAN IV

Scar·pa's fascia \ˈskär-pəz-\ *n* : the deep layer of the superficial fascia of the anterior abdominal wall

Scarpa, Antonio (1752–1832), Italian anatomist and surgeon.

Scarpa's triangle *n* : FEMORAL TRIANGLE

scar tissue *n* : the connective tissue forming a scar and composed chiefly of fibroblasts in recent scars and largely of dense collagenous fibers in old scars

ScD *abbr* doctor of science

Schatz·ki ring \ˈshats-kē-\ *or* **Schatzki's ring** \-kēz-\ *n* : a local narrowing in the lower part of the esophagus that may cause dysphagia

Schatzki, Richard (1901–1992), American radiologist.

sched·ule \ˈske-ˌjül, -jəl; ˈshe-jü-wəl\ *n* **1** : a program or plan that indicates the sequence of each step or procedure; *esp* : REGIMEN **2** *often cap* : an official list of drugs that are subject to the same legal controls and restrictions — usu. used with a Roman numeral from I to V indicating decreasing potential for abuse or addiction ⟨the Drug Enforcement Administration classifies heroin as a ∼ I drug while diazepam is on ∼ IV⟩

Scheie syndrome \ˈshī-\ *n* : an autosomal recessive mucopolysaccharidosis similar to Hurler syndrome but less severe that is characterized by clouding of the cornea, slight deformity of the extremities, and disease of the aorta but not by intellectual disability or early death

Scheie, Harold Glendon (1909–1990), American ophthalmologist.

sche·ma \ˈskē-mə\ *n, pl* **sche·ma·ta** \-mə-tə\ *also* **sche·mas** **1** : a nonconscious adjustment of the brain to the afferent impulses indicative of bodily posture that is a prerequisite of appropriate bodily movement and of spatial perception **2** : a mental codification of experience that includes a particular organized way of perceiving cognitively and responding to a complex situation or set of stimuli — **sche·mat·ic** \ski-ˈma-tik\ *adj*

scheme \ˈskēm\ *n* : SCHEMA

Scheuer•mann's disease \ˈshȯi-ər-ˌmänz-\ *n* : osteochondrosis of the vertebrae associated in the active state with pain and kyphosis

Scheuermann, Holger Werfel (1877–1960), Danish orthopedist.

Schick test \ˈshik-\ *n* : a serological test for susceptibility to diphtheria by cutaneous injection of a diluted diphtheria toxin that causes an area of reddening and induration in susceptible individuals

Schick, Béla (1877–1967), American pediatrician.

Schiff's reagent \ˈshifs-\ *or* **Schiff reagent** \ˈshif-\ *n* : a solution of fuchsin decolorized by treatment with sulfur dioxide that gives a useful test for aldehydes because they restore the reddish-violet color of the dye — compare FEULGEN REACTION

Schiff, Hugo Josef (1834–1915), German chemist.

Schil•der's disease \ˈshil-dərz-\ *n* : ADRENOLEUKODYSTROPHY

Schilder, Paul Ferdinand (1886–1940), Austrian psychiatrist.

Schil•ler's test \ˈshi-lərz-\ *n* : a preliminary test for cancer of the uterine cervix in which the cervix is painted with an aqueous solution of iodine and potassium iodide and which shows up healthy tissue by staining it brown and possibly cancerous tissue as white or yellow

Schiller, Walter (1887–1960), American pathologist.

Schil•ling test \ˈshi-liŋ-\ *n* : a test for gastrointestinal absorption of vitamin B_{12} in which a dose of the radioactive vitamin is taken orally, a dose of the nonradioactive vitamin is given by injection to impede uptake of the absorbed radioactive dose by the liver, and the proportion of the radioactive dose absorbed is determined by measuring the radioactivity of the urine

Schilling, Robert Frederick (1919–2014), American hematologist.

schin•dy•le•sis \ˌskin-də-ˈlē-səs\ *n, pl* **-le•ses** \-ˌsēz\ : an articulation in which one bone is received into a groove or slit in another

Schiotz tonometer \ˈshyu̇ts-, ˈshy-ərts-\ *n* : a tonometer used to measure intraocular pressure in millimeters of mercury

Schiøtz, Hjalmar (1850–1927), Norwegian ophthalmologist.

-schi•sis \skə-səs\ *n comb form, pl* **-schi•ses** \skə-ˌsēz\ *also* **-schi•sis•es** : breaking up of attachments or adhesions : fissure ⟨gastro*schisis*⟩ ⟨cranio*schisis*⟩

schisto- *comb form* : cleft : divided ⟨*schisto*cyte⟩

schis•to•cyte \ˈshis-tə-ˌsīt, ˈskis-\ *n* : a hemoglobin-containing fragment of a red blood cell

schis•to•so•ma \ˌshis-tə-ˈsō-mə, ˌskis-\ *n* **1** *cap* : a genus of elongated digenetic trematode worms (family Schistosomatidae) that parasitize the blood vessels of birds and mammals and include species (as *S. haematobium*, *S. japonicum*, and *S. mansoni*) causing human schistosomiasis **2** : any trematode of the genus *Schistosoma* : SCHISTOSOME

schis•to•some \ˈshis-tə-ˌsōm, ˈskis-\ *n* : any trematode worm of the genus *Schistosoma* or of the family (Schistosomatidae) to which it belongs — called also *blood fluke* — **schis•to•so•mal** \ˌshis-tə-ˈsō-məl, ˌskis-\ *adj*

schistosome dermatitis *n* : SWIMMER'S ITCH

schis•to•so•mi•a•sis \ˌshis-tə-sō-ˈmī-ə-səs, ˌskis-\ *n, pl* **-a•ses** \-ˌsēz\ : infestation with or disease caused by schistosomes; *specif* : a severe endemic disease of humans in much of Asia, Africa, and So. America that is caused by any of three trematode worms of the genus *Schistosoma* (*S. haematobium, S. mansoni,* and *S. japonicum*) which multiply in snail intermediate hosts and are disseminated into freshwaters as cercariae that bore into the body, migrate through the tissues to the visceral venous plexuses (as of the bladder or intestine) where they attain maturity, and cause much of their injury through hemorrhage and damage to tissues resulting from the passage of the usu. spiny eggs to the intestine and bladder — called also *bilharzia, bilharziasis, snail fever;* compare SWIMMER'S ITCH

schistosomiasis hae•ma•to•bi•um \-ˌhē-mə-ˈtō-bē-əm\ *n* : schistosomiasis caused by a schistosome (*Schistosoma haematobium*) occurring over most of Africa and in Asia Minor and predominantly involving infestation of the veins of the urinary bladder

schistosomiasis ja•pon•i•ca \-jə-ˈpä-ni-kə\ *n* : schistosomiasis caused by a schistosome (*Schistosoma japonicum*) occurring chiefly in eastern Asia and the Pacific islands and predominantly involving infestation of the portal and mesenteric veins — see KATAYAMA SYNDROME

schistosomiasis man•soni \-ˈman-sə-ˌnī\ *n* : schistosomiasis caused by a schistosome (*Schistosoma mansoni*) occurring chiefly in central Africa and eastern So. America and predominantly involving infestation of the mesenteric and portal veins — called also *Manson's disease*

P. Manson — see MANSONELLA

schis•to•som•u•lum \ˌshis-tə-ˈsäm-yə-ləm, ˌskis-\ *n, pl* **-la** \-lə\ : an immature schistosome in the body of the definitive host

schiz- *or* **schizo-** *comb form* **1** : characterized by or involving cleavage ⟨*schizo*gony⟩ **2** : schizophrenia ⟨*schiz*oid⟩

schizo \ˈskit-(ˌ)sō\ *n, pl* **schiz•os** : SCHIZOPHRENIC

schizo–af•fec•tive \-a-ˈfek-tiv\ *adj* : relating to, characterized by, or exhibiting symptoms of both schizophrenia and a mood disorder (as major depression or bipolar disorder)

schi•zog•o•ny \ski-ˈzä-gə-nē, skit-ˈsä-\ *n, pl* **-nies** : asexual reproduction by multiple segmentation characteristic of sporozoans (as the malaria parasite) — **schizo•gon•ic** \ˌskit-sə-ˈgä-nik\ *or* **schi•zog•o•nous** \ski-ˈzä-gə-nəs, skit-ˈsä-\ *adj*

[1]**schiz•oid** \ˈskit-ˌsȯid\ *adj* : characterized by, resulting from, tending toward, or suggestive of schizophrenia

[2]**schizoid** *n* : a schizoid individual

schizoid personality *n* **1** : a personality disorder characterized by shyness, withdrawal, inhibition of emotional expression, and apparent diminution of affect — called also *schizoid personality disorder* **2** : an individual with a schizoid personality

schiz•ont \ˈski-ˌzänt, ˈskit-ˌsänt\ *n* : a multinucleate sporozoan (as a malaria parasite) that reproduces by schizogony

schi•zon•ti•cide \ski-ˈzän-tə-ˌsīd, skit-ˈsän-\ *n* : an agent selectively destructive of the schizont of a sporozoan parasite — **schi•zon•ti•ci•dal** \ski-ˌzän-tə-ˈsīd-ᵊl, skit-ˌsän-\ *adj*

schizo•phrene \ˈskit-sə-ˌfrēn\ *n* : SCHIZOPHRENIC

schizo•phre•nia \ˌskit-sə-ˈfrē-nē-ə\ *n* : a mental illness characterized by loss of contact with the environment, by noticeable deterioration in the level of functioning in everyday life, and by disintegration of personality expressed as disorder of feeling, thought (as in delusions), perception (as in hallucinations), and behavior — called also *dementia praecox;* see PARANOID SCHIZOPHRENIA

[1]**schizo•phren•ic** \-ˈfre-nik\ *adj* : relating to, characteristic of, or affected with schizophrenia ⟨~ behavior⟩

[2]**schizophrenic** *n* : an individual affected with schizophrenia

schizophrenic reaction *n* : SCHIZOPHRENIA

schiz•o•phren•i•form \ˌskit-sə-ˈfre-nə-ˌfȯrm\ *adj* : resembling schizophrenia in appearance or manifestations but tending to last less than six months but more than one month ⟨~ disorder⟩

schiz•o•phreno•gen•ic \ˌskit-sə-ˌfre-nə-ˈje-nik\ *adj* : tending to produce schizophrenia ⟨~ factors⟩

schizos *pl of* SCHIZO

schizo•ty•pal \ˌskit-sə-ˈtī-pəl\ *adj* : characterized by, exhibiting, or being patterns of thought, perception, communication, and behavior suggestive of schizophrenia but not of sufficient severity to warrant a diagnosis of schizophrenia ⟨~ personality disorder⟩

Schlemm's canal \ˈshlemz-\ *n* : CANAL OF SCHLEMM

Schön•lein–Hen•och \ˈshœn-līn-ˈhe-nək\ *adj* : being a form of purpura that is characterized by swelling and pain of the joints in association with gastrointestinal bleeding and pain

Schönlein, Johann Lucas (1793–1864), German physician.

Henoch, Eduard Heinrich (1820–1910), German pediatrician.

Schönlein's disease *n* : Schönlein-Henoch purpura that is characterized esp. by swelling and pain of the joints — compare HENOCH'S PURPURA

Schüff•ner's dots \ˈshu̇f-nərz-\ *n pl* : punctate granulations present in red blood cells invaded by the tertian malaria parasite

Schüff•ner \ˈshuef-nər\, **Wilhelm August Paul (1867–1949),** German pathologist.

Schüller–Christian disease *n* : HAND-SCHÜLLER-CHRISTIAN DISEASE

Schwann cell \ˈshwän-\ *n* : a myelin-secreting glial cell that spirally wraps around an axon of the peripheral nervous system to form the myelin sheath

Schwann \ˈshvän\, **Theodor Ambrose Hubert (1810–1882),** German anatomist and physiologist.

schwan•no•ma \shwä-ˈnō-mə\ *n, pl* **-mas** \-məz\ *or* **-ma•ta** \-mə-tə\ : NEURILEMMOMA

Schwann's sheath *n* : NEURILEMMA

sci•at•ic \sī-ˈa-tik\ *adj* **1** : of, relating to, or situated near the hip **2** : of, relating to, or caused by sciatica ⟨~ pains⟩

sci•at•i•ca \sī-ˈa-ti-kə\ *n* : pain along the course of a sciatic nerve esp. in the back of the thigh caused by compression, inflammation, or reflex mechanisms; *broadly* : pain in the lower back, buttocks, hips, or adjacent parts

sciatic foramen *n* : either of two foramina on each side of the pelvis that are formed by the hip bone, the sacrospinous ligament, and the sacrotuberous ligament: **a** : one giving passage to the piriformis muscle and to the sciatic, superior and inferior gluteal, and pudendal nerves together with their associated arteries and veins — called also *greater sciatic foramen* **b** : one giving passage to the tendon of the obturator internus muscle and its nerve, to the internal pudendal artery and veins, and to the pudendal nerve — called also *lesser sciatic foramen*

sciatic nerve *n* : either of the pair of largest nerves in the body that arise one on each side from the sacral plexus and that pass out of the pelvis through the greater sciatic foramen and down the back of the thigh to its lower third where division into the tibial and common peroneal nerves occurs

sciatic notch *n* : either of two notches on the dorsal border of the hip bone on each side that when closed off by ligaments form the corresponding sciatic foramina: **a** : a relatively large notch just above the ischial spine that is converted into the greater sciatic foramen by the sacrospinous ligament — called also *greater sciatic notch* **b** : a smaller notch just below the ischial spine that is converted to the lesser sciatic foramen by the sacrospinous ligament and the sacrotuberous ligament — called also *lesser sciatic notch*

SCID *abbr* severe combined immunodeficiency

sci•ence \ˈsī-əns\ *n* : knowledge or a system of knowledge covering general truths or the operation of general laws esp. as obtained and tested through the scientific method and concerned with the physical world and its phenomena — **sci•en•tif•ic** \ˌsī-ən-ˈti-fik\ *adj* — **sci•en•tif•i•cal•ly** *adv*

scientific method *n* : principles and procedures for the systematic pursuit of knowledge involving the recognition and formulation of a problem, the collection of data through observation and experiment, and the formulation and testing of hypotheses

sci•en•tist \ˈsī-ən-tist\ *n* : one learned in science and esp. natural science : a scientific investigator

scin•ti•gram \ˈsin-tə-ˌgram\ *n* : a picture produced by scintigraphy

scin•tig•ra•phy \sin-ˈti-grə-fē\ *n, pl* **-phies** : a diagnostic technique in which a two-dimensional picture of internal body tissue is produced through the detection of radiation emitted by a radioactive substance administered into the body — **scin•ti•graph•ic** \ˌsin-tə-ˈgra-fik\ *adj*

scintillating scotoma *n* : a blind spot in the visual field that is bordered by shimmering or flashing light and that is often a premonitory symptom of migraine attack

scin•til•la•tion \ˌsint-ᵊl-ˈā-shən\ *n, often attrib* : a flash of light produced in a phosphorescent substance by an ionizing event — **scin•til•late** \ˈsint-ᵊl-ˌāt\ *vb*

scintillation counter *n* : a device for detecting and registering individual scintillations (as in radioactive emission) — called also *scintillometer*

scin•til•la•tor \ˈsint-ᵊl-ˌā-tər\ *n* **1** : a phosphorescent substance in which scintillations occur (as in a scintillation counter) **2** : a device for sending out scintillations of light **3** : SCINTILLATION COUNTER

scin•til•lom•e•ter \ˌsint-ᵊl-ˈä-mə-tər\ *n* : SCINTILLATION COUNTER

scin•ti•scan \ˈsin-ti-ˌskan\ *n* : a two-dimensional representation of radioisotope radiation from a bodily organ (as the spleen or kidney)

scirrhi *pl of* SCIRRHUS

scir•rhous \ˈsir-əs, ˈskir-\ *adj* : of, relating to, or being a scirrhous carcinoma ⟨~ infiltration⟩

scirrhous carcinoma *n* : a hard slow-growing malignant tumor having a preponderance of fibrous tissue

scir•rhus \ˈsir-əs, ˈskir-\ *n, pl* **scir•rhi** \ˈsir-ˌī, ˈskir-, -ˌē\ : SCIRRHOUS CARCINOMA

scler- *or* **sclero-** *comb form* **1** : hard ⟨*sclero*derma⟩ **2** : sclera ⟨*scler*itis⟩

sclera \ˈskler-ə\ *n* : the dense fibrous opaque white outer coat enclosing the eyeball except the part covered by the cornea — called also *sclerotic, sclerotic coat* — **scler•al** \ˈskler-əl\ *adj*

sclerae — see SINUS VENOSUS SCLERAE

scle•rec•to•my \sklə-ˈrek-tə-mē\ *n, pl* **-mies** : surgical removal of a part of the sclera

scle•re•ma neo•na•to•rum \sklə-ˈrē-mə-ˌnē-ə-nə-ˈtōr-əm\ *n* : hardening of the cutaneous and subcutaneous tissues in newborn infants

scle•ri•tis \sklə-ˈrī-təs\ *n* : inflammation of the sclera

sclero•cor•ne•al \ˌskler-ō-ˈkȯr-nē-əl\ *adj* : of or involving both sclera and cornea

sclero•dac•ty•ly \-ˈdak-tə-lē\ *n, pl* **-lies** : scleroderma of the fingers and toes

sclero•der•ma \ˌskler-ə-ˈdər-mə\ *n, pl* **-mas** *also* **-ma•ta** \-mə-tə\ : a usu. slowly progressive disease marked by the deposition of fibrous connective tissue in the skin and often in internal organs and structures, by hand and foot pain upon exposure to cold, and by tightening and thickening of the skin — **sclero•der•ma•tous** \-təs\ *adj*

scle•ro•ma \sklə-ˈrō-mə\ *n, pl* **-mas** *also* **-ma•ta** \-mə-tə\ : hardening of tissues

sclero•pro•tein \ˌskler-ō-ˈprō-ˌtēn\ *n* : any of various proteins (as collagen and keratin) that occur esp. in connective and skeletal tissues, are usu. insoluble in aqueous solvents, and are resistant to chemical reagents — called also *albuminoid*

scle•rose \sklə-ˈrōs, -ˈrōz\ *vb* **-rosed; -ros•ing** **1** : to cause sclerosis in **2** : to undergo or become affected with sclerosis

scle•ros•ing *adj* : causing or characterized by sclerosis ⟨~ agents⟩ — see SUBACUTE SCLEROSING PANENCEPHALITIS

scle•ro•sis \sklə-ˈrō-səs\ *n, pl* **-ro•ses** \-ˌsēz\ **1** : a pathological condition in which a tissue has become hard and which is produced by overgrowth of fibrous tissue and other changes (as in arteriosclerosis) or by increase in interstitial tissue and other changes (as in multiple sclerosis) — called also *hardening* **2** : any of various diseases characterized by sclerosis — usu. used in combination; see ARTERIOSCLEROSIS, MULTIPLE SCLEROSIS

scle•ro•stome \ˈskler-ə-ˌstōm\ *n* : STRONGYLE

sclerosus — see LICHEN SCLEROSUS ET ATROPHICUS

sclero•ther•a•py \ˌskler-ō-ˈther-ə-pē\ *n, pl* **-pies** : the injection of a sclerosing agent (as saline) into a varicose vein to produce inflammation and scarring which closes the lumen and is followed by shrinkage; *also* : PROLOTHERAPY

[1]**scle•rot•ic** \sklə-ˈrä-tik\ *adj* **1** : being or relating to the sclera ⟨the ~ layer of the eye⟩ **2** : of, relating to, or affected with sclerosis ⟨~ arteries⟩

[2]**sclerotic** *n* : SCLERA

sclerotic coat *n* : SCLERA

scle•ro•tium \sklə-ˈrō-shəm, -shē-əm\ *n, pl* **-tia** \-shə, -shē-ə\ : a compact mass of hardened mycelium of a fungus — **scle•ro•tial** \-shəl\ *adj*

sclero•tome \ˈskler-ə-ˌtōm\ *n* : the ventral and mesial portion of a somite that proliferates mesenchyme which migrates about the notochord to form the axial skeleton and ribs — **sclero•tom•ic** \ˌskler-ə-ˈtō-mik, -ˈtä-\ *adj*

scle•rot•o•my \sklə-ˈrä-tə-mē\ *n, pl* **-mies** : surgical cutting of the sclera

ScM *abbr* master of science

SCM *abbr* state certified midwife

SCN *abbr* suprachiasmatic nucleus

sco•lex \ˈskō-ˌleks\ *n, pl* **sco•li•ces** \ˈskō-lə-ˌsēz\ *also* **scol•e•ces** \ˈskä-lə-ˌsēz, ˈskō-\ *or* **scolexes** : the head of a tapeworm from which the proglottids are produced by budding

sco•li•o•sis \ˌskō-lē-ˈō-səs\ *n, pl* **-o•ses** \-ˌsēz\ : a lateral curvature of the spine — compare KYPHOSIS, LORDOSIS 2 — **sco•li•ot•ic** \-ˈä-tik\ *adj*

scoop \ˈsküp\ *n* : a spoon-shaped surgical instrument used in extracting various materials (as debris and pus)

scope \ˈskōp\ *n* : any of various instruments (as an arthroscope or endoscope) for viewing or observing — **scope** *vb*

-scope \ˌskōp\ *n comb form* : means (as an instrument) for viewing or observing ⟨micro*scope*⟩ ⟨laparo*scope*⟩

-scop•ic \ˈskä-pik\ *adj comb form* : viewing or observing ⟨laparo*scopic*⟩

sco•pol•amine \skō-ˈpä-lə-ˌmēn, -mən\ *n* : a poisonous alkaloid $C_{17}H_{21}NO_4$ similar to atropine that is found in various plants (as jimsonweed) of the nightshade family (Solanaceae) and is used chiefly in the form of its hydrated hydrobromide $C_{17}H_{21}NO_4 \cdot HBr \cdot 3H_2O$ for its anticholinergic effects (as preventing nausea in motion sickness and inducing mydriasis) — called also *hyoscine*

sco•po•phil•ia \ˌskō-pə-ˈfi-lē-ə\ *also* **scop•to•phil•ia** \ˌskäp-tə-ˈfi-lē-ə\ *n* : a desire to look at sexually stimulating scenes esp. as a substitute for actual sexual participation — **sco•po•phil•ic** *or* **scop•to•phil•ic** \-ˈfi-lik\ *adj*

sco•po•phil•i•ac *also* **scop•to•phil•i•ac** \-ˈfi-lē-ˌak\ *n* : an individual affected with scopophilia — **scopophiliac** *also* **scoptophiliac** *adj*

-s•co•py \s-kə-pē\ *n comb form, pl* **-s•co•pies** : viewing : observation ⟨laparo*scopy*⟩

scor•bu•tic \skȯr-ˈbyü-tik\ *adj* : of, relating to, producing, or affected with scurvy ⟨a ~ diet⟩

scor•pi•on \ˈskȯr-pē-ən\ *n* : any of an order (Scorpionida) of arachnids that have an elongated body and a narrow segmented tail bearing a venomous stinger at the tip

sco•to•ma \skə-ˈtō-mə\ *n, pl* **-mas** *or* **-ma•ta** \-mə-tə\ : a spot in the visual field in which vision is absent or deficient

sco•to•pic \skə-ˈtō-pik, -ˈtä-\ *adj* : of, relating to, being, or suitable for scotopic vision ⟨~ sensitivity⟩

scotopic vision *n* : vision in dim light with dark-adapted eyes that involves only the retinal rods as light receptors

scour \ˈskau̇r\ *n sing or pl* : diarrhea or dysentery occurring esp. in young domestic animals

scra•pie \ˈskrā-pē\ *n* : a usu. fatal prion disease of sheep and goats that is characterized by twitching, excitability, intense itching, excessive thirst, emaciation, weakness, and finally paralysis

scrap•ing \ˈskrā-piŋ\ *n* : material scraped esp. from diseased tissue for microscopic examination

scratch test *n* : a test for allergic susceptibility made by rubbing an extract of an allergy-producing substance into small breaks or scratches in the skin — compare INTRADERMAL TEST, PATCH TEST, PRICK TEST

screen \ˈskrēn\ *vb* : to test or examine for the presence of something (as a disease) ⟨~ patients for cancer⟩

screen — see INTENSIFYING SCREEN, SUNSCREEN

screen memory *n* : a recollection of early childhood that may be falsely recalled or magnified in importance and that masks another memory of deep emotional significance

screw•fly \ˈskrü-ˌflī\ *n, pl* **-flies** : SCREWWORM FLY

screw•worm \ˈskrü-ˌwərm\ *n* **1** : either of two dipteran flies of the genus *Cochliomyia*: **a** : one (*C. hominivorax*) of the warmer parts of America whose larva develops in sores or wounds or in the nostrils of mammals including humans; *esp* : its larva **b** : SECONDARY SCREWWORM **2** : a dipteran fly (*Chrysomya bezziana*) that causes myiasis in Africa and southern Asia

screwworm fly *n* : the adult of a screwworm — called also *screwfly*

scrip \ˈskrip\ *n* : PRESCRIPTION 1

script \ˈskript\ *n* : PRESCRIPTION 1

scroful- *or* **scrofulo-** *comb form* : scrofula ⟨*scrofulo*derma⟩

scrof•u•la \ˈskrȯ-fyə-lə, ˈskrä-\ *n* : tuberculosis of lymph nodes esp. in the neck — called also *king's evil*

scrof•u•lo•der•ma \ˌskrȯ-fyə-lō-ˈdər-mə, ˌskrä-\ *n* : a disease of the skin of tuberculous origin

scrot- *or* **scroti-** *or* **scroto-** *comb form* : scrotum ⟨*scroto*plasty⟩

scro•tal \ˈskrōt-ᵊl\ *adj* **1** : of or relating to the scrotum **2** : lying in or having descended into the scrotum ⟨~ testes⟩

scro•to•plas•ty \ˈskrō-tə-ˌplas-tē\ *n, pl* **-ties** : plastic surgery performed on the scrotum

scro•tum \ˈskrō-təm\ *n, pl* **scro•ta** \-tə\ *or* **scrotums** : the external pouch that in most mammals contains the testes

scrub \ˈskrəb\ *vb* **scrubbed; scrub•bing** : to clean and disinfect (the hands and forearms) before participating in surgery — **scrub** *n*

scrub nurse *n* : a nurse who assists the surgeon in an operating room

scrub suit *n* : a loose-fitting two-piece garment worn by hospital staff

scrub typhus *n* : an acute febrile disease that is caused by a rickettsial bacterium (*Orientia tsutsugamushi* syn. *Rickettsia tsutsugamushi*) transmitted by mite larvae, resembles louse-borne typhus, and is widespread in the western Pacific area — called also *tsutsugamushi disease*

scru•ple \ˈskrü-pəl\ *n* : a unit of apothecaries' weight equal to 20 grains or $^1/_3$ dram or 1.296 grams

scurf \ˈskərf\ *n* : thin dry scales detached from the epidermis esp. in an abnormal skin condition; *specif* : DANDRUFF — **scurfy** \ˈskər-fē\ *adj*

scur•vy \ˈskər-vē\ *n, pl* **scur•vies** : a disease that is characterized by spongy gums, loosening of the teeth, and a bleeding into the skin and mucous membranes and that is caused by a lack of vitamin C

Se *symbol* selenium

sea•bath•er's eruption \ˈsē-ˌbā-thərz-\ *n* : acute pruritic dermatitis that occurs on parts of the body covered by a swimsuit within 24 hours after exposure to seawater containing certain tiny coelenterate larvae (as of thimble jellyfishes or sea anemones)

sea•borg•i•um \sē-ˈbȯr-gē-əm\ *n* : a short-lived radioactive element that is artificially produced — symbol *Sg;* see ELEMENT table

seal \ˈsēl\ *vb* : to apply dental sealant to

seal•ant \ˈsē-lənt\ *n* : a plastic material that is applied to parts of teeth with imperfections (as pits and fissures) usu. to prevent dental decay

seal finger *n* : a painful swollen finger that results from infection esp. with a bacterium of the genus *Mycoplasma* transmitted to individuals handling marine mammals and typically seals or sealskins

sea lice *n pl* : tiny coelenterate larvae that cause seabather's eruption; *also* : SEABATHER'S ERUPTION

sea•sick•ness \ˈsē-ˌsik-nəs\ *n* : motion sickness experienced on the water — called also *mal de mer* — **seasick** *adj*

sea snake *n* : any of a family (Hydrophidae) of numerous venomous snakes inhabiting the tropical parts of the Pacific and Indian oceans

seasonal affective disorder *n* : depression that tends to recur each year chiefly during the late fall and winter and is associated with shorter hours of daylight — abbr. *SAD*

Sea•so•nale \ˌsē-zə-ˈnäl\ *trademark* — used for a preparation of ethinyl estradiol and levonorgestrol

Sea•so•nique \ˌsē-zə-ˈnēk\ *trademark* — used for a preparation of ethinyl estradiol and levonorgestrol

[1]seat \ˈsēt\ *n* : a part or surface esp. in dentistry on or in which another part or surface rests — see REST SEAT

[2]seat *vb* : to provide with or position on a dental seat

seat•worm \-ˌwərm\ *n* : a pinworm of the genus *Enterobius* (*E. vermicularis*) that is parasitic in humans

sea wasp *n* : any of various jellyfishes (order or suborder Cubomedusae of the class Scyphozoa) of tropical waters that inflict a painful and sometimes fatal sting — called also *box jellyfish*

se•ba•ceous \si-ˈbā-shəs\ *adj* **1** : secreting sebum **2** : of, relating to, or being fatty material ⟨a ~ exudate⟩

sebaceous cyst *n* : a cyst filled with sebaceous matter and formed by distension of a sebaceous gland as a result of obstruction of its excretory duct

sebaceous gland *n* : any of the small sacculated glands that are lodged in the substance of the dermis, usu. open into the hair follicles, and secrete sebum

sebi- *or* **sebo-** *comb form* : fat : grease : sebum ⟨*sebo*rrhea⟩

seb•or•rhea \ˌse-bə-ˈrē-ə\ *n* : abnormally increased secretion and discharge of sebum producing an oily appearance of the skin and the formation of greasy scales

seb•or•rhe•al \ˌse-bə-ˈrē-əl\ *adj* : SEBORRHEIC

seb•or•rhe•ic \-ˈrē-ik\ *adj* : of, relating to, or characterized by seborrhea

seborrheic dermatitis *n* : a red, scaly, itchy dermatitis chiefly affecting areas (as of the face, scalp, or chest) with many large sebaceous glands

seborrheic keratosis *n* : a benign hyperkeratotic tumor that occurs singly or in clusters on the surface of the skin, is usu. brown or black in color, and typically has a warty texture often with a waxy appearance

se•bor•rhoea, se•bor•rhoe•al, se•bor•rhoe•ic *chiefly Brit var of* SEBORRHEA, SEBORRHEAL, SEBORRHEIC

se•bum \ˈsē-bəm\ *n* : fatty lubricant matter that is secreted by sebaceous glands of the skin and acts to soften and protectively coat the hair and skin

seco•bar•bi•tal \ˌse-kō-ˈbär-bə-ˌtȯl\ *n* : a barbiturate used chiefly in the form of its sodium salt $C_{12}H_{17}N_2NaO_3$ as a hypnotic and sedative — called also *quinalbarbitone;* see SECONAL

Sec•o•nal \ˈse-kə-ˌnȯl, -ˌnal, -nəl\ *trademark* — used for a preparation of the sodium salt of secobarbital

sec·ond·ary \ˈse-kən-ˌder-ē\ *adj* **1** : not first in order of occurrence or development: as **a** : dependent or consequent on another disease ⟨~ diabetes⟩ **b** : occurring or being in the second stage ⟨~ symptoms of syphilis⟩ **c** : occurring some time after the original injury ⟨a ~ hemorrhage⟩ **2** : characterized by or resulting from the substitution of two atoms or groups in a molecule ⟨a ~ salt⟩ **3** : relating to or being the three-dimensional coiling of the polypeptide chain of a protein esp. in the form of an alpha-helix — compare PRIMARY 3, TERTIARY 2 — **sec·ond·ari·ly** \ˌse-kən-ˈder-ə-lē\ *adv*

secondary amenorrhea *n* : the temporary or permanent cessation of menstruation in a woman who has previously experienced normal menses

secondary care *n* : medical care that is provided by a specialist or facility upon referral by a primary care physician and that requires more specialized knowledge, skill, or equipment than the primary care physician can provide — compare PRIMARY CARE, TERTIARY CARE

secondary dentin *n* : dentin formed following the loss (as by erosion or abrasion) of original dentin

secondary gain *n* : a benefit (as sympathetic attention) associated with a physical or psychological disorder

secondary hypertension *n* : hypertension that results from an underlying identifiable cause

secondary infection *n* : infection occurring at the site of a preexisting infection

secondary oocyte *n* : an oocyte that is produced by division of a primary oocyte in the first meiotic division

secondary screwworm *n* : a screwworm of the genus *Cochliomyia* (*C. macellaria*) chiefly of warmer parts of America whose larva develops in dead tissue (as of wounds); *esp* : its larva

secondary sex characteristic *n* : a physical characteristic (as the breasts of a female) that appears in members of one sex at puberty or in seasonal breeders at the breeding season and is not directly concerned with reproduction — called also *secondary sex character, secondary sexual characteristic*

secondary spermatocyte *n* : a spermatocyte that is produced by division of a primary spermatocyte in the first meiotic division and that divides in the second meiotic division to give rise to two haploid spermatids

secondary syphilis *n* : the second stage of syphilis that appears from 2 to 6 months after primary infection, that is marked by lesions esp. in the skin but also in organs and tissues, and that lasts from 3 to 12 weeks

secondary tympanic membrane *n* : a membrane closing the round window and separating the scala tympani from the middle ear

second cranial nerve *n* : OPTIC NERVE

second–degree burn *n* : a burn marked by pain, blistering, and superficial destruction of dermis with edema and hyperemia of the tissues beneath the burn

secondhand smoke *n* : tobacco smoke that is exhaled by a smoker or given off by burning tobacco (as of a cigarette) and is inhaled by persons nearby — called also *passive smoke*

second in·ten·tion \-in-ˈten-chən\ *n* : the healing of an incised wound by granulations that bridge the gap between skin edges — compare FIRST INTENTION

sec·ond–line \ˈse-kənd-ˈlīn\ *adj* : being or using a drug that is not the usual or preferred choice — compare FIRST-LINE

second messenger *n* : an intracellular substance (as cyclic AMP) that mediates cell activity by relaying a signal from an extracellular molecule (as of a hormone or neurotransmitter) bound to the cell's surface

second polar body *n* : POLAR BODY b

second wind *n* : recovered full power of respiration after the first exhaustion during exertion due to improved heart action

secret- *or* **secreto-** *comb form* : secretion ⟨*secret*in⟩

se·cre·ta·gogue \si-ˈkrē-tə-ˌgäg\ *n* : a substance that stimulates secretion

se·cre·tase \si-ˈkrē-ˌtās\ *n* : any of several transmembrane proteases that are capable of cleaving amyloid precursor protein and include two forms that function in the generation of beta-amyloid

se·cre·tin \si-ˈkrēt-ᵊn\ *n* : an intestinal proteinaceous hormone capable of stimulating secretion by the pancreas and liver

se·cre·tion \si-ˈkrē-shən\ *n* **1** : the process of segregating, elaborating, and releasing some material either functionally specialized (as saliva) or isolated for excretion (as urine) **2** : a product of secretion formed by an animal or plant; *esp* : one performing a specific useful function in the organism — **se·crete** \si-ˈkrēt\ *vb* — **se·cre·to·ry** \ˈsē-krə-ˌtōr-ē, si-ˈkrē-tə-rē\ *adj*

se·cre·tor \si-ˈkrē-tər\ *n* : an individual of blood group A, B, or AB who secretes the antigens characteristic of these blood groups in bodily fluids (as saliva)

secretory otitis media *n* : SEROUS OTITIS MEDIA

-sect \ˌsekt\ *vb comb form* : cut : divide ⟨hemi*sect*⟩ ⟨tran*sect*⟩

sec·tion \ˈsek-shən\ *n* **1** : the action or an instance of cutting or separating by cutting; *esp* : the action of dividing (as tissues) surgically ⟨abdominal ~⟩ — see CESAREAN SECTION **2** : a very thin slice (as of tissue) suitable for microscopic examination — **section** *vb*

Sec·tral \ˈsek-ˌtral\ *trademark* — used for a preparation of the hydrochloride of acebutolol

se·cun·di·grav·id \si-ˌkən-dē-ˈgra-vəd\ *adj* : pregnant for the second time

se·cun·di·grav·i·da \-ˈgra-vi-də\ *n, pl* **-dae** \-ˌdē, -ˌdī\ *also* **-das** : a woman in her second pregnancy

sec·un·dines \ˈse-kən-ˌdēnz, -ˌdīnz; se-ˈkən-dənz\ *n pl* : AFTERBIRTH

sec·un·dip·a·ra \ˌse-kən-ˈdi-pə-rə\ *n, pl* **-ras** *or* **-rae** \-ˌrē, -ˌrī\ : a woman who has borne children in two separate pregnancies

security blanket *n* : a blanket carried by a child as a protection against anxiety

se·date \si-ˈdāt\ *vb* **se·dat·ed; se·dat·ing** : to dose with sedatives

se·da·tion \si-ˈdā-shən\ *n* **1** : the inducing of a relaxed easy state esp. by the use of sedatives **2** : a state resulting from sedation — see CONSCIOUS SEDATION, DEEP SEDATION

[1]**sed·a·tive** \ˈse-də-tiv\ *adj* : tending to calm, moderate, or tranquilize nervousness or excitement

[2]**sedative** *n* : a sedative agent or drug

[1]**sed·i·ment** \ˈse-də-mənt\ *n* : the matter that settles to the bottom of a liquid

[2]**sed·i·ment** \-ˌment\ *vb* : to deposit as sediment

sed·i·men·ta·tion \ˌse-də-(ˌ)men-ˈtā-shən\ *n* **1** : the action or process of depositing sediment **2** : the depositing esp. by mechanical means of matter suspended in a liquid

sedimentation rate *n* : the speed at which red blood cells settle to the bottom of a column of citrated blood measured in millimeters deposited per hour and which is used esp. in diagnosing the progress of various abnormal conditions

sed rate \ˈsed-\ *n* : SEDIMENTATION RATE

[1]**seed** \ˈsēd\ *n, pl* **seed** *or* **seeds 1 a** : the fertilized ripened ovule of a flowering plant **b** : a propagative animal structure; *esp* : SEMEN **2** : a small usu. glass and gold or platinum capsule used as a container for a radioactive substance (as radium or radon) to be applied usu. interstitially in the treatment of cancer — **seed·ed** \ˈsē-dəd\ *adj*

[2]**seed** *adj* : selected or used to produce a new crop or stock ⟨~ virus⟩

Seeing Eye *trademark* — used for a guide dog trained to lead the blind

[1]**seg·ment** \ˈseg-mənt\ *n* : one of the constituent parts into which a body, entity, or quantity is divided or marked off by or as if by natural boundaries — **seg·men·tal** \seg-ˈment-ᵊl\ *adj* — **seg·men·tal·ly** *adv*

[2]**seg·ment** \ˈseg-ˌment\ *vb* **1** : to cause to undergo segmentation by division or multiplication of cells **2** : to separate into segments

segmental resection *n* : excision of a segment of an organ; *specif* : excision of a portion of a lobe of a lung — called also *segmentectomy;* compare PNEUMONECTOMY

seg·men·ta·tion \ˌseg-(ˌ)men-ˈtā-shən\ *n* **1** : the act or process of dividing into segments; *esp* : the formation of many cells from a single cell (as in a developing egg) **2** : annular contraction of smooth muscle (as of the intestine) that seems to cut the part affected into segments

segmentation cavity *n* : BLASTOCOEL

seg·men·tec·to·my \ˌseg-mən-ˈtek-tə-mē\ *n, pl* **-mies** : SEGMENTAL RESECTION

seg·ment·ed \ˈseg-ˌmen-təd, seg-ˈ\ *adj* **1** : having or made up of segments **2** : being a cell in which the nucleus is divided into lobes connected by a fine filament ⟨~ neutrophils⟩

seg·re·gant \ˈse-gri-gənt\ *n* : SEGREGATE

[1]**seg·re·gate** \ˈse-gri-ˌgāt\ *vb* **-gat·ed; -gat·ing** : to undergo genetic segregation

[2]**seg·re·gate** \-gət\ *n* : an individual or class of individuals differing in one or more genetic characters from the parental line usu. because of segregation of genes

seg·re·ga·tion \ˌse-gri-ˈgā-shən\ *n* : the separation of allelic genes that occurs typically during meiosis

Sei·gnette salt \sen-ˈyet-\ *or* **Sei·gnette's salt** \-ˈyets-\ *n* : ROCHELLE SALT

Seignette, Pierre (1660–1719), French pharmacist.

sei·zure \ˈsē-zhər\ *n* **1** : a sudden attack (as of disease); *esp* : the physical manifestations (as convulsions, sensory disturbances, or loss of consciousness) resulting from abnormal electrical discharges in the brain (as in epilepsy) **2** : an abnormal electrical discharge in the brain

Sel·dane \ˈsel-ˌdān\ *n* : a preparation of terfenadine — formerly a U.S. registered trademark

se·lec·tin \sə-ˈlek-tin\ *n* : any of a various sugar-binding proteins found on the surface of cells that are involved in the calcium-dependent adhesion of cells (as white blood cells) to other cells (as endothelial cells) and that mediate the migration of cells to sites of inflammation

se·lec·tion \sə-ˈlek-shən\ *n* : a natural or artificial process that results or tends to result in the survival and propagation of some individuals or organisms but not of others with the result that the inherited traits of the survivors are perpetuated

se·lec·tive \sə-ˈlek-tiv\ *adj* **1** : of, relating to, or characterized by selection : selecting or tending to select **2** : highly specific in activity or effect — **se·lec·tive·ly** *adv* — **se·lec·tiv·i·ty** \sə-ˌlek-ˈti-və-tē, ˌsē-\ *n*

selective estrogen receptor modulator *n* : any of a class of drugs (as raloxifene or tamoxifen) that bind with estrogen receptors and act as agonists to enhance estrogen activity in some tissues and as antagonists to inhibit estrogen activity in other tissues — called also *SERM*

selective mutism *n* : an anxiety disorder of childhood characterized by consistent failure to speak in specific social settings (as at school) despite having the ability to speak normally in other settings (as at home) — called also *elective mutism*

selective reduction *n* : abortion of one or more but not all embryos in a pregnancy with multiple embryos — called also *selective termination*

selective serotonin–norepinephrine reuptake inhibitor *n* : SNRI

selective serotonin reuptake inhibitor *n* : SSRI

se•leg•i•line \si-ˈle-jə-ˌlēn\ *n* : the levorotatory form of deprenyl that is administered in the form of its hydrochloride $C_{13}H_{17}N{\cdot}HCl$ esp. as an adjuvant to therapy using the combination of L-dopa and carbidopa in the treatment of Parkinson's disease

sel•e•nif•er•ous \ˌse-lə-ˈni-fə-rəs\ *adj* : containing or yielding selenium

se•le•ni•um \sə-ˈlē-nē-əm\ *n* : a nonmetallic element that is an essential trace element found esp. in grains and meat — symbol *Se;* see ELEMENT table, SELENOSIS

selenium sulfide *n* : the sulfide SeS_2 of selenium usu. in the form of an orange powder that is used in preparations for treating dandruff and seborrheic dermatitis of the scalp

sel•e•no•me•thi•o•nine \ˌse-lə-nō-mə-ˈthī-ə-ˌnēn\ *n* : a selenium analog $C_5H_{11}NO_2Se$ of methionine that is used as a diagnostic aid in scintigraphy esp. of the pancreas and as a dietary supplement

sel•e•no•sis \ˌse-lə-ˈnō-səs\ *n* : poisoning due to excessive intake of selenium; *esp* : poisoning of livestock by high levels of selenium consumed in plants grown in seleniferous soils — see BLIND STAGGERS

self \ˈself\ *n, pl* **selves** \ˈselvz\ **1** : the union of elements (as body, emotions, thoughts, and sensations) that constitute the individuality and identity of a person **2** : material that is part of an individual organism ⟨the immune system distinguishes ~ from nonself⟩

self–abuse \ˌself-ə-ˈbyüs\ *n* : MASTURBATION

self–ac•tu•al•ize \ˈself-ˈak-chə-wə-ˌlīz\ *vb* **-ized; -iz•ing** : to realize fully one's potential — **self–ac•tu•al•iza•tion** \-ˌak-chə-wə-lə-ˈzā-shən\ *n*

self–ad•min•i•ster \-əd-ˈmi-nə-stər\ *vb* : to administer to oneself ⟨~*ed* an analgesic⟩ — **self–ad•min•i•stra•tion** \-ˌmi-nə-ˈstrā-shən\ *n*

self–anal•y•sis \-ə-ˈna-lə-səs\ *n, pl* **-y•ses** \-ˌsēz\ : a systematic attempt by an individual to understand his or her own personality without the aid of another person — **self–an•a•lyt•i•cal** \-ˌa-nə-ˈli-ti-kəl\ *also* **self–an•a•lyt•ic** \-tik\ *adj*

self–an•ti•gen \-ˈan-ti-jən\ *n* : any molecule or chemical group of an organism which acts as an antigen in inducing antibody formation in another organism but to which the healthy immune system of the parent organism is tolerant

self–as•sem•bly \-ə-ˈsem-blē\ *n, pl* **-blies** : the process by which a complex macromolecule (as collagen) or a supramolecular system (as a virus) spontaneously assembles itself from its components — **self–as•sem•ble** \-bəl\ *vb*

self–aware•ness \-ə-ˈwer-nəss\ *n* : an awareness of one's own personality or individuality — **self–aware** *adj*

self–care \-ˈker\ *n* : care for oneself : SELF-TREATMENT

self–con•cept \ˈself-ˈkän-ˌsept\ *n* : the mental image one has of oneself

self–de•struc•tion \-di-ˈstrək-shən\ *n* : destruction of oneself; *esp* : SUICIDE

self–de•struc•tive \-ˈstrək-tiv\ *adj* : acting or tending to harm or destroy oneself ⟨~ behavior⟩; *also* : SUICIDAL — **self–de•struc•tive•ly** *adv* — **self–de•struc•tive•ness** *n*

self–ex•am•i•na•tion \-ig-ˌza-mə-ˈnā-shən\ *or* **self–ex•am** \-ig-ˈzam\ *n* : examination of one's body esp. for evidence of disease ⟨~ for detection of breast cancer⟩

self–hyp•no•sis \ˌself-hip-ˈnō-səs\ *n, pl* **-no•ses** \-ˌsēz\ : hypnosis of oneself : AUTOHYPNOSIS

self–im•age \-ˈi-mij\ *n* : one's conception of oneself or of one's role

self–in•duced \-in-ˈdüst, -ˈdyüst\ *adj* : induced by oneself ⟨a ~ abortion⟩

self–in•flict•ed \-in-ˈflik-təd\ *adj* : inflicted by oneself ⟨~ vomiting⟩

self–in•ject \-in-ˈjekt\ *vb* : to inject oneself with a drug or other substance — **self–in•ject•able** \-ˈjek-tə-bəl\ *adj* — **self–in•jec•tion** \-ˈjek-shən\ *n*

self•ish \ˈsel-fish\ *adj* : being an actively replicating repetitive sequence of nucleic acid that serves no known function ⟨~ DNA⟩; *also* : being genetic material solely concerned with its own replication ⟨~ genes⟩

self–lim•it•ed \-ˈli-mə-təd\ *adj* : limited by one's or its own nature; *specif* : running a definite and limited course

self–lim•it•ing *adj* : SELF-LIMITED

self–med•i•ca•tion \-ˌme-də-ˈkā-shən\ *n* : medication of oneself esp. without the advice of a physician : SELF-TREATMENT — **self–med•i•cate** \-ˈme-də-ˌkāt\ *vb*

self–mu•ti•la•tion \-ˌmyü-tə-ˈlā-shən\ *n* : injury or disfigurement of oneself

self–re•ac•tive \-rē-ˈak-tiv\ *adj* : capable of participating in an autoimmune response ⟨~ T cells⟩

self–rec•og•ni•tion \-ˌre-kəg-ˈni-shən\ *n* : the process by which the immune system of an organism distinguishes between the body's own chemicals, cells, and tissues and those of foreign organisms or agents — compare SELF-TOLERANCE

self–re•fer•ral \-ri-ˈfər-əl\ *n* : the referral of a patient to a specialized medical facility (as a medical imaging center) in which the referring physician has a financial interest — **self–re•fer** \-ri-ˈfər\ *vb*

self–rep•li•cat•ing \-ˈre-plə-ˌkā-tiŋ\ *adj* : reproducing itself autonomously ⟨DNA is a ~ molecule⟩ — **self–rep•li•ca•tion** \-ˌre-plə-ˈkā-shən\ *n*

self–stim•u•la•tion \-ˌstim-yə-ˈlā-shən\ *n* : stimulation of oneself as a result of one's own activity or behavior; *esp* : MASTURBATION — **self–stim•u•la•to•ry** \-ˈstim-yə-lə-ˌtōr-ē\ *adj*

self–tan•ner \-ˈta-nər\ *n* : a product (as one containing dihydroxyacetone) that when applied to the skin reacts chemically with its surface layer to give the appearance of a tan

self–tol•er•ance \-ˈtä-lə-rəns\ *n* : the physiological state that exists in a developing organism when its immune system has proceeded far enough in the process of self-recognition to lose the capacity to attack and destroy its own bodily constituents — called also *horror autotoxicus*

self–treat•ment \-ˈtrēt-mənt\ *n* : medication of oneself or treatment of one's own disease without medical supervision or prescription

sel•la \ˈse-lə\ *n, pl* **sellas** *or* **sel•lae** \-lē\ : SELLA TURCICA

sellae — see DIAPHRAGMA SELLAE

sel•lar \ˈse-lər, -ˌlär\ *adj* : of, relating to, or involving the sella turcica

sella tur•ci•ca \-ˈtər-ki-kə, -si-\ *n, pl* **sellae tur•ci•cae** \-ki-ˌkī, -si-ˌsē\ : a depression in the middle line of the upper surface of the sphenoid bone in which the pituitary gland is lodged

SEM *abbr* scanning electron microscope; scanning electron microscopy

se•man•tic memory \si-ˌman-tik-\ *n* : long-term memory of facts, information, and meanings that is not related to any specific event personally experienced in the past — compare EPISODIC MEMORY

se•men \ˈsē-mən\ *n* : a viscid whitish fluid of the male reproductive tract consisting of spermatozoa suspended in secretions of the accessory glands (as of the prostate and Cowper's glands)

semi•cir•cu•lar canal \ˌse-mē-ˈsər-kyə-lər-, ˌse-ˌmī-\ *n* : any of the loop-shaped tubular parts of the labyrinth of the ear that together constitute a sensory organ associated with the maintenance of bodily equilibrium, that consist of an inner membranous canal of the membranous labyrinth and a corresponding outer bony canal of the bony labyrinth, and that form a group of three in each ear usu. in planes nearly at right angles to each other — see SEMICIRCULAR DUCT

semicircular duct *n* : any of the three loop-shaped membranous inner tubular parts of the semicircular canals that are about one-fourth the diameter of the corresponding outer bony canals, that communicate at each end with the utricle, and that have near one end an expanded ampulla containing the crista

semi•co•ma \-ˈkō-mə\ *n* : a semicomatose state from which a person can be aroused

semi•co•ma•tose \-ˈkō-mə-ˌtōs\ *adj* : marked by or affected with stupor and disorientation but not complete coma ⟨a ~ state⟩ ⟨~ patients⟩

semi•con•scious \-ˈkän-chəs\ *adj* : incompletely conscious : imperfectly aware or responsive — **semi•con•sci•ous•ness** *n*

semi•con•ser•va•tive \-kən-ˈsər-və-tiv\ *adj* : relating to or being genetic replication in which a double-stranded molecule of nucleic acid separates into two single strands each of which serves as a template for the formation of a complementary strand that together with the template forms a complete molecule — **semi•con•ser•va•tive•ly** *adv*

semi•dom•i•nant \-ˈdä-mi-nənt\ *adj* : producing an intermediate phenotype in the heterozygous condition

semi•flu•id \-ˈflü-əd\ *adj* : having the qualities of both a fluid and a solid : VISCOUS — **semifluid** *n*

semi•lu•nar \-ˈlü-nər\ *adj* : shaped like a crescent

semilunar bone *n* : LUNATE BONE

semilunar cartilage *n* : MENISCUS a(2)

semilunar cusp *n* : any of the crescentic cusps making up the semilunar valves

semilunares — see LINEA SEMILUNARIS, PLICA SEMILUNARIS

semilunar ganglion *n* : TRIGEMINAL GANGLION

semilunaris — see HIATUS SEMILUNARIS, LINEA SEMILUNARIS, PLICA SEMILUNARIS

semilunar line *n* : LINEA SEMILUNARIS

semilunar lobule *n* : either of a pair of crescent-shaped lobules situated one on each side in the posterior and ventral part of the cerebellum

semilunar notch *n* : TROCHLEAR NOTCH

semilunar valve *n* **1** : either of two valves of which one is situated at the opening between the heart and the aorta and the other at the opening between the heart and the pulmonary artery, which prevent regurgitation of blood into the ventricles, and each of which is made up of three crescent-shaped cusps **2** : SEMILUNAR CUSP

semi•mem•bra•no•sus \ˌse-mē-ˌmem-brə-ˈnō-səs, ˌse-ˌmī-\ *n, pl* **-no•si** \-ˌsī\

: a large muscle of the inner part and back of the thigh that arises by a thick tendon from the back part of the tuberosity of the ischium, is inserted into the medial condyle of the tibia, and acts to flex the leg and rotate it medially and to extend the thigh

sem•i•nal \ˈse-mən-ᵊl\ *adj* : of, relating to, or consisting of semen

seminal duct *n* : a tube or passage serving esp. or exclusively as an efferent duct of the testis and in humans being made up of the tubules of the epididymis, the vas deferens, and the ejaculatory duct

seminal fluid *n* **1** : SEMEN **2** : the part of the semen that is produced by various accessory glands (as the prostate gland and seminal vesicles) : semen excepting the spermatozoa

seminal vesicle *n* : either of a pair of glandular pouches that lie one on either side of the male reproductive tract and that in human males secrete a sugar- and protein-containing fluid into the ejaculatory duct

sem•i•nif•er•ous \ˌse-mə-ˈni-fə-rəs\ *adj* : producing or bearing semen

seminiferous tubule *n* : any of the coiled threadlike tubules that make up the bulk of the testis and are lined with a layer of epithelial cells from which the spermatozoa are produced

sem•i•no•ma \ˌse-mi-ˈnō-mə\ *n, pl* **-mas** *also* **-ma•ta** \-mə-tə\ : a germinoma of the testis

semi•per•me•able \ˌse-mē-ˈpər-mē-ə-bəl, ˌse-ˌmī-\ *adj* : partially but not freely or wholly permeable; *specif* : permeable to some usu. small molecules but not to other usu. larger particles ⟨~ membranes⟩ — **semi•per•me•abil•i•ty** \-ˌpər-mē-ə-ˈbi-lə-tē\ *n*

semi•pri•vate \-ˈprī-vət\ *adj* : of, receiving, or associated with hospital service giving a patient more privileges than a ward patient but fewer than a private patient ⟨a ~ room⟩

semi•spi•na•lis \-ˌspī-ˈnā-ləs\ *n, pl* **-les** \-ˌlēz\ : any of three muscles of the cervical and thoracic parts of the spinal column: **a** : SEMISPINALIS THORACIS **b** : SEMISPINALIS CERVICIS **c** : SEMISPINALIS CAPITIS

semispinalis cap•i•tis \-ˈka-pi-təs\ *n* : a deep longitudinal muscle of the back that arises esp. from the transverse processes of the upper six or seven thoracic and the seventh cervical vertebrae, is inserted on the outer surface of the occipital bone between two ridges behind the foramen magnum, and acts to extend and rotate the head — called also *complexus*

semispinalis cer•vi•cis \-ˈsər-vi-sis\ *n* : a deep longitudinal muscle of the back that arises from the transverse processes of the upper five or six thoracic vertebrae, is inserted into the cervical spinous processes from the axis to the fifth cervical vertebra, and with the semispinalis thoracis acts to extend the spinal column and rotate it toward the opposite side

semispinalis tho•ra•cis \-thō-ˈrā-səs\ *n* : a deep longitudinal muscle of the back that arises from the transverse processes of the lower five thoracic vertebrae, is inserted into the spinous processes of the upper four thoracic and lower two cervical vertebrae, and with the semispinalis cervicis acts to extend the spinal column and rotate it toward the opposite side

semi•syn•thet•ic \-sin-ˈthe-tik\ *adj* **1** : produced by chemical alteration of a natural starting material ⟨~ penicillins⟩ **2** : containing both chemically identified and complex natural ingredients ⟨a ~ diet⟩ — **semi•syn•thet•i•cal•ly** \-ti-k(ə-)lē\ *adv*

sem•i•ten•di•no•sus \-ˌten-də-ˈnō-səs\ *n, pl* **-no•si** \-ˌsī\ : a fusiform muscle of the posterior and inner part of the thigh that arises from the ischial tuberosity along with the biceps femoris, that is inserted by a long round tendon into the inner surface of the upper part of the shaft of the tibia, and that acts to flex the leg and rotate it medially and to extend the thigh

Sem•li•ki For•est virus \ˈsem-lē-kē-ˈfór-əst-\ *n* : a virus of the genus *Alphavirus* (species *Semliki Forest virus*) isolated from mosquitoes in a Ugandan forest and capable of infecting humans and laboratory animals

Sen•dai virus \ˈsen-ˌdī-\ *n* : a paramyxovirus (species *Sendai virus* of the genus *Respirovirus*) that infects swine, mice, and humans

se•ne•cio \si-ˈnē-shē-ˌō, -shō\ *n, pl* **-cios** **1** *cap* : a genus of widely distributed plants (family Compositae) including some containing various alkaloids which are poisonous to livestock **2** *pl* **-cios** : any plant of the genus *Senecio*

se•ne•ci•o•sis \se-ˌnē-sē-ˈō-səs\ *n, pl* **-o•ses** \-ˌsēz\ : a frequently fatal intoxication esp. of livestock feeding on plants of the genus *Senecio*

se•nes•cence \si-ˈnes-ᵊns\ *n* : the state of being old : the process of becoming old — **se•nes•cent** \-ᵊnt\ *adj*

se•nile \ˈsē-ˌnīl\ *adj* **1** : of, relating to, exhibiting, or characteristic of old age; *esp* : exhibiting a loss of cognitive abilities (as memory) associated with old age **2** : being a cell that cannot undergo mitosis and is in a stage of declining function prior to the time of death ⟨~ red blood cells⟩

senile cataract *n* : a cataract of a type that occurs in the aged and is characterized by an initial opacity in the lens, subsequent swelling of the lens, and final shrinkage with complete loss of transparency

senile dementia *n* : dementia of old age esp. of the degenerative type associated with Alzheimer's disease

senile psychosis *n* : SENILE DEMENTIA
senilis — see ARCUS SENILIS, LENTIGO SENILIS
se•nil•i•ty \si-ˈni-lə-tē, se-\ *n, pl* **-ties** : the quality or state of being senile
se•ni•um \ˈsē-nē-əm\ *n* : the final period in the normal life span
sen•na \ˈse-nə\ *n* **1** : any of a genus (*Cassia* syn. *Senna*) of leguminous plants; *esp* : one used medicinally **2** : the dried leaflets or pods of various sennas (esp. *Cassia angustifolia* syn. *Senna alexandrina*) used as a purgative
sen•sa•tion \sen-ˈsā-shən, sən-\ *n* **1 a** : a mental process (as hearing or smelling) resulting from the immediate external stimulation of a sense organ often as distinguished from a conscious awareness of the sensory process — compare PERCEPTION **b** : awareness (as of pain) due to stimulation of a sense organ **c** : a state of consciousness due to internal bodily changes ⟨a ~ of hunger⟩ **2** : something (as a physical stimulus or pain) that causes or is the object of sensation
[1]**sense** \ˈsens\ *n* **1 a** : the faculty of perceiving by means of sense organs **b** : a specialized function or mechanism (as sight, hearing, smell, taste, or touch) by which an animal receives and responds to external or internal stimuli **c** : the sensory mechanisms constituting a unit distinct from other functions (as movement or thought) **2** : a particular sensation or kind or quality of sensation ⟨a good ~ of balance⟩
[2]**sense** *vb* **sensed; sens•ing** : to perceive by the senses
sense–da•tum \-ˈdā-təm, -ˈda-, -ˈdä-\ *n, pl* **sense–da•ta** \-tə\ : the immediate private perceived object of sensation as distinguished from the objective material object itself
sense organ *n* : a bodily structure that receives a stimulus (as heat or sound waves) and is affected in such a manner as to initiate a wave of excitation in associated sensory nerve fibers : RECEPTOR
sen•si•bil•i•ty \ˌsen-sə-ˈbi-lə-tē\ *n, pl* **-ties** **1** : ability to receive sensations ⟨tactile ~⟩ **2** : awareness of and responsiveness toward something
sen•si•ble \ˈsen-sə-bəl\ *adj* **1** : perceptible to the senses or to reason or understanding **2** : capable of receiving sensory impressions ⟨~ to pain⟩
Sen•si•par \ˈsen(t)-sə-ˌpär\ *trademark* — used for a preparation of cinacalcet
sen•si•tive \ˈsen-sə-tiv\ *adj* **1** : SENSORY 2 ⟨~ nerves⟩ **2 a** : receptive to sense impressions **b** : capable of being stimulated or excited by external agents **3** : highly responsive or susceptible: as **a** : easily hurt or damaged ⟨~ skin⟩; *esp* : easily hurt emotionally **b** : excessively or abnormally susceptible : HYPERSENSITIVE **c** : capable of indicating minute differences — **sen•si•tive•ness** *n* — **sen•si•tiv•i•ty** \ˌsen-sə-ˈti-və-tē\ *n*
sensitivity training *n* : training in a small interacting group that is designed to increase each individual's awareness of his or her own feelings and the feelings of others and to enhance interpersonal relations
sen•si•ti•za•tion \ˌsen-sə-tə-ˈzā-shən\ *n* **1** : the action or process of making sensitive or hypersensitive ⟨allergic ~ of the skin⟩ **2** : the process of becoming sensitive or hypersensitive (as to an antigen); *also* : the resulting state **3** : a form of nonassociative learning characterized by an increase in responsiveness upon repeated exposure to a stimulus — compare HABITUATION 3 — **sen•si•tize** \ˈsen-sə-ˌtīz\ *vb*
sen•si•tiz•er \-ˌtī-zər\ *n* : a substance that sensitizes the skin on first contact so that subsequent contact causes inflammation
sen•sor \ˈsen-ˌsȯr, -sər\ *n* : a device that responds to a physical stimulus (as heat, light, sound, or motion) and transmits a resulting impulse; *also* : SENSE ORGAN
sensori- *also* **senso-** *comb form* : sensory : sensory and ⟨*sensori*motor⟩
sen•so•ri•al \sen-ˈsōr-ē-əl\ *adj* : SENSORY
sen•so•ri•mo•tor \ˌsen-sə-rē-ˈmō-tər\ *adj* : of, relating to, or functioning in both sensory and motor aspects of bodily activity ⟨~ disturbances⟩
sen•so•ri•neu•ral \-ˈnu̇r-əl, -ˈnyu̇r-\ *adj* : of, relating to, or involving the aspects of sense perception mediated by nerves ⟨~ hearing loss⟩
sen•so•ri•um \sen-ˈsōr-ē-əm\ *n, pl* **-ri•ums** *or* **-ria** \-ē-ə\ **1** : the parts of the brain or the mind concerned with the reception and interpretation of sensory stimuli; *broadly* : the entire sensory apparatus **2 a** : ability of the brain to receive and interpret sensory stimuli **b** : the state of consciousness judged in terms of this ability
sen•so•ry \ˈsen-sə-rē\ *adj* **1** : of or relating to sensation or the senses **2** : conveying nerve impulses from the sense organs to the nerve centers : AFFERENT ⟨~ nerve fibers⟩
sensory aphasia *n* : inability to understand spoken, written, or tactile speech symbols that results from damage (as by a brain lesion) to an area of the brain (as Wernicke's area) concerned with language — called also *Wernicke's aphasia*
sensory area *n* : an area of the cerebral cortex that receives afferent nerve fibers from lower sensory or motor areas
sensory cell *n* **1** : a peripheral nerve cell (as an olfactory cell) located at a sensory receiving surface and being the primary receptor of a sensory impulse **2** : a nerve cell (as a spinal ganglion cell) transmitting sensory impulses

sensory neuron *n* : a neuron that transmits nerve impulses from a sense organ towards the central nervous system — compare INTERNEURON, MOTOR NEURON

sensory root *n* : a nerve root containing only sensory fibers; *specif* : DORSAL ROOT — compare MOTOR ROOT

sen·ti·nel \ˈsent-ᵊn-əl\ *adj* : being an individual or part of a population potentially susceptible to an infection or infestation that is being monitored for the appearance or recurrence of the causative pathogen or parasite

sentinel node *n* : the first lymph node to receive lymphatic drainage from the site of a primary tumor — called also *sentinel lymph node*

sep·a·ra·tion \ˌse-pə-ˈrā-shən\ *n* **1** : the process of isolating or extracting from or of becoming isolated from a mixture; *also* : the resulting state **2** : DISLOCATION — see SHOULDER SEPARATION — **sep·a·rate** \ˈse-pə-ˌrāt\ *vb*

separation anxiety *n* : a form of anxiety experienced by a child or adolescent that is caused by separation from a significant nurturant figure and typically a parent or from familiar surroundings

sep·a·ra·tor \ˈse-pə-ˌrā-tər\ *n* : a dental appliance for separating adjoining teeth to give access to their surfaces

sep·sis \ˈsep-səs\ *n, pl* **sep·ses** \ˈsep-ˌsēz\ : a systemic response typically to a serious usu. localized infection (as of the abdomen or lungs) esp. of bacterial origin that is usu. marked by abnormal body temperature and white blood cell count, tachycardia, and tachypnea; *specif* : systemic inflammatory response syndrome induced by a documented infection — see MULTIPLE ORGAN DYSFUNCTION SYNDROME, SEPTIC SHOCK

sept- *or* **septo-** *also* **septi-** *comb form* : septum ⟨*sept*al⟩ ⟨*septo*plasty⟩

septa *pl of* SEPTUM

sep·tal \ˈsept-ᵊl\ *adj* : of or relating to a septum ⟨~ defects⟩

septal cartilage *n* : the cartilage of the nasal septum

septa pellucida *pl of* SEPTUM PELLUCIDUM

sep·tate \ˈsep-ˌtāt\ *adj* : divided by or having a septum — **sep·ta·tion** \sep-ˈtā-shən\ *n*

septa transversa *pl of* SEPTUM TRANSVERSUM

sep·tec·to·my \sep-ˈtek-tə-mē\ *n, pl* **-mies** : surgical excision of a septum

sep·tic \ˈsep-tik\ *adj* **1** : of, relating to, or causing putrefaction **2** : relating to, involving, caused by, or affected with sepsis ⟨~ arthritis⟩ ⟨~ patients⟩

septic abortion *n* : spontaneous or induced abortion associated with bacterial infection (as by E. coli, beta-hemolytic streptococci, or *Clostridium perfringens*)

sep·ti·cae·mia *chiefly Brit var of* SEPTICEMIA

sep·ti·ce·mia \ˌsep-tə-ˈsē-mē-ə\ *n* : invasion of the bloodstream by virulent microorganisms from a focus of infection that is accompanied by acute systemic illness — called also *blood poisoning;* see PYEMIA; compare SEPSIS — **sep·ti·ce·mic** \-ˈsē-mik\ *adj*

septic shock *n* : a life-threatening severe form of sepsis that usu. results from the presence of bacteria and their toxins in the bloodstream and is characterized esp. by persistent hypotension with reduced blood flow to organs and tissues and often organ dysfunction

septic sore throat *n* : STREP THROAT

septo- — see SEPT-

sep·to·plas·ty \ˈsep-tə-ˌplas-tē\ *n, pl* **-ties** : surgical repair of the nasal septum

sep·tos·to·my \sep-ˈtäs-tə-mē\ *n, pl* **-mies** : the surgical creation of an opening through the interatrial septum

Sep·tra \ˈsep-trə\ *trademark* — used for a preparation of sulfamethoxazole and trimethoprim

sep·tum \ˈsep-təm\ *n, pl* **sep·ta** \-tə\ : a dividing wall or membrane esp. between bodily spaces or masses of soft tissue; *esp* : NASAL SEPTUM

septum pel·lu·ci·dum \-pə-ˈlü-sə-dəm\ *n, pl* **septa pel·lu·ci·da** \-də\ : the thin double partition extending vertically from the lower surface of the corpus callosum to the fornix and neighboring parts and separating the lateral ventricles of the brain

septum trans·ver·sum \-tranz-ˈvər-səm\ *n, pl* **septa trans·ver·sa** \-sə\ : the diaphragm or the embryonic structure from which it in part develops

sep·tup·let \sep-ˈtə-plət, -ˈtü-plət, -ˈtyü-; ˈsep-tə-\ *n* **1** : one of seven offspring born at one birth **2 septuplets** *pl* : a group of seven such offspring

se·quel \ˈsē-kwəl, -ˌkwel\ *n* : SEQUELA

se·quela \si-ˈkwe-lə\ *n, pl* **se·quel·ae** \-(ˌ)lē\ : a negative aftereffect ⟨neurological *sequelae* of bacterial meningitis⟩

[1]**se·quence** \ˈsē-kwəns, -ˌkwens\ *n* **1** : a continuous or connected series; *specif* : the exact order of bases in a nucleic acid or of amino acids in a protein **2** : a consequence, result, or subsequent development (as of a disease)

[2]**sequence** *vb* **se·quenced; se·quenc·ing** : to determine the sequence of chemical constituents (as amino acid residues in a protein or bases in a strand of DNA)

se·quenc·er \ˈsē-kwən-sər, -ˌkwen-\ *n* : one that sequences; *esp* : a device for determining the order of occurrence of amino acids in a protein or of bases in a nucleic acid

se·quen·tial \si-ˈkwen-chəl\ *adj* **1** : occurring as a sequela of disease or injury **2** : of, relating to, forming, or taken or administered in a sequence ⟨~ chemotherapy⟩ — **sequential** *n*

se•ques•ter \si-ˈkwes-tər\ *vb* : to hold (as a metallic ion) in solution esp. for the purpose of suppressing undesired chemical or biological activity

se•ques•trant \-trənt\ *n* : a sequestering agent (as citric acid)

se•ques•tra•tion \ˌsē-kwəs-ˈtrā-shən, ˌse-, si-ˌkwes-\ *n* **1** : the formation of a sequestrum **2** : the process of sequestering or result of being sequestered

se•ques•trec•to•my \ˌsē-ˌkwe-ˈstrek-tə-mē\ *n, pl* **-mies** : the surgical removal of a sequestrum

se•ques•trum \si-ˈkwes-trəm\ *n, pl* **-trums** *also* **-tra** \-trə\ : a fragment of dead bone detached from adjoining sound bone

Ser *abbr* serine; seryl

sera *pl of* SERUM

serial section *n* : any of a series of sections cut in sequence by a microtome from a prepared specimen — **serially sectioned** *adj* — **serial sectioning** *n*

ser•ine \ˈser-ˌēn\ *n* : a nonessential amino acid $C_3H_7NO_3$ that occurs esp. as a structural part of many proteins and phosphatidylethanolamines and is a precursor of glycine — abbr. *Ser*

se•ri•ous \ˈsir-ē-əs\ *adj* : having important or dangerous possible consequences ⟨a ~ injury⟩

SERM \ˈsərm\ *n* : SELECTIVE ESTROGEN RECEPTOR MODULATOR

sero- *comb form* **1** : serum ⟨*sero*logy⟩ ⟨*sero*diagnosis⟩ **2** : serous and ⟨*sero*purulent⟩

se•ro•con•ver•sion \ˌsir-ō-kən-ˈvər-zhən, ˌser-\ *n* : the production of antibodies in response to an antigen — **se•ro•con•vert** \-ˈvərt\ *vb*

se•ro•con•vert•er \-kən-ˈvər-tər\ *n* : one that is undergoing or has undergone seroconversion

se•ro•di•ag•no•sis \-ˌdī-ig-ˈnō-səs\ *n, pl* **-no•ses** \-ˌsēz\ : diagnosis by the use of serum (as in the Wassermann test) — **se•ro•di•ag•nos•tic** \-ˈnäs-tik\ *adj*

se•ro•ep•i•de•mi•o•log•ic \-ˌe-pə-ˌdē-mē-ə-ˈlä-jik\ *or* **se•ro•ep•i•de•mi•o•log•i•cal** \-ji-kəl\ *adj* : of, relating to, or being epidemiological investigations involving the identification of antibodies to specific antigens in populations of individuals — **se•ro•ep•i•de•mi•ol•o•gy** \-mē-ˈä-lə-jē\ *n*

se•ro•group \ˈsir-ō-ˌgrüp\ *n* : a group of serotypes having one or more antigens in common

se•rol•o•gist \si-ˈrä-lə-jist\ *n* : a specialist in serology

se•rol•o•gy \si-ˈrä-lə-jē\ *n, pl* **-gies** : a medical science dealing with blood serum esp. in regard to its immunological reactions and properties; *also* : the testing of blood serum to detect the presence of antibodies against a specific antigen — **se•ro•log•i•cal** \ˌsir-ə-ˈlä-ji-kəl\ *or* **se•ro•log•ic** \-jik\ *adj* — **se•ro•log•i•cal•ly** *adv*

se•ro•neg•a•tive \ˌsir-ō-ˈne-gə-tiv, ˌser-ō-\ *adj* : having or being a negative serum reaction esp. in a test for the presence of an antibody ⟨a ~ patient⟩ — **se•ro•neg•a•tiv•i•ty** \-ˌne-gə-ˈti-və-tē\ *n*

se•ro•pos•i•tive \-ˈpä-zə-tiv\ *adj* : having or being a positive serum reaction esp. in a test for the presence of an antibody ⟨a ~ donor⟩ — **se•ro•pos•i•tiv•i•ty** \-ˌpä-zə-ˈti-və-tē\ *n*

se•ro•prev•a•lence \-ˈpre-və-ləns\ *n* : the frequency of individuals in a population that have a particular element (as antibodies to HIV) in their blood serum

se•ro•pu•ru•lent \-ˈpyu̇r-ə-lənt, -ˈpyu̇r-yə-\ *adj* : consisting of a mixture of serum and pus ⟨a ~ exudate⟩

Ser•o•quel \ˈser-ə-ˌkwel\ *trademark* — used for a preparation of quetiapine

se•ro•re•ac•tiv•i•ty \-(ˌ)rē-ˌak-ˈti-və-tē\ *n, pl* **-ties** : reactivity of blood serum — **se•ro•re•ac•tion** \ˌsir-ō-rē-ˈak-shən, ˌser-\ *n* — **se•ro•re•act•ive** \-rē-ˈak-tiv\ *adj*

se•ro•sa \sə-ˈrō-zə\ *n, pl* **-sas** *also* **-sae** \-zē\ : a usu. enclosing serous membrane — **se•ro•sal** \-zəl\ *adj*

se•ro•san•guin•e•ous \ˌsir-ō-san-ˈgwi-nē-əs, ˌser-ō-, -saŋ-\ *adj* : containing or consisting of both blood and serous fluid ⟨a ~ discharge⟩

se•ro•si•tis \ˌsir-ō-ˈsī-təs, ˌser-\ *n* : inflammation of one or more serous membranes ⟨peritoneal ~⟩

se•ro•sta•tus \ˈsir-ə-ˌstā-təs, ˈser-, -ˌsta-\ *n* : status with respect to being seropositive or seronegative for a particular antibody ⟨HIV ~⟩

se•ro•sur•vey \ˈsir-ō-ˌsər-ˌvā, ˈser-\ *n* : a test of blood serum from a group of individuals to determine seroprevalence (as of antibodies to HIV)

se•ro•ther•a•py \ˌsir-ō-ˈther-ə-pē, ˌser-ō-\ *n, pl* **-pies** : the treatment of a disease with specific immune serum

se•ro•to•ner•gic \ˌsir-ə-tə-ˈnər-jik\ *or* **se•ro•to•nin•er•gic** \ˌsir-ə-ˌtō-nə-ˈnər-jik\ *adj* : liberating, activated by, or involving serotonin in the transmission of nerve impulses

se•ro•to•nin \ˌsir-ə-ˈtō-nən, ˌser-\ *n* : a phenolic amine neurotransmitter $C_{10}H_{12}N_2O$ that is a powerful vasoconstrictor and is found esp. in the brain, blood serum, and gastric mucous membrane of mammals — called also *5-HT, 5-hydroxytryptamine*

serotonin–norepinephrine reuptake inhibitor *n* : SNRI

[1]**se•ro•type** \ˈsir-ə-ˌtīp, ˈser-\ *n* **1** : a group of intimately related microorganisms distinguished by a common set of antigens **2** : the set of antigens characteristic of a serotype — **se•ro•typ•ic** \ˌsir-ə-ˈti-pik\ *adj*

[2]**serotype** *vb* **-typed; -typ•ing** : to determine the serotype of ⟨~ streptococci⟩

se•rous \ˈsir-əs\ *adj* : of, relating to, producing, or resembling serum; *esp* : having a thin watery constitution

serous cavity *n* : a cavity (as the peritoneal cavity, pleural cavity, or pericardial cavity) that is lined with a serous membrane

serous cell *n* : a cell (as of the parotid gland) that secretes a serous fluid

serous gland *n* : a gland secreting a serous fluid

serous membrane *n* : any of various thin membranes (as the peritoneum, pericardium, or pleurae) that consist of a single layer of thin flat mesothelial cells resting on a connective-tissue stroma, secrete a serous fluid, and usu. line bodily cavities or enclose the organs contained in such cavities — compare MUCOUS MEMBRANE

serous otitis media *n* : a form of otitis media that is characterized by the accumulation of serous exudate in the middle ear and that typically results from an unresolved attack of acute otitis media — called also *secretory otitis media*

ser•o•var \ˈsir-ə-ˌvär, ˈser-, -ˌvar\ *n* : SEROTYPE 1

Ser•pa•sil \ˈsər-pə-ˌsil\ *n* : a preparation of reserpine — formerly a U.S. registered trademark

ser•pig•i•nous \(ˌ)sər-ˈpi-jə-nəs\ *adj* : slowly spreading; *esp* : healing over in one portion while continuing to advance in another ⟨∼ ulcer⟩

ser•pin \ˈsir-pən, ˈser-\ *n* [*ser*ine *p*roteinase *in*hibitor] : any of a group of structurally related proteins (as antithrombin and antitrypsin) that are typically inhibitors of proteases having serine as the main functional group and that include some (as angiotensinogen) which have lost their inhibitory action

serrata — see ORA SERRATA

ser•ra•ted \sə-ˈrā-təd, ˈser-ˌā-\ *or* **serrate** \ˈser-ˌāt, sə-ˈrāt\ *adj* : notched or toothed on the edge

Ser•ra•tia \se-ˈrā-shə, -shē-ə\ *n* : a genus of aerobic saprophytic flagellated rod-shaped bacteria (family Enterobacteriaceae) including one (*S. marcescens*) associated with some human opportunistic infections

Ser•ra•ti \se-ˈrä-tē\, **Serafino,** Italian boatman.

ser•ra•tus \se-ˈrā-təs\ *n, pl* **ser•ra•ti** \-ˈrā-ˌtī\ : any of three muscles of the thorax that have complex origins but arise chiefly from the ribs or vertebrae: **a** : SERRATUS ANTERIOR **b** : SERRATUS POSTERIOR INFERIOR **c** : SERRATUS POSTERIOR SUPERIOR

serratus anterior *n* : a thin muscular sheet of the thorax that arises from the first eight or nine ribs and from the intercostal muscles between them, is inserted into the ventral side of the medial margin of the scapula, and acts to stabilize the scapula by holding it against the chest wall and to rotate it in raising the arm

serratus posterior inferior *n* : a thin quadrilateral muscle at the junction of the thoracic and lumbar regions that arises chiefly from the spinous processes of the lowest two thoracic and first two or three lumbar vertebrae, is inserted into the lowest four ribs, and acts to counteract the pull of the diaphragm on the ribs to which it is attached

serratus posterior superior *n* : a thin quadrilateral muscle of the upper and dorsal part of the thorax that arises chiefly from the spinous processes of the lowest cervical and the first two or three thoracic vertebrae, is inserted into the second to fifth ribs, and acts to elevate the upper ribs

Ser•to•li cell \ˈser-tə-lē-, ser-ˈtō-lē-\ *also* **Ser•to•li's cell** \-lēz-\ *n* : any of the elongated striated cells in the seminiferous tubules of the testis to which the spermatids become attached and from which they apparently derive nourishment

Sertoli, Enrico (1842–1910), Italian physiologist.

ser•tra•line \ˈsər-trə-ˌlēn\ *n* : a drug that functions as an SSRI and is administered orally in the form of its hydrochloride $C_{17}H_{17}NCl_2{\cdot}HCl$ esp. to treat depression, anxiety, panic disorder, and obsessive-compulsive disorder — see ZOLOFT

[1]**se•rum** \ˈsir-əm\ *n, pl* **se•ra** \-ə\ *or* **serums** : the watery portion of an animal fluid remaining after coagulation: **a** (1) : the clear yellowish fluid that remains from blood plasma after fibrinogen, prothrombin, and other clotting factors have been removed by clot formation — called also *blood serum* (2) : ANTISERUM **b** : a normal or pathological serous fluid (as in a blister)

[2]**serum** *adj* : occurring or found in the serum of the blood ⟨∼ cholesterol⟩

serum albumin *n* : a crystallizable albumin or mixture of albumins that normally constitutes more than half of the protein in blood serum, serves to maintain the osmotic pressure of the blood, and is used in transfusions esp. for the treatment of shock

serum globulin *n* : a globulin or mixture of globulins occurring in blood serum and containing most of the antibodies of the blood

serum hepatitis *n* : HEPATITIS B

serum sickness *n* : an allergic reaction to the injection of foreign serum manifested by hives, swelling, eruption, arthritis, and fever

ser•vice \ˈsər-vis\ *n* : a branch of a hospital medical staff devoted to a particular specialty ⟨pediatric ∼⟩

se•ryl \ˈsir-əl, ˈser-\ *n* : the amino acid radical or residue $HOCH_2CH(NH_2)$-CO– of serine — abbr. *Ser*

[1]**ses•a•moid** \ˈse-sə-ˌmȯid\ *adj* : of, relating to, or being a nodular mass of bone or cartilage in a tendon esp. at a joint or bony prominence

[2]**sesamoid** *n* : a sesamoid bone (as the patella) or cartilage

ses•a•moid•itis \ˌse-sə-ˌmȯi-ˈdī-təs\ *n* **1** : pain and inflammation of either of the two small sesamoid bones or surrounding tendons of the ball of the foot at the base of the big toe **2** : inflammation of the navicular bone and adjacent structures in the horse

ses•sile \ˈse-sīl, -səl\ *adj* **1** : attached directly by a broad base : not pedunculated ⟨a ∼ tumor⟩ **2** : firmly attached : not free to move about

[1]**set** \ˈset\ *vb* **set; set•ting** : to restore to normal position or connection when dislocated or fractured ⟨∼ a broken bone⟩

[2]**set** *n* : a state of psychological preparedness usu. of limited duration for action in response to an anticipated stimulus or situation

Se•tar•ia \se-ˈtar-ē-ə\ *n* : a genus of filarial worms parasitic in various ungulate mammals (as cattle and deer)

se•ton \ˈsēt-ᵊn\ *n* : one or more threads or horsehairs or a strip of linen introduced beneath the skin by a knife or needle to provide drainage

set•tle \ˈset-ᵊl\ *vb* **set•tled; set•tling** *of an animal* **1** : IMPREGNATE 1a **2** : CONCEIVE

se•vel•a•mer \sə-ˈvel-ə-mər\ *n* : a phosphate-binding drug that is a polymer containing amine groups taken orally in the form of its hydrochloride or carbonate in the treatment of hyperphosphatemia in patients with end-stage renal disease and who are on dialysis — see RENAGEL, RENVELA

seventh cranial nerve *n* : FACIAL NERVE

seventh nerve *n* : FACIAL NERVE

severe acute respiratory syndrome *n* : SARS

severe combined immunodeficiency *n* : a rare congenital disorder of the immune system that is characterized by inability to produce a normal complement of antibodies and T cells and that results usu. in early death — abbr. *SCID;* called also *severe combined immune deficiency, severe combined immunodeficiency disease;* see ADENOSINE DEAMINASE

[1]**sex** \ˈseks\ *n* **1** : either of the two major forms of individuals that occur in many species and that are distinguished respectively as male or female **2** : the sum of the structural, functional, and behavioral characteristics of living things that are involved in reproduction by two interacting parents and that distinguish males and females **3 a** : sexually motivated phenomena or behavior **b** : SEXUAL INTERCOURSE

[2]**sex** *vb* : to identify the sex of

sex cell *n* : GAMETE; *also* : its cellular precursor

sex chromatin *n* : BARR BODY

sex chromosome *n* : a chromosome (as the X chromosome or the Y chromosome in humans) that is directly concerned with the inheritance of sex and that contains the genes governing the inheritance of various sex-linked and sex-limited characters

sex gland *n* : GONAD

sex hormone *n* : a steroid hormone (as estradiol, progesterone, androstenedione, or testosterone) that is produced esp. by the ovaries, testes, or adrenal cortex and that exerts estrogenic, progestational, or androgenic activity on the growth or function of the reproductive organs or the development of secondary sex characteristics

sex–limited *adj* : expressed in the phenotype of only one sex ⟨∼ traits⟩

sex–linked *adj* **1** : located in a sex chromosome ⟨a ∼ gene⟩ **2** : mediated by a sex-linked gene ⟨a ∼ character⟩ — **sex–linkage** *n*

sex object *n* : a person regarded esp. exclusively as an object of sexual interest

sex•ol•o•gy \sek-ˈsä-lə-jē\ *n, pl* **-gies** : the study of sex or of the interaction of the sexes esp. among human beings — **sex•ol•o•gist** \-jist\ *n*

sex ratio *n* : the proportion of males to females in a population esp. as expressed by the number of males per hundred females

sex•tu•plet \sek-ˈstə-plət, -ˈstü-, -ˈstyü-; ˈsek-stə-\ *n* **1** : any of six offspring born at one birth **2 sextuplets** *pl* : a group of six offspring born at one birth

sex•u•al \ˈsek-shə-wəl\ *adj* **1** : of, relating to, or associated with sex or the sexes ⟨∼ differentiation⟩ ⟨∼ conflict⟩ **2** : having or involving sex ⟨∼ reproduction⟩ — **sex•u•al•ly** *adv*

sexual assault *n* : illegal sexual contact that usu. involves force upon a person without consent or is inflicted upon a person who is incapable of giving consent (as because of age or mental incapacity) or who places the assailant (as a family friend) in a position of trust or authority

sexual intercourse *n* **1** : heterosexual intercourse involving penetration of the vagina by the penis : COITUS **2** : intercourse (as anal or oral intercourse) that does not involve penetration of the vagina by the penis

sex•u•al•i•ty \ˌsek-shə-ˈwa-lə-tē\ *n, pl* **-ties** : the quality or state of being sexual: **a** : the condition of having sex **b** : sexual activity **c** : expression of sexual receptivity or interest esp. when excessive

sexually transmitted disease *n* : any of various diseases or infections that can be transmitted by direct sexual contact including some (as syphilis, gonorrhea, chlamydia, and genital herpes) chiefly spread by sexual means and others (as hepatitis B and AIDS) often contracted by nonsexual means — called also *STD*

sexual orientation *n* : the inclination of an individual with respect to heterosexual, homosexual, and bisexual behavior — called also *sexual preference*

sexual relations *n pl* : COITUS

Se•za•ry syndrome \ˌsā-zä-ˈrē-\ *or* **Se•za•ry's syndrome** \-ˈrēz-\ *n* : cutaneous T-cell lymphoma characterized by exfoliative dermatitis with intense itching and by the presence in the peripheral blood and in the skin of numerous large malignant mononuclear T cells with irregularly shaped nuclei

Sézary, Albert (1880–1956), French physician.

SFA \ˌes-ˌef-ˈā\ *n* : a saturated fatty acid

Sg *symbol* seaborgium

SGOT *abbr* serum glutamic-oxaloacetic transaminase

SGPT *abbr* serum glutamic-pyruvic transaminase

SH *abbr* serum hepatitis

shad•ow \ˈsha-(ˌ)dō\ *n* **1** : a dark outline or image on an X-ray photograph where the X-rays have been blocked by a radiopaque mass (as a tumor) **2** : a colorless or slightly pigmented or stained body (as a degenerate cell or empty membrane) only faintly visible under the microscope

shaft \ˈshaft\ *n* : a long slender cylindrical body or part: as **a** : the cylindrical part of a long bone between the enlarged ends **b** : HAIR SHAFT

shaft louse *n* : a biting louse of the genus *Menopon* (*M. gallinae*) that commonly infests domestic fowls

shaken baby syndrome *n* : one or more of a group of symptoms (as limb paralysis, lethargy, seizures, or loss of consciousness) that tend to occur in an infant which has been severely shaken but that may also result from other actions (as tossing) causing internal trauma (as hemorrhage, hematoma, or contusions) esp. to the brain region, and that may ultimately result in permanent brain damage or death — called also *shaken infant syndrome*

shakes \ˈshāks\ *n sing or pl* **1** : a condition of trembling; *specif* : DELIRIUM TREMENS **2** : MALARIA 1

shaking palsy *n, dated* : PARKINSON'S DISEASE

shal•low \ˈsha-(ˌ)lō\ *adj* : displacing comparatively little air ⟨~ breathing⟩

sham \ˈsham\ *adj* : being a treatment or procedure that is performed as a control and that is similar to but omits a key therapeutic element of the treatment or procedure under investigation ⟨a ~ injection of saline solution⟩

shank \ˈshaŋk\ *n* : the part of the leg between the knee and the ankle in humans or a corresponding part in other vertebrates

shape \ˈshāp\ *vb* **shaped; shap•ing** : to modify (behavior) by rewarding changes that tend toward a desired response

sharp \ˈshärp\ *n* : a medical instrument (as a scalpel, lancet, or syringe needle) that is sharp or may produce sharp pieces by shattering — usu. used in pl.

Shar•pey's fiber \ˈshär-pēz-\ *n* : any of the thready processes of the periosteum that penetrate the tissue of the superficial lamellae of bones

Sharpey, William (1802–1880), British anatomist and physiologist.

sheath \ˈshēth\ *n, pl* **sheaths** \ˈshēthz, ˈshēths\ **1** : an investing cover or case of a plant or animal body or body part: as **a** : the tubular fold of skin into which the penis of many mammals is retracted **b** : the connective tissue of an organ or part that binds together its component elements and holds it in place **2** : CONDOM 1 — **sheathed** *adj*

sheath of Schwann \-ˈshwän\ *n* : NEURILEMMA

T. A. H. Schwann — see SCHWANN CELL

shed \ˈshed\ *vb* **shed; shed•ding** : to give off or out: as **a** : to lose as part of a natural process ⟨~ the milk teeth⟩ **b** : to discharge usu. gradually from the body ⟨~ a virus in the urine⟩

Shee•han's syndrome \ˈshē-ənz-\ *also* **Shee•han syndrome** \-ən-\ *n* : necrosis of the pituitary gland with associated hypopituitarism resulting from postpartum hemorrhage

Sheehan, Harold Leeming (1900–1988), British pathologist.

sheep botfly *n* : a dipteran fly of the genus *Oestrus* (*O. ovis*) whose larvae parasitize sheep and lodge esp. in the nasal passages and frontal sinuses

sheep ked *n* : a wingless bloodsucking dipteran fly of the genus *Melophagus* (*M. ovinus*) that feeds chiefly on sheep and is a vector of sheep trypanosomiasis — called also *ked, sheep tick*

sheep pox *n* : a disease of sheep that is caused by a poxvirus (species *Sheeppox virus* of the genus *Capripoxvirus*)

sheep tick *n* : SHEEP KED

shell•fish poisoning \ˈshel-ˌfish-\ *n* : food poisoning that results from consumption of shellfish and esp. two-shelled mollusks (as clams, oysters, or mussels) contaminated with toxic dinoflagellates typically found in red tides — see AMNESIC SHELLFISH POISONING, DIARRHEAL SHELLFISH POISONING, NEUROTOXIC SHELLFISH POISONING, PARALYTIC SHELLFISH POISONING

shell shock *n* : COMBAT FATIGUE — **shell–shocked** \ˈshel-ˌshäkt\ *adj*

shi•at•su *also* **shi•at•zu** \shē-ˈät-sü\ *n, often cap* : acupressure esp. of a form that originated in Japan

Shi•ga bacillus \ˈshē-gə-\ *n* : a widely distributed but chiefly tropical bacterium of the genus *Shigella* (*S. dysenteriae*) that causes dysentery

Shiga, Kiyoshi (1870–1957), Japanese bacteriologist.

shi•gel•la \shi-ˈge-lə\ *n* **1** *cap* : a genus of nonmotile aerobic enterobacteria that form acid but no gas on many carbohydrates and that cause dysenteries in animals and esp. humans **2** *pl* **-gel·lae** \-ˌlē\ *also* **-gellas** : any bacterium of the genus *Shigella* **3** : SHIGELLOSIS

shig·el·lo·sis \ˌshi-gə-ˈlō-səs\ *n, pl* **-lo·ses** \-ˈlō-ˌsēz\ : infection with or dysentery caused by bacteria of the genus *Shigella*

shin \ˈshin\ *n* : the front part of the leg below the knee

shin·bone \ˈshin-ˌbōn\ *n* : TIBIA

shin·er \ˈshī-nər\ *n* : BLACK EYE

shin·gles \ˈshiŋ-gəlz\ *n* : an acute viral inflammation of the sensory ganglia of spinal and cranial nerves associated with a vesicular eruption and neuralgic pain and caused by reactivation of the herpesvirus causing chicken pox — called also *herpes zoster, zona, zoster*

shin splints *n sing or pl* : painful injury to and inflammation of the tibial and toe extensor muscles or their fasciae that is caused by repeated minimal traumas (as by running on a hard surface)

shipping fever *n* : an often fatal febrile disease esp. of young cattle and sheep that occurs under highly stressful conditions (as crowding in feedlots) and is caused by a bacterium (esp. *Mannheimia haemolytica* syn. *Pasteurella haemolytica*) usu. in association with a virus

shiv·er \ˈshi-vər\ *vb* : to undergo trembling : experience rapid involuntary muscular twitching esp. in response to cold — **shiver** *n*

shivering *n* **1** : an act or action of one that shivers **2** : a constant abnormal twitching of various muscles in the horse that is prob. due to sensory nerve derangement

shock \ˈshäk\ *n* **1** : a sudden or violent disturbance in the mental or emotional faculties **2** : a state of profound depression of the vital processes of the body that is characterized by pallor, rapid but weak pulse, rapid and shallow respiration, reduced total blood volume, and low blood pressure and that is caused usu. by severe esp. crushing injuries, hemorrhage, burns, or major surgery **3** : sudden stimulation of the nerves or convulsive contraction of the muscles accompanied by a feeling of concussion that is caused by the discharge of electricity through the body — compare ELECTROCONVULSIVE THERAPY — **shock** *vb*

shock lung *n* : a condition of severe pulmonary edema associated with shock

shock therapy *n* : the treatment of mental illness by the artificial induction of coma or convulsions through use of drugs or electric current — called also *convulsive therapy, shock treatment;* see ELECTROCONVULSIVE THERAPY

shoot \ˈshüt\ *vb* **shot** \ˈshät\; **shoot·ing** **1** : to give an injection to **2** : to take or administer (as a drug) by hypodermic needle

shoot·ing *adj* : characterized by sudden sharp piercing sensations ⟨~ pains⟩

short bone *n* : a bone (as of the tarsus or carpus) that is of approximately equal length in all dimensions

short bowel syndrome *n* : malabsorption from the small intestine that is marked by diarrhea, malnutrition, and steatorrhea and that results from resection of the small intestine — called also *short gut syndrome*

short ciliary nerve *n* : any of 6 to 10 delicate nerve filaments of parasympathetic, sympathetic, and general sensory function that arise in the ciliary ganglion and innervate the smooth muscles and tunics of the eye — compare LONG CILIARY NERVE

shortness of breath *n* : difficulty in drawing sufficient breath : labored breathing

short posterior ciliary artery *n* : any of 6 to 10 arteries that arise from the ophthalmic artery or its branches and supply the choroid and the ciliary processes — compare LONG POSTERIOR CILIARY ARTERY

short saphenous vein *n* : SAPHENOUS VEIN b

short·sight·ed \ˈshȯrt-ˈsī-təd\ *adj* : NEARSIGHTED

short·sight·ed·ness *n* : MYOPIA

short–term memory *n* : memory that involves recall of information for a relatively short time (as a few seconds) — abbr. *STM*

shot \ˈshät\ *n* : an injection of a drug, immunizing substance, nutrient, or medicament ⟨a tetanus ~⟩ — see BOOSTER SHOT, FLU SHOT

shoul·der \ˈshōl-dər\ *n* **1** : the laterally projecting part of the body formed of the bones and joints with their covering tissue by which the arm is connected with the trunk **2** : the two shoulders and the upper part of the back — usu. used in pl.

shoulder blade *n* : SCAPULA

shoulder girdle *n* : the bony or cartilaginous arch supporting the forelimbs of a vertebrate that corresponds to the pelvic girdle of the hind limbs — called also *pectoral girdle*

shoulder–hand syndrome *n* : reflex sympathetic dystrophy affecting the upper extremities and characterized by pain in and stiffening of the shoulder followed by swelling and stiffening of the hand and fingers

shoulder joint *n* : the ball-and-socket joint of the humerus and the scapula

shoulder separation *n* : a dislocation of the shoulder at the acromioclavicular joint

show \ˈshō\ *n* **1** : a discharge of mucus streaked with blood from the vagina at the onset of labor **2** : the first appearance of blood in a menstrual period

shrink \ˈshriŋk\ *n* : a clinical psychiatrist or psychologist

shud·der \ˈshə-dər\ *vb* **shud·dered; shud·der·ing** : to tremble convulsively : SHIVER — **shudder** *n*

shunt \ˈshənt\ *n* **1** : a passage by which a bodily fluid (as blood) is diverted from one channel, circulatory path, or part to another; *esp* : such a passage established by surgery or occurring as an abnormality ⟨an arteriovenous ~⟩ **2 a** : a surgical procedure for the establishment of an artificial shunt — see PORTACAVAL SHUNT **b** : a device (as a narrow tube) used to establish an artificial shunt — **shunt** *vb*

[1]**shut–in** \ˈshət-ˌin\ *n* : a person who is confined to home, a room, or bed because of illness or incapacity

[2]**shut–in** \ˈshət-ˈin\ *adj* **1** : confined to one's home or an institution by illness or incapacity **2** : tending to avoid social contact : WITHDRAWN

Shy–Dra·ger syndrome \ˈshī-ˈdrā-gər-\ *n* : multiple system atrophy in which autonomic dysfunction predominates — called also *Shy-Drager disease*

Shy, George Milton (1919–1967), and **Drager, Glenn Albert (1917–1967),** American neurologists.

Si *symbol* silicon

SI *abbr* [French *Système International d'Unités*] International System of Units

sial- *or* **sialo-** *comb form* : saliva ⟨*sialo*lith⟩ ⟨*sialo*rrhea⟩

si·al·ad·e·ni·tis \ˌsī-ə-ˌlad-ᵊn-ˈī-təs\ *n* : inflammation of a salivary gland

si·al·a·gogue \sī-ˈa-lə-ˌgäg\ *n* : an agent that promotes the flow of saliva — called also *sialogogue*

si·al·ic acid \sī-ˈa-lik-\ *n* : any of a group of reducing amido acids that are essentially carbohydrates and are found esp. as components of blood glycoproteins and mucoproteins

si·alo·ad·e·nec·to·my \ˌsī-ə-lō-ˌad-ᵊn-ˈek-tə-mē\ *n, pl* **-mies** : surgical excision of a salivary gland

si·alo·gly·co·pro·tein \-ˌglī-kō-ˈprō-ˌtēn\ *n* : a glycoprotein (as of blood) having sialic acid as a component

si·al·o·gogue \sī-ˈa-lə-ˌgäg\ *n* : SIALAGOGUE

si·al·o·gram \sī-ˈa-lə-ˌgram\ *n* : a radiograph of the salivary tract made by sialography

si·a·log·ra·phy \ˌsī-ə-ˈlä-grə-fē\ *n, pl* **-phies** : radiography of the salivary tract after injection of a radiopaque substance

si·al·o·lith \sī-ˈa-lə-ˌlith\ *n* : a calculus occurring in a salivary gland

si·al·o·li·thi·a·sis \ˌsī-ə-lō-li-ˈthī-ə-səs\ *n, pl* **-a·ses** \-ˌsēz\ : the formation or presence of a calculus or calculi in a salivary gland

si·al·or·rhea \ˌsī-ə-lə-ˈrē-ə\ *n* : excessive salivation : HYPERSALIVATION — called also *ptyalism*

si·al·or·rhoea *chiefly Brit var of* SIALORRHEA

Si·a·mese twin \ˈsī-ə-ˌmēz-, -ˌmēs-\ *n* : either of a pair of conjoined twins

sib \ˈsib\ *n* : a brother or sister considered irrespective of sex

sib·i·lant \ˈsi-bə-lənt\ *adj* : having, containing, or producing the sound of or a sound resembling that of the *s* or *sh* in *sash* ⟨~ breathing⟩

sib·ling \ˈsi-bliŋ\ *n* : SIB; *also* : one of two or more individuals having one common parent

sibling rivalry *n* : competition between siblings esp. for the attention, affection, and approval of their parents

si·bu·tra·mine \sə-ˈbyü-trə-ˌmēn\ *n* : an appetite suppressant $C_{17}H_{26}ClN \cdot HCl \cdot H_2O$ used to treat obesity by inhibiting the reuptake of norepinephrine, serotonin, and dopamine but has been withdrawn from sale by the manufacturer due to its link to cardiovascular events (as heart attack and stroke)

sicca — see KERATOCONJUNCTIVITIS SICCA

sic·ca syndrome \ˈsi-kə-\ *n* : SJÖGREN'S SYNDROME

sick \ˈsik\ *adj* **1 a** : affected with disease or ill health **b** : of, relating to, or intended for use in sickness **c** : affected with nausea : inclined to vomit or being in the act of vomiting **2** : mentally or emotionally unsound or disordered

sick bay *n* : a compartment in a ship used as a dispensary and hospital; *broadly* : a place for the care of the sick or injured

sick·bed \ˈsik-ˌbed\ *n* : the bed upon which one lies sick

sick building syndrome *n* : a set of symptoms (as headache, fatigue, eye irritation, and breathing difficulties) that typically affect workers in modern airtight office buildings, that are believed to be caused by indoor pollutants (as formaldehyde fumes, particulate matter, or microorganisms), and that tend to disappear when affected individuals leave the building — abbr. *SBS*

sick call *n* : a scheduled time at which individuals (as soldiers) may report as sick to a medical officer

sick·en \ˈsi-kən\ *vb* : to make or become sick

sick·en·ing *adj* : causing sickness or nausea ⟨a ~ odor⟩

sick headache *n* : MIGRAINE

sick·lae·mia *chiefly Brit var of* SICKLEMIA

[1]**sick·le** \ˈsi-kəl\ *n* : a dental scaler with a curved 3-sided point

[2]**sickle** *adj* : of, relating to, or characteristic of sickle cell anemia or sickle-cell trait ⟨~ hemoglobin⟩

[3]**sickle** *vb* **sick·led; sick·ling** : to change (a red blood cell) into a sickle cell

sick leave *n* **1** : an absence from work permitted because of illness **2** : the number of days per year for which an employer agrees to pay employees who are sick

sickle cell *n* **1** : an abnormal red blood cell of crescent shape **2** : a condition characterized by sickle cells : SICKLE CELL ANEMIA, SICKLE-CELL TRAIT

sickle cell anemia *n* : a chronic anemia that occurs in individuals (as those of African or Mediterranean descent) who are homozygous for the gene controlling hemoglobin S and that is characterized by destruction of red blood cells and by episodic blocking of blood vessels by the adherence of sickle cells to the vascular endothelium which causes the serious complications of the disease (as organ failure) — abbr. *SCA*

sickle cell disease *n* : SICKLE CELL ANEMIA

sickle–cell trait *n* : a usu. asymptomatic blood condition in which some red blood cells tend to sickle but usu. not enough to produce anemia and which occurs in individuals (as those of African or Mediterranean descent) who are heterozygous for the gene controlling hemoglobin S

sick·le·mia \si-ˈklē-mē-ə\ *n* : SICKLE-CELL TRAIT — **sick·le·mic** \-mik\ *adj*

sick·ler \ˈsi-klər\ *n* : a person with sickle-cell trait or sickle cell anemia

sick·ly \ˈsi-klē\ *adj* **1** : somewhat unwell; *also* : habitually ailing **2** : produced by or associated with sickness **3** : producing or tending to produce disease **4** : tending to produce nausea

sick·ness \ˈsik-nəs\ *n* **1** : the condition of being ill : ill health **2** : a specific disease **3** : NAUSEA

sick·room \ˈsik-ˌrüm, -ˌru̇m\ *n* : a room in which a person is confined by sickness

sick sinus syndrome *n* : a cardiac disorder typically characterized by alternating tachycardia and bradycardia

side \ˈsīd\ *n* **1** : the right or left part of the wall or trunk of the body ⟨a pain in the ~⟩ **2** : a lateral half or part of an organ or structure ⟨the right ~ of one leg⟩

side·bone \-ˌbōn\ *n* **1** *or* **sidebones** : abnormal ossification of the cartilages in the lateral posterior part of a horse's hoof (as of a forefoot) often causing lameness — used with a sing. verb **2** : one of the bony structures characteristic of sidebone

side chain *n* : a branched chain of atoms attached to the principal chain or to a ring in a molecule

side effect *n* : a secondary and usu. adverse effect (as of a drug) — called also *side reaction*

sider- *or* **sidero-** *comb form* : iron ⟨*sidero*penia⟩

sid·ero·blast \ˈsi-də-rə-ˌblast\ *n* : an erythroblast containing cytoplasmic iron granules — **sid·ero·blas·tic** \ˌsi-də-rə-ˈblas-tik\ *adj*

sid·ero·cyte \ˈsi-də-rə-ˌsīt\ *n* : an atypical red blood cell containing iron not bound in hemoglobin

sid·ero·pe·nia \ˌsi-də-rə-ˈpē-nē-ə\ *n* : iron deficiency in the blood serum — **sid·ero·pe·nic** \-ˈpē-nik\ *adj*

sid·er·o·sis \ˌsi-də-ˈrō-səs\ *n, pl* **-o·ses** \-ˌsēz\ *also* **-o·sis·es** **1** : pneumoconiosis occurring in iron workers from inhalation of particles of iron **2** : deposit of iron pigment in a bodily tissue — **sid·er·ot·ic** \ˌsi-də-ˈrä-tik\ *adj*

side·stream \ˈsīd-ˌstrēm\ *adj* : relating to or being tobacco smoke that is emitted from the lit end of a cigarette or cigar — compare MAINSTREAM

side·wind·er \ˈsīd-ˌwīn-dər\ *n* : a small pale-colored venomous rattlesnake of the genus *Crotalus* (*C. cerastes*) of the southwestern U.S. that moves by thrusting its body diagonally forward in a series of S-shaped curves — called also *horned rattlesnake*

SIDS *abbr* sudden infant death syndrome

sie·vert \ˈsē-vərt\ *n* : an SI unit for the dosage of ionizing radiation equal to 100 rems — abbr. *Sv*

Sievert, Rolf Maximilian (1896–1966), Swedish physicist.

Sig *abbr* signa — used to introduce the signature in writing a prescription

sight \ˈsīt\ *n* **1** : something that is seen **2** : the process, power, or function of seeing; *specif* : the sense by which light stimuli received by the eye are interpreted by the brain in the construction of a representation of the position, shape, brightness, and usu. color of objects in space **3 a** : a perception of an object by the eye **b** : the range of vision

sight·ed \ˈsī-təd\ *adj* : having sight : not blind

sight·less \ˈsīt-ləs\ *adj* : lacking sight : BLIND — **sight·less·ness** *n*

¹sig·moid \ˈsig-ˌmȯid\ *adj* **1 a** : curved like the letter C **b** : curved in two directions like the letter S **2** : of, relating to, or being the sigmoid colon of the intestine ⟨~ lesions⟩

²sigmoid *n* : SIGMOID COLON

sigmoid artery *n* : any of several branches of the inferior mesenteric artery that supply the sigmoid colon

sigmoid colon *n* : the contracted and crooked part of the colon immediately above the rectum — called also *pelvic colon, sigmoid flexure*

sig·moid·ec·to·my \ˌsig-mȯi-ˈdek-tə-mē\ *n, pl* **-mies** : surgical excision of part of the sigmoid colon

sigmoid flexure *n* : SIGMOID COLON

sigmoid notch *n* **1** : MANDIBULAR NOTCH **2** : TROCHLEAR NOTCH

sig·moid·o·scope \sig-ˈmȯi-də-ˌskōp\ *n* : an endoscope designed to be passed through the anus in order to permit inspection, diagnosis, treatment, and photography esp. of the sigmoid colon — called also *proctosigmoidoscope*

sig·moid·os·co·py \ˌsig-ˌmȯi-ˈdäs-kə-pē\ *n, pl* **-pies** : the process of using a sigmoidoscope — called also *proctosigmoidoscopy* — **sig·moid·o·scop·ic** \-də-ˈskä-pik\ *adj*

sigmoid sinus *n* : a sinus on each side of the brain that is a continuation of the transverse sinus on the same side, follows an S-shaped course to the jugular foramen, and empties into the internal jugular vein

sigmoid vein *n* : any of several veins that drain the sigmoid colon and empty into the superior rectal vein

sign \ˈsīn\ *n* **1** : one of a set of gestures used to represent language **2** : an objective evidence of disease esp. as observed and interpreted by the physician — compare SYMPTOM

sig·na \ˈsig-nə\ *vb* : write on label — used to introduce the signature in writing a prescription; abbr. *S, Sig*

signal node *n* : a supraclavicular lymph node which when tumorous is often a secondary sign of gastrointestinal cancer — called also *Virchow's node*

sig·na·ture \ˈsig-nə-ˌchu̇r, -chər, -ˌtyu̇r, -ˌtu̇r\ *n* : the part of a medical prescription which contains the directions to the patient

sig·net ring cell \ˈsig-nət-\ *n* : a cell that has its nucleus shifted to one side by a large cytoplasmic vacuole and that occurs esp. in mucin-producing adenocarcinomas esp. of the stomach — called also *signet cell*

sign language *n* : a formal language employing a system of hand gestures for communication (as by the deaf) — compare FINGER SPELLING

Si·las·tic \si-ˈlas-tik\ *trademark* — used for a soft pliable plastic

sil·den·a·fil \sil-ˈde-nə-ˌfil\ *n* : a drug that is used in the form of its citrate $C_{22}H_{30}N_6O_4S \cdot C_6H_8O_7$ chiefly to treat erectile dysfunction in males and hypertension of the lungs by increasing levels of cyclic GMP in the body which promotes relaxation of smooth muscle allowing for increased blood flow to the lungs to lower blood pressure and to the corpus cavernosum to produce an erection during sexual arousal — see REVATIO, VIAGRA

si·lence \ˈsī-ləns\ *vb* **si·lenced; si·lenc·ing** : to block the genetic expression of : SUPPRESS

si·lent \ˈsī-lənt\ *adj* **1** : not exhibiting the usual signs or symptoms of presence ⟨a ~ infection⟩ ⟨~ ischemia⟩ **2** : yielding no detectable response to stimulation — used esp. of an association area of the brain ⟨~ cortex⟩ **3** : having no detectable function or effect ⟨~ genes⟩ — **si·lent·ly** *adv*

silic- *or* **silico-** *comb form* **1** : relating to or containing silicon or its compounds ⟨*silic*one⟩ **2** : silicosis and ⟨*silico*tuberculosis⟩

sil·i·ca \ˈsi-li-kə\ *n* : the dioxide of silicon SiO_2

silica gel *n* : colloidal silica possessing many fine pores and therefore extremely adsorbent

silicate cement *n* : a dental cement used in restorations

sil·i·con \ˈsi-li-kən, -ˌkän\ *n* : a nonmetallic element that occurs combined as the most abundant element next to oxygen in the earth's crust — symbol *Si;* see ELEMENT table

silicon dioxide *n* : SILICA

sil·i·cone \ˈsi-lə-ˌkōn\ *n* : any of various polymeric organic silicon compounds some of which have been used as surgical implants

sil·i·co·sis \ˌsi-lə-ˈkō-səs\ *n, pl* **-co·ses** \-ˌsēz\ : pneumoconiosis characterized by massive fibrosis of the lungs resulting in shortness of breath and caused by prolonged inhalation of silica dusts

[1]**sil·i·cot·ic** \ˌsi-lə-ˈkä-tik\ *adj* : relating to, caused by, or affected with silicosis ⟨~ patients⟩ ⟨~ lungs⟩

[2]**silicotic** *n* : an individual affected with silicosis

sil·i·co·tu·ber·cu·lo·sis \ˌsi-li-kō-tu̇-ˌbər-kyə-ˈlō-səs, -tyu̇-\ *n, pl* **-lo·ses** \-ˌsēz\ : silicosis and tuberculosis in the same lung

silk \ˈsilk\ *n* **1** : a lustrous tough elastic fiber produced by silkworms **2** : strands of silk thread of various thicknesses used as suture material in surgery ⟨surgical ~⟩

sil·ver \ˈsil-vər\ *n* : a white metallic element that has the highest thermal and electric conductivity of any substance — symbol *Ag;* see ELEMENT table

silver iodide *n* : a compound AgI that darkens on exposure to light and is used in medicine as a local antiseptic

silver nitrate *n* : an irritant compound $AgNO_3$ used in medicine esp. as an antiseptic and caustic

silver protein *n* : any of several colloidal light-sensitive preparations of silver and protein used in aqueous solution on mucous membranes as antiseptics and classified by their efficacy and irritant properties: as **a** : a preparation containing 19 to 23 percent of silver — called also *mild silver protein* **b** : a more irritant preparation containing 7.5 to 8.5 percent of silver — called also *strong silver protein*

sil·y·marin \ˌsi-li-ˈmar-ən\ *n* : an antioxidant flavonoid $C_{25}H_{22}O_{10}$ isolated from seeds of the milk thistle that is held to protect the liver from or clear it of toxins and is used in dietary supplements and herbal remedies

si·meth·i·cone \si-ˈme-thi-ˌkōn\ *n* : a liquid mixture of silicone polymers used as an antiflatulent — see MYLICON

sim•i•an crease \ˈsi-mē-ən-\ *n* : a deep crease extending across the palm that results from the fusion of the two normally occurring horizontal palmar creases and is found esp. in individuals with Down syndrome

simian immunodeficiency virus *n* : SIV

simian virus 40 \-ˈfȯr-tē\ *n* : a virus of the genus *Polyomavirus* (species *Simian virus 40*) that infects monkeys and has been shown experimentally to cause tumors in laboratory rodents — called also *SV40*

Sim•monds' disease \ˈsi-məndz-\ *n* : a disease characterized by panhypopituitarism that causes progressive emaciation, atrophy of the gonads, thyroid, and adrenal cortex, and loss of body hair and that results from atrophy or destruction of the anterior lobe of the pituitary gland

Simmonds, Morris (1855–1925), German physician.

[1]**sim•ple** \ˈsim-pəl\ *adj* **sim•pler; sim•plest 1** : free from complexity or difficulty: as **a** : easily treated or cured **b** : controlled by a single gene ⟨~ inherited characters⟩ **2** : of, relating to, or being an epithelium in which the cells are arranged in a single layer

[2]**simple** *n* **1** : a medicinal plant **2** : a vegetable drug having only one ingredient

simple fracture *n* : a bone fracture that does not form an open wound in the skin — compare COMPOUND FRACTURE

simple mastectomy *n* : TOTAL MASTECTOMY

simple ointment *n* : WHITE OINTMENT

simple sugar *n* : MONOSACCHARIDE

simplex — see EPIDERMOLYSIS BULLOSA SIMPLEX, GENITAL HERPES SIMPLEX, HERPES SIMPLEX, LICHEN SIMPLEX CHRONICUS

Sim•plex•vi•rus \ˈsim-ˌpleks-ˌvī-rəs\ *n* : a genus of herpesviruses that usu. infect primates and that includes two (HSV-1 and HSV-2) which are specific for humans and tend to persist in the human host as latent infections in neurons

Sim•po•ni \ˈsim-pə-nē\ *trademark* — used for a preparation of golimumab

sim•u•late \ˈsim-yə-ˌlāt\ *vb* **-lat•ed; -lat•ing** : to have or produce a symptomatic resemblance to — **sim•u•la•tion** \ˌsim-yə-ˈlā-shən\ *n*

Si•mu•li•um \si-ˈmyü-lē-əm\ *n* : a genus of dark-colored bloodsucking dipteran flies (family Simuliidae) of which some are vectors of onchocerciasis or of protozoan diseases of birds — see BLACKFLY

sim•va•stat•in \ˈsim-və-ˌsta-tᵊn\ *n* : a statin $C_{25}H_{38}O_5$ that inhibits the synthesis of cholesterol and is used orally to lower high levels of cholesterol in the blood — see VYTORIN, ZOCOR

si•nal \ˈsī-nᵊl\ *adj* : of, relating to, or coming from a sinus ⟨a ~ discharge⟩

Sind•bis virus \ˈsind-bis-\ *n* : a virus of the genus *Alphavirus* (species *Sindbis virus*) transmitted by mosquitoes and causing a febrile disease marked by joint pain, rash, and malaise in parts of Africa, the Middle East, Europe, Asia, and Australia

Sin•e•met \ˈsi-nə-ˌmet\ *trademark* — used for a preparation containing carbidopa and L-dopa

Sin•e•quan \ˈsi-nə-ˌkwan\ *trademark* — used for a preparation of the hydrochloride of doxepin

sin•ew \ˈsin-yü\ *n* : TENDON

single–blind *adj* : of, relating to, or being an experimental procedure in which the experimenters but not the subjects know the makeup of the test and control groups during the actual course of the experiments — compare DOUBLE-BLIND, OPEN-LABEL

single bond *n* : a chemical bond in which one pair of electrons is shared by two atoms in a molecule and which is usu. represented in chemical formulas by a single line

single nucleotide polymorphism *n* : SNP

single photon absorptiometry *n* : a scanning technique using photons of a single energy to measure the density of a material and esp. bone

single photon emission computed tomography *n* : a medical imaging technique that is used esp. for mapping brain function and that is similar to positron-emission tomography in using the photons emitted by the agency of a radioactive tracer to create an image but that differs in being able to detect only a single photon for each nuclear disintegration and in generating a lower-quality image — abbr. *SPECT*

sin•gle•ton \ˈsiŋ-gəl-tən\ *n* : an offspring born singly

Sin•gu•lair \ˌsiŋ-gyə-ˈler\ *trademark* — used for a preparation of the sodium salt of montelukast

[1]**si•nis•tral** \ˈsi-nəs-trəl, sə-ˈnis-\ *adj* : of, relating to, or inclined to the left; *esp* : LEFT-HANDED

[2]**sinistral** *n* : a person exhibiting dominance of the left hand and eye : a left-handed person

sin•is•tral•i•ty \ˌsi-nə-ˈstra-lə-tē\ *n, pl* **-ties** : the quality or state of having the left side or one or more of its parts (as the hand or eye) different from and usu. more efficient than the right or its corresponding parts; *also* : LEFT-HANDEDNESS

sino- *also* **sinu-** *comb form* : relating to a sinus or sinuses and ⟨*sino*atrial node⟩

si•no•atri•al \ˌsī-nō-ˈā-trē-əl\ *or* **si•nu•atri•al** \ˌsī-n(y)ü-\ *adj* : of, involving, or being the sinoatrial node

sinoatrial node *n* : a small mass of tissue that is made up of Purkinje fibers, ganglion cells, and nerve fibers, that is embedded in the musculature of the right atrium, and that originates the impulses stimulating the heartbeat — called also *S-A node, sinus node*

si•no•au•ric•u•lar \-ō-ˈri-kyə-lər\ *adj* : SINOATRIAL

si•no•pul•mo•nary \ˌsī-nō-ˈpu̇l-mə-ˌner-ē, -ˈpəl-\ *adj* : of, relating to, involving, or affecting the paranasal sinuses and the airway of the lungs

sin•se•mil•la \ˌsin-sə-ˈmē-lə, -ˈmi-, -yə, -lyə\ *n* : highly potent marijuana from female plants having a high resin content; *also* : a female hemp plant grown to produce sinsemilla

si•nus \ˈsī-nəs\ *n* : a cavity or hollow in the body: as **a** : a narrow elongated tract extending from a focus of suppuration and serving for the discharge of pus ⟨a tuberculous ~⟩ **b** (1) : a cavity in the substance of a bone of the skull that usu. communicates with the nostrils and contains air (2) : a channel for venous blood (3) : a dilatation in a bodily canal or vessel

sinus bradycardia *n* : abnormally slow sinus rhythm; *specif* : sinus rhythm at a rate lower than 60 beats per minute

si•nus•itis \ˌsī-nə-ˈsī-təs, -nyə-\ *n* : inflammation of a sinus of the skull

sinus node *n* : SINOATRIAL NODE

sinus of the dura mater *n* : any of numerous venous channels (as the sagittal sinuses) that are situated between the two layers of the dura mater and drain blood from the brain and the bones forming the cranium and empty it into the internal jugular vein — called also *dural sinus*

sinus of Val•sal•va \-väl-ˈsäl-və\ *n* : any one of the pouches of the aorta and pulmonary artery which are located behind the flaps of the semilunar valves and into which the blood in its regurgitation toward the heart enters and thereby closes the valves — called also *aortic sinus*

Valsalva, Antonio Maria (1666–1723), Italian anatomist.

si•nu•soid \ˈsī-nə-ˌsȯid, -nyə-\ *n* : a minute endothelium-lined space or passage for blood in the tissues of an organ (as the liver) — **si•nu•soi•dal** \ˌsī-nə-ˈsȯid-ᵊl, -nyə-\ *adj* — **si•nu•soi•dal•ly** *adv*

si•nus•ot•o•my \ˌsī-nə-ˈsä-tə-mē, -nyə-\ *n, pl* **-mies** : surgical incision into a sinus of the skull

sinus rhythm *n* : the rhythm of the heart produced by impulses from the sinoatrial node

sinus tachycardia *n* : abnormally rapid sinus rhythm; *specif* : sinus rhythm at a rate greater than 100 beats per minute

si•nus ve•no•sus \ˌsī-nəs-vi-ˈnō-səs\ *n* : an enlarged pouch that adjoins the heart, is formed by the union of the large systemic veins, and is the passage through which venous blood enters the embryonic heart

sinus venosus scle•rae \-ˈsklē-rē\ *n* : CANAL OF SCHLEMM

si•pho•no•phore \sī-ˈfä-nə-ˌfōr, ˈsī-fə-nə-\ *n* : any of an order (Siphonophora) of compound free-swimming or floating oceanic coelenterates — see PORTUGUESE MAN-OF-WAR

si•re•no•me•lia \ˌsī-rə-nō-ˈmē-lē-ə\ *n* : a congenital malformation in which the lower limbs are fused

si•ro•li•mus \si-ˈrō-li-məs\ *n* : an immunosuppressive drug $C_{51}H_{79}NO_{13}$ obtained from a soil bacterium of the genus *Streptomyces* (*S. hygroscopicus*) and taken orally esp. to prevent rejection of transplanted organs — called also *rapamycin;* see RAPAMUNE

SIRS *abbr* systemic inflammatory response syndrome

sirup *var of* SYRUP

sis•ter \ˈsis-tər\ *n, chiefly Brit* : a head nurse in a hospital ward or clinic; *broadly* : NURSE

sister chromatid *n* : any of the chromatids formed by replication of one chromosome during interphase of the cell cycle esp. while they are still joined by a centromere

Sis•tru•rus \si-ˈstru̇r-əs\ *n* : a genus of small rattlesnakes having the top of the head covered with scales

si•ta•glip•tin \ˌsī-tə-ˈglip-tən\ *n* : a hypoglycemic drug taken orally in the form of its phosphate $C_{16}H_{15}F_6N_5O \cdot H_3PO_4 \cdot H_2O$ to treat type 2 diabetes — see JANUMET, JANUVIA

site \ˈsīt\ *n* : the place, scene, or point of something — see ACTIVE SITE

si•to•sta•nol \ˌsī-tō-ˈsta-nᵊl\ *n* : a plant sterol $C_{29}H_{52}O$ that is derived from sitosterol and has been shown to reduce serum cholesterol by inhibiting cholesterol absorption

si•tos•ter•ol \sī-ˈtäs-tə-ˌrȯl, sə-, -ˌrōl\ *n* : any of several sterols that occur widely in plant products (as wheat germ) and are used in the synthesis of steroid hormones; *esp* : BETA-SITOSTEROL

situ — see IN SITU

sit•u•a•tion•al \ˌsi-chə-ˈwā-shə-nəl\ *adj* : of, relating to, or occurring in a particular set of circumstances ⟨~ impotence⟩ ⟨~ hypertension⟩

si•tus \ˈsī-təs\ *n* : the place where something exists or originates : SITE

situs in•ver•sus \-in-ˈvər-səs\ *n* : a congenital abnormality characterized by lateral transposition of the viscera (as of the heart or the liver)

sitz bath \ˈsits-\ *n* **1** : a tub in which one bathes in a sitting posture **2** : a bath in which the hips and buttocks are immersed in hot water for the therapeutic effect of moist heat in the perineal and anal regions

SIV \ˌes-ˌī-ˈvē\ *n* : a retrovirus of the genus *Lentivirus* (species *Simian immunodeficiency virus*) that causes a disease in monkeys similar to AIDS and that is closely related to HIV-2 of humans — called also *simian immunodeficiency virus*

six–o–six *or* **606** \ˌsiks-ˌō-ˈsiks\ *n* : ARSPHENAMINE

sixth cranial nerve *n* : ABDUCENS NERVE

six–year molar *n* : one of the first permanent molar teeth of which there are four including one on each side of the upper and lower jaws and which erupt at about six years of age — called also *sixth-year molar;* compare TWELVE-YEAR MOLAR

Sjö•gren's syndrome \ˈshœ̄-ˌgrenz-\ *also* **Sjögren syndrome** \-ˌgren-\ *n* : a chronic inflammatory autoimmune disease that affects esp. older women, that is characterized by dryness of mucous membranes esp. of the eyes and mouth and by infiltration of the affected tissues by lymphocytes, and that is often associated with rheumatoid arthritis — called also *sicca syndrome, Sjögren's, Sjögren's disease*

Sjögren, Henrik Samuel Conrad (1899–1986), Swedish ophthalmologist.

Ske•lax•in \skə-ˈlak-sin\ *trademark* — used for a preparation of metaxalone

skelet- *or* **skeleto-** *comb form* **1** : skeleton ⟨*skelet*al⟩ **2** : skeletal and ⟨*skeleto*muscular⟩

skel•e•tal \ˈske-lət-ᵊl\ *adj* : of, relating to, forming, attached to, or resembling a skeleton ⟨~ structures⟩

skeletal muscle *n* : striated muscle that is usu. attached to the skeleton and is usu. under voluntary control

skel•e•to•mus•cu•lar \ˌske-lə-tō-ˈməs-kyə-lər\ *adj* : constituting, belonging to, or dependent upon the skeleton and the muscles that move it

skel•e•ton \ˈske-lət-ᵊn\ *n* : a usu. rigid supportive or protective structure or framework of an organism; *esp* : the bony or more or less cartilaginous framework supporting the soft tissues and protecting the internal organs of a vertebrate

Skene's gland \ˈskēnz-\ *n* : PARAURETHRAL GLAND

Skene, Alexander Johnston Chalmers (1838–1900), American gynecologist.

skia•gram \ˈskī-ə-ˌgram\ *n* : RADIOGRAPH

skia•graph \-ˌgraf\ *n* : RADIOGRAPH

skilled nursing facility *n* : a health-care institution that meets specific federal criteria (as the supervision of the care of every patient by a physician and the employment full-time of at least one registered nurse) for Medicaid and Medicare reimbursement for nursing care

skim milk *n* : milk from which the cream has been taken — called also *skimmed milk*

¹skin \ˈskin\ *n* : the 2-layered covering of the body consisting of an outer ectodermal epidermis that is more or less cornified and penetrated by the openings of sweat and sebaceous glands and an inner mesodermal dermis that is composed largely of connective tissue and is richly supplied with blood vessels and nerves

²skin *vb* **skinned; skin•ning** : to cut or scrape the skin of ⟨*skinned* his knee⟩

skin•fold \ˈskin-ˌfōld\ *n, often attrib* : a fold of skin formed by pinching or compressing the skin and subcutaneous layers esp. in order to estimate the amount of body fat

skinfold caliper *n* : a pair of calipers used to form and measure the thickness of skinfolds in order to estimate the amount of body fat — usu. used in pl.

skin graft *n* : a piece of skin that is taken from a donor area to replace skin in a defective or denuded area (as one that has been burned); *also* : the procedure by which such a piece of skin is removed and transferred to a new area

skinned \ˈskind\ *adj* : having skin esp. of a specified kind — usu. used in combination ⟨dark-*skinned*⟩

Skin•ner box \ˈski-nər-ˌbäks\ *n* : a laboratory apparatus in which an animal is caged for experiments in operant conditioning and which typically contains a lever that must be pressed by the animal to gain reward or avoid punishment

Skinner, Burrhus Frederic (1904–1990), American psychologist.

Skin•ner•ian \ski-ˈnir-ē-ən, -ˈner-\ *adj* : of, relating to, or suggestive of the behavioristic theories of B. F. Skinner

skin patch *n* : PATCH 1b

skin tag \-ˌtag\ *n* : a small soft pendulous growth on the skin esp. around the eyes or on the neck, armpits, or groin — called also *acrochordon*

skin test *n* : a test (as a scratch test or a tuberculin test) for an allergic or immune response to a substance that is performed by administering the substance to or through the skin and is used esp. in detecting allergic hypersensitivity — **skin testing** *n*

skull \ˈskəl\ *n* : the skeleton of the head forming a bony case that encloses and protects the brain and chief sense organs and supports the jaws

skull•cap \ˈskəl-ˌkap\ *n* : the upper portion of the skull : CALVARIUM

SLE *abbr* systemic lupus erythematosus

sleep \ˈslēp\ *n* **1** : the natural periodic suspension of consciousness during which the powers of the body are restored — compare REM SLEEP, SLOW-WAVE SLEEP **2** : a state resembling sleep: as **a** : DEATH 1 ⟨put a pet cat to ~⟩ **b** : a state marked by a diminution of feeling followed by tingling ⟨his foot went to ~⟩ — **sleep** *vb* — **sleep•i•ness** \ˈslē-pē-nəs\ *n* — **sleepy** *adj*

sleep apnea *n* : brief periods of recurrent cessation of breathing during sleep that is caused esp. by obstruction of the airway or a disturbance in the brain's respiratory center and is associated esp. with excessive daytime sleepiness

sleeping pill *n* : a drug and esp. a barbiturate that is taken as a tablet or capsule to induce sleep — called also *sleeping tablet*

sleeping sickness *n* **1** : a serious disease that is prevalent in much of tropical Africa, is marked by fever, headache, protracted lethargy, confusion, sleep disturbances, tremors, and loss of weight, and is caused by either of two trypanosomes (*Trypanosoma brucei gambiense* and *T. b. rhodesiense*) transmitted by tsetse flies — called also *African sleeping sickness* **2** : any of various viral encephalitides or encephalomyelitides of which lethargy or somnolence is a prominent feature; *esp* : EQUINE ENCEPHALITIS

sleep·less \ˈslē-pləs\ *adj* : not able to sleep : INSOMNIAC — **sleep·less·ness** *n*

sleep spindle *n* : a burst of synchronous alpha waves that occurs during light sleep

sleep·walk·er \ˈslēp-ˌwȯ-kər\ *n* : one who is subject to somnambulism : one who walks while sleeping — called also *somnambulist* — **sleep·walk** \-ˌwȯk\ *vb*

sleepy sickness *n, Brit* : ENCEPHALITIS LETHARGICA

slide \ˈslīd\ *n* : a flat piece of glass or plastic on which an object is mounted for microscopic examination

sliding filament hypothesis *n* : a theory in physiology holding that muscle contraction occurs when the actin filaments next to the Z line at each end of a sarcomere are drawn toward each other between the thicker myosin filaments more centrally located in the sarcomere by the projecting globular heads of myosin molecules that form temporary attachments to the actin filaments — called also *sliding filament theory;* see CROSSBRIDGE

slim disease \ˈslim-\ *n* : AIDS; *also* : severe wasting of the body in the later stages of AIDS

sling \ˈsliŋ\ *n* : a hanging bandage suspended from the neck to support an arm or hand

slipped disk *n* : a protrusion of an intervertebral disk and its nucleus pulposus that produces pressure upon spinal nerves resulting in low-back pain and often sciatic pain

slipped tendon *n* : PEROSIS

slit lamp \ˈslit-ˌlamp\ *n* : a lamp for projecting a narrow beam of intense light that is used in conjunction with a biomicroscope for examining the anterior parts (as of the conjunctiva or cornea) of an eye; *also* : a unit consisting of both the lamp and biomicroscope

[1]**slough** \ˈsləf\ *n* : dead tissue separating from living tissue; *esp* : a mass of dead tissue separating from an ulcer

[2]**slough** \ˈsləf\ *vb* : to separate in the form of dead tissue from living tissue

slow infection *n* : a degenerative disease caused by a slow virus

slow–reacting substance *n* : SLOW-REACTING SUBSTANCE OF ANAPHYLAXIS — abbr. *SRS*

slow–reacting substance of anaphylaxis *n* : a mixture of three leukotrienes produced in anaphylaxis that causes contraction of smooth muscle after minutes in contrast to histamine which acts in seconds and that is prob. responsible for the bronchoconstriction occurring in anaphylaxis — abbr. *SRS-A*

slow–release \ˌslō-ri-ˈlēs\ *adj* : SUSTAINED-RELEASE; *also* : EXTENDED-RELEASE

slow–twitch \ˈslō-ˌtwich\ *adj* : of, relating to, or being muscle fiber that contracts slowly esp. during sustained physical activity requiring endurance — compare FAST-TWITCH

slow virus *n* : any of various viruses (as a lentivirus) or prions having a long incubation period between infection and the clinical appearance of the slowly progressive serious or fatal disease (as scrapie or Creutzfeldt-Jakob disease) associated with it

slow wave *n* : DELTA WAVE

slow–wave sleep *n* : a state of deep usu. dreamless sleep that occurs regularly during a normal period of sleep with intervening periods of REM sleep and that is characterized by delta waves and a low level of autonomic physiological activity — called also *non-REM sleep, NREM sleep, orthodox sleep, S sleep, synchronized sleep*

slug·gish \ˈslə-gish\ *adj* : markedly slow in movement, progression, or response ⟨~ healing⟩ — **slug·gish·ly** *adv* — **slug·gish·ness** *n*

Sm *symbol* samarium

small bowel *n* : SMALL INTESTINE

small calorie *n* : CALORIE 1a

small–cell lung cancer *n* : cancer of a highly malignant form that affects the lungs, tends to metastasize to other parts of the body, and is characterized by small round or oval cells which resemble oat grains and have little cytoplasm — called also *oat-cell cancer, oat-cell carcinoma, small-cell carcinoma, small-cell lung carcinoma*

small intestine *n* : the part of the intestine that lies between the stomach and colon, consists of duodenum, jejunum, and ileum, secretes digestive enzymes, and is the chief site of the absorption of digested nutrients — called also *small bowel*

small·pox \ˈsmȯl-ˌpäks\ *n* : an acute contagious febrile disease of humans that is caused by a poxvirus of the genus *Orthopoxvirus* (species *Variola virus*), is characterized by skin eruption with pustules, sloughing, and scar formation, and is believed to have been eradicated globally by widespread vaccination — called also *variola;* see VARIOLA MAJOR, VARIOLA MINOR

small saphenous vein *n* : SAPHENOUS VEIN b

smart \ˈsmärt\ *vb* : to cause or be the cause or seat of a sharp poignant pain; *also* : to feel or have such a pain

smart drug *n* : NOOTROPIC

smear \ˈsmir\ *n* : material spread on a surface (as of a microscopic slide); *also* : a preparation made by spreading material on a surface — see PAP SMEAR, VAGINAL SMEAR — **smear** *vb*

smeg•ma \ˈsmeg-mə\ *n* : the secretion of a sebaceous gland; *specif* : the cheesy sebaceous matter that collects between the glans penis and the foreskin or around the clitoris and labia minora

[1]**smell** \ˈsmel\ *vb* **smelled** \ˈsmeld\ *or* **smelt** \ˈsmelt\; **smell•ing** : to perceive the odor or scent of through stimuli affecting the olfactory nerves : get the odor or scent of with the nose

[2]**smell** *n* **1** : the property of a thing that affects the olfactory organs : ODOR **2** : the special sense concerned with the perception of odor

smell brain *n* : RHINENCEPHALON

smelling salts *n pl* : a usu. scented aromatic preparation of ammonium carbonate and ammonia water used as a stimulant and restorative

Smith fracture \ˈsmith-\ *or* **Smith's fracture** \ˈsmiths-\ *n* : a fracture of the lower portion of the radius with forward displacement of the lower fragment — compare COLLES' FRACTURE

Smith, Robert William (1807–1873), British surgeon.

Smith–Pe•ter•sen nail \ˈsmith-ˈpē-tər-sən-\ *n* : a metal nail used to fix the femoral head in fractures of the neck of the femur

Smith–Petersen, Marius Nygaard (1886–1953), American orthopedic surgeon.

smog \ˈsmäg, ˈsmȯg\ *n* : a fog made heavier and darker by smoke and chemical fumes; *also* : a photochemical haze caused by the action of solar ultraviolet radiation on atmosphere polluted with hydrocarbons and oxides of nitrogen esp. from automobile exhaust

smoke \ˈsmōk\ *vb* **smoked; smok•ing** : to inhale and exhale the fumes of burning plant material and esp. tobacco; *esp* : to smoke tobacco habitually

smok•er \ˈsmō-kər\ *n* : a person who smokes habitually

smooth \ˈsmüth\ *adj* : forming or being a colony with a flat shiny surface usu. made up of organisms that form no chains or filaments, show characteristic internal changes, and tend toward marked increase in capsule formation and virulence — used of dissociated strains of bacteria; compare ROUGH

smooth muscle *n* : muscle tissue that lacks cross striations, that is made up of elongated spindle-shaped cells having a central nucleus, and that is found esp. in hollow organs and structures (as the small intestine and bladder) as thin sheets performing functions not subject to direct voluntary control — called also *nonstriated muscle, unstriated muscle;* compare CARDIAC MUSCLE, STRIATED MUSCLE

Sn *symbol* tin

snail \ˈsnāl\ *n* : any of various gastropod mollusks and esp. those having an external enclosing spiral shell including some which serve as intermediate hosts of trematodes

snail fever *n* : SCHISTOSOMIASIS

snake \ˈsnāk\ *n* : any of numerous limbless scaled reptiles (suborder Serpentes syn. Ophidia) with a long tapering body and with salivary glands often modified to produce venom which is injected through grooved or tubular fangs

snake•bite \-ˌbīt\ *n* : the bite of a snake; *also* : the condition resulting from the bite of a venomous snake characterized by variable symptoms (as pain and swelling at the puncture site, blurred vision, difficulty in breathing, or internal bleeding)

snare \ˈsnar\ *n* : a surgical instrument consisting usu. of a wire loop constricted by a mechanism in the handle and used for removing tissue masses (as tonsils or polyps)

sneeze \ˈsnēz\ *vb* **sneezed; sneez•ing** : to make a sudden violent spasmodic audible expiration of breath through the nose and mouth esp. as a reflex act following irritation of the nasal mucous membrane — **sneeze** *n*

Snel•len chart \ˈsne-lən-\ *n* : the chart used in the Snellen test with black letters of various sizes against a white background

Snellen, Hermann (1834–1908), Dutch ophthalmologist.

Snellen test *n* : a test for visual acuity presenting letters of graduated sizes to determine the smallest size that can be read at a standard distance

SNF *abbr* skilled nursing facility

snif•fles \ˈsni-fəlz\ *n pl* **1** : a head cold marked by nasal discharge **2** : BULLNOSE — usu. used with a sing. verb

snore \ˈsnōr\ *vb* **snored; snor•ing** : to breathe during sleep with a rough hoarse noise due to vibration of the soft palate — **snore** *n* — **snor•er** *n*

snort \ˈsnȯrt\ *vb* : to inhale (a narcotic drug in powdered form) through the nostrils <~ cocaine>

snow \ˈsnō\ *n, slang* **1** : COCAINE **2** : HEROIN

snow blindness *n* : inflammation and photophobia caused by exposure of the eyes to ultraviolet rays reflected from snow or ice — **snow–blind** \-ˌblīnd\ *or* **snow–blind•ed** \-ˌblīn-dəd\ *adj*

SNP \ˈsnip\ *n* : a variant DNA sequence in which the purine or pyrimidine base (as cytosine) of a single nucleotide has been replaced by another such base (as thymine) — called also *single nucleotide polymorphism*

SNRI \ˌes-ˌen-ˌär-ˈī\ *n* : any of a class of drugs (as desvenlafaxine and duloxetine) that inhibit the inactivation of serotonin and norepinephrine by blocking their reuptake by presynaptic nerve cell endings and are typically used to treat depression, anxiety, and chronic pain — called also *selective serotonin norepinephrine reuptake inhibitor, serotonin-norepinephrine reuptake inhibitor, SSNRI;* compare SSRI

snuff \ˈsnəf\ *n* : a preparation of pulverized tobacco to be inhaled through the nostrils, chewed, or placed against the gums; *also* : a preparation of a powdered drug to be inhaled through the nostrils

snuf•fles \ˈsnə-fəlz\ *n pl* **1** : SNIFFLES 1 **2** : a respiratory disorder (as bullnose) in animals marked esp. by catarrhal inflammation and sniffling — usu. used with a sing. verb

soak \ˈsōk\ *n* : an often hot medicated solution with which a body part is soaked usu. long or repeatedly esp. to promote healing, relieve pain, or stimulate local circulation

soap \ˈsōp\ *n* **1** : a cleansing and emulsifying agent made usu. by action of alkali on fat or fatty acids and consisting essentially of sodium or potassium salts of such acids **2** : a salt of a fatty acid and a metal

SOB *abbr* short of breath

so•cial \ˈsō-shəl\ *adj* **1** : tending to form cooperative and interdependent relationships with others of one's kind **2** : of or relating to human society, the interaction of the individual and the group, or the welfare of human beings as members of society ⟨immature ∼ behavior⟩ — **so•cial•ly** *adv*

social anxiety *n* : a form of anxiety that is brought about by social situations in which an individual fears being embarrassed or negatively judged by others; *esp* : SOCIAL ANXIETY DISORDER

social anxiety disorder *n* : an anxiety disorder in which an individual has persistent and exaggerated fears of being embarrassed or negatively judged by others in various social situations (as meeting strangers or public speaking) and that causes significant distress, avoidance of anxiety-producing situations, and impairment of normal social or occupational interpersonal relationships and activities

social disease *n* **1** : VENEREAL DISEASE **2** : a disease (as tuberculosis) whose incidence is directly related to social and economic factors

so•cial•i•za•tion \ˌsō-shə-lə-ˈzā-shən\ *n* : the process by which a human being beginning at infancy acquires the habits, beliefs, and accumulated knowledge of society through education and training for adult status — **so•cial•ize** \ˈsō-shə-ˌlīz\ *vb*

socialized medicine *n* : medical and hospital services for the members of a class or population administered by an organized group (as a state agency) and paid for from funds obtained usu. by assessments, philanthropy, or taxation

social phobia *n* : SOCIAL ANXIETY

social psychiatry *n* **1** : a branch of psychiatry that deals in collaboration with related specialties (as sociology and anthropology) with the influence of social and cultural factors on the causation, course, and outcome of mental illness **2** : the application of psychodynamic principles to the solution of social problems

social psychology *n* : the study of the manner in which the personality, attitudes, motivations, and behavior of the individual influence and are influenced by social groups — **social psychologist** *n*

social recovery *n* : a return to effective social functioning (as following stroke, a traumatic event, or treatment for mental illness)

social work *n* : any of various professional services, activities, or methods concretely concerned with the investigation, treatment, and material aid of the economically, physically, mentally, or socially disadvantaged — **social worker** *n*

socio- *comb form* **1** : society : social ⟨*socio*path⟩ **2** : social and ⟨*socio*psychological⟩

so•cio•cul•tur•al \ˌsō-sē-ō-ˈkəl-chə-rəl, ˌsō-shē-\ *adj* : of, relating to, or involving a combination of social and cultural factors — **so•cio•cul•tur•al•ly** *adv*

so•ci•ol•o•gy \ˌsō-sē-ˈä-lə-jē, ˌsō-shē-\ *n, pl* **-gies** : the science of society, social institutions, and social relationships; *specif* : the systematic study of the development, structure, interaction, and collective behavior of organized groups of human beings — **so•cio•log•i•cal** \ˌsō-sē-ə-ˈlä-ji-kəl, ˌsō-shē-ə-\ *also* **so•cio•log•ic** \-jik\ *adj* — **so•cio•log•i•cal•ly** *adv* — **so•ci•ol•o•gist** \ˌsō-sē-ˈä-lə-jist, -shē-\ *n*

so•cio•med•i•cal \ˌsō-sē-ō-ˈme-di-kəl, ˌsō-shē-\ *adj* : of or relating to the interrelations of medicine and social welfare

so·cio·path \ˈsō-sē-ə-ˌpath, ˈsō-shē-ə-\ *n* : a sociopathic person : PSYCHOPATH

so·cio·path·ic \ˌsō-sē-ə-ˈpa-thik, ˌsō-shē-ə-\ *adj* : of, relating to, or characterized by antisocial behavior or an antisocial personality — **so·ci·op·a·thy** \ˌsō-sē-ˈä-pə-thē, ˌsō-shē-\ *n*

so·cio·psy·cho·log·i·cal \ˌsō-sē-ō-ˌsī-kə-ˈlä-ji-kəl, ˌsō-shē-\ *adj* **1** : of, relating to, or involving a combination of social and psychological factors **2** : of or relating to social psychology

so·cio·sex·u·al \-ˈsek-shə-wəl\ *adj* : of or relating to the interpersonal aspects of sexuality

sock·et \ˈsä-kət\ *n* : an opening or hollow that forms a holder for something: as **a** : any of various hollows in body structures in which some other part normally lodges ⟨the bony ~ of the eye⟩ ⟨an inflamed tooth ~⟩; *esp* : the depression in a bone with which the rounded head of another bone fits in a ball-and-socket joint **b** : a cavity terminating an artificial limb into which the bodily stump fits

SOD *abbr* superoxide dismutase

so·da \ˈsō-də\ *n* : SODIUM CARBONATE; *also* : SODIUM BICARBONATE

soda lime *n* : a granular mixture of calcium hydroxide with sodium hydroxide or potassium hydroxide or both used to absorb moisture and acid gases and esp. carbon dioxide (as in gas masks and in oxygen therapy)

sod disease \ˈsäd-\ *n* : VESICULAR DERMATITIS

so·di·um \ˈsō-dē-əm\ *n* : a silver white soft waxy ductile element — symbol *Na;* see ELEMENT table

sodium ascorbate *n* : the sodium salt $C_6H_7NaO_6$ of vitamin C

sodium benzoate *n* : a crystalline or granular salt $C_7H_5O_2Na$ used chiefly as a food preservative

sodium bicarbonate *n* : a white crystalline weakly alkaline salt $NaHCO_3$ used in medicine esp. as an antacid — called also *baking soda, bicarb, bicarbonate of soda*

sodium bromide *n* : a crystalline salt NaBr having a biting saline taste that is used in medicine as a sedative, hypnotic, and anticonvulsant

sodium caprylate *n* : the sodium salt $C_8H_{15}O_2Na$ of caprylic acid used esp. in the topical treatment of fungal infections

sodium carbonate *n* : any of several salts (as Na_2CO_3) of carbonic acid

sodium chloride *n* : SALT 1a

sodium citrate *n* : a crystalline salt $C_6H_5Na_3O_7$ used chiefly as an expectorant, a systemic and urinary alkalizer, and in combination as an anticoagulant (as in stored blood)

sodium cro·mo·gly·cate \-ˌkrō-mō-ˈglī-ˌkāt\ *n* : CROMOLYN

sodium di·hy·dro·gen phosphate \-ˌdī-ˈhī-drə-jən-\ *n* : SODIUM PHOSPHATE 1

sodium fluoride *n* : a poisonous crystalline salt NaF that is used in trace amounts in the fluoridation of water, toothpastes, and oral rinses and as an antiseptic — see LURIDE

sodium glutamate *n* : MONOSODIUM GLUTAMATE

sodium hydroxide *n* : a white brittle solid NaOH that dissolves readily in water to form a strongly alkaline and caustic solution and that is used in pharmacy as an alkalizing agent

sodium hypochlorite *n* : an unstable salt NaOCl produced usu. in aqueous solution and used as a bleaching and disinfecting agent

sodium iodide *n* : a crystalline salt NaI used as an iodine supplement and expectorant

sodium io·do·hip·pu·rate \-ī-ˌō-dō-ˈhi-pyə-ˌrāt\ *n* : HIPPURAN

sodium lactate *n* : a hygroscopic syrupy salt $C_3H_5NaO_3$ used chiefly as an antacid in medicine and as a substitute for glycerol

sodium lau·ryl sulfate \-ˌlȯ-ril-\ *n* : a crystalline sodium salt $C_{12}H_{25}NaO_4S$; *also* : a mixture of sulfates of sodium consisting principally of this salt and used as a detergent, wetting, and emulsifying agent (as in toothpastes, ointments, and shampoos)

sodium mor·rhu·ate \-ˈmȯr-ü-ˌāt\ *n* : MORRHUATE SODIUM

sodium nitrate *n* : a crystalline salt $NaNO_3$ used in curing meat — called also *saltpeter*

sodium nitrite *n* : salt $NaNO_2$ that is used as a meat preservative and in medicine as a vasodilator and an antidote for cyanide poisoning

sodium ni·tro·prus·side \-ˌnī-trō-ˈprə-ˌsīd\ *n* : a red crystalline salt $C_5FeN_6Na_2O$ administered intravenously as a vasodilator esp. in hypertensive emergencies — see NIPRIDE

sodium pentobarbital *n* : the sodium salt of pentobarbital

sodium pentobarbitone *n, Brit* : SODIUM PENTOBARBITAL

sodium per·bor·ate \-pər-ˈbōr-ˌāt\ *n* : a white crystalline powder $NaBO_3 \cdot 4H_2O$ used as an oral antiseptic

sodium phosphate *n* **1** : a phosphate NaH_2PO_4 of sodium containing one sodium atom per molecule that with the phosphate containing two sodium atoms per molecule constitutes the principal buffer system of the urine — called also *sodium dihydrogen phosphate* **2** : a phosphate Na_2HPO_4 of sodium containing two sodium atoms per molecule that is used in medicine as a laxative and antacid

sodium potassium tartrate *n* : ROCHELLE SALT

sodium pump *n* **1** : a molecular mechanism by which sodium ions move across a cell membrane by active transport; *esp* : one that is controlled by a specialized cell membrane protein by which a high concentration of potassium ions and a low concentration of sodium ions are maintained within a cell **2** : the specialized cell membrane protein that controls the sodium pump mechanism

sodium salicylate *n* : a crystalline salt $NaC_7H_5O_3$ that has a sweetish saline taste and is used chiefly as an analgesic, antipyretic, and antirheumatic

sodium secobarbital *n* : the sodium salt $C_{12}H_{17}N_2NaO_3$ of secobarbital

sodium stearate *n* : a white powdery water-soluble salt $C_{18}H_{35}NaO_2$ used esp. in glycerin suppositories, cosmetics, and some toothpastes

sodium sulfate *n* : a bitter salt Na_2SO_4 used in its hydrated form as a cathartic — see GLAUBER'S SALT

sodium thiosulfate *n* : a hygroscopic crystalline salt $Na_2O_3S_2$ used as an antidote in poisoning esp. by cyanides and as an antifungal agent

sodium valproate *n* : the sodium salt $C_8H_{15}NaO_2$ of valproic acid used as an anticonvulsant

so•do•ku \ˈsō-də-ˌkü\ *n* : RAT-BITE FEVER b

sod•omy \ˈsä-də-mē\ *n, pl* **-om•ies** : anal or oral copulation with a member of the same or opposite sex; *also* : copulation with an animal — **sod•om•ize** \ˈsä-də-ˌmīz\ *vb*

so•fos•bu•vir \sō-ˈfäs-bu̇-ˌvir\ *n* : an antiviral drug $C_{22}H_{29}FN_3O_9P$ that is a nucleotide analog taken orally with other antiretroviral agents (as ribavirin or ledipasvir) to treat hepatitis C infection — see HARVONI, SOVALDI

soft \ˈsȯft\ *adj* **1** : yielding to physical pressure **2** : deficient in or free from substances (as calcium and magnesium salts) that prevent lathering of soap ⟨~ water⟩ **3** : having relatively low energy ⟨~ X-rays⟩ **4** : BIODEGRADABLE **5** *of a drug* : considered less detrimental than a hard narcotic ⟨marijuana is usually regarded as a ~ drug⟩ **6** : being or based on interpretive or speculative data ⟨~ evidence⟩

soft chancre *n* : CHANCROID

soft contact lens *n* : a contact lens made of soft water-absorbing plastic that adheres closely and with minimal discomfort to the eye

soft•gel \ˈsȯft-ˌjel\ *n* : a pliable soft gelatin capsule containing a liquid preparation (as a medicine)

soft lens *n* : SOFT CONTACT LENS

soft palate *n* : the membranous and muscular fold suspended from the posterior margin of the hard palate and partially separating the mouth cavity from the pharynx

soft spot *n* : a fontanel of a fetal or young skull

soft tissue *n* : body tissue that is not hardened or calcified; *specif* : tissue (as tendon, muscle, skin, fat, and fascia) that typically connects, supports, or surrounds bone and internal organs ⟨*soft tissue* sarcoma⟩

sol \ˈsäl, ˈsȯl\ *n* : a fluid colloidal system; *esp* : one in which the medium is a liquid

so•la•nine *or* **so•la•nin** \ˈsō-lə-ˌnēn, -nən\ *n* : a bitter poisonous crystalline alkaloid $C_{45}H_{72}NO_{15}$ from several plants (as some potatoes or tomatoes) of the nightshade family (Solanaceae)

so•la•num \sə-ˈlā-nəm, -ˈlä-, -ˈla-\ *n* **1** *cap* : a genus of often spiny herbs, shrubs, and trees of the nightshade family (Solanaceae) that have white, purple, or yellow flowers and a fruit that is a berry **2** : any plant of the genus *Solanum*

so•lar•i•um \sō-ˈlar-ē-əm, sə-\ *n, pl* **-ia** \-ē-ə\ *also* **-ums** : a room (as in a hospital) used esp. for sunbathing or therapeutic exposure to light

so•lar plex•us \ˈsō-lər-ˈplek-səs\ *n* **1** : CELIAC PLEXUS **2** : the part of the abdomen including the stomach and celiac plexus that is particularly vulnerable to the effects of a blow to the body wall in front of it — not used technically

soldier's heart *n* : NEUROCIRCULATORY ASTHENIA

sole \ˈsōl\ *n* : the undersurface of a foot

So•le•nop•sis \ˌsō-lə-ˈnäp-səs\ *n* : a genus of small stinging ants including several tropical and subtropical forms (as the imported fire ants)

so•le•us \ˈsō-lē-əs\ *n, pl* **so•lei** \-lē-ˌī\ *also* **soleuses** : a broad flat muscle of the calf of the leg that lies deep to the gastrocnemius, arises from the back and upper part of the tibia and fibula and from a tendinous arch between them, inserts by a tendon that unites with that of the gastrocnemius to form the Achilles tendon, and acts to flex the foot

[1]**sol•id** \ˈsä-ləd\ *adj* **1** : being without an internal cavity : not hollow ⟨~ tumors⟩ **2** : possessing or characterized by the properties of a solid

[2]**solid** *n* **1** : a substance that does not flow perceptibly under moderate stress and under ordinary conditions retains a definite size and shape **2** : the part of a solution or suspension that when freed from solvent or suspending medium has the qualities of a solid — usu. used in pl. ⟨milk ~*s*⟩

so•li•fen•a•cin \ˌsō-lə-ˈfen-ə-sən\ *n* : an antimuscarinic drug taken orally in the form of its succinate $C_{23}H_{26}N_2O_2 \cdot C_4H_6O_4$ to treat urge incontinence, frequent urination, and urinary urgency associated with an overactive bladder — see VESICARE

solitarius — see TRACTUS SOLITARIUS

sol•i•tary \ˈsä-lə-ˌter-ē\ *adj* : occurring singly and not as part of a group

sol•u•bil•i•ty \ˌsäl-yə-ˈbi-lə-tē\ *n, pl* **-ties** **1** : the quality or state of being soluble **2** : the amount of a substance that will dissolve in a given amount of another substance

sol•u•ble \'säl-yə-bəl\ *adj* **1** : susceptible of being dissolved in or as if in a fluid **2** : capable of being emulsified

soluble RNA *n* : TRANSFER RNA

sol•ute \'säl-ˌyüt\ *n* : a dissolved substance

so•lu•tion \sə-'lü-shən\ *n* **1 a** : an act or the process by which a solid, liquid, or gaseous substance is homogeneously mixed with a liquid or sometimes a gas or solid **b** : a homogeneous mixture formed by this process **2 a** : a liquid containing a dissolved substance ⟨an aqueous ~⟩ **b** : a liquid and usu. aqueous medicinal preparation with the solid ingredients soluble **c** : the condition of being dissolved ⟨a substance in ~⟩

[1]**sol•vent** \'säl-vənt, 'sȯl-\ *adj* : that dissolves or can dissolve ⟨~ fluids⟩ ⟨~ action of water⟩

[2]**solvent** *n* : a usu. liquid substance capable of dissolving or dispersing one or more other substances

so•ma \'sō-mə\ *n, pl* **so•ma•ta** \'sō-mə-tə\ *or* **somas** **1** : the body of an organism **2** : all of an organism except the germ cells **3** : CELL BODY

So•ma \'sō-mə\ *trademark* — used for a preparation of carisoprodol

som•aes•thet•ic *chiefly Brit var of* SOMESTHETIC

somat- *or* **somato-** *comb form* **1** : body ⟨*somato*sensory⟩ **2** : somatic and ⟨*somato*psychic⟩

so•mat•ic \sō-'ma-tik, sə-\ *adj* **1 a** : of, relating to, or affecting the body esp. as distinguished from the germplasm or psyche : PHYSICAL **b** : of, relating to, supplying, or involving skeletal muscles ⟨the ~ nervous system⟩ **2** : of or relating to the wall of the body as distinguished from the viscera : PARIETAL — **so•mat•i•cal•ly** *adv*

somatic cell *n* : any of the cells of the body that compose the tissues, organs, and parts of that individual other than the germ cells

somatic mutation *n* : a mutation occurring in a somatic cell

so•ma•ti•za•tion \ˌsō-mə-tə-'zā-shən\ *n* : conversion of a mental state (as depression or anxiety) into physical symptoms; *also* : the existence of physical bodily complaints in the absence of a known medical condition

somatization disorder *n* : a somatoform disorder characterized by multiple and recurring physical complaints for which the patient has sought medical treatment over several years without any organic or physiological basis for the symptoms being found

so•ma•to•form disorder \'sō-mə-tə-ˌfȯrm-, sə-'ma-tə-\ *n* : any of a group of psychological disorders (as body dysmorphic disorder or hypochondriasis) marked by physical complaints for which no organic or physiological explanation is found and for which there is a strong likelihood that psychological factors are involved

so•ma•to•mam•mo•tro•pin \ˌsō-mə-tə-ˌma-mə-'trō-pᵊn, sə-ˌma-tə-\ *n* : any of several hormones (as growth hormone and prolactin) having lactogenic and somatotropic properties; *esp* : PLACENTAL LACTOGEN

so•ma•to•me•din \sō-ˌma-tə-'mēd-ᵊn, ˌsō-mə-tə-\ *n* : any of several endogenous peptides produced esp. in the liver that are dependent on and mediate growth hormone activity; *specif* : INSULIN-LIKE GROWTH FACTOR

so•ma•to•pause \sō-'ma-tə-ˌpȯz, 'sō-mə-tə-\ *n* : a gradual and progressive decrease in growth hormone secretion that occurs normally with increasing age during adult life and is associated with an increase in adipose tissue and LDL levels and a decrease in lean body mass

so•ma•to•plasm \sō-'ma-tə-ˌpla-zəm, 'sō-mət-ə-\ *n* **1** : protoplasm of somatic cells as distinguished from that of germ cells **2** : somatic cells as distinguished from germ cells

so•ma•to•pleure \sō-'ma-tə-ˌplu̇r, 'sō-mə-tə-\ *n* : a complex fold of tissue in the embryo that consists of an outer layer of mesoderm together with the ectoderm ensheathing it and that gives rise to the amnion and chorion — compare SPLANCHNOPLEURE

so•ma•to•psy•chic \sō-ˌma-tə-'sī-kik, ˌsō-mə-tə-\ *adj* : of or relating to the body and the mind

so•ma•to•sen•so•ry \sō-ˌma-tə-'sens-ə-rē, ˌsō-mə-tə-\ *adj* : of, relating to, or being sensory activity having its origin elsewhere than in the special sense organs (as eyes and ears) and conveying information about the state of the body proper and its immediate environment ⟨~ pathways⟩

somatosensory cortex *n* : either of two regions in the postcentral gyrus that receive and process somatosensory stimuli — called also *somatosensory area*

so•mato•stat•in \sō-ˌma-tə-'stat-ᵊn\ *n* : a polypeptide neurohormone that is found esp. in the hypothalamus, is composed of a chain of 14 amino acid residues, and inhibits the secretion of several other hormones (as growth hormone, insulin, and gastrin)

so•ma•to•ther•a•py \ˌsō-mə-tə-'ther-ə-pē, sō-ˌma-tə-\ *n, pl* **-pies** : therapy for psychological problems that uses physiological intervention (as by drugs or surgery) to modify behavior — **so•ma•to•ther•a•peu•tic** \-ˌther-ə-'pyü-tik\ *adj*

so•ma•to•top•ic \-'tä-pik\ *adj* : of, relating to, or mediating the orderly and specific relation between particular body regions (as a hand or the face) and corresponding motor areas of the brain — **so•ma•to•top•i•cal•ly** *adv*

so•ma•to•trope \sō-'ma-tə-ˌtrōp, 'sō-mə-tə-\ *n* : SOMATOTROPH

so•ma•to•troph \-ˌtrōf, -ˌträf\ *n* : any of various cells of the adenohypophysis of the pituitary gland that secrete growth hormone — called also *somatotrope*

so•ma•to•trop•ic \-ˈtrō-pik, -ˈträ-\ *or* **so•ma•to•tro•phic** \-ˈtrō-fik\ *adj* : promoting growth ⟨~ activity⟩

somatotropic hormone *n* : GROWTH HORMONE

so•ma•to•tro•pin \-ˈtrō-pən\ *also* **so•ma•to•tro•phin** \-fən\ *n* : GROWTH HORMONE

so•ma•to•type \ˈsō-mə-tə-ˌtīp, sō-ˈma-tə-\ *n* : a body type or physique esp. in a system of classification based on the relative development of ectomorphic, endomorphic, and mesomorphic components — **somatotype** *vb*

so•ma•tro•pin \sō-ˈma-trə-pən, ˌsō-mə-ˈtrō-\ *n* : HUMAN GROWTH HORMONE; *esp* : a recombinant version of human growth hormone

-some \ˌsōm\ *n comb form* **1** : body ⟨chromo*some*⟩ **2** : chromosome ⟨mono*some*⟩

som•es•thet•ic \ˌsō-mes-ˈthe-tik\ *adj* : of, relating to, or concerned with bodily sensations ⟨the ~ area of the brain⟩

-so•mia \ˈsō-mē-ə\ *n comb form* : condition of having (such) a body ⟨micro*somia*⟩

-som•ic \ˌsō-mik\ *adj comb form* : having or being a chromosome complement of which one or more but not all chromosomes or genomes exhibit (such) a degree of reduplication ⟨mono*somic*⟩

so•mite \ˈsō-ˌmīt\ *n* : one of the longitudinal series of segments into which the body of many animals is divided : METAMERE

somnambul- *comb form* : sleep in which motor acts are performed ⟨*somnambul*ist⟩

som•nam•bu•lant \säm-ˈnam-byə-lənt\ *adj* : walking or tending to walk while asleep

som•nam•bu•late \-ˌlāt\ *vb* **-lat•ed; -lat•ing** : to walk while asleep — **som•nam•bu•la•tion** \-ˌnam-byə-ˈlā-shən\ *n*

som•nam•bu•lism \säm-ˈnam-byə-ˌli-zəm\ *n* **1** : an abnormal condition of sleep in which motor acts (as walking) are performed **2** : actions characteristic of somnambulism — **som•nam•bu•lis•tic** \-ˌnam-byə-ˈlis-tik\ *adj*

som•nam•bu•list \säm-ˈnam-byə-list\ *n* : SLEEPWALKER

somni- *comb form* : sleep ⟨*somni*facient⟩

[1]**som•ni•fa•cient** \ˌsäm-nə-ˈfā-shənt\ *adj* : inducing sleep : HYPNOTIC 1

[2]**somnifacient** *n* : a somnifacient agent (as a drug) : HYPNOTIC 1

som•nif•er•ous \säm-ˈni-fə-rəs\ *adj* : SOPORIFIC

som•no•lence \ˈsäm-nə-ləns\ *n* : the quality or state of being drowsy — **som•no•lent** \-lənt\ *adj*

So•mo•gyi effect \ˈsō-mō-jē-\ *n* : hyperglycemia following an episode of hypoglycemia; *esp* : hyperglycemia that occurs after breakfast following nocturnal hypoglycemia and that may occur in type 1 diabetes esp. when too much insulin has been taken the day before — called also *Somogyi phenomenon;* compare DAWN PHENOMENON

Somogyi, Michael (1883–1971), American biochemist.

son- *or* **sono-** *comb form* : sound ⟨*sono*gram⟩

So•na•ta \sō-ˈnä-tə\ *trademark* — used for a preparation of zaleplon

sono•gram \ˈsä-nə-ˌgram\ *n* : an image produced by ultrasound — called also *echogram, ultrasonogram*

so•nog•ra•pher \sō-ˈnä-grə-fər\ *n* : a person trained in the use of ultrasound — called also *ultrasonographer*

so•nog•ra•phy \sō-ˈnä-grə-fē\ *n, pl* **-phies** : ULTRASOUND 2 — **sono•graph•ic** \ˌsä-nə-ˈgra-fik\ *adj* — **sono•graph•i•cal•ly** \-fi-k(ə-)lē\ *adv*

so•po•rif•er•ous \ˌsä-pə-ˈri-fə-rəs, ˌsō-\ *adj* : SOPORIFIC

[1]**so•po•rif•ic** \-ˈri-fik\ *adj* : causing or tending to cause sleep

[2]**soporific** *n* : a soporific agent (as a drug)

sorb \ˈsȯrb\ *vb* : to take up and hold by either adsorption or absorption

sor•bic acid \ˈsȯr-bik-\ *n* : a crystalline acid $C_6H_8O_2$ obtained from the unripe fruits of the mountain ash (genus *Sorbus*) or synthesized and used esp. as a fungicide and food preservative

sor•bi•nil \ˈsȯr-bə-ˌnil\ *n* : a drug $C_{11}H_{19}FN_2O_3$ that has been used experimentally in the treatment of diabetic neuropathy

sor•bi•tol \ˈsȯr-bə-ˌtȯl, -ˌtōl\ *n* : a faintly sweet alcohol $C_6H_{14}O_6$ that occurs esp. in fruits of the mountain ash (genus *Sorbus*), is made synthetically, and is used esp. as a humectant, a softener, and a sweetener and in making ascorbic acid

sor•des \ˈsȯr-(ˌ)dēz\ *n, pl* **sordes** : the crusts that collect on the teeth and lips in debilitating diseases with protracted low fever

[1]**sore** \ˈsōr\ *adj* **sor•er; sor•est** **1** : causing pain or distress ⟨a ~ wound⟩ **2** : painful esp. from overuse, injury, or inflammation ⟨~ muscles⟩ — **sore•ly** *adv* — **sore•ness** *n*

[2]**sore** *n* : a localized sore spot on the body; *esp* : one (as an ulcer) with the tissues ruptured or abraded and usu. with infection

sore mouth *n* **1** : a highly contagious disease of sheep and goats that is caused by a poxvirus (species *Orf virus* of the genus *Parapoxvirus*) and is characterized by extensive vesiculation and subsequent ulceration about the lips, gums, and tongue — called also *scabby mouth* **2** : necrobacillosis affecting the mouth; *esp* : CALF DIPHTHERIA

sore•muz•zle \-ˌməz-ᵊl\ *n* : BLUETONGUE

sore throat *n* : painful throat due to inflammation of the fauces and pharynx

So•ri•a•tane \ˈsȯr-ē-ə-ˌtān\ *trademark* — used for a preparation of acitretin

SOS *abbr* [Latin *si opus sit*] if occasion require; if necessary — used in writing prescriptions

so•ta•lol \ˈsō-tə-ˌlȯl, -ˌlōl\ *n* : a beta-adrenergic blocking agent administered in the form of its hydrochloride $C_{12}H_{20}N_2O_3S·HCl$ to treat ventricular arrhythmias

souf•fle \ˈsü-fəl\ *n* : a blowing sound heard on auscultation ⟨the uterine ~ heard in pregnancy⟩

[1]**sound** \ˈsau̇nd\ *adj* **1** : free from injury or disease : exhibiting normal health **2** : deep and undisturbed ⟨a ~ sleep⟩ — **sound•ness** *n*

[2]**sound** *n* **1** : a particular auditory impression ⟨heart ~*s* heard by auscultation⟩ **2** : the sensation perceived by the sense of hearing **3** : mechanical radiant energy that is transmitted by waves of pressure in a material medium (as air) and is the objective cause of hearing

[3]**sound** *vb* : to explore or examine (a body cavity) with a sound

[4]**sound** *n* : an elongated instrument for exploring or examining body cavities ⟨a uterine ~⟩

sound pollution *n* : NOISE POLLUTION

sound wave *n* **1** : SOUND 1 **2** *pl* : longitudinal pressure waves esp. when transmitting audible sound

sour \ˈsau̇r\ *adj* : causing, characterized by, or being the one of the four basic taste sensations that is produced chiefly by acids — compare BITTER, SALT, SWEET — **sour•ness** *n*

South American blastomycosis *n* : blastomycosis caused by a fungus of the genus *Paracoccidioides* (*P. brasiliensis* syn. *Blastomyces brasiliensis*) and characterized by formation of ulcers on the mucosal surfaces of the mouth that spread to lips, nose, and cheeks, by great enlargement of lymph nodes esp. of the throat and chest, and by involvement of the gastrointestinal tract — called also *paracoccidioidomycosis*

South•ern blot \ˈsə-t͟hərn-\ *n* : a blot consisting of a sheet of a cellulose derivative or nylon that contains spots of DNA for identification by a suitable molecular probe — compare NORTHERN BLOT, WESTERN BLOT — **Southern blotting** *n*

Southern, Edwin M. (*fl* 1975), British biologist.

So•val•di \sō-ˈväl-dē\ *trademark* — used for a preparation of sofosbuvir

spa \ˈspä, ˈspȯ\ *n* **1 a** : a mineral spring **b** : a resort with mineral springs **2** : a commercial establishment (as a resort) providing facilities devoted esp. to health, fitness, weight loss, beauty, and relaxation

space maintainer *n* : a temporary orthodontic appliance used following the loss or extraction of a tooth (as a milk tooth) to prevent the shifting of adjacent teeth into the resulting space — called also *space retainer*

space medicine *n* : a branch of medicine concerned with the physiological and biological effects on the human body of spaceflight

space perception *n* : the perception of the properties and relationships of objects in space esp. with respect to direction, size, distance, and orientation

spac•er \ˈspā-sər\ *n* : a region of chromosomal DNA between genes that is not transcribed into messenger RNA and is of uncertain function

space retainer *n* : SPACE MAINTAINER

space sickness *n* : sickness and esp. nausea and dizziness that occurs under the conditions of sustained spaceflight — **space•sick** \ˈspās-ˌsik\ *adj*

Spanish flu *n* : influenza that is caused by a subtype (H1N1) of the orthomyxovirus causing influenza A and that was responsible for about 500,000 deaths in the U.S. in the influenza pandemic of 1918–1919 — called also *Spanish influenza;* compare ASIAN FLU, HONG KONG FLU

Spanish fly *n* **1** : a green beetle (*Lytta vesicatoria* of the family Meloidae) of southern Europe that is the source of cantharides **2** : CANTHARIS 2

spar•ga•no•sis \ˌspär-gə-ˈnō-səs\ *n, pl* **-no•ses** \-ˌsēz\ : the condition of being infected with spargana

spar•ga•num \ˈspär-gə-nəm\ *n, pl* **-na** \-nə\ *also* **-nums** : an intramuscular or subcutaneous vermiform parasite that is the larva of a tapeworm (as *Spirometra mansoni*)

Spar•ine \ˈspär-ˌēn\ *n* : a preparation of promazine — formerly a U.S. registered trademark

spar•te•ine \ˈspär-tē-ən, ˈspär-ˌtēn\ *n* : a liquid alkaloid used esp. formerly in medicine in the form of its hydrated sulfate $C_{15}H_{26}N_2·H_2SO_4·5H_2O$

spasm \ˈspa-zəm\ *n* **1** : an involuntary and abnormal contraction of muscle or muscle fibers or of a hollow organ (as the esophagus) that consists largely of involuntary muscle fibers **2** : the state or condition of a muscle or organ affected with spasms — **spas•mod•ic** \spaz-ˈmä-dik\ *adj* — **spas•mod•i•cal•ly** *adv*

spasmodic dysmenorrhea *n* : dysmenorrhea associated with painful contractions of the uterus

spasmodic torticollis *n* : CERVICAL DYSTONIA

spas•mo•gen•ic \ˌspaz-mə-ˈje-nik\ *adj* : inducing spasm ⟨a ~ drug⟩

spas•mo•lyt•ic \ˌspaz-mə-ˈli-tik\ *adj* : ANTISPASMODIC ⟨~ drugs⟩ — **spasmolytic** *n*

spas•mo•phil•ia \ˌspaz-mə-ˈfi-lē-ə\ *n* : an abnormal tendency to convulsions, tetany, or spasms from even slight mechanical or electrical stimulation ⟨~ associated with rickets⟩

[1]**spas·tic** \ˈspas-tik\ *adj* **1** : of, relating to, or characterized by spasm **2** : affected with or marked by spasticity or spastic paralysis ⟨a ~ patient⟩ ⟨~ hemiplegia⟩ — **spas·ti·cal·ly** *adv*

[2]**spastic** *n* : an individual affected with spastic paralysis

spastic cerebral palsy *n* : the most common form of cerebral palsy marked by hypertonic muscles and stiff and jerky movements

spastic colon *n* : IRRITABLE BOWEL SYNDROME; *also* : a colon affected with spasms

spas·ti·ci·ty \spa-ˈsti-sə-tē\ *n, pl* **-ties** : a spastic state or condition; *esp* : muscular hypertonicity with increased tendon reflexes

spastic paralysis *n* : paralysis with tonic spasm of the affected muscles and with increased tendon reflexes

spat *past and past part of* SPIT

spa·tial \ˈspā-shəl\ *adj* **1** : relating to, occupying, or having the character of space ⟨~ disorientation⟩ **2** : of or relating to facility in perceiving relations (as of objects) in space ⟨~ ability⟩ — **spa·tial·ly** \-sh(ə-)lē\ *adv*

spatial summation *n* : sensory summation that involves stimulation of several spatially separated neurons at the same time

spat·u·la \ˈspa-chə-lə\ *n* : a flat thin instrument used for spreading or mixing soft substances, scooping, lifting, or scraping

spav·in \ˈspa-vən\ *n* : osteoarthritis of the hock of a horse — **spav·ined** \-vənd\ *adj*

spay \ˈspā\ *vb* **spayed**; **spay·ing** : to remove the ovaries and uterus of (a female animal)

SPCA *abbr* Society for the Prevention of Cruelty to Animals

spe·cial·ist \ˈspe-shə-list\ *n* : a medical practitioner whose practice is limited to a particular class of patients (as children) or of diseases (as skin diseases) or of technique (as surgery); *esp* : a physician who is qualified by advanced training and certification by a specialty examining board to so limit his or her practice

Spe·cial K \ˈspe-shəl-ˈkā\ *n, slang* : the anesthetic ketamine used illicitly

special needs *n pl* : the individual requirements (as for education) of a person with a disadvantaged background or a mental, emotional, or physical disability or a high risk of developing one — **special–needs** *adj*

special sense *n* : any of the senses of sight, hearing, equilibrium, smell, taste, or touch

spe·cial·ty \ˈspe-shəl-tē\ *n, pl* **-ties** : something (as a branch of medicine) in which one specializes

spe·cies \ˈspē-(ˌ)shēz, -(ˌ)sēz\ *n, pl* **species 1 a** : a category of biological classification ranking immediately below the genus or subgenus, comprising related organisms or populations potentially capable of interbreeding, and being designated by a binomial that consists of the name of the genus followed by an uncapitalized noun or adjective that is Latin or has a Latin form and agrees grammatically with the genus name **b** : an individual or kind belonging to a biological species **2** : a particular kind of atomic nucleus, atom, molecule, or ion

[1]**spe·cif·ic** \spi-ˈsi-fik\ *adj* **1 a** : restricted by nature to a particular individual, situation, relation, or effect **b** : exerting a distinctive influence (as on a body part or a disease) ⟨~ antibodies⟩ **2** : of, relating to, or constituting a species and esp. a biological species

[2]**specific** *n* : a drug or remedy having a specific mitigating effect on a disease

specific epithet *n* : a noun or adjective that is Latin or has a Latin form and follows the genus name in a taxonomic binomial

specific gravity *n* : the ratio of the density of a substance to the density of some substance (as pure water) taken as a standard when both densities are obtained by weighing in air

spec·i·fic·i·ty \ˌspe-sə-ˈfi-sə-tē\ *n, pl* **-ties** : the quality or condition of being specific: as **a** : the condition of being peculiar to a particular individual or group of organisms ⟨host ~ of a parasite⟩ **b** : the condition of participating in or catalyzing only one or a few chemical reactions ⟨enzyme ~⟩

spec·i·men \ˈspe-sə-mən\ *n* **1** : an individual, item, or part typical of a group, class, or whole **2** : a portion or quantity of material for use in testing, examination, or study ⟨a urine ~⟩

SPECT *abbr* single photon emission computed tomography

spec·ta·cles \ˈspek-ti-kəlz\ *n pl* : GLASSES

spec·ti·no·my·cin \ˌspek-tə-nō-ˈmīs-ᵊn\ *n* : a white crystalline broad-spectrum antibiotic derived from a bacterium of the genus *Streptomyces* (*S. spectabilis*) that is used clinically esp. in the form of its hydrated dihydrochloride $C_{14}H_{24}N_2O_7·2HCl·5H_2O$ to treat gonorrhea — called also *actinospectacin;* see TROBICIN

spec·tral \ˈspek-trəl\ *adj* : of, relating to, or made by a spectrum

spec·trin \ˈspek-trən\ *n* : a large cytoskeletal protein that is found on the inner cell membrane of red blood cells and that functions esp. in maintaining cell shape

spec·trom·e·ter \spek-ˈträ-mə-tər\ *n* **1** : an instrument used for measuring wavelengths of light spectra **2** : any of various analytical instruments in which an emission (as of particles or radiation) is dispersed according to some property (as mass or energy) of the emission and the amount of dispersion is measured ⟨nuclear magnetic resonance ~⟩ — **spec•tro•met•ric** \ˌspek-trə-ˈme-trik\ *adj* — **spec•trom•e•try** \spek-ˈträ-mə-trē\ *n*

spec•tro•pho•tom•e•ter \ˌspek-trō-fə-ˈtä-mə-tər\ *n* : a photometer for measuring the relative intensities of the light in different parts of a spectrum — **spec•tro•pho•to•met•ric** \-trə-ˌfō-tə-ˈme-trik\ *adj* — **spec•tro•pho•to•met•ri•cal•ly** *adv* — **spec•tro•pho•tom•e•try** \ˌspek-(ˌ)trō-fə-ˈtä-mə-trē\ *n*

spec•tro•scope \ˈspek-trə-ˌskōp\ *n* : an instrument for forming and examining optical spectra — **spec•tro•scop•ic** \ˌspek-trə-ˈskä-pik\ *adj* — **spec•tro•scop•i•cal•ly** *adv* — **spec•tros•co•pist** \spek-ˈträs-kə-pist\ *n* — **spec•tros•co•py** \spek-ˈträs-kə-pē\ *n*

spec•trum \ˈspek-trəm\ *n, pl* **spec•tra** \-trə\ *or* **spectrums** **1** : an array of the components of an emission or wave separated and arranged in the order of some varying characteristic (as wavelength, mass, or energy) **2** : a continuous sequence or range; *specif* : a range of effectiveness against pathogenic organisms — see BROAD-SPECTRUM, NARROW-SPECTRUM

spec•u•lum \ˈspe-kyə-ləm\ *n, pl* **-la** \-lə\ *also* **-lums** : any of various instruments for insertion into a body passage to facilitate visual inspection or medication ⟨a vaginal ~⟩ ⟨a nasal ~⟩ — **spec•u•lar** \-lər\ *adj*

speech \ˈspēch\ *n* : the communication or expression of thoughts in spoken words

speech center *n* : a brain center exerting control over speech : BROCA'S AREA

speech therapist *n* : a specialist in speech therapy

speech therapy *n* : therapeutic treatment of impairments and disorders of speech, voice, language, communication, and swallowing

speed \ˈspēd\ *n* : METHAMPHETAMINE; *also* : a related stimulant drug and esp. an amphetamine

spell \ˈspel\ *n* : a period of bodily or mental distress or disorder ⟨fainting ~*s*⟩

sperm \ˈspərm\ *n, pl* **sperm** *or* **sperms** **1** : SEMEN **2** : a male gamete : SPERMATOZOON — **sper•mat•ic** \(ˌ)spər-ˈma-tik\ *adj*

sperm- *or* **spermo-** *or* **sperma-** *or* **spermi-** *comb form* : seed : germ : sperm ⟨*spermi*cidal⟩

spermat- *or* **spermato-** *comb form* : seed : spermatozoon ⟨*spermat*id⟩

spermatic artery — see INTERNAL SPERMATIC ARTERY

spermatic cord *n* : a cord that suspends the testis within the scrotum, contains the vas deferens and vessels and nerves of the testis, and extends from the deep inguinal ring through the inguinal canal and superficial inguinal ring downward into the scrotum

spermatic duct *n* : VAS DEFERENS

spermatic plexus *n* : a nerve plexus that receives fibers from the renal plexus and a plexus associated with the aorta and that passes with the testicular artery to the testis

spermatic vein *n* : TESTICULAR VEIN

sper•ma•tid \ˈspər-mə-tid\ *n* : one of the haploid cells that are formed by division of the secondary spermatocytes and that differentiate into spermatozoa — compare OOTID

sper•mato•cele \(ˌ)spər-ˈma-tə-ˌsēl\ *n* : a cystic swelling of the ducts in the epididymis or in the rete testis usu. containing spermatozoa

sper•mato•cide \(ˌ)spər-ˈma-tə-ˌsīd\ *n* : SPERMICIDE — **sper•mato•cid•al** \-ˌma-tə-ˈsīd-ᵊl\ *adj*

sper•mato•cyte \(ˌ)spər-ˈma-tə-ˌsīt\ *n* : a cell giving rise to sperm; *esp* : a cell that is derived from a spermatogonium and ultimately gives rise to four haploid spermatids

sper•mato•gen•e•sis \(ˌ)spər-ˌma-tə-ˈje-nə-səs\ *n, pl* **-e•ses** \-ˌsēz\ : the process of male gamete formation including formation of a primary spermatocyte from a spermatogonium, meiotic division of the spermatocyte, and transformation of the four resulting spermatids into spermatozoa — **sper•mato•gen•ic** \-ˈje-nik\ *adj*

sper•mato•go•ni•um \-ˈgō-nē-əm\ *n, pl* **-nia** \-nē-ə\ : a primitive male germ cell that gives rise to primary spermatocytes in spermatogenesis — **sper•mato•go•ni•al** \-nē-əl\ *adj*

sper•ma•tor•rhea \ˌspər-mə-tə-ˈrē-ə, (ˌ)spər-ˌma-\ *n* : abnormally frequent or excessive emission of semen without orgasm

sper•ma•tor•rhoea *chiefly Brit var of* SPERMATORRHEA

spermatozoa *pl of* SPERMATOZOON

sper•ma•to•zo•al \ˌspər-mə-tə-ˈzō-əl, (ˌ)spər-ˌma-\ *adj* : of or relating to spermatozoa

sper•ma•to•zo•an \(ˌ)spər-ˌma-tə-ˈzō-ən, ˌspər-mə-\ *n* : SPERMATOZOON — **spermatozoan** *adj*

sper•ma•to•zo•on \-ˈzō-ˌän, -ˈzō-ən\ *n, pl* **-zoa** \-ˈzō-ə\ : a motile male gamete of an animal usu. with rounded or elongate head and a long posterior flagellum

sperm cell *n* : SPERM 2

sperm duct *n* : VAS DEFERENS

spermi- *or* **spermo-** — see SPERM-

-sper•mia \ˈspər-mē-ə\ *n comb form* : condition of having or producing (such) sperm ⟨*aspermia*⟩

-sper•mic \ˈspər-mik\ *adj comb form* : being the product of (such) a number of spermatozoa : resulting from (such) a multiple fertilization ⟨poly*spermic*⟩

sper·mi·cide \ˈspər-mə-ˌsīd\ *n* : a preparation or substance (as nonoxynol-9) used to kill sperm — called also *spermatocide* — **sper·mi·cid·al** \ˌspər-mə-ˈsīd-ᵊl\ *adj* — **sper·mi·cid·al·ly** *adv*

sper·mio·gen·e·sis \ˌspər-mē-ō-ˈje-nə-səs\ *n, pl* **-e·ses** \-ˌsēz\ **1** : SPERMATOGENESIS **2** : transformation of a spermatid into a spermatozoon

-sper·my \ˈspər-mē\ *n comb form, pl* **-sper·mies** : state of exhibiting or resulting from (such) a fertilization ⟨poly*spermy*⟩

SPF \ˌes-(ˌ)pē-ˈef\ *n* : a number assigned to a sunscreen that is the factor by which the time required for unprotected skin to become sunburned is increased when the sunscreen is used — called also *sun protection factor*

S phase *n* : the period in the cell cycle during which DNA replication takes place — compare G_1 PHASE, G_2 PHASE, M PHASE

sphen- *or* **spheno-** *comb form* : sphenoid and ⟨*spheno*palatine⟩

sphe·no·eth·moid recess \ˌsfē-nō-ˈeth-ˌmȯid-\ *n* : a small space between the sphenoid bone and the superior nasal concha into which the sphenoid sinus opens

[1]**sphe·noid** \ˈsfē-ˌnȯid\ *or* **sphe·noi·dal** \sfē-ˈnȯid-ᵊl\ *adj* : of, relating to, or being a compound bone of the base of the cranium formed by the fusion of several bony elements with the basisphenoid and in humans consisting of a median body from whose sides extend a pair of broad curved winglike expansions in front of which is another pair of much smaller triangular lateral processes while ventrally two large deeply cleft processes extend downward — see GREATER WING, LESSER WING

[2]**sphenoid** *n* : a sphenoid bone

sphenoid sinus *or* **sphenoidal sinus** *n* : either of two irregular cavities in the body of the sphenoid bone that communicate with the nasal cavities

sphe·no·man·dib·u·lar ligament \ˌsfē-nō-man-ˈdi-byə-lər-\ *n* : a flat thin band of fibrous tissue derived from Meckel's cartilage which extends downward from the sphenoid bone to the lingula of the mandibular foramen

sphe·no·max·il·lary fissure \ˌsfē-nō-ˈmak-sə-ˌler-ē-, -mak-ˈsi-lə-re-\ *n* : ORBITAL FISSURE b

[1]**sphe·no·pal·a·tine** \ˌsfē-nō-ˈpa-lə-ˌtīn\ *adj* : of, relating to, lying in, or distributed to the vicinity of the sphenoid and palatine bones

[2]**sphenopalatine** *n* : a sphenopalatine part; *specif* : PTERYGOPALATINE GANGLION

sphenopalatine foramen *n* : a foramen between the sphenoidal and orbital parts of the vertical plate of the palatine bone; *also* : a deep notch between these parts that by articulation with the sphenoid bone is converted into a foramen

sphenopalatine ganglion *n* : PTERYGOPALATINE GANGLION

sphe·no·pa·ri·etal sinus \ˌsfē-nō-pə-ˈrī-ət-ᵊl-\ *n* : a venous sinus of the dura mater on each side of the cranium arising at a meningeal vein near the apex of the lesser wing of the sphenoid bone and draining into the anterior part of the cavernous sinus

spher- *or* **sphero-** *comb form* : spherical ⟨*sphero*cyte⟩

sphe·ro·cyte \ˈsfir-ə-ˌsīt, ˈsfer-\ *n* : a more or less globular red blood cell that is characteristic of some hemolytic anemias — **sphe·ro·cyt·ic** \ˌsfir-ə-ˈsi-tik, ˌsfer-\ *adj*

sphe·ro·cy·to·sis \ˌsfir-ō-sī-ˈtō-səs, ˌsfer-\ *n* : the presence of spherocytes in the blood; *esp* : HEREDITARY SPHEROCYTOSIS

sphinc·ter \ˈsfiŋk-tər\ *n* : an annular muscle surrounding and able to contract or close a bodily opening — see ANAL SPHINCTER, CARDIAC SPHINCTER, PRECAPILLARY SPHINCTER, PYLORIC SPHINCTER — **sphinc·ter·al** \-tə-rəl\ *adj*

sphincter ani ex·ter·nus \-ˈā-ˌnī-ik-ˈstər-nəs\ *n* : ANAL SPHINCTER a

sphincter ani in·ter·nus \-in-ˈtər-nəs\ *n* : ANAL SPHINCTER b

sphinc·ter·ic \sfiŋk-ˈter-ik\ *adj* : of, relating to, or being a sphincter

sphincter of Od·di \-ˈä-dē\ *n* : a complex sphincter closing the duodenal orifice of the common bile duct

Oddi, Ruggero (1864–1913), Italian physician.

sphinc·tero·plas·ty \ˈsfiŋk-tər-ə-ˌplas-tē\ *n, pl* **-ties** : plastic surgery of a sphincter ⟨anal ~⟩

sphinc·ter·ot·o·my \ˌsfiŋk-tər-ˈä-tə-mē\ *n, pl* **-mies** : surgical incision of a sphincter

sphincter pu·pil·lae \-pyü-ˈpi-lē\ *n* : a broad flat band of smooth muscle in the iris that surrounds the pupil of the eye

sphincter ure·thrae \-yu̇-ˈrē-thrē\ *n* : a muscle composed of fibers that arise from the inferior ramus of the ischium and that interdigitate with those from the opposite side of the body to form in the male a narrow ring of muscle around the urethra — called also *urethral sphincter*

sphincter va·gi·nae \-və-ˈjī-nē\ *n* : the bulbocavernosus of the female

sphingo- *comb form* : sphingomyelin ⟨*sphingo*sine⟩

sphin·go·lip·id \ˌsfiŋ-gō-ˈli-pəd\ *n* : any of a group of lipids (as sphingomyelins and cerebrosides) that yield sphingosine or one of its derivatives as one product of hydrolysis

sphin·go·lip·i·do·sis \-ˌli-pə-ˈdō-səs\ *n, pl* **-do·ses** \-ˌsēz\ : any of various usu. hereditary disorders (as Gaucher disease and Tay-Sachs disease) characterized by abnormal metabolism and storage of sphingolipids

sphin·go·my·elin \ˌsfiŋ-gō-ˈmī-ə-lən\ *n* : any of a group of crystalline phosphatides that are obtained esp. from nerve tissue and that on hydrolysis yield a fatty acid, sphingosine, choline, and phosphoric acid

sphin·go·my·elin·ase \-ˈmī-ə-lə-ˌnās, -ˌnāz\ *n* : any of several enzymes that catalyze the hydrolysis of sphingomyelin and are lacking in some metabolic deficiency diseases (as Niemann-Pick disease)

sphin·go·sine \ˈsfiŋ-gə-ˌsēn, -sən\ *n* : an unsaturated amino alcohol $C_{18}H_{37}NO_2$ containing two hydroxyl groups and obtained by hydrolysis of various sphingomyelins, cerebrosides, and gangliosides

sphygmo- *comb form* : pulse ⟨*sphygmo*gram⟩

sphyg·mo·gram \ˈsfig-mə-ˌgram\ *n* : a tracing made by a sphygmograph and consisting of a series of curves that correspond to the beats of the heart

sphyg·mo·graph \ˈsfig-mə-ˌgraf\ *n* : an instrument that records graphically the movements or character of the pulse — **sphyg·mo·graph·ic** \ˌsfig-mə-ˈgra-fik\ *adj*

sphyg·mo·ma·nom·e·ter \ˌsfig-mō-mə-ˈnä-mə-tər\ *n* : an instrument for measuring blood pressure and esp. arterial blood pressure — **sphyg·mo·mano·met·ric** \-ˌma-nə-ˈme-trik\ *adj* — **sphyg·mo·ma·nom·e·try** \-mə-trē\ *n*

spi·ca \ˈspī-kə\ *n, pl* **spi·cae** \-ˌkē\ *or* **spicas** : a bandage that is applied in successive V-shaped crossings and is used to immobilize a limb esp. at a joint; *also* : such a bandage impregnated with plaster of paris

spic·ule \ˈspi-(ˌ)kyül\ *n* : a minute slender pointed usu. hard body (as of bone)

spi·der \ˈspī-dər\ *n* **1** : any of an order (Araneae syn. Araneida) of arachnids having a body with two main divisions, four pairs of walking legs, and two or more pairs of abdominal organs for spinning threads of silk used esp. in making webs for catching prey **2** : SPIDER NEVUS ⟨an arterial ~⟩

spider nevus *n* : a pigmented area on the skin formed of dilated capillaries or arterioles radiating from a central point like the legs of a spider — called also *spider angioma*

spider vein *n* : a telangiectasia (as on the legs or face) often appearing as a central area with outward radiations resembling the legs of a spider

Spiel·mey·er–Vogt disease \ˈshpēl-ˌmī-ər-ˈfōkt-\ *n* : BATTEN DISEASE

Spielmeyer, Walter (1879–1935), and **Vogt, Heinrich** (1875–1957), German neurologists.

spi·ge·lian hernia \spī-ˈjē-lē-ən-\ *n, often cap S* : a hernia occurring along the linea semilunaris

Spie·ghel \ˈspē-gəl\, **Adriaan van den** (1578–1625), Flemish anatomist.

spigelian lobe *n, often cap S* : CAUDATE LOBE

[1]**spike** \ˈspīk\ *n* **1** : the pointed element in the wave tracing in an electroencephalogram **2** : a sharp increase in body temperature followed by a rapid fall **3** : a momentary sharp increase and fall in the record of an action potential; *also* : ACTION POTENTIAL

[2]**spike** *vb* **spiked; spik·ing** : to undergo a sudden sharp increase in (temperature or fever) usu. up to an indicated level ⟨her fever *spiked* to 103°⟩

spike potential *n* **1** : SPIKE 3 **2** : ACTION POTENTIAL

spik·ing *adj* : characterized by recurrent sharp rises in body temperature ⟨a ~ fever⟩; *also* : resulting from a sharp rise in body temperature ⟨a ~ temperature of 105°⟩

spin- *or* **spini-** *or* **spino-** *comb form* **1** : spinal column : spinal cord ⟨*spino*tectal tract⟩ **2** : of, relating to, or involving the spinal cord and ⟨*spino*cerebellar⟩

spi·na \ˈspī-nə\ *n, pl* **spi·nae** \-ˌnē\ : an anatomical spine or spinelike process

spina bi·fi·da \-ˈbi-fə-də, -ˈbī-\ *n* : a neural tube defect marked by congenital cleft of the spinal column usu. with hernial protrusion of the meninges and sometimes the spinal cord — see MENINGOCELE, MYELOCELE, MYELOMENINGOCELE

spina bifida oc·cul·ta \-ə-ˈkəl-tə\ *n* : a mild often asymptomatic form of spina bifida in which there is no hernial protrusion of the meninges of the spinal cord

spinae — see ERECTOR SPINAE

[1]**spi·nal** \ˈspīn-ᵊl\ *adj* **1** : of, relating to, or situated near the spinal column **2 a** : of, relating to, or affecting the spinal cord ⟨~ reflexes⟩ **b** : having the spinal cord functionally isolated (as by surgical section) from the brain ⟨experiments on ~ animals⟩ **c** : used for spinal anesthesia ⟨a ~ anesthetic⟩ **3** : made for or fitted to the spinal column ⟨a ~ brace⟩ — **spi·nal·ly** *adv*

[2]**spinal** *n* : a spinal anesthetic

spinal accessory nerve *n* : ACCESSORY NERVE

spinal accessory nucleus *n* : a cluster of motor neurons in the ventral horn of the cervical region of the spinal cord that give rise to the accessory nerve

spinal and bulbar muscular atrophy *n* : KENNEDY'S DISEASE

spinal anesthesia *n* : anesthesia produced by injection of an anesthetic into the subarachnoid space of the spine

spinal artery *n* **:** any of three arteries that supply the spinal cord and its membranes and adjacent structures: **a :** a single unpaired artery that is formed by the anastomosis of a branch of the vertebral artery on each side — called also *anterior spinal artery* **b :** either of two arteries of which one arises from a vertebral artery on each side below the level at which the corresponding branch of the anterior spinal artery arises — called also *posterior spinal artery*

spinal canal *n* **:** VERTEBRAL CANAL

spinal column *n* **:** the articulated series of vertebrae connected by ligaments and separated by more or less elastic intervertebral fibrocartilages that forms the supporting axis of the body and a protection for the spinal cord and that extends from the hind end of the skull through the median dorsal part of the body to the coccyx — called also *backbone, spine, vertebral column*

spinal cord *n* **:** the thick longitudinal cord of nervous tissue that in vertebrates extends along the back dorsal to the bodies of the vertebrae and is enclosed in the vertebral canal formed by their neural arches, is continuous anteriorly with the medulla oblongata, gives off at intervals pairs of spinal nerves to the various parts of the trunk and limbs, serves not only as a pathway for nerve impulses to and from the brain but as a center for carrying out and coordinating many reflex actions independently of the brain, and is composed largely of white matter arranged in columns and tracts of longitudinal fibers about a large central core of gray matter — called also *medulla spinalis*

spinales *pl of* SPINALIS

spinal fluid *n* **:** CEREBROSPINAL FLUID

spinal fusion *n* **:** surgical fusion of two or more vertebrae for remedial immobilization of the spine

spinal ganglion *n* **:** a ganglion on the dorsal root of each spinal nerve that is one of a series of ganglia containing cell bodies of sensory neurons — called also *dorsal root ganglion*

spi•na•lis \spī-ˈnā-ləs, spi-ˈna-lis\ *n, pl* **spi•na•les** \-(ˌ)lēz\ **:** the most medial division of the sacrospinalis situated next to the spinal column and acting to extend it or any of the three muscles making up this division: **a :** SPINALIS THORACIS **b :** SPINALIS CERVICIS **c :** SPINALIS CAPITIS

spinalis ca•pi•tis \-ˈka-pə-təs\ *n* **:** a muscle that arises with, inserts with, and is intimately associated with the semispinalis capitis

spinalis cer•vi•cis \-ˈsər-və-səs\ *n* **:** an inconstant muscle that arises esp. from the spinous processes of the lower cervical and upper thoracic vertebrae and inserts esp. into the spinous process of the axis

spinalis tho•ra•cis \-thō-ˈrā-səs\ *n* **:** an upward continuation of the sacrospinalis that is situated medially to and blends with the longissimus thoracis, arises from the spinous processes of the first two lumbar and last two thoracic vertebrae, and inserts into the spinous processes of the upper thoracic vertebrae

spinal meningitis *n* **:** inflammation of the meninges of the spinal cord; *also* **:** CEREBROSPINAL MENINGITIS

spinal muscular atrophy *n* **:** any of several inherited disorders (as Kugelberg-Welander disease) that are characterized by the degeneration of motor neurons in the spinal cord resulting in muscular weakness and atrophy and that in some forms (as Werdnig-Hoffmann disease) are fatal

spinal nerve *n* **:** any of the paired nerves which leave the spinal cord, supply muscles of the trunk and limbs, and connect with the nerves of the sympathetic nervous system, which arise by a short motor ventral root and a short sensory dorsal root, and of which there are 31 pairs in humans classified according to the part of the spinal cord from which they arise into 8 pairs of cervical nerves, 12 pairs of thoracic nerves, 5 pairs of lumbar nerves, 5 pairs of sacral nerves, and one pair of coccygeal nerves

spinal puncture *n* **:** LUMBAR PUNCTURE

spinal shock *n* **:** a temporary condition following transection of the spinal cord that is characterized by muscular flaccidity and loss of motor reflexes in all parts of the body below the point of transection

spinal stenosis *n* **:** narrowing of the lumbar spinal column that produces pressure on the nerve roots resulting in sciatica and a condition resembling intermittent claudication and that usu. occurs in middle or old age

spinal tap *n* **:** LUMBAR PUNCTURE

spin•dle \ˈspind-ᵊl\ *n* **1 :** something shaped like a round stick or pin with tapered ends: as **a :** a network of chiefly microtubular fibers along which the chromosomes are distributed during mitosis and meiosis **b :** MUSCLE SPINDLE **2 :** SLEEP SPINDLE

spindle cell *n* **:** a spindle-shaped cell (as in some tumors)

spindle–cell sarcoma *n* **:** a sarcoma (as a fibrosarcoma) composed chiefly or entirely of spindle cells

spindle fiber *n* **:** any of the filaments constituting a mitotic spindle

spine \ˈspīn\ *n* **1 :** SPINAL COLUMN **2 :** a pointed prominence or process (as on a bone)

spin echo *n* **:** a signal that is detected in a nuclear magnetic resonance spectrometer and is produced by a planned series of radio-frequency pulses — usu. used attributively; compare GRADIENT ECHO

spine of the scapula *n* : a projecting triangular bony process on the dorsal surface of the scapula that divides it obliquely into the area of origin of parts of the supraspinatus and infraspinatus muscles and that terminates in the acromion

spini- *or* **spino-** — see SPIN-

spinn•bar•keit \ˈspin-ˌbär-ˌkīt, ˈshpin-\ *n* : the elastic quality that is characteristic of mucus of the uterine cervix esp. shortly before ovulation

spi•no•cer•e•bel•lar \ˌspī-nō-ˌser-ə-ˈbel-ər\ *adj* : of or relating to the spinal cord and cerebellum ⟨~ pathways⟩

spinocerebellar ataxia *n* : any of a group of inherited neurodegenerative disorders that are characterized by cerebellar dysfunction manifested esp. by progressive ataxia — abbr. *SCA*

spinocerebellar tract *n* : any of four nerve tracts which pass from the spinal cord to the cerebellum and of which two are situated on each side external to the crossed corticospinal tracts: **a** : a posterior tract on each side that begins at the level of the attachments of the second or third lumbar spinal nerves and ascends to the inferior cerebellar peduncle and vermis of the cerebellum — called also *dorsal spinocerebellar tract, posterior spinocerebellar tract* **b** : an anterior tract on each side that arises from cells mostly in the dorsal horn of gray matter on the same or opposite side and passes through the medulla oblongata and pons to the superior cerebellar peduncle and vermis — called also *ventral spinocerebellar tract*

spi•no–ol•i•vary \-ˈä-lə-ˌver-ē\ *adj* : connecting the spinal cord with the olivary nuclei ⟨~ fibers⟩

spi•nose ear tick \ˈspī-ˌnōs-\ *n* : an ear tick of the genus *Otobius* (*O. megnini*) that is a serious pest of cattle, horses, sheep, and goats

spinosum — see FORAMEN SPINOSUM, STRATUM SPINOSUM

spi•no•tec•tal tract \ˌspī-nō-ˈtekt-ᵊl-\ *n* : an ascending tract of nerve fibers in each lateral funiculus of white matter of the spinal cord that passes upward and terminates in the superior colliculus of the opposite side

spi•no•tha•lam•ic \ˌspī-nō-thə-ˈla-mik\ *adj* : of, relating to, comprising, or associated with the spinothalamic tracts ⟨the ~ system⟩

spinothalamic tract *n* : any of four tracts of nerve fibers of the spinal cord that are arranged in pairs with one member of a pair on each side and that ascend to the thalamus by way of the brain stem: **a** : one on each side of the anterior median fissure that carries nerve impulses relating to the sense of touch — called also *anterior spinothalamic tract, ventral spinothalamic tract* **b** : one on each lateral part of the spinal cord that carries nerve impulses relating to the senses of touch, pain, and temperature — called also *lateral spinothalamic tract*

spi•nous \ˈspī-nəs\ *adj* : slender and pointed like a spine

spinous process *n* : SPINE 2; *specif* : the median spinelike or platelike dorsal process of the neural arch of a vertebra

spiny–headed worm *n* : ACANTHOCEPHALAN

spi•ral \ˈspī-rəl\ *adj* **1 a** : winding around a center or pole and gradually receding from or approaching it **b** : HELICAL ⟨the ~ structure of DNA⟩ **2** : being a fracture in which the break is produced by twisting apart the bone — **spiral** *n* — **spi•ral•ly** *adv*

spiral ganglion *n* : a mass of bipolar cell bodies occurring in the modiolus of the organ of Corti and giving off axons which comprise the cochlear nerve

spiralis — see LAMINA SPIRALIS

spiral lamina *n* : a twisting shelf of bone which projects from the modiolus into the canal of the cochlea — called also *lamina spiralis*

spiral ligament *n* : the thick periosteum that forms the outer wall of the cochlear duct

spiral organ *n* : ORGAN OF CORTI

spiral valve *n* : a series of crescentic folds of mucous membrane somewhat spirally arranged on the interior of the gallbladder and continuing into the cystic duct

spi•ra•my•cin \ˌspī-rə-ˈmīs-ᵊn\ *n* : a mixture of macrolide antibiotics produced by a soil bacterium of the genus *Streptomyces* (*S. ambofaciens*) and having antibacterial activity

spi•ril•lum \spī-ˈri-ləm\ *n* **1** *cap* : a genus of gram-negative bacteria having tufts of flagella at both poles and usu. living in stagnant water rich in organic matter — see RAT-BITE FEVER **2** *pl* **-ril•la** \-ˈri-lə\ : any bacterium of the genus *Spirillum*

spir•it \ˈspir-ət\ *n* **1 a** : the liquid containing ethyl alcohol and water that is distilled from an alcoholic liquid or mash — often used in pl. **b** : a usu. volatile organic solvent (as an alcohol, ester, or hydrocarbon) **2** : an alcoholic solution of a volatile substance ⟨~ of camphor⟩

spirit of harts•horn *or* **spirits of harts•horn** \-ˈhärts-ˌhȯrn\ *n* : AMMONIA WATER

Spi•ri•va \spi-ˈrē-və\ *trademark* — used for a preparation of tiotropium

spiro- *comb form* : respiration ⟨*spi*rometer⟩

Spi•ro•cer•ca \ˌspī-rō-ˈsər-kə\ *n* : a genus of red filarial worms (family Thelaziidae) forming nodules in the walls of the digestive tract and sometimes the aorta of canines

spi•ro•chaet•ae•mia, spi•ro•chaete, spi•ro•chae•ti•ci•dal, spi•ro•chaet•osis *chiefly Brit var of* SPIROCHETEMIA, SPIROCHETE, SPIROCHETICIDAL, SPIROCHETOSIS

spi•ro•chete \ˈspī-rə-ˌkēt\ *n* : any of an order (Spirochaetales) of slender spirally undulating bacteria including those causing syphilis, yaws, Lyme disease, and relapsing fever — **spi•ro•chet•al** \ˌspī-rə-ˈkēt-ᵊl\ *adj*

spi•ro•chet•emia \ˌspī-rə-ˌkē-ˈtē-mē-ə\ *n* : the abnormal presence of spirochetes in the circulating blood

spi•ro•che•ti•ci•dal \ˌspī-rə-ˌkē-tə-ˈsīd-ᵊl\ *adj* : destructive to spirochetes ⟨a ~ drug⟩ — **spi•ro•che•ti•cide** \ˌspī-rə-ˈkē-tə-ˌsīd\ *n*

spi•ro•chet•osis \ˌspī-rə-ˌkē-ˈtō-səs\ *n, pl* **-oses** \-ˌsēz\ : infection with or a disease caused by spirochetes

spi•ro•gram \ˈspī-rə-ˌgram\ *n* : a graphic record of respiratory movements traced on a revolving drum

spi•ro•graph \ˈspī-rə-ˌgraf\ *n* : an instrument for recording respiratory movements — **spi•ro•graph•ic** \ˌspī-rə-ˈgra-fik\ *adj* — **spi•rog•ra•phy** \spī-ˈrä-grə-fē\ *n*

spi•rom•e•ter \spi-ˈrä-mə-tər\ *n* : an instrument used in spirometry for measuring the air entering and leaving the lungs — **spi•ro•met•ric** \ˌspī-rə-ˈme-trik\ *adj*

Spi•rom•e•tra \spī-ˈrä-mə-trə, spi-\ *n* : a genus of pseudophyllidean tapeworms including several (as *S. mansoni* of Asia and *S. mansonoides* of the southern U.S.) which sometimes cause sparganosis in humans

spi•rom•e•try \spi-ˈrä-mə-trē\ *n, pl* **-tries** : measurement by means of a spirometer of the volume of air entering and leaving the lungs (as to determine lung function in diagnosing pulmonary disease)

spi•ro•no•lac•tone \ˌspī-rə-nō-ˈlak-ˌtōn, spi-ˌrō-nə-\ *n* : an aldosterone antagonist $C_{24}H_{32}O_4S$ that promotes diuresis and sodium excretion and is used to treat essential hypertension, edema with congestive heart failure, hepatic cirrhosis with ascites, nephrotic syndrome, and idiopathic edema

[1]**spit** \ˈspit\ *vb* **spit** *or* **spat** \ˈspat\; **spit•ting** : to eject (as saliva) from the mouth

[2]**spit** *n* : SALIVA

spitting cobra *n* : any of several cobras (as *Naja nigrocollis* and *Hemachatus haemachatus* of Africa) that in defense typically eject their venom toward the victim without striking

spit•tle \ˈspit-ᵊl\ *n* : SALIVA

splanch•nic \ˈsplaŋk-nik\ *adj* : of or relating to the viscera : VISCERAL

splanch•ni•cec•to•my \ˌsplaŋk-nə-ˈsek-tə-mē\ *n, pl* **-mies** : surgical excision of a segment of one or more splanchnic nerves to relieve hypertension

splanchnic ganglion *n* : a small ganglion on the greater splanchnic nerve that is usu. located near the eleventh or twelfth thoracic vertebra

splanchnic nerve *n* : any of three nerves situated on each side of the body and formed by the union of branches from the six or seven lower thoracic and first lumbar ganglia of the sympathetic system: **a** : a superior one ending in the celiac ganglion — called also *greater splanchnic nerve* **b** : a middle one ending in a detached ganglionic mass of the celiac ganglion — called also *lesser splanchnic nerve* **c** : an inferior one ending in the renal plexus — called also *least splanchnic nerve, lowest splanchnic nerve*

splanchno- *comb form* : viscera ⟨*splanchno*logy⟩

splanch•nol•o•gy \splaŋk-ˈnä-lə-jē\ *n, pl* **-gies** : a branch of anatomy concerned with the viscera

splanch•no•pleure \ˈsplaŋk-nə-ˌplu̇r\ *n* : a layer of tissue that consists of the inner of the two layers into which the unsegmented sheet of mesoderm splits in the embryo together with the endoderm internal to it and that forms most of the walls and substance of the visceral organs — compare SOMATOPLEURE

splay•foot \ˈsplā-ˌfu̇t, -ˈfu̇t\ *n* : a foot abnormally flattened and spread out; *specif* : FLATFOOT — **splay•foot•ed** \-ˈfu̇-təd\ *adj*

spleen \ˈsplēn\ *n* : a highly vascular ductless organ that plays a role in the final destruction of red blood cells, filtration and storage of blood, and production of lymphocytes, and that in humans is a dark purplish flattened oblong object of a soft fragile consistency lying in the upper left part of the abdominal cavity near the cardiac end of the stomach and which is divisible into a loose friable red pulp in intimate connection with the blood supply and with red blood cells free in its interstices and a denser white pulp chiefly of lymphoid tissue condensed in masses about the small arteries

splen- *or* **spleno-** *comb form* : spleen ⟨*splen*ectomy⟩ ⟨*spleno*megaly⟩

sple•nec•to•my \spli-ˈnek-tə-mē\ *n, pl* **-mies** : surgical excision of the spleen — **sple•nec•to•mize** \spli-ˈnek-tə-ˌmīz\ *vb*

splen•ic \ˈsple-nik\ *adj* : of, relating to, or located in the spleen

splenic artery *n* : the branch of the celiac artery that carries blood to the spleen and sends branches also to the pancreas and the cardiac end of the stomach

splenic fever *n* : ANTHRAX

splenic flexure *n* : the sharp bend of the colon under the spleen where the transverse colon joins the descending colon — called also *left colic flexure*

splenic flexure syndrome *n* : pain in the upper left quadrant of the abdomen that may radiate upward to the left shoulder and inner aspect of the left arm and that sometimes mimics angina pectoris but is caused by bloating and gas in the colon

splenic pulp *n* : the characteristic tissue of the spleen

splenic vein *n* : the vein that carries blood away from the spleen and that joins the superior mesenteric vein to form the portal vein — called also *lienal vein*

sple•ni•um \ˈsplē-nē-əm\ *n, pl* **-nia** \-nē-ə\ : the thick rounded fold that forms the posterior border of the corpus callosum and is continuous by its undersurface with the fornix

sple•ni•us \-nē-əs\ *n, pl* **-nii** \-nē-ˌī\ : either of two flat oblique muscles on each side of the back of the neck and upper thoracic region: **a** : SPLENIUS CAPITIS **b** : SPLENIUS CERVICIS

splenius cap•i•tis \-ˈka-pi-təs\ *n* : a flat muscle on each side of the back of the neck and the upper thoracic region that arises from the caudal half of the ligamentum nuchae and the spinous processes of the seventh cervical and the first three or four thoracic vertebrae, that is inserted into the occipital bone and the mastoid process of the temporal bone, and that rotates the head to the side on which it is located and with the help of the muscle on the opposite side extends it

splenius cer•vi•cis \-ˈsər-vi-kəs\ *n* : a flat narrow muscle on each side of the back of the neck and the upper thoracic region that arises from the spinous processes of the third to sixth thoracic vertebrae, is inserted into the transverse processes of the first two or three cervical vertebrae, and acts to rotate the head to the side on which it is located and with the help of the muscle on the opposite side to extend and arch the neck

spleno- — see SPLEN-

sple•no•cyte \ˈsplē-nə-ˌsīt, ˈsple-\ *n* : a macrophage of the spleen

spleno•meg•a•ly \ˌsple-nō-ˈme-gə-lē\ *n, pl* **-lies** : abnormal enlargement of the spleen

spleno•re•nal \ˌsple-nō-ˈrēn-ᵊl\ *adj* : of, relating to, or joining the splenic and renal veins or arteries

sple•no•sis \splē-ˈnō-səs\ *n, pl* **-no•ses** \-ˌsēz\ *or* **-no•sis•es** : a rare condition in which fragments of tissue from a ruptured spleen become implanted throughout the peritoneal cavity and often undergo regeneration and vascularization

splice \ˈsplīs\ *vb* **spliced; splic•ing** : to join together or insert (as segments of RNA or DNA) to form new genetic combinations ⟨~ a human gene for insulin into a bacterium⟩ — see GENE-SPLICING

spli•ce•o•some \ˈsplī-sē-ə-ˌsōm\ *n* : a ribonucleoprotein complex that is the site in the cell nucleus where introns are excised from precursor messenger RNA and exons are joined together to form functional messenger RNA — **spli•ce•o•som•al** \ˌsplī-sē-ə-ˈsō-məl\ *adj*

[1]**splint** \ˈsplint\ *n* **1** : material or a device used to protect and immobilize a body part **2** : a bony enlargement on the upper part of the cannon bone of a horse usu. on the inside of the leg

[2]**splint** *vb* **1** : to support and immobilize (as a broken bone) with a splint **2** : to protect against pain by reducing the motion of

splin•ter \ˈsplin-tər\ *n* : a thin piece (as of wood) split or broken off lengthwise; *esp* : such a piece embedded in the skin — **splinter** *vb*

split \ˈsplit\ *vb* **split; split•ting** : to divide or break down (a chemical compound) into constituents; *also* : to remove by such separation

split–brain \ˈsplit-ˌbrān\ *adj* : of, relating to, concerned with, or having undergone separation of the two cerebral hemispheres by surgical division of the optic chiasma and corpus callosum ⟨~ patients⟩

split personality *n* **1** : SCHIZOPHRENIA — not used technically **2** : MULTIPLE PERSONALITY DISORDER — not used technically

spondyl- *or* **spondylo-** *comb form* : vertebra : vertebrae ⟨*spondyl*osis⟩

spon•dyl•ar•thri•tis \ˌspän-di-lär-ˈthrī-təs\ *n, pl* **-thrit•i•des** \-ˈthri-tə-ˌdēz\ : arthritis of the spine

spon•dy•li•tis \ˌspän-də-ˈlī-təs\ *n* : inflammation of the vertebrae ⟨tuberculous ~⟩ — see ANKYLOSING SPONDYLITIS — **spon•dy•lit•ic** \-ˈli-tik\ *adj*

spon•dy•lo•ar•throp•a•thy \ˌspän-də-lō-är-ˈthrä-pə-thē\ *also* **spon•dyl•ar•throp•a•thy** \ˌspän-də-lär-ˈthrä-\ *n, pl* **-thies** : any of several diseases (as ankylosing spondylitis) affecting the joints of the spine

spon•dy•lo•lis•the•sis \ˌspän-də-lō-lis-ˈthē-səs\ *n* : forward displacement of a lumbar vertebra on the one below it and esp. of the fifth lumbar vertebra on the sacrum producing pain by compression of nerve roots

spon•dy•lol•y•sis \ˌspän-də-ˈlä-lə-səs\ *n, pl* **-y•ses** \-ˌsēz\ : disintegration or dissolution of a vertebra

spon•dy•lop•a•thy \ˌspän-də-ˈlä-pə-thē\ *n, pl* **-thies** : any disease or disorder of the vertebrae

spon•dy•lo•sis \ˌspän-də-ˈlō-səs\ *n, pl* **-lo•ses** \-ˌsēz\ *or* **-lo•sis•es** : any of various degenerative diseases of the spine

sponge \ˈspənj\ *n* **1 a** : a pad (as of folded gauze) used in surgery and medicine (as to remove discharge or apply medication) **b** : a porous dressing (as of fibrin or gelatin) applied to promote wound healing **c** : a plastic prosthesis used in chest cavities following lung surgery **2** : an absorbent contraceptive device impregnated with spermicide that is inserted into the vagina before sexual intercourse to cover the cervix and act as a barrier to sperm — **sponge** *vb*

sponge bath *n* : a bath in which water is applied to the body without actual immersion

spongi- *or* **spongio-** *comb form* : spongy ⟨*spongio*blast⟩

spon·gi·form \ˈspən-ji-ˌfȯrm\ *adj* : of, relating to, or being a spongiform encephalopathy ⟨~ lesions⟩

spongiform encephalopathy *n* : any of various degenerative diseases of the brain characterized by the development of porous spongelike lesions in brain tissue and by deterioration in neurological functioning; *specif* : PRION DISEASE

spon·gi·o·blas·to·ma \ˌspən-jē-ō-(ˌ)bla-ˈstō-mə, ˌspän-\ *n, pl* **-mas** *also* **-ma·ta** \-mə-tə\ : GLIOBLASTOMA

spon·gi·o·cyte \ˈspən-jē-ō-ˌsīt, ˈspän-\ *n* : any of the cells of the adrenal cortex that have a spongy appearance due to lipid vacuoles the contents of which have been dissolved out

spon·gi·o·sa \ˌspən-jē-ˈō-sə, ˌspän-\ *n* : the part of a bone (as much of the epiphyseal area of long bones) made up of spongy cancellous bone

spon·gi·o·sis \ˌspən-jē-ˈō-səs, ˌspän-\ *n* : swelling localized in the epidermis and often occurring in eczema

spongiosum — see CORPUS SPONGIOSUM, STRATUM SPONGIOSUM

spongy \ˈspən-jē\ *adj* **spong·i·er; -est** : resembling a sponge; *esp* : full of cavities : CANCELLOUS ⟨~ bone⟩

spon·ta·ne·ous \spän-ˈtā-nē-əs\ *adj* **1** : proceeding from natural feeling or native tendency without external constraint **2** : developing without apparent external influence, force, cause, or treatment ⟨a ~ nosebleed⟩ — **spon·ta·ne·ous·ly** *adv*

spontaneous abortion *n* : naturally occurring expulsion of a nonviable fetus

spontaneous recovery *n* : reappearance of an extinguished conditioned response without positive reinforcement

spoon nails \ˈspün-\ *n* : KOILONYCHIA

spor- *or* **spori-** *or* **sporo-** *comb form* : seed : spore ⟨*sporo*cyst⟩

spo·rad·ic \spə-ˈra-dik\ *adj* **1** : occurring occasionally, singly, or in scattered instances ⟨~ diseases⟩ — compare ENDEMIC, EPIDEMIC 1 **2** : arising or occurring randomly with no known cause ⟨~ Creutzfeldt-Jakob disease⟩ — **spo·rad·i·cal·ly** *adv*

Spor·a·nox \ˈspȯr-ə-ˌnäks\ *trademark* — used for a preparation of itraconazole

spore \ˈspōr\ *n* : a primitive usu. unicellular often environmentally resistant dormant or reproductive body produced by plants, fungi, and some microorganisms and capable of development into a new individual either directly or after fusion with another spore — **spore** *vb*

spo·ro·blast \ˈspō-rə-ˌblast\ *n* : a cell of a sporozoan resulting from sexual reproduction and producing spores and sporozoites

spo·ro·cyst \-ˌsist\ *n* **1** : a case or cyst secreted by some sporozoans preliminary to sporogony; *also* : a sporozoan encysted in such a case **2** : a saccular body that is the first asexual reproductive form of a digenetic trematode, develops from a miracidium, and buds off cells from its inner surface which develop into rediae

spo·ro·gen·e·sis \ˌspōr-ə-ˈje-nə-səs\ *n, pl* **-e·ses** \-ˌsēz\ **1** : reproduction by spores **2** : spore formation — **spo·rog·e·nous** \spə-ˈrä-jə-nəs, spȯ-\ *also* **spo·ro·gen·ic** \ˌspōr-ə-ˈje-nik\ *adj*

spo·rog·o·ny \spə-ˈrä-gə-nē\ *n, pl* **-nies** : reproduction by spores; *specif* : formation of spores containing sporozoites that is characteristic of some sporozoans and that results from the encystment and subsequent division of a zygote — **spo·ro·gon·ic** \ˌspōr-ə-ˈgä-nik\ *adj*

spo·ront \ˈspōr-ˌänt\ *n* : a sporozoan that engages in sporogony

spo·ro·phore \ˈspōr-ə-ˌfōr\ *n* : the spore-producing organ esp. of a fungus

spo·ro·thrix \-ˌthriks\ *n* **1** *cap* : a genus of imperfect fungi (family Moniliaceae) that includes the causative agent (*S. schenckii*) of sporotrichosis **2** : any fungus of the genus *Sporothrix*

spo·ro·tri·cho·sis \spə-ˌrä-tri-ˈkō-səs; ˌspōr-ə-tri-\ *n, pl* **-cho·ses** \-ˌsēz\ : infection with or disease caused by a fungus of the genus *Sporothrix* (*S. schenckii* syn. *Sporotrichum schenckii*) that is characterized by often ulcerating or suppurating nodules in the skin, subcutaneous tissues, and nearby lymph nodes and that is usu. transmitted by entry of the fungus through a skin abrasion or wound

spo·ro·zo·an \ˌspōr-ə-ˈzō-ən\ *n* : any of a class (Sporozoa) of strictly parasitic protozoans that have a complex life cycle usu. involving both asexual and sexual generations often in different hosts and that include many serious pathogens (as malaria parasites and babesias) — **sporozoan** *adj*

spo·ro·zo·ite \-ˈzō-ˌīt\ *n* : a usu. motile infective form of some sporozoans (as the malaria parasite) that is a product of sporogony and initiates an asexual cycle in the new host

sports medicine *n* : a medical specialty concerned with the prevention and treatment of injuries and disorders that are related to participation in sports

spor·u·la·tion \ˌspōr-ə-ˈlā-shən, ˌspōr-yə-\ *n* : the formation of spores; *esp* : division into many small spores (as after encystment) — **spor·u·late** \ˈspōr-ə-ˌlāt, ˈspōr-yə-\ *vb*

[1]**spot** \ˈspät\ *n* : a circumscribed mark or area: as **a** : a circumscribed surface lesion of disease (as measles) **b** : a circumscribed abnormality in an organ seen by means of X-rays or an instrument ⟨a ~ on the lung⟩

[2]**spot** *vb* **spot·ted; spot·ting** : to experience abnormal and sporadic bleeding in small amounts from the uterus

spot film *n* : a radiograph of a restricted area in the body

spotted cow·bane \-ˈkau̇-ˌbān\ *n* : a tall biennial No. American herb (*Cicuta maculata*) of the carrot family (Umbelliferae) with clusters of tuberous roots that resemble small sweet potatoes and are extremely poisonous — called also *spotted hemlock*

spotted fever *n* : any of various eruptive fevers; *esp* : ROCKY MOUNTAIN SPOTTED FEVER

sprain \ˈsprān\ *n* : a sudden or violent twist or wrench of a joint causing the stretching or tearing of ligaments and often rupture of blood vessels with hemorrhage into the tissues; *also* : the condition resulting from a sprain that is usu. marked by swelling, inflammation, hemorrhage, and discoloration — compare [3]STRAIN b — **sprain** *vb*

sprain fracture *n* : AVULSION FRACTURE

[1]**spray** \ˈsprā\ *n* : a jet of vapor or finely divided liquid; *specif* : a jet of fine medicated vapor used as an application to a diseased part or to charge the air of a room with a disinfectant or deodorant

[2]**spray** *vb* : to emit a stream or spray of urine ⟨a cat ~*s* to mark its territory⟩

spreading factor *n* : HYALURONIDASE

Spreng·el's deformity \ˈshpreŋ-əlz-, -gəlz-\ *n* : a congenital elevation of the scapula

Sprengel, Otto Gerhard Karl (1852–1915), German surgeon.

spring \ˈspriŋ\ *n* : any of various elastic orthodontic devices used esp. to apply constant pressure to misaligned teeth

spring ligament *n* : PLANTAR CALCANEONAVICULAR LIGAMENT

[1]**sprout** \ˈsprau̇t\ *vb* : to send out new growth : produce sprouts

[2]**sprout** *n* : a new outgrowth (as of nerve tissue)

sprue \ˈsprü\ *n* **1** : CELIAC DISEASE **2** : TROPICAL SPRUE

spud \ˈspəd\ *n* : any of various small surgical instruments with a shape resembling that of a spade

spu·ma·vi·rus \ˈspü-mə-ˌvī-rəs\ *n* : FOAMY VIRUS

spur \ˈspər\ *n* **1** : a projection from an anatomical part : CALCAR **2** : BONE SPUR ⟨painful heel ~*s*⟩ — **spurred** \ˈspərd\ *adj*

spur cell *n* : ACANTHOCYTE

spu·ri·ous \ˈspyu̇r-ē-əs\ *adj* : simulating a symptom or condition without being pathologically or morphologically genuine ⟨~ labor pains⟩

spu·tum \ˈspü-təm, ˈspyü-\ *n, pl* **spu·ta** \-tə\ : matter expectorated from the respiratory system and esp. the lungs that is composed of mucus but may contain pus, blood, fibrin, or microorganisms (as bacteria) in diseased states

squa·la·mine \ˈskwä-lə-ˌmēn\ *n* : a steroid broad-spectrum antibiotic $C_{34}H_{67}N_3O_5S$ that has been shown to inhibit angiogenesis in tumors

squa·ma \ˈskwā-mə, ˈskwä-\ *n, pl* **squa·mae** \ˈskwā-ˌmē, ˈskwä-ˌmī\ : a structure resembling a scale or plate: as **a** : the curved platelike posterior portion of the occipital bone **b** : the vertical portion of the frontal bone that forms the forehead **c** : the thin anterior upper portion of the temporal bone

squame \ˈskwām\ *n* : a scale or flake (as of skin)

squa·mous \ˈskwā-məs\ *adj* **1 a** : covered with or consisting of scales **b** : of, relating to, or being a stratified epithelium that consists at least in its outer layers of small scalelike cells **2** : resembling a scale or plate; *esp* : of, relating to, or being the thin anterior upper portion of the temporal bone

squamous carcinoma *n* : SQUAMOUS CELL CARCINOMA

squamous cell *n* : a cell of or derived from squamous epithelium

squamous cell carcinoma *n* : a carcinoma made up of or arising from squamous cells and usu. occurring in areas of the body exposed to strong sunlight over a period of many years

squash bite \ˈskwäsh-, ˈskwȯsh-\ *n* : an impression of the teeth and mouth made by closing the teeth on modeling composition or wax

squill \ˈskwil\ *n* **1** : a Mediterranean bulbous herb of the genus *Urginea* (esp. *U. maritima*) **2** : the dried sliced bulb of a white-bulbed form of the squill (*Urginea maritima*) used esp. formerly as an expectorant, cardiac stimulant, and diuretic — called also *white squill*

[1]**squint** \ˈskwint\ *vb* **1** : to be cross-eyed **2** : to look or peer with eyes partly closed

[2]**squint** *n* **1** : STRABISMUS **2** : an instance or habit of squinting

squir·rel corn \ˈskwər-əl-\ *n* : a poisonous No. American herb (*Dicentra canadensis* of the family Fumariaceae)

Sr *symbol* strontium

SR *abbr* slow-release; sustained-release

sRNA \ˈes-ˌär-(ˌ)en-ˈā\ *n* : TRANSFER RNA
SRS *abbr* slow-reacting substance
SRS–A *abbr* slow-reacting substance of anaphylaxis
ss *abbr* [Latin *semis*] one half — used in writing prescriptions
S sleep *n* : SLOW-WAVE SLEEP
SSNRI \ˌes-ˌes-ˌen-ˌär-ˈī\ *n* : SNRI
SSPE *abbr* subacute sclerosing panencephalitis
SSRI \ˌes-ˌes-ˌär-ˈī\ *n* : any of a class of antidepressants (as fluoxetine or sertraline) that inhibit the inactivation of serotonin by blocking its reuptake by presynaptic nerve cell endings — called also *selective serotonin reuptake inhibitor;* compare SNRI
SSSS *abbr* staphylococcal scalded skin syndrome
ST \ˌes-ˈtē\ *n* : ST SEGMENT
stab \ˈstab\ *n* : a wound produced by a pointed weapon — **stab** *vb*
stab•bing *adj* : having a sharp piercing quality ⟨~ pain⟩
stab cell *n* : BAND CELL
sta•bil•i•ty \stə-ˈbi-lə-tē\ *n, pl* **-ties** : the quality, state, or degree of being stable ⟨emotional ~⟩
sta•bi•lize \ˈstā-bə-ˌlīz\ *vb* **-lized; -liz•ing** : to make or become stable ⟨~ a patient's condition⟩ — **sta•bi•li•za•tion** \ˌstā-bə-lə-ˈzā-shən\ *n* — **sta•bi•liz•er** \ˈstā-bə-ˌlī-zər\ *n*
sta•ble \ˈstā-bəl\ *adj* **sta•bler; sta•blest 1** : not changing or fluctuating ⟨~ condition⟩ **2** : not subject to insecurity or emotional illness ⟨a ~ personality⟩ **3 a** : not readily altering in chemical makeup or physical state **b** : not spontaneously radioactive
stable factor *n* : FACTOR VII
stable fly *n* : a biting dipteran fly of the genus *Stomoxys* (*S. calcitrans*) that is common in stables
stachy•bot•ryo•tox•i•co•sis \ˌsta-ki-ˌbä-trē-ō-ˌtäk-sə-ˈkō-səs\ *n, pl* **-co•ses** \-ˌsēz\ : a serious and sometimes fatal intoxication chiefly affecting domestic animals (as horses) that is due to ingestion of a toxin produced by a mold (*Stachybotrys chartarum*)
sta•di•om•e•ter \ˌstā-dē-ˈä-mə-tər\ *n* : a device for measuring height that typically consists of a vertical ruler with a sliding horizontal rod or paddle which is adjusted to rest on the top of the head
Sta•dol \ˈstā-ˌdȯl\ *trademark* — used for a preparation of the tartrate of butorphanol
staff \ˈstaf\ *n* : the doctors and surgeons regularly attached to a hospital and helping to determine its policies and guide its activities
staff nurse *n* : a registered nurse employed by a medical facility who does not assist in surgery
staff of Aes•cu•la•pi•us \-ˌes-kyə-ˈlā-pē-əs\ *n* : a conventionalized representation of a staff branched at the top with a single snake twined around it that is used as a symbol of medicine and as the official insignia of the American Medical Association — called also *Aesculapian staff*
[1]**stage** \ˈstāj\ *n* **1** : a period or step in a process, activity, or development: as **a** : one of the distinguishable periods of growth and development of a plant or animal **b** : a period or phase in the course of a disease; *also* : the degree of involvement or severity of a disease **c** : one of two or more operations performed at different times but constituting a single procedure ⟨a two-*stage* thoracoplasty⟩ **d** : any of the four degrees indicating depth of general anesthesia **2** : the small platform of a microscope on which an object is placed for examination
[2]**stage** *vb* **staged; stag•ing** : to determine the phase or severity of (a disease) based on a classification of established symptomatic criteria; *also* : to evaluate (a patient) to determine the phase, severity, or progression of a disease
stag•gers \ˈsta-gərz\ *n pl* **1** : any of various disorders of domestic animals associated with damage to the central nervous system — used with a sing. or pl. verb; see BLIND STAGGERS **2** : vertigo occurring as a symptom of decompression sickness
stag•horn calculus \ˈstag-ˌhȯrn-\ *n* : a large renal calculus with multiple irregular branches
stag•ing \ˈstā-jiŋ\ *n* : the classification of the severity of a disease in distinct stages on the basis of established symptomatic criteria
[1]**stain** \ˈstān\ *vb* **1 a** : to cause discoloration of **b** : to color by processes affecting chemically or otherwise the material itself ⟨~ bacteria with a fluorescent dye⟩ **2** : to receive a stain
[2]**stain** *n* **1** : a discolored spot or area (as on the skin or teeth) — see PORT-WINE STAIN **2** : a dye or mixture of dyes used in microscopy to make minute and transparent structures visible, to differentiate tissue elements, or to produce specific chemical reactions
stair•case effect \ˈstar-ˌkās-\ *n* : TREPPE
Sta•le•vo \stə-ˈlē-vō\ *trademark* — used for a preparation containing carbidopa, L-dopa, and entacapone
stalk \ˈstȯk\ *n* : a slender supporting or connecting part : PEDUNCLE ⟨the pituitary ~⟩ — **stalked** \ˈstȯkt\ *adj* — **stalk•less** *adj*
stam•i•na \ˈsta-mi-nə\ *n* : the strength or vigor of bodily constitution : capacity for standing fatigue or resisting disease
stam•mer \ˈsta-mər\ *vb* **stam•mered; stam•mer•ing** : to make involuntary stops and repetitions in speaking

: STUTTER — **stammer** *n* — **stam·mer·er** \ˈsta-mər-ər\ *n*

stammering *n* **1** : the act of one who stammers **2** : a speech disorder characterized by involuntary stops and repetitions or blocking of utterance : STUTTERING

stanch *also* **staunch** \ˈstȯnch, ˈstänch\ *vb* : to check or stop the flowing of ⟨∼ bleeding⟩; *also* : to stop the flow of blood from ⟨∼ a wound⟩

stand·still \ˈstand-ˌstil\ *n* : a state characterized by absence of motion or of progress : ARREST ⟨cardiac ∼⟩

Stan·ford–Bi·net test \ˈstan-fərd-bi-ˈnā-\ *n* : an intelligence test prepared at Stanford University as a revision of the Binet-Simon scale and commonly employed with children — called also *Stanford-Binet*

A. Binet — see BINET AGE

stan·nous fluoride \ˈsta-nəs-\ *n* : a white compound SnF_2 of tin and fluorine used in toothpastes and oral rinses to combat tooth decay

sta·nol \ˈsta-ˌnȯl, ˈstā-\ *n* : any of the fully saturated phytosterols — see SITOSTANOL

stan·o·lone \ˈsta-nə-ˌlōn\ *n* : a semisynthetic dihydrotestosterone derivative $C_{19}H_{30}O_2$ used esp. in the treatment of breast cancer

stan·o·zo·lol \ˈsta-nə-zō-ˌlȯl\ *n* : an anabolic steroid $C_{21}H_{32}N_2O$

sta·pe·dec·to·my \ˌstā-pi-ˈdek-tə-mē\ *n, pl* **-mies** : surgical removal and prosthetic replacement of part or all of the stapes to relieve deafness

sta·pe·di·al \stā-ˈpē-dē-əl, stə-\ *adj* : of, relating to, or located near the stapes

sta·pe·di·us \stə-ˈpē-dē-əs\ *n, pl* **-dii** \-dē-ˌī\ : a small muscle of the middle ear that arises from the wall of the tympanum, is inserted into the neck of the stapes by a tendon that sometimes contains a slender spine of bone, and serves to check and dampen vibration of the stapes — called also *stapedius muscle*

sta·pes \ˈstā-(ˌ)pēz\ *n, pl* **stapes** *or* **sta·pe·des** \stə-ˈpē-ˌdēz\ : the innermost of the chain of three ossicles in the middle ear which has the form of a stirrup, a base occupying the oval window, and a head connected with the incus — called also *stirrup*

staph \ˈstaf\ *n* : STAPHYLOCOCCUS 2; *also* : an infection with staphylococci

staphyl- *or* **staphylo-** *comb form* : staphylococcal ⟨*staphylo*toxin⟩

staph·y·lo·coc·cal \ˌsta-fə-lō-ˈkä-kəl\ *also* **staph·y·lo·coc·cic** \-ˈkä-kik, -ˈkäk-sik\ *adj* : of, relating to, caused by, or being a staphylococcus

staphylococcal scalded skin syndrome *n* : an acute skin disorder esp. of infants and immunocompromised individuals that is characterized by widespread erythema, peeling, and necrosis of the skin, that is caused by a toxin produced by a bacterium of the genus *Staphylococcus* (*S. aureus*), and that exposes the affected individual to serious infections but is rarely fatal if diagnosed and treated promptly — abbr. *SSSS;* compare TOXIC EPIDERMAL NECROLYSIS

staph·y·lo·coc·co·sis \ˌsta-fə-lō-kä-ˈkō-səs\ *n* : infection with or disease caused by staphylococci

staph·y·lo·coc·cus \ˌsta-fə-lō-ˈkä-kəs\ *n* **1** *cap* : a genus of nonmotile gram-positive spherical bacteria that is placed in either of two families (Staphylococcaceae or Micrococcaceae), contains forms occurring singly, in pairs or tetrads, or in irregular clusters, and includes causative agents of various diseases (as skin infections, food poisoning, and endocarditis) **2** *pl* **-coc·ci** \-ˈkäk-ˌsī\ : any bacterium of the genus *Staphylococcus; broadly* : MICROCOCCUS 2

staph·y·lo·ki·nase \-ˈkī-ˌnās, -ˌnāz\ *n* : a protease from some pathogenic staphylococci that converts plasminogen to plasmin

staph·y·lo·ma \ˌsta-fə-ˈlō-mə\ *n* : a protrusion of the cornea or sclera of the eye

staph·y·lo·tox·in \ˌsta-fə-lō-ˈtäk-sən\ *n* : a toxin produced by staphylococci

sta·ple \ˈstā-pəl\ *n* : a usu. U-shaped and typically metal surgical fastener used to hold layers of tissue together (as in the closure of an incision) — **staple** *vb* — **sta·pler** \-plər\ *n*

starch \ˈstärch\ *n* : a white odorless tasteless granular or powdery complex carbohydrate $(C_6H_{10}O_5)_x$ that is the chief storage form of carbohydrate in plants, is an important foodstuff, has demulcent and absorbent properties, and is used in pharmacy esp. as a dusting powder and as a constituent of ointments and pastes — **starchy** \ˈstär-chē\ *adj*

Star·ling's hypothesis \ˈstär-liŋz-\ *also* **Star·ling hypothesis** \-liŋ-\ *n* : a hypothesis in physiology: the flow of fluids across capillary walls depends on the balance between the force of blood pressure on the walls and the osmotic pressure across the walls so that the declining gradient in blood pressure from the arterial to the venous end of the capillary results in an outflow of fluids at its arterial end with an increasing inflow toward its venous end

E. H. Starling — see FRANK-STARLING LAW

Starling's law of the heart *n* : a statement in physiology: the strength of the heart's systolic contraction is directly proportional to its diastolic expansion with the result that under normal physiological conditions the heart pumps out of the right atrium all the blood returned to it without letting any back up in the veins —

called also *Frank-Starling law, Frank-Starling law of the heart, Starling's law*

start codon *n* : a genetic codon in messenger RNA that stimulates the binding of a transfer RNA which starts protein synthesis — called also *initiation codon;* compare STOP CODON

starve \ˈstärv\ *vb* **starved; starv·ing** **1 a** : to perish from lack of food **b** : to suffer extreme hunger **2** : to deprive of nourishment — **star·va·tion** \stär-ˈvā-shən\ *n*

sta·sis \ˈstā-səs, ˈsta-\ *n, pl* **sta·ses** \ˈstā-ˌsēz, ˈsta-\ : a slowing or stoppage of the normal flow of a bodily fluid or semifluid ⟨biliary ~⟩: as **a** : slowing of the current of circulating blood **b** : reduced motility of the intestines with retention of feces

stasis ulcer *n* : an ulcer (as on the lower leg) caused by localized slowing or stoppage of blood flow

stat \ˈstat\ *adv* : STATIM

-stat \ˌstat\ *n comb form* : agent causing inhibition of growth without destruction ⟨bacterio*stat*⟩

state \ˈstāt\ *n* : mode or condition of being: as **a** : condition of mind or temperament ⟨a manic ~⟩ **b** : a condition or stage in the physical being of something ⟨the gaseous ~ of water⟩

state hospital *n* : a hospital for the mentally ill that is run by a state

stat·im \ˈsta-tim\ *adv* : immediately or without delay

stat·in \ˈsta-tᵊn\ *n* : any of a group of lipid-lowering drugs (as lovastatin and simvastatin) that function by inhibiting a liver enzyme which controls the synthesis of cholesterol and by promoting the production of LDL-binding receptors in the liver resulting in usu. marked decrease in the level of LDL and a modest increase in the level of HDL circulating in blood plasma

sta·tion \ˈstā-shən\ *n* **1** : the place at which someone is positioned or is assigned to remain ⟨the nurse's ~ on a hospital ward⟩ **2** : the act or manner of standing : POSTURE

sta·tion·ary \ˈstā-shə-ˌner-ē\ *adj* **1** : fixed in position : not moving **2** : characterized by a lack of change

stato- *comb form* : balance : equilibrium ⟨*stato*lith⟩

stato·co·nia \ˌsta-tə-ˈkō-nē-ə\ *n pl* : OTOCONIA

stato·lith \ˈstat-ᵊl-ˌith\ *n* : OTOLITH

sta·tus \ˈstā-təs, ˈsta-\ *n, pl* **sta·tus·es** : a particular state or condition

status asth·mat·i·cus \-az-ˈma-ti-kəs\ *n* : a prolonged severe attack of asthma that is unresponsive to initial standard therapy, is characterized esp. by dyspnea, dry cough, wheezing, and hypoxemia, and that may lead to respiratory failure

status ep·i·lep·ti·cus \-ˌe-pə-ˈlep-ti-kəs\ *n* : a state in epilepsy in which the attacks occur in rapid succession without recovery of consciousness

stat·u·to·ry rape \ˈsta-chə-ˌtōr-ē-\ *n* : sexual intercourse with a person who is below the age of consent as defined by law

staunch *var of* STANCH

stav·u·dine \ˈsta-vyü-ˌdēn\ *n* : a synthetic antiretroviral nucleoside drug $C_{10}H_{12}N_2O_4$ that is an analog of thymidine and is administered orally in the treatment of HIV infection — called also *d4T*

STD \ˌes-(ˌ)tē-ˈdē\ *n* : SEXUALLY TRANSMITTED DISEASE

steady state *n* : a state of physiological equilibrium esp. in connection with a specified metabolic relation or activity

steal \ˈstēl\ *n* : abnormal circulation characterized by deviation (as through collateral vessels or by backward flow) of blood to tissues where the normal flow of blood has been cut off by occlusion of an artery

ste·ap·sin \stē-ˈap-sən\ *n* : the lipase in pancreatic juice

stea·rate \ˈstē-ə-ˌrāt, ˈstir-ˌāt\ *n* : a salt or ester of stearic acid

stea·ric acid \stē-ˈar-ik-, ˈstir-ik-\ *n* : a white crystalline fatty acid $C_{18}H_{36}O_2$ obtained from tallow and some other hard fats; *also* : a commercial mixture of stearic and palmitic acids

stea·rin \ˈstē-ə-rən, ˈstir-ən\ *n* : an ester of glycerol and stearic acid $C_3H_5(C_{18}H_{35}O_2)_3$ that is a predominant constituent of many hard fats

steat- *or* **steato-** *comb form* : fat ⟨*stea*toma⟩

ste·a·ti·tis \ˌstē-ə-ˈtī-təs\ *n* : inflammation of fatty tissue; *esp* : YELLOW FAT DISEASE

ste·a·to·ma \ˌstē-ə-ˈtō-mə\ *n, pl* **-mas** *or* **-ma·ta** \-mə-tə\ : SEBACEOUS CYST

ste·ato·py·gia \ˌstē-ə-tə-ˈpi-jē-ə, stē-ˌa-tō-, -ˈpī-\ *n* : an accumulation of a large amount of fat on the buttocks — **ste·ato·py·gous** \-ˈpī-gəs\ *or* **ste·ato·py·gic** \-ˈpi-jik, -ˈpī-\ *adj*

ste·at·or·rhea \(ˌ)stē-ˌa-tə-ˈrē-ə\ *n* : an excess of fat in the stools

ste·at·or·rhoea *chiefly Brit var of* STEATORRHEA

ste·a·to·sis \ˌstē-ə-ˈtō-səs\ *n, pl* **-to·ses** \-ˌsēz\ : FATTY DEGENERATION

Stein–Lev·en·thal syndrome \ˈstīn-ˈlev-ᵊn-ˌthäl-\ *n* : POLYCYSTIC OVARY SYNDROME

Stein, Irving Freiler (1887–1976), and **Leventhal, Michael Leo (1901–1971),** American gynecologists.

Stein·mann pin \ˈstīn-mən-\ *n* : a stainless steel spike used for the internal fixation of fractures of long bones

Steinmann, Fritz (1872–1932), Swiss surgeon.

Ste·lara \stə-ˈlär-ə\ *trademark* — used for a preparation of ustekinumab

Stel·a·zine \ˈste-lə-ˌzēn\ *trademark* — used for a preparation of the hydrochloride of trifluoperazine

stel·late \ˈste-ˌlāt\ *adj* : shaped like a star ⟨a ∼ ulcer⟩

stellate cell *n* : a cell (as a Kupffer cell) with radiating cytoplasmic processes

stellate ganglion *n* : a composite ganglion formed by fusion of the most inferior of the three cervical ganglia with the first thoracic ganglion of the sympathetic chain

stellate ligament *n* : RADIATE LIGAMENT

stellate reticulum *n* : a loosely-connected mass of stellate epithelial cells that in early developmental stages makes up a large portion of the enamel organ

stem cell *n* : an unspecialized cell capable of perpetuating itself through cell division and having the potential to give rise to differentiated cells with specialized functions ⟨hematopoietic *stem cells*⟩

ste·nosed \ste-ˈnōst, -ˈnōzd\ *adj* : affected with stenosis : abnormally constricted ⟨a ∼ eustachian tube⟩

ste·nos·ing \ste-ˈnō-siŋ, -ziŋ\ *adj* : causing or characterized by stenosis (as of a tendon sheath)

ste·no·sis \stə-ˈnō-səs\ *n, pl* **-no·ses** \-ˌsēz\ : a narrowing or constriction of the diameter of a bodily passage or orifice ⟨esophageal ∼⟩ — see AORTIC STENOSIS, MITRAL STENOSIS, PULMONARY STENOSIS, SPINAL STENOSIS, SUBAORTIC STENOSIS

ste·not·ic \stə-ˈnä-tik\ *adj* : of, relating to, characterized by, or causing stenosis ⟨∼ lesions⟩

Sten·sen's duct *also* **Sten·son's duct** \ˈsten-sənz-\ *n* : PAROTID DUCT

Sten·sen *or* **Steen·sen** \ˈstān-sən\, **Niels** (*Latin* **Nicolaus Steno) (1638–1686),** Danish anatomist and geologist.

stent \ˈstent\ *also* **stint** \ˈstint\ *n* **1** : a mold formed from a resinous compound and used for holding a surgical graft in place; *also* : something (as a pad of gauze immobilized by sutures) used like a stent **2** : a short narrow metal or plastic tube often in the form of a mesh that is inserted into the lumen of an anatomical vessel (as an artery or bile duct) esp. to keep a previously blocked passageway open

Stent, Charles R. (1845–1901), British dentist.

stent·ing \ˈsten-tiŋ\ *n* : a surgical procedure or operation for inserting a stent into an anatomical vessel — **stent** *vb*

Steph·a·no·fi·lar·ia \ˌste-fə-ˌnō-fi-ˈlar-ē-ə\ *n* : a genus of filarial worms parasitic in the skin and subcutaneous tissues of ruminants and horses

Steph·a·nu·rus \ˌste-fə-ˈnu̇r-əs, -ˈnyu̇r-\ *n* : a genus of strongylid nematode worms that includes the kidney worm (*S. dentatus*) of swine

ster·co·ra·ceous \ˌstər-kə-ˈrā-shəs\ *adj* : of, relating to, containing, produced by, or being feces : FECAL

ster·cu·lia gum \stər-ˈkül-yə-, -ˈkyül-\ *n* : KARAYA GUM

stere- *or* **stereo-** *comb form* **1** : stereoscopic ⟨*stere*opsis⟩ **2** : having or dealing with three dimensions of space ⟨*stereo*taxic⟩

ste·reo·acui·ty \ˌster-ē-ō-ə-ˈkyü-ə-tē, ˌstir-\ *n, pl* **-ties** : the ability to detect differences in distance using stereoscopic cues that is measured by the smallest difference in the images presented to the two eyes that can be detected reliably

ste·reo·cil·i·um \ˌster-ē-ō-ˈsi-lē-əm, ˌstir-\ *n, pl* **-cil·ia** \-lē-ə\ : a microvillus that resembles cilia and projects from the surface of certain cells (as the auditory hair cells) — see KINOCILIUM

ste·re·og·no·sis \ˌster-ē-äg-ˈnō-səs, ˌstir-\ *n* : ability to perceive or the perception of material qualities (as shape) of an object by handling or lifting it : tactile recognition

ste·reo·iso·mer \ˌster-ē-ō-ˈī-sə-mər, ˌstir-\ *n* : any of a group of isomers in which atoms are linked in the same order but differ in their spatial arrangement — **ste·reo·iso·mer·ic** \-ˌī-sə-ˈmer-ik\ *adj* — **ste·reo·isom·er·ism** \-ī-ˈsä-mə-ˌri-zəm\ *n*

ste·re·op·sis \ˌster-ē-ˈäp-səs, ˌstir-\ *n* : stereoscopic vision

ste·reo·scope \ˈster-ē-ə-ˌskōp, ˈstir-\ *n* : an optical instrument with two eyepieces for helping the observer to combine the images of two pictures taken from points of view a little way apart and thus to get the effect of solidity or depth

ste·reo·scop·ic \ˌster-ē-ə-ˈskä-pik, ˌstir-\ *adj* **1** : of or relating to the stereoscope or the production of three-dimensional images **2** : characterized by the seeing of objects in three dimensions ⟨∼ vision⟩ — **ste·reo·scop·i·cal·ly** *adv* — **ste·re·os·co·py** \ˌster-ē-ˈäs-kə-pē, ˌstir-; ˈster-ē-ə-ˌskō-pē, ˈstir-\ *n*

ste·reo·tac·tic \ˌster-ē-ə-ˈtak-tik, ˌstir-\ *adj* : involving, being, utilizing, or used in a surgical technique for precisely directing the tip of a delicate instrument (as a needle) or beam of radiation in three planes using coordinates provided by medical imaging (as computed tomography) in order to reach a specific locus in the body — **ste·reo·tac·ti·cal·ly** *adv*

stereotactic radiosurgery *n* : a surgical technique involving the use of narrow beams of radiation (as gamma rays) that are precisely targeted by stereotactic methods to destroy tumors or lesions esp. of the brain

ste·reo·tax·ic \ˌster-ē-ə-ˈtak-sik, ˌstir-\ *adj* : STEREOTACTIC — **ste·reo·tax·i·cal·ly** *adv*

ste·reo·tax·is \-ˈtak-səs\ *n, pl* **-tax·es** \-ˌsēz\ : a stereotactic technique or procedure

[1]**ste·reo·type** \ˈster-ē-ə-ˌtīp, ˈstir-\ *vb* **-typed; -typ·ing** **1** : to repeat without variation ⟨*stereotyped* behavior⟩ **2** : to develop a mental stereotype about

[2]**stereotype** *n* : something conforming to a fixed or general pattern; *esp* : an often oversimplified or biased mental picture held to characterize the typical individual of a group — **ste·reo·typ·i·cal** \ˌster-ē-ə-ˈti-pi-kəl\ *also* **ste·reo·typ·ic** \-pik\ *adj*

ste·reo·ty·py \ˈster-ē-ə-ˌtī-pē, ˈstir-\ *n, pl* **-pies** : frequent almost mechanical repetition of the same posture, movement, or form of speech (as in schizophrenia or autism)

ster·il·ant \ˈster-ə-lənt\ *n* : a sterilizing agent

ster·ile \ˈster-əl\ *adj* **1** : failing to produce or incapable of producing offspring ⟨a ~ hybrid⟩ **2** : free from living organisms and esp. microorganisms ⟨a ~ cyst⟩ — **ster·ile·ly** *adv* — **ste·ril·i·ty** \stə-ˈri-lə-tē\ *n*

ster·il·ize \ˈster-ə-ˌlīz\ *vb* **-ized; -iz·ing** : to make sterile: **a** : to deprive of the power of reproducing **b** : to free from living microorganisms (as by the use of physical or chemical agents) — **ster·il·i·za·tion** \ˌster-ə-lə-ˈzā-shən\ *n* — **ster·il·iz·er** \ˈster-ə-ˌlī-zər\ *n*

stern- *or* **sterno-** *comb form* **1** : breast : sternum : breastbone ⟨*sterno*tomy⟩ **2** : sternal and ⟨*sterno*costal⟩

ster·nal \ˈstərn-ᵊl\ *adj* : of or relating to the sternum

ster·ne·bra \ˈstər-nə-brə\ *n, pl* **-brae** \-ˌbrē, -ˌbrī\ : any of the four segments into which the body of the sternum is divided in childhood and which fuse to form the gladiolus

ster·no·cla·vic·u·lar \ˌstər-nō-kla-ˈvi-kyə-lər\ *adj* : of, relating to, or being articulation of the sternum and the clavicle ⟨~ dislocation⟩

ster·no·clei·do·mas·toid \ˌstər-nō-ˌklī-də-ˈmas-ˌtȯid\ *n* : a thick superficial muscle on each side that arises by one head from the first segment of the sternum and by a second from the inner part of the clavicle, that inserts into the mastoid process and occipital bone, and that acts esp. to bend, rotate, flex, and extend the head — **sternocleidomastoid** *adj*

ster·no·clei·do·mas·toi·de·us \-ˌmas-ˈtȯi-dē-əs\ *n, pl* **-dei** \-dē-ˌī\ : STERNOCLEIDOMASTOID

ster·no·cos·tal \ˌstər-nō-ˈkäst-ᵊl\ *adj* : of, relating to, or situated between the sternum and ribs

ster·no·hy·oid \ˌstər-nō-ˈhī-ˌȯid\ *n* : an infrahyoid muscle on each side of the midline that arises from the medial end of the clavicle and the first segment of the sternum, inserts into the body of the hyoid bone, and acts to depress the hyoid bone and the larynx — **sternohyoid** *adj*

ster·no·hy·oi·de·us \-hī-ˈȯi-dē-əs\ *n, pl* **-dei** \-dē-ˌī\ : STERNOHYOID

ster·no·mas·toid muscle \-ˈmas-ˌtȯid-\ *n* : STERNOCLEIDOMASTOID

ster·no·thy·roid \ˌstər-nō-ˈthī-ˌrȯid\ *n* : an infrahyoid muscle on each side of the body below the sternohyoid that arises from the sternum and from the cartilage of the first and sometimes of the second ribs, inserts into the thyroid cartilage, and acts to draw the larynx downward by depressing the thyroid cartilage — **sternothyroid** *adj*

ster·no·thy·roi·de·us \-thī-ˈrȯi-dē-əs\ *n, pl* **-dei** \-dē-ˌī\ : STERNOTHYROID

ster·not·o·my \stər-ˈnä-tə-mē\ *n, pl* **-mies** : surgical incision through the sternum

ster·num \ˈstər-nəm\ *n, pl* **-nums** *or* **-na** \-nə\ : a compound ventral bone or cartilage that lies in the median central part of the body of most vertebrates other than fishes and that in humans is about seven inches (18 centimeters) long, consists in the adult of three parts, and connects with the clavicles and the cartilages of the upper seven pairs of ribs — called also *breastbone*

ster·nu·ta·tion \ˌstər-nyə-ˈtā-shən\ *n* : the act, fact, or noise of sneezing

ster·nu·ta·tor \ˈstər-nyə-ˌtā-tər\ *n* : an agent that induces sneezing and often lacrimation and vomiting

ste·roid \ˈster-ˌȯid, ˈstir-\ *n* : any of numerous natural or synthetic compounds containing a 17-carbon 4-ring system and including the sterols and various hormones and glycosides — see ANABOLIC STEROID — **steroid** *or* **ste·roi·dal** \stə-ˈrȯid-ᵊl\ *adj*

steroid hormone *n* : any of numerous hormones (as estrogen, testosterone, cortisone, and aldosterone) having the characteristic ring structure of steroids and formed in the body from cholesterol

ste·roido·gen·e·sis \stə-ˌrȯi-də-ˈje-nə-səs; ˌstir-ˌȯi-, ˌster-\ *n, pl* **-e·ses** \-ˌsēz\ : synthesis of steroids ⟨adrenal ~⟩ — **ste·roido·gen·ic** \-ˈje-nik\ *adj*

ste·rol \ˈstir-ˌȯl, ˈster-, -ˌōl\ *n* : any of various solid steroid alcohols (as cholesterol) widely distributed in animal and plant lipids

ster·to·rous \ˈstər-tə-rəs\ *adj* : characterized by a harsh snoring or gasping sound — **ster·to·rous·ly** *adv*

stetho·scope \ˈste-thə-ˌskōp\ *n* : an instrument used to detect and study sounds produced in the body that are conveyed to the ears of the listener through rubber tubing connected with a usu. cup-shaped piece placed upon the area to be examined — **stetho·scop·ic** \ˌste-thə-ˈskä-pik\ *adj* — **stetho·scop·i·cal·ly** *adv*

Ste·vens–John·son syndrome \ˈstē-vənz-ˈjän-sən-\ *n* : a severe and sometimes fatal form of erythema multiforme marked esp. by erosive lesions of the skin and mucous membranes (as of the mouth, nose, eye, and anus) that usu. occurs following an infectious illness or adverse drug reaction but often has no identifiable cause

Stevens, Albert Mason (1884–1945), and **Johnson, Frank Chambliss (1894–1934),** American pediatricians.

ste•via \ˈstē-vē-ə\ *n* : a very sweet noncaloric glycoside-containing substance that is obtained from the leaves of a So. American shrub (*Stevia rebaudiana* of the family Compositae)

STH *abbr* somatotropic hormone

sthen•ic \ˈsthe-nik\ *adj* **1** : notably or excessively vigorous or active ⟨~ fever⟩ ⟨~ emotions⟩ **2** : PYKNIC

stib•o•phen \ˈsti-bə-ˌfen\ *n* : a crystalline antimony compound $C_{12}H_4Na_5O_{16}S_4Sb \cdot 7H_2O$ used in the treatment of various tropical diseases

Stick•ler syndrome \ˈstik-lər-\ *n* : a variable disorder of connective tissue that is characterized by myopia, retinal detachment, cleft palate, micrognathia, flat facies, premature arthritis, hip deformity, and hyperextensibility of the large joints and is inherited as an autosomal dominant trait

Stickler, Gunnar B. (*fl* 1965–67), American pediatrician.

stick•tight flea \ˈstik-ˌtīt-\ *n* : a flea of the genus *Echidnophaga* (*E. gallinacea*) that is parasitic esp. on the heads of chickens

sties *pl of* STY

stiff \ˈstif\ *adj* : lacking in suppleness ⟨~ muscles⟩ — **stiff•ness** *n*

stiff–lamb disease \ˈstif-ˌlam-\ *n* : white muscle disease of lambs

stiff–person syndrome *n* : an uncommon neurological disorder of unknown cause that is marked by progressive muscle stiffness in the spine and limbs and esp. the legs and by episodes of painful muscle spasms which occur spontaneously or are triggered by various external stimuli (as a sudden loud noise) — called also *stiff-man syndrome*

sti•fle \ˈstī-fəl\ *n* : the joint next above the hock in the hind leg of a quadruped (as a horse or a dog) corresponding to the human knee

stig•ma \ˈstig-mə\ *n, pl* **stig•ma•ta** \stig-ˈmä-tə, ˈstig-mə-tə\ *or* **stigmas** **1** : an identifying mark or characteristic; *specif* : a specific diagnostic sign of a disease ⟨the *stigmata* of syphilis⟩ **2** : PETECHIA **3** : a small spot, scar, or opening on a plant or animal

stilb•am•i•dine \stil-ˈba-mə-ˌdēn\ *n* : a drug used chiefly in the form of one of its salts $C_{20}H_{28}N_4O_8S_2$ in treating various fungal infections

stil•bes•trol \stil-ˈbes-ˌtrȯl, -ˌtrōl\ *n* : DIETHYLSTILBESTROL

sti•let \ˈstī-lət\ *or* **sti•lette** \sti-ˈlet\ *n* : STYLET

still•birth \ˈstil-ˌbərth\ *n* : the birth of a dead fetus — compare LIVE BIRTH

still•born \-ˌbȯrn\ *adj* : dead at birth — compare LIVE-BORN — **stillborn** *n*

Still's disease \ˈstilz-\ *n* : rheumatoid arthritis esp. in children

Still, Sir George Frederic (1868–1941), British pediatrician.

stim•u•lant \ˈstim-yə-lənt\ *n* **1** : an agent (as a drug) that produces a temporary increase of the functional activity or efficiency of an organism or any of its parts **2** : STIMULUS 2

stim•u•late \-ˌlāt\ *vb* **-lat•ed; -lat•ing** **1** : to excite to activity or growth or to greater activity **2 a** : to function as a physiological stimulus to (as a nerve or muscle) **b** : to arouse or affect by a stimulant (as a drug) — **stim•u•la•tion** \ˌstim-yə-ˈlā-shən\ *n* — **stim•u•la•tive** \ˈstim-yə-ˌlā-tiv\ *adj* — **stim•u•la•to•ry** \-lə-ˌtōr-ē\ *adj*

stim•u•la•tor \ˈstim-yə-ˌlā-tər\ *n* : one that stimulates or provides a stimulus

stim•u•lus \ˈstim-yə-ləs\ *n, pl* **-li** \-ˌlī, -ˌlē\ **1** : STIMULANT 1 **2** : an agent (as an environmental change) that directly influences the activity of living protoplasm (as by exciting a sensory organ or evoking muscular contraction or glandular secretion)

stimulus–response *adj* : of, relating to, or being a reaction to a stimulus; *also* : representing the activity of an organism as composed of such reactions ⟨~ psychology⟩

sting \ˈstiŋ\ *vb* **stung** \ˈstəŋ\; **sting•ing** **1** : to prick painfully: as **a** : to pierce or wound with a poisonous or irritating process **b** : to affect with sharp quick pain **2** : to feel or cause a keen burning pain or smart — **sting** *n*

sting•er \ˈstiŋ-ər\ *n* **1** : a sharp organ (as of a bee or scorpion) that is usu. connected with a poison gland or otherwise adapted to wound by piercing and injecting a poison **2** : a usu. sports-related injury of the brachial plexus marked by a painful burning sensation that radiates from the neck down the arm and is often accompanied by weakness or numbness of the affected area — called also *burner*

stinging nettle *n* : NETTLE 1; *esp* : a Eurasian nettle (*Urtica dioica*) widely naturalized in No. America and having numerous hairs that are extremely irritating to the skin

sting•ray \ˈstiŋ-ˌrā\ *n* : any of numerous large flat cartilaginous fishes (order Rajiformes and esp. family Dasyatidae) with one or more large sharp barbed dorsal spines near the base of the whiplike tail capable of inflicting severe wounds

stint *var of* STENT

stip•pling \ˈstip-liŋ\ *n* : the appearance of spots : a spotted condition (as in basophilic red blood cells)

stir•rup \ˈstər-əp, ˈstir-əp\ *n* **1** : STAPES **2** : an attachment to an examining or operating table designed to raise and spread the legs of a patient

stitch \ˈstich\ *n* **1** : a local sharp and sudden pain esp. in the side **2 a** : one in-and-out movement of a threaded needle in suturing **b** : a portion of a suture left in the tissue after one stitch ⟨removal of ~*es*⟩ — **stitch** *vb*

STM *abbr* short-term memory

stock \ˈstäk\ *n* : a population, colony, or culture of organisms used for scientific research or medical purposes

Stock•holm syndrome \ˈstäk-ˌhō(l)m-\ *n* : the psychological tendency of a hostage to bond with, identify with, or sympathize with his or her captor

stock•ing \ˈstäk-iŋ\ — see ELASTIC STOCKING

Stokes–Ad•ams syndrome \ˈstōks-ˈa-dəmz-\ *n* : fainting sometimes accompanied by seizures that is induced by complete heart block with a pulse rate of 40 beats per minute or less — called also *Adams-Stokes syndrome, Stokes-Adams attack, Stokes-Adams disease*

W. Stokes — see CHEYNE-STOKES RESPIRATION

Adams, Robert (1791–1875), British physician.

sto•ma \ˈstō-mə\ *n, pl* **-mas** : an artificial permanent opening esp. in the abdominal wall made in surgical procedures ⟨a colostomy ~⟩

stom•ach \ˈstə-mik\ *n* **1 a** : a saclike expansion of the digestive tract communicating anteriorly with the esophagus and posteriorly with the duodenum and being typically a simple often curved sac with an outer serous coat, a strong complex muscular wall that contracts rhythmically, and a mucous lining membrane that contains gastric glands **b** : one of the compartments of a ruminant stomach **2** : the part of the body that contains the stomach : BELLY, ABDOMEN

stom•ach•ache \-ˌāk\ *n* : pain in or in the region of the stomach

sto•mach•ic \stə-ˈma-kik\ *n* : a stimulant or tonic for the stomach

stomach pump *n* : a suction pump with a flexible tube for removing the contents of the stomach

stomach tube *n* : a flexible tube passed into the stomach (as by way of the nasal passages and esophagus or through a surgical opening in the abdominal wall) for introduction of material (as food) or removal of gastric contents

stomach worm *n* : any of various nematode worms parasitic in the stomach of mammals or birds; *esp* : a worm of the genus *Haemonchus* (*H. contortus*) common in ruminants (as sheep) but rare in humans

sto•mal \ˈstō-məl\ *adj* : of, relating to, or situated near a surgical stoma

stomat- *or* **stomato-** *comb form* : mouth ⟨*stomat*itis⟩ ⟨*stomato*logy⟩

sto•ma•ti•tis \ˌstō-mə-ˈtī-təs\ *n, pl* **-tit•i•des** \-ˈti-tə-ˌdēz\ *or* **-ti•tis•es** \ˌtī-tə-səz\ : any of numerous inflammatory diseases of the mouth — see APHTHOUS STOMATITIS, GANGRENOUS STOMATITIS, VESICULAR STOMATITIS

sto•ma•to•gnath•ic \ˌstō-mə-(ˌ)täg-ˈna-thik\ *adj* : of or relating to the jaws and the mouth

sto•ma•tol•o•gist \ˌstō-mə-ˈtä-lə-jist\ *n* : a specialist in stomatology

sto•ma•tol•o•gy \ˌstō-mə-ˈtä-lə-jē\ *n, pl* **-gies** : a branch of medical science dealing with the mouth and its disorders — **sto•ma•to•log•i•cal** \ˌstō-mət-ᵊl-ˈä-ji-kəl\ *also* **sto•ma•to•log•ic** \-jik\ *adj*

-sto•mia \ˈstō-mē-ə\ *n comb form* : mouth exhibiting (such) a condition ⟨xero*stomia*⟩

sto•mo•de•um *or* **sto•mo•dae•um** \ˌstō-mə-ˈdē-əm\ *n, pl* **-dea** *or* **-daea** \-ˈdē-ə\ *also* **-deums** *or* **-daeums** : the embryonic anterior ectodermal part of the digestive tract — **sto•mo•de•al** *or* **sto•mo•dae•al** \-ˈdē-əl\ *adj*

Sto•mox•ys \stə-ˈmäk-səs\ *n* : a genus of bloodsucking dipteran flies (family Muscidae) that includes the stable fly

-s•to•my \s-tə-mē\ *n comb form, pl* **-s•to•mies** : surgical operation establishing a usu. permanent opening into (such) a part ⟨entero*stomy*⟩

stone \ˈstōn\ *n* : CALCULUS 1

stoned \ˈstōnd\ *adj* : being drunk or under the influence of a drug (as marijuana) taken esp. for pleasure : HIGH

stone man syndrome *n* : FIBRODYSPLASIA OSSIFICANS PROGRESSIVA

stool \ˈstül\ *n* : a discharge of fecal matter

stop codon *n* : a genetic codon in messenger RNA that signals the termination of protein synthesis during translation — called also *termination codon;* compare START CODON

storage disease *n* : the abnormal accumulation in the body of one or more specific substances and esp. substances (as cerebrosides in Gaucher disease) that are normally broken down by the body— see GLYCOGEN STORAGE DISEASE, LIPOFUSCINOSIS

sto•rax \ˈstōr-ˌaks\ *n* **1** : a fragrant balsam obtained from the bark of an Asian tree of the genus *Liquidambar* (*L. orientalis*) that is used as an expectorant — called also *Levant storax* **2** : a balsam similar to storax that is obtained from a No. American tree of the genus *Liquidambar* (*L. styraciflua*) — called also *liquidambar*

storm \ˈstȯrm\ *n* : a crisis or sudden increase in the symptoms of a disease — see THYROID STORM

stormy \ˈstȯr-mē\ *adj* **storm•i•er; -est** : having alternating exacerbations and remissions of symptoms

STP \ˌes-(ˌ)tē-ˈpē\ *n* : a hallucinogenic drug chemically related to mescaline and amphetamine — called also *DOM*

stra•bis•mus \strə-ˈbiz-məs\ *n* : inability of one eye to attain binocular vision with the other because of imbalance of the muscles of the eyeball — called also *heterotropia, squint;* compare CROSS-EYE — **stra•bis•mic** \strə-ˈbiz-mik\ *adj*

straightjacket *var of* STRAITJACKET

straight sinus *n* : a venous sinus of the brain that is located along the line of junction of the falx cerebri and tentorium cerebelli and passes posteriorly to terminate in the confluence of sinuses

[1]**strain** \ˈstrān\ *n* : a group of presumed common ancestry with clear-cut physiological but usu. not morphological distinctions ⟨a ~ of bacteria⟩

[2]**strain** *vb* **1 a** : to exert (as oneself) to the utmost **b** : to injure by overuse, misuse, or excessive pressure **2** : to contract the muscles forcefully in attempting to defecate — often used in the phrase *strain at stool*

[3]**strain** *n* : an act of straining or the condition of being strained: as **a** : excessive physical or mental tension; *also* : a force, influence, or factor causing such tension **b** : bodily injury from excessive tension, effort, or use ⟨heart ~⟩; *esp* : one resulting from a wrench or twist and involving undue stretching of muscles or ligaments ⟨back ~⟩ — compare SPRAIN

strait•jack•et *also* **straight•jack•et** \ˈstrāt-ˌja-kət\ *n* : a cover or garment of strong material (as canvas) used to bind the body and esp. the arms closely in restraining a violent prisoner or patient

stra•mo•ni•um \strə-ˈmō-nē-əm\ *n* **1** : the dried leaves of the jimsonweed (*Datura stramonium*) or of a related plant of the genus *Datura* containing the alkaloids atropine, hyoscyamine, and scopolamine and used esp. formerly in medicine (as to treat asthma) **2** : JIMSONWEED

strand \ˈstrand\ *n* : something (as a molecular chain) resembling a thread

strand•ed \ˈstran-dəd\ *adj* : having a strand or strands esp. of a specified kind or number — usu. used in combination ⟨double-*stranded* DNA⟩ — **strand•ed•ness** *n*

stran•gle \ˈstraŋ-gəl\ *vb* **stran•gled; stran•gling** **1** : to choke to death **2** : to obstruct seriously or fatally the normal breathing of

stran•gles \-gəlz\ *n sing or pl* : an infectious febrile disease of horses and other equines that is caused by a bacterium of the genus *Streptococcus* (*S. equi*)

stran•gu•lat•ed hernia \ˈstraŋ-gyə-ˌlā-təd-\ *n* : a hernia in which the blood supply of the herniated viscus is so constricted by swelling and congestion as to arrest its circulation

stran•gu•la•tion \ˌstraŋ-gyə-ˈlā-shən\ *n* **1** : the action or process of strangling or of becoming constricted so as to stop circulation **2** : the state or condition resulting from strangulation; *esp* : excessive or pathological constriction or compression of a bodily tube (as a blood vessel or a loop of intestine) that interrupts its ability to act as a passage — **stran•gu•late** \ˈstraŋ-gyə-ˌlāt\ *vb*

stran•gu•ry \ˈstraŋ-gyə-rē, -ˌgyu̇r-ē\ *n, pl* **-ries** : a slow and painful discharge of urine drop by drop produced by spasmodic muscular contraction of the urethra and bladder

[1]**strap** \ˈstrap\ *n* : a flexible band or strip

[2]**strap** *vb* **strapped; strap•ping** **1** : to secure with or attach by means of a strap **2** : to support (as a sprained joint) with overlapping strips of adhesive plaster

strapping *n* : the application of adhesive plaster in overlapping strips upon or around a part (as a sprained ankle) to serve as a splint or to hold surgical dressings in place; *also* : material so used

strat•i•fied \ˈstra-tə-ˌfīd\ *adj* : arranged in layers; *esp* : of, relating to, or being an epithelium consisting of more than one layer of cells — **strat•i•fi•ca•tion** \ˌstra-tə-fə-ˈkā-shən\ *n*

Strat•tera \strə-ˈter-ə\ *trademark* — used for a preparation of the hydrochloride of atomoxetine

stra•tum \ˈstrā-təm, ˈstra-\ *n, pl* **stra•ta** \ˈstrā-tə, ˈstra-\ : a layer of tissue

stratum ba•sa•le \-bā-ˈsā-lē\ *n, pl* **strata ba•sa•lia** \-lē-ə\ **1** : the basal layer of the epidermis consisting of a single row of columnar or cuboidal epithelial cells that continually divide and replace the rest of the epidermis as it wears away — called also *stratum germinativum;* see MALPIGHIAN LAYER **2** : the deep layer of the endometrium between the stratum spongiosum and the myometrium that is retained during menstruation

stratum com•pac•tum \-kəm-ˈpak-təm\ *n, pl* **strata com•pac•ta** \-ˈpak-tə\ : the relatively dense superficial layer of the endometrium

stratum corneum *n, pl* **strata cornea** : the outer more or less horny part of the epidermis

stratum ger•mi•na•ti•vum \-ˌjər-mə-nə-ˈtī-vəm\ *n, pl* **strata ger•mi•na•ti•va** \-və\ : STRATUM BASALE 1

stratum gran•u•lo•sum \-ˌgran-yə-ˈlō-səm\ *n, pl* **strata gran•u•lo•sa** \-sə\ : a layer of granular cells lying immediately above the stratum basale in most parts of the epidermis

stratum in•ter•me•di•um \-ˌin-tər-ˈmē-dē-əm\ *n, pl* **strata in•ter•me•dia** \-dē-ə\ : the cell layer of the enamel organ next to the layer of ameloblasts

stratum lu•ci•dum \-ˈlü-si-dəm\ *n, pl* **strata lu•ci•da** \-də\ : a thin somewhat translucent layer of cells lying under the stratum corneum esp. in thickened epidermis

stratum spi•no•sum \-spi-ˈnō-səm\ *n, pl* **strata spi•no•sa** \-sə\ : the layers of prickle cells over the layer of the stratum basale capable of undergoing mitosis — called also *prickle cell layer;* see MALPIGHIAN LAYER

stratum spon•gi•o•sum \-ˌspən-jē-ˈō-səm\ *n, pl* **strata spon•gi•o•sa** \-sə\ : the middle layer of the endometrium between the stratum basale and stratum compactum that contains dilated and tortuous portions of the uterine glands

strawberry gallbladder *n* : an abnormal condition characterized by the deposition of cholesterol in the lining of the gallbladder in a pattern resembling the surface of a strawberry

strawberry mark *n* : a tumor of the skin filled with small blood vessels and appearing usu. as a red and elevated birthmark

strawberry tongue *n* : a tongue that is red from swollen congested papillae and that occurs esp. in scarlet fever and Kawasaki disease

[1]**streak** \ˈstrēk\ *n* **1** : a usu. irregular line or stripe — see PRIMITIVE STREAK **2** : inoculum implanted in a line on a solid medium

[2]**streak** *vb* : to implant (inoculum) in a line on a solid medium

stream \ˈstrēm\ *n* : an unbroken current or flow (as of a bodily fluid) — see BLOODSTREAM, MIDSTREAM

stream of consciousness *n* : the continuous unedited flow of conscious experience through the mind

street virus *n* : a naturally occurring rabies virus as distinguished from virus attenuated in the laboratory

strength \ˈstreŋth, ˈstrenth\ *n, pl* **strengths** **1** : the quality or state of being strong : capacity for exertion or endurance **2** : degree of potency of effect or of concentration **3** : degree of ionization of a solution — used of acids and bases

strength training *n* : a system of physical conditioning in which muscles are exercised by being worked against an opposing force (as by lifting weights) to increase strength

strep \ˈstrep\ *n, often attrib* : STREPTOCOCCUS ⟨a ~ infection⟩

strepho•sym•bo•lia \ˌstre-fō-sim-ˈbō-lē-ə\ *n* : a learning disorder in which symbols and esp. phrases, words, or letters appear to be reversed or transposed in reading

strep throat *n* : an inflammatory sore throat caused by hemolytic Group A streptococci and marked by fever, prostration, and toxemia — called also *septic sore throat, strep sore throat*

strepto- *comb form* **1** : twisted : twisted chain ⟨*strepto*coccus⟩ **2** : streptococcus ⟨*strepto*kinase⟩

strep•to•ba•cil•lus \ˌstrep-tō-bə-ˈsi-ləs\ *n* **1** *cap* : a genus of facultatively anaerobic gram-negative rod-shaped bacteria (family Fusobacteriaceae) in which the individual cells are often joined in a chain **2** *pl* **-li** \-ˌlī\ : any bacterium of the genus *Streptobacillus; esp* : one (*S. moniliformis*) that is the causative agent of one form of rat-bite fever — **strep•to•ba•cil•la•ry** \-ˈba-sə-ˌler-ē, -bə-ˈsi-lə-rē\ *adj*

strep•to•coc•cal \ˌstrep-tə-ˈkä-kəl\ *also* **strep•to•coc•cic** \-ˈkä-kik, -ˈkäk-sik\ *adj* : of, relating to, caused by, or being streptococci ⟨~ gingivitis⟩

strep•to•coc•cus \-ˈkä-kəs\ *n* **1** *cap* : a genus of spherical or ovoid chiefly nonmotile and parasitic gram-positive bacteria (family Streptococcaceae) that divide only in one plane, occur in pairs or chains, and include important pathogens of humans and domestic animals **2** *pl* **-coc•ci** \-ˈkä-ˌkī, -ˈkäk-ˌsī\ : any bacterium of the genus *Streptococcus; broadly* : a coccus occurring in chains

strep•to•dor•nase \ˌstrep-tō-ˈdȯr-ˌnās, -ˌnāz\ *n* : a deoxyribonuclease from hemolytic streptococci that dissolves pus and is usu. administered in a mixture with streptokinase — see VARIDASE

strep•to•gram•in \ˌstrep-tō-ˈgra-mən\ *n* : an antibiotic complex produced by a bacterium of the genus *Streptomyces* (*S. graminofaciens*)

strep•to•ki•nase \ˌstrep-tō-ˈkī-ˌnās, -ˌnāz\ *n* : a proteolytic enzyme produced by hemolytic streptococci that promotes the dissolution of blood clots by activating plasminogen to produce plasmin — see VARIDASE

strep•to•ly•sin \ˌstrep-tə-ˈlīs-ᵊn\ *n* : any of various antigenic hemolysins produced by streptococci

strep•to•my•ces \-ˈmī-ˌsēz\ *n* **1** *cap* : a genus of mostly soil streptomycetes including some that form antibiotics as by-products of their metabolism **2** *pl* **streptomyces** : any bacterium of the genus *Streptomyces*

strep•to•my•cete \-ˈmī-ˌsēt, -ˌmī-ˈsēt\ *n* : any of a family (Streptomycetaceae) of actinomycetes that are typically aerobic soil saprophytes but include a few parasites of plants and animals

strep•to•my•cin \-ˈmīs-ᵊn\ *n* : an antibiotic $C_{21}H_{39}N_7O_{12}$ that is produced by a soil actinomycete of the genus *Streptomyces* (*S. griseus*), is active against bacteria, and is used esp. in the treatment of infections (as tuberculosis) by gram-negative bacteria

strep•to•ni•grin \-ˈnī-grən\ *n* : a toxic antibiotic $C_{25}H_{22}N_4O_8$ from an actinomycete of the genus *Streptomyces* (*S. flocculus*) that is used as an antineoplastic agent

strep•to•zo•cin \ˌstrep-tə-ˈzō-sən\ *n* : STREPTOZOTOCIN

strep•to•zot•o•cin \ˌstrep-tə-ˈzä-tə-sən\ *n* : a broad-spectrum antibiotic $C_8H_{15}N_3O_7$ with antineoplastic and diabetogenic properties that has been isolated from a bacterium of the genus *Streptomyces* (*S. achromogenes*)

stress \ˈstres\ *n* **1 a :** a force exerted when one body or body part presses on, pulls on, pushes against, or tends to compress or twist another body or body part **b :** the deformation caused in a body by such a force **2 a :** a physical, chemical, or emotional factor that causes bodily or mental tension and may be a factor in disease causation **b :** a state of bodily or mental tension resulting from factors that tend to alter an existent equilibrium **3 :** the force exerted between teeth of the upper and lower jaws during mastication — **stress** *vb* — **stress•ful** \ˈstres-fəl\ *adj* — **stress•ful•ly** *adv*

stress breaker *n* **:** a flexible dental device used to lessen the occlusal forces exerted on teeth to which a partial denture is attached

stress fracture *n* **:** a usu. hairline fracture of a bone (as of the foot) that has been subjected to repeated stress

stress incontinence *n* **:** involuntary leakage of urine from the bladder accompanying physical activity (as in laughing or coughing) which places increased pressure on the abdomen — compare URGE INCONTINENCE

stress•or \ˈstre-sər, -ˌsȯr\ *n* **:** a stimulus that causes stress

stress test *n* **:** an electrocardiographic test of heart function before, during, and after a controlled period of increasingly strenuous exercise (as on a treadmill)

[1]**stretch** \ˈstrech\ *vb* **1 :** to extend or become extended in length or breadth **2 :** to enlarge or distend esp. by force

[2]**stretch** *n* **:** the act of stretching **:** the state of being stretched

stretch•er \ˈstre-chər\ *n* **:** a device for carrying a sick, injured, or dead person

stretch•er–bear•er \-ˌbar-ər\ *n* **:** a person who carries one end of a stretcher

stretch marks *n pl* **:** striae on the skin (as of the hips, abdomen, and breasts) from excessive stretching and rupture of elastic fibers esp. due to pregnancy or obesity

stretch receptor *n* **:** MUSCLE SPINDLE

stretch reflex *n* **:** a spinal reflex involving reflex contraction of a muscle in response to stretching — called also *myotatic reflex*

stria \ˈstrī-ə\ *n, pl* **stri•ae** \ˈstrī-ˌē\ **1 :** STRIATION 2 **2 :** a narrow structural band esp. of nerve fibers **3 :** a stripe or line (as in the skin) distinguished from surrounding tissue by color, texture, or elevation — see STRETCH MARKS

striata *pl of* STRIATUM

stri•a•tal \strī-ˈāt-ᵊl\ *adj* **:** of or relating to the corpus striatum ⟨∼ neurons⟩

stri•ate cortex \ˈstrī-ət-, -ˌāt-\ *n* **:** an area of the brain that receives visual impulses, contains a conspicuous band of myelinated fibers, and is located mostly in the walls and along the edges of the calcarine sulcus of the occipital lobe — called also *visual projection area*

stri•at•ed \ˈstrī-ˌā-təd\ *adj* **1 :** marked with striae **2 :** of, relating to, or being striated muscle

striated muscle *n* **:** muscle tissue that is marked by transverse dark and light bands, that is made up of elongated fibers, and that includes skeletal and usu. cardiac muscle — compare SMOOTH MUSCLE, VOLUNTARY MUSCLE

stria ter•mi•na•lis \-ˌtər-mə-ˈnā-ləs\ *n* **:** a bundle of nerve fibers that passes from the amygdala mostly to the anterior part of the hypothalamus with a few fibers crossing the anterior commissure to the amygdala on the opposite side

stri•a•tion \strī-ˈā-shən\ *n* **1 :** the fact or state of being striated **2 :** a minute groove, scratch, or channel esp. when one of a parallel series **3 :** any of the alternate dark and light cross bands of a myofibril of striated muscle

stri•a•to•ni•gral \strī-ˌā-tə-ˈnī-grəl\ *adj* **:** connecting the corpus striatum and substantia nigra ⟨∼ axons⟩

stri•a•tum \strī-ˈā-təm\ *n, pl* **stri•a•ta** \-ˈā-tə\ **1 :** CORPUS STRIATUM **2 :** NEOSTRIATUM

stria vas•cu•la•ris \-ˌvas-kyə-ˈler-əs\ *n* **:** the upper part of the spiral ligament of the cochlear duct that contains numerous small blood vessels

Stri•bild \ˈstrī-ˌbild\ *trademark* — used for a preparation of cobicistat, elvitegravir, emtricitabine, and the fumarate of tenofovir

stric•ture \ˈstrik-chər\ *n* **:** an abnormal narrowing of a bodily passage (as from inflammation or the formation of scar tissue); *also* **:** the narrowed part

stri•dor \ˈstrī-dər, -ˌdȯr\ *n* **:** a harsh vibrating sound heard during respiration in cases of obstruction of the air passages ⟨laryngeal ∼⟩ — **strid•u•lous** \ˈstri-jə-ləs\ *adj*

stridulus — see LARYNGISMUS STRIDULUS

strike \ˈstrīk\ *n* **:** cutaneous myiasis (as of sheep) ⟨body ∼⟩ ⟨blowfly ∼⟩

string•halt \ˈstriŋ-ˌhȯlt\ *n* **:** a condition of lameness in the hind legs of a horse caused by muscular spasms — **string•halt•ed** \-ˌhȯl-təd\ *adj*

strip \ˈstrip\ *vb* **stripped** \ˈstript\ *also* **stript; strip•ping :** to remove (a vein) by means of a stripper

strip•per \ˈstri-pər\ *n* **:** a surgical instrument used for removal of a vein

stroke \ˈstrōk\ *n* **:** sudden impairment or loss of consciousness, sensation, and voluntary motion that is caused by rupture or obstruction (as by a clot) of a blood vessel supplying the brain and is accompanied by permanent damage of brain tissue — called also *apoplexy, brain attack, cerebral accident, cerebrovascular accident;* see HEMORRHAGIC STROKE, ISCHEMIC STROKE, TRANSIENT ISCHEMIC ATTACK

stroke volume *n* : the volume of blood pumped from a ventricle of the heart in one beat

stro•ma \ˈstrō-mə\ *n, pl* **stro•ma•ta** \-mə-tə\ **1** : the supporting framework of an animal organ typically consisting of connective tissue **2** : the spongy protoplasmic framework of some cells (as a red blood cell) — **stro•mal** \-məl\ *adj*

strong silver protein *n* : SILVER PROTEIN b

stron•gyle \ˈsträn-ˌjīl\ *n* : STRONGYLID; *esp* : a worm of the genus *Strongylus* parasitic esp. in the intestines and tissues of the horse

stron•gy•lid \ˈsträn-jə-lid\ *n* : any of a family (Strongylidae) of nematode worms that are parasites of vertebrates — **strongylid** *adj*

stron•gy•li•do•sis \ˌsträn-jə-lə-ˈdō-səs\ *n* : STRONGYLOSIS

stron•gy•loid \ˈsträn-jə-ˌlȯid\ *n* : any of a superfamily (Strongyloidea) of nematode worms including the hookworms, strongyles, and related forms — **strongyloid** *adj*

Stron•gy•loi•des \ˌsträn-jə-ˈlȯi-ˌdēz\ *n* : a genus of nematode worms (family Strongyloididae) having both free-living males and females and parthenogenetic females parasitic in the intestine of various vertebrates and including some medically and economically important pests of humans

stron•gy•loi•di•a•sis \ˌsträn-jə-ˌlȯi-ˈdī-ə-səs\ *n, pl* **-a•ses** \-ə-ˌsēz\ : infestation with or disease caused by nematodes of the genus *Strongyloides*

stron•gy•loi•do•sis \-ˈdō-səs\ *n* : STRONGYLOIDIASIS

stron•gy•lo•sis \ˌsträn-jə-ˈlō-səs\ *n* : infestation with or disease caused by strongyles — called also *strongylidosis*

Stron•gy•lus \ˈsträn-jə-ləs\ *n* : a genus of strongylid nematode worms including gastrointestinal parasites of the horse

stron•tium \ˈsträn-chəm, -chē-əm, -tē-əm\ *n* : a soft malleable ductile bivalent metallic element — symbol *Sr;* see ELEMENT table

strontium 90 *n* : a heavy radioactive isotope of strontium having the mass number 90 that is present in the fallout from nuclear explosions and is hazardous because like calcium it can be assimilated in biological processes and deposited in the bones — called also *radiostrontium*

stro•phan•thin \strō-ˈfan-thən\ *n* : a bitter toxic glycoside $C_{36}H_{54}O_{14}$ from a woody vine of the genus *Strophanthus* (*S. kombé*) used similarly to digitalis; *also* : a related glycoside (as ouabain)

stro•phan•thus \-thəs\ *n* **1** *cap* : a genus of Asian and African trees, shrubs, or woody vines of the dogbane family (Apocynaceae) including one (*S. kombé*) that yields strophanthin **2** : the dried seeds of any of several plants of the genus *Strophanthus* (as *S. kombé* and *S. hispidus*) that contain strophanthin and are in moderate doses a cardiac stimulant but in larger doses a violent poison

struc•tur•al \ˈstrək-chə-rəl\ *adj* **1** : of or relating to the physical makeup of a plant or animal body ⟨~ defects of the heart⟩ — compare FUNCTIONAL 1a **2** : of, relating to, or affecting structure ⟨~ stability⟩ — **struc•tur•al•ly** *adv*

structural formula *n* : an expanded molecular formula (as H-O-H for water) showing the arrangement within the molecule of atoms and of bonds

structural gene *n* : a gene that codes for the amino acid sequence of a protein (as an enzyme) or for a ribosomal RNA or transfer RNA

struc•tur•al•ism \ˈstrək-chə-rə-ˌli-zəm\ *n* : psychology concerned esp. with resolution of the mind into structural elements

struc•ture \ˈstrək-chər\ *n* **1** : something (as an anatomical part) arranged in a definite pattern of organization **2 a** : the arrangement of particles or parts in a substance or body ⟨molecular ~⟩ **b** : organization of parts as dominated by the general character of the whole ⟨personality ~⟩ **3** : the aggregate of elements of an entity in their relationships to each other

stru•ma \ˈstrü-mə\ *n, pl* **-mae** \-(ˌ)mē\ *or* **-mas** : GOITER

struma lym•pho•ma•to•sa \-lim-ˌfō-mə-ˈtō-sə\ *n* : HASHIMOTO'S THYROIDITIS

stru•vite \ˈstrü-ˌvīt\ *n* : a hydrated magnesium-containing mineral $Mg(NH_4)(PO_4)\cdot 6H_2O$ which is found in kidney stones associated with bacteria that cleave urea

strych•nine \ˈstrik-ˌnīn, -nən, -ˌnēn\ *n* : a bitter poisonous alkaloid $C_{21}H_{22}N_2O_2$ that is obtained from nux vomica and related plants of the genus *Strychnos* and is used as a poison (as for rodents) and medicinally as a stimulant of the central nervous system

Strych•nos \ˈstrīk-nəs, -ˌnäs\ *n* : a large genus of tropical trees and woody vines (family Loganiaceae) — see CURARE, NUX VOMICA, STRYCHNINE

STS *abbr* serologic test for syphilis

ST segment *or* **S–T segment** \ˌes-ˈtē-\ *n* : the part of an electrocardiogram between the QRS complex and the T wave

Stu•art–Prow•er factor \ˈstü-ərt-ˈprau̇-ər-, -ˈstyü-\ *n* : FACTOR X

Stuart and **Prower,** 20th-century hospital patients.

stuff \ˈstəf\ *vb* : to choke or block up (as nasal passages) ⟨a ~*ed* up nose⟩ — **stuff•i•ness** \ˈstə-fē-nəs\ *n* — **stuffy** \ˈstəf-ē\ *adj*

stump \ˈstəmp\ *n* **1** : the basal portion of a bodily part (as a limb) remaining after the rest is removed **2** : a rudimentary or vestigial bodily part

stung *past and past part of* STING

stunt \ˈstənt\ *vb* : to hinder the normal growth, development, or progress of ⟨an emotionally ~*ed* child⟩

stupe \ˈstüp, ˈstyüp\ *n* : a hot wet often medicated cloth applied externally (as to stimulate circulation)

stu•pe•fy \ˈstü-pə-ˌfī, ˈstyü-\ *vb* **-fied; -fy•ing** : to make stupid, groggy, or insensible ⟨a patient *stupefied* by anesthesia⟩ — **stu•pe•fac•tion** \ˌstü-pə-ˈfak-shən, ˌstyü-\ *n*

stu•por \ˈstü-pər, ˈstyü-\ *n* : a condition of greatly dulled or completely suspended sense or sensibility ⟨a drunken ~⟩; *specif* : a chiefly mental condition marked by absence of spontaneous movement, greatly diminished responsiveness to stimulation, and usu. impaired consciousness — **stu•por•ous** \ˈstü-pə-rəs, ˈstyü-\ *adj*

stur•dy \ˈstər-dē\ *n, pl* **sturdies** : GID

Sturge–Web•er syndrome \ˈstərj-ˈwe-bər-\ *n* : a rare congenital condition that is characterized by a port-wine stain affecting the facial skin on one side in the area innervated by the first branch of the trigeminal nerve and by malformed blood vessels in the brain that may cause progressive intellectual disability, epilepsy, and glaucoma in the eye on the affected side — called also *Sturge-Weber disease*

Sturge, William Allen (1850–1919), and **Weber, Frederick Parkes (1863–1962),** British physicians.

stut•ter \ˈstə-tər\ *vb* : to speak with involuntary disruption or blocking of speech (as by abnormal repetition or prolongation of vocal sounds) — **stutter** *n* — **stut•ter•er** \ˈstə-tər-ər\ *n*

stuttering *n* **1** : the act of one who stutters **2** : a disorder of vocal communication that is marked esp. by involuntary disruption or blocking of speech (as by abnormal repetition, prolongation, or stoppage of vocal sounds)

sty *or* **stye** \ˈstī\ *n, pl* **sties** *or* **styes** : an inflamed swelling of a sebaceous gland at the margin of an eyelid — called also *hordeolum*

styl- *or* **stylo-** *comb form* : styloid process ⟨*stylo*glossus⟩

sty•let \stī-ˈlet, ˈstī-lət\ *also* **sty•lette** \stī-ˈlet\ *n* **1** : a slender surgical probe **2** : a thin wire inserted into a catheter to maintain rigidity or into a hollow needle to maintain patency

sty•lo•glos•sus \ˌstī-lō-ˈglä-səs, -ˈglò-\ *n, pl* **-glos•si** \-ˈglä-ˌsī, -ˈglò-\ : a muscle that arises from the styloid process of the temporal bone, inserts along the side and underpart of the tongue, and functions to draw the tongue upwards

sty•lo•hy•oid \ˌstī-lō-ˈhī-ˌòid\ *n* : STYLOHYOID MUSCLE

sty•lo•hy•oi•de•us \-hī-ˈòi-dē-əs\ *n, pl* **-dei** \-dē-ˌī\ : STYLOHYOID MUSCLE

stylohyoid ligament *n* : a band of fibrous tissue connecting the tip of the styloid process of the temporal bone to the ceratohyal of the hyoid bone

stylohyoid muscle *n* : a slender muscle that arises from the posterior surface of the styloid process of the temporal bone, inserts into the body of the hyoid bone, and acts to elevate and retract the hyoid bone resulting in elongation of the floor of the mouth — called also *stylohyoid, stylohyoideus*

sty•loid \ˈstī-ˌlòid\ *adj* : having a slender pointed shape

styloid process *n* : any of several long slender pointed bony processes: as **a** : a sharp spine that projects downward and forward from the inferior surface of the temporal bone just in front of the stylomastoid foramen **b** : an eminence on the distal extremity of the ulna giving attachment to a ligament of the wrist joint **c** : a conical prolongation of the lateral surface of the distal extremity of the radius that gives attachment to several tendons and ligaments

sty•lo•man•dib•u•lar ligament \ˌstī-lō-man-ˈdi-byə-lər\ *n* : a band of deep fascia that connects the styloid process of the temporal bone to the gonial angle

sty•lo•mas•toid foramen \-ˈmas-ˌtòid-\ *n* : a foramen that occurs on the lower surface of the temporal bone between the styloid and mastoid processes

sty•lo•pha•ryn•ge•us \ˌstī-lō-fə-ˈrin-jē-əs, -ˌfar-ən-ˈjē-əs\ *n, pl* **-gei** \-jē-ˌī\ : a slender muscle that arises from the base of the styloid process of the temporal bone, inserts into the side of the pharynx, and acts with the contralateral muscle in swallowing to increase the transverse diameter of the pharynx by drawing its sides upward and laterally

[1]**styp•tic** \ˈstip-tik\ *adj* : tending to check bleeding; *esp* : having the property of arresting oozing of blood (as from a shallow surface injury) when applied to a bleeding part ⟨~ agent⟩

[2]**styptic** *n* : an agent (as a drug) having a styptic effect

styptic pencil *n* : a cylindrical stick of a medicated styptic substance used esp. in shaving to stop the bleeding from small cuts

sub- *prefix* **1** : under : beneath : below ⟨*sub*coastal⟩ **2** : subordinate portion of : subdivision of ⟨*sub*species⟩ **3** : less than completely or perfectly ⟨*sub*normal⟩

sub•acro•mi•al \ˌsəb-ə-ˈkrō-mē-əl\ *adj* : of, relating to, or affecting the subacromial bursa ⟨~ bursitis⟩

subacromial bursa *n* : a bursa lying between the acromion and the capsule of the shoulder joint

sub•acute \ˌsəb-ə-ˈkyüt\ *adj* **1** : falling between acute and chronic in character esp. when closer to acute ⟨~ endocarditis⟩ **2** : less marked in severity or duration than a corresponding acute state ⟨~ pain⟩ — **sub•acute•ly** *adv*

subacute sclerosing panencephalitis *n* : a usu. fatal neurological disease of children and young adults that is caused by infection of the brain by a previously latent morbillivirus causing measles and that is marked esp. by behavioral changes, myoclonic seizures, progressive deterioration of motor and mental functioning, and coma — abbr. *SSPE*

sub•aor•tic stenosis \ˌsəb-ā-ˈȯr-tik-\ *n* : aortic stenosis produced by an obstruction in the left ventricle below the aortic valve

sub•arach•noid \ˌsəb-ə-ˈrak-ˌnȯid\ *also* **sub•arach•noid•al** \-rak-ˈnȯid-ᵊl\ *adj* **1** : situated or occurring under the arachnoid membrane ⟨~ hemorrhage⟩ **2** : of, relating to, or involving the subarachnoid space and the fluid within it ⟨~ meningitis⟩

subarachnoid space *n* : the space between the arachnoid and the pia mater through which the cerebrospinal fluid circulates

sub•are•o•lar \ˌsəb-ə-ˈrē-ə-lər\ *adj* : situated or occurring beneath an areola of the breast ⟨a ~ abscess⟩

sub•cal•lo•sal \ˌsəb-ka-ˈlō-səl\ *adj* : situated below the corpus callosum

subcallosal area *n* : a small area of cortex in each cerebral hemisphere below the genu of the corpus callosum

sub•cap•su•lar \ˌsəb-ˈkap-sə-lər\ *adj* : situated or occurring beneath or within a capsule ⟨~ cataracts⟩

subcarbonate — see BISMUTH SUBCARBONATE

sub•cel•lu•lar \ˌsəb-ˈsel-yə-lər\ *adj* **1** : of less than cellular scope or level of organization **2** : relating to or being local or restricted area within a cell

sub•chon•dral \-ˈkän-drəl\ *adj* : situated beneath cartilage ⟨~ bone⟩

sub•cho•roi•dal \ˌsəb-kə-ˈrȯid-ᵊl\ *adj* : situated or occurring between the choroid and the retina ⟨~ fluid⟩

sub•class \ˈsəb-ˌklas\ *n* : a category in biological classification ranking below a class and above an order

subclavia — see ANSA SUBCLAVIA

[1]**sub•cla•vi•an** \ˌsəb-ˈklā-vē-ən\ *adj* : of, relating to, being, performed on, or inserted into a part (as an artery or vein) located under the clavicle ⟨a ~ catheter⟩

[2]**subclavian** *n* : a subclavian part

subclavian artery *n* : the proximal part of the main artery of the arm that arises on the right side from the brachiocephalic artery and on the left side from the arch of the aorta and that supplies or gives off branches supplying the brain, neck, anterior wall of the thorax, and shoulder

subclavian trunk *n* : a large lymphatic vessel on each side of the body that receives lymph from the axilla and arms and that on the right side empties into the right lymphatic duct and on the left side into the thoracic duct

subclavian vein *n* : the proximal part of the main vein of the arm that is a continuation of the axillary vein and extends from the level of the first rib to the sternal end of the clavicle where it unites with the internal jugular vein to form the brachiocephalic vein

sub•cla•vi•us \ˌsəb-ˈklā-vē-əs\ *n, pl* **-vii** \-vē-ˌī\ : a small muscle on each side of the body that arises from the junction of the first rib and its cartilage, inserts into the inferior surface of the clavicle, and acts to stabilize the clavicle by depressing and drawing forward its lateral end during movements of the shoulder joint

sub•clin•i•cal \-ˈkli-ni-kəl\ *adj* : not detectable or producing effects that are not detectable by the usual clinical tests ⟨a ~ infection⟩ ⟨~ cancer⟩ — **sub•clin•i•cal•ly** *adv*

sub•con•junc•ti•val \ˌsəb-ˌkän-ˌjəŋk-ˈtī-vəl\ *adj* : situated or occurring beneath the conjunctiva ⟨~ hemorrhage⟩ — **sub•con•junc•ti•val•ly** *adv*

[1]**sub•con•scious** \ˌsəb-ˈkän-chəs\ *adj* **1** : existing in the mind but not immediately available to consciousness : affecting thought, feeling, and behavior without entering awareness **2** : imperfectly conscious : partially but not fully aware — **sub•con•scious•ly** *adv* — **sub•con•scious•ness** *n*

[2]**subconscious** *n* : the mental activities just below the threshold of consciousness; *also* : the aspect of the mind concerned with such activities — compare UNCONSCIOUS

sub•cor•a•coid \-ˈkȯr-ə-ˌkȯid\ *adj* : situated or occurring under the coracoid process of the scapula

sub•cor•ti•cal \-ˈkȯr-ti-kəl\ *adj* : of, relating to, involving, or being nerve centers below the cerebral cortex ⟨~ lesions⟩ — **sub•cor•ti•cal•ly** *adv*

sub•cos•tal \-ˈkäs-təl, -ˈkȯs-\ *adj* : situated or performed below a rib

subcostal artery *n* : either of a pair of arteries that are the most posterior branches of the thoracic aorta and follow a course beneath the last pair of ribs

sub·cos·ta·lis \-käs-ˈtā-ləs, -kȯs-\ *n, pl* **-ta·les** \-ˌlēz\ : any of a variable number of small muscles that arise on the inner surface of a rib, are inserted into the inner surface of the second or third rib below, and prob. function to draw adjacent ribs together

subcostal vein *n* : either of two veins: **a** : one that arises on the right side of the anterior abdominal wall and joins in the formation of the azygos vein — called also *right subcostal vein* **b** : one on the left side of the body that usu. empties into the hemiazygos vein — called also *left subcostal vein*

sub·cul·ture \ˈsəb-ˌkəl-chər\ *n* **1** : a culture (as of bacteria) derived from another culture **2** : an act or instance of producing a subculture — **subculture** *vb*

subcutanea — see TELA SUBCUTANEA

sub·cu·ta·ne·ous \ˌsəb-kyu̇-ˈtā-nē-əs\ *adj* : being, living, used, or made under the skin ⟨~ parasites⟩ — **sub·cu·ta·ne·ous·ly** *adv*

subcutaneous bursa *n* : a bursa lying between the skin and a bony process or a ligament

subcutaneous emphysema *n* : the presence of a gas and esp. air in the subcutaneous tissue

sub·cu·tic·u·lar \-kyu̇-ˈti-kyə-lər\ *adj* : situated or occurring beneath a cuticle ⟨~ sutures⟩ ⟨~ tissues⟩

sub·cu·tis \ˌsəb-ˈkyü-təs\ *n* : SUPERFICIAL FASCIA

sub·del·toid \ˌsəb-ˈdel-ˌtȯid\ *adj* : situated underneath or inferior to the deltoid muscle ⟨~ calcareous deposits⟩

subdeltoid bursa *n* : the bursa that lies beneath the deltoid muscle

sub·der·mal \-ˈdər-məl\ *adj* : SUBCUTANEOUS — **sub·der·mal·ly** *adv*

sub·di·a·phrag·ma·tic \ˌsəb-ˌdī-ə-frə-ˈma-tik, -ˌfrag-\ *adj* : situated, occurring, or performed below the diaphragm ⟨a ~ abscess⟩

subdivision *n* : a category in botanical classification ranking below a division and above a class

sub·du·ral \ˌsəb-ˈdu̇r-əl, -ˈdyu̇r-\ *adj* : situated, occurring, or performed under the dura mater or between the dura mater and thc arachnoid ⟨~ empyema⟩ — **sub·du·ral·ly** *adv*

subdural hematoma *n* : a hematoma that occurs between the dura mater and arachnoid in the subdural space

subdural space *n* : a fluid-filled space or potential space between the dura mater and the arachnoid

sub·en·do·car·di·al \ˌsəb-ˌen-dō-ˈkär-dē-əl\ *adj* : situated or occurring beneath the endocardium or between the endocardium and myocardium

sub·en·do·the·li·al \-ˌen-dō-ˈthē-lē-əl\ *adj* : situated under an endothelium

sub·ep·en·dy·mal \-e-ˈpen-də-məl\ *adj* : situated under the ependyma

sub·epi·der·mal \ˌsəb-ˌe-pə-ˈdər-məl\ *adj* : lying beneath or constituting the innermost part of the epidermis

sub·epi·the·li·al \-ˌe-pə-ˈthē-lē-əl\ *adj* : situated or occurring beneath an epithelial layer; *also* : SUBCUTANEOUS

sub·fam·i·ly \ˈsəb-ˌfam-lē\ *n* : a category in biological classification ranking below a family and above a genus

sub·fas·cial \-ˈfa-shəl, -shē-əl\ *adj* : situated, occurring, or performed below a fascia ⟨a ~ tumor⟩ ⟨~ suturing⟩

sub·fe·brile \-ˈfe-ˌbrīl, -ˈfē-\ *adj* : of, relating to, or constituting a body temperature very slightly above normal but not febrile

sub·fer·til·i·ty \-fər-ˈti-lə-tē\ *n, pl* **-ties** : the condition of being less than normally fertile though still capable of effecting fertilization — **sub·fer·tile** \-ˈfərt-ᵊl\ *adj*

sub·ge·nus \ˈsəb-ˌjē-nəs\ *n, pl* **-gen·e·ra** \-ˌje-nər-ə\ : a category in biological classification ranking below a genus and above a species

sub·gin·gi·val \ˌsəb-ˈjin-jə-vəl\ *adj* : situated, performed, or occurring beneath the gums and esp. between the gums and the basal part of the crowns of the teeth — **sub·gin·gi·val·ly** *adv*

sub·glot·tic \-ˈglä-tik\ *adj* : situated or occurring below the glottis

su·bic·u·lum \sə-ˈbi-kyə-ləm\ *n, pl* **-la** \-lə\ : a part of the parahippocampal gyrus that is a ventral continuation of the hippocampus and is situated ventrally and medially to the dentate gyrus; *also* : a section of this that borders the hippocampal sulcus — **su·bic·u·lar** \-lər\ *adj*

sub·in·tern \-ˈin-ˌtərn\ *n* : a medical student in the last year of medical school who performs work supervised by interns and residents in a hospital

sub·in·ti·mal \-ˈin-tə-məl\ *adj* : situated beneath an intima and esp. between the intima and media of an artery

sub·in·vo·lu·tion \-ˌin-və-ˈlü-shən\ *n* : partial or incomplete involution

sub·ja·cent \səb-ˈjās-ᵊnt\ *adj* : lying immediately under or below ⟨~ tissue⟩

sub·ject \ˈsəb-jikt\ *n* **1** : an individual whose reactions or responses are studied **2** : a dead body for anatomical study and dissection

sub·jec·tive \(ˌ)səb-ˈjek-tiv\ *adj* **1 a** : relating to or determined by the mind as the subject of experience ⟨~ reality⟩ **b** : characteristic of or belonging to reality as perceived rather than as independent of mind **c** : relating to or being experience or knowledge as conditioned by personal mental characteristics or states **2 a** : arising from conditions within the brain or sense organs and not directly caused by external stimuli ⟨~ sensations⟩ **b** : arising out of or identified by means of one's perception of one's own states and processes and not observable by an examiner ⟨a ~ symptom of disease⟩ — compare OBJECTIVE 2 — **sub·jec·tive·ly** *adv*

subjective vertigo *n* : vertigo characterized by a sensation that one's body is revolving in space

sub·le·thal \ˌsəb-ˈlē-thəl\ *adj* : less than but usu. only slightly less than lethal ⟨a ~ dose⟩

sub·li·ma·tion \ˌsə-blə-ˈmā-shən\ *n* : the process of converting and expressing a primitive instinctual desire or impulse to a form that is socially or culturally acceptable — **sub·li·mate** \ˈsə-blə-ˌmāt\ *vb*

sub·lim·i·nal \(ˌ)səb-ˈli-mə-nəl\ *adj* **1** : inadequate to produce a sensation or a perception **2** : existing or functioning below the threshold of consciousness ⟨the ~ mind⟩ ⟨~ advertising⟩ — **sub·lim·i·nal·ly** *adv*

[1]**sub·lin·gual** \ˌsəb-ˈliŋ-gwəl, -gyə-wəl\ *adj* **1** : situated or administered under the tongue ⟨~ tablets⟩ **2** : of or relating to the sublingual glands — **sub·lin·gual·ly** *adv*

[2]**sublingual** *n* : SUBLINGUAL GLAND

sublingual gland *n* : a small salivary gland on each side of the mouth lying beneath the mucous membrane in a fossa in the mandible near the symphysis — called also *sublingual salivary gland*

sub·lob·u·lar vein \ˌsəb-ˈlä-byə-lər-\ *n* : one of several veins in the liver into which the central veins empty and which in turn empty into the hepatic veins

sub·lux·a·tion \ˌsəb-ˌlək-ˈsā-shən\ *n* : partial dislocation (as of one of the bones in a joint) — **sub·lux·at·ed** \ˈsəb-ˌlək-ˌsā-təd\ *adj*

[1]**sub·man·dib·u·lar** \ˌsəb-man-ˈdi-byə-lər\ *adj* **1** : of, relating to, situated, or performed in the region below the lower jaw **2** : of, relating to, or associated with the submandibular glands

[2]**submandibular** *n* : a submandibular part (as an artery or bone)

submandibular ganglion *n* : an autonomic ganglion that is situated on the hyoglossus muscle above the deep part of the submandibular gland, receives preganglionic fibers from the facial nerve, and sends postganglionic fibers to the submandibular and sublingual glands — called also *submaxillary ganglion*

submandibular gland *n* : a salivary gland inside of and near the lower edge of the mandible on each side and discharging by Wharton's duct into the mouth under the tongue — called also *submandibular salivary gland, submaxillary gland, submaxillary salivary gland*

sub·max·il·lary \ˌsəb-ˈmak-sə-ˌler-ē\ *adj or n* : SUBMANDIBULAR

submaxillary ganglion *n* : SUBMANDIBULAR GANGLION

submaxillary gland *n* : SUBMANDIBULAR GLAND

submaxillary salivary gland *n* : SUBMANDIBULAR GLAND

sub·max·i·mal \ˌsəb-ˈmak-sə-məl\ *adj* : being less than the maximum of which an individual is capable

sub·men·tal \-ˈment-ᵊl\ *adj* : located in, affecting, or performed on the area under the chin

submental artery *n* : a branch of the facial artery that branches off near the submandibular gland and is distributed to the muscles of the jaw

sub·meta·cen·tric \ˌsəb-ˌme-tə-ˈsen-trik\ *adj* : having the centromere situated so that one chromosome arm is somewhat shorter than the other — **submetacentric** *n*

sub·mi·cro·scop·ic \ˌsəb-ˌmī-krə-ˈskä-pik\ *adj* : too small to be seen in an ordinary light microscope ⟨~ particles⟩ — compare MICROSCOPIC 2 — **sub·mi·cro·scop·i·cal·ly** *adv*

sub·mis·sion \səb-ˈmi-shən\ *n* : the condition of being submissive

sub·mis·sive \-ˈmi-səv\ *adj* : characterized by tendencies to yield to the will or authority of others ⟨a ~ personality⟩ — **sub·mis·sive·ness** *n*

sub·mu·co·sa \ˌsəb-myü-ˈkō-sə\ *n* : a supporting layer of loose connective tissue directly under a mucous membrane — **sub·mu·co·sal** \-zəl\ *adj*

sub·mu·cous \ˌsəb-ˈmyü-kəs\ *adj* : lying under or involving the tissues under a mucous membrane

subnitrate — see BISMUTH SUBNITRATE

sub·nor·mal \ˌsəb-ˈnȯr-məl\ *adj* **1** : lower or smaller than normal ⟨a ~ temperature⟩ **2** : having less of something and esp. of intelligence than is normal — **sub·nor·mal·i·ty** \ˌsəb-nȯr-ˈma-lə-tē\ *n*

sub·oc·cip·i·tal \-äk-ˈsi-pət-ᵊl\ *adj* **1** : situated or performed below the occipital bone **2** : situated or performed below the occipital lobe of the brain

suboccipital nerve *n* : the first cervical nerve that supplies muscles around the suboccipital triangle and that sends branches to the rectus capitis posterior minor and semispinalis capitis

suboccipital triangle *n* : a space of the suboccipital region on each side of the dorsal cervical region that is bounded superiorly and medially by a muscle arising by a tendon from a spinous process of the axis and inserting into the inferior nuchal line and the adjacent inferior region of the occipital bone, that is bounded superiorly and laterally by the obliquus capitis superior, and that is bounded inferiorly and laterally by the obliquus capitis inferior

sub·op·ti·mal \ˌsəb-ˈäp-tə-məl\ *adj* : less than optimal ⟨a ~ dose⟩

sub•or•der \ˈsəb-ˌȯr-dər\ *n* : a category in biological classification ranking below an order and above a family

Sub•ox•one \ˌsəb-ˈäk-ˌsōn\ *trademark* — used for a preparation of the hydrochloride of buprenorphine and naloxone administered sublingually

sub•peri•os•te•al \-ˌper-ē-ˈäs-tē-əl\ *adj* : situated or occurring beneath the periosteum — **sub•peri•os•te•al•ly** *adv*

sub•phren•ic \ˌsəb-ˈfre-nik\ *adj* : situated or occurring below the diaphragm

subphrenic space *n* : a space on each side of the falciform ligament between the underside of the diaphragm and the upper side of the liver

sub•phy•lum \ˈsəb-ˌfī-ləm\ *n, pl* **-la** \-lə\ : a category in biological classification ranking below a phylum and above a class

sub•pleu•ral \-ˈplu̇r-əl\ *adj* : situated or occurring between the pleura and the body wall — **sub•pleu•ral•ly** *adv*

sub•pop•u•la•tion \ˌsəb-ˌpä-pyə-ˈlā-shən\ *n* : an identifiable fraction or subdivision of a population

sub•po•tent \ˌsəb-ˈpōt-ᵊnt\ *adj* : less potent than normal ⟨~ drugs⟩ — **sub•po•ten•cy** \-ˈpōt-ᵊn-sē\ *n*

sub•pu•bic angle \ˌsəb-ˈpyü-bik-\ *n* : the angle that is formed just below the pubic symphysis by the meeting of the inferior ramus of the pubis on one side with the corresponding part on the other side

sub•ret•i•nal \-ˈret-ᵊn-əl\ *adj* : situated or occurring beneath the retina

sub•sa•lic•y•late \-sə-ˈli-sə-ˌlāt\ *n* : a basic salicylate (as bismuth subsalicylate)

sub•sar•co•lem•mal \-ˌsär-kə-ˈle-məl\ *adj* : situated or occurring beneath a sarcolemma ⟨~ mitochondria⟩

sub•scap•u•lar \ˌsəb-ˈska-pyə-lər\ *adj* : situated under the scapula

subscapular artery *n* : an artery that is usu. the largest branch of the axillary artery, that arises opposite the lower border of the subscapularis muscle, and that passes down and back to the lower part of the scapula where it forms branches and anastomoses with arteries in that region

subscapular fossa *n* : the concave depression of the anterior surface of the scapula

sub•scap•u•lar•is \ˌsəb-ˌska-pyə-ˈlar-əs\ *n* : a large triangular muscle that fills up the subscapular fossa, that arises from the surface of the scapula, that is inserted into the lesser tubercle of the humerus, and that stabilizes the shoulder joint as part of the rotator cuff and rotates the humerus medially when the arm is held by the side of the body

sub•scrip•tion \səb-ˈskrip-shən\ *n* : a part of a prescription that contains directions to the pharmacist

sub•se•rous \ˌsəb-ˈsir-əs\ *or* **sub•se•ro•sal** \-sə-ˈrō-zəl\ *adj* : situated or occurring under a serous membrane

sub•side \səb-ˈsīd\ *vb* **sub•sid•ed; sub•sid•ing** : to lessen in severity : become diminished — **sub•si•dence** \səb-ˈsīd-ᵊns, ˈsəb-səd-əns\ *n*

sub•spe•cial•ist \ˌsəb-ˈspe-shə-list\ *n* : a physician having a subspecialty

sub•spe•cial•ty \ˌsəb-ˈspe-shəl-tē\ *n, pl* **-ties** : a subordinate field of specialization

sub•spe•cies \ˈsəb-ˌspē-shēz, -sēz\ *n* : a subdivision of a species: as **a** : a category in biological classification that ranks immediately below a species and designates a population of a particular geographical region genetically distinguishable from other such populations of the same species and capable of interbreeding successfully with them where its range overlaps theirs **b** : a named subdivision (as a race or variety) of a species — **sub•spe•cif•ic** \ˌsəb-spi-ˈsi-fik\ *adj*

sub•stage \ˈsəb-ˌstāj\ *n* : an attachment to a microscope by means of which accessories (as mirrors or condensers) are held in place beneath the stage of the instrument

sub•stance \ˈsəb-stəns\ *n* : something (as alcohol, cocaine, or marijuana) deemed harmful and usu. subject to legal restriction ⟨heroin is a controlled ~⟩ ⟨~ abuse⟩

substance P *n* : a neuropeptide that consists of 11 amino acid residues, that is widely distributed in the brain, spinal cord, and peripheral nervous system, and that acts across nerve synapses to produce prolonged postsynaptic excitation

sub•stan•tia gel•a•ti•no•sa \səb-ˈstan-chə-ˌje-lə-tə-ˈnō-sə\ *n* : a mass of gelatinous gray matter that lies on the dorsal surface of the dorsal horn and extends the entire length of the spinal cord into the medulla oblongata and that functions in the transmission of painful sensory information

substantia in•nom•i•na•ta \-i-ˌnä-mə-ˈnā-tə\ *n* : a band of large cells of indeterminate function that lie just under the surface of the globus pallidus

sub•stan•tia ni•gra \səb-ˈstan-chə-ˈnī-grə, -ˈni-\ *n, pl* **sub•stan•ti•ae ni•grae** \-chē-ˌē-ˈnī-ˌgrē, -ˈni-\ : a layer of deeply pigmented gray matter situated in the midbrain and containing the cell bodies of a tract of dopamine-producing nerve cells whose secretion tends to be deficient in Parkinson's disease

substantia pro•pria \-ˈprō-prē-ə\ *n, pl* **substantiae pro•pri•ae** \-prē-ˌē\ : the layer of lamellated transparent fibrous connective tissue that makes up the bulk of the cornea of the eye

sub•ster•nal \ˌsəb-ˈstər-nəl\ *adj* : situated or perceived behind or below the sternum ⟨~ pain⟩

sub·stit·u·ent \səb-ˈsti-chə-wənt\ *n* : an atom or group that replaces another atom or group in a molecule — **substituent** *adj*

sub·sti·tute \ˈsəb-stə-ˌtüt, -ˌtyüt\ *n* : a person or thing that takes the place or function of another — **substitute** *adj*

sub·sti·tu·tion \ˌsəb-stə-ˈtü-shən, -ˈtyü-\ *n* **1** : the turning from an obstructed desire to another desire whose gratification is socially acceptable **2** : the turning from an obstructed form of behavior to a different and often more primitive expression of the same tendency

sub·strate \ˈsəb-ˌstrāt\ *n* **1** : the base on which an organism lives **2** : a substance acted upon (as by an enzyme)

sub·stra·tum \ˈsəb-ˌstrā-təm, -ˌstra-\ *n, pl* **-stra·ta** \-tə\ : SUBSTRATE 1

sub·struc·ture \ˈsəb-ˌstrək-chər\ *n* : an underlying or supporting structure — **sub·struc·tur·al** \-chə-rəl\ *adj*

sub·syn·dro·mal \ˌsəb-sin-ˈdrō-məl\ *adj* : characterized by or exhibiting symptoms that are not severe enough for diagnosis as a clinically recognized syndrome ⟨∼ depression⟩

sub·ta·lar \ˌsəb-ˈtā-lər\ *adj* : situated or occurring beneath the talus; *specif* : of, relating to, or being the articulation formed between the posterior facet of the inferior surface of the talus and the posterior facet of the superior surface of the calcaneus

sub·tem·po·ral decompression \-ˈtem-pə-rəl-\ *n* : relief of intracranial pressure by excision of a portion of the temporal bone

sub·tha·lam·ic \ˌsəb-thə-ˈla-mik\ *adj* : of or relating to the subthalamus

subthalamic nucleus *n* : an oval mass of gray matter that is located in the caudal part of the subthalamus and when affected with lesions is associated with hemiballismus of the contralateral side of the body

sub·thal·a·mus \ˌsəb-ˈtha-lə-məs\ *n, pl* **-mi** \-ˌmī\ : the ventral part of the thalamus

sub·ther·a·peu·tic \-ˌther-ə-ˈpyü-tik\ *adj* : not producing a therapeutic effect ⟨∼ doses of penicillin⟩

sub·thresh·old \ˌsəb-ˈthresh-ˌhōld\ *adj* : inadequate to produce a response ⟨∼ dosages⟩ ⟨a ∼ stimulus⟩

sub·to·tal \ˌsəb-ˈtōt-ᵊl\ *adj* : somewhat less than complete : nearly total ⟨∼ thyroidectomy⟩

sub·tro·chan·ter·ic \ˌsəb-ˌtrō-kən-ˈter-ik, -ˌkan-\ *adj* : situated or occurring below a trochanter

sub·un·gual \ˌsəb-ˈəŋ-gwəl, -ˈən-\ *adj* : situated or occurring under a fingernail or toenail ⟨a ∼ abscess⟩

Sub·u·tex \ˈsəb-yu̇-ˌteks\ *trademark* — used for a preparation of the hydrochloride of buprenorphine administered sublingually

sub·val·vu·lar \ˌsəb-ˈval-vyə-lər\ *adj* : situated or occurring below a valve (as a semilunar valve) ⟨∼ stenosis⟩

sub·vi·ral \ˌsəb-ˈvī-rəl\ *adj* : relating to, being, or caused by a piece or a structural part (as a protein) of a virus

sub·xi·phoid \ˌsəb-ˈzī-ˌfȯid, -ˈzi-\ *adj* : situated, occurring, or performed below the xiphoid process

succedaneum — see CAPUT SUCCEDANEUM

suc·ci·nate \ˈsək-sə-ˌnāt\ *n* : a salt or ester of succinic acid

succinate dehydrogenase *n* : an iron-containing flavoprotein enzyme that catalyzes often reversibly the dehydrogenation of succinic acid to fumaric acid — called also *succinic dehydrogenase*

suc·cin·ic acid \(ˌ)sək-ˈsi-nik-\ *n* : a crystalline acid $C_4H_6O_4$ containing two carboxyl groups that is formed in the Krebs cycle and in various fermentation processes

suc·ci·nyl·cho·line \ˌsək-sə-nəl-ˈkō-ˌlēn, -ˌnil-\ *n* : a basic compound that acts similarly to curare and is used intravenously chiefly in the form of its chloride salt as a short-term relaxant of skeletal muscle in surgery — called also *suxamethonium;* see ANECTINE

suc·ci·nyl·sul·fa·thi·a·zole \ˌsək-sə-nəl-ˌsəl-fə-ˈthī-ə-ˌzōl, -ˌnil-\ *n* : a sulfa drug $C_{13}H_{13}N_3O_5S_2$ used esp. for treating gastrointestinal infections

suc·cus en·ter·i·cus \ˌsə-kəs-en-ˈter-i-kəs\ *n* : INTESTINAL JUICE

suc·cus·sion \sə-ˈkə-shən\ *n* : the action or process of shaking or the condition of being shaken esp. with violence: **a** : a shaking of the body to ascertain if fluid is present in a cavity and esp. in the thorax **b** : the splashing sound made by succussion

suck \ˈsək\ *vb* **1** : to draw (as liquid) into the mouth through a suction force produced by movements of the lips and tongue **2** : to draw out by suction

suck·er \ˈsə-kər\ *n* **1** : an organ in various animals (as a trematode or tapeworm) used for adhering or holding **2** : a mouth (as of a leech) adapted for sucking or adhering

sucking louse *n* : any of an order (Anoplura) of wingless insects comprising the true lice with mouthparts adapted for sucking body fluids

suck·le \ˈsə-kəl\ *vb* **suck·led; suck·ling** **1** : to give milk to from the breast or udder **2** : to draw milk from the breast or udder of

su·cral·fate \sü-ˈkral-ˌfāt\ *n* : an aluminum complex $C_{12}H_mAl_{16}O_nS_8$ where *m* and *n* are approximately 54 and 75 that is taken orally in the treatment of duodenal ulcers — see CARAFATE

su·cra·lose \ˈsü-krə-ˌlōs\ *n* : a white crystalline powder $C_{12}H_{19}Cl_3O_8$ that is derived from sucrose and is used as a low-calorie sweetener

su·crase \ˈsü-ˌkrās, -ˌkrāz\ *n* : INVERTASE

su•crose \ˈsü-ˌkrōs, -ˌkrōz\ *n* : a sweet crystalline dextrorotatory disaccharide sugar $C_{12}H_{22}O_{11}$ that occurs naturally in most plants and is obtained commercially esp. from sugarcane or sugar beets

[1]**suc•tion** \ˈsək-shən\ *n* **1** : the act or process of sucking **2 a** : the act or process of exerting a force upon a solid, liquid, or gaseous body by reason of reduced air pressure over part of its surface **b** : force so exerted **3** : the act or process of removing secretions or fluids from hollow or tubular organs or cavities by means of a tube and a device (as a suction pump) that operates on negative pressure

[2]**suction** *vb* : to remove (as from a body cavity or passage) by suction

suction lipectomy *n* : LIPOSUCTION

suction pump *n* : a common pump in which the liquid to be raised is pushed by atmospheric pressure into the partial vacuum under a retreating valved piston on the upstroke and reflux is prevented by a valve in the pipe that permits flow in only one direction — see STOMACH PUMP

su•dam•i•na \sü-ˈda-mə-nə\ *n pl* : a transient eruption of minute translucent vesicles caused by retention of sweat in the sweat glands and in the corneous layer of the skin and occurring after profuse perspiration — called also *miliaria crystallina* — **su•dam•i•nal** \-nəl\ *adj*

Su•dan \sü-ˈdan\ *n* : any of several azo solvent dyes including some which have a specific affinity for fatty substances

Sudan IV \-ˈfōr\ *n* : a red dye used chiefly as a biological stain and in ointments for promoting the growth of epithelium (as in the treatment of burns, wounds, or ulcers) — called also *scarlet red*

su•dan•o•phil•ia \sü-ˌda-nə-ˈfi-lē-ə\ *n* : the quality or state of being sudanophilic

su•dan•o•phil•ic \sü-ˌda-nə-ˈfi-lik\ *also* **su•dan•o•phil** \sü-ˈda-nə-ˌfil\ *adj* : staining selectively with Sudan dyes; *also* : containing lipids

sudden cardiac arrest *n* : CARDIAC ARREST — abbr. *SCA*

sudden cardiac death *n* : death occurring within minutes or hours following onset of acute symptoms of cardiac arrest resulting esp. from an arrhythmia

sudden death *n* : unexpected death that is instantaneous or occurs within minutes from any cause other than violence; *esp* : SUDDEN CARDIAC DEATH

sudden infant death syndrome *n* : death of an apparently healthy infant usu. before one year of age that is of unknown cause and occurs esp. during sleep — abbr. *SIDS;* called also *cot death, crib death*

su•do•mo•tor \ˈsü-də-ˌmō-tər\ *adj* : of, relating to, or being nerve fibers controlling the activity of sweat glands

su•do•rif•er•ous gland \ˌsü-də-ˈri-fə-rəs-\ *n* : SWEAT GLAND

[1]**su•do•rif•ic** \-ˈri-fik\ *adj* : causing or inducing sweat : DIAPHORETIC

[2]**sudorific** *n* : a sudorific agent or medicine

su•fen•ta•nil \sü-ˈfen-tə-ˌnil\ *n* : an opioid analgesic that is administered intravenously in the form of its citrate $C_{22}H_{30}N_2O_2S{\cdot}C_6H_8O_7$ as an anesthetic or an anesthetic adjuvant

suf•fo•cate \ˈsə-fə-ˌkāt\ *vb* **-cat•ed; -cat•ing 1** : to stop the respiration of (as by strangling or asphyxiation) **2** : to deprive of oxygen **3** : to die from being unable to breathe — **suf•fo•ca•tion** \ˌsə-fə-ˈkā-shən\ *n* — **suf•fo•ca•tive** \ˈsə-fə-ˌkā-tiv\ *adj*

suf•fuse \sə-ˈfyüz\ *vb* **suf•fused; suf•fus•ing** : to flush or spread over or through in the manner of a fluid and esp. blood — **suf•fu•sion** \sə-ˈfyü-zhən\ *n*

sug•ar \ˈshu̇-gər\ *n* **1** : a sweet substance that is colorless or white when pure, consists chiefly of sucrose, and is obtained esp. from sugarcane or sugar beets **2** : any of various water-soluble compounds that vary widely in sweetness and comprise the saccharides of smaller molecular size including sucrose

sugar diabetes *n* : DIABETES MELLITUS

sugar pill *n* : a pharmacologically inert pill : PLACEBO

sui•cide \ˈsü-ə-ˌsīd\ *n* **1** : the act or an instance of taking one's own life voluntarily and intentionally **2** : a person who commits or attempts suicide — **sui•cid•al** \ˌsü-ə-ˈsīd-ᵊl\ *adj* — **sui•cid•al•ly** \-ᵊl-ē\ *adv* — **suicide** *vb*

sui•cid•ol•o•gy \ˌsü-ə-ˌsī-ˈdä-lə-jē\ *n, pl* **-gies** : the study of suicide and suicide prevention — **sui•cid•ol•o•gist** \-jist\ *n*

suit — see G SUIT, PRESSURE SUIT

suite \ˈswēt\ *n* : a group of rooms in a medical facility dedicated to a specified function or specialty <surgical ~>

sul•bac•tam \səl-ˈbak-ˌtam, -təm\ *n* : a beta-lactamase inhibitor that is usu. administered in the form of its sodium salt $C_8H_{10}NNaO_5S$ in combination with a beta-lactam antibiotic (as ampicillin)

sul•cus \ˈsəl-kəs\ *n, pl* **sul•ci** \-ˌkī, -ˌsī\ : FURROW, GROOVE; *esp* : a shallow furrow on the surface of the brain separating adjacent convolutions — compare FISSURE 1c — **sul•cal** \ˈsəl-kəl\ *adj*

sulcus ter•mi•na•lis \-ˌtər-mə-ˈnā-ləs\ *n, pl* **sulci ter•mi•na•les** \-ˌlēz\ **1** : a V-shaped groove separating the anterior two thirds of the tongue from the posterior third and containing the circumvallate papillae **2** : a shallow groove on the outside of the right atrium of the heart

sulf- *or* **sulfo-** *comb form* : sulfur : containing sulfur <*sulf*arsphenamine>

[1]**sul·fa** \ˈsəl-fə\ *adj* **1** : related chemically to sulfanilamide **2** : of, relating to, employing, or containing sulfa drugs <~ therapy>

[2]**sulfa** *n* : SULFA DRUG

sul·fa·cet·a·mide *also* **sul·fa·cet·i·mide** \ˌsəl-fə-ˈse-tə-ˌmīd, -məd\ *n* : a sulfa drug $C_8H_{10}N_2O_3S$ that is used chiefly for treating infections of the urinary tract and in the form of its sodium salt $C_8H_9N_2NaO_3S$ to treat infections of the eye and acne vulgaris

sul·fa·di·a·zine \ˌsəl-fə-ˈdī-ə-ˌzēn\ *n* : a sulfa drug $C_{10}H_{10}N_4O_2S$ used esp. in the treatment of toxoplasmosis

sulfa drug *n* : any of various synthetic organic bacteria-inhibiting drugs that are sulfonamides closely related chemically to sulfanilamide — called also *sulfa*

sul·fa·gua·ni·dine \ˌsəl-fə-ˈgwä-nə-ˌdēn\ *n* : a sulfa drug $C_7H_{10}N_4O_2S$ used esp. in veterinary medicine — called also *sulfanilylguanidine*

sul·fa·mer·a·zine \ˌsəl-fə-ˈmer-ə-ˌzēn\ *n* : a sulfa drug $C_{11}H_{12}N_4O_2S$ that is a derivative of sulfadiazine and is used similarly

sul·fa·meth·a·zine \-ˈme-thə-ˌzēn\ *n* : a sulfa drug $C_{12}H_{14}N_4O_2S$ that is a derivative of sulfadiazine and is used similarly

sul·fa·meth·ox·a·zole \-ˌme-ˈthäk-sə-ˌzōl\ *n* : an antibacterial sulfonamide $C_{10}H_{11}N_3O_3S$ used alone or in combination with trimethoprim (as in the treatment of urinary tract infections or acute otitis media) — see BACTRIM, SEPTRA

sul·fa·mez·a·thine \-ˈme-zə-ˌthēn\ *n* : SULFAMETHAZINE

Sul·fa·my·lon \ˌsəl-fə-ˈmī-ˌlän\ *trademark* — used for a preparation of the acetate of mafenide

sul·fa·nil·amide \ˌsəl-fə-ˈni-lə-ˌmīd, -məd\ *n* : a crystalline sulfonamide $C_6H_8N_2O_2S$ that is the amide of sulfanilic acid and the parent compound of most of the sulfa drugs

sul·fan·i·lyl·gua·ni·dine \səl-ˌfa-ni-ˌlil-ˈgwä-nə-ˌdēn\ *n* : SULFAGUANIDINE

sul·fa·pyr·i·dine \ˌsəl-fə-ˈpir-ə-ˌdēn\ *n* : a sulfa drug $C_{11}H_{11}N_3O_2S$ that is derived from pyridine and sulfanilamide and is used in small doses in the treatment of dermatitis herpetiformis and esp. formerly against pneumococcal and gonococcal infections

sul·fa·qui·nox·a·line \-kwi-ˈnäk-sə-ˌlēn\ *n* : a sulfa drug $C_{14}H_{12}N_4O_2S$ used esp. in veterinary medicine

sulf·ars·phen·a·mine \ˌsəl-ˌfärs-ˈfe-nə-ˌmēn, -mən\ *n* : an orange-yellow powder $C_{14}H_{14}As_2N_2Na_2O_8S_2$ formerly used to treat syphilis

sul·fa·sal·a·zine \ˌsəl-fə-ˈsa-lə-ˌzēn\ *n* : a sulfonamide $C_{18}H_{14}N_4O_5S$ used in the treatment of chronic ulcerative colitis — called also *salicylazosulfapyridine*

[1]**sul·fate** \ˈsəl-ˌfāt\ *n* **1** : a salt or ester of sulfuric acid **2** : a bivalent group or anion SO_4 characteristic of sulfuric acid and the sulfates

[2]**sulfate** *vb* **sul·fat·ed; sul·fat·ing** : to treat or combine with sulfuric acid or a sulfate

sul·fa·thi·a·zole \ˌsəl-fə-ˈthī-ə-ˌzōl\ *n* : a sulfa drug $C_9H_9N_3O_2S_2$ derived from thiazole and sulfanilamide but seldom prescribed due to its toxicity

sul·fa·tide \ˈsəl-fə-ˌtīd\ *n* : any of the sulfates of cerebrosides that often accumulate in the central nervous systems of individuals affected with metachromatic leukodystrophy

sulf·he·mo·glo·bin \ˌsəlf-ˈhē-mə-ˌglō-bən\ *n* : a green pigment formed from hemoglobin and found in putrefied organs and cadavers

sulf·he·mo·glo·bi·ne·mia \ˌsəlf-ˌhē-mə-ˌglō-bə-ˈnē-mē-ə\ *n* : the presence of sulfhemoglobin in the blood

sulf·hy·dryl \ˌsəlf-ˈhī-drəl\ *n* : THIOL 2 — used chiefly in molecular biology

sul·fide \ˈsəl-ˌfīd\ *n* **1** : any of various organic compounds characterized by a sulfur atom attached to two carbon atoms **2** : a binary compound (as CuS) of sulfur usu. with a more electrically positive element or group

sul·fin·py·ra·zone \ˌsəl-fən-ˈpī-rə-ˌzōn\ *n* : a uricosuric drug $C_{23}H_{20}N_2O_3S$ used in the treatment of chronic gout

sul·fi·sox·a·zole \ˌsəl-fə-ˈsäk-sə-ˌzōl\ *n* : a sulfa drug $C_{11}H_{13}N_3O_3S$ derived from sulfanilamide that is less likely than other sulfanilamide derivatives to produce renal damage because of its greater solubility

sulfo- — see SULF-

sul·fo·bro·mo·phtha·lein \ˌsəl-fə-ˌbrō-mō-ˈtha-lē-ən, -ˈthā-ˌlēn\ *n* : a diagnostic material used in the form of its disodium salt $C_{20}H_8Br_4Na_2O_{10}S_2$ in a liver function test

sul·fon·amide \ˌsəl-ˈfä-nə-ˌmīd, -məd; -ˈfō-nə-ˌmīd\ *n* : any of various amides (as sulfanilamide) of a sulfonic acid; *also* : SULFA DRUG

sul·fon·eth·yl·meth·ane \ˌsəl-ˌfō-ˌne-thəl-ˈme-ˌthān\ *n* : a crystalline hypnotic $C_8H_{18}O_4S_2$ that is an ethyl analog of sulfonmethane

sul·fon·ic acid \ˌsəl-ˈfä-nik-, -ˈfō-\ *n* : any of numerous acids that contain the SO_3H group

sul·fon·meth·ane \ˌsəl-ˌfōn-ˈme-ˌthān\ *n* : a crystalline hypnotic $C_5H_{10}O_4S_2$

sul·fo·nyl·urea \ˌsəl-fə-ˌnil-ˈyůr-ē-ə, -ˌni-ˈlůr-\ *n* : any of several hypoglycemic compounds related to the sulfonamides and used in the oral treatment of type 2 diabetes

sul·fo·raph·ane \ˌsəl-fō-ˈra-ˌfān\ *n* : a compound $C_6H_{11}NOS_2$ found in vegetables (as broccoli and cauliflower) of the mustard family that stimulates the production of enzymes in the body which initiate antioxidant activity

sul•fo•sal•i•cyl•ic acid \ˌsəl-fō-ˌsa-lə-ˈsi-lik-\ *n* : a sulfonic acid derivative $C_7H_6O_6S_3$ used esp. to detect and precipitate proteins (as albumin) from urine

sulf•ox•one sodium \ˌsəl-ˈfäk-ˌsōn-\ *n* : a crystalline salt $C_{14}H_{14}N_2Na_2O_6S_3$ used in the treatment of leprosy

sul•fur \ˈsəl-fər\ *n* : a nonmetallic element that occurs either free or combined esp. in sulfides and sulfates — symbol *S;* see ELEMENT table — **sulfur** *adj*

sulfurated potash *n* : a mixture composed principally of sulfurated potassium compounds that is used in treating skin diseases

sulfur dioxide *n* : a heavy pungent toxic gas SO_2 that is a major air pollutant esp. in industrial areas

sul•fu•ric \ˌsəl-ˈfyu̇r-ik\ *adj* : of, relating to, or containing sulfur esp. with a higher valence than sulfurous compounds

sulfuric acid *n* : a heavy corrosive oily strong acid H_2SO_4 having two replaceable hydrogen atoms

sulfur mustard *n* : MUSTARD GAS

sul•fu•rous \ˈsəl-fə-rəs, -fyə-; ˌsəl-ˈfyu̇r-əs\ *adj* **1** : of, relating to, or containing sulfur esp. with a lower valence than sulfuric compounds **2** : resembling or emanating from sulfur and esp. burning sulfur

sulfurous acid *n* : a weak unstable acid H_2SO_3 used in medicine as an antiseptic

su•lin•dac \sə-ˈlin-ˌdak\ *n* : an NSAID $C_{20}H_{17}FO_3S$ used esp. in the treatment of rheumatoid arthritis

sul•i•so•ben•zone \ˌsə-li-sō-ˈben-ˌzōn\ *n* : a sunscreening agent $C_{14}H_{12}O_6S$

sulph- *or* **sulpho-** *chiefly Brit var of* SULF-

sul•pha, sul•phate, sul•phide, sul•phur, sul•phu•ric *chiefly Brit var of* SULFA, SULFATE, SULFIDE, SULFUR, SULFURIC

sul•pir•ide \ˈsəl-(ˌ)pir-īd\ *n* : an antipsychotic drug $C_{15}H_{23}N_3O_4S$ used esp in the treatment of schizophrenia

su•mac *also* **su•mach** \ˈsü-ˌmak, ˈshü-\ *n* **1** : any plant of the genus *Rhus* **2** : POISON SUMAC

su•ma•trip•tan \ˌsü-mə-ˈtrip-ˌtan, -tən\ *n* : a triptan $C_{14}H_{21}N_3O_2S$ administered as a nasal spray or in the form of its succinate $C_{14}H_{21}N_3O_2S{\cdot}C_4H_6O_4$ either as an oral tablet or by injection to treat migraine attacks — see IMITREX

sum•ma•tion \(ˌ)sə-ˈmā-shən\ *n* : cumulative action or effect; *esp* : the process by which a sequence of stimuli that are individually inadequate to produce a response are cumulatively able to induce a nerve impulse — see SPATIAL SUMMATION, TEMPORAL SUMMATION

summer complaint *n* : SUMMER DIARRHEA

summer diarrhea *n* : diarrhea esp. of children that is prevalent in hot weather and is usu. caused by ingestion of food contaminated by various microorganisms

sun•block \ˈsən-ˌbläk\ *n* : a preparation (as a lotion) applied to the skin to prevent sunburn (as by physically blocking out ultraviolet radiation); *also* : its active ingredient (as titanium dioxide) — compare SUNSCREEN

sun•burn \ˈsən-ˌbərn\ *n* : inflammation of the skin caused by overexposure to ultraviolet radiation esp. from sunlight — **sunburn** *vb*

sun•down•ing \ˈsən-dau̇-niŋ\ *n* : a state of increased agitation, confusion, disorientation, and anxiety that typically occurs in the late afternoon or evening in some individuals affected with dementia

sun•glass•es \-ˌgla-səs\ *n pl* : glasses used to protect the eyes from the sun

sun•lamp \ˈsən-ˌlamp\ *n* : an electric lamp designed to emit radiation of wavelengths from ultraviolet to infrared and used esp. for therapeutic purposes or for producing tan artificially

sun protection factor *n* : SPF

sun•screen \-ˌskrēn\ *n* : a preparation (as a lotion) applied to the skin to prevent sunburn (as by chemically absorbing ultraviolet radiation); *also* : its active ingredient (as benzophenone) — compare SUNBLOCK — **sun•screen•ing** *adj*

sunshine vitamin *n* : VITAMIN D

sun•stroke \-ˌstrōk\ *n* : heatstroke caused by direct exposure to the sun; *broadly* : HEATSTROKE

sun•tan \-ˌtan\ *n* : a browning of the skin from exposure to the rays of the sun — **sun•tanned** \-ˌtand\ *adj*

super- *prefix* **1** : greater than normal : excessive ⟨*super*ovulation⟩ **2** : situated or placed above, on, or at the top of ⟨*super*ciliary⟩; *specif* : situated on the dorsal side of

su•per•bug \ˈsü-pər-ˌbəg\ *n* : a pathogenic microorganism and esp. a bacterium that has developed resistance to the medications normally used against it

su•per•cil•i•ary \ˌsü-pər-ˈsi-lē-ˌer-ē\ *adj* : of, relating to, or adjoining the eyebrow : SUPRAORBITAL

superciliary ridge *n* : SUPRAORBITAL RIDGE — called also *superciliary arch*

su•per•coil \ˈsü-pər-ˌkȯil\ *n* : a double helix (as of DNA) that has undergone additional twisting in the same or in the opposite direction as the turns in the original helix — **supercoil** *vb*

su•per•ego \ˌsü-pər-ˈē-(ˌ)gō, ˈsü-pər-ˌ, -ˈe-(ˌ)gō\ *n* : the one of the three divisions of the psyche in psychoanalytic theory that is only partly conscious, represents internalization of parental conscience and the rules of society, and functions to reward and punish through a system of moral attitudes, conscience, and a sense of guilt — compare EGO, [1]ID

su·per·fam·i·ly \ˈsü-pər-ˌfam-lē\ *n, pl* **-lies** : a category of taxonomic classification between a family and an order

su·per·fat·ted \ˈsü-pər-ˌfa-təd\ *adj* : containing extra oil or fat ⟨~ soap⟩

su·per·fe·cun·da·tion \ˌsü-pər-ˌfe-kən-ˈdā-shən, -ˌfē-\ *n* : successive fertilization of two or more ova from the same ovulation esp. by different mates

su·per·fe·ta·tion \ˌsü-pər-fē-ˈtā-shən\ *n* : successive fertilization of two or more ova of different ovulations resulting in the presence of embryos of unlike ages in the same uterus

su·per·fi·cial \ˌsü-pər-ˈfi-shəl\ *adj* **1** : of, relating to, or located near the surface ⟨~ blood vessels⟩ **2** : lying on, not penetrating below, or affecting only the surface ⟨~ wounds⟩ — **su·per·fi·cial·ly** *adv*

superficial external pudendal artery *n* : EXTERNAL PUDENDAL ARTERY a

superficial fascia *n* : the thin layer of loose fatty connective tissue underlying the dermis and binding it to the parts beneath — called also *hypodermis, tela subcutanea;* compare DEEP FASCIA

superficial inguinal ring *n* : the inguinal ring that is the external opening of the inguinal canal — called also *external inguinal ring;* compare DEEP INGUINAL RING

superficialis — see FLEXOR DIGITORUM SUPERFICIALIS, TRANSVERSUS PERINEI SUPERFICIALIS

superficial palmar arch *n* : PALMAR ARCH b

superficial peroneal nerve *n* : a nerve that arises as a branch of the common peroneal nerve and that innervates or supplies branches innervating the muscles of the anterior part of the leg and the skin on the lower anterior part of the leg, on the dorsum of the foot, on the lateral and medial sides of the foot, and between the toes — called also *musculocutaneous nerve;* compare DEEP PERONEAL NERVE

superficial temporal artery *n* : the one of the two terminal branches of each external carotid artery that arises in the substance of the parotid gland, passes upward over the zygomatic process of the temporal bone, and is distributed by way of branches esp. to the more superficial parts of the side of the face and head

superficial temporal vein *n* : TEMPORAL VEIN a(1)

superficial transverse metacarpal ligament *n* : a transverse ligamentous band across the palm of the hand in the superficial fascia at the base of the fingers — called also *superficial transverse ligament*

superficial transverse perineal muscle *n* : TRANSVERSUS PERINEI SUPERFICIALIS

su·per·fuse \ˌsü-pər-ˈfyüz\ *vb* **-fused; -fus·ing** : to maintain the metabolic or physiological activity of (as an isolated organ) by submitting to a continuous flow of a sustaining medium over the outside — **su·per·fu·sion** \-ˈfyü-zhən\ *n*

su·per·gene \ˈsü-pər-ˌjēn\ *n* : a group of linked genes acting as an allelic unit esp. when due to the suppression of crossing-over

su·per·he·lix \ˈsü-pər-ˌhē-liks\ *n* : SUPERCOIL — **su·per·he·li·cal** \ˌsü-pər-ˈhe-li-kəl, -ˈhē-\ *adj*

su·per·in·fec·tion \ˌsü-pər-in-ˈfek-shən\ *n* : a second infection superimposed on an earlier one esp. by a different microbial agent of exogenous or endogenous origin that is resistant to the treatment used against the first infection — **su·per·in·fect** \-in-ˈfekt\ *vb*

su·pe·ri·or \sů-ˈpir-ē-ər\ *adj* **1** : situated toward the head and further away from the feet than another and esp. another similar part — compare INFERIOR 1 **2** : situated in a more anterior or dorsal position in the body of a quadruped — compare INFERIOR 2

superior alveolar nerve *n* : any of the branches of the maxillary nerve or of the infraorbital nerve that supply the teeth and gums of the upper jaw

superior articular process *n* : ARTICULAR PROCESS a

superior cerebellar artery *n* : an artery that arises from the basilar artery just before it divides to form the posterior cerebral arteries and supplies or gives off branches supplying the superior part of the cerebellum, midbrain, pineal gland, and choroid plexus of the third ventricle

superior cerebellar peduncle *n* : CEREBELLAR PEDUNCLE a

superior colliculus *n* : either member of the anterior and higher pair of corpora quadrigemina that together constitute a primitive center for vision — called also *optic lobe, optic tectum;* compare INFERIOR COLLICULUS

superior concha *n* : NASAL CONCHA c

superior constrictor *n* : a 4-sided muscle of the pharynx that acts to constrict part of the pharynx in swallowing — called also *constrictor pharyngis superior, superior pharyngeal constrictor muscle;* compare INFERIOR CONSTRICTOR, MIDDLE CONSTRICTOR

superior extensor retinaculum *n* : EXTENSOR RETINACULUM 1b

superior ganglion *n* **1** : the upper and smaller of the two sensory ganglia of the glossopharyngeal nerve that may be absent but when present is situated in a groove in which the nerve passes through the jugular foramen — called also *jugular ganglion;* compare INFERIOR GANGLION 1 **2 :** the upper of the two ganglia of the vagus nerve that is situated at the point where it exits through the jugular foramen — called also *jugular ganglion, superior vagal ganglion;* compare INFERIOR GANGLION 2

superior gluteal artery *n* **:** GLUTEAL ARTERY a

superior gluteal nerve *n* **:** GLUTEAL NERVE a

superior gluteal vein *n* **:** any of several veins that accompany the superior gluteal artery and empty into the internal iliac vein

superior hemorrhoidal artery *n* **:** RECTAL ARTERY c

superior hemorrhoidal vein *n* **:** RECTAL VEIN c

superior intercostal vein *n* **:** a vein on each side formed by the union of the veins draining the first two or three intercostal spaces of which the one on the right usu. empties into the azygos vein but sometimes into the right brachiocephalic vein and the one on the left empties into the left innominate vein after crossing the arch of the aorta

superioris — see LEVATOR LABII SUPERIORIS, LEVATOR LABII SUPERIORIS ALAEQUE NASI, LEVATOR PALPEBRAE SUPERIORIS, QUADRATUS LABII SUPERIORIS

superiority complex *n* **:** an excessive striving for or pretense of superiority to compensate for supposed inferiority

superior laryngeal artery *n* **:** LARYNGEAL ARTERY b

superior laryngeal nerve *n* **:** LARYNGEAL NERVE a — called also *superior laryngeal*

superior longitudinal fasciculus *n* **:** a large bundle of association fibers in the white matter of each cerebral hemisphere that extends above the insula from the frontal lobe to the occipital lobe where it curves downward and forward into the temporal lobe

su•pe•ri•or•ly \sú-ˈpir-ē-ər-lē\ *adv* **:** in or to a more superior position or direction

superior meatus *n* **:** a curved relatively short anteroposterior passage on each side of the nose that occupies the middle third of the lateral wall of a nasal cavity between the superior and middle nasal conchae — compare INFERIOR MEATUS, MIDDLE MEATUS

superior mesenteric artery *n* **:** MESENTERIC ARTERY b

superior mesenteric ganglion *n* **:** MESENTERIC GANGLION b

superior mesenteric plexus *n* **:** MESENTERIC PLEXUS b

superior mesenteric vein *n* **:** MESENTERIC VEIN b

superior nasal concha *n* **:** NASAL CONCHA c

superior nuchal line *n* **:** NUCHAL LINE a

superior oblique *n* **:** OBLIQUE b(1) — called also *superior oblique muscle*

superior olive *n* **:** a small gray nucleus situated on the dorsolateral aspect of the trapezoid body — called also *superior olivary nucleus;* compare INFERIOR OLIVE

superior ophthalmic vein *n* **:** OPHTHALMIC VEIN a

superior orbital fissure *n* **:** ORBITAL FISSURE a

superior pancreaticoduodenal artery *n* **:** PANCREATICODUODENAL ARTERY b

superior pectoral nerve *n* **:** PECTORAL NERVE a

superior peroneal retinaculum *n* **:** PERONEAL RETINACULUM a

superior petrosal sinus *n* **:** PETROSAL SINUS a

superior pharyngeal constrictor muscle *n* **:** SUPERIOR CONSTRICTOR

superior phrenic artery *n* **:** PHRENIC ARTERY a

superior phrenic vein *n* **:** PHRENIC VEIN a

superior ramus *n* **:** RAMUS b(1)

superior rectal artery *n* **:** RECTAL ARTERY c

superior rectal vein *n* **:** RECTAL VEIN c

superior rectus *n* **:** RECTUS 2a

superior sagittal sinus *n* **:** SAGITTAL SINUS a

superior temporal gyrus *n* **:** TEMPORAL GYRUS a

superior thyroid artery *n* **:** THYROID ARTERY a

superior turbinate *n* **:** NASAL CONCHA c

superior turbinate bone *n* **:** NASAL CONCHA c

superior ulnar collateral artery *n* **:** a long slender artery that arises from the brachial artery or one of its branches just below the middle of the upper arm, descends to the elbow following the course of the ulnar nerve, and terminates under the flexor carpi ulnaris — compare INFERIOR ULNAR COLLATERAL ARTERY

superior vagal ganglion *n* **:** SUPERIOR GANGLION 2

superior vena cava *n* **:** a vein that is the second largest vein in the human body, is formed by the union of the two brachiocephalic veins at the level of the space between the first two ribs, and returns blood to the right atrium of the heart from the upper half of the body

superior vena cava syndrome *n* : a condition characterized by elevated venous pressure of the upper extremities with accompanying distension of the affected veins and swelling of the face and neck and caused by blockage (as by a thrombus) or compression (as by a tumor) of the superior vena cava

superior vermis *n* : VERMIS 1a

superior vesical *n* : VESICAL ARTERY a

superior vesical artery *n* : VESICAL ARTERY a

superior vestibular nucleus *n* : the one of the four vestibular nuclei on each side of the medulla oblongata that sends ascending fibers to the oculomotor and trochlear nuclei in the cerebrum on the same side of the brain

superior vocal cords *n pl* : FALSE VOCAL CORDS

su·per·na·tant \ˌsü-pər-ˈnāt-ᵊnt\ *n* : the usu. clear liquid overlying material deposited by settling, precipitation, or centrifugation — **supernatant** *adj*

su·per·nu·mer·ary \ˌsü-pər-ˈnü-mə-ˌrer-ē, -ˈnyü-\ *adj* : exceeding the usual or normal number ⟨~ teeth⟩

supero- *comb form* : situated above ⟨*supero*lateral⟩

su·pero·lat·er·al \ˌsü-pə-rō-ˈla-tə-rəl\ *adj* : situated above and toward the side

su·per·ovu·la·tion \-ˌä-vyə-ˈlā-shən\ *n* : ovulation marked by the production of more than the normal number of mature eggs at one time — **su·per·ovu·late** \-ˈä-vyə-ˌlāt\ *vb*

su·per·ox·ide \-ˈäk-ˌsīd\ *n* : the monovalent anion O_2^- or a compound containing it ⟨potassium ~ KO_2⟩

superoxide dis·mu·tase \-dis-ˈmyü-ˌtās, -ˌtāz\ *n* : a metal-containing antioxidant enzyme that reduces potentially harmful free radicals of oxygen formed during normal metabolic cell processes to oxygen and hydrogen peroxide — abbr. *SOD*

su·per·po·tent \ˌsü-pər-ˈpōt-ᵊnt\ *adj* : of greater than normal or acceptable potency ⟨~ topical corticosteroids⟩ — **su·per·po·ten·cy** \-ᵊn-sē\ *n*

su·per·scrip·tion \ˌsü-pər-ˈskrip-shən\ *n* : the part of a pharmaceutical prescription which contains or consists of the Latin word *recipe* or the sign ℞

su·per·son·ic \-ˈsä-nik\ *adj* : ULTRASONIC 1 — **su·per·son·i·cal·ly** *adv*

su·per·vene \ˌsü-pər-ˈvēn\ *vb* **-vened; -ven·ing** : to follow or result as an additional, adventitious, or unlooked-for development (as in the course of a disease)

su·pi·na·tion \ˌsü-pə-ˈnā-shən\ *n* **1** : rotation of the forearm and hand so that the palm faces forward or upward and the radius lies parallel to the ulna; *also* : a corresponding movement of the foot and leg **2** : the position resulting from supination — **su·pi·nate** \ˈsü-pə-ˌnāt\ *vb*

su·pi·na·tor \ˈsü-pə-ˌnā-tər\ *n* : a muscle that produces the motion of supination; *specif* : a deeply situated muscle of the forearm that arises in two layers from the lateral epicondyle of the humerus and adjacent parts of the ligaments and bones of the elbow and that passes over the head of the radius to insert into its neck and the lateral surface of its shaft

supinator crest *n* : a bony ridge on the upper lateral surface of the shaft of the ulna that is the origin for part of the supinator muscle

su·pine \su̇-ˈpīn, ˈsü-ˌpīn\ *adj* **1** : lying on the back or with the face upward **2** : marked by supination

[1]**sup·ple·ment** \ˈsə-plə-mənt\ *n* **1** : something that completes or makes an addition **2** : DIETARY SUPPLEMENT

[2]**sup·ple·ment** \-ˌment\ *vb* : to add a supplement to : serve as a supplement for — **sup·ple·men·ta·tion** \ˌsə-plə-ˌmen-ˈtā-shən, -mən-\ *n*

sup·ple·men·tal \ˌsə-plə-ˈment-ᵊl\ *adj* : serving to supplement : SUPPLEMENTARY

supplemental air *n* : the air that can still be expelled from the lungs after an ordinary expiration — compare RESIDUAL AIR

sup·ple·men·ta·ry \ˌsə-plə-ˈmen-tə-rē\ *adj* : added or serving as a supplement ⟨~ vitamins⟩

sup·ply \sə-ˈplī\ *vb* **sup·plied; sup·ply·ing** : to furnish (organs, tissues, or cells) with a vital element (as blood or nerve fibers) — used of nerves and blood vessels

[1]**sup·port** \sə-ˈpōrt\ *vb* **1** : to hold up or serve as a foundation or prop for **2** : to maintain in condition, action, or existence ⟨~ life⟩ — **sup·por·tive** \-ˈpōr-tiv\ *adj*

[2]**support** *n* **1** : the act or process of supporting : the condition of being supported ⟨respiratory ~⟩ **2** : SUPPORTER

sup·port·er *n* : a woven or knitted band or elastic device supporting a part; *esp* : ATHLETIC SUPPORTER

support group *n* : a group of people with common experiences and concerns who provide emotional and moral support for one another

support hose *n* : stockings (as elastic stockings) worn to supply mild compression to assist the veins of the legs — usu. used with a pl. verb; called also *support hosiery*

sup·pos·i·to·ry \sə-ˈpä-zə-ˌtōr-ē\ *n, pl* **-ries** : a solid but readily melting cone or cylinder of usu. medicated material for insertion into a bodily passage or cavity (as the rectum)

sup·press \sə-ˈpres\ *vb* **1** : to exclude from consciousness ⟨~*ed* anxiety⟩ **2** : to restrain from a usual course or action ⟨~ a cough⟩ **3** : INHIBIT 2; *esp* : to inhibit the genetic expression of ⟨~ a mutation⟩ — **sup·press·ible** \-ˈpre-sə-bəl\ *adj*

¹sup·press·ant \sə-ˈpres-ᵊnt\ *adj* : SUPPRESSIVE

²suppressant *n* : an agent (as a drug) that tends to suppress or reduce in intensity rather than eliminate something

sup·pres·sion \sə-ˈpre-shən\ *n* : an act or instance of suppressing: as **a** : stoppage of a bodily function or a symptom **b** : the failure of development of a bodily part or organ **c** : the conscious intentional exclusion from consciousness of a thought or feeling — compare REPRESSION 2a

sup·pres·sive \sə-ˈpre-siv\ *adj* : tending or serving to suppress something (as the symptoms of a disease) ⟨~ drugs⟩

sup·pres·sor \sə-ˈpre-sər\ *n* : one that suppresses; *esp* : a mutant gene that suppresses the expression of another nonallelic mutant gene when both are present

suppressor T cell *n* : a T cell that suppresses the immune response of B cells and other T cells to an antigen — called also *suppressor cell, suppressor lymphocyte, suppressor T lymphocyte;* compare CYTOTOXIC T CELL, HELPER T CELL

sup·pu·ra·tion \ˌsə-pyə-ˈrā-shən\ *n* : the formation of, conversion into, or process of discharging pus — **sup·pu·rate** \ˈsə-pyə-ˌrāt\ *vb* — **sup·pu·ra·tive** \ˈsə-pyə-ˌrā-tiv\ *adj*

suppurativa — see HIDRADENITIS SUPPURATIVA

supra- *prefix* **1** : SUPER- 2 ⟨*supra*orbital⟩ **2** : transcending ⟨*supra*molecular⟩

su·pra·cer·vi·cal hysterectomy \ˌsü-prə-ˈsər-vi-kəl-\ *n* : a hysterectomy in which the uterine cervix is not removed

su·pra·chi·as·mat·ic \-ˌkī-əz-ˈma-tik\ *adj* : SUPRAOPTIC

suprachiasmatic nucleus *n* : either of a pair of neuron clusters in the hypothalamus directly above the optic chiasma that receive photic input from the retina via the optic nerve and that regulate the body's circadian rhythms — abbr. *SCN*

su·pra·cla·vic·u·lar \-kla-ˈvi-kyə-lər, -klə-\ *adj* : situated or occurring above the clavicle ⟨~ lymph nodes⟩

supraclavicular nerve *n* : any of three nerves that are descending branches of the cervical plexus arising from the third and fourth cervical nerves and that supply the skin over the upper chest and shoulder

su·pra·clu·sion \ˌsü-prə-ˈklü-zhən\ *n* : SUPRAOCCLUSION

su·pra·con·dy·lar \ˌsü-prə-ˈkän-də-lər, -ˌprä-\ *adj* : of, relating to, affecting, or being the part of a bone situated above a condyle ⟨a ~ fracture⟩

supracondylar ridge *n* : either of two ridges above the condyle of the humerus of which one is situated laterally and the other medially and which give attachment to muscles

su·pra·gin·gi·val \-ˈjin-jə-vəl\ *adj* : located on the surface of a tooth not surrounded by gingiva ⟨~ calculus⟩

su·pra·gle·noid \-ˈgle-ˌnȯid, -ˈglē-\ *adj* : situated or occurring superior to the glenoid cavity

su·pra·glot·tic \-ˈglä-tik\ *adj* : situated or occurring above the glottis

su·pra·hy·oid \-ˈhī-ˌȯid\ *adj* : situated or occurring superior to the hyoid bone ⟨~ lymphadenectomy⟩

suprahyoid muscle *n* : any of several muscles (as the mylohyoid and geniohyoid) passing upward to the jaw and face from the hyoid bone

su·pra·mar·gi·nal gyrus \-ˌmär-jən-ᵊl-\ *n* : a gyrus of the inferior part of the parietal lobe that is continuous in front with the postcentral gyrus and posteriorly and inferiorly with the superior temporal gyrus

su·pra·mo·lec·u·lar \-mə-ˈle-kyə-lər\ *adj* : more complex than a molecule; *also* : composed of many molecules

su·pra·nu·cle·ar \-ˈnü-klē-ər, -ˈnyü-\ *adj* : situated, occurring, or produced by a lesion superior or cortical to a nucleus esp. of the brain

supranuclear palsy *n* : PROGRESSIVE SUPRANUCLEAR PALSY

su·pra·oc·clu·sion \-ə-ˈklü-zhən\ *n* : the projection of a tooth beyond the plane of occlusion

su·pra·op·tic \-ˈäp-tik\ *adj* : situated or occurring above the optic chiasma

supraoptic nucleus *n* : a small nucleus of closely packed neurons that overlies the optic chiasma and is intimately connected with the neurohypophysis

su·pra·or·bit·al \-ˈȯr-bət-ᵊl\ *adj* : situated or occurring above the orbit of the eye

supraorbital artery *n* : a branch of the ophthalmic artery supplying the orbit and parts of the forehead

supraorbital fissure *n* : ORBITAL FISSURE a

supraorbital foramen *n* : SUPRAORBITAL NOTCH

supraorbital nerve *n* : a branch of the frontal nerve supplying the forehead, scalp, cranial periosteum, and adjacent parts

supraorbital notch *n* : a notch or foramen in the bony border of the upper inner part of the orbit serving for the passage of the supraorbital nerve, artery, and vein

supraorbital ridge *n* : a prominence of the frontal bone above the eye caused by the projection of the frontal sinuses — called also *brow ridge, superciliary ridge*

supraorbital vein *n* : a vein that drains the supraorbital region and unites with the frontal vein to form the angular vein

su·pra·phys·i·o·log·i·cal \-ˌfi-zē-ə-ˈlä-ji-kəl\ *also* **su·pra·phys·i·o·log·ic** \-ˈlä-jik\ *adj* : greater than normally present in the body

su·pra·pu·bic \-ˈpyü-bik\ *adj* : situated, occurring, or performed from above the pubis ⟨~ prostatectomy⟩ — **su·pra·pu·bi·cal·ly** *adv*

[1]**su·pra·re·nal** \-ˈrēn-ᵊl\ *adj* : situated above or anterior to the kidneys; *specif* : ADRENAL

[2]**suprarenal** *n* : a suprarenal part; *esp* : ADRENAL GLAND

suprarenal artery *n* : any of three arteries on each side of the body that supply the adrenal gland located on the same side and that arise from the inferior phrenic artery, the abdominal aorta, or the renal artery

suprarenal gland *n* : ADRENAL GLAND

suprarenal vein *n* : either of two veins of which one arises from the right adrenal gland and empties directly into the inferior vena cava while the other arises from the left adrenal gland, passes behind the pancreas, and empties into the renal vein on the left side

su·pra·scap·u·lar \ˌsü-prə-ˈska-pyə-lər, -ˌprä-\ *adj* : situated or occurring superior to the scapula

suprascapular artery *n* : a branch of the thyrocervical trunk that passes over the suprascapular ligament to the back of the scapula

suprascapular ligament *n* : a thin flat ligament that is attached at one end to the coracoid process and at the other end to the upper margin of the scapula on its dorsal surface

suprascapular nerve *n* : a branch of the brachial plexus that supplies the supraspinatus and infraspinatus muscles

suprascapular notch *n* : a deep notch in the upper border of the scapula at the base of the coracoid process giving passage to the suprascapular nerve

su·pra·sel·lar \-ˈse-lər\ *adj* : situated or rising above the sella turcica — used chiefly of tumors of the pituitary gland

su·pra·spi·nal \-ˈspī-nəl\ *adj* : situated or occurring above a spine

supraspinal ligament *n* : a fibrous cord that joins the tips of the spinous processes of the vertebrae from the seventh cervical vertebra to the sacrum and that continues forward to the skull as the ligamentum nuchae — called also *supraspinous ligament*

su·pra·spi·na·tus \-ˌspī-ˈnā-təs\ *n* : a muscle of the back of the shoulder that arises from the supraspinous fossa of the scapula, that inserts into the top of the greater tubercle of the humerus, that is one of the muscles making up the rotator cuff of the shoulder, and that rotates the humerus laterally and helps to abduct the arm

su·pra·spi·nous fossa \ˌsü-prə-ˈspī-nəs-\ *n* : a smooth concavity above the spine on the dorsal surface of the scapula that gives origin to the supraspinatus muscle

supraspinous ligament *n* : SUPRASPINAL LIGAMENT

su·pra·ster·nal \-ˈstərn-ᵊl\ *adj* : situated above or measured from the top of the sternum ⟨~ height⟩

suprasternal notch *n* : the depression in the top of the sternum between its articulations with the two clavicles

suprasternal space *n* : a long narrow space in the lower part of the deep fascia of the cervical region containing areolar tissue, the sternal part of the sternocleidomastoid muscles, and the lower part of the anterior jugular veins

su·pra·ten·to·ri·al \-ten-ˈtōr-ē-əl\ *adj* : relating to, occurring in, affecting, or being the tissues overlying the tentorium cerebelli ⟨a ~ glioma⟩

su·pra·thresh·old \-ˈthresh-ˌhōld\ *adj* : of sufficient strength or quantity to produce a perceptible physiological effect ⟨~ stimuli⟩

su·pra·troch·le·ar artery \-ˈträ-klē-ər-\ *n* : one of the terminal branches of the ophthalmic artery that ascends upon the forehead from the inner angle of the orbit

supratrochlear nerve *n* : a branch of the frontal nerve supplying the skin of the forehead and the upper eyelid

su·pra·val·vu·lar \-ˈval-vyə-lər\ *adj* : situated or occurring above a valve ⟨~ aortic stenosis⟩

su·pra·ven·tric·u·lar \-ven-ˈtri-kyə-lər\ *adj* : relating to or being a rhythmic abnormality of the heart caused by impulses originating above the ventricles (as in the atrioventricular node) ⟨~ tachycardia⟩

su·pra·vi·tal \-ˈvīt-ᵊl\ *adj* : constituting or relating to the staining of living tissues or cells surviving after removal from a living body by dyes that penetrate living substance but induce more or less rapid degenerative changes — compare INTRAVITAL 2 — **su·pra·vi·tal·ly** *adv*

supreme thoracic artery *n* : THORACIC ARTERY 1a

su·ral nerve \ˈsu̇r-əl-\ *n* : any of several nerves in the region of the calf of the leg; *esp* : one formed by the union of a branch of the tibial nerve with a branch of the common peroneal nerve that supplies branches to the skin of the back of the leg and sends a continuation to the little toe by way of the lateral side of the foot

sur·a·min \ˈsu̇r-ə-mən\ *n* : a trypanocidal drug $C_{51}H_{34}N_6Na_6O_{23}S_6$ administered intravenously in the early stages of African sleeping sickness — called also *germanin, suramin sodium*

surface–active *adj* : altering the properties and esp. lowering the tension at the surface of contact between phases ⟨soaps are typical ~ substances⟩

surface tension *n* : the attractive force exerted upon the surface molecules of a liquid by the molecules beneath that tends to draw the surface molecules into the bulk of the liquid and makes the liquid assume the shape having the least surface area

sur·fac·tant \(ˌ)sər-ˈfak-tənt, ˈsər-ˌ\ *n* : a surface-active substance; *specif* : a surface-active lipoprotein mixture which coats the alveoli and which prevents collapse of the lungs by reducing the surface tension of pulmonary fluids — **surfactant** *adj*

surg *abbr* **1** surgeon **2** surgery **3** surgical

sur·geon \ˈsər-jən\ *n* **1** : a medical specialist who performs surgery : a physician qualified to treat those diseases that are amenable to or require surgery — compare INTERNIST **2** : the senior medical officer of a military unit

surgeon general *n, pl* **surgeons general** : the chief medical officer of a branch of the armed services or of a public health service

sur·gery \ˈsər-jə-rē\ *n, pl* **-ger·ies** **1** : a branch of medicine concerned with diseases and conditions requiring or amenable to operative or manual procedures **2 a** *Brit* : a physician's or dentist's office **b** : a room or area where surgery is performed **3 a** : the work done by a surgeon **b** : OPERATION

sur·gi·cal \ˈsər-ji-kəl\ *adj* **1** : of, relating to, or concerned with surgeons or surgery **2** : requiring surgical treatment ⟨a ~ appendix⟩ **3** : used in or in connection with surgery ⟨~ gauze⟩ **4** : following or resulting from surgery ⟨~ fevers⟩

sur·gi·cal·ly \ˈsər-ji-klē, -kə-lē\ *adv* : by means of surgery

surgical neck *n* : a slightly narrowed part of the humerus below the greater and lesser tubercles that is frequently the site of fractures

sur·gi·cen·ter \ˈsər-jə-ˌsen-tər\ *n* : a medical facility that performs minor surgery on an outpatient basis

sur·ra \ˈsu̇r-ə\ *n* : a severe febrile and hemorrhagic disease of tropical or subtropical domestic animals that is caused by a protozoan of the genus *Trypanosoma* (*T. evansi*)

sur·ro·ga·cy \ˈsər-ə-gə-sē\ *n, pl* **-cies** : the practice of serving as a surrogate mother

sur·ro·gate \-gət\ *n* : one that serves as a substitute: as **a** : a representation of a person substituted through symbolizing (as in a dream) for conscious recognition of the person **b** : a drug substituted for another drug **c** : SURROGATE MOTHER

surrogate mother *n* : a woman who becomes pregnant usu. by artificial insemination or surgical implantation of a fertilized egg for the purpose of carrying the fetus to term for another woman — **surrogate motherhood** *n*

sur·veil·lance \sər-ˈvā-ləns, -lyəns\ *n* : close and continuous observation or testing ⟨serological ~⟩ — see IMMUNOLOGICAL SURVEILLANCE

sur·vi·vor·ship \sər-ˈvī-vər-ˌship\ *n* **1** : the state of being a survivor **2** : the probability of surviving to a particular age; *also* : the number or proportion of survivors (as of an age group)

[1]**sus·cep·ti·ble** \sə-ˈsep-tə-bəl\ *adj* **1** : having little resistance to a specific infectious disease : capable of being infected **2** : predisposed to develop a noninfectious disease ⟨~ to diabetes⟩ **3** : abnormally reactive to various drugs — **sus·cep·ti·bil·i·ty** \sə-ˌsep-tə-ˈbi-lə-tē\ *n*

[2]**susceptible** *n* : one that is susceptible (as to a disease)

suspended animation *n* : temporary suspension of the vital functions

sus·pen·sion \sə-ˈspen-chən\ *n* **1 a** : the state of a substance when its particles are mixed with but undissolved in a fluid or solid **b** : a substance in this state — see ORAL SUSPENSION **2** : a system consisting of a solid dispersed in a solid, liquid, or gas usu. in particles of larger than colloidal size

[1]**sus·pen·so·ry** \sə-ˈspen-sə-rē\ *adj* : serving to suspend : providing support

[2]**suspensory** *n, pl* **-ries** : something that suspends or holds up; *esp* : a fabric supporter for the scrotum

suspensory ligament *n* : a ligament or fibrous membrane suspending an organ or part: as **a** : a ringlike fibrous membrane connecting the ciliary body and the lens of the eye and holding the lens in place **b** : FALCIFORM LIGAMENT

suspensory ligament of the ovary *n* : a fold of peritoneum that consists of a part of the broad ligament that is attached to the ovary near the end joining the fallopian tube and that contains blood and lymph vessels passing to and from the ovary — called also *infundibulopelvic ligament;* compare LIGAMENT OF THE OVARY

sustained–release *adj* : designed to slowly release a drug in the body over an extended period of time esp. to sustain therapeutic levels

sus·ten·tac·u·lar cell \ˌsəs-tən-ˈta-kyə-lər-\ *n* : a supporting epithelial cell (as of the olfactory epithelium) that lacks a specialized function

sustentacular fiber of Müller *n* : MÜLLER CELL

sus·ten·tac·u·lum ta·li \ˌsəs-tən-ˈta-kyə-ləm-ˈtā-ˌlī\ *n* : a medial process of the calcaneus supporting part of the talus

Sus·ti·va \sə-ˈstē-və\ *trademark* — used for a preparation of efavirenz

su·ture \ˈsü-chər\ *n* **1 a** : a stitch made with a suture **b** : a strand or fiber used to sew parts of the living body **c** : the act or process of sewing with sutures **2 a** : the line of union in an immovable articulation (as between the bones of the skull); *also* : such an articulation **b** : a furrow at the junction of adjacent bodily parts — **su·tur·al** \ˈsü-chə-rəl\ *adj* — **suture** *vb*

suxa·me·tho·ni·um \ˌsu̇k-sə-mə-ˈthō-nē-əm\ *n, chiefly Brit* : SUCCINYLCHOLINE

Sv *abbr* sievert

sved·berg \ˈsfed-ˌbərg, -ˌber-ē\ *n* : a unit of time amounting to 10^{-13} second that is used to measure the sedimentation velocity of a colloidal solution (as of a protein) in an ultracentrifuge and to determine molecular weight by substitution in an equation — called also *svedberg unit*

Svedberg, Theodor (1884–1971), Swedish chemist.

SV40 \ˌes-ˌvē-ˈfȯr-tē\ *n* : SIMIAN VIRUS 40

SVT *abbr* supraventricular tachycardia

swab \ˈswäb\ *n* **1** : a wad of absorbent material usu. wound around one end of a small stick and used for applying medication or for removing material from an area **2** : a specimen taken with a swab ⟨a throat ~⟩ — **swab** *vb*

swamp fever *n* : EQUINE INFECTIOUS ANEMIA

Swan–Ganz catheter \ˈswän-ˈganz-\ *n* : a soft catheter with a balloon tip that is used for measuring blood pressure in the pulmonary artery

Swan, Harold James Charles (1922–2005), and **Ganz, William (1919–2009),** American cardiologists.

S wave \ˈes-ˌ\ *n* : the negative downward deflection in the QRS complex of an electrocardiogram that follows the R wave

sway·back \ˈswā-ˌbak\ *n* **1** : LORDOSIS 2 **2** : an abnormal sagging of the back found esp. in horses **3** : a copper-deficiency disease of young or newborn lambs — **sway·backed** \-ˌbakt\ *adj*

¹sweat \ˈswet\ *vb* **sweat** *or* **sweat·ed; sweat·ing** : to excrete moisture in visible quantities through the opening of the sweat glands : PERSPIRE

²sweat *n* **1** : the fluid excreted from the sweat glands of the skin : PERSPIRATION **2** : abnormally profuse sweating — often used in pl. ⟨soaking ~*s*⟩ — **sweaty** \-ē\ *adj*

sweat duct *n* : the part of a sweat gland which extends through the dermis to the surface of the skin

sweat gland *n* : a simple tubular gland of the skin that secretes perspiration and in humans is widely distributed in nearly all parts of the skin — called also *sudoriferous gland*

sweat test *n* : a test for cystic fibrosis that involves measuring the subject's sweat for abnormally high sodium chloride content

swee·ny \ˈswē-nē\ *n, pl* **sweenies** : an atrophy of the shoulder muscles of a horse; *broadly* : any muscular atrophy of a horse

sweet \ˈswēt\ *adj* : being or inducing the one of the four basic taste sensations that is typically induced by disaccharides and is mediated esp. by receptors in taste buds at the front of the tongue — compare BITTER, SALT 2, SOUR — **sweet·ness** *n*

Sweet's syndrome \ˈswēts-\ *or* **Sweet syndrome** *n* : a disease that occurs esp. in middle-aged women, that is characterized by red raised often painful patches on the skin and by fever and neutrophilia in the peripheral blood, that responds to treatment with corticosteroids, and that is of unknown cause but is sometimes associated with an underlying malignant disorder — called also *acute febrile neutrophilic dermatosis*

Sweet, Robert Douglas (1917–2001), British dermatologist.

swell \ˈswel\ *vb* **swelled; swelled** *or* **swol·len** \ˈswō-lən\; **swell·ing** : to become distended or puffed up

swell·ing \ˈswel-iŋ\ *n* : an abnormal bodily protuberance or localized enlargement ⟨an inflammatory ~⟩

Swift's disease \ˈswifts-\ *n* : ACRODYNIA

Swift, H. (*fl* 1918), Australian physician.

swimmer's ear *n* : inflammation of the canal in the outer ear that is characterized by itching, redness, swelling, pain, discharge, and sometimes hearing loss and that typically occurs when water trapped in the outer ear during swimming becomes infected usu. with a bacterium

swimmer's itch *n* : an itching inflammation that is a reaction to the invasion of the skin by schistosomes that are not normally parasites of humans — called also *schistosome dermatitis*

swine dysentery \ˈswīn-\ *n* : an acute infectious hemorrhagic dysentery of swine

swine erysipelas *n* : a destructive contagious disease of various mammals and birds caused by a bacterium of the genus *Erysipelothrix* (*E. rhusiopathiae*) — called also *erysipelas*

swine fever *n* **1** : HOG CHOLERA **2** : AFRICAN SWINE FEVER

swine flu : SWINE INFLUENZA; *also* : influenza of humans that is caused by a subtype (H1N1) of an orthomyxovirus (species *Influenza A virus* of the genus *Influenzavirus A*) originating in swine and is marked esp. by fever, sore throat, cough, chills, body aches, fatigue, and sometimes diarrhea and vomiting — see H1N1

swineherd's disease *n* : a form of leptospirosis contracted from swine

swine influenza *n* : influenza of swine that is marked by fever, lethargy, labored breathing, coughing, and anorexia, is caused by infection with a subtype (as H1N1 or N3N2) of the orthomyxovirus causing influenza A, and has been transmitted to humans sometimes causing outbreaks — see SWINE FLU

swine•pox \ˈswīn-ˌpäks\ *n* : a mild virus disease of young pigs that is marked by fever, loss of appetite, lethargy, and formation of skin lesions and that is caused by a poxvirus (species *Swinepox virus* of the genus *Suipoxvirus*) transmitted esp. by the hog louse

swol•len *adj* : protuberant or abnormally distended (as by injury or disease)

sy•co•sis \sī-ˈkō-səs\ *n, pl* **sy•co•ses** \-ˌsēz\ : a chronic inflammatory disease involving the hair follicles esp. of the bearded part of the face and marked by papules, pustules, and tubercles perforated by hairs with crusting

sycosis bar•bae \-ˈbär-bē\ *n* : sycosis of the bearded part of the face

Syd•en•ham's chorea \ˈsid-ᵊn-əmz-\ *n* : chorea following infection (as rheumatic fever) and occurring usu. in children and adolescents — called also *Saint Vitus' dance*

Sydenham, Thomas (1624–1689), British physician.

syl•vat•ic \sil-ˈva-tik\ *adj* : occurring in, affecting, or transmitted by wild animals ⟨∼ diseases⟩

sylvatic plague *n* : a form of plague of which wild rodents and their fleas are the reservoirs and vectors and which is widely distributed in western No. and So. America though rarely affecting humans

syl•vi•an \ˈsil-vē-ən\ *adj, often cap* : of or relating to the sylvian fissure

Du•bois \dᵫ-ˈbwä\ *or* **De Le Boë** \ˌdā-lā-ˈbō-ā\, **François** *or* **Franz** (*Latin* **Franciscus Sylvius) (1614–1672),** Dutch anatomist, physician, and chemist.

sylvian fissure *n, often cap 1st S* : a deep fissure of the lateral aspect of each cerebral hemisphere that divides the temporal from the parietal and frontal lobes — called also *fissure of Sylvius, lateral fissure, lateral sulcus*

sym- — see SYN-

Sym•bi•cort \ˈsim-bə-ˌkȯrt\ *trademark* — used for a preparation of budesonide and formoterol for oral inhalation

sym•bi•ont \ˈsim-ˌbī-ˌänt, -bē-\ *n* : an organism living in symbiosis; *esp* : the smaller member of a symbiotic pair — called also *symbiote*

sym•bi•o•sis \ˌsim-ˌbī-ˈō-səs, -bē-\ *n, pl* **-bi•o•ses** \-ˌsēz\ **1** : the living together in more or less intimate association or close union of two dissimilar organisms **2** : the intimate living together of two dissimilar organisms in a mutually beneficial relationship — **sym•bi•ot•ic** \ˌsim-ˌbī-ˈä-tik, -bē-\ *adj* — **sym•bi•ot•i•cal•ly** *adv*

sym•bi•ote \ˈsim-ˌbī-ˌōt, -bē-\ *n* : SYMBIONT

sym•bleph•a•ron \sim-ˈble-fə-rän\ *n* : adhesion between an eyelid and the eyeball

sym•bol \ˈsim-bəl\ *n* : something that stands for or suggests something else; *esp* : an object or act representing something in the unconscious mind that has been repressed ⟨phallic ∼*s*⟩ — **sym•bol•ic** \sim-ˈbä-lik\ *adj* — **sym•bol•i•cal•ly** *adv*

Syme's amputation \ˈsīmz-\ *or* **Syme amputation** \ˈsīm-\ *n* : amputation of the foot through the articulation of the ankle with removal of the malleoli of the tibia and fibula — compare PIROGOFF'S AMPUTATION

Syme, James (1799–1870), British surgeon.

Sym•lin \ˈsim-lin\ *trademark* — used for a preparation of the acetate of pramlintide

Sym•met•rel \ˈsi-mə-ˌtrel\ *trademark* — used for a preparation of the hydrochloride of amantadine

sym•me•try \ˈsi-mə-trē\ *n, pl* **-tries** : correspondence in size, shape, and relative position of parts on opposite sides of a dividing line or median plane or about a center or axis — see BILATERAL SYMMETRY, RADIAL SYMMETRY — **sym•met•ri•cal** \sə-ˈme-tri-kəl\ *or* **sym•met•ric** \-trik\ *adj* — **sym•met•ri•cal•ly** *adv*

sympath- *or* **sympatho-** *comb form* : sympathetic nerve : sympathetic nervous system ⟨*sympatho*lytic⟩

sym•pa•thec•to•my \ˌsim-pə-ˈthek-tə-mē\ *n, pl* **-mies** : surgical interruption of sympathetic nerve pathways — **sym•pa•thec•to•mized** \-ˌmīzd\ *adj*

[1]**sym•pa•thet•ic** \ˌsim-pə-ˈthe-tik\ *adj* **1** : of or relating to the sympathetic nervous system **2** : mediated by or acting on the sympathetic nerves — **sym•pa•thet•i•cal•ly** *adv*

[2]**sympathetic** *n* : a sympathetic structure; *esp* : SYMPATHETIC NERVOUS SYSTEM

sympathetic chain *n* : either of the pair of ganglionated longitudinal cords of the sympathetic nervous system of which one is situated on each side of the spinal column — called also *sympathetic trunk;* compare VERTEBRAL GANGLION

sympathetic nerve *n* : a nerve of the sympathetic nervous system

sympathetic nervous system *n* : the part of the autonomic nervous system that contains chiefly adrenergic fibers and tends to depress secretion, decrease the tone and contractility of smooth muscle, and increase heart rate and that consists of preganglionic fibers arising in the thoracic and upper lumbar parts of the spinal cord and passing through white rami communicantes to ganglia located in a pair of sympathetic chains situated one on each side of the spinal column or to more peripheral ganglia or ganglionated plexuses and postganglionic fibers passing typically through gray rami communicantes to spinal nerves with which they are distributed to various end organs — called also *sympathetic system;* compare PARASYMPATHETIC NERVOUS SYSTEM

sympathetico- *comb form* : SYMPATH- ⟨*sympathetico*mimetic⟩

sym•pa•thet•i•co•mi•met•ic \ˌsim-pə-ˈthe-ti-kō-mə-ˈme-tik\ *adj or n* : SYMPATHOMIMETIC

sympathetic ophthalmia *n* : inflammation in an uninjured eye as a result of injury and inflammation of the other

sym•pa•thet•i•co•to•nia \ˌsim-pə-ˌthe-ti-kə-ˈtō-nē-ə\ *n* : SYMPATHICOTONIA

sympathetic system *n* : SYMPATHETIC NERVOUS SYSTEM

sympathetic trunk *n* : SYMPATHETIC CHAIN

sympathico- *comb form* : SYMPATH- ⟨*sympathico*tonia⟩

sym•path•i•co•lyt•ic \sim-ˌpa-thi-kō-ˈli-tik\ *adj or n* : SYMPATHOLYTIC

sym•path•i•co•mi•met•ic \-mə-ˈme-tik, -mī-\ *adj or n* : SYMPATHOMIMETIC

sym•path•i•co•to•nia \sim-ˌpa-thi-kō-ˈtō-nē-ə\ *n* : a condition produced by relatively great activity or stimulation of the sympathetic nervous system and characterized by goose bumps, vascular spasm, and abnormally high blood pressure — called also *sympatheticotonia;* compare VAGOTONIA — **sym•path•i•co•ton•ic** \-ˈtä-nik\ *adj*

sym•pa•thin \ˈsim-pə-thən\ *n* : a substance (as norepinephrine) that is secreted by sympathetic nerve endings and acts as a chemical mediator

sym•pa•tho•ad•re•nal \ˌsim-pə-thō-ə-ˈdrē-nəl\ *adj* : relating to or involving the sympathetic nervous system and the adrenal medulla

sym•pa•tho•go•nia \ˌsim-pə-thō-ˈgō-nē-ə\ *n* : precursor cells of the sympathetic nervous system

sym•pa•tho•go•ni•o•ma \-ˌgō-nē-ˈō-mə\ *n, pl* **-mas** *also* **-ma•ta** \-mə-tə\ : a tumor derived from sympathogonia; *also* : NEUROBLASTOMA

¹sym•pa•tho•lyt•ic \ˌsim-pə-thō-ˈli-tik\ *adj* : tending to oppose the physiological results of sympathetic nervous activity or of sympathomimetic drugs — compare PARASYMPATHOLYTIC

²sympatholytic *n* : a sympatholytic agent

¹sym•pa•tho•mi•met•ic \-mə-ˈme-tik, -(ˌ)mī-\ *adj* : simulating sympathetic nervous action in physiological effect — compare PARASYMPATHOMIMETIC

²sympathomimetic *n* : a sympathomimetic agent

sym•phal•an•gism \(ˌ)sim-ˈfa-lən-ˌji-zəm\ *n* : ankylosis of the joints of one or more digits

sym•phy•se•al \ˌsim-fə-ˈsē-əl\ *adj* : of, relating to, or constituting a symphysis

sym•phy•si•ot•o•my \ˌsim-fə-zē-ˈä-tə-mē, sim-ˌfi-zē-\ *n, pl* **-mies** : the operation of dividing the pubic symphysis

sym•phy•sis \ˈsim-fə-səs\ *n, pl* **-phy•ses** \-ˌsēz\ **1** : an immovable or more or less movable articulation of various bones in the median plane of the body **2** : an articulation (as between the bodies of vertebrae) in which the bony surfaces are connected by pads of fibrous cartilage without a synovial membrane

symphysis pubis *n* : PUBIC SYMPHYSIS

symp•tom \ˈsimp-təm\ *n* : subjective evidence of disease or physical disturbance observed by the patient; *broadly* : something that indicates the presence of a physical disorder — compare SIGN 2

symp•tom•at•ic \ˌsimp-tə-ˈma-tik\ *adj* **1 a** : being a symptom of a disease **b** : having the characteristics of a particular disease but arising from another cause ⟨~ epilepsy resulting from brain damage⟩ **2** : concerned with or affecting symptoms ⟨~ treatment⟩ **3** : having symptoms ⟨a ~ patient⟩ — **symp•tom•at•i•cal•ly** *adv*

symp•tom•atol•o•gy \ˌsimp-tə-mə-ˈtä-lə-jē\ *n, pl* **-gies** **1** : SYMPTOM COMPLEX **2** : a branch of medical science concerned with symptoms of diseases — **symp•tom•at•o•log•i•cal** \-ˌmat-ᵊl-ˈä-ji-kəl\ *or* **symp•tom•at•o•log•ic** \-ˈä-jik\ *adj* — **symp•tom•at•o•log•i•cal•ly** *adv*

symptom complex *n* : a group of symptoms occurring together and characterizing a particular disease

symp•tom•less \ˈsimp-təm-ləs\ *adj* : exhibiting no symptoms

syn- *or* **sym-** *prefix* **1** : with : along with : together ⟨*sym*biosis⟩ **2** : at the same time ⟨*syn*esthesia⟩

syn·aes·the·sia *chiefly Brit var of* SYNESTHESIA

syn·an·throp·ic \ˌsi-nan-ˈthrä-pik\ *adj* : ecologically associated with humans ⟨~ flies⟩ — **syn·an·thro·py** \sin-ˈan-thrə-pē\ *n*

[1]**syn·apse** \ˈsi-ˌnaps, sə-ˈnaps\ *n* **1** : the place at which a nerve impulse passes from one neuron to another **2** : SYNAPSIS

[2]**synapse** *vb* **syn·apsed; syn·aps·ing** : to form a synapse or come together in synapsis

syn·ap·sis \sə-ˈnap-səs\ *n, pl* **-ap·ses** \-ˌsēz\ : the association of homologous chromosomes with chiasma formation that is characteristic of the first meiotic prophase and is held to be the mechanism for genetic crossing-over

syn·ap·tic \si-ˈnap-tik\ *adj* **1** : of, relating to, or participating in synapsis ⟨~ chromosomes⟩ **2** : of or relating to a synapse ⟨~ transmission⟩ — **syn·ap·ti·cal·ly** *adv*

synaptic cleft *n* : the space between neurons at a nerve synapse across which a nerve impulse is transmitted by a neurotransmitter — called also *synaptic gap*

synaptic vesicle *n* : a small secretory vesicle that contains a neurotransmitter, is found inside an axon near the presynaptic membrane, and releases its contents into the synaptic cleft after fusing with the membrane

syn·ap·to·gen·e·sis \sə-ˌnap-tə-ˈje-nə-səs\ *n, pl* **-e·ses** \-ˌsēz\ : the formation of nerve synapses

syn·ap·tol·o·gy \ˌsi-nap-ˈtä-lə-jē\ *n, pl* **-gies** : the scientific study of nerve synapses

syn·ap·to·phy·sin \si-ˈnap-tə-ˌfī-sᵊn\ *n* : a transmembrane glycoprotein found chiefly in presynaptic vesicles of neurons and neurosecretory granules of neuroendocrine cells

syn·ap·to·some \sə-ˈnap-tə-ˌsōm\ *n* : a nerve ending that is isolated from homogenized nerve tissue — **syn·ap·to·som·al** \-ˌnap-tə-ˈsō-məl\ *adj*

syn·ar·thro·sis \ˌsi-när-ˈthrō-səs\ *n, pl* **-thro·ses** \-ˌsēz\ : an immovable articulation in which the bones are united by intervening fibrous connective tissues

syn·chon·dro·sis \ˌsin-ˌkän-ˈdrō-səs\ *n, pl* **-dro·ses** \-ˌsēz\ : an immovable skeletal articulation in which the union is cartilaginous

syn·cho·ri·al \ˌsin-ˈkōr-ē-əl, siŋ-\ *adj* : having a common placenta — used of multiple fetuses

syn·chro·nic·i·ty \ˌsiŋ-krə-ˈni-sə-tē\ *n, pl* **-ties** : the coincidental occurrence of events and esp. psychic events (as similar thoughts in widely separated persons) that seem related but are not explained by conventional mechanisms of causality — used esp. in the psychology of C. G. Jung

syn·chro·nized sleep \ˈsiŋ-krə-ˌnīzd-, ˈsin-\ *n* : SLOW-WAVE SLEEP

syn·co·pe \ˈsiŋ-kə-pē, ˈsin-\ *n* : loss of consciousness resulting from insufficient blood flow to the brain : FAINT — **syn·co·pal** \ˈsiŋ-kə-pəl, ˈsin-\ *adj*

syn·cy·tial \sin-ˈsi-shəl, -shē-əl\ *adj* : of, relating to, or constituting syncytium

syn·cy·tio·tro·pho·blast \sin-ˌsi-shē-ō-ˈtrō-fə-ˌblast\ *n* : the outer syncytial layer of the trophoblast that actively invades the uterine wall forming the outermost fetal component of the placenta — called also *syntrophoblast;* compare CYTOTROPHOBLAST

syn·cy·tium \sin-ˈsi-shəm, -shē-əm\ *n, pl* **-tia** \-shə, -shē-ə\ : a multinucleate mass of protoplasm resulting from fusion of cells

syn·dac·tyl \ˌsin-ˈdakt-ᵊl\ *adj* : having two or more digits wholly or partly united

syn·dac·ty·lism \sin-ˈdak-tə-ˌli-zəm\ *n* : SYNDACTYLY

syn·dac·ty·lous \sin-ˈdak-tə-ləs\ *adj* : SYNDACTYL

syn·dac·ty·ly \-lē\ *n, pl* **-lies** : a union of two or more digits that occurs in humans often as a hereditary disorder marked by the joining or webbing of two or more fingers or toes

syndesm- *or* **syndesmo-** *comb form* : ligament ⟨*syndesm*osis⟩

syn·des·mo·sis \ˌsin-ˌdez-ˈmō-səs, -ˌdes-\ *n, pl* **-mo·ses** \-ˌsēz\ : an articulation in which the contiguous surfaces of the bones are rough and are bound together by a ligament

syn·drome \ˈsin-ˌdrōm\ *n* : a group of signs and symptoms that occur together and characterize a particular abnormality

syndrome X *n* **1** : angina pectoris of a usu. benign form in which the coronary arteriogram is normal **2** : METABOLIC SYNDROME

syn·drom·ic \sin-ˈdrō-mik, -ˈdrä-\ *adj* : occurring as a syndrome or part of a syndrome ⟨~ deafness⟩

syn·e·chia \si-ˈne-kē-ə, -ˈnē-\ *n, pl* **-chiae** \-kē-ˌē, -ˌī\ : an adhesion of parts and esp. one involving the iris of the eye: as **a** : adhesion of the iris to the cornea — called also *anterior synechia* **b** : adhesion of the iris to the crystalline lens — called also *posterior synechia*

syn·eph·rine \sə-ˈne-frən\ *n* : a crystalline sympathomimetic amine $C_9H_{13}NO_2$ isomeric with phenylephrine

syn·er·gic \si-ˈnər-jik\ *adj* : working together ⟨~ muscle contraction⟩ — **syn·er·gi·cal·ly** *adv*

syn·er·gism \ˈsi-nər-ˌji-zəm\ *n* : interaction of discrete agents (as drugs) such that the total effect is greater than the sum of the individual effects

— called also *synergy;* compare ANTAGONISM b — **syn•er•gis•tic** \ˌsi-nər-ˈjis-tik\ *adj* — **syn•er•gis•ti•cal•ly** *adv*

syn•er•gist \-jist\ *n* **1** : an agent that increases the effectiveness of another agent when combined with it; *esp* : a drug that acts in synergism with another **2** : an organ (as a muscle) that acts in concert with another to enhance its effect — compare AGONIST 1, ANTAGONIST a

syn•er•gize \ˈsi-nər-ˌjīz\ *vb* **-gized; -giz•ing 1** : to act as synergists : exhibit synergism **2** : to increase the activity of (a substance)

syn•er•gy \-jē\ *n, pl* **-gies** : SYNERGISM

syn•es•the•sia \ˌsi-nəs-ˈthē-zhə, -zhē-ə\ *n* : a concomitant sensation and esp. a subjective sensation or image of a sense (as of color) other than the one (as of sound) being stimulated; *also* : the condition marked by the experience of such sensations — **syn•es•thet•ic** \-ˈthe-tik\ *adj*

Syn•ga•mus \ˈsiŋ-gə-məs\ *n* : a genus (family Syngamidae) of nematode worms that are parasitic in the trachea or esophagus of various birds and mammals and include the gapeworm (*S. trachea*)

syn•ga•my \ˈsiŋ-gə-mē\ *n, pl* **-mies** : sexual reproduction by union of gametes

syn•ge•ne•ic \ˌsin-jə-ˈnē-ik\ *adj* : genetically identical esp. with respect to antigens or immunological reactions ⟨~ tumor cells⟩ — compare ALLOGENEIC, XENOGENEIC

syn•kary•on \sin-ˈkar-ē-ˌän, -ē-ən\ *n* : a cell nucleus formed by the fusion of two preexisting nuclei

syn•ki•ne•sia \ˌsin-kə-ˈnē-zhə, -ˌkī-, -zhē-ə\ *n* : SYNKINESIS

syn•ki•ne•sis \-ˈnē-səs\ *n, pl* **-ne•ses** \-ˌsēz\ : involuntary movement in one part when another part is moved : an associated movement — **syn•ki•net•ic** \-ˈne-tik\ *adj*

syn•os•to•sis \ˌsi-ˌnäs-ˈtō-səs\ *n, pl* **-to•ses** \-ˌsēz\ : union of two or more separate bones to form a single bone; *also* : the union so formed — **syn•os•tot•ic** \-ˈtä-tik\ *adj*

syn•o•vec•to•my \ˌsi-nə-ˈvek-tə-mē\ *n, pl* **-mies** : surgical removal of a synovial membrane

sy•no•via \sə-ˈnō-vē-ə, sī-\ *n* : SYNOVIAL FLUID

sy•no•vi•al \-vē-əl\ *adj* : of, relating to, or secreting synovial fluid ⟨~ effusion⟩; *also* : lined with synovial membrane ⟨a ~ bursa⟩

synovial cyst *n* : a cyst (as a Baker's cyst) containing synovial fluid

synovial fluid *n* : a transparent viscid lubricating fluid secreted by a membrane of an articulation, bursa, or tendon sheath — called also *joint fluid, synovia*

synovial joint *n* : DIARTHROSIS

synovial membrane *n* : the dense connective-tissue membrane that secretes synovial fluid and that lines the ligamentous surfaces of joint capsules, tendon sheaths where free movement is necessary, and bursae

sy•no•vi•tis \ˌsī-nə-ˈvī-təs\ *n* : inflammation of a synovial membrane usu. with pain and swelling of the joint

sy•no•vi•um \sə-ˈnō-vē-əm, sī-\ *n* : SYNOVIAL MEMBRANE

syn•the•sis \ˈsin-thə-səs\ *n, pl* **-the•ses** \-ˌsēz\ **1** : the composition or combination of parts or elements so as to form a whole **2** : the production of a substance by the union of chemical elements, groups, or simpler compounds or by the degradation of a complex compound ⟨protein ~⟩ — **syn•the•size** \-ˌsīz\ *vb*

syn•the•tase \ˈsin-thə-ˌtās, -ˌtāz\ *n* : an enzyme that catalyzes the linking together of two molecules esp. by using the energy derived from the concurrent splitting off of a group from a triphosphate (as ATP) — called also *ligase*

[1]**syn•thet•ic** \sin-ˈthe-tik\ *adj* : of, relating to, or produced by chemical or biochemical synthesis; *esp* : produced artificially ⟨~ drugs⟩ — **syn•thet•i•cal•ly** *adv*

[2]**synthetic** *n* : a product (as a drug) of chemical synthesis

Syn•throid \ˈsin-ˌthrȯid\ *trademark* — used for a preparation of the sodium salt of levothyroxine

syn•tro•pho•blast \sin-ˈtrō-fə-ˌblast\ *n* : SYNCYTIOTROPHOBLAST

syphil- *or* **syphilo-** *comb form* : syphilis ⟨*syphilo*ma⟩

syph•i•lid \ˈsi-fə-lid\ *n* : a skin eruption caused by syphilis

syph•i•lis \ˈsi-fə-ləs\ *n* : a chronic contagious usu. venereal and often congenital disease that is caused by a spirochete of the genus *Treponema* (*T. pallidum*) and if left untreated produces chancres, rashes, and systemic lesions in a clinical course with three stages continued over many years — called also *lues;* see PRIMARY SYPHILIS, SECONDARY SYPHILIS, TERTIARY SYPHILIS

[1]**syph•i•lit•ic** \ˌsi-fə-ˈli-tik\ *adj* : of, relating to, or infected with syphilis — **syph•i•lit•i•cal•ly** *adv*

[2]**syphilitic** *n* : a person infected with syphilis

syph•i•lo•ma \ˌsi-fə-ˈlō-mə\ *n, pl* **-mas** *or* **-ma•ta** \-mə-tə\ : a syphilitic tumor : GUMMA ⟨a testicular ~⟩

sy•rette \sə-ˈret\ *n, often cap* : a small collapsible tube fitted with a hypodermic needle for injecting a single dose of a medicinal agent

syring- *or* **syringo-** *comb form* : tube : fistula ⟨*syringo*bulbia⟩

sy•ringe \sə-ˈrinj, ˈsir-inj\ *n* : a device used to inject fluids into or withdraw them from something (as the body or its cavities): as **a** : a device that consists of a nozzle of varying length and a compressible rubber bulb and is used for injection or irrigation ⟨an ear ~⟩ **b** : an instrument (as for the injection of medicine or the withdrawal of bodily fluids) that consists of a hollow barrel fitted with a plunger and a hollow needle **c** : a gravity device consisting of a reservoir fitted with a long rubber tube ending with an exchangeable nozzle that is used for irrigation of the vagina or bowel — **syringe** *vb*

sy·rin·go·bul·bia \sə-ˌriŋ-gō-ˈbəl-bē-ə\ *n* : the presence of abnormal cavities in the medulla oblongata

sy·rin·go·my·elia \sə-ˌriŋ-gō-mī-ˈē-lē-ə\ *n* : a chronic progressive disease of the spinal cord associated with sensory disturbances, muscle atrophy, and spasticity

syr·inx \ˈsir-iŋks\ *n, pl* **sy·rin·ges** \sə-ˈriŋ-ˌgēz, -ˈrin-ˌjēz\ *or* **syr·inx·es** : a pathological cavity in the brain or spinal cord esp. in syringomyelia

syr·o·sin·go·pine \ˌsir-ō-ˈsiŋ-gə-ˌpēn, -ˌpīn\ *n* : an antihypertensive agent $C_{35}H_{42}N_2O_{11}$ that is closely related to reserpine

syr·up *also* **sir·up** \ˈsər-əp, ˈsir-əp\ *n* : a thick sticky liquid consisting of a concentrated solution of sugar and water with or without the addition of a flavoring agent or medicinal substance — **syr·upy** \-ə-pē\ *adj*

syrup of ipecac *n* : IPECAC SYRUP

sys·tem \ˈsis-təm\ *n* **1** : a group of body organs that together perform one or more vital functions — see CIRCULATORY SYSTEM, DIGESTIVE SYSTEM, ENDOCRINE SYSTEM, LIMBIC SYSTEM, NERVOUS SYSTEM, REPRODUCTIVE SYSTEM, RESPIRATORY SYSTEM **2** : the body considered as a functional unit

[1]**sys·tem·ic** \sis-ˈte-mik\ *adj* : of, relating to, or common to a system: as **a** : affecting the body generally — compare LOCAL **b** : supplying those parts of the body that receive blood through the aorta rather than through the pulmonary artery **c** : being a pesticide that as used is harmless to a higher animal or a plant but when absorbed into the bloodstream or the sap makes the whole organism toxic to pests (as an insect or fungus) — **sys·tem·i·cal·ly** *adv*

[2]**systemic** *n* : a systemic pesticide

systemic circulation *n* : the passage of arterial blood from the left atrium of the heart through the left ventricle, the systemic arteries, and the capillaries to the organs and tissues that receive much of its oxygen in exchange for carbon dioxide and the return of the carbon-dioxide carrying blood via the systemic veins to enter the right atrium of the heart and to participate in the pulmonary circulation

systemic inflammatory response syndrome *n* : a severe systemic response to a condition (as trauma, an infection, or a burn) that provokes an acute inflammatory reaction indicated by the presence of two or more of a group of symptoms including abnormally increased or decreased body temperature, heart rate greater than 90 beats per minute, respiratory rate greater than 20 breaths per minute or a reduced concentration of carbon dioxide in the arterial blood, and the white blood cell count greatly decreased or increased or consisting of more than ten percent immature neutrophils — abbr. *SIRS;* see SEPSIS

systemic lupus erythematosus *n* : a chronic inflammatory autoimmune disease of connective tissue that occurs chiefly in women and is typically characterized by fever, skin rash, fatigue, and joint pain and often by disorders of the blood, kidneys, heart, lungs, and brain (as hemolytic anemia, nephritis, pleurisy, pericarditis, cognitive dysfunction, or meningitis) — abbr. *SLE;* called also *systemic lupus*

systemic necrotizing vasculitis *n* : NECROTIZING VASCULITIS

sys·to·le \ˈsis-tə-(ˌ)lē\ *n* : the contraction of the heart by which the blood is forced onward and the circulation kept up — compare DIASTOLE — **sys·tol·ic** \sis-ˈtä-lik\ *adj*

systolic blood pressure *n* : the highest arterial blood pressure of a cardiac cycle occurring immediately after systole of the left ventricle of the heart — abbr. *SBP;* called also *systolic pressure;* compare DIASTOLIC BLOOD PRESSURE

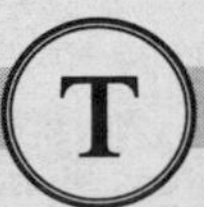

T *abbr* **1** thoracic — used with a number from 1 to 12 to indicate a vertebra or segment of the spinal cord ⟨a fracture of *T-12*⟩ **2** thymine

T *symbol* tritium

2,4,5–T — see entry alphabetized as TWO, FOUR, FIVE-T in the letter *t*

Ta *symbol* tantalum

TA *abbr* transactional analysis

tab \ˈtab\ *n* : TABLET

ta•bel•la \tə-ˈbe-lə\ *n, pl* **-lae** \-ˌlē\ : a medicated lozenge or tablet

ta•bes \ˈtā-(ˌ)bēz\ *n, pl* **tabes 1** : wasting accompanying a chronic disease **2** : TABES DORSALIS

tabes dor•sa•lis \-dȯr-ˈsā-ləs, -ˈsa-\ *n* : a syphilitic disorder that involves the dorsal horns of the spinal cord and the sensory nerve trunks and that is marked by wasting, pain, lack of coordination of voluntary movements and reflexes, and disorders of sensation, nutrition, and vision — called also *locomotor ataxia*

ta•bet•ic \tə-ˈbe-tik\ *adj* : of, relating to, or affected with tabes and esp. tabes dorsalis ⟨~ pains⟩ ⟨a ~ joint⟩

ta•ble•spoon \ˈtā-bəl-ˌspün\ *n* : a unit of measure equal to 4 fluid drams or $^1/_2$ fluid ounce or 15 milliliters

ta•ble•spoon•ful \ˌtā-bəl-ˈspün-ˌfu̇l, ˈtā-bəl-ˌ\ *n, pl* **tablespoonfuls** \-ˌfu̇lz\ *also* **ta•ble•spoons•ful** \-ˈspünz-ˌfu̇l, -ˌspünz-\ : TABLESPOON

tab•let \ˈta-blət\ *n* : a small mass of medicated material (as in the shape of a disk) ⟨an aspirin ~⟩

tabo- *comb form* : progressive wasting : tabes ⟨*tabo*paresis⟩

ta•bo•pa•re•sis \ˌtā-bō-pə-ˈrē-səs, -ˈpar-ə-səs\ *n, pl* **-re•ses** \-ˌsēz\ : paresis occurring with tabes and esp. with tabes dorsalis

tache noire \ˈtäsh-ˈnwär\ *n, pl* **taches noires** *same or* -ˈnwärz\ : a small dark-centered ulcer that appears at the site of a tick bite and is the primary lesion of boutonneuse fever

ta•chis•to•scope \tə-ˈkis-tə-ˌskōp-, ta-\ *n* : an apparatus for the brief exposure of visual stimuli that is used in the study of learning, attention, and perception — **ta•chis•to•scop•ic** \-ˌkis-tə-ˈskä-pik\ *adj* — **ta•chis•to•scop•i•cal•ly** *adv*

tachy- *comb form* : rapid : accelerated ⟨*tachy*cardia⟩

tachy•ar•rhyth•mia \ˌta-kē-ā-ˈrit͟h-mē-ə\ *n* : arrhythmia characterized by a rapid irregular heartbeat

tachy•car•dia \ˌta-ki-ˈkär-dē-ə\ *n* : relatively rapid heart action whether physiological (as after exercise) or pathological — see JUNCTIONAL TACHYCARDIA, PAROXYSMAL TACHYCARDIA, SINUS TACHYCARDIA, VENTRICULAR TACHYCARDIA; compare BRADYCARDIA — **tachy•car•di•ac** \-dē-ˌak\ *adj*

tachy•phy•lax•is \ˌta-ki-fi-ˈlak-səs\ *n, pl* **-lax•es** \-ˌsēz\ : diminished response to later increments in a sequence of applications of a physiologically active substance — **tachy•phy•lac•tic** \-fi-ˈlak-tik\ *adj*

tachy•pnea \ˌta-kip-ˈnē-ə\ *n* : increased rate of respiration — **tachy•pne•ic** \-ˈnē-ik\ *adj*

tachy•pnoea *chiefly Brit var of* TACHYPNEA

tac•rine \ˈta-ˌkrēn, -ˌkrīn\ *n* : an anticholinesterase used in the form of its hydrochloride $C_{13}H_{14}N_2 \cdot HCl$ esp. in the palliative treatment of cognitive deficits in learning, memory, and mood associated with Alzheimer's disease — called also *tetrahydroaminoacridine, THA*

[1]**tac•tile** \ˈtak-təl, -ˌtīl\ *adj* **1** : of, relating to, mediated by, or affecting the sense of touch **2** : having or being organs or receptors for the sense of touch — **tac•tile•ly** *adv*

[2]**tactile** *n* : a person whose prevailing mental imagery is tactile rather than visual, auditory, or motor — compare AUDILE, VISUALIZER

tactile corpuscle *n* : one of the numerous minute bodies (as a Meissner's corpuscle) in the skin and some mucous membranes that usu. consist of a group of cells enclosed in a capsule, contain nerve terminations, and are held to be end organs of touch

tactile receptor *n* : an end organ (as a Meissner's corpuscle or a Pacinian corpuscle) that responds to light touch

tac•toid \ˈtak-ˌtȯid\ *n* : an elongated particle (as in a sickle cell) that appears as a spindle-shaped body under a polarizing microscope

tac•tual \ˈtak-chə-wəl\ *adj* : of or relating to the sense or the organs of touch : derived from or producing the sensation of touch : TACTILE ⟨a ~ sense⟩

ta•da•la•fil \tə-ˈda-lə-ˌfil\ *n* : a drug $C_{22}H_{19}N_3O_4$ taken orally to treat erectile dysfunction, benign prostatic hyperplasia, and hypertension of the lungs and that functions similarly to sildenafil — see ADCIRCA, CIALIS

taen- *or* **taeni-** *also* **ten-** *or* **teni-** *comb form* : tapeworm ⟨*taen*iasis⟩

tae•nia \ˈtē-nē-ə\ *n* **1 a** *also* **te•nia** \ˈtē-nē-ə\ *pl* **taenias** *also* **tenias** : TAPEWORM **b** *cap* : a genus of taeniid tapeworms that comprises forms usu. occurring as adults in the intestines of carnivores and as larvae in various ruminants, and that includes the beef tapeworm (*T. saginata*) and the pork tapeworm (*T. solium*) of humans **2** *also* **tenia** *pl* **tae•ni•ae** \-nē-ˌē, -ˌī\ *or* taenias *also* **te•ni•ae** *or* **tenias** : a band of nervous tissue or of muscle

taenia co•li *also* **tenia coli** \-ˈkō-ˌlī\ *n, pl* **taeniae coli** *also* **teniae coli** : any of three external longitudinal muscle bands of the large intestine

tae•ni•a•sis *also* **te•ni•a•sis** \tē-ˈnī-ə-səs\ *n, pl* **-a•ses** : infestation with or disease caused by tapeworms

tae•ni•id \ˈtē-nē-əd\ *n* : any of a family (Taeniidae) of tapeworms that includes numerous forms of medical or veterinary importance — **taeniid** *adj*

tae•ni•oid \ˈtē-nē-ˌȯid\ *adj* : resembling or related to the taeniid tapeworms

[1]**tag** \ˈtag\ *n* **1 a** : a shred of flesh or muscle **b** : a small abnormal projecting piece of tissue esp. when potentially or actually neoplastic in character **2** : LABEL

[2]**tag** *vb* **tagged; tag•ging** : LABEL

Tag•a•met \ˈta-gə-ˌmet\ *trademark* — used for a preparation of cimetidine

tai chi *also* **t'ai chi** \ˈtī-ˈjē, -ˈchē\ *n, often cap T&C* : an ancient Chinese discipline involving a continuous series of controlled usu. slow movements designed to improve physical and mental well-being — called also *t'ai chi ch'uan, tai chi chuan* \-chü-ˈän\

tail \ˈtāl\ *n, often attrib* **1** : the rear end or a process or prolongation of the rear end of the body of an animal **2** : any of various parts of bodily structures that are terminal: as **a** : the distal tendon of a muscle **b** : the slender left end of the human pancreas **c** : the common convoluted tube that forms the lower part of the epididymis **3** : the motile part of a sperm that extends from the middle portion to the end and that comprises the flagellum

tail•bone \-ˈbōn\ *n* **1** : a caudal vertebra **2** : COCCYX

tail bud *n* : a knob of embryonic tissue that contributes to the formation of the posterior part of the vertebrate body — called also *end bud*

Ta•ka•ya•su's arteritis \ˌtä-kə-ˈyä-süz-\ *n* : a chronic inflammatory disease esp. of the aorta and its major branches that results in progressive stenosis, occlusion, and aneurysm formation and is marked esp. by diminution or loss of the pulse (as in the arm) and by ischemic symptoms (as visual disturbances or pain or weakness of the extremities) — called also *pulseless disease, Takayasu's disease*

Takayasu, Michishige (1872—1938), Japanese physician.

[1]**take** \ˈtāk\ *vb* **took** \ˈtu̇k\; **tak•en** \ˈtā-kən\; **tak•ing** **1** : to establish a take esp. by uniting or growing **2** *of a vaccine or vaccination* : to produce a take

[2]**take** *n* **1** : a local or systemic reaction indicative of successful vaccination **2** : a successful union (as of a graft)

take up *vb* : to absorb or incorporate into itself — **take–up** *n*

tali *pl of* TALUS

tali•pes \ˈta-lə-ˌpēz\ *n* : CLUBFOOT 1

talipes equi•no•var•us \-ˌe-kwi-nō-ˈvar-əs\ *n* : a congenital deformity of the foot in which both talipes equinus and talipes varus occur so that walking is done on the toes and outer side of the sole

talipes equi•nus \-ˈe-kwi-nəs\ *n* : a congenital deformity of the foot in which the sole is permanently flexed so that walking is done on the toes without touching the heel to the ground

talipes valgus *n* : a congenital deformity of the foot in which it is rotated inward so that walking is done on the inner side of the sole

talipes varus *n* : a congenital deformity of the foot in which it is rotated outward so that walking is done on the outer side of the sole

talk therapy *n* : psychotherapy emphasizing conversation between therapist and patient

talo- *comb form* : astragalar and ⟨*talo*tibial⟩

ta•lo•cru•ral \ˌtā-lō-ˈkru̇r-əl\ *adj* : relating to or being the ankle joint

ta•lo•na•vic•u•lar \ˌtā-lō-nə-ˈvi-kyə-lər\ *adj* : of or relating to the talus and the navicular of the tarsus

ta•lo•tib•i•al \ˌtā-lō-ˈti-bē-əl\ *adj* : of or relating to the talus and the tibia

ta•lus \ˈtā-ləs\ *n, pl* **ta•li** \ˈtā-ˌlī\ **1** : the human astragalus that bears the weight of the body and together with the tibia and fibula forms the ankle joint — called also *anklebone* **2** : the entire ankle

Tal•win \ˈtal-ˌwin\ *trademark* — used for a preparation of pentazocine

Tam•i•flu \ˈta-mi-ˌflü\ *trademark* — used for a preparation of the phosphate of oseltamivir

ta•mox•i•fen \ta-ˈmäk-si-ˌfen\ *n* : a selective estrogen receptor modulator that acts as an estrogen antagonist in breast tissue and is administered orally in the form of its citrate $C_{26}H_{29}NO{\cdot}C_6H_8O_7$ esp. to treat breast cancer or reduce the risk of its development or reoccurrence— see NOLVADEX

[1]**tam•pon** \ˈtam-ˌpän\ *n* : a wad of absorbent material (as of cotton) introduced into a body cavity or canal usu. to absorb secretions (as from menstruation) or to arrest hemorrhaging

[2]**tampon** *vb* : to place or insert a tampon into

tam•pon•ade \ˌtam-pə-ˈnād\ *n* **1** : the closure or blockage (as of a wound) by or as if by a tampon esp. to stop bleeding **2** : CARDIAC TAMPONADE

tam•su•lo•sin \tam-ˈsü-lə-sən\ *n* : an alpha-adrenergic blocking agent administered orally in the form of its hydrochloride $C_{20}H_{28}N_2O_5S{\cdot}HCl$ to treat benign prostatic hyperplasia — see FLOMAX

tan \ˈtan\ *n* : a brown color imparted to the skin by exposure to the sun or wind — **tan** *vb*

T and A *abbr* tonsillectomy and adenoidectomy

tan•dem repeat \ˈtan-dəm-\ *n* : any of several identical DNA segments lying one after the other in a sequence

tan•gle \ˈtaŋ-gəl\ *n* : NEUROFIBRILLARY TANGLE

tan•ta•lum \ˈtant-ᵊl-əm\ *n* : a hard ductile gray-white acid-resisting metallic element sometimes used in surgical implants and sutures — symbol *Ta;* see ELEMENT table

T antigen \ˈtē-\ *n* : any of several proteins produced by some DNA viruses (as simian virus 40) that induce tumor formation and play a role in viral replication

tap \ˈtap\ *n* : the procedure of removing fluid (as from a body cavity) — see LUMBAR PUNCTURE — **tap** *vb*

[1]**tape** \ˈtāp\ *n* : a narrow band of woven fabric; *esp* : ADHESIVE TAPE

[2]**tape** *vb* **taped; tap•ing** : to fasten, tie, bind, cover, or support with tape and esp. adhesive tape

ta•pe•tum \tə-ˈpē-təm\ *n, pl* **ta•pe•ta** \-ˈpē-tə\ **1** : any of various membranous layers or areas esp. of the choroid and retina of the eye **2** : a layer of nerve fibers derived from the corpus callosum and forming part of the roof of each lateral ventricle of the brain — **ta•pe•tal** \-təl\ *adj*

tape•worm \ˈtāp-ˌwərm\ *n* : any of a class (Cestoda) of flatworms that are parasitic esp. in the digestive tract of vertebrates and that typically consist of a head bearing an attachment organ usu. with suckers or hooks for adhering to the host's intestine followed by an undifferentiated growth region from which buds off a chain of proglottids — called also *cestode;* see BEEF TAPEWORM, CAT TAPEWORM, DOG TAPEWORM, FISH TAPEWORM, FRINGED TAPEWORM, PORK TAPEWORM

ta•pote•ment \tə-ˈpōt-mənt\ *n* : PERCUSSION 2

tar \ˈtär\ *n* **1** : any of various dark brown or black viscous liquids obtained by distillation of organic material (as wood or coal); *esp* : one used medicinally (as to treat skin diseases) **2** : a substance in some respects resembling tar; *esp* : a residue present in smoke from burning tobacco that contains combustion by-products (as resins and phenols)

ta•ran•tu•la \tə-ˈran-chə-lə, -tə-lə\ *n, pl* **-las** *also* **-lae** \-ˌlē\ : any of a family (Theraphosidae) of large hairy American spiders that are typically rather sluggish and capable of biting sharply though most forms are not significantly poisonous to humans

tarda — see OSTEOGENESIS IMPERFECTA TARDA

tar•dive \ˈtär-div\ *adj* : tending to or characterized by lateness esp. in development or maturity

tardive dyskinesia *n* : a neurological disorder characterized by involuntary uncontrollable movements esp. of the mouth, tongue, trunk, and limbs and occurring esp. as a side effect of prolonged use of antipsychotic drugs (as phenothiazine) — abbr. *TD*

tar•get \ˈtär-gət\ *n* **1** : something to be affected by an action or development; *specif* : an organ, part, or tissue that is affected by the action of a hormone **2** : a body, surface, or material bombarded with nuclear particles or electrons **3** : the thought or object that is to be recognized (as by telepathy) or affected (as by psychokinesis) in a parapsychological experiment

target cell *n* : a cell that is acted on selectively by a specific agent (as a virus, drug, or hormone)

tar•ry stool \ˈtar-ē-\ *n* : an evacuation from the bowels having the color of tar caused esp. by hemorrhage in the stomach or upper intestines

[1]**tar•sal** \ˈtär-səl\ *adj* **1** : of or relating to the tarsus **2** : being or relating to plates of dense connective tissue that serve to stiffen the eyelids

[2]**tarsal** *n* : a tarsal part (as a bone)

tarsal gland *n* : MEIBOMIAN GLAND

tarsal plate *n* : the plate of strong dense fibrous connective tissue that forms the supporting structure of the eyelid

tarso- *comb form* **1** : tarsus ⟨*tarso*metatarsal⟩ **2** : tarsal plate ⟨*tarso*rrhaphy⟩

tar•so•meta•tar•sal \ˌtär-sō-ˌme-tə-ˈtär-səl\ *adj* : of or relating to the tarsus and metatarsus ⟨~ articulations⟩

tar•sor•rha•phy \tär-ˈsȯr-ə-fē\ *n, pl* **-phies** : the operation of suturing the eyelids together entirely or in part

tar•sus \ˈtär-səs\ *n, pl* **tar•si** \-ˌsī, -ˌsē\ **1** : the part of the foot between the metatarsus and the leg; *also* : the small bones that support this part of the limb **2** : TARSAL PLATE

tar•tar \ˈtär-tər\ *n* : an incrustation on the teeth consisting of plaque that has become hardened by the deposition of mineral salts (as calcium carbonate)

tartar emetic *n* : a poisonous crystalline salt $KSbOC_4H_4O_6 \cdot {}^1/_2H_2O$ of sweetish metallic taste used esp. formerly in medicine as an expectorant, anthelmintic, and emetic — called also *antimony potassium tartrate, potassium antimonyltartrate*

tar•tar•ic acid \(ˌ)tär-ˈtar-ik-\ *n* : a strong acid $C_4H_6O_6$ of plant origin that contains two carboxyl groups and occurs in three isomeric forms

tar•trate \ˈtär-ˌtrāt\ *n* : a salt or ester of tartaric acid

tar•tra•zine \ˈtär-trə-ˌzēn, -zən\ *n* : a yellow azo dye used in coloring foods and drugs that sometimes causes bronchoconstriction in individuals with asthma

[1]**taste** \ˈtāst\ *vb* **tast·ed; tast·ing** **1** : to ascertain the flavor of by taking a little into the mouth **2** : to have a specific flavor

[2]**taste** *n* **1** : the special sense that is concerned with distinguishing the sweet, sour, bitter, or salty quality of a dissolved substance and is mediated by taste buds on the tongue **2** : the objective sweet, sour, bitter, or salty quality of a dissolved substance as perceived by the sense of taste **3** : a sensation obtained from a substance in the mouth that is typically produced by the stimulation of the sense of taste combined with those of touch and smell

taste bud *n* : an end organ mediating the sensation of taste and lying chiefly in the epithelium of the tongue and esp. in the walls of the circumvallate papillae

taste cell *n* : a neuroepithelial cell that is located in a taste bud and is the actual receptor of the sensation of taste

taste hair *n* : the hairlike free end of a taste cell

tast·er \ˈtās-tər\ *n* : a person able to taste the chemical phenylthiocarbamide

tat \ˈtat\ *n, often cap* **1** : a protein produced by a lentivirus (as HIV) that greatly increases the rate of viral transcription and replication and enhances the susceptibility of T cells to infection — called also *tat protein* **2** : the viral gene that codes for the tat protein

TAT *abbr* thematic apperception test

tat·too \ta-ˈtü\ *n, pl* **tattoos** : an indelible mark or figure fixed upon the body by insertion of pigment under the skin or by production of scars — **tattoo** *vb*

tau \ˈtau̇, ˈtȯ\ *n* : a protein that binds to and regulates the assembly and stability of neuronal microtubules and that is found in an abnormal form as the major component of neurofibrillary tangles — called also *tau protein*

tau·rine \ˈtȯ-ˌrēn\ *n* : a colorless crystalline acid $C_2H_7NO_3S$ that is synthesized in the body from cysteine and methionine, is similar to amino acids but is not a component of proteins, and is involved in various physiological functions (as bile acid conjugation and cell membrane stabilization)

tau·ro·cho·lic acid \ˌtȯr-ə-ˈkō-lik-, -ˈkä-\ *n* : a deliquescent acid occurring in the form of its sodium salt $C_{26}H_{44}NNaO_7S$ in bile

tax·ane \ˈtak-ˌsān\ *n* : any of various compounds (as docetaxel and paclitaxel) with anticancer activity that are obtained from yew trees (genus *Taxus*) or are made synthetically and that inhibit cell division

tax·is \ˈtak-səs\ *n, pl* **tax·es** \-ˌsēz\ **1** : the manual restoration of a displaced body part; *specif* : the reduction of a hernia manually **2 a** : reflex movement by a freely moving and usu. simple organism in relation to a source of stimulation (as a light) **b** : a reflex reaction involving a taxis

Tax·ol \ˈtak-ˌsȯl\ *trademark* — used for a preparation of paclitaxel

tax·on \ˈtak-ˌsän\ *n, pl* **taxa** \-sə\ *also* **tax·ons** **1** : a taxonomic group or entity **2** : the name applied to a taxonomic group in a formal system of nomenclature

tax·on·o·my \tak-ˈsä-nə-mē\ *n, pl* **-mies** **1** : the study of the general principles of scientific classification **2** : orderly classification of plants and animals according to their presumed natural relationships — **tax·o·nom·ic** \ˌtak-sə-ˈnä-mik\ *adj* — **tax·o·nom·i·cal·ly** *adv* — **tax·on·o·mist** \-mist\ *n*

Tax·o·tere \ˈtak-sə-ˌter, -ˌtir\ *trademark* — used for a preparation of docetaxel

Tay–Sachs disease \ˈtā-ˈsaks-\ *n* : a hereditary disorder of lipid metabolism typically affecting individuals of eastern European Jewish ancestry that is marked by the accumulation of lipids esp. in nervous tissue due to a deficiency of hexosaminidase A, that is characterized by weakness, macrocephaly, red retinal spots, hyperacusis, retarded development, blindness, convulsions, paralysis, and death in early childhood, and that is inherited as an autosomal recessive trait — called also *Tay-Sachs;* see SANDHOFF'S DISEASE

Tay, Warren (1843–1927), British physician.

Sachs, Bernard (1858–1944), American neurologist.

Tb *symbol* terbium

TB \ˌtē-ˈbē\ *n* : TUBERCULOSIS

TB *abbr* tubercle bacillus

TBE *abbr* tick-borne encephalitis

TBG *abbr* thyroid-binding globulin; thyroxine-binding globulin

TBI *abbr* traumatic brain injury

Tc *symbol* technetium

TCA *abbr* tricyclic antidepressant

TCDD \ˌtē-(ˌ)sē-(ˌ)dē-ˈdē\ *n* : a carcinogenic dioxin $C_{12}H_4O_2Cl_4$ found esp. as a contaminant in 2,4,5-T — called also *2,3,7,8-tetrachlorodibenzo-para-dioxin, 2,3,7,8-tetrachlorodibenzo-p-dioxin*

TCE *abbr* trichloroethylene

T cell *n* : any of several lymphocytes (as a helper T cell) that differentiate in the thymus, possess highly specific cell-surface antigen receptors, and include some that control the initiation or suppression of cell-mediated and humoral immunity (as by the regulation of T and B cell maturation and proliferation) and others that lyse antigen-bearing cells — called also *T lymphocyte;* see CYTOTOXIC T CELL, HELPER T CELL, KILLER CELL, SUPPRESSOR T CELL, T4 CELL

T–cell leukemia — see ADULT T-CELL LEUKEMIA

T–cell lymphoma *n* — see CUTANEOUS T-CELL LYMPHOMA

TCR *abbr* T cell (antigen) receptor — used for the receptor on an immunoreactive T cell that enables it to bind and react with a specific antigen

Td *abbr* tetanus diphtheria — used for a vaccine containing toxoids of the bacteria causing tetanus and diphtheria

TD *abbr* tardive dyskinesia

Tdap *abbr* tetanus, diphtheria, acellular pertussis (vaccine)

tds *abbr* [Latin *ter die sumendum*] to be taken three times a day — used in writing prescriptions

Te *symbol* tellurium

TEA *abbr* tetraethylammonium

teaching hospital *n* : a hospital that is affiliated with a medical school and provides the means for medical education to students, interns, residents, and sometimes postgraduates

[1]**tear** \ˈtir\ *n* **1** : a drop of clear saline fluid secreted by the lacrimal gland and diffused between the eye and eyelids to moisten the parts and facilitate their motion **2** *pl* : a secretion of profuse tears that overflow the eyelids and dampen the face

[2]**tear** *vb* : to fill with tears : shed tears

[3]**tear** \ˈtar\ *vb* **tore** \ˈtōr\; **torn** \ˈtōrn\; **tear•ing** : to wound by or as if by pulling apart by force ⟨~ the skin⟩

[4]**tear** *n* : a wound made by tearing a bodily part ⟨a muscle ~⟩

tear duct *n* : LACRIMAL DUCT

tear gas *n* : a solid, liquid, or gaseous substance that on dispersion in the atmosphere irritates mucous membranes resulting esp. in blinding of the eyes with tears

tear gland *n* : LACRIMAL GLAND

tease \ˈtēz\ *vb* **teased; teas•ing** : to tear in pieces; *esp* : to shred (a tissue or specimen) for microscopic examination

tea•spoon \ˈtē-ˌspün\ *n* : a unit of measure equal to 1/6 fluid ounce or 1/3 tablespoon or 5 milliliters

tea•spoon•ful \-ˌfu̇l\ *n, pl* **teaspoonfuls** \-ˌfu̇lz\ *also* **tea•spoons•ful** \-ˌspünz-ˌfu̇l\ : TEASPOON

teat \ˈtit, ˈtēt\ *n* : the protuberance through which milk is drawn from an udder or breast : NIPPLE

tea tree oil *n* : an essential oil derived from an Australian tree (*Melaleuca alternifolia*) and used esp. as an antiseptic

Tec•fi•dera \ˌtek-fə-ˈder-ə\ *trademark* — used for a preparation of dimethyl fumarate

tech *abbr* technician

tech•ne•tium \tek-ˈnē-shəm, -shē-əm\ *n* : a radioactive metallic element obtained esp. from nuclear fuel as a product of uranium fission and used in medicine in the preparation of radiopharmaceuticals — symbol *Tc;* see ELEMENT table, PERTECHNETATE

tech•nic \ˈtek-nik\ *n* : TECHNIQUE

tech•ni•cian \tek-ˈni-shən\ *n* : a specialist in the technical details of a subject or occupation ⟨a medical ~⟩

tech•nique \tek-ˈnēk\ *n* : a method or body of methods for accomplishing a desired end ⟨new surgical ~*s*⟩

tecta *pl of* TECTUM

tec•tal \ˈtek-təl\ *adj* : of or relating to a tectum

tec•to•ri•al membrane \tek-ˈtōr-ē-əl-\ *n* : a membrane having the consistency of jelly that covers the surface of the organ of Corti

tec•to•spi•nal \ˌtek-tō-ˈspīn-ᵊl\ *adj* : of, relating to, or being a tract of myelinated nerve fibers that mediate various visual and auditory reflexes and that originate in the superior colliculus, cross to the opposite side, and terminate in the ventral horn of gray matter in the cervical region of the spinal cord

tec•tum \ˈtek-təm\ *n, pl* **tec•ta** \-tə\ **1** : a bodily structure resembling or serving as a roof **2** : the dorsal part of the midbrain including the corpora quadrigemina

teeth *pl of* TOOTH

teethe \ˈtēth\ *vb* **teethed; teeth•ing** : to cut one's teeth : grow teeth

teeth•ing \ˈtē-thiŋ\ *n* **1** : the first growth of teeth **2** : the phenomena accompanying the growth of teeth through the gums

teg•men \ˈteg-mən\ *n, pl* **teg•mi•na** \-mə-nə\ : an anatomical layer or cover; *specif* : TEGMEN TYMPANI

teg•men•tum \teg-ˈmen-təm\ *n, pl* **-men•ta** \-tə\ : an anatomical covering : TEGMEN; *esp* : the part of the ventral midbrain above the substantia nigra — **teg•men•tal** \-təl\ *adj*

tegmen tym•pa•ni \-ˈtim-pə-ˌnī\ *n* : a thin plate of bone that covers the middle ear

tegmina *pl of* TEGMEN

Teg•o•pen \ˈte-gə-ˌpen\ *trademark* — used for a preparation of cloxacillin

Teg•re•tol \ˈte-grə-ˌtȯl\ *trademark* — used for a preparation of carbamazepine

tel- *or* **telo-** *also* **tele-** *comb form* : end ⟨*tel*angiectasia⟩

te•la \ˈtē-lə\ *n, pl* **te•lae** \-ˌlē\ : an anatomical tissue or layer of tissue

tela cho•roi•dea \-kō-ˈrȯi-dē-ə\ *n* : a fold of pia mater roofing a ventricle of the brain

tel•an•gi•ec•ta•sia \ˌte-ˌlan-jē-ˌek-ˈtā-zhə, ˌtē-, tə-, -zhē-ə\ *or* **tel•an•gi•ec•ta•sis** \-ˈek-tə-səs\ *n, pl* **-ta•sias** *or* **-ta•ses** \-tə-ˌsēz\ : an abnormal dilation of red, blue, or purple superficial capillaries, arterioles, or venules typically located just below the skin's surface (as on the face) — see ATAXIA TELANGIECTASIA, HEREDITARY HEMORRHAGIC TELANGIECTASIA, SPIDER VEIN — **tel•an•gi•ec•tat•ic** \-ˌek-ˈta-tik\ *adj*

te•la sub•cu•ta•nea \ˈtē-lə-ˌsəb-kyü-ˈtā-nē-ə\ *n* : SUPERFICIAL FASCIA

tele·di·ag·no·sis \ˌte-lə-ˌdī-əg-ˈnō-səs\ *n, pl* **-no·ses** \-ˌsēz\ : medical diagnosis made by means of telemedicine

tele·ki·ne·sis \ˌte-lə-kə-ˈnē-səs, -kī-\ *n, pl* **-ne·ses** \-ˌsēz\ : the apparent production of motion in objects (as by a spiritualistic medium) without contact or other physical means — compare PRECOGNITION, PSYCHOKINESIS — **tele·ki·net·ic** \-ˈne-tik\ *adj* — **tele·ki·net·i·cal·ly** *adv*

tele·med·i·cine \-ˈme-də-sən\ *n* : the practice of medicine when the doctor and patient are widely separated using two-way voice and visual communication (as by satellite, computer, or closed-circuit television) — **tele·med·i·cal** \-di-kəl\ *adj*

1**tele·me·ter** \ˈte-lə-ˌmē-tər\ *n* : an electrical apparatus for measuring a quantity (as pressure or temperature), transmitting the result esp. by radio to a distant station, and there indicating or recording the quantity measured

2**telemeter** *vb* : to transmit by telemeter

te·lem·e·try \tə-ˈle-mə-trē\ *n, pl* **-tries** **1** : the science or process of telemetering data **2** : data transmitted by telemetry **3** : BIOTELEMETRY — **tele·met·ric** \ˌte-lə-ˈme-trik\ *adj*

tel·en·ceph·a·lon \ˌte-len-ˈse-fə-ˌlän, -lən\ *n, pl* **-la** \-lə\ *or* **-lons** : the anterior subdivision of the embryonic forebrain or the corresponding part of the adult forebrain that includes the cerebral hemispheres and associated structures — **tel·en·ce·phal·ic** \-ˌen-sə-ˈfa-lik\ *adj*

te·lep·a·thy \tə-ˈle-pə-thē\ *n, pl* **-thies** : apparent communication from one mind to another by extrasensory means — **tele·path·ic** \ˌte-lə-ˈpa-thik\ *adj* — **tele·path·i·cal·ly** *adv*

tele·ra·di·ol·o·gy \ˌte-lə-ˌrā-dē-ˈä-lə-jē\ *n* : radiology concerned with the transmission of digitized medical images over electronic networks and with the interpretation of the transmitted images for diagnostic purposes

tele·ther·a·py \-ˈther-ə-pē\ *n, pl* **-pies** : the treatment of diseased tissue with high-intensity radiation (as gamma rays from radioactive cobalt)

tel·lu·ri·um \tə-ˈlu̇r-ē-əm, te-\ *n* : a semimetallic element related to selenium and sulfur — symbol *Te;* see ELEMENT table

tel·mi·sar·tan \ˌtel-mə-ˌsär-ˌtan\ *n* : an antihypertensive drug $C_{33}H_{30}N_4O_2$ that is taken orally and blocks the action of angiotensin II — see MICARDIS

telo- — see TEL-

telo·cen·tric \ˌte-lə-ˈsen-trik, ˌtē-\ *adj* : having the centromere terminally situated so that there is only one chromosomal arm ⟨a ~ chromosome⟩ — compare ACROCENTRIC, METACENTRIC — **telocentric** *n*

te·lo·gen \ˈtē-lə-ˌjen\ *n* : the resting phase of the hair growth cycle following anagen and catagen and preceding shedding

te·lo·me·rase \te-ˈlō-mə-ˌrās, -ˌrāz\ *n* : a DNA polymerase that is a ribonucleoprotein catalyzing the elongation of chromosomal telomeres in eukaryotic cell division and is particularly active in cancer cells

telo·mere \ˈte-lə-ˌmir, ˈtē-\ *n* : the natural end of a eukaryotic chromosome composed of a usu. repetitive DNA sequence and serving to stabilize the chromosome — **telo·mer·ic** \ˌte-lə-ˈmer-ik\ *adj*

telo·phase \ˈte-lə-ˌfāz, ˈtē-\ *n* **1** : the final stage of mitosis and of the second division of meiosis in which the spindle disappears and the nuclear envelope reforms around each set of chromosomes **2** : the final stage in the first division of meiosis that may be missing in some organisms and that is characterized by the gathering at opposite poles of the cell of half the original number of chromosomes including one from each homologous pair

TEM \ˌtē-(ˌ)ē-ˈem\ *n* : TRIETHYLENEMELAMINE

TEM *abbr* transmission electron microscope; transmission electron microscopy

te·maz·e·pam \tə-ˈma-zə-ˌpam\ *n* : a benzodiazepine $C_{16}H_{13}ClN_2O_2$ used for its sedative and tranquilizing effects in the treatment of insomnia — see RESTORIL

temp \ˈtemp\ *n* : TEMPERATURE

tem·per·ate \ˈtem-pə-rət\ *adj* : existing as a prophage in infected cells and rarely causing lysis ⟨~ bacteriophages⟩

tem·per·a·ture \ˈtem-pər-ˌchu̇r, -pə-rə-, -chər, -ˌtyu̇r\ *n* **1** : degree of hotness or coldness measured on a definite scale — see THERMOMETER **2 a** : the degree of heat that is natural to a living body **b** : a condition of abnormally high body heat

tem·plate \ˈtem-plət\ *n* : a molecule (as of DNA) that serves as a pattern for the synthesis of another macromolecule (as messenger RNA)

tem·ple \ˈtem-pəl\ *n* **1** : the flattened space on each side of the forehead **2** : one of the side supports of a pair of glasses jointed to the bows and passing on each side of the head

1**tem·po·ral** \ˈtem-pə-rəl\ *n* : a temporal part (as a bone or muscle)

2**temporal** *adj* : of or relating to the temples or the sides of the skull behind the orbits

temporal arteritis *n* : GIANT CELL ARTERITIS

temporal artery *n* **1** : either of two branches of the maxillary artery that supply the temporalis and anastomose with the middle temporal artery — called also *deep temporal artery* **2 a** : SUPERFICIAL TEMPORAL ARTERY **b** : a branch of the superficial temporal artery that arises just above the zygomatic arch and sends branches to the temporalis — called also *middle temporal artery* **3** : any of three branches of the middle cerebral artery: **a** : one that supplies the anterior parts of the superior, middle, and inferior temporal gyri — called also *anterior temporal artery* **b** : one that supplies the middle parts of the superior and middle temporal gyri — called also *intermediate temporal artery* **c** : one that supplies the middle and posterior parts of the superior temporal gyrus and the posterior parts of the middle and inferior temporal gyri — called also *posterior temporal artery*

temporal bone *n* : a compound bone of the side of the skull that has four principal parts including the squamous, petrous, and tympanic portions and the mastoid process

temporal fossa *n* : a broad fossa on the side of the skull behind the orbit that contains muscles for raising the lower jaw and that in humans is occupied by the temporalis muscle

temporal gyrus *n* : any of three major convolutions of the external surface of the temporal lobe: **a** : the one that is uppermost and borders the sylvian fissure — called also *superior temporal gyrus* **b** : one lying in the middle between the other two — called also *middle temporal gyrus* **c** : the lowest of the three — called also *inferior temporal gyrus*

tem•po•ral•is \ˌtem-pə-ˈrā-ˌləs\ *n* : a large muscle in the temporal fossa that serves to raise the lower jaw — called also *temporalis muscle, temporal muscle*

temporal line *n* : either of two nearly parallel ridges or lines on each side of the skull

temporal lobe *n* : a large lobe of each cerebral hemisphere that is situated in front of the occipital lobe and contains a sensory area associated with the organ of hearing

temporal lobe epilepsy *n* : epilepsy characterized by partial rather than generalized seizures that typically originate in the temporal lobe and are marked by impairment of consciousness, automatisms, unusual changes in behavior, and hallucinations (as of odors) — abbr. *TLE;* called also *psychomotor epilepsy*

temporal muscle *n* : TEMPORALIS

temporal nerve — see AURICULOTEMPORAL NERVE, DEEP TEMPORAL NERVE

temporal process *n* : a process of the zygomatic bone that forms part of the zygomatic arch

temporal summation *n* : sensory summation that involves the addition of single stimuli over a short period of time

temporal vein *n* : any of several veins draining the temporal region: as **a** (1) : a large vein on each side of the head that unites with the maxillary vein to form a vein that contributes to the formation of the external jugular vein (2) : a vein that drains the lateral orbital region and empties into the superficial temporal vein just above the zygomatic arch — called also *middle temporal vein* **b** : any of several veins arising from behind the temporalis and emptying into the pterygoid plexus — called also *deep temporal vein*

temporo- *comb form* : temporal and ⟨*temporo*mandibular⟩

tem•po•ro•man•dib•u•lar \ˈtem-pə-rō-man-ˈdi-byə-lər\ *adj* : of, relating to, or affecting the temporomandibular joint ⟨~ dysfunction⟩

temporomandibular disorder *n* : TEMPOROMANDIBULAR JOINT SYNDROME — abbr. *TMD*

temporomandibular joint *n* : the diarthrosis between the temporal bone and mandible that includes the condyloid process below separated by an articular disk from the glenoid fossa above and that allows for the opening, closing, protrusion, retraction, and lateral movement of the mandible — abbr. *TMJ*

temporomandibular joint syndrome *n* : a group of symptoms that may include pain or tenderness in the temporomandibular joint or surrounding muscles, headache, earache, neck, back, or shoulder pain, limited jaw movement, or a clicking or popping sound in the jaw and that are caused either by dysfunction of the temporomandibular joint or another problem affecting the region of the temporomandibular joint — called also *temporomandibular disorder, temporomandibular joint disorder, temporomandibular joint dysfunction, TMJ syndrome*

tem•po•ro•pa•ri•etal \-pə-ˈrī-ət-ᵊl\ *adj* : of or relating to the temporal and parietal bones or lobes

TEN *abbr* toxic epidermal necrolysis

ten- — see TAEN-

te•na•cious \tə-ˈnā-shəs\ *adj* : tending to adhere or cling esp. to another substance : VISCOUS ⟨~ sputum⟩

te•nac•u•lum \tə-ˈna-kyə-ləm\ *n, pl* **-la** \-lə\ *or* **-lums** : a slender sharp-pointed hook attached to a handle and used mainly in surgery for seizing and holding parts (as arteries)

ten•der \ˈten-dər\ *adj* : sensitive to touch or palpation ⟨~ skin⟩ — **ten•der•ness** *n*

ten•di•ni•tis *or* **ten•don•itis** \ˌten-də-ˈnī-təs\ *n* : inflammation of a tendon

ten•di•nous *also* **ten•do•nous** \ˈten-də-nəs\ *adj* **1** : consisting of tendons ⟨~ tissue⟩ **2** : of, relating to, or resembling a tendon

tendinous arch *n* : a thickened arch of fascia which gives origin to muscles or ligaments or through which pass vessels or nerves; *esp* : a thickening in the pelvic fascia that gives attachment to supporting ligaments

ten•do cal•ca•ne•us \ˈten-dō-kal-ˈkā-nē-əs\ *n* : ACHILLES TENDON

ten·don \ˈten-dən\ *n* : a tough cord or band of dense white fibrous connective tissue that unites a muscle with some other part, transmits the force which the muscle exerts, and is continuous with the connective-tissue epimysium and perimysium of the muscle and when inserted into a bone with the periosteum of the bone

tendonitis *var of* TENDINITIS

tendon of Achil·les \-ə-ˈki-lēz\ *n* : ACHILLES TENDON

tendon of Zinn \-ˈtsin\ *n* : LIGAMENT OF ZINN

tendon organ *n* : GOLGI TENDON ORGAN

tendon reflex *n* : a reflex act (as a knee jerk) in which a muscle is made to contract by a blow upon its tendon

tendon sheath *n* : a synovial sheath covering a tendon (as in the hand)

[1]**-tene** \ˌtēn\ *adj comb form* : having (such or so many) chromosomal filaments ⟨poly*tene*⟩ ⟨pachy*tene*⟩

[2]**-tene** *n comb form* : stage of meiotic prophase characterized by (such) chromosomal filaments ⟨diplo*tene*⟩

tenens, tenentes — see LOCUM TENENS

te·nes·mus \tə-ˈnez-məs\ *n* : a distressing but ineffectual urge to evacuate the rectum or urinary bladder

Ten·ex \ˈte-ˌneks\ *trademark* — used for a preparation of guanfacine

teni- — see TAEN-

tenia, tenia coli, teniasis *var of* TAENIA, TAENIA COLI, TAENIASIS

te·nip·o·side \tə-ˈni-pə-ˌsīd\ *n* : an antineoplastic agent $C_{32}H_{32}O_{13}S$ that is a semisynthetic derivative of podophyllotoxin

tennis elbow *n* : inflammation and pain over the outer side of the elbow involving the lateral epicondyle of the humerus and usu. resulting from excessive strain on and twisting of the forearm — called also *lateral humeral epicondylitis*

teno- *comb form* : tendon ⟨*teno*synovitis⟩

te·no·de·sis \ˌte-nə-ˈdē-səs\ *n, pl* **-de·ses** \-ˌsēz\ : the operation of suturing the end of a tendon to a bone

te·no·fo·vir \tə-ˌnō-fə-ˌvir\ *n* : a reverse transcriptase inhibitor $C_9H_{14}N_5O_4P$ that is orally administered esp. in the form of its fumarate $C_{19}H_{30}N_5O_{10}$-$P{\cdot}C_4H_4O_4$ usu. in conjunction with other antiretroviral drugs to treat hepatitis B and HIV infection — see ATRIPLA, COMPLERA, STRIBILD, TRUVADA, VIREAD

tenofovir di·so·prox·il fumarate \-ˌdī-sō-ˈpräk-sil-\ *n* : the fumarate C_{19}-$H_{30}N_5O_{10}P{\cdot}C_4H_4O_4$ of tenofovir — called also *tenofovir DF*

te·nol·y·sis \te-ˈnä-lə-səs\ *n, pl* **-y·ses** \-ˌsēz\ : a surgical procedure to free a tendon from surrounding adhesions

teno·my·ot·o·my \ˌte-nō-mī-ˈä-tə-mē\ *n, pl* **-mies** : surgical excision of a portion of a tendon and muscle

Te·non's capsule \tə-ˈnōnz-, ˈte-nənz-\ *n* : a thin connective-tissue membrane ensheathing the eyeball behind the conjunctiva

Te·non \tə-ˈnōⁿ\, **Jacques René (1724–1816)**, French surgeon.

Ten·or·min \ˈte-nər-ˌmin\ *trademark* — used for preparation of atenolol

teno·syn·o·vi·tis \ˌte-nō-ˌsi-nə-ˈvī-təs\ *n* : inflammation of a tendon sheath

te·not·o·my \te-ˈnä-tə-mē\ *n, pl* **-mies** : surgical division of a tendon

TENS \ˈtenz\ *abbr or n* **1** TRANSCUTANEOUS ELECTRICAL NERVE STIMULATION **2** : a device used for transcutaneous electrical nerve stimulation : TRANSCUTANEOUS ELECTRICAL NERVE STIMULATOR

tense \ˈtens\ *adj* **tens·er; tens·est** **1** : stretched tight : made taut or rigid **2** : feeling or showing nervous tension — **tense** *vb* — **tense·ness** *n*

Ten·si·lon \ˈten-si-ˌlän\ *trademark* — used for a preparation of edrophonium

ten·sion \ˈten-chən\ *n* **1 a** : the act or action of stretching or the condition or degree of being stretched to stiffness ⟨muscular ~⟩ **b** : STRESS 1b **2 a** : either of two balancing forces causing or tending to cause extension **b** : the stress resulting from the elongation of an elastic body **3** : inner striving, unrest, or imbalance often with physiological indication of emotion **4** : PARTIAL PRESSURE — **ten·sion·al** \ˈten-chə-nəl\ *adj* — **ten·sion·less** *adj*

tension headache *n* : headache marked by mild to moderate pain of variable duration that affects both sides of the head and is typically accompanied by contraction of the neck and scalp muscles

tension pneumothorax *n* : pneumothorax resulting from a wound in the chest wall which acts as a valve that permits air to enter the pleural cavity but prevents its escape

tension–time index *n* : a measure of ventricular work and oxygen demand that is found by multiplying the average pressure in the ventricle during the period in which it ejects blood by the time it takes to do this

ten·sor \ˈten(t)-sər, ˈten-ˌsȯ(ə)r\ *n* : a muscle that stretches a part or makes it tense — called also *tensor muscle*

tensor fas·ci·ae la·tae \-ˈfa-shē-ē-ˈlā-tē\ *or* **tensor fas·cia la·ta** \-ˈfa-shē-ə-ˈlā-tə\ *n* : a muscle that arises esp. from the anterior part of the iliac crest and from the anterior superior iliac spine, is inserted into the iliotibial band of the fascia lata, and acts to flex and abduct the thigh

tensor pa·la·ti \-ˈpa-lə-ˌtī\ *n* : TENSOR VELI PALATINI

tensor tym·pa·ni \-ˈtim-pə-ˌnī\ *n* : a small muscle of the middle ear that is located in the bony canal just above the bony part of the eustachian tube and that serves to adjust the tension of the tympanic membrane — called also *tensor tympani muscle*

tensor ve·li pa·la·ti·ni \-ˈvē-ˌlī-ˌpa-lə-ˈtī-ˌnī\ *n* : a ribbonlike muscle of the palate that acts esp. to tense the soft palate

tent \ˈtent\ *n* : a canopy or enclosure placed over the head and shoulders to retain vapors or oxygen during medical administration

tenth cranial nerve *n* : VAGUS NERVE

ten·to·ri·al \ten-ˈtōr-ē-əl\ *adj* : of, relating to, or involving the tentorium cerebelli ⟨a ~ meningioma⟩

tentorial notch *n* : an oval opening that is bounded by the anterior border of the tentorium cerebelli, that surrounds the midbrain, and that gives passage to the posterior cerebral arteries — called also *tentorial incisure*

ten·to·ri·um \-ē-əm\ *n, pl* **-ria** \-ē-ə\ : TENTORIUM CEREBELLI

tentorium ce·re·bel·li \-ˌser-ə-ˈbe-ˌlī\ *n* : an arched fold of dura mater that covers the upper surface of the cerebellum and supports the occipital lobes of the cerebrum

Ten·u·ate \ˈten-yə-ˌwāt\ *trademark* — used for a preparation of the hydrochloride of diethylpropion

te·pa \ˈtē-pə\ *n* : a soluble crystalline compound $C_6H_{12}N_3OP$ used esp. as a chemical sterilizing agent of insects and in medicine as a palliative in some kinds of cancer — see THIOTEPA

TEPP \ˌtē-ˌē-ˌpē-ˈpē\ *n* : a liquid organophosphate $C_8H_{20}O_7P_2$ that is a powerful anticholinesterase and is used esp. as an insecticide — called also *tetraethyl pyrophosphate*

terat- *or* **terato-** *comb form* : developmental malformation ⟨*terato*genic⟩

te·rato·car·ci·no·ma \ˌter-ə-tō-ˌkärs-ᵊn-ˈō-mə\ *n, pl* **-mas** *also* **-ma·ta** \-mə-tə\ : a malignant teratoma; *esp* : one involving germinal cells of the testis or ovary

te·rato·gen \tə-ˈra-tə-jən\ *n* : a teratogenic agent (as a drug or virus)

ter·a·to·gen·e·sis \ˌter-ə-tə-ˈje-nə-səs\ *n, pl* **-e·ses** \-ˌsēz\ : production of developmental malformations

ter·a·to·gen·ic \-ˈje-nik\ *adj* : of, relating to, or causing developmental malformations ⟨a ~ agent⟩ ⟨~ effects⟩ — **ter·a·to·ge·nic·i·ty** \-jə-ˈni-sə-tē\ *n*

ter·a·to·log·i·cal \ˌter-ət-ᵊl-ˈä-ji-kəl\ *or* **ter·a·to·log·ic** \-jik\ *adj* **1** : abnormal in growth or structure **2** : of or relating to teratology

ter·a·tol·o·gy \ˌter-ə-ˈtä-lə-jē\ *n, pl* **-gies** : the study of malformations or serious deviations from the normal type in organisms — **ter·a·tol·o·gist** \-jist\ *n*

ter·a·to·ma \ˌter-ə-ˈtō-mə\ *n, pl* **-mas** *also* **-ma·ta** \-mə-tə\ : a tumor derived from more than one embryonic layer and made up of a heterogeneous mixture of tissues (as epithelium, bone, cartilage, or muscle)

te·ra·zo·sin \tə-ˈrā-zə-ˌsin\ *n* : an alpha-adrenergic blocking agent administered orally in the form of its hydrated hydrochloride $C_{19}H_{25}N_5O_4 \cdot HCl \cdot 2H_2O$ esp. in the treatment of benign prostatic hyperplasia and hypertension — see HYTRIN

ter·bin·a·fine \tər-ˈbi-nə-ˌfēn\ *n* : an antifungal agent used in the form of its hydrochloride $C_{21}H_{25}N \cdot HCl$ orally in the treatment of onychomycosis and topically in the treatment of tinea corporis, tinea cruris, and athlete's foot — see LAMISIL

ter·bi·um \ˈtər-bē-əm\ *n* : a usu. trivalent metallic element — symbol *Tb;* see ELEMENT table

ter·bu·ta·line \tər-ˈbyü-tə-ˌlēn\ *n* : a bronchodilator used esp. in the form of its sulfate $(C_{12}H_{19}NO_3)_2 \cdot H_2SO_4$

ter·e·bene \ˈter-ə-ˌbēn\ *n* : a mixture of terpenes that has been used as an expectorant

teres — see LIGAMENTUM TERES, PRONATOR TERES

te·res major \ˈter-ēz-, ˈtir-\ *n* : a thick somewhat flattened muscle that arises from the lower axillary border of the scapula, inserts on the medial border of the bicipital groove of the humerus, and functions in opposition to the muscles comprising the rotator cuff by extending the arm when it is in the flexed position and by rotating it medially

teres minor *n* : a long cylindrical muscle that arises from the upper axillary border of the scapula, inserts chiefly on the greater tubercle of the humerus, contributes to the formation of the rotator cuff of the shoulder, and acts to rotate the arm laterally and draw the humerus toward the glenoid fossa

ter·fen·a·dine \(ˌ)tər-ˈfe-nə-ˌdēn\ *n* : a drug $C_{32}H_{41}NO_2$ formerly used as a nonsedating antihistamine but now withdrawn from U.S. markets because of its link to cardiac arrhythmias — see SELDANE

¹**term** \ˈtərm\ *n* : the time at which a pregnancy of normal length terminates ⟨had her baby at full ~⟩

²**term** *adj* : carried to, occurring at, or associated with full term

¹**ter·mi·nal** \ˈtər-mə-nəl\ *adj* **1** : of, relating to, or being at an end, extremity, boundary, or terminus ⟨the ~ phalanx of a finger⟩ **2 a** : leading ultimately to death : FATAL ⟨~ cancer⟩ **b** : approaching or close to death : being in the final stages of a fatal disease ⟨a ~ patient⟩ **3** : being at or near the end of a chain of atoms making up a molecule — **ter·mi·nal·ly** *adv*

²**terminal** *n* : a part that forms an end; *esp* : NERVE ENDING

terminale — see FILUM TERMINALE

terminal ganglion *n* : a usu. parasympathetic ganglion situated on or close to an innervated organ and being the site where preganglionic nerve fibers terminate

terminalis — see LAMINA TERMINALIS, NERVUS TERMINALIS, STRIA TERMINALIS, SULCUS TERMINALIS
terminal nerve *n* : NERVUS TERMINALIS
ter•mi•na•tion codon \ˌtər-mə-ˈnā-shən-\ *n* : STOP CODON — called also *ter•mi•na•tor* \ˈtər-mə-ˌnāt-ər\, *terminator codon*
ter•pene \ˈtər-ˌpēn\ *n* : any of various isomeric hydrocarbons $C_{10}H_{16}$ found in essential oils; *broadly* : any of numerous hydrocarbons $(C_5H_8)_n$ found esp. in essential oils, resins, and balsams
ter•pin hydrate \ˈtər-pin-\ *n* : a crystalline or powdery compound $C_{10}H_{18}(OH)_2 \cdot H_2O$ used as an expectorant for coughs
Ter•ra•my•cin \ˌter-ə-ˈmīs-ᵊn\ *trademark* — used for a preparation of oxytetracycline
[1]**ter•tian** \ˈtər-shən\ *adj* : recurring at approximately 48-hour intervals — used chiefly of vivax malaria; compare QUARTAN
[2]**tertian** *n* : a tertian fever; *specif* : VIVAX MALARIA
ter•tia•ry \ˈtər-shē-ˌer-ē, -shə-rē\ *adj* **1** : of third rank, importance, or value **2 a** : involving or resulting from the substitution of three atoms or groups ⟨~ amines⟩ **b** : of, relating to, or being the normal folded structure of the coiled chain of a protein or of a DNA or RNA — compare PRIMARY 3, SECONDARY 3 **3** : occurring in or being a third stage **4** : providing tertiary care
tertiary care *n* : highly specialized health care usu. over an extended period of time that involves advanced and complex procedures and treatments performed by medical specialists in state-of-the-art facilities — compare PRIMARY CARE, SECONDARY CARE
tertiary syphilis *n* : the third stage of syphilis that develops after the disappearance of the secondary symptoms and is marked by ulcers in and gummas under the skin and commonly by involvement of the skeletal, cardiovascular, and nervous systems
tertius — see PERONEUS TERTIUS
Tesch•en disease \ˈte-shən-\ *n* : a mild to severe encephalomyelitis of swine caused by a picornavirus (species *Porcine teschovirus* of the genus *Teschovirus*)
test \ˈtest\ *n* **1** : a critical examination, observation, evaluation, or trial **2** : a means of testing: as **a** (1) : a procedure or reaction used to identify or characterize a substance or constituent (2) : a reagent used in such a test **b** : a diagnostic procedure for determining the nature of a condition or disease or for revealing a change in function **c** : something (as a series of questions) for measuring the skill, knowledge, intelligence, capacities, or aptitudes of an individual or group **3** : a result or value determined by testing — **test** *adj or vb*
test•cross \ˈtest-ˌkrȯs\ *n* : a genetic cross between a homozygous recessive individual and a corresponding suspected heterozygote to determine the genotype of the latter — **testcross** *vb*
testes *pl of* TESTIS
tes•ti•cle \ˈtes-ti-kəl\ *n* : TESTIS; *esp* : one usu. with its enclosing structures
tes•tic•u•lar \tes-ˈti-kyə-lər\ *adj* : of, relating to, or derived from the testes
testicular artery *n* : either of a pair of arteries which supply blood to the testes and of which one arises on each side from the front of the aorta a little below the corresponding renal artery and passes downward to the spermatic cord of the same side and along it to the testis — called also *internal spermatic artery*
testicular feminization *n* : ANDROGEN INSENSITIVITY SYNDROME — called also *testicular feminization syndrome*
testicular vein *n* : any of the veins leading from the testes, forming with tributaries from the epididymis the pampiniform plexus in the spermatic cord, and thence accompanying the testicular artery and eventually uniting to form a single trunk which on the right side opens into the vena cava and on the left into the renal vein — called also *spermatic vein*
tes•tis \ˈtes-təs\ *n, pl* **tes•tes** \ˈtes-ˌtēz\ : a typically paired male reproductive gland that usu. consists largely of seminiferous tubules from the epithelium of which spermatozoa develop and that descends into the scrotum before the attainment of sexual maturity and in many cases before birth
tes•tos•ter•one \te-ˈstäs-tə-ˌrōn\ *n* : a hormone that is a hydroxy steroid ketone $C_{19}H_{28}O_2$ produced by the testes or made synthetically and that is responsible for inducing and maintaining male secondary sex characteristics — see ANDROGEL, AXIRON
testosterone enan•thate \-ē-ˈnan-ˌthāt\ *n* : a white or whitish crystalline ester $C_{26}H_{40}O_3$ of testosterone that is administered chiefly by intramuscular injection esp. in the treatment of conditions (as hypogonadism) associated with deficient or absent endogenous testosterone or in the palliative treatment of metastatic breast cancer
testosterone propionate *n* : a white or whitish crystalline ester $C_{22}H_{32}O_3$ of testosterone that is administered and used similarly to testosterone enanthate
test–tube *adj* **1** : IN VITRO ⟨~ experiments⟩ **2** : produced by in vitro fertilization ⟨~ babies⟩
test tube *n* : a plain or lipped tube usu. of thin glass closed at one end

te•tan•ic \te-ˈta-nik\ *adj* : of, relating to, being, or tending to produce tetany or tetanus ‹a ~ condition›

tet•a•nize \ˈtet-ᵊn-ˌīz\ *vb* **-nized; -niz•ing** : to induce tetanus in

tet•a•nus \ˈtet-ᵊn-əs, ˈtet-nəs\ *n* **1 a** : an acute infectious disease characterized by tonic spasm of voluntary muscles and esp. of the muscles of the jaw and caused by an exotoxin produced by a bacterium of the genus *Clostridium* (*C. tetani*) which is usu. introduced through a wound — compare LOCKJAW **b** : TETANUS BACILLUS **2** : prolonged contraction of a muscle resulting from a series of motor impulses following one another too rapidly to permit intervening relaxation of the muscle

tetanus bacillus *n* : the bacterium of the genus *Clostridium* (*C. tetani*) that causes tetanus

tet•a•ny \ˈtet-ᵊn-ē, ˈtet-nē\ *n, pl* **-nies** : a condition of physiological calcium imbalance that is marked by intermittent tonic spasm of the voluntary muscles and is associated with deficiencies of parathyroid secretion or other disturbances (as vitamin D deficiency)

tet•ra•ben•a•zine \ˌte-trə-ˈbe-nə-ˌzēn\ *n* : a serotonin antagonist $C_{19}H_{27}NO_3$ that is used esp. in the treatment of psychosis and anxiety

tet•ra•caine \ˈte-trə-ˌkān\ *n* : a crystalline basic ester that is closely related chemically to procaine and is used chiefly in the form of its hydrochloride $C_{15}H_{24}N_2O_2{\cdot}HCl$ as a local anesthetic — called also *amethocaine, pantocaine;* see PONTOCAINE

tet•ra•chlo•ride \ˌte-trə-ˈklōr-ˌīd\ *n* : a chloride containing four atoms of chlorine

2,3,7,8–tet•ra•chlo•ro•di•ben•zo–para–di•ox•in \ˌtü-ˌthrē-ˌse-vən-ˌāt-ˌte-trə-ˌklōr-ō-dī-ˌben-zō-ˌpar-ə-dī-ˈäk-sən\ *n* : TCDD

2,3,7,8–tet•ra•chlo•ro•di•ben•zo–p–di•ox•in \-ˈpē-dī-ˈäk-sən\ *n* : TCDD

tet•ra•cy•cline \ˌte-trə-ˈsī-ˌklēn\ *n* : a yellow crystalline broad-spectrum antibiotic that is produced by a soil actinomycete of the genus *Streptomyces* (*S. virdifaciens*) or made synthetically and that is administered chiefly in the form of its hydrochloride $C_{22}H_{24}N_2O_8{\cdot}HCl$; *also* : any of several chemically related antibiotics

tet•rad \ˈte-ˌtrad\ *n* : a group or arrangement of four: as **a** : a group of four cells produced by the successive divisions of a mother cell **b** : a group of four synapsed chromatids that become visibly evident in the pachytene stage of meiotic prophase

tet•ra•eth•yl•am•mo•ni•um \ˌte-trə-ˌe-thə-lə-ˈmō-nē-əm\ *n* : a quaternary ammonium ion $(C_2H_5)_4N^+$ containing four ethyl groups; *also* : a salt of this ion (as the crystalline chloride used as a ganglionic blocking agent) — abbr. *TEA*

tet•ra•eth•yl py•ro•phos•phate \ˌte-trə-ˌe-thəl-ˌpī-rō-ˈfäs-ˌfāt\ *n* : TEPP

tet•ra•eth•yl•thi•u•ram di•sul•fide \ˌte-trə-ˌe-thəl-ˈthī-yu̇-ˌram-ˌdī-ˈsəl-ˌfīd\ *n* : DISULFIRAM

tet•ra•hy•dro•ami•no•ac•ri•dine \ˌte-trə-ˌhī-drə-ə-mē-nō-ˈa-krə-ˌdēn\ *n* : TACRINE

tet•ra•hy•dro•can•nab•i•nol \-ˌhī-drə-kə-ˈna-bə-ˌnȯl, -ˌnōl\ *n* : THC; *esp* : THC a

te•tral•o•gy of Fal•lot \te-ˈtra-lə-jē-əv-fä-ˈlō\ *n* : a congenital abnormality of the heart characterized by pulmonary stenosis, an opening in the interventricular septum, malposition of the aorta over both ventricles, and hypertrophy of the right ventricle

Fallot, Étienne–Louis–Arthur (1850–1911), French physician.

tetranitrate — see ERYTHRITYL TETRANITRATE, PENTAERYTHRITOL TETRANITRATE

tet•ra•pa•re•sis \ˌte-trə-pə-ˈrē-səs\ *n, pl* **-re•ses** \-ˌsēz\ : QUADRIPARESIS

tet•ra•pa•ret•ic \-pə-ˈre-tik\ *adj* : QUADRIPARETIC

tet•ra•ple•gia \ˌte-trə-ˈplē-jə, -jē-ə\ *n* : QUADRIPLEGIA

tet•ra•ple•gic \-ˈplē-jik\ *adj or n* : QUADRIPLEGIC

tet•ra•ploid \ˈte-trə-ˌplȯid\ *adj* : having or being a chromosome number four times the monoploid number ‹a ~ cell› — **tet•ra•ploi•dy** \-ˌplȯi-dē\ *n*

tet•ra•zo•li•um \ˌte-trə-ˈzō-lē-əm\ *n* : a cation or group CH_3N_4 that is analogous to ammonium; *also* : any of several derivatives used esp. as electron acceptors to test for metabolic activity in living cells

te•tro•do•tox•in \te-ˌtrō-də-ˈtäk-sən\ *n* : a neurotoxin $C_{11}H_{17}N_3O_8$ that is found esp. in puffer fishes and that blocks nerve conduction by suppressing permeability of the nerve fiber to sodium ions

te•trox•ide \te-ˈträk-ˌsīd\ *n* : a compound of an element or group with four atoms of oxygen — see OSMIUM TETROXIDE

Texas fever *n* : a tick-borne disease of cattle caused by a sporozoan of the genus *Babesia* (*B. bigemina*) that destroys red blood cells — called also *Texas cattle fever*

T4 *or* **T_4** \ˌtē-ˈfōr\ *n* : THYROXINE

T4 cell *n* : any of the T cells (as a helper T cell) that bear the CD4 molecule on their surface and become severely depleted in AIDS — called also *helper/inducer T cell, T4 lymphocyte*

TGF *abbr* transforming growth factor

T–group \ˈtē-ˌgrüp\ *n* : a group of people under the leadership of a trainer who seek to develop self-awareness and sensitivity to others by verbalizing feelings uninhibitedly at group sessions — compare ENCOUNTER GROUP

Th *symbol* thorium

THA \ˌtē-ˌāch-ˈā\ *n* : TACRINE

thalam- *or* **thalamo-** *comb form* **1** : thalamus ⟨*thalamo*tomy⟩ **2** : thalamic and ⟨*thalamo*cortical⟩

tha•lam•ic \thə-ˈla-mik\ *adj* : of, relating to, or involving the thalamus

thal•a•mo•cor•ti•cal \ˌtha-lə-mō-ˈkȯr-ti-kəl\ *adj* : of, relating to, or connecting the thalamus and the cerebral cortex

thal•a•mot•o•my \ˌtha-lə-ˈmä-tə-mē\ *n, pl* **-mies** : a surgical operation involving electrocoagulation of areas of the thalamus to interrupt pathways of nervous transmission through the thalamus for relief of certain mental and psychomotor disorders

thal•a•mus \ˈtha-lə-məs\ *n, pl* **-mi** \-ˌmī, -ˌmē\ : the largest subdivision of the diencephalon that consists chiefly of an ovoid mass of nuclei in each lateral wall of the third ventricle and serves to relay impulses and esp. sensory impulses to and from the cerebral cortex

thal•as•sae•mia, thal•as•sae•mic *chiefly Brit var of* THALASSEMIA, THALASSEMIC

thal•as•se•mia \ˌtha-lə-ˈsē-mē-ə\ *n* : any of a group of inherited hypochromic anemias and esp. Cooley's anemia controlled by a series of allelic genes that cause reduction in or failure of synthesis of one of the globin chains making up hemoglobin and that tend to occur esp. in individuals of Mediterranean, African, or southeastern Asian ancestry — sometimes used with a prefix (as alpha-, beta-, or delta-) to indicate the hemoglobin chain affected; called also *Mediterranean anemia;* see ALPHA-THALASSEMIA, BETA-THALASSEMIA

thalassemia major *n* : COOLEY'S ANEMIA

thalassemia minor *n* : a mild form of thalassemia associated with the heterozygous condition for the gene involved

[1]**thal•as•se•mic** \ˌtha-lə-ˈsē-mik\ *adj* : of, relating to, or affected with thalassemia

[2]**thalassemic** *n* : an individual affected with thalassemia

tha•las•so•ther•a•py \thə-ˌla-so-ˈther-ə-pē\ *n, pl* **-pies** : exposure to seawater (as in a hot tub) or application of sea products (as seaweed or sea salt) to the body for health or beauty benefits

tha•lid•o•mide \thə-ˈli-də-ˌmīd, -məd\ *n* : a sedative, hypnotic, and antiemetic drug $C_{13}H_{10}N_2O_4$ that was formerly used chiefly in Europe during the late 1950s and early 1960s esp. to treat morning sickness but was withdrawn after being shown to cause serious malformations (as missing or severely shortened arms or legs) in infants born to mothers using it during the first trimester of pregnancy and that is now used as an immunomodulatory agent chiefly in the treatment of cutaneous complications of leprosy and in combination with dexamethasone in the treatment of multiple myeloma

thal•li•um \ˈtha-lē-əm\ *n* : a sparsely but widely distributed poisonous metallic element — symbol *Tl;* see ELEMENT table

thanat- *or* **thanato-** *comb form* : death ⟨*thanato*logy⟩

than•a•tol•o•gy \ˌtha-nə-ˈtä-lə-jē\ *n, pl* **-gies** : the description or study of the phenomena of death and of psychological mechanisms for coping with them — **than•a•to•log•i•cal** \ˌtha-nə-tə-ˈlä-ji-kəl\ *adj* — **than•a•tol•o•gist** \ˌtha-nə-ˈtä-lə-jist\ *n*

than•a•to•pho•ric \ˌtha-nə-tə-ˈfȯr-ik\ *adj* : relating to, affected with, or being a severe form of congenital dwarfism which results in early death

Than•a•tos \ˈtha-nə-ˌtäs\ *n* : DEATH INSTINCT

THC \ˌtē-(ˌ)āch-ˈsē\ *n* : either of two physiologically active isomers $C_{21}H_{30}O_2$ that occur naturally in hemp plant resin or are synthetically prepared: **a** : one that is the chief intoxicant in marijuana and is used medicinally — called also *delta-9-tetrahydrocannabinol, delta-9-THC;* see DRONABINOL **b** : one that is present in marijuana only in minute quantities

the•ater *or* **the•atre** \ˈthē-ə-tər\ *n* **1** : a room often with rising tiers of seats for assemblies (as for lectures or surgical demonstrations) **2** *usu theatre, Brit* : a hospital operating room

the•ba•ine \thə-ˈbā-ˌēn\ *n* : a poisonous crystalline alkaloid $C_{19}H_{21}NO_3$ found in opium in small quantities

The•be•sian vein \thə-ˈbē-zhən-\ *n* : any of the minute veins of the heart wall that drain directly into the cavity of the heart — called also *Thebesian vessel*

The•be•si•us \te-ˈbā-zē-əs\, **Adam Christian (1686–1732),** German anatomist.

the•ca \ˈthē-kə\ *n, pl* **the•cae** \ˈthē-ˌsē, -ˌkē\ : an enveloping case or sheath of an anatomical part — **the•cal** \-kəl\ *adj*

theca cell *n* **1** : THECA LUTEIN CELL **2** : a cell of the columnar epithelium lining the gastric pits of the stomach

theca ex•ter•na \-ek-ˈstər-nə\ *n* : the outer layer of the theca folliculi that is composed of fibrous and muscular tissue

theca fol•lic•u•li \-fə-ˈli-kyə-ˌlī\ *n* : the outer covering of a graafian follicle that is made up of the theca externa and theca interna

theca in•ter•na \-in-ˈtər-nə\ *n* : the inner layer of the theca folliculi that is highly vascular and that contributes theca lutein cells to the formation of the corpus luteum

the•cal sac \ˈthē-kəl-\ *n* : the membranous sac of dura mater covering the spinal cord and cauda equina and containing cerebrospinal fluid

theca lutein cell *n* : a cell of the corpus luteum that is derived from cells of the theca interna and secretes estrone and estradiol as well as progesterone — called also *theca cell*

thei•le•ria \thī-ˈlir-ē-ə\ *n* **1** *cap* : a genus of protozoans (family Theileriidae) that includes a parasite (*T. parva*) causing east coast fever of cattle **2** *pl* **-ri•ae** \-ē-ˌē\ *also* **-rias** : any organism of the genus *Theileria* — **thei•le•ri•al** \-ē-əl\ *adj*

Thei•ler \ˈtī-lər\, **Sir Arnold (1867–1936)**, South African veterinary bacteriologist.

thei•le•ri•a•sis \thī-lə-ˈrī-ə-səs\ *n, pl* **-a•ses** \-ˌsēz\ : THEILERIOSIS

thei•le•ri•o•sis \thī-ˌlir-ē-ˈō-səs\ *n, pl* **-o•ses** \-ˌsēz\ *or* **-osises** : infection with or disease caused by a protozoan of the genus *Theileria; esp* : EAST COAST FEVER

the•lar•che \thē-ˈlär-kē\ *n* : the beginning of breast development at the onset of puberty ⟨premature ~⟩

The•la•zia \thə-ˈlā-zē-ə\ *n* : a genus of nematode worms (family Thelaziidae) that includes various eye worms

T–help•er cell \ˌtē-ˈhel-pər-\ *n* : HELPER T CELL

T–helper lymphocyte *n* : HELPER T CELL

thematic apperception test *n* : a projective psychological test that is used in clinical psychology to make personality, psychodynamic, and diagnostic assessments based on the subject's verbal responses to a series of black and white pictures — abbr. *TAT*

the•nar \ˈthē-ˌnär, -nər\ *adj* : of, relating to, involving, or constituting the thenar eminence or the thenar muscles

thenar eminence *n* : the ball of the thumb

thenar muscle *n* : any of the muscles that comprise the intrinsic musculature of the thumb and include the abductor pollicis brevis, adductor pollicis, flexor pollicis brevis, and opponens pollicis

the•o•bro•ma oil \ˌthē-ə-ˈbrō-mə-\ *n* : COCOA BUTTER — used esp. in pharmacy

theo•bro•mine \ˌthē-ə-ˈbrō-ˌmēn, -mən\ *n* : a bitter alkaloid $C_7H_8N_4O_2$ closely related to caffeine that is used as a diuretic, myocardial stimulant, and vasodilator

the•oph•yl•line \thē-ˈä-fə-lən\ *n* : a feebly basic bitter crystalline compound $C_7H_8N_4O_2$ that is present in small amounts in tea, is isomeric with theobromine, and is used in medicine esp. as a bronchodilator

theophylline ethylenediamine *n* : AMINOPHYLLINE

the•o•ry \ˈthir-ē\ *n, pl* **-ries** **1** : the general or abstract principles of a body of fact, a science, or an art **2** : a plausible or scientifically acceptable general principle or body of principles offered to explain natural phenomena **3** : a working hypothesis that is considered probable based on experimental evidence of factual or conceptual analysis and is accepted as a basis for experimentation — **the•o•ret•i•cal** \ˌthē-ə-ˈre-ti-kəl\ *also* **the•o•ret•ic** \-tik\ *adj* — **the•o•ret•i•cal•ly** *adv*

ther•a•peu•sis \ˌther-ə-ˈpyü-səs\ *n, pl* **-peu•ses** \-ˌsēz\ : THERAPEUTICS

ther•a•peu•tic \-ˈpyü-tik\ *adj* **1** : of, relating to, or used in the treatment of disease or disorders by remedial agents or methods : CURATIVE, MEDICINAL **2** : having a beneficial effect on the body or mind — **ther•a•peu•ti•cal•ly** *adv*

therapeutic abortion *n* : abortion induced when pregnancy constitutes a threat to the physical or mental health of the mother

therapeutic index *n* : a measure of the relative desirability of a drug for the attaining of a particular medical end that is usu. expressed as the ratio of the largest dose producing no toxic symptoms to the smallest dose routinely producing cures

ther•a•peu•tics \ˌther-ə-ˈpyü-tiks\ *n sing or pl* : a branch of medical science dealing with the application of remedies to diseases ⟨cancer ~⟩ — called also *therapeusis*

therapeutic touch *n* : a technique often included in alternative medicine in which the practitioner passes his or her hands over the body of the person being treated and that is held to induce relaxation, reduce pain, and promote healing

therapeutic window *n* **1** : the range of dosage of a drug or of its concentration in a bodily system that provides safe effective therapy **2** : a usu. short time interval (as after clinical onset of stroke) during which a particular therapy can be given safely and effectively

ther•a•peu•tist \-ˈpyü-tist\ *n* : a person skilled in therapeutics

ther•a•py \ˈther-ə-pē\ *n, pl* **-pies** : therapeutic treatment esp. of bodily, mental, or behavioral disorder — **ther•a•pist** \ˈther-ə-pist\ *n*

the•rio•ge•nol•o•gy \ˌthir-ē-ō-jə-ˈnä-lə-jē\ *n, pl* **-gies** : a branch of veterinary medicine concerned with veterinary obstetrics and with the diseases and physiology of animal reproductive systems — **the•rio•gen•o•log•i•cal** \ˌthir-ē-ō-ˌje-nə-ˈlä-ji-kəl\ *adj* — **the•rio•ge•nol•o•gist** \ˌthir-ē-ō-jə-ˈnä-lə-jist\ *n*

therm- *or* **thermo-** *comb form* : heat ⟨*thermo*receptor⟩

ther•mal \ˈthər-məl\ *adj* **1** : of, relating to, or caused by heat **2** : being or involving a state of matter dependent upon temperature — **ther•mal•ly** *adv*

-ther•mia \ˈthər-mē-ə\ *or* **-ther•my** \ˌthər-mē\ *n comb form, pl* **-thermias** *or* **-thermies** : state of heat : generation of heat ⟨hypo*thermia*⟩

ther·mo·co·ag·u·la·tion \ˌthər-mō-kō-ˌa-gyə-ˈlā-shən\ *n* : surgical coagulation of tissue by the application of heat

ther·mo·di·lu·tion \ˌthər-mō-dī-ˈlü-shən\ *adj* : relating to or being a method of determining cardiac output by measurement of the change in temperature in the bloodstream after injecting a measured amount of cool fluid (as saline)

ther·mo·gen·e·sis \ˌthər-mō-ˈje-nə-səs\ *n, pl* **-e·ses** \-ˌsēz\ : the production of heat esp. in the body — **ther·mo·gen·ic** \-ˈje-nik\ *adj*

ther·mo·gram \ˈthər-mə-ˌgram\ *n* **1** : the record made by a thermograph **2** : a photographic record made by thermography

ther·mo·graph \-ˌgraf\ *n* **1** : THERMOGRAM **2** : the apparatus used in thermography **3** : a thermometer that produces an automatic record

ther·mog·ra·phy \(ˌ)thər-ˈmä-grə-fē\ *n, pl* **-phies** : a technique for detecting and measuring variations in the heat emitted by various regions of the body and transforming them into visible signals that can be recorded photographically — **ther·mo·graph·ic** \ˌthər-mə-ˈgra-fik\ *adj* — **ther·mo·graph·i·cal·ly** *adv*

ther·mo·la·bile \ˌthər-mō-ˈlā-ˌbīl, -bəl\ *adj* : unstable when heated — **ther·mo·la·bil·i·ty** \-lā-ˈbi-lə-tē\ *n*

ther·mol·y·sis \(ˌ)thər-ˈmä-lə-səs\ *n, pl* **-y·ses** \-ˌsēz\ **1** : the dissipation of heat from the living body **2** : decomposition by heat

ther·mom·e·ter \thər-ˈmä-mə-tər\ *n* : an instrument for determining temperature

ther·mo·met·ric \ˌthər-mə-ˈme-trik\ *adj* : of or relating to a thermometer or to thermometry

ther·mom·e·try \thər-ˈmä-mə-trē\ *n, pl* **-tries** : the measurement of temperature

ther·mo·plas·tic \ˌthər-mə-ˈplas-tik\ *adj* : capable of softening or fusing when heated and of hardening again when cooled ⟨~ resins⟩ — **thermoplastic** *n*

ther·mo·re·cep·tor \ˌthər-mō-ri-ˈsep-tər\ *n* : a sensory end organ that is stimulated by heat or cold

ther·mo·reg·u·la·tion \-ˌre-gyə-ˈlā-shən\ *n* : the maintenance or regulation of temperature; *specif* : the maintenance of a particular temperature of the living body — **ther·mo·reg·u·late** \-ˈre-gyə-ˌlāt\ *vb* — **ther·mo·reg·u·la·to·ry** \-ˈre-gyə-lə-ˌtōr-ē\ *adj*

ther·mo·sta·ble \ˌthər-mō-ˈstā-bəl\ *adj* : stable when heated — **ther·mo·sta·bil·i·ty** \-stə-ˈbi-lə-tē\ *n*

ther·mo·ther·a·py \ˌthər-mō-ˈther-ə-pē\ *n, pl* **-pies** : treatment of disease by heat (as by hot air or hot baths)

-thermy — see -THERMIA

the·ta rhythm \ˈthā-tə-ˌri*th*-əm\ *n* : a relatively high amplitude brain wave pattern between approximately 4 and 9 hertz that is characteristic esp. of the hippocampus but occurs in many regions of the brain including the cortex — called also *theta, theta wave*

thi- *or* **thio-** *comb form* : containing sulfur ⟨*thi*amine⟩ ⟨*thio*pental⟩

thia·ben·da·zole \ˌthī-ə-ˈben-də-ˌzōl\ *n* : a drug $C_{10}H_7N_3S$ used in the control of parasitic nematodes and in the treatment of fungus infections

thi·acet·azone \ˌthī-ə-ˈse-tə-ˌzōn\ *n* : a bitter pale yellow crystalline tuberculostatic drug $C_{10}H_{12}N_4OS$

thi·ami·nase \thī-ˈa-mə-ˌnās, ˈthī-ə-mə-, -ˌnāz\ *n* : an enzyme that catalyzes the breakdown of thiamine

thi·a·mine \ˈthī-ə-mən, -ˌmēn\ *also* **thi·a·min** \-mən\ *n* : a vitamin $C_{12}H_{17}N_4OSCl$ of the vitamin B complex that is a water-soluble salt occurring widely both in plants and animals and that is essential for carbohydrate metabolism and for normal functioning of the nervous system — called also *vitamin* B_1

Thi·ara \thī-ˈar-ə\ *n* : a genus of freshwater snails (family Thiaridae) that includes several forms (as *T. granifera*) which are intermediate hosts of medically important trematodes

thi·a·zide \ˈthī-ə-ˌzīd, -zəd\ *n* : any of a group of drugs used as oral diuretics esp. in the control of hypertension

thi·a·zine \ˈthī-ə-ˌzēn\ *n* : any of various compounds that are characterized by a ring composed of four carbon atoms, one sulfur atom, and one nitrogen atom and include some that are important as tranquilizers — see PHENOTHIAZINE

thi·a·zole \ˈthī-ə-ˌzōl\ *n* **1** : a colorless basic liquid C_3H_3NS; *also* : any of various thiazole derivatives

thi·a·zol·i·dine·di·one \ˌthī-ə-ˌzō-lə-ˌdēn-ˈdī-ˌōn\ *n* : any of a class of drugs (as pioglitazone and rosiglitazone) used to reduce insulin resistance in the treatment of type 2 diabetes — abbr. *TZD;* called also *glitazone*

thick filament *n* : a myofilament of one of the two types making up myofibrils that is 10 to 12 nanometers (100 to 120 angstroms) in width and is composed of the protein myosin — compare THIN FILAMENT

Thiersch graft \ˈtirsh-\ *n* : a skin graft that consists of thin strips or sheets of epithelium with the tops of the dermal papillae and that is split off with a sharp knife

Thiersch, Carl (1822–1895), German surgeon.

thigh \ˈthī\ *n* : the proximal segment of the leg extending from the hip to the knee and supported by a single large bone — compare FEMUR

thigh bone *n* : FEMUR

thimble jellyfish *n* : a small jellyfish (*Linuche unguiculata*) whose tiny larvae cause seabather's eruption esp. in coastal waters of southern Florida and the Caribbean

thi·mer·o·sal \thī-ˈmer-ə-ˌsal\ *n* : a crystalline mercurial antiseptic C_9H_9-

$HgNaO_2S$ used esp. for its antifungal and bacteriostatic properties — see MERTHIOLATE

thin filament *n* : a myofilament of the one of the two types making up myofibrils that is about 5 nanometers (50 angstroms) in width and is composed chiefly of the protein actin — compare THICK FILAMENT

thio \ˈthī-ō\ *adj* : relating to or containing sulfur esp. in place of oxygen

thio- — see THI-

thio acid *n* : an acid in which oxygen is partly or wholly replaced by sulfur

thio•amide \ˌthī-ō-ˈa-ˌmīd, -məd\ *n* : an amide of a thio acid

thio•car•ba•mide \ˌthī-ō-ˈkär-bə-ˌmīd, -kär-ˈba-ˌmīd\ *n* : THIOUREA

thi•oc•tic acid *also* **6,8–thi•oc•tic acid** \(ˌsiks-ˌāt-)thī-ˈäk-tik-\ *n* : a lipoic acid $C_8H_{14}O_2S_2$ that has been reported to ameliorate the effects of poisoning by mushrooms (as the death cap) of the genus *Amanita*

thio•cy•a•nate \ˌthī-ō-ˈsī-ə-ˌnāt, -nət\ *n* : a compound that consists of the chemical group SCN bonded by the sulfur atom to a group or an atom other than a hydrogen atom

thiocyanoacetate — see ISOBORNYL THIOCYANOACETATE

thio•es•ter \ˌthī-ō-ˈes-tər\ *n* : an ester formed by uniting a carboxyl group of one compound (as acetic acid) with a sulfhydryl group of another (as coenzyme A)

thio•gua•nine \-ˈgwä-ˈnēn\ *n* : a crystalline compound $C_5H_5N_5S$ that is an antimetabolite and has been used in the treatment of leukemia

thi•ol \ˈthī-ˌȯl, -ˌōl\ *n* **1** : any of various compounds having the general formula RSH which are analogous to alcohols but in which sulfur replaces the oxygen of the hydroxyl group and which have disagreeable odors **2** : the functional group –SH characteristic of thiols — **thi•o•lic** \thī-ˈō-lik\ *adj*

thio•pen•tal \ˌthī-ō-ˈpen-ˌtal, -ˌtȯl\ *n* : a barbiturate used in the form of its sodium salt $C_{11}H_{17}N_2NaO_2S$ esp. as an intravenous anesthetic — see PENTOTHAL

thio•pen•tone \-tōn\ *n, Brit* : THIOPENTAL

thio•rid•a•zine \ˌthī-ə-ˈri-də-ˌzēn, -zən\ *n* : a phenothiazine tranquilizer used in the form of its hydrochloride $C_{21}H_{26}N_2S_2 \cdot HCl$ for relief of anxiety states and in the treatment of psychotic disorders and severe childhood behavioral problems — see MELLARIL

thio•te•pa \ˌthī-ə-ˈtē-pə\ *n* : a sulfur analog $C_6H_{12}N_3PS$ of tepa that is used esp. as an antineoplastic agent and is less toxic than tepa

thio•thix•ene \ˌthī-ō-ˈthik-ˌsēn\ *n* : an antipsychotic drug $C_{23}H_{29}N_3O_2S_2$ used esp. in the treatment of schizophrenia — see NAVANE

thio•ura•cil \ˌthī-ō-ˈyu̇r-ə-ˌsil\ *n* : a bitter crystalline compound $C_4H_4N_2OS$ that depresses the function of the thyroid gland

thio•urea \-yu̇-ˈrē-ə\ *n* : a colorless bitter compound $CS(NH_2)_2$ analogous to and resembling urea that is used esp. in medicine as an antithyroid drug — called also *thiocarbamide*

thio•xan•thene \ˌthī-ō-ˈzan-ˌthēn\ *n* : a compound $C_{13}H_{10}S$ that is the parent compound of various antipsychotic drugs (as thiothixene); *also* : a derivative of thioxanthene

third cranial nerve *n* : OCULOMOTOR NERVE

third–degree burn *n* : a severe burn characterized by destruction of the skin through the depth of the dermis and possibly into underlying tissues, loss of fluid, and sometimes shock

third eyelid *n* : NICTITATING MEMBRANE

third ventricle *n* : the median unpaired ventricle of the brain bounded by parts of the telencephalon and diencephalon

thirst \ˈthərst\ *n* : a sensation of dryness in the mouth and throat associated with a desire for liquids; *also* : the bodily condition (as of dehydration) that induces this sensation — **thirsty** \ˈthər-stē\ *adj*

Thom•as splint \ˈtä-məs-\ *n* : a metal splint for fractures of the arm or leg that consists of a ring at one end to fit around the upper arm or leg and two metal shafts extending down the sides of the limb in a long U with a crosspiece at the bottom where traction is applied

Thomas, Hugh Owen (1834–1891), British orthopedic surgeon.

Thom•sen's disease \ˈtȯm-sənz-, ˈtäm-\ *n* : MYOTONIA CONGENITA

Thomsen, Asmus Julius Thomas (1815–1896), Danish physician.

thon•zyl•a•mine \thän-ˈzi-lə-ˌmēn, -mən\ *n* : an antihistamine derived from pyrimidine and used in the form of its hydrochloride $C_{16}H_{22}N_4O \cdot HCl$

thorac- *or* **thoraci-** *or* **thoraco-** *comb form* **1** : chest : thorax ⟨*thoracoplasty*⟩ **2** : thoracic and ⟨*thoracolumbar*⟩

tho•ra•cen•te•sis \ˌthō-rə-sen-ˈtē-səs\ *n, pl* **-te•ses** \-ˌsēz\ : aspiration of fluid from the chest (as in empyema) — called also *thoracocentesis*

thoraces *pl of* THORAX

tho•rac•ic \thə-ˈra-sik\ *adj* : of, relating to, located within, or involving the thorax — **tho•rac•i•cal•ly** *adv*

thoracic aorta *n* : the part of the aorta that lies in the thorax and extends from the arch to the diaphragm

thoracic artery *n* : either of two arteries that branch from the axillary artery or from one of its branches: **a** : a small artery that supplies or sends branches to the two pectoralis muscles and the walls of the chest — called also *supreme thoracic artery* **b** : an artery that supplies both pectoralis muscles and the serratus anterior and sends branches to the lymph nodes of the axilla and to the subscapularis muscle — called also *lateral thoracic artery;* compare INTERNAL MAMMARY ARTERY

thoracic cage *n* : RIB CAGE

thoracic cavity *n* : the division of the body cavity that lies above the diaphragm, is bounded peripherally by the wall of the chest, and contains the heart and lungs

thoracic duct *n* : the main trunk of the system of lymphatic vessels that lies along the front of the spinal column and receives chyle from the intestine and lymph from the abdomen, the lower limbs, and the entire left side of the body — called also *left lymphatic duct*

thoracic ganglion *n* : any of the ganglia of the sympathetic chain in the thoracic region that occur in 12 or fewer pairs

thoracic nerve *n* : any of the spinal nerves of the thoracic region that consist of 12 pairs of which one pair emerges just below each thoracic vertebra

thoracic outlet syndrome *n* : any of a group of neurovascular disorders that are marked by the compression of nerves (as the brachial plexus) or blood vessels (as the subclavian artery or vein) as they pass from the neck toward the armpit or proximal arm through a space in the upper thorax between the clavicle and the first rib, that typically result in pain, numbness, weakness, or intolerance to cold, and that are usu. caused by a congenital anatomical anomaly, traumatic injury, or repetitive motion of the shoulder and arm

thoracic vertebra *n* : any of the 12 vertebrae dorsal to the thoracic region and characterized by articulation with the ribs

thoracis — see ILIOCOSTALIS THORACIS, LONGISSIMUS THORACIS, SEMISPINALIS THORACIS, SPINALIS THORACIS, TRANSVERSUS THORACIS

thoraco- — see THORAC-

tho•ra•co•ab•dom•i•nal \ˌthō-rə-ˌkō-ab-ˈdä-mə-nəl\ *also* **tho•rac•i•co•ab•dom•i•nal** \thə-ˌra-si-ˌkō-\ *adj* : of, relating to, involving, or affecting the thorax and the abdomen

tho•ra•co•acro•mi•al artery \ˌthō-rə-ˌkō-ə-ˈkrō-mē-əl-\ *n* : a short branch of the axillary artery that divides into four branches supplying the region of the pectoralis muscles, deltoid, subclavius, and sternoclavicular joint

tho•ra•co•cen•te•sis \-sen-ˈtē-səs\ *n, pl* **-te•ses** \-ˌsēz\ : THORACENTESIS

tho•ra•co•dor•sal artery \ˌthō-rə-kō-ˈdȯr-səl-\ *n* : an artery that is continuous with the axillary artery and supplies or gives off branches supplying the subscapularis muscle, latissimus dorsi, serratus anterior, and the intercostal muscles

thoracodorsal nerve *n* : a branch of the posterior cord of the brachial plexus that supplies the latissimus dorsi

tho•ra•co•lum•bar \-ˈləm-bər, -ˌbär\ *adj* **1** : of, relating to, arising in, or involving the thoracic and lumbar regions ⟨~ spine fractures⟩ **2** : SYMPATHETIC 1 ⟨~ nerve fibers⟩

tho•ra•co•plas•ty \ˈthōr-ə-kō-ˌplas-tē\ *n, pl* **-ties** : the surgical operation of removing or resecting one or more ribs so as to obliterate the pleural cavity and collapse a diseased lung

tho•ra•co•scope \thə-ˈrā-kə-ˌskōp, -ˈra-\ *n* : an endoscope that is inserted through a puncture in the chest wall in an intercostal space (as for visual examination of the chest cavity) — **tho•ra•co•scop•ic** \thə-ˌrä-kə-ˈskä-pik\ *adj*

tho•ra•cos•co•py \ˌthōr-ə-ˈkäs-kə-pē\ *n, pl* **-pies** : examination of the chest and esp. the pleural cavity by means of a thoracoscope — called also *pleuroscopy*

tho•ra•cos•to•my \ˌthōr-ə-ˈkäs-tə-mē\ *n, pl* **-mies** : surgical opening of the chest (as for drainage)

tho•ra•cot•o•my \ˌthōr-ə-ˈkä-tə-mē\ *n, pl* **-mies** : surgical incision of the chest wall

tho•rax \ˈthōr-ˌaks\ *n, pl* **tho•rax•es** *or* **tho•ra•ces** \ˈthōr-ə-ˌsēz\ **1** : the part of the body that is situated between the neck and the abdomen and is supported by the ribs, costal cartilages, and sternum; *also* : THORACIC CAVITY **2** : the middle of the three chief divisions of the body of an insect; *also* : the corresponding part of a crustacean or an arachnid

Tho•ra•zine \ˈthōr-ə-ˌzēn\ *n* : a preparation of the hydrochloride of chlorpromazine — formerly a U.S. registered trademark

tho•ri•um \ˈthōr-ē-əm\ *n* : a radioactive metallic element — symbol *Th;* see ELEMENT table

thorn–headed worm *or* **thorny–headed worm** *n* : ACANTHOCEPHALAN

Thr *abbr* threonine

thread lungworm *n* : a slender lungworm of the genus *Dictyocaulus* (*D. filaria*) that parasitizes sheep

thread•worm \ˈthred-ˌwərm\ *n* : any long slender nematode worm

thready pulse \ˈthre-dē-\ *n* : a scarcely perceptible and commonly rapid pulse that feels like a fine mobile thread under a palpating finger

three–day fever *n* : a fever or febrile state lasting three days: as **a** : SANDFLY FEVER **b** : ROSEOLA INFANTUM

3TC \ˌthrē-(ˌ)tē-ˈsē\ *trademark* — used for a preparation of lamivudine

thre•o•nine \ˈthrē-ə-ˌnēn\ *n* : a colorless crystalline essential amino acid $C_4H_9NO_3$ — abbr. *Thr*

thresh•old \ˈthresh-ˌhōld\ *n* : the point at which a physiological or psychological effect begins to be produced (as the degree of stimulation of a nerve which just produces a response) — called also *limen*

thrill \ˈthril\ *n* : an abnormal fine tremor or vibration in the respiratory or circulatory systems felt on palpation

throat \ˈthrōt\ *n* **1** : the part of the neck in front of the spinal column **2** : the passage through the throat to the stomach and lungs containing the pharynx and upper part of the esophagus, the larynx, and the trachea

throat botfly *n* : a botfly of the genus *Gasterophilus* (*G. nasalis*) that lays its eggs on the hairs about the mouth and throat of the horse from where the larvae migrate to the stomach and intestine — called also *throat fly*

[1]**throb** \ˈthräb\ *vb* **throbbed; throbbing** : to pulsate or pound esp. with abnormal force or rapidity

[2]**throb** *n* : a single pulse of a pulsating movement or sensation

throe \ˈthrō\ *n* : PANG, SPASM — usu. used in pl. ⟨death ~*s*⟩

thromb- *or* **thrombo-** *comb form* **1** : blood clot : clotting of blood ⟨*thrombin*⟩ **2** : marked by or associated with thrombosis ⟨*thrombo*angiitis⟩

throm•base \ˈthräm-ˌbās\ *n* : THROMBIN

throm•bas•the•nia \ˌthräm-bəs-ˈthē-nē-ə\ *n* : a blood disorder marked by platelet dysfunction; *esp* : GLANZMANN THROMBASTHENIA

throm•bec•to•my \thräm-ˈbek-tə-mē\ *n, pl* **-mies** : surgical excision of a thrombus

thrombi *pl of* THROMBUS

throm•bin \ˈthräm-bən\ *n* : a proteolytic enzyme formed from prothrombin that facilitates the clotting of blood by catalyzing conversion of fibrinogen to fibrin — called also *thrombase*

throm•bo•an•gi•i•tis \ˌthräm-bō-ˌan-jē-ˈī-təs\ *n, pl* **-it•i•des** \-ˈi-tə-ˌdēz\ : inflammation of the lining of a blood vessel with thrombus formation

thromboangiitis ob•lit•er•ans \-ə-ˈbli-tə-ˌranz\ *n* : BUERGER'S DISEASE

throm•bo•cyte \ˈthräm-bə-ˌsīt\ *n* : PLATELET — **throm•bo•cyt•ic** \ˌthräm-bə-ˈsi-tik\ *adj*

throm•bo•cy•the•mia \ˌthräm-bō-sī-ˈthē-mē-ə\ *n* : a myeloproliferative disorder marked esp. by an abnormal chronic increase in the number of circulating platelets

throm•bo•cy•top•a•thy \ˌthräm-bə-ˌsī-ˈtä-pə-thē\ *n, pl* **-thies** : any of various functional disorders of platelets

throm•bo•cy•to•pe•nia \ˌthräm-bə-ˌsī-tə-ˈpē-nē-ə, -nyə\ *n* : persistent decrease in the number of blood platelets that is often associated with hemorrhagic conditions — called also *thrombopenia* — **throm•bo•cy•to•pe•nic** \-nik\ *adj*

thrombocytopenic purpura *n* : an autoimmune blood disorder that is marked by bleeding from small blood vessels esp. into the skin and mucous membranes resulting in purplish bruises, petechiae, hematomas, nosebleeds, and bleeding from the gums, is caused by a reduction in circulating blood platelets, and typically arises spontaneously but may occur secondary to a preexisting condition (as hepatitis C) ⟨idiopathic *thrombocytopenic purpura*⟩ — called also *purpura hemorrhagica, Werlhof's disease;* compare THROMBOTIC THROMBOCYTOPENIC PURPURA

throm•bo•cy•to•sis \ˌthräm-bə-ˌsī-ˈtō-səs\ *n, pl* **-to•ses** \-ˈtō-sēz\ : increase and esp. abnormal increase in the number of platelets in the blood that typically occurs in association with a myeloproliferative disorder (as thrombocythemia or chronic myelogenous leukemia) or as a nonspecific response to an underlying disorder or disease (as a systemic infection); *also* : THROMBOCYTHEMIA

throm•bo•em•bo•lism \ˌthräm-bō-ˈem-bə-ˌli-zəm\ *n* : the blocking of a blood vessel by a particle that has broken away from a blood clot at its site of formation — **throm•bo•em•bol•ic** \-em-ˈbä-lik\ *adj*

throm•bo•end•ar•te•rec•to•my \ˌthräm-bō-ˌen-ˌdär-tə-ˈrek-tə-mē\ *n, pl* **-mies** : surgical excision of a thrombus and the adjacent arterial lining

throm•bo•gen•e•sis \ˌthräm-bō-ˈje-nə-səs\ *n, pl* **-e•ses** \-ˌsēz\ : the formation of a thrombus

throm•bo•gen•ic \ˌthräm-bə-ˈje-nik\ *adj* : tending to produce a thrombus — **throm•bo•ge•nic•i•ty** \-jə-ˈni-sə-tē\ *n*

throm•bo•ki•nase \ˌthräm-bō-ˈkī-ˌnās, -ˌnāz\ *n* : THROMBOPLASTIN

[1]**throm•bo•lyt•ic** \ˌthräm-bə-ˈli-tik\ *adj* : destroying or breaking up a thrombus ⟨a ~ agent⟩ ⟨~ therapy⟩ — **throm•bol•y•sis** \ˌthräm-ˈbä-lə-səs\ *n*

[2]**thrombolytic** *n* : a thrombolytic drug (as streptokinase or urokinase) : CLOT-BUSTER

throm•bo•pe•nia \ˌthräm-bō-ˈpē-nē-ə\ *n* : THROMBOCYTOPENIA — **throm•bo•pe•nic** \-ˈpē-nik\ *adj*

throm•bo•phil•ia \-ˈfi-lē-ə\ *n* : a hereditary or acquired disorder (as factor V Leiden) marked by an abnormal increase in the tendency of blood to clot and higher than normal risk of thrombosis

throm•bo•phle•bi•tis \-fli-ˈbī-təs\ *n, pl* **-bit•i•des** \-ˈbi-tə-ˌdēz\ : inflammation of a vein with formation of a thrombus — compare PHLEBOTHROMBOSIS

throm•bo•plas•tic \ˌthräm-bō-ˈplas-tik\ *adj* : initiating or accelerating the clotting of blood ⟨a ~ substance⟩

throm•bo•plas•tin \ˌthräm-bō-ˈplas-tən\ *n* : a complex enzyme that is found esp. in blood platelets and functions in the conversion of prothrombin to thrombin in the clotting of blood — called also *thrombokinase*

throm•bo•plas•tin•o•gen \-plas-ˈti-nə-jən\ *n* : FACTOR VIII

throm•bo•poi•e•tin \-ˈpȯi-ə-tən\ *n* : a hormone that regulates blood platelet production by promoting the proliferation and maturation of megakaryocyte progenitor cells and the development of megakaryocytes into blood platelets

throm•bo•sis \thräm-ˈbō-səs, thrəm-\ *n, pl* **-bo•ses** \-ˌsēz\ : the formation or presence of a blood clot within a blood vessel — see CORONARY THROMBOSIS, DEEP VEIN THROMBOSIS — **throm•bose** \ˈthräm-ˌbōs, -ˌbōz\ *vb* — **throm•bot•ic** \thräm-ˈbä-tik\ *adj*

thrombotic thrombocytopenic purpura *n* : a rare serious blood disorder chiefly of adults that is characterized by hemolytic anemia, low platelet count, mild to severe neurological abnormalities (as confusion and paresthesias), fever, and sometimes renal dysfunction, is sometimes considered a form of hemolytic uremic syndrome, and is typically associated with an enzyme deficiency which inhibits the cleavage of von Willebrand factor — abbr. *TTP;* compare THROMBOCYTOPENIC PURPURA

throm•box•ane \thräm-ˈbäk-ˌsān\ *n* : any of several substances that are produced esp. by platelets, are formed from endoperoxides, cause constriction of vascular and bronchial smooth muscle, and promote blood clotting

throm•bus \ˈthräm-bəs\ *n, pl* **throm•bi** \-ˌbī, -ˌbē\ : a clot of blood formed within a blood vessel and remaining attached to its place of origin — compare EMBOLUS

throw up *vb* : VOMIT

thrush \ˈthrəsh\ *n* **1** : a disease that is caused by a fungus of the genus *Candida* (*C. albicans*), occurs esp. in infants and children, and is marked by white patches in the oral cavity; *broadly* : CANDIDIASIS ⟨vaginal ~⟩ **2** : a suppurative disorder of the feet in various animals (as the horse)

thu•li•um \ˈthü-lē-əm, ˈthyü-\ *n* : a metallic element — symbol *Tm;* see ELEMENT table

thumb \ˈthəm\ *n* : the short and thick first or most preaxial digit of the human hand that differs from the other fingers in having only two phalanges, in having greater freedom of movement, and in being opposable to the other fingers

thumb–suck•ing \-ˌsə-kiŋ\ *n* : the habit esp. of infants and young children of sucking a thumb — **thumb–suck•er** *n*

thym- *or* **thymo-** *comb form* : thymus ⟨*thym*ic⟩ ⟨*thymo*cyte⟩

thy•mec•to•my \thī-ˈmek-tə-mē\ *n, pl* **-mies** : surgical excision of the thymus — **thy•mec•to•mize** \-ˌmīz\ *vb*

thyme oil \ˈtīm-, ˈthīm-\ *n* : a fragrant essential oil that is obtained from various thymes (genus *Thymus* of the mint family, Labiatae) and is used chiefly as an antiseptic in pharmaceutical and dental preparations

-thy•mia \ˈthī-mē-ə\ *n comb form* : condition of mind and will ⟨dys*thymia*⟩

thy•mic \ˈthī-mik\ *adj* : of or relating to the thymus ⟨a ~ tumor⟩

thymic corpuscle *n* : HASSALL'S CORPUSCLE

thy•mi•co•lym•phat•ic \ˌthī-mi-(ˌ)kō-lim-ˈfa-tik\ *adj* : of, relating to, or affecting both the thymus and the lymphatic system ⟨~ involution⟩

thy•mi•dine \ˈthī-mə-ˌdēn\ *n* : a nucleoside $C_{10}H_{14}N_2O_5$ that is composed of thymine and deoxyribose and occurs as a structural part of DNA

thymidine kinase *n* : an enzyme that catalyzes the phosphorylation of thymidine in a pathway leading to DNA synthesis, that is active esp. in tissues undergoing growth or regeneration, and that is the key enzyme mediating replication in certain viruses (as the herpesvirus causing herpes simplex)

thy•mine \ˈthī-ˌmēn\ *n* : a pyrimidine base $C_5H_6N_2O_2$ that is one of the four bases coding genetic information in the polynucleotide chain of DNA — compare ADENINE, CYTOSINE, GUANINE, URACIL

thy•mo•cyte \ˈthī-mə-ˌsīt\ *n* : a cell of the thymus; *esp* : a thymic lymphocyte

thy•mol \ˈthī-ˌmȯl, -ˌmōl\ *n* : a crystalline phenol $C_{10}H_{14}O$ of aromatic odor and antiseptic properties found esp. in thyme oil or made synthetically and used chiefly as a fungicide and preservative

thy•mo•ma \thī-ˈmō-mə\ *n, pl* **-mas** *also* **-ma•ta** \-mə-tə\ : a tumor that arises from the tissue elements of the thymus

thy•mo•sin \ˈthī-mə-sən\ *n* : a mixture of polypeptides isolated from the thymus; *also* : any of these polypeptides

thy•mus \ˈthī-məs\ *n, pl* **thy•mus•es** *also* **thy•mi** \-ˌmī\ : a glandular structure of largely lymphoid tissue that functions in cell-mediated immunity by being the site where T cells develop, that is present in the young of most vertebrates typically in the upper anterior chest or at the base of the neck, and that gradually decreases in size and activity after puberty — called also *thymus gland*

thyr- *or* **thyro-** *comb form* **1** : thyroid ⟨*thyro*globulin⟩ **2** : thyroid and ⟨*thyro*arytenoid⟩

thy•ro•ac•tive \ˌthī-rō-ˈak-tiv\ *adj* **1** : capable of entering into the thyroid metabolism and of being incorporated into the thyroid hormone ⟨~ iodine⟩ **2** : simulating the action of the thyroid hormone ⟨~ iodinated casein⟩

thy•ro•ar•y•te•noid \-ˌar-ə-ˈtē-ˌnȯid, -ə-ˈrit-ᵊn-ˌȯid\ *n* : a broad thin muscle that arises esp. from the thyroid cartilage, inserts into the arytenoid cartilage, and that functions to relax and shorten the vocal cords — called also *thyroarytenoid muscle;* see INFERIOR THYROARYTENOID LIGAMENT

thy·ro·ar·y·te·noi·de·us \-ˌar-ə-tə-ˈnȯi-dē-əs\ *n* : THYROARYTENOID

thy·ro·cal·ci·to·nin \ˌthī-rō-ˌkal-sə-ˈtō-nən\ *n* : CALCITONIN 1

thy·ro·cer·vi·cal \-ˈsər-vi-kəl\ *adj* : of, relating to, or being the thyrocervical trunk ⟨the ~ artery⟩

thyrocervical trunk *n* : a short thick branch of the subclavian artery that divides into the inferior thyroid, suprascapular, and transverse cervical arteries

thy·ro·epi·glot·tic ligament \ˌthī-rō-ˌe-pə-ˈglä-tik-\ *n* : a long narrow ligamentous cord connecting the thyroid cartilage and epiglottis

thy·ro·glob·u·lin \ˌthī-rō-ˈglä-byə-lən\ *n* : an iodine-containing protein of the thyroid gland that on proteolysis yields thyroxine and triiodothyronine

thy·ro·glos·sal \ˌthī-rō-ˈglä-səl\ *adj* : of, relating to, or originating in the thyroglossal duct ⟨~ cysts⟩

thyroglossal duct *n* : a temporary duct connecting the embryonic thyroid gland and the tongue

thy·ro·hy·al \ˌthī-rō-ˈhī-əl\ *n* : the larger and more lateral of the two lateral projections on each side of the human hyoid bone — called also *greater cornu;* compare CERATOHYAL

¹thy·ro·hy·oid \-ˈhī-ˌȯid\ *adj* : of, relating to, or supplying the thyrohyoid muscle

²thyrohyoid *n* : a thyrohyoid part; *esp* : THYROHYOID MUSCLE

thyrohyoid membrane *n* : a broad fibroelastic sheet that connects the upper margin of the thyroid cartilage and the upper margin of the back of the hyoid bone

thyrohyoid muscle *n* : a small quadrilateral muscle that arises from the thyroid cartilage, inserts into the thyrohyal of the hyoid bone, and functions to depress the hyoid bone and to elevate the thyroid cartilage — called also *thyrohyoid*

¹thy·roid \ˈthī-ˌrȯid\ *also* **thy·roi·dal** \thī-ˈrȯid-ᵊl\ *adj* **1** : of, relating to, or being the thyroid gland ⟨~ disorders⟩ **2** : of, relating to, or being the thyroid cartilage

²thyroid *n* **1** : a large bilobed endocrine gland that arises as a median ventral outgrowth of the pharynx, lies in the anterior base of the neck, and produces esp. the hormones thyroxine and triiodothyronine — called also *thyroid gland* **2** : a preparation of the thyroid gland of various domestic animals (as pigs) used in treating thyroid disorders — called also *thyroid extract*

thyroid artery *n* : either of two arteries supplying the thyroid gland and nearby structures at the front of the neck: **a** : one that branches from the external carotid artery or sometimes from the common carotid artery — called also *superior thyroid artery* **b** : one that branches from the thyrocervical trunk — called also *inferior thyroid artery*

thyroid–binding globulin *n* : THYROXINE-BINDING GLOBULIN

thyroid cartilage *n* : the chief cartilage of the larynx that consists of two broad lamellae joined at an angle and that forms the Adam's apple

thy·roid·ec·to·my \ˌthī-ˌrȯi-ˈdek-tə-mē\ *n, pl* **-mies** : surgical excision of thyroid gland tissue — **thy·roid·ec·to·mize** \-ˌmīz\ *vb*

thyroid extract *n* : THYROID 2

thyroid gland *n* : THYROID 1

thyroid hormone *n* : any of several closely related metabolically active compounds (as triiodothyronine) that are stored in the thyroid gland in the form of thyroglobulin or circulate in the blood usu. bound to plasma protein; *esp* : THYROXINE

thy·roid·itis \ˌthī-ˌrȯi-ˈdī-təs\ *n* : inflammation of the thyroid gland

thy·roid·ol·o·gy \-ˈdä-lə-jē\ *n, pl* **-gies** : the study of the thyroid gland — **thy·roid·ol·o·gist** \-jəst\ *n*

thyroid–stimulating hormone *n* : a hormone secreted by the adenohypophysis of the pituitary gland that regulates the formation and secretion of thyroid hormone — called also *thyrotropic hormone, thyrotropin, TSH*

thyroid storm *n* : a sudden life-threatening exacerbation of the symptoms (as high fever, tachycardia, weakness, or extreme restlessness) of hyperthyroidism that is brought on by various causes (as infection, surgery, or stress)

thyroid vein *n* : any of several small veins draining blood from the thyroid gland and nearby structures in the front of the neck

thy·ro·nine \ˈthī-rə-ˌnēn, -nən\ *n* : a phenolic amino acid $C_{15}H_{15}NO_4$ of which thyroxine is a derivative; *also* : any of various derivatives and esp. iodine-containing derivatives of this

thy·rot·o·my \thī-ˈrä-tə-mē\ *n, pl* **-mies** : surgical incision or division of the thyroid cartilage

thy·ro·tox·ic \ˌthī-rō-ˈtäk-sik\ *adj* : of, relating to, induced by, or affected with hyperthyroidism

thy·ro·tox·i·co·sis \ˈthī-rō-ˌtäk-sə-ˈkō-səs\ *n, pl* **-co·ses** \-ˌsēz\ : HYPERTHYROIDISM

thy·ro·tro·pic \ˌthī-rə-ˈtrō-pik, -ˈträ-\ *also* **thy·ro·tro·phic** \-ˈtrō-fik\ *adj* : exerting or characterized by a direct influence on the secretory activity of the thyroid gland ⟨~ functions⟩

thyrotropic hormone *n* : THYROID-STIMULATING HORMONE

thy·ro·tro·pin \ˌthī-rə-ˈtrō-pən\ *also* **thy·ro·tro·phin** \-fən\ *n* **1** : THYROID-STIMULATING HORMONE **2** : a recombinant form of thyroid-stimulating hormone used esp. as a diagnostic agent (as in the detection of thyroid cancer) — called also *thyrotropin alfa*

thyrotropin–releasing hormone *n* : a tripeptide hormone synthesized in the hypothalamus that stimulates secretion of thyrotropin by the anterior lobe of the pituitary gland — abbr. *TRH;* called also *protirelin, thyrotropin-releasing factor*

thy•rox•ine *or* **thy•rox•in** \thī-ˈräk-ˌsēn, -sən\ *n* : an iodine-containing hormone $C_{15}H_{11}I_4NO_4$ that is an amino acid produced by the thyroid gland as a product of the cleavage of thyroglobulin, that increases the metabolic rate, and that is used to treat thyroid disorders — called also *T4*

thyroxine–binding globulin *n* : a blood serum glycoprotein that is synthesized in the liver and that binds tightly to thyroxine and less firmly to triiodothyronine preventing their removal from the blood by the kidneys and releasing them as needed at sites of activity — abbr. *TBG;* called also *thyroid-binding globulin*

Thysa•no•so•ma \ˌthī-sə-nō-ˈsō-mə\ *n* : a genus of tapeworms (family Anoplocephalidae) including the common fringed tapeworm of ruminants

Ti *symbol* titanium

TIA *abbr* transient ischemic attack

tib•ia \ˈti-bē-ə\ *n, pl* **-i•ae** \-bē-ˌē, -bē-ˌī\ *also* **-i•as** : the inner and usu. larger of the two bones of the leg between the knee and ankle that articulates above with the femur and below with the talus — called also *shinbone* — **tib•i•al** \-bē-əl\ *adj*

tibial artery *n* : either of the two arteries of the lower leg formed by the bifurcation of the popliteal artery: **a** : a larger posterior artery that divides into the lateral and medial plantar arteries — called also *posterior tibial artery* **b** : a smaller anterior artery that continues beyond the ankle joint into the foot as the dorsalis pedis artery — called also *anterior tibial artery*

tibial collateral ligament *n* : MEDIAL COLLATERAL LIGAMENT 1

tib•i•a•lis \ˌti-bē-ˈā-ləs\ *n, pl* **tib•i•a•les** \-(ˌ)lēz\ : either of two muscles of the calf of the leg: **a** : a muscle arising chiefly from the lateral condyle and part of the shaft of the tibia, inserting by a long tendon into the first cuneiform and first metatarsal bones, and acting to flex the foot dorsally and to invert it — called also *tibialis anterior, tibialis anticus* **b** : a deeply situated muscle that arises from the tibia and fibula, interosseous membrane, and intermuscular septa, that is inserted by a tendon passing under the medial malleolus into the navicular and first cuneiform bones, and that flexes the foot in the direction of the sole and tends to invert it — called also *tibialis posterior, tibialis posticus*

tibialis anterior *n* : TIBIALIS a

tibialis an•ti•cus \-an-ˈtī-kəs\ *n* : TIBIALIS a

tibialis pos•ti•cus \-pōs-ˈtī-kəs\ *n* : TIBIALIS b

tibial nerve *n* : the large nerve in the back of the leg that is a continuation of the sciatic nerve and terminates at the medial malleolus in the lateral and medial plantar nerves — called also *medial popliteal nerve*

tibial plateau *n* : the smooth bony surface of either the lateral condyle or the medial condyle of the tibia that articulates with the corresponding condylar surface of the femur

tibial vein *n* : any of several veins that accompany the corresponding tibial arteries and that unite to form the popliteal vein: **a** : one accompanying the posterior tibial artery — called also *posterior tibial vein* **b** : one accompanying the anterior tibial artery — called also *anterior tibial vein*

tibio- *comb form* : tibial and ⟨*tibio*femoral⟩

tib•io•fem•o•ral \ˌti-bē-ō-ˈfe-mə-rəl\ *adj* : relating to or being the articulation occurring between the tibia and the femur ⟨the ~ joint⟩

tib•io•fib•u•lar \-ˈfi-byə-lər\ *adj* : of, relating to, or connecting the tibia and fibula ⟨the proximal ~ joint⟩

tib•io•tar•sal \-ˈtar-səl\ *adj* : of, relating to, or affecting the tibia and the tarsus

tic \ˈtik\ *n* **1** : local and habitual spasmodic motion of particular muscles esp. of the face : TWITCHING **2** : a habitual usu. unconscious quirk of behavior or speech

ti•car•cil•lin \ˌtī-kär-ˈsi-lən\ *n* : a semisynthetic antibiotic used esp. in the form of its disodium salt $C_{15}H_{14}N_2Na_2O_6S_2$

tic dou•lou•reux \ˈtik-ˌdü-lə-ˈrü, -ˈrœ\ *n* : TRIGEMINAL NEURALGIA

tick \ˈtik\ *n* **1** : any of a superfamily (Ixodoidea of the order Acarina) of bloodsucking arachnids that are larger than the closely related mites, attach themselves to warm-blooded vertebrates to feed, and include important vectors of various infectious diseases **2** : any of various usu. wingless parasitic dipteran flies (as the sheep ked)

tick–bite fever *n* : boutonneuse fever esp. as it occurs in South Africa

tick–borne *adj* : capable of being transmitted by the bites of ticks

tick–borne encephalitis *n* : any encephalitis transmitted by ticks; *specif* : a mild to fatal virus disease of humans of Europe and Asia that is characterized most often by meningitis or encephalitis or both or sometimes only by a mild fever and that is caused by the tick-borne encephalitis virus — abbr. *TBE;* see RUSSIAN SPRING-SUMMER ENCEPHALITIS

tick–borne encephalitis virus *n* : a virus of the genus *Flavivirus* (species *Tick-borne encephalitis virus*) that causes tick-borne encephalitis in Europe and Asia

tick–borne fever *n* : a usu. mild rickettsial disease of ruminant mammals (as sheep and cattle) esp. in Europe that is caused by a bacterium of the genus *Anaplasma* (*A. phagocytophilum* syn. *Ehrlichia phagocytophila*) which is transmitted by a tick of the genus *Ixodes* and that is marked by fever, listlessness, and anorexia

tick fever *n* **1** : TEXAS FEVER **2** : a febrile disease (as Rocky Mountain spotted fever or relapsing fever) transmitted by the bites of ticks

tick paralysis *n* : a progressive spinal paralysis that moves upward toward the brain and is caused by a neurotoxin secreted by some ticks (as *Dermacentor andersoni*)

tick typhus *n* : any of various tick-borne rickettsial spotted fevers (as Rocky Mountain spotted fever or boutonneuse fever)

ti•cryn•a•fen \tī-ˈkri-nə-ˌfen\ *n* : a diuretic, uricosuric, and antihypertensive agent $C_{13}H_8Cl_2O_4S$ withdrawn from use because of its link to hepatic disorders

tid *abbr* [Latin *ter in die*] three times a day — used in writing prescriptions

tid•al \ˈtīd-ᵊl\ *adj* : of, relating to, or constituting tidal air

tidal air *n* : the air that passes in and out of the lungs in an ordinary breath

tidal volume *n* : the volume of the tidal air

tide \ˈtīd\ *n* : a temporary increase or decrease in a specified substance or quality in the body or one of its systems ⟨an acid ~ during fasting⟩

tie off *vb* **tied off; ty•ing off** *or* **tie•ing off** : to close by means of an encircling or enveloping ligature ⟨*tie off* a bleeding vessel⟩

Tie•tze's syndrome \ˈtēt-səz-\ *n* : a condition of unknown origin that is characterized by inflammation of costochondral cartilage — called also *costochondritis, Tietze's disease*

Tietze, Alexander (1864–1927), German surgeon.

tiger mosquito *n* **1** : YELLOW-FEVER MOSQUITO **2** : ASIAN TIGER MOSQUITO

tiger rattlesnake *n* : a rather small venomous rattlesnake of the genus *Crotalus* (*C. tigris*) that occurs in mountainous deserts of western No. America

ti•groid substance \ˈtī-ˌgrȯid-\ *n* : NISSL BODIES

TIL \ˌtē-(ˌ)ī-ˈel\ *n* : TUMOR-INFILTRATING LYMPHOCYTE

timber rattlesnake *n* : a moderate-sized venomous rattlesnake of the genus *Crotalus* (*C. horridus*) widely distributed through the eastern half of the U.S.

time \ˈtīm\ *n* : the measured or measurable period during which an action, process, or condition exists or continues — see BLEEDING TIME, COAGULATION TIME, PROTHROMBIN TIME, REACTION TIME

timed–release *or* **time–release** *adj* : SUSTAINED-RELEASE; *also* : DELAYED RELEASE

ti•mo•lol \ˈtī-mə-ˌlōl\ *n* : a beta-blocker used esp. in the form of its maleate $C_{13}H_{24}N_4O_3S{\cdot}C_4H_4O_4$ to treat hypertension, to reduce the risk of reinfarction, to prevent migraine headaches, and to lower intraocular pressure associated esp. with open-angle glaucoma and ocular hypertension — see COMBIGAN, TIMOPTIC

Ti•mop•tic \tə-ˈmäp-tik\ *trademark* — used for an ophthalmic preparation of the maleate of timolol

tin \ˈtin\ *n* : a soft white crystalline metallic element malleable at ordinary temperatures — symbol *Sn;* see ELEMENT table

Ti•nac•tin \ti-ˈnak-tən\ *trademark* — used for a preparation of tolnaftate

tinc•to•ri•al \tiŋk-ˈtōr-ē-əl\ *adj* : of or relating to dyeing or staining

tinc•tu•ra \tiŋk-ˈtu̇r-ə, -ˈtyu̇r-\ *n, pl* **-rae** \-rē\ : TINCTURE

tinc•ture \ˈtiŋk-chər\ *n* : a solution of a medicinal substance in an alcoholic menstruum — compare LIQUOR

tin•ea \ˈti-nē-ə\ *n* : any of several fungal diseases of the skin; *esp* : RINGWORM

tinea ca•pi•tis \-ˈka-pə-təs\ *n* : an infection of the scalp caused by fungi of the genera *Trichophyton* and *Microsporum* and characterized by scaly patches penetrated by a few dry brittle hairs

tinea cor•po•ris \-ˈkȯr-pə-rəs\ *n* : a fungal infection involving parts of the body not covered with hair — called also *body ringworm*

tinea cru•ris \-ˈkru̇r-əs\ *n* : a fungal infection involving esp. the groin and perineum — called also *jock itch*

tinea pe•dis \-ˈpe-dəs\ *n* : ATHLETE'S FOOT

tinea ver•si•col•or \-ˈvər-si-ˌkə-lər\ *n* : a common chronic infection of the skin esp. of the trunk and shoulders that is caused by a lipophilic fungus (esp. *Melassezia furfur* and *M. globosa*), is marked by the formation of irregular often scaly patches of discolored skin, and that occurs esp. in warm humid climates — called also *pityriasis versicolor*

Ti•nel's sign \ti-ˈnelz-\ *n* : a tingling sensation felt in the distal portion of a limb upon percussion of the skin over a regenerating nerve in the limb

Tinel, Jules (1879–1952), French neurologist.

tine test \ˈtīn-\ *n* : a tuberculin test in which the tuberculin is introduced intradermally by means of four tines on a stainless steel disk

tin·ni·tus \ˈti-nə-təs, ti-ˈnī-təs\ *n* : a sensation of noise (as a ringing or roaring) that is caused by a bodily condition (as a disturbance of the auditory nerve or wax in the ear) and typically is of subjective form which can only be heard by the one affected

ti·o·tro·pi·um \ˌtī-ō-ˈtrō-pē-əm\ *n* : an anticholinergic drug administered by oral inhalation in the form of its bromide $C_{19}H_{22}NO_4S_2Br·H_2O$ as a bronchodilator in the treatment of chronic obstructive pulmonary disease — called also *tiotropium bromide;* see SPIRIVA

tis·sue \ˈti-(ˌ)shü\ *n* : an aggregate of cells usu. of a particular kind together with their intercellular substance that form one of the structural materials of a plant or an animal and that in animals include connective tissue, epithelium, muscle tissue, and nerve tissue

tissue culture *n* : the process or technique of making body tissue grow in a culture medium outside the organism; *also* : a culture of tissue

tissue fluid *n* : a fluid that permeates the spaces between individual cells, is in osmotic contact with the blood and lymph, and serves in interstitial transport of nutrients and waste

tissue plasminogen activator *n* : a clot-dissolving enzyme that has an affinity for fibrin, that catalyzes the conversion of plasminogen to plasmin, that is produced naturally in blood vessel linings, and that is used in a genetically engineered form to prevent damage to heart muscle following a heart attack and to reduce neurological damage following ischemic stroke — abbr. *TPA*

tissue typing *n* : the determination of the degree of compatibility of tissues or organs from different individuals based on the similarity of histocompatibility antigens esp. on lymphocytes and used esp. as a measure of potential rejection in an organ transplant procedure

tis·su·lar \ˈti-shyə-lər\ *adj* : of, relating to, or affecting organismic tissue

ti·ta·ni·um \tī-ˈtā-nē-əm, -ˈta-\ *n* : a silvery gray metallic element — symbol *Ti;* see ELEMENT table

titanium dioxide *n* : an oxide TiO_2 of titanium that is used in sunblocks

ti·ter \ˈtī-tər\ *n* **1** : the strength of a solution or the concentration of a substance in solution as determined by titration **2** : the dilution of a serum containing a specific antibody at which the solution just retains a specific activity (as neutralizing an antigen) which it loses at any greater dilution — **ti·tered** \-tərd\ *adj*

ti·tra·tion \tī-ˈtrā-shən\ *n* : a method or the process of determining the concentration of a dissolved substance in terms of the smallest amount of a reagent of known concentration required to bring about a given effect in reaction with a known volume of the test solution — **ti·trate** \ˈtī-ˌtrāt\ *vb*

ti·tre *chiefly Brit var of* TITER

tit·u·ba·tion \ˌti-chə-ˈbā-shən\ *n* : a staggering gait or a swaying or shaking of the trunk or head that is observed esp. in individuals affected with a disease of the cerebellum

Tl *symbol* thallium

TLE *abbr* temporal lobe epilepsy

T lymphocyte \ˈtē-\ *n* : T CELL

Tm *symbol* thulium

TMD *abbr* temporomandibular disorder

TMJ *abbr* temporomandibular joint

TMJ syndrome \ˌtē-ˌem-ˈjā-\ *n* : TEMPOROMANDIBULAR JOINT SYNDROME

TMS *abbr* transcranial magnetic stimulation

TNF *abbr* tumor necrosis factor

toad·stool \ˈtōd-ˌstül\ *n* : a fungus having an umbrella-shaped spore-bearing structure : MUSHROOM; *esp* : a poisonous or inedible one as distinguished from an edible mushroom

to·bac·co \tə-ˈba-(ˌ)kō\ *n, pl* **-cos** **1** : any of a genus (*Nicotiana*) of plants of the nightshade family (Solanaceae); *esp* : an annual So. American herb (*N. tabacum*) cultivated for its leaves **2** : the leaves of cultivated tobacco prepared for use in smoking or chewing or as snuff **3** : manufactured products of tobacco; *also* : the use of tobacco as a practice

to·bra·my·cin \ˌtō-brə-ˈmī-sᵊn\ *n* : a colorless water-soluble antibiotic $C_{18}H_{37}N_5O_9$ isolated from a soil bacterium of the genus *Streptomyces* (*S. tenebrarius*) and effective esp. against gram-negative bacteria — see ZYLET

tocodynamometer *var of* TOKODYNAMOMETER

to·col·y·sis \tō-ˈkä-lə-səs\ *n, pl* **-y·ses** \-ˌsēz\ : inhibition of uterine contractions

¹to·co·lyt·ic \ˌtō-kə-ˈli-tik\ *adj* : inhibiting uterine contractions

²tocolytic *n* : a tocolytic drug

to·coph·er·ol \tō-ˈkä-fə-ˌrȯl, -ˌrōl\ *n* : any of several fat-soluble oily phenolic compounds with varying degrees of antioxidant vitamin E activity; *esp* : ALPHA-TOCOPHEROL

to·co·tri·en·ol \ˌtō-kō-ˈtrī-ə-ˌnōl, -nȯl\ *n* : any of several compounds that are structurally similar to the tocopherols

Todd's paralysis \ˈtädz-\ *n* : temporary weakness or paralysis of one limb or one side of the body that occurs following a seizure

Todd, Robert Bentley (1809–1860), British physician.

toe \ˈtō\ *n* : one of the terminal members of a foot

toed \ˈtōd\ *adj* : having a toe or toes esp. of a specified kind or number — usu. used in combination ⟨five-*toed*⟩

toe·nail \ˈtō-ˌnāl\ *n* : a nail of a toe

to·fa·ci·ti·nib \ˌtō-fə-ˈsi-tə-ˌnib\ *n* : a drug that inhibits enzymes involved in mediating inflammatory immune responses and is taken orally in the form of its citrate $C_{16}H_{20}N_6O·C_6H_8O_7$

esp. to treat rheumatoid arthritis — see XELJANZ

To·fra·nil \tō-ˈfrā-nil\ *trademark* — used for a preparation of imipramine

to·ga·vi·rus \ˈtō-gə-ˌvī-rəs\ *n* : any of a family (*Togaviridae*) of single-stranded RNA viruses that have a spherical virion and include the causative agents of German measles and the three forms of equine encephalitis — see ALPHAVIRUS, RUBIVIRUS

toi·let \ˈtȯi-lət\ *n* : cleansing in preparation for or in association with a medical or surgical procedure ⟨pulmonary ~⟩

toilet training *n* : the process of training a child to control bladder and bowel movements and to use the toilet — **toilet train** \-ˌtrān\ *vb*

token economy *n* : a system of operant conditioning used for behavior therapy that involves rewarding desirable behaviors with tokens which can be exchanged for items or privileges and punishing undesirable behaviors by taking away tokens

to·ko·dy·na·mom·e·ter *or* **to·co·dy·na·mom·e·ter** \ˌtō-kō-ˌdī-nə-ˈmä-mə-tər\ *n* : an instrument by means of which the force of uterine puerperal contractions can be measured

to·laz·amide \tō-ˈla-zə-ˌmīd\ *n* : a sulfonylurea $C_{14}H_{21}N_3O_3S$ used orally to lower blood sugar in the treatment of type 2 diabetes — see TOLINASE

to·laz·o·line \tō-ˈla-zə-ˌlēn\ *n* : a weak alpha-adrenergic blocking agent used in the form of its hydrochloride $C_{10}H_{12}N_2{\cdot}HCl$ to produce peripheral vasodilation

tol·bu·ta·mide \täl-ˈbyü-tə-ˌmīd\ *n* : a sulfonylurea $C_{12}H_{18}N_2O_3S$ used orally to lower blood sugar in the treatment of type 2 diabetes

Tol·ec·tin \ˈtä-lek-tin\ *trademark* — used for a preparation of the hydrated sodium salt of tolmetin

tol·er·ance \ˈtä-lə-rəns\ *n* **1** : the capacity of the body to endure or become less responsive to a substance (as a drug) or a physiological insult with repeated use or exposure ⟨developed a ~ to painkillers⟩ **2** : the immunological state marked by unresponsiveness to a specific antigen — **tol·er·ant** \-rənt\ *adj* — **tol·er·ate** \-ˌrāt\ *vb*

tol·er·a·tion \ˌtä-lə-ˈrā-shən\ *n* : TOLERANCE

tol·ero·gen \ˈtä-lə-rə-jən\ *n* : a tolerogenic antigen

tol·ero·gen·ic \ˌtä-lə-rə-ˈje-nik\ *adj* : capable of producing immunological tolerance ⟨~ antigens⟩

To·li·nase \ˈtō-lə-ˌnās, ˈtä-lə-ˌnāz\ *n* : a preparation of tolazamide — formerly a U.S. registered trademark

tol·met·in \ˈtäl-mə-tən\ *n* : an anti-inflammatory drug administered esp. in the form of its hydrated sodium salt $C_{15}H_{14}NNaO_3{\cdot}2H_2O$ — see TOLECTIN

tol·naf·tate \täl-ˈnaf-ˌtāt\ *n* : a topical antifungal drug $C_{19}H_{17}NOS$ — see TINACTIN

tol·ter·o·dine \ˌtäl-ˈter-ə-ˌdēn\ *n* : an anticholinergic drug administered in the form of its tartrate $C_{22}H_{31}NO{\cdot}C_4H_6O_6$ to treat urge incontinence, frequent urination, and urinary urgency associated with an overactive bladder — see DETROL

to·lu \tə-ˈlü, tō-\ *n* : BALSAM OF TOLU

tolu balsam *n* : BALSAM OF TOLU

tol·u·ene·sul·fon·ic acid \ˌtäl-yə-ˌwēn-səl-ˈfä-nik-\ *n* : any of three isomeric crystalline oily liquid strong acids $CH_3C_6H_4SO_3H$

-tome \ˌtōm\ *n comb form* **1** : part : segment ⟨myo*tome*⟩ **2** : cutting instrument ⟨micro*tome*⟩

Tomes' fiber \ˈtōmz-\ *n* : any of the fibers extending from the odontoblasts into the alveolar canals : a dentinal fiber — called also *Tomes' process*

Tomes, Sir John (1815–1895), British dental surgeon.

Tom·my John surgery \ˈtä-mē-ˈjän-\ *n* : ULNAR COLLATERAL LIGAMENT RECONSTRUCTION

John, Thomas Edward (*b* 1943), American baseball player.

to·mo·gram \ˈtō-mə-ˌgram\ *n* : a radiograph made by tomography

to·mo·graph \-ˌgraf\ *n* : an X-ray machine used for tomography

to·mog·ra·phy \tō-ˈmä-grə-fē\ *n, pl* **-phies** : a method of producing a three-dimensional image of the internal structures of a solid object (as the human body) by the observation and recording of the differences in the effects on the passage of waves of energy impinging on those structures — see COMPUTED TOMOGRAPHY, POSITRON-EMISSION TOMOGRAPHY — **to·mo·graph·ic** \ˌtō-mə-ˈgra-fik\ *adj*

-t·o·my \t-ə-mē\ *n comb form, pl* **-t·o·mies** : incision : section ⟨blepharo*tomy*⟩ ⟨laparo*tomy*⟩

¹tone \ˈtōn\ *n* **1** : a sound of definite pitch and vibration **2 a** : the state of a living body or of any of its organs or parts in which the functions are healthy and performed with due vigor **b** : normal tension or responsiveness to stimuli; *specif* : TONUS 2

²tone *vb* **toned; ton·ing** : to impart tone to

tone–deaf \ˈtōn-ˌdef\ *adj* : relatively insensitive to differences in musical pitch — **tone deafness** *n*

ton·er \ˈtō-nər\ *n* : one that tones; *esp* : a liquid cosmetic for cleansing the skin and contracting the pores

tongue \ˈtəŋ\ *n* : a process of the floor of the mouth that is attached basally to the hyoid bone, that consists essentially of a mass of extrinsic muscle attaching its base to other parts, intrinsic muscle by which parts of the structure move in relation to each other, and an epithelial covering rich in sensory end organs and small glands, and that functions esp. in taking and swallowing food and as a speech organ

tongue depressor *n* : a thin wooden blade rounded at both ends that is used to depress the tongue to allow for inspection of the mouth and throat — called also *tongue blade*

tongue roll•er \-ˌrō-lər\ *n* : a person who carries a dominant gene which confers the capacity to roll the tongue into the shape of a U

tongue thrust \-ˌthrəst\ *n* : the thrusting of the tongue against or between the incisors during the act of swallowing which if persistent in early childhood can lead to various dental abnormalities

tongue–tie *n* : a congenital defect characterized by limited mobility of the tongue due to shortness of the frenulum : ANKYLOGLOSSIA — **tongue–tied** *adj*

tongue worm *n* : any of a taxonomic group (Pentastomida) of invertebrates that are parasites of the respiratory passages of reptiles, birds, and mammals — see HALZOUN

-to•nia \ˈtō-nē-ə\ *n comb form* : condition or degree of tonus ⟨myo*tonia*⟩

[1]**ton•ic** \ˈtä-nik\ *adj* **1 a** : characterized by tonus ⟨~ contraction of muscle⟩; *also* : marked by or being prolonged muscular contraction ⟨~ convulsions⟩ **b** : producing or adapted to produce healthy muscular condition and reaction of organs (as muscles) **2 a** : increasing or restoring physical or mental tone **b** : yielding a tonic substance — **ton•i•cal•ly** *adv*

[2]**tonic** *n* : an agent (as a drug) that increases body tone

tonic–clonic *adj* : relating to, marked by, or being a seizure that affects both cerebral hemispheres and is characterized by the abrupt loss of consciousness with initially tonic muscle contractions followed by clonic muscle spasms

to•nic•i•ty \tō-ˈni-sə-tē\ *n, pl* **-ties** **1** : the property of possessing tone; *esp* : healthy vigor of body or mind **2** : TONUS 2

ton•i•co•clon•ic \ˌtä-ni-kō-ˈklä-nik\ *adj* : TONIC-CLONIC

tono- *comb form* **1** : tone ⟨*tono*topic⟩ **2** : pressure ⟨*tono*meter⟩

tono•clon•ic \ˌtä-nō-ˈklä-nik\ *adj* : TONIC-CLONIC

tono•fi•bril \-ˈfī-brəl, -ˈfi-\ *n* : a thin fibril made up of tonofilaments

tono•fil•a•ment \-ˈfi-lə-mənt\ *n* : a slender cytoplasmic organelle found esp. in some epithelial cells

to•nog•ra•phy \tō-ˈnä-grə-fē\ *n, pl* **-phies** : the procedure of recording measurements (as of intraocular pressure) with a tonometer — **to•no•graph•ic** \ˌtō-nə-ˈgra-fik, ˌtä-\ *adj*

to•nom•e•ter \tō-ˈnä-mə-tər\ *n* : an instrument for measuring tension or pressure and esp. intraocular pressure — **to•no•met•ric** \ˌtō-nə-ˈme-trik, ˌtä-\ *adj* — **to•nom•e•try** \tō-ˈnä-mə-trē\ *n*

to•no•top•ic \ˌtō-nə-ˈtä-pik\ *adj* : relating to or being the anatomic organization by which specific sound frequencies are received by specific receptors in the inner ear with nerve impulses traveling along selected pathways to specific sites in the brain

ton•sil \ˈtän-səl\ *n* **1 a** : either of a pair of prominent masses of lymphoid tissue that lie one on each side of the throat between the anterior and posterior pillars of the fauces and are composed of lymph follicles grouped around one or more deep crypts — called also *palatine tonsil* **b** : PHARYNGEAL TONSIL **c** : LINGUAL TONSIL **2** : a rounded prominence situated medially on the lower surface of each lateral hemisphere of the cerebellum — **ton•sil•lar** \ˈtän-sə-lər\ *adj*

tonsill- *or* **tonsillo-** *comb form* : tonsil ⟨*tonsill*ectomy⟩

tonsillar crypt *n* : any of the deep invaginations occurring on the surface of the palatine and pharyngeal tonsils

ton•sil•lec•to•my \ˌtän-sə-ˈlek-tə-mē\ *n, pl* **-mies** : surgical excision of the tonsils

ton•sil•li•tis \ˌtän-sə-ˈlī-təs\ *n* : inflammation of the tonsils and esp. the palatine tonsils typically due to viral or bacterial infection and marked by red enlarged tonsils usu. with sore throat, fever, difficult swallowing, hoarseness or loss of voice, and tender or swollen lymph nodes

ton•sil•lo•phar•yn•geal \ˌtän-sə-lō-ˌfar-ən-ˈjē-əl; -fə-ˈrin-jəl, -jē-əl\ *adj* : of, relating to, or involving the tonsils and pharynx ⟨the ~ area⟩

ton•sil•lo•phar•yn•gi•tis \-ˌfar-ən-ˈjī-təs\ *n, pl* **-git•i•des** \-ˈji-tə-ˌdēz\ : inflammation of the tonsils and pharynx

to•nus \ˈtō-nəs\ *n* **1** : TONE 2a **2** : a state of partial contraction that is characteristic of normal muscle, is maintained at least in part by a continuous bombardment of motor impulses originating reflexly, and serves to maintain body posture — called also *muscle tone;* compare CLONUS

-to•ny \ˌtō-nē, tᵊn-ē\ *n comb form, pl* **-to•nies** : -TONIA ⟨hypo*tony*⟩

tooth \ˈtüth\ *n, pl* **teeth** \ˈtēth\ : any of the hard bony appendages that are borne on the jaws and serve esp. for the prehension and mastication of food — see MILK TOOTH, PERMANENT TOOTH

tooth•ache \ˈtüth-ˌāk\ *n* : pain in or about a tooth — called also *odontalgia*

tooth•brush \-ˌbrəsh\ *n* : a brush for cleaning the teeth — **tooth•brush•ing** *n*

tooth bud *n* : a mass of tissue having the potentiality of differentiating into a tooth

tooth germ *n* : TOOTH BUD

tooth·less \ˈtüth-ləs\ *adj* : having no teeth
tooth·paste \ˈtüth-ˌpāst\ *n* : a paste for cleaning the teeth
tooth·pick \-ˌpik\ *n* : a pointed instrument (as a slender tapering piece of wood) used for removing food particles lodged between the teeth
top- *or* **topo-** *comb form* : local ⟨*top*ectomy⟩ ⟨*topo*gnosia⟩
to·pec·to·my \tə-ˈpek-tə-mē\ *n, pl* **-mies** : surgical excision of selected portions of the frontal cortex of the brain esp. for the relief of medically intractable epilepsy
to·pha·ceous \tə-ˈfā-shəs\ *adj* : relating to, being, or characterized by the occurrence of tophi ⟨~ gout⟩
to·phus \ˈtō-fəs\ *n, pl* **to·phi** \ˈtō-ˌfī, -ˌfē\ : a deposit of urates in tissues (as cartilage) characteristic of gout
top·i·cal \ˈtä-pi-kəl\ *adj* : designed for or involving application to or action on the surface of a part of the body ⟨applied a ~ anesthetic to numb the skin⟩ — **top·i·cal·ly** *adv*
top·og·no·sia \ˌtä-ˌpäg-ˈnō-zhə, ˌtō-, -zhē-ə\ *n* : recognition of the location of a stimulus on the skin or elsewhere in the body
topo·graph·i·cal \ˌtä-pə-ˈgra-fi-kəl\ *or* **topo·graph·ic** \-fik\ *adj* **1** : of, relating to, or concerned with topography **2** : of or relating to a mind made up of different strata and esp. of the conscious, preconscious, and unconscious — **topo·graph·i·cal·ly** *adv*
topographic anatomy *n* : REGIONAL ANATOMY
to·pog·ra·phy \tə-ˈpä-grə-fē\ *n, pl* **-phies** **1** : the physical or natural features of an object or entity and their structural relationships ⟨the ~ of the abdomen⟩ **2** : REGIONAL ANATOMY
topo·isom·er·ase \ˌtō-pō-ī-ˈsä-mə-ˌrās\ *n* : any of a class of enzymes that reduce supercoiling in DNA by breaking and rejoining one or both strands of the DNA molecule
To·prol \ˈtō-ˌprōl\ *trademark* — used for a preparation of the succinate of metoprolol
TORCH \ˈtȯrch\ *n* [*to*xoplasma, *r*ubella virus, *c*ytomegalovirus, *h*erpes simplex virus] : a group of pathological agents that cause similar symptoms in newborns and that include esp. a toxoplasma (*Toxoplasma gonii*), cytomegalovirus, herpes simplex virus, and the togavirus causing German measles
TORCH infection *n* : a group of symptoms esp. of newborn infants that include hepatosplenomegaly, jaundice, and thrombocytopenia, and are caused by infection with one or more of the TORCH agents — called also *TORCH syndrome*
tori *pl of* TORUS
to·ric \ˈtōr-ik\ *adj* : of, relating to, or shaped like a torus or segment of a torus; *specif* : being a simple lens having for one of its surfaces a segment of an equilateral zone of a torus and consequently having different refracting power in different meridians
tor·pid \ˈtȯr-pəd\ *adj* : sluggish in functioning or acting : characterized by torpor — **tor·pid·i·ty** \tȯr-ˈpi-də-tē\ *n*
tor·por \ˈtȯr-pər\ *n* : a state of mental and motor inactivity with partial or total insensibility : extreme sluggishness or stagnation of function
¹torque \ˈtȯrk\ *n* : a force that produces or tends to produce rotation or torsion; *also* : a measure of the effectiveness of such a force
²torque *vb* **torqued; torqu·ing** : to impart torque to : cause to twist
torr \ˈtȯr\ *n, pl* **torr** : a unit of pressure equal to $^{1}/_{760}$ of an atmosphere or about 0.019 pounds per square inch
tor·sades de pointes \tȯr-ˌsäd(z)-də-ˈpwant\ *or* **tor·sade de pointes** \-ˌsäd-\ *n* : ventricular tachycardia that is characterized by fluctuation of the QRS complexes around the electrocardiographic baseline, is typically caused by a long QT interval, and may lead to life-threatening ventricular fibrillation
tor·sion \ˈtȯr-shən\ *n* **1** : the twisting of a bodily organ or part on its own axis ⟨intestinal ~⟩ **2** : the twisting or wrenching of a body by the exertion of forces tending to turn one end or part about a longitudinal axis while the other is held fast or turned in the opposite direction; *also* : the state of being twisted — **tor·sion·al** \ˈtȯr-shə-nəl\ *adj*
torsion dystonia *n* : DYSTONIA MUSCULORUM DEFORMANS
tor·so \ˈtȯr-(ˌ)sō\ *n, pl* **torsos** *or* **tor·si** \ˈtȯr-ˌsē\ : the human trunk
tort·ed \ˈtȯr-təd\ *adj, chiefly Brit* : marked by torsion
tor·ti·col·lis \ˌtȯr-tə-ˈkä-ləs\ *n* : a twisting of the neck to one side that results in abnormal carriage of the head and is usu. caused by muscle spasms — called also *wryneck*
tor·tu·ous \ˈtȯr-chə-wəs\ *adj* : marked by repeated twists, bends, or turns ⟨a ~ blood vessel⟩ — **tor·tu·os·i·ty** \ˈtȯr-chə-ˈwä-sə-tē\ *n*
tor·u·la \ˈtȯr-yə-lə, ˈtär-\ *n* **1** *pl* **-lae** \-ˌlē, -ˌlī\ *also* **-las** : CRYPTOCOCCOSIS **2** *cap* : a genus of yeasts including pathogens (as *T. histolytica* syn. *Cryptococcus neoformans* that causes cryptococcosis) usu. placed in the genus *Cryptococcus*
Tor·u·lop·sis \ˌtȯr-yə-ˈläp-səs, ˌtär-\ *n* : a genus of round, oval, or cylindrical yeasts that include forms which in other classifications are placed either in the genus *Torula* or *Cryptococcus*
tor·u·lo·sis \ˌtȯr-yə-ˈlō-səs, ˌtär-\ *n* : CRYPTOCOCCOSIS
to·rus \ˈtōr-əs\ *n, pl* **to·ri** \ˈtōr-ˌī, -ˌē\ : a smooth rounded anatomical protuberance (as a bony ridge on the skull)

torus tu•ba•ri•us \-tü-ˈber-ē-əs, -tyü-\ *n* : a protrusion on the lateral wall of the nasopharynx marking the pharyngeal end of the cartilaginous part of the eustachian tube

torus ure•ter•i•cus \-ˌyu̇r-ə-ˈter-i-kəs\ *n* : a band of smooth muscle joining the orifices of the ureter and forming the base of the trigone of the bladder

tos•yl•ate \ˈtä-sə-ˌlāt\ *n* : an ester of the para isomer of toluenesulfonic acid

total hysterectomy *n* : PANHYSTERECTOMY

total mastectomy *n* : a mastectomy in which the breast tissue, associated skin, nipple, and areola are removed — called also *simple mastectomy*

to•ti•po•ten•cy \ˌtō-tə-ˈpōt-ᵊn-sē\ *n, pl* **-cies** : ability of a cell or bodily part to generate or regenerate the whole organism

to•ti•po•tent \tō-ˈti-pə-tənt\ *adj* : capable of developing into a complete organism or differentiating into any of its cells or tissues ⟨~ blastomeres⟩

touch \ˈtəch\ *n* **1** : the special sense by which pressure or traction exerted on the skin or mucous membrane is perceived **2** : a light attack ⟨a ~ of fever⟩

Tou•rette's syndrome \tu̇r-ˈets-\ *or* **Tou•rette syndrome** \-ˈet-\ *n* : a familial neurological disorder of variable expression that is characterized by recurrent involuntary tics involving body movements (as eye blinks or grimaces) and vocalizations (as grunts or utterance of inappropriate words), often has one or more associated conditions (as obsessive-compulsive disorder), is more common in males than females, and usu. has an onset in childhood and often stabilizes or ameliorates in adulthood — abbr. *TS;* called also *Gilles de la Tourette syndrome, Tourette's disease, Tourette's disorder*

Gilles de la Tourette \ˈzhēl-də-lä-ˈtür-et\, **Georges (1857–1904),** French physician.

tour•ni•quet \ˈtu̇r-ni-kət, ˈtər-\ *n* : a device (as a bandage twisted tight with a stick) to check bleeding or blood flow

tower head *n* : OXYCEPHALY

tower skull *n* : OXYCEPHALY

tox- *or* **toxi-** *or* **toxo-** *comb form* **1** : toxic : poisonous ⟨*tox*in⟩ **2** : toxin : poison ⟨*toxi*genic⟩

tox•ae•mia *chiefly Brit var of* TOXEMIA

Tox•as•ca•ris \täk-ˈsas-kə-rəs\ *n* : a genus of ascarid roundworms that infest the small intestine of the dog and cat and related wild animals

tox•e•mia \täk-ˈsē-mē-ə\ *n* : an abnormal condition associated with the presence of toxic substances in the blood: as **a** : a generalized intoxication due to absorption and systemic dissemination of bacterial toxins from a focus of infection **b** : intoxication due to dissemination of toxic substances (as some by-products of protein metabolism) that cause functional or organic disturbances (as in the kidneys) — **tox•e•mic** \-mik\ *adj*

toxemia of pregnancy *n* : a disorder of unknown cause that is peculiar to pregnancy, is usu. of sudden onset, is marked by hypertension, albuminuria, edema, headache, and visual disturbances, and may or may not be accompanied by convulsions

toxi- — see TOX-

[1]**tox•ic** \ˈtäk-sik\ *adj* **1** : containing or being poisonous material esp. when causing serious injury or death ⟨~ gas⟩ ⟨~ drugs⟩ **2** : of, relating to, or caused by a poison or toxin ⟨~ liver damage⟩ **3 a** : affected by a poison or toxin **b** : affected with toxemia of pregnancy — **tox•ic•i•ty** \täk-ˈsi-sə-tē\ *n*

[2]**toxic** *n* : a toxic substance

toxic- *or* **toxico-** *comb form* : poison ⟨*toxico*logy⟩ ⟨*toxic*osis⟩

toxic epidermal necrolysis *n* : a skin disorder characterized by widespread erythema and the formation of flaccid bullae and later by skin that is scalded in appearance and separates from the body in large sheets — abbr. *TEN;* called also *epidermal necrolysis, Lyell's syndrome, scalded-skin syndrome;* compare STAPHYLOCOCCAL SCALDED SKIN SYNDROME

Tox•i•co•den•dron \ˌtäk-si-kō-ˈden-ˌdrän\ *n* : a genus of shrubs and trees of the cashew family (Anacardiaceae) that includes some plants (as poison ivy, poison oak, and poison sumac) producing irritating oils that cause dermatitis

tox•i•co•gen•ic \ˌtäk-si-kō-ˈje-nik\ *adj* : producing toxins or poisons

tox•i•co•log•i•cal \ˌtäk-si-kə-ˈlä-ji-kəl\ *or* **tox•i•co•log•ic** \-jik\ *adj* : of or relating to toxicology or toxins — **tox•i•co•log•i•cal•ly** *adv*

tox•i•col•o•gy \ˌtäk-si-ˈkä-lə-jē\ *n, pl* **-gies:** the scientific study of the adverse effects of chemical substances on the living organism — **tox•i•col•o•gist** *n*

tox•i•co•sis \ˌtäk-sə-ˈkō-səs\ *n, pl* **-co•ses** \-ˌsēz\ : a pathological condition caused by the action of a poison or toxin

toxic shock *n* : TOXIC SHOCK SYNDROME

toxic shock syndrome *n* : an acute and sometimes fatal disease that is characterized by fever, nausea, diarrhea, diffuse erythema, and shock, is associated esp. with the presence of a bacterium of the genus *Staphylococcus* (*S. aureus*), and occurs esp. in menstruating females using tampons — called also *toxic shock*

toxi•gen•ic \ˌtäk-sə-ˈje-nik\ *adj* : producing toxin ⟨~ bacteria⟩ — **toxi•ge•nic•i•ty** \ˌtäk-si-jə-ˈni-sə-tē\ *n*

tox•in \ˈtäk-sən\ *n* : a poisonous substance that is a specific product of the metabolic activities of a living organism and is usu. very unstable, notably toxic when introduced into the tissues, and typically capable of inducing antibody formation

tox·in–antitoxin *n* : a mixture of toxin and antitoxin used esp. formerly in immunizing against a disease (as diphtheria) for which they are specific

toxo- — see TOX-

Tox·o·cara \ˌtäk-sə-ˈkar-ə\ *n* : a genus of nematode worms including the common ascarids (*T. canis* and *T. cati*) of the dog and cat

tox·o·ca·ri·a·sis \ˌtäk-sə-ka-ˈrī-ə-səs\ *n, pl* **-a·ses** \-ˌsēz\ : infection with or disease caused by nematode worms of the genus *Toxocara*

tox·oid \ˈtäk-ˌsȯid\ *n* : a toxin of a pathogenic organism treated so as to destroy its toxicity but leave it capable of inducing the formation of antibodies on injection ⟨diphtheria ~⟩ — called also *anatoxin*

toxo·plas·ma \ˌtäk-sə-ˈplaz-mə\ *n* **1** *cap* : a genus of sporozoans that are typically serious pathogens of vertebrates **2** *pl* **-mas** *or* **-ma·ta** \-mə-tə\ *also* **-ma** : any sporozoan of the genus *Toxoplasma* — **toxo·plas·mic** \-mik\ *adj*

toxo·plas·mo·sis \-ˌplaz-ˈmō-səs\ *n, pl* **-mo·ses** \-ˌsēz\ : infection with or disease caused by a sporozoan of the genus *Toxoplasma* (*T. gondii*) that invades the tissues and may seriously damage the central nervous system esp. of infants

tPA *abbr* tissue plasminogen activator

TPI *abbr* Treponema pallidum immobilization (test)

TPN \ˌtē-(ˌ)pē-ˈen\ *n* : NADP

TPN *abbr* total parenteral nutrition

TPR *abbr* temperature, pulse, respiration

tra·bec·u·la \trə-ˈbe-kyə-lə\ *n, pl* **-lae** \-ˌlē\ *also* **-las** **1** : a small bar, rod, bundle of fibers, or septal membrane in the framework of a bodily organ or part (as the spleen) **2** : any of the intersecting osseous bars occurring in cancellous bone — **tra·bec·u·lar** \-lər\ *adj* — **tra·bec·u·la·tion** \trə-ˌbe-kyə-ˈlā-shən\ *n*

trabecular meshwork *n* : trabecular tissue that separates the angle of the anterior chamber from the canal of Schlemm and that contains spaces through which aqueous humor normally drains from the anterior chamber into the canal of Schlemm

tra·bec·u·lec·to·my \trə-ˌbe-kyə-ˈlek-tə-mē\ *n, pl* **-mies** : surgical excision of a small portion of the trabecular meshwork in order to facilitate drainage of aqueous humor for the relief of glaucoma

tra·bec·u·lo·plas·ty \trə-ˈbe-kyə-lō-ˌplas-tē\ *n, pl* **-ties** : plastic surgery of a trabecula; *specif* : laser surgery to create small openings in the trabecular meshwork of the eye from which the aqueous humor can drain to reduce intraocular pressure caused by open-angle glaucoma

trace \ˈtrās\ *n* **1** : the marking made by a recording instrument (as a kymograph) **2** : an amount of a chemical constituent not always quantitatively determinable because of minuteness **3** : ENGRAM — **trace** *vb* — **trace·able** \ˈtrā-sə-bəl\ *adj*

trace element *n* : a chemical element present in minute quantities; *esp* : a micronutrient (as iodine, iron, and zinc) with an optimum daily intake of typically less than 100 milligrams

trac·er \ˈtrā-sər\ *n* : a substance used to trace the course of a process; *specif* : a labeled element or atom that can be traced throughout chemical or biological processes by its radioactivity or its unusual isotopic mass

trache- *or* **tracheo-** *comb form* **1** : trachea ⟨*tracheo*scopy⟩ **2** : tracheal and ⟨*tracheo*bronchial⟩

tra·chea \ˈtrā-kē-ə\ *n, pl* **tra·che·ae** \-kē-ˌē\ *also* **tra·che·as** : the main trunk of the system of tubes by which air passes to and from the lungs that is about four inches (10 centimeters) long and somewhat less than an inch (2.5 centimeters) in diameter, extends down the front of the neck from the larynx, divides in two to form the bronchi, has walls of fibrous and muscular tissue stiffened by incomplete cartilaginous rings which keep it from collapsing, and is lined with mucous membrane whose epithelium is composed of columnar ciliated mucus-secreting cells — called also *windpipe* — **tra·che·al** \-əl\ *adj*

tracheal node *n* : any of a group of lymph nodes arranged along each side of the thoracic part of the trachea

tracheal ring *n* : any of the 16 to 20 C-shaped bands of highly elastic cartilage which are found as incomplete rings in the anterior two-thirds of the tracheal wall and of which there are usu. 6 to 8 in the right bronchus and 9 to 12 in the left

tra·che·itis \ˌtrā-kē-ˈī-təs\ *n* : inflammation of the trachea

trachel- *or* **trachelo-** *comb form* **1** : neck ⟨*trachelo*mastoid muscle⟩ **2** : uterine cervix ⟨*trachelo*plasty⟩

trach·e·lec·to·my \ˌtra-kə-ˈlek-tə-mē\ *n, pl* **-mies** : CERVICECTOMY

trach·e·lo·mas·toid muscle \ˌtra-kə-lō-ˈmas-ˌtȯid-\ *n* : LONGISSIMUS CAPITIS

trach·e·lo·plas·ty \ˈtra-kə-lō-ˌplas-tē\ *n, pl* **-ties** : plastic surgery on the uterine cervix

trach·e·lor·rha·phy \ˌtra-kə-ˈlȯr-ə-fē\ *n, pl* **-phies** : the operation of sewing up a laceration of the uterine cervix

tra·cheo·bron·chi·al \ˌtrā-kē-ō-ˈbräŋ-kē-əl\ *adj* : of, relating to, affecting, or produced in the trachea and bronchi ⟨~ secretion⟩ ⟨~ lesions⟩

tracheobronchial node *n* : any of the lymph nodes arranged in four or five groups along the trachea and bronchi — called also *tracheobronchial lymph node*

tracheobronchial tree *n* : the trachea and bronchial tree considered together

tra•cheo•bron•chi•tis \ˌtrā-kē-ō-bräŋ-ˈkī-təs\ *n, pl* **-chit•i•des** \-ˈki-tə-ˌdēz\ : inflammation of the trachea and bronchi

tra•cheo•esoph•a•ge•al \-i-ˌsä-fə-ˈjē-əl\ *adj* : relating to or connecting the trachea and the esophagus <a ~ fistula>

tra•cheo•plas•ty \ˈtrā-kē-ə-ˌplas-tē\ *n, pl* **-ties** : plastic surgery on the trachea

tra•che•os•co•py \ˌtrā-kē-ˈäs-kə-pē\ *n, pl* **-pies** : inspection of the interior of the trachea (as by a bronchoscope)

tra•cheo•sto•ma \ˌtrā-kē-ˈäs-tə-mə\ *n* : an opening into the trachea created by tracheostomy

tra•che•os•to•my \ˌtrā-kē-ˈäs-tə-mē\ *n, pl* **-mies** : the surgical formation of an opening into the trachea through the neck esp. to allow the passage of air; *also* : the opening itself

tra•che•ot•o•my \ˌtrā-kē-ˈä-tə-mē\ *n, pl* **-mies** **1** : the surgical operation of cutting into the trachea esp. through the skin **2** : the opening created by a tracheotomy

tra•cho•ma \trə-ˈkō-mə\ *n* : a chronic contagious conjunctivitis marked by inflammatory granulations on the conjunctival surfaces, caused by a bacterium of the genus *Chlamydia* (*C. trachomatis*), and commonly resulting in blindness if left untreated — **tra•cho•ma•tous** \trə-ˈkō-mə-təs, -ˈkä-\ *adj*

trac•ing \ˈtrā-siŋ\ *n* : a graphic record made by an instrument (as an electrocardiograph) that registers some movement

tract \ˈtrakt\ *n* **1** : a system of body parts or organs that act together to perform some function <the digestive ~> — see GASTROINTESTINAL TRACT, LOWER RESPIRATORY TRACT, UPPER RESPIRATORY TRACT **2** : a bundle of nerve fibers having a common origin, termination, and function and esp. one within the spinal cord or brain — called also *fiber tract;* see CORTICOSPINAL TRACT, OLFACTORY TRACT, OPTIC TRACT, SPINOTHALAMIC TRACT; compare FASCICULUS b

trac•tion \ˈtrak-shən\ *n* **1** : the pulling of or tension established in one body part by another **2** : a pulling force exerted on a skeletal structure (as in a fracture) by means of a special device or apparatus <a ~ splint>; *also* : a state of tension created by such a pulling force <a leg in ~>

tract of Burdach *n* : FASCICULUS CUNEATUS

K. F. Burdach — see COLUMN OF BURDACH

tract of Lissauer *n* : DORSOLATERAL TRACT

Lissauer, Heinrich (1861—1891), German neurologist.

trac•tot•o•my \trak-ˈtä-tə-mē\ *n, pl* **-mies** : surgical division of a nerve tract

trac•tus \ˈtrak-təs\ *n, pl* **tractus** : TRACT 2

tractus sol•i•ta•ri•us \-ˌsä-li-ˈtar-ē-əs\ *n* : a descending tract of nerve fibers that is situated near the dorsal surface of the medulla oblongata, mediates esp. the sense of taste, and includes fibers from the facial, glossopharyngeal, and vagus nerves

Trad•jen•ta \trə-ˈjen-tə\ *trademark* — used for a preparation of linagliptin

trag•a•canth \ˈtra-jə-ˌkanth, -gə-, -kənth; ˈtra-gə-ˌsanth\ *n* : a gum obtained from various Asian or East European plants (genus *Astragalus* and esp. *A. gummifer*) of the legume family (Leguminosae) and is used as an emulsifying, suspending, and thickening agent and as a demulcent — called also *gum tragacanth*

tra•gus \ˈtrā-gəs\ *n, pl* **tra•gi** \-ˌgī, -ˌjī\ : a small projection in front of the external opening of the ear

train•able \ˈtrā-nə-bəl\ *adj* : affected with moderate intellectual disability and capable of being trained in self-care and in simple social and work skills in a sheltered environment — compare EDUCABLE

trained nurse *n* : GRADUATE NURSE

trait \ˈtrāt\ *n* : an inherited characteristic

TRALI *abbr* transfusion-related acute lung injury

tram•a•dol \ˈtra-mə-ˌdȯl\ *n* : a synthetic opioid analgesic administered orally in the form of its hydrochloride $C_{16}H_{25}NO_2{\cdot}HCl$ to treat moderate to severe pain — see ULTRAM

trance \ˈtrans\ *n* **1** : a sleeplike altered state of consciousness (as of deep hypnosis) usu. characterized by partly suspended animation with diminished or absent sensory and motor activity and subsequent lack of recall **2** : a state of profound abstraction or absorption — **trance•like** \-ˌlīk\ *adj*

tran•do•la•pril \tran-ˈdō-lə-ˌpril\ *n* : an ACE inhibitor $C_{24}H_{34}N_2O_5$ taken orally to treat hypertension or to treat heart failure or left ventricular dysfunction following heart attack — see MAVIK

tran•ex•am•ic acid \ˌtra-nek-ˈsa-mik-\ *n* : an antifibrinolytic drug $C_8H_{15}NO_2$

tran•quil•ize *also* **tran•quil•lize** \ˈtraŋ-kwə-ˌlīz, ˈtran-\ *vb* **-ized** *also* **-lized; -iz•ing** *also* **-liz•ing** : to relieve of mental tension and anxiety by means of drugs — **tran•quil•i•za•tion** \ˌtraŋ-kwə-lə-ˈzā-shən, ˌtran-\ *n*

tran•quil•iz•er *also* **tran•quil•liz•er** \-ˌlī-zər\ *n* : a drug used to reduce mental disturbance (as anxiety and tension) — see ANTIPSYCHOTIC

trans \ˈtrans, ˈtranz\ *n* : characterized by or having certain groups of atoms on opposite sides of the longitudinal axis of a double bond or of the plane of a ring in a molecule

trans•ab•dom•i•nal \ˌtrans-ab-ˈdä-mə-nəl, ˌtranz-\ *adj* : passing through or performed by passing through the abdomen or the abdominal wall ⟨~ amniocentesis⟩

trans·ac·tion·al analysis \-ˌak-shə-nəl-\ *n* : a system of psychotherapy involving analysis of individual episodes of social interaction for insight that will aid communication — abbr. *TA*

trans·am·i·nase \-ˈa-mə-ˌnās, -ˌnāz\ *n* : an enzyme promoting transamination

trans·am·i·na·tion \-ˌa-mə-ˈnā-shən\ *n* : a reversible oxidation-reduction reaction in which an amino group is transferred typically from an alpha-amino acid to an alpha-keto acid

trans·bron·chi·al \-ˈbräŋ-kē-əl\ *adj* : occurring or performed by way of a bronchus; *specif* : involving the passage of a bronchoscope through the lumen of a bronchus

trans·cap·il·lary \-ˈka-pə-ˌler-ē\ *adj* : existing or taking place across the capillary walls

trans·cath·e·ter \-ˈka-thə tər\ *adj* : performed through the lumen of a catheter ⟨~ embolization⟩

trans·cer·vi·cal \-ˈsər-vi-kəl\ *adj* : performed by way of the uterine cervix

trans·con·dy·lar \-ˈkän-də-lər\ *adj* : passing through a pair of condyles ⟨a ~ fracture of the humerus⟩

trans·cor·ti·cal \-ˈkȯr-ti-kəl\ *adj* : crossing the cortex of the brain; *esp* : passing from the cortex of one hemisphere to that of the other

trans·cor·tin \-ˈkȯrt-ᵊn\ *n* : an alpha globulin produced in the liver that binds with and transports cortisol in the blood

trans·cra·ni·al \-ˈkrā-nē-əl\ *adj* : passing or performed through the skull ⟨~ Doppler ultrasound⟩

transcranial magnetic stimulation *n* : a noninvasive technique for stimulating brain neurons that uses an electromagnetic coil usu. placed on the scalp to produce magnetic fields which generate electric currents in specific areas of the brain esp. to measure and map brain function and to treat depression and neuropathic pain — abbr. *TMS*

tran·scribe \trans-ˈkrīb\ *vb* **tran·scribed; tran·scrib·ing** : to cause (as DNA) to undergo genetic transcription

tran·script \ˈtrans-ˌkript\ *n* : a sequence of RNA produced by transcription from a DNA template

tran·scrip·tase \tran-ˈskrip-ˌtās, -ˌtāz\ *n* : RNA POLYMERASE; *also* : REVERSE TRANSCRIPTASE

tran·scrip·tion \trans-ˈkrip-shən\ *n* : the process of constructing a messenger RNA molecule using a DNA molecule as a template with resulting transfer of genetic information to the messenger RNA — compare REVERSE TRANSCRIPTION, TRANSLATION — **tran·scrip·tion·al** \-shə-nəl\ *adj* — **tran·scrip·tion·al·ly** *adv*

transcription factor *n* : any of various proteins that bind to DNA and play a role in the regulation of gene expression by promoting transcription

tran·scrip·tion·ist \-shə-nist\ *n* : one that transcribes; *esp* : MEDICAL TRANSCRIPTIONIST

trans·cu·ta·ne·ous \ˌtrans-kyu̇-ˈtā-nē-əs\ *adj* : passing, entering, or made by penetration through the skin

transcutaneous electrical nerve stimulation *n* : electrical stimulation of the skin to relieve pain by interfering with the neural transmission of signals from underlying pain receptors — called also *TENS, transcutaneous nerve stimulation* — **transcutaneous electrical nerve stimulator** *n*

trans·der·mal \ˌtrans-ˈdər-məl, ˌtranz-\ *adj* : relating to, being, or supplying a medication in a form for absorption through the skin into the bloodstream ⟨~ drug delivery⟩ ⟨a ~ nicotine patch⟩ ⟨~ nitroglycerin⟩ — **trans·der·mal·ly** *adv*

trans·dia·phrag·mat·ic \-ˌdī-ə-frəg-ˈma-tik, -ˌfrag-\ *adj* : occurring, passing, or performed through the diaphragm ⟨~ hernia⟩

trans·duce \-ˈdüs, -ˈdyüs\ *vb* **trans·duced; trans·duc·ing** **1** : to convert (as energy) into another form **2** : to cause (genetic material) to undergo transduction; *also* : to introduce genetic material into (a cell) by transduction

trans·duc·tion \-ˈdek-shən\ *n* : the action or process of transducing; *esp* : the transfer of genetic material from one organism (as a bacterium) to another by a genetic vector and esp. a bacteriophage — compare TRANSFORMATION 2 — **trans·duc·tion·al** \-shə-nəl\ *adj*

trans·du·o·de·nal \-ˌdü-ə-ˈdē-nəl, -ˌdyü-; -dü-ˈäd-ᵊn-əl, -dyü-\ *adj* : performed by cutting across or through the duodenum

tran·sect \tran-ˈsekt\ *vb* : to cut transversely — **tran·sec·tion** \-ˈsek-shən\ *n*

trans·epi·the·li·al \ˌtrans-ˌe-pə-ˈthē-lē-əl, ˌtranz-\ *adj* : existing or taking place across an epithelium

transeptal *var of* TRANSSEPTAL

trans·esoph·a·ge·al \-i-ˌsä-fə-ˈjē-əl\ *adj* : passing through or performed by way of the esophagus ⟨~ echocardiography⟩

transexual *var of* TRANSSEXUAL

trans fat *n* : a fat containing trans-fatty acids

trans–fat·ty acid \ˈtrans-ˈfa-tē, ˈtranz-\ *n* : an unsaturated fatty acid characterized by a trans arrangement of alkyl chains that is formed esp. during the hydrogenation of vegetable oils and has been linked to an increase in blood cholesterol

trans·fec·tant \trans-ˈfek-tənt\ *n* : a cell that has incorporated foreign nucleic acid and esp. DNA through a process of transfection

trans·fec·tion \trans-ˈfek-shən\ *n* : infection of a cell with isolated viral nucleic acid followed by production of the complete virus in the cell; *also* : the incorporation of exogenous DNA into a cell — **trans·fect** \-ˈfekt\ *vb*

trans·fem·o·ral \-ˈfe-mə-rəl\ *adj* **1** : passing through or performed by way of the femoral artery ⟨~ angiography⟩ **2 a** : occurring across or involving the femur ⟨~ amputation⟩ **b** : having undergone transfemoral amputation; *also* : suitable for use following transfemoral amputation

trans·fer \ˈtrans-ˌfər\ *n* **1** : TRANSFERENCE **2** : the carryover or generalization of learned responses from one type of situation to another — see NEGATIVE TRANSFER

trans·fer·ase \ˈtrans-(ˌ)fər-ˌās, -ˌāz\ *n* : an enzyme that promotes transfer of a group from one molecule to another

trans·fer·ence \trans-ˈfər-əns, ˈtrans-(ˌ)\ *n* : the redirection of feelings and desires and esp. of those unconsciously retained from childhood toward a new object (as a psychoanalyst conducting therapy)

transference neurosis *n* : a neurosis developed in the course of psychoanalytic treatment and manifested by the reliving of infantile experiences in the presence of the analyst

transfer factor *n* : a substance that is produced and secreted by a lymphocyte functioning in cell-mediated immunity and that upon incorporation into a lymphocyte which has not been sensitized confers on it the same immunological specificity as the sensitized cell

trans·fer·rin \trans-ˈfer-ən\ *n* : a beta globulin in blood plasma capable of combining with ferric ions and transporting iron in the body

transfer RNA *n* : a relatively small RNA that transfers a particular amino acid to a growing polypeptide chain at the ribosomal site of protein synthesis during translation — called also *soluble RNA, tRNA;* compare MESSENGER RNA

trans·fix·ion \trans-ˈfik-shən\ *n* : a piercing of a part of the body (as by a suture or pin) in order to fix it in position — **trans·fix** \-ˈfiks\ *vb*

trans·form \trans-ˈfȯrm\ *vb* **1** : to change or become changed in structure, appearance, or character **2** : to cause (a cell) to undergo genetic transformation

trans·for·ma·tion \ˌtrans-fər-ˈmā-shən, -fȯr-\ *n* **1** : an act, process, or instance of transforming or being transformed **2 a** : genetic modification of a bacterium by incorporation of free DNA from another ruptured bacterial cell — compare TRANSDUCTION **b** : genetic modification of a cell by the uptake and incorporation of exogenous DNA

transforming growth factor *n* : any of a group of polypeptides that are secreted by a variety of cells (as monocytes, T cells, or blood platelets) and have diverse effects (as inducing angiogenesis, stimulating fibroblast proliferation, or inhibiting T cell proliferation) on the division and activity of cells — abbr. *TGF*

trans·fuse \trans-ˈfyüz\ *vb* **trans·fused; trans·fus·ing** **1** : to transfer (as blood) into a vein or artery of a human being or an animal **2** : to subject (a patient) to transfusion — **trans·fus·able** *or* **trans·fus·ible** \trans-ˈfyü-zə-bəl\ *adj*

trans·fu·sion \trans-ˈfyü-zhən\ *n* **1** : the process of transfusing fluid (as blood) into a vein or artery **2** : something transfused — **trans·fu·sion·al** \-zhə-nəl\ *adj*

trans·fu·sion·ist \-zhə-nist\ *n* : one skilled in performing transfusions

transfusion–related acute lung injury *n* : a sometimes fatal complication of blood transfusion that is characterized by pulmonary edema and may be accompanied by fever, dyspnea, hypoxemia, hypotension, or hypertension followed by hypotension, that usu. starts one to two hours after blood is transfused and is usu. resolved within 96 hours, and is believed to be caused in susceptible individuals either by antibodies introduced into the blood pool by donors or by biologically active substances generated in stored blood — abbr. *TRALI*

trans·gen·der \-ˈjen-dər\ *or* **trans·gen·dered** \-dərd\ *adj* : of, relating to, or being a person (as a transsexual or a transvestite) who identifies with or expresses a gender identity that differs from the one which corresponds to the person's sex at birth — **trans·gen·der·ism** \-də-ˌri-zəm\ *n*

trans·gene \ˈtrans-ˌjēn, ˈtranz\ *n* : a gene that is taken from the genome of one organism and introduced into the genome of another organism by artificial techniques

[1]**trans·gen·ic** \ˌtrans-ˈje-nik, ˌtranz-\ *adj* : being or used to produce an organism or cell of one species into which one or more genes of other species have been incorporated ⟨~ crops⟩; *also* : produced by or composed of transgenic plants or animals

[2]**transgenic** *n* **1 transgenics** *pl* : a branch of biotechnology concerned with the production of transgenic plants, animals, and foods **2** : a transgenic plant or animal

trans·glu·ta·min·ase \-ˈglü-tə-mə-ˌnās, -glü-ˈta-mə-ˌnāz\ *n* : any of various enzymes that form strong bonds between glutamine and lysine residues in proteins including one that is the active form of clotting factor VIII promoting the formation of cross-links between strands of fibrin

trans•he•pat•ic \-hi-ˈpa-tik\ *adj* : passing through or performed by way of the bile ducts; *specif* : involving direct injection (as of a radiopaque medium) into the bile ducts

tran•sient \ˈtran-zē-ənt, -shənt, -chənt\ *adj* : passing away in time : existing temporarily ⟨~ symptoms⟩

transient global amnesia *n* : temporary amnesia of short duration (as several hours) that is marked by sudden onset, by loss of past memories, and by an inability to form new memories

transient ischemic attack *n* : a brief episode of cerebral ischemia that is usu. characterized by temporary blurring of vision, slurring of speech, numbness, paralysis, or syncope and that is often predictive of a serious stroke — abbr. *TIA;* called also *little stroke, ministroke*

trans•il•lu•mi•nate \ˌtrans-ə-ˈlü-mə-ˌnāt, ˌtranz-\ *vb* **-nat•ed; -nat•ing** : to pass light through (a body part) for medical examination — **trans•il•lu•mi•na•tion** \-ə-ˌlü-mə-ˈnā-shən\ *n*

tran•si•tion•al \tran-ˈsi-shə-nəl, -ˈzi-\ *adj* : of, relating to, or being an epithelium (as in the urinary bladder) that consists of several layers of soft cuboidal cells which become flattened when stretched

trans•la•tion \trans-ˈlā-shən, tranz-\ *n* : the process of forming a protein molecule at a ribosomal site of protein synthesis from information contained in messenger RNA — compare TRANSCRIPTION — **trans•late** \-ˈlāt\ *vb* — **trans•la•tion•al** \-ˈlā-shə-nəl\ *adj*

translational research *n* : medical research that is concerned with facilitating the practical application of scientific discoveries to the development and implementation of new ways to prevent, diagnose, and treat disease — called also *translational medicine*

trans•lo•ca•tion \ˌtrans-lō-ˈkā-shən, ˌtranz-\ *n* **1** : transfer of part of a chromosome to a different position esp. on a nonhomologous chromosome; *esp* : the exchange of parts between nonhomologous chromosomes **2** : a chromosome or part of a chromosome that has undergone translocation — **trans•lo•cate** \-ˈlō-ˌkāt\ *vb*

trans•lum•bar \ˌtrans-ˈləm-bər, ˌtranz-, -ˌbär\ *adj* : passing through or performed by way of the lumbar region; *specif* : involving the injection of a radiopaque medium through the lumbar region ⟨~ aortography⟩

trans•lu•mi•nal \-ˈlü-mə-nəl\ *adj* : passing across or performed by way of a lumen; *specif* : involving the passage of an inflatable catheter along the lumen of a blood vessel ⟨~ angioplasty⟩

trans•mem•brane \-ˈmem-ˌbrān\ *adj* : taking place, existing, or arranged from one side to the other of a membrane ⟨~ proteins⟩ ⟨a ~ potential⟩

trans•mis•si•ble \trans-ˈmi-sə-bəl, tranz-\ *adj* : capable of being transmitted ⟨~ diseases⟩ — **trans•mis•si•bil•i•ty** \-ˌmi-sə-ˈbi-lə-tē\ *n*

transmissible mink encephalopathy *n* : a prion disease of mink that resembles scrapie

transmissible spongiform encephalopathy *n* : PRION DISEASE — abbr. *TSE*

trans•mis•sion \trans-ˈmi-shən, tranz-\ *n* : an act, process, or instance of transmitting ⟨~ of HIV⟩

transmission deafness *n* : CONDUCTION DEAFNESS

transmission electron microscope *n* : a conventional electron microscope which produces an image of a cross-sectional slice of a specimen all points of which are illuminated by the electron beam at the same time — **transmission electron microscopy** *n*

trans•mit \trans-ˈmit, tranz-\ *vb* **trans•mit•ted; trans•mit•ting** : to pass, transfer, or convey from one person or place to another: as **a** : to pass or convey by heredity ⟨~ a genetic abnormality⟩ **b** : to convey (infection) abroad or to another ⟨mosquitoes ~ malaria⟩ **c** : to cause (energy) to be conveyed through space or a medium ⟨substances that ~ nerve impulses⟩

trans•mit•ta•ble \-ˈmi-tə-bəl\ *adj* : TRANSMISSIBLE

trans•mit•ter \-ˈmi-tər\ *n* : one that transmits; *specif* : NEUROTRANSMITTER

trans•mu•co•sal \ˌtran(t)s-myü-ˈkō-zəl, ˌtranz-\ *adj* : relating to, being, or supplying a medication that enters through or across a mucous membrane (as of the mouth)

trans•mu•ral \-ˈmyu̇r-əl\ *adj* : passing or administered through an anatomical wall ⟨~ stimulation of the ileum⟩; *also* : involving the whole thickness of a wall ⟨~ myocardial infarction⟩ — **trans•mu•ral•ly** *adv*

trans•neu•ro•nal \-nu̇-ˈrōn-əl, -nyu̇-; -ˈnu̇r-ən-əl, -ˈnyu̇r-\ *adj* : TRANSSYNAPTIC ⟨~ cell atrophy⟩

trans•or•bit•al \-ˈȯr-bət-əl\ *adj* : passing through or performed by way of the eye socket

trans•ovar•i•al \-ō-ˈvar-ē-əl\ *adj* : relating to or being transmission of a pathogen from an organism (as a tick) to its offspring by infection of eggs in its ovary — **trans•ovar•i•al•ly** *adv*

trans•ovar•i•an \-ē-ən\ *adj* : TRANSOVARIAL

trans•par•ent \trans-ˈpar-ənt\ *adj* **1** : having the property of transmitting light so that bodies lying beyond are seen clearly **2** : allowing the passage of a specified form of radiation (as X-rays)

trans·pep·ti·dase \trans-ˈpep-tə-ˌdās, tranz-, -ˌdāz\ *n* : an enzyme that catalyzes the transfer of an amino acid residue or a peptide residue from one amino compound to another

trans·peri·to·ne·al \-ˌper-ə-tə-ˈnē-əl\ *adj* : passing or performed through the peritoneum

trans·per·son·al \-ˈpərs-nəl\ *adj* : of, relating to, or being psychology or psychotherapy concerned esp. with esoteric mental experience (as mysticism and altered states of consciousness) beyond the usual limits of ego and personality

trans·pla·cen·tal \ˌtrans-plə-ˈsent-ᵊl\ *adj* : relating to, involving, or being passage (as of an antibody) between mother and fetus through the placenta — **trans·pla·cen·tal·ly** *adv*

[1]**trans·plant** \trans-ˈplant\ *vb* : to transfer from one place to another; *esp* : to transfer (an organ or tissue) from one part or individual to another — **trans·plant·abil·i·ty** \-ˌplan-tə-ˈbi-lə-tē\ *n* — **trans·plant·able** \-ˈplan-tə-bəl\ *adj* — **trans·plan·ta·tion** \ˌtrans-ˌplan-ˈtā-shən\ *n*

[2]**trans·plant** \ˈtrans-ˌplant\ *n* **1** : something (as an organ or part) that is transplanted **2** : the act or process of transplanting ⟨a liver ~⟩

trans·pleu·ral \-ˈplu̇r-əl\ *adj* : passing through or requiring passage through the pleura ⟨a ~ surgical procedure⟩

[1]**trans·port** \trans-ˈpōrt, ˈtrans-ˌ\ *vb* : to transfer or convey from one place to another

[2]**trans·port** \ˈtrans-ˌpōrt\ *n* : an act or process of transporting; *specif* : ACTIVE TRANSPORT

transposable element *n* : a segment of genetic material that is capable of changing its location in the genome or in some bacteria of undergoing transfer between an extrachromosomal plasmid and a chromosome — called also *transposable genetic element*

trans·pose \trans-ˈpōz\ *vb* **trans·posed; trans·pos·ing** : to transfer from one place or period to another; *specif* : to subject to or undergo genetic transposition — **trans·pos·able** \-ˈpō-zə-bəl\ *adj*

trans·po·si·tion \ˌtrans-pə-ˈzi-shən\ *n* : an act, process, or instance of transposing or being transposed: as **a** : the displacement of a viscus to a side opposite from that which it normally occupies ⟨~ of the heart⟩ **b** : the transfer of a segment of DNA from one site to another in the genome either between chromosomal sites or between an extrachromosomal site (as on a plasmid) and a chromosome — **trans·po·si·tion·al** \-ˈzi-shə-nəl\ *adj*

trans·po·son \ˌtrans-ˈpō-ˌzän\ *n* : a transposable element esp. when it contains genetic material controlling functions other than those related to its relocation

trans·py·lor·ic \-pī-ˈlōr-ik\ *adj* : relating to or being the transverse plane or the line marking its intersection with the surface of the abdomen that passes below the rib cage cutting the pylorus of the stomach and the first lumbar vertebra and that is one of the four planes marking off the nine abdominal regions

trans·rec·tal \-ˈrekt-ᵊl\ *adj* : passing through or performed by way of the rectum ⟨~ prostatic biopsy⟩

trans·sep·tal *also* **tran·sep·tal** \-ˈsept-ᵊl\ *adj* **1** : passing across a septum ⟨~ fibers between teeth⟩ **2** : passing or performed through a septum ⟨~ cardiac catheterization⟩

trans·sex·u·al *also* **tran·sex·u·al** \-ˈsek-shə-wəl\ *n* : a person who psychologically identifies with the opposite sex and may seek to live as a member of this sex esp. by undergoing surgery and hormone therapy to obtain the necessary physical appearance (as by changing the external sex organs) — **transsexual** *also* **transexual** *adj* — **trans·sex·u·al·ism** *also* **tran·sex·u·al·ism** \-wə-ˌli-zəm\ *n* — **trans·sex·u·al·i·ty** *also* **tran·sexu·al·ity** \-ˌsek-shə-ˈwa-lə-tē\ *n*

trans·sphe·noi·dal \-sfi-ˈnȯid-ᵊl\ *adj* : performed by entry through the sphenoid bone ⟨~ hypophysectomy⟩

trans·syn·ap·tic \-sə-ˈnap-tik\ *adj* : occurring or taking place across nerve synapses ⟨~ degeneration⟩

trans·tho·rac·ic \-thə-ˈra-sik\ *adj* **1** : performed or made by way of the thoracic cavity **2** : crossing or having connections that cross the thoracic cavity ⟨a ~ pacemaker⟩ — **trans·tho·rac·i·cal·ly** *adv*

trans·thy·re·tin \-ˈthī-rə-tin\ *n* : a protein component of blood serum that functions esp. in the transport of thyroxine — called also *prealbumin*

trans·tib·i·al \-ˈti-bē-əl\ *adj* **1** : occurring across or involving the tibia ⟨~ amputation⟩ **2** : having undergone transtibial amputation; *also* : suitable for use following transtibial amputation ⟨a ~ prosthesis⟩

trans·tra·che·al \-ˈtrā-kē-əl\ *adj* : passing through or administered by way of the trachea ⟨~ anesthesia⟩

tran·su·date \ˌtran-ˈsü-dət, -ˈsyü-, -ˈzü-, -ˈzyü-, -ˌdāt\ *n* : a transuded substance

tran·su·da·tion \ˌtran-sü-ˈdā-shən, -syü-, -zü-, -zyü-\ *n* **1** : the act or process of transuding or being transuded **2** : TRANSUDATE

tran·sude \tran-ˈsüd, -ˈsyüd, -ˈzüd, -ˈzyüd\ *vb* **tran·sud·ed; tran·sud·ing** : to pass or permit passage of through a membrane or permeable substance

trans·ure·tero·ure·ter·os·to·my \ˌtrans-yu̇-ˌrē-tə-ˌrō-yu̇-ˌrē-tə-ˈräs-tə-mē\ *n, pl* **-mies** : anastomosis of a ureter to the contralateral ureter

trans•ure•thral \-yu̇-ˈrē-thrəl\ *adj* : passing through or performed by way of the urethra ⟨~ prostatectomy⟩

trans•vag•i•nal \-ˈva-jən-ᵊl\ *adj* : passing through or performed by way of the vagina ⟨~ laparoscopy⟩

trans•ve•nous \-ˈvē-nəs\ *adj* : relating to or involving the use of an intravenous catheter containing an electrode carrying electrical impulses from an extracorporeal source to the heart

trans•ven•tric•u•lar \-ven-ˈtri-kyə-lər, -vən-\ *adj* : passing through or performed by way of a ventricle

transversa, transversum — see SEPTUM TRANSVERSUM

trans•ver•sa•lis cer•vi•cis \ˌtrans-vər-ˈsā-ləs-ˈsər-vi-səs\ *n* : LONGISSIMUS CERVICIS

transversalis fascia *n* : the whole deep layer of fascia lining the abdominal wall; *also* : the part of this covering the inner surface of the transversus abdominis and separating it from the peritoneum

trans•verse \trans-ˈvərs, tranz-, ˈtrans-ˌ, ˈtranz-ˌ\ *adj* **1** : acting, lying, or being across : set crosswise **2** : made at right angles to the long axis of the body ⟨a ~ section⟩ — **trans•verse•ly** *adv*

transverse carpal ligament *n* : FLEXOR RETINACULUM 2

transverse cervical artery *n* : an inconstant branch of the thyrocervical trunk or of the subclavian artery that supplies the region at the base of the neck and the muscles of the scapula

transverse colon *n* : the part of the large intestine that extends across the abdominal cavity joining the ascending colon to the descending colon

transverse crural ligament *n* : EXTENSOR RETINACULUM 1b

transverse facial artery *n* : a large branch of the superficial temporal artery that arises in the parotid gland and supplies the parotid gland, masseter muscle, and adjacent parts

transverse fissure *n* : PORTA HEPATIS

transverse foramen *n* : a foramen in each transverse process of a cervical vertebra through which the vertebral artery and vertebral vein pass in each cervical vertebra except the seventh

transverse ligament *n* : any of various ligaments situated transversely with respect to a bodily axis or part: as **a** : the transverse part of the cruciate ligament of the atlas **b** : one in the anterior part of the knee connecting the anterior margins of the lateral and medial menisci

transverse process *n* : a process that projects on the dorsolateral aspect of each side of the neural arch of a vertebra

transverse sinus *n* : either of two large venous sinuses of the cranium that begin at the bony protuberance on the middle of the inner surface of the occipital bone at the intersection of its bony ridges and that terminate at the jugular foramen on either side to become the internal jugular vein

transverse thoracic muscle *n* : TRANSVERSUS THORACIS

transverse tubule *n* : T TUBULE

trans•ver•sion \trans-ˈvər-zhən, tranz-\ *n* : the eruption of a tooth in an abnormal position on the jaw

transversum — see SEPTUM TRANSVERSUM

trans•ver•sus ab•dom•i•nis \trans-ˈvər-səs-əb-ˈdä-mə-nəs\ *n* : a flat muscle with transverse fibers that forms the innermost layer of the anterolateral wall of the abdomen and that acts to constrict the abdominal viscera and assist in expulsion of the contents of various abdominal organs (as in defecation, vomiting, and childbirth)

transversus pe•rin•ei su•per•fi•ci•a•lis \-pe-ˈri-nē-ˌī-ˌsü-pər-ˌfi-shē-ˈā-ləs\ *n* : a small band of muscle of the urogenital region of the perineum that arises from the ischial tuberosity and that with the contralateral muscle inserts into and acts to stabilize the mass of tissue in the midline between the anus and the penis or vagina — called also *superficial transverse perineal muscle*

transversus tho•ra•cis \-thə-ˈrā-səs\ *n* : a thin flat sheet of muscle and tendon fibers of the anterior wall of the chest that arises esp. from the xiphoid process and lower third of the sternum, inserts into the costal cartilages of the second to sixth ribs, and acts to draw the ribs downward — called also *transverse thoracic muscle*

trans•ves•i•cal \trans-ˈve-si-kəl, tranz-\ *adj* : passing through or performed by way of the urinary bladder

trans•ves•tism \trans-ˈves-ˌti-zəm, tranz-\ *n* : the practice of adopting the dress, manner and sometimes the sexual role of the opposite sex — **trans•ves•tite** \-ˌtīt\ *n or adj*

Tran•xene \ˈtran-ˌzēn\ *trademark* — used for a preparation of the dipotassium salt of clorazepate

tran•yl•cy•pro•mine \ˌtran-ᵊl-ˈsī-prə-ˌmēn\ *n* : an antidepressant drug that is an inhibitor of monoamine oxidase and is administered in the form of its sulfate $(C_9H_{11}N)_2 \cdot H_2SO_4$

tra•pe•zi•um \trə-ˈpē-zē-əm, tra-\ *n, pl* **-zi•ums** *or* **-zia** \-zē-ə\ : a bone in the distal row of the carpus at the base of the thumb — called also *greater multangular*

tra•pe•zi•us \trə-ˈpē-zē-əs, tra-\ *n, pl* **-zii** \-zē-ˌī\ *also* **-zi•us•es** : a large flat triangular superficial muscle of each side of the upper back that arises from the occipital bone, the ligamentum nuchae, and the spinous processes of the last cervical and all the thoracic vertebrae, is inserted into the outer part of the clavicle, the acromion, and the spine of the scapula, and serves chiefly to rotate the scapula so as to present the glenoid cavity upward

trap•e•zoid \ˈtra-pə-ˌzȯid\ *n* : a bone in the distal row of the carpus at the base of the index finger — called also *lesser multangular, trapezoid bone, trapezoideum*

trapezoid body *n* : a bundle of transverse fibers in the dorsal part of the pons

trap•e•zoi•de•um \ˌtra-pə-ˈzȯi-dē-əm\ *n* : TRAPEZOID

tras•tu•zu•mab \ˌtras-ˈtü-zü-ˌmab\ *n* : a genetically engineered monoclonal antibody administered by injection to slow or inhibit tumor growth in some advanced breast cancers — see HERCEPTIN

Tras•y•lol \ˈtra-sə-ˌlȯl\ *trademark* — used for a preparation of aprotinin

trau•ma \ˈtrau̇-mə, ˈtrȯ-\ *n, pl* **traumas** *also* **trau•ma•ta** \-mə-tə\ **1 a** : an injury (as a wound) to living tissue caused by an extrinsic agent ⟨surgical ~⟩ — see BLUNT TRAUMA **b** : a disordered psychological or behavioral state resulting from mental or emotional stress or physical injury **2** : an agent, force, or mechanism that causes trauma — **trau•mat•ic** \trə-ˈma-tik, trȯ-, trau̇-\ *adj* — **trau•mat•i•cal•ly** *adv*

trauma center *n* : a hospital unit specializing in the treatment of patients with acute and esp. life-threatening traumatic injuries

traumat- *or* **traumato-** *comb form* : wound : trauma ⟨*traumat*ism⟩

traumatic brain injury *n* : an acquired brain injury caused by external force (as a blow to the head sustained in a motor vehicle accident or a bullet entering through the skull); *broadly* : ACQUIRED BRAIN INJURY — abbr. *TBI*

trau•ma•tism \ˈtrau̇-mə-ˌti-zəm, ˈtrȯ-\ *n* : the development or occurrence of trauma; *also* : TRAUMA

trau•ma•tize \-ˌtīz\ *vb* **-tized; -tiz•ing** : to inflict a trauma upon ⟨*traumatized* tissues⟩ ⟨children *traumatized* by physical abuse⟩ — **trau•ma•ti•za•tion** \ˌtrau̇-mə-tə-ˈzā-shən, ˌtrȯ-\ *n*

trau•ma•tol•o•gist \ˌtrau̇-mə-ˈtä-lə-jəst, ˈtrȯ-\ *n* : a surgeon who practices traumatology or who is on duty at a trauma center

trau•ma•tol•o•gy \ˌtrau̇-mə-ˈtä-lə-jē, ˌtrȯ-\ *n, pl* **-gies** : the surgical treatment of wounds ⟨pediatric ~⟩

Trav•a•tan \ˈtra-və-ˌtan\ *trademark* — used for an ophthalmic preparation containing travoprost

traveler's diarrhea *n* : intestinal sickness and diarrhea affecting a traveler and typically caused by ingestion of pathogenic microorganisms (as some E. coli) — compare MONTEZUMA'S REVENGE

travel sickness *n* : MOTION SICKNESS

trav•o•prost \ˈtra-vō-ˌpräst\ *n* : a synthetic prostaglandin analog $C_{26}H_{35}F_3O_6$ that reduces intraocular pressure and is used in a solution applied as eye drops to treat ocular hypertension and open-angle glaucoma — see TRAVATAN

tray \ˈtrā\ *n* : an appliance consisting of a rimmed body and a handle for use in holding plastic material against the gums or teeth in making negative impressions for dentures

traz•o•done \ˈtra-zə-ˌdōn\ *n* : an antidepressant drug that is administered in the form of its hydrochloride $C_{19}H_{22}ClN_5O{\cdot}HCl$ and inhibits the uptake of serotonin by the brain

Trea•cher Col•lins syndrome \ˈtrē-chər-ˈkä-lənz-\ *n* : MANDIBULOFACIAL DYSOSTOSIS

Collins, Edward Treacher (1862–1932), British ophthalmologist.

tread•mill \ˈtred-ˌmil\ *n* : a device having an endless belt on which an individual walks or runs in place that is used for exercise and in tests of physiological functions — see STRESS TEST

Tre•an•da \trē-ˈan-də\ *trademark* — used for a preparation of bendamustine

treat \ˈtrēt\ *vb* : to care for or deal with medically or surgically : deal with by medical or surgical means ⟨~*ed* their diseases⟩ — **treat•abil•i•ty** \ˌtrē-tə-ˈbi-lə-tē\ *n* — **treat•able** \ˈtrē-tə-bəl\ *adj* — **treat•ment** \ˈtrēt-mənt\ *n*

tree \ˈtrē\ *n* : an anatomical system or structure having many branches — see BILIARY TREE, BRONCHIAL TREE, TRACHEOBRONCHIAL TREE

-tre•ma \ˈtrē-mə\ *n comb form, pl* **-tremas** *or* **-tre•ma•ta** \ˈtrē-mə-tə\ : hole : orifice : opening ⟨helico*trema*⟩

trem•a•tode \ˈtre-mə-ˌtōd\ *n* : any of a class (Trematoda) of parasitic flatworms including the flukes — **trematode** *adj*

trem•bles \ˈtrem-bəlz\ *n* : poisoning of livestock and esp. cattle by a toxic alcohol present in white snakeroot and rayless goldenrod

tremens — see DELIRIUM TREMENS

trem•or \ˈtre-mər\ *n* : a trembling or shaking usu. from physical weakness, emotional stress, or disease

trem•u•lous \ˈtrem-yə-ləs\ *adj* : characterized by or affected with trembling or tremors — **trem•u•lous•ness** *n*

trench fever *n* : a disease that is marked by fever and pain in muscles, bones, and joints and that is caused by a bacterium (*Bartonella quintana* syn. *Rochalimaea quintana*) transmitted by the human body louse (*Pediculus humanus humanus*)

trench foot *n* : a painful foot disorder resembling frostbite and resulting from exposure to cold and wet

trench mouth *n* : ACUTE NECROTIZING ULCERATIVE GINGIVITIS; *also* : VINCENT'S ANGINA

Tren•de•len•burg position \ˈtrend-ᵊl-ən-ˌbərg-\ *n* : a position of the body for medical examination or operation in which the patient is placed head down on a table inclined at about 45 degrees from the floor with the knees uppermost and the legs hanging over the end of the table

Trendelenburg, Friedrich (1844–1924), German surgeon.

Tren•tal \ˈtren-ˌtal\ *trademark* — used for a preparation of pentoxifylline

treph•i•na•tion \ˌtre-fə-ˈnā-shən\ *n* : an act or instance of using a trephine (as to perforate the skull)

tre•phine \ˈtrē-ˌfīn\ *n* : a surgical instrument for cutting out circular sections (as of bone or corneal tissue) — **tre•phine** \ˈtrē-ˌfīn, tri-ˈ\ *vb*

trep•o•ne•ma \ˌtre-pə-ˈnē-mə\ *n* **1** *cap* : a genus of anaerobic spirochetes (family Spirochaetaceae) that are pathogenic in humans and other warm-blooded animals and include one (*T. pallidum*) causing syphilis and another (*T. pertenue*) causing yaws **2** *pl* **-ma•ta** \-mə-tə\ *or* **-mas** : any spirochete of the genus *Treponema* — **trep•o•ne•mal** \-ˈnē-məl\ *adj*

Treponema pal•li•dum immobilization test \-ˈpa-lə-dəm-\ *n* : a serological test for syphilis — abbr. *TPI*

trepo•ne•ma•to•sis \ˌtre-pə-ˌnē-mə-ˈtō-səs, -ˌne-\ *n, pl* **-to•ses** \-ˌsēz\ : infection with or disease caused by spirochetes of the genus *Treponema*

trepo•neme \ˈtre-pə-ˌnēm\ *n* : TREPONEMA 2

trep•pe \ˈtre-pə\ *n* : the graduated series of increasingly vigorous contractions that results when a corresponding series of identical stimuli is applied to a rested muscle — called also *staircase effect*

tre•tin•o•in \tre-ˈti-nō-ən, ˈtre-tə-ˌnȯin\ *n* : a trans isomer of retinoic acid that is applied topically to the skin to treat acne vulgaris and to reduce facial wrinkles, roughness, and pigmented spots and that is administered orally to treat acute myelogenous leukemia in which more than half the cells are malignant promyelocytes — called also *all-trans-retinoic acid, retinoic acid;* see ISOTRETINOIN, RETIN-A

TRF *abbr* thyrotropin-releasing factor

TRH *abbr* thyrotropin-releasing hormone

tri•ac•e•tyl•ole•an•do•my•cin \(ˌ)trī-ˌa-sət-ᵊl-ˌō-lē-ˌan-dō-ˈmīs-ᵊn\ *n* : TROLEANDOMYCIN

tri•ad \ˈtrī-ˌad\ *n* : a union or group of three ⟨a ~ of symptoms⟩

tri•age \trē-ˈäzh, ˈtrē-ˌ\ *n* **1** : the sorting of and allocation of treatment to patients and esp. battle and disaster victims according to a system of priorities designed to maximize the number of survivors **2** : the sorting of patients (as in an emergency room) according to the urgency of their need for care — **triage** *vb*

tri•al \ˈtrī-əl\ *n* **1** : a tryout or experiment to test quality, value, or usefulness — see CLINICAL TRIAL **2** : one of a number of repetitions of an experiment

tri•am•cin•o•lone \ˌtrī-ˌam-ˈsin-ᵊl-ˌōn\ *n* : a glucocorticoid drug $C_{21}H_{27}FO_6$ that has anti-inflammatory and immunosuppressant effects and is used chiefly in the treatment of skin disorders, asthma, and allergic rhinitis — see AZMACORT, NASACORT

tri•am•ter•ene \trī-ˈam-tər-ˌēn\ *n* : a diuretic drug $C_{12}H_{11}N_7$ that promotes potassium retention — see DYAZIDE, MAXZIDE

tri•an•gle \ˈtrī-ˌaŋ-gəl\ *n* : a three-sided region or space and esp. an anatomical one — see ANTERIOR TRIANGLE, CAROTID TRIANGLE, FEMORAL TRIANGLE, POSTERIOR TRIANGLE, SUBOCCIPITAL TRIANGLE

tri•an•gu•lar \trī-ˈaŋ-gyə-lər\ *n* : TRIQUETRAL BONE

triangular bone *n* : TRIQUETRAL BONE

triangular fossa *n* : a shallow depression in the anterior part of the top of the ear's auricle between the two crura into which the antihelix divides

tri•an•gu•la•ris \trī-ˌaŋ-gyə-ˈlar-əs\ *n, pl* **-la•res** \-ˈlar-ˌēz\ **1** : a flat triangular muscle that extends from the base of the mandible to the angle formed by the joining of the upper and lower lips and that acts to depress this angle **2** : TRIQUETRAL BONE

triangular ridge *n* : a triangular surface that slopes downward from the tip of a cusp of a molar or premolar toward the center of its occlusal surface

tri•at•o•ma \trī-ˈa-tə-mə\ *n* **1** *cap* : a genus of large blood-sucking bugs (family Reduviidae) that feed on mammals and sometimes transmit Chagas disease to their hosts — see CONENOSE **2** : any bug of the genus *Triatoma*

[1]**tri•at•o•mid** \trī-ˈa-tə-mid\ *adj* : belonging to the genus *Triatoma*

[2]**triatomid** *n* : TRIATOMA 2

tri•az•i•quone \trī-ˈa-zə-ˌkwōn\ *n* : an antineoplastic drug $C_{12}H_{13}N_3O_2$

tri•azo•lam \trī-ˈa-zə-ˌlam\ *n* : a benzodiazepine $C_{17}H_{12}Cl_2N_4$ used as a sleep-inducing agent in the short-term treatment of insomnia — see HALCION

tri•azole \ˈtrī-ə-ˌzōl\ *n* : any of a group of compounds that are characterized by a ring composed of two carbon atoms and three nitrogen atoms and that include a number of antifungal agents (as fluconazole)

trib•a•dism \ˈtri-bə-ˌdi-zəm\ *n* : a homosexual practice among women in which the external genitalia are rubbed together

Tri•ben•zor \trī-ˈben-ˌzȯr\ *trademark* — used for a preparation of amlodipine, hydrochlorothiazide, and olmesartan

tri•bro•mo•eth•a•nol \ˌtrī-ˌbrō-mō-ˈe-thə-ˌnȯl, -ˌnōl\ *n* : a crystalline bromine derivative $C_2H_3Br_3O$ of ethyl alcohol used as a basal anesthetic

trib•u•tary \ˈtri-byə-ˌter-ē\ *n, pl* **-tar•ies** : a vein that empties into a larger vein

tri•car•box•yl•ic acid cycle \ˌtrī-ˌkär-ˌbäk-ˈsi-lik-\ *n* : KREBS CYCLE

tri•ceps \ˈtrī-ˌseps\ *n, pl* **triceps** : a muscle that arises from three heads: **a** : the large extensor muscle that is situated along the back of the upper arm, arises by the long head from the infraglenoid tubercle of the scapula and by two heads from the shaft of the humerus, is inserted into the olecranon at the elbow, and extends the forearm at the elbow joint — called also *triceps brachii* **b** : the gastrocnemius and soleus muscles viewed as constituting together one muscle

triceps bra•chii \-ˈbrā-kē-ˌī\ *n* : TRICEPS a

trich \ˈtrik\ *n* **1** : TRICHOMONIASIS **2** : TRICHOTILLOMANIA

trich- *or* **tricho-** *comb form* : hair : filament ⟨*tricho*bezoar⟩

-trich•ia \ˈtri-kē-ə\ *n comb form* : condition of having (such) hair ⟨a*trichia*⟩

tri•chi•a•sis \tri-ˈkī-ə-səs\ *n* : a turning inward of the eyelashes often causing irritation of the eyeball

tri•chi•na \tri-ˈkī-nə\ *n, pl* **-nae** \-(ˌ)nē\ *also* **-nas** : a small slender nematode worm of the genus *Trichinella* (*T. spiralis*) that as an adult is a short-lived parasite of the intestines of a flesh-eating mammal where it produces immense numbers of larvae which migrate to the muscles, become encysted, may persist for years, and if consumed by a new host in raw or insufficiently cooked meat are liberated by the digestive processes and rapidly become adult to initiate a new parasitic cycle — see TRICHINOSIS

Trichina *n, syn of* TRICHINELLA

trich•i•nel•la \ˌtri-kə-ˈne-lə\ *n* **1** *cap* : a genus of nematode worms (family Trichinellidae) comprising the trichinae **2** *pl* **-lae** \-lē\ : TRICHINA

trich•i•ni•a•sis \ˌtri-kə-ˈnī-ə-səs\ *n, pl* **-a•ses** \-ˌsēz\ : TRICHINOSIS

trich•i•no•sis \ˌtri-kə-ˈnō-səs\ *n, pl* **-noses** \-ˌsēz\ : infestation with or disease caused by trichinae contracted by eating raw or insufficiently cooked infested food and esp. pork and marked initially by abdominal pain, nausea, and diarrhea and later by muscular pain, dyspnea, fever, and edema — called also *trichiniasis*

tri•chlor•fon *also* **tri•chlor•phon** \(ˈ)trī-ˈklōr-ˌfän\ *n* : an organophosphate $C_4H_8Cl_3O_4P$ used as a parasiticide in veterinary medicine

tri•chlor•me•thi•a•zide \ˌtrī-ˌklȯr-me-ˈthī-ə-ˌzīd\ *n* : a diuretic and antihypertensive drug $C_8H_8Cl_3N_3O_4S_2$ — see METAHYDRIN, NAQUA

tri•chlo•ro•ace•tic acid \ˌtrī-ˌklōr-ō-ə-ˈsē-tik-\ *also* **tri•chlor•ace•tic** \-ˌklōr-ə-ˈsē-tik\ *n* : a strong acid $C_2Cl_3HO_2$ used in medicine as a caustic and astringent

tri•chlo•ro•eth•y•lene \-ˈe-thə-ˌlēn\ *also* **tri•chlor•eth•y•lene** \-ˌklōr-ˈe-thə-ˌlēn\ *n* : a nonflammable liquid C_2HCl_3 used in medicine as an anesthetic and analgesic — abbr. *TCE*

tri•chlo•ro•meth•ane \-ˈme-ˌthān\ *n* : CHLOROFORM

tri•chlo•ro•phe•nol \-ˈfē-ˌnōl, -ˌnȯl, -fi-ˈ\ *n* : a bactericide and fungicide $C_6H_3Cl_3O$ that is a major constituent of hexachlorophene

tri•chlo•ro•phen•oxy•ace•tic acid \(ˌ)tri-ˌklōr-ō-fə-ˌnäk-sē-ə-ˈsē-tik-\ *n* : 2,4,5-T

tricho•be•zoar \ˌtri-kō-ˈbē-ˌzōr\ *n* : HAIR BALL

Tricho•bil•har•zia \ˌtri-kō-bil-ˈhär-zē-ə, -ˈhärt-sē-ə\ *n* : a genus of digenetic trematode worms (family Schistosomatidae) including forms that normally parasitize aquatic birds and cause swimmer's itch in humans

Tricho•dec•tes \ˌtri-kə-ˈdek-ˌtēz\ *n* : a genus of biting lice (family Trichodectidae) of domesticated mammals

tricho•epi•the•li•o•ma \ˌtri-kō-ˌe-pə-ˌthē-lē-ˈō-mə\ *n, pl* **-mas** *also* **-ma•ta** \-mə-tə\ : a benign epithelial tumor developing from the hair follicles esp. on the face

tri•chol•o•gy \tri-ˈkä-lə-jē\ *n, pl* **-gies** : the scientific study of the hair and scalp — **tri•chol•o•gist** \tri-ˈkä-lə-jist\ *n*

tricho•mo•na•cide \ˌtri-kə-ˈmō-nə-ˌsīd\ *n* : an agent used to destroy trichomonads — **tricho•mo•na•cid•al** \-ˌmō-nə-ˈsīd-ᵊl\ *adj*

[1]**tricho•mo•nad** \ˌtri-kə-ˈmō-ˌnad, -nəd\ *n* : any protozoan of the genus *Trichomonas*

[2]**trichomonad** *adj* : TRICHOMONAL

tricho•mo•nal \ˌtri-kə-ˈmō-nəl\ *adj* : of, relating to, or caused by flagellated protozoans of the genus *Trichomonas*

trich•o•mo•nas \ˌtri-kə-ˈmō-nəs\ *n* **1** *cap* : a genus of flagellated protozoans (family Trichomonadidae) that are parasites of the digestive or genitourinary tracts of numerous vertebrate and invertebrate hosts including one (*T. vaginalis*) causing human vaginitis **2** : a protozoan of the genus *Trichomonas* : TRICHOMONAD

tricho•mo•ni•a•sis \ˌtri-kə-mə-ˈnī-ə-səs\ *n, pl* **-a•ses** \-ˌsēz\ : infection with or disease caused by trichomonads: as **a** : a human sexually transmitted disease occurring esp. as vaginitis with a persistent discharge and caused by a trichomonad (*Trichomonas vaginalis*) that may also invade the male urethra and bladder **b** : a venereal disease of domestic cattle caused by a trichomonad (*T. foetus*) and marked by abortion and sterility **c** : one or more diseases of various birds caused by trichomonads (esp. *T. gallinae*) and resembling blackhead — called also *roup*

tricho•phy•ton \ˌtri-kə-ˈfī-ˌtän, tri-ˈkä-fə-ˌtän\ *n* **1** *cap* : a genus of fungi (family Moniliaceae) that are parasitic in the skin and hair follicles and include several causing ringworm — see EPIDERMOPHYTON **2** : any fungus of the genus *Trichophyton*

Tricho•spo•ron \ˌtri-kə-ˈspōr-ˌän, tri-ˈkäs-pə-ˌrän\ *n* : a genus of imperfect fungi (order Moniliales) found esp. in the soil that includes the causative agents of white piedra and several forms which occur as commensals (as on the skin and in the gastrointestinal and respiratory tracts) but which may disseminate (as to the lungs or liver) in the body to cause serious infection esp. in immunocompromised individuals

tricho•stron•gyle \ˌtri-kə-ˈsträn-ˌjīl\ *n* : any worm of the genus *Trichostrongylus*

tricho•stron•gy•lo•sis \ˌtri-kō-ˌsträn-jə-ˈlō-səs\ *n* : infestation with or disease caused by roundworms of the genus *Trichostrongylus* chiefly in young sheep and cattle

Tricho•stron•gy•lus \ˌtri-kō-ˈsträn-jə-ləs\ *n* : a genus of nematode worms (family Trichostrongylidae) parasitic in birds and mammals including humans that comprises forms formerly placed in the genus *Strongylus*

tricho•til•lo•ma•nia \-ˌti-lə-ˈmā-nē-ə\ *n* : abnormal desire to pull out one's hair — called also *hairpulling, trich* — **tricho•til•lo•man•ic** \-ˈma-nik\ *adj*

tri•chro•mat \ˈtrī-krō-ˌmat, (ˌ)trī-ˈ\ *n* : an individual with trichromatism

tri•chro•mat•ic \ˌtrī-krō-ˈma-tik\ *adj* **1** : of, relating to, or consisting of three colors ⟨~ light⟩ **2 a** : relating to or being the theory that human color vision involves three types of retinal sensory receptors **b** : characterized by trichromatism ⟨~ vision⟩

tri•chro•ma•tism \(ˌ)trī-ˈkrō-mə-ˌti-zəm\ *n* : color vision based on the perception of three primary colors and esp. red, green, and blue — compare DEUTERANOMALY, PROTANOMALY

trich•u•ri•a•sis \ˌtri-kyə-ˈrī-ə-səs\ *n, pl* **-a•ses** \-ˌsēz\ : infestation with or disease caused by nematode worms of the genus *Trichuris*

Trich•u•ris \tri-ˈkyůr-əs\ *n* : a genus of nematode worms (family Trichuridae) comprising the whipworms

tri•clo•car•ban \ˌtrī-ˌklō-ˈkär-ˌban\ *n* : an antiseptic $C_{13}H_9Cl_3N_2O$ used esp. in soaps

tri•clo•san \trī-ˈklō-ˌsan\ *n* : a whitish crystalline powder $C_{12}H_7Cl_3O_2$ used esp. as a broad-spectrum antibacterial agent (as in soaps, deodorants, and mouthwash)

Tri•Cor \ˈtrī-ˌkȯr\ *trademark* — used for a preparation of fenofibrate

tri•cus•pid \(ˌ)trī-ˈkəs-pəd\ *adj* **1** : having three cusps ⟨~ molars⟩ **2** : of, relating to, or involving the tricuspid valve of the heart ⟨~ disease⟩

tricuspid valve *n* : a valve that is situated at the opening of the right atrium of the heart into the right ventricle and that resembles the mitral valve in structure but consists of three triangular membranous flaps — called also *right atrioventricular valve*

[1]**tri•cy•clic** \(ˌ)trī-ˈsī-klik, -ˈsi-\ *adj* : being a chemical with three usu. fused rings in the molecular structure and esp. a tricyclic antidepressant

[2]**tricyclic** *n* : TRICYCLIC ANTIDEPRESSANT

tricyclic antidepressant *n* : any of a group of antidepressant drugs (as imipramine and amitriptyline) that contain three fused benzene rings, potentiate the action of catecholamines (as norepinephrine and serotonin) by inhibiting their uptake by nerve endings, and do not inhibit the action of monoamine oxidase

tri•di•hex•eth•yl chloride \ˌtrī-ˌdī-ˌheks-ˈeth-ᵊl-\ *n* : a quaternary ammonium compound $C_{21}H_{36}ClNO$ used as an anticholinergic drug — see PATHILON

Tri•di•one \trī-ˈdī-ˌōn\ *trademark* — used for a preparation of trimethadione

triethiodide — see GALLAMINE TRIETHIODIDE

tri•eth•yl•ene gly•col \(ˌ)trī-ˈe-thə-ˌlēn-ˈglī-ˌkȯl, -ˌkōl\ *n* : a hygroscopic liquid alcohol $C_6H_{14}O_4$ that is used in medicine as an air disinfectant

tri•eth•yl•ene•mel•amine \(ˌ)trī-ˌe-thə-ˌlēn-ˈme-lə-ˌmēn, -mən\ *n* : a cytotoxic crystalline compound $C_9H_{12}N_6$ used as an antineoplastic drug — called also *TEM*

tri•fa•cial nerve \ˌtrī-ˈfā-shəl-\ *n* : TRIGEMINAL NERVE

trifacial neuralgia *n* : TRIGEMINAL NEURALGIA

tri•fluo•per•a•zine \ˌtrī-ˌflü-ō-ˈper-ə-ˌzēn, -zən\ *n* : a phenothiazine tranquilizer used in the form of its hydrochloride $C_{21}H_{24}F_3N_3S{\cdot}HCl$ to treat psychotic disorders and esp. schizophrenia — see STELAZINE

tri•flu•pro•ma•zine \ˌtrī-ˌflü-ˈprō-mə-ˌzēn, -zən\ *n* : a phenothiazine tranquilizer used in the form of its hydrochloride $C_{18}H_{19}F_3N_2S{\cdot}HCl$ esp. in the treatment of psychotic disorders and as an antiemetic — see VESPRIN

[1]**tri•fo•cal** \(ˌ)trī-ˈfō-kəl\ *adj, of an eyeglass lens* : having one part that corrects for near vision, one for intermediate vision (as at arm's length), and one for distant vision

[2]**tri•fo•cal** \ˈtrī-ˌfō-kəl\ *n* **1** : a trifocal glass or lens **2** *pl* : eyeglasses with trifocal lenses

[1]**tri•gem•i•nal** \trī-ˈje-mə-nəl\ *adj* : of or relating to the trigeminal nerve

[2]**trigeminal** *n* : TRIGEMINAL NERVE

trigeminal ganglion *n* : the large flattened sensory root ganglion of the trigeminal nerve that lies within the skull and behind the orbit — called also *gasserian ganglion, semilunar ganglion*

trigeminal nerve *n* : either of the fifth pair of cranial nerves that are mixed nerves and in humans are the largest of the cranial nerves and that arise by a small motor root and a larger sensory root which both emerge from the side of the pons with the sensory root bearing the trigeminal ganglion and dividing into ophthalmic, maxillary, and mandibular nerves and the motor root supplying fibers to the mandibular nerve and through this to the muscles of mastication — called also *fifth cranial nerve, trifacial nerve, trigeminus*

trigeminal neuralgia *n* : an intense paroxysmal neuralgia involving one or more branches of the trigeminal nerve — called also *tic douloureux*

trigger finger *n* : an abnormal condition in which flexion or extension of a finger may be momentarily obstructed by spasm followed by a snapping into place

trigger point *n* : a localized usu. tender or painful area of the body and esp. of a muscle that when stimulated gives rise to pain elsewhere in the body — called also *trigger area, trigger zone*

trigger zone *n* **1** : TRIGGER POINT **2** : CHEMORECEPTOR TRIGGER ZONE **3** : the site on an axon where action potentials are initiated and that typically occupies the same region as the axon hillock

Tri•glide \ˈtrī-ˌglīd\ *trademark* — used for a preparation of fenofibrate

tri•glyc•er•ide \(ˌ)trī-ˈgli-sə-ˌrīd\ *n* : any of a group of lipids that are esters formed from one molecule of glycerol and three molecules of one or more fatty acids, are widespread in adipose tissue, and commonly circulate in the blood in the form of lipoproteins — called also *neutral fat*

tri•gone \ˈtrī-ˌgōn\ *also* **tri•gon** \-ˌgän\ *n* : a triangular body part; *specif* : a smooth triangular area on the inner surface of the bladder limited by the apertures of the ureters and urethra

tri•go•ni•tis \ˌtrī-gə-ˈnī-təs\ *n* : inflammation of the trigone of the bladder

tri•go•no•ceph•a•ly \ˌtri-gə-nə-ˈse-fə-lē, ˌtrī-ˌgō-nō-\ *n, pl* **-lies** : a congenital deformity in which the head is somewhat triangular and flat

tri•go•num \trī-ˈgō-nəm\ *n, pl* **-nums** *or* **-na** \-nə\ : a triangular anatomical part : TRIGONE

trigonum ha•ben•u•lae \-hə-ˈben-yə-ˌlē\ *n* : a triangular area on the dorsomedial surface of the lateral geniculate body rostral to the pineal gland

trigonum ves•i•cae \-ˈve-si-kē\ *n* : the trigone of the urinary bladder

tri•halo•meth•ane \ˌtrī-ˌhā-lə-ˈme-ˌthān\ *n* : any of various derivatives CHX_3 of methane (as chloroform) having three halogen atoms per molecule and formed esp. during the chlorination of drinking water

tri•io•do•thy•ro•nine \ˌtrī-ˌī-ə-dō-ˈthī-rə-ˌnēn\ *n* : a crystalline iodine-containing hormone $C_{15}H_{12}I_3NO_4$ that is an amino acid derived from thyroxine and is used esp. in the form of its soluble sodium salt $C_{15}H_{11}I_3NNaO_4$ in the treatment of hypothyroidism and metabolic insufficiency — called also *liothyronine, T3*

Tri•lip•ix \trī-ˈlip-iks\ *trademark* — used for a preparation of the choline salt of fenofibric acid

tri•mep•ra•zine \trī-ˈme-prə-ˌzēn\ *n* : a phenothiazine used esp. in the form of its tartrate $(C_{18}H_{22}N_2S)_2 \cdot C_4H_6O_6$ as an antipruritic

tri•mes•ter \(ˌ)trī-ˈmes-tər, ˈtrī-ˌ\ *n* : a period of three or about three months; *esp* : any of three periods of approximately three months each into which a human pregnancy is divided

tri•metha•di•one \ˌtrī-ˌme-thə-ˈdī-ˌōn\ *n* : a crystalline anticonvulsant $C_6H_9NO_3$ used chiefly in the treatment of absence seizures — see TRIDIONE

tri•meth•a•phan \trī-ˈme-thə-ˌfan\ *n* : a ganglionic blocking agent used as a salt $C_{32}H_{40}N_2O_5S_2$ to lower blood pressure esp. in hypertensive emergencies

tri•metho•ben•za•mide \ˌtrī-ˌme-thə-ˈben-zə-ˌmīd\ *n* : an antiemetic drug used esp. in the form of its hydrochloride $C_{21}H_{28}N_2O_5 \cdot HCl$

tri•meth•o•prim \trī-ˈme-thə-ˌprim\ *n* : a synthetic antibacterial drug $C_{14}H_{18}N_4O_3$ used alone esp. to treat urinary tract infections and Pneumocystis carinii pneumonia and in combination with sulfamethoxazole to treat these as well as other infections (as shigellosis or acute otitis media) — see BACTRIM, SEPTRA

tri•me•trex•ate \ˌtrī-mi-ˈtrek-ˌsāt\ *n* : a toxic drug structurally related to methotrexate that is administered intravenously in the form of its salt $C_{19}H_{23}N_5O_3 \cdot C_6H_{10}O_7$ with concurrent administration of leucovorin to reduce toxicity and is used esp. in the treatment of Pneumocystis carinii pneumonia and certain carcinomas

Tri•mox \ˈtrī-ˌmäks\ *trademark* — used for a preparation of amoxicillin

tri•ni•tro•phe•nol \(ˌ)trī-ˌnī-trō-ˈfē-ˌnōl, -ˌnȯl, -fi-ˈnōl\ *or* **2,4,6–trinitrophenol** \ˌtü-ˌfȯr-ˌsiks-\ *n* : PICRIC ACID

tri•no•mi•al \trī-ˈnō-mē-əl\ *n* : a biological taxonomic name of three terms of which the first designates the genus, the second the species, and the third the subspecies or variety

tri•nu•cle•o•tide \(ˌ)trī-ˈnü-klē-ə-ˌtīd, -ˈnyü-\ *n* : a nucleotide consisting of three mononucleotides in combination : CODON

tri•or•tho•cre•syl phosphate \ˌtrī-ˌȯr-thō-ˌkre-səl-, -ˌkrē-\ *n* : a usu. colorless, odorless, tasteless neurotoxin $C_{21}H_{21}O_4P$

tri•ox•sa•len \ˌtrī-ˈäk-sə-lən\ *n* : a synthetic psoralen $C_{14}H_{12}O_3$ that promotes tanning of the skin

tri•par•a•nol \trī-ˈpar-ə-ˌnȯl, -ˌnōl\ *n* : a drug $C_{27}H_{32}ClNO_2$ formerly used to inhibit the formation of cholesterol but now withdrawn from use because of its link to toxic side effects

tri•pel•en•na•mine \ˌtrī-pe-ˈle-nə-ˌmēn, -mən\ *n* : an antihistamine drug used in the form of its citrate $C_{16}H_{21}N_3 \cdot C_6H_8O_7$ or hydrochloride $C_{16}H_{21}N_3 \cdot HCl$

tri•pep•tide \(ˌ)trī-ˈpep-ˌtīd\ *n* : a peptide that yields three amino acid residues on hydrolysis

tri•phe•nyl•meth•ane \ˌtrī-ˌfen-ᵊl-ˈme-ˌthān, -ˌfēn-\ *n* : a crystalline hydrocarbon $CH(C_6H_5)_3$ from which various dyes are derived

tri•phos•pha•tase \(ˌ)trī-ˈfäs-fə-ˌtās, -ˌtāz\ *n* : an enzyme that catalyzes hydrolysis of a triphosphate — see ATPASE

tri•phos•phate \(ˌ)trī-ˈfäs-ˌfāt\ *n* : a salt or acid that contains three phosphate groups — see ATP, GTP

tri•phos•pho•pyr•i•dine nucleotide \ˌtrī-ˌfäs-fō-ˈpir-ə-ˌdēn-\ *n* : NADP

triple bond *n* : a chemical bond in which three pairs of electrons are shared by two atoms in a molecule and which is usu. represented in chemical formulas by three lines

triple E *n* : EASTERN EQUINE ENCEPHALITIS

tri•ple•gia \(ˌ)trī-ˈplē-jə, -jē-ə\ *n* : hemiplegia plus paralysis of a limb on the opposite side

triple point *n* : the condition of temperature and pressure under which the gaseous, liquid, and solid phases of a substance can exist in equilibrium

triple screen *n* : a blood test for pregnant women for alpha-fetoprotein, human chorionic gonadotropin, and estriol in order to assess the risk of fetal abnormality (as Down syndrome, anencephaly, and spina bifida) — called also *triple test*

trip•let \ˈtri-plət\ *n* **1 a** : a combination, set, or group of three **b** : CODON **2 a** : one of three children or offspring born at one birth **b triplets** *pl* : a group of three offspring born at one birth

[1]**trip•loid** \ˈtri-ˌplȯid\ *adj* : having or being a chromosome number three times the monoploid number — **trip•loi•dy** \-ˌplȯi-dē\ *n*

[2]**triploid** *n* : a triploid individual

trip•tan \ˈtrip-ˌtan, -tən\ *n* : any of a class of drugs (as sumatriptan) that bind to and are agonists of serotonin receptors and are used to treat migraine attacks

tri•que•tral bone \trī-ˈkwē-trel-\ *n* : the bone in the proximal row of the carpus that is third counting from the thumb side of the wrist, has a pyramidal shape, and is situated between the lunate and pisiform bones — called also *triangular, triangular bone, triangularis, triquetral*

tri•que•trum \trī-ˈkwē-trəm\ *n, pl* **tri•que•tra** \-trə\ : TRIQUETRAL BONE

tris \ˈtris\ *n, often cap* : a white crystalline powder $C_4H_{11}NO_3$ used as a buffer (as in the treatment of acidosis) — called also *tris buffer, tromethamine*

tri•sac•cha•ride \(ˌ)trī-ˈsa-kə-ˌrīd\ *n* : a sugar that yields on complete hydrolysis three monosaccharide molecules

tris•kai•deka•pho•bia \ˌtris-ˌkī-ˌde-kə-ˈfō-bē-ə, ˌtris-kə-\ *n* : fear of the number 13

tris•mus \ˈtriz-məs\ *n* : spasm of the muscles of mastication resulting from any of various abnormal conditions or diseases (as tetanus)

[1]**tri•so•mic** \(ˌ)trī-ˈsō-mik\ *adj* : relating to, caused by, or characterized by trisomy ⟨~ cells⟩

[2]**trisomic** *n* : a trisomic individual

tri•so•my \ˈtrī-ˌsō-mē\ *n, pl* **-mies** : the condition (as in Down syndrome) of having one or a few chromosomes triploid in an otherwise diploid set

trisomy 18 *n* : a congenital condition that is characterized esp. by intellectual disability and by craniofacial, cardiac, gastrointestinal, and genitourinary abnormalities, is caused by trisomy of the human chromosome numbered 18, and is typically fatal esp. within the first year of life — called also *Edwards syndrome*

trisomy 13 *n* : a congenital condition that is characterized esp. by usu. severe intellectual disability and by craniofacial, cardiac, ocular, and cerebral abnormalities, is caused by trisomy of the human chromosome numbered 13, and is typically fatal esp. within the first six months of life — called also *Patau syndrome*

trisomy 21 *n* : DOWN SYNDROME

trit•an•ope \ˈtrīt-ᵊn-ˌōp, ˈtrit-\ *n* : an individual affected with tritanopia

trit•an•opia \ˌtrīt-ᵊn-ˈō-pē-ə, ˌtrit-\ *n* : dichromatism in which the spectrum is seen in tones of red and green — **trit•an•opic** \ˌtrīt-ᵊn-ˈō-pik, ˌtrit-ᵊn-ˈä-\ *adj*

tri•ti•um \ˈtri-tē-əm, -shəm, -shē-əm\ *n* : a radioactive isotope of hydrogen that has three times the mass of ordinary hydrogen — symbol *T*

[1]**trit•u•rate** \ˈtri-chə-ˌrāt\ *vb* **-rat•ed; -rat•ing** : to pulverize thoroughly by rubbing or grinding — **trit•u•ra•tion** \ˌtri-chə-ˈrā-shən\ *n*

[2]**trit•u•rate** \-rət\ *n* : a triturated substance

tri•va•lent \(ˌ)trī-ˈvā-lənt\ *adj* : conferring immunity to three different pathogenic strains or species ⟨a ~ influenza vaccine⟩

tRNA \ˌtē-ˌär-ˌen-ˈā\ *n* : TRANSFER RNA

Tro•bi•cin \trō-ˈbīs-ᵊn\ *trademark* — used for a preparation of the hydrated dihydrochloride of spectinomycin

tro•car *also* **tro•char** \ˈtrō-ˌkär\ *n* : a sharp-pointed surgical instrument fitted with a cannula and used esp. to insert the cannula into a body cavity as a drainage outlet

tro•chan•ter \trō-ˈkan-tər\ *n* : a rough prominence or process at the upper part of the femur serving usu. for the attachment of muscles and being usu. two on each femur: **a** : a larger one situated on the outer part of the upper end of the shaft at its junction with the neck — called also *greater trochanter* **b** : a smaller one situated at the lower back part of the junction of the shaft and neck — called also *lesser trochanter* — **tro•chan•ter•ic** \ˌtrō-kən-ˈter-ik, -ˌkan-\ *adj*

trochanteric fossa *n* : a depression at the base of the internal surface of the greater trochanter of the femur for the attachment of the tendon of the obturator externus

tro•che \ˈtrō-kē\ *n* : LOZENGE

troch•lea \ˈträ-klē-ə\ *n* : an anatomical structure resembling a pulley: as **a** : the articular surface on the medial condyle of the humerus that articulates with the ulna **b** : the fibrous ring in the inner upper part of the orbit through which the tendon of the superior oblique muscle of the eye passes

troch•le•ar \-ər\ *adj* **1** : of, relating to, or being a trochlea **2** : of, relating to, or being a trochlear nerve ⟨~ fibers⟩

trochlear fovea *n* : a depression located in the orbital surface of each bony plate of the frontal bone and forming a point of attachment for the superior oblique muscle of the eye

trochlear nerve *n* : either of the fourth pair of cranial nerves that arise from the dorsal aspect of the brain stem just below the inferior colliculus and supply the superior oblique muscle of the eye with motor fibers

trochlear notch *n* : the deep depression in the proximal end of the ulna by which the ulna articulates with the trochlea of the humerus at the elbow — called also *semilunar notch, sigmoid notch*

trochlear nucleus *n* : a nucleus that is situated behind the oculomotor nucleus and is the source of the motor fibers of the trochlear nerve

tro•choid \ˈtrō-ˌkȯid\ *n* : PIVOT JOINT

tro•glit•a•zone \trō-ˈgli-tə-ˌzōn\ *n* : a drug $C_{24}H_{27}NO_5S$ formerly used to treat type 2 diabetes but now withdrawn from use because of its link to serious hepatic reactions

tro•land \ˈtrō-lənd\ *n* : PHOTON 1

Troland, Leonard Thompson (1889–1932), American psychologist and physicist.

tro•le•an•do•my•cin \ˌtrō-lē-ˌan-də-ˈmīs-ᵊn\ *n* : an antibacterial drug $C_{41}H_{67}NO_{15}$ used chiefly against bacteria of the genus *Streptococcus* (esp. *S. pneumoniae* and *S. pyogenes*) — called also *triacetyloleandomycin*

trol•ley *also* **trol•ly** \ˈträ-lē\ *n, pl* **trolleys** *also* **trollies** *Brit* : GURNEY

trol•ni•trate \ˌträl-ˈnī-ˌtrāt\ *n* : an organic nitrate with vasodilator activity that is used in the form of its diphosphate salt $C_6H_{12}N_4O_9{\cdot}2H_3PO_4$ to prevent attacks of angina pectoris

Trom•bic•u•la \träm-ˈbi-kyə-lə\ *n* : a genus of mites (family Trombiculidae) including some forms that in Asia transmit scrub typhus

tro•meth•a•mine \trō-ˈme-thə-ˌmēn\ *n* : TRIS

troph- *or* **tropho-** *comb form* : nutritive ⟨*tropho*blast⟩

troph•ec•to•derm \ˌtrō-ˈfek-tə-ˌdərm\ *n* : TROPHOBLAST; *esp* : the outer layer of the blastocyst after differentiation of the ectoderm, mesoderm, and endoderm when the outer layer is continuous with the embryonic ectoderm

tro•phic \ˈtrō-fik\ *adj* **1** : of or relating to nutrition : NUTRITIONAL ⟨~ disorders⟩ **2** : TROPIC **3** : promoting cellular growth, differentiation, and survival — **tro•phi•cal•ly** *adv*

-tro•phic \ˈtrō-fik\ *adj comb form* **1** : of, relating to, or characterized by (such) nutrition or growth ⟨hyper*trophic*⟩ **2** : -TROPIC ⟨gonado*trophic*⟩

trophic ulcer *n* : an ulcer (as a bedsore) caused by faulty nutrition in the affected part

tro•pho•blast \ˈtrō-fə-ˌblast\ *n* : the outer layer of the blastocyst that supplies nutrition to the embryo, facilitates implantation by eroding away the tissues of the uterus with which it comes in contact, and differentiates into the extraembryonic membranes surrounding the embryo — called also *trophoderm* — **tro•pho•blas•tic** \ˌtrō-fə-ˈblas-tik\ *adj*

troph•o•derm \ˈtrō-fə-ˌdərm\ *n* : TROPHOBLAST

tro•pho•zo•ite \ˌtrō-fə-ˈzō-ˌīt\ *n* : a protozoan of a vegetative form as distinguished from one of a reproductive or resting form

-tro•phy \trə-fē\ *n comb form, pl* **-tro•phies** : nutrition : nurture : growth ⟨hypo*trophy*⟩

tro•pia \ˈtrō-pē-ə\ *n* : deviation of an eye from the normal position with respect to the line of vision when the eyes are open : STRABISMUS — see ESOTROPIA, HYPERTROPIA

tro•pic \ˈtrō-pik\ *adj* **1** : of, relating to, or characteristic of tropism or of a tropism **2** *of a hormone* : influencing the activity of a specified gland

-tro•pic \ˈtrō-pik\ *adj comb form* : attracted to or acting upon (something specified) ⟨neuro*tropic*⟩

tropical medicine *n* : a branch of medicine dealing with tropical diseases and other medical problems of tropical regions

tropical oil *n* : any of several oils (as coconut oil) that are high in saturated fatty acids

tropical sprue *n* : a disease of tropical regions that is of unknown cause and is characterized by fatty diarrhea, malabsorption of nutrients, and weight loss — called also *sprue*

tropical ulcer *n* : a chronic sloughing sore of unknown cause occurring usu. on the legs and prevalent in wet tropical regions

tro•pic•amide \trə-ˈpi-kə-ˌmīd\ *n* : a synthetic anticholinergic $C_{17}H_{20}N_2O_2$ used esp. to dilate pupils in ophthalmological examinations — see MYDRIACYL

-tro•pin \ˈtrō-pən\ *or* **-tro•phin** \-fən\ *n comb form* : hormone ⟨lipo*tropin*⟩

tro•pism \ˈtrō-ˌpi-zəm\ *n* : involuntary orientation by an organism or one of its parts (as by differential growth) toward or away from a source of stimulation; *also* : a reflex reaction involving a tropism

tro•po•col•la•gen \ˌträ-pə-ˈkä-lə-jən, ˌtrō-\ *n* : a subunit of collagen fibrils consisting of three polypeptide strands arranged in a helix

tro•po•my•o•sin \ˌträ-pə-ˈmī-ə-sən, ˌtrō-\ *n* : a protein of muscle that forms a complex with troponin regulating the interaction of actin and myosin in muscular contraction

tro•po•nin \ˈtrō-pə-nən, ˈträ-, -ˌnin\ *n* : a protein of muscle that together with tropomyosin forms a regulatory protein complex controlling the interaction of actin and myosin and that when combined with calcium ions permits muscular contraction

trough — see GINGIVAL TROUGH

troy \ˈtrȯi\ *adj* : expressed in troy weight ⟨a ~ ounce⟩

troy weight *n* : a series of units of weight based on a pound of 12 ounces and an ounce of 480 grains or 31.103 grams

Trp *abbr* tryptophan

true conjugate *n* : CONJUGATE DIAMETER

true pelvis *n* : the lower more contracted part of the pelvic cavity — called also *true pelvic cavity;* compare FALSE PELVIS

true rib *n* : any of the ribs having costal cartilages connected directly with the sternum and in humans constituting the first seven pairs — called also *vertebrosternal rib*

true vocal cords *n pl* : the lower pair of vocal cords each of which encloses a vocal ligament, extends from the inner surface of one side of the thyroid cartilage near the median line to a process of the corresponding arytenoid cartilage on the same side of the larynx, and when drawn taut, approximated to the contralateral member of the pair, and subjected to a flow of breath produces the voice — called also *inferior vocal cords, vocal folds*

trun•cal \ˈtrəŋ-kəl\ *adj* : of or relating to the trunk of the body or of a bodily part (as a nerve) ⟨~ obesity⟩

trun•cus \ˈtrəŋ-kəs\ *n* : TRUNK 2

truncus bra•chio•ce•phal•i•cus \-ˌbrā-kē-(ˌ)ō-se-ˈfa-li-kəs\ *n* : BRACHIOCEPHALIC ARTERY

truncus ce•li•a•cus \-se-ˈlī-ə-kəs\ *n* : CELIAC ARTERY

trunk \ˈtrəŋk\ *n* **1** : the human body apart from the head and appendages : TORSO **2** : the main body of an anatomical part (as a nerve or blood vessel) that divides into branches

truss \ˈtrəs\ *n* : a device worn to reduce a hernia by pressure

truth serum *n* : a hypnotic or anesthetic (as thiopental) held to induce a subject under questioning to talk freely

Tru•va•da \trü-ˈvä-də\ *trademark* — used for a preparation of emtricitabine and the fumarate of tenofovir

trypan- *or* **trypano-** *comb form* : trypanosome ⟨*trypano*cidal⟩

try•pano•ci•dal \tri-ˌpa-nə-ˈsīd-ᵊl\ *adj* : destroying trypanosomes ⟨a ~ drug⟩ — **try•pano•cide** \tri-ˈpa-nə-ˌsīd\ *n*

try•pano•so•ma \tri-ˌpa-nə-ˈsō-mə\ *n* **1** *cap* : a genus of parasitic flagellate protozoans (family Trypanosomatidae) that infest the blood of various vertebrates including humans, are usu. transmitted by the bite of an insect, and include some that cause serious diseases (as Chagas disease, African sleeping sickness, and surra) **2** *pl* **-mas** *or* **-ma•ta** \-mə-tə\ : TRYPANOSOME

try•pano•some \tri-ˈpa-nə-ˌsōm\ *n* : any flagellate of the genus *Trypanosoma* — **try•pano•so•mal** \-ˌpa-nə-ˈsō-məl\ *adj*

try•pano•so•mi•a•sis \tri-ˌpa-nə-sə-ˈmī-ə-səs\ *n, pl* **-a•ses** \-ˌsēz\ : infection with or disease caused by flagellates of the genus *Trypanosoma*

tryp•ars•amide \tri-ˈpär-sə-ˌmīd\ *n* : an arsenical $C_8H_{10}AsN_2O_4Na \cdot {}^1/_2H_2O$ used esp. formerly to treat African sleeping sickness and syphilis

tryp•sin \ˈtrip-sən\ *n* **1** : a crystallizable proteolytic enzyme that is produced and secreted in the pancreatic juice in the form of inactive trypsinogen and activated in the intestine — compare CHYMOTRYPSIN **2** : a preparation from the pancreatic juice containing principally proteolytic enzymes and used chiefly as a digestive and lytic agent

tryp•sin•ize \ˈtrip-sə-ˌnīz\ *vb* **-ized; -iz•ing** : to subject to the action of trypsin ⟨*trypsinized* tissue cells⟩ — **tryp•sin•i•za•tion** \ˌtrip-sə-nə-ˈzā-shən\ *n*

tryp•sin•o•gen \trip-ˈsi-nə-jən\ *n* : the inactive substance released by the pancreas into the duodenum to form trypsin

tryp•tase \ˈtrip-ˌtās, -ˌtāz\ *n* : a protease of human mast cells that has been implicated as a pathological mediator of numerous allergic and inflammatory conditions (as asthma, rhinitis, and conjunctivitis)

tryp·tic \ˈtrip-tik\ *adj* : of, relating to, or produced by trypsin or its action

tryp·to·phan \ˈtrip-tə-ˌfan\ *also* **tryp·to·phane** \-ˌfān\ *n* : a crystalline essential amino acid $C_{11}H_{12}N_2O_2$ that is widely distributed in proteins — abbr. *Trp*

L–tryptophan — see entry alphabetized in the letter *l*

TS *abbr* Tourette's syndrome; Tourette syndrome

TSE *abbr* transmissible spongiform encephalopathy

tset·se \ˈtset-sē, ˈtsēt-, ˈtet-, ˈtēt-\ *n, pl* **tsetse** *or* **tsetses** : TSETSE FLY

tsetse fly *n* : any of several dipteran flies of the genus *Glossina* that occur in sub-Saharan Africa and include vectors of human and animal trypanosomes (as those causing sleeping sickness) — called also *tsetse*

TSH \ˌtē-(ˌ)es-ˈāch\ *n* : THYROID-STIMULATING HORMONE

TSS *abbr* toxic shock syndrome

T suppressor cell *n* : SUPPRESSOR T CELL

tsu·tsu·ga·mu·shi disease \ˌtsüt-sə-gə-ˈmü-shē-, ˌtüt-, ˌsüt-, -ˈgä-mu̇-shē-\ *n* : SCRUB TYPHUS

T system *n* : the system of T tubules in striated muscle

T3 *or* T_3 \ˌtē-ˈthrē\ *n* : TRIIODOTHYRONINE

TTP *abbr* thrombotic thrombocytopenic purpura

T–tube *n* : a narrow flexible tube in the form of a T that is used for drainage esp. of the common bile duct

T tubule *n* : any of the small tubules which run transversely through a striated muscle fiber and through which electrical impulses are transmitted from the sarcoplasm to the fiber's interior

tub·al \ˈtü-bəl, ˈtyü-\ *adj* : of, relating to, or involving a tube and esp. a fallopian tube ⟨a ~ infection⟩

tubal abortion *n* : spontaneous abortion of an ectopic pregnancy in a fallopian tube

tubal ligation *n* : ligation of the fallopian tubes that by preventing passage of ova from the ovaries to the uterus serves as a method of female sterilization

tubal pregnancy *n* : ectopic pregnancy in a fallopian tube

tubarius — see TORUS TUBARIUS

[1]**tube** \ˈtüb, ˈtyüb\ *n* **1** : a slender channel within a plant or animal body : DUCT — see BRONCHIAL TUBE, EUSTACHIAN TUBE, FALLOPIAN TUBE **2 a** : a piece of laboratory or technical apparatus usu. serving to isolate or convey a product of reaction **b** : TEST TUBE **3** : a hollow cylindrical device (as a cannula) used for insertion into bodily passages or hollow organs for removal or injection of materials

[2]**tube** *vb* **tubed; tub·ing** : to furnish with, enclose in, or pass through a tube

tubed *adj* : having the sides sewn together so as to form a tube

tuberalis — see PARS TUBERALIS

tu·ber ci·ne·re·um \ˈtü-bər-si-ˈnir-ē-əm, ˈtyü-\ *n* : an eminence of gray matter which lies on the lower surface of the brain and of which the upper surface forms part of the floor of the third ventricle and the lower surface bears the infundibulum to which the pituitary gland is attached

tu·ber·cle \ˈtü-bər-kəl, ˈtyü-\ *n* **1** : a small knobby prominence or excrescence: as **a** : a prominence on the crown of a molar tooth **b** : a small rough prominence (as the greater tubercle or adductor tubercle) on a bone usu. being smaller than a tuberosity and serving for the attachment of one or more muscles or ligaments **c** : an eminence near the head of a rib that articulates with the transverse process of a vertebra **d** : any of several prominences (as the acoustic tubercle) in the central nervous system that mark the nuclei of various nerves **2** : a small discrete lump in the substance of an organ or in the skin; *esp* : the specific lesion of tuberculosis consisting of a packed mass of epithelioid cells, giant cells, disintegration products of white blood cells and bacilli, and usu. a necrotic center

tubercle bacillus *n* : a bacterium of the genus *Mycobacterium* (*M. tuberculosis*) that is a causative agent of tuberculosis; *also* : a related mycobacterium (*M. bovis*) that causes tuberculosis in cattle and sometimes humans esp. in underdeveloped countries

tubercul- *or* **tuberculo-** *comb form* **1** : tubercle ⟨*tubercul*ar⟩ **2** : tubercle bacillus ⟨*tubercul*in⟩ **3** : tuberculosis ⟨*tubercul*oid⟩

[1]**tu·ber·cu·lar** \tu̇-ˈbər-kyə-lər, tyu̇-\ *adj* **1 a** : of, relating to, or affected with tuberculosis : TUBERCULOUS **b** : caused by the tubercle bacillus ⟨~ meningitis⟩ **2** : characterized by lesions that are or resemble tubercles ⟨~ leprosy⟩ **3** : relating to, resembling, or constituting a tubercle

[2]**tubercular** *n* : an individual affected with tuberculosis

tu·ber·cu·lid \tu̇-ˈbər-kyə-lid, tyu̇-\ *n* : a tuberculous lesion of the skin; *esp* : one that is an id

tu·ber·cu·lin \tu̇-ˈbər-kyə-lən, tyu̇-\ *n* : a sterile solution containing the growth products of or specific substances extracted from the tubercle bacillus and used in the diagnosis of tuberculosis — see PURIFIED PROTEIN DERIVATIVE

tuberculin reaction *n* : a skin reaction that occurs at the site of a tuberculin test

tuberculin test *n* : a test (as the Mantoux test or tine test) for hypersensitivity to tuberculin in which tuberculin is introduced (as by injection) usu. into the skin of the individual tested and the appearance of inflammation or induration at the site of introduction is construed as indicating past or present tubercular infection — called also *tuberculin skin test*

tu•ber•cu•loid \tü-ˈbər-kyə-ˌlȯid, tyü-\ *adj* **1** : resembling tuberculosis and esp. the tubercles characteristic of it **2** : of, relating to, characterized by, or affected with tuberculoid leprosy

tuberculoid leprosy *n* : the one of the two major forms of leprosy that is characterized by the presence of few or no Hansen's bacilli in the lesions and by the loss of sensation in affected areas of the skin — compare LEPROMATOUS LEPROSY

tu•ber•cu•lo•ma \tü-ˌbər-kyə-ˈlō-mə, tyü-\ *n, pl* **-mas** \-məz\ *also* **-ma•ta** \-mə-tə\ : a large solitary caseous tubercle of tuberculous character occurring esp. in the brain

tu•ber•cu•lo•sis \tü-ˌbər-kyə-ˈlō-səs, tyü-\ *n, pl* **-lo•ses** \-ˌsēz\ : a usu. chronic highly variable disease that is caused by a bacterium of the genus *Mycobacterium* (*Mycobacterium tuberculosis*) and rarely in the U.S. by a related mycobacterium (*M. bovis*), is usu. communicated by inhalation of the airborne causative agent, affects esp. the lungs but may spread to other areas (as the kidney or spinal column) from local lesions or by way of the lymph or blood vessels, and is characterized by fever, cough, difficulty in breathing, inflammatory infiltrations, formation of tubercles, caseation, pleural effusion, and fibrosis — called also *TB*

[1]**tu•ber•cu•lo•stat•ic** \tü-ˌbər-kyə-lō-ˈsta-tik, tyü-\ *adj* : inhibiting the growth of the tubercle bacillus

[2]**tuberculostatic** *n* : a tuberculostatic agent

tu•ber•cu•lous \tü-ˈbər-kyə-ləs, tyü-\ *adj* **1** : constituting or affected with tuberculosis **2** : caused by or resulting from the presence or products of the tubercle bacillus ⟨~ peritonitis⟩

tu•ber•os•i•ty \ˌtü-bə-ˈrä-sə-tē, ˌtyü-\ *n, pl* **-ties** : a rounded prominence; *esp* : a large prominence on a bone usu. serving for the attachment of muscles or ligaments ⟨ischial *tuberosities*⟩

tuberous sclerosis *n* : a genetic disorder of the skin and nervous system that is typically characterized by epilepsy and intellectual disability, by a facial rash resembling acne, and by multiple hamartomas of the brain, kidney, retina, skin, and heart and that is inherited as an autosomal dominant trait or results from spontaneous mutation — called also *epiloia*

tu•bo•cu•ra•rine \ˌtü-bō-kyü-ˈrär-ən, -ˌēn, ˌtyü-\ *n* : a toxic alkaloid that is obtained chiefly from the bark and stems of a So. American vine (*Chondrodendron tomentosum* of the family Menispermaceae), that in its dextrorotatory form constitutes the chief active constituent of curare, and that is used in the form of its hydrated hydrochloride $C_{37}H_{41}ClN_2O_6·HCl·5H_2O$ esp. as a skeletal muscle relaxant

tu•bo–ovar•i•an \ˌtü-bō-ō-ˈvar-ē-ən, ˌtyü-\ *adj* : of, relating to, or affecting a fallopian tube and ovary

tu•bu•lar \ˈtü-byə-lər, ˈtyü-\ *adj* **1** : having the form of or consisting of a tube **2** : of, relating to, or sounding as if produced through a tube or tubule

tu•bule \ˈtü-(ˌ)byül, ˈtyü-\ *n* : a small tube; *esp* : a slender elongated anatomical channel

tu•bu•lin \ˈtü-byə-lən, ˈtyü-\ *n* : a globular protein that polymerizes to form microtubules

tu•bu•lo•ac•i•nar \ˌtü-byə-lō-ˈa-sə-nər, ˌtyü-\ *or* **tu•bu•lo•ac•i•nous** \-nəs\ *adj* : TUBULOALVEOLAR

tu•bu•lo•al•ve•o•lar \ˌtü-byə-lō-al-ˈvē-ə-lər, ˌtyü-\ *adj* : of, relating to, or being a gland having branching tubules which end in secretory alveoli

tu•bu•lo•in•ter•stit•ial \ˌtü-byə-lō-ˌin-tər-ˈsti-shəl, ˌtyü-\ *adj* : affecting or involving the tubules and interstitial tissue of the kidney ⟨~ disease⟩

tu•bu•lus \ˈtü-byə-ləs, ˈtyü-\ *n, pl* **tu•bu•li** \-ˌlī\ : TUBULE

tuck \ˈtək\ *n* : a cosmetic surgical operation for the removal of excess skin or fat from a body part — see TUMMY TUCK

Tu•i•nal \ˈtü-i-ˌnäl\ *trademark* — used for a preparation of amobarbital and secobarbital

tu•lar•ae•mia *chiefly Brit var of* TULAREMIA

tu•la•re•mia \ˌtü-lə-ˈrē-mē-ə, ˌtyü-\ *n* : an infectious disease esp. of wild rabbits, rodents, some domestic animals, and humans that is caused by a bacterium (*Francisella tularensis*), is transmitted esp. by the bites of insects, and in humans is marked by symptoms (as fever) of toxemia — called also *rabbit fever* — **tu•la•re•mic** \-mik\ *adj*

tulle gras \ˌtül-ˈgrä\ *n* : fine-meshed gauze impregnated with a fatty substance (as soft paraffin)

tu•me•fa•cient \ˌtü-mə-ˈfā-shənt, ˌtyü-\ *adj* : producing swelling

tu•me•fac•tion \-ˈfak-shən\ *n* **1** : an action or process of swelling or becoming tumorous **2** : SWELLING

tu•me•fac•tive \-ˈfak-tiv\ *adj* : producing swelling ⟨~ lesions⟩

tu•mes•cence \tü-ˈmes-ᵊns, tyü-\ *n* : the quality or state of being tumescent; *esp* : readiness for sexual activity marked esp. by vascular congestion of the sex organs

tu·mes·cent \-ˈmes-ᵊnt\ *adj* : somewhat swollen ⟨~ tissue⟩
tummy tuck *n* : ABDOMINOPLASTY
tu·mor \ˈtü-mər, ˈtyü-\ *n* : an abnormal benign or malignant new growth of tissue that possesses no physiological function and arises from uncontrolled usu. rapid cellular proliferation — see CANCER 1, CARCINOMA, SARCOMA — **tu·mor·al** \-mə-rəl\ *adj* — **tu·mor-like** \-ˌlīk\ *adj*
tu·mor·i·cid·al \ˌtü-mə-rə-ˈsīd-ᵊl, ˌtyü-\ *adj* : destroying tumor cells
tu·mor·i·gen·ic \-ˈje-nik\ *adj* : producing or tending to produce tumors; *also* : CARCINOGENIC — **tu·mor·i·gen·e·sis** \-ˈje-nə-səs\ *n* — **tu·mor·i·ge·nic·i·ty** \-jə-ˈni-sə-tē\ *n*
tumor–infiltrating lymphocyte *n* : a T cell that infiltrates a malignant tumor and when cultured with interleukin-2 in adoptive immunotherapy possesses greater cytotoxicity than a lymphokine-activated killer cell — called also *TIL*
tumor necrosis factor *n* : a protein that is produced chiefly by monocytes and macrophages in response esp. to endotoxins, that mediates inflammation, and that induces the destruction of some tumor cells and the activation of white blood cells — abbr. *TNF*
tu·mor·ous \ˈtü-mə-rəs, ˈtyü-\ *adj* : of, relating to, or resembling a tumor
tumor suppressor gene *n* : any of a class of genes (as p53) that act in normal cells to inhibit unrestrained cell division and that when inactivated (as by mutation) place the cell at increased risk for malignant proliferation — called also *anti-oncogene*
tumor virus *n* : a virus (as Rous sarcoma virus) that causes neoplastic or cancerous growth
tu·mour *chiefly Brit var of* TUMOR
Tums \ˈtəmz\ *trademark* — used for an antacid preparation containing calcium carbonate
Tun·ga \ˈtəŋ-gə\ *n* : a genus of fleas (family Tungidae) that include the chigoe (*T. penetrans*)
tung·sten \ˈtəŋ-stən\ *n* : a gray-white high-melting ductile metallic element — symbol *W;* called also *wolfrum;* see ELEMENT table
tu·nic \ˈtü-nik, ˈtyü-\ *n* : an enclosing or covering membrane or tissue : TUNICA ⟨the ~*s* of the eye⟩
tu·ni·ca \ˈtü-ni-kə, ˈtyü-\ *n, pl* **tu·ni·cae** \-nə-ˌkē, -ˌkī, -ˌsē\ : an enveloping membrane or layer of body tissue
tunica adventitia *n* : ADVENTITIA
tunica al·bu·gin·ea \-ˌal-bu̇-ˈji-nē-ə, -byu̇-\ *n, pl* **tunicae al·bu·gin·e·ae** \-ˈji-nē-ˌē, -ˌī\ : a white fibrous capsule esp. of the testis
tunica intima *n* : INTIMA
tunica media *n* : MEDIA
tunica mucosa *n* : mucous membrane and esp. that lining the digestive tract
tunica muscularis *n* : MUSCULAR COAT
tunica pro·pria \-ˈprō-prē-ə\ *n* : LAMINA PROPRIA
tunica va·gi·na·lis \-ˌva-jə-ˈnā-ləs, -ˈna-\ *n, pl* **tunicae va·gi·na·les** \-(ˌ)lez\ : a pouch of serous membrane covering the testis and derived from the peritoneum
tuning fork *n* : a 2-pronged metal implement that gives a fixed tone when struck
tun·nel \ˈtən-ᵊl\ *n* : a bodily channel — see CARPAL TUNNEL
tunnel of Cor·ti \-ˈkȯr-tē\ *n* : a spiral passage in the organ of Corti
tunnel vision *n* : constriction of the visual field resulting in loss of peripheral vision
tur·bel·lar·i·an \ˌtər-bə-ˈlar-ē-ən\ *n* : any of a class (Turbellaria) of mostly aquatic and free-living flatworms — **turbellarian** *adj*
tur·bid \ˈtər-bəd\ *adj* : thick or opaque with matter in suspension : cloudy or muddy in appearance ⟨~ urine⟩ — **tur·bid·i·ty** \ˌtər-ˈbi-də-tē\ *n*
tur·bi·dim·e·ter \ˌtər-bə-ˈdi-mə-tər\ *n* **1** : an instrument for measuring and comparing the turbidity of liquids by viewing light through them and determining how much light is transmitted **2** : NEPHELOMETER — **tur·bi·di·met·ric** \ˌtər-bə-də-ˈme-trik, ˌtər-ˌbi-\ *adj* — **tur·bi·dim·e·try** \ˌtər-bə-ˈdi-mə-trē\ *n*
[1]**tur·bi·nate** \ˈtər-bə-nət, -ˌnāt\ *adj* : of, relating to, or being a nasal concha
[2]**turbinate** *n* : NASAL CONCHA
turbinate bone *also* **tur·bi·nat·ed bone** \ˈtər-bə-ˌnā-təd-\ *n* : NASAL CONCHA
turcica — see SELLA TURCICA
turf toe *n* : a minor but painful usu. sports-related injury involving hyperextension of the big toe that results in spraining or tearing of the ligament of the metatarsophalangeal joint
tur·ges·cent \ˌtər-ˈjes-ᵊnt\ *adj* : becoming turgid, distended, or swollen — **tur·ges·cence** \-ˈjes-ᵊns\ *n*
tur·gid \ˈtər-jəd\ *adj* : being in a normal or abnormal state of distension : SWOLLEN ⟨~ limbs⟩ ⟨~ living cells⟩ — **tur·gid·i·ty** \ˌtər-ˈji-də-tē\ *n*
tur·gor \ˈtər-gər, -ˌgȯr\ *n* : the normal state of turgidity and tension in living cells
tu·ris·ta \tu̇-ˈrē-stə\ *n* : TRAVELER'S DIARRHEA
tur·mer·ic \ˈtər-mə-rik\ *n* : the powdered ground yellow rhizome of an Indian herb (*Curcuma longa*) of the ginger family used in dietary supplements and herbal remedies and as a spice — see CURCUMIN
turn \ˈtərn\ *vb* : to injure by twisting or wrenching ⟨~*ed* his ankle⟩
Tur·ner's syndrome \ˈtər-nərz-\ *or* **Tur·ner syndrome** \-nər-\ *n* : a genetically determined condition that is typically associated with the presence of only one complete X chromosome

and no Y chromosome and is characterized esp. by a female phenotype, underdeveloped and usu. infertile ovaries, absence of menstrual onset, and short stature

Turner, Henry Hubert (1892–1970), American endocrinologist.

turn•over \ˈtərn-ˌō-vər\ *n* : the continuous process of loss and replacement of a constituent (as a neurotransmitter, cell, or tissue) of a living system

TURP *abbr* transurethral resection of the prostate

tur•ri•ceph•a•ly \ˌtər-ə-ˈse-fə-lē\ *n, pl* **-lies** : OXYCEPHALY

tus•sive \ˈtə-siv\ *adj* : of, relating to, or involved in coughing ⟨~ force⟩

T wave \ˈtē-ˌwāv\ *n* : the deflection in an electrocardiogram that represents the electrical activity produced by ventricular repolarization — compare P WAVE, QRS COMPLEX

Tween \ˈtwēn\ *trademark* — used for any of several preparations of polysorbates

twee•zers \ˈtwē-zərz\ *n sing or pl* : any of various small metal instruments that are usu. held between the thumb and index finger, are used for plucking, holding, or manipulating, and consist of two legs joined at one end

twelfth cranial nerve *n* : HYPOGLOSSAL NERVE

12–step \ˈtwelv-ˌstep\ *adj* : of, relating to, or characteristic of a program that is designed esp. to help an individual overcome an addiction, compulsion, serious shortcoming, or traumatic experience by adherence to 12 tenets emphasizing personal growth and dependence on a higher spiritual being

twelve–year molar *n* : any of the second permanent molar teeth which erupt at about 12 years of age and include four of which one is located on each side of the upper and lower jaws — compare SIX-YEAR MOLAR

twenty–twenty *or* **20/20** *adj* : having the normal visual acuity of the human eye that according to one common scale can distinguish at a distance of 20 feet characters one-third inch in diameter ⟨~ vision⟩

twig \ˈtwig\ *n* : a minute branch of a nerve or artery

twi•light sleep \ˈtwī-ˌlīt-\ *n* : a state in which awareness of pain is dulled and memory of pain is dimmed or effaced and which is produced by hypodermic injection of morphine and scopolamine and used esp. formerly chiefly in childbirth

twilight state *n* : a dreamy state lacking touch with present reality, occurring in epilepsy, hysteria, and schizophrenia, and sometimes induced with narcotics

[1]**twin** \ˈtwin\ *adj* : born with one other or as a pair at one birth ⟨~ girls⟩

[2]**twin** *n* **1** : either of two offspring produced at a birth **2 twins** *pl* : a group of two offspring born at one birth — **twin•ship** \-ˌship\ *n*

twinge \ˈtwinj\ *n* : a sudden sharp stab of pain

twin•ning \ˈtwi-niŋ\ *n* : the bearing of twins

twitch \ˈtwich\ *n* : a brief spasmodic contraction of muscle fibers; *also* : a slight jerk of a body part caused by such a contraction — **twitch** *vb*

two–egg *adj* : DIZYGOTIC ⟨~ twins⟩

2,4–D \ˌtü-ˌfōr-ˈdē\ *n* : a white crystalline irritant compound $C_8H_6Cl_2O_3$ used as a weed killer — called also *2,4-dichlorophenoxyacetic acid;* see AGENT ORANGE

2,4,5–T \-ˌfīv-ˈtē\ *n* : an irritant compound $C_8H_5Cl_3O_3$ used esp. formerly as an herbicide and defoliant — called also *trichlorophenoxyacetic acid;* see AGENT ORANGE

Tx *abbr* treatment

ty•ba•mate \ˈtī-bə-ˌmāt\ *n* : a tranquilizing drug $C_{13}H_{26}N_2O_4$

Ty•bost \ˈtī-ˌbäst\ *trademark* — used for a preparation of cobicistat

ty•lec•to•my \tī-ˈlek-tə-mē\ *n, pl* **-mies** : LUMPECTOMY

Ty•le•nol \ˈtī-lə-ˌnȯl\ *trademark* — used for a preparation of acetaminophen

ty•lo•sin \ˈtī-lə-sən\ *n* : an antibacterial antibiotic $C_{45}H_{77}NO_{17}$ from an actinomycete of the genus *Streptomyces* (*S. fradiae*) used in veterinary medicine and as a feed additive

ty•lo•sis \tī-ˈlō-səs\ *n, pl* **ty•lo•ses** \-ˈlō-sēz\ : a thickening and hardening of the skin : CALLOSITY

tympani — see CHORDA TYMPANI, SCALA TYMPANI, TEGMEN TYMPANI, TENSOR TYMPANI

tym•pan•ic \tim-ˈpa-nik\ *adj* : of, relating to, or being a tympanum

tympanic antrum *n* : a large air-containing cavity in the mastoid process communicating with the tympanum and often being the location of dangerous inflammation — called also *mastoid antrum*

tympanic canal *n* : SCALA TYMPANI

tympanic cavity *n* : MIDDLE EAR

tympanic membrane *n* : a thin membrane separating the middle ear from the inner part of the external auditory canal that vibrates in response to sound waves and transmits the resulting mechanical vibrations to the ossicles of the middle ear — called also *eardrum, tympanum*

tympanic nerve *n* : a branch of the glossopharyngeal nerve arising from the petrosal ganglion and entering the middle ear where it takes part in forming the tympanic plexus — called also *Jacobson's nerve*

tympanic plate *n* : a curved platelike bone that is part of the temporal bone and forms the floor and anterior wall of the external auditory canal

tympanic plexus *n* : a nerve plexus of the middle ear that is formed by the tympanic nerve and two or three filaments from the carotid plexus, sends fibers to the mucous membranes of the middle ear, the eustachian tube, and the mastoid cells, and gives off the lesser petrosal nerve to the otic ganglion

tym•pa•ni•tes \ˌtim-pə-ˈnī-tēz\ *n* : a distension of the abdomen caused by accumulation of gas in the intestinal tract or peritoneal cavity

tym•pa•nit•ic \ˌtim-pə-ˈni-tik\ *adj* **1** : of, relating to, or affected with tympanites ⟨a ~ abdomen⟩ **2** : resonant on percussion : hollow-sounding

tym•pa•no•plas•ty \ˈtim-pə-nō-ˌplas-tē\ *n, pl* **-ties** : a reparative surgical operation performed on the middle ear

tym•pa•nos•to•my \ˌtim-pə-ˈnäs-tə-mē\ *n, pl* **-mies** : MYRINGOTOMY

tym•pa•not•o•my \ˌtim-pə-ˈnä-tə-mē\ *n, pl* **-mies** : MYRINGOTOMY

tym•pa•num \ˈtim-pə-nəm\ *n, pl* **-na** \-nə\ *also* **-nums** **1** : TYMPANIC MEMBRANE **2** : MIDDLE EAR

tym•pa•ny \-nē\ *n, pl* **-nies** **1** : TYMPANITES **2** : a resonant sound heard in percussion (as of the abdomen)

[1]**type** \ˈtīp\ *n* : a particular kind, class, or group ⟨cell ~*s*⟩; *specif* : a group distinguishable on physiological or serological bases ⟨salmonella ~*s*⟩

[2]**type** *vb* **typed; typ•ing** : to determine the type of (as a sample of blood or a culture of bacteria)

type A *adj* : relating to, characteristic of, having, or being a personality that is marked by impatience, aggressiveness, and competitiveness and that is held to be associated with increased risk of cardiovascular disease

type B *adj* : relating to, characteristic of, having, or being a personality that is marked by a lack of excessive aggressiveness and tension and that is held to be associated with reduced risk of cardiovascular disease

type 1 diabetes *n* : diabetes of a form that usu. develops during childhood or adolescence and is characterized by a severe deficiency of insulin secretion resulting from atrophy of the islets of Langerhans and causing hyperglycemia and a marked tendency toward ketoacidosis — called also *insulin-dependent diabetes, insulin-dependent diabetes mellitus, juvenile diabetes, juvenile-onset diabetes, type 1 diabetes mellitus*

type 2 diabetes *n* : diabetes mellitus of a common form that develops esp. in adults and most often in obese individuals and that is characterized by hyperglycemia resulting from impaired insulin utilization coupled with the body's inability to compensate with increased insulin production — called also *adult-onset diabetes, late-onset diabetes, maturity-onset diabetes, non-insulin-dependent diabetes, non-insulin-dependent diabetes mellitus, type 2 diabetes mellitus*

[1]**ty•phoid** \ˈtī-ˌfȯid, (ˌ)tī-ˈ\ *adj* **1** : of, relating to, or suggestive of typhus **2** : of, relating to, affected with, or constituting typhoid fever

[2]**typhoid** *n* **1** : TYPHOID FEVER **2** : any of several diseases of domestic animals resembling human typhus or typhoid fever

ty•phoi•dal \tī-ˈfȯid-ᵊl\ *adj* : of, relating to, or resembling typhoid fever

typhoid fever *n* : a communicable disease marked by fever, diarrhea, prostration, headache, splenomegaly, eruption of rose-colored spots, leukopenia, and intestinal inflammation and caused by a bacterium of the genus *Salmonella* (*S. typhi*)

ty•phus \ˈtī-fəs\ *n* : any of various bacterial diseases caused by rickettsiae: as **a** : a severe human febrile disease that is caused by one (*Rickettsia prowazekii*) transmitted esp. by body lice and is marked by high fever, stupor alternating with delirium, intense headache, and a dark red rash — called also *louse-borne typhus* **b** : MURINE TYPHUS **c** : SCRUB TYPHUS

typhus fever *n* : TYPHUS

Tyr *abbr* tyrosine

ty•ra•mine \ˈtī-rə-ˌmēn\ *n* : a phenolic amine $C_8H_{11}NO$ that is found in various foods and beverages (as cheese and red wine), has a sympathomimetic action, and is derived from tyrosine

ty•ro•ci•dine *also* **ty•ro•ci•din** \ˌtī-rə-ˈsīd-ᵊn\ *n* : a basic polypeptide antibiotic produced by a soil bacterium of the genus *Bacillus* (*B. brevis*) — see TYROTHRICIN

Ty•rode solution \ˈtī-ˌrōd-\ *or* **Ty•rode's solution** \-ˌrōdz-\ *n* : physiological saline containing sodium chloride 0.8, potassium chloride 0.02, calcium chloride 0.02, magnesium chloride 0.01, sodium bicarbonate 0.1, and sodium dihydrogen phosphate 0.005 percent

Tyrode, Maurice Vejux (1878–1930), American pharmacologist.

ty•ro•sin•ae•mia *chiefly Brit var of* TYROSINEMIA

ty•ro•sine \ˈtī-rə-ˌsēn\ *n* : a phenolic amino acid $C_9H_{11}NO_3$ that is a precursor of several important substances (as epinephrine and melanin) — abbr. *Tyr*

tyrosine hydroxylase *n* : an enzyme that catalyzes the first step in the biosynthesis of catecholamines (as dopamine and norepinephrine)

tyrosine kinase *n* : any of a group of enzymes of protein kinase that catalyze the transfer of a phosphate group from ATP to a tyrosine residue in a protein's side chain and include some that act as cell membrane receptors and others that regulate intracellular processes

ty·ro·sin·emia \ˌtī-rō-si-ˈnē-mē-ə\ *n* : a rare inherited disorder of tyrosine metabolism that is characterized by abnormally high concentrations of tyrosine in the blood and urine with associated abnormalities esp. of the liver and kidneys

ty·ro·sin·osis \ˌtī-rō-si-ˈnō-səs\ *n* : a condition of faulty metabolism of tyrosine marked by the excretion of unusual amounts of tyrosine in the urine

ty·ro·sin·uria \ˌtī-rō-si-ˈnu̇r-ē-ə, -ˈnyu̇r-\ *n* : the excretion of tyrosine in the urine

ty·ro·thri·cin \ˌtī-rə-ˈthrīs-ᵊn\ *n* : an antibiotic mixture that consists chiefly of tyrocidine and gramicidin, is obtained from a soil bacterium of the genus *Bacillus* (*B. brevis*), and is used in the topical treatment of infections esp. of the skin and mouth caused by gram-positive bacteria

Ty·son's gland \ˈtī-sᵊnz-\ *n* : PREPUTIAL GLAND

E. Tyson — see GLAND OF TYSON

TZD *abbr* thiazolidinedione

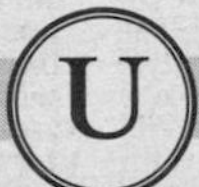

U *abbr* uracil

U *symbol* uranium

ubi·qui·none \yü-ˈbi-kwə-ˌnōn, ˌyü-bi-kwi-ˈnōn\ *n* : any of a group of lipid-soluble quinones that are found esp. in mitochondria and function in oxidative phosphorylation as electron-carrying coenzymes in electron transport; *esp* : COENZYME Q10

ubiq·ui·tin \yü-ˈbi-kwə-tən\ *n* : a chiefly eukaryotic protein that when bound to other cellular proteins marks them for proteolytic degradation

Ucer·is \yü-ˈser-əs\ *trademark* — used for a preparation of budesonide

UCL \ˌyü-ˌsē-ˈel\ *n* : ULNAR COLLATERAL LIGAMENT

ud·der \ˈə-dər\ *n* : a large pendulous organ (as of a cow) consisting of two or more mammary glands enclosed in a common envelope and each provided with a single nipple

[1]**ul·cer** \ˈəl-sər\ *n* : a break in skin or mucous membrane with loss of surface tissue, disintegration and necrosis of epithelial tissue, and often pus ⟨a stomach ~⟩

[2]**ulcer** *vb* **ul·cered; ul·cer·ing** : ULCERATE

ul·cer·ate \ˈəl-sə-ˌrāt\ *vb* **-at·ed; -at·ing** : to become affected with or as if with an ulcer — **ul·cer·ation** \ˌəl-sə-ˈrā-shən\ *n*

ul·cer·a·tive \ˈəl-sə-ˌrā-tiv, -rə-\ *adj* : of, relating to, or characterized by an ulcer or by ulceration ⟨~ gingivitis⟩

ulcerative colitis *n* : a chronic inflammatory disease of the colon that is of unknown cause and is characterized by diarrhea with discharge of mucus and blood, cramping abdominal pain, and inflammation and edema of the mucous membrane with patches of ulceration

ulcero- *comb form* **1** : ulcer ⟨*ulcero*genic⟩ **2** : ulcerous and ⟨*ulcero*glandular⟩

ul·cero·gen·ic \ˌəl-sə-rō-ˈje-nik\ *adj* : tending to produce or develop into ulcers or ulceration ⟨an ~ drug⟩

ul·cero·glan·du·lar \ˌəl-sə-rō-ˈglan-jə-lər\ *adj* : being a type of tularemia in which the place of infection is the skin where a papule and then an ulcer develops with enlargement of the lymph nodes in the associated region

ul·cer·ous \ˈəl-sə-rəs\ *adj* **1** : characterized or caused by ulceration **2** : affected with an ulcer

ul·cus \ˈəl-kəs\ *n, pl* **ul·cera** \ˈəl-sə-rə\ : ULCER

ul·na \ˈəl-nə\ *n, pl* **ul·nae** \-nē\ *or* **ul·nas** : the bone on the little-finger side of the forearm that forms with the humerus the elbow joint and serves as a pivot in rotation of the hand

[1]**ul·nar** \ˈəl-nər\ *adj* **1** : of or relating to the ulna **2** : located on the same side of the forearm as the ulna

[2]**ulnar** *n* : an ulnar anatomical part

ulnar artery *n* : an artery that is the larger of the two terminal branches of the brachial artery, runs along the ulnar side of the forearm, and gives off near its origin the anterior and posterior ulnar recurrent arteries

ulnar collateral artery — see INFERIOR ULNAR COLLATERAL ARTERY, SUPERIOR ULNAR COLLATERAL ARTERY

ulnar collateral ligament *n* **1** : a triangular ligament of the elbow that connects the medial epicondyle of the humerus with the medial edge of the coronoid process and the olecranon of the ulna, that helps to stabilize the elbow joint, and that is often injured in sports (as baseball) which involve repeated overhand throwing — called also *medial collateral ligament, UCL;* compare RADIAL COLLATERAL LIGAMENT 1 **2** : a ligament of the wrist on the little finger side that connects the distal end of the ulna of the arm with the triquetral and pisiform bones and helps to stabilize the wrist joint — called also *UCL;* compare RADIAL COLLATERAL LIGAMENT 2 **3** : a ligament of the inner middle joint of the thumb that connects the head of the metacarpal bone with the adjacent phalanx — called also *UCL;* compare RADIAL COLLATERAL LIGAMENT 3

ulnar collateral ligament reconstruction *n* : a surgical procedure in which a torn ulnar collateral ligament of the elbow is replaced with a tendon graft typically obtained from the palmaris longus — called also *Tommy John surgery*

ulnaris — see EXTENSOR CARPI ULNARIS, FLEXOR CARPI ULNARIS

ulnar nerve *n* : a large superficial nerve of the arm that is a continuation of the medial cord of the brachial plexus, passes around the elbow superficially in a groove between the olecranon and the medial epicondyle of the humerus, and continues down the inner side of the forearm to supply the skin and muscles of the little-finger side of the forearm and hand — see FUNNY BONE

ulnar notch *n* : the narrow medial concave surface on the lower end of the radius that articulates with the ulna

ulnar recurrent artery *n* : either of the two small branches of the ulnar artery arising from its medial side: **a** : one that arises just below the elbow and supplies the brachialis muscle and the pronator teres — called also *anterior ulnar recurrent artery* **b** : one that is larger, arises lower on the arm, and supplies the elbow and associated muscles — called also *posterior ulnar recurrent artery*

ulnar vein *n* : any of several deep veins of the forearm that accompany the ulnar artery and unite at the elbow with the radial veins to form the brachial veins

Ulor·ic \yü-ˈlȯr-ik\ *trademark* — used for a preparation of febuxostat

ul·tra·cen·tri·fuge \ˌəl-trə-ˈsen-trə-ˌfyüj\ *n* : a high-speed centrifuge able to sediment colloidal and other very small particles (as proteins or nucleic acids) — **ul·tra·cen·trif·u·gal** \-ˌsen-ˈtri-fyə-gəl, -fi-\ *adj* — **ul·tra·cen·tri·fu·ga·tion** \-ˌsen-trə-fyu̇-ˈgā-shən\ *n* — **ultracentrifuge** *vb*

ul·tra·di·an \əl-ˈtrād-ē-ən\ *adj* : being, characterized by, or occurring in periods or cycles (as of biological activity) of less than 24 hours and often repeated frequently (as every 90 minutes) throughout a 24-hour period

ul·tra·fil·tra·tion \ˌəl-trə-fil-ˈtrā-shən\ *n* : filtration through a medium (as a semipermeable capillary wall) which allows small molecules (as of water) to pass but holds back larger ones (as of protein) — **ul·tra·fil·tra·ble** \-ˈfil-trə-bəl\ *adj* — **ul·tra·fil·trate** \-ˈfil-ˌtrāt\ *n*

ul·tra·len·te insulin \ˌəl-trə-ˈlen-tā-\ *n, often cap* : insulin zinc suspension that contains insulin in a predominantly crystalline form and is of long-acting duration — formerly a U.S. registered trademark; called also *ultralente*

Ul·tram \ˈəl-ˌtram\ *trademark* — used for a preparation of the hydrochloride of tramadol

ul·tra·mi·cro·scope \ˌəl-trə-ˈmī-krə-ˌskōp\ *n* : an apparatus for making visible by scattered light particles too small to be perceived by the ordinary microscope — called also *dark-field microscope* — **ul·tra·mi·cros·co·py** \-mī-ˈkräs-kə-pē\ *n*

ul·tra·mi·cro·scop·ic \-ˌmī-krə-ˈskä-pik\ *also* **ul·tra·mi·cro·scop·i·cal** \-pi-kəl\ *adj* **1** : SUBMICROSCOPIC **2** : of or relating to an ultramicroscope — **ul·tra·mi·cro·scop·i·cal·ly** *adv*

ul·tra·mi·cro·tome \-ˈmī-krə-ˌtōm\ *n* : a microtome for cutting extremely thin sections for electron microscopy — **ul·tra·mi·crot·o·my** \-mī-ˈkrä-tə-mē\ *n*

ul·tra·son·ic \-ˈsä-nik\ *adj* **1 a** : having a frequency above the human ear's audibility limit of about 20,000 hertz — used of waves and vibrations **b** : utilizing, produced by, or relating to ultrasonic waves or vibrations ⟨an ~ scaler for tartar removal⟩ **2** : ULTRASOUND — **ul·tra·son·i·cal·ly** *adv*

ul·tra·sono·gram \-ˈsä-nə-ˌgram\ *n* : SONOGRAM

ul·tra·so·nog·ra·pher \ˌəl-trə-sə-ˈnä-grə-fər\ *n* : SONOGRAPHER

ul·tra·so·nog·ra·phy \-fē\ *n, pl* **-phies** : ULTRASOUND 2 — **ul·tra·so·no·graph·ic** \-ˌsä-nə-ˈgra-fik, -ˌsō-\ *adj*

[1]**ul·tra·sound** \ˈəl-trə-ˌsau̇nd\ *n* **1** : vibrations of the same physical nature as sound but with frequencies above the range of human hearing **2** : the diagnostic or therapeutic use of ultrasound and esp. a noninvasive technique involving the formation of a two-dimensional image used for the examination and measurement of internal body structures and the detection of bodily abnormalities — called also *echography, sonography, ultrasonography* **3** : a diagnostic examination using ultrasound

[2]**ultrasound** *adj* : of, relating to, performed by, using, or specializing in ultrasound ⟨an ~ technician⟩

ul·tra·vi·o·let \ˌəl-trə-ˈvī-ə-lət\ *adj* **1** : situated beyond the visible spectrum at its violet end — used of radiation having a wavelength shorter than wavelengths of visible light and longer than those of X-rays **2** : relating to, producing, or employing ultraviolet radiation — **ultraviolet** *n*

ultraviolet A *n* : UVA

ultraviolet B *n* : UVB

ultraviolet microscope *n* : a microscope equipped to irradiate material under examination with ultraviolet radiation in order to detect or study fluorescent components — called also *fluorescence microscope*

uma·mi \ü-ˈmä-mē\ *n* : a taste sensation that is meaty or savory and is produced by several amino acids and nucleotides (as aspartate, inosinate, and glutamate) — **umami** *adj*

um·bi·lec·to·my \ˌəm-bi-ˈlek-tə-mē\ *n, pl* **-mies** : OMPHALECTOMY

um·bil·i·cal \ˌəm-ˈbi-li-kəl\ *adj* **1** : of, relating to, or used at the navel **2** : of or relating to the central abdominal region that is situated between the right and left lumbar regions and between the epigastric region above and the hypogastric region below

umbilical artery *n* : either of a pair of arteries that arise from the fetal hypogastric arteries and pass through the umbilical cord to the placenta to which they carry the deoxygenated blood from the fetus

umbilical cord *n* : a cord arising from the navel that connects the fetus with the placenta and contains the two umbilical arteries and the umbilical vein

umbilical hernia *n* : a hernia of abdominal viscera at the navel

umbilical ligament — see MEDIAL UMBILICAL LIGAMENT, MEDIAN UMBILICAL LIGAMENT

umbilical vein *n* : a vein that passes through the umbilical cord to the fetus and returns the oxygenated and nutrient blood from the placenta to the fetus

umbilical vesicle *n* : the yolk sac of a mammalian embryo having a transitory connection with the digestive tract by way of the omphalomesenteric duct

um·bil·i·cat·ed \ˌəm-ˈbi-lə-ˌkā-təd\ *or* **um·bil·i·cate** \-kət\ *adj* : having a small depression that resembles a navel ⟨~ vesicles⟩ — **um·bil·i·cate** \-ˌkāt\ *vb*

um·bi·li·cus \ˌəm-bə-ˈlī-kəs, ˌəm-ˈbi-li-\ *n, pl* **um·bi·li·ci** \ˌəm-bə-ˈlī-ˌkī, -ˌsī; ˌəm-ˈbi-lə-ˌkī, -ˌkē\ *or* **um·bi·li·cus·es** : NAVEL

um·bo \ˈəm-(ˌ)bō\ *n, pl* **um·bo·nes** \ˌəm-ˈbō-(ˌ)nēz\ *or* **um·bos** : an elevation in the tympanic membrane of the ear

ume·cli·din·i·um \ˌyü-mə-klə-ˈdi-nē-əm\ *n* : an anticholinergic bronchodilator $C_{29}H_{34}NO_2 \cdot Br$ administered by oral inhalation to treat chronic obstructive pulmonary disease

un·anes·the·tized \ˌən-ə-ˈnes-thə-ˌtīzd\ *adj* : not having been subjected to an anesthetic ⟨an ~ patient⟩

un·bal·anced \ˌən-ˈba-lənst\ *adj* : mentally disordered : affected with mental illness

un·blind·ed \-ˈblīn-dəd\ *adj* : made or done with knowledge of significant facts by the participants : not blind ⟨~ studies of a drug's effectiveness⟩

un·born \-ˈbȯrn\ *adj* : not yet born : existing in utero ⟨~ children⟩

un·bro·ken \-ˈbrō-kən\ *adj* : not broken ⟨~ skin⟩ ⟨an ~ blister⟩

un·cal \ˈəŋ-kəl\ *adj* : of or relating to the uncus ⟨the ~ region⟩

un·cal·ci·fied \ˌən-ˈkal-sə-ˌfīd\ *adj* : not calcified ⟨~ osteoid tissue⟩

uncal herniation *n* : downward displacement of the uncus and adjacent structures into the tentorial notch

unci *pl of* UNCUS

un·ci·form \ˈən-sə-ˌfȯrm\ *n* : HAMATE

unciform bone *n* : HAMATE

Un·ci·nar·ia \ˌən-sə-ˈnar-ē-ə\ *n* : a genus of hookworms (family Ancylostomatidae) that are parasites of carnivorous mammals and includes one (*U. stenocephala*) infecting dogs, foxes, cats, and rarely humans

un·ci·nate fasciculus \ˈən-sə-ˌnāt-\ *n* : a hook-shaped bundle of long association fibers connecting the frontal lobe with the anterior portion of the temporal lobe

uncinate process *n* : a hooklike body part: as **a** : an irregular downwardly and backwardly directed process of each lateral mass of the ethmoid bone that articulates with the inferior nasal conchae **b** : a bony upward projection arising from each side of the upper surface of any of the cervical vertebrae numbered three to seven and forming a raised lateral margin **c** : the portion of the pancreas that wraps behind the superior mesenteric artery and superior mesenteric vein

un·cir·cum·cised \ˌən-ˈsər-kəm-ˌsīzd\ *adj* : not circumcised

un·com·pen·sat·ed \-ˈkäm-pən-ˌsā-təd, -ˌpen-\ *adj* **1** : accompanied by a change in the pH of the blood ⟨~ acidosis⟩ ⟨~ alkalosis⟩ — compare COMPENSATED **2** : not corrected or affected by physiological compensation ⟨~ congestive heart failure⟩

un·com·pli·cat·ed \ˌən-ˈkäm-plə-ˌkā-təd\ *adj* : not involving or marked by complications ⟨~ peptic ulcer⟩

un·con·di·tion·al \ˌən-kən-ˈdi-shə-nəl\ *adj* : UNCONDITIONED 2

un·con·di·tioned \-ˈdi-shənd\ *adj* **1** : not dependent on or subjected to conditioning or learning **2** : producing an unconditioned response

[1]**un·con·scious** \ˌən-ˈkän-chəs\ *adj* **1** : not marked by conscious thought, sensation, or feeling ⟨~ motivation⟩ **2** : of or relating to the unconscious **3** : having lost consciousness ⟨was ~ for three days⟩ — **un·con·scious·ly** *adv* — **un·con·scious·ness** *n*

[2]**unconscious** *n* : the part of mental life that is not ordinarily integrated or available to consciousness yet may be manifested as a motive force in overt behavior (as in neurosis) and is often revealed (as through dreams, slips of the tongue, or dissociated acts) — compare SUBCONSCIOUS

un·con·trolled \ˌən-kən-ˈtrōld\ *adj* **1** : not being under control ⟨~ hypertension⟩ **2** : not incorporating suitable experimental controls ⟨~ drug trials⟩

un•co•or•di•nat•ed \-kō-ˈȯrd-ᵊn-ˌā-təd\ *adj* : not coordinated : lacking proper or effective coordination ⟨~ muscles⟩
un•crossed \-ˈkrȯst\ *adj* : not forming a decussation ⟨~ nerve fibers⟩
unc•tu•ous \ˈəŋk-chə-wəs, -shə-\ *adj* : rich in oil or fat : FATTY
un•cur•able \ˌən-ˈkyu̇r-ə-bəl\ *adj* : INCURABLE
un•cus \ˈəŋ-kəs\ *n, pl* **un•ci** \ˈən-ˌsī\ : a hooked anatomical part or process; *specif* : the anterior curved end of the parahippocampal gyrus
un•dec•y•le•nic acid \ˌən-ˌde-sə-ˈle-nik-, -ˌlē-\ *n* : an acid $C_{11}H_{20}O_2$ used in the treatment of fungus infections (as ringworm) of the skin
[1]**un•der** \ˈən-dər\ *adv* : in or into a condition of unconsciousness ⟨put the patient ~ prior to surgery⟩
[2]**under** *prep* : receiving or using the action or application of ⟨an operation performed ~ local anesthesia⟩
[3]**under** *adj* : being in an induced state of unconsciousness
un•der•achiev•er \ˌən-dər-ə-ˈchē-vər\ *n* : a person (as a student) who fails to attain a predicted level of achievement or does not do as well as expected — **un•der•achieve** \-ˈchēv\ *vb* — **un•der•achieve•ment** \-mənt\ *n*
un•der•ac•tive \-ˈak-tiv\ *adj* : characterized by an abnormally low level of activity ⟨an ~ thyroid gland⟩ — **un•der•ac•tiv•i•ty** \-ak-ˈti-və-tē\ *n*
un•der•arm \ˈən-dər-ˌärm\ *n* : ARMPIT
un•der•cut \ˈən-dər-ˌkət\ *n* : the part of a tooth lying between the gum and the points of maximum outward bulge on the tooth's surfaces
un•der•de•vel•oped \ˌən-dər-di-ˈve-ləpt\ *adj* : not normally or adequately developed ⟨~ muscles⟩ — **un•der•de•vel•op•ment** \-əp-mənt\ *n*
un•der•di•ag•nose \-ˈdī-ig-ˌnōs, -ˌnōz\ *vb* **-nosed; -nos•ing** : to diagnose (a condition or disease) less often than it is actually present
un•der•do•sage \-ˈdō-sij\ *n* : the administration or taking of an underdose
[1]**un•der•dose** \-ˈdōs\ *vb* **-dosed; -dos•ing** : to take or administer an insufficient dose
[2]**un•der•dose** \-ˌdōs\ *n* : an insufficient dose
un•der•feed \ˌən-dər-ˈfēd\ *vb* **-fed** \-ˈfed\; **-feed•ing** : to feed with too little food
un•der•nour•ished \ˌən-dər-ˈnər-isht\ *adj* : supplied with less than the minimum amount of the foods essential for sound health and growth — **un•der•nour•ish•ment** \-ˈnər-ish-mənt\ *n*
un•der•nu•tri•tion \-nu̇-ˈtri-shən, -nyu̇-\ *n* : deficient bodily nutrition due to inadequate food intake or faulty assimilation — **un•der•nu•tri•tion•al** \-shə-nəl\ *adj*
un•der•sexed \-ˈsekst\ *adj* : deficient in sexual desire
un•der•shot \ˈən-dər-ˌshät\ *adj* : having the lower incisor teeth or lower jaw projecting beyond the upper when the mouth is closed — used chiefly of animals
un•der•tak•er \ˈən-dər-ˌtā-kər\ *n* : one whose business is to prepare the dead for burial and to arrange and manage funerals — called also *mortician*
un•der•treat \-ˈtrēt\ *vb* : to treat (as a condition, disease, or patient) inadequately — **un•der•treat•ment** \-mənt\ *n*
un•der•ven•ti•la•tion \ˌən-dər-ˌven-ti-ˈlā-shən\ *n* : HYPOVENTILATION
un•der•weight \-ˈwāt\ *adj* : weighing less than the normal amount for one's age, height, and build
un•de•scend•ed \ˌən-di-ˈsen-dəd\ *adj* : retained within the iliac region rather than descending into the scrotum ⟨an ~ testis⟩
un•de•vel•oped \ˌən-di-ˈve-ləpt\ *adj* : lacking in development : not developed ⟨physiologically ~⟩
un•di•ag•nos•able \-ˌdī-ig-ˈnō-sə-bəl\ *adj* : not capable of being diagnosed
un•di•ag•nosed \-ˈnōst\ *adj* : not diagnosed : eluding diagnosis ⟨~ disease⟩
un•dif•fer•en•ti•at•ed \-ˌdi-fə-ˈren-chē-ˌā-təd\ *adj* : not differentiated ⟨an ~ sarcoma⟩
un•di•gest•ed \ˌən-dī-ˈjes-təd\ *adj* : not digested ⟨~ food⟩
un•di•gest•ible \-dī-ˈjes-tə-bəl\ *adj* : not capable of being digested
un•du•lant fever \ˈən-jə-lənt-, -dyə-\ *n* : BRUCELLOSIS 2
un•erupt•ed \ˌən-i-ˈrəp-təd\ *adj, of a tooth* : not yet having emerged through the gum
un•fer•til•ized \-ˈfərt-ᵊl-ˌīzd\ *adj* : not fertilized ⟨an ~ egg⟩
ung *abbr* [Latin *unguentum*] ointment — used in writing prescriptions
un•gual \ˈəŋ-gwəl, ˈən-\ *adj* : of or relating to a fingernail or toenail
un•guent \ˈəŋ-gwənt, ˈən-jənt\ *n* : a soothing or healing salve : OINTMENT
un•guis \ˈəŋ-gwəs, ˈən-\ *n, pl* **un•gues** \-ˌgwēz\ : a fingernail or toenail
un•gu•late \ˈəŋ-gyə-lət, ˈən-, -ˌlāt\ *n* : a hoofed typically herbivorous quadruped mammal (as a ruminant, swine, camel, or horse) of a group formerly considered a major mammalian taxon (Ungulata) — **ungulate** *adj*
Unh *symbol* unnilhexium
un•healed \ˌən-ˈhēld\ *adj* : not healed
un•health•ful \-ˈhelth-fəl\ *adj* : detrimental to good health ⟨~ working conditions⟩ — **un•health•ful•ness** *n*
un•healthy \-ˈhel-thē\ *adj* **un•health•i•er; -est** **1** : not conducive to health ⟨an ~ climate⟩ **2** : not in good health : SICKLY — **un•health•i•ness** *n*
un•hy•gi•en•ic \ˌən-ˌhī-ˈje-nik, -ˈjē-, -jē-ˈe-\ *adj* : not healthful or sanitary — **un•hy•gi•en•i•cal•ly** \-ni-k(ə-)lē\ *adv*
uni•cel•lu•lar \ˌyü-ni-ˈsel-yə-lər\ *adj* : having or consisting of a single cell ⟨~ microorganisms⟩ — **uni•cel•lu•lar•i•ty** \-ˌsel-yə-ˈlar-ə-tē\ *n*

uni•fo•cal \ˌyü-ni-ˈfō-kəl\ *adj* : arising from or occurring in a single focus or location ⟨~ infection⟩

uni•la•mel•lar \ˌyü-ni-lə-ˈme-lər\ *adj* : composed of, having, or involving a single lamella or layer

uni•lat•er•al \ˌyü-ni-ˈla-tə-rəl\ *adj* : occurring on, performed on, or affecting one side of the body or one of its parts ⟨~ exophthalmos⟩ — **uni•lat•er•al•ly** *adv*

uni•loc•u•lar \ˌyü-ni-ˈlä-kyə-lər\ *adj* : containing a single cavity

un•im•mu•nized \(ˌ)ən-ˈi-myə-ˌnīzd\ *adj* : not immunized

un•in•fect•ed \ˌən-in-ˈfek-təd\ *adj* : free from infection ⟨an ~ fracture⟩

uni•nu•cle•ate \ˌyü-ni-ˈnü-klē-ət, -ˈnyü-\ *also* **uni•nu•cle•at•ed** \-ˌā-təd\ *adj* : having a single nucleus : MONONUCLEAR

union \ˈyü-nyən\ *n* : an act or instance of uniting or joining two or more things into one: as **a** : the growing together of severed parts ⟨~ of a fractured bone⟩ **b** : the joining of two germ cells in the process of fertilization

uni•ovu•lar \ˌyü-nē-ˈä-vyə-lər\ *adj* : MONOZYGOTIC ⟨~ twins⟩

unip•a•ra \yü-ˈni-pə-rə\ *n, pl* **-ras** *or* **-rae** \-ˌrē\ : a woman who has borne one child

uni•pa•ren•tal \ˌyü-ni-pə-ˈren-tᵊl\ *adj* : having, involving, or derived from a single parent; *specif* : involving or being inheritance in which an offspring's complete genotype or all copies of one or more genes, chromosome parts, or whole chromosomes are derived from a single parent ⟨~ disomy⟩ — **uni•pa•ren•tal•ly** \-ē\ *adv*

uni•pen•nate \ˌyü-ni-ˈpe-ˌnāt\ *adj* : having the fibers arranged obliquely and inserting into a tendon only on one side ⟨a ~ muscle⟩

uni•po•lar \ˌyü-ni-ˈpō-lər\ *adj* **1** : involving or being an electrode or lead attached to the surface of a bodily site (as the chest) for recording the difference in electrical potential between the site and that of another electrode or lead having zero potential **2** *of a neuron* : having but one process **3** : relating to or being a manic-depressive disorder in which there is a depressive phase only ⟨~ depression⟩ — compare BIPOLAR

un•ir•ra•di•at•ed \ˌun-ir-ˈā-dē-ˌā-təd\ *adj* : not having been exposed to radiation ⟨~ lymphocytes⟩

unit \ˈyü-nət\ *n* **1** : an amount of a biologically active agent (as a drug or antigen) required to produce a specific result under strictly controlled conditions ⟨a ~ of penicillin⟩ **2** : a small molecule esp. when combined in a larger molecule **3** : an area in a medical facility and esp. a hospital that is specially staffed and equipped to provide a particular type of care

unit•age \ˈyü-nə-tij\ *n* **1** : specification of the amount constituting a unit (as of a vitamin) **2** : amount in units ⟨a ~ of 50,000 per capsule⟩

unit membrane *n* : the membrane of cells and various organelles viewed formerly as a 3-layered structure with an inner lipid layer and two outer protein layers and currently as a fluid phospholipid bilayer with intercalated proteins

[1]**uni•va•lent** \ˌyü-ni-ˈvā-lənt\ *n* : a chromosome that lacks a synaptic mate

[2]**univalent** *adj* **1** : MONOVALENT 1 **2** : being a chromosomal univalent **3** *of an antibody* : capable of agglutinating or precipitating but not both : having only one combining group

Uni•vasc \ˈyü-ni-ˌvask\ *trademark* — used for a preparation of the hydrochloride of moexipril

universal antidote *n* : an antidote for ingested poisons having activated charcoal as its principal ingredient

universal donor *n* **1** : a person who has Rh-negative blood of the blood group O and whose blood can be donated to any recipient; *broadly* : a person with blood group O blood **2** : the blood or blood group of a universal donor

universal recipient *n* **1** : a person who has Rh-positive blood of the blood group AB and who can receive blood from any donor; *broadly* : a person with blood group AB blood **2** : the blood or blood group of a universal recipient

un•la•beled *or* **un•la•belled** \ˌən-ˈlā-bəld\ *adj* : not labeled esp. with an isotopic label ⟨~ DNA⟩

un•la•bored \ˌən-ˈlā-bərd\ *adj* : produced without exertion, pain, or undue effort ⟨~ breathing⟩

un•li•censed \-ˈlī-sᵊnst\ *adj* : not licensed; *esp, of a drug* : not approved for use by the appropriate regulating authority (as the Food and Drug Administration in the U.S.)

un•linked \-ˈliŋkt\ *adj* : not belonging to the same genetic linkage group ⟨~ genes⟩

un•my•elin•at•ed \-ˈmī-ə-lə-ˌnā-təd\ *adj* : lacking a myelin sheath ⟨~ axons⟩

Un•na's boot \ˈü-nəz-\ *or* **Un•na boot** \-nə-\ *n* : a compression dressing for varicose veins or ulcers consisting of a paste made of zinc oxide, gelatin, glycerin, and water

Unna, Paul Gerson (1850–1929), German dermatologist.

Unna's paste boot *n* : UNNA'S BOOT

un•nil•hex•i•um \ˌyün-ᵊl-ˈhek-sē-əm\ *n* : SEABORGIUM — symbol *Unh*

un•nil•pen•ti•um \ˌyün-ᵊl-ˈpen-tē-əm\ *n* : DUBNIUM — symbol *Unp*

un•nil•qua•di•um \ˌyün-ᵊl-ˈkwä-dē-əm\ *n* : RUTHERFORDIUM — symbol *Unq*

un•of•fi•cial \ˌən-ə-ˈfi-shəl\ *adj* : not official; *specif* : of, relating to, or being a drug not described in the *U.S. Pharmacopeia* and *National Formulary* — compare NONOFFICIAL, OFFICIAL

un•op•posed \-ə-ˈpōzd\ *adj* : being or relating to estrogen replacement therapy in which a progestin (as medroxyprogesterone acetate) is not coadministered to reduce the potential risks (as endometrial cancer) associated with estrogen used alone

un•os•si•fied \-ˈä-sə-ˌfīd\ *adj* : not ossified

un•ox•y•gen•at•ed \-ˈäk-si-jə-ˌnā-təd, -äk-ˈsi-jə-\ *adj* : not oxygenated ⟨~ blood⟩

Unp *symbol* unnilpentium

un•paired \-ˈpard\ *adj* **1** : not paired: as **a** : not matched or mated **b** : being an electron that does not share its orbital with another electron **2** : situated in the median plane of the body; *also* : not matched by a corresponding part on the opposite side

un•pig•ment•ed \-ˈpig-mən-təd\ *adj* : not pigmented : having no pigment

un•pro•tect•ed \-prə-ˈtek-təd\ *adj* : not protected; *esp* : performed without measures to prevent pregnancy or sexually transmitted disease ⟨~ sex⟩

Unq *symbol* unnilquadium

un•re•ac•tive \-rē-ˈak-tiv\ *adj* : not reactive ⟨pupils ~ to light⟩

un•re•sect•able \-ri-ˈsek-tə-bəl\ *adj* : not capable of being surgically removed ⟨an ~ tumor⟩

un•re•solved \-ri-ˈzälvd, -ˈzȯlvd\ *adj* : not resolved : not having undergone resolution ⟨~ pneumonia⟩

un•re•spon•sive \ˌən-ri-ˈspän-siv\ *adj* : not responsive (as to a treatment or stimulus) — **un•re•spon•sive•ness** *n*

un•san•i•tary \-ˈsa-nə-ˌter-ē\ *adj* : not sanitary : INSANITARY ⟨~ facilities⟩

un•sat•u•rate \-ˈsa-chə-rət\ *n* : an unsaturated chemical compound

un•sat•u•rat•ed \-ˈsa-chə-ˌrā-təd\ *adj* : not saturated: as **a** : capable of absorbing or dissolving more of something ⟨an ~ solution⟩ **b** : able to form products by chemical addition; *esp* : containing double or triple bonds between carbon atoms ⟨~ oils⟩ — **un•sat•u•ra•tion** \-ˌsa-chə-ˈrā-shən\ *n*

un•seg•ment•ed \-ˈseg-ˌmen-təd\ *adj* : not divided into or made up of segments

un•sound \-ˈsau̇nd\ *adj* : not sound: as **a** : not healthy or whole ⟨an ~ limb⟩ **b** : not mentally normal : not wholly sane ⟨of ~ mind⟩ **c** : not fit to be eaten ⟨~ food⟩ — **un•sound•ness** *n*

un•sta•ble \-ˈstā-bəl\ *adj* : not stable: as **a** : characterized by frequent or unpredictable changes ⟨a patient in ~ condition⟩ **b** : readily changing in chemical composition or biological activity **c** : characterized by the lack of emotional control or stability

unstable angina *n* : angina pectoris characterized by sudden changes (as an increase in the severity or length of anginal attacks or a decrease in the exertion required to precipitate an attack) esp. when symptoms were previously stable

un•stri•at•ed muscle \ˌən-ˈstrī-ˌā-təd-\ *n* : SMOOTH MUSCLE

un•struc•tured \-ˈstrək-chərd\ *adj* : lacking structure : not formally organized ⟨~ psychological tests⟩

un•trau•ma•tized \-ˈtrau̇-mə-ˌtīzd, -ˈtrȯ-\ *adj* : not subjected to trauma

un•treat•ed \-ˈtrē-təd\ *adj* : not subjected to treatment ⟨an ~ disease⟩ — **un•treat•able** \-ˈtrē-tə-bəl\ *adj*

un•vac•ci•nat•ed \-ˈvak-sə-ˌnā-təd\ *adj* : not vaccinated ⟨~ children⟩

un•well \-ˈwel\ *adj* : being in poor health : SICK

up•grade \ˈəp-ˌgrād\ *vb* **-grad•ed; -grad•ing 1** : to assign a less serious status to **2** : to reclassify (as a cancer or concussion) to a more serious grade when the grades are numbered from least to most serious

¹up•per \ˈə-pər\ *n* : an upper tooth or denture

²upper *n* : a stimulant drug; *esp* : AMPHETAMINE

upper airway *n* : any or all of the air-conducting passages of the respiratory system that extend to the larynx from the two external openings of the nose and from the lips through the mouth

upper GI series *n* : fluoroscopic and radiographic examination (as for the detection of gastroesophageal reflux, hiatal hernia, or ulcers) of the esophagus, stomach, and duodenum during and following oral ingestion of a solution of barium sulfate — called also *upper gastrointestinal series*

upper jaw *n* : JAW 1a

upper respiratory *adj* : of, relating to, or affecting the upper respiratory tract ⟨*upper respiratory* infection⟩

upper respiratory tract *n* : the part of the respiratory system including the nose, nasal passages, and nasopharynx — compare LOWER RESPIRATORY TRACT

up•reg•u•la•tion \ˈəp-ˌre-gyə-ˈlā-shən, -gə-\ *n* : the process of increasing the response to a stimulus; *specif* : increase in a cellular response to a molecular stimulus due to increase in the number of receptors on the cell surface — **up•reg•u•late** \-ˈre-gyə-ˌlāt\ *vb*

up•set \ˈəp-ˌset\ *n* **1** : a minor physical disorder ⟨a stomach ~⟩ **2** : an emotional disturbance — **up•set** \(ˌ)əp-ˈset\ *vb* — **up•set** \ˈəp-ˌset\ *adj*

up•stream \ˌəp-ˈstrēm\ *adv or adj* **1** : in a direction along a molecule of DNA or RNA opposite to that in which transcription and translation take place and toward the end having a hydroxyl group attached to the position labeled 5′ in the terminal nucleotide — compare DOWNSTREAM 1 **2** : toward the beginning of series of cellular processes : preceding a molecular sequence — compare DOWNSTREAM 2

up·take \ˈəp-ˌtāk\ *n* : an act or instance of absorbing and incorporating something esp. into a living organism, tissue, or cell ⟨oxygen ~⟩

ur- *or* **uro-** *comb form* **1** : urine ⟨*ur*ic⟩ **2** : urinary tract ⟨*uro*logy⟩ **3** : urinary and ⟨*uro*genital⟩ **4** : urea ⟨*ur*acil⟩

ura·chal \ˈyu̇r-ə-kəl\ *adj* : of or relating to the urachus ⟨a ~ cyst⟩

ura·chus \-kəs\ *n* : a cord of fibrous tissue extending from the bladder to the navel and constituting the functionless remnant of a part of the duct of the allantois of the embryo

ura·cil \ˈyu̇r-ə-ˌsil, -səl\ *n* : a pyrimidine base $C_4H_4N_2O_2$ that is one of the four bases coding genetic information in the polynucleotide chain of RNA — compare ADENINE, CYTOSINE, GUANINE, THYMINE

ur·ae·mia *chiefly Brit var of* UREMIA

ura·ni·um \yu̇-ˈrā-nē-əm\ *n* : a silvery heavy radioactive metallic element that exists naturally as a mixture of three isotopes of mass number 234, 235, and 238 — symbol *U;* see ELEMENT table

uranium 235 *n* : a light isotope of uranium of mass number 235 that when bombarded with slow neutrons undergoes rapid fission into smaller atoms with the release of neutrons and energy

urate \ˈyu̇r-ˌāt\ *n* : a salt of uric acid

ure- *or* **ureo-** *comb form* : urea ⟨*ure*ase⟩

urea \yu̇-ˈrē-ə\ *n* : a soluble weakly basic nitrogenous compound CH_4N_2O that is the chief solid component of mammalian urine and an end product of protein decomposition and that is administered intravenously as a diuretic drug

urea cycle *n* : a sequence of metabolic reactions occurring in the liver by which ammonia is converted to urea

urea·plas·ma \yu̇-ˈrē-ə-ˌplaz-mə\ *n* **1** *cap* : a genus of mycoplasmas (family Mycoplasmataceae) that are able to hydrolyze urea with the formation of ammonia and that include one (*U. urealyticum*) found in the human genitourinary tract, oropharynx, and anal canal **2** : a mycoplasma of the genus *Ureaplasma*

ure·ase \ˈyu̇r-ē-ˌās, -ˌāz\ *n* : an enzyme that catalyzes the hydrolysis of urea into ammonia and carbon dioxide

Ure·cho·line \ˌyu̇r-ə-ˈkō-ˌlēn\ *trademark* — used for a preparation of the chloride of bethanechol

ure·mia \yu̇-ˈrē-mē-ə\ *n* **1** : accumulation in the blood of constituents normally eliminated in the urine that produces a severe toxic condition and usu. occurs in severe kidney disease **2** : the toxic bodily condition associated with uremia — **ure·mic** \-mik\ *adj*

ure·ter \ˈyu̇r-ə-tər, yu̇-ˈrē-tər\ *n* : either of the paired ducts that carry away urine from a kidney to the bladder or cloaca and that in humans are slender membranous epithelium-lined flat tubes about sixteen inches (41 centimeters) long which open above into the pelvis of a kidney and below into the back part of the same side of the bladder — **ure·ter·al** \yu̇-ˈrē-tə-rəl\ *also* **ure·ter·ic** \ˌyu̇r-ə-ˈter-ik\ *adj*

ure·ter·ec·ta·sis \ˌyu̇r-ə-tər-ˈek-tə-səs, yu̇-ˌrē-tər-\ *n, pl* **-ta·ses** \-ˌsēz\ : dilation of a ureter

ure·ter·ec·to·my \ˌyu̇r-ə-tər-ˈek-tə-mē, yu̇-ˌrē-tər-\ *n, pl* **-mies** : surgical excision of all or part of a ureter

uretericus — see TORUS URETERICUS

ure·ter·itis \ˌyu̇r-ə-tər-ˈī-təs, yu̇-ˌrē-tər-\ *n* : inflammation of a ureter

uretero- *comb form* **1** : ureter ⟨*uretero*graphy⟩ **2** : ureteral and ⟨*uretero*ileal⟩

ure·ter·o·cele \yu̇-ˈrē-tə-rə-ˌsēl\ *n* : cystic dilation of the lower part of a ureter into the bladder

ure·tero·en·ter·os·to·my \yu̇-ˌrē-tə-rō-ˌen-tə-ˈräs-tə-mē\ *n, pl* **-mies** : surgical formation of an artificial opening between a ureter and the intestine

ure·ter·o·gram \yu̇-ˈrē-tə-rə-ˌgram\ *n* : an X-ray photograph of the ureters after injection of a radiopaque substance — **ure·ter·og·ra·phy** \yu̇-ˌrē-tə-ˈrä-grə-fē, ˌyu̇r-ə-tə-\ *n*

ure·tero·il·e·al \yu̇-ˌrē-tə-rō-ˈi-lē-əl\ *adj* : relating to or connecting a ureter and the ileum

ure·tero·li·thot·o·my \yu̇-ˌrē-tə-rō-li-ˈthä-tə-mē\ *n, pl* **-mies** : removal of a calculus by incision of a ureter

ure·ter·ol·y·sis \ˌyu̇r-ə-tər-ˈä-lə-səs, yu̇-ˌrē-tər-\ *n, pl* **-y·ses** \-ˌsēz\ : a surgical procedure to free a ureter from abnormal adhesions or surrounding tissue (as in retroperitoneal fibrosis)

ure·tero·neo·cys·tos·to·my \yu̇-ˌrē-tər-ō-ˌnē-ō-sis-ˈtäs-tə-mē\ *n, pl* **-mies** : surgical reimplantation of a ureter into the bladder

ure·tero·pel·vic \yu̇-ˌrē-tə-rō-ˈpel-vik\ *adj* : of, relating to, or involving a ureter and the adjoining renal pelvis ⟨~ obstruction⟩

ure·tero·plas·ty \yu̇-ˈrē-tə-rə-ˌplas-tē\ *n, pl* **-ties** : plastic surgery performed on a ureter

ure·tero·py·elog·ra·phy \yu̇-ˌrē-tə-rō-ˌpī-ə-ˈlä-grə-fē\ *n, pl* **-phies** : X-ray photography of a renal pelvis and a ureter following the injection of a radiopaque medium

ure·tero·py·elo·ne·os·to·my \yu̇-ˌrē-tə-rō-ˌpī-ə-lō-nē-ˈäs-tə-mē\ *n, pl* **-mies** : surgical creation of a new channel joining a renal pelvis to a ureter

ure·tero·py·e·los·to·my \-ˌpī-ə-ˈläs-tə-mē\ *n, pl* **-mies** : URETEROPYELONEOSTOMY

ure·ter·or·rha·phy \yu̇-ˌrē-tə-ˈrȯr-ə-fē, ˌyu̇r-ə-tə-\ *n, pl* **-phies** : the surgical operation of suturing a ureter

ure·tero·scope \yu̇-ˈrē-tə-rō-ˌskōp\ *n* : an endoscope for visually examining and passing instruments into the interior of the ureter

ure·ter·os·co·py \yu̇-ˌrē-tə-ˈräs-kə-pē, ˌyu̇r-ə-tə-\ *n, pl* **-pies** : visual examination of the interior of a ureter

ure·tero·sig·moid·os·to·my \yu̇-ˌrē-tə-rō-ˌsig-ˌmȯi-ˈdäs-tə-mē\ *n, pl* **-mies** : surgical implantation of a ureter in the sigmoid colon

ure·ter·os·to·my \ˌyu̇r-ə-tər-ˈäs-tə-mē, yu̇-ˌrē-tər-\ *n, pl* **-mies** : surgical creation of an opening on the surface of the body for the ureters

ure·ter·ot·o·my \ˌyu̇r-ə-tər-ˈä-tə-mē, yu̇-ˌrē-tər-\ *n, pl* **-mies** : the operation of cutting into a ureter

ure·tero·ure·ter·os·to·my \yu̇-ˌrē-tə-rō-yu̇-ˌrē-tər-ˈäs-tə-mē\ *n, pl* **-mies** : surgical establishment of an artificial communication between two ureters or between different parts of the same ureter

ure·tero·ves·i·cal \yu̇-ˌrē-tə-rō-ˈve-si-kəl\ *adj* : of or relating to the ureters and the urinary bladder

ure·thane \ˈyu̇r-ə-ˌthān\ *or* **ure·than** \-ˌthan\ *n* : a crystalline compound $C_3H_7NO_2$ that is used esp. as a solvent and in anesthetizing laboratory animals — called also *ethyl carbamate*

urethr- *or* **urethro-** *comb form* : urethra ⟨*urethr*itis⟩ ⟨*urethro*scope⟩

ure·thra \yu̇-ˈrē-thrə\ *n, pl* **-thras** *or* **-thrae** \-(ˌ)thrē\ : the canal that carries off the urine from the bladder and in the male serves also as a passageway for semen — **ure·thral** \-thrəl\ *adj*

urethrae — see SPHINCTER URETHRAE

urethral crest *n* : a narrow longitudinal fold or ridge along the posterior wall or floor of the female urethra or the prostatic portion of the male urethra

urethral gland *n* : any of the small mucous glands in the wall of the urethra — see GLAND OF LITTRÉ

urethral sphincter *n* : SPHINCTER URETHRAE

urethral syndrome *n* : a group of symptoms (as urinary frequency, dysuria, and suprapubic pain) that resemble those of a urinary tract infection but for which no significant bacteriuria exists

ure·threc·to·my \ˌyu̇r-i-ˈthrek-tə-mē\ *n, pl* **-mies** : total or partial surgical excision of the urethra

ure·thri·tis \ˌyu̇r-i-ˈthrī-təs\ *n* : inflammation of the urethra

ure·thro·cele \yə-ˈrē-thrə-ˌsēl\ *n* : a pouched protrusion of urethral mucous membrane in the female

ure·thro·cu·ta·ne·ous \yu̇-ˌrē-thrō-kyu̇-ˈtā-nē-əs\ *adj* : of, relating to, or joining the urethra and the skin

ure·thro·cys·tog·ra·phy \yu̇-ˌrē-thrō-sis-ˈtä-grə-fē\ *n, pl* **-phies** : radiography of the urethra and bladder that utilizes a radiopaque substance

ure·throg·ra·phy \ˌyu̇r-i-ˈthrä-grə-fē\ *n, pl* **-phies** : radiography of the urethra after injection of a radiopaque substance

ure·thro·pexy \yu̇-ˈrē-thrə-ˌpek-sē\ *n, pl* **-pex·ies** : surgical fixation to nearby tissue of a displaced urethra that is causing incontinence by placing stress on the opening from the bladder

ure·thro·plas·ty \yu̇-ˈrē-thrə-ˌplas-tē\ *n, pl* **-ties** : plastic surgery of the urethra

ure·thro·rec·tal \yu̇-ˌrē-thrō-ˈrekt-ᵊl\ *adj* : of, relating to, or joining the urethra and the rectum ⟨a ~ fistula⟩

ure·thror·rha·phy \ˌyu̇r-ə-ˈthrȯr-ə-fē\ *n, pl* **-phies** : suture of the urethra for an injury or fistula

ure·thro·scope \yu̇-ˈrē-thrə-ˌskōp\ *n* : an endoscope for viewing the interior of the urethra — **ure·thro·scop·ic** \yu̇-ˌrē-thrə-ˈskä-pik\ *adj* — **ure·thros·co·py** \ˌyu̇r-ə-ˈthräs-kə-pē\ *n*

ure·thros·to·my \ˌyu̇r-ə-ˈthräs-tə-mē\ *n, pl* **-mies** : the creation of a surgical opening between the perineum and the urethra

ure·throt·o·my \ˌyu̇r-ə-ˈthrä-tə-mē\ *n, pl* **-mies** : surgical incision into the urethra esp. for the relief of stricture

ure·thro·vag·i·nal \yu̇-ˌrē-thrō-ˈva-jən-ᵊl\ *adj* : of, relating to, or joining the urethra and the vagina ⟨a ~ fistula⟩

urge incontinence *n* : involuntary leakage of urine from the bladder when a sudden strong need to urinate is felt — compare STRESS INCONTINENCE

ur·gen·cy \ˈər-jən-sē\ *n, pl* **-cies** : a sudden compelling desire to urinate or defecate

ur·gin·ea \ər-ˈji-nē-ə\ *n* **1** *cap* : a genus of bulbous herbs native to the Old World and esp. to the Mediterranean region — see SQUILL **2** *often cap* : the sliced young bulb of an Asian plant of the genus *Urginea* (*U. indica*) with the same properties and uses as those of squill (*U. maritima*)

URI *abbr* upper respiratory infection

-uria \ˈyu̇r-ē-ə, ˈu̇r-\ *n comb form* **1** : presence of (a specified substance) in urine ⟨albumin*uria*⟩ **2** : condition of having (such) urine ⟨poly*uria*⟩; *esp* : abnormal or diseased condition marked by the presence of (a specified substance) ⟨py*uria*⟩

uric \ˈyu̇r-ik\ *adj* : of, relating to, or found in urine

uric- *or* **urico-** *comb form* : uric acid ⟨*urico*suric⟩

uric acid *n* : a white odorless and tasteless nearly insoluble acid $C_5H_4N_4O_3$ that is present in small quantity in human urine and occurs pathologically in renal calculi and the tophi of gout

uric•ac•id•uria \ˌyu̇r-ik-ˌa-sə-ˈdu̇r-ē-ə, -ˈdyu̇r-\ *n* : the presence of excess uric acid in the urine

uri•cae•mia *chiefly Brit var of* URICEMIA

uri•ce•mia \ˌyu̇r-ə-ˈsē-mē-ə\ *n* : HYPERURICEMIA — **uri•ce•mic** \-mik\ *adj*

uri•co•su•ria \ˌyu̇r-i-kə-ˈsu̇r-ē-ə, -ˈshu̇r-\ *n* : the excretion of uric acid in the urine esp. in excessive amounts

uri•co•su•ric \ˌyu̇r-i-kə-ˈsu̇r-ik, -ˈshu̇r-\ *adj* : relating to or promoting uricosuria — **uricosuric** *n*

uri•dine \ˈyu̇r-ə-ˌdēn\ *n* : a ribonucleoside $C_9H_{12}N_2O_6$ containing uracil in the form of phosphate derivatives that plays an important role in carbohydrate metabolism

urin- *or* **urino-** *comb form* : UR- ⟨*urinary*⟩

urinae — see DETRUSOR URINAE

uri•nal \ˈyu̇r-ən-ᵊl\ *n* **1** : a vessel into which a bedridden person urinates **2** : a container worn by a person with urinary incontinence

uri•nal•y•sis \ˌyu̇r-ə-ˈna-lə-səs\ *n, pl* **-y•ses** \-ˌsēz\ : chemical analysis of urine

uri•nary \ˈyu̇r-ə-ˌner-ē\ *adj* **1** : relating to, occurring in, or constituting the organs concerned with the formation and discharge of urine ⟨~ infections⟩ **2** : of, relating to, or used for urine **3** : excreted as or in urine

urinary bladder *n* : a distensible membranous sac that serves for the temporary retention of the urine, is situated in the pelvis in front of the rectum, receives the urine from the two ureters and discharges it at intervals into the urethra through an orifice closed by a sphincter

urinary calculus *n* : a calculus occurring in any portion of the urinary tract and esp. in the pelvis of the kidney — called also *urinary stone, urolith*

urinary system *n* : the organs of the urinary tract comprising the kidneys, ureters, urinary bladder, and urethra

urinary tract *n* : the tract through which urine passes and which consists of the renal tubules and renal pelvis, the ureters, the bladder, and the urethra

uri•nate \ˈyu̇r-ə-ˌnāt\ *vb* **-nat•ed; -nat•ing** : to discharge urine

uri•na•tion \ˌyu̇r-ə-ˈnā-shən\ *n* : the act of urinating — called also *micturition*

urine \ˈyu̇r-ən\ *n* : waste material that is secreted by the kidney, is rich in end products (as urea, uric acid, and creatinine) of protein metabolism together with salts and pigments, and forms a clear amber and usu. slightly acid fluid

uri•nif•er•ous tubule \ˌyu̇r-ə-ˈni-fə-rəs-\ *n* : a tubule of the kidney that collects or conducts urine

uri•no•ma \ˌyu̇r-ə-ˈnō-mə\ *n, pl* **-mas** *also* **-ma•ta** \-mə-tə\ : a cyst that contains urine

uri•nom•e•ter \ˌyu̇r-ə-ˈnä-mə-tər\ *n* : a small hydrometer for determining the specific gravity of urine

uro- — see UR-

uro•bi•lin \ˌyu̇r-ə-ˈbī-lən\ *n* : any of several brown bile pigments formed from urobilinogens and found in normal feces, in normal urine in small amounts, and in pathological urines in larger amounts

uro•bi•lin•o•gen \ˌyu̇r-ə-bī-ˈli-nə-jən, -ˌjen\ *n* : any of several chromogens that are reduction products of bilirubin

uro•ca•nic acid \ˌyu̇r-ə-ˈkā-nik-, -ˈka-\ *n* : a crystalline acid $C_6H_6N_2O_2$ normally present in human skin that is held to act as a screening agent for ultraviolet radiation

uro•dy•nam•ics \ˌyu̇r-ə-dī-ˈna-miks\ *n* : the hydrodynamics of the urinary tract — **uro•dy•nam•ic** \-mik\ *adj* — **uro•dy•nam•i•cal•ly** \-mi-k(ə-)lē\ *adv*

uro•ep•i•the•li•um \ˌyu̇r-ō-ˌe-pə-ˈthē-lē-əm\ *n* : UROTHELIUM — **uro•ep•i•the•li•al** \-əl\ *adj*

uro•er•y•thrin \ˌyu̇r-ō-ˈer-ə-thrən\ *n* : a pink or reddish pigment found in many pathological urines and also frequently in normal urine in very small quantity

uro•gas•trone \ˌyu̇r-ə-ˈgas-ˌtrōn\ *n* : a polypeptide that has been isolated from urine and inhibits gastric secretion

uro•gen•i•tal \ˌyu̇r-ō-ˈje-nə-tᵊl\ *adj* : of, relating to, affecting, treating, or being the organs or functions of excretion and reproduction : GENITOURINARY

urogenital diaphragm *n* : a double layer of pelvic fascia with its included muscle that is situated between the ischial and pubic rami, supports the prostate in the male, is traversed by the vagina in the female, gives passage to the membranous part of the urethra, and encloses the sphincter urethrae

urogenital sinus *n* : the ventral part of the embryonic mammalian cloaca that eventually forms the neck of the bladder and some of the more distal portions of the genitourinary tract

urogenital system *n* : GENITOURINARY TRACT

urogenital tract *n* : GENITOURINARY TRACT

uro•gram \ˈyu̇r-ə-ˌgram\ *n* : a radiograph made by urography

urog•ra•phy \yu̇-ˈrä-grə-fē\ *n, pl* **-phies** : radiography of a part of the urinary tract (as a kidney or ureter) after injection of a radiopaque substance — **uro•graph•ic** \ˌyu̇r-ə-ˈgra-fik\ *adj*

uro•gy•ne•col•o•gist \ˌyu̇r-ō-ˌgī-nə-ˈkä-lə-jəst\ *n* : a specialist in urogynecology

uro•gy•ne•col•o•gy \-ˈkä-lə-jē\ *n, pl* **-gies** : a branch of medicine concerned with the urological problems (as urinary incontinence) of women — **uro·gy·ne·co·log·ic** \-kə-ˈlä-jik\ *or* **uro·gy·ne·co·log·i·cal** \-ji-kəl\ *adj*

uro·ki·nase \ˌyu̇r-ō-ˈkī-ˌnās, -ˌnāz\ *n* : an enzyme that is produced by the kidney and is found in urine, that activates plasminogen, and that is used therapeutically to dissolve blood clots (as in the heart)

uro·lag·nia \ˌyu̇r-ō-ˈlag-nē-ə\ *n* : sexual excitement associated with urine or with urination

uro·lith \ˈyu̇r-ə-ˌlith\ *n* : URINARY CALCULUS

uro·lith·ia·sis \ˌyu̇r-ə-li-ˈthī-ə-səs\ *n, pl* **-ia·ses** \-ˌsēz\ : a condition that is characterized by the formation or presence of calculi in the urinary tract

urol·o·gist \yu̇-ˈrä-lə-jist\ *n* : a physician who specializes in urology

urol·o·gy \-jē\ *n, pl* **-gies** : a branch of medicine dealing with the urinary or urogenital organs — **uro·log·i·cal** \ˌyu̇r-ə-ˈlä-ji-kəl\ *also* **uro·log·ic** \-ˈlä-jik\ *adj*

uro·patho·gen·ic \ˌyu̇r-ō-ˌpa-thə-ˈje-nik\ *adj* : of, relating to, or being a pathogen (as some strains of E. coli) of the urinary tract — **uro·patho·gen** \-ˈpa-thə-jən\ *n*

urop·a·thy \yu̇-ˈrä-pə-thē\ *n, pl* **-thies** : a disease of the urinary or urogenital organs — **uro·path·ic** \ˌyu̇r-ə-ˈpa-thik\ *adj*

uro·pep·sin \ˌyu̇r-ō-ˈpep-sən\ *n* : a proteolytic hormone found in urine esp. in cases of peptic ulcers and other disorders of the digestive tract

uro·por·phy·rin \ˌyu̇r-ō-ˈpȯr-fə-rən\ *n* : any of four isomeric porphyrins $C_{40}H_{38}N_4O_{16}$ closely related to the coproporphyrins

uro·ra·di·ol·o·gy \ˌyu̇r-ō-ˌrā-dē-ˈä-lə-jē\ *n, pl* **-gies** : radiology of the urinary tract — **uro·ra·dio·log·ic** \-ˌrā-dē-ə-ˈlä-jik\ *adj*

uros·co·py \yu̇r-ˈäs-kə-pē\ *n, pl* **-pies** : examination or analysis of the urine

uro·sep·sis \ˌyu̇r-ō-ˈsep-səs\ *n, pl* **-sep·ses** \-ˌsēz\ : sepsis caused by an infection originating in the urinary tract that is typically associated with gram-negative bacteria (as E. coli) and may become life-threatening

uros·to·my \yu̇-ˈräs-tə-mē\ *n, pl* **-mies** : an ostomy for the elimination of urine from the body

uro·the·li·um \ˌyu̇r-ə-ˈthē-lē-əm\ *n* : the transitional epithelium that lines most structures of the urinary tract — called also *uroepithelium* — **uro·the·li·al** \-əl\ *adj*

ur·so·de·oxy·cho·lic acid \ˌər-sō-dē-ˌäk-sē-ˈkō-lik-\ *n* : URSODIOL

ur·so·di·ol \ˌər-sō-ˈdī-ˌȯl, -ˌōl\ *n* : a bile acid $C_{24}H_{40}O_4$ stereoisomeric with chenodeoxycholic acid that is taken orally to dissolve uncalcified radiolucent gallstones and to treat primary biliary cirrhosis — called also *ursodeoxycholic acid*

ur·ti·ca \ˈər-ti-kə\ *n* **1** *cap* : a genus of widely distributed plants (family Urticaceae, the nettle family) comprising the nettles with leaves having stinging hairs **2** : NETTLE 1

ur·ti·car·ia \ˌər-tə-ˈkar-ē-ə\ *n* : HIVES — **ur·ti·car·i·al** \-ē-əl\ *adj*

urticaria pig·men·to·sa \-ˌpig-mən-ˈtō-sə, -(ˌ)men-, -zə\ *n* : a skin disorder usu. occurring in children that is caused by the proliferation of mast cells and is marked by small itchy reddish-brown spots or bumps on the skin

urticata — see ACNE URTICATA

uru·shi·ol \yu̇-ˈrü-shē-ˌȯl, -ˌōl\ *n* : an oily toxic irritant mixture present in poison ivy and some related plants of the genus *Rhus*

USAN *abbr* United States Adopted Names — used to designate officially recognized nonproprietary names of drugs as established by a joint committee of medical and pharmaceutical professionals

Ush·er syndrome \ˈə-shər-\ *also* **Ush·er's syndrome** \-shərz-\ *n* : a genetic disease that is characterized by congenital deafness or progressive hearing loss during childhood and by retinitis pigmentosa and that is inherited chiefly as an autosomal recessive trait

Usher, Charles Howard (1865–1942), British ophthalmologist.

us·nic acid \ˈəs-nik-\ *n* : a yellow crystalline antibiotic $C_{18}H_{16}O_7$ that is obtained from various lichens (as *Usnea barbata*)

USP *abbr* United States Pharmacopeia

USPSTF *abbr* U.S. Preventive Services Task Force

uste·kin·u·mab \ˌyü-stə-ˈkin-ü-ˌmab\ *n* : an immunosuppressive drug that is a genetically engineered monoclonal antibody administered by injection to treat psoriasis and psoriatic arthritis — see STELARA

uta \ˈü-tə\ *n* : mucocutaneous leishmaniasis occurring in the highlands of Peru and Argentina — compare ESPUNDIA

ut dict *abbr* [Latin *ut dictum*] as directed — used in writing prescriptions

uter- *or* **utero-** *for 2,* ˌyü-tə-rō\ *comb form* **1** : uterus ⟨*utero*salpingography⟩ **2** : uterine and ⟨*utero*placental⟩

uteri *pl of* UTERUS

uteri — see CERVIX UTERI, CORPUS UTERI

uter·ine \ˈyü-tə-rən, -ˌrīn\ *adj* : of, relating to, occurring in, or affecting the uterus ⟨~ tissue⟩ ⟨~ cancer⟩

uterine artery *n* : an artery that arises from the internal iliac artery and supplies the uterus and adjacent parts and during pregnancy the placenta

uterine gland *n* : any of the branched tubular glands in the mucous membrane of the uterus

uterine plexus *n* : a plexus of veins tributary to the internal iliac vein by which blood is returned from the uterus

uterine tube *n* : FALLOPIAN TUBE

uterine vein *n* : any of the veins that make up the uterine plexus

utero–ovar·ian \ˌyü-tə-(ˌ)rō-ō-ˈvar-ē-ən\ *adj* : of or relating to the uterus and the ovary ⟨~ blood flow⟩

utero·pla·cen·tal \-plə-ˈsent-ᵊl\ *adj* : of or relating to the uterus and the placenta ⟨~ circulation⟩

utero·sa·cral ligament \ˌyü-tə-rō-ˈsa-krəl-, -ˈsā-\ *n* : a fibrous fascial band on each side of the uterus that passes along the lateral wall of the pelvis from the uterine cervix to the sacrum and that serves to support the uterus and hold it in place — called also *sacrouterine ligament*

utero·sal·pin·gog·ra·phy \-ˌsal-ˌpiŋ-ˈgä-grə-fē\ *n, pl* **-phies** : HYSTEROSALPINGOGRAPHY

utero·ton·ic \ˌyü-tə-rō-ˈtä-nik\ *adj* : stimulating muscular tone in the uterus ⟨a ~ substance⟩

utero·tub·al \-ˈtü-bəl, -ˈtyü-\ *adj* : of or relating to the uterus and fallopian tubes ⟨the ~ junction⟩

utero·vag·i·nal \-ˈva-jən-ᵊl\ *adj* : of or relating to the uterus and the vagina

utero·ves·i·cal pouch \-ˈve-si-kəl-\ *n* : a pouch formed by the peritoneum between the uterus and the bladder

uter·us \ˈyü-tə-rəs\ *n, pl* **uteri** \-ˌrī\ *also* **uter·us·es** : an organ in female mammals for containing and usu. for nourishing the young during development prior to birth that has thick walls consisting of an outer serous layer, a very thick middle layer of smooth muscle, and an inner mucous layer containing numerous glands — called also *womb;* see CERVIX 2a, CORPUS UTERI, FUNDUS c

UTI \ˌyü-ˌtē-ˈī\ *n or abbr* : a urinary tract infection

utilization review *n* : the critical evaluation (as by a physician or nurse) of health-care services provided to patients that is made esp. for the purpose of controlling costs and monitoring quality of care

utri·cle \ˈyü-tri-kəl\ *n* : a small anatomical pouch: as **a** : the part of the membranous labyrinth of the ear into which the semicircular canals open and that contains the macula utriculi — called also *utriculus* **b** : PROSTATIC UTRICLE — **utric·u·lar** \yu̇-ˈtri-kyə-lər\ *adj*

utriculi — see MACULA UTRICULI

utric·u·lo·sac·cu·lar duct \yu̇-ˌtri-kyə-lō-ˈsa-kyə-lər-\ *n* : a narrow tube connecting the utricle to the saccule in the membranous labyrinth of the ear

utric·u·lus \yu̇-ˈtri-kyə-ləs\ *n, pl* **-li** \-ˌlī\ : UTRICLE a

UV *abbr* ultraviolet

UVA \ˌyü-ˌvē-ˈā\ *n* : radiation that is in the region of the ultraviolet spectrum which is nearest to visible light and extends from about 320 to 400 nm in wavelength and from which comes the radiation that causes tanning and contributes to aging of the skin

UVB \-ˈbē\ *n* : radiation that is in the region of the ultraviolet spectrum which extends from about 280 to 320 nm in wavelength and that is primarily responsible for sunburn, aging of the skin, and the development of skin cancer

UVC \-ˈsē\ *n* : radiation that is in the region of the ultraviolet spectrum which extends from about 200 to 280 nm in wavelength and that is more hazardous than UVB but is mostly absorbed by the earth's upper atmosphere

uvea \ˈyü-vē-ə\ *n* : the middle layer of the eye consisting of the iris and ciliary body together with the choroid coat — called also *vascular tunic* — **uve·al** \ˈyü-vē-əl\ *adj*

uve·itis \ˌyü-vē-ˈī-təs\ *n, pl* **uve·it·i·des** \-ˈi-tə-ˌdēz\ : inflammation of the uvea

uveo·pa·rot·id fever \ˌyü-vē-ō-pə-ˈrä-təd-\ *n* : chronic inflammation of the parotid gland and uvea that is typically associated with sarcoidosis and is marked esp. by low-grade fever, facial swelling, and paralysis of the facial nerves — called also *Heerfordt's syndrome*

UV index *n* : a number on a scale which extends indefinitely upward from a baseline of 0 and whose values express the intensity of solar ultraviolet radiation at noon on a given day for a particular location with 0 indicating negligible ultraviolet exposure and values over 10 indicating very high ultraviolet exposure

uvu·la \ˈyü-vyə-lə\ *n, pl* **-las** \-ləz\ *or* **-lae** \-ˌlē\ **1** : the pendent fleshy lobe in the middle of the posterior border of the soft palate **2** : a lobe of the inferior vermis of the cerebellum located in front of the pyramid — **uvu·lar** \-lər\ *adj*

uvu·lec·to·my \ˌyü-vyə-ˈlek-tə-mē\ *n, pl* **-mies** : surgical excision of the uvula

U wave \ˈyü-ˌ\ *n* : a positive wave following the T wave on an electrocardiogram

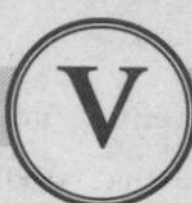

V *symbol* vanadium
vac·ci·nal \ˈvak-sən-ᵊl, vak-ˈsēn-\ *adj* : of or relating to vaccine or vaccination ⟨∼ control of a disease⟩
vac·ci·nate \ˈvak-sə-ˌnāt\ *vb* **-nat·ed; -nat·ing** : to administer a vaccine to usu. by injection — **vac·ci·na·tor** \-ˌnā-tər\ *n*
vac·ci·na·tion \ˌvak-sə-ˈnā-shən\ *n* **1** : the act of vaccinating **2** : the scar left by vaccinating
vac·cine \vak-ˈsēn, ˈvak-ˌ\ *n* : a preparation of killed microorganisms, living attenuated organisms, or living fully virulent organisms that is administered to produce or artificially increase immunity to a particular disease; *also* : a mixture of several such vaccines
vac·ci·nee \ˌvak-sə-ˈnē\ *n* : a vaccinated individual
vac·cin·ia \vak-ˈsi-nē-ə\ *n* **1 a** : COWPOX **b** : a reaction to smallpox vaccine prepared from live vaccinia virus that may involve a rash, fever, headache, and body pain **2** : a poxvirus of the genus *Orthopoxvirus* (species *Vaccinia virus*) that differs from but is closely related to the viruses causing smallpox and cowpox and that includes a strain of uncertain natural origin used in making vaccines against smallpox — called also *vaccinia virus* — **vac·cin·i·al** \-nē-əl\ *adj*
vac·u·o·lat·ed \ˈva-kyü-ō-ˌlā-təd\ *or* **vac·u·o·late** \-ˌlāt\ *adj* : containing one or more vacuoles
vac·u·o·la·tion \ˌva-kyü-ō-ˈlā-shən\ *n* : the development or formation of vacuoles ⟨neuronal ∼⟩
vac·u·ole \ˈva-kyü-ˌōl\ *n* **1** : a small cavity or space in the tissues of an organism containing air or fluid **2** : a cavity or vesicle in the cytoplasm of a cell usu. containing fluid — **vac·u·o·lar** \ˌva-kyü-ˈō-lər, -ˌlär\ *adj*
vac·u·ol·i·za·tion \ˌva-kyü-ˌō-lə-ˈzā-shən\ *n* : VACUOLATION
vac·uum aspiration \ˈva-(ˌ)kyüm-, -kyəm-\ *n* : a method of abortion performed in the later half of the first trimester of pregnancy by aspiration of the contents of the uterus through a narrow tube — **vacuum aspirator** *n*
VAD \ˌvē-(ˌ)ā-ˈdē\ *abbr or n* : VENTRICULAR ASSIST DEVICE
vag- *or* **vago-** *comb form* : vagus nerve ⟨*vago*tomy⟩ ⟨*vago*tonia⟩
va·gal \ˈvā-gəl\ *adj* : of, relating to, mediated by, or being the vagus nerve — **va·gal·ly** *adv*
vagal escape *n* : resumption of the heartbeat that takes place after stimulation of the vagus nerve has caused it to stop and that occurs despite the continuing of such stimulation
vagal tone *n* : impulses from the vagus nerve producing inhibition of the heartbeat
vagi *pl of* VAGUS
vagin- *also* **vagini-** *comb form* : vagina ⟨*vagin*ectomy⟩
va·gi·na \və-ˈjī-nə\ *n, pl* **-nae** \-(ˌ)nē\ *or* **-nas** : a canal in a female mammal that leads from the uterus to the external orifice opening into the vestibule between the labia minora
vaginae — see SPHINCTER VAGINAE
va·gi·nal \ˈva-jən-ᵊl, və-ˈjī-nᵊl\ *adj* **1** : of, relating to, or resembling a vagina : THECAL **2 a** : of, relating to, or affecting the genital vagina ⟨∼ discharge⟩ ⟨∼ infection⟩ **b** : occurring through the birth canal ⟨a ∼ delivery⟩ ⟨a ∼ birth⟩ — **va·gi·nal·ly** *adv*
vaginal artery *n* : any of the several arteries that supply the vagina and that usu. arise from the internal iliac artery or the uterine artery
vaginal hysterectomy *n* : a hysterectomy performed through the vagina
Vaginalis — see PROCESSUS VAGINALIS, TUNICA VAGINALIS
vaginal process *n* **1** : a projecting lamina of bone on the inferior surface of the petrous portion of the temporal bone that is continuous with the tympanic plate and surrounds the root of the styloid process **2** : either of a pair of projecting laminae on the inferior surface of the sphenoid that articulate with the alae of the vomer
vaginal smear *n* : a smear taken from the vaginal mucosa for cytological diagnosis
vaginal thrush *n* : candidiasis of the vagina or vulva
vag·i·nec·to·my \ˌva-jə-ˈnek-tə-mē\ *n, pl* **-mies** : partial or complete surgical excision of the vagina — called also *colpectomy*
vag·i·nis·mus \ˌva-jə-ˈniz-məs\ *n* : a painful spasmodic contraction of the vagina
vag·i·ni·tis \ˌva-jə-ˈnī-təs\ *n, pl* **-nit·i·des** \-ˈni-tə-ˌdēz\ **1** : inflammation of the vagina (as from bacterial or fungal infection, allergic reaction, or hormone deficiency) that may be marked by irritation and vaginal discharge — see ATROPHIC VAGINITIS, BACTERIAL VAGINOSIS, TRICHOMONIASIS **2** : inflammation of a sheath (as a tendon sheath)
vag·i·no·plas·ty \ˈva-jə-nə-ˌplas-tē\ *n, pl* **-ties** : plastic surgery of the vagina
vag·i·no·sis \ˌva-jə-ˈnō-səs\ *n, pl* **-no·ses** \-ˌsēz\ : an abnormal or diseased condition of the vagina; *specif* : BACTERIAL VAGINOSIS
vago- — see VAG-
va·go·lyt·ic \ˌvā-gə-ˈli-tik\ *adj* : PARASYMPATHOLYTIC ⟨∼ effects⟩
va·got·o·my \vā-ˈgä-tə-mē\ *n, pl* **-mies** : surgical division of the vagus nerve — **va·got·o·mize** \-ˌmīz\ *vb*
va·go·to·nia \ˌvā-gə-ˈtō-nē-ə\ *n* : excessive excitability of the vagus nerve

resulting typically in vasomotor instability, constipation, and sweating — compare SYMPATHICOTONIA — **va·go·ton·ic** \-ˈtä-nik\ *adj*

va·go–va·gal \ˌvā-gō-ˈvā-gəl\ *adj* : relating to or arising from both afferent and efferent impulses of the vagus nerve ⟨a ~ reflex⟩

va·gus \ˈvā-gəs\ *n, pl* **va·gi** \ˈvā-ˌgī, -ˌjī\ : VAGUS NERVE

vagus nerve *n* : either of the tenth pair of cranial nerves that arise from the medulla and supply chiefly the viscera esp. with autonomic sensory and motor fibers — called also *pneumogastric nerve, tenth cranial nerve, vagus*

Val *abbr* valine

val·a·cy·clo·vir \ˌva-lə-ˈsī-klō-ˌvir\ *n* : a prodrug of acyclovir that is administered orally in the form of its hydrochloride $C_{13}H_{20}N_6O_4·HCl$ to treat shingles, genital herpes, and cold sores — see VALTREX

val·de·cox·ib \ˌval-də-ˈkäk-sib\ *n* : a COX-2 inhibitor $C_{16}H_{14}N_2O_3S$ used esp. to treat osteoarthritis, rheumatoid arthritis, and primary dysmenorrhea but withdrawn from sale by the manufacturer because of its link to cardiovascular events (as heart attack) and severe skin rashes — see BEXTRA

va·lence \ˈvā-ləns\ *n* **1** : the degree of combining power of an atom as shown by the number of electrons in its outermost energy level that are lost, gained, or shared in the formation of chemical bonds **2** : relative capacity to unite, react, or interact (as with antigens or a biological substrate)

-va·lent \ˈvā-lənt\ *adj comb form* : having (so many) chromosomal strands or homologous chromosomes ⟨bi*valent*⟩

va·le·ri·an \və-ˈlir-ē-ən\ *n* : a preparation of the dried rhizome and roots of a perennial herb (*Valeriana officinalis* of the family Valerianaceae, the valerian family) that is used as an herbal remedy esp. to relieve insomnia and anxiety — called also *valerian root*

valgum — see GENU VALGUM

val·gus \ˈval-gəs\ *adj* **1** : turned outward; *esp* : of, relating to, or being a deformity in which an anatomical part is turned outward away from the midline of the body to an abnormal degree ⟨~ deformity of the big toe⟩ ⟨a ~ heel⟩ — see CUBITUS VALGUS, HALLUX VALGUS, TALIPES VALGUS; compare GENU VALGUM, GENU VARUM **2** : VARUS 1 — used esp. in orthopedics of the knee — **valgus** *n*

va·line \ˈvā-ˌlēn, ˈva-\ *n* : a crystalline essential amino acid $C_5H_{11}NO_2$ — abbr. *Val*

val·in·o·my·cin \ˌva-lə-nō-ˈmīs-ᵊn\ *n* : an antibiotic $C_{54}H_{90}N_6O_{18}$ produced by a bacterium of the genus *Streptomyces* (*S. fulvissimus*)

Val·ium \ˈva-lē-əm, ˈval-yəm\ *trademark* — used for a preparation of diazepam

val·late \ˈva-ˌlāt\ *adj* : having a raised edge surrounding a depression

vallate papilla *n* : CIRCUMVALLATE PAPILLA

val·lec·u·la \va-ˈle-kyə-lə\ *n, pl* **-lae** \-ˌlē\ : an anatomical groove, channel, or depression: as **a** : a groove between the base of the tongue and the epiglottis **b** : a fossa on the underside of the cerebellum separating the hemispheres and including the inferior vermis — **val·lec·u·lar** \-lər\ *adj*

valley fever *n* : COCCIDIOIDOMYCOSIS

val·pro·ate \val-ˈprō-ˌāt\ *n* : a salt or ester of valproic acid; *esp* : SODIUM VALPROATE

val·pro·ic acid \val-ˈprō-ik-\ *n* : a carboxylic acid $C_8H_{16}O_2$ used as an anticonvulsant often in the form of its sodium salt $C_8H_{15}NaO_2$ — see DEPAKENE, SODIUM VALPROATE

Val·sal·va maneuver \val-ˈsal-və-\ *also* **Val·sal·va's maneuver** \-vəz-\ *n* : a forceful attempt at expiration when the airway is closed at some point; *esp* : a conscious effort made while holding the nostrils closed and keeping the mouth shut (as for the purpose of adjusting middle ear pressure or aborting supraventricular tachycardia) — called also *Valsalva*

A. M. Valsalva — see SINUS OF VALSALVA

val·sar·tan \val-ˈsär-ˌtan\ *n* : an antihypertensive drug $C_{24}H_{29}N_5O_3$ that is taken orally and blocks the action of angiotensin II — see DIOVAN, EXFORGE

Val·trex \ˈval-ˌtreks\ *trademark* — used for a preparation of the hydrochloride of valacyclovir

val·va \ˈval-və\ *n, pl* **val·vae** \-ˌvē\ : VALVE

valve \ˈvalv\ *n* **1** : a bodily structure (as the mitral valve) that closes temporarily a passage or orifice or permits movement of fluid in one direction only **2** : any of various mechanical devices by which the flow of liquid (as blood) may be started, stopped, or regulated by a movable part that opens, shuts, or partially obstructs one or more ports or passageways; *also* : the movable part of such a device

valves of Kerk·ring *or* **valves of Kerck·ring** \-ˈker-kriŋ\ *n pl* : PLICAE CIRCULARES

Kerck·ring \ˈker-kriŋ\, **Theodor (1640–1693)**, Dutch anatomist.

val·vot·o·my \val-ˈvä-tə-mē\ *n, pl* **-mies** : VALVULOTOMY

valvul- *or* **valvulo-** *comb form* : small valve : fold ⟨*valvul*itis⟩ ⟨*valvulo*tome⟩

val·vu·la \ˈval-vyə-lə\ *n, pl* **-lae** \-ˌlē, -ˌlī\ : a small valve or fold

valvulae con·ni·ven·tes \-ˌkä-nə-ˈven-ˌtēz\ *n pl* : PLICAE CIRCULARES

val·vu·lar \ˈval-vyə-lər\ *adj* **1** : resembling or functioning as a valve **2** : of, relating to, or affecting a valve esp. of the heart ⟨~ heart disease⟩

val•vu•li•tis \ˌval-vyə-ˈlī-təs\ *n* : inflammation of a valve esp. of the heart

val•vu•lo•plas•ty \ˈval-vyə-lō-ˌplas-tē\ *n, pl* **-ties** : plastic surgery performed on a heart valve

val•vu•lo•tome \ˈval-vyə-lō-ˌtōm\ *n* : a surgical blade designed for valvulotomy or commissurotomy

val•vu•lot•o•my \ˌval-vyə-ˈlä-tə-mē\ *n, pl* **-mies** : surgical incision of a valve; *specif* : the operation of enlarging a narrowed heart valve by cutting through the mitral commissures with a knife or by a finger thrust to relieve the symptoms of mitral stenosis

vampire bat *n* : any of several Central and So. American bats (*Desmodus rotundus*, *Diaemus youngi*, and *Diphylla ecaudata*) that feed on the blood of birds and mammals and esp. domestic animals and that are sometimes vectors of disease and esp. of rabies; *also* : any of several other bats that do not feed on blood but are sometimes reputed to do so

va•na•di•um \və-ˈnā-dē-əm\ *n* : a grayish malleable ductile metallic element — symbol *V*; see ELEMENT table

Van•ce•nase \ˈvan-sə-ˌnāz\ *trademark* — used for a preparation of the dipropionate of beclomethasone administered as a nasal spray

Van•ce•ril \ˈvan-sə-ˌril\ *trademark* — used for a preparation of the dipropionate of beclomethasone for oral inhalation

Van•co•cin \ˈvan-kə-ˌsin\ *trademark* — used for a preparation of vancomycin

van•co•my•cin \ˌvaŋ-kə-ˈmīs-ᵊn\ *n* : an antibiotic $C_{66}H_{75}Cl_2N_9O_{24}$ derived from an actinomycete (*Amycolatopsis orientalis* syn. *Streptomyces orientalis* syn. *Nocardia orientalis*) that is effective against gram-positive bacteria and is used chiefly in the form of its hydrochloride $C_{66}H_{75}Cl_2N_9O_{24}{\cdot}HCl$ against staphylococci resistant to methicillin — see VANCOCIN

vancomycin–resistant enterococcus *n* : any of several bacteria of the genus *Enterococcus* (as *E. faecalis* and *E. faecium*) that are resistant to vancomycin and other commonly used antibiotics (as cephalosporin and tetracycline), are typically benign colonizers of the gastrointestinal tract and female genital tract but may cause severe infections (as of the urinary tract or bloodstream) esp. in hospitalized patients with weakened immune systems and in individuals who are on long-term regimens of antibiotics, and are usu. spread by direct contact with contaminated hands, surfaces, or medical equipment — abbr. *VRE*

van den Bergh test \ˈvan-dən-ˌbərg-\ *also* **van den Bergh's test** \-ˌbərgz-\ *n* : a test indicating presence of bilirubin in the blood (as in jaundice)

Van den Bergh, Albert Abraham Hijmans (1869–1943), Dutch physician.

van•il•lyl•man•de•lic acid \ˌva-nə-ˌlil-man-ˈdē-lik-\ *n* : a principal catecholamine metabolite $C_9H_{10}O_5$ whose presence in excess in the urine is used as a test for pheochromocytoma — abbr. *VMA*

van•il•man•de•lic acid \ˌvan-ᵊl-man-ˈdē-lik-\ *n* : VANILLYLMANDELIC ACID

vape \ˈvāp\ *vb* **vaped; vap•ing** : to inhale vapor through the mouth from a usu. battery-operated electronic device that heats up and vaporizes a physiologically-active substance (as nicotine or THC) contained in a solution or as a constituent of solid material (as marijuana)

va•por \ˈvā-pər\ *n* : a substance in the gaseous state as distinguished from the liquid or solid state — **va•por•ize** \ˈvā-pə-ˌrīz\ *vb* — **va•por•iz•able** \ˌvā-pə-ˈrī-zə-bəl\ *adj*

va•por•iz•er \ˈvā-pə-ˌrī-zər\ *n* : one that vaporizes: as **a** : ATOMIZER **b** : a device for converting water or a medicated liquid into a vapor for inhalation

va•pour *chiefly Brit var of* VAPOR

Va•quez's disease \vä-ˈke-zəz-\ *n* : POLYCYTHEMIA VERA

Vaquez, Louis Henri (1860–1936), French physician.

Var \ˈvär\ *n* : a vaccine that protects against chicken pox — see VARIVAX

var•den•a•fil \vär-ˈde-nə-ˌfil\ *n* : a drug that is used in the form of its hydrated hydrochloride $C_{23}H_{32}N_6O_4S{\cdot}HCl{\cdot}3H_2O$ to treat erectile dysfunction and that functions similarly to sildenafil — see LEVITRA

va•ren•i•cline \və-ˈre-nə-klən\ *n* : a drug taken orally in the form of its tartrate $C_{13}H_{13}N_3{\cdot}C_4H_6O_6$ that is used as an aid to stop smoking and that blocks the activity of nicotine as well as reduces nicotine cravings and withdrawal symptoms — see CHANTIX

variable region *n* : the part of the polypeptide chain of a light or heavy chain of an antibody that ends in a free amino group $-NH_2$, that varies greatly in its sequence of amino acid residues from one antibody to another, and that prob. determines the conformation of the combining site which confers the specificity of the antibody for a particular antigen — called also *variable domain;* compare CONSTANT REGION

variant Creutzfeldt–Jakob disease *n* : a fatal prion disease that is held to be a variant of Creutzfeldt-Jakob disease caused by the prion associated with bovine spongiform encephalopathy and contracted by consuming infected beef or beef products — abbr. *vCJD;* called also *new variant Creutzfeldt-Jakob disease, variant CJD*

varic- *or* **varico-** *comb form* : varix ⟨*varico*sis⟩ ⟨*varico*cele⟩

var•i•ce•al \ˌvar-ə-ˈsē-əl, və-ˈri-sē-əl\ *adj* : of, relating to, or caused by varices ⟨∼ hemorrhage⟩

var·i·cel·la \ˌvar-ə-ˈse-lə\ *n* : CHICKEN POX
varicella zoster *n* : a herpesvirus that causes chicken pox and shingles — called also *varicella-zoster virus*
var·i·cel·li·form \ˌvar-ə-ˈse-lə-ˌfȯrm\ *adj* : resembling chicken pox
Var·i·cel·lo·vi·rus \ˌvar-ə-ˈse-lə-ˌvī-rəs\ *n* : a genus of herpesviruses that includes the causative agents of chicken pox, infectious bovine rhinotracheitis, pseudorabies, rhinopneumonitis, and shingles
varices *pl of* VARIX
var·i·co·cele \ˈvar-i-kō-ˌsēl\ *n* : a varicose enlargement of the veins of the spermatic cord producing a soft compressible tumor mass in the scrotum
var·i·co·cel·ec·to·my \ˌvar-i-kō-sē-ˈlek-tə-mē\ *n, pl* **-mies** : surgical treatment of varicocele by excision of the affected veins often with removal of part of the scrotum
var·i·cose \ˈvar-ə-ˌkōs\ *also* **var·i·cosed** \-ˌkōst\ *adj* **1** : abnormally swollen or dilated ⟨~ lymph vessels⟩ **2** : affected with varicose veins ⟨~ legs⟩
varicose vein *n* : an abnormal swelling and tortuosity esp. of a superficial vein of the legs — usu. used in pl.
var·i·co·sis \ˌvar-ə-ˈkō-səs\ *n, pl* **-co·ses** \-ˌsēz\ : the condition of being varicose or of having varicose vessels
var·i·cos·i·ty \ˌvar-ə-ˈkä-sə-tē\ *n, pl* **-ties** **1** : the quality or state of being abnormally or markedly swollen or dilated **2** : VARIX
Var·i·dase \ˈvar-ə-ˌdās\ *n* : a preparation containing a mixture of streptodornase and streptokinase — formerly a U.S. registered trademark
va·ri·ety \və-ˈrī-ə-tē\ *n, pl* **-et·ies** : any of various groups of plants or animals ranking below a species : SUBSPECIES
va·ri·o·la \və-ˈrī-ə-lə\ *n* : SMALLPOX; *also* : the poxvirus of the genus *Orthopoxvirus* (species *Variola virus*) that causes smallpox
variola major *n* : a severe form of smallpox characterized historically by a death rate of about 30 percent
variola minor *n* : a mild form of smallpox of low mortality — called also *alastrim*
var·i·o·la·tion \ˌvar-ē-ə-ˈlā-shən\ *n* : the deliberate inoculation of an uninfected person with the smallpox virus (as by contact with pustular matter) that was widely practiced before the era of vaccination as prophylaxis against the severe form of smallpox
variola vac·cin·ia \-vak-ˈsi-nē-ə\ *n* : COWPOX
var·i·ol·i·form \ˌvar-ē-ˈō-lə-ˌfȯrm\ *adj* : resembling smallpox
varioliformis — see PITYRIASIS LICHENOIDES ET VARIOLIFORMIS ACUTA
va·ri·o·loid \ˈvar-ē-ə-ˌlȯid, və-ˈrī-ə-ˌlȯid\ *n* : a modified mild form of smallpox occurring in persons who have been vaccinated or who have had smallpox
Var·i·vax \ˈvar-ə-ˌvaks\ *trademark* — used for a vaccine against chicken pox containing live attenuated varicella zoster
var·ix \ˈvar-iks\ *n, pl* **var·i·ces** \ˈvar-ə-ˌsēz\ : an abnormally dilated and lengthened vein, artery, or lymph vessel; *esp* : VARICOSE VEIN
Varolii — see PONS VAROLII
varum — see GENU VARUM
var·us \ˈvar-əs\ *adj* **1** : of, relating to, or being a deformity in which an anatomical part is turned inward toward the midline of the body to an abnormal degree ⟨a ~ heel⟩ — see CUBITUS VARUS, TALIPES VARUS; compare GENU VALGUM, GENU VARUM **2** : VALGUS 1 — used esp. in orthopedics of the knee — **varus** *n*
vas \ˈvas\ *n, pl* **va·sa** \ˈvā-zə\ : an anatomical vessel : DUCT
VAS *abbr* visual analog scale
vas- *or* **vaso-** *comb form* **1** : vessel: as **a** : blood vessel ⟨*vaso*motor⟩ **b** : vas deferens ⟨*vas*ectomy⟩ **2** : vascular and ⟨*vaso*vagal⟩
vasa ab·er·ran·tia \-ˌa-bə-ˈran-chə, -chē-ə\ *n pl* : slender arteries that are only occas. present and that connect the axillary or brachial artery with an artery (as the radial artery) of the forearm or with its branches
vas ab·er·rans of Hal·ler \-ˈa-bə-ˌranz . . . -ˈhä-lər\ *n, pl* **vasa ab·er·ran·tia of Haller** \-ˌa-bə-ˈran-chə-, -chē-ə-\ : a blind tube occas. present parallel to the first part of the vas deferens
Haller, Albrecht von (1708–1777), Swiss biologist.
vasa deferentia *pl of* VAS DEFERENS
vasa ef·fer·en·tia \-ˌe-fə-ˈren-chə, -chē-ə\ *n pl* : the 12 to 20 ductules that lead from the rete testis to the vas deferens and except near their commencement are greatly convoluted and form the compact head of the epididymis
va·sal \ˈvā-zəl\ *adj* : of, relating to, or constituting an anatomical vessel
vasa rec·ta \-ˈrek-tə\ *n pl* **1** : numerous small vessels that arise from the terminal branches of arteries supplying the intestine, encircle the intestine, and divide into more branches between its layers **2** : hairpin-shaped vessels that arise from the arteriole leading away from a renal glomerulus, descend into the renal pyramids, reunite as they ascend, and play a role in the concentration of urine
vasa va·so·rum \-vā-ˈsōr-əm\ *n pl* : small blood vessels that supply or drain the walls of the larger arteries and veins and connect with a branch of the same vessel or a neighboring vessel
vascul- *or* **vasculo-** *comb form* : vessel; *esp* : blood vessel ⟨*vasculo*toxic⟩
vas·cu·lar \ˈvas-kyə-lər\ *adj* **1** : of, relating to, constituting, or affecting a tube or a system of tubes for the conveyance of a body fluid (as blood or

lymph) **2** : supplied with or containing ducts and esp. blood vessels — **vas·cu·lar·i·ty** \ˌvas-kyə-ˈlar-ə-tē\ *n*

vascular bed *n* : an intricate network of minute blood vessels that ramifies through the tissues of the body or of one of its parts

vascular dementia *n* : dementia (as multi-infarct dementia) of abrupt or gradual onset that is caused by cerebrovascular disease

vascular endothelial growth factor *n* : a protein that promotes the growth of new blood vessels — abbr. *VEGF*

vascularis — see STRIA VASCULARIS

vas·cu·lar·i·za·tion \ˌvas-kyə-lə-rə-ˈzā-shən\ *n* : the process of becoming vascular; *also* : abnormal or excessive formation of blood vessels (as in the retina or on the cornea) — **vas·cu·lar·ize** \ˈvas-kyə-lə-ˌrīz\ *vb*

vascular resistance *n* : resistance to blood flow through blood vessels and esp. arterioles — see PERIPHERAL VASCULAR RESISTANCE

vascular tunic *n* : UVEA

vas·cu·la·ture \ˈvas-kyə-lə-ˌchu̇r, -ˌtyu̇r, -ˌtu̇r\ *n* : the arrangement of blood vessels in an organ or part

vas·cu·li·tis \ˌvas-kyə-ˈlī-təs\ *n, pl* **-lit·i·des** \-ˈli-tə-ˌdēz\ : inflammation of a blood or lymph vessel — **vas·cu·lit·ic** \ˌvas-kyə-ˈli-tik\ *adj*

vas·cu·lo·gen·ic \ˌvas-kyə-lō-ˈje-nik\ *adj* : caused by disorder or dysfunction of the blood vessels ⟨~ impotence⟩ ⟨~ migraine⟩

vas·cu·lo·tox·ic \ˌvas-kyə-lō-ˈtäk-sik\ *adj* : destructive to blood vessels or the vascular system ⟨~ effects⟩

vas def·er·ens \-ˈde-fə-rənz, -ˌrenz\ *n, pl* **vasa def·er·en·tia** \-ˌde-fə-ˈren-chə, -chē-ə\ : a sperm-carrying duct that is a small but thick-walled tube about two feet (0.6 meter) long that begins at and is continuous with the tail of the epididymis, runs in the spermatic cord through the inguinal canal, and descends into the pelvis where it joins the duct of the seminal vesicle to form the ejaculatory duct — called also *ductus deferens, spermatic duct*

va·sec·to·my \və-ˈsek-tə-mē, vā-ˈzek-\ *n, pl* **-mies** : surgical division or resection of all or part of the vas deferens usu. to induce sterility — **va·sec·to·mize** \-ˌmīz\ *vb*

Vas·e·line \ˌva-sə-ˈlēn\ *trademark* — used for a preparation of petroleum jelly

vaso- — see VAS-

va·so·ac·tive \ˌvā-zō-ˈak-tiv\ *adj* : affecting the blood vessels esp. in respect to the degree of their relaxation or contraction — **va·so·ac·tiv·i·ty** \-ak-ˈti-və-tē\ *n*

vasoactive intestinal peptide *n* : a protein hormone that consists of a chain of 28 amino acid residues, has been implicated as a neurotransmitter, and has a wide range of physiological activities (as stimulation of secretion by the pancreas and small intestine, vasodilation, and inhibition of gastric juice production) — abbr. *VIP;* called also *vasoactive intestinal polypeptide*

va·so·con·stric·tion \ˌvā-zō-kən-ˈstrik-shən\ *n* : narrowing of the lumen of blood vessels esp. as a result of vasomotor action — **va·so·con·stric·tive** \-ˈstrik-tiv\ *adj*

va·so·con·stric·tor \ˌvā-zō-kən-ˈstrik-tər\ *n* : an agent (as a sympathetic nerve fiber or a drug) that induces or initiates vasoconstriction — **vasoconstrictor** *adj*

va·so·de·pres·sor \ˌvā-zō-di-ˈpre-sər\ *adj* : causing or characterized by vasomotor depression resulting in lowering of the blood pressure

va·so·di·la·tion \ˌvā-zo-dī-ˈlā-shən\ *or* **va·so·di·la·ta·tion** \-ˌdi-lə-ˈtā-shən, -ˌdī-\ *n* : widening of the lumen of blood vessels

va·so·di·la·tor \ˌvā-zō-ˈdī-ˌlā-tər\ *n* : an agent (as a parasympathetic nerve fiber or a drug) that induces or initiates vasodilation — **vasodilator** *also* **va·so·di·la·to·ry** \-ˈdi-lə-ˌtōr-ē, -ˈdī-\ *adj*

va·so·for·ma·tive \ˌvā-zō-ˈfȯr-mə-tiv\ *adj* : functioning in the development and formation of vessels and esp. blood vessels ⟨~ cells⟩

va·sog·ra·phy \vā-ˈzä-grə-fē\ *n, pl* **-phies** : radiography of blood vessels

va·so·li·ga·tion \ˌvā-zō-lī-ˈgā-shən\ *n* : surgical ligation of a vessel and esp. of the vas deferens

va·so·mo·tion \ˌvā-zō-ˈmō-shən\ *n* : alteration in the caliber of blood vessels

va·so·mo·tor \ˌvā-zō-ˈmō-tər\ *adj* : of, relating to, affecting, or being nerves or the centers (as in the medulla and spinal cord) from which they arise that supply the muscle fibers of the walls of blood vessels, include sympathetic vasoconstrictors and parasympathetic vasodilators, and by their effect on vascular diameter regulate the amount of blood passing to a particular body part or organ

vasomotor rhinitis *n* : chronic rhinitis that is not attributable to allergy or infection and is marked by runny nose, nasal congestion, postnasal drip, and sometimes sneezing triggered or exacerbated by various potentially irritating stimuli (as strong odors, smoke, alcohol, or sudden temperature changes)

va·so–oc·clu·sive \-ə-ˈklü-siv\ *adj* : relating to, resulting from, or caused by occlusion of a blood vessel ⟨a ~ crisis characteristic of sickle cell anemia⟩

va·so·pres·sin \ˌvā-zō-ˈpres-ᵊn\ *n* : a polypeptide hormone that is secreted together with oxytocin by the posterior lobe of the pituitary gland, is also obtained synthetically, and increases blood pressure and exerts an antidiuretic effect — called also *antidiuretic hormone;* see ARGININE VASOPRESSIN, LYSINE VASOPRESSIN, PITRESSIN

[1]**va•so•pres•sor** \-ˈpre-sər\ *adj* : causing a rise in blood pressure by exerting a vasoconstrictor effect

[2]**vasopressor** *n* : a vasopressor agent

[1]**va•so•re•lax•ant** \-ri-ˈlak-sənt\ *adj* : relating to or producing vasorelaxation

[2]**vasorelaxant** *n* : a vasorelaxant agent

va•so•re•lax•ation \-ˌrē-ˌlak-ˈsā-shən\ *n* : reduction of vascular tension

vasorum — see VASA VASORUM

va•so•spasm \ˈvā-zō-ˌspa-zəm\ *n* : sharp and often persistent contraction of a blood vessel reducing its caliber and blood flow — **va•so•spas•tic** \ˌvā-zō-ˈspas-tik\ *adj*

Va•so•tec \ˈvā-zō-ˌtek\ *trademark* — used for a preparation of enalaprilat or the maleate of enalapril

va•sot•o•my \vā-ˈzä-tə-mē\ *n, pl* **-mies** : surgical incision of the vas deferens

va•so•va•gal \ˌvā-zō-ˈvā-gəl\ *adj* : of, relating to, or involving both vascular and vagal factors

vasovagal syncope *n* : a usu. transitory condition that is marked esp. by fainting associated with hypotension, peripheral vasodilation, and bradycardia resulting from increased stimulation of the vagus nerve — called also *neurocardiogenic syncope*

va•so•va•sos•to•my \ˌvā-zō-vā-ˈzäs-tə-mē\ *n, pl* **-mies** : surgical anastomosis of a divided vas deferens to reverse a previous vasectomy

vas•tus in•ter•me•di•us \ˈvas-təs-ˌin-tər-ˈmē-dē-əs\ *n* : the division of the quadriceps muscle that arises from and covers the front of the shaft of the femur

vastus in•ter•nus \-in-ˈtər-nəs\ *n* : VASTUS MEDIALIS

vastus lat•er•a•lis \-ˌla-tər-ˈā-ləs, -ˈa-\ *n* : the division of the quadriceps muscle that covers the outer anterior aspect of the femur, arises chiefly from the femur, and inserts into the outer border of the patella by a flat tendon — called also *vastus externus*

vastus me•di•a•lis \-ˌmē-de-ˈā-ləs, -ˈa-\ *n* : the division of the quadriceps muscle that covers the inner anterior aspect of the femur, arises chiefly from the femur and the adjacent intermuscular septum, inserts into the inner border of the patella and into the tendon of the other divisions of the muscle, sends also a tendinous expansion to the capsule of the knee joint, and is closely and in the upper part often inseparably united with the vastus intermedius — called also *vastus internus*

vault \ˈvȯlt\ *n* : an arched or dome-shaped anatomical structure: as **a** : SKULLCAP, CALVARIUM ⟨the cranial ~⟩ **b** : FORNIX d

VBAC \ˈvē-ˌbak\ *n* [*v*aginal *b*irth *a*fter *c*esarean] : delivery through the birth canal in a pregnancy subsequent to one in which delivery was by cesarean section

VCG *abbr* vectorcardiogram

vCJD *abbr* variant Creutzfeldt-Jakob disease

VD *abbr* venereal disease

VDRL \ˌvē-(ˌ)dē-(ˌ)är-ˈel\ *n* : VDRL TEST

VDRL *abbr* venereal disease research laboratory

VDRL slide test *n* : VDRL TEST

VDRL test *n* : a flocculation test for syphilis employing cardiolipin in combination with lecithin and cholesterol

[1]**vec•tor** \ˈvek-tər\ *n* **1** : a quantity that has magnitude and direction and that is usu. represented by part of a straight line with the given direction and with a length representing the magnitude **2** : an organism (as an insect) that transmits a pathogen from one organism to another ⟨fleas are ~*s* of plague⟩ — compare CARRIER 1a **3** : an agent (as a plasmid or virus) that contains or carries modified genetic material (as recombinant DNA) and can be used to introduce exogenous genes into the genome of an organism — **vec•to•ri•al** \vek-ˈtōr-ē-əl\ *adj*

[2]**vector** *vb* **vec•tored; vec•tor•ing** : to transmit (a pathogen or disease) from one organism to another : act as a vector for ⟨a disease ~*ed* by flies⟩

vec•tor•car•dio•gram \ˌvek-tər-ˈkär-dē-ə-ˌgram\ *n* : a graphic record made by vectorcardiography — abbr. *VCG*

vec•tor•car•di•og•ra•phy \-ˌkär-dē-ˈä-grə-fē\ *n, pl* **-phies** : a method of recording the direction and magnitude of the electrical forces of the heart by means of a continuous series of vectors that form a curving line around a center — **vec•tor•car•dio•graph•ic** \-dē-ə-ˈgra-fik\ *adj*

VEE *abbr* Venezuelan equine encephalitis; Venezuelan equine encephalomyelitis

veg•an \ˈvē-gən\ *n* : a strict vegetarian who consumes no animal food or dairy products — **vegan** *adj* — **veg•an•ism** \ˈvē-gə-ˌni-zəm\ *n*

veg•e•ta•ble \ˈvej-tə-bəl\ *n* : a person whose mental and physical functioning is severely impaired and esp. one who requires supportive measures (as mechanical ventilation) to survive

veg•e•tar•i•an•ism \ˌve-jə-ˈter-ē-ə-ˌni-zəm\ *n* : the theory or practice of living on a diet made up of vegetables, fruits, grains, nuts, and sometimes eggs or dairy products — **veg•e•tar•i•an** \-ˈter-ē-ən\ *n or adj*

veg•e•ta•tion \ˌve-jə-ˈtā-shən\ *n* : an abnormal outgrowth upon a body part; *specif* : any of the warty excrescences on the valves of the heart that are composed of various tissue elements including fibrin and collagen and that are typical of endocarditis

veg•e•ta•tive \ˈve-jə-ˌtā-tiv\ *adj* **1 a** (1) : growing or having the power of growing (2) : of, relating to, or engaged in nutritive and growth functions as contrasted with reproductive functions ⟨a ~ nucleus⟩ **b :** of, relating to, or involving propagation by nonsexual processes or methods **2 :** affecting, arising from, or relating to involuntary bodily functions **3 :** characterized by, resulting from, or being a state in which there is a total loss of cognitive functioning typically indicated by a lack of awareness of oneself or one's environment and in which only involuntary bodily functions (as breathing or blinking of the eyes) are sustained ⟨a ~ state⟩ — **veg•e•ta•tive•ly** *adv*

VEGF *abbr* vascular endothelial growth factor

ve•hi•cle \ˈvē-i-kəl, -ˌhi-\ *n* **1 :** an inert medium in which a medicinally active agent is administered **2 :** an agent of transmission ⟨a ~ of infection⟩

vein \ˈvān\ *n* **:** any of the tubular branching vessels that carry blood from the capillaries toward the heart and have thinner walls than the arteries and often valves at intervals to prevent reflux of the blood which flows in a steady stream and is in most cases dark-colored due to the presence of reduced hemoglobin — **veiny** \ˈvā-nē\ *adj*

vein•ous \ˈvā-nəs\ *adj* **1 :** having veins that are esp. prominent ⟨~ hands⟩ **2 :** VENOUS

vela *pl of* VELUM

Vel•cade \ˈvel-ˌkād\ *trademark* — used for a preparation of bortezomib

veli — see LEVATOR VELI PALATINI, TENSOR VELI PALATINI

ve•lo•pha•ryn•geal \ˌvē-lō-ˌfar-ən-ˈjē-əl, -fə-ˈrin-jəl, -jē-əl\ *adj* **:** of or relating to the soft palate and the pharynx

Vel•peau bandage \vel-ˈpō-\ *or* **Vel•peau's bandage** \-ˈpōz-\ *n* **:** a bandage used to support and immobilize the arm when the clavicle is fractured

Velpeau, Alfred–Armand–Louis–Marie (1795–1867), French surgeon.

ve•lum \ˈvē-ləm\ *n, pl* **ve•la** \-lə\ **:** a membrane or membranous part resembling a veil or curtain: as **a :** SOFT PALATE **b :** SEMILUNAR CUSP

ven- *or* **veni-** *or* **veno-** *comb form* **:** vein ⟨*veni*puncture⟩

ve•na ca•va \ˌvē-nə-ˈkā-və\ *n, pl* **ve•nae ca•vae** \ˌvē-nē-ˈkā-(ˌ)vē\ **:** either of two large veins by which the blood is returned to the right atrium of the heart: **a :** INFERIOR VENA CAVA **b :** SUPERIOR VENA CAVA — **vena ca•val** \-vəl\ *adj*

vena co•mi•tans \-ˈkō-mə-ˌtanz\ *n, pl* **venae co•mi•tan•tes** \-ˌkō-mə-ˈtan-ˌtēz\ **:** a vein accompanying an artery

venae cor•dis min•i•mae \-ˈkȯr-dəs-ˈmi-nə-ˌmē\ *n pl* **:** minute veins in the wall of the heart that empty into the atria or ventricles

vena vor•ti•co•sa \-ˌvȯr-tə-ˈkō-sə\ *n, pl* **venae vor•ti•co•sae** \-(ˌ)sē\ **:** any of the veins of the outer layer of the choroid of the eye — called also *vorticose vein*

ve•neer \və-ˈnir\ *n* **:** a plastic or porcelain coating bonded to the surface of a cosmetically imperfect tooth

ve•ne•re•al \və-ˈnir-ē-əl\ *adj* **1 :** resulting from or contracted during sexual intercourse ⟨~ infections⟩ **2 :** of, relating to, or affected with venereal disease ⟨a high ~ rate⟩ **3 :** involving the genital organs ⟨~ sarcoma⟩ — **ve•ne•re•al•ly** *adv*

venereal disease *n* **:** a contagious disease (as gonorrhea or syphilis) that is typically acquired in sexual intercourse — abbr. *VD;* compare SEXUALLY TRANSMITTED DISEASE

venereal wart *n* **:** GENITAL WART

ve•ne•re•ol•o•gy \və-ˌnir-ē-ˈä-lə-jē\ *also* **ven•er•ol•o•gy** \ˌve-nə-ˈrä-lə-jē\ *n, pl* **-gies :** a branch of medical science concerned with venereal diseases — **ve•ne•re•o•log•i•cal** \və-ˌnir-ē-ə-ˈlä-ji-kəl\ *adj* — **ve•ne•re•ol•o•gist** \və-ˌnir-ē-ˈä-lə-jist\ *n*

venereum — see LYMPHOGRANULOMA VENEREUM, LYMPHOPATHIA VENEREUM

veneris — see MONS VENERIS

vene•sec•tion \ˈve-nə-ˌsek-shən, ˈvē-\ *n* **:** PHLEBOTOMY

Venezuelan equine encephalitis *n* **:** EQUINE ENCEPHALITIS C

Venezuelan equine encephalomyelitis *n* **:** EQUINE ENCEPHALITIS C

veni- — see VEN-

ve•ni•punc•ture \ˈvē-nə-ˌpəŋk-chər, ˈve-\ *n* **:** surgical puncture of a vein esp. for the withdrawal of blood or for administration of intravenous fluids or drugs

venisection *var of* VENESECTION

ven•la•fax•ine \ˌven-lə-ˈfak-ˌsēn\ *n* **:** a drug that functions as an SNRI and is used in the form of its hydrochloride $C_{17}H_{27}NO_2 \cdot HCl$ esp. to treat depression, anxiety, and panic disorder — see EFFEXOR

veno- — see VEN-

ve•no•ar•te•ri•al \ˌvē-nō-är-ˈtir-ē-əl\ *adj* **:** relating to or involving an artery and vein

ve•noc•ly•sis \vē-ˈnä-klə-səs\ *n, pl* **-ly•ses** \-ˌsēz\ **:** clysis into a vein

ve•no•con•stric•tion \ˌvē-nō-kən-ˈstrik-shən\ *n* **:** constriction of a vein

ve•no•gram \ˈvē-nə-ˌgram\ *n* **:** a radiograph made by venography

ve•nog•ra•phy \vi-ˈnä-grə-fē, vā-\ *n, pl* **-phies :** radiography of a vein after injection of an opaque substance — **ve•no•graph•ic** \ˌvē-nə-ˈgra-fik\ *adj*

ven•om \ˈve-nəm\ *n* **:** a toxic substance produced by some animals (as snakes, scorpions, or bees) that is injected into prey or an enemy by biting or stinging and has an injurious or lethal effect; *broadly* **:** a substance that is poisonous

ven•om•ous \ˈve-nə-məs\ *adj* **1 :** POISONOUS **2 :** producing venom in a specialized gland and capable of inflicting injury or death ⟨~ snakes⟩

ve•no–oc•clu•sive \ˌvē-nō-ə-ˈklü-siv\ *adj* : marked by occlusion or compression of small veins ⟨~ disease⟩

venosum — see LIGAMENTUM VENOSUM

venosus — see DUCTUS VENOSUS, SINUS VENOSUS, SINUS VENOSUS SCLERAE

ve•not•o•my \vi-ˈnä-tə-mē\ *n, pl* **-mies** : PHLEBOTOMY

ve•nous \ˈvē-nəs\ *adj* **1 a** : full of or characterized by veins **b** : made up of or carried on by veins ⟨the ~ circulation⟩ **2** : of, relating to, or performing the functions of a vein ⟨a ~ inflammation⟩ **3** *of blood* : having passed through the capillaries and given up oxygen for the tissues and become charged with carbon dioxide and ready to pass through the respiratory organs to release its carbon dioxide and renew its oxygen supply : dark red from reduced hemoglobin — compare ARTERIAL 2

venous hum *n* : a humming sound sometimes heard during auscultation of the veins of the neck esp. in anemia

venous return *n* : the flow of blood from the venous system into the right atrium of the heart

venous sinus *n* **1** : a large vein or passage (as the canal of Schlemm) for venous blood **2** : SINUS VENOSUS

vent \ˈvent\ *n* : the external opening of the rectum or cloaca : ANUS

ven•ti•late \ˈvent-ᵊl-ˌāt\ *vb* **-lat•ed; -lat•ing 1** : to expose to air and esp. to a current of fresh air for purifying or refreshing **2 a** : OXYGENATE, AERATE ⟨~ blood in the lungs⟩ **b** : to subject the lungs of (an individual) to ventilation **3** : to give verbal expression to (as mental or emotional conflicts)

ven•ti•la•tion \ˌvent-ᵊl-ˈā-shən\ *n* **1** : the act or process of ventilating **2** : the circulation and exchange of gases in the lungs or gills that is basic to respiration — **ven•ti•la•to•ry** \ˈvent-ᵊl-ə-ˌtōr-ē\ *adj*

ven•ti•la•tor \ˈvent-ᵊl-ˌā-tər\ *n* : RESPIRATOR 2

Ven•to•lin \ˈven-tᵊl-ən\ *trademark* — used for a preparation of albuterol

ventr- *or* **ventri-** *or* **ventro-** *comb form* **1** : abdomen ⟨*ventral*⟩ **2** : ventral and ⟨*ventro*medial⟩

ven•tral \ˈven-trəl\ *adj* **1** : of or relating to the belly : ABDOMINAL **2 a** : being or located near, on, or toward the lower surface of an animal (as a quadruped) opposite the back or dorsal surface **b** : being or located near, on, or toward the front or anterior part of the human body — **ven•tral•ly** *adv*

ventral column *n* : VENTRAL HORN

ventral corticospinal tract *n* : a band of nerve fibers that descends in the ventrolateral part of the spinal cord and consists of fibers arising in the motor cortex of the brain on the same side of the body — called also *anterior corticospinal tract, direct pyramidal tract*

ventral funiculus *n* : a longitudinal division on each side of the spinal cord comprising white matter between the anterior median fissure and the ventral root — called also *anterior funiculus;* compare LATERAL FUNICULUS, POSTERIOR FUNICULUS

ventral gray column *n* : VENTRAL HORN

ventral horn *n* : a longitudinal subdivision of gray matter in the anterior part of each lateral half of the spinal cord that contains neurons giving rise to motor fibers of the ventral roots of the spinal nerves — called also *anterior column, anterior gray column, anterior horn, ventral column, ventral gray column;* compare DORSAL HORN, LATERAL COLUMN 1

ventralis — see SACROCOCCYGEUS VENTRALIS

ventral median fissure *n* : ANTERIOR MEDIAN FISSURE

ventral mesogastrium *n* : MESOGASTRIUM 1

ventral root *n* : the one of the two roots of a spinal nerve that passes anteriorly from the spinal cord separating the anterior and lateral funiculi and that consists of motor fibers — called also *anterior root;* compare DORSAL ROOT

ventral spinocerebellar tract *n* : SPINOCEREBELLAR TRACT b

ventral spinothalamic tract *n* : SPINOTHALAMIC TRACT a

ventral tegmental area *n* : an area of the midbrain lying adjacent to the substantia nigra that contains the cell bodies of dopaminergic neurons projecting esp. to the nucleus accumbens, amygdala, and olfactory tubercle as part of the mesolimbic system — abbr. *VTA;* called also *ventral tegmentum*

ventri- — see VENTR-

ven•tri•cle \ˈven-tri-kəl\ *n* : a cavity of a bodily part or organ: as **a** : a chamber of the heart which receives blood from a corresponding atrium and from which blood is forced into the arteries **b** : any of a system of communicating cavities in the brain that are continuous with the central canal of the spinal cord — see FOURTH VENTRICLE, LATERAL VENTRICLE, THIRD VENTRICLE **c** : a fossa or pouch on each side of the larynx between the false vocal cords above and the true vocal cords below

ven•tric•u•lar \ven-ˈtri-kyə-lər, vən-\ *adj* : of, relating to, or being a ventricle esp. of the heart or brain

ventricular assist device *n* : a device that is implanted in the chest or upper abdomen to assist the left or right ventricle in pumping blood in a damaged or weakened heart — called also *VAD*

ventricular fibrillation *n* : very rapid uncoordinated fluttering contractions of the ventricles of the heart resulting in loss of synchronization between heartbeat and pulse beat — abbr. *VF, V-fib*

ventricular folds *n pl* : FALSE VOCAL CORDS

ventricular septal defect *n* : a congenital defect in the interventricular septum — abbr. *VSD*

ventricular tachycardia *n* : tachycardia that is associated with the generation of electrical impulses within the ventricles and is characterized by an electrocardiogram having a broad QRS complex — abbr. *VT;* called also *V-tach*

ven•tric•u•li•tis \ven-ˌtri-kyə-ˈlī-təs\ *n* : inflammation of the ventricles of the brain

ven•tric•u•lo•atri•al \ven-ˌtri-kyə-lō-ˈā-trē-əl\ *adj* **1** : of, relating to, or being an artificial shunt between a ventricle of the brain and an atrium of the heart esp. to drain cerebrospinal fluid (as in hydrocephalus) **2** : of, relating to, or being conduction from the ventricle to the atrium of the heart

ven•tric•u•lo•atri•os•to•my \-ˌā-trē-ˈäs-tə-mē\ *n, pl* **-mies** : surgical establishment of a shunt to drain cerebrospinal fluid (as in hydrocephalus) from a ventricle of the brain to the right atrium

ven•tric•u•lo•cis•ter•nos•to•my \-ˌsis-tər-ˈnäs-tə-mē\ *n, pl* **-mies** : the surgical establishment of a communication between a ventricle of the brain and the subarachnoid space and esp. the cisterna magna to drain cerebrospinal fluid esp. in hydrocephalus

ven•tric•u•lo•gram \ven-ˈtri-kyə-lə-ˌgram\ *n* : an X-ray photograph made by ventriculography

ven•tric•u•log•ra•phy \ven-ˌtri-kyə-ˈlä-grə-fē\ *n, pl* **-phies** **1** : the act or process of making an X-ray photograph of the ventricles of the brain after withdrawing fluid from the ventricles and replacing it with air or a radiopaque substance **2** : the act or process of making an X-ray photograph of a ventricle of the heart after injecting a radiopaque substance — **ven•tric•u•lo•graph•ic** \-kyə-lō-ˈgra-fik\ *adj*

ven•tric•u•lo•peri•to•ne•al \ven-ˌtri-kyə-lō-ˌper-ə-tə-ˈnē-əl\ *adj* : relating to or serving to communicate between a ventricle of the brain and the peritoneal cavity ⟨a ∼ shunt⟩

ven•tric•u•los•to•my \ven-ˌtri-kyə-ˈläs-tə-mē\ *n, pl* **-mies** : the surgical establishment of an opening in a ventricle of the brain to drain cerebrospinal fluid esp. in hydrocephalus

ven•tric•u•lot•o•my \ven-ˌtri-kyə-ˈlä-tə-mē\ *n, pl* **-mies** : surgical incision of a ventricle (as of the heart)

ventro- — see VENTR-

ven•tro•lat•er•al \ˌven-ˌtrō-ˈla-tə-rəl\ *adj* : ventral and lateral — **ven•tro•lat•er•al•ly** *adv*

ven•tro•me•di•al \-ˈmē-dē-əl\ *adj* : ventral and medial — **ven•tro•me•di•al•ly** *adv*

ventromedial nucleus *n* : a medially located nucleus of the hypothalamus situated between the lateral wall of the third ventricle and the fornix

ve•nule \ˈvēn-(ˌ)yül, ˈven-\ *n* : a small vein; *esp* : any of the minute veins connecting the capillaries with the larger systemic veins — **ven•u•lar** \ˈven-yə-lər\ *adj*

vera — see ALOE VERA, DECIDUA VERA, POLYCYTHEMIA VERA

ve•rap•am•il \və-ˈra-pə-ˌmil\ *n* : a calcium channel blocker used in the form of its hydrochloride $C_{27}H_{38}N_2O_4{\cdot}HCl$ esp. to treat hypertension and angina pectoris — see CALAN

ver•a•trine \ˈver-ə-ˌtrēn\ *n* : a mixture of poisonous alkaloids that is obtained from the seeds of a Mexican plant (*Schoenocaulon officinalis*) of the lily family (Liliaceae) and has been used as a counterirritant in neuralgia and arthritis

ve•ra•trum \və-ˈrā-trəm\ *n* **1 a** *cap* : a genus of herbs having short poisonous rootstocks **b** : any hellebore of the genus *Veratrum* **2** : HELLEBORE 2b

ver•big•er•a•tion \(ˌ)vər-ˌbi-jə-ˈrā-shən\ *n* : continual repetition of stereotyped phrases (as in some forms of mental illness)

verge — see ANAL VERGE

ver•gence \ˈvər-jəns\ *n* : a movement of one eye in relation to the other

vermes *pl of* VERMIS

vermi- *comb form* : worm ⟨*vermi*cide⟩ ⟨*vermi*form⟩

ver•mi•cide \ˈvər-mə-ˌsīd\ *n* : an agent that destroys worms; *esp* : ANTHELMINTIC

ver•mi•form \ˈvər-mə-ˌfórm\ *adj* : resembling a worm in shape

vermiform appendix *n* : a narrow blind tube usu. about three or four inches (7.6 to 10.2 centimeters) long that extends from the cecum in the lower right-hand part of the abdomen and represents an atrophied terminal part of the cecum

ver•mi•fuge \ˈvər-mə-ˌfyüj\ *n* : an agent that serves to destroy or expel parasitic worms : ANTHELMINTIC — **ver•mif•u•gal** \vər-ˈmi-fyə-gəl, ˌvər-mə-ˈfyü-gəl\ *adj*

ver•mil•ion border \vər-ˈmil-yən-\ *n* : the exposed pink or reddish margin of a lip

ver•mil•ion•ec•to•my \vər-ˌmil-yə-ˈnek-tə-mē\ *n, pl* **-mies** : surgical excision of the vermilion border

ver•min \ˈvər-mən\ *n, pl* **vermin** : small common harmful or objectionable animals (as lice or fleas) that are difficult to control

ver•min•ous \ˈvər-mə-nəs\ *adj* **1** : consisting of, infested with, or being vermin **2** : caused by parasitic worms

ver•mis \ˈvər-mis\ *n, pl* **ver•mes** \-ˌmēz\ **1** : either of two parts of the median lobe of the cerebellum: **a** : one slightly prominent on the upper surface — called also *superior vermis* **b** : one on the lower surface sunk in the vallecula — called also *inferior* *vermis* **2** : the median lobe or part of the cerebellum

vernal conjunctivitis *n* : conjunctivitis occurring in warm seasons as a result of exposure to allergens

Ver•ner–Mor•ri•son syndrome \ˈvər-nər-ˈmȯr-ə-sən-, -ˈmär-\ *n* : a syndrome characterized esp. by severe watery diarrhea and hypokalemia that is often due to an excessive secretion of vasoactive intestinal peptide from a vipoma esp. of the pancreas — called also *pancreatic cholera*

Verner, John Victor (1927–2008), American physician.

Morrison, Ashton Byrom (*b* 1922), American pathologist.

ver•ni•er acuity \ˈvər-nē-ər\ *n* : the aspect of visual acuity that involves the ability to detect the alignment or lack of alignment of the two parts of a broken line

ver•nix \ˈvər-niks\ *n* : VERNIX CASEOSA

vernix ca•se•o•sa \-ˌka-sē-ˈō-sə\ *n* : a pasty covering chiefly of dead cells and sebaceous secretions that protects the skin of the fetus

ver•o•nal \ˈver-ə-ˌnȯl, -nəl\ *n, often cap* : a preparation of the sodium salt of barbital

ver•ru•ca \və-ˈrü-kə\ *n, pl* **-cae** \-(ˌ)kē\ : a wart or warty skin lesion

verruca acu•mi•na•ta \-ə-ˌkyü-mə-ˈnā-tə\ *n* : GENITAL WART

verruca pla•na \-ˈplä-nə\ *n* : FLAT WART

verruca plan•ta•ris \-ˌplan-ˈtar-əs\ *n* : PLANTAR WART

verruca vul•ga•ris \-ˌvəl-ˈgar-əs\ *n* : WART 1; *esp* : one occurring on the back of the fingers and hands

ver•ru•cose \və-ˈrü-ˌkōs\ *adj* **1** : covered with warty elevations **2** : having the form of a wart ⟨a ~ nevus⟩

ver•ru•cous \və-ˈrü-kəs\ *adj* **1** : VERRUCOSE **2** : characterized by the formation of warty lesions ⟨~ dermatitis⟩

verrucous endocarditis *n* : endocarditis marked by the formation or presence of warty nodules of fibrin on the lips of the heart valves

ver•ru•ga \və-ˈrü-gə\ *n* **1** : VERRUCA **2** : VERRUGA PERUANA

verruga per•u•a•na \-ˌper-ə-ˈwä-nə\ *also* **verruga pe•ru•vi•ana** \-pə-ˌrü-vē-ˈa-nə\ *n* : the second stage of bartonellosis characterized by warty nodules tending to ulcerate and bleed

versicolor — see PITYRIASIS VERSICOLOR, TINEA VERSICOLOR

ver•sion \ˈvər-zhən, -shən\ *n* **1** : a condition in which an organ and esp. the uterus is turned from its normal position **2** : manual turning of a fetus in the uterus to aid delivery

ver•te•bra \ˈvər-tə-brə\ *n, pl* **-brae** \-ˌbrā, -(ˌ)brē\ *or* **-bras** : any of the bony or cartilaginous segments composing the spinal column that have a short more or less cylindrical body whose ends articulate by pads of elastic or cartilaginous tissue with those of adjacent vertebrae and a bony arch that encloses the spinal cord

¹ver•te•bral \(ˌ)vər-ˈtē-brəl, ˈvər-tə-\ *adj* **1** : of, relating to, or being vertebrae or the spinal column : SPINAL **2** : composed of or having vertebrae

²vertebral *n* : a vertebral part or element (as an artery)

vertebral arch *n* : NEURAL ARCH

vertebral artery *n* : a large branch of the subclavian artery that ascends through the foramina in the transverse processes of each of the cervical vertebrae except the last one or two, enters the cranium through the foramen magnum, and unites with the corresponding artery of the opposite side to form the basilar artery

vertebral body *n* : the main anterior bony part of a vertebra that consists of the centrum, the ossified posterolateral joints linking the centrum and each half of the neural arch, and part of the neural arch

vertebral canal *n* : a canal that contains the spinal cord and is delimited by the neural arches on the dorsal side of the vertebrae — called also *spinal canal*

vertebral column *n* : SPINAL COLUMN

vertebral foramen *n* : the opening formed by a neural arch through which the spinal cord passes

vertebral ganglion *n* : any of a group of sympathetic ganglia which form two chains extending from the base of the skull to the coccyx along the sides of the spinal column — compare SYMPATHETIC CHAIN

vertebral notch *n* : either of two concave constrictions of which one occurs on the inferior surface and one on the superior surface of the pedicle on each side of a vertebra and which are arranged so that the superior notches of one vertebra and the corresponding inferior notches of a contiguous vertebra combine to form an intervertebral foramen on each side

vertebral plexus *n* : a plexus of veins associated with the spinal column

vertebral vein *n* : a tributary of the brachiocephalic vein that is formed by the union of branches originating in the occipital region and forming a plexus about the vertebral artery in its passage through the foramina of the cervical vertebrae

vertebra pro•mi•nens \-ˈprä-mi-ˌnenz\ *n* : the seventh cervical vertebra characterized by a prominent spinous process which can be felt at the base of the neck

ver•te•brate \ˈvər-tə-brət, -ˌbrāt\ *n* : any of a subphylum (Vertebrata) of animals with a spinal column including the mammals, birds, reptiles, amphibians, and fishes — **vertebrate** *adj*

ver•te•bro•ba•si•lar \ˌvər-tə-brō-ˈbā-sə-lər\ *adj* : of, relating to, or being the vertebral and basilar arteries

ver·te·bro·chon·dral rib \ˌvər-tə-brō-ˈkän-drəl-\ *n* : any of the three false ribs that are located above the floating ribs and that are attached to each other by costal cartilages

ver·te·bro·plas·ty \vər-tə-brō-ˌplas-tē\ *n, pl* **-ties** : a medical procedure for reducing pain caused by a vertebral compression fracture (as that associated with osteoporosis) that involves injection of an acrylic cement into the body of the fractured vertebra for stabilization — compare KYPHOPLASTY

ver·te·bro·ster·nal rib \-ˈstər-nəl-\ *n* : TRUE RIB

ver·tex \ˈvər-ˌteks\ *n, pl* **ver·ti·ces** \ˈvər-tə-ˌsēz\ *also* **ver·tex·es** **1** : the top of the head **2** : the highest point of the skull

vertex presentation *n* : normal obstetric presentation in which the fetal occiput lies at the opening of the uterus

ver·ti·cal \ˈvər-ti-kəl\ *adj* : relating to or being transmission (as of a disease) by genetic inheritance or by a congenital or perinatal route — compare HORIZONTAL 2 — **ver·ti·cal·ly** *adv*

vertical dimension *n* : the distance between two arbitrarily chosen points on the face above and below the mouth when the teeth are in occlusion

vertical nystagmus *n* : nystagmus characterized by up-and-down movement of the eyes

ver·tig·i·nous \(ˌ)vər-ˈti-jə-nəs\ *adj* : of, relating to, characterized by, or affected with vertigo or dizziness

ver·ti·go \ˈvər-ti-ˌgō\ *n, pl* **-goes** *or* **-gos** **1** : a sensation of motion which is associated with various disorders (as of the inner ear) and in which the individual or the individual's surroundings seem to whirl dizzily — see SUBJECTIVE VERTIGO **2** : disordered vertiginous movement as a symptom of disease in lower animals; *also* : a disease (as gid) causing this

ver·vet \ˈvər-vət\ *n* : GREEN MONKEY

very–low–density lipoprotein *n* : VLDL

vesicae — see TRIGONUM VESICAE, UVULA VESICAE

ves·i·ca fel·lea \ˈve-si-kə-ˈfe-lē-ə\ *n* : GALLBLADDER

[1]**ves·i·cal** \ˈve-si-kəl\ *adj* : of or relating to a bladder and esp. to the urinary bladder ⟨~ burning⟩

[2]**vesical** *n* : VESICAL ARTERY

vesical artery *n* : any of several arteries that arise from the internal iliac artery or one of its branches and that supply the urinary bladder and adjacent parts: as **a** : any of several arteries that arise from the umbilical artery and supply the upper part of the bladder — called also *superior vesical, superior vesical artery* **b** : one that arises from the internal iliac artery or the internal pudendal artery and that supplies the bladder, prostate, and seminal vesicles — called also *inferior vesical, inferior vesical artery*

vesical plexus *n* : a plexus of nerves that comprises preganglionic fibers derived chiefly from the hypogastric plexus and postganglionic neurons whose fibers are distributed to the bladder and adjacent parts

vesical venous plexus *n* : a plexus of veins surrounding the neck of the bladder and the base of the prostate gland

ves·i·cant \ˈve-si-kənt\ *adj* : producing or tending to produce blisters ⟨~ chemotherapy drugs⟩ — **vesicant** *n*

VESI·care \ˈves-i-ˌker\ *trademark* — used for a preparation of the succinate of solifenacin

vesica uri·nar·ia \-ˌyu̇r-i-ˈnar-ē-ə\ *n* : URINARY BLADDER

ves·i·cle \ˈve-si-kəl\ *n* **1 a** : a membranous and usu. fluid-filled pouch (as a cyst or cell) in a plant or animal **b** : SYNAPTIC VESICLE **2** : a small abnormal elevation of the outer layer of skin enclosing a watery liquid : BLISTER **3** : a pocket of embryonic tissue that is the beginning of an organ — see BRAIN VESICLE, OPTIC VESICLE

vesico- *comb form* : of or relating to the urinary bladder and ⟨*vesico*uterine⟩

ves·i·co·en·ter·ic \ˌve-si-kō-en-ˈter-ik\ *adj* : of, relating to, or connecting the urinary bladder and the intestinal tract ⟨a ~ fistula⟩

ves·i·cos·to·my \ˌve-si-ˈkäs-tə-mē\ *n, pl* **-mies** : CYSTOSTOMY

ves·i·co·ure·ter·al reflux \ˌve-si-kō-yu̇-ˈrē-tə-rəl-\ *n* : reflux of urine from the bladder into a ureter

ves·i·co·ure·ter·ic reflux \-tə-rik-\ *n* : VESICOURETERAL REFLUX

ves·i·co·uter·ine \ˌve-si-kō-ˈyü-tə-ˌrīn, -rən\ *adj* : of, relating to, or connecting the urinary bladder and the uterus

ves·i·co·vag·i·nal \ˌve-si-kō-ˈva-jən-ᵊl\ *adj* : of, relating to, or connecting the urinary bladder and vagina

vesicul- *or* **vesiculo-** *comb form* **1** : vesicle ⟨*vesicul*ectomy⟩ **2** : vesicular and ⟨*vesiculo*bullous⟩

ve·sic·u·lar \və-ˈsi-kyə-lər, ve-\ *adj* **1** : characterized by the presence or formation of vesicles ⟨a ~ rash⟩ **2** : having the form of a vesicle

vesicular breathing *n* : normal breathing that is soft and low-pitched when heard in auscultation

vesicular dermatitis *n* : a severe dermatitis esp. of young chickens and turkeys — called also *sod disease*

vesicular exanthema *n* : an acute virus disease primarily of swine that is caused by a calicivirus (species *Vesicular exanthema of swine virus* of the genus *Vesivirus*) and closely resembles foot-and-mouth disease

vesicular ovarian follicle *n* : GRAAFIAN FOLLICLE

vesicular stomatitis *n* : an acute virus disease esp. of horses and cows that resembles foot-and-mouth disease, is marked by erosive blisters in and about the mouth, and is caused by any of three rhabdoviruses (species *Vesicular stomatitis Alagoas virus, Ve-*

sicular stomatitis Indiana virus, and *Vesicular stomatitis New Jersey virus* of the genus *Vesiculovirus*) which sometimes infect humans producing symptoms resembling influenza

ve•sic•u•la•tion \və-ˌsi-kyə-ˈlā-shən\ *n* **1** : the presence or formation of vesicles **2** : the process of becoming vesicular ⟨~ of a papule⟩

ve•sic•u•lec•to•my \və-ˌsi-kyə-ˈlek-tə-mē\ *n, pl* **-mies** : surgical excision of a seminal vesicle

ve•sic•u•li•tis \və-ˌsi-kyə-ˈlī-təs\ *n* : inflammation of a vesicle and esp. a seminal vesicle

ve•sic•u•lo•bul•lous \və-ˌsi-kyə-lō-ˈbu̇-ləs\ *adj* : of, relating to, or being both vesicles and bullae ⟨a ~ rash⟩

ve•sic•u•lo•gram \və-ˈsi-kyə-lə-ˌgram\ *n* : a radiograph produced by vesiculography

ve•sic•u•log•ra•phy \və-ˌsi-kyə-ˈlä-grə-fē\ *n, pl* **-phies** : radiography of the seminal vesicles following the injection of a radiopaque medium

ve•sic•u•lo•pus•tu•lar \və-ˌsi-kyə-lō-ˈpəs-chə-lər\ *adj* : of, relating to, or marked by both vesicles and pustules

ve•sic•u•lot•o•my \və-ˌsi-kyə-ˈlä-tə-mē\ *n, pl* **-mies** : surgical incision of a seminal vesicle

Ves•prin \ˈves-prən\ *trademark* — used for a preparation of triflupromazine

ves•sel \ˈve-səl\ *n* : a tube or canal (as an artery, vein, or lymphatic) in which a body fluid (as blood or lymph) is contained and conveyed or circulated

ves•tib•u•lar \ve-ˈsti-byə-lər\ *adj* **1** : of or relating to the vestibule of the inner ear, the vestibular system, the vestibular nerve, or the vestibular sense **2** : lying within or facing the vestibule of the mouth ⟨the ~ side of a tooth⟩ — **ves•tib•u•lar•ly** *adv*

vestibular apparatus *n* : VESTIBULAR SYSTEM

vestibular folds *n pl* : FALSE VOCAL CORDS

vestibular ganglion *n* : a sensory ganglion in the trunk of the vestibular nerve in the internal auditory canal that contains cell bodies supplying nerve fibers comprising the vestibular nerve

vestibular gland *n* : any of the glands (as Bartholin's glands) that open into the vestibule of the vagina

vestibular ligament *n* : the narrow band of fibrous tissue contained in each of the false vocal cords and stretching between the thyroid and arytenoid cartilages

vestibular membrane *n* : a thin cellular membrane separating the cochlear duct and scala vestibuli — called also *Reissner's membrane*

vestibular nerve *n* : a branch of the auditory nerve that consists of bipolar neurons with cell bodies collected in the vestibular ganglion, with peripheral processes passing to the semicircular canals, utricle, and saccule, and with central processes passing to the vestibular nuclei of the medulla oblongata

vestibular neuronitis *n* : a disorder of uncertain etiology that is characterized by transitory attacks of severe vertigo

vestibular nucleus *n* : any of four nuclei in the medulla oblongata on each side of the floor of the fourth ventricle of the brain in which fibers of the vestibular nerve terminate — see INFERIOR VESTIBULAR NUCLEUS, LATERAL VESTIBULAR NUCLEUS, MEDIAL VESTIBULAR NUCLEUS, SUPERIOR VESTIBULAR NUCLEUS

vestibular sense *n* : a complex sense concerned with the perception of bodily position and motion, mediated by end organs in the vestibular system, and stimulated by alterations in the pull of gravity and by head movements — called also *labyrinthine sense*

vestibular system *n* : a complex system of the inner ear that functions in mediating the vestibular sense and consists of the saccule, utricle, and semicircular canals — called also *vestibular apparatus*

ves•ti•bule \ˈves-tə-ˌbyül\ *n* : any of various bodily cavities esp. when serving as or resembling an entrance to some other cavity or space: as **a** (1) : the central cavity of the bony labyrinth of the ear (2) : the parts of the membranous labyrinth comprising the utricle and the saccule and contained in the cavity of the bony labyrinth **b** : the space between the labia minora containing the orifice of the urethra **c** : the part of the left ventricle of the heart immediately below the aortic orifice **d** : the part of the mouth cavity outside the teeth and gums

vestibuli — see FENESTRA VESTIBULI, SCALA VESTIBULI

ves•tib•u•lo•co•chle•ar nerve \ve-ˌsti-byə-lō-ˈkō-klē-ər-, -ˈkä-\ *n* : AUDITORY NERVE

ves•tib•u•lo•plas•ty \ve-ˈsti-byə-lō-ˌplas-tē\ *n, pl* **-ties** : plastic surgery of the vestibular region of the mouth

ves•tib•u•lo•spi•nal tract \ve-ˌsti-byə-lō-ˈspī-nəl-\ *n* : a nerve tract on each side of the central nervous system containing nerve fibers that arise from cell bodies in the lateral vestibular nucleus on one side of the medulla oblongata and that descend on the same side in the lateral and anterior funiculi of the spinal cord to synapse with motor neurons in the ventral roots

ves•tige \ˈves-tij\ *n* : a bodily part or organ that is small and degenerate or imperfectly developed in comparison to one more fully developed in an earlier stage of the individual, in a past generation, or in closely related forms — **ves•tig•ial** \ve-ˈsti-jəl, -jē-əl\ *adj*

vestigial fold of Mar•shall \-ˈmär-shəl\ *n* : a fold of endocardium that extends from the left pulmonary artery to the more superior of the two left pulmonary veins

J. Marshall — see OBLIQUE VEIN OF MARSHALL

vet \ˈvet\ *n* : VETERINARIAN

vet•er•i•nar•i•an \ˌve-tə-rə-ˈner-ē-ən, ˌve-trə-\ *n* : a person qualified and authorized to practice veterinary medicine

[1]**vet•er•i•nary** \ˈve-tə-rə-ˌner-ē, ˈve-trə-\ *adj* : of, relating to, or being the science and art of prevention, cure, or alleviation of disease and injury in animals and esp. domestic animals

[2]**veterinary** *n, pl* **-nar•ies** : VETERINARIAN

veterinary surgeon *n, Brit* : VETERINARIAN

VF *abbr* ventricular fibrillation

V–fib *abbr* ventricular fibrillation

vi•a•ble \ˈvī-ə-bəl\ *adj* **1** : capable of living ⟨~ cancer cells⟩; *esp* : having attained such form and development of organs as to be normally capable of surviving outside the uterus ⟨a 26-week old ~ fetus⟩ **2** : capable of growing or developing ⟨~ eggs⟩ — **vi•a•bil•i•ty** \ˌvī-ə-ˈbi-lə-tē\ *n*

Vi•ag•ra \vī-ˈa-grə\ *trademark* — used for a preparation of the citrate of sildenafil

vi•al \ˈvī-əl, ˈvīl\ *n* : a small closed or closable vessel esp. for liquids — called also *phial*

Vi antigen \ˈvē-ˈī-\ *n* : a heat-labile somatic antigen associated with virulence in some bacteria (as of the genus *Salmonella*) and esp. in the typhoid fever bacterium

Vi•bra•my•cin \ˌvī-brə-ˈmīs-ᵊn\ *trademark* — used for a preparation of doxycycline

vibration white finger *n, chiefly Brit* : Raynaud's disease esp. when caused by severe vibration

vi•bra•tor \ˈvī-ˌbrā-tər\ *n* : a vibrating electrical apparatus used in massage or for sexual stimulation

vib•rio \ˈvi-brē-ō\ *n* **1** *cap* : a genus of motile gram-negative bacteria (family Vibrionaceae) that are straight or curved rods and include pathogens (as *V. cholerae*) causing esp. gastrointestinal disease (as cholera) **2** : any bacterium of the genus *Vibrio; broadly* : a curved rod-shaped bacterium

vib•ri•o•sis \ˌvi-brē-ˈō-səs\ *n, pl* **-o•ses** \-ˌsēz\ **1** : infection with or disease caused by a bacterium of the genus *Vibrio; esp* : a gastrointestinal illness of humans that is caused by consuming raw or undercooked fish or shellfish contaminated with a vibrio (as *V. parahaemolyticus*) **2** : an infectious disease of sheep and cattle caused by a bacterium of the genus *Campylobacter* (*C. fetus* syn. *Vibrio fetus*) and marked esp. by infertility and abortion

vi•bris•sa \vī-ˈbri-sə, və-\ *n, pl* **vi•bris•sae** \vī-ˈbri-(ˌ)sē; və-ˈbri-(ˌ)sē, -sī\ : any of the coarse hairs growing within the nostrils that serve to impede the inhalation of particulate matter

vi•car•i•ous \vī-ˈkar-ē-əs, və-\ *adj* : occurring in an unexpected or abnormal part of the body instead of the usual one ⟨~ menstruation manifested by bleeding from the nose⟩

vice \ˈvīs\ *n* : an abnormal behavior pattern in a domestic animal detrimental to its health or usefulness

Vi•co•din \ˈvī-kō-dən\ *trademark* — used for a preparation of acetaminophen and the bitartrate of hydrocodone

Vic•to•za \vik-ˈtō-zə\ *trademark* — used for a preparation of liraglutide

vid•ar•a•bine \vi-ˈdär-ə-ˌbēn\ *n* : an antiviral agent $C_{10}H_{13}N_5O_4 \cdot H_2O$ derived from adenine and arabinoside and used esp. to treat keratitis and encephalitis caused by the herpes simplex virus — called also *adenine arabinoside, ara-A*

Vi•dex \ˈvī-ˌdeks\ *trademark* — used for a preparation of ddI

Vid•i•an artery \ˈvi-dē-ən-\ *n* : a branch of the maxillary artery passing through the pterygoid canal of the sphenoid bone

Gui•di \ˈgwē-dē\, **Guido** (*Latin* **Vidus Vidius**) **(1508–1569)**, Italian anatomist and surgeon.

Vidian canal *n* : PTERYGOID CANAL

Vidian nerve *n* : a nerve formed by the union of the greater petrosal and the deep petrosal nerves that passes forward through the pterygoid canal in the sphenoid bone and joins the pterygopalatine ganglion

vi•gab•a•trin \vī-ˈga-bə-trən\ *n* : an anticonvulsant drug $C_6H_{11}NO_2$

Vii•bryd \ˈvī-brəd\ *trademark* — used for a preparation of the hydrochloride of vilazodone

vi•lan•te•rol \vī-ˈlan-tə-ˌrȯl\ *n* : a beta-agonist bronchodilator $C_{22}H_{33}Cl_2NO_5 \cdot C_{20}H_{16}O_2$ administered by oral inhalation usu. in combination with another drug to treat asthma and chronic obstructive pulmonary disease

vi•laz•o•done \və-ˈlaz-ə-ˌdōn\ *n* : an antidepressant drug that functions as an SSRI and is taken orally in the form of its hydrochloride $C_{26}H_{27}N_5O_2 \cdot HCl$ to treat major depressive disorder — see VIIBRYD

vil•lo•nod•u•lar \ˌvi-lō-ˈnä-jə-lər\ *adj* : characterized by villous and nodular thickening (as of a synovial membrane) ⟨~ synovitis⟩

vil•lus \ˈvi-ləs\ *n, pl* **vil•li** \-ˌlī\ : a small slender vascular process: as **a** : one of the minute fingerlike processes of the mucous membrane of the small intestine that serve in the absorption of nutriment **b** : one of the branching processes of the surface of the chorion of the developing embryo of most mammals that help to form the placenta — **vil•lous** \ˈvi-ləs\ *adj*

vin•blas•tine \(ˌ)vin-ˈblas-ˌtēn\ *n* : an alkaloid that is obtained from the rosy periwinkle and is used esp. in the form of its sulfate $C_{46}H_{58}N_4O_9 \cdot H_2SO_4$ to treat neoplastic diseases (as Hodgkin's lymphoma and testicular carcinoma) — called also *vincaleukoblastine;* see ABVD

vin•ca \ˈviŋ-kə\ *n* : PERIWINKLE

vin•ca•leu•ko•blas•tine \ˌviŋ-kə-ˌlü-kə-ˈblas-ˌtēn\ *n* : VINBLASTINE

Vin•cent's angina \ˈvin-sənts-, (ˌ)vaⁿ-ˈsäⁿz-\ *n* : acute necrotizing ulcerative gingivitis in which the ulceration has spread to surrounding tissues (as of the pharynx and tonsils) — called also *trench mouth*

Vincent, Jean Hyacinthe (1862–1950), French bacteriologist.

Vincent's infection *n* : ACUTE NECROTIZING ULCERATIVE GINGIVITIS

Vincent's organisms *n pl* : a bacterium of the genus *Fusobacterium* (*F. nucleatum*) and a spirochete of the genus *Treponema* (*T. vincentii*) that are sometimes found in necrotic tissue (as that of acute necrotizing ulcerative gingivitis or tropical ulcer)

vin•cris•tine \(ˌ)vin-ˈkris-ˌtēn\ *n* : an alkaloid that is obtained from the rosy periwinkle and is used esp. in the form of its sulfate $C_{46}H_{56}N_4O_{10} \cdot H_2SO_4$ to treat some neoplastic diseases (as acute leukemia) — called also *leurocristine;* see ONCOVIN

Vine•berg procedure \ˈvīn-ˌbərg-\ *n* : surgical implantation of an internal mammary artery into the myocardium

Vineberg, Arthur Martin (1903–1988), Canadian surgeon.

vi•nyl chloride \ˈvīn-ᵊl-\ *n* : a flammable gaseous carcinogenic compound C_2H_3Cl

vinyl ether *n* : a volatile flammable liquid unsaturated ether C_4H_6O formerly used as an inhalation anesthetic

vi•o•my•cin \ˌvī-ə-ˈmīs-ᵊn\ *n* : a polypeptide antibiotic that is produced by several soil actinomycetes of the genus *Streptomyces* and is administered intramuscularly in the form of its sulfate $C_{25}H_{43}N_{13}O_{10} \cdot xH_2SO_4$ to treat tuberculosis esp. in combination with other antituberculous drugs

vi•os•ter•ol \vī-ˈäs-tə-ˌrȯl, -ˌrōl\ *n* : CALCIFEROL

Vi•oxx \ˈvī-ˌäks\ *trademark* — used for a preparation of rofecoxib

VIP *abbr* vasoactive intestinal peptide; vasoactive intestinal polypeptide

vi•per \ˈvī-pər\ *n* : a common Eurasian venomous snake of the genus *Vipera* (*V. berus*) whose bite is usu. not fatal to humans; *broadly* : any of a family (Viperidae) of venomous snakes that includes Old World snakes (subfamily Viperinae) and the pit vipers

Vi•pera \ˈvī-pə-rə\ *n* : a genus of Old World venomous snakes (family Viperidae)

vi•po•ma \vī-ˈpō-mə, vi-\ *n* : a tumor of endocrine tissue esp. in the pancreas that secretes vasoactive intestinal peptide

Vi•ra•cept \ˈvī-rə-ˌsept\ *trademark* — used for a preparation of the mesylate of nelfinavir

vi•rae•mia *chiefly Brit var of* VIREMIA

vi•ral \ˈvī-rəl\ *adj* : of, relating to, or caused by a virus — **vi•ral•ly** *adv*

Vir•chow–Ro•bin space \ˈfir-ˌkō-rō-ˈbaⁿ-\ *n* : any of the spaces that surround blood vessels as they enter the brain and that communicate with the subarachnoid space

Virchow, Rudolf Ludwig Karl (1821–1902), German pathologist, anthropologist, and statesman.

Robin, Charles–Philippe (1821–1885), French anatomist and histologist.

Virchow's node *n* : SIGNAL NODE

Vir•e•ad \ˈvir-ē-ˌad\ *trademark* — used for a preparation of the fumarate of tenofovir

vi•re•mia \vī-ˈrē-mē-ə\ *n* : the presence of virus in the blood of a host — **vi•re•mic** \-mik\ *adj*

vir•gin \ˈvər-jən\ *n* : a person who has not had sexual intercourse — **vir•gin•i•ty** \(ˌ)vər-ˈji-nə-tē\ *n*

vi•ri•ci•dal \ˌvī-rə-ˈsīd-ᵊl\ *adj* : VIRUCIDAL

vi•ri•cide \ˈvī-rə-ˌsīd\ *n* : VIRUCIDE

vir•ile \ˈvir-əl, -ˌīl\ *adj* **1** : having the nature, properties, or qualities of an adult male; *specif* : capable of functioning as a male in copulation **2** : characteristic of or associated with men : MASCULINE — **vi•ril•i•ty** \və-ˈri-lə-tē\ *n*

vir•il•ism \ˈvir-ə-ˌli-zəm\ *n* **1** : precocious development of secondary sex characteristics in the male **2** : the appearance of secondary sex characteristics of the male in a female

vir•il•ize \ˈvir-ə-ˌlīz\ *vb* **-ized; -iz•ing** : to make virile; *esp* : to cause or produce virilism in — **vir•il•i•za•tion** \ˌvir-ə-lə-ˈzā-shən\ *n*

vi•ri•on \ˈvī-rē-ˌän, ˈvir-ē-\ *n* : a complete virus particle that consists of an RNA or DNA core with a protein coat sometimes with external envelopes and that is the extracellular infective form of a virus

vi•rol•o•gy \vī-ˈrä-lə-jē\ *n, pl* **-gies** : a branch of science that deals with viruses — **vi•ro•log•i•cal** \ˌvī-rə-ˈlä-ji-kəl\ *or* **vi•ro•log•ic** \-jik\ *adj* — **vi•ro•log•i•cal•ly** *adv* — **vi•rol•o•gist** \vī-ˈrä-lə-jist\ *n*

vi•ro•pause \ˈvī-rə-ˌpȯz\ *n* : ANDROPAUSE

virtual colonography *n* : COLONOGRAPHY

virtual colonoscopy *n* : COLONOGRAPHY

virtual dead space *n* : PHYSIOLOGICAL DEAD SPACE

vi•ru•cid•al \ˌvī-rə-ˈsīd-ᵊl\ *adj* : having the capacity to or tending to destroy or inactivate viruses ⟨∼ activity⟩

vi•ru•cide \ˈvī-rə-ˌsīd\ *n* : an agent having the capacity to destroy or inactivate viruses — called also *viricide*

vir•u•lence \ˈvir-yə-ləns, ˈvir-ə-\ *n* : the quality or state of being virulent: as **a**

: relative severity and malignancy **b** : the relative capacity of a pathogen to overcome body defenses — compare INFECTIVITY

vir•u•len•cy \-lən-sē\ *n, pl* **-cies** : VIRULENCE

vir•u•lent \-lənt\ *adj* **1 a** : marked by a rapid, severe, and malignant course ⟨a ~ infection⟩ **b** : able to overcome bodily defense mechanisms ⟨a ~ pathogen⟩ **2** : extremely poisonous or venomous : NOXIOUS

vi•rus \ˈvī-rəs\ *n* **1** : the causative agent of an infectious disease **2** : any of a large group of submicroscopic infective agents that are usu. regarded as nonliving extremely complex molecules or sometimes as very simple microorganisms, that typically contain a protein coat surrounding an RNA or DNA core of genetic material but no semipermeable membrane, that are capable of growth and multiplication only in living cells, and that cause various important diseases — see FILTERABLE VIRUS **3** : a disease caused by a virus

virus pneumonia *n* : pneumonia caused or thought to be caused by a virus; *esp* : PRIMARY ATYPICAL PNEUMONIA

viscer- *or* **visceri-** *or* **viscero-** *comb form* : visceral : viscera ⟨*viscero*tropic⟩

viscera *pl of* VISCUS

vis•cer•al \ˈvi-sə-rəl\ *adj* : of, relating to, or located on or among the viscera — compare PARIETAL 1 — **vis•cer•al•ly** *adv*

visceral arch *n* : BRANCHIAL ARCH

visceral leishmaniasis *n* : KALA-AZAR

visceral muscle *n* : smooth muscle esp. in visceral structures

visceral pericardium *n* : EPICARDIUM

visceral peritoneum *n* : the part of the peritoneum that lines the abdominal viscera — compare PARIETAL PERITONEUM

visceral reflex *n* : a reflex mediated by autonomic nerves and initiated in the viscera

vis•cero•meg•a•ly \ˌvi-sə-rō-ˈme-gə-lē\ *n, pl* **-lies** : ORGANOMEGALY

vis•cero•mo•tor \ˌvi-sə-rō-ˈmō-tər\ *adj* : causing or concerned in the functional activity of the viscera

vis•cer•op•to•sis \ˌvi-sə-räp-ˈtō-səs\ *n, pl* **-to•ses** \-ˌsēz\ : downward displacement of the abdominal viscera

vis•cer•o•trop•ic \ˌvi-sə-rə-ˈträ-pik\ *adj* : tending to affect or having an affinity for the viscera ⟨~ leishmaniasis⟩ — **vis•cer•ot•ro•pism** \ˌvi-sə-ˈrä-trəˌpi-zəm\ *n*

vis•cid \ˈvi-səd\ *adj* **1** : having an adhesive quality **2** : having a glutinous consistency

vis•com•e•ter \vis-ˈkä-mə-tər\ *n* : an instrument used to measure viscosity — **vis•co•met•ric** \ˌvis-kə-ˈme-trik\ *adj*

vis•co•sim•e•ter \ˌvis-kə-ˈsi-mə-tər\ *n* : VISCOMETER — **vis•cos•i•met•ric** \vis-ˌkä-sə-ˈme-trik\ *adj*

vis•cos•i•ty \vis-ˈkä-sə-tē\ *n, pl* **-ties** : the quality of being viscous; *esp* : the property of resistance to flow in a fluid

vis•cous \ˈvis-kəs\ *adj* **1** : having a glutinous consistency and the quality of sticking or adhering : VISCID **2** : having or characterized by viscosity

vis•cus \ˈvis-kəs\ *n, pl* **vis•cera** \ˈvi-sə-rə\ : an internal organ of the body; *esp* : one (as the heart, liver, or intestine) located in the large cavity of the trunk

vis•i•ble \ˈvi-zə-bəl\ *adj* **1** : capable of being seen : perceptible to vision **2** : situated in the visible spectrum

visible spectrum *n* : the part of the electromagnetic spectrum to which the human eye is sensitive extending from a wavelength of about 400 nm for violet light to about 700 nm for red light

vi•sion \ˈvi-zhən\ *n* **1** : the act or power of seeing **2** : the special sense by which the qualities of an object (as color, shape, and size) constituting its appearance are perceived through a process in which light rays entering the eye are transformed by the retina into electrical signals that are transmitted to the brain via the optic nerve

vis•it \ˈvi-zət\ *n* **1** : a professional call (as by a physician to treat a patient) **2** : a call upon a professional person (as a physician or dentist) for consultation or treatment — **visit** *vb*

visiting nurse *n* : a nurse employed (as by a hospital or social-service agency) to perform public health services and esp. to visit and provide care for sick persons in a community — called also *public health nurse*

vis•na \ˈvis-nə\ *n* : ovine progressive pneumonia esp. as manifested by neurological symptoms

Vis•ta•ril \ˈvis-tə-ˌril\ *trademark* — used for a preparation of hydroxyzine

Vis•tide \ˈvis-ˌtīd\ *trademark* — used for a preparation of cidofovir

vi•su•al \ˈvi-zhə-wəl\ *adj* **1** : of, relating to, or used in vision ⟨~ organs⟩ **2** : attained or maintained by sight ⟨~ impressions⟩ — **vi•su•al•ly** *adv*

visual acuity *n* : the relative ability of the visual organ to resolve detail

visual agnosia *n* : a form of agnosia characterized by inability to recognize familiar objects observed by sight — see PROSOPAGNOSIA

visual analog scale *n* : a testing technique for measuring subjective or behavioral phenomena (as pain) in which a subject selects from a gradient of alternatives (as from "no pain" to "worst imaginable pain") arranged in linear fashion — abbr. *VAS*

visual cortex *n* : a sensory area of the occipital lobe of the cerebral cortex receiving afferent projection fibers concerned with the sense of sight — called also *visual area*

visual field *n* : the entire expanse of space visible at a given instant without moving the eyes — called also *field of vision*

vi·su·al·i·za·tion \ˌvi-zhə-wə-lə-ˈzā-shən\ *n* **1** : formation of mental visual images **2** : the process of making an internal organ visible by the introduction (as by swallowing, by an injection, or by an enema) of a radiopaque substance followed by radiography — **vi·su·al·ize** \ˈvi-zhə-wə-ˌlīz\ *vb*

vi·su·al·iz·er \-ˌlī-zər\ *n* : one that visualizes; *esp* : a person whose mental imagery is prevailingly visual — compare AUDILE, TACTILE

visual projection area *n* : STRIATE CORTEX

visual purple *n* : RHODOPSIN

vi·suo·mo·tor \ˌvi-zhə-wō-ˈmō-tər\ *adj* : of or relating to vision and muscular movement ⟨~ coordination⟩

vi·suo·spa·tial \-ˈspā-shəl\ *adj* : of or relating to thought processes that involve visual and spatial awareness

vi·tal \ˈvīt-ᵊl\ *adj* **1 a** : existing as a manifestation of life **b** : concerned with or necessary to the maintenance of life ⟨~ organs⟩ **2** : characteristic of life or living beings **3** : recording data relating to lives **4** : of, relating to, or constituting the staining of living tissues — **vi·tal·ly** *adv*

vital capacity *n* : the breathing capacity of the lungs expressed as the number of cubic inches or cubic centimeters of air that can be forcibly exhaled after a full inspiration

vital function *n* : a function of the body (as respiration) on which life is directly dependent

vi·tal·i·ty \vī-ˈta-lə-tē\ *n, pl* **-ties** : capacity to live and develop; *also* : physical or mental vigor esp. when highly developed

Vi·tal·li·um \vī-ˈta-lē-əm\ *trademark* — used for a cobalt-chromium alloy of platinum-white color used esp. for cast dentures and prostheses

vi·tals \ˈvīt-ᵊlz\ *n pl* : vital organs (as the heart, liver, lungs, and brain)

vital signs *n pl* : signs of life; *specif* : the pulse rate, respiratory rate, body temperature, and often blood pressure of a person

vital statistics *n pl* : statistics relating to births, deaths, marriages, health, and disease

vi·ta·min \ˈvī-tə-mən\ *n* : any of various organic substances that are essential in minute quantities to the nutrition of most animals and some plants, act esp. as coenzymes and precursors of coenzymes in the regulation of metabolic processes but do not provide energy or serve as building units, and are present in natural foodstuffs or sometimes produced within the body

vitamin A *n* : any of several fat-soluble vitamins or a mixture of two or more of them whose lack in the animal body causes keratinization of epithelial tissues (as in the eye with resulting night blindness and xerophthalmia): as **a** : a pale yellow crystalline alcohol $C_{20}H_{29}OH$ that is found in animal products (as egg yolk, milk, and butter) and esp. in marine fish-liver oils (as of cod, halibut, and shark) — called also *retinol, vitamin A_1* **b** : a yellow viscous liquid alcohol $C_{20}H_{27}OH$ that contains one more double bond in a molecule than vitamin A_1 and is less active biologically in mammals and that occurs esp. in the liver oil of freshwater fish — called also *vitamin A_2*

vitamin A aldehyde *n* : RETINAL

vitamin A_1 \-ˌā-ˈwən\ *n* : VITAMIN A a

vitamin A palmitate *n* : RETINYL PALMITATE

vitamin A_2 \-ˌā-ˈtü\ *n* : VITAMIN A b

vitamin B *n* **1** : VITAMIN B COMPLEX **2** : any of numerous members of the vitamin B complex; *esp* : THIAMINE

vitamin B_c \-ˌbē-ˈsē\ *n* : FOLIC ACID

vitamin B complex *n* : a group of water-soluble vitamins (as biotin, niacin, and thiamine) found esp. in yeast, seed germs, eggs, meat, and green vegetables that have varied metabolic functions and include coenzymes and growth factors — called also *B complex*

vitamin B_1 \-ˌbē-ˈwən\ *n* : THIAMINE

vitamin B_{17} \-ˌbē-ˌse-vən-ˈtēn\ *n* : LAETRILE

vitamin B_6 \-ˌbē-ˈsiks\ *n* : pyridoxine or a closely related compound found widely in combined form and considered essential to vertebrate nutrition

vitamin B_T \-ˌbē-ˈtē\ *n* : CARNITINE

vitamin B_3 \-ˌbē-ˈthrē\ *n* : NIACIN

vitamin B_{12} \-ˌbē-ˈtwelv\ *n* **1** : a complex cobalt-containing compound $C_{63}H_{88}CoN_{14}O_{14}P$ found in animal products (as meat and eggs) that is essential to normal blood formation, neural function, and growth, and is used esp. in treating pernicious and related anemias and in animal feed as a growth factor — called also *cyanocobalamin* **2** : any of several compounds similar to vitamin B_{12} in action but having different chemistry

vitamin B_2 \-ˌbē-ˈtü\ *n* : RIBOFLAVIN

vitamin C *n* : a water-soluble vitamin $C_6H_8O_6$ found in plants and esp. in fruits and leafy vegetables or made synthetically and used in the prevention and treatment of scurvy and as an antioxidant for foods — called also *ascorbic acid*

vitamin D *n* : any or all of several fat-soluble vitamins chemically related to steroids, essential for normal bone and tooth structure, and found esp. in fish-liver oils, egg yolk, and milk or produced by activation (as by ultraviolet irradiation) of sterols: as **a** : CALCIFEROL **b** : CHOLECALCIFEROL — called also *sunshine vitamin*

vitamin D_3 \-ˌdē-ˈthrē\ *n* : CHOLECALCIFEROL

vitamin D_2 \-ˌdē-ˈtü\ *n* : CALCIFEROL

vitamin E *n* : any of several fat-soluble vitamins that are chemically tocopherols, are essential in nutrition, are found esp. in wheat germ, vegetable oils, egg yolk, and green leafy vegetables or are made synthetically, and are used chiefly in animal feeds and as antioxidants; *esp* : ALPHA-TOCOPHEROL

vitamin G *n* : RIBOFLAVIN

vitamin H *n* : BIOTIN

vitamin K *n* **1** : either of two naturally occurring fat-soluble vitamins that are essential for the clotting of blood because of their role in the production of prothrombin in the liver and that are used in preventing and treating hypoprothrombinemia and hemorrhage: **a** : an oily naphthoquinone $C_{31}H_{46}O_2$ that is obtained esp. from alfalfa or made synthetically and that has a fast, potent, and prolonged biological effect — called also *phylloquinone, phytonadione, vitamin* K_1; see MEPHYTON **b** : a crystalline naphthoquinone $C_{41}H_{56}O_2$ that is obtained esp. from putrefied fish meal and is synthesized by various bacteria (as in the intestines) and that is slightly less active biologically than vitamin K_1 — called also *menaquinone, vitamin* K_2 **2** : any of several synthetic compounds that are closely related chemically to vitamins K_1 and K_2 but are simpler in structure; *esp* : MENADIONE

vitamin K_1 \-ˌkā-ˈwən\ *n* : VITAMIN K 1a

vitamin K_3 \-ˌkā-ˈthrē\ *n* : MENADIONE

vitamin K_2 \-ˌkā-ˈtü\ *n* : VITAMIN K 1b

vitamin M *n* : FOLIC ACID

vi•ta•min•ol•o•gy \ˌvī-tə-mə-ˈnä-lə-jē\ *n, pl* **-gies** : a branch of knowledge dealing with vitamins, their nature, action, and use

vitamin PP \-ˌpē-ˈpē\ *n* : NIACIN

Vi•tek•ta \vī-ˈtek-tə\ *trademark* — used for a preparation of elvitegravir

vitell- *or* **vitello-** *comb form* : yolk : vitellus ⟨*vitello*genesis⟩

vi•tel•lin \vī-ˈte-lən, və-\ *n* : a phosphoprotein in egg yolk — called also *ovovitellin*

vi•tel•line \-ˈte-lən, -ˌlēn, -ˌlīn\ *adj* : of, relating to, or producing yolk

vitelline duct *n* : OMPHALOMESENTERIC DUCT

vitelline membrane *n* : a membrane enclosing the egg proper and corresponding to the plasma membrane of an ordinary cell

vi•tel•lo•gen•e•sis \vī-ˌte-lō-ˈje-nə-səs, və-\ *n, pl* **-e•ses** \-ˌsēz\ : yolk formation — **vi•tel•lo•gen•ic** \-ˈje-nik\ *adj*

vi•tel•lus \vī-ˈte-ləs, və-\ *n* : the egg cell proper including the yolk but excluding any albuminous or membranous envelopes; *also* : YOLK

vit•i•li•go \ˌvi-tə-ˈlī-gō, -ˈlē-\ *n* : a progressive skin disorder that is a form of leukoderma caused by the localized or generalized destruction of melanocytes and marked by sharply circumscribed white spots of skin

vit•rec•to•my \və-ˈtrek-tə-mē\ *n, pl* **-mies** : surgical removal of all or part of the vitreous body

¹vit•re•ous \ˈvi-trē-əs\ *adj* : of, relating to, constituting, or affecting the vitreous body ⟨~ hemorrhages⟩

²vitreous *n* : VITREOUS BODY

vitreous body *n* : the clear colorless transparent jelly that fills the eyeball posterior to the lens and is enclosed by a delicate hyaloid membrane

vitreous chamber *n* : the space in the eyeball between the lens and the retina that is occupied by the vitreous body

vitreous detachment *n* : separation of the posterior part of the vitreous body from the retina due to contraction of the vitreous body that typically occurs as part of the process of aging, that is usu. accompanied by the presence of floaters, and that may result in a torn retina or in retinal detachment — called also *posterior vitreous detachment*

vitreous humor *n* : VITREOUS BODY

vitro — see IN VITRO

vit•ro•nec•tin \ˌvi-trō-ˈnek-tən\ *n* : a glycoprotein of blood plasma that promotes cell adhesion and migration and is similar to fibronectin

Vi•vac•til \vī-ˈvak-til\ *trademark* — used for a preparation of protriptyline

vi•vax malaria \ˈvī-ˌvaks-\ *n* : malaria caused by a plasmodium (*Plasmodium vivax*) that induces paroxysms at 48-hour intervals — compare FALCIPARUM MALARIA

vivi- *comb form* : alive : living ⟨*vivi*section⟩

vi•vip•a•rous \vī-ˈvi-pə-rəs, və-\ *adj* : producing living young instead of eggs from within the body in the manner of nearly all mammals, many reptiles, and a few fishes — compare OVIPAROUS, OVOVIVIPAROUS — **vi•vi•par•i•ty** \ˌvī-və-ˈpar-ə-tē, ˌvi-\ *n*

vivi•sec•tion \ˌvi-və-ˈsek-shən, ˈvi-və-ˌ\ *n* : the cutting of or operation on a living animal usu. for physiological or pathological investigation; *broadly* : animal experimentation esp. if considered to cause distress or result in injury or death to the subject — **vivi•sect** \-ˈsekt\ *vb* — **vivi•sec•tion•ist** \ˌvi-və-ˈsek-sh(ə-)nəst\ *n*

vivo — see IN VIVO

VLDL \ˌvē-(ˌ)el-(ˌ)dē-ˈel\ *n* : a plasma lipoprotein that is produced primarily by the liver with lesser amounts contributed by the intestine, that contains relatively large amounts of triglycerides compared to protein, and that leaves a residue of cholesterol in the tissues during the process of conversion to LDL — called also *very-low-density lipoprotein;* compare HDL, LDL

VMA *abbr* vanillylmandelic acid

VMD *abbr* doctor of veterinary medicine

VNA *abbr* Visiting Nurse Association

VNTR \ˌvē-ˌen-ˌtē-ˈär\ *n, often attrib* [*v*ariable *n*umber *t*andem *r*epeat] : a tandem repeat from a single genetic locus in which the number of repeated DNA segments varies from individual to individual and is used for identification purposes (as in DNA fingerprinting)

vo•cal \ˈvō-kəl\ *adj* **1** : uttered by the voice : ORAL **2** : having or exercising the power of producing voice, speech, or sound **3** : of, relating to, or resembling the voice — **vo•cal•ly** *adv*

vocal cord *n* **1** *pl* : either of two pairs of folds of mucous membrane of which each member of each pair stretches from the thyroid cartilage in front to the arytenoid cartilage in back, contains a band of fibrous or elastic tissue, and has a free edge projecting into the cavity of the larynx toward the contralateral member of the same pair forming a cleft which can be opened or closed: **a** : FALSE VOCAL CORDS **b** : TRUE VOCAL CORDS **2** : VOCAL LIGAMENT

vocal folds *n pl* : TRUE VOCAL CORDS

vo•ca•lis \vō-ˈkā-ləs\ *n* : a small muscle that is the medial part of the thyroarytenoid, originates in the lamina of the thyroid cartilage, inserts in the vocal process of the arytenoid cartilage, and modulates the tension of the true vocal cords

vo•cal•i•za•tion \ˌvō-kə-lə-ˈzā-shən\ *n* : the act or process of producing sounds with the voice; *also* : a sound thus produced — **vo•cal•ize** *vb*

vocal ligament *n* : the band of yellow elastic tissue contained in each true vocal cord and stretching between the thyroid and arytenoid cartilages — called also *inferior thyroarytenoid ligament*

vocal process *n* : the anterior angle of the arytenoid cartilage on each side of the larynx to which the vocal ligament of the corresponding side is attached

voice \ˈvȯis\ *n* **1** : sound produced esp. by means of lungs or larynx; *esp* : sound so produced by human beings **2** : the faculty of utterance : SPEECH

voice box *n* : LARYNX

void \ˈvȯid\ *vb* : to discharge or emit ⟨~ urine⟩

vol *abbr* volume

vo•lar \ˈvō-lər, -ˌlär\ *adj* : relating to the palm of the hand or the sole of the foot; *specif* : located on the same side as the palm of the hand

vol•a•tile \ˈvä-lə-təl, -ˌtīl\ *adj* : readily vaporizable at a relatively low temperature — **vol•a•til•i•ty** \ˌvä-lə-ˈti-lə-tē\ *n*

volatile oil *n* : an oil that vaporizes readily; *esp* : ESSENTIAL OIL

volitantes — see MUSCAE VOLITANTES

vo•li•tion \vō-ˈli-shən, və-\ *n* **1** : an act of making a choice or decision; *also* : a choice or decision made **2** : the power of choosing or determining — **vo•li•tion•al** \-ˈli-shə-nəl\ *adj*

Volk•mann's canal \ˈfōlk-mənz-\ *n* : any of the small channels in bone that transmit blood vessels from the periosteum into the bone and that lie perpendicular to and communicate with the haversian canals

Volkmann, Alfred Wilhelm (1800–1877), German physiologist.

Volkmann's contracture *or* **Volkmann contracture** *n* : ischemic contracture of an extremity and esp. of a hand

volt \ˈvōlt\ *n* : the practical mks unit of electrical potential difference and electromotive force equal to the difference of potential between two points in a conducting wire carrying a constant current of one ampere when the power dissipated between these two points is equal to one watt

Vol•ta \ˈvȯl-tä\, **Alessandro Giuseppe Antonio Anastasio (1745–1827),** Italian physicist.

volt•age \ˈvōl-tij\ *n* : electrical potential or potential difference expressed in volts

voltage clamp *n* : stabilization of a membrane potential by depolarization and maintenance at a given potential by means of an electric current from a source outside the living system — **voltage clamp** *vb*

voltage–gat•ed \-ˌgā-təd\ *adj* : permitting or blocking passage through a cell membrane in response to an electrical stimulus (as a potential difference across a cell membrane)

Vol•ta•ren \ˈvōl-tə-rən\ *trademark* — used for a preparation of the sodium salt of diclofenac

vol•un•tary \ˈvä-lən-ˌter-ē\ *adj* **1** : proceeding from the will or from one's own choice or consent **2** : of, relating to, subject to, or regulated by the will ⟨~ behavior⟩ — **vol•un•tari•ly** *adv*

voluntary hospital *n* : a private nonprofit hospital that is operated under individual, partnership, or corporation control

voluntary muscle *n* : muscle (as most striated muscle) under voluntary control

vol•vu•lus \ˈväl-vyə-ləs\ *n* : a twisting of the intestine upon itself that causes obstruction — compare ILEUS

vo•mer \ˈvō-mər\ *n* : a bone of the skull that in humans forms the posterior and inferior part of the nasal septum comprising a vertical plate pointed in front and expanding at the upper back part into lateral wings

vom•ero•na•sal \ˌvä-mə-rō-ˈnā-zəl, ˌvō-\ *adj* : of or relating to the vomer and the nasal region and esp. to the vomeronasal organ or the vomeronasal cartilage

vomeronasal cartilage *n* : a narrow process of cartilage between the vomer and the cartilage of the nasal septum

vomeronasal organ *n* : either of a pair of small blind pouches or tubes in many vertebrates that are situated one on either side of the nasal septum or in the buccal cavity and that are reduced to rudimentary pits in adult humans but are developed in reptiles, amphibians, and some mammals as chemoreceptors — called also *Jacobson's organ*

vomica — see NUX VOMICA

[1]**vom·it** \ˈvä-mət\ *n* **1** : VOMITING **2** : stomach contents disgorged through the mouth — called also *vomitus*

[2]**vomit** *vb* : to disgorge the contents of the stomach through the mouth

vomiting *n* : an act or instance of disgorging the contents of the stomach through the mouth — called also *emesis*

vomiting center *n* : a nerve center in the medulla oblongata that initiates the act of vomiting when stimulated

vom·i·tus \ˈvä-mə-təs\ *n* : VOMIT 2

von Gier·ke disease \vän-ˈgir-kə-\ *or* **von Gier·ke's disease** \-kəz-\ *n* : a glycogen storage disease that is caused by a deficiency of glucose-6-phosphate, has a clinical onset at birth or during infancy, is characterized esp. by enlargement of the liver and kidney, hypoglycemia, hyperlipidemia, and stunted growth, and is inherited as an autosomal recessive trait

Gierke, Edgar Otto Konrad von (1877–1945), German pathologist.

von Grae·fe's sign \ˌvän-ˈgrā-fəz-\ *n* : the failure of the upper eyelid to follow promptly and smoothly the downward movement of the eyeball that is seen in Graves' disease

von Grae·fe \fȯn-ˈgre-fə\, **Albrecht Friedrich Wilhelm Ernst (1828–1870),** German ophthalmologist.

von Hip·pel–Lin·dau disease \vän-ˈhi-pəl-ˈlin-ˌdau̇-\ *n* : a rare genetic disease that is characterized by hemangiomas of the retina and cerebellum and often by cysts or tumors of the liver, pancreas, and kidneys and that is typically inherited as an autosomal dominant trait — called also *Lindau's disease*

von Hippel, Eugen (1867–1939), German ophthalmologist.

Lindau, Arvid Vilhelm (1892–1958), Swedish pathologist.

von Reck·ling·hau·sen's disease \-ˈre-kliŋ-ˌhau̇-zənz-\ *n* : NEUROFIBROMATOSIS 1

F. D. Recklinghausen — see RECKLINGHAUSEN'S DISEASE

von Wil·le·brand disease \vän-ˈvi-lə-ˌbränt-\ *also* **von Willebrand's disease** *n* : a genetic blood disorder marked by prolonged, excessive, or abnormal bleeding that commonly results in recurrent nosebleeds, heavy menstrual flow, and bleeding from the gums, is caused by deficient or defective von Willebrand factor, typically occurs in a mild form that is less serious than hemophilia, and is inherited chiefly as an autosomal dominant trait

Willebrand, Erick Adolf von (1870–1949), Finnish physician.

von Willebrand factor *n* : a large glycoprotein clotting factor circulating in blood plasma that mediates platelet adhesion to collagen at sites of vascular injury, that binds to and protects factor VIII from degradation, and that is deficient or defective in individuals affected with von Willebrand disease

vorticosa — see VENA VORTICOSA

vor·ti·cose vein \ˈvȯr-tə-ˌkōs-\ *n* : VENA VORTICOSA

VO$_2$ max \ˌvē-ō-ˈtü-ˈmaks\ *n* : the maximum amount of oxygen the body can use during a specified period of usu. intense exercise that depends on body weight and the strength of the lungs — called also *maximal oxygen consumption, maximal oxygen uptake, max VO$_2$*

voy·eur \vȯi-ˈyər, vwä-\ *n* : one obtaining sexual gratification from observing unsuspecting individuals who are partly undressed, naked, or engaged in sexual acts; *broadly* : one who habitually seeks sexual stimulation by visual means — **voy·eur·ism** \-ˌi-zəm\ *n* — **voy·eur·is·tic** \ˌvwä-(ˌ)yər-ˈis-tik, ˌvȯi-ər-\ *adj*

VRE \ˌvē-ˌär-ˈē\ *abbr or n* : VANCOMYCIN-RESISTANT ENTEROCOCCUS

VS *abbr* vesicular stomatitis

VSD *abbr* ventricular septal defect

VT *abbr* ventricular tachycardia

VTA *abbr* ventral tegmental area

V–tach \ˈvē-ˌtak\ *n* : VENTRICULAR TACHYCARDIA

vulgaris — see ACNE VULGARIS, ICHTHYOSIS VULGARIS, LUPUS VULGARIS, PEMPHIGUS VULGARIS, VERRUCA VULGARIS

vul·ner·a·ble \ˈvəl-nə-rə-bəl\ *adj* : capable of being hurt : susceptible to injury or disease — **vul·ner·a·bil·i·ty** \ˌvəl-nə-rə-ˈbi-lə-tē\ *n*

vul·sel·lum \vəl-ˈse-ləm\ *n, pl* **-sel·la** \-ˈse-lə\ : a surgical forceps with serrated, clawed, or hooked blades

vulv- *or* **vulvo-** *comb form* **1** : vulva ⟨*vulv*itis⟩ **2** : vulvar and ⟨*vulvo*vaginal⟩

vul·va \ˈvəl-və\ *n, pl* **vul·vae** \-ˌvē, -ˌvī\ : the external parts of the female genital organs comprising the mons pubis, labia majora, labia minora, clitoris, vestibule of the vagina, bulb of the vestibule, and Bartholin's glands — **vul·val** \ˈvəl-vəl\ *or* **vul·var** \-vər\ *adj*

vulvae — see KRAUROSIS VULVAE, PRURITUS VULVAE

vul·vec·to·my \ˌvəl-ˈvek-tə-mē\ *n, pl* **-mies** : surgical excision of the vulva

vul·vi·tis \ˌvəl-ˈvī-təs\ *n* : inflammation of the vulva

vul·vo·dyn·ia \ˌvəl-vō-ˈdin-ē-ə\ *n* : chronic discomfort of the vulva of uncertain cause that is experienced as burning or shooting pain, stinging, or irritation

vul•vo•vag•i•nal \ˌvəl-vō-ˈva-jən-ᵊl\ *adj* : of or relating to the vulva and the vagina ⟨~ hematoma⟩

vul•vo•vag•i•ni•tis \ˌvəl-vō-ˌva-jə-ˈnī-təs\ *n, pl* **-nit•i•des** \-ˈni-tə-ˌdēz\ : coincident inflammation of the vulva and vagina

VX \ˈvē-ˈeks\ *n* : an extremely toxic persistent chemical warfare agent $C_{11}H_{26}NO_2PS$ that is used esp. as a nerve gas and that in large doses typically causes convulsions, loss of consciousness, paralysis, and failure of the respiratory system leading to death

Vy•tor•in \vī-ˈtȯr-ən\ *trademark* — used for a preparation of ezetimibe and simvastatin

Vy•vanse \ˈvī-ˌvan(t)s\ *trademark* — used for a preparation of lisdexamfetamine dimesylate

W *symbol* [German *wolfram*] tungsten

Waar•den•burg syndrome \ˈvär-dᵊn-ˌbərg-\ *or* **Waar•den•burg's syndrome** \-ˌbərgz-\ *n* : a highly variable genetic disorder inherited as an autosomal dominant trait and marked esp. by hearing loss, white hair and esp. a white forelock, widely spaced eyes, and heterochromia of the irises

Waardenburg, Petrus Johannes (1886–1979), Dutch ophthalmologist.

Wa•da test \ˈwä-də-\ *n* : a procedure for identifying which hemisphere of the brain is dominant for language and memory function and that typically involves anesthetizing one hemisphere at a time (as by injection of amobarbital into the internal carotid artery) and having the patient perform several cognitive tasks (as identifying words or counting backwards)

Wada, Juhn Atsushi (*b* 1924), Canadian (Japanese-born) neurologist.

wad•ding \ˈwä-diŋ\ *n* : a soft absorbent sheet of cotton, wool, or cellulose used esp. in hospitals for surgical dressings

WAIS *abbr* Wechsler Adult Intelligence Scale

waist \ˈwāst\ *n* : the typically narrowed part of the body between the thorax and hips

waist•line \ˈwāst-ˌlīn\ *n* : body circumference at the waist

wake•ful \ˈwāk-fəl\ *adj* : not sleeping or able to sleep : SLEEPLESS — **wake•ful•ness** *n*

Wal•den•ström's macroglobulinemia \ˈväl-dən-ˌstremz-\ *n* : lymphoplasmacytic lymphoma marked by an elevated serum concentration of a monoclonal antibody of the class IgM and characterized esp. by hyperviscosity of blood, lymphadenopathy, hepatosplenomegaly, anemia, and peripheral neuropathy

Waldenström, Jan Gosta (1906–1996), Swedish physician.

Wal•dey•er's ring \ˈväl-ˌdī-ərz-\ *n* : a ring of lymphatic tissue formed by the two palatine tonsils, the pharyngeal tonsil, the lingual tonsil, and intervening lymphoid tissue

Wal•dey•er–Hartz \ˈväl-ˌdī-ər-ˈhärts\, **Heinrich Wilhelm Gottfried von (1836–1921),** German anatomist.

walk•er \ˈwȯ-kər\ *n* : a framework designed to support a baby learning to walk or an infirm or physically disabled person

[1]**walk–in** \ˈwȯk-ˌin\ *adj* : providing medical services to ambulatory patients without an appointment ⟨a ~ clinic⟩; *also* : being an individual who uses such services

[2]**walk–in** *n* : a walk-in patient

walk•ing \ˈwȯ-kiŋ\ *adj* : able to walk : AMBULATORY ⟨the ~ wounded⟩

walking cast *n* : a cast that is worn on a patient's leg and has a stirrup with a heel or other supporting device embedded in the plaster to facilitate walking

walking pneumonia *n* : a usu. mild pneumonia caused by a bacterium of the genus *Mycoplasma* (*M. pneumoniae*) and characterized by malaise, cough, and often fever

wall \ˈwȯl\ *n* : a structural layer surrounding a cavity, hollow organ, or mass of material ⟨the abdominal ~⟩ — **walled** \ˈwȯld\ *adj*

Wal•le•ri•an degeneration \wä-ˈlir-ē-ən-\ *n* : degeneration of nerve fibers that occurs following injury or disease and that progresses from the place of injury along the axon away from the cell body while the part between the place of injury and the cell body remains intact

Wal•ler \ˈwä-lər\, **Augustus Volney (1816–1870),** British physiologist.

wall•eye \ˈwȯ-ˌlī\ *n* **1 a** : an eye with a whitish or bluish-white iris **b** : an eye with an opaque white cornea **2 a** : strabismus in which the eye turns outward away from the nose — called also *exotropia;* compare CROSS-EYE 1 **b** *pl* : eyes affected with divergent strabismus — **wall•eyed** \-ˈlīd\ *adj*

[1]**wan•der•ing** \ˈwän-də-riŋ\ *adj* : FLOATING ⟨a ~ spleen⟩

[2]**wandering** *n* : movement of a tooth out of its normal position esp. as a result of periodontal disease

wandering cell *n* : any of various amoeboid phagocytic tissue cells

wandering pacemaker *n* : a back-and-forth shift in the location of cardiac pacemaking esp. from the sinoatrial node to or near the atrioventricular node

Wan·gen·steen apparatus \ˈwaŋ-ən-ˌstēn-, -gən-\ *n* : the apparatus used in Wangensteen suction — called also *Wangensteen appliance*

Wangensteen, Owen Harding (1898–1981), American surgeon.

Wangensteen suction *n* : a method of draining fluid or secretions from body cavities (as the stomach) by means of an apparatus that operates on negative pressure

war·ble \ˈwȯr-bəl\ *n* **1** : a swelling under the hide esp. of cattle and horses caused by the maggot of a botfly or warble fly **2** : the maggot of a warble fly — **war·bled** \-bəld\ *adj*

warble fly *n* : any of various dipteran flies (family Oestridae) whose larvae live under the skin of cattle and other mammals and cause warbles

ward \ˈwȯrd\ *n* : a division in a hospital; *esp* : a large room in a hospital where a number of patients often requiring similar treatment are accommodated ⟨a diabetic ~⟩

war·fa·rin \ˈwȯr-fə-rən\ *n* : an anticoagulant coumarin derivative $C_{19}H_{16}O_4$ related to dicumarol that inhibits the production of prothrombin by vitamin K and is used as a rodent poison and in medicine; *also* : its sodium salt $C_{19}H_{15}NaO_4$ used esp. in the prevention or treatment of thromboembolic disease — see COUMADIN

warm–blood·ed \ˈwȯrm-ˈblə-dəd\ *adj* : having a relatively high and constant body temperature relatively independent of the surroundings — **warm–blood·ed·ness** *n*

warm up *vb* : to engage in preliminary exercise (as to stretch the muscles) — **warm–up** \ˈwȯr-ˌməp\ *n*

war neurosis *n* : COMBAT FATIGUE

wart \ˈwȯrt\ *n* **1** : a horny projection on the skin usu. of the extremities produced by proliferation of the skin papillae and caused by any of numerous genotypes of the human papillomaviruses — called also *verruca vulgaris;* see FLAT WART, GENITAL WART, PLANTAR WART **2** : a skin lesion having the form of a wart but not caused by a human papillomavirus — **warty** \ˈwär-tē\ *adj*

War·thin–Star·ry stain \ˈwȯr-thən-ˈstär-ē-\ *n* : a silver nitrate stain used to show the presence of bacilli

Warthin, Aldred Scott (1866–1931), and **Starry, Allen Chronister (1890–1973),** American pathologists.

War·thin's tumor \ˈwȯr-thənz-\ *n* : ADENOLYMPHOMA

[1]**wash** \ˈwȯsh, ˈwäsh\ *vb* **1** : to cleanse by or as if by the action of liquid (as water) **2** : to flush or moisten (a bodily part or injury) with a liquid **3** : to pass through a liquid to carry off impurities or soluble components

[2]**wash** *n* : a liquid medicinal preparation used esp. for cleansing or antisepsis — see EYEWASH, MOUTHWASH

wash·able \ˈwȯ-shə-bəl, ˈwä-\ *adj* **1** : capable of being washed without damage **2** : soluble in water

washings *n pl* : material collected by the washing of a bodily cavity

wash·out \ˈwȯsh-ˌau̇t, ˈwäsh-\ *n* : the action or process of progressively reducing the concentration of a substance (as a dye injected into the left ventricle of the heart)

wasp \ˈwäsp, ˈwȯsp\ *n* : any of numerous social or solitary winged hymenopteran insects (esp. families Sphecidae and Vespidae) that usu. have a slender smooth body with the abdomen attached by a narrow stalk, biting mouthparts, and in the females and workers an often painful sting

Was·ser·mann \ˈwä-sər-mən, ˈvä-\ *n* : WASSERMANN TEST

Wassermann reaction *n* : the complement-fixing reaction that occurs in a positive complement fixation test for syphilis using the serum of an infected individual

Wassermann, August Paul von (1866–1925), German bacteriologist.

Wassermann test *n* : a test for the detection of syphilitic infection using the Wassermann reaction — called also *Wassermann*

[1]**waste** \ˈwāst\ *n* **1** : loss through breaking down of bodily tissue **2** *pl* : bodily waste materials : EXCREMENT

[2]**waste** *vb* **wast·ed; wast·ing** : to lose or cause to lose weight, strength, or vitality : EMACIATE — often used with *away*

[3]**waste** *adj* : excreted from or stored in inert form in a living body as a by-product of vital activity

[1]**wast·ing** \ˈwās-tiŋ\ *adj* : undergoing or causing decay or loss of strength

[2]**wasting** *n* : unintended loss of weight and lean body tissue characteristic of many diseases (as cancer, tuberculosis, and AIDS) : gradual loss of strength or substance : ATROPHY

wa·ter \ˈwȯ-tər, ˈwä-\ *n* **1** : the liquid that descends from the clouds as rain, is a major constituent of all living matter and that when pure is an odorless, tasteless, very slightly compressible liquid oxide of hydrogen H_2O, and freezes at 0°C (32°F) and boils at 100°C (212°F) **2** : liquid containing or resembling water: as **a** (1) : a pharmaceutical or cosmetic preparation made with water (2) : a watery solution of a gaseous or readily volatile substance — see AMMONIA WATER **b** : a watery fluid (as tears or urine) formed or circulating in a living body **c** : AMNIOTIC FLUID — often used in pl.; *also* : BAG OF WATERS

water balance *n* : the ratio between the water assimilated into the body and that lost from the body; *also* : the condition of the body when this ratio approximates unity

water blister *n* : a blister with a clear watery content that is not purulent or sanguineous

wa•ter•borne \ˈwȯ-tər-ˌbōrn, ˈwä-\ *adj* : carried or transmitted by water and esp. by drinking water

water brash *n* : regurgitation of an excessive accumulation of saliva from the lower part of the esophagus often with some acid material from the stomach — compare HEARTBURN

water–hammer pulse *n* : CORRIGAN'S PULSE

water hemlock *n* : a tall poisonous Eurasian perennial herb (*Cicuta virosa*) of the carrot family (Umbelliferae); *also* : any of several poisonous No. American plants of the same genus — compare POISON HEMLOCK

Wa•ter•house–Frid•er•ich•sen syndrome \ˈwȯ-tər-ˌhau̇s-ˈfri-də-rik-sən-\ *n* : acute and severe meningococcemia with hemorrhage into the adrenal glands

Waterhouse, Rupert (1873–1958), British physician.

Friderichsen, Carl (1886–1979), Danish physician.

wa•ter•logged \-ˌlägd\ *adj* : containing excess fluid : EDEMATOUS

water moc•ca•sin \-ˈmä-kə-sən\ *n* : a venomous pit viper (*Agkistrodon piscivorus*) chiefly of the southeastern U.S. closely related to the copperhead — called also *cottonmouth, cottonmouth moccasin*

water on the brain *n* : HYDROCEPHALUS

water on the knee *n* : an accumulation of synovial fluid in the knee joint (as from injury or disease) marked esp. by swelling

water pick \-ˌpik\ *n* : a device that cleans teeth by directing a stream of water over and between the teeth

water pill *n* : a diuretic pill

water–soluble *adj* : soluble in water

Wa•ters' view \ˈwȯ-tərz-\ *n* : a radiographic image obtained by passing a beam of X-rays through the chin at an angle and used esp. to obtain diagnostic information in a single X-ray image about the bony structures of the front of the head

Waters, Charles Alexander (1888–1961), American radiologist.

wa•tery \ˈwȯ-tə-rē, ˈwä-\ *adj* **1** : consisting of or filled with water **2** : containing, sodden with, or yielding water or a thin liquid ⟨∼ stools⟩

Wat•son–Crick \ˈwät-sən-ˈkrik\ *adj* : of or relating to the Watson-Crick model ⟨the *Watson-Crick* helix⟩

Watson, James Dewey (*b* 1928), American molecular biologist.

Crick, Francis Harry Compton (1916–2004), British molecular biologist.

Watson–Crick model *n* : a model of DNA structure in which the molecule is a double-stranded helix, each strand is composed of alternating links of phosphate and deoxyribose, and the strands are linked by pairs of purine and pyrimidine bases projecting inward from the deoxyribose sugars and joined by hydrogen bonds with adenine paired with thymine and with cytosine paired with guanine — compare DOUBLE HELIX

watt \ˈwät\ *n* : the mks unit of power equal to the work done at the rate of one joule per second or to the power produced by a current of one ampere across a potential difference of one volt

Watt, James (1736–1819), British engineer and inventor.

wave \ˈwāv\ *n* **1 a** : a disturbance or variation that transfers energy progressively from point to point in a medium and that may take the form of an elastic deformation or of a variation of pressure, electrical or magnetic intensity, electrical potential, or temperature **b** : one complete cycle of such a disturbance **2** : an undulating or jagged line constituting a graphic representation of an action ⟨an electroencephalographic ∼⟩

wave•form \ˈwāv-ˌfȯrm\ *n* : a usu. graphic representation of the shape of a wave that indicates its characteristics (as frequency and amplitude) — called also *waveshape*

wave•length \-ˌleŋkth\ *n* : the distance in the line of advance of a wave from any one point to the next point of corresponding phase — symbol λ

wave•shape \ˈwāv-ˌshāp\ *n* : WAVEFORM

wax \ˈwaks\ *n* **1** : a substance secreted by bees that is a dull yellow solid plastic when warm — called also *beeswax* **2** : any of various substances resembling beeswax: as **a** : any of numerous substances of plant or animal origin that differ from fats in being less greasy, harder, and more brittle and in containing principally compounds of high molecular weight **b** : a pliable or liquid composition used esp. in uniting surfaces, making patterns or impressions, or producing a polished surface ⟨dental ∼*es*⟩ **3** : a waxy secretion; *esp* : EARWAX

wax•ing *n* : the process of removing body hair with a depilatory wax

waxy \ˈwak-sē\ *adj* **wax•i•er; -est 1** : made of, abounding in, or covered with wax **2** : resembling wax ⟨∼ secretions⟩ ⟨a ∼ complexion⟩

waxy flexibility *n* : a condition in which a patient's limbs retain any position into which they are manipulated by another person and which occurs esp. in catatonic schizophrenia

WBC *abbr* white blood cell

weal \ˈwēl\ *n* : WELT

wean \ˈwēn\ *vb* **1** : to accustom (as an infant or young child) to take food otherwise than by nursing **2 :** to detach usu. gradually from a cause of dependence or form of treatment ⟨being *~ed* off the medication⟩

web \ˈweb\ *n* **:** a tissue or membrane of an animal or plant; *esp* **:** that uniting fingers or toes at their bases — **webbed** \ˈwebd\ *adj*

Web•er–Chris•tian disease \ˈwe-bər-ˈkris-chən-\ *also* **Web•er–Chris•tian's disease** \-chənz-\ *n* **:** PANNICULITIS 2

Weber, Frederick Parkes (1863–1962), British physician.

H. A. Christian — see HAND-SCHÜLLER-CHRISTIAN DISEASE

We•ber–Fech•ner law \ˈwe-bər-ˈfek-nər-, ˈvā-bər-ˈfek-nər-\ *n* **:** an approximately accurate generalization in psychology: the intensity of a sensation is proportional to the logarithm of the intensity of the stimulus causing it — called also *Fechner's law*

Weber, Ernst Heinrich (1795–1878), German anatomist and physiologist.

Fechner, Gustav Theodor (1801–1887), German physicist and psychologist.

We•ber's law \ˈwe-bərz-, ˈvā-bərz-\ *n* **:** an approximately accurate generalization in psychology: the smallest change in the intensity of a stimulus capable of being perceived is proportional to the intensity of the original stimulus

E. H. Weber — see WEBER-FECHNER LAW

We•ber test \ˈwe-bər-, ˈvā-\ *or* **We•ber's test** \-bərz-\ *n* **:** a test to determine the nature of unilateral hearing loss in which a vibrating tuning fork is held against the forehead at the midline and conduction deafness is indicated if the sound is heard more loudly in the affected ear and nerve deafness is indicated if it is heard more loudly in the normal ear

We•ber–Liel \ˈvā-bər-ˈlēl\, **Friedrich Eugen (1832–1891),** German otologist.

Wechs•ler Adult Intelligence Scale \ˈweks-lər-\ *n* **:** an updated version of the Wechsler-Bellevue test having the same structure but standardized against a different population to more accurately reflect the general population — abbr. *WAIS*

Wechsler, David (1896–1981), American psychologist.

Wechs•ler–Belle•vue test \-ˈbel-ˌvyü-\ *n* **:** a test of general intelligence and coordination in adults that involves both verbal and nonverbal tests and is now superseded by the Wechsler Adult Intelligence Scale — called also *Wechsler-Bellevue scale*

Wechsler Intelligence Scale for Children *n* **:** an intelligence test for children of elementary- and secondary-school age that involves verbal ability tests (as vocabulary and comprehension tests) and nonverbal performance tests (as assembly of an object given its parts) — abbr. *WISC*

wedge biopsy *n* **:** a biopsy in which a wedge-shaped sample of tissue is obtained ⟨*wedge biopsy* of the liver⟩; *also* **:** the tissue sample itself

wedge pressure \ˈwej-\ *n* **:** intravascular pressure that is measured by means of a catheter wedged into the pulmonary artery so as to block the flow of blood and that is equivalent to the pressure in the left atrium — called also *pulmonary capillary wedge pressure, pulmonary wedge pressure*

wedge resection *n* **:** any of several surgical procedures for removal of a wedge-shaped mass of tissue

WEE *abbr* western equine encephalitis; western equine encephalomyelitis

weep \ˈwēp\ *vb* **wept** \ˈwept\; **weep•ing 1 :** to pour forth (tears) from the eyes **2 :** to exude (a fluid) slowly ⟨a *~ing* burn⟩

Weg•e•ner's granulomatosis \ˈve-gə-nərz-\ *n, esp formerly* **:** an uncommon disease of unknown cause that is characterized chiefly by inflammation of small blood vessels and granuloma formation esp. in the respiratory tract and kidneys **:** GRANULOMATOSIS WITH POLYANGIITIS

Wegener, F. (1907–1990), German pathologist.

weigh \ˈwā\ *vb* **1 :** to find the heaviness of **2 :** to measure or apportion (a definite quantity) on or as if on a scale **3 :** to have weight or a specified weight

weight \ˈwāt\ *n* **1 :** the amount that a thing weighs **2 :** a unit of weight or mass

weight•less•ness \ˈwāt-ləs-nəs\ *n* **:** the state or condition of having little or no weight due to lack of apparent gravitational pull — **weight•less** *adj*

Weil–Fe•lix reaction \ˈvīl-ˈfā-liks-\ *n* **:** an agglutination test for various rickettsial infections (as typhus and Rocky Mountain spotted fever) using particular strains of bacteria of the genus *Proteus* that have antigens in common with the rickettsiae to be identified — called also *Weil-Felix test*

Weil, Edmund (1880–1922), and **Felix, Arthur (1887–1956),** Austrian bacteriologists.

Weil's disease \ˈvīlz-, ˈwīlz-\ *n* **:** a severe form of leptospirosis that is characterized by jaundice, chills, fever, muscle pain, shortness of breath, and chest pain, is caused by a spirochete of the genus *Leptospira* (*L. interrogans*, esp. serotype *icterohaemorrhagiae*), and if left untreated may cause life-threatening damage to the brain, kidneys, lungs, liver, or heart — called also *Weil's syndrome*

Weil, Adolf (1848–1916), German physician.

Wel•chol \ˈwel-ˌkōl\ *trademark* — used for a preparation of colesevelam

well \ˈwel\ *adj* **1** : free or recovered from infirmity or disease : HEALTHY **2** : completely cured or healed

well–adjusted *adj* : WELL-BALANCED 2

well–balanced *adj* **1** : nicely or evenly balanced, arranged, or regulated ⟨a ~ diet⟩ **2** : emotionally or psychologically untroubled

Well•bu•trin \ˌwel-ˈbyü-trin\ *trademark* — used for a preparation of the hydrochloride of bupropion

well•ness *n* : the quality or state of being in good health esp. as an actively sought goal

welt \ˈwelt\ *n* : a ridge or lump raised on the body (as by a blow or an allergic reaction)

wen \ˈwen\ *n* : SEBACEOUS CYST; *broadly* : an abnormal growth or a cyst protruding from a surface esp. of the skin

Wencke•bach period \ˈweŋ-kə-ˌbäk-\ *n* : WENCKEBACH PHENOMENON

Wenckebach, Karel Frederik (1864–1940), Dutch internist.

Wenckebach phenomenon *n* : heart block in which a pulse from the atrium periodically does not reach the ventricle and which is characterized by progressive prolongation of the P-R interval until a pulse is skipped

Werd•nig–Hoff•mann disease \ˈvert-nik-ˈhȯf-ˌmän-\ *n* : muscular atrophy that is caused by degeneration of the ventral horn cells of the spinal cord, is inherited as an autosomal recessive trait, becomes symptomatic during early infancy, is characterized by hypotonia and flaccid paralysis, and is often fatal during childhood — called also *Werdnig-Hoffmann syndrome;* compare KUGELBERG-WELANDER SYNDROME

Werdnig, Guido (1844–1919), Austrian neurologist, and **Hoffmann, Johann (1857–1919),** German neurologist.

Werl•hof's disease \ˈverl-ˌhōfs-\ *n* : THROMBOCYTOPENIC PURPURA

Werlhof, Paul Gottlieb (1699–1767), German physician.

Wer•ner syndrome \ˈver-nər-\ *or* **Wer•ner's syndrome** \-nərz-\ *n* : a rare genetic disorder with onset during adolescence or early adulthood that is characterized by cessation of growth at puberty and by premature and accelerated aging with associated abnormalities (as muscle wasting, cataracts, osteoporosis, and hypogonadism) and that is inherited as an autosomal recessive trait

Werner, Otto (1879–1936), German physician.

Wer•nicke's aphasia \ˈver-nə-kəz-\ *n* : SENSORY APHASIA; *specif* : sensory aphasia in which the affected individual speaks words fluently but without meaningful content

Wernicke, Carl (1848–1905), German neurologist.

Wernicke's area *n* : an area located in the posterior part of the superior temporal gyrus that plays an important role in the comprehension of language

Wernicke's encephalopathy *n* : an acute inflammatory hemorrhagic encephalopathy that is caused by thiamine deficiency (as that associated with chronic alcoholism or malnutrition) and is characterized by loss of muscle coordination, visual disturbances (as diplopia), and confusion and memory loss — see KORSAKOFF SYNDROME

Wert•heim operation \ˈvert-ˌhīm-\ *or* **Wert•heim's operation** \-ˌhīmz-\ *n* : radical hysterectomy performed by way of an abdominal incision

Wertheim, Ernst (1864–1920), Austrian gynecologist.

Wes•ter•gren erythrocyte sedimentation rate \ˈves-tər-grən-\ *n* : sedimentation rate of red blood cells determined by the Westergren method — called also *Westergren sedimentation rate*

Westergren, Alf Vilhelm (1891–1968), Swedish physician.

Westergren method *n* : a method for estimating the sedimentation rate of red blood cells in fluid blood

western black–legged tick *n* : a tick of the genus *Ixodes* (*I. pacificus*) that is found in the western U.S. and British Columbia and is a vector of several diseases (as Lyme disease) — called also *black-legged tick*

Western blot *n* : a blot consisting of a sheet of a cellulose derivative or nylon that contains spots of protein for identification by a suitable molecular probe and is used esp. for the detection of antibodies — compare NORTHERN BLOT, SOUTHERN BLOT — **Western blotting** *n*

western equine encephalitis *n* : EQUINE ENCEPHALITIS b

western equine encephalomyelitis *n* : EQUINE ENCEPHALITIS b

West Nile \ˈwest-ˈnīl\ *n* : WEST NILE VIRUS

West Nile encephalitis *n* : a severe form of West Nile virus marked by encephalitis

West Nile fever *n* : WEST NILE VIRUS 2

West Nile virus *n* **1** : a virus of the genus *Flavivirus* (species *West Nile virus*) that causes an illness marked by fever, headache, muscle ache, skin rash, and sometimes encephalitis or meningitis, that is spread esp. from birds to humans by mosquitoes chiefly of the genus *Culex*, and that is closely related to the viruses causing Japanese B encephalitis and Saint Louis encephalitis **2** : the illness caused by West Nile virus — called also *West Nile fever;* see WEST NILE ENCEPHALITIS

wet \ˈwet\ *adj* : marked by the presence or abundance of fluid (as secretions or effusions)

wet dream *n* : an erotic dream culminating in orgasm and in the male accompanied by seminal emission

wet mount *n* : a glass slide holding a specimen suspended in a drop of liquid (as water) for microscopic examination; *also* : a specimen mounted in this way — **wet–mount** *adj*

wet nurse *n* : a woman who cares for and suckles young not her own

wetting agent *n* : a substance that promotes the spreading of a liquid on a surface or the penetration of a liquid into a material esp. by becoming adsorbed in such a way that the liquid is no longer repelled

Whar•ton's duct \ˈhwȯrt-ᵊnz-, ˈwȯrt-\ *n* : the duct of the submandibular gland that opens into the mouth on a papilla at the side of the frenulum of the tongue

Wharton, Thomas (1614–1673), British anatomist.

Wharton's jelly *n* : a soft connective tissue that occurs in the umbilical cord and consists of large stellate fibroblasts and a few wandering cells and macrophages embedded in a homogeneous jellylike intercellular substance

wheal \ˈhwēl, ˈwēl\ *n* : a suddenly formed elevation of the skin surface: as **a** : WELT; *esp* : a flat burning or itching eminence on the skin **b** : the transient lump occurring at the site of injection of a solution before the solution is normally dispersed — **whealing** *n*

wheat germ *n* : the embryo of the wheat kernel separated in milling and used esp. as a source of vitamins and protein

wheel•chair \ˈhwēl-ˌchar, ˈwēl-\ *n* : a chair mounted on wheels esp. for the use of disabled individuals

¹**wheeze** \ˈhwēz, ˈwēz\ *vb* **wheezed; wheez•ing** : to breathe with difficulty usu. with a whistling sound

²**wheeze** *n* : a sibilant whistling sound caused by difficult or obstructed respiration

whey \ˈhwā, ˈwā\ *n* : the serum or watery part of milk that is separated from the coagulable part or curd, is rich in lactose, minerals, and vitamins, and contains lactalbumin and traces of fat

whip•lash \ˈhwip-ˌlash, ˈwip-\ *n* : injury resulting from a sudden sharp whipping movement of the neck and head (as of a person in a vehicle that is struck head-on or from the rear by another vehicle)

Whip•ple operation \ˈhwi-pəl-, ˈwi-\ *or* **Whip•ple's operation** \-pəlz-\ *n* : WHIPPLE PROCEDURE

Whipple procedure *or* **Whipple's procedure** *n* : PANCREATICODUODENECTOMY; *esp* : one in which there is complete excision of the pancreas and partial excision of the duodenum

Whipple, Allen Oldfather (1881–1963), American surgeon.

Whipple's disease *also* **Whipple disease** *n* : a rare malabsorption syndrome that is caused by an actinomycetous fungus (*Tropheryma whippelli*) in the mucous membrane of the intestine, that affects primarily the small intestine but becomes more generalized affecting esp. the joints, brain, liver, and heart, and that is marked by the accumulation of lipid deposits in the intestinal lymphatic tissues, diarrhea, weight loss, joint pain, mental confusion, and generalized lymphadenopathy — called also *intestinal lipodystrophy*

Whipple, George Hoyt (1878–1976), American pathologist.

whip•worm \ˈhwip-ˌwərm, ˈwip-\ *n* : a parasitic nematode worm of the genus *Trichuris* having a body that is thickened posteriorly and is very long and slender anteriorly; *esp* : one (*T. trichiura*) of the human intestine

whirl•pool bath \ˈhwərl-ˌpül-, ˈwərl-\ *n* : a therapeutic bath in which all or part of the body is exposed to forceful whirling currents of hot water — called also *whirlpool*

white blood cell *n* : any of the blood cells of the immune system that are colorless, lack hemoglobin, contain a nucleus, and include the lymphocytes, monocytes, neutrophils, eosinophils, and basophils along with their precursors and derivatives (as macrophages) : LEUKOCYTE — abbr. *WBC;* called also *white blood corpuscle, white cell, white corpuscle;* compare RED BLOOD CELL

white coat hypertension *n* : a temporary elevation in a patient's blood pressure that occurs when measured in a medical setting (as a physician's office) and that is usu. due to anxiety on the part of the patient — called also *white coat effect*

white count *n* : the count or the total number of white blood cells in the blood usu. stated as the number in one cubic millimeter — compare DIFFERENTIAL BLOOD COUNT

white fat *n* : normal fat tissue that replaces brown fat in infants during the first year of life

white•head \ˈhwīt-ˌhed, ˈwīt-\ *n* : MILIUM

white light *n* : light that is composed of a wide range of electromagnetic frequencies and that appears colorless to the eye

white lotion *n* : a preparation made of sulfurated potash and zinc sulfate that is applied topically in the treatment of various skin disorders

white matter *n* : neural tissue esp. of the brain and spinal cord that consists largely of myelinated nerve fibers bundled into tracts, has a whitish color, and typically underlies the gray matter

white muscle disease *n* : a degenerative muscle disease of young domestic animals caused by a dietary deficiency of selenium or vitamin E — see STIFF-LAMB DISEASE

white noise *n* : a heterogeneous mixture of sound waves extending over a wide frequency range that has been used to mask out unwanted noise interfering with sleep — called also *white sound*

white ointment *n* : an ointment consisting of 5 percent white wax and 95 percent white petrolatum — called also *simple ointment*

white petrolatum *n* : decolorized petroleum jelly — called also *white petroleum jelly*

white piedra *n* : a form of piedra that affects esp. the facial hairs and is caused by fungi of the genus *Trichosporon* (*T. ovoides* and *T. inkin*)

white pulp *n* : a parenchymatous tissue of the spleen that consists of compact masses of lymphatic cells and that forms the Malpighian corpuscles — compare RED PULP

white ramus *n* : RAMUS COMMUNICANS a

white ramus communicans *n* : RAMUS COMMUNICANS a

whites *n pl* : LEUKORRHEA

white shark *n* : GREAT WHITE SHARK

white snake•root \-ˈsnāk-ˌrüt, -ˌru̇t\ *n* : a poisonous No. American herb (*Eupatorium rugosum* of the family Compositae) that is a cause of trembles and milk sickness

white sound *n* : WHITE NOISE

white squill *n* : SQUILL 2

Whit•field's ointment \ˈhwit-ˌfēldz-, ˈwit-\ *also* **Whit•field ointment** \-ˌfēld-\ *n* : an ointment that contains benzoic acid and salicylic acid and is used for its keratolytic effect in treating fungus skin diseases (as ringworm)

Whitfield, Arthur (1868–1947), British dermatologist.

whit•low \ˈhwit-(ˌ)lō, ˈwit-\ *n* **1** : an infection of the finger and esp. the fingertip that is typically caused by infection of a virus (as the herpes simplex virus) and is marked by redness, tenderness, and fluid-filled blisters — compare PARONYCHIA **2** : FELON

WHO *abbr* World Health Organization

whole \ˈhōl\ *adj* : containing all its natural constituents, components, or elements

whole blood *n* : blood with all its components (as white and red blood cells, platelets, and plasma) intact that has been withdrawn from a donor into an anticoagulant solution, that may be used in transfusions to restore blood volume esp. after traumatic blood loss, and that is often subjected to centrifugation to separate blood components for use in transfusion or for specimen testing

whole–body *adj* : of, relating to, or affecting the entire body ⟨~ radiation⟩

whole food *n* : a natural food and esp. an unprocessed one

whoop \ˈhüp, ˈhu̇p, ˈhwu̇p\ *n* : the crowing intake of breath following a paroxysm in whooping cough — **whoop** *vb*

whooping cough *n* : an infectious disease esp. of children caused by a bacterium of the genus *Bordetella* (*B. pertussis*) and marked by a convulsive spasmodic cough sometimes followed by a crowing intake of breath — called also *pertussis*

whorl \ˈhwȯrl, ˈwȯrl, ˈhwərl, ˈwərl\ *n* : a fingerprint in which the central papillary ridges turn through at least one complete turn

Wi•dal reaction \vē-ˈdäl-\ *also* **Widal's reaction** \-ˈdälz-\ *n* : a specific reaction consisting in agglutination of typhoid bacilli or other salmonellae when mixed with serum from a patient having typhoid fever or other salmonella infection and constituting a test for the disease

Widal, Georges–Fernand–Isidore (1862–1929), French physician and bacteriologist.

Widal test *also* **Widal's test** *n* : a test for detecting typhoid fever and other salmonella infections using the Widal reaction — compare AGGLUTINATION TEST

wide–spectrum *adj* : BROAD-SPECTRUM

wid•ow–mak•er \ˈwi-(ˌ)dō-ˌmā-kər\ *n* : a blockage in a branch of the left coronary artery that commonly causes a fatal heart attack; *also* : the branch of the left coronary artery susceptible to fatal blockage

wild type *n* : a phenotype, genotype, or gene that predominates in a natural population of organisms or strain of organisms in contrast to that of natural or laboratory mutant forms; *also* : an organism or strain displaying the wild type — **wild–type** *adj*

Wil•liams syndrome \ˈwil-yəmz-\ *also* **Williams–Beu•ren syndrome** \-ˈbȯi-rən-\ *n* : a rare genetic disorder marked esp. by hypercalcemia of infants, heart defects, characteristic facial features (as an upturned nose and pointed chin), a sociable personality, and mild to moderate intellectual disability but a high verbal aptitude

Williams, J. C. P. (*fl* 1961), New Zealand cardiologist.

Beuren, Alois J. (1919–1984), German cardiologist.

Wilms' tumor \ˈvilmz-\ *also* **Wilms's tumor** \ˈvilm-zəz-\ *n* : a malignant tumor of the kidney that primarily affects children and is made up of embryonic elements — called also *nephroblastoma*

Wilms, Max (1867–1918), German surgeon.

Wil•son's disease \ˈwil-sənz-\ *n* : a genetic disease that is characterized by the accumulation of copper in the body (as in the liver or brain) due to abnormal copper metabolism associated with ceruloplasmin deficiency, that is inherited as an autosomal recessive trait, and that is marked esp. by liver dysfunction and disease and neurologic or psychiatric symptoms (as tremors or dementia) — called also *hepatolenticular degeneration;* see KAYSER-FLEISCHER RING

Wilson, Samuel Alexander Kinnier (1877–1937), British neurologist.

wind•burn \ˈwind-ˌbərn\ *n* : irritation of the skin caused by wind — **wind•burned** \-ˌbərnd\ *adj*

wind•chill \-ˌchil\ *n* : a still-air temperature that would have the same cooling effect on exposed human skin as a given combination of temperature and wind speed — called also *chill factor, windchill factor, windchill index*

win•dow \ˈwin-(ˌ)dō\ *n* **1** : FENESTRA 1 **2** : a small surgically created opening : FENESTRA 2a **3** : a usu. narrow interval of time or range of values for which a certain condition or an opportunity exists — see THERAPEUTIC WINDOW

wind•pipe \ˈwind-ˌpīp\ *n* : TRACHEA

wing \ˈwiŋ\ *n* **1** : one of the movable feathered or membranous paired appendages by means of which a bird, bat, or insect is able to fly **2** : a winglike anatomical part or process : ALA; *esp* : any of the four winglike processes of the sphenoid bone — see GREATER WING, LESSER WING — **winged** \ˈwiŋd, ˈwiŋ-əd\ *adj*

win•ter•green \ˈwin-tər-ˌgrēn\ *n* **1** : a low white-flowered evergreen plant (*Gaultheria procumbens* of the heath family, Ericaceae) with spicy red berries **2** : OIL OF WINTERGREEN

wintergreen oil *n* : OIL OF WINTERGREEN

winter itch *n* : an itching disorder caused by prolonged exposure to cold dry air

winter tick *n* : an ixodid tick of the genus *Dermacentor* (*D. albipictus*) that is actively parasitic during the winter months on animals (as deer and moose) in parts of Canada and the northern and western U.S.

wire \ˈwīr\ *n* : metal thread or a rod used in surgery to suture soft tissue or transfix fractured bone and in orthodontic dentistry to position teeth — **wire** *vb*

Wir•sung's duct \ˈvir-ˌsu̇ŋz-\ *n* : PANCREATIC DUCT a

J. G. Wirsung — see DUCT OF WIRSUNG

WISC *abbr* Wechsler Intelligence Scale for Children

wisdom tooth *n* : the third molar that is the last tooth to erupt on each side of the upper and lower jaws

wish–fulfillment *n* : the gratification of a desire esp. symbolically (as in dreams or neurotic symptoms)

Wis•kott–Al•drich syndrome \ˈvis-ˌkät-ˈȯl-ˌdrich-\ *n* : a usu. fatal immunodeficiency disease of male children that is inherited as an X-linked recessive trait and is characterized esp. by thrombocytopenia, leukopenia, recurrent infections, eczema, and abnormal bleeding

Wiskott, Alfred (1898–1978), German pediatrician.

Aldrich, Robert Anderson (1917–1998), American pediatrician.

witch ha•zel \ˈwich-ˌhā-zəl\ *n* **1** : a small tree or shrub (*Hamamelis virginiana* of the family Hamamelidaceae) of eastern No. America **2** : an alcoholic solution of a distillate of the bark of the witch hazel used as a soothing and mildly astringent lotion

with•draw•al \wit͟h-ˈdrȯ-əl, with-\ *n* **1 a** : a pathological retreat from objective reality (as in some schizophrenic states) **b** : social or emotional detachment **2 a** : the discontinuance of administration or use of a drug **b** : the syndrome of often painful physical and psychological symptoms that follows discontinuance of an addicting substance **3** : COITUS INTERRUPTUS — **with•draw** \-ˈdrȯ\ *vb*

withdrawal symptom *n* : one of a group of symptoms (as nausea, sweating, or depression) produced by deprivation of an addictive substance

with•drawn \wit͟h-ˈdrȯn\ *adj* : socially detached and unresponsive : exhibiting withdrawal : INTROVERTED

with•ers \ˈwi-t͟hərz\ *n pl* **1** : the ridge between the shoulder bones of a horse **2** : a part corresponding to the withers in a quadruped other than a horse

Wit•zel•sucht \ˈvit-səl-ˌzu̇kt\ *n* : excessive facetiousness and inappropriate or pointless humor esp. when considered as part of an abnormal condition

wohl•fahr•tia \ˌvōl-ˈfär-tē-ə\ *n* **1** *cap* : a genus of dipteran flies (family Sarcophagidae) that deposit their larvae in wounds or on the intact skin of humans and domestic animals causing severe cutaneous myiasis **2** : any fly of the genus *Wohlfahrtia*

Wol•fart \ˈvōl-ˌfärt\, **Peter (1675–1726),** German physician.

Wolff•ian body \ˈwu̇l-fē-ən-\ *n* : MESONEPHROS

Wolff \ˈvȯlf\, **Caspar Friedrich (1734–1794),** German anatomist and embryologist.

Wolffian duct *n* : the duct of the mesonephros that persists in the female chiefly as part of the epoophoron and in the male as the duct system leaving the testis and including the epididymis, vas deferens, seminal vesicle, and ejaculatory duct — called also *mesonephric duct*

Wolff–Par•kin•son–White syndrome \ˈwu̇lf-ˈpär-kən-sən-ˈhwīt-, -ˈwīt-\ *n* : an abnormal heart condition characterized by preexcitation of the ventricle and an electrocardiographic tracing with a shortened P-R interval and a widened QRS complex — called also *WPW syndrome*

Wolff, Louis (1898–1972), and **White, Paul Dudley (1886–1973),** American cardiologists.
Parkinson, Sir John (1885–1976), British cardiologist.

wol•fram \ˈwu̇l-frəm\ *n* : TUNGSTEN

Wol•fram syndrome *or* **Wolfram's syndrome** \ˈwu̇l-frəm-\ *n* : a rare hereditary disorder that is characterized esp. by type 1 diabetes, diabetes insipidus, optic atrophy, sensorineural deafness, and bladder dysfunction and that is inherited as an autosomal recessive trait
Wolfram, D. J. (*fl* 1938), American physician.

womb \ˈwüm\ *n* : UTERUS

wonder drug *n* : MIRACLE DRUG

wood alcohol *n* : METHANOL

Wood's lamp \ˈwu̇dz-\ *also* **Wood lamp** \ˈwu̇d-\ *n* : a lamp for producing ultraviolet radiation that is used to detect various skin conditions (as some fungus infections) by the fluorescence induced in the affected areas by ultraviolet radiation
Wood, Robert Williams (1868–1955), American physicist.

Wood's light *also* **Wood light** *n* : WOOD'S LAMP; *also* : ultraviolet radiation produced by a Wood's lamp

wood tick *n* : any of several ixodid ticks: as **a** : ROCKY MOUNTAIN WOOD TICK **b** : AMERICAN DOG TICK

wool fat \ˈwu̇l-\ *n* : wool grease esp. after refining : LANOLIN

wool grease *n* : a fatty slightly sticky wax coating the surface of the fibers of sheep's wool that is used as a source of lanolin

wool•sort•er's disease \ˈwu̇l-ˌsȯr-tərz-\ *n* : pulmonary anthrax resulting esp. from inhalation of bacterial spores from contaminated wool or hair

word–association test *n* : a test of personality and mental function in which the subject is required to respond to each of a series of words with the first word that comes to mind or with a word of a specified class of words

word blindness *n* : ALEXIA

word salad *n* : a jumble of extremely incoherent speech as sometimes observed in schizophrenia

working memory *n* : memory that involves storing, focusing attention on, and manipulating information for a relatively short period of time (as a few seconds)

work–related musculoskeletal disorder *n* : REPETITIVE STRAIN INJURY

work•up \ˈwər-ˌkəp\ *n* : an intensive diagnostic study ⟨a gastrointestinal ~⟩

work up \ˌwər-ˈkəp, ˈwər-\ *vb* : to perform a diagnostic workup upon

[1]**worm** \ˈwərm\ *n* **1** : any of various relatively small elongated usu. naked and soft-bodied parasitic animals (as a grub, pinworm, or tapeworm) **2** : HELMINTHIASIS — usu. used in pl. ⟨a dog with ~*s*⟩ — **worm•like** *adj*

[2]**worm** *vb* : to treat (an animal) with a drug to destroy or expel parasitic worms

worm•er \ˈwər-mər\ *n* : a worming agent used in veterinary medicine

Wor•mi•an bone \ˈwȯr-mē-ən-\ *n* : a small irregular inconstant plate of bone interposed in a suture between large cranial bones
Worm \ˈwȯrm\, **Ole** (*Latin* **Olaus Wormius**) **(1588–1654),** Danish physician.

worm•seed \ˈwərm-ˌsēd\ *n* : any of various plants (as of the genera *Artemisia* or *Chenopodium*) whose seeds possess anthelmintic properties

worm•wood \ˈwərm-ˌwu̇d\ *n* : any of various aromatic shrubs and herbs (genus *Artemisia* and esp. *A. absinthium* of the family Compositae)

wound \ˈwünd\ *n* **1 a** : a physical injury to the body consisting of a laceration or breaking of the skin or mucous membrane often with damage to underlying tissues **b** : an opening made in the skin or a membrane of the body incidental to a surgical operation or procedure **2** : a mental or emotional hurt or blow — **wound** *vb*

WPW syndrome \ˌdə-bəl-yü-ˌpē-ˈdə-bəl-yü-\ *n* : WOLFF-PARKINSON-WHITE SYNDROME

wrench \ˈrench\ *n* : a sharp twist or sudden jerk straining muscles or ligaments; *also* : the resultant injury (as of a joint) — **wrench** *vb*

Wright's stain \ˈrīts-\ *n* : a stain used in staining blood and parasites living in blood
Wright, James Homer (1869–1928), American pathologist.

wrin•kle \ˈriŋ-kəl\ *n* : a small ridge or furrow in the skin esp. when due to age, worry, or fatigue — **wrinkle** *vb*

wrist \ˈrist\ *n* : the joint or the region of the joint between the human hand and the arm

wrist•bone \-ˌbōn\ *n* **1** : a carpal bone **2** : the styloid process of the human radius that forms a prominence on the outer side of the wrist above the thumb

wrist–drop \-ˌdräp\ *n* : paralysis of the extensor muscles of the hand causing the hand to hang down at the wrist

wrist joint *n* : the articulation at the wrist

writer's cramp *n* : a painful spasmodic cramp of muscles of the hand or fingers brought on by excessive writing — called also *graphospasm*

wry•neck \ˈrī-ˌnek\ *n* : TORTICOLLIS

wt *abbr* weight

Wuch•er•e•ria \ˌwu̇-kə-ˈrir-ē-ə\ *n* : a genus of filarial worms (family Dipetalonematidae) including a parasite (*W. bancrofti*) that causes elephantiasis
Wu•cher•er \ˈvu̇-k̲ər-ər\, **Otto Eduard Heinrich (1820–1873),** German physician.

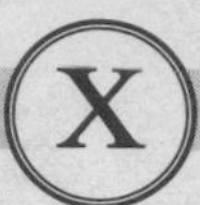

x \ˈeks\ *n, pl* **x's** *or* **xs** \ˈek-səz\ : the basic or haploid number of chromosomes of a polyploid series : the number contained in a single genome — compare N 1
x *symbol* power of magnification
Xal•a•tan \ˈza-lə-ˌtan\ *trademark* — used for a preparation of latanoprost
Xan•ax \ˈza-ˌnaks\ *trademark* — used for a preparation of alprazolam
xanth- *or* **xantho-** *comb form* : yellow ⟨*xanth*oma⟩
xan•than gum \ˈzan-thən-\ *n* : a polysaccharide produced by fermentation of carbohydrates by a bacterium (*Xanthomonas campestris*) and used as a thickening and suspending agent in pharmaceuticals and prepared foods — called also *xanthan*
xan•the•las•ma \ˌzan-thə-ˈlaz-mə\ *n* : xanthoma of the eyelid
xanthelasma pal•pe•bra•rum \-ˌpal-ˌpē-ˈbrar-əm\ *n* : XANTHELASMA
xan•thene dye \ˈzan-ˌthēn-\ *n* : any of various brilliant fluorescent yellow to pink to bluish-red dyes
xan•thine \ˈzan-ˌthēn\ *n* : a feebly basic compound $C_5H_4N_4O_2$ that occurs esp. in animal or plant tissue, is derived from guanine and hypoxanthine, and yields uric acid on oxidation; *also* : any of various derivatives of this
xan•tho•chro•mia \ˌzan-thə-ˈkrō-mē-ə\ *n* : xanthochromic discoloration
xan•tho•chro•mic \-ˈkrō-mik\ *adj* : having a yellowish discoloration
xan•tho•ma \zan-ˈthō-mə\ *n, pl* **-mas** *also* **-ma•ta** \-mə-tə\ : a fatty irregular yellow patch or nodule on the skin that is associated esp. with disturbances of cholesterol metabolism
xan•tho•ma•to•sis \(ˌ)zan-ˌthō-mə-ˈtō-səs\ *n, pl* **-to•ses** \-ˌsēz\ : a condition marked by the presence of multiple xanthomas
xan•tho•ma•tous \zan-ˈthō-mə-təs\ *adj* : of, relating to, marked by, or characteristic of a xanthoma or xanthomatosis ⟨~ lesions⟩
xan•tho•phyll \ˈzan-thə-ˌfil\ *n* : any of several neutral yellow to orange carotenoid pigments that are oxygen derivatives of carotenes; *esp* : LUTEIN
xan•thop•sia \zan-ˈthäp-sē-ə\ *n* : a visual disturbance in which objects appear yellow
xan•tho•tox•in \ˈzan-thə-ˌtäk-sən\ *n* : METHOXSALEN
xanth•uren•ic acid \ˌzanth-yə-ˈre-nik-\ *n* : a yellow crystalline phenolic acid $C_{10}H_7NO_4$ that is a tryptophan metabolite excreted in the urine
Xa•rel•to \zə-ˈrel-tō\ *trademark* — used for a preparation of rivaroxaban
X chromosome *n* : a sex chromosome that usu. occurs paired in each female cell and single in each male cell in species in which the male typically has two unlike sex chromosomes — compare Y CHROMOSOME
X–disease *n* : any of various usu. virus diseases of obscure etiology and relationships; *esp* : MURRAY VALLEY ENCEPHALITIS
XDR *abbr* extensively drug-resistant
Xe *symbol* xenon
Xel•janz \ˈzel-ˌjanz\ *trademark* — used for a preparation of the citrate of tofacitinib
Xel•o•da \ˈzel-ə-də\ *trademark* — used for a preparation of capecitabine
xen- *or* **xeno-** *comb form* **1** : strange : foreign ⟨*xeno*biotic⟩ **2** : HETER- ⟨*xeno*graft⟩
Xen•i•cal \ˈze-ni-ˌkal\ *trademark* — used for a preparation of orlistat
xe•no•bi•ot•ic \ˌze-nō-bī-ˈä-tik, ˌzē-, -bē-\ *n* : a chemical compound (as a drug or pesticide) that is foreign to a living organism — **xenobiotic** *adj*
xe•no•di•ag•no•sis \ˌze-nō-ˌdī-ig-ˈnō-səs, ˌzē-\ *n, pl* **-no•ses** \-ˌsēz\ : the detection of a parasite (as of humans) by feeding supposedly infected material (as blood) to a suitable intermediate host (as an insect) and later examining the intermediate host for the parasite — **xe•no•di•ag•nos•tic** \-ˈnäs-tik\ *adj*
xe•no•ge•ne•ic \ˌze-nō-jə-ˈnē-ik, ˌzē-\ *also* **xe•no•gen•ic** \-ˈje-nik\ *adj* : derived from, originating in, or being a member of another species — compare ALLOGENEIC, SYNGENEIC
xe•no•graft \ˈze-nə-ˌgraft, ˈzē-\ *n* : a graft of tissue taken from a donor of one species and grafted into a recipient of another species — called also *heterograft, heterotransplant, xenotransplant;* compare HOMOGRAFT — **xenograft** *vb*
xe•non \ˈzē-ˌnän, ˈze-\ *n* : a heavy, colorless, and relatively inert gaseous element — symbol *Xe;* see ELEMENT table
xe•no•phobe \ˈze-nə-ˌfōb, ˈzē-\ *n* : one unduly fearful of what is foreign and esp. of people of foreign origin — **xe•no•pho•bic** \ˌze-nə-ˈfō-bik, ˌzē-\ *adj*
xe•no•pho•bia \ˌze-nə-ˈfō-bē-ə, ˌzē-\ *n* : fear and hatred of strangers or foreigners or of anything that is strange or foreign
Xen•op•syl•la \ˌze-näp-ˈsi-lə\ *n* : a genus of fleas (family Pulicidae) including several (as the oriental rat flea) that are vectors of plague
xe•no•trans•plant \ˌze-nə-ˈtrans-ˌplant, ˌzē-\ *n* : XENOGRAFT — **xenotransplant** *vb*
xe•no•trans•plan•ta•tion \-ˌtrans-ˌplan-ˈtā-shən\ *n* : transplantation of an organ, tissue, or cells between two different species
xe•no•tro•pic \ˌze-nə-ˈträ-pik, ˌzē-nə-ˈtrō-pik\ *adj* : replicating or reproduc-

ing only in cells other than those of the host species ⟨~ viruses⟩

xer- *or* **xero-** *comb form* : dry : arid ⟨*xero*derma⟩

xe•ro•der•ma \ˌzir-ə-ˈdər-mə\ *n* : a disease of the skin characterized by dryness and roughness and a fine scaly desquamation

xeroderma pig•men•to•sum \-ˌpig-mən-ˈtō-səm, -ˌmen-\ *n* : a genetic condition inherited chiefly as a recessive autosomal trait that is caused by a defect in mechanisms that repair DNA damaged by ultraviolet light and is characterized by the development of pigment abnormalities and multiple skin cancers in body areas exposed to the sun — abbr. *XP*

xe•rog•ra•phy \zə-ˈrä-grə-fē, zir-ˈä-\ *n, pl* **-phies** **1** : a process for copying graphic matter by the action of light on an electrically charged surface in which the latent image is developed with a resinous powder **2** : XERORADIOGRAPHY — **xe•ro•graph•ic** \ˌzir-ə-ˈgra-fik\ *adj* — **xe•ro•graph•i•cal•ly** *adv*

xe•ro•mam•mog•ra•phy \ˌzir-ō-ma-ˈmä-grə-fē\ *n, pl* **-phies** : xeroradiography of the breast — **xe•ro•mam•mo•gram** \-ˈma-mə-ˌgram\ *n*

xe•roph•thal•mia \ˌzir-ˌäf-ˈthal-mē-ə, -ˌäp-ˈthal-\ *n* : a dry thickened lusterless condition of the eyeball resulting esp. from a severe deficiency of vitamin A — compare KERATOMALACIA — **xe•roph•thal•mic** \-mik\ *adj*

xe•ro•ra•di•og•ra•phy \ˌzir-ō-ˌrā-dē-ˈä-grə-fē\ *n, pl* **-phies** : radiography used esp. in mammographic screening for breast cancer that produces an image using X-rays in a manner similar to the way an image is produced by light in xerography — **xe•ro•ra•dio•graph•ic** \-ˌrā-dē-ō-ˈgra-fik\ *adj*

xe•ro•sis \zi-ˈrō-səs\ *n, pl* **xe•ro•ses** \-ˌsēz\ : abnormal dryness of a body part or tissue (as the skin)

xe•ro•sto•mia \ˌzir-ə-ˈstō-mē-ə\ *n* : abnormal dryness of the mouth due to insufficient secretions — called also *dry mouth*

Xge•va \eks-ˈjē-və\ *trademark* — used for a preparation of denosumab

xiph- *or* **xiphi-** *or* **xipho-** *comb form* : sword-shaped ⟨*xiphi*sternum⟩

xi•phi•ster•num \ˌzī-fə-ˈstər-nəm, ˌzi-\ *n, pl* **-na** \-nə\ : XIPHOID PROCESS

xi•phoid \ˈzī-ˌfȯid, ˈzi-\ *n* : XIPHOID PROCESS — **xiphoid** *adj*

xiphoid process *n* : the smallest and lowest division of the human sternum that is cartilaginous early in life but becomes more or less ossified during adulthood — called also *ensiform cartilage, ensiform process*

x–ir•ra•di•a•tion \ˈeks-\ *n, often cap X* : X-RADIATION 1 — **x–ir•ra•di•ate** *vb, often cap X*

XL *abbr* extended-release

X–linked *adj* : located on an X chromosome ⟨an ~ gene⟩; *also* : transmitted by an X-linked gene ⟨an ~ disease⟩

Xo•lair \ˈzō-ˌler\ *trademark* — used for a preparation of omalizumab

Xo•pe•nex \ˈzō-pə-ˌneks\ *trademark* — used for a preparation of levalbuterol

XP *abbr* xeroderma pigmentosum

XR *abbr* extended-release

x–ra•di•a•tion *n, often cap X* **1** : exposure to X-rays **2** : radiation composed of X-rays

x–ra•di•og•ra•phy *n, pl* **-phies** *often cap X* : radiography by means of X-rays

x–ray \ˈeks-ˌrā\ *vb, often cap X* : to examine, treat, or photograph with X-rays

X-ray *n* **1** : any of the electromagnetic radiations of the same nature as visible radiation but of an extremely short wavelength that has the properties of ionizing a gas upon passage through it, of penetrating various thicknesses of all solids, of producing secondary radiations by impinging on material bodies, of acting on photographic films and plates as light does, and of causing fluorescent screens to emit light — called also *roentgen ray* **2** : a photograph obtained by use of X-rays ⟨a chest *X-ray*⟩ — **X–ray** *adj*

X–ray therapy *n* : medical treatment (as of cancer) by controlled application of X-rays

XTC \ˈek-stə-sē\ *n* : ECSTASY 2

xy•la•zine \ˈzī-lə-ˌzēn\ *n* : a veterinary sedative, analgesic, and muscle relaxant administered in the form of its hydrochloride $C_{12}H_{16}N_2S{\cdot}HCl$

xy•lene \ˈzī-ˌlēn\ *n* : any of three toxic flammable oily isomeric aromatic hydrocarbons C_8H_{10}

xy•li•tol \ˈzī-lə-ˌtȯl, -ˌtōl\ *n* : a crystalline alcohol $C_5H_{12}O_5$ that is a derivative of xylose and is used as a sweetener

Xy•lo•caine \ˈzī-lə-ˌkān\ *trademark* — used for a preparation of lidocaine

xy•lo•met•a•zo•line \ˌzī-lə-ˌme-tə-ˈzō-ˌlēn\ *n* : a sympathomimetic agent with vasoconstrictive activity that is used in the form of its hydrochloride $C_{16}H_{24}N_2{\cdot}HCl$ esp. as a topical nasal decongestant

xy•lose \ˈzī-ˌlōs, -ˌlōz\ *n* : a crystalline aldose sugar $C_5H_{10}O_5$

xy•lu•lose \ˈzīl-yu̇-ˌlōs, ˈzī-lu̇-, -ˌlōz\ *n* : a ketose sugar $C_5H_{10}O_5$ of the pentose class that plays a role in carbohydrate metabolism and is found in the urine in cases of pentosuria

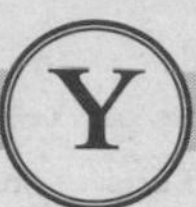

Y *symbol* yttrium
YAC *abbr* yeast artificial chromosome
yage \ˈyä-ˌhā\ *n* : AYAHUASCA
Yas·min \ˈyaz-min\ *trademark* — used for a preparation of drospirenone and ethinyl estradiol
yaw \ˈyȯ\ *n* : one of the lesions characteristic of yaws
yawn \ˈyȯn, ˈyän\ *n* : an opening of the mouth wide while taking a deep breath often as an involuntary reaction to fatigue or boredom — **yawn** *vb*
yaws \ˈyȯz\ *n sing or pl* : an infectious contagious tropical disease that is caused by a spirochete of the genus *Treponema* (*T. pertenue*) and that is characterized by a primary ulcerating lesion on the skin followed by a secondary stage in which ulcers develop all over the body and by a third stage in which the bones are involved — called also *frambesia, pian*
Yaz \ˈyaz\ *trademark* — used for a preparation of drospirenone and ethinyl estradiol
Yb *symbol* ytterbium
Y chromosome \ˈwī-\ *n* : a sex chromosome that is characteristic of male cells in species in which the male typically has two unlike sex chromosomes — compare X CHROMOSOME
yeast \ˈyēst\ *n* **1** : a unicellular chiefly ascomycetous fungus (as of the family Saccharomycetaceae) that has usu. little or no mycelium, that typically reproduces asexually by budding, and that includes forms (as *Saccharomyces cerevisiae*) which cause alcoholic fermentation and are used esp. in the making of alcoholic beverages and leavened bread **2** : a yellowish surface froth or sediment that occurs esp. in sugary fermenting liquids (as fruit juices) and consists chiefly of yeast cells and carbon dioxide **3** : a commercial product containing yeast cells in a moist or dry medium — **yeast·like** \-ˌlīk\ *adj*
yeast artificial chromosome *n* : a chromosome that is used esp. to clone DNA segments longer than those capable of being cloned in bacteria and that is introduced for cloning into a yeast of the genus *Saccharomyces* (*S. cerevisiae*) — abbr. *YAC*
yeast infection *n* : an infection of the vagina with an overgrowth of a yeastlike fungus of the genus *Candida* (*C. albicans*) normally present in the vaginal flora that is characterized by vaginal discharge and vulvovaginitis; *broadly* : an infection (as thrush) caused by a yeast or yeastlike fungus
yellow body *n* : CORPUS LUTEUM
yellow fat disease *n* : a disease esp. of swine, cats, and mink that is associated with a deficiency of vitamin E and is marked by inflammation of the fatty tissue, subcutaneous edema, and varied visceral lesions — called also *steatitis, yellow fat*
yellow fever *n* : an infectious disease of sudden onset that is endemic in sub-Saharan Africa and tropical So. America, that is marked by acute symptoms (as fever, muscle pain, and headache) which typically resolve within a few days but are sometimes followed by more serious symptoms (as jaundice, high fever, and hemorrhage), and that is caused by a flavivirus (species *Yellow fever virus*) transmitted esp. by the yellow-fever mosquito
yellow–fever mosquito *n* : a small dark-colored mosquito of the genus *Aedes* (*A. aegypti*) that is the usual vector of yellow fever — called also *tiger mosquito*
yellow jacket *n* **1** : any of various yellow-marked social wasps (esp. genus *Vespula* of the family Vespidae) that usu. nest in the ground and can sting repeatedly and painfully **2** *slang* : pentobarbital esp. in a yellow capsule — usu. used in pl.
yellow marrow *n* : BONE MARROW a
yellow petrolatum *n* : petroleum jelly that has not been wholly or mostly decolorized
yel·lows \ˈye-(ˌ)lōz\ *n sing or pl* : any of several diseases of domestic animals (as sheep) marked by jaundice
yellow wax *n* : a wax obtained as a yellow to brown solid by melting a honeycomb with boiling water, straining, and cooling — called also *beeswax*
yer·ba san·ta \ˈyer-bə-ˈsän-tə, ˈyər-, -ˈsan-\ *n* : an evergreen shrub (*Eriodictyon californicum* of the family Hydrophyllaceae) of California with aromatic leaves; *also* : ERIODICTYON
yer·sin·ia \yər-ˈsi-nē-ə\ *n* **1** *cap* : a genus of enterobacteria that includes several important pathogens (as the plague bacterium, *Y. pestis*) formerly included in the genus *Pasteurella* — see PLAGUE 2 **2** : any bacterium of the genus *Yersinia*
Yer·sin \yer-ˈsan\, **Alexandre–Émile–John (1863–1943),** French bacteriologist.
yer·sin·i·o·sis \yər-ˌsi-nē-ˈō-səs\ *n* : infection with or disease caused by a bacterium of the genus *Yersinia; esp* : an infectious disease that is caused by a yersinia (*Y. enterocolitica*) transmitted chiefly in contaminated water and food (as raw or undercooked pork products) and is marked esp. by fever, abdominal pain, and diarrhea

Y ligament *n* : ILIOFEMORAL LIGAMENT

yo•ga \ˈyō-gə\ *n* **1** *cap* : a Hindu theistic philosophy teaching the suppression of all activity of body, mind, and will in order that the self may realize its distinction from them and attain liberation **2** : a system of physical postures, breathing techniques, and meditation derived from Yoga but often practiced independently to promote bodily or mental control and well-being — see HATHA YOGA — **yogic** \-gik\ *adj*

yo•gurt *also* **yo•ghurt** \ˈyō-gərt\ *n* : a fermented slightly acid often flavored semisolid food made of milk and milk solids to which cultures of bacteria of the genus *Lactobacillus* (*L. bulgarius*) and *Streptococcus* (*S. thermophilus*) have been added

yo•him•be \yō-ˈhim-bā\ *n* : a tropical African tree (*Pausinystalia yohimbe* syn. *Corynanthe yohimbe*) of the madder family (Rubiaceae) whose bark yields yohimbine; *also* : a preparation of the bark that is used esp. as an aphrodisiac

yo•him•bine \yō-ˈhim-ˌbēn, -bən\ *n* : an alkaloid obtained from the bark of yohimbe that is a weak blocker of alpha-adrenergic receptors and has been used in the form of its hydrochloride $C_{21}H_{26}N_2O_3·HCl$ as a mydriatic and aphrodisiac and to treat impotence

yolk \ˈyōk\ *n* : material stored in an ovum that supplies food to the developing embryo and consists chiefly of proteins, lecithin, and cholesterol

yolk sac *n* : a membranous sac of most vertebrates that encloses the yolk, is continuous in most forms (as in humans) through the omphalomesenteric duct with the intestinal cavity of the embryo, and is supplied with blood vessels that transport nutritive yolk products to the developing embryo

yolk stalk *n* : OMPHALOMESENTERIC DUCT

Young–Helm•holtz theory \ˈyəŋ-ˈhelm-ˌhōlts-\ *n* : a theory in color vision: the eye has three separate elements each of which is stimulated by a different primary color

Young, Thomas (1773–1829), British physician, physicist, and archaeologist.

Helmholtz, Hermann Ludwig Ferdinand von (1821–1894), German physicist and physiologist.

yo–yo dieting *n* : the practice of repeatedly losing weight by dieting and subsequently regaining it

yt•ter•bi•um \i-ˈtər-bē-əm\ *n* : a bivalent or trivalent metallic element — symbol *Yb;* see ELEMENT table

yt•tri•um \ˈi-trē-əm\ *n* : a trivalent metallic element — symbol *Y;* see ELEMENT table

yup•pie flu \ˈyə-pē-\ *n* : CHRONIC FATIGUE SYNDROME

Z

za·fir·lu·kast \zə-ˈfir-lü-ˌkast\ *n* : a leukotriene antagonist $C_{31}H_{33}N_3O_6S$ that is administered orally to inhibit bronchoconstriction in the treatment of asthma

zal·cit·a·bine \zal-ˈsi-tə-ˌbēn, -ˌbīn\ *n* : DDC

zal·e·plon \ˈza-lə-ˌplän\ *n* : a sedative and hypnotic drug $C_{12}H_{15}N_5O$ used in the treatment of insomnia — see SONATA

za·nam·i·vir \zə-ˈna-mə-ˌvir\ *n* : a neuraminidase inhibitor $C_{12}H_{20}N_4O_7$ used in the form of an inhalant against influenza A and B to prevent the spread of influenza virus from cell to cell in the lungs — see RELENZA

Zan·tac \ˈzan-ˌtak\ *trademark* — used for a preparation of the hydrochloride of ranitidine

Z–DNA \ˈzē-\ *n* : the left-handed uncommon form of double helix DNA in which the chains twist up and to the left around the front of the axis of the helix — compare B-DNA

ZDV \ˌzē-dē-ˈvē\ *n* : AZT

Ze·be·ta \ze-ˈbā-tə\ *trademark* — used for a preparation of the fumarate of bisoprolol

Zei·gar·nik effect \zī-ˈgär-nik-\ *n* : the psychological tendency to remember an uncompleted task rather than a completed one

Zeigarnik, Bluma (1900–1988), Russian psychologist.

Zen·ker's diverticulum \ˈzeŋ-kərz-, ˈtseŋ-\ *n* : an abnormal pouch in the upper part of the esophagus in which food may become trapped causing bad breath, irritation, difficulty in swallowing, and regurgitation — called also *pharyngoesophageal diverticulum*

Zenker, Friedrich Albert von (1825–1898), German pathologist and anatomist.

Zeph·i·ran \ˈze-fə-ˌran\ *trademark* — used for a preparation of benzalkonium chloride

Zes·tril \ˈzes-tril\ *trademark* — used for a preparation of lisinopril

Zet·ia \ˈze-tē-ə\ *trademark* — used for a preparation of ezetimibe

Ze·ton·na \zi-ˈtō-nə\ *trademark* — used for a preparation of ciclesonide administered as a nasal aerosol

zi·con·o·tide \zī-ˈkä-nə-ˌtīd\ *n* : an analgesic $C_{102}H_{172}N_{36}O_{32}S_7$ that is a synthetic analog of a peptide found in a marine snail (*Conus magus*) and that is administered intrathecally to relieve chronic intractable pain

zi·do·vu·dine \zī-ˈdō-vü-ˌdēn, -vyü-\ *n* : AZT

Ziehl–Neel·sen stain \ˈtsēl-ˈnāl-sən-\ *n* : a stain used esp. for detecting the tubercle bacillus

Ziehl, Franz (1857–1926), German bacteriologist.

Neelsen, Friedrich Carl Adolf (1854–1894), German pathologist.

ZIFT *abbr* zygote intrafallopian transfer

Zi·ka virus \ˈzē-kə-\ *or* **Zika 1** : a flavivirus (species *Zika virus* of the genus *Flavivirus*) typically transmitted by aedes mosquitoes that causes a usually mild illness marked chiefly by fever, joint pain, rash, and conjunctivitis and that has been associated with an increased incidence of microcephaly in infants born to pregnant women infected with the virus **2** : the illness caused by Zika virus

zi·leu·ton \zī-ˈlü-tᵊn\ *n* : an anti-asthma drug $C_{11}H_{12}N_2O_2S$ that is administered orally and acts by inhibiting the lipoxygenase catalyzing the formation of leukotrienes

zi·mel·i·dine \zi-ˈme-lə-ˌdēn\ *n* : a compound $C_{16}H_{17}BrN_2$ that functions as an SSRI but was withdrawn from use as an antidepressant because of its link to Guillain-Barré syndrome

zinc \ˈziŋk\ *n* : a bluish-white crystalline bivalent metallic element that is an essential micronutrient for both plants and animals — symbol *Zn;* see ELEMENT table

zinc carbonate *n* : a crystalline salt $ZnCO_3$ having astringent and antiseptic properties

zinc chloride *n* : a poisonous caustic salt $ZnCl_2$ that is used as a disinfectant and astringent

zinc finger *n* : any of a class of proteins that typically possess fingerlike loops of amino acids with each loop containing a zinc-binding site that regulates transcription by binding to specific regions of a gene's DNA; *also* : one of the fingerlike amino acid loops of such a protein

zinc ointment *n* : ZINC OXIDE OINTMENT

zinc oxide *n* : a white solid ZnO used in pharmaceutical and cosmetic preparations (as ointments and sunblocks)

zinc oxide ointment *n* : an ointment containing about 20 percent of zinc oxide and used in treating skin disorders

zinc peroxide *n* : any of various white to yellowish-white powders that have the peroxide ZnO_2 of zinc as their chief ingredient and are used chiefly as disinfectants, astringents, and deodorants

zinc picolinate *n* : a biologically active salt $C_{12}H_8N_2O_4Zn$ of zinc complexed with picolinic acid that is used as a dietary supplement

zinc pyr·i·thi·one \-ˌpir-i-ˈthī-ˌōn\ *n* : an antibacterial and antifungal compound $C_{10}H_8N_2O_2S_2Zn$ that is nearly insoluble in water, possesses cytostatic activity against epidermal cells, and is the active ingredient in various shampoos used to control dandruff and seborrheic dermatitis — called also *pyrithione zinc*

zinc stearate *n* : an insoluble salt usu. of commercial stearic acid and usu. containing some zinc oxide that has astringent and antiseptic properties and is used as a constituent of ointments and powders

zinc sulfate *n* : a crystalline salt $ZnSO_4$ used in medicine as an astringent, emetic, and weak antiseptic

zinc un•dec•y•len•ate \-ˌən-ˌde-si-ˈle-ˌnāt\ *n* : a fine white powder $C_{22}H_{38}O_4Zn$ used as a fungistatic agent

zinc white *n* : ZINC OXIDE

zir•co•ni•um \ˌzər-ˈkō-nē-əm\ *n* : a strong ductile metallic element — symbol *Zr;* see ELEMENT table

zit \ˈzit\ *n, slang* : PIMPLE 1

Zith•ro•max \ˈzī-thrō-ˌmaks\ *trademark* — used for a preparation of azithromycin

Z line *n* : any of the dark thin lines across a striated muscle fiber that mark the junction of actin filaments in adjacent sarcomeres

Zn *symbol* zinc

zo- *or* **zoo-** *comb form* : animal ⟨*zoo*nosis⟩

Zo•cor \ˈzō-ˌkȯr\ *trademark* — used for a preparation of simvastatin

Zo•fran \ˈzō-ˌfran\ *trademark* — used for a preparation of ondansetron

-zo•ic \ˈzō-ik\ *adj comb form* : having a (specified) animal mode of existence ⟨sapro*zoic*⟩

Zol•ling•er–El•li•son syndrome \ˈzä-liŋ-ər-ˈe-li-sən-\ *n* : a syndrome consisting of fulminant intractable peptic ulcers, gastric hypersecretion and hyperacidity, and the occurrence of gastrinomas of the pancreatic cells of the islets of Langerhans

Zollinger, Robert Milton (1903–1992), American surgeon.

Ellison, Edwin Homer (1918–1970), American surgeon.

zol•mi•trip•tan \ˌzōl-mi-ˈtrip-ˌtan\ *n* : a triptan $C_{16}H_{21}N_3O_2$ administered as an oral tablet or as a nasal spray to treat migraine headaches

Zo•loft \ˈzō-ˌlȯft\ *trademark* — used for a preparation of the hydrochloride of sertraline

zol•pi•dem \ˈzōl-pə-ˌdem\ *n* : a sedative and hypnotic drug administered orally in the form of its tartrate $(C_{19}H_{21}N_3O)_2{\cdot}C_4H_6O_6$ in the short-term treatment of insomnia — called also *zolpidem tartrate;* see AMBIEN

Zo•max \ˈzō-ˌmaks\ *n* : a preparation of zomepirac — formerly a U.S. registered trademark

zo•me•pir•ac \ˌzō-mə-ˈpir-ˌak\ *n* : a compound $C_{15}H_{13}ClNNaO_3{\cdot}2H_2O$ formerly used as an anti-inflammatory and analgesic agent but now withdrawn from use because of its link to life-threatening anaphylactic reactions — see ZOMAX

zo•na \ˈzō-nə\ *n, pl* **zo•nae** \-ˌnē, -nī\ *or* **zonas** **1** : an anatomical zone or layer; *esp* : ZONA PELLUCIDA **2** : SHINGLES

zona fas•cic•u•la•ta \-fa-ˌsi-kyə-ˈlā-tə\ *n* : the middle of the three layers of the adrenal cortex that consists of radially arranged columnar epithelial cells

zona glo•mer•u•lo•sa \-glō-ˌmer-yə-ˈlō-sə\ *n* : the outermost of the three layers of the adrenal cortex that consists of round masses of granular epithelial cells that stain deeply — called also *glomerulosa*

zona pel•lu•ci•da \-pə-ˈlü-sə-də\ *n* : the transparent more or less elastic noncellular outer layer or envelope of a mammalian ovum that is composed of glycoproteins

zona re•tic•u•lar•is \-re-ˌti-kyə-ˈlar-əs\ *n* : the innermost of the three layers of the adrenal cortex that consists of irregularly arranged cylindrical masses of epithelial cells

zone \ˈzōn\ *n* **1** : an encircling anatomical structure **2** : a region or area set off as distinct

zo•nu•la \ˈzōn-yə-lə\ *n, pl* **-lae** \-ˌlē\ *or* **-las** : ZONULE OF ZINN

zonula cil•i•ar•is \-ˌsi-lē-ˈar-əs\ *n* : ZONULE OF ZINN

zo•nu•lar \ˈzōn-yə-lər\ *adj* : of or relating to the zonule of Zinn

zon•ule \ˈzōn-ˌyül\ *n* : ZONULE OF ZINN

zonule of Zinn \-ˈtsin\ *n, pl* **zonules of Zinn** : the suspensory ligament of the crystalline lens of the eye — called also *zonula, zonula ciliaris*

J. G. Zinn — see LIGAMENT OF ZINN

zoo- — see ZO-

zo•ol•o•gy \zō-ˈäl-ə-jē\ *n, pl* **-gies** **1** : a branch of biology that deals with the classification and the properties and vital phenomena of animals **2** : the properties and vital phenomena exhibited by an animal, animal type, or group — **zoo•log•i•cal** \ˌzō-ə-ˈläj-i-kəl\ *also* **zoo•log•ic** \-ik\ *adj* — **zo•ol•o•gist** \zō-ˈäl-ə-jəst\ *n*

-zo•on \ˈzō-ˌän, -ən\ *n comb form* : animal ⟨spermato*zoon*⟩

zoo•no•sis \ˌzō-ə-ˈnō-səs, zō-ˈä-nə-səs\ *n, pl* **-no•ses** \-ˌsēz\ : a disease communicable from animals to humans under natural conditions — **zoo•not•ic** \ˌzō-ə-ˈnä-tik\ *adj*

zoo•par•a•site \ˌzō-ə-ˈpar-ə-ˌsīt\ *n* : a parasitic animal

zoo•phil•ia \ˌzō-ə-ˈfil-ē-ə\ *n* : an erotic fixation on animals that may result in sexual excitement through real or imagined contact

zoo•pho•bia \ˌzō-ə-ˈfō-bē-ə\ *n* : abnormal fear of animals

Zor•tress \ˈzȯr-ˌtres\ *trademark* — used for a preparation of everolimus

Zos•ta•vax \ˈzäs-tə-ˌvaks\ *trademark* — used for a vaccine against shingles containing live attenuated varicella zoster virus

zos•ter \ˈzäs-tər\ *n* : SHINGLES

zos•ter•i•form \zäs-ˈter-ə-ˌfȯrm\ *adj* : resembling shingles ⟨a ∼ rash⟩

Zos•trix \ˈzäs-triks\ *trademark* — used for a preparation containing capsaicin

Zo•vi•rax \zō-ˈvī-ˌraks\ *trademark* — used for a preparation of acyclovir

zox•a•zol•amine \ˌzäk-sə-ˈzä-lə-ˌmēn\ *n* : a drug $C_7H_5ClN_2O$ used esp. formerly as a skeletal muscle relaxant and uricosuric agent

Z–PAK \ˈzē-ˌpak\ *trademark* — used for a blister pack containing six tablets of azithromycin

ZPG *abbr* zero population growth

Z–plas•ty \ˈzē-ˌplas-tē\ *n, pl* **-ties** : a surgical procedure for the repair of constricted scar tissue in which a Z-shaped incision is made in the skin and the two resulting flaps are interposed

Zr *symbol* zirconium

Zub•solv \ˈzəb-ˌsälv\ *trademark* — used for a preparation of the hydrochloride of buprenorphine and naloxone administered sublingually

Zy•ban \ˈzī-ˌban\ *trademark* — used for a preparation of the hydrochloride of bupropion

zyg- *or* **zygo-** *comb form* **1** : pair ⟨*zyg*apophysis⟩ **2** : union : fusion ⟨*zygo*genesis⟩

zyg•apoph•y•sis \ˌzī-gə-ˈpä-fə-səs\ *n, pl* **-y•ses** \-ˌsēz\ : any of the articular processes of the neural arch of a vertebra of which there are usu. two anterior and two posterior

zy•go•gen•e•sis \ˌzī-gō-ˈje-nə-səs\ *n, pl* **-e•ses** \-ˌsēz\ : reproduction by means of specialized germ cells or gametes : sexual reproduction

zy•go•ma \zī-ˈgō-mə\ *n, pl* **-ma•ta** \-mə-tə\ *also* **-mas** **1** : ZYGOMATIC ARCH **2** : ZYGOMATIC BONE

[1]**zy•go•mat•ic** \ˌzī-gə-ˈma-tik\ *adj* : of, relating to, constituting, or situated in the region of the zygomatic bone and the zygomatic arch

[2]**zygomatic** *n* : ZYGOMATIC BONE

zygomatic arch *n* : the arch of bone that extends along the front or side of the skull beneath the orbit and that is formed by the union of the temporal process of the zygomatic bone in front with the zygomatic process of the temporal bone behind

zygomatic bone *n* : a bone of the side of the face below the eye that forms part of the zygomatic arch and part of the orbit and articulates with the temporal, sphenoid, and frontal bones and with the maxilla of the upper jaw — called also *cheekbone, jugal, malar bone, zygoma*

zygomatic nerve *n* : a branch of the maxillary nerve that divides into a facial branch supplying the skin of the prominent part of the cheek and a temporal branch supplying the skin of the anterior temporal region

zygomatico- *comb form* : zygomatic and ⟨*zygomatico*facial⟩

zy•go•mat•i•co•fa•cial \ˌzī-gə-ˌma-ti-kō-ˈfā-shəl\ *adj* **1** : of, relating to, or being the branch of the zygomatic nerve that supplies the skin of the prominent part of the cheek **2** : of, relating to, or being a foramen in the zygomatic bone that gives passage to the zygomaticofacial branch of the zygomatic nerve

zy•go•mat•i•co•max•il•lary \-ˈmak-sə-ˌler-ē\ *adj* : of, relating to, or uniting the zygomatic bone and the maxilla of the upper jaw ⟨the ~ suture⟩

zy•go•mat•i•co•tem•po•ral \-ˈtem-pə-rəl\ *adj* **1** : of, relating to, or uniting the zygomatic arch and the temporal bone ⟨the ~ suture⟩ **2 a** : of, relating to, or being the branch of the zygomatic nerve that supplies the skin of the anterior temporal region **b** : of, relating to, or being a foramen in the zygomatic bone that gives passage to the zygomaticotemporal branch of the zygomatic nerve

zygomatic process *n* : any of several bony processes that articulate with the zygomatic bone: as **a** : a long slender process of the temporal bone helping to form the zygomatic arch **b** : a narrow process of the frontal bone articulating with the zygomatic bone **c** : a rough triangular eminence of the maxilla of the upper jaw articulating with the zygomatic bone

zy•go•mat•i•cus \ˌzī-gə-ˈma-ti-kəs\ *n* **1** : ZYGOMATICUS MAJOR **2** : ZYGOMATICUS MINOR

zygomaticus major *n* : a slender band of muscle on each side of the face that arises from the zygomatic bone, inserts into the orbicularis oris and skin at the corner of the mouth, and acts to pull the corner of the mouth upward and backward

zygomaticus minor *n* : a slender band of muscle on each side of the face that arises from the zygomatic bone, inserts into the upper lip between the zygomaticus major and the levator labii superioris, and acts to raise the upper lip upward and laterally

zy•gos•i•ty \zī-ˈgä-sə-tē\ *n, pl* **-ties** : the makeup or characteristics of a particular zygote

zy•gote \ˈzī-ˌgōt\ *n* : a cell formed by the union of two gametes; *broadly* : the developing individual produced from such a cell — **zy•got•ic** \zī-ˈgä-tik\ *adj* — **zy•got•i•cal•ly** *adv*

zygote intrafallopian transfer *n* : a method of assisting reproduction in cases of infertility in which eggs obtained from an ovary are fertilized in vitro with sperm and some of the resulting fertilized eggs are deposited into a fallopian tube by a laparoscope — abbr. *ZIFT;* compare GAMETE INTRAFALLOPIAN TRANSFER

zy•go•tene \ˈzī-gə-ˌtēn\ *n* : the stage of meiotic prophase which immediately follows the leptotene and during which synapsis of homologous chromosomes occurs — **zygotene** *adj*

-zy·gous \ˈzī-gəs\ *adj comb form* : having (such) a zygotic constitution ⟨hetero*zygous*⟩

Zy·let \ˈzī-ˌlet\ *trademark* — used for a preparation of loteprednol and tobramycin

zym- *or* **zymo-** *comb form* : enzyme ⟨*zymo*gen⟩

-zyme \ˌzīm\ *n comb form* : enzyme ⟨lyso*zyme*⟩

zy·mo·gen \ˈzī-mə-jən\ *n* : an inactive protein precursor of an enzyme secreted by living cells and converted (as by a kinase or an acid) into an active form — called also *proenzyme*

zy·mo·gram \ˈzī-mə-ˌgram\ *n* : an electrophoretic strip (as of starch gel) or a representation of it exhibiting the pattern of separated enzymes and esp. isoenzymes after electrophoresis

zy·mo·san \ˈzī-mə-ˌsan\ *n* : an insoluble largely polysaccharide fraction of yeast cell walls

Zy·prexa \zī-ˈprek-sə\ *trademark* — used for a preparation of olanzapine

Zyr·tec \ˈzər-ˌtek\ *trademark* — used for a preparation of the dihydrochloride of cetirizine

SIGNS AND SYMBOLS

BIOLOGY

○ an individual, specif., a female—used chiefly in inheritance charts

□ an individual, specif., a male—used chiefly in inheritance charts

♀ female

♂ *or* ♂ male

× crossed with; hybrid

+ wild type

CHEMISTRY AND PHYSICS

(for element symbols see ELEMENT table)

α alpha particle

β beta particle, beta ray

λ wavelength

\+ signifies "plus," "and," "together with"—used between the symbols of substances brought together for, or produced by, a reaction;

signifies a unit charge of positive electricity when placed to the right of a symbol as a superscript: Ca^{2+} or Ca^{++} denotes the ion of calcium, which carries two positive charges;

signifies a dextrorotatory compound when preceding in parentheses a compound name [as in (+)-tartaric acid]

– signifies removal or loss of a part from a compound during a reaction (as in $-CO_2$);

signifies a unit charge of negative electricity when placed to the right of a symbol as a superscript: Cl^- denotes a chlorine ion carrying a negative charge;

signifies a levorotatory compound when preceding in parentheses a compound name [as in (–)-quinine]

- signifies a single bond—used between the symbols of elements or groups which unite to form a compound (as in H–Cl for HCl and H–O–H for H_2O)

> signifies separate single bonds from an atom to two other atoms or groups (as in the group >C=NNHR characteristic of hydrazone)

· used to separate parts of a substance regarded as loosely joined (as in $CuSO_4{\cdot}5H_2O$);

also used to denote the presence of a single unpaired electron (as in H·)

= indicates a double bond;

signifies two unit charges of negative electricity when placed to the right of a symbol as a superscript (as in $SO_4^{=}$, the negative ion of sulfuric acid)

≡ signifies a triple bond or a triple negative charge

: signifies a pair of electrons belonging to an atom that are not shared with another atom (as in $:NH_3$);

sometimes signifies a double bond (as in $CH_2:CH_2$)

( ) marks groups within a compound [as in $(CH_3)_2SO$, the formula for dimethyl sulfoxide which contains two methyl groups (CH_3)]

—*or*— joins attached atoms or groups in structural formulas for cyclic compounds, as that for glucose

——O——

$CH_2OHCH(CHOH)_3CHOH$

1-, 2-, etc. used in names to indicate the positions of substituting groups, attached to the first, second, etc., of the numbered atoms of the parent compound (as in 5-fluorouracil or glucose-6-phosphate)

x, m, n used as subscripts following an atom or group in a chemical formula to indicate that the number of times the atom or group occurs is indefinite [as in $(C_6H_{10}O_5)_x$ for glycogen] or approximate [as in $C_{12}H_mAl_{16}O_nS_8$ for sucralfate where *m* and *n* are approximately 54 and 75]

R group—used esp. of an organic group

′ used to distinguish between different substituents of the same kind (as R′, R″, R‴ to indicate different organic groups)

MEDICINE

℞ take—used on prescriptions; prescription; treatment

☠ poison

☣ biohazard, biohazardous materials

☢ *or* ☢ radiation, radioactivity, radioactive materials

APOTHECARIES' MEASURES

℥ ounce

f℥ fluid ounce

*f*ʒ fluid dram

min *or* ♍ minim

APOTHECARIES' WEIGHTS

℔ pound

℥ ounce: as

℥ i or ℥ j, one ounce;

℥ ss, half an ounce;

℥ iss *or* ℥ jss, one ounce and a half;

℥ ij, two ounces

ʒ dram

℈ scruple